PEDIATRIC RESPIRATORY DISEASE

PEDIATRIC RESPIRATORY DISEASE:

Diagnosis and Treatment

Bettina C. Hilman, M.D.
Louisiana State University
School of Medicine in Shreveport
Shreveport, Louisiana

W.B. SAUNDERS COMPANY

A Division of
Harcourt Brace & Company
Philadelphia   London   Toronto   Montreal   Sydney   Tokyo

W.B. SAUNDERS COMPANY
A Division of
Harcourt Brace & Company

The Curtis Center
Independence Square West
Philadelphia, Pennsylvania 19106

Library of Congress Cataloging-in-Publication Data

Pediatric respiratory disease : diagnosis and treatment /
[edited by]   Bettina C. Hilman.
　　　　p.　cm.

　　ISBN 0-7216-4683-2

　　1. Pediatric respiratory diseases. I. Hilman, Bettina C.
　　[DNLM: 1. Respiration Disorders—diagnosis.
2. Respiration Disorders—in infancy & childhood.
3. Respiration Disorders—therapy.　　WS 280 P3672]
　　RJ431.P397　1993
　　618.92′2—dc20
　　DNLM/DLC　　　　　　　　　　　　92-13383

Pediatric Respiratory Disease: Diagnosis and Treatment　　　　　　　　　　　ISBN 0-7216-4683-2

Printed in the United States of America.

Last digit is the print number:　　　9　8　7　6　5　4　3　2　1

CONTRIBUTORS

ROSALIND S. ABERNATHY, M.D.
Associate Professor of Pediatrics,
University of Arkansas for Medical
Sciences, and Arkansas Children's
Hospital, Little Rock, Arkansas
Sarcoidosis

JULIAN L. ALLEN, M.D.
Associate Professor of Pediatrics, Temple
University School of Medicine;
Pulmonary Director, Pulmonary Function
Laboratory, St. Christopher's Hospital for
Children, Philadelphia, Pennsylvania
*Clinical Applications of Pulmonary
Function Testing in Children and
Adolescents; Bronchopulmonary Dysplasia*

BRAD E. ALPERT, M.D.
Associate Professor of Pediatrics, Division
of Pulmonary and Critical Care Medicine,
University of Texas Health Science Center
at Houston, Houston, Texas
Bronchopulmonary Dysplasia

DANIEL R. AMBRUSO, M.D.
Associate Professor of Pediatrics and
Pathology, University of Colorado School
of Medicine; The Children's Hospital;
Associate Medical Director, Belle Bonfils
Memorial Blood Center, Denver,
Colorado
Chronic Granulomatous Disease

ROBERT C. BECKERMAN, M.D.
Professor of Pediatrics and Physiology,
Section Chief, Pediatric Pulmonology, and
Director, Constance Kaufman Center for
Study of Breathing Disorders in Infants
and Children, Tulane University Medical
Center; Tulane University Hospital,
Charity Hospital of New Orleans, and
Ochsner Foundation Clinic, New Orleans,
Louisiana
*Obstructive Sleep Apnea Syndrome;
Sudden Infant Death Syndrome*

PHILIP BLACK, M.D.
Associate Professor of Pediatrics,
University of Missouri at Kansas City
School of Medicine; Chief, Section of
Pulmonology, Children's Mercy Hospital,
Kansas City, Missouri
Evaluation of Chronic or Recurrent Cough

CYNTHIA BLACK-PAYNE, M.D.
Assistant Professor of Pediatrics, Section
of Pediatric Infectious Diseases, Louisiana
State University School of Medicine;
Louisiana State University Hospital,
Shreveport, Louisiana
Bronchiolitis

JOANN BLESSING-MOORE, M.D.
Clinical Assistant Professor, Stanford
University Hospital, Palo Alto, California
*Self-Management Programs in Pediatric
Respiratory Diseases*

JOSEPH A. BOCCHINI, JR., M.D.
Professor of Pediatrics and Acting
Chairman, Department of Pediatrics, and
Chief, Pediatric Infectious Disease Section,
Louisiana State University Medical
Center—Shreveport, Shreveport,
Louisiana
The Chlamydiae

RICHARD J. BONFORTE, M.D.
Professor of Pediatrics, Mount Sinai
School of Medicine; Director of Pediatrics,
Beth Israel Medical Center, New York
City, New York
Pneumonia of Infancy

BRIAN A. BRENNAN, M.D.
McFarland Clinic, Ames, Iowa
*Bronchial Challenge Techniques in
Children: Methacholine, Histamine,
Hyperventilation, and Osmolar*

RICHARD BRYARLY, JR., M.D.
Clinical Assistant Professor, Louisiana
State University Medical School,
Shreveport, Louisiana
Pediatric Rigid Bronchoscopy

PRESTON W. CAMPBELL III, M.D.
Assistant Professor, Vanderbilt University
School of Medicine; Medical Director,
Cystic Fibrosis Center, Vanderbilt Medical
Center, Nashville, Tennessee
Lung Abscess

WALDEMAR CARLO, M.D.
Professor of Pediatrics; Director, Division of Neonatology; and Director, Newborn Nurseries, University of Alabama at Birmingham, Birmingham, Alabama
Mechanical Ventilation in Newborns

ANTONINO CATANZARO, M.D.
Associate Professor of Medicine, University of California, San Diego (UCSD), School of Medicine; Department of Medicine, Division of Pulmonary and Critical Care Medicine, UCSD Medical Center, San Diego, California
Diagnosis and Treatment of Coccidioidomycosis

TERRY W. CHIN, M.D.
Assistant Professor of Pediatrics, University of California, Irvine; Director, Allergy-Immunology-Rheumatology, and Assistant Director, Pediatric Pulmonary, Memorial Miller Children's Hospital, Long Beach, California
Bacterial Pneumonia

KEITH CLARK, M.D.
Associate Professor, Otolaryngology, University of Oklahoma Health Sciences Center; Children's Hospital of Oklahoma, Oklahoma Memorial Hospital, Oklahoma City, Oklahoma
Airway Management; Tracheotomy

ALLAN L. COATES, M.D.CM., B.ENG. (ELECT)
Professor, Department of Pediatrics, McGill University; Director, Division of Respiratory Medicine, Montreal Children's Hospital, Montreal, Québec, Canada
Pulmonary Mechanics

JOHN L. COLOMBO, M.D.
Associate Professor of Pediatrics and Chief, Pediatric Pulmonology, University of Nebraska Medical Center and Children's Memorial Hospital, Omaha, Nebraska
Pulmonary Aspiration

ELIZABETH CRAVEN, M.D.
Clinical Professor of Pediatrics, Jefferson Medical College, Philadelphia, Pennsylvania; Alfred I. du Pont Institute and Medical Center of Delaware, Wilmington, Delaware
Recurrent and Persistent Pneumonia

NIKHIL K. DAVE, M.D.
Private Practice, Pittsburgh, Pennsylvania
Bronchial Challenge Techniques in Children: Methacholine, Histamine, Hyperventilation, and Osmolar

G. MICHAEL DAVIS, MB.ChB.
Assistant Professor, Department of Pediatrics, McGill University; Division of Respiratory Medicine, Montreal Children's Hospital, Montreal, Québec, Canada
Pulmonary Mechanics

SCOTT DAVIS, M.D.
Associate Professor of Pediatrics, Tulane University School of Medicine; Director of Cystic Fibrosis Center, Tulane University Hospital and Clinic, New Orleans, Louisiana
Home Intravenous Antibiotic Use

LOUIS P. DEHNER, M.D.
Professor of Pathology and Professor of Pathology in Pediatrics, Washington University; Director of Anatomic Pathology and Surgical Pathology and Surgical Pathologist-in-Chief, Barnes Hospital; Pathologist-in-Chief, St. Louis Children's Hospital, St. Louis, Missouri
Thoracopulmonary Neoplasia and Lung Complications of Childhood Cancer

PENELOPE H. DENNEHY, M.D.
Assistant Professor of Pediatrics, Brown University School of Medicine; Associate Director, Pediatric Infectious Diseases, Rhode Island Hospital, Providence, Rhode Island
Rapid Diagnosis of Viral Respiratory Infections

JAVIER DIAZ-BLANCO, M.D.
Director of Neonatology, Wuesthoff Hospital, Rockledge, Florida
Continuous Noninvasive Monitoring of Blood Gases

JOHN S. DONOVAN, M.D.
Associate, Salem Hospital, Salem, Oregon
Airway Management; Tracheotomy

MAYNARD C. DYSON, M.D.
Assistant Professor, Baylor College of Medicine; Texas Children's Hospital and Ben Taub Hospital, Houston, Texas
Obstructive Sleep Apnea Syndrome

HOWARD EIGEN, M.D.
Professor of Pediatrics, Indiana University School of Medicine; Director, Section of Pediatric Pulmonology and Pediatric Intensive Care, Riley Hospital for Children, Indianapolis, Indiana
Childhood Near-Drowning; Pulmonary Edema

GREG R. ELLIOTT, M.D.
Associate Professor of Pediatrics, Medical College of Virginia; Division of Pediatric Pulmonology, Medical College of Virginia, Richmond, Virginia
Bronchoalveolar Lavage

ELLIOT F. ELLIS, M.D.
Professor Emeritus, State University of New York at Buffalo; Chief, Clinical Pharmacology Division, Nemours Children's Clinic; Jacksonville-Wolfson Children's Hospital, Jacksonville, Florida
Theophylline Use in Pediatric Pulmonary Disease

LORRY ROBERT FRANKEL, M.D.
Associate Professor of Pediatrics and Chief, Division of Intensive Care, Stanford University Medical Center, Palo Alto, California
Cardiopulmonary Resuscitation in the Pediatric Patient

MARTHA FRANZ, M.D.
Clinical Professor of Pediatrics, Emeritus, Wright State University School of Medicine; Children's Medical Center, Dayton, Ohio
Evaluation of Chest Pain in Childhood and Adolescence

RALPH C. FRATES, JR., M.D.
Associate Professor of Pediatrics and Co-Director, Pediatric Intensive Care Unit, University of Texas Medical Branch, Galveston, Texas
Respiratory Mucus

LINDA GAGE-WHITE, M.D.
Clinical Associate Professor of Otolaryngology, Louisiana State University Medical Center in Shreveport; Schumpert Medical Center, Shreveport, Louisiana
Upper Respiratory Tract Disease in Cystic Fibrosis

A. JOANNE GATES, M.D., M.B.A.
Clinical Associate Professor of Pediatrics, Tulane University School of Medicine and Louisiana State University School of Medicine; Associate Medical Director, Medical Director of Respiratory Care, Children's Hospital, New Orleans, Louisiana
Home Ventilation

PETE GOYCO, M.D.
Chief of Service, Pediatrics, Lallie Kemp Regional Hospital, Independence, Louisiana
Sudden Infant Death Syndrome

RONI GRAD, M.D.
Assistant Professor of Pediatrics, University of New Mexico; University Hospital, Albuquerque, New Mexico
Pulmonary Involvement in Collagen Vascular Disorders

NEIL J. GROSSMAN, M.D.
Associate Professor of Clinical Pediatrics, Ohio State University College of Medicine; Pediatric Hematologist, Columbus Children's Hospital, Columbus, Ohio
Venous Thrombosis and Pulmonary Embolus in Childhood

KAREN HARDY, M.D.
Chief, Pediatric Pulmonary and Cystic Fibrosis Center, California Pacific Medical Center, San Francisco, California
Obliterative Bronchiolitis

THOMAS ARTHUR HAZINSKI, M.D.
Department of Pediatrics, Vanderbilt University School of Medicine, Director, Division of Pediatric Pulmonary Medicine, Vanderbilt University Hospital, Nashville, Tennessee
Pulmonary Oxygen Toxicity

JOHN J. HERBST, M.D.
Professor of Pediatrics and Chief, Pediatric Gastroenterology, Louisiana State University School of Medicine—Shreveport, Shreveport, Louisiana
Gastroesophageal Reflux and Respiratory Sequelae

BETTINA C. HILMAN, M.D.
Professor of Pediatrics and Chief, Pulmonary/Allergy, Louisiana State University Medical Center in Shreveport; Director of Cystic Fibrosis Center, Director of Pediatric Pulmonary Function Laboratory, and Director of Allergy Clinic, Shreveport; Clinical Professor of Pediatrics, Tulane Medical Center, New Orleans; Clinical Professor of Pediatrics, Louisiana State University, New Orleans, Louisiana
Clinical Assessment of Pulmonary Disease in Infants and Children; Clinical Applications of Pulmonary Function Testing in Children and Adolescents; Recurrent and Persistent Pneumonia; Pulmonary Tuberculosis and Tuberculous Infection in Infants, Children, and Adolescents; Interstitial Lung Disease in Children; Gastroesophageal Reflux and Respiratory Sequelae; Clinical Manifestations of Cystic Fibrosis

RONALD HIROKAWA, M.D.
Assistant Professor of Surgery, Section of Otolaryngology, Yale University; Section of Otolaryngology, Hospital of Saint Raphael, New Haven; Chief of Otolaryngology, Department of Surgery, Griffin Hospital, Derby, Connecticut
Pediatric Rigid Bronchoscopy

ROBERT HOPKINS, M.D.
Associate Professor of Pediatrics, Tulane University School of Medicine; Director, Pediatric Intensive Care Unit, Tulane University Hospital, New Orleans, Louisiana
Thoracic Trauma

RUSSELL JAMES HOPP, D.O.
Associate Professor, Pediatrics, Creighton University; St. Joseph's Hospital, Omaha, Nebraska
Bronchial Challenge Techniques in Children: Methacholine, Histamine, Hyperventilation, and Osmolar

WALTER T. HUGHES, M.D.
Professor of Pediatrics and Professor of Biostatistics and Epidemiology, University of Tennessee Center for Health Sciences; Chairman, Department of Infectious Diseases, St. Jude Children's Research Hospital, Memphis, Tennessee
Pneumonia in the Immunosuppressed Host

LAURA S. INSELMAN, M.D.
Associate Professor of Pediatrics, Jefferson Medical College of Thomas Jefferson University, Philadelphia, Pennsylvania; Associate Pulmonologist and Medical Director, Respiratory Care Department and Pulmonary Function Laboratory, and Attending Pediatrician, Alfred I. du Pont Institute of the Nemours Foundation, Wilmington, Delaware
Pediatric Human Immunodeficiency Virus Infection

HILLEL JANAI, M.D.
Assistant Clinical Professor, Pediatrics, Ohio State University; Hocking Valley Community Hospital and Columbus Children's Hospital, Columbus, Ohio
Antibiotics in Pediatric Pulmonary Infections

RICHARD B. JOHNSTON, JR., M.D.
Adjunct Professor, Department of Pediatrics, Yale University School of Medicine, New Haven, Connecticut
Chronic Granulomatous Disease

JOHN A. KAFKA, M.D.
Assistant Clinical Professor, Pediatrics, University of California, San Diego (UCSD); UCSD Medical Center, Children's Hospital, Sharp Memorial Hospital, and Mercy Hospital, San Diego, California
Diagnosis and Treatment of Coccidioidomycosis

JAMSHED KANGA, M.D.
Associate Professor of Pediatrics and Chief, Division of Pediatric Pulmonology, University of Kentucky; University of Kentucky Medical Center, Lexington, Kentucky
Histoplasmosis

KARL. H. KARLSON, JR., M.D.
Associate Professor of Pediatrics, University of Arkansas for Medical Sciences; Director, Arkansas Cystic Fibrosis Center, and Associate Medical Director, Respiratory Care, Arkansas Children's Hospital, Little Rock, Arkansas
Atelectasis

ROBERT KATZ, M.D.
Associate Professor, Pediatrics, University of New Mexico School of Medicine; Director, Pediatric Intensive Care Unit, University of New Mexico Hospital, Albuquerque, New Mexico
Cardiopulmonary Resuscitation in the Pediatric Patient

SHEILA M. KATZ, M.D., M.B.A.
Professor of Pathology and Laboratory Medicine and Associate University Dean for Academic Coordination, Hahnemann University School of Medicine, Philadelphia, Pennsylvania
The Immotile Cilia Syndrome

H. WILLIAM KELLY, PHARM.D.
Professor of Pharmacy and Associate Professor of Pediatrics, College of Pharmacy and School of Medicine, University of New Mexico; Clinical Pharmacist, Pediatric Intensive Care Unit, Children's Hospital of New Mexico, Albuquerque, New Mexico
The Management of Acute Exacerbation of Childhood Asthma; Glucocorticoids

KATHLEEN KENNEDY, M.D.
Assistant Professor of Pediatrics, University of Texas Southwestern Medical Center; Medical Director of Nurseries, St. Paul Medical Center, Dallas, Texas
Pulmonary Oxygen Toxicity

DANA G. KETCHUM, M.D., M.P.H.
Major, Medical Corps, United States Air
Force; AFSC Regional Hospital, Eglin Air
Force Base, Florida
Viral Pneumonia

KATHERINE W. KLINGER, Ph.D.
Adjunct Assistant Professor, Department
of Molecular Biology and Microbiology,
Case Western Reserve University School
of Medicine, Cleveland, Ohio; Vice
President, Science Integrated Genetics,
Framingham, Massachusetts
Genetic Aspects of Cystic Fibrosis

ANN M. KOSLOSKE, M.D., M.P.H.
Professor of Surgery and Pediatrics, The
Ohio State University College of
Medicine; Chief, Section of Pediatric
Surgery, Children's Hospital, Columbus,
Ohio
Respiratory Foreign Body

RICHARD M. KRAVITZ, M.D.
Assistant Professor of Pediatrics,
Children's Hospital of Philadelphia;
University of Pennsylvania School of
Medicine, Philadelphia, Pennsylvania
*Allergic Bronchopulmonary
Aspergillosis*

PAUL KUBIC, M.D.
Instructor, Division of Pediatric
Pulmonology, Department of Pediatrics,
University of Minnesota; Director,
Pediatric Pulmonology, Children's
Hospital, St. Paul, Minnesota
*Thoracopulmonary Neoplasia and Lung
Complications of Childhood Cancer*

GEOFFREY KURLAND, M.D.
Associate Professor of Pediatrics,
University of Pittsburgh School of
Medicine; Children's Hospital of
Pittsburgh, Pittsburgh, Pennsylvania
Adaptation to High Altitude

LOURDES R. LARAYA-CUASAY, M.D.
Professor of Clinical Pediatrics, University
of Medicine and Dentistry of New
Jersey—Robert Wood Johnson Medical
School; Director, Pediatric Pulmonary and
Cystic Fibrosis Division, Robert Wood
Johnson University Hospital; St. Peter's
Medical Center and Point Pleasant
Hospital; Attending Physician, Jersey
Shore Medical Center and Robert Wood
Johnson University Hospital, New
Brunswick, New Jersey
Respiratory Sequelae of Viral Infections

RICHARD J. LEMEN, M.D.
Professor of Pediatrics, University of
Arizona College of Medicine; University
Medical Center, Tucson, Arizona
*Pulmonary Involvement in Collagen
Vascular Disorders*

LUCILLE A. LESTER, M.D.
Associate Professor of Clinical Pediatrics,
The University of Chicago, Pritzker
School of Medicine; Associate Professor of
Clinical Pediatrics, Section of Pulmonary
Medicine, and Co-Director, Cystic
Fibrosis Center, The University of
Chicago Medical Center, Chicago,
Illinois
Oxygen Therapy

STEPHEN D. LEVINE, M.D.
Clinical Associate Professor of Pediatrics,
Tulane University; Clinical Assistant
Professor of Pediatrics, Louisiana State
University; Director, Pediatric Critical
Care, Children's Hospital, New Orleans,
Louisiana
Croup and Epiglottitis

JACOV LEVY, M.D.
Senior Lecturer, Faculty of Health
Sciences, Ben Gurion University;
Director, Department of Pediatrics "A,"
Foroka Medical Center, Beer Sheva,
Israel
Pulmonary Hemosiderosis

NORMAN J. LEWISTON, M.D. [DECEASED]
Professor of Pediatrics, Stanford
University School of Medicine; Lucile
Salter Packard Children's Hospital at
Stanford and Stanford University
Hospital, Palo Alto, California
*Bronchiectasis; Clinical Manifestations of
Cystic Fibrosis; Heart-Lung and Lung
Transplantation*

MICHELLE LIERL, M.D.
Assistant Professor of Clinical Pediatrics,
Division of Allergy and Immunology,
Children's Hospital Medical Center, and
University of Cincinnati College of
Medicine, Cincinnati, Ohio
Congenital Abnormalities

HAILEN MAK, M.D., M.P.H.
Clinical Assistant Professor, Department
of Pediatrics, Stanford University School
of Medicine, Palo Alto; Chairman,
Pediatric Quality Assurance Committee,
O'Connor Hospital, San Jose,
California
Mycoplasma Pneumoniae Infections

GEORGE B. MALLORY, JR., M.D.
Assistant Professor of Pediatrics,
Washington University School of
Medicine; Medical Director, Pediatric
Lung Transplant Program, and Director,
Pediatric Pulmonology Fellowship
Training Program, St. Louis Children's
Hospital, St. Louis, Missouri
*Respiratory Muscle Disease and
Dysfunction*

HERBERT C. MANSMANN, JR., M.D.
Professor of Pediatrics and Associate
Professor of Medicine, Thomas Jefferson
University, Philadelphia, Pennsylvania
*Environmental Control as a Modality of
Management for the Pulmonary Patient*

STEPHEN MARKER, M.D.
Pediatric Clinical Faculty, University of
Minnesota; Department of Infectious
Disease, Minneapolis Children's Medical
Center, Minneapolis, Minnesota
Influenza

MELVIN I. MARKS, M.D.
Professor and Vice Chair of Pediatrics,
University of California, Irvine; Medical
Director, Memorial Miller Children's
Hospital, Long Beach, California
Bacterial Pneumonia

RICHARD J. MARTIN, M.D.
Professor of Pediatrics, Case Western
Reserve University; Co-Director of
Neonatology, Rainbow Babies and
Children's Hospital, Cleveland, Ohio
Mechanical Ventilation in Newborns

JAMES W. MATHEWSON, M.D.
Division of Cardiology, and Director,
Cardiovascular Stress Laboratory,
Children's Hospital of San Diego,
San Diego, California
*Cardiovascular-Related Respiratory
Disease*

KAREN S. McCOY, M.D.
Assistant Professor of Pediatrics,
Pulmonary Division, Ohio State
University; Chief, Section of Pulmonary
Medicine, Columbus Children's Hospital,
Columbus, Ohio
*Venous Thrombosis and Pulmonary
Embolus in Childhood*

BENNIE McWILLIAMS, M.D.
Associate Professor of Pediatrics,
University of New Mexico; University of
New Mexico Hospital, Albuquerque,
New Mexico
Mechanical Ventilation in Pediatric Patients

SUSAN MILLARD, M.D.
Assistant Professor, Children's Hospital of
Buffalo, State University of New York at
Buffalo; Pediatric Pulmonologist,
Children's Hospital of Buffalo, Buffalo,
New York
*Pulmonary Involvement in Collagen
Vascular Disorders*

RICHARD B. MOSS, M.D.
Associate Professor of Pediatrics, Stanford
University School of Medicine; Chief,
Division of Allergy, Immunology and
Respiratory Medicine, Lucile Salter
Packard Children's Hospital at Stanford;
Stanford University Hospital, Palo Alto,
California
*Pulmonary Defenses;
Immunopathogenesis of Cystic Fibrosis
Lung Disease*

PATRICIA C. MOYNIHAN, M.D.
Professor, James H. Quillen College of
Medicine, East Tennessee State
University; Director, Division of Pediatric
Surgery, and Staff, Johnson City Medical
Center, Johnson City, Tennessee
Surgical Aspects of Pulmonary Diseases

DENISE MULVIHILL, M.D.
Assistant Professor, Department of
Radiology, Medical University of South
Carolina, Charleston, South Carolina
*Application of Diagnostic Imaging
Techniques in Pediatric Pulmonary Diseases*

SHIRLEY MURPHY, M.D.
Professor of Pediatrics and Director,
Pediatric Pulmonary/Critical Care
Division, University of New Mexico
School of Medicine; University of New
Mexico Hospital/Children's Hospital,
Albuquerque, New Mexico
*Asthma: An Inflammatory Disease; The
Management of Acute Exacerbation of
Childhood Asthma; Cromolyn Sodium:
Basic Mechanisms and Clinical Usage*

J. LAWRENCE NAIMAN, M.D.
Clinical Professor of Pediatrics, Stanford
University School of Medicine, Stanford;
Medical Director, Central California
Region, American Red Cross Blood
Services, San Jose, California
*Pulmonary Complications of Sickle Cell
Disease*

ELIEZER NUSSBAUM, M.D.
Professor of Pediatrics, University of
California, Irvine; Medical Director,
Pediatric Pulmonary and Pediatric Critical
Care, Memorial Miller Children's

Hospital, Long Beach, California
Bacterial Pneumonia

JUDY PALMER, M.D.
Clinical Associate Professor of Pediatrics, Stanford University School of Medicine; Lucile Salter Packard Children's Hospital at Stanford, Palo Alto, California
Pulmonary Complications of Sickle Cell Disease

HOWARD PANITCH, M.D.
Assistant Professor of Pediatrics, Temple University School of Medicine; St. Christopher's Hospital for Children, Philadelphia, Pennsylvania
The Immotile Cilia Syndrome

SUNG MIN PARK, M.D.
Clinical Professor of Pediatrics, University of California, San Diego, School of Medicine, La Jolla; Chief, Division of Pulmonary Medicine, Children's Hospital and Health Center, San Diego, California
Cardiovascular-Related Respiratory Disease

ARUN K. PRAMANIK, M.D.
Associate Professor of Pediatrics, Louisiana State University Medical School; Chief of Neonatology, Louisiana State University Medical Center, Shreveport, Louisiana
Continuous Noninvasive Monitoring of Blood Gases

JOHN R. PRIEST, M.D.
Assistant Professor, Department of Pediatrics, University of Minnesota Hospitals, Minneapolis; Director, Pediatric Hematology and Oncology, Children's Hospital, St. Paul, Minnesota
Thoracopulmonary Neoplasia and Lung Complications of Childhood Cancer

ROBERT W. PRYOR, M.D.
Medical Director, Pediatric Intensive Care Unit, Medical City, Dallas, Texas
Adult Respiratory Distress Syndrome

GREGORY J. REDDING, M.D.
Associate Professor, Department of Pediatrics, University of Washington; Chief, Pulmonary Medicine, and Medical Director of Respiratory Care, Children's Hospital and Medical Center, Seattle, Washington
Pulmonary Hypertension and Cor Pulmonale in Children

WARREN E. REGELMANN, M.D.
Associate Professor of Pediatrics and Infectious Diseases, University of Minnesota Medical School, Minneapolis; University of Minnesota Hospital, Minneapolis; Minneapolis Children's Hospital, Minneapolis, and St. Paul Children's Hospital, St. Paul, Minnesota
Bronchoalveolar Lavage

SANTIAGO-R. REYES DE LA ROCHA, M.D.
Clinical Associate Professor, University of Oklahoma; Director, Pediatric Pulmonary Section, Baptist Medical Center; The Children's Hospital, Oklahoma City, Oklahoma
Adult Respiratory Distress Syndrome

BERYL J. ROSENSTEIN, M.D.
Professor of Pediatrics, Johns Hopkins University School of Medicine; Director, Cystic Fibrosis Center, Johns Hopkins Hospital; Medical Director, Mt. Washington Pediatric Hospital, Baltimore, Maryland
Hemoptysis

RICHARD R. ROSENTHAL, M.D.
Assistant Professor of Medicine, Johns Hopkins University School of Medicine, Baltimore, Maryland; Johns Hopkins Hospital, Baltimore, Maryland, and Fairfax Hospital, Fairfax, Virginia
Bronchoprovocation by Inhalation Challenge With Antigen in Children

DAVID ROSS, M.D.
Assistant Professor of Medicine, University of California, Los Angeles; Medical Director, Lung Transplant Program, Cedars-Sinai Medical Center, Los Angeles, California
Heart-Lung and Lung Transplantation

JONATHAN M. SAMET, M.D.
Professor of Medicine and Chief, Pulmonary and Critical Care Division, University of New Mexico School of Medicine, Albuquerque, New Mexico
Epidemiology and the Pediatric Pulmonologist

DANIEL V. SCHIDLOW, M.D.
Professor and Deputy Chairman, Department of Pediatrics, Temple University School of Medicine; Chief, Section of Pediatric Pulmonology, St. Christopher's Hospital for Children, Philadelphia, Pennsylvania
Bronchopulmonary Dysplasia; The Immotile Cilia Syndrome

DIANE E. SCHULLER, M.D.
Clinical Professor of Pediatrics, Thomas Jefferson Medical College, Philadelphia;

Director, Department of Pediatric Allergy, Immunology and Pulmonary Diseases, Geisinger Medical Center, Danville, Pennsylvania
Antihistamines

ROBERT H. SCHWARTZ, M.D.
Clinical Professor of Pediatrics, University of Rochester Medical Center; Director, Clinical Allergy, Division of Immunology, Allergy and Rheumatology and Department of Pediatrics, Strong Memorial Hospital, University of Rochester Medical Center, Rochester, New York
Alpha₁-Antitrypsin Deficiency

GAIL G. SHAPIRO, M.D.
Clinical Professor of Pediatrics, School of Medicine, University of Washington; Children's Hospital and Medical Center, Seattle, Washington
Glucocorticoids

R. MICHAEL SLY, M.D.
Professor of Pediatrics, The George Washington University School of Medicine and Health Sciences; Chairman of Allergy and Immunology, Children's National Medical Center, Washington, D.C.
Exercise-Induced Asthma; Beta-Adrenergic Agonists in the Treatment of Asthma

MARK SMITH, M.D.
Associate, Division of Pediatric Surgery, M.D. Anderson Hospital; Clinical Instructor, Herman Hospital; Clinical Instructor, Lyndon B. Johnson Hospital, Houston, Texas
Surgical Aspects of Pulmonary Diseases

MARGARET ANN SPRINGER, M.D.
Instructor in Pediatrics, Louisiana State University School of Medicine, Shreveport; Louisiana State University Medical Center, Shreveport, Louisiana
Croup and Epiglottitis

VAUGHN STARNES, M.D.
Professor of Surgery, University of Southern California (USC) School of Medicine; USC University Hospital, Los Angeles County and USC Medical Center, and Children's Hospital—Los Angeles, Los Angeles, California
Heart-Lung and Lung Transplantation

JOHN STEVENS, M.D.
Clinical Associate Professor of Pediatrics,

Indiana University School of Medicine; James Whitcomb Riley Hospital for Children, Indianapolis, Indiana
Pulmonary Edema

HARRIS R. STUTMAN, M.D.
Assistant Professor, Department of Pediatrics, University of California, Irvine; Director, Pediatric Infectious Diseases, Memorial Miller Children's Hospital, Long Beach, California
Antibiotics in Pediatric Pulmonary Infections

MARGARET M. SULLIVAN, M.D.
Assistant Professor of Pediatrics, New York Medical College, Valhalla; St. Vincent's Hospital and Medical Center, New York City, New York
Pulmonary Manifestations of Neurologic Disease

ROBERT S. TEPPER, M.D., PH.D.
Associate Professor of Pediatrics, Department of Pediatrics, Indiana University Medical Center; James Whitcomb Riley Hospital for Children, Indianapolis, Indiana
Pulmonary Function Testing in Infants

JAMES THEODORE, M.D.
Associate Professor of Medicine, Stanford University School of Medicine; Stanford University Hospital, and Lucile Salter Packard Children's Hospital at Stanford, Palo Alto, California
Heart-Lung and Lung Transplantation

ROBERT TOWNLEY, M.D.
Professor of Medicine, Creighton University; St. Joseph Hospital, Omaha, Nebraska
Bronchial Challenge Techniques in Children: Methacholine, Histamine, Hyperventilation, and Osmolar

WILLIAM Y. TUCKER, M.D.
Assistant Professor of Cardiothoracic Surgery, Bowman Gray School of Medicine, Winston-Salem; North Carolina Baptist Hospital, Winston-Salem, and High Point Regional Hospital, High Point, North Carolina
Thoracentesis and Tube Thoracostomy

DALE T. UMETSU, M.D., PH.D.
Assistant Professor of Pediatrics, Stanford University; Lucile Salter Packard Children's Hospital at Stanford, Palo Alto, California
Immunodeficiency and Lung Disease

LAIRTON VALENTIM, M.D.
Pediatric Pulmonologist, Joinville
Community Hospital, Santa Catarina,
Brazil
*Pulmonary Involvement in Collagen
Vascular Disorders*

RUSSELL B. VAN DYKE, M.D.
Associate Professor and Head, Section of
Infectious Diseases, Department of
Pediatrics, Tulane University School of
Medicine; Tulane Medical Center
Hospital, Charity Hospital of New
Orleans, and Children's Hospital of New
Orleans, New Orleans, Louisiana
*Viral Pneumonia; Antiviral Therapy for
Pulmonary Infections*

JOHN E. VAN WYE, M.D.
Former Fellow, Division of Allergy,
Immunology and Respiratory Diseases,
Department of Pediatrics, Stanford
University School of Medicine, Palo Alto,
California; Regional Allergy and Asthma
Consultants; Memorial Mission Hospital
and St. Joseph's Hospital, Asheville, North
Carolina
Passive Smoking

SUSANNAH B. WALKER, M.D.
Clinical Assistant Professor of Pediatrics,
University of Washington; Children's
Hospital and Medical Center, Seattle,
Washington
Glucocorticoids

WILLIAM W. WARING, M.D.
Jane B. Aron Professor of Pediatrics,
Section of Pulmonary Diseases,
Department of Pediatrics, Tulane
University School of Medicine; Tulane
Medical Center Hospital, Charity Hospital
of New Orleans, and Children's Hospital
of New Orleans, New Orleans, Louisiana
Lung Sounds and Phonopneumography

WARREN J. WARWICK, M.D.
Annalisa Marzotto Professor of Cystic
Fibrosis, Pediatrics, Bioengineering, and
Biophysics, Department of Pediatrics,
University of Minnesota Medical School;
Attending Staff, University of Minnesota

Hospital and Clinics, Minneapolis,
Minnesota
Pneumothorax

JAN WATTERSON, B.A.
Research Assistant, Children's Hospital,
St. Paul, Minnesota
*Thoracopulmonary Neoplasia and Lung
Complications of Childhood Cancer*

DAVID F. WESTENKIRCHNER, M.D.
Clinical Associate Professor of Pediatrics,
Indiana University Medical Center;
Medical Director, Emergency
Department, and Associate Medical
Director, Intensive Care Unit, Riley
Hospital for Children, Indianapolis, Indiana
Childhood Near-Drowning

ROBERT W. WILMOTT, M.D.
Associate Professor, Department of
Pediatrics, University of Cincinnati
College of Medicine; Director, Division of
Pulmonary Medicine, Children's Hospital
Medical Center, Cincinnati, Ohio
*Pulmonary Hemosiderosis; Allergic
Bronchopulmonary Aspergillosis*

H. DAVID WILSON, M.D.
Professor of Pediatrics and Chief, Pediatric
Infectious Diseases, University of
Kentucky Medical Center; Attending
Physician, University of Kentucky
Medical Center, Lexington, Kentucky
Histoplasmosis

GLENNA B. WINNIE, M.D.
Associate Professor of Pediatrics, Albany
Medical College; Director, Pediatric
Pulmonary and Cystic Fibrosis Center,
Albany Medical Center Hospital, Albany,
New York
*Perioperative Management of Pediatric
Patients: Physiologic Considerations*

ROBERT E. WOOD, PH.D., M.D.
Professor of Pediatrics, University of
North Carolina; Chief, Pediatric
Pulmonary Medicine, North Carolina
Children's Hospital, Chapel Hill, North
Carolina
Flexible Bronchoscopy in Children

FOREWORD

Although the subspecialty of pediatric pulmonology was not officially recognized by certification boards until 1986, it could be considered one of the oldest as well as one of the newest subspecialties in pediatrics. Many of the common respiratory disorders of children were known to Hippocrates. Today, respiratory disorders of children and newborns account for more hospital days than do disorders of any other organ system. Certainly bronchial asthma has emerged as the most common admission diagnosis in many urban hospitals today.

Pulmonology is one of the disciplines of pediatrics that did not parallel the pathway of its counterparts in internal medicine. Pulmonary internists, many of whom initially directed most of their efforts to the treatment of patients with tuberculosis, staked out their "claim" to all parts of the region between the larynx and diaphragm, except the heart and great vessels, with their subspecialty of pulmonary and critical care medicine. This implied that they claimed competence in all aspects of breathing, infectious disease, critical care, and even the newly established discipline of sleep disorders.

The development of pediatric pulmonology was much more fragmented. The neonatologists were the first to establish their pulmonary related subspecialty; they included all sick newborns under their discipline and promoted the development of neonatal intensive care units and step-down care units under their supervision. Patients with asthma were initially managed predominantly by subspecialists in allergy; now pediatric allergists and pulmonologists share in their management. Pediatric gastroenterologists, infectious disease subspecialists, and pulmonologists continue to share in the treatment of pediatric patients with cystic fibrosis. Common respiratory infections and tuberculosis overlap the domain of the subspecialties in infectious disease and pediatric pulmonary medicine.

The emergence of the current discipline of pediatric pulmonology can be dated to the development of technologies that provide unique means of studying the organ of interest. Among these are the flexible fiberoptic bronchoscope, pioneered by Dr. Robert Wood, and infant pulmonary function testing equipment, developed by Drs. Simon Godfrey, Lynn Taussig, and Mary Ellen Wohl and developed later by other physicians such as Drs. Wayne Morgan, Robert Tepper, Peter LeSouef, and Janet Stocks. The allergists have expanded their horizon into clinical immunology. The neonatologists have pioneered technology to provide life support and transport capability for very small, immature infants. Pediatricians in the field of infectious disease helped in the development of rapid viral diagnosis by immunologic methods and effective, safe antiviral agents such as acyclovir, ganciclovir, and ribavirin. Once pediatric pulmonology was firmly established in 1986, this new subspecialty represented a coalescence of many overlapping subspecialty areas, focusing on disorders of the respiratory system.

Many of us who have contributed to this book have had the good fortune to witness the development of pediatric pulmonology. In the past, we watched helplessly while children struggled with the cough of pertussis or when children died of the pulmonary complications of measles, a common childhood viral disorder. We have observed the development of artificial surfactant and its use in the immature lungs of infants with respiratory distress. We have seen the increased survival of patients with cystic fibrosis and the cloning of the cystic fibrosis gene and its impact in our understanding of the pathophysiology of this disorder. We are beginning to see the application of this discovery in the development of new therapies, both in pharmacology and in genetic engineering with the potential of gene replacement therapy. Many pediatric pulmonologists work with or refer patients with end-stage lung disease for heart-lung or double-lung transplants.

Some of the dark sides of our subspecialty that sadden us are the increase in pulmonary disease and other complications of children with acquired immunodeficiency syndrome (AIDS) and the increased number of premature births of babies addicted to crack cocaine. We anguish over ways and means of providing routine immunizations to large populations of children in many countries. We wonder how society is going to pay for major organ transplants, extracorporeal membrane oxygenation (ECMO) therapy, and even the regular infusions of intravenous immunoglobulin that seem to be helpful for some immunodeficiencies. Solving the issue of costs and benefits of new and expensive treatments is just another hurdle for the future physicians interested in pediatric pulmonary medicine to conquer. Pediatric pulmonologists and other physicians interested in pediatric pulmonary medicine will become increasingly involved in new areas of medicine, including molecular biology, organ transplantation, and the expanding field of clinical immunology.

I think that Dr. Hilman and her co-authors have met their stated goal in producing a successful textbook. I believe that you will enjoy the book; more important, I think that you will use the book in your daily practice of medicine.

———Norman J. Lewiston, M.D.

PREFACE

Physicians keep up with changes in the field of medicine in a number of ways. There are a variety of continuing education seminars, professional conventions, journals, audiotapes, and even a television cable channel devoted to health education. Most health care workers, however, find a need to consult a readily available source such as a textbook. Books come in a variety of shapes and sizes from encyclopedic tomes to pocket handbooks. Both of these have value: the encyclopedic book provides the background necessary for a comprehensive understanding of a subject, and the pocket reference supplies tables and formulas for rapid bedside use. The most frequently used type of book, however, is the textbook, which is somewhere between the two extremes. It is my hope that this textbook on pediatric pulmonary medicine will be useful in the hospital, in the home, and in the clinic.

This book represents contributions from clinicians and scientists from many disciplines who have been very generous in their time and efforts in writing chapters and responding to my requests for updated material. We have tried to provide pathophysiologic background for many clinical problems along with discussions of techniques and pharmacologic agents used in pediatric pulmonary medicine.

As a clinician who has practiced in two subspecialty areas, I have drawn from my peers in both pediatric pulmonology and in allergy/clinical immunology. No single volume textbook can include all appropriate topics in these two overlapping areas. My goal and that of my contributors included a special effort not to duplicate other existing textbooks, but to bring a combined clinical approach to the existing, newly defined area of pediatric respiratory medicine. I have been fortunate to practice clinical pediatric pulmonology and train young physicians in this area while the subspecialty has been developing. I appreciate the opportunity of seeing pediatric pulmonary patients, from whom we have learned so much about the effects of dysfunction of the respiratory system.

I hope this book will be helpful to clinicians in pediatrics and the various overlapping subspecialty areas of infectious disease, allergy/immunology, intensive care, and neonatology as well as thoracic, general, and otolaryngologic surgery and radiology who have interests in pediatric pulmonary subjects. As a teacher, I hope this will be a good resource for medical students, physicians in training, and other health care professionals who assist in the management of pediatric respiratory patients.

I would like to thank my mentor, who introduced me to and trained me in pediatric respiratory medicine, Dr. William Waring. I am also grateful to Dr. Judy Palmer for her assistance in editing and to my office and technical and professional staff who helped make this book possible.

———Bettina C. Hilman, M.D.

CONTENTS

I General Information

1 PULMONARY MECHANICS

G. MICHAEL DAVIS, MB.ChB. / ALLAN L. COATES, M.D.CM, B.Eng. (Elect)

GENERAL PRINCIPLES

The basic purpose of ventilation is the adequate exchange of oxygen and carbon dioxide by the movement of gas into and out of the lungs. The expansion of the lungs (the inspiratory movement) is driven by the respiratory muscles and is opposed primarily by the elastic and resistive forces of the lung. Expiration is usually passive, driven by the elastic recoil forces from energy stored during inspiration. These elastic forces are a combination of surface active forces and the elastic recoil of the tissues; surface forces predominate at low lung volumes, and tissue forces predominate at high volumes.[1] These factors are related through Laplace's law, which states that for a given surface tension (T), the pressure (P) required to hold a given spherical structure open is inversely proportional to the radius (R):

$$P = 2T/R.$$

Hence when the radius is small, the pressure is high but diminishes with increasing volume. As volume increases, the connective tissue infrastructure plays an increasing role in expansion, eventually limiting the maximal volume. If Laplace's law is the only factor, it intuitively seems impossible for large alveoli to coexist with smaller ones because the small ones would collapse into the large ones. Pulmonary surfactant, which generally reduces the surface tension of the air-liquid interface, is unique among surface active agents because as the surface area of the alveolus decreases during exhalation or emptying, the surfactant effect increases, thereby reducing the pressure necessary to keep the alveolus open.[2] This allows the coexistence of populations of alveoli of varying sizes in free communication with each other and with the atmosphere. Overall, the pressure required for expanding the lung against the elastic forces is considered linearly proportional to lung volume (although this is not strictly correct) and is called *compliance,* expressed as the change in volume per unit change in pressure ($C = \Delta V/\Delta P$).

The resistive forces inherent in the lung that oppose the movement of gas and tissues are properties of the airways and the parenchyma. The resistance to the flow of gas is generally much higher than the nonelastic viscous resistance of the tissue. The element of airflow resistance[3] has two components: resistance during laminar airflow, which predominates in the small airways, and resistance during turbulent flow, which predominates in the large central airways; the latter component is by far the major factor determining resistance in older children and adults. In streamlined or laminar flow, the resistance (R) is directly proportional to the length of the airway (l) and the viscosity (n) of the gas and inversely proportional to the fourth power of the radius (r) of the airway (Poiseuille's law):[4]

$$R = 8\eta l/\pi r^4.$$

Because the total cross-sectional area of the airways diminishes as gas moves from the alveoli to the mouth, gas must be accelerated in order to achieve the same bulk flow within a smaller cross section. This gives rise to the second, or turbulent, resistive factor, which is proportional to the velocity of the gas and its density. For clinical measurements, resistance during normal breathing is calculated as the ratio of driving pressure to velocity. Because the diameter of the airways increases with increasing lung volume, this measurement is volume dependent.

The resistance of the respiratory system (R_{rs}) represents the frictional forces opposing airflow through the airways and the energy dissipated within the lung by tissues moving against tissues. Resistance is the measure of the change in pressure required for a unit change in flow ($R = \Delta P/\Delta \dot{V}$), the resistance of the respiratory system (R_{rs}) being the sum of the airway resistance (R_{aw}), lung tissue resistance (R_{LT}), and chest wall resistance (R_W). Each of these resistances from specific areas in the lung may be separately derived according to exactly which pressure is being used with the same flow signal. Thus the accurate definition of the pressure being measured depends on what property of the lung is being examined. In general, R_{aw} is both the major component of R_{rs} and the one most likely to change in disease states. Because most parameters need

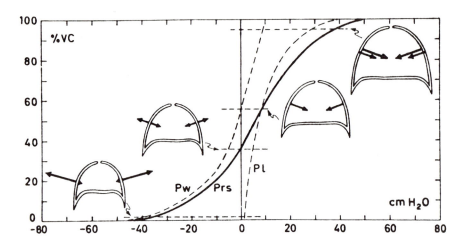

Figure 1-1. Static volume-pressures of the lungs (P_L), the chest wall (P_W), and the total respiratory system (P_{rs}) during relaxation in sitting posture. Large arrows indicate static forces of the lungs and the chest wall (dimensions of arrows are not to scale). Horizontal broken lines indicate volume for each drawing. Volume is expressed as a percentage of vital capacity. The compliance of the lungs, the chest wall, and the respiratory system is the slope of the respective pressure-volume curve. (From Agostoni E, Hyatt RE: Static behavior of the respiratory system. *In* Macklem PT, Mead J (eds): Handbook of Physiology: The Respiratory System, Section 3, Vol. 3, Part I, pp. 113–130. New York: Oxford University Press, 1986.

to be normalized for the size of the child in order to derive normal values, there is a problem with resistance in that it falls as the airway becomes larger. To circumvent this problem, *Conductance* (G) is defined as the reciprocal of the resistance. When the conductance is specified for the lung volume at which it is measured (functional residual capacity, or FRC), it is then called the *specific conductance* (SGaw) with units of $1 \cdot s^{-1} \cdot cmH_2O/1$ FRC for which normal values exist over a wide range of size.

The combination of resistive and elastic forces is expressed as

$$P = V/C + dV/dt \times R + d^2V/dt^2 \times I,$$

where P is the pressure difference between the pleural surface and the mouth (transpulmonary pressure, P_{tp}), V the lung volume, C the compliance of the lung, dV/dt the flow (usually notated as $\dot{V}$), R the resistance, d^2V/dt^2 the acceleration component of the change in volume, and I the inertial component of the lung. In practice, it is common to ignore the last term and compute only the resistive and compliance terms. In other words, the pressure required to move gas through the system is the sum of the pressures required to overcome both the resistive and elastic forces at a given flow and volume.

Thus far, the mechanical properties of the lung (airways and parenchyma) have been considered in isolation. However, the respiratory system includes both the chest wall and the lung. Although function is related primarily to the mechanical properties of the lung in both health and most disease states during quiet breathing, the effect of the chest wall cannot be totally ignored. The respiratory system compliance (C_{rs}) can be divided into two components: that of the chest wall (C_W) and that of the lungs (C_L). The relationship between them is expressed by reciprocals:

$$1/C_{rs} = 1/C_L + 1/C_W.$$

This is more conveniently expressed as the reciprocal of the compliance, the *Elastance* (E), where

$$E = \Delta P/\Delta V \text{ and } E_{rs} = E_L + E_W.$$

The elastic recoil of the lung is always inward, whereas that of the chest wall is outward at low volumes and

inward at high volumes[5] (Fig. 1–1). At a certain point, the inward recoil of the lung is equal and opposite to the outward recoil of the chest wall. This equilibrium point represents the lung volume of the relaxed system and is known as the FRC.

DYNAMICS OF BREATHING

Ventilation is achieved by the action of the muscles of the respiratory system, which causes a change in volume of the thoracic cavity. The principal respiratory muscle groups are the diaphragm, the intercostal muscles, the abdominal wall muscles, and the accessory muscles of the neck, all of which act on the chest wall. Furthermore, the laryngeal muscles control the glottis, which dilates during inspiration and constricts during expiration. The inspiratory muscles act to enlarge the capacity of the thorax through descent of the diaphragm and stabilization with lifting of the rib cage by the intercostal muscles (the so-called bucket-handle movement of the ribs). This action results in a decrease in the intrathoracic pressure (the pressure becomes negative), and airflow from the mouth to the alveoli occurs because of the pressure gradient generated. At times of increased respiratory work, the accessory muscles assist the intercostal muscles.

The action of inspiration requires integration of the diaphragm, the intercostal muscles, and the laryngeal muscles. Contraction of the diaphragm, through its insertion at the borders of the seventh to eleventh ribs, causes the volume of the thorax to increase. In adults, the chest wall is rigid, and therefore the small horizontal component of the muscle force is resisted by the osseous construction of the ribs (Fig. 1–2, left panel). This is not the case in infants and children under 3 years of age, in whom the rib cage is pliable. Hence the horizontal vector of the muscular force may cause inward distortion because newborns do not have a rigid anterior chest wall. During quiet breathing, when the intercostal muscles are stabilizing the rib cage, diaphragmatic contraction in a normal term infant results in effective transmission of the tension generated into a downward displacement of the diaphragm. With increasing force of diaphragmatic contraction, the horizontal tension vector that develops becomes larger and exceeds the structural rigidity of the chest wall, which

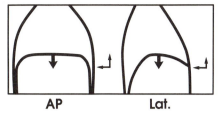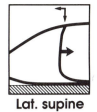

Figure 1–2. Anteroposterior (AP) and lateral (Lat.) schematic of the attachment of the diaphragm to the thorax. *Left panel:* in adults, bold arrows indicate the force applied by the diaphragm during inspiration; light arrows indicate the force applied to the rib cage. *Right panel:* lateral schematic in a supine infant. The potential inward or paradoxical motion of the anterior chest wall during inspiration is resisted by the stiffness of the chest wall. Bold and light arrows have the same meaning as in the left panel.

leads to subcostal retractions and distortion of the anterior chest wall, thereby minimizing the effectiveness of the increase in volume of the thorax (Fig. 1–2, right panel). This volume loss caused by distortion varies with the C_W, which decreases with increasing age. Thus in the premature newborn with lung disease in which the dynamic compliance of the lung is very low (e.g., hyaline membrane disease), the chest wall may be more compliant than the lung, which leads to chest wall distortion.

Such chest wall pliability (increased compliance) also exists in the term infant, but to a lesser degree, and persists after birth because the rib cage, which is primarily cartilaginous at birth, takes many years to become fully ossified and rigid. Even in adults, the loss of the stabilizing effect of the intercostal muscles during inspiration, as is seen in cervical spinal cord injuries, leads to chest wall distortion from the unopposed action of the diaphragm. In infants and young children, C_W is greater than C_L.[6] Because each breath requires approximately 10 cm H_2O pressure for expanding the lungs of a normal infant, the chest wall muscles must augment the rigidity of the pliable rib cage by their tonic contraction in order to fixate the chest wall when the diaphragmatic contraction pulls it

inwards. Otherwise, the pressure generated by the diaphragm would "suck in the chest wall rather than fresh air."[7] This is illustrated in Figure 1–3, which shows progressive chest wall distortion in an infant with progressive laryngeal obstruction due to edema. The tone of the chest wall muscles increases during contraction of the diaphragm in concert with the increase in respiratory drive from the respiratory center and with changes in sleep state. Studies in which C_W has been measured have shown a value of approximately three times the C_L in unmedicated 32-week preterm neonates.[6] C_W then decreases progressively with increasing age; by adolescence, the chest is more rigid, and at midlung volumes, C_W is approximately the same as C_L.[8,9] (see Fig. 1–1).

UPPER AIRWAY

The structures normally included in a description of the upper airway are the larynx, the pharynx, and the nasal and oral cavities. Because of the treelike branching structure of the lungs, the smallest cross section is at the vocal cords, where airflow is highest through the narrowest aperture. The integration of normal inspiration includes dilatation of the larynx with abduction of the vocal cords, in order to facilitate inspiratory airflow.

Investigations of the function of the upper airway have indicated an active role of the airway in the modulation of respiratory pattern, particularly in expiration. Limiting expiratory flow by increasing expiratory resistance is associated with higher lung volume and elevation of the FRC. This phenomenon may explain the advantage to the neonate of expiratory grunting in response to hypoxia.

Under dynamic conditions, the action of the upper airway is paradoxical to that of the intrathoracic airway. During inspiration, the pleural pressure surrounding the trachea and the bronchi is lower than the pressure in the airway, which leads to dilatation of these structures. In the extrathoracic airway, the negative intraluminal pressure of inspiration is augmented by the positive tissue pressure

Figure 1–3. Contribution of the two compartments of the respiratory tract to each breath with the movement of the rib cage (V_{RC}) and abdomen (V_{ABD}) separately measured by Respitrace, and the ventilatory tidal volumes (V_T) simultaneously measured by pneumotachograph. *A,* quiet breathing with synchronous movements. *B,* a mild distortion of the rib cage early in inspiration. *C,* severe sustained rib cage distortion throughout inspiration with a concomitant decrease in V_T. (From Davis GM, Bureau MA: Pulmonary and chest wall mechanics in the control of respiration in the newborn. Clin Perinatol 14:551–579, 1987.)

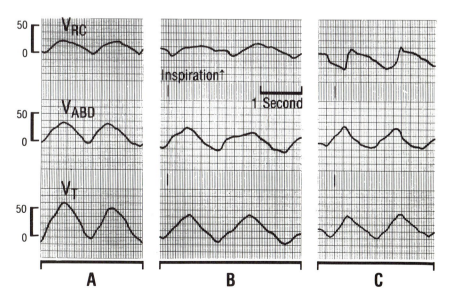

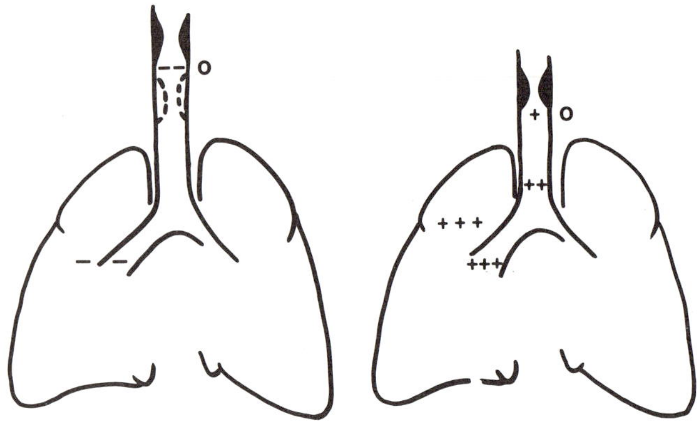

Figure 1-4. The negative intraluminal pressure of the extrathoracic airway favors further collapse of a narrowed segment during inspiration in laryngotracheobronchitis ("croup"). On expiration, the elastic recoil of the lung generates a positive intraluminal pressure that tends to open the airway.

INSPIRATION   **EXPIRATION**

in order to increase the transtracheal pressure and facilitate tracheal narrowing. The converse is true during expiration, so that increased inspiratory resistance is almost always extrathoracic, and an increase in expiratory resistance is usually caused by intrathoracic disease. These differences in pressure have serious consequences in diseases that result in airway narrowing, and the manifestations depend on the location of the disease. In laryngotracheobronchitis (or croup), the upper airway is the predominant site of obstruction. During inspiration there is a pressure drop across the subglottic area, and the pressure in the trachea becomes extremely negative in relation to the surrounding tissue. This results in increased obstruction during inspiration (Fig. 1-4). Conversely, during expiration, the pressure in the trachea becomes positive and hence forces the airway to open.

LARYNGEAL FUNCTION

The expiratory noise associated with vocal cord closure, or the grunting of neonates with hyaline membrane disease, has been recognized as a dynamic braking of expiration by the larynx.[8,10] Proper understanding of the grunting phenomenon led to mimicking the physiologic phenomenon by continuous positive airway pressure (CPAP) or positive end-expiratory pressure (PEEP) in intubated patients.[8,11] Expiratory braking, CPAP, and PEEP are all believed to enhance gas exchange by favoring homogeneous emptying of the lung between the high- and low-compliance alveoli and by increasing the lung volume, thereby augmenting the gas exchange surface through recruitment of new alveoli.

In the absence of audible grunting, the larynx still maintains a dynamic but less apparent role in the slowing down of expiration. This effect, often referred to as intrinsic PEEP, tends to augment lung stability at low lung volume, with minimal cost of energy expenditure. High levels of intrinsic PEEP have been reported in adults with chronic lung disease.[8,12]

DYNAMIC CONTROL OF FRC

In infants, the FRC level is dynamically determined; the FRC is kept above the passive resting volume of totally relaxed expiration.[8,13] This may be achieved by postinspiratory inspiratory muscle activity of the diaphragm, by starting the next inspiration before the relaxed FRC is reached through laryngeal braking during expiration, or by a combination of these actions. Laryngeal braking can be seen as an alternative to the postinspiratory activity of the diaphragm in slowing expiratory flow.[14] These two mechanisms are complementary in that laryngeal braking may relieve the diaphragm of its expiratory work and, conversely, in intubated or tracheotomized patients who lack laryngeal function, may be compensated by the diaphragm to brake expiration.

The dynamic elevation of FRC is not always present. Also, the FRC may change from breath to breath. This concept of a dynamically determined FRC is supported by the fall in FRC that occurs during rapid eye movement (REM) sleep, in which tonic muscle activity is decreased.[8,15,16] Low lung volume is associated with a reduced compliance, and therefore, increased pressure is required for increasing the volume of the alveolus. In other words, the dynamically determined FRC minimizes the work of breathing, optimizes the compliance profile of the system, and maintains an oxygen gas reservoir to minimize changes in arterial oxygenation during expiration.

PRINCIPLES IN THE ASSESSMENT OF PULMONARY FUNCTION

The functional evaluation of the respiratory system in children depends on several factors, the two most important of which are whether the subject is able to cooperate during the measurement procedure and the degree of invasiveness. Because of the requirement to perform practiced ventilatory maneuvers reproducibly, children less than 6 years of age and, often, those who are older but uncooperative have difficulty with some of the basic tests that are necessary for evaluation of pulmonary function.

In normal lungs in adults and in children past the neonatal age range, the FRC is determined passively by the balanced forces of inward elastic recoil of the lung and the outward elastic recoil of the chest wall. The volume of a maximal expiration from FRC is the expired reserve volume (ERV). The volume remaining in the lung is the residual volume (RV). A maximal inspiration from FRC is the inspiratory capacity (IC), and the total volume in the lung at that point is the total lung capacity (TLC) (Fig. 1-5). In normal children, the RV is determined by the outward recoil of the chest wall, which is opposing the maximal contraction of the expiratory muscles. In disease states, it is frequently determined by the closure of narrowed or diseased airways with gas trapping distal to the airway closure.

During forced expiration, when the critical positive driving pressure (P_{dr}) is reached, further increases in P_{dr} do not result in an increase in flow. At this point, part of the P_{dr} is transmitted to the alveoli and across the airway wall,

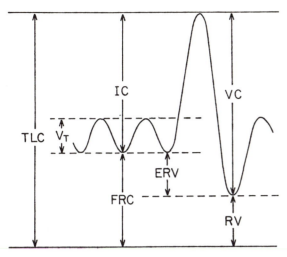

Figure 1–5. The subdivisions of lung volume. The maximal total volume excursion is the vital capacity (VC), the resting lung volume, the functional residual capacity (FRC), the normal volume during tidal breathing (V_T), the inspiratory capacity from FRC (IC), and the expiratory reserve volume from FRC (ERV). The residual volume (RV) remains in the lung after a maximal expiration, and the maximal volume is the total lung capacity (TLC). (From Bates DV, Macklem PT, Christie RV: Respiratory Function in Disease, Chap. 2, pp. 11–35. Philadelphia: WB Saunders, 1971.)

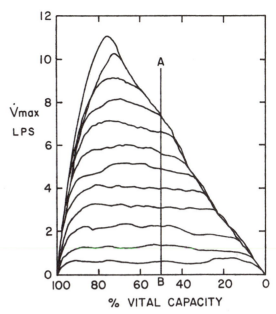

Figure 1–6. Flow-volume curves in which expiratory flow in liters per second (LPS) is plotted against volume as a percentage of vital capacity. These are obtained when a subject performs a series of vital capacity expirations of graded effort, varying from a very slow breath out to one of maximal speed and effort. If the driving pressure (the static elastic recoil pressure plus pleural pressure) for each flow intersected by the line A-B (at 50% vital capacity) is plotted against flow, it can be seen that the four largest efforts achieved a critical driving pressure, above which increased effort does not result in increased flow. $\dot{V}_{max}$, maximal flow. (From Bates DV, Macklem PT, Christie RV: Respiratory Function in Disease, Chap. 2, pp. 11–35. Philadelphia: WB Saunders, 1971.)

causing dynamic compression and resulting in an increase in resistance as P_{dr} increases. This gives rise to the concepts of *flow limitation* and *effort independence* of flow in the maximal expiratory flow-volume curve (MEFVC).[17] The MEFVC consists of expiratory flow plotted against lung volume (Fig. 1–6). Evidence suggests that at lung volumes below 50% of vital capacity, the flow is dependent on (1) lung volume (becoming less as volume decreases); (2) lung elastic recoil, which is the inverse of compliance at any given lung volume and is itself dependent on lung volume; and (3) the tone of the airways. Because the first two factors are less likely to change in most disease states, the MEFVC has gained popularity in the assessment of airway disease.

The measurement of lung compliance requires the measurement of the pressure in the pleural space (P_{pl}). In most clinical settings, this is not feasible, and an indirect method is to use the pressure in the lower third of the esophagus (P_{es}) as a reflection of P_{pl}. This requires a measuring device in the esophagus, a procedure that is somewhat unpleasant but not associated with significant risk. In infants and children unable to cooperate, flow and volume can be measured during normal tidal breathing with a face mask attached to a flow-measuring device. Flow is then integrated with tidal volume (V_T). If P_{pl} is measured simultaneously, compliance and resistance can be calculated. Less invasive methods are used to measure the total respiratory system compliance (C_{rs}), and it is assumed that the compliance of the chest wall is normal and that only lung compliance is affected by any disease process.

The measurement of resistance is more complicated than that of compliance. The respiratory system resistance (R_{rs}) can be partitioned into its contributing elements, and these elements can be independently deter-

mined by a variety of techniques, such as measurement by a plethysmograph of the airway resistance (R_{aw}) alone during quiet breathing.[18] Both R_{aw} and R_{rs} are measured during quiet breathing and behave as fixed resistances over a small range in volume close to FRC, so that an increase in the respiratory driving pressure (P_{dr}), in this case P_{pl}, causes a proportional increase in flow.

Before specific pulmonary function testing in children is considered, it is necessary to examine techniques for measurement because the properties of the respiratory system vary with the part being examined. It is important to know whether the measurement in question is pleural pressure, transpulmonary pressure, or pressure across the whole respiratory system. The flow or volume of the gas exchanged may be measured either by displacement of the body surface or by actual measurement of the gas at the mouth.

The measurement of tidal volume is usually performed in one of three manners: volume displacement with the use of a water or dry rolling seal spirometer, change in volume of the whole body during each respiratory cycle (plethysmography), or integration of airflow measured at the mouth.

1. The *spirometer* measures tidal volume directly by determining the expired breath volume by physical displacement. This is the most precise and reproducible technique, and the results are the standard measurements against which all comparisons of measurements are made.

2. *Body plethysmography* is based on the change in the total body volume with each respiratory effort. The pressure plethysmograph is an airtight container into which the patient (an infant or an older child) is placed with only the head, the face, or the airway in communication with the outside. Each inspiration changes the volume of the thorax, leading to a compression of gas in the box surrounding the subject, and a rise in the pressure inside the box is measured by a pressure transducer. The volume change is calculated according to Boyle's law. For older patients, a volume displacement plethysmograph can be used if changes in volume are measured by a spirometer connected to the plethysmograph.

3. The *pneumotachograph* is the most common and practical method of measuring the resting ventilation. The technique depends on laminar airflow through a known resistance. The pressure differential across a resistance is measured and the flow calculated ($\dot{V} = \Delta P/R$). To obtain tidal volume, the flow signal is integrated with time and requires calibration for gas concentration, humidity, and temperature.

TECHNIQUES FOR COOPERATIVE CHILDREN

Spirometry

The FVC maneuver is the crux of spirometry, and the ability to perform it reliably and consistently is the basis of tests that require active cooperation. During the maneuver, the relationship between expired lung volume from TLC to RV is plotted against time (Fig. 1–7). Clinically useful are both the actual FVC and the volume that

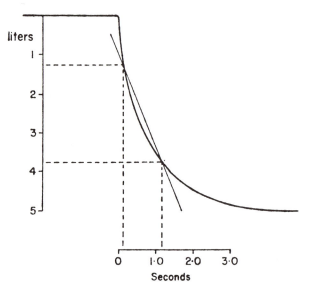

Figure 1–7. Forced expiration from total lung capacity. The maximal volume excursion is the forced vital capacity (FVC); the volume emerging in the first second is the forced expiratory volume in 1 sec (FEV$_1$). The slope of the fine line drawn between the points at 25% and 75% of the FVC is the forced expiratory flow at 25% and 75% of vital capacity (FEF$_{25-75}$). (From Bates DV, Macklem PT, Christie RV: Respiratory Function in Disease, Chap. 2, pp. 11–35. Philadelphia: WB Saunders, 1971.)

comes out during the first second (the forced expiratory volume in 1 sec, or FEV$_1$). Both indices have been shown to be reproducible for a given subject through the use of a wide range of measuring devices, and normal reference standards are available for age, sex, and race.[19–21] More important, in a growing number of disease states, prognostic and pathophysiologic interpretations are possible. A decreased FVC with normal flow indices is suggestive of restrictive lung disease, whereas a decreased FEV$_1$ with a normal FVC is suggestive of obstructive airway disease.

Less precise measures, both physiologically and epidemiologically, are the peak expiratory flow rate (PEFR) and the forced expiratory flow between 25% and 75% of vital capacity (FEF$_{25-75}$). Both tests, particularly the PEFR, are less reproducible than either the FVC or the FEV$_1$ and thus normal values have a larger range. Furthermore, the measuring devices do not have the same interapparatus reproducibility for the flow parameters as for measurement of the FEV$_1$ or the FVC. Consequently, the recommendations of the American Thoracic Society[22] are that emphasis be placed on the FEV$_1$ and the FVC, for which standards are better defined and normal values better developed.

Flow-Volume Curves

The MEFVC is the plot of expiratory flow against volume instead of volume against time, as shown by spirometry (Fig. 1–8). Not only can the FVC and the FEV$_1$ be determined but, as mentioned earlier, the maneuver also becomes effort independent after the first 50% of expired volume.[17] The clinical use of the MEFVC depends on the measurement of maximal flow at specific lung volumes, usually 25% and 50% of VC or 60% of TLC (measuring from RV) which, in order to normalize for size, are frequently expressed as TLC/sec. Clinical use also depends on the ability to accurately measure lung volume. During the MEFVC, the lung volume depends on both the expired volume of gas from the lungs and the volume of gas that has been compressed by transpulmonary pressure; the latter is extremely effort dependent because it is directly related to the magnitude of P$_{dr}$. The theory of flow limitation was developed through the use of data derived from MEFVC performed in a volume displacement plethysmograph, which measured both the expired volume and the compressed volume. Subsequently, many centers have used an MEFVC in which volume is derived only from the expired gas and have thereby ignored the volume of gas compression. This causes only minor errors in normal subjects, but in patients with significant lung disease, the errors can be large and extremely effort dependent,[23] hence diminishing the physiologic basis of the assessment.

Assessment of Lung Volumes

Measurement of lung volume—that is, the amount of gas inside the thoracic cavity—is critical for the description of the physical properties of the respiratory system. The lung is unable to completely empty, and therefore, an unknown amount of residual gas is always present within the thorax at RV or at maximal end expiration. Because

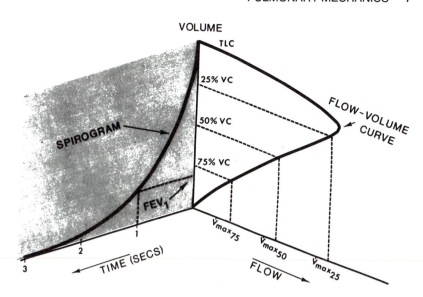

Figure 1–8. The forced expiratory maneuver is represented as a volume-time plot *(left)* and as a maximal expiratory flow volume (MEFV) curve *(right.)* Volume is represented as a percentage of vital capacity (VC). In this illustration, the percentage of VC is given as a percentage of expired volume so that flows at high lung volumes are represented as flows of 25% of VC. Another convention, often used when MEFV curves are examined, is to consider volume in terms of the fraction of the VC remaining in the lung. Thus 25% of expired VC is equivalent to 75% of VC; that is, 75% of VC is the volume in the lung. MEFV curves are frequently represented with volume on the horizontal axis (see Fig. 1–3). Total lung capacity (TLC), or 100% of VC, may be represented on the left or right side of the volume axis. FEV_1, forced expiratory volume in 1 second. $\dot{V}_{max_{25}}$, $\dot{V}_{max_{50}}$, and $\dot{V}_{max_{75}}$ represent the maximal airflow at 25%, 50%, and 75% of the expired VC. (From McBride JT, Wohl ME: Pulmonary function tests. Pediatr Clin North Am 26:537–551, 1979.)

it is difficult to perform respiratory maneuvers at RV, the relaxed volume at the end of expiration during quiet ventilation (FRC) is generally the volume determined. The two principal techniques for measuring lung volumes are (1) gas dilution with the use of an inert gas and (2) body plethysmography. In order to denote a plethysmographic measurement, the volume measured is referred to as the thoracic gas volume (V_{tg}).

To measure FRC by gas dilution, the subject commences rebreathing at FRC from a circuit with a known volume and concentration of the inert marker gas (usually helium) mixed with oxygen and nitrogen. Carbon dioxide is scrubbed from the system and oxygen added as it is taken up in order to keep the overall total volume the same. At equilibration, when inspired and expired helium concentrations are the same, the final concentration of the helium marker (He) is decreased in proportion to the unknown lung volume that was added to the known volume of the system. This is most commonly performed with an initial helium concentration of approximately 20%. Because the total amount of helium is the same at the initial $[He_i]$ and final $[He_f]$, the FRC is determined as follows:

$$V_1 \times He_i = (V_1 + FRC) \times He_f$$

An alternative but similar technique is to displace the nitrogen within the lung by breathing pure oxygen; this method is referred to as the *nitrogen washout technique.* In this method, the total nitrogen content expired after the switch to oxygen is proportional to the total volume of gas within the lung at the beginning of the test. This method was used by Bancalari[24] in newborns to estimate FRC by determining the integrated nitrogen content during conditions of constant flow.

Both helium dilution and nitrogen washout techniques measure the gas that is in direct continuity with the central airway. In diseases associated with gas trapping and in poorly communicating regions where gas is inaccessible for exchange, the FRC is underestimated in these tech-

niques. In addition, leaks in the circuit or at the mouth are a potential source of error. In the nitrogen washout technique, the use of 100% oxygen may cause significant amount of absorption atelectasis and alteration in ventilation perfusion ratios.

Plethysmography

In an effort to measure the total volume of air in the lungs, including the volume of gas not in direct communication with the airway opening, Dubois and colleagues[25] described the use of a gas-compression technique based on Boyle's law. In this technique, the subject is seated within the plethysmograph and performs a series of forced inspiratory and expiratory maneuvers (panting) against an occluded airway, which causes gas rarefaction and compression to occur in the lungs. The resultant change in total body volume can be related to pressure changes at the airway opening, thus enabling the measurement of the total volume of gas in the lungs (or the thorax), which is denoted the V_{tg}. The V_{tg}, the ERV, and a slow vital capacity (VC) can be used to derive the TLC (Fig. 1–5). This maneuver has traditionally involved panting against a shutter valve at the mouth, a procedure that some young children find difficult. An alternative method has been proposed,[26] in which the child makes a single inspiratory effort against the shutter valve, causing rarefaction of gas in the lungs. According to Boyle's law,

$$V_1 P_1 = V_2 P_2$$

or

$$V_{tg} \times (P_{bar} - 47) = (V_{tg} + \Delta V) \times (P_{bar} - 47 - \Delta P),$$

where P_{bar} is the barometric pressure, 47 is the saturated water vapor pressure (in millimeters of mercury), and ΔV and ΔP are the changes in volume and pressure.

Three assumptions underlie this method. The first is that the maneuver is isothermal within the lungs, a premise supported by fairly strong experimental evidence. The second is that the pressure measured at the airway opening is identical to the pressure in the alveolus; in other words, there are no flow-resistive losses, and the pressure is transmitted either directly or through a negligible barrier. Third, the change in gas volume applies only to thoracic gas. If the frequency of panting is high, the upper airway may act as a capacitive element, and flow-resistive losses may occur as gas flows back and forth through narrowed airways into and out of the upper airway. These flow-resistive pressure losses can be avoided through the use of a panting frequency of 1 Hz or less[27] and by the placement of hands on the subject's cheeks to provide support and reduce the capacitance. The transmission of pressure to all alveoli has been recognized as a problem in neonates and small infants[28] but not in older children or adults. At present, the usefulness of this method in infants and neonates does not rest on firm experimental evidence. Finally, although abdominal gas theoretically may undergo volume change, experimental evidence suggests that this is not a major concern.[25]

In addition to measuring lung volume, the plethysmograph is useful in the measurement of R_{aw} and the MEFVC. The measurement of R_{aw} is predicated on the basis that differences in alveolar pressure and ambient pressure give rise to slight but measurable changes in total body volume as pulmonary gas is compressed and rarefied during quiet breathing. Because the relationship between changes in volume and alveolar pressure has already been established during the measurement of V_{tg} with the measurement of flow at the airway opening and with changes in body volume, R_{aw} can be calculated.[18] Specifically, after the measurement of V_{tg}, the subject breathes quietly through the pneumotachograph within the plethysmograph so that the only change in the volume of the plethysmograph is caused by compression and rarefaction of alveolar gas. From this change in volume, the alveolar pressure in relationship to flow can be derived and the resistance calculated.

Measurement of Static Compliance

Quasi-static compliance of the lung means that the elastic recoil pressures are measured in the absence of any airflow or movement of the respiratory system. With an esophageal pressure–measuring device in place (usually a balloon attached to a catheter), the subject makes a slow inspiration followed by a slow expiration with multiple pauses in which, with the glottis open, the pressure difference between the mouth and the esophagus is measured. The maneuver is performed so that volume can be measured simultaneously, usually by a pneumotachograph or a spirometer. The pressure in the esophagus, taken to represent P_{pl}, is plotted against volume, and a pressure-volume curve is created. The slope of the curve in the region of FRC is the compliance. The pressure at any given lung volume is the static elastic recoil pressure (P_{st}). Although during the maneuver the pressure at airway opening (P_{ao}) (or mouth) traditionally is atmospheric, this does not have to be the case. In the more general approach, under static conditions, P_{st} is the transpulmonary pressure (P_{tp}), which is by definition $P_{pl} - P_{ao}$.

TECHNIQUES IN INFANTS

A major barrier to the measurement of lung function in infants, newborns, and preschool children is the lack of coordination and cooperation from the subjects in the performance of respiratory maneuvers. In addition, there are physiologic differences, the most important being variation in FRC (V_{tg}) as a result of the changes in the stability of the airway and the chest wall under respiratory loads. Thus most investigators have found difficulty in obtaining reproducible results, and values reported in normal infants vary widely according to the techniques and whether sedation was used. Sedation is sometimes used to attain quiet regular respiration and improve reproducibility. The simplest measurements performed on preschool children and newborns is the measurement of tidal volumes (V_T) either during quiet spontaneous breathing or during mechanical ventilation. Although volume-displacement spirometry and plethysmography are possible, the most commonly used technique is tidal volume measurements with a pneumotachograph. A pneumotachograph suitable for a sick or small infant must be of low mass, small dead space, and low resistance.

Measurement of Volumes

The use of a pneumotachograph of low resistance and small dead space to measure airflow in newborns is widespread. The device is either coupled directly to an endotracheal tube if one is in place or used in conjunction with a face mask of appropriate size. The flow signal is then integrated to V_T in order to give breath-by-breath information about the pattern of respiration.

There are technical problems with these techniques. First, an appropriate pneumotachograph of small dead space must be used to avoid disturbing the pattern of respiration by increasing dead space (V_D). In intubated infants the fit of the endotracheal tube in the trachea is important because air leakage negates the precision of the measurement. This is apparent in the V_T tracing because there is a large discrepancy between the inspiratory and expiratory limb of the trace, which leads to an unstable base line. Air leakage, which is most apparent on expiration, can be minimized by gentle tracheal pressure.

The use of a face mask also introduces errors into the measurement. First, an increase in V_D is contributed by the pneumotachograph and the face mask in an effort to increase ventilatory efforts. Furthermore, positioning of the face mask is associated with trigeminal nerve stimulation, a potent inducer of vagal reflexes that may alter the pattern of respiration. Despite these limitations, face mask recordings remain a popular method of determining breath-by-breath ventilation in infants.

Partial Flow Volume Curves

In an attempt to assess the maximal flow characteristics of the respiratory system in infants, techniques for forcing expiration have been developed. The externally applied positive pressure ("hugging") technique of Taussig and associates[29] and the negative tracheal pressure technique of Motoyama[30] are two examples of this approach for accelerating expiration to maximal flow pattern. After normal inspiration occurs, an external force is applied in order to maximize expiratory flow and to extend the expiratory limb beyond FRC. The results are expressed as flow at FRC ($\dot{V}_{max}$ FRC), previously established as a constant volume in the quiet-breathing flow-volume curve. This technique is used to measure flow characteristics and is most useful in the assessment of diseases associated with altered resistance.

A number of issues with these techniques remain unresolved. In the "hugging" technique, the external force applied varies and is not necessarily fully transmitted to the pleural space, so that flow rates achieved may be related to the magnitude and the mode of inflation of the external cuff.[31,32] The sudden application of negative tracheal pressure may avoid these problems, but this technique requires intubation and usually anesthesia, which thereby limits its applicability. Finally, normal values are extremely variable, although there is strong correlation within the same subject before and after the use of bronchodilators.

Compliance and Resistance

In the classic *Mead-Whittenberger method*, techniques developed for the measurement of both dynamic C_L and R_L in adults are used in infants; esophageal pressure (P_{es}) and pressure of the airway opening (P_{ao}) are used to derive P_{tp} (the difference between the two), and flow, which is integrated into volume, is measured. That P_{es} reflects the change in pleural pressure can be validated with an occlusion test[33,34] in which the airway is occluded during inspiration so that under conditions of no flow, if $\Delta P_{es} = \Delta P_{ao}$, then $P_{pl} = P_{es}$.

P_{es} has been successfully measured in neonates either by an esophageal balloon[35] or by water-filled catheter,[33,36] according to well-described techniques. Conflicting findings suggest that the pleural pressure may not be uniform throughout the pleural space under all conditions and that during REM sleep or with chest wall distortion, validation of the occlusion test may be impossible.[37] However, results of one study[36] suggested that a fluid-filled catheter in intubated neonates with obvious chest wall distortion can yield valid measurements of P_{pl}. The technique requires an intact pleural-esophageal interaction, and thus measurements are suspect in patients who have undergone thoracic or abdominal surgery.

The technique is based on the general equation of the lung

$$P_{tp} = (V_T \times 1/C) + (\dot{V} \times R_L),$$

where P_{tp} is the pressure generated by the respiratory muscles on inspiration and by the elastic recoil on expiration. At points of no flow ($\dot{V} = 0$), resistive forces are negligible and the pressure is directly related to volume. Hence the compliance is

$$C_L \text{ (dyn)} = \Delta V_T / \Delta P,$$

where ΔV_T is taken from end inspiration to end expiration in which $\dot{V} = 0$. Similarly, at the points of equal vol-

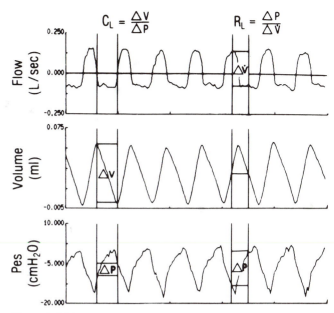

Figure 1–9. Measurement of dynamic lung compliance (C_L) and dynamic lung resistance (R_L) by continuous measurement of flow (V), tidal volume (V_T), and esophageal pressure (here, Pes), which, because the airway is open to the atmosphere, represents transpulmonary pressure (P_{tp}). (From Davis GM, Coates AL, Dalle D, Bureau MA: Measurement of pulmonary mechanics in the newborn lamb: A comparison of three techniques. J Appl Physiol 64:972–981, 1988.)

ume, one on inspiration and the other on expiration, the elastic tissue forces are assumed to be equal and opposite (Fig. 1–9). Resistance is

$$R_L = \Delta P / \Delta \dot{V}$$

There are limitations to this method. The first is that the subject must have slow, regular respiration with a constant volume in order to accurately determine compliance, and these conditions occur mainly during quiet sleep. Second, the measurements include only two points within the respiratory cycle, and it is assumed that the system is linear. In fact, there is strong physiologic evidence of a difference in the inspiratory and expiratory resistances, especially in the presence of expiratory laryngeal braking. This variable may be excluded by intubation to control the role of the upper airway.

A number of techniques[13,38,39] involving airway pressure (P_{ao}) have been developed to avoid placing an intraesophageal measuring device by using P_{ao} as a reflection of the pressure at the alveolus (P_{alv}) under conditions of occlusion. Because these techniques entail measuring the pressure across the whole respiratory system, the C_{rs} and R_{rs} (the combination of lung and chest wall resistances and compliances) can be obtained.

Occlusion of the airway at end inspiration invokes the expiratory Hering-Breuer reflex in young infants. This vagally mediated reflex leads to a cessation of respiratory muscle activity and relaxation of the chest wall against the occluded airway, generating a positive expiratory pressure plateau that represents the elastic recoil of the system towards FRC.[34,39] The combination of tidal volume at occlusion (V_{occ}) and the airway pressure (ΔP_{ao}) represents

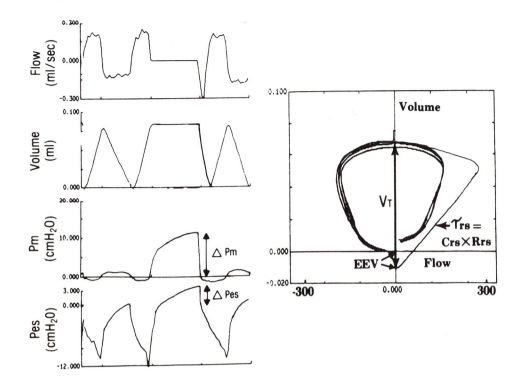

Figure 1–10. Occlusion at end inspiration. The pressure at the mouth rises as the system relaxes *(left panel).* The occlusion is released, resulting in a partial flow volume curve *(single line, right panel).* From the change in mouth pressure (ΔP_m) and total expired volume, respiratory system compliance (C_{rs}) can be calculated. The slope of the flow volume curve is the time constant (τ), which is $C_{rs} \times R_{rs}$ (respiratory system resistance), enabling the calculation of R_{rs}. (From Davis GM, Coates AL, Dalle D, Bureau MA: Measurement of pulmonary mechanics in the newborn lamb: A comparison of three techniques. J Appl Physiol 64:972–981, 1988.)

the static compliance of the respiratory system ($C_{rs(stat)}$), where

$$C_{rs(stat)} = V_{occ}/\Delta P_{ao}.$$

At various times after this relaxation, depending on respiratory drive from chemoreceptors, the next respiratory effort is another inspiration. Release of the occlusion before the termination of the Hering-Breuer reflex leads to passive deflation of the lungs, which is not influenced by respiratory muscle activity. The slope of the linear portion of the flow-volume curve generated by this passive deflation (Fig. 1–10) represents the passive time constant (τ_{rs}), where

$$\tau_{rs} = C_{rs} \times R_{rs},$$

and thus the passive respiratory system resistance (R_{rs}) may be determined from a single expiratory occlusion.

Variations in this technique have been used to extend the validity of the results. In the "volume clamping" technique,[40] measurements of successive inspirations are stacked one on top of another to give values for $C_{rs(stat)}$ over a larger volume range, and occlusions at different points in tidal breathing.[41] The technique may be used to determine the dynamic elevation of FRC, inasmuch as the passive expired volume is below the previous FRC level. Extrapolation yields a new lower resting volume, which is considered the relaxed equilibrium volume (see Fig. 1–10) or the volume at which outward chest wall recoil balances inward recoil of the lungs. Because the change in pressure is the pressure at end-inspiratory occlusion minus atmospheric pressure, it is essential that the change in volume, or V_{occ}, be the volume at end inspiration minus the equilibrium volume. If FRC is dynamically deter-

mined and the relaxed volume not measured, C_{rs} is too low.[34]

Several assumptions are inherent in this method. First, all respiratory muscles are relaxed by the Hering-Breuer reflex. It is known that the laryngeal muscles act independently of the Hering-Breuer reflex, and therefore the technique may be inaccurate in the nonintubated subject. Second, sleep state alters the sensitivity to the Hering-Breuer reflex and therefore may not be reliably evoked during REM sleep. Furthermore, the assumption of a linear P/V relationship is probably correct over tidal volume range, but the variability of FRC in REM sleep makes the measurement of V_{occ} difficult. Finally, the assumption of a single time constant (τ) for the respiratory system is questionable, especially in infants with lung disease.

Mortola and Saetta[38] used inspiratory occlusion as a means of determining dynamic respiratory system mechanics with P_{ao}. The assumptions of this technique include a constant respiratory drive and pattern, a stable FRC, and the ability to time respiratory events precisely. If the respiratory pattern is stable, the pressure-time profile to produce $\dot{V}$ and V_T is the same from breath to breath. Thus the driving pressure from an occluded breath is identical to that from a nonoccluded breath when $\dot{V}$ and V_T are measured (Fig. 1–11). In this technique, the changes in P_{ao} during an occluded breath are matched to the $\dot{V}$ and V_T from the previous nonoccluded breath. In practice, this technique is extremely difficult to perform. The timing of the occlusions is critical, and reflex mechanoreceptor feedback is induced by the pressure gradient with lung expansion to alter the pressure-time profile. If the data obtained in the first 150 msec of occlusion are used (before the feedback alters the respiratory strategy), dynamic respiratory system compliance and resistance can be calculated. Again, however, a small portion of each

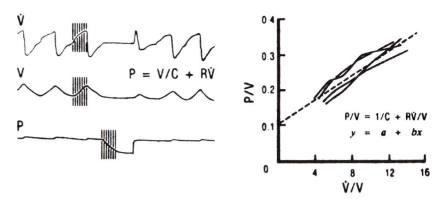

Figure 1–11. Graphic illustration of analytic methods. Measurement of dynamic lung compliance (C) and dynamic lung resistance by continuous measurement of flow ($\dot{V}$), tidal volume (V_T), and esophageal pressure (P). The end-expiratory occlusion technique with linear regression of mouth pressure (P_m) divided by V_T versus $\dot{V}/V_T$ to give dynamic respiratory system resistance as the slope of the regression line and dynamic respiratory system compliance as the reciprocal of the intercept of the ordinate. V, volume. (From Davis GM, Coates AL, Dalle D, Bureau MA: Measurement of pulmonary mechanics in the newborn lamb: A comparison of three techniques. J Appl Physiol 64:972–981, 1988.)

respiration is used to determine the respiratory mechanics and may not be truly representative of the whole breath.

The multiple-occlusion interrupter technique has been reintroduced as a method of describing theoretical models of the lung[42] by utilizing a rapidly closing valve (10 to 15 msec) that transiently interrupts airflow. Occlusion of the airflow above FRC leads to a recoil of the respiratory system and the generation of pressure transients. The pressure transient has two components: a rapidly achieved ΔP_{init}, which is thought to represent the resistive pressure gradient across the airways (and perhaps a component of the chest wall), and the more slowly achieved plateau of ΔP_{ss}, which represents stress recovery of the tissues of the lung and chest wall.

R_{init}, represented by $\Delta P_{init}/\dot{V}$ at the time of valve closure, appears to represent the resistance and elastance of the conducting airways, whereas the later ΔP_{ss} may represent the viscoelastic properties of the tissues. In animal studies and in a limited number of human studies, it appears that this technique has considerable promise in providing detailed physiologic information in ventilated subjects, but further assessment of the limitations of the technique are needed.

Forced oscillation, in contrast with most pulmonary function tests in children, does not require cooperation and therefore is potentially useful in young children, usually over 4 years of age. In this technique, the subject breathes through a pneumotachograph, and an oscillatory pressure signal at various frequencies (but at least at several times the respiratory rate) is applied to the respiratory system. From the changes in magnitude and phase relationship of flow to the superimposed pressure signal, it is possible to calculate total respiratory system resistance, the in-phase component of the pressure-flow relationship, and the reactance (the 90-degree out-of-phase component).[4] This resistance (R_{rs}) represents the combination of airway, tissue, and chest wall resistance, whereas the reactance (X_{rs}) is the combination of elastic and inertial components. The total impedance of the system (Z_{rs}) is equal to the square root of ($R_{rs}^2 + X_{rs}^2$). Although this technique appears reliable in experimental conditions, it may be influenced by several variables not always easily controlled in small children. In particular, it is essential to support the subject's cheeks in order to reduce the capacitance of the upper airway, to limit movement of the tongue or the neck, and to prevent changes in the glottic aperture, all of which are not always easy to achieve and may influence the results obtained. Nevertheless, this technique has been shown to yield results equivalent to the FEV_1 in asthmatics undergoing a bronchial provocation test.[43]

REFERENCES

1. Rodarte JR, Rehder K: Dynamics of Respiration. *In* Macklem PT, Mead J (eds): Handbook of Physiology: The Respiratory System, Section 3, vol. 3, pt. I, pp. 131–144. Bethesda, MD: American Physiological Society, 1986.
2. Notter RH, Shapiro DL: Lung surfactant in an era of replacement therapy. Pediatrics 68:781–789, 1981.
3. Pedley TJ, Drazen JM: Aerodynamic theory. *In* Macklem PT, Mead J (eds): Handbook of Physiology: The Respiratory System, Section 3, vol. 3, pt. I, pp. 41–54. Bethesda, MD: American Physiological Society, 1986.
4. Peslin R, Fredberg JJ: Oscillation mechanics of the respiratory system. *In* Macklem PT, Mead J (eds): Handbook of Physiology: The Respiratory System, Section 3, vol. 3, pt. I, pp. 145–177. Bethesda, MD: American Physiological Society, 1986.
5. Agostoni E, Hyatt RE: Static behavior of the respiratory system. *In* Macklem PT, Mead J (eds): Handbook of Physiology: The Respiratory System, Section 3, vol. 3, pt. I, pp. 113–130. Bethesda, MD: American Physiological Society, 1986.
6. Davis GM, Coates AL, Papageorgiou A, Bureau MA: Direct measurement of static chest wall compliance in animal and human neonates. J Appl Physiol 65:1093–1098, 1988.
7. Muller, NL, Bryan AC: Chest wall mechanics and respiratory muscles in infants. Pediatr Clin North Am 26:503–516, 1979.
8. Davis GM, Bureau MA: Pulmonary and chest wall mechanics in the control of respiration in the newborn. Clinics in Perinatology, 14:551–579, 1987.
9. Sharp M, Druz W, Balgot R, et al: Total respiratory compliance in infants. J Appl Physiol 29:775–779, 1970.
10. Hjalmarson O: Mechanics of breathing in RDS. *In* Raivo KO, Hallmann N, Kouralainen K, et al (eds): Respiratory Distress Syndrome, pp. 171–185. London: Academic Press, 1984.
11. Harrison VC, de Hesse E, Klein M: The significance of grunting in hyaline membrane disease. Pediatr 41:549–559, 1968.
12. Milic-Emili J: Is weaning an art or a science? [Editorial] Am Rev Respir Dis 134:1107–1108, 1986.
13. Mortola JP, Fisher JT, Smith B: Dynamics of breathing in infants. J Appl Physiol 52:1209–1215, 1982.
14. England SJ, Bartlett D, Knutt SM: Comparison of human vocal cord movements during isocapneic hypoxia and hypercapnea. J Appl Physiol 53:81–86, 1982.
15. Henderson-Smart DJ, Reid DJC: Depression of intercostal and abdominal muscle activity and vulnerability to asphyxia during active sleep in the newborn. *In* Guilleminault C, Dement WC (eds): Sleep Apnea Syndromes, pp. 93–117. New York: Liss, 1978.
16. Lopes J, Muller NL, Bryan MH, et al: Importance of inspiratory muscle tone in maintenance of FRC in the newborn. J Appl Physiol 51:830–834, 1981.
17. Mead J, Turner JM, Macklem PT, Little JB: Significance of the relationship between lung recoil and maximum expiratory flow. J Appl Physiol 22:95–108, 1967.

18. Dubois AB, Botelho SY, Comroe JH: A new method for measuring airway resistance in man using a body plethysmograph: Values in normal subjects and patients with respiratory disease. J Clin Invest 35:327–335, 1956.
19. Hsi BP, Hsu KHK, Jenkins DE: Ventilatory functions of normal children and young adults: Mexican-American, white and black. III: Sitting height as a predictor. J Pediatr 102:860–865, 1983.
20. Knudson RJ, Lebowitz MD, Holberg CJ, Burrows B: Changes in the maximum expiratory flow-volume curve with growth and aging. Am Rev Respir Dis 127:725–734, 1983.
21. Schwartz J, Katz SA, Fegley RW, Tockman MS: Sex and race differences in the development of lung function. Am Rev Respir Dis 138:1415–1421, 1988.
22. American Thoracic Society: Lung function testing: Selection of reference values and interpretive strategies. Am Rev Respir Dis 144:1202–1218, 1991..
23. Coates AL, Desmond KJ, Demizio D, et al: Sources of error in flow-volume curves: Effect of expired volume measured at the mouth vs. that measured in a body plethysmograph. Chest 94:976–982, 1988.
24. Bancalari E: Pulmonary function testing and other diagnostic laboratory procedures. In Thibeault DW, Gregory GA (eds): Neonatal Respiratory Care, pp. 195–234. Norwalk, CT: Appleton-Century-Crofts, 1986.
25. Dubois AB, Botelho SY, Bedell GN, et al: A rapid plethysmographic method for measuring thoracic gas volume: Comparison with nitrogen washout method for measuring functional residual capacity in normal subjects. J Clin Invest 35:322–326, 1956.
26. Desmond KJ, Demizio DL, Allen PD, et al: An alternate method for the determination of functional residual capacity in a plethysmograph. Am Rev Respir Dis 137:273–276, 1988.
27. Shore S, Milic-Emili J, Martin J: Reassessment of body plethysmographic technique for the measurement of thoracic gas volume in asthmatics. Am Rev Respir Dis 126:515–520, 1982.
28. Godfrey S, Beardsmore S, Maayan C, Bar-Yishay E: Can thoracic gas volume be measured in infants with airways obstruction? Am Rev Respir Dis 133:245–251, 1986.
29. Taussig LM, Landau LI, Godfrey S, Arad I: Determinations of forced expiratory flows in newborn infants. J Appl Physiol 53:1270–1277, 1982.
30. Motoyama EK: Respiratory mechanics during early postnatal years. Pediatr Res 11:220–223, 1977.
31. Castile RG, Laflamme MJ, Dorkin HL, et al: Changes in intrathoracic pressure during partial expiratory flow-volume manoeuvres in infants [Abstract]. Pediatr Res 23:562A, 1988.
32. Lesouëf PN, Hughes DM, Landau LI: Effect of compression pressure on forced expiratory flow in infants. J Appl Physiol 61:1639–1646, 1986.
33. Asher MI, Coates AL, Milic-Emili J: Measurement of pleural pressure in neonates. J Appl Physiol 52:491–494, 1982.
34. Davis GM, Coates AL, Dalle D, Bureau MA: Measurement of pulmonary mechanics in the newborn lamb: A comparison of three techniques. J Appl Physiol 64:972–981, 1988.
35. Beardsmore CS, Helms P, Stocks J, et al: Improved esophageal balloon techniques for use in infants. J Appl Physiol 49:735–742, 1980.
36. Coates AL, Davis GM, Vallinis P, Outerbridge EO: The use of a liquid filled esophageal catheter to measure pleural pressure in the preterm neonate with lung disease. J Appl Physiol 67:889–893, 1989.
37. Lesouëf PN, Lopes JM, England SJ, et al: Influence of chest wall distortion on esophageal pressure. J Appl Physiol 55:353–358, 1983.
38. Mortola JP, Saetta M: Measurements of respiratory mechanics in the newborn: A simple approach. Pediatr Pulmonol 3:123–130, 1987.
39. Zin WA, Pengelly DL, Milic-Emili J: Single-breath method for the measurement of respiratory mechanics in anesthetised animals. J Appl Physiol 52:1266–1271, 1982.
40. Grunstein MM, Springer C, Godfrey S, et al: Expiratory volume clamping: A new method to assess respiratory mechanics in sedated infants. J Appl Physiol 62:2107–2114, 1987.
41. Gottfried SB, Rossi A, Calferley PMA, et al: Interrupter technique for measurement of respiratory mechanics in anesthetized cats. J Appl Physiol 56:681–690, 1984.
42. Bates JHT, Baconnier P, Milic-Emili J: A theoretical analysis of the interrupter technique for measuring respiratory mechanics. J Appl Physiol 64:2204–2214, 1988.
43. Lebecque P, Spier S, Lapierre JG, et al: Histamine challenge test in children using forced oscillation to measure total airway resistance. Chest 92:313–318, 1987.

2 PULMONARY DEFENSES

RICHARD B. MOSS, M.D.

The interface in the respiratory tract between the individual human and the environment is large, dynamic, and critical. Sixteen generations of conducting airways lead to three generations of respiratory bronchioles, which branch into three generations of alveolar ducts and finally end in the alveolar sacs.[1] The average adult respiratory tract and pulmonary parenchyma include an air-tissue surface area of 50 to 100 sq m, much of which consists of about 150,000 gossamer-thin (<0.5 μm) gas exchange units in alveolar epithelial–vascular endothelial terminals; each of these units contains approximately 100 alveolar ducts and 2000 alveolar sacs. Although about 5×10^7 alveoli are formed at full-term birth, 80% to 90% of the final adult number are added by alveolar multiplication in the first year or two of life,[2] a fact that stresses the potentially devastating impact of early lung disease on long-term lung function and outcome. Inhaled or aspirated foreign substances—microorganisms, organic or inorganic particulates, gases, and soluble macromolecules—enter into this maze. How are they disposed of? They must be removed, degraded or metabolized, or isolated; otherwise, injury or infection results. A complex network of host defenses serves to maintain virtual sterility of the entire system below the vocal cords with extreme efficiency.

There are several ways to conceptualize this network.

Table 2–1. FUNCTIONAL ORGANIZATION OF
PULMONARY DEFENSES

Mechanical Defenses
Filtration, impaction
Sneeze, cough reflexes
Mucus, epithelial barrier
Mucociliary transport

Phagocytic Defenses
Resident pulmonary macrophages
Recruited polymorphonuclear neutrophils

Immune Defenses
Antigen Sampling, Presentation
Specialized epithelial cells
Pulmonary macrophages
Humoral Immunity
B cell/plasmacyte lineage
Antibody-mediated effector functions
   Complement activation
   Opsonization
   Neutralization
   Immune complex formation
   Antibody-dependent cell-mediated cytotoxicity
Cellular Immunity
T cell lineage
   CD4+ helper/inducer subsets
   CD8+ suppressor/cytotoxic subsets
Lymphokine or cell-to-cell contact effector functions
   Cytotoxicity
   Immunoregulation
   Amplification

One is to classify the defenses into three broad categories on the basis of functional attributes: mechanical, phagocytic (nonspecific), and immunologic (antigen-specific) mechanisms (Table 2–1). A second way to view the network is based on a concept of defense in depth, a division into primary and secondary mechanisms of defense. This categorization is considered later in this chapter after discussion of the functional components of the system.

A full understanding of the lung host defense system requires familiarity with the various cell types present in normal human lung and their function. Because this important topic is well beyond the scope of this chapter, the interested reader is referred to reviews in other sources.[3,4]

MECHANICAL DEFENSES

The upper airways contribute to pulmonary defenses primarily through mechanical mechanisms such as particle filtration and mucociliary clearance. The velocity of incoming air and the anatomic structure of the nares combine to cause impaction of most particles larger than 5 to 10 μm in diameter; they are then swept into the oropharynx at an average rate of 6 mm/min by the mucociliary apparatus, or sometimes they are pushed out whence they came by the forceful expression of a sneeze. (An exception to this general rule appears to be certain cylinder-shaped particles, such as asbestos fibers, which can penetrate to the alveoli by longitudinal orientation along the airstream.) Particles 2 to 5 μm in diameter often penetrate variably into the succeeding generations of con-

ducting airways, and particles <2 μm in diameter may gain access to the gas exchange units (acini). Most particles >1 μm are deposited by inertial impaction, whereas smaller particles may come to rest by gravitational sedimentation in peripheral regions of low flow or, for very small particles <0.5 μm, by Brownian diffusion with gas molecules and tissue walls. Between the larynx and the terminal bronchioles at the 16th generation of airways, the major operative defense mechanism is mucociliary clearance, aided by cough if the irritative stimulus is sufficient.

MUCUS

Airway mucus is a variable mix of water (95%), a small amount of low-molecular-weight material, and macromolecules (about 5%; mainly mucus glycoproteins [4%] but also proteins [1%] and lipids [<1%]). The origins of the various macromolecules in mucus are listed in Table 2–2. At least 4 of the 10 cell types lining the airway—goblet, mucous, serous, and Clara cells—have been shown to contribute glycoproteins to mucus.[5] The predominant sources of mucus are mucous and serous cell–containing submucosal glands, which are more than fortyfold more common than the intraepithelial goblet cells. Submucosal gland development appears to continue postnatally through middle childhood.[6]

Mucus glycoproteins are an incompletely understood, heterogeneous mix of mostly acid molecules that are huge (molecular weight up to 2×10^4 kD) and line up in interconnecting sheets swelled by water, which results in the

Table 2–2. COMPOSITION OF MUCUS

Constituents of Mucus
Water: 95%
Dialyzable constituents: 1%
Macromolecules: 4%
   Mucus glycoproteins: 25%–50%
   Proteins: 10%–25%
   Lipids: 20%–30%

Origin of Mucus Macromolecules
Mucus Glycoproteins
   Surface epithelium: mucous cell, ciliated cell
   Submucosal glands: mucous cell, serous cell
Proteins
Locally produced
   Mucous/serous cells: secretory component, lysozyme, lactoferrin
   Plasmacytes: IgA, IgG, IgE, IgM
   Clara cell (?): low-molecular-weight bronchial protease inhibitor
   Mast cells: mediators (histamine, leukotrienes)
   Lung macrophages: complement components, cytokines, mediators
Tissue fluid transudate: albumin, immunoglobulins, haptoglobin, α1-protease inhibitor, α_1-antichymotrypsin, α_2-macroglobulin, transferrin, α_1-acid glycoprotein, complement components, water, electrolytes, other substances
Lipids
Locally produced
   Type II pneumocyte: alveolar surfactant
   Clara cell
   Mucus granule membrane
Tissue fluid transudate

Modified from Lopez-Vidriero MT, Reid L: Bronchial mucus in health and disease. Br Med Bull 34:63–74, 1978.

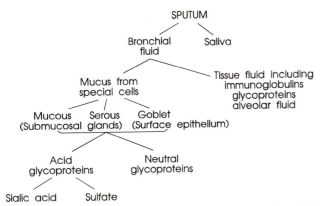

Figure 2–1. Sputum is a pathologically excessive mixture of bronchial fluids and saliva.

peculiar viscoelastic properties characteristic of mucus. Oligosaccharide side chains of 1 to 20 sugars are linked via *O*-glycosidic bonds to hydroxyl groups of serine and threonine residues on the peptide backbone of mucus glycoproteins, in contrast to the predominantly *N*-glycosidic links from *N*-acetylglucosamine to the amide nitrogen of asparagine in most serum glycoproteins.[7] At least 15 nonserum proteins have been detected in mucus, including secretory IgA, lysozyme, lactoferrin, and peroxidase. In addition, the sieving characteristics of the alveolar endothelial-epithelial barrier allow serum proteins of <150 kD to diffuse into the bronchoalveolar fluid. Prominent among these proteins are alpha$_1$-protease inhibitor (alpha$_1$-antitrypsin), albumin, transferrin, IgG, and C3.

Mucus performs a number of protective functions independent of its host defense role: namely, lubrication, humidification, and insulation. It also serves as a trap for particles, a sieve for foreign molecules, a surface for the actions of defense molecules, and a covering sheet for removal of trapped materials by ciliary action and cough. Baseline mucus secretion averages about 0.5 ml/kg/day.[6] Mucus secretion is modulated by a wide variety of endogenous and potential exogenous pharmacologic agents, including sympathomimetics, histamine, cyclic nucleotides, and arachidonate metabolites. Important pathophysiologic mucus secretagogues appear to include mast cell–derived anaphylactic mediators, autonomic neurohormones (especially cholinergic and perhaps peptidergic), and partly characterized lung macrophage–derived products.[8]

Sputum is a pathologic excess of bronchial fluid containing mucus that is mixed with variable amounts of saliva and extracellular tissue fluid transudate (Fig. 2–1). The presence of sputum is often a reflection of airway inflammation with or without infection (e.g., cystic fibrosis or asthma, respectively), and host inflammatory cell DNA contributes heavily to the purulent appearance and increased viscosity. Normal mucus production does not exceed the capacity of a healthy person to more or less unconsciously swallow whatever is brought up to the larynx.[9] The normal mucus blanket appears to consist of discontinuous islands moving along the shifting sea of ciliary action, which takes place in the micromilieu of a continuous coat of serous periciliary fluid (Fig. 2–2).

CILIA

Ciliated epithelial cells are found not only in the respiratory tract but also in the genital tract and parts of the central nervous system (ependyma and spinal cord). The respiratory tract is ciliated for 17 generations of conducting airways; in these regions, ciliated cells outnumber goblet cells by about four to one. Each ciliated cell contains approximately 200 cilia, each 6 μm long and 0.25 μm in diameter. More than 3×10^{12} cilia cover a net area of 0.5 sq m of respiratory surface. Ciliary structure has been extensively studied at the morphologic and biochemical levels. Figure 2–3 is a diagram of the basic ciliary structure. The axenome, or the projecting part of the cilium, contains more than 180 polypeptides.[10] Nine pairs of peripheral microtubules surround the central microtubule pair. The tubules are composed mostly of tubulin, a structural protein devoid of enzymatic activity but containing binding sites for dynein. Dynein, found in inner and outer arms of the outer microtubules, is a high-molecular-weight protein rich in ATPase. The ciliary membrane is an extension of the cell membrane, and its mass is half that of the cilia. At the base, a ciliary necklace of proteins circles the axenome base and regulates calcium flux. Below the cell surface, the basal body anchors the cilium to the cytosol (Fig. 2–4). At the top, a ciliary crown claws the mucus forward (Fig. 2–5).

Ciliary beating is effected by the action of dynein arms on one outer microtubule sliding along the side of another that belongs to an adjacent outer pair of microtubules. Microtubule doublets are held together by elastic nexin links. Radial spokes limit the sliding but also transduce it into coordinated bending by detaching and reattaching to the central sheath. Average ciliary beat frequency in the airways, determined by high-speed stroboscopic cinematography or laser-scattering spectroscopy, is 13 Hz (range is 11 to 17); the frequency is somewhat higher in central than in peripheral regions.[11] There is little evidence of endogenous regulation, but tracheal mucus velocity can be increased by supraphysiologic doses of adrenergic agents and can be slowed by atropine. Disorders of ciliary motility, usually caused by one or more of a variety of ultrastructural defects, affect approximately 1 in 20,000 persons.[10]

COUPLING OF CILIARY ACTION TO MUCUS CLEARANCE

The mucus blanket consists of two distinct layers: a 5 to 6 μm serous periciliary fluid, which bathes the cilia and corresponds in depth to the exact height of fully extended cilia, and a 2 to 3 μm mucous layer with gel-like characteristics (Fig. 2–2).[12] Histologic and pharmacologic studies have established the critical interaction between ciliary tips and the mucous gel layer in mucociliary clearance (Fig. 2–6). Ciliary beating itself is coordinated in a metachronal (discontinuous and wavelike) fashion to propel the mucus cephalad. Wave propagation and coordination seem to be the result of the intrinsic properties of individual ciliary beating frequencies and their spatial movement characteristics.[13] Linear velocity of mucus

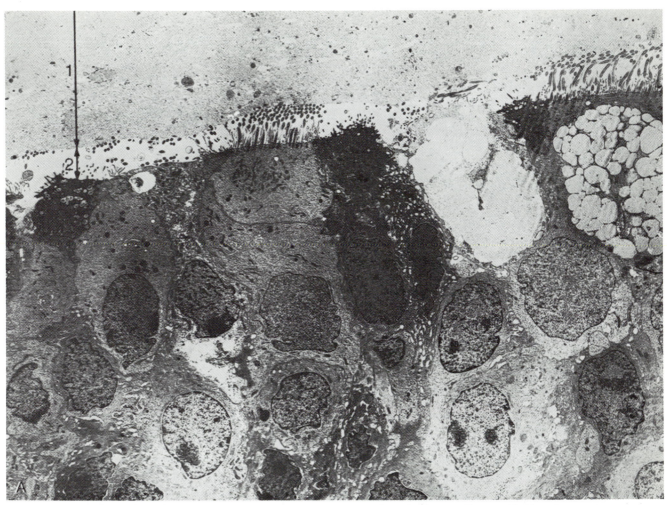

Figure 2–2. *A,* Transmission electron micrograph of normal human bronchial epithelial surface at magnification of 2400×, showing physiologic relationship of ciliated epithelium to mucus layer (1). The depth of the serous periciliary fluid bathing the luminal surface is normally equal to that of fully extended cilia (2), so that tips with clawlike projections just barely contact the mucus gel, propelling it cephalad along the mucociliary escalator. Several mucus-secreting cells can also be seen in the epithelium at right.

Illustration continued on following page

transport in the human lung ranges between 0.5 to 1 mm/min in peripheral airways and 5 to 20 mm/min in the trachea.[14] Particles deposited in large airways are therefore cleared within about 1 h, whereas peripherally placed particles take several hours.

The importance of mucus-ciliary interaction was illustrated in experiments in which particle transport was abolished by removal of mucus and restored by replacement of mucus on ciliated epithelium. The interaction seems to be heavily influenced by hydration state, rheology, and thickness of the mucus layer.[15] The critical nature of the depth of the periciliary layer becomes evident in view of the fact that too much periciliary fluid results in detachment of cilia from mucus during the stroke, which leads to slowed transport; conversely, loss of periciliary depth results in matting of cilia in mucus and slowed transport. At present, despite increasing study, little is known about the regulatory factors that work to maintain the critical periciliary fluid composition and depth within finely controlled limits.[13]

Mucociliary function can be assessed by measuring either the clearance of inhaled aerosols or the transport of

marker particles placed on the mucosa. The two methods do not necessarily involve measuring the same thing, inasmuch as the latter relies on larger markers (such as radioactively labeled microspheres or radiopaque polytef [Teflon] disks) that are usually centrally placed, do not penetrate the mucus layer, and reflect mucus transport more than ciliary activity or periciliary fluid effects. Radioisotope aerosols, in contrast, penetrate airways more peripherally, less regionally, and deeper toward the epithelium.

Pharmacologic modulation of mucociliary clearance is of obvious interest with regard to several disease states. It is known that parasympathetic drugs increase mucus secretion by mucus cells and are antagonized by atropine and its congeners. Alpha-adrenergic drugs appear to increase secretion from submucosal serous cells, and beta-adrenergic drugs increase mucus cell secretion. All these may indirectly increase clearance by means of the increase in mucus secretion. Beta-adrenergic agents may directly stimulate ciliary beating;[13] methylxanthines may also stimulate ciliary activity.[15] Depression of mucociliary clearance by general anesthetics (especially barbiturates)

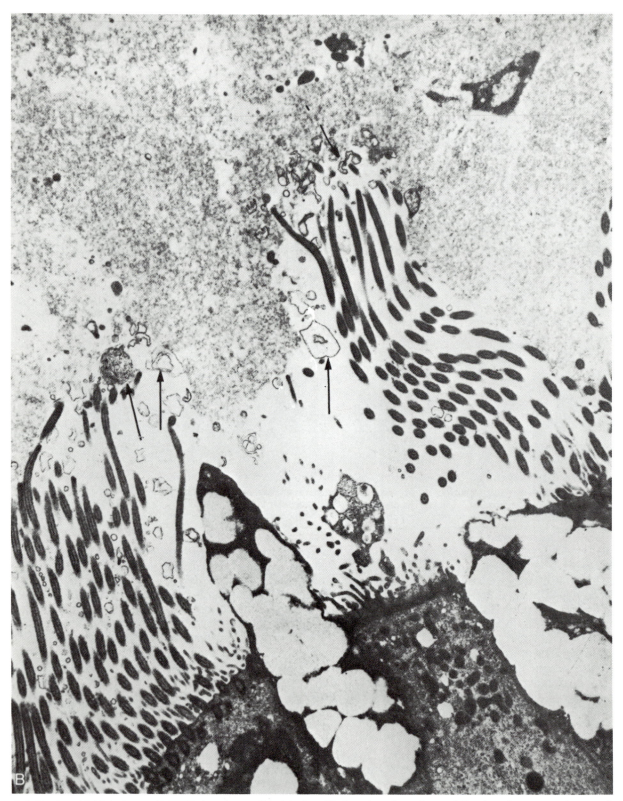

Figure 2–2 *Continued B,* Higher power (×9500) view of mucociliary interface. The low-viscosity, watery periciliary layer is seen as a clear zone below the granular mucus layer. Several phospholipid membranous vesicles containing surfactant can be seen in the periciliary layer *(arrows)*. Microvilli covering the surface of epithelial cells between cilia probably perform absorptive and possibly ionic secretory functions. Apical portions of several mucous goblet cells are also seen. (From Morgenroth K, Newhouse MT: Bronchitis. Munich: Pharmazentische Verlagsgesellschaft, 1983.)

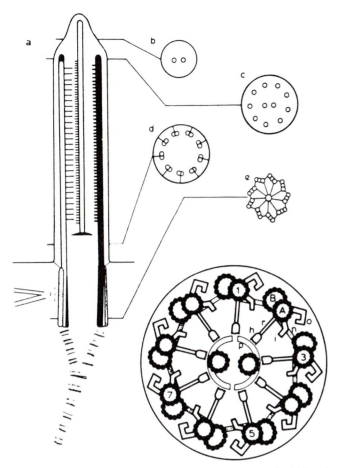

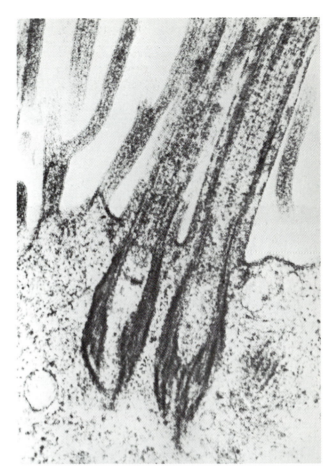

Figure 2-3. Schematic structure of cilia seen in longitudinal (*a*) and transverse (*f*) sections. The ciliary basal body is seen arising from the cell, where striated roots penetrate the cytosol. The microtubules of the axenomal shaft extend from the basal body. Note different cross-sectional structure at various levels of transection (*b* to *e*). Section *f* shows the classical appearance at midaxenomal level, illustrating the nine pairs of peripheral microtubules (B and A) surrounding the central pair, which carry lateral projections (p). Outer doublets are connected to each other via nexin links (n) and to the central doublet by radial spokes (r) carrying dilated heads (h). The outer microtubules (A) carry outer (o) and inner (i) dynein arms, which are responsible for ciliary beat. Bending of the axenome occurs by sliding of the outer microtubule (A) along the inner microtubule (B) of the adjacent doublet. (From Brain JD, Proctor DR, Reid LM (eds): Respiratory Defense Mechanisms: Lung Biology in Health and Disease, vol 5, p. 256. New York: Marcel Dekker, 1977.)

Figure 2-4. Transmission electron micrograph ($\times$115,000) of ciliary basal bodies. Axenomal microtubules can be seen arising from the basal bodies. The membrane of the cilium can be seen arising directly from the apical cell membrane. (From Morgenroth K, Newhouse MT: Bronchitis. Munich: Pharmazentische Verlagsgesellschaft, 1983.)

COUGH

Cough is both an important physiologic component of the lung defense network and a cardinal indicator of disease. It performs two major physiologic functions: defense against aspiration and clearance of inhaled particulates large enough, or gases irritative enough, to trigger the cough reflex. The metamorphosis of coughing from a normal to a pathologic event occurs along a gradient that must include an increase in frequency and a change in character. Other subjective and objective factors, such as accompanying respiratory symptoms and signs, also play a role in the significance of cough. In bronchorrhea, the trigger to cough is the endogenous buildup of mucus or injury to the epithelium, and the cough becomes the major mechanism of mucus clearance, whereas in health the mucociliary escalator performs the majority of the work.[17]

The cough mechanism involves a deep inspiration followed by forced expiration against a closed glottis, resulting in a buildup of intrathoracic pressure to $\geq$50 mm Hg, which is suddenly relieved by opening of the glottis. Expiratory flow during the cough may reach 12 l/sec; beyond this, compression of the large airways causes up to 80%

and local anesthetics, the latter at least in part by ciliotoxic effects, has been well documented. Opiates and alcohol also depress mucus transport.[15]

The physiologic effect of a given pharmacologic agent cannot be predicted from its action on either cilia or mucus secretion independently. For example, certain products (such as leukotrienes) of allergen-induced lung mast cell degranulation released during local anaphylaxis have been shown to stimulate ciliary beat frequency and independently stimulate mucus secretion, and yet overall mucociliary transport is decreased.[16] This paradoxical effect can probably be attributed to uncoupling of the normal ciliary-mucus gel layer interaction by a change in the depth of the periciliary fluid or in the physical characteristics of the secreted mucus.

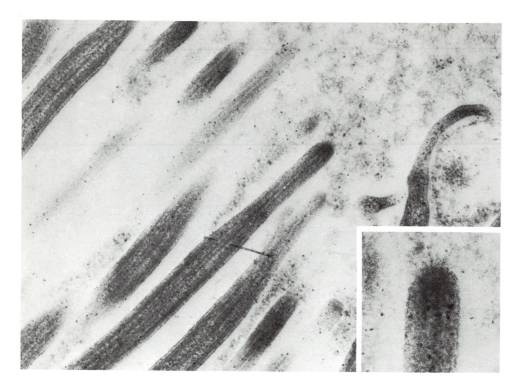

Figure 2–5. Transmission electron micrograph (×30,000) of cilia in longitudinal section. At the extreme tip of the dome-shaped end of the cilia, filamentous claw-like projections can be seen. *Inset:* high-power (×90,000) closeup. (From Morgenroth K, Newhouse MT: Bronchitis. Munich: Pharmazentische Verlagsgesellschaft, 1983.)

reduction in tracheal cross section, resulting in air velocities nearing 25,000 cm/sec, or 75% of the speed of sound.[18]

The cough reflex is initiated by stimulation of vagal, trigeminal, glossopharyngeal, or phrenic nerve irritant receptors present in the airways epithelium from the pharynx to terminal bronchioles. Cough receptors are most dense in areas of highest anticipated particle impaction: the larynx, the carina, and the bifurcation of larger bronchi. Afferent impulses are carried to the cough center in the upper brainstem and the pons, and efferent signals are transmitted down vagal, phrenic, and spinal motor nerves to laryngeal, diaphragmatic, thoracic, and abdominal muscles.[19]

The clinical evaluation of cough in children has been reviewed.[18,20] It is particularly important that the clinician focus on the common symptom complex of persistent (>1 month) or recurrent productive cough caused by interrelated mucosal injury, inflammation, and bronchial hyperreactivity, which occurs in 2% to 20% of children.[21]

Table 2–3 lists considerations in the differential diagnosis for persistent cough in children.

Age has an important bearing on the likelihood that a particular kind of disorder will be a cause of cough. In infancy, congenital malformations, congenital or neonatal infections, aspiration, and cystic fibrosis must be strongly considered. In the preschool years, foreign bodies, suppurative lung diseases, and bronchitis associated with upper respiratory infection are common. In the school years, active or passive smoking, mycoplasmal infections, and psychogenic causes should be considered.[20]

PHAGOCYTIC DEFENSES

Particles that succeed in breaching the mechanical defenses of the lung are usually ingested, inactivated, and removed by phagocytic cells in or near the airways and the gas exchange units. The composition of the cells of the

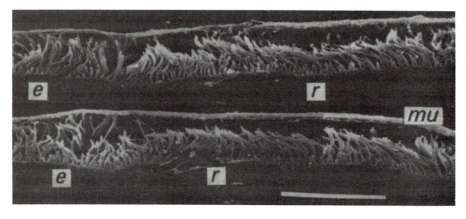

Figure 2–6. Scanning electron micrograph (scale bar, 10 μm) of two adjacent sections of cultured rabbit tracheal epithelium (e) showing mucociliary interface. A layer of exogenously added mucus (mu) is transported by the tips of cilia in fully extended effective strokes (e) while recovery strokes (r) take place in the periciliary fluid layer. (From Sleigh MA, Blake JR, Liron N: The propulsion of mucus by cilia. Am Rev Respir Dis 137:726–741, 1988.)

Table 2-3. DIFFERENTIAL DIAGNOSIS OF CHRONIC OR RECURRENT COUGH

Phase One: Specific Etiologies

Asthma (Reactive Airways Disease)
Most likely diagnosis; often follows a viral infection
Pre-Existing Lung Disease
Bronchopulmonary dysplasia (mild)
Posttraumatic or postinfectious bronchiectasis
Cystic Fibrosis
Especially in infants and children with failure to thrive
Aspiration Syndromes
Abnormal enteropulmonary communications (e.g., tracheoesophageal fistula or laryngeal cleft)
Gastroesophageal reflux
Swallowing dysfunction
Poor infant feeding practices
Airway Compression
Extrinsic compression (e.g., abnormal vessels or hilar adenopathy)
Weakened wall (e.g., tracheomalacia or bronchomalacia)
Foreign Body
Intrathoracic or extrathoracic airway
Esophageal
Congenital Heart Disease
Periairway edema, bronchospasm, or both; pulmonary congestion
Large airway compression by enlarged vessels or enlarged left atrium
Infection
Increased exposure to viral infection (e.g., day care)
Chlamydial, mycoplasmal, or ureaplasmal infection in young infant
Granulomatous disease (e.g., tuberculosis or fungal infection)
Primary Ciliary Abnormalities
With situs inversus (Kartagener's syndrome) or without other abnormalities
Immunodeficiency
IgA deficiency
Alpha$_1$-Antitrypsin Deficiency
Rarely causes pulmonary disease in childhood

Phase Two: Nonspecific Airway Irritation

Cigarette Smoke
Passive exposure
Active use of tobacco and other smoking materials
Air Pollution
Outdoor secondary to automobile exhaust, industry, etc.
Indoor secondary to exposure to irritants and chemicals, e.g., housepaint, dusts

Modified from Morgan WJ, Taussig LM: The chronic bronchitis complex in children. Pediatr Clin North Am 31:851–864, 1984.

Table 2-4. PULMONARY CELLS RECOVERED BY BRONCHOALVEOLAR LAVAGE OF NORMAL NONSMOKING ADULT SUBJECTS

Differential Cell Count	%
Macrophages	85–90
Neutrophils	1–2
Ciliated cells	1–5
Eosinophils/basophils	<1
Erythrocytes	<5
Lymphocytes	7–12
Subsets (% total lymphs)	
T cells	70
CD4+* (% of T cells)	50
CD8+*	30
B cells/plasmacytes†	5–10
Killer cells	7
Untypable	~5

From Reynolds HY: Bronchoalveolar lavage. Am Rev Respir Dis 135:250–263, 1987.
Total cell count, 15 × 10^6, obtained after 100- to 300-ml lavage.
*CD4+, helper/inducer subset; CD8+, suppressor/cytotoxic subset.
†Secretion of immunoglobulin IgG = IgA > IgM > IgE.

sue, the pulmonary vascular bed, and the pleura. Because surface antigenic differences between PMOs taken from various lung regions have been described, functional heterogeneity cannot be excluded as well.[24]

PMOs are fully differentiated cells of monocytic lineage and thus derive ultimately from the bone marrow. The differentiation process includes increases in cell size, cytosolic organelles, phagocytic capacity, surface phagocytic receptors (secondary to the increase in cell size), and response to activating lymphokines.[25,26] However, there is continued uncertainty as to how many PMOs arise from migrating blood-borne monocytes and how many arise from local replication of resident cells in the pulmonary interstitium.[27]

PMOs normally do not appear to be present at term birth. Presumably, their population of the lung is driven by sudden emergence of the respiratory function of the lungs at birth, inasmuch as they are present 48 h after birth.[28] In addition, PMOs obtained from BAL in neonatal rhesus monkeys show deficient chemotaxis, phagocytosis, and candidicidal activities in comparison with BAL PMOs from older (infant, juvenile, or adult) monkeys,[29] which suggests that similar deficiencies may exist in human neonates. This would be consistent with similar data obtained from human neonatal blood monocytes[30] and with a reduced ability of human neonatal PMOs to efficiently kill ingested bacteria.[31]

PMOs function in the pulmonary host defense network in three general ways:

1. They perform *effector* functions as phagocytic cells, either directly and independently, or as a result of nonspecific activation by antigen-stimulated T lymphocytes.

2. They perform an *accessory cell* role in initiating specific immune responses by ingestion, degradation, and presentation (cell surface re-expression) of antigens to T lymphocytes.

3. They perform a *regulatory* role on the activity of the immune system by secretion of soluble factors, such as

lung in contact with external particles has been assessed in histologic studies and by extensive use of bronchoalveolar lavage (BAL), which was made feasible by the advent of fiberoptic technology in the early to mid-1970s.[22] The normal composition of cells accessible by BAL from healthy, nonsmoking adults is given in Table 2-4. Smoking causes a four- to five-fold increase in average total BAL cells, with an increased proportion of phagocytic cells, both macrophages and neutrophils, in comparison with lymphocytes.[23] It is obvious that the resident phagocyte in the lung is a specialized tissue macrophage (MO), which has been termed the *alveolar* or *pulmonary macrophage* (PMO). Since only the late 1980s has it been appreciated that besides alveolar MOs, some PMOs recovered by BAL are truly residents of conducting airways, present either on or in the epithelium, presumably achieving their position by conduction along the mucociliary escalator or migration into the airways; moreover, PMOs have also been found in connective tis-

prostaglandins, that suppress primarily lymphocyte functions.[32]

PHAGOCYTOSIS

PMOs are avidly phagocytic cells.[33] Their highly ruffled plasma membranes offer wide surface areas for contact, and they have a well-developed ability to deform and move to chemotactic stimuli via footlike extensions called lamellipodia or filopodia (Fig. 2–7). Their organelles contain a wide variety of degradative enzymes packaged in cytosolic inclusion bodies (primary lysosomes) that fuse with phagocytic vesicles after ingestion to form the secondary lysosome or phagolysosome (Fig. 2–8). PMOs show a high resting oxidative metabolism that is appropriate for the highly aerobic airspace environment and does not greatly increase with phagocytosis, in contrast to neutrophils or MOs from other tissues. Glycolytic metabolism is, however, also important for effective phagocytosis and killing. Although the respiratory oxidative burst is thought to be critical to the killing function of PMOs, they also employ a number of nonoxidative mechanisms to kill ingested microorganisms, such as lysosomal proteolytic enzymes, phagolysosomal acidification, and microbicidal cationic proteins.[34]

Lung macrophages can ingest certain particles without opsonins by means of surface receptors that recognize lectinlike carbohydrate moieties. Phagocytosis and intracellular killing by PMOs is usually greatly enhanced, however, by opsonization of microbes with antibody or complement or both, inasmuch as the PMO is further abundantly equipped with receptors for the Fc fragment

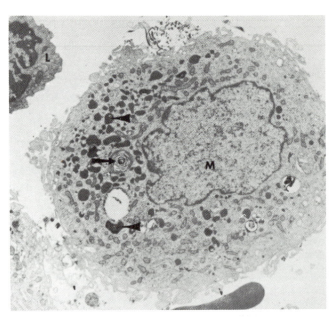

Figure 2–8. Transmission electron micrograph (×8500) of pulmonary macrophage. Arrowheads indicate phagolysosomes. Note the ruffled cytoplasmic membrane and the numerous cytosolic organelles, which include many mitochondria and a few myelin bodies *(arrow)*. Lymphocyte (L) is at upper left. (From Green GM, Jakab GJ, Low RB, Davis GS: Defense mechanism of the respiratory membrane. Am Rev Respir Dis 115:479–514, 1977.)

of IgG and the C3b/C3d fragments of the complement component C3.[35] Among the four IgG subclasses, Fc receptors on freshly isolated PMOs bind IgG_3, IgG_1, and IgG_4.[36] In addition to antibody and complement, other nonspecific enhancers of PMO phagocytic activity with probable biologic significance, including fibronectin and surfactant, have been described.[37,38]

PMO phagocytic activity can also be stimulated by activated T lymphocytes, primarily through the action of secreted lymphokines such as interferon-γ.[39] Thus a specific immune stimulus that activates lymphocytes through antigen processing and presentation by an accessory cell ultimately leads to a nonspecific amplification of host defense capacity. In this way, PMOs may become an effector arm of the immune response mediated by T lymphocytes, as well as front-line nonspecific scavengers of foreign material entering the lungs. Activation can be assessed in numerous ways, such as an increase in various cellular enzyme levels, in metabolic rates, or in secretory, phagocytic, and bactericidal activities.[40] Activated PMOs appear to be especially critical to successful host defense against facultative and obligate intracellular pathogens.[41]

ACCESSORY CELL/ANTIGEN PRESENTATION

In the lung, as elsewhere, MOs have the ability to ingest, degrade, and re-express antigen on their surface in physical association with class II major histocompatibility proteins, the immune-associated (I_a) complex, or the human leukocyte antigen (HLA-DR) complex. Such presentation is essential for recognition by and activation of helper

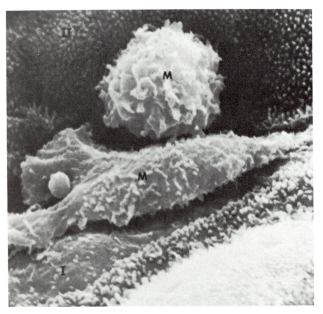

Figure 2–7. Scanning electron micrograph (×6000) of pulmonary macrophages (M). The upper macrophage appears to be at rest on the alveolar surface atop the microvilli of a type II pneumocyte (II); the lower macrophage shows typical morphologic activation changes in executing the chemotactic and phagocytic response to *Staphylococcus* microbe being ingested at left. Surface of type I pneumocyte (I) is at lower left. (From Green GM, Jakab GJ, Low RB, Davis GS: Defense mechanisms of the respiratory membrane. Am Rev Respir Dis 115:479–514, 1977.)

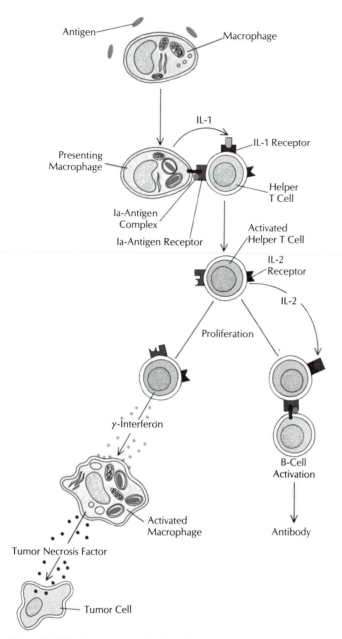

Figure 2-9. Antigen presentation by pulmonary macrophage occurs by phagocytosis and partial degradation of ingested antigen, followed by re-expression on macrophage surface in physical association with class II major histocompatibility antigens (Ia), where it is recognized by the antigen-specific receptor on the T cell surface. The cell-to-cell contact stimulates macrophage secretion of interleukin-1 (IL-1), which binds to a specific receptor on the T cell, inducing activation and secretion. Among the key lymphokines of the now-activated T cell is interleukin-2 (IL-2), which, as a proliferative stimulus to T cells, thereby amplifies the clonal response. The expanded population of helper T cells interacts with B cells, causing them to differentiate into specific antibody-producing plasmacytes *(lower right)*. Another key lymphokine, interferon-γ, feeds back on macrophages to activate them, resulting in enhanced microbicidal activity and secretion of macrophage cytokines such as tumor necrosis factor *(lower left)*. (From Unanue ER, Allen PM: The basis for the immunoregulatory role of macrophages and other accessory cells. Science 236:551–557, 1987. Copyright 1987 by the American Association for the Advancement of Science.)

T lymphocytes, which result in the generation of an effective specific immune response to that antigen.[42] This process and the related positive feedback loop action of the activated lymphocytes back on the MOs are illustrated in

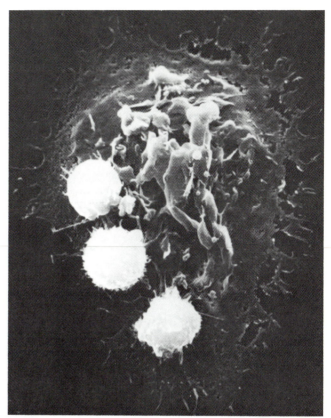

Figure 2-10. Scanning electron micrograph (×6000) of pulmonary macrophage with three adherent T lymphocytes obtained from bronchoalveolar lavage. This adherence presumably portrays the antigen presentation process. (From Herscowitz HB: In defense of the lung: Paradoxical role of the pulmonary alveolar macrophage. Ann Allergy 55:634–648, 1985.)

Figures 2–9 and 2–10. The accessory cell role of the PMO has received extensive attention; results have been very confusing, revealing quite a complicated picture. In general, it does appear that at high PMO-to-lymphocyte ratios, which ostensibly most closely mimic the physiologic conditions in the lungs, PMOs are poor accessory cells and generally suppress immune responses.[43] This appears to be a result, not of abnormal antigen processing or display of HLA-DR antigens on the PMO surface, but of secretion of suppressor substances, which might include prostaglandin inhibitors of interleukin-1, a macrophage-derived cytokine crucial for initiating lymphocyte responses.[44] A teleologic rationale for these observations has been offered: that low accessory cell activity by PMOs serves to suppress inflammatory responses in the lung. This rationale is supported by observed increases in PMO accessory activity in T cell–mediated hypersensitivity inflammatory diseases of the lung, such as sarcoidosis.[45]

IMMUNOREGULATION

Besides an obvious regulatory role in the antigen presentation process, PMOs also regulate later phases of the immune response by affecting lymphocyte proliferation, differentiation, and effector activities. As mentioned

Table 2–5. SECRETORY PRODUCTS OF
PULMONARY MACROPHAGES

Host Defense Modulators/Mediators

Chemotactic factors
Neutrophil activating factor
Complement components: C1, C4, C2, C3, C5, B, D, properdin, C3b
    inactivator, β-1H
Leukotrienes: B4, C, D, E, HETE
Prostaglandins: E_2, $F_{2\alpha}$, prostacyclin, thromboxane
Interleukin-1
Tumor necrosis factor α
Interferon-α
Oxygen metabolites: superoxide, peroxide, hydroxyl radical,
    hypohalous acids
Platelet activating factor
Natural peptide antibiotics
Cationic microbiocidal proteins
Protease inhibitors: α_1-protease inhibitor, α_2-macroglobulin,
    plasminogen activator inhibitor, collagenase inhibitor, phospholipase
    inhibitor (lipomodulin/macrocortin)
Histamine-releasing factor

Enzymes

Lysozyme
Acid hydrolases: proteases, lipase, DNAase, phosphatase,
    glycosidase, sulfatase
Glucuronidase
Neutral proteases: elastase, collagenase, angiotensin convertase,
    plasminogen activator
Superoxide dismutase
Catalase
Esterase
5'-Nucleotidase
Lipases: lipoprotein lipase, phospholipase A_2

Coagulation Factors

Factors V, IX, X, VII; prothrombin; tissue factor; prothrombinase;
    plasminogen activator

Growth and Differentiation Factors

Fibroblast growth and activating factors
Erythropoietin
Insulinlike activity
Transforming growth factor β
Colony-stimulating factor for granulocytes
Erythrocyte colony–stimulating factor

Adhesion Factors

Fibronectin, proteoglycans, avidin, transferrin

Other Products

β-Endorphin, ACTH, thymidine, uric acid, macrophage-derived mucus
    secretagogue, 1α,25-dihydroxyvitamin D_3

HETE, hydroxyeicosatetraenoic acid; ACTH, adrenocorticotropic hormone.

earlier, a number of secretory products of PMOs, including prostaglandin E_2 and other interleukin-1 inhibitors, have potential regulatory features, mostly suppressive.[44] Other PMO secretory products such as opsonizing complement proteins and fibronectin may act nonspecifically to enhance defenses. Still other PMO products are pleiotropic, such as the cytokines interleukin-1, tumor necrosis factor α, and interferon-α. In fact, the secretory products of PMOs are so numerous and have such diverse potential effects that the task of defining what they actually mean and do *in vivo* is just beginning. An incomplete list of secretory products of PMOs is given in Table 2–5; a more extensive discussion was given by Nathan.[46]

The other major phagocytic cell of the lung, the polymorphonuclear neutrophil, is rarely seen in normal lung tissue, although very large numbers (0.5 to 3.0 times the total circulating pool) are marginated in the pulmonary vascular bed and can quickly arrive in lung parenchyma and airways in response to inflammatory chemotactic stimuli.[47] They are therefore considered later in the chapter, in conjunction with discussion of secondary (inflammatory) defense mechanisms.

SPECIFIC IMMUNITY

ORGANIZATION OF IMMUNE TISSUE IN THE LUNG

Lymphocytes, the linchpin of the immune system, are organized in lung tissue at all levels, from nasopharynx to alveoli and from airway surface to interstitium. Several discrete organizational structures can be observed[48] (Fig. 2–11):

1. Hilar tracheobronchial lymph nodes serve to monitor both lymphatic drainage from the lung parenchyma and antigens penetrating the epithelium to submucosal lymphoid or accessory cells.

2. Submucosal lymphocytes are organized in nodules within and below the epithelium along the bronchi in a functional unit, termed the *bronchus-associated lym-*

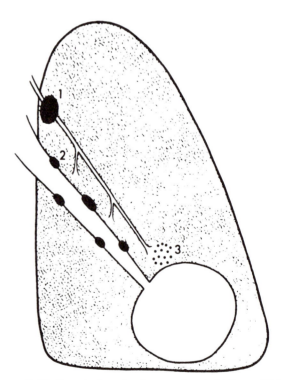

Figure 2–11. Organization of pulmonary lymphoid tissue. (1) Lymph nodes draining lymphatic channels from lung parenchyma. (2) Bronchus-associated lymphoid tissue (BALT) along airway mucosa, especially at major bifurcation points in larger bronchi. (3) Lymphoreticular aggregates in lung parenchyma, which are often at origin of lymphatic channels. (From Jeffrey PK, Corrin B: Structural analysis of the respiratory tract. *In* Bienenstock J [ed]: Immunology of the Lung and Upper Respiratory Tract, p. 15. New York: McGraw-Hill, 1984.)

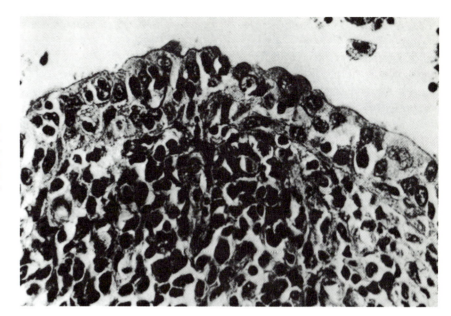

Figure 2–12. Histologic section (×800) of BALT, showing lymphoepithelial layer with lymphoid aggregate below. The lymphoepithelial cells are flattened, without cilia, and possess a highly microvillous apical surface. (From Meuwissen HJ, Hussain M: Bronchus-associated lymphoid tissue in human lung. Clin Immunol Immunopathol 23:548–561, 1982.)

phoid tissue (BALT), in a manner analogous to that in the gastrointestinal tract[49] (Fig. 2–12). BALT is most dense at bifurcations of bronchi, where antigen impact is likely to be highest. There is strong evidence that antigen intake in BALT occurs through specialized lymphoepithelial cells overlying these nodules, presumably for processing and initiation of immune responses (Fig. 2–13). BALT appears to be a homing target for IgA precursor cells (to be described later in this chapter).

3. Lymphoreticular aggregates are small groups of lymphocytes and plasmacytes scattered throughout lung tissues, including airways, alveoli, and pleura. They are placed at points where lymphatics commence, presumably in order to monitor tissue fluid and cells that drain airspaces and parenchyma.

4. Lymphoid cells are normally present in the airspaces, which are accessible by BAL (Table 2–4). In view of the high PMO-to-lymphocyte ratios normally present (see earlier section on phagocytic defenses), it is currently thought that the BAL lymphocytes do not exert high-efficiency effector activities.[50] This notion is supported by evidence that cells obtained by BAL are generally incapable of *de novo* immunoglobulin synthesis and secretion, in contrast to cells obtained from lung parenchyma.[51]

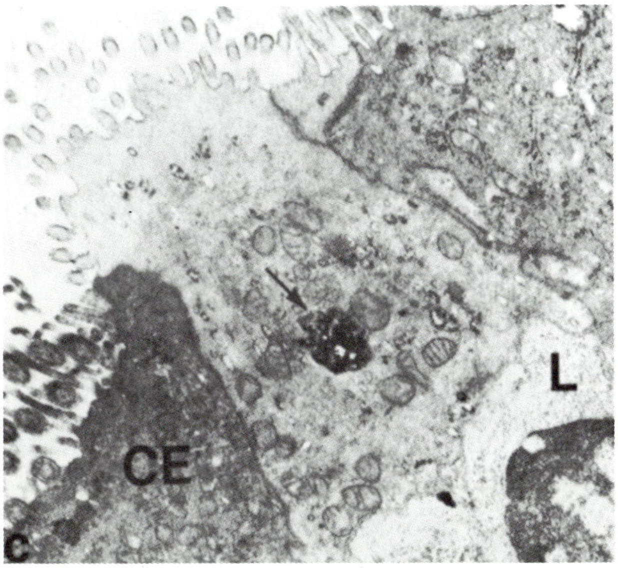

ANTIGEN UPTAKE IN THE LUNG

Antigens entering the lower respiratory tract may encounter a number of fates (Fig. 2–14):

1. Most inhaled antigen is transported up the mucociliary escalator without penetration to the immune system and is swallowed; immune response in the gut, if there is any, is generally low and secondary to efficient breakdown and disposal.[52]

2. Antigens may be phagocytosed by PMOs. Degradation may be followed by presentation to lymphoid cells (Fig. 2–9).

3. Antigens may penetrate the epithelium through paracellular pores or by cellular endocytosis and transport. They may then encounter accessory or lymphoid cells in the submucosa or parenchyma, or they may continue until their absorption in the blood stream for dissemination to systemic lymphoid tissues.[53]

4. Antigens may be endocytosed by the lymphoepithelium of BALT or submucosal lymphoreticular aggregates (Fig. 2–13).

All these potential routes of antigen immunogenicity have been demonstrated under certain conditions in various mammalian species, but how they relate to each

Figure 2–13. Transmission electron micrograph (×10,000) showing pinocytotic uptake of experimental antigen (horseradish peroxidase, *arrow*) by lymphoepithelial cell (L) of BALT in the rabbit. Note microvillous luminal membrane of lymphoepithelial cell. A lymphocyte (L) is in direct contact with lymphoepithelial cell. Ciliated epithelial cells (CE) are adjacent to BALT. (From Rácz P, Tenner-Rácz K, Myrvick QN, et al: Functional architecture of bronchial associated lymphoid tissue and lymphoepithelium in pulmonary cell-mediated reactions in the rabbit. J. Reticuloendothel Soc 22:59–83, 1977.)

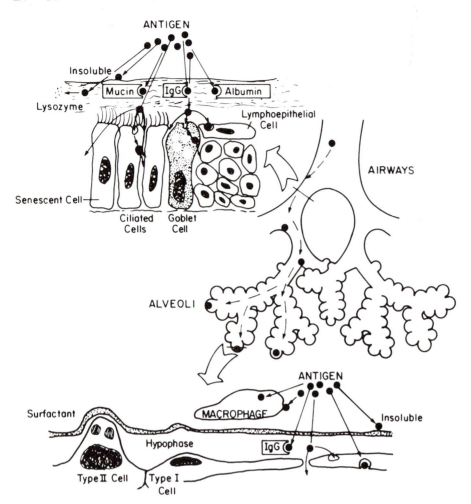

Figure 2-14. Potential mechanisms of antigen uptake in the lung include deposition in respiratory secretions for mucociliary clearance into the gastrointestinal tract, phagocytic uptake by resident macrophages or recruited neutrophils, passage across epithelium via paracellular or cellular paths, and processing by lymphoepithelium of bronchus-associated lymphoid tissue. (From Boucher RC, Ranga V: Fate and handling of antigens by the lung. *In* Daniele RP [ed]: Immunology and Immunologic Diseases of the Lung, pp. 55–78. Boston: Blackwell Scientific, 1988.)

other and to the overall handling of antigens physiologically is not known.

CELLULAR IMMUNITY IN THE LUNG

Effector actions of activated T lymphocytes are known to be critical in the expression of delayed hypersensitivity reactions such as the skin tuberculin response and tissue granuloma formation, in resistance to intracellular microbial pathogens and many viruses, and in tumor surveillance. Lymphocytes are relatively rare within lung tissue; however, upon antigen penetration into lung parenchyma, a T cell response is initiated by entry of sensitized lymphocytes into the lung from the systemic circulation.[47] The speed and magnitude of this T cell response depend largely on the history of exposure of the host, because previous antigen exposure results in the presence of clones of reactive T cells in the circulation, whereas in initial exposure, the sensitization and the clonal expansion of such reactive cells require time.

Once present in sufficient numbers, these activated T cells are capable of arming lung macrophages for effective killing (see earlier section on phagocytic activities of PMO), performing direct defense functions through direct T cell–mediated cytotoxicity, and enhancing inflammatory responses by additional cell types by lymphokine secretion. Cytotoxic T cells usually express the CD8 surface antigen marker and recognize their target cell antigen in the context of major histocompatibility complex class I antigens (HLA-DR) on the target cell surface.[54] Cytotoxicity is considered to be of paramount importance in lung defense against viral infection of the parenchyma. Defects in T cell function may be associated with a variety of viral as well as opportunistic bacterial, fungal, and protozoan infections of the lung.

ANTIBODY-MEDIATED IMMUNITY IN THE LUNG

IgG, IgA, IgM, and IgE can be detected in bronchoalveolar lavage fluid; most of the immunoglobulins detected are IgG (Table 2–6). However, centrally and cephalad from the alveoli to the upper respiratory tract, the concentration of IgG relative to IgA drops, so that in nasal wash, IgA is present in three to eight times the concentration of IgG (Table 2–7). The distribution of IgG subclasses in BAL fluid differs from that in serum, in that the BAL is relatively enriched with IgG_4 (Table 2–8), which is suggestive of enhanced local synthesis.[55] The significance of this modest alteration is unknown. Local synthesis of IgG probably occurs in parenchymal cells rather than in cells obtained by BAL.[51] Most IgG in the airways

Table 2–6. IMMUNOLOGIC SUBSTANCES IN NORMAL LOWER AIRWAY AND ALVEOLAR LINING FLUIDS AS SAMPLED BY BRONCHOALVEOLAR LAVAGE

Component	Estimated % of Total Protein in BAL Sample
Serum derived	
Albumin	30
Transferrin	0.1
Immunologic proteins	
IgA: 11S dimeric (with bound secretory component and J-chain constitutes about 90% of IgA)	5
Monomeric IgA (<10%)	
IgG	14
IgE	0.00001
IgM	<0.1
IgD	Unknown
Complement components	
Properdin factor B, C4, C3, C6	—
Lactoferrin	
Carcinoembryonic antigen	
Epithelial cell products	
Free secretory component	1.0
Enzyme inhibitors	
α_1-Antitrypsin	0.7
α_2-Macroglobulin	0
Low-molecular-weight trypsin inactivator	—
Enzymes (metalloprotease, serine proteases, collagenase, angiotensin convertase, lysozyme)	—
Vasoactive mediators	
Surfactant	
Structural proteins	
Fibronectin	—
% of total protein identified	~52

From Young KR, Reynolds HY: Bronchoalveolar washings. *In* Bienenstock J (ed): Immunology of the Lung and Upper Respiratory Tract, pp. 157–173. New York: McGraw-Hill, 1984.

BAL, Bronchoalveolar lavage

secretions and lung tissue, however, is probably derived by transudation from the vascular space, a process obviously markedly enhanced by inflammation and increased permeability.[47,50] IgG antibodies contribute to lung defense in the same way they do to systemic defenses: by opsonization, immune complex formation, complement activation, agglutination, neutralization, and triggering of various cellular responses. IgM antibodies are present in no more than trace amounts, which indicates lack of local synthesis and size-limited impermeability to diffusion into the airways, and they probably play little if any role in the uninflamed lung. IgE antibodies are present in lung secretions in amounts sufficient to sensitize local mast cells and thereby initiate pulmonary allergic reactions. There is evidence that at least some IgE is locally synthesized.[55,56]

NONSPECIFIC SOLUBLE MEDIATORS OF LUNG DEFENSES

In addition to antigen-specific antibody formation, a number of soluble proteins detectable in BAL fluid aid in lung defense.[12,57] Lysozyme, synthesized by lung macrophages and epithelial cells, has variable bactericidal activity. In addition, there is some evidence that lysozyme may

Table 2–7. IMMUNOGLOBULIN CONCENTRATIONS IN RESPIRATORY FLUIDS

Source	Total Protein (mg/ml)	Albumin	Secretory A	IgG	IgM	IgE*
Upper tract						
Parotid gland (n = 10)	1.34	10	12	0.1	0	0
Nasal wash (n = 16)	0.21	10	10	2.9	0	0
Lower tract						
Bronchoalveolar lavage (n = 14)	1.30	40	2.6	5.6	0.5	0.3

From Fick RB, Hunninghake GW: Antimicrobial defense of the lung. *In* Simmons DN (ed): Current Pulmonology, vol 8, pp. 165–198. Boston: Houghton Mifflin, 1986.

Albumin, sIgA, IgG, IgM expressed as % of total protein. n, Number of subjects tested.

*Expressed in units per milligram of total protein.

Table 2–8. IgG SUBCLASSES IN SERUM AND
BRONCHOALVEOLAR LAVAGE (BAL) FLUID OF NORMAL
SMOKERS AND NONSMOKERS

	Nonsmokers (n = 19)		Smokers (n = 12)	
Subclass	Serum*	BAL	Serum*	BAL
IgG$_1$	67 ± 2.4	65 ± 2.4	80 ± 2.4	79 ± 2.0
IgG$_2$	31 ± 0.1	28 ± 0.9	18 ± 0.6	13 ± 0.5
IgG$_3$	0.4 ± 0.01	1.8 ± 0.2	0.5 ± 0.2	3.7 ± 0.3
IgG$_4$	1.3 ± 0.02	5.2 ± 0.6	1.0 ± 0.03	4.6 ± 0.1

From Reynolds HY: Lung immunology and its contribution to the immunopathogenesis of certain respiratory diseases. J Allergy Clin Immunol 78:833–847, 1986.
*Percentage of total IgG, presented as mean ± standard error of the mean.

enhance lysis of bacteria by aggregated IgA in the presence of complement. Lactoferrin is a product of both epithelial cells and neutrophils. By chelating iron, lactoferrin often inhibits growth of bacteria that require this mineral. Alpha$_1$-protease inhibitor (alpha$_1$-antitrypsin) is an important inhibitor of both bacterial and host proteolytic activity; in central airways, a distinct low-molecular-weight bronchial protease inhibitor, or antileukoprotease, also affords protection against proteolytic injury. Fibronectin, a large glycoprotein produced by a number of cells, including PMO and fibroblasts, probably aids host defense as both an antiadhesive factor and a nonspecific opsonin.

Perhaps most important of the soluble nonspecific host mediators in the lung are proteins of the complement system. Although they are present in low amounts, their importance is attested to both in animal models of complement deficiencies, which result in delayed lung clearance of some bacterial species, and in clinical cases of complement deficiencies, which sometimes result in recurrent respiratory infection. Complement proteins have a number of biologic activities, including opsonization, chemotaxis, viral neutralization, bacteriolysis, and immunoregulation, each of which may be important in a given challenge. Components of both the classical and the alternate complement pathways have been detected in BAL, and total hemolytic complement activity proportional to that expected according to transudation of serum complement is present in the noninflamed lung.[58] In addition, the capacity of lung macrophages to secrete numerous complement components (Table 2–5) suggests that under activated conditions, additional complement-mediated processes may be enhanced.[59]

SECRETORY IMMUNITY: THE RESPIRATORY TRACT IgA SYSTEM

The mucosal IgA humoral immune system has been studied broadly and intensively since its descriptive discovery in 1965.[60] The high levels of IgA in respiratory, gastrointestinal, and other mucosal secretions are now known to be derived from a complex and fascinating secretory process involving cooperation among different cell types.[61] IgA-secreting plasmacytes present in the submucosa of the respiratory tract are often the end products of a complicated process; they often begin as undifferentiated lymphoid cells at distal mucosal sites such as Peyer's patches in the gastrointestinal tract. After antigenic stimulation, B lymphocytes in these sites differentiate into IgA-committed B cells bearing membrane-bound surface IgA molecules. These IgA cells arrive at their final destination—whether elsewhere in the gastrointestinal tract, breast milk, the genitourinary system, or the respiratory tract—through an incompletely understood process of homing in that involves interactions with specific ligands on endothelial cells in the target tissues.[62–64] The organization of the mucosal immune system is illustrated in Figure 2–15.

The history and travels of these B cells of the mucosal immune system are beyond the scope of this chapter,[64–66] but their final destiny and function are germane. In the respiratory and gastrointestinal mucosal lamina propria, after antigenic stimulation and terminal differentiation into plasmacytes, B cells secrete immunoglobulins that are distinctive in at least three ways from the analogous immunoglobulins in the central lymphoid system accessed through analysis of blood:

- There is substantial enrichment of the IgA class isotype in comparison with the other classes of immunoglobulin (IgG, IgM, IgD, and IgE).[67] Table 2–6 lists the concentration and distribution of soluble proteins, including the immunoglobulin isotypes, in the lower respiratory tract of normal adults, as obtained from BAL.
- There is enrichment of the IgA$_2$ subclass isotype. About 50% of all IgA produced submucosally is IgA$_2$, in contrast to ≤15% to 20% of the IgA produced in central lymphoid tissue.[68,69] Table 2–9 summarizes the differences between the two IgA subclass isotypes.
- There is enrichment of J chain–containing polymeric IgA (pIgA), primarily 11S-sized dimers; pIgA constitutes about 95% of the IgA in secretions but only about 10% in serum.[70] The secretion of J chains (molecular weight, 15 kD) by the plasmacyte along with the immunoglobulin heavy and light chains is thought to be essential for the polymerization process;[71] most J chain–containing plasmacytes are located in submucosal sites.[72] Interestingly, there is a dissociation between the processes of polymerization and isotype switch, which indicates that this is a complex and clearly well-regulated system, albeit poorly understood at present.

Polymeric (but not monomeric) IgA secreted by local submucosal IgA plasmacytes is then selectively taken up into epithelial cells, which produce and display on their basolateral cell membrane a specific, high-affinity membrane-bound receptor for polymerized immunoglobulin. The internalization process is one of specific receptor-mediated endocytosis. Internalized pIgA is subsequently sorted away from the epithelial cell's lysosomal degradative endosomal pathway, unidirectionally transported across the cell in endocytotic vesicles to the apical membrane, and released into the lumen along with an extracellular portion of the receptor, which is termed *secretory component* (SC; 80 kD).[67,73,74] The SC-pIgA transport system is summarized diagrammatically in Figure 2–16, and

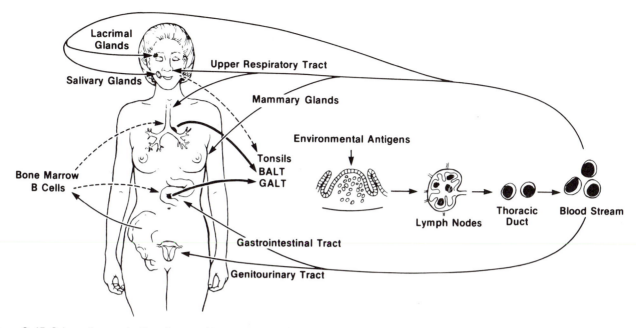

Figure 2-15. Schematic organization of mucosal immune system. Lymphoid precursor cells produced in the bone marrow enter Peyer's patches of the gut-associated lymphoid tissue (GALT) and possibly the tonsils, where differentiation to IgA-bearing B cells occurs under the influence of regulatory T lymphocytes and accessory cells (stromal cells, dendritic cells, or macrophages). Antigen exposure via specialized antigen-presenting cells in these epithelia interact with the accessory, T, and B cells. Then the IgA-committed cells leave Peyer's patches and enter regional lymphatic tissue, lymph ducts, and eventually the circulation. These cells ultimately home in on various mucosal target sites, where terminal differentiation into IgA-secreting plasmacytes occurs. (From Mestecky J: The common mucosal immune system and current strategies for induction of immune responses in external secretions. J Clin Immunol 7:265–276, 1987.)

the molecular structure of secretory IgA (sIgA; 415 kD) is depicted in Figure 2–17. In the lower respiratory tract, the polymeric immunoglobulin receptor is present on non-ciliated respiratory epithelial cells in bronchioles and on type II alveolar epithelial cells.[75]

Polymeric IgM, which incorporates J chains, may also undergo this process, but there are few IgM-secreting plas-macytes in mucosal tissues. However, in persons with selective IgA deficiency,[76] secretory IgM is often able to compensate for the absence of IgA and appears to provide partial and, in some patients, even complete functional replacement of the missing IgA.[61,77] In the minority of IgA-deficient persons who suffer from repeated lower respiratory tract infections, concomitant dysregulation of

Table 2-9. CHARACTERISTICS OF IgA SUBCLASSES

Property	IgA₁	IgA₂
Serum concentration	1.8 mg/ml	0.2 mg/ml
Serum proportion	75%–93%	7%–25%
Proportion in bone marrow, spleen	79%–88%	8%–12%
Proportion in secretory tissues (salivary, lacrimal glands, intestine)	39%–56%	44%–61%
Proportion in external secretions (saliva, tears, milk, intestine)	50%–67%	33%–50%
Proportion in bronchoalveolar lavage fluid (82% polymeric)	66%–69%	31%–33%
Antibody response in secretions		
Proteins	+ to +++	± to ++
Carbohydrates	++	0 to ++
Amphophilic (LPS, lipoteichoic acid)	+	++
Electrophoretic mobility	Slower	Faster (anodal)
Hinge region	Intact	Deletion (12-13 aa residu
Susceptibility to bacterial protease	Yes	No
Serum half-life	6 Days	4.5 Days
Fractional catabolic rate	24%	32%
Synthetic rate	24 mg/kg/day	4 mg/kg/day
Total body pool*	185 mg/kg	25 mg/kg
Allotypes	Absent	A₂m(1) or A₂m(2)
Glycosylation	6.1%	8.2%
Monomer combines with secretory component	No	Yes: A₂m(1)
		No: A₂m(2)

LPS, lipopolysaccharide.
*Total daily production of IgA in normal adult is 3.5–9.2 g vs 3 g/day for IgG.

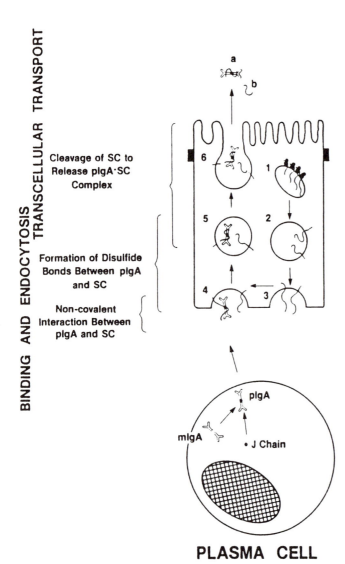

EPITHELIAL CELL

BINDING AND ENDOCYTOSIS   TRANSCELLULAR TRANSPORT

Cleavage of SC to
Release pIgA·SC
Complex

Formation of Disulfide
Bonds Between pIgA
and SC

Non-covalent
Interaction Between
pIgA and SC

a

b

6   1

5   2

4   3

pIgA

mIgA   • J Chain

PLASMA CELL

Figure 2–16. Transport system for secretory IgA in mucosal tissues. Secretory immunoglobulin (mostly polymerized IgA, but also some IgM) is produced by isotype-committed, J chain–producing submucosal plasmacytes. Secretory component (SC) is manufactured in rough endoplasmic reticulum of epithelial cells (1). After glycosylation in the Golgi apparatus (2), SC vesicles are selectively transported to and fuse with the basolateral membrane (3). Membrane-bound SC forms complexes with polymerized IgA or IgM on the basolateral surface (4). The complexes are endocytosed in pinocytotic vesicles (5), where the extracellular portion of SC is probably cleaved, and are transported to the apical surface (6). Secretory IgA (a) is released by fusion of the vesicle with the apical membrane. Excess secretion of free SC (b) also occurs. (Modified from Mestecky J, McGhee JR: Immunoglobulin A (IgA): Molecular and cellular interactions involved in IgA biosynthesis and immune response. Adv Immunol 40:153–245, 1987.)

other isotypes, such as an IgG subclass abnormality or deficient secretory IgM response, may be responsible for the increased risk of infection.[78]

In contrast to IgA or IgM, IgG—which does not incorporate J chains—is not endocytosed by epithelium expressing the polymeric immunoglobulin receptor, and

consequently IgG that is present in secretions apparently gets there either by local secretion or by passive transudation from serum.[50] The latter is especially likely once antigenic penetration into the mucosa occurs and phlogistic mechanisms are activated. One physiologic exception is the presence of high levels of IgG and albumin in saliva near birth, which is suggestive of increased mucosal permeability in the postnatal period. Complete mucosal immunocompetence cannot be assumed until a child reaches about 5 years of age.[79]

As mentioned earlier, the ectocytoplasmic portion of the polymeric immunoglobulin receptor is proteolytically cleaved from its transmembrane and cytosolic portions during endocytotic transit or at the apical surface and is released in covalent complex with its polymerized immunoglobulin ligand as the complete sIgA molecule.[80,81] There is constitutive synthesis of the polymerized immunoglobulin receptor; therefore, if there is an excess of receptor over pIgA (the stoichiometry is 1:1), unbound or free secretory component (fSC) is released into the lumen. The ratio of fSC to pIgA-bound SC presumably depends on both the availability of pIgA ligand and the level of constitutive production of receptor by the epithelial cells. It appears that there is always an excess of receptor production over pIgA availability, and hence the normal presence of fSC (8% to 60% of the total SC) in mucosal secretions.[67,82] In contrast to secretions, SC is detectable in serum only when it is bound to pIgA—that is, as part of sIgA.[83] The normal level of sIgA in serum is 5 to 10 μg/ml.[84]

Several remarkable aspects of this process are noted as follows:

- There is no other known transport process in which a receptor is *permanently* bound to its ligand.[85] Thus the ligand (pIgA) is not ultimately sorted to lysosomal endosomes, the receptor-ligand complex is not dissociated after endocytosis, the receptor is not recycled, and the ligand is released covalently bound to a portion of the receptor.[86] Hence SC has been called the "sacrificial receptor."[87] The fate of the remaining transmembrane and intracellular portions of the polymeric immunoglobulin receptor is not yet known with certainty. Presumably, they are degraded shortly after proteolytic release of fSC or sIgA.
- Secretory component is a member of the immunoglobulin gene superfamily,[88] containing five discrete repeating regions homologous to immunoglobulin light chain variable domains.[89] Yet it is expressed exclusively in differentiated polarized exocrine epithelial tissues and not in lymphocytes or other cell types.
- Production of the polymerized immunoglobulin receptor is constitutive and not regulated by level or availability of ligand.[67,87] Thus in IgA deficiency, elevated levels of fSC are found in mucosal secretions. However, receptor production can be modulated by hormonal factors such as sex steroids and is affected by the degree of cell differentiation as well as by cell transformation.[73] Receptor level is also responsive to interferon-γ, a broad regulator of translational expression of many products of the immunoglobulin

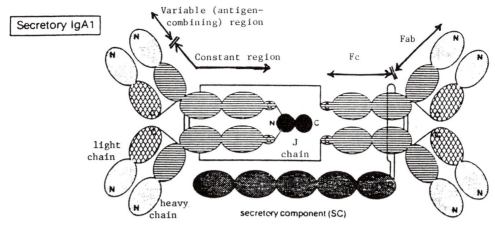

Figure 2–17. Molecular structure of secretory IgA (IgA₁ is shown). Secretory IgA consists of an IgA polymer (a dimer, the most common polymer, is shown), a J chain, and a secretory component (SC). IgA shares general features of the immunoglobulin superfamily unit structure of 10- to 15-kD double β–pleated sheet domains (ellipses), which are stabilized by one or two internal disulfide bonds. Monomer tertiary structure is stabilized by both covalent and noncovalent bonds. The J chain, which is essential for polymerization, may bind to one 160-kD IgA monomer, as shown, or to both. The dimer is held together by disulfide bonds. SC is another immunoglobulin superfamily member of five domains homologous to immunoglobulin light chain variable domains. SC binds only to polymerized IgA, probably by initial noncovalent interaction with both monomers simultaneously and subsequently by disulfide binding to the third heavy chain domain of one IgA monomer, as shown, although binding to the other monomer is possible. The completed molecule is well suited, as is IgM, for neutralizing and agglutinating effector functions, whereas complement-activating and opsonic activities are poor. Priming of monocytes and macrophages with receptors for the Fc region of IgA for antibody-dependent cell-mediated cytotoxicity may occur, as may priming of neutrophils with similar receptors for bactericidal activity. (Modified from Underdown BJ, Schiff MJ: Immunoglobulin A: Strategic defense initiative at the mucosal surface. Annu Rev Immunol 4:389–417, 1986. Reproduced, with permission, from the Annual Review of Immunology, Vol. 4, © 1986 by Annual Reviews Inc.)

supergene family.[90] Regulation of epithelial polymerized immunoglobulin receptor display by cytokines such as interferon-γ and tumor necrosis factor α[91] is a newly discovered and unexplored aspect of feedback cycles between the immune system and the respiratory epithelium.

- SC processing exhibits distinct and rigid subcellular topographic sequencing. After synthesis and core glycosylation in the rough endoplasmic reticulum, terminal glycosylation (the end product is approximately 25% carbohydrate) occurs in the Golgi apparatus. Transport, presumably vesicular, is then routed to the basolateral membrane. Receptor-mediated endocytosis of pIgA is followed by unidirectional transport to the apical membrane, fusion, and luminal release of vesicle contents.[92,93] This process is not well understood, although a model has been proposed whereby vesicle acidification promotes preferential pIgA-receptor binding over pIgA binding to other receptors, such as hepatic binding protein (the asialoglycoprotein receptor) in the rat hepatocyte.[94] The relatively long carboxy-terminal intracytoplasmic "tail" of the receptor (molecular weight, 15 to 20 kD) may play a key role in the unidirectional sorting of pIgA in its journey across the cell, but how this occurs is unknown.[85,86]

The primary physiologic function of sIgA, *immune exclusion,* is a broad, noninflammatory antiadhesive function based on neutralizing and agglutinating properties against viral and bacterial mucosal pathogens and against soluble macromolecular antigens.[60–62,70] By binding soluble or particulate foreign antigens without much complement activation, chemotactic activity, or opsonophagocytic potential, as seems to be the case in most studies of effector function, sIgA antibodies may function pri-

marily as a sort of "antiseptic paint" on mucosal surfaces. The IgA₂ subclass is of particular interest in view of its increased representation in secretions, its resistance to bacterial IgA₁ proteases,[69] and IgA₂-restricted immune responses to bacterial surface polysaccharides,[69] which may be analogous to IgG₂-restricted systemic responses to similar or identical pathogenic bacterial antigens.[95,96]

Failure of this first line of immunologic pulmonary defense results in penetration of foreign antigens into the epithelium and submucosal regions. This penetration, besides causing direct toxic tissue damage in many instances, also causes activation of phlogistic host defense mechanisms, which form a secondary line of defense. These mechanisms, which increase clearance but can also lead to inflammatory tissue damage if the challenge is not rapidly and completely terminated, are illustrated in Figure 2–18 and discussed further in the next section.

Thus the secretory immune process culminating in luminal sIgA incorporates diverse elements of cell cooperation, membrane function at both ends of polarized epithelial cells, intracellular glycosylation, intracellular sorting and traffic, and intercellular feedback loops of great complexity. It ultimately involves synthesis of the key molecule of the mucosal immune system, sIgA, which might provide a link between normal cell physiologic processes and clinical pathophysiologic processes of many respiratory diseases.

Further progress in understanding the secretory immune system will undoubtedly result from the most recent advances in molecular biology. The primary structures of both IgA₁ and IgA₂ subclasses have been determined.[64,69] A given IgA molecule carries one of three distinct, mutually exclusive, genetically determined heavy-chain allotype antigens of uncertain functional significance.[97] The gene for the polymeric immunoglobulin receptor has been cloned and sequenced in rabbits.[89] The

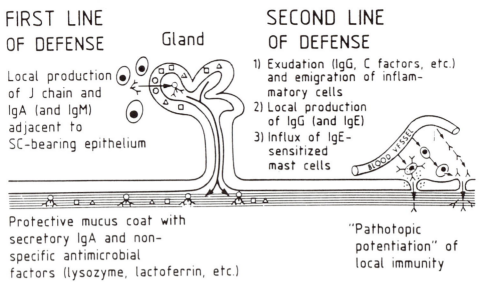

FIRST LINE OF DEFENSE

Gland

Local production of J chain and IgA (and IgM) adjacent to SC-bearing epithelium

Protective mucus coat with secretory IgA and non-specific antimicrobial factors (lysozyme, lactoferrin, etc.)

SECOND LINE OF DEFENSE

1) Exudation (IgG, C factors, etc.) and emigration of inflammatory cells
2) Local production of IgG (and IgE)
3) Influx of IgE-sensitized mast cells

BLOOD VESSEL

"Pathotopic potentiation" of local immunity

Figure 2–18. Concept of "defense in depth" of the mucosa is illustrated. Mucosal immune system, with secretory IgA as linchpin, is the first line of defense. Besides IgA, physical properties of mucus, ciliary transport, and nonspecific antimicrobial factors such as lysozyme and lactoferrin contribute to clearance of most inhaled particulate and soluble antigens. However, if the system is breached, secondary immunologic mechanisms are called into play. These may involve the IgE mast cell–dependent mediator release system, IgG-mediated reactions such as complement activation, or cell-mediated reactions, all of which are proinflammatory and serve to quickly amplify the recruitment and concentration of defense molecules and cells. This enhancement by inflammation has been termed *pathotopic potentiation* of local immunity by P. Brandtzaeg, but it also provides the seeds of host tissue damage if the challenge is not quickly and efficiently ended. (From Brandtzaeg P: Immune functions of human nasal mucosa and tonsils in health and disease. *In* Bienenstock J [ed]: Immunology of the Lung and Upper Respiratory Tract, pp. 28–95. New York: McGraw-Hill, 1984.)

primary amino acid sequence of purified human SC has been determined.[73] The tertiary structure of bovine SC has been elucidated.[98] The fine glycosylation structures of both IgA and SC have also been worked out.[69,73] Finally, a number of reliable monoclonal and monospecific polyclonal antibodies to various sIgA and SC epitopes are now available.[99,100] Once better understanding of the mucosal immune system is achieved, dramatic advances can be expected in mucosal immunization and other forms of local immunotherapy.[101]

SECONDARY DEFENSES OF THE LUNG: PULMONARY INJURY AND INFLAMMATION

Mild or brief injury to lung tissue is usually healed completely by a complex process of epithelial repair, which depends on the integrity of the basement membrane; on endothelial repair, regulation of which is poorly understood; and on fibroblast proliferation, which is at least partly regulated by PMO-derived mediators, including fibronectin and a fibroblast growth factor.[102] However, in settings of severe or prolonged challenge to the normal network of resident lung defenses, amplifying mechanisms are activated and result in a phlogistic inflammatory response. These inflammatory components unleash powerful destructive forces that offer the double-edged prospect of enhanced removal or destruction of the foreign material and possible damage to normal host lung tissue as well.

A helpful mechanistic general classification of inflammatory responses into four types of immune-mediated hypersensitivity reactions, as listed and modified for the lung in Figure 2–19, was proposed by Gell and Coombs in the 1960s and has stood the test of time.[103] Many pulmonary inflammatory reactions can be categorized according to this schema and assigned priority in the pathophysiologic processes of a given disease state or host response.

A key element of the lung's amplifying machinery is the potential ensemble of chemoattractant factors available for recruiting nonresident phagocytes by processes of directed migration (chemotaxis). The resulting composition of the inflammatory cell infiltrate in various pathologic states is determined largely by the nature, proportion, and activities of the chemoattractants elaborated. For example, acute extracellular bacterial infection is most likely to lead to release of chemotactic formyl peptides from bacterial surfaces, release of complement-derived chemotaxins from activation of the alternate complement pathway in the nonimmune host, or antigen-antibody immune complex–induced activation of the classical complement pathway in immune hosts.[104] The most potent of the complement-derived chemotactic factors are C5a and its metabolite $C5a_{des\ arg}$, split products of activated complement component C5. These chemotactic factors tend to preferentially attract neutrophils.[105]

In contrast, mast cell activation and degranulation (e.g., induced by inhalation of allergen in an allergic asthmatic) leads to release of arachidonate-derived leukotrienes and preformed chemotactic peptides that preferentially attract eosinophils.[106]

In addition, PMOs have been shown to elaborate an approximately 10-kD chemotactic peptide that preferentially attracts neutrophils.[107] PMOs also may secrete a

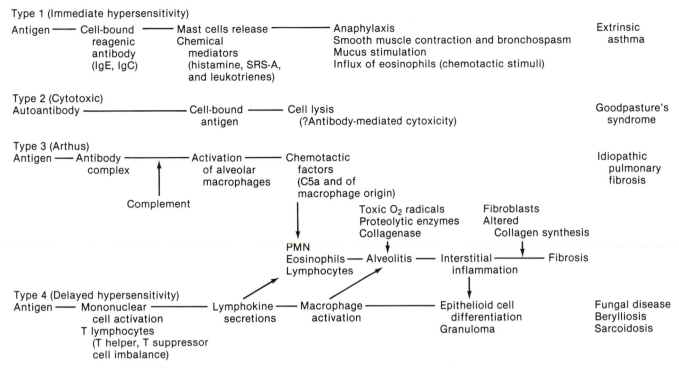

Figure 2–19. Gell and Coombs' classification of immune-mediated hypersensitivity reactions.

variety of other products with chemotactic activities. Prominent among these is leukotriene B₄, a potent chemoattractant for neutrophils.[108]

Finally, elements of the clotting, fibrinolytic, and kinin systems (e.g., plasminogen activator, kallikrein) have been found to have chemoattractant activity and may play a role in amplification of the inflammatory response.[58] The stimuli that initiate activation of these

cascade systems and their biologic role in the lung have not been elucidated. Figure 2–20 illustrates how a bacterial stimulus may interact with these amplifying and recruitment systems to enhance the inflammatory response in the lung.

Chemoattractant activity is only one of several mechanisms of amplification of the inflammatory response. Many of the inflammatory mediators mentioned earlier,

AIRWAY – ALVEOLAR SURFACE

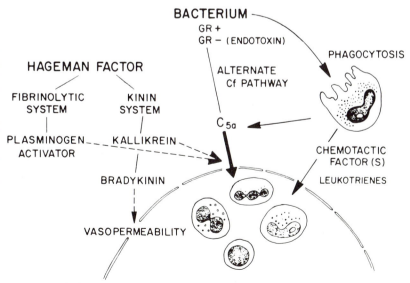

Figure 2–20. Generation of an inflammatory response by interaction of a stimulus (here, bacterial infection) with one or more of several potential amplifying mechanisms present in the airways and gas exchange units. These amplifying mechanisms include activation pathways for the complement, kinin, or fibrinolytic cascades, each of which is capable of generating chemotactic factors or elaboration of chemotactic factors by activated resident phagocytes. Through increases in vasopermeability and through chemotaxis, the host response is quickly multiplied and localized. (From Reynolds HY: Lung inflammation: Role of endogenous chemotactic factors in attracting polymorphonuclear granulocytes. Am Rev Respir Dis 127:S16–S25, 1983.)

CAPILLARY – ENDOTHELIAL SURFACE

as well as a number of others, may have narrow or broad cell-activation properties, vasopermeability activities, or neural reflex irritant activities.[58,106,109-112] The molecular mechanisms underlying chemotaxis, inflammatory cell activation, and inflammatory cell effector functions (e.g., phagocytosis, killing, secretion) all are incompletely understood areas under intensive study by contemporary cell biologists. Overall, inflammatory responses do seem designed to deliver increased quantities of cellular and soluble defense components to the site of challenge; such a design supports the hypothesis of pathotopic potentiation of immunity by inflammation (see Fig. 2–18).

The by-products of the inflammatory response, however, are largely nonspecific in target activity and may produce "innocent bystander" tissue damage by a variety of mechanisms,[113,114] especially when extracellular release of toxic molecules that are probably intended for intracellular action occurs. The extent and nature of the resulting tissue damage will depend largely on the general type of inflammatory cell response evoked, and on which hypersensitivity reaction mechanism predominates, in a given pathologic state. Two general mechanisms in particular are receiving extensive study:

- The effects of mast cell–mediated anaphylactic reactions, which prominently involve tissue effects of the mast cell mediators themselves, and those subsequently derived from recruited eosinophils.[115,116]
- Neutrophil-mediated damage that may result from direct recruitment (e.g., by bacterial chemotactic peptides), activation of complement pathways, or immune complex formation after the initiation of the specific humoral immune response. In these cases, most attention is being directed to the ability of the neutrophil to secrete toxic oxygen metabolites and proteases (Fig. 2–21).[14,117,118]

Understanding the role that various types of inflammation play in the pathophysiologic processes of particular lung diseases will lead to more rational and focused therapies that are based on the profile of host responses, especially for the many lung diseases in which basic pathogenetic stimuli remain undefined and thereby unamenable to prophylaxis or early intervention. Thus, for example, diseases such as chronic asthma that are characterized by predominantly eosinophilic infiltrates and by eosinophil-derived toxic products will be treated with therapies increasingly targeted to blunting the deleterious effects of defined eosinophil products (e.g., inhibitors of platelet activating factor or major basic protein), whereas diseases such as cystic fibrosis that are characterized by predominantly neutrophilic infiltrates will be treated with corresponding strategies (e.g., antielastases, antioxidants) aimed at countering potential neutrophil-mediated damage.

DEVELOPMENTAL ASPECTS OF PULMONARY DEFENSES

Previous sections have alluded to the dramatic impact of normal lung development on defense capabilities. The postnatal effects of simple anatomic growth on airway cal-

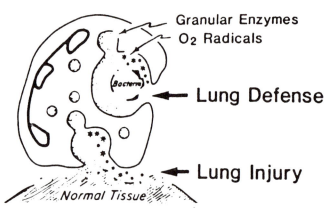

Figure 2–21. The potential for both immunity and hypersensitivity inflammatory injury exists with the arrival of activated neutrophils in the lung (a similar schema would apply for eosinophils). The same mechanisms used for intracellular killing could cause tissue damage if extracellular release occurs in amounts exceeding local buffering capacities. The latter is especially likely to occur when the phagocytic stimulus is too large to be adequately engulfed; this leads to a state of "frustrated phagocytosis." Proteolytic enzymes and toxic oxygen metabolites are leading candidates for mediators of neutrophil-associated inflammation. (From Harada RN, Repine JE: Pulmonary host defense mechanisms. Chest 87:247–252, 1985.)

iber and subsequent vulnerability to obstruction, multiplication of gas exchange units, differentiation of macrophages and population of lung tissue, maturation of intrinsic cellular competency, and responsiveness to regulatory nervous and humoral inputs all undoubtedly play important roles in overall defensive action. Although there is a large body of information on the ontogeny and postnatal development of elements of the systemic immune and inflammatory systems, very little is known about compartmental pulmonary expression of these components.

MACROPHAGES

Studies of neonatal blood monocytes have shown a paucity of cells carrying class II histocompatibility antigens (HLA-DR) in comparison with adult monocytes, which makes poor antigen presentation a likely cause of defective immune responses in early life. This depressed expression of HLA-DR may in turn be mediated by suppressive factors, which possibly include prostaglandin E_2 and alpha-fetoprotein, which is present in highest concentrations in fetal and neonatal serum.[119] In the lung, antigen presentation is probably also defective early in life, whereas cytotoxic function may be comparable to adult PMO, but data are scanty.[27]

The population of airspaces by PMO soon after birth may be mediated by the release of type II pneumocytes and surfactant into the newly created air-lung interface at birth. Subsequent scavenging of excess surfactant by PMO may play a role in depressed killing ability.[27] Adaptive responses of monocytes and macrophages in late gestation and at term must also include rapid and dramatic increases in oxidative metabolism and production of antioxidant enzymes such as superoxide dismutase, catalase, and glutathione peroxidase.[120]

T CELLS

Systemic T cell functions become manifest close to or at birth; response magnitudes are usually close to adult levels.[121] However, functions dependent on antigen presentation (e.g., B cell help) are depressed, presumably secondary to the maturational defect in accessory cell HLA-DR expression noted earlier. In addition, nonspecific suppressor cells (of both immature T cell and non–T cell lineages by criteria of surface differentiation antigen expression) are present in the early neonatal period and depress certain *in vitro* responses. These suppressor cells may also be activated by alpha-fetoprotein.[122] Suppressor activity may persist throughout the first year of life.[123] In addition, neonatal lymphocytes are deficient in production of lymphokines such as interferon-γ.[124] There are no data on how these systemic responses might apply to pulmonary T cell activities.

B CELLS

Antibody production by the fetus has been detected as early as 20 weeks. There is clear evidence from molecular genetic studies that clonal diversity (the antigen-responsive repertoire) of antibody-secreting cells is well established at birth, although clonal expansion continues well into childhood. However, cell maturation and differentiation, and immunoglobulin class and subclass switching processes, appear to be deficient in early life. Immunoglobulin secretion follows a sequence of IgM→IgG→IgA both *in vitro* and *in vivo*. At birth and through the first few months of infancy, there are increased numbers of functionally immature B cells bearing surface IgM or IgD.[121] Normal adult serum levels of IgM are achieved by about the first birthday, IgG levels reach maturity at 5 to 8 years, and IgA levels reach maturity in late childhood (10 to 12 years). IgG subclasses are further distinguished by a lag of IgG_2 and IgG_4 responsiveness behind that of IgG_1 and IgG_3. Because polysaccharide antigen-antibody responses are largely IgG_2, poor infantile responses to these antigens may be based on the slow maturation of the IgG_2 B cell response. B cells from neonates are not only partially suppressed but also intrinsically deficient in ability to secrete IgG and IgA.[125]

With regard to pulmonary expression of humoral immunity, it is of interest that the secretory IgA system appears to mature more quickly than the systemic IgA system; sIgA appears in the neonatal period, and its concentrations attain adult levels by ages 2 to 4 years.[123] Secretory IgA antibody responses to mucosal and systemic antigens appear early in infancy, albeit at lower titers than in later life.[126] In the serum, polymeric IgA levels are high in early infancy and reach adult levels by 1 year; in contrast, monomeric IgA levels are low and rise gradually.[121]

INFLAMMATORY RESPONSES

Neonates display a wide gamut of depressed inflammatory responses as measured by numerous *in vivo* and *in vitro* assays, including depressed rates of skin sensitization to injected antigens; slowed rejection of skin homografts; depression of monocyte and neutrophil chemotaxis; deficient neutrophil random mobility, adherence, deformability, phagocytosis, oxidative metabolism, and killing; low levels of complement and complement-dependent opsonins; low levels of certain components of the clotting-kinin-fibrinolytic cascades; and depressed neutrophil and monocyte entry into Rebuck's skin windows.[27,124,127,128] Deficient adherence may underlie poor antibody-dependent cell-mediated cytotoxicity by neonatal monocytes and natural killer cells.[121]

The consequences of this array of inflammatory deficiencies for defense of the lung in term neonates and young infants—and even more so for premature or low-birth-weight infants—remain virtually unknown. With regard to pulmonary defense mechanisms, a National Institutes of Health workshop on postnatal lung development reached this conclusion: "There is a lack of knowledge, even at a descriptive level, about developmental aspects of the local generation of opsonins and the competence of phagocytes in the lung . . . developmental biology of the pulmonary host defenses should be an extremely fruitful area for future research."[129]

REFERENCES

General References

Bienenstock J (ed): Immunology of the Lung and Upper Respiratory Tract. New York: McGraw-Hill, 1984.

Brain JD, Proctor DR, Reid LM (eds): Respiratory Defense Mechanisms: Lung Biology in Health and Disease, vol. 5. New York: Marcel Dekker, 1977.

Daniele RP (ed): Immunology and Immunologic Diseases of the Lung. Boston: Blackwell Scientific, 1988.

Gallin JI, Fauci AS (eds): Mucosal Immunity: Advances in Host Defense Mechanisms, vol. 4. New York: Raven Press, 1984.

Greene GM, Jakab GJ, Low RB, Davis GS: Defense mechanisms of the respiratory membrane. Am Rev Respir Dis 115:479–514, 1977.

Hanson LA, Brandtzaeg P: The mucosal defense system. *In* Stiehm ER (ed): Immunologic Disorders in Infants and Children, 3rd ed, pp. 116–155. Philadelphia: WB Saunders, 1989.

Murray JF, Nadel JA: Defense mechanisms and immunology. *In* Murray JF, Nadel JA (eds): Textbook of Respiratory Medicine, pp. 313–388. Philadelphia: WB Saunders, 1988.

Literature Cited

1. Weibel ER: Morphometry of the Human Lung. New York, Academic Press, 1963.
2. Thurlbeck WM: Postnatal human lung growth. Thorax 37:564–571, 1982.
3. Breeze RG, Wheeldon EB: The cells of the pulmonary airways. Ann Rev Respir Dis 116:705–777, 1977.
4. Gail DB, Lenfant CJM: Cells of the lung: Biology and clinical implications. Am Rev Respir Dis 127:366–387, 1983.
5. Jones R, Reid L: Secretory cells and their glycoproteins in health and disease. Br Med Bull 34:9–16, 1978.
6. Sturgess JM: Mucous secretions in the respiratory tract. Pediatr Clin North Am 26:481–501, 1979.
7. Kornfeld R, Kornfeld S: Comparative aspects of glycoprotein structure. Annu Rev Biochem 45:217–237, 1976.
8. Kaliner M, Shelhamer JH, Borson B, et al: Human respiratory mucus. Am Rev Respir Dis 134:612–621, 1986.
9. Lopez-Vidriero MT, Reid L: Bronchial mucus in health and disease. Br Med Bull 34:63–74, 1978.
10. Palmblad J, Mossberg B, Afzelius BA: Ultrastructural, cellular, and clinical features of the immotile-cilia syndrome. Annu Rev Med 35:481–492, 1984.

11. Greenstone M, Cole PJ: Ciliary function in health and disease. Br J Dis Chest 79:9–26, 1985.

12. Newhouse M, Sanchis J, Bienenstock J: Lung defense mechanisms. N Engl J Med 295:990–998, 1045–1052, 1976.

13. Sleigh MA, Blake JR, Liron N: The propulsion of mucus by cilia. Am Rev Respir Dis 137:726–741, 1988.

14. Harada RN, Repine JE: Pulmonary host defense mechanisms. Chest 87:247–252, 1985.

15. Wanner A: Clinical aspects of mucociliary transport. Am Rev Respir Dis 116:73–125, 1977.

16. Wanner A: Allergic mucociliary dysfunction. J Allergy Clin Immunol 72:347–350, 1983.

17. Loudon RG: Cough: A symptom and a sign. Basics RD 9:19–24, 1981.

18. Eigen H: The clinical evaluation of cough. Pediatr Clin North Am 29:67–78, 1982.

19. Leith DE: Cough. *In* Brain JD, Proctor DR, Reid LM (eds): Respiratory Defense Mechanisms: Lung Biology in Health and Disease, vol. 5, pp. 545–592. New York: Marcel Dekker, 1977.

20. Mellis CM: Evaluation and treatment of chronic cough in children. Pediatr Clin North Am 26:553–564, 1979.

21. Morgan WJ, Taussig LM: The chronic bronchitis complex in children. Pediatr Clin North Am 31:851–864, 1984.

22. Hunninghake GW, Gadek JE, Kawanami O, et al: Inflammatory and immune processes in the human lung in health and disease: Evaluation by bronchoalveolar lavage. Am J Pathol 97:149–206, 1979.

23. Daniele RP, Elias JA, Epstein PE, Rossman MD: Bronchoalveolar lavage: Role in the pathogenesis, diagnosis, and management of interstitial lung disease. Ann Intern Med 102:93–108, 1985.

24. Brain JD: Lung macrophages: How many kinds are there? What do they do? Am Rev Respir Dis 137:507–509, 1988.

25. Rossman MD, Chien P, Cassizzi-Cprek A, et al: The binding of monomeric IgG to human blood monocytes and alveolar macrophages. Am Rev Respir Dis 133:292–297, 1986.

26. Nakashima H, Ando M, Sugimotot M, et al: Receptor-mediated O₂ release by alveolar macrophages and peripheral blood monocytes from smokers and nonsmokers. Am Rev Respir Dis 136:310–315, 1987.

27. Fick RB: Cell-mediated antibacterial defenses of the distal airways. Am Rev Respir Dis 131:S43–S48, 1985.

28. Alenghat E, Esterly JR: Alveolar macrophages in perinatal infants. Pediatrics 74:221–223, 1984.

29. Kurland G, Cheung ATW, Miller ME, et al: The ontogeny of pulmonary defenses: Alveolar macrophage function in neonatal and juvenile rhesus monkeys. Pediatr Res 23:293–297, 1988.

30. Miller ME: The inflammatory and natural defense systems. *In* Stiehm ER, Fulginiti VA (eds): Immunologic Disorders in Infants and Children, pp. 165–180. Philadelphia: WB Saunders, 1980.

31. Bellanti JA, Nerukar LS, Zeligs BJ: Host defenses in the fetus and neonate: Studies of the alveolar macrophage during maturation. Pediatrics 64:726–739, 1979.

32. Kaltreider HB: Alveolar macrophages: Enhancers or suppressors of pulmonary immune reactivity? Chest 82:261–263, 1982.

33. Goldstein E, Lippert W, Warshauer D: Pulmonary alveolar macrophage: Defender against bacterial infection of the lung. J Clin Invest 54:519–528, 1974.

34. Hocking WG, Golde DW: The pulmonary-alveolar macrophage. N Engl J Med 301:580–587, 639–645, 1979.

35. Reynolds HY, Atkinson JP, Newball HH, Frank MM: Receptors for immunoglobulin and complement on human alveolar macrophages. J Immunol 114:1813–1819, 1975.

36. Naegel GP, Young KR, Reynolds HY: Receptors for human IgG subclasses on human alveolar macrophages. Am Rev Respir Dis 129:413–418, 1984.

37. Czop JK, McGowan SE, Center DM: Opsonin-independent phagocytosis by human alveolar macrophages: Augmentation by human plasma fibronectin. Am Rev Respir Dis 125:607–609, 1982.

38. O'Neill SJ, Lesperance E, Klass DJ: Human lung lavage surfactant enhances staphylococcal phagocytosis by alveolar macrophages. Am Rev Respir Dis 130:1177–1179, 1984.

39. Nathan CF, Prendergast TJ, Wiebe ME, et al: Activation of human macrophages: Comparison of other cytokines with interferon-γ. J Exp Med 160:600–605, 1984.

40. Adams DO, Hamilton TA: The cell biology of macrophage activation. Annu Rev Immunol 2:283–318, 1984.

41. Nathan CF, Murray HW, Wiebe ME, Rubin BY: Identification of interferon-γ as the lymphokine that activates human macrophage oxidative metabolism and antimicrobial activity. J Exp Med 158:670–689, 1983.

42. Unanue ER, Allen PM: The basis for the immunoregulatory role of macrophages and other accessory cells. Science 236:551–557, 1987.

43. Herscowitz HB: In defense of the lung: Paradoxical role of the pulmonary alveolar macrophage. Ann Allergy 55:634–648, 1985.

44. Hunninghake GW: Immunoregulatory functions of human alveolar macrophages. Am Rev Respir Dis 136:253–254, 1987.

45. Holt PG: Down regulation of immune responses in the lower respiratory tract: The role of alveolar macrophages. Clin Exp Immunol 63:261–270, 1986.

46. Nathan CF: Secretory products of macrophages. J Clin Invest 79:319–326, 1987.

47. Kaltreider HB: Phagocytic, antibody and cell-mediated immune mechanisms. *In* Murray NF, Nadel JA (eds): Textbook of Respiratory Medicine, pp. 332–357. Philadelphia: WB Saunders, 1988.

48. Gil J, Daniele RP: Morphology of the lung's immune system. *In* Daniele RP (ed): Immunology and Immunologic Diseases of the Lung, pp. 21–54. Boston: Blackwell Scientific, 1988.

49. Bienenstock J: Bronchus-associated lymphoid tissue. *In* Bienenstock J (ed): Immunology of the Lung and Upper Respiratory Tract, pp. 96–118. New York: McGraw-Hill, 1984.

50. Kaltreider HB: Local immunity. *In* Bienenstock J (ed): Immunology of the Lung and Upper Respiratory Tract, pp. 191–215. New York: McGraw-Hill, 1984.

51. Hance AJ, Saltini C, Crystal RG: Does *de novo* immunoglobulin synthesis occur on the epithelial surface of the human lower respiratory tract? Am Rev Respir Dis 137:17–24, 1988.

52. Willoughby WF, Willoughby JB: Antigen handling. *In* Bienenstock J (ed): Immunology of the Lung and Upper Respiratory Tract, pp. 174–190. New York: McGraw-Hill, 1984.

53. Boucher RC, Ranga V: Fate and handling of antigens by the lung. *In* Daniele RP (ed): Immunology and Immunologic Diseases of the Lung, pp. 55–78. Boston: Blackwell Scientific, 1988.

54. Meuer SC, Acuto O, Hercend T, et al: The human T-cell receptor. Annu Rev Immunol 2:23–50, 1984.

55. Merrill WW, Naegel GP, Olchowski JJ, Reynolds HY: Immunoglobulin G subclass proteins in serum and lavage fluid of normal subjects: Quantitation and comparison with immunoglobulins A and E. Am Rev Respir Dis 131:584–587, 1985.

56. Bienenstock J: The lung as an immunologic organ. Annu Rev Med 35:49–62, 1984.

57. Murphy S, Florman AL: Lung defenses against infection: A clinical correlation. Pediatrics 72:1–15, 1983.

58. Reynolds HY, Merrill WW: Lung immunology: The inflammatory response in lung parenchyma. *In* Simmons DH (ed): Current Pulmonology, vol. 2, pp. 299–322. Boston: Houghton Mifflin, 1980.

59. Auerbach HS, Colten HR: The secretion of components of complement by alveolar macrophages. *In* Daniele RP (ed): Immunology and Immunologic Diseases of the Lung, pp. 159–165. Boston: Blackwell Scientific, 1988.

60. Tomasi TB, Tan EM, Solomon A, Prendergast RA: Characteristics of an immune system common to certain external secretions. J Exp Med 121:101–124, 1965.

61. Mestecky J, Russell MW, Jackson S, Brown TA: The human IgA system: A reassessment. Clin Immunol Immunopathol 40:105–114, 1986.

62. Tomasi TB, Plaut AG: Humoral aspects of mucosal immunity. *In* Gallin JI, Fauci AS (eds): Mucosal Immunity: Advances in Host Defense Mechanisms, vol. 4, pp. 31–61. New York: Raven Press, 1985.

63. Underdown BJ, Schiff MJ: Immunoglobulin A: Strategic defense initiative at the mucosal surface. Annu Rev Immunol 4:389–417, 1986.

64. Mestecky J, McGhee JR: Immunoglobulin A (IgA): Molecular and cellular interactions involved in IgA biosynthesis and immune response. Adv Immunol 40:153–245, 1987.

65. Strober W, Jacobs D: Cellular differentiation, migration, and function in the mucosal immune system. *In* Gallin JI, Fauci AS (eds):

Mucosal Immunity: Advances in Host Defense Mechanisms, vol. 4, pp. 1–30. New York: Raven Press, 1985.

66. Word CA, Crago SS, Tomasi TB: Regulation of IgA expression by isotype-specific T cells and soluble binding factors. Annu Rev Microbiol 40:503–524, 1986.

67. Brandtzaeg P: Role of J chain and secretory component in receptor-mediated glandular and hepatic transport of immunoglobulins in man. Scand J Immunol 22:111–146, 1985.

68. Kett K, Brandtzaeg P, Radi R, Haaijman JJ: Different subclass distribution of IgA-producing cells in human lymphoid organs and various secretory tissues. J Immunol 136:3631–3635, 1986.

69. Mestecky J, Russell MW: IgA subclasses. Monogr Allergy 19:277–301, 1986.

70. Conley ME, Delacroix DL: Intravascular and mucosal immunoglobulin A; two separate but related systems of immune defense? Ann Intern Med 106:892–899, 1987.

71. Brandtzaeg P, Prydz H: Direct evidence for an integrated function of J chain and secretory component in epithelial transport of immunoglobulins. Nature 311:71–73, 1984.

72. Crago SS, Kutteh WH, Moro I, et al: Distribution of IgA1-, IgA2-, and J chain–containing cells in human tissues. J Immunol 132:16–18, 1984.

73. Ahnen DJ, Brown WR, Kloppel TM: Secretory component. Gastroenterology 89:667–682, 1985.

74. Mostov KE, Deitcher DL: Polymeric immunoglobulin receptor expressed in MDCK cells transcytoses IgA. Cell 46:613–621, 1986.

75. Haimoto H, Nsgura H, Imaizumi M, et al: Immunoelectronmicrocopic study on the transport of secretory IgA in the lower respiratory tract and alveoli. Virchows Arch [Pathol Anat] 404:369–380, 1984.

76. Burks AW, Steele RW: Selective IgA deficiency. Ann Allergy 57:3–8, 1986.

77. Kvale D, Brandtzaeg P: An enzyme-linked immunosorbent assay for differential quantitation of secretory immunoglobulins of the A and M isotypes in human serum. J Immunol Methods 86:107–114, 1986.

78. Hanson LA, Bjorklander J, Carlson B, et al: The heterogeneity of IgA deficiency. J Clin Immunol 8:159–162, 1988.

79. Cripps AW, Clancy RL, Gleeson M, et al: Mucosal immunocompetence in man—the first five years. Adv Exp Med Biol 216B:1369–1375, 1987.

80. Mostov KE, Blobel G: A transmembrane precursor of secretory component: The receptor for transcellular transport of polymeric immunoglobulins. J Biol Chem 257:11816–11821, 1982.

81. Mostov KE, Blobel G: Biosynthesis, processing, and function of secretory component. Meth Enzymol 98:458–466, 1983.

82. Merrill WW, Goodenberger D, Strober W, et al: Free secretory component and other proteins in human lung lavage. Am Rev Respir Dis 122:156–161, 1980.

83. Iscaki S, Geneste C, Pillot J: Molecular state of secretory component in human serum. Immunol Lett 1:217–221, 1980.

84. Wood GM, Trejdosiewicz LK, Losowsky MS: ELISA for measurement of secretory IgA distinct from monomeric IgA. J Immunol Methods 97:269–274, 1987.

85. Farquhar MG: Intracellular membrane traffic: pathways, carriers, and sorting devices. Meth Enzymol 98:1–13, 1983.

86. Mostov KE, Simister NE: Transcytosis. Cell 43:389–390, 1985.

87. Solari R, Kraehenbuhl J-P: The biosynthesis of secretory component and its role in the transepithelial transport of IgA dimer. Immunol Today 6:17–20, 1985.

88. Williams AF, Barclay AN: The immunoglobulin superfamily—Domains for cell surface recognition. Annu Rev Immunol 6:381–405, 1988.

89. Mostov KE, Friedlander M, Blobel G: The receptor for transepithelial transport of IgA and IgM contains multiple immunoglobulin-like domains. Nature 308:37–43, 1984.

90. Sollid LM, Kvale D, Brandtzaeg P, et al: Interferon-gamma enhances expression of secretory component, the epithelial receptor for polymeric immunoglobulins. J Immunol 138:4303–4306, 1987.

91. Kvale D, Lovhaug D, Sollid LM, Brandtzaeg P: Tumor necrosis factor-α up-regulates expression of secretory component, the epithelial receptor for polymeric Ig. J Immunol 140:3086–3089, 1988.

92. Goodman MR, Link DW, Brown WR, Nakane PK: Ultrastruc-

tural evidence of transport of secretory IgA across bronchial epithelium. Am Rev Respir Dis 123:115–119, 1981.

93. Solari R, Kraehenbuhl J-P: Biosynthesis of the IgA antibody receptor: A model for the transepithelial sorting of a membrane glycoprotein. Cell 36:61–71, 1984.

94. Schiff JM, Fisher MM, Jones AL, Underdown BJ: Human IgA as a heterovalent ligand: Switching from the asialoglycoprotein receptor to secretory component during transport across the rat hepatocyte. J Cell Biol 102:920–931, 1986.

95. Hammarstrom L, Smith CIE: IgG subclasses in bacterial infections. Monogr Allergy 19:122–133, 1986.

96. Hammarstrom L, Smith CIE: IgG subclass changes in response to vaccination. Monogr Allergy 19:241–252, 1986.

97. Van Loghem E, Biewenga J: Allotypic and isotypic aspects of human immunoglobulin A. Mol Immunol 20:1001–1007, 1983.

98. Beale D, Coadwell J: Tertiary structures for the extracellular domains of the epithelial polyimmunoglobulin receptor (secretory component) derived by primary structure comparisons with immunoglobulins. Comp Biochem Physiol 86B:365–372, 1987.

99. Delacroix DL, Van Snick J, Vaerman JP, et al: Monoclonal antibodies against isotypic and isoallotypic determinants of human IgA1 and IgA2. Molec Immunol 23:367–375, 1986.

100. Russell MW, Brown TA, Radl J, et al: Assay of human IgA subclass antibodies in serum and secretions by means of monoclonal antibodies. J Immunol Methods 87:87–93, 1986.

101. Mestecky J: The common mucosal immune system and current strategies for induction of immune responses in external secretions. J Clin Immunol 7:265–276, 1987.

102. Rennard SI, Bitterman PB, Crystal RG: Response of the lower respiratory tract to injury: Mechanisms of repair of the parenchymal cells of the alveolar wall. Chest 84:735–739, 1983.

103. Roitt I: Essential Immunology, pp. 193–214. Oxford, England: Blackwell Scientific, 1988.

104. Frank MM: Complement in the pathophysiology of human disease. N Engl J Med 316:1525–1530, 1987.

105. Fearon DT: Complement. J Allergy Clin Immunol 71:520–529, 1983.

106. Serafin WE, Austen KF: Mediators of immediate hypersensitivity reactions. N Engl J Med 317:30–34, 1987.

107. Reynolds HY: Lung inflammation: Role of endogenous chemotactic factors in attracting polymorphonuclear granulocytes. Am Rev Respir Dis 127:S16–S25, 1983.

108. Martin TR, Altman LC, Albert RK, Henderson WR: Leukotriene B4 production by the human alveolar macrophage: a potential mechanism for amplifying inflammation in the lung. Am Rev Respir Dis 129:106–111, 1984.

109. Wasserman SI: Mediators of immediate hypersensitivity. J Allergy Clin Immunol 72:101–118, 1983.

110. Barnes PJ: Neural control of human airways in health and disease. Am Rev Respir Dis 134:1289–1314, 1986.

111. Barnes PJ: Neuropeptides in the lung. J Allergy Clin Immunol 79:285–295, 1987.

112. Henderson WR: Eicosanoids and lung inflammation. Am Rev Respir Dis 135:1176–1185, 1987.

113. Cohen AB: Potential adverse effects of lung macrophages and neutrophils. Fed Proceed 38:2644–2647, 1979.

114. Johnson KJ, Ward PA: Mechanisms of acute and chronic immune inflammatory responses in the lung. In Daniele RP (ed): Immunology and Immunologic Diseases of the Lung, pp. 193–214. Boston: Blackwell Scientific, 1988.

115. Holgate ST, Hardy C, Robinson C, et al: The mast cell as a primary effector cell in the pathogenesis of asthma. J Allergy Clin Immunol 77:274–282, 1986.

116. Frigras E, Gleich GJ: The eosinophil and the pathology of asthma. J Allergy Clin Immunol 77:527–537, 1986.

117. Janoff A, White R, Carp H, et al: Lung injury induced by leukocytic proteases. Am J Pathol 97:111–136, 1979.

118. Schraufstatter IU, Revak SD, Cochrane CG: Proteases and oxidants in experimental pulmonary inflammatory injury. J Clin Invest 73:1175–1184, 1984.

119. Lu CY, Unanue ER: Macrophage ontogeny: Implications for host defense, T lymphocyte differentiation, and the acquisition of self-tolerance. Clinic Immunol Allergy 5:253–270, 1985.

120. Frank L, Sosenk IRS: Development of lung antioxidant enzyme

system in late gestation: Possible implications for the prematurely born infant. J Pediatr 110:9–14, 1987.

121. Goldman AS, Pong AJH, Golblum RM: Host defenses: Development and maternal contributions. *In* Barness LA (ed): Advances in Pediatrics, vol. 32, pp. 71–100. Chicago: Year Book Medical, 1985.

122. Stutman O: Ontogeny of T cells. Clinic Immunol Allergy 5:191–234, 1985.

123. Wilson M: Immunology of the fetus and newborn: Lymphocyte phenotype and function. Clinic Immunol Allergy 5:271–286, 1985.

124. Stiehm ER: Human neonatal immune capacity: The B, T, and monocyte/macrophage systems. *In* Hodes H, Kagan BM (eds): Pediatric Immunology, pp. 75–88. New York: Science & Medicine Publishing, 1979.

125. Vogler LB, Lawton AR: Ontogeny of B cells and humoral immune functions. Clin Immunol Allergy 5:235–252, 1985.

126. Hanson LA, Carlsson B, Dahlsen U, et al: Vaccination and the ontogeny of secretory IgA responses. Adv Exp Med Biol 216B:1353–1358, 1987.

127. Miller ME: The neonatal inflammatory response. *In* Hodes H, Kagan BM (eds): Pediatric Immunology, pp. 89–112. New York: Science & Medicine Publishing, 1979.

128. Wilson CB: Immunologic basis for increased susceptibility of the neonate to infection. J Pediatr 108:1–12, 1986.

129. Motoyama EK, Brody JS, Colten HR, Warshaw JB: NHBLI Workshop summary: Postnatal lung development in health and disease. Am Rev Respir Dis 137:742–746, 1988.

3 RESPIRATORY MUCUS

RALPH C. FRATES, JR., M.D.

The word *mucus* is Latin and means "nasal discharge."[1] The Romans may have taken the word from the Greek word μνδδεδθαι or the Sanskrit word *muñcati,* meaning "slippery substance."[2] Hoppe-Seyler as early as 1877 defined mucus as "schliemstoff," a "jelly-like slippery viscous mass . . . dispersed but not dissolved in water . . . the product of epithelial cells of mucous membranes and salivary glands.[3] In this chapter, *mucus* means "the total secretion from mucous membranes."[4] The subject of mucus is complex, and the literature is voluminous and changing rapidly. The object of this discussion is to offer the reader a survey of contemporary thought, emphasizing the aspects related to pediatric pulmonology. A more comprehensive review is available in *Mucus in Health and Disease,* Volume 2.[5]

APPROACHES TO THE STUDY OF MUCUS

Respiratory tract mucus is difficult to study because healthy people do not produce samples sufficient for analysis. Even if expectorated samples were obtainable from a normal person, they would be contaminated with saliva and mouth flora. Any attempt to bypass the mouth in order to obtain uncontaminated respiratory mucus involves instrumentation, which entails risk, discomfort, and the introduction of other variables. Insertion of an endotracheal tube causes local inflammation; insertion of a bronchoscope and lavage with saline result in dilution of recovered samples and probably cause transudation of serum proteins across damaged alveolar-capillary membranes into the very small amount of mucus recovered.

Many investigators have sought to answer questions about mucus by focusing their efforts at the tissue or cellular and molecular level. These approaches avoid problems of contamination that are inherent in working with intact animals or humans and possibly offer a more detailed understanding of mucus.

Both *in vivo* and *in vitro* techniques are used to study mucus. One interesting new *in vivo* method is the measurement of tracheal submucosal gland output. There are two means of making such measurements. In both, the animal is anesthetized and paralyzed, and the cervical trachea is opened. Using neutral red dye, the investigator can identify gland ducts on the mucosa and insert a micropipette.[6] Alternatively, fine tantalum can be dusted onto the mucosa and an electrical stimulus applied to the trachea. The resultant gland secretions appear as hillocks, which are photographically recorded.[7,8] As discussed by Widdicombe,[9] these methods make possible the measurement of submucosal gland flow rates under basal and stimulated conditions, and the pipette method enables some valuable chemical and physical measurements of gland output.[10,11] The limitations are the necessary equipment and skill and the nanoliter volumes of mucus obtained.[10,11]

The hillock experiments provide more abundant secretions, but they can be analyzed only for their total volume.[9] Both these whole animal systems yield systemic effects when drugs are injected intravenously; more localized effects may be obtained by injection into a tracheal artery.[12] Among the *in vitro* models used is the isolated whole trachea, usually from a ferret.[13] Large volumes of secretions can be collected, and electrodes may be inserted or placed on the mucosa to measure ion flux and serosal-luminal potential voltage differences. Drugs may be applied to the epithelium as well as into the bath around the serosa because the inside of the trachea is filled with air. Most ferret tracheal secretions probably come from the submucosal glands.[14]

On a smaller scale, airway tissue explants have long been used to study secretion of mucus[15] or ciliary motion.[16] Because such a small amount of tissue is needed, biopsies may be taken from healthy human volunteers. In addition, relatively little equipment is required for work with tissue explants. A disadvantage of this method is that the amount of secretion obtained is quite small, and heterogeneous cells with many interactions may be involved in secretion. There may be a heightened possibility of injury artifact with the use of small explants because the ratio of the area of cut tissue to that of unperturbed tissue is high. In the case of explants that include tracheal cartilage, there has been concern that the proteoglycans detected in the wash or bath could be products of cartilage rather than of epithelial secretory cells.[17] Mixing of secretions from the luminal or the epithelial side with those from the submucosal side of the explant is unavoidable, and the equilibrium of radiolabeled material is lost.[18]

Another approach to the use of tissue explants is the use of Ussing's chamber. Epithelial explant tissue may be mounted as a semipermeable diaphragm between two fluid-filled compartments. This technique enables radiolabeled precursors to equilibrate between the submucosal and epithelial sides of the explant. Electrical potential difference measurements and ion fluxes can then be studied. The macromolecular secretions from the luminal side of the epithelium may be produced by cells other than those in submucosal glands.[18]

The next step in the study of mucus is scrutiny of the individual cell or cell types. Light microscopy with periodic acid-Schiff staining enables identification of neutral mucin; Alcian blue stains mucins with sialic acid or sulfate residues.[19] Immunocytologic staining techniques extend the range of the light microscope to include intracellular localization of other mucus components such as lactoferrin[20] and lysozyme.[21] The ability to study that degree of specificity of cell and molecular structure and function has been improved by the electron microscope. Basbaum[22] used electron microphotographs with autoradiography and morphometry to demonstrate that ferret tracheal submucosal-gland mucus cells respond to beta-adrenergic stimulation but not to alpha-adrenergic stimulation, whereas the response of serous cells was the reverse.

Electron microscopy has also been used to view mucin molecules.[23-25] Electron photomicrographs showed mucins as intertwined linear threads; these results were similar to those from laser light analyses of scattering by mucins in solution (i.e., laser correlational spectroscopy).[26] Dehydration of mucin molecules for electron microscopy adds a degree of uncertainty with regard to how well these images reflect nature. Electron microscopy, together with autoradiography, morphometry, and immunochemistry, can better show the correspondence of anatomy to function. The use of primary cultures in which all cells are apparently the same type and in which monoclonal antibodies bind to specific protein or carbo-hydrate antigens on mucus secretions helps determine which type of cell produces a specific secretory product in response to a given stimulus. Cell monolayers are used for studying secretions of both ions and organic molecules. Monoclonal antibodies have labeled cell-specific mucus molecules in histologic specimens in human[27] and non-human primates[28] and other animals.[29,30]

CLINICAL ASPECTS OF MUCUS

Estimates of the volume of mucus production in healthy humans were made from two studies. Toremaln[31] found that mucus production in laryngectomy patients, whose airways were kept properly humidified, was 0.2 to 0.3 ml/kg of body weight per day. Hilding[32] found that one laryngectomized patient produced 1.16 g of mucus in 3 h, which was extrapolated to 9.28 g per 24 h. As Kilburn[33] observed, the relationship of the volumes of respiratory tract fluid produced, reabsorbed, and expelled is unknown. Bronchorrhea, or excessive mucus secretion, (which usually means expectorated sputa), is said to involve more than 100 ml per day.[34]

The composition of mucus is complex. Normal mucus is 95% to 98% water by weight.[35,36] Lipids, proteins (including glycoconjugates), and electrolytes make up the remainder of mucus.

Mucus is segregated in the larger airways into an electrolucent watery sol phase, which covers the epithelium from its luminal aspect to the tips of the cilia, and an electron-dense gel phase at or above the cilia tips on the luminal side. Gil and Weibel,[37] in an electron microscopic study of rat bronchioles, found the cilia to be covered by an osmophilic layer possibly consisting of surfactant, rather than by a sol-gel biphasic layer of mucus. The depth of mucus on the respiratory epithelium measured in rat tracheas was found to be 5 μm by Dalhamm[38] and 5 to 10 μm by Yoneda,[39] and the depth of mucus in guinea pig tracheas and bronchi was found to be 10 μm by Hulbert and associates.[40] Hulbert and associates' method,[40] which involved rapid perfusion of the bronchial circulations with fixative plus aerosolized fixative via a tracheal tube, was specifically chosen to stabilize both respiratory mucus and epithelium in relation to one another. Electron microphotographs of guinea pig tracheas after 100 puffs of cigarette smoke showed a tenfold increase in the thickness of the electron-dense gel layer and the absence of the electrolucent sol layer in the area of inflamed epithelium. This severe diminution of the sol layer, in which the cilia must move, suggested that the cilia could not perform their job under those circumstances. Sanderson and Sleigh[41] photographed rabbit tracheal cilia in motion. They noted that the depth of the sol layer was critical: too deep a sol layer caused the gel to float above cilia tips, unable to be propelled, whereas too shallow a sol layer flattened the cilia. Sturgess,[36] on the basis of electron microphotographs in freeze-fracture studies, summarized respiratory mucus thickness for humans as follows: 5 to 10 μm in larger airways, 1 to 4 μm in bronchioles, and 0.1 μm in terminal bronchioles.

The question of whether mucus travels as a continuous blanket or as discrete, separate particles atop cilia is not yet answered. Van As and Webster,[42,43] basing their conclusions on both *in vivo* and scanning electron microscopic studies of healthy and bronchitic rat airways, concluded that mucus normally moved as separate particles that coalesced into "droplets," then "flakes," and later "plaques" as mucus moved cranially, finally joining streams in the principal bronchi and trachea.[44] On the other hand, scanning electron microphotographs of human airways by Sturgess[36] demonstrated rather smooth mucus sheets in tracheas, thinning to "open networks" of "fibrils" in lobar bronchi and finally to "plaques" in distal airways.

Rheology is the study of the flow and deformation of liquids. The mathematics and methods used in mucus rheology have been reviewed in detail.[45] Most of the attention to the rheology of mucus has focused on measuring its viscosity, or resistance to flow, and its elasticity, or ability to stretch and then resume its previous length. Mucus is a non-Newtonian substance, which means that at high shear rates or stresses, the application of force causes the molecules of mucus to deform without resuming their shape and original mechanical properties. Difficulties in studying mucus rheology include (1) the small amount of mucus available for study, (2) dehydration, and (3) contamination with saliva, serum transudates, or products of infection or inflammation.

Despite these difficulties, a general consensus among investigators has emerged over the years. Charman and Reid,[46] using a Ferranti-Shirley cone-and-plate viscometer, found that increase in viscosity of sputum was attributable to its purulence rather than to the diagnosis of the patient who provides the specimen. Interestingly, mucoid sputum from asthmatic patients was more viscous than sputa from cystic fibrosis (CF) patients, which had the same appearance. From the same center and using the same technique as in the previous study, Picot and colleagues[47] demonstrated that the *in vivo* DNA content of sputum did not correlate significantly with increased viscosity, although viscosity was increased by the addition of DNA to sputum *in vitro*. Picot and colleagues suggested that the breakdown of mucus *in vivo* by inflammatory products such as enzymes offsets any increase in viscosity that results from higher DNA concentrations.

More recent work has reinforced these conclusions. King,[48] using a small steel sphere 10 μm in diameter that was vibrated by an electromagnet, was able to calculate viscosity, elasticity, and the ratio of viscosity to elasticity from 5- to 10-μl aliquots of either tracheal secretions from healthy dogs or sputum from CF patients. Only when the CF patients' sputa was purulent did it have higher viscosity and elasticity and a lower viscosity/elasticity ratio. When CF sputa were mucoid or mucopurulent in appearance, the viscosity/elasticity ratio was the same as that of dogs' tracheal secretions. Puchelle and co-workers[49] found that CF sputa, collected free of saliva, were viscous only when the patients were sick and had low Shwachman clinical scores when the sputa had high concentrations of bacteria and white blood cells.

Rheologic properties other than viscosity and elasticity may also play a role in mucociliary transport. Puchelle and Zahm[50] found a significant positive correlation between "spinnability" of human respiratory mucus (the ability to draw mucus into long threads) and the rate at which cilia on a mucus-depleted frog palate would beat when loaded with human respiratory mucus. In brief, the greater the "spinnability" of mucus and the lower its viscosity and elasticity, the more quickly the frog palate cilia beat.[49-51]

Purulent mucus contains a number of substances besides DNA that affect its rheology and transport. For example, Sanderson and Sleigh[52] measured the effects of immunoglobulin M (IgM) on the ciliary action measured in a biologic system (sea mussels). In these experiments, IgM caused disorganization of the ciliary beat and agglutination of cilia. The effect was the same regardless of whether IgM was from sera of healthy humans, CF patients, dogs, cattle, or sheep. Mian and collaborators[53] performed a comprehensive investigation on the effects of many different agents on the viscosity of three types of mucus from chicken tracheas. Using the Ferranti-Shirley cone-and-plate viscometer, they found that treatment of mucus with thiol reagents or enzymes, including papain, pronase, or sulfatase, had no effect, but sonication, agents which reduced hydrogen binding, and various salt solutions all decreased viscosity. Neuraminidase treatment reduced the viscosity of aqueous, or soluble, mucus by half but did not affect fibrillar or gelatinous mucus. Of particular note was their finding that less thick native mucus became more viscous with increased concentrations of *N*-acetylneuraminic acid, whereas the most viscous native mucus had relatively high sulfate concentrations; the sulfate concentration increased directly with viscosity. The latter point is of particular interest because heavily sulfated, high-molecular-weight glycoconjugates were known to be secreted by CF airways,[54] organ culture,[55,56] and nasal epithelial cell cultures.[57] Cheng and co-authors[57] suggested that the high degree of sulfation of airway macromolecules was a primary phenotypic defect of the airway epithelium of CF patients, one that increased the viscosity of mucus. This somehow enabled the characteristic airway pathogens of CF, such as *Staphylococcus aureus* and *Pseudomonas aeruginosa*, to establish chronic colonization and infection.

COMPOSITION AND FUNCTION OF MUCUS

WATER

Water is the main constituent of respiratory mucus and perhaps the most important one. By weight, water accounts for 95% to 98% of mucus.[35,36] Water in mucus is vital for at least three functions: (1) regulating heat and humidity in the respiratory tract (air conditioning), (2) mucociliary clearing, and (3) dissolving noxious gases, which are then neutralized by mucus or carried away by the mucociliary escalator.

The air-conditioning function of water in mucus is extremely efficient. For example, the nasal mucosa, a rather small part of the total respiratory epithelial area, can add 3 g of water to each cubic meter of inhaled air.[58] This is about 10% of all water vapor added by the mucosa. Proctor[59] found human nasal passages adjusted inhaled

Table 3–1. SOME DIFFERENCES AMONG GLYCOCONJUGATE PROTEINS IN MUCUS

Characteristic	Mucus Glycoprotein (Mucin)	Serum Glycoprotein	Proteoglycan
Linkage	O-glycosidic: N-acetylgalactosamine to serine/threonine	N-glycosidic (major): N-acetylglucosamine to asparagine O-glycosidic (minor)	O-glycosidic: (1) xylose to serine; (2) N-acetylgalactosamine to serine/threonine; (3) mannose to serine/threonine N-glycosidic: N-acetylglucosamine to asparagine
Oligosaccharide unit size	Fewer than 25 monosaccharides (average 8 to 10)	Fewer than 25 monosaccharides	More than 50 monosaccharides and a few small oligosaccharides
Repeating structure	Commonly: GalNAc β1-4 N-acetylglucosamine β1-3$_n$	None	Repeating disaccharides with hexosamine residues (glycosaminoglycans)
Uronic acid	None	None	Present
Shape	Branched	Branched	Linear unbranched
Monosaccharides: fucose, galactose, N-acetylglucosamine	Present	Present	N-acetylglucosamine $\gg$ fucose, galactose
N-acetylneuraminic acid	Present	Present	Low levels
Mannose	Absent	Present	Low levels
N-acetylgalactosamine	Present	Low levels or absent	May be present
Xylose	Absent	Absent	May be present

Modified from Clamp JR: Mucus in Health and Disease. New York: Plenum Press, 1977.

air to within 10°C of body temperature despite environment air temperatures ranging from −20°C to 55°C. McFadden and co-workers[60,61] pointed out that hyperventilation of cold air could temporarily tax the air-conditioning system. In their study, volunteers breathed 60 l/min of air at 17°C, decreasing their right lower lobe temperatures from 37°C to 27°C. The high specific heat content of water, most of which is in the sol layer of mucus, prevents freeze injury and stores heat for the respiratory tract.[60] It is possible that in humans, as in camels[62] and dogs,[63] water loss and recovery by respiratory mucus accounts for humidity control and probably a great deal of the thermal regulation of intraluminal air.[64]

The respiratory cilia beat in the watery sol, their tips touching the overlying gel layer to sweep mucus toward the pharynx. Changes in the depth or composition of the aqueous sol layer or in the viscoelasticity of the gel or the mucus layer in its entire thickness probably affect human mucociliary transport.[41] Experimental pathology studies of animals exposed to noxious gases show disruption of the respiratory epithelium,[65] including a drastic reduction in the depth of the sol layer.[40] Chopra and associates[66] measured tracheal transport velocity of radiolabeled albumin microspheres in anesthetized dogs and measured the velocity again 24 h after withholding fluids. They then rehydrated dogs with saline and repeated the same measurements. The mean tracheal transport rate dropped significantly with dehydration but returned to normal again after intravenous rehydration. Baetjer[67] similarly found that 72 h of dehydration decreased clearance of radioactive droplets on chicken tracheas. The amount of water loss from mucus needed to compromise mucociliary clearance is unknown.

A third function of water in mucus is its action as a solvent. An example is its ability to absorb sulfur dioxide, a common industrial noxious gas. This gas is so well absorbed in the water of mucus that its penetration beyond the upper airways ranges from less than 1% to no more than 4%, despite a tenfold increase in the concentration of the sulfur dioxide inhaled.[68,69] In contrast, ozone is relatively insoluble in water and is able to escape entrapment in upper airway mucus to penetrate deep into the lung.[69]

MUCINS

Mucins are the second most important component of mucus. These glycoproteins have been scrutinized by investigators for decades because of their prominent role in mucociliary clearance and in the pathologic processes of cystic fibrosis. According to Rose's reviews on mucins,[70] carbohydrates account for 50% to 85% of mucins' molecular mass, which is generally more than 1 $\times$ 10^6 D. The carbohydrate oligosaccharide side chains are 1 to 15 or more sugars in length and are covalently linked through an oxygen atom to a polypeptide backbone. The primary sugar is N-acetylgalactosamine, which is attached to either serine or threonine. The oligosaccharides may be branched or linear. Monosaccharides in mucins are galactose, fucose, N-acetylneuraminic acid, N-acetylglucosamine, and N-acetylgalactosamine..[71,72] After glycosylation, mucins are packaged into granules in specialized epithelial cells. More recent information provided by studies of dog tracheal epithelial cell cultures that were free of either submucosal gland cells or goblet cells demonstrated high molecular weight secretion without intracellular granules.[73]

It is increasingly clear that mucins are only one of the types of macromolecules in mucus. Other high-molecular-weight glycoconjugates found in mucus include proteoglycans and serum glycoproteins. A comparison of the properties of these types of proteins is given in Table 3–1.

Mucins have several functions in mucus. Litt,[74] using

the frog palate model and mucin from the human middle ear, clearly demonstrated that the rate of mucociliary transport effectiveness depended mainly on mucin concentration. Carson and collaborators[75] similarly observed mucostasis in cat tracheas when mucus viscosity was too high. The concentration of mucin in mucus seems to be critical for mucociliary clearance.

On the other hand, mucins may participate in other processes that are more important than mucociliary clearance. Since Eliasson and associates[76] described the immotile cilia syndrome, it has become clear that humans can survive without normal mucociliary clearance, despite some sinopulmonary disease and male sterility.

There are several other examples of the putative functions of mucins. Mucins are probably the foremost defense in preventing water loss from airway mucus. Although only 5% of water available may be bound to mucins,[77] they form a viscous coating over the watery sol layer, thereby preventing dehydration of evaporation. At a biologic level, mucins may influence ion flux. Lee and Nicholls[77] compared the rates of diffusion of ionized potassium through both pig gastric mucin and a neutral starch gel and concluded that the mucus gel, a polyanion, repelled some of the potassium cation. Cross and colleagues[78] determined the effects of various oxidizing agents on pig tracheal and gastric mucins. The mucin products of the reaction were degraded by oxygen radicals and became smaller and less viscous. Cross and colleagues speculated that mucins, by reducing the number of oxygen radicals that attacked the mucins' protein backbone, could protect the mucosa from oxidants in cigarette smoke or polluted air. Finally, Ramphal and associates[79–81] demonstrated that *Pseudomonas aeruginosa*, a common bacterial colonizer and pathogen in the airways of patients with CF, adheres to the same receptors on both human tracheal cells and human tracheobronchial mucins. Ramphal and associates suggested mucin may protect tracheal cells from binding with *Pseudomonas aeruginosa*. (However, many bacteria bind to carbohydrate structures not found on mucins, including mannose and Gal alpha 1-4 Gal, and to the carbohydrate structures in lipids identified by Krivan and co-workers.[82,83]) In summary, mucins may do more than form the steps of the mucociliary escalator.

Mucins have been reported in the sera of humans who have diseases.[84] Many CF patients have high levels of mucin-associated serum antigens in comparison with healthy volunteers and with patients with bronchiectasis.[85] Preliminary information indicated that the rise in serum mucin–associated antigen levels in CF patients was directly correlated with increase in age and severity of illness. Unfortunately, the monoclonal antibody 19-9, which detected the mucin-associated sialyl Lewis bloodgroup antigen, either underestimated or could not detect mucin-associated antigen levels of many CF patients whose Lewis blood group types were (a−b+) or (a−b−). Martin and co-authors[86] described the monoclonal antibody 17Q2 whose epitope is a linear lacto-*N*-tetraose oligosaccharide and is not a blood group antigen. Using this antibody in a "double-sandwich" enzyme-linked immunosorbent assay (ELISA) system with purified human respiratory mucin as their standard, Lin and

associates[87] confirmed by other means that mean serum mucin concentrations of adult CF patients were much higher than those of non-CF patients with bronchitis or those of normal volunteers. These new methods of quantifying mucin in patients' sera or in culture preparations should prove useful to clinical and laboratory investigators.

LIPIDS

There is a general lack of knowledge concerning the origin and function of pulmonary lipids. Examples of lipids in the respiratory tract include the surfactant phospholipid, which is responsible for reducing alveolar surface tension.[88,89] Woodward and colleagues[90] reported that the total weight percentage of lipids associated with void-volume mucins filtered from bronchial aspirates of patients who were free of respiratory disease ranged from 5% to 15%. Sahu and Lynn[91] found that lipids make up 30% to 40% of the weight of the nonaqueous fraction of lung lavage secretions from patients with CF or asthma. Coles and co-authors[92] partially analyzed lipids purified from human bronchial and canine tracheal explants and suggested that lipids are yet another compound synthesized and secreted by airway tissue.

The lipid composition of mucus varies a great deal. Woodward and colleagues[90] reported that neutral lipids accounted for 56% of total lipid weight from Sepharose CL-4B void volume material. Both phospholipids and glycolipids were present. These results are similar to those of Lewis,[93] who analyzed the lipid content of expectorated sputum from an asthmatic adult. Slomiany and collaborators,[94] working with mucus obtained from tracheal aspirates of intubated patients free of respiratory disease, found that mucus lipid from normal patients was 40% neutral, 22% phospholipids, 25% glycosphingolipids, and 13% glyceroglycolipids. CF patients' expectorated mucus had a 33% higher lipid content than did mucus from the patients free of respiratory disease; other quantitative differences in the distribution of types of lipids were also noted.

Slomiany and collaborators[95] more recently suggested that mucins from CF patients were covalently bound to increased amounts of lipids, making those patients' mucus abnormally sticky. However, Houdret and associates[96] found that the amount of lipid associated with mucins was about the same for bronchitic patients as for CF patients and concluded the association was attributable to the purulence of sputum rather than the diagnosis of CF. In another study, Lethem and Marriot[97] mixed ^{14}C-labeled palmitic acid with mucins, removing lipids and 98% of the radioactive marker by chloroform-methanol extraction. Using gas-liquid chromatography to determine the amount of lipid in the small amount of material that remained, they concluded that no detectable amount of lipid could be covalently bound to mucin *in vitro*.

Krivan and co-workers[82,83] found the carbohydrate structure GalNAc beta 1-4 in human whole-lung glycolipid extracts to be a selective receptor for many human respiratory pathogens. The sulfatide whose carbohydrate structure is Gal (3SO) beta 1, however, was a receptor specifically for *Mycoplasma pneumoniae*. Both of the carbohydrate structures on glycolipids bind their respective radiolabeled pathogens in much greater numbers than do the partially characterized oligosaccharide receptor or receptors on human tracheobronchial mucin.[79-81] However, Krivan and co-workers' structures[82,83] have not yet been localized by histopathologic or other methods in either human airways or secretions, so the biologic relevance of their findings is not clear.

PROTEOGLYCANS

Proteoglycans are complex carbohydrates. The primary unit of proteoglycans is the glycosaminoglycan. Glycosaminoglycans, according to Hascall,[98] are "polyionic polysaccharide chains of variable length that consist of repeating disaccharide units each of which contains a hexosamine and usually a negatively charged sulfate ester and/or carboxylate group." The three classes of mammalian glysosaminoglycans are chondroitin sulfate or dermatan sulfate, heparan sulfate or heparin, and keratan sulfate.[99] One or more glycosaminoglycan chains are covalently attached to a protein core to form the proteoglycan macromolecule. A comparison of proteoglycans with the other two glycoconjugate proteins in mucus is provided in Table 3–1.

Proteoglycans that appeared in respiratory secretions were traditionally thought to be the result of injury to cartilage underlying animal airway explants.[17,100] In 1982, Coles and co-authors[101] found xylose and uronic acid in cesium bromide ultracentrifugation fractions from human bronchial mucosal explant secretions. The tissue preparations were free of cartilage, and so Coles and co-authors concluded that the major macromolecular secretion from unstimulated mucosa was proteoglycan, although typical mucins were the primary macromolecular secretion from methacholine-stimulated tissue. In subsequent experiments, they found glycosaminoglycans in endoscopic aspirates from the tracheas or bronchi of normal nonsmoking volunteers. They also found a mixture of glycosaminoglycans and epithelial glycoproteins in aspirates obtained from tracheostomy tubes of neurologically impaired patients.[102] Similar findings were obtained from bronchial lavages of dogs before and after chronic sulfur dioxide exposure. Xylose, uronic acid, and iduronic acid—all found in proteoglycans—and sugars of glycoprotein were identified in pre-exposure ultracentrifuged lavage fluid fractions. In the postexposure ultracentrifuged fractions, which had a higher density, the compositional analysis revealed higher percentages of glycolipid and of glycoprotein carbohydrates and a lower percentage of glycosaminoglycans.[103] Coles and co-authors concluded that proteoglycans were the major macromolecular epithelial secretions in normal airways but that glycoproteins and lipids are predominant in irritated and inflamed airways. On the other hand, Woodward and colleagues[90] found no evidence of proteoglycans in human tracheobronchial mucus.

Glycosaminoglycans were also identified in secretions from cultured human nasal epithelium[104] and primary respiratory epithelial cell cultures of swine,[105] rabbits,[106] and hamsters.[107] Paul and collatorators[108] identified chondroitin sulfate and hyaluronic acid and glycoproteins in cultured serous cells from the bovine tracheal submucosal gland. Kim[106] found that rabbit tracheal epithelial cells secreted hyaluronic acid-rich, high-molecular-weight products when grown on plastic surfaces, but when the cells were grown on collagen gel, a mixture of this product and mucinlike glycoproteins was secreted.

The function or effect of proteoglycans in respiratory mucus is unknown. However, Basbaum and co-authors[109] speculated that glycosaminoglycans in bovine tracheal gland serous cells were copackaged with cationic proteins to reduce osmotic pressure in secretory granules of epithelial cells.

ADDITIONAL PROTEINS

A number of proteins released from various cell types found in human or other mammalian respiratory epithelium have been identified. These include lysozyme, lactoferrin, kallikrein, secretory IgA, and antiproteases.[110] Small concentrations of typical serum proteins customarily thought to be transudates are also present in normal mucus. Mucus from diseased lungs may have high concentrations of serum proteins, DNA, and other cell breakdown products.

Only three of these proteins are considered here: lysozyme, lactoferrin, and secretory IgA. Immunocytochemical studies of human bronchial submucosal glands have localized lactoferrin and lysozyme to serous cells.[20,21] Not all of these proteins, which are found in normal mucus, are produced exclusively by respiratory epithelium. For example, lactoferrin in mucus could also come from contamination with saliva or from polymorphonuclear cells.[111]

IgA is the product of plasma cells in the lamina propria of mucosal epithelium. It becomes secretory IgA after the epithelial cells attach a polypeptide secretory component to the dimeric IgA molecule provided by the plasma cells. The secretory IgA molecule travels through the epithelial cells vesicles to the apex of the cell, where exocytosis expels the secretory IgA with its cleaved secretory component onto the mucosa.[112]

These three proteins seem to protect the epithelium underneath the mucus. Lysozyme can destroy cell walls of certain bacteria. Creeth and associates[113] demonstrated that lysozyme binds to mucins, probably as a result of charge,[114] so that mucus could carry the lysozyme to kill susceptible inhaled bacteria on first contact. Jennsen and colleagues[115] suggested that lysozyme binding to mucus might increase mucus viscosity. Lactoferrin may also have more than one role in mucus function. One widely accepted theory is that lactoferrin binds free iron, aiding in bacteriostasis of at least the iron-dependent bacteria.[116] Clamp and Creeth[114] also suggested that lactoferrin's chelation of free iron would prevent attack by hydroxyl radicals on mucus glycoproteins. Prevention of mucin degradation by oxidation may be important to the health of the underlying epithelium, particularly in people who smoke.[117] Secretory IgA in the respiratory tract may have two functions: blocking the viral and bacterial adherence to the mucosa[118-120] and promoting bacterial adherence to mucins,[121] thereby preventing bacterial attachment to the respiratory mucosa.

CONTROL OF SECRETION

Water, ions, proteins, and probably lipids are secreted into the lumen of the airways. There must be control mechanisms for ensuring that the airways are neither drowned nor desiccated. At least six types of cells contribute secretions that aid in this regulation: ciliated respiratory epithelial cells, goblet cells, Clara cells, alveolar type II cells, the serous cells, and mucous cells. The ciliated epithelial cells produce water, sodium, and chloride ions and high-molecular-weight glycoconjugates. The net osmotic force of chloride draws water across cell membranes. Osmotic force of as little as 1 mmol/kg of tissue weight can cause water movement across epithelia.[122] A number of hormones and inflammatory mediators promote chloride secretion and hence water movement in vitro to the luminal side of epithelia.[123] Ciliated epithelial cells from dog tracheas in vitro have also been found to secrete sulfated macromolecular glycoconjugates, which were probably proteoglycans.[73] The output of the macromolecules increased when the cultured cells were treated with enzymes,[73] including some from the airway bacterial pathogens Pseudomonas aeruginosa and Staphylococcus aureus. These cells apparently secrete macromolecules from their cell surfaces without using granules in the customary exocytosis mechanism.

Goblet cells seem to secrete macromolecules by exocytosis in response to irritants. These cells, which are found mainly in large and small airways but not bronchioles of humans,[124] pack tightly into a mass of electrolucent secretory granules.[125] These granules are discharged on contact with gases, such as those in tobacco smoke,[126] bacterial proteinases,[127] elastases,[128] and particulate matter.[129] It is unlikely that the goblet cells are under neural control.[130,131]

Clara cells remain something of a mystery. These nonciliated epithelial or secretory cells are located primarily in terminal bronchioles, at least in humans.[132] They are perhaps best characterized by the projection of the cellular apex into the airway lumen.[133-137] There is considerable species variation in cell structure. This intra- and interspecies cell variation is important because most of the evidence that Clara cells are secretory depends on (1) interpretation of histochemical and morphologic variation before and after stimulation and (2) metabolic studies in which presumed secretory precursors are taken up by the cells in question.[133] Using such ultrastructure morphometric measurements in an isolated perfused mouse lung, Massaro and co-workers[138,139] found that murine secretion by Clara cells was induced by increased tidal ventilation through prostaglandins rather than by autonomic nervous system chemical mediators. The nature of the secretion of Clara cells remains controversial. Widdecombe and Pack[133] concluded that Clara cells produced (1) lipids but not surfactant, (2) proteins but not glycoproteins, except for those bound to cell membranes, and perhaps (3) enzymes.

In contrast with neighboring Clara cells, the alveolar type II pneumocytes have been well studied and understood for years. They produce and secrete surfactant, a lipoprotein mixture that reduces alveolar surface tension, thus helping prevent alveolar collapse. Relatively little or no surfactant is generally found upstream from the terminal bronchioles, and so whether it should be considered part of mucus is questionable.

The tracheal and bronchial submucosal glands produce most of respiratory tract secretions.[123] In Reid's studies of human respiratory mucosa, the gland structures occupied 40 times more volume than did goblet cells.[140,141] The histologic and anatomic features of these glands in humans were described by Meyrick and Reid.[142-144] Each gland has a ciliated duct leading down from the epithelial surface to a central collecting duct, which branches into many secretory tubules lined either with serous cells full of electrondense secretory granules or with mucus cells full of electrolucent granules. Gland secretion was found to be regulated by the parasympathetic and sympathetic nervous systems and by noncholinergic nonadrenergic nerves. The physical characteristics and biochemical composition of secretions varied with the species tested and the type of neurochemical stimulation applied, inasmuch as the two principal secretory cell types have different neurochemical receptors and contents.

Verdugo[145] proposed a "jack-in-the-box" model for part of the exocytosis mechanism of intracellular mucins. In this model, mucins or other macromolecules packed inside granules rapidly expand and swell out of the cell when hydrated. Water movement into the mucin gel was dependent on ion concentration and on pH, as Tam and Verdugo[146] demonstrated in vitro; hence, this was a process of Donnan's equilibrium.

EFFECT OF THERAPY ON MUCUS

The soundest advice about therapy of conditions resulting from excessive or abnormal respiratory mucus is to treat the underlying problem. Beyond this, the physician must depend largely on anecdotal information.

Kaliner and associates described their approach to the treatment of excess respiratory mucus in adult patients.[147] They noted that treatment with antihistamines was "generally disappointing" but that topical and systemic steroids were "very effective." It is of interest that some of these authors were among those who described "lipocortin," an inhibitor of phospholipases that contributes to the activation of inflammatory arachidonic acid metabolites and therefore inhibits respiratory glycoconjugate secretion in vitro.[148] Lipocortin is stimulated by corticosteroids.

Removal of excess airway mucus by mechanical means is also a standard approach. Chest percussion and bronchial drainage mobilize secretions so that patients can cough them out. This "ketchup-bottle method," as Murray[149] called it, of thumping and draining mucus out of the airway clearly improved patients' pulmonary function test results in the short term,[150,151] if those patients had plenty of "ketchup" in their "bottles" to begin with.[149]

Another avenue of attack on the problem of excessive or abnormal airway mucus is the manipulation of the proposed human respiratory mucin gene and its protein products. Toward that end, several investigators have used antibodies against the polypeptide backbones of deglycosylated human respiratory mucins to identify complementary DNA clones from expression libraries derived from lung tissue. Partial amino acid sequences have now been deduced from these complementary DNA clones.[152] As is the case for the CF gene and its protein, it is hoped this new knowledge of mucin genes will eventually lead to effective therapies. It is clear that definitive therapies for life-threatening mucus airway obstruction rest on the success of these efforts.

REFERENCES

1. Murray JAH, Bradley HK, Craigie WA, Onions CT (eds): Oxford English Dictionary, vol. 7, p. 739. Oxford, England: Oxford University Press, 1970.
2. Gove PB (ed): Webster's Third New International Dictionary, p. 1482. Springfield, MA: Merriam-Webster, 1981.
3. Gottschalk A: Historical introduction. In Gottschalk A (ed): Glycoproteins: Their Composition, Structure, and Function, pp. 1–23. New York: Elsevier, 1972.
4. Clamp JR: Mucus in health and disease. In Elstein M, Parke D (eds): Mucus in Health and Disease, pp. 1–15. New York: Plenum Press, 1977.
5. Chantler EN, Elder JB, Elstein M (eds): Mucus in Health and Disease II: Advances in Experimental Medicine and Biology, vol. 144. New York: Plenum Press, 1982.
6. Ueki I, German VF, Nadel JA: Micropipette measurement of airway submucosal gland secretion: Autonomic effects. Am Rev Respir Dis 121:351–357, 1980.
7. Davis B, Marin M, Fischer S, et al: New method for study of canine mucous gland secretion in vivo: Cholinergic regulation [Abstract]. Am Rev Respir Dis 113:257, 1976.
8. Davis B, Chinn R, Gold J, et al: Hypoxemia reflexly increases secretion from tracheal submucosal glands in dogs. J Appl Physiol 52:1416–1419, 1982.
9. Widdicombe JG: Methods for collecting and measuring mucus from specific sources. In Braga PC, Allegra L (eds): Methods in Bronchial Mucology, pp. 21–30. New York: Raven Press, 1988.
10. Ueki I, German VF, Nadel J: Differences in total protein concentration in submucosal gland fluid: Alpha-adrenergic vs. cholinergic [Abstract]. Fed Proc 40:622, 1981.
11. Leikauf GD, Ueki IF, Nadel J: Autonomic regulation of viscoelasticity of cat tracheal gland secretions. J Appl Physiol 56:426–430, 1984.
12. Johnson HG, McNee ML: Secretagogue responses of leukotriene C$_4$, D$_4$: Comparison of potency in canine trachea in vivo. Prostaglandins 25:237–243, 1983.
13. Robinson N, Widdicombe JG, Xie C-C: In vitro collection of mucus from the ferret trachea. J Physiol 340:7P–8P, 1983.
14. Robinson NP, Venning L, Kyle H, Widdicombe JG: Quantitation of secretory cells of the ferret tracheobronchial tree. J Anat 145:173–188, 1986.
15. Sturgess J, Reid L: Secretory activity of a human bronchial mucous gland in vitro. Exper Molec Path 16:362–381, 1972.
16. Dulfano MJ, Luk CK, Beckage M, Wooten O: Ciliary beat frequency in human respiratory explants. Am Rev Respir Dis 123:139–140, 1981.
17. Kent PW, Daniel PF, Gallagher JT: Metabolism of respiratory tissue: Secretion of mucosubstances by organ culture of mammalian trachea. Biochem J 124:59P–60P, 1971.
18. Borson DB, Gashi AA, Nadel JA: Methods for studying secretions from airways. In Braga PC, Allegra L (eds): Methods in Bronchial Mucology, pp. 303–334. New York: Raven Press, 1988.
19. Barbolini G, Bisetti A, Moretti M: Histochemical methods and light microscopy. In Braga PC, Allegra L (eds): Methods in Bronchial Mucology, pp. 229–244. New York: Raven Press, 1988.
20. Bowes D, Clark AE, Corrin B: Ultrastructural localization of lactoferrin and glycoprotein in human bronchial glands. Thorax 36:108–115, 1981.
21. Bowes D, Corrin B: Ultrastructural immunocytochemical localization of lysozyme in human bronchial glands. Thorax 32:163–170, 1977.
22. Basbaum CB: Regulation of secretion from serous and mucous cells in the trachea. In Nugent J, O'Connor M (eds): Mucus and Mucosa: Ciba Foundation Symposium 109, pp. 4–19. Bath, England: Pittman, 1984.
23. Sheehan JK, Oates K, Carlstedt I: Electron microscopy of cervical, gastric and bronchial mucus glycoproteins. Biochem J 239:147–153, 1986.
24. Rose MC, Voter WA, Brown CF, Kaufman B: Structural features of human tracheobronchial mucus glycoprotein. Biochem J 222:371–377, 1984.
25. Slayter HS, Lamblin G, LeTreut A, et al: Complex structure of human bronchial mucus glycoproteins. Eur J Biochem 142:209–218, 1984.
26. Verdugo P, Tam PY, Butler J: Conformational structure of respiratory mucus studied by laser correlation spectroscopy. Biorheol 20:223–230, 1983.
27. Finkbeiner WE, Basbaum CB: Monoclonal antibodies directed against human sputum: Localization and periodate sensitivity of tracheal antigens [Abstract]. Am Rev Respir Dis 137:77, 1986.
28. St. George JA, Cranz DL, Zicker SC, et al: An immunochemical characterization of rhesus monkey respiratory secretions using monoclonal antibodies. Am Rev Respir Dis 132:556–563, 1985.
29. St George JA, Plopper CG, Etchison JR, Dungworth DL: An immunocytochemical/histochemical approach to tracheobronchial mucin characterization in the rabbit. Am Rev Rerspir Dis 130:124–127, 1984.
30. Basbaum CB, Mann J, Chow A, et al: Monoclonal antibodies as probes for unique antigens in secretory cells of mixed exocrine organs. Proc Natl Acad Sci USA 81:4419–4423, 1984.
31. Toremaln NG: The daily amount of tracheo-bronchial secretions in man, a method for continuous tracheal aspiration in laryngectomized and tracheostomized patients. Acta Otolaryngol (Stockh) 158(Suppl):43–53, 1960.
32. Hilding AC: Experimental studies on some little understood aspects of the physiology of the respiratory tract and their clinical importance. Trans Am Acad Ophthalmol Otol 65:475–495, 1961.
33. Kilburn KH: A hypothesis for pulmonary clearance and its implications. Am Rev Respir Dis 98:449–463, 1968.
34. Lopez-Vidriero M, Charman J, Keal E, Reid L: Bronchorrhoea. Thorax 30:624–630, 1975.
35. Potter JL, Matthews LW, Lemm J, Spector S: Human pulmonary secretions in health and disease. Ann N Y Acad Sci 106:692–697, 1963.
36. Sturgess JM: Electron microscopy investigation of mucus. In Braga PC, Allegra L (eds): Methods in Bronchial Mucology, pp. 245–253. New York: Raven Press, 1988.
37. Gil J, Weibel ER: Extracellular lining of bronchioles after perfusion-fixation of rat lungs for electron microscopy. Anat Rec 169:185–199, 1971.
38. Dalhamn T: Mucus flow and ciliary activity in the trachea of healthy rats and rats exposed to respiratory irritant gases (SO$_2$,H$_3$N,HCHO). Acta Physiol Scand 36(Suppl 123):5–161, 1956.
39. Yoneda K: Mucous blanket of rat bronchus: An ultrastructure study. Am Rev Respir Dis 114:837–842, 1976.
40. Hulbert WC, Forster BB, Laird W, et al: An improved method for the fixation of the respiratory epithelial surface with mucous and surfactant layers. Lab Invest 47:354–363, 1982.
41. Sanderson MJ, Sleigh MA: Ciliary activity of cultured rabbit tracheal epithelium: Beat pattern and metachrony. J Cell Sci 47:331–347, 1981.
42. Van As A, Webster I: The morphology of mucus in mammalian pulmonary airway. Environ Res 79:1–12, 1974.
43. Van As A, Webster I: The organization of ciliary activity and mucus transport in pulmonary airways. S Afr Med J 46:347–350, 1972.
44. Iravani J, Van As A: Mucus transport in the tracheobronchial tree of normal and bronchitic rats. J Pathol 106:81–93, 1972.
45. Davis SS: Mathematical description. In Braga PC, Allegra L (eds):

Methods in Bronchial Mucology, pp. 33–49. New York: Raven Press, 1988.

46. Charman J, Reid L: Sputum viscosity in chronic bronchitis, bronchiectasis, asthma, and cystic fibrosis. Biorheol 9:185–199, 1972.

47. Picot R, Das I, Reid L: Pus, deoxyribonucleic acid, and sputum viscosity. Thorax 33:235–242, 1978.

48. King M: Is cystic fibrosis mucus abnormal? Pediatr Res 15:120–122, 1981.

49. Puchelle E, Jacquot J, Beck G, et al: Rheological and transport properties of airway secretions of cystic fibrosis—Relationships with the degree of infection and severity of the disease. Eur J Clin Invest 15:389–394, 1985.

50. Puchelle E, Zahm JM: Influence of rheological properties of human bronchial secretions on the ciliary beat frequency. Biorheol 21:265–272, 1984.

51. Puchelle E, Zahm JM, Duvivier C: Spinnability of bronchial mucus: Relationship with viscoelasticity and mucous transport properties. Biorheol 20:239–249, 1983.

52. Sanderson MJ, Sleigh MA: Serum proteins agglutinate cilia and modify ciliary coordination. Pediatr Res 15:219–228, 1981.

53. Mian N, Pope AJ, Anderson CE, Kent PW: Factors influencing the viscous properties of chicken tracheal mucins. Biochim Biophys Acta 717:41–48, 1982.

54. Boat TF, Cheng P-W, Iyer RN, et al: Human respiratory tract secretion. Arch Biochem Biophys 177:95–104, 1976.

55. Boat TF, Kleinerman JI, Carlson DM, et al: Human respiratory tract secretions: 1. Mucus glycoproteins secreted by cultured nasal polyp epithelium from subjects with allergic rhinitis and with cystic fibrosis. Am Rev Respir Dis 110:428–441, 1974.

56. Frates RC Jr, Kaizu TT, Last JA: Mucous glycoproteins secreted by respiratory epithelial tissue from cystic fibrosis patients. Pediatr Res 17:30–34, 1983.

57. Cheng P-W, Boat TF, Cranfill K, et al: Increased sulfation of glycoconjugates by cultured nasal epithelial cells from patients with cystic fibrosis. J Clin Invest 84:68–72, 1989.

58. Liese W, Joshi R, Cumming G: Humidification of respired gas by nasal mucosa. Ann Oto Rhino Laryngol 82:330–332, 1973.

59. Proctor DF: The upper airways: I. Nasal physiology and defense of the lungs. Am Rev Respir Dis 115:97–129, 1977.

60. McFadden ER Jr: Respiratory heat and water exchange: Physiological and clinical implications. J Appl Physiol 54:331–336, 1983.

61. McFadden ER Jr, Denison DM, Waller JR, et al: Direct recordings of the temperatures in the tracheobronchial tree in normal man. J Clin Invest 69:700–705, 1982.

62. Schmidt-Nielsen K, Schroter RC, Shkolnick A: Desaturation of exhaled air in camels. Proc R Soc Lond [Biol] 211:305–319, 1981.

63. Boucher RC, Stutts MJ, Bromberg PA, Gatzy JT: Regional differences in airway surface liquid composition. J Appl Physiol 50:613–620, 1981.

64. Hanna LM, Scherer PW: Regional control of local airway heat and water vapor losses. J Appl Physiol 61:624–632, 1986.

65. Dalhamn T, Rhodin J: Mucous flow and ciliary activity in the trachea of rats exposed to pulmonary irritant gas. Br J Ind Med 13:110–113, 1956.

66. Chopra SK, Taplin GV, Simmons DH, et al: Effects of hydration and physical therapy on tracheal transport velocity. Am Rev Respir Dis 115:1009–1014, 1977.

67. Baetjer AM: Effect of ambient temperature and vapor pressure on cilia-mucus clearance rate. J Appl Physiol 23:498–504, 1967.

68. Frank NR, Yoder RE, Brain JD, Yokoyama E: SO_2 (^{38}S labelled) absorption by the nose and mouth under conditions of varying concentration and flow. Arch Environ Health 18:315–322, 1969.

69. Hanna LM, Frank R, Scherer PW: Absorption of soluble gases and vapors in the respiratory system. In Chang HK, Paiva M (eds): Respiratory Physiology: An Analytical Approach. Lung Biology in Health and Disease, vol. 40, pp. 233–316. New York: Dekker, 1989.

70. Rose MC: Epithelial mucous glycoproteins and cystic fibrosis. Horm Metab Res 20:601–608, 1988.

71. Schachter H, Williams D: Biosynthesis of mucus glycoproteins. In Chantler EN, Elder JB, Elstein M (eds): Mucus in Health and Disease: II. Advances in Experimental Medicine and Biology, vol. 144, pp. 3–28. New York: Plenum Press, 1982.

72. Snider MD: Biosynthesis of glycoproteins: Formation of O-linked oligosaccharides. In Ginsburg V, Robbins PW (eds): Biology of Carbohydrates, vol. 2, pp. 163–198. New York: Wiley, 1984.

73. Varsano S, Basbaum CB, Forsbergh LS, et al: Dog tracheal epithelial cells in culture synthesize sulfated macromolecular glycoconjugates and release them from the cell surface upon exposure to extracellular proteinases. Exp Lung Res 13:157–184, 1987.

74. Litt M: Comparative studies of mucus and mucin physiochemistry. In Nugent J, O'Connor M (eds): Mucus and Mucosa: Ciba Foundation Symposium 109, pp. 196–211. Bath, England: Pittman, 1984.

75. Carson S, Goldhamer R, Weinberg MS: Characterization of physical, chemical, and biological properties of mucus in the intact animal. Ann N Y Acad Sci 130:935–943, 1966.

76. Eliasson R, Mossberg B, Cammer P, Afzelius BA: The immotile cilia syndrome: A congenital ciliary abnormality as an etiological factor in chronic airway infections and male sterility. N Engl J Med 297:1–6, 1977.

77. Lee SP, Nicholls JF: Diffusion of charged ions in mucus gel: Effect of net charge. Biorheol 24:565–569, 1987.

78. Cross CE, Allen A, Pearson JP, et al: Studies of the degradation behavior of native and partially purified stomach and tracheal mucus by oxygen radical and oxidation. In Chester MA, Heinegård XX, Lundblad A, et al (eds): Proceedings of the Seventh International Symposium on Glycoconjugates, pp. 578–579. Stockholm: Råhmsi-Lund, 1983.

79. Ramphal R, Pyle M: Adherence of mucoid and nonmucoid *Pseudomonas aeruginosa* to acid-injured tracheal epithelium. Infect Immun 41:345–351, 1983.

80. Ramphal R, Pyle M: Evidence for mucins and sialic acid as receptors for *Pseudomonas aeruginosa* in the lower respiratory tract. Infect Immun 41:339–344, 1983.

81. Visthwanath S, Ramphal R: Tracheobronchial mucin receptor for *Pseudomonas aeruginosa*: Predominance of amino sugars in binding sites. Infect Immun 48:331–334, 1985.

82. Krivan HC, Roberts DD, Ginsburg V: Many pulmonary pathogenic bacteria bind specifically to the carbohydrate sequence GalNAc beta 1-4 Gal found in some glycolipids. Proc Natl Acad Sci USA 85:6157–6161, 1988.

83. Krivan HC, Olson LD, Barile MF, et al: Adhesion of *Mycoplasma pneumoniae* to sulfated glycolipid and inhibition by dextran sulfate. J Biol Chem 264:9283–9288, 1989.

84. Magnani JL, Steplewski Z, Koprowski H, Ginsburg V: The identification of the gastrointestinal and pancreatic cancer–associated antigen detected by monoclonal antibody 19-9 in the sera of patients as a mucin. Cancer Res 43:5489–5492, 1983.

85. Frates RC Jr, Fink RJ, Chernick MS, et al: Serum mucin–associated antigen levels of cystic fibrosis patients are related to their ages and clinical statuses. Pediatr Res 25:49–54, 1989.

86. Martin WR, Cross CE, Wu R: Elevated levels of serum mucin-associated antigen in adult cystic fibrosis patients [Abstract]. Am Rev Respir Dis 141(Suppl):A84, 1990.

87. Lin H, Carlson DM, St. George JA, et al.: An ELISA method for the quantitation of tracheal mucins from human and nonhuman primates. Am J Respir Cell Molec Biol 1:41–48, 1989.

88. Goerke J: Lung surfactant. Biochim Biophys Acta 344:241–261, 1974.

89. King RJ: Composition and metabolism of apolipoproteins of pulmonary surfactant. Annu Rev Physiol 47:775–788, 1985.

90. Woodward H, Horsey B, Bhavanandan VP, Davidson EA: Isolation, purification, and properties of respiratory mucus glycoproteins. Biochem 21:694–701, 1982.

91. Sahu S, Lynn WS: Lipid composition of airway secretions from patients with asthma and patients with cystic fibrosis. Am Rev Respir Dis 115:233–239, 1977.

92. Coles SJ, Bhaskar KR, O'Sullivan DD, et al: Airway mucus: composition and regulation of its secretion by neuropeptides in vitro. In Nugent J, O'Connor M (eds): Mucus and Mucosa: Ciba Foundation Symposium 109, pp. 40–50. Bath, England: Pittman, 1984.

93. Lewis RW: Lipid composition of human bronchial mucus. Lipids 6:859–861, 1971.

94. Slomiany A, Murty VL, Aono M, et al: Lipid composition of tracheobronchial secretions from normal individuals and patients with cystic fibrosis. Biochim Biophys Acta 710:106–111, 1982.

95. Slomiany A, Witas H, Aono M, Slomiany BL: Covalently linked

fatty acids in gastric mucus glycoprotein of cystic fibrosis patients. J Biol Chem 258:8535–8538, 1983.

96. Houdret N, Perini J-M, Galabert C, et: The high lipid content of respiratory mucins in cystic fibrosis is related to infection. Biochim Biophys Acta 880:54–61, 1986.

97. Lethem MI, Marriot C: The relationship between covalently and non-covalently associated lipid in mucus glycoproteins [Abstract]. Pediatr Pulmonol 2(Suppl):112, 1988.

98. Hascall VC: Proteoglycans: Structure and function. In Ginsburg V, Robbin P (eds): Biology of Carbohydrates, vol. 1, pp. 1–49. New York: Wiley, 1981.

99. Yanagashita M, Midura J, Hascall VC: Proteoglycans: Isolation and purification from tissue cultures. In Ginsburg V (ed): Methods in Enzymology, vol. 138, pp. 279–289. New York: Academic Press, 1987.

100. Gallagher JT, Kent PW: Glycoproteins and acid mucopolysaccharides (glycosaminoglycans) in rabbit trachea: A study in organ culture. Biochem Soc Trans 1:842–844, 1973.

101. Coles SJ, Bhaskar KR, O'Sullivan DD, Reid LM: Macromolecular composition of secretions produced by human bronchial explants. In Chantler E, Elder JB, Elstein M (eds): Mucus in Health and Disease: II. Advances in Experimental Medicine and Biology, vol. 144, pp. 357–360. New York: Plenum Press, 1982.

102. Bhaskar KR, O'Sullivan DD, Seltzer J, et al: Density gradient study of bronchial mucus aspirates from healthy volunteers (smokers and nonsmokers) and from patients with tracheostomy. Exp Lung Res 9:289–308, 1985.

103. Bhaskar KR, Drazen JM, O'Sullivan DD, et al: Transition from normal to hypersecretory bronchial mucus in a canine model of bronchitis: Changes in yield and composition. Exp Lung Res 14:101–120, 1988.

104. Wu R, Yankaskas J, Cheng E, et al: Growth and differentiation of human nasal epithelial cells in culture: Serum-free, hormone-supplemented medium and proteoglycan synthesis. Am Rev Respir Dis 132:311–320, 1985.

105. DeBuysscher E, Kennedy J, Mendicino J: Synthesis of mucin glycoproteins by epithelial cells isolated from swine trachea by specific proteolysis. In Vitro Cell Dev Biol 20:433–446, 1984.

106. Kim KC: Possible requirement of collagen gel substratum for production of mucus-like glycoproteins by primary rabbit tracheal epithelial cells in culture. In Vitro 21:617–621, 1985.

107. Kim KC, Opaskar-Hincman HJ, Bhaskar K: Secretion from primary hamster tracheal surface epithelial cells in culture: mucin-like glycoproteins, proteoglycans, and lipids. Exp Lung Res 15:299–314, 1989.

108. Paul A, Picard J, Mergey M, et al: Glycoconjugates secreted by bovine tracheal serous cells in culture. Arch Biochem Biophys 260:75–84, 1988.

109. Basbaum CB, Forsberg LS, Paul A, et al: Studies of tracheal secretion using serous cell cultures and monoclonal antibodies. Biorheol 24:585–588, 1987.

110. Basbaum CB, Finkbeiner WE: Airway secretion: A cell-specific analysis. Horm Metabol Res 20:661–667, 1988.

111. Maginlevsky N, Retegui LA, Masson PL: Comparison of human lactoferrins from milk and neutrophilic leukocytes: Relative molecular mass, isoelectric point, iron-binding properties and uptake by the liver. Biochem J 229:353–359, 1985.

112. Bienenstock J: Mucosal immuological protection mechanisms in the airways. Eur J Resp Dis 69(Suppl 147):62–71, 1986.

113. Creeth JM, Bridge JL, Horton Jr: An interaction between lysozyme and mucus glycoproteins. Biochem J 181:717–724, 1979.

114. Clamp JR, Creeth J: Some non-mucin components of mucus and their possible biological roles: Implications for density-gradient separations. In Nugent J, O'Connor M (eds): Mucus and Mucosa: Ciba Foundation Symposium 109, pp. 121–136. Bath, England: Pittman Press, 1984.

115. Jennsen AO, Smidsrod O, Harbitz O: The importance of lysozyme for the viscosity of sputum from patients with chronic obstructive lung disease. Scand J Clin Lab Invest 40:727–731, 1980.

116. Aisen P, Liebman A: Lactoferrin and transferrin: A comparative study. Biochim Biophys Acta 257:314–323, 1972.

117. Cross CE, Halliwell B, Allen A: Antioxidant protection: A function of tracheobronchial and gastrointestinal mucus. Lancet 1:1328–1330, 1984.

118. Brown TA, Clements ML, Murphy BR, et al: Molecular form and subclass distribution of IgA antibodies after immunization with live and inactivated influenza A vaccines. Adv Exp Med Biol 216B:1691–1700, 1987.

119. Kurono Y, Mogi G: Otitis media with effusion and the nasopharynx: A bacteriological and immunological study. Acta Otolaryngol Suppl (Stockh) 454:214–217, 1988.

120. Kurono Y, Mogi G: Secretory IgA and serum type IgA in nasal secretion and antibody activity against the M protein. Ann Otol Rhinol Laryngol 96:419–424, 1987.

121. Magnusson KE, Stjernström I: Mucosal barrier mechanisms: Interplay between secretory IgA (SIgA), IgG and mucins on the surface properties and association of Salmonellae with intestine and granulocytes. Immunology 45:239–248, 1982.

122. Cotton CU, Reuss L: Measurement of hydraulic water permeability (L_p) of the apical membrane of Necturus gallbladder epithelium [Abstract]. Fed Proc 45:891, 1986.

123. Nadel JA, Borson DB: Secretion and ion transport in airways during inflammation. Biorheol 24:541–549, 1987.

124. Bucher U, Reid L: Development of the mucus-secreting elements in human lung. Thorax 16:219–225, 1961.

125. Rhodin JA: The ciliated cell: Ultrastructure and function of the human tracheal mucosa. Am Rev Respir Dis Suppl 93:1–15, 1966.

126. Jones R, Phil M, Reid L: Secretory cell hyperplasia and modification of intracellular glycoprotein in rat airways induced by short periods of exposure to tobacco smoke and the effect of the anti-inflammatory agent phenylmethyloxyadiazite. Lab Invest 39:41–49, 1978.

127. Klinger JD, Tandler B, Liedtke CM, Boat TF: Proteinases of Pseudomonas aeruginosa evoke mucin release by tracheal epithelium. J Clin Invest 74:1669–1678, 1984.

128. Kim KC, Wasano K, Niles RM, et al: Human neutrophil elastase releases cell surface mucins from primary cultures of hamster tracheal epithelial cells. Proc Natl Acad Sci USA 84:9304–9308, 1987.

129. Florey H, Carleton HM, Wells AQ: Mucus secretion in the trachea. Br J Exp Pathol 13:269–284, 1932.

130. Widdicombe JG: Control of secretions of tracheobronchial mucus. Br Med Bull 34:57–61, 1978.

131. Spicer SS, Martinez JR: Mucin biosynthesis and secretion in the respiratory tract. Environ Health Perspect 55:193–204, 1984.

132. Cutz E, Conen PE: Ultrastructure and cytochemistry of Clara cells. Am J Pathol 62:127–141, 1971.

133. Widdicombe JG, Pack RJ: The Clara cell. Eur J Respir Dis 63:202–220, 1982.

134. Plopper CG, Mariassy AT, Hill LH: Ultrastructure of the nonciliated bronchiolar epithelial (Clara) cell of mammalian lung: I. A comparison of rabbit, guinea pig, rat, hamster, and mouse. Exp Lung Res 1:139–154, 1980.

135. Plopper CG, Mariassy AT, Hill LH: Ultrastructure of the nonciliated bronchiolar epithelial (Clara) cell of mammalian lung: II. A comparison of horse, steer, sheep, dog, and cat. Exp Lung Res 1:155–169, 1980.

136. Plopper CG, Mahony JL, Serabjit-Singh CJ, Philpot RM: Cytodifferentiation of the nonciliated bronchiolar lung epithelial (Clara) cell in the rabbit lung. Anat Rec 199:204A, 1981.

137. Plopper CG, Mariassy AT, Hill LH: Ultrastructure of the nonciliated bronchiolar epithelial (Clara) cell of mammalian lung: III. A study of man with comparison of 15 mammalian species. Exp Lung Res 1:171–180, 1980.

138. Massaro GD, Amado O, Clerch L, Massaro D: Studies on the regulation of secretion in Clara cells with evidence for chemical non-autononide mediation of the secretory response to increased ventilation in rat lungs. J Clin Invest 70:608–613, 1982.

139. Massaro GD, Fischman M, Chiang MJ, et al: Regulation of secretion in Clara cells: Studies using the isolated perfused rat lung. J Clin Invest 67:345–351, 1981.

140. Reid LM: Measurement of bronchial mucous gland layer: Diagnostic yardstick in chronic bronchitis. Thorax 15:132–141, 1960.

141. Reid LM: Pathology of chronic bronchitis. Lancet 1:275–278, 1954.

142. Meyrick B: Mucus-producing cells of the tracheobronchial tree. In Elstein M, Parke DV (eds): Mucus in Health and Disease, pp. 61–76. New York: Plenum Press, 1977.

143. Meyrick B, Reid L: Ultrastructure of cells in the human bronchial submucosal glands. J Anat 107:281–299, 1970.
144. Meyrick B, Reid L: In vitro incorporation of (^{3}H) threonine and (^{3}H) glucose by the mucous and serous cells of the human bronchial submucosal gland: A quantitative electron microscope study. J Cell Biol 67:320–344, 1975.
145. Verdugo P: Molecular biophysics of mucin secretion in cervical goblet cells: New evidence for the jack-in-the-box theory of exocytosis. [Abstract 515.1]. Biorheol 26:510, 1989.
146. Tam PY, Verdugo P: Control of mucus hydration as a Donnan equilibrium process. Nature 292:340–342, 1981.
147. Kaliner M, Marom Z, Patow C, Shelhamer J: Human respiratory mucus. J Allergy Clin Immunol 73:318–323, 1984.
148. Lundgren JD, Hirata F, Marom Z, et al.: Dexamethasone inhibits respiratory glycoconjugate secretion from feline airways in vitro by the induction of lipocortin (lipomodulin) synthesis. Am Rev Respir Dis 137:353–357, 1988.
149. Murray JF: The ketchup-bottle method. N Engl J Med 300:1155–1157, 1979.
150. Feldman J, Traver GA, Taussig LM: Maximal expiratory flows after postural drainage. Am Rev Respir Dis 119:239–245, 1979.
151. Desmond KJ, Schwenk WF, Thomas E, et al: Immediate and long-term effects of chest physiotherapy in patients with cystic fibrosis. J Pediatr 103:538–542, 1983.
152. Aubert JP, Porchet M, Crepin M, et al: cDNAs coding for human tracheal mucins: Characterization by immunochemistry and DNA sequences [Abstract S 15.3]. Biorheol 26:511, 1989.

4 EPIDEMIOLOGY AND THE PEDIATRIC PULMONOLOGIST

JONATHAN M. SAMET, M.D.

In pediatric pulmonology, as in other clinical specialties, epidemiologic evidence is used to identify the causes of disease as a basis for prevention; in addition, clinical practice routinely draws from epidemiologic data on risk factors, diagnostic testing, efficacy of treatment, and prognosis. Many of the central research questions in pediatric pulmonology can best be addressed by epidemiologic methods (Table 4–1). Epidemiologic studies have already provided insights concerning the causes and natural history of childhood asthma, the effects of involuntary exposure to tobacco smoke on children's lungs, and the sequelae of respiratory infections. Clinical practice should be firmly based in clinical epidemiology; quantitative reasoning is inherent in the care of patients. The diagnosis and treatment of a child with a respiratory disease follows a sequence of steps that implicitly requires the comparison of options for gathering information for establishing a diagnosis and for identifying optimal treatment. Thus in treating an ill patient, the physician collects data, synthesizes the information in order to develop diagnostic hypotheses, and selects the most suitable modalities for diagnosis and treatment.

The role of epidemiology in pediatric pulmonology can be illustrated by asthma, the most common chronic disease of children. The frequency or prevalence of childhood asthma has been documented through surveys both of national samples[1] and of children in specific locations.[2] Mortality statistics provide an index of the severity of the disease in the population. The causes of childhood asthma have been examined in cross-sectional studies and in cohort or longitudinal studies.[2] Factors that exacerbate asthma have been evaluated in case-control and cross-sectional studies, and the natural history of the disease has been described in cohort studies.[2] Clinical studies have assessed the sensitivity and specificity of diagnostic tests for asthma[2,3] and the efficacy of various therapeutic modalities.[4]

This chapter provides an introduction to epidemiology for pediatric pulmonologists. The study designs used for epidemiologic research are reviewed, and their application is illustrated by the example of childhood asthma.

Table 4–1. TOPICAL QUESTIONS IN PEDIATRIC PULMONOLOGY AND THE STUDY DESIGN FOR ANSWERING EACH QUESTION

Question	Study Design
What factors determine the rate of lung growth?	Prospective cohort study
What is the natural history of childhood asthma?	Prospective cohort study
Is childhood asthma mortality increasing?	Descriptive study of mortality rates
What factors exacerbate asthma?	Cohort or case-control study
What is the optimal treatment for asthma?	Clinical trial
What are the sequelae of lower respiratory illness?	Cohort or case-control study
What is the natural history of bronchopulmonary dysplasia?	Prospective cohort study
What are the health effects of indoor air pollution?	Cross-sectional, prospective cohort, and case-control studies

DEFINITIONS

Epidemiology comprises the scientific methods used to study disease occurrence in human populations; the emphasis on human populations separates epidemiology from clinical research.[5] Epidemiology has been considered to have two distinct components: (1) description of patterns of disease occurrence, primarily by person, place, and time, and (2) the identification of risk factors for disease.[6] The scope of epidemiology also includes evaluation methods, such as clinical trials and the quasi-experimental designs often used in health services research.

The term *clinical epidemiology* is increasingly used to describe the extension of epidemiologic methods for addressing problems in clinical medicine. Clinical epidemiology can be defined as the scientific method used to translate the results of clinical and epidemiologic studies into appropriate care and treatment for individual patients.[7]

ASSOCIATION AND CAUSE

Etiologic investigations determine whether disease occurrence differs in exposed populations (e.g., those exposed to a particular environmental characteristic or possessing a certain host characteristic) and nonexposed populations and provide a measure of the degree of association between exposure and disease. In etiologic research, the objective is generally to establish or exclude a causal association between exposure and disease. In general, this goal cannot be achieved with just one study. The associations found in multiple investigations must be evaluated together and weighed, along with other relevant biologic data, against criteria for causality.[8] For example, the determination in the 1964 Surgeon General's Report that smoking caused lung cancer was based on such criteria.[9]

The criteria include the strength of association, evidence of a dose-response relationship, an appropriate temporal sequence between exposure and disease, consistency of the association, and biologic coherence and plausibility.[8,10] Of these criteria, only the demonstration of an appropriate time sequence between exposure and disease is requisite,[11] although meeting the other criteria may strengthen the argument for causality. The first criterion implies that a causal relationship becomes more likely as the strength of an association increases; bias is a less likely explanation for strong associations than for weak associations. Increasing effect with increasing exposure, a dose-response relationship, also strengthens the argument for causality, although linear dose-response relationships may not always be biologically appropriate. Exposure must always precede the effect. Consistency among multiple studies of the same exposure-disease relationship also favors causality. Specificity of association—that is, a unique exposure-disease relationship—is generally not relevant because most diseases are miltifactorial in origin. Finally, the exposure-disease relationship should be consistent with other relevant biologic knowledge.

METHODS OF EPIDEMIOLOGY

DESCRIPTIVE EPIDEMIOLOGY

The occurrence of disease in a population is described in terms of incidence, mortality, and prevalence rates.

The incidence rate is the occurrence of new cases of disease; it is calculated as the ratio of the number of new cases during a specified time period to the size of the population at risk during that period. Mortality is calculated similarly, but the number of deaths is the numerator. In the prevalence ratio, the numerator is the proportion of persons with disease at a particular time.

Estimates of the incidence of childhood asthma have been obtained by following cohorts of infants from birth, with monitoring for new cases. For example, in the Christchurch (New Zealand) Child Development Study, 1056 children were enrolled at birth as a cohort.[12] The children were evaluated periodically, and the occurrence of illnesses and of other events was recorded. A diagnosis of childhood asthma was based on the child's having two medical consultations for wheezing or associated symptoms that were labeled as asthma or wheezy bronchitis. By age 6 years, 10.3% of the cohort met this definition of incident asthma. However, methods for determining the incidence of asthma in large, representative population samples are lacking.

The mortality rate for childhood ashtma can be calculated from counts of deaths routinely reported in U.S. vital statistics. In the currently applicable (ninth) Revision of the International Classification of Diseases (ICD) deaths from asthma are coded to ICD 493. The U.S. mortality rate for childhood asthma can be calculated as the ratio of the number of deaths in this category (e.g., 90 deaths in children younger than 15 years in 1980) to the number of children in that age group. If the cause of death is not correctly classified, mortality rates may be biased, either upwards or downwards. The ratio of the number of deaths to the estimated number of children with asthma is the case/fatality ratio.

The prevalence of childhood asthma has been described in numerous population surveys. In these surveys, a parental report is typically used to establish the presence of asthma in a child. The prevalence rate is simply the ratio of the number of children reported to have asthma to the total number of children surveyed. Alternatively, the presence of asthma might be based on a physician's diagnosis or on results of testing for nonspecific airway hyperresponsiveness to cold air or a pharmacologic agent.

Prevalence estimates for childhood asthma in the United States range from about 4% to 10%.[2] The National Center for Health Statistics periodically surveys random samples of the U.S. population for the prevalence of selected diseases and symptoms. One report described the prevalence of childhood asthma in surveys conducted between 1963 and 1980.[1] The diagnosis of asthma was based on a report of diagnosis by a physician or of frequent wheezing during the previous year. Overall, 6.7% of subjects had asthma, and the rates were higher in blacks, in boys, and in children living in urban areas. Descriptive surveys, however, cannot be used to draw causal inference about exposure-disease relationships, although survey results may identify hypotheses for subsequent testing. For example, the relationship between maternal smoking and childhood asthma might be biased if mothers of asthmatic children stopped smoking in order to improve their children's health.

ANALYTICAL EPIDEMIOLOGY

Epidemiologists use other study designs to test for association between exposure and disease. The nonexperimental approaches are the case-control and cohort studies. Clinical trials are an experimental design; the investigator randomly assigns subjects to exposed and nonexposed groups or to treated and untreated groups. The clinical trial is the proper design for evaluating drugs and other therapies. At a minimum, case-control and cohort studies provide a measure of association between exposure and disease.

In a cohort study, subjects are followed from exposure through the development of disease. The study is labeled *prospective* if the disease events occur in the future and *retrospective* if they have already taken place. The cohort design is optimal for studying the effects of rare exposure. Other advantages of the cohort design include the direct estimation of disease rates for exposed and nonexposed persons (Table 4–2) and the capability of accumulating exposure information in a prospective study.

The study of respiratory diseases in 1056 infants followed from birth in Christchurch, New Zealand, exemplifies the prospective cohort design.[12] In this study, household characteristics, including parental smoking, were documented at the time of a child's birth and at subsequent annual follow-up visits. The incidences of asthma, of other illnesses involving wheezing, and of lower respiratory illnesses was assessed in relation to maternal and paternal smoking and other factors. The investigators found that maternal but not paternal smoking increased the rate of lower respiratory illness during the first 2 years of life.[13] The incidence rates of bronchitis/pneumonia during the first 2 years of life were 15.3% among children of nonsmoking mothers, 19.5% among children of mothers who smoked 10 or fewer cigarettes daily, and 24.5% among children of mothers who smoked 11 or more cigarettes daily. In contrast, parental smoking did not increase the incidence of asthma.[12]

The retrospective cohort design can be used to evaluate rapidly the effects of an exposure because both exposure and disease have already occurred. This design was used effectively to examine sequelae of lower respiratory infection, including asthma. Cohorts of children who had previously been hospitalized for severe lower respiratory illness were identified; the children were traced, and their

Table 4–2. DATA IN A HYPOTHETICAL COHORT STUDY OR CLINICAL TRIAL WITH TWO EXPOSURE CATEGORIES

Involvement	Exposed	Nonexposed
*Population Time**		
New cases during follow-up	a	b
Population time (person years)	PY_1	PY_0
Cumulative Risk†		
Disease during follow-up	a	b
No disease during follow-up	c	d

*Measure of association: ratio of incidence rates in exposed and nonexposed = $(a/PY_1)/(b/PY_0)$.

†Measure of association: risk ratio comparing exposed to nonexposed = $[a/(a + c)]/[b/(b + d)]$.

Table 4–3. DATA IN A HYPOTHETICAL CASE-CONTROL STUDY*

Population	Exposed	Not Exposed
Case	a	b
Control	c	d

*The measure of association is the relative risk of disease in exposed compared with nonexposed estimated as the exposure odds ratio: a/b ÷ c/d, or ad/bc.

clinical and physiologic statuses were assessed.[14] For example, Kattan and co-workers[15] conducted a retrospective cohort study to assess long-term sequelae of bronchiolitis in infancy. Hospital records were used to identify children who had been hospitalized at 1 to 18 months of age, approximately 10 years earlier. The children were located, and their lung function was assessed at a mean age of 11 years. Thus Kattan and co-workers were able to examine the functional sequelae of bronchiolitis without waiting for years to pass, as would have been necessary with a prospective cohort design.

In a case-control study, the exposures of "cases" (patients) with the disease of interest are contrasted with those of "controls," persons without the disease of interest who would become "cases" on developing the disease (Table 4–3). Cases may be selected from a hospital, clinic, or practice or from the general population. The exposure histories of cases and controls are assessed by record review, interview, serologic testing or other techniques. In general, the advantages of case-control studies, in comparison with cohort studies, are lower cost, more feasibility, and shorter time frame. The case-control study is the best method for studying a rare disease. Bias from the retrospective assessment of exposure and, in some circumstances, from the selection of cases and controls may limit this design.

The case-control approach has been used to assess determinants of death from asthma, an uncommon event that could not be feasibly studied in a cohort approach. Strunk and colleagues[16] conducted a case-control study of children who had died of asthma at some time after admission to the National Jewish Center, Denver, Colorado. From a 10-year period, 21 cases were identified. The controls were randomly selected from discharged children who were known to be alive. The characteristics of the cases and controls, documented during the admission to the National Jewish Center, were compared. The results suggested that psychological factors, as well as indicators of severity, may be associated with death from childhood asthma. The case-control design was also recently used to examine risk factors for death from asthma in the population of Auckland, New Zealand.[17]

Clinical trials have been used primarily to assess therapeutic modalities, such as drugs and other clinical treatments. The clinical trial might also be used for evaluating potentially beneficial changes in the environment, such as control of house dust mites or cockroaches in the homes of asthmatic patients.

The results of each of these analytic designs may be affected by bias. Case-control studies involving subjects from special populations are particularly vulnerable to bias that may be introduced by the method used to identify cases and controls. Selection bias is the distortion of the exposure-disease association as a result of differential patterns of participation by subjects in relation to exposure and disease status.[10] Berkson[18] first demonstrated that differing rates of hospitalization for different diseases could result in biased measures of association when a study was carried out in a hospital-based population. Selection bias may arise in cohort studies from losses at the time of follow-up and in cross-sectional studies from survival of certain types of persons with disease.[10]

Error in measurement of exposure or disease status results in misclassification. If the error is equally common in cases and controls in a case-control study or in exposed and nonexposed subjects in a cohort study, the resulting bias, termed *nondifferential* or *random misclassification,* always reduces associations toward the null value (i.e., toward showing no effect). If the misclassification is differential, associations may be increased or decreased. Such bias is of particular concern in case-control studies in which interviews are used to assess exposures; diseased and nondiseased persons may not provide comparable responses, and in some instances, subjects may be aware of the hypotheses of a study. For example, publicity about passive smoking may introduce bias into case-control studies of the association between passive smoking and disease.

Bias introduced by confounding is also of particular concern in assessing the origins of multifactorial chronic diseases. Confounding bias occurs when the effect of the exposure of interest is altered by the effect of another risk factor. For example, in investigations of passive smoking, failure to consider the possibility that schoolchildren engage in active smoking might introduce confounding, because children of smokers are more likely to be smokers than are children of nonsmokers.

These biases may strongly influence the interpretation of the findings of epidemiologic studies of childhood respiratory illness, particularly when weak associations are found or anticipated. Selection or information bias and uncontrolled confounding may introduce associations of significant magnitude from the public health perspective. In contrast, random errors in the assessment of exposure reduce the likelihood of finding an association. Studies with apparently "negative" findings must be interpreted within this constraint.

EPIDEMIOLOGY AND CLINICAL PRACTICE

RISK FACTORS

Clinicians use the word *risk* frequently in caring for patients; they talk about risk factors for disease, being at risk for a complication, and being at risk for death. Patients and their parents ask about information concerning risk factors and risk reduction. The parents of a child newly diagnosed with asthma may ask about the causes of the disease and the steps that could be taken to reduce disease risk. Physicians and patients frequently use language about risk in a loose fashion; the concepts are often too

vague, and terms are used interchangeably and inappropriately.

Risk means the probability of some event: for example, an illness of the lower respiratory tract, a surgical complication or death. Risk can be expressed in different ways: as a percentage or ratio (e.g., a 20% risk of a severe infection of the lower respiratory tract during the first 2 years of life) or as an absolute incidence rate (e.g., two episodes of lower respiratory tract illness per 100 children during the first year of life). A *risk factor* is a characteristic of a person that increases or decreases the probability of developing disease. A risk factor may be an endogenous characteristic, such as alpha$_1$-antitrypsin deficiency, or an exogenous exposure, such as cigarette smoking by a parent. The *relative risk* is used to express the quantitative effect of a risk factor, or the occurrence of disease in persons with a particular risk factor in relation to those without the risk factor. Relative risk estimates are obtained from the results of case-control and cohort studies.

Both preventive care of healthy children and management of ill children inherently require the consideration of risk factors of individual patients. Children at high risk for a disease are selected for screening on the basis of the presence of risk factors. Candidates for risk factor modification are identified from risk factor profiles, which contain such items as activity level, obesity, hypertension, smoking, and levels of lipids for coronary artery disease (in adults) and parental smoking (in children). Risk factors are also used to establish differential diagnoses and to rank the alternative diagnoses. For example, the diagnosis of childhood asthma might be pursued more vigorously if a parent or another sibling has asthma.

TESTING

Testing is pervasive in the care of patients with pediatric lung disease, as in other specialties. Tests are used to provide information that indicates which diagnosis should be selected from the alternatives that are included in a differential diagnosis. Screening tests are used to identify patients at risk for disease (e.g., alpha$_1$-antitrypsin deficiency) or who have early or preclinical disease (e.g., lung function abnormality without frank impairment). Even the routine history and physical examination should be considered a form of testing; in fact, symptoms and signs probably remain the findings that are most important for clinical diagnosis. Thus an understanding of the characteristics of tests is essential for the practice of pediatric pulmonology.

The utility of a test is determined by its accuracy, which has two components: reliability and validity. *Reliability* refers to the repeatability of the test; that is, does the test produce the same results when applied on two occasions? *Validity* refers to the ability of the test to measure the characteristics that it is intended to measure. Validity of a test is described by sensitivity and specificity as measured against some accepted gold standard (Table 4–4). For example, a new screening test for cystic fibrosis might be evaluated against a conventional sweat test.

Ideally, both sensitivity and specificity should be 100%, and corresponding false-negative and false-positive

Table 4–4. EVALUATION OF A DIAGNOSTIC TEST AGAINST A GOLD STANDARD

Test	Gold Standard	
	Positive	Negative
Positive	a	b
Negative	c	d

Sensitivity = a/(a+c), the proportion of subjects positive by the gold standard that is also positive by the test under evaluation.
Specificity = d/(b+d), the proportion of subjects negative by the gold standard that is also negative by the test under evaluation.
False negatives = c, 1-sensitivity gives the false negative rate.
False positives = b, 1-specificity gives the false positive rate.

rates should be 0%. However, sensitivity and specificity are well below 100% for most tests; in general, as test sensitivity increases, specificity declines, and as specificity increases, sensitivity declines. Use of a highly sensitive test is indicated when the consequences of missing the disease are serious, as in cystic fibrosis; a highly sensitive test is optimal for ruling out disease because the false-negative rate is low. Use of a highly specific test is indicated when the consequences of incorrectly diagnosing disease are serious; a highly specific test is optimal for ruling in disease because the false-positive rate is low.

In the evaluation of information on the sensitivity and specificity of a diagnostic test, consideration should be given to the choice of the gold standard, the population used for the evaluation, and potential bias in judging the performance of the test. With regard to the gold standard, the validity of the standard itself should be queried; a new test that is actually better than the gold standard may seem worse than the gold standard. The population of patients used to evaluate the new test may also influence test sensitivity and specificity. The performance of a test in patients with advanced disease followed at a referral center may not be adequately predictive of the performance of the test in patients with milder disease in a community setting. Moreover, the patients without disease should be representative of patients with symptoms and signs that are likely to be confused with the disease of interest.

Although satisfactory sensitivity and specificity are essential test characteristics, the results of a test must be interpreted according to the prevalence of disease in the populations to which the test is applied. In the extreme stuation of applying a test to a population in which no one has disease, all persons with a positive test result would represent false-positive findings. Similarly, if all persons had disease, all negative results would represent false-negative findings. The positive and negative predictive values describe the yield of diagnostic testing in a population, whether it consists of patients seen at a clinic or residents of a particular community. The relationship of positive and negative predictive value with disease prevalence, test sensitivity, and test specificity is described by Bayes' theorem.

For example, a diagnosis of childhood asthma might be made on the basis of a parent's report of the child's wheezing and dyspnea, the finding of wheezing on chest auscul-

tation, the results of spirometry, or the results of inhalation challenge testing. Parents' reports might have a high false-positive rate because airway sounds associated with disease of the lower respiratory tract might be misinterpreted as wheezing associated with asthma. The predictive value of a parent's report would be particularly low for children with a high rate of lower respiratory infection. Spirometry is potentially insensitive because a particular test may show children with asthma to have normal ventilatory function. Inhalation challenge testing is highly sensitive (in virtually all children with asthma, test results are positive for methacholine or other agents) but nonspecific (not all children with positive test results have asthma).[19]

TREATMENT

Pediatric pulmonologists must constantly evaluate information about new approaches to treatment and about therapies that are considered established. New drugs for asthma regularly reach the market, and other therapeutic modalities for pediatric respiratory diseases have proliferated. Information on the effectiveness of treatment comes from various lines of investigation. Basic laboratory work may lead to new pharmacologic agents. Surgical procedures may proceed from animal models to human trials. Technologic advances may offer new opportunities. The extent of evidence needed for documenting the efficacy of a new therapy has been controversial. Many therapeutic approaches have been advocated on the basis of descriptive case series that seem to show efficacy. However, in some instances, more formally designed evaluations have not shown efficacy.

Although clinical series have provided many important observations on the efficacy of new and old therapies, the controlled clinical trial is the most appropriate (and, in some instances, the only) design for evaluating a new therapy. A clinical trial has two essential elements: (1) a treatment group and a comparison group and (2) random assignment of potential subjects to either the treatment group or the comparison group. Although there are many options in design (such as crossovers, multiple random assignments, and multiple treatment arms), a study must incorporate random assignment and one or more comparison groups in order to be classified as a clinical trial.

Investigators select subjects for a clinical trial in order to obtain a study population that represents the reference population to which the study results are meant to be applicable (Fig. 4–1). Conversely, in considering the results of a clinical trial, the clinician should question the applicability of the findings to the patients. Findings at a particular referral center may not be predictive of the outcome at another referral center or in the community. The study population may not represent the reference population because of inappropriate exclusions or a high rate of refusal by subjects to participate in the study.

In a clinical trial, subjects must be randomly assigned to treatment or control status; other methods such as haphazard assignment or investigator-controlled assignment may introduce bias. For example, a physician may prefer that only the healthiest patients receive the experimental

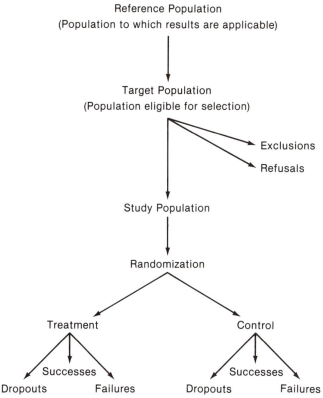

Reference Population
(Population to which results are applicable)

Target Population
(Population eligible for selection)

→ Exclusions

→ Refusals

Study Population

Randomization

Treatment   Control

Successes   Successes

Dropouts   Failures   Dropouts   Failures

Figure 4–1. Structure of a clinical trial.

drug. Random selection of patients is accomplished to ensure that the treatment and control groups are comparable with regard to factors that may influence response and prognosis, such as age, extent of disease, and the presence of other diseases. Random selection does not necessarily ensure comparability of treatment and control groups; in some studies, random selection does not work, and treatment and control groups may differ in important ways.

For some outcomes, it may be necessary to conduct the trial in a "blinded" manner, in which patients or the evaluators are unaware of the assignment of the subjects. Blinding is indicated particularly if the therapeutic benefit is of a subjective nature, such as relief of symptoms in a child with asthma. In a single-blind study, the subjects are unaware of their assignments; in a double-blind study, neither the subjects nor the observers are aware of the assignment.

The analysis and presentation of the findings of a clinical trial involve comparison of the responses in the treatment and control groups (see Table 4–2). In the interpretation of a clinical trial the representativeness of the target population in relation to the reference population should always be considered, as should the comparability of the target population with the clinician's own patients. High dropout rates compromise validity, and data from dropouts should be retained in the analysis. "Negative" findings should be interpreted with caution, and the possibility of type II or beta error should be considered. Many clinical trials have involved populations that were too small and have not had sufficient power to detect therapeutic effects of interest. In many journals, reports on neg-

ative clinical trials routinely include power calculations or confidence limits.

PROGNOSIS

Physicians use information on prognosis routinely as they practice medicine. In making decisions concerning therapy, they often balance toxicity against the potential gain in survival. Information concerning prognostic factors is also used in the assessment of outcome for a particular patient. *Prognosis* means the course of the disease. Prognostic factors are determinants of the course of the disease after it has developed; risk factors are determinants of the likelihood of developing disease. Age, for example, is typically a prognostic factor; cigarette smoking is a risk factor for many diseases but a relatively unimportant prognostic factor.

Information on prognosis is obtained from descriptive observation of persons who have developed disease. In a consideration of the information from a study of prognosis, the value of the data depends on the characteristics of the observed cases, the approach taken for identifying the onset of disease, and the completeness with which the cases are observed. With regard to the case series, the methods used for diagnosing disease and the homogeneity of the cases should be examined. Even a carefully assembled case series may not be relevant if the patients are not comparable with a particular clinician's own patients. Identifying the onset of illness may be problematic. If the series was ascertained with several approaches that identify different stages of disease, a clear description of survival may not be obtained. For example, children with asthma who are identified by screening physical examinations for school athletics may have a different prognosis than those identified through presentation to a physician's office. The validity of any series is threatened by losses to follow-up.

The techniques used to describe prognosis are referred to as *survival analysis.* Survival curves are used to describe the death of subjects or some other outcome over time (Fig. 4–2). Such curves represent the proportion of

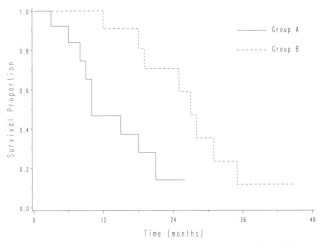

Figure 4–2. Example of survival plots for two groups, A and B.

subjects living through each successive interval of follow-up time. Separate survival curves may be presented for specific groups of patients.

Prognostic factors are determinants of survival; the effects of prognostic factors can be gauged by examination of survival curves and by more complicated mathematical analyses (e.g., Kaplan-Meier method, Cox's proportional hazard model). The effect of a prognostic factor is expressed as a ratio (the hazard ratio), in which the probability of death in persons with the factor is compared with the probability of death in persons without the factor. Through the use of more advanced mathematical models, the effects of multiple prognostic factors can be considered simultaneously.

REFERENCES

1. Gergen PJ, Mullally DI, Evans R III: National survey of prevalence of asthma among children in the United States, 1976 to 1980. Pediatrics 81:1–7, 1988.
2. Coultas DB, Samet JM: Epidemiology and natural history of childhood asthma. *In* Tinkelman DG, Falliers CJ, Naspitz CK (eds): Childhood Asthma: Pathophysiology and Treatment, pp. 131–157. New York: Marcel Dekker, 1987.
3. Samet JM: Epidemiologic approaches for the identification of asthma. Chest 91 (June Suppl):74S–78S, 1987.
4. Ellis EF: Bronchodilator treatment of children. *In* Jenne JW, Murphy S (eds): Drug Therapy for Asthma, pp. 837–868. New York: Marcel Dekker, 1987.
5. Lilienfeld D: Definitions of epidemiology. Am J Epidemiol 107:87–90, 1979.
6. MacMahon B, Pugh TF: Epidemiology: Principles and Methods, p. 1. Boston: Little, Brown, 1970.
7. Fletcher RH, Fletcher SW, Wagner EH: Clinical Epidemiology: The Essentials, pp. 1–6. Baltimore: Williams & Wilkins, 1988.
8. Susser M: Causal Thinking in the Health Sciences: Concepts and Strategies in Epidemiology. New York: Oxford University Press, 1973.
9. U.S. Public Health Service: Smoking and Health: Report of the Advisory Committee to the Surgeon General of the Public Health Service, DHEW Publication No. (PHS) 1103, pp. 17–22. Washington, DC: U.S. Government Printing Office, 1964.
10. Kleinbaum DG, Kupper LL, Morganstern H: Epidemiologic Research: Principles and Quantitative Methods, pp. 26–34. Belmont, CA: Lifetime Learning Publication, 1983.
11. Rothman KJ: Modern Epidemiology, pp. 7–21. Boston: Little, Brown, 1986.
12. Horwood LJ, Fergusson DM, Shannon FT: Social and familial factors in the development of early childhood asthma. Pediatrics 75:859–868, 1985.
13. Fergusson DM, Hons BA, Horwood LJ: Parental smoking and respiratory illness during early childhood: A six-year longitudinal study. Pediatr Pulmonol 1:99–106, 1985.
14. Samet JM, Tager IB, Speizer FE: The relationship between respiratory illness in childhood and chronic airflow obstruction in adulthood. Am Rev Respir Dis 127:508–523, 1983.
15. Kattan M, Keens TG, Lapierre J-G, et al: Pulmonary function abnormalities in symptom-free children after bronchiolitis. Pediatrics 59:683–688, 1977.
16. Strunk RC, Mrazek DA, Fuhrmann GS, LaBrecque JF: Physiologic and psychological characteristics associated with deaths due to asthma in childhood: A case-controlled study. JAMA 254:1193–1198, 1985.
17. Rea HH, Scragg R, Jackson R, et al: A case-control study of deaths from asthma. Thorax 41:833–839, 1986.
18. Berkson J: Limitations of the application of fourfold table analysis to hospital data. Biometrics 2:47–53, 1946.
19. Hopp RJ, Bewtra AK, Nair NM, Townley RG: Specificity and sensitivity of methacholine inhalation challenge in normal and asthmatic children. J Allergy Clin Immunol 74:154–158, 1984.

5 SELF-MANAGEMENT PROGRAMS IN PEDIATRIC RESPIRATORY DISEASES

JOANN BLESSING-MOORE, M.D.

The 1980s was a period of a renaissance of scientific interest in research into health education and programs of self-management, especially those that apply to the control of chronic disease.[1] Self-management programs are actually comanagement programs involving the patient, the family, the physician, the nurse, and other health care providers. Such programs are designed to complement and enhance traditional care by teaching patients how to make informed decisions with the assistance of their health care providers.[2] Implicit in this concept is the premise that patients can benefit from becoming more involved in their own care.

Engaging effectively in such a program entails two important steps: (1) the diagnosis and the treatment must be recognized and accepted by the patient and the medical team, and (2) the patient has to be willing to participate actively in the health care plan.[3] Once the patient is willing, the medical team is responsible for knowing what programs and materials are available and how to gain access to (and, if necessary, help support) appropriate local programs.

Health care educational programs have received little attention in training programs for health care professionals. Despite the rapid expansion in education programs for patients during the 1980s, health care providers are still often unaware of materials available or how to gain

Table 5–1. SELF-MANAGEMENT PROGRAMS FOR CHILDHOOD ASTHMA

A.C.T. for Kids
Asthma and Allergy Foundation, Suite 203, 1717 Massachusetts Ave, Washington, DC 20036

Air Wise
American Institute of Research, Palo Alto, CA

Air Power
American Institute of Research, Palo Alto, CA

Living With Asthma
National Asthma Center, Denver, CO

Open Airways
Columbia University, New York, NY

Superstuff
American Lung Association, 1740 Broadway, New York, NY 10019

Camp Wheeze
Joann Blessing-Moore, M.D., 770 Welch Road, #232, Palo Alto, CA 94304

Teaching My Parents About Asthma and Teaching Myself About Asthma
Health Education Associates, 14 North Lake Road, Columbia, SC 29223

Winning Over Wheezing
William H. Rorer, Inc., 500 Virginia Drive, Fort Washington, PA 19304

A.C.T., asthma care training.

access to such materials. They are easily frustrated by the lack of resources for implementation of such programs.

In this chapter, the educational needs of specific populations of children with pulmonary disease are explored, and some of the existing programs that may meet these needs are identified. Three disease categories are considered: asthma, chronic lung disease of childhood, and cystic fibrosis.

ASTHMA

Asthma affects 3 million persons in the United States who are less than 18 years of age. Approximately 7% of American children have asthma.[4] Of all children with asthma, 23% experience significant limitation in activity, with an annual loss of 16 million school days.[4]

To enhance early recognition of asthma and appropriate treatment, The National Heart, Lung, and Blood Institue (NHLBI) established a National Asthma Educational Program in 1991, "The Year of Asthma." The first publication includes guidelines for physicians for the care of the asthmatic patient in various settings (acute to chronic). The NHLBI program also includes education for the public and patient as well as school health programs.[5]

Asthma comanagement programs have been shown to improve health management skills, to improve school attendance and performance, and to reduce emergency health care services for program participants.[6] Programs have been developed for a variety of settings and populations (Table 5–1). Some of these are discussed as follows.

CAMP AND SEMINAR PROGRAMS

These programs involve patients who have gathered solely for the educational (and recreational) experience.

The programs may include sleep-over or day camp designed for asthmatic children only or special programs for asthmatic children within a general camp setting. There are also educational meetings or seminars sponsored by a variety of agencies such as the Asthma and Allergy Foundation of America, the American Lung Association, local hospitals, clinics, and schools. There are several advantages to these programs: they can be tailored to the educational and socioeconomic needs of the community, they serve a large population base, repeated sessions can incorporate new materials, and they can serve a number of patients not reachable through other avenues.[7]

As a result of a National Institute of Allergy and Immunologic Diseases–sponsored workshop, a number of programs were developed, known as the National Institutes of Health (NIH) Childhood Asthma Self-Management Programs. *Open Airways,* developed by Columbia University, was designed for children aged 4 to 7 years and 7 to 14 years from inner-city families of low income and low educational level. Materials are available both in English and in Spanish. The program consists of six sessions in which group dynamics are used to teach problem solving. Parents and children learn to recognize signs of respiratory difficulty and to determine when to seek medical care. Evaluation of this program suggested that participants could demonstrate the use of relaxation techniques to control wheezing and had an improved ability to set appropriate activity guidelines. The program developers reported a significant reduction in emergency service use and hospitalization for the acute care of asthma.[8,9]

The National Asthma Center in Denver produced a program called *Living With Asthma.* This provides eight sessions for children 8 to 13 years of age. Discussion and problem-solving techniques are enhanced with the use of check sheets, situation cards, and specific questions. Children and their parents are seen in separate sessions. Initial evaluation of the program revealed a significant decrease in the frequency of asthma attacks and revealed changes in attitude, self-concept, locus of control, and general medical information. A decrease in absenteeism from school was coupled with a reduction in costs for direct and indirect medical care.[10]

The American Institute of Research in Palo Alto, California, developed a program, *Air Power,* aimed at children aged 9 to 13 years. *Air Power* consists of four 1-h sessions for parents with separate sessions for children. The format for children includes discussion, informal sharing of experiences, and demonstration of relaxation techniques. Parents, in evaluating this program, noted an increase in self-management behaviors in their children, although there was no change in health care use.[11,12]

ACT (Asthma Care Training) was developed at the University of California, Los Angeles, and now is distributed by the Asthma and Allergy Foundation of America. This consists of five 1-h sessions for children aged 8 to 12 years and separate sessions for parents. Parents and children join together at the end of each session for discussion. This program focuses on family dynamics as well as management skills. The experimental group demonstrated a significant reduction in the numbers of hospitalizations and emergency room visits.[13]

The Family Asthma Program (produced by the American Lung Association of Buffalo) is designed for children aged 6 to 14 years; 12 h are devoted to education, discussion, and exercise. On evaluation, it was noted that there was an increase in the total number of activities in which the children participated in and out of school. There was also a decrease in the number of unscheduled health-care visits and in school absenteeism.[14]

Camp Wheeze is another seminar-based program that provides a core educational health care program, small-group discussion with role play, and recreation with other asthmatic children. Parents noted an increase in compliance, improvement in peer relationships, and a slight decrease in the use of emergency facilities for asthma.[15]

Many other programs have been used in a seminar setting. *Superstuff,* produced by the American Lung Association, is a packaged program that can be used individually or in a group setting.[16] Detailed parameters for the operation of camps for children with asthma are available,[7, 16] as is a listing of many of the camps in the United States.[17]

REHABILITATION PROGRAMS FOR ASTHMATICS

Rehabilitation programs are well established for adult patients with chronic lung disease. Physical conditioning programs are equally important for asthmatic patients of all ages and levels of disease severity. Goals of rehabilitation include (1) participation in age-appropriate physical conditioning activities with peers; (2) maximizing school or work attendance, participation, and productivity; and (3) promotion of self-esteem and self-confidence and a decrease in anxiety about the illness.[18–20]

Several programs have been established and can serve as models:

1. "Breathing Buddies" (Ft. Collins, Colorado) was established by a parents' support group. For participation, children are given bogus $1 bills that can be redeemed for prizes. In addition, special rates are available at local swimming pools, skating rinks, and other facilities.

2. Similar programs have been established by the Young Men's Christian Association and by church and school leaders in several communities. Intense training of asthmatic patients has been the subject of many reports, and new information is being gained about the appropriate level of intensity.[21]

The goals of all these programs have been to minimize restrictions from this chronic illness and its treatment and to help patients live a normal life. Rehabilitation programs are an important part of the total management program for asthmatic patients.

OFFICE-BASED PROGRAMS

These programs are designed for individual application to the patient and the family through the office of the caregiver. Several books have focused on home management, or the ability to adjust medications before contact with a physician. Such publications are useful for physicians who desire to share much of the responsibility for asthma management with the parents and the patients. The use of such tools as the peak flow meter for monitoring has been central to many of these self-management programs.

The program developed at the University of Pittsburgh is conducted in the office setting by a nurse educator. There are four sessions of individual instruction and two sessions with other patients. Access to the health care provider by phone and monitoring of daily asthma activity with a diary are part of this program. Twenty-six children followed for 13 months showed improved compliance with medication regimens, a decrease in the number of absences from school, and a decrease in the number of emergency room and hospital visits.[22] A number of other programs involving the use of video cassettes and computers and adaptations of packaged programs are available for use in the office setting.

EMERGENCY ROOM PROGRAMS

Some of the office programs such as the video cassettes can be used in an acute care situation. Taggert and co-authors described their experience at directing patients from episodic emergency care to a total care program.[23]

SCHOOL PROGRAMS

Parcel and associates studied the effectiveness of asthma educational programs delivered to children at school. Their program consists of 24 weekly sessions for children ages 5 to 10 years. Included in this endeavor are teachers, nurses, psychologists, and a pediatrician. Parents are invited to participate with their children. The text for this program is a book called *Teaching Myself About Asthma* and can be used for group sessions with the younger children.[24]

Since this pioneering work began, a number of other programs have become available for presentation through the school system, including a Columbia University school program,[8] a program from the University of Rochester that entails peer teaching,[25] a Utah Lung Association program for preschoolers,[26] and several other American Lung Association programs.

CHRONIC LUNG DISEASE OF CHILDHOOD

Perinatal and infant mortality rates decreased significantly during the 1980s; however, this decrease has been associated with the development of increased pulmonary sequelae.[27, 28] One percent of all births are premature, and 80% of all infants weighing 750 to 1000 g are expected to survive.[29] It is estimated that 13,000 infants per year develop significant chronic lung disease.[30] Although most of these infants improve in health as new lung tissue is grown, studies have revealed an increase in airway reactivity, an increased number of episodes of respiratory illness, and an increased incidence of airway obstruction at age 10 years.[31] The care of these infants involves a co-management program between family and health care providers that begins in the nursery and may continue through adolescence. The early need is for the understanding of procedures related to home care, such as apnea monitors and nasogastric tubes. Later needs require consideration of possible impairments of sight and hearing, developmental impairment, and the likelihood of hyperreactive airway disease.

Many neonatal intensive care units (NICUs) have classes and support groups conducted by staff and parents of infants who are graduates of NICUs.[32] There also are a number of packaged materials containing reviews of medical and psychosocial issues related to hospital and home care.[33, 34] Follow-up programs are essential, and yet some centers have reported a loss to follow-up rate as high as 70%. An increase in awareness in the general pediatric community of the potential physical and developmental problems of these children, as well as an accomplishment of comanagement developed during the transition from hospital to home care, may do much to improve continuity of care.[35]

CYSTIC FIBROSIS

Of the 20,000 known patients who have cystic fibrosis (CF) in the United States, 30% are now adults. As patients become older, they need to learn about their medical care management, and self-management becomes increasingly important. New advances in chest physiotherapy and in a variety of vascular access devices have decreased the amount of hospital-based care required. Home delivery of intravenous antimicrobial agents is a well-accepted practice (see Chapter 78). Patients with a new diagnosis of CF are managed as outpatients if there are no urgent health needs. This means that all information about CF must be provided to the patient and the family in the outpatient setting. Martin and Seilheimer identified eight performance variables that define CF self-management behavior:[36] respiratory infection, respiratory obstruction, nutrition, availability of health care services, communication with peers, communication with the community as a whole, coping with health problems, and choosing activities that are appropriate for the level of health.[26]

The CF Center at Baylor Medical College in Houston, Texas performed a needs assessment for parents and patients with CF. The assessment revealed that parents performed high level of home care with confidence. A generalized need for more information was also reported, and patients felt frustrated in that they had to take an active role in obtaining this information and training. Teenage and adult patients reported that their primary concern was disruption of work and school because of health limitations. Spinelli and colleagues used this information to devise a program aimed at older CF patients and their parents.[37]

Support and counseling groups have been extremely popular among CF patients. Problems cited by persons conducting the groups have included distance to travel for meetings and the stress of meeting other people with the disease.[38] Much of the success of one particular group has been attributed to peer counseling and support.[39]

There is no shortage of educational materials for a variety of pulmonary conditions. What generally is lacking is a uniformly accepted set of criteria for evaluation of the educational value and performance outcome of each of these programs.

REFERENCES

1. Goldstein RA, Green LW, Parker S: Self-management of childhood asthma. J Allergy Clin Immunol 72:522–525, 1983.
2. Conboy K: Self-management skills for cooperative care in asthma. J Pediatrics 115:863–866, 1989.
3. Hindi-Alexander M: Decision making in asthma self-management. Chest 87:100S–104S, 1985.
4. Evans D, Clark N, Feldman C, et al: A school health education program for children with asthma aged 8–11 years. Health Educ Q 14:267–279, 1987.
5. Shaffer A: Natural asthma education vocational program, attacks asthma [Editorial]. J Allergy Clin Immunol 87:468–469, 1991.
6. Blessing-Moore J, Fritz G, Lewiston N: Self-management programs for childhood asthma. Chest 87:1075–1105, 1985.
7. Holbreich M, Weisberg SC: Asthma camps: Whom to send, what to look for. J Respir Dis 11:366–376, 1991.
8. Clark N, Feldman C, Evans D, et al: The impact of health education on frequency and cost of health care use by low income children with asthma. J Allergy Clin Immunol 78:108–115, 1986.
9. Feldman C, Clark N: Development and evaluation of a self-management program for children with asthma. In Self-Management Educational Programs for Childhood Asthma, pp. 53–104. Washington, DC: National Institute of Allergy and Immunologic Diseases, 1981.
10. Creer T, Backial M, Burns K, et al: Living with asthma: I. Genesis and development of a self-management program for childhood asthma. J Asthma 25:335–362, 1988.
11. Wilson-Pessano S, McNabb W: The role of patient education in the management of childhood asthma. Prevent Med 14:670–687, 1985.
12. McNabb W, Wilson-Pessano S, Highes G, Scamagas P: Self-management education of children with asthma. Am J Pub Health 75:1219–1220, 1985.
13. Lewis CE, Rachelfsky G, Lewis MA, et al: A randomized trial of A.C.T. (asthma care training) for kids. Pediatrics 74:478–486, 1984.
14. Hindi-Alexander M, Cropp G: Evaluation of a family asthma program. J Allergy Clin Immunol 74:505–510, 1984.
15. Blessing-Moore J, Landon M, Miya A, Bergman A: Camp wheeze: An educational/recreational program for asthmatic children and their parents. In Self-Management Educational Programs for Childhood Asthma, pp. 151–198. Washington, DC: National Institute of Allergy and Immunologic Diseases, 1981.
16. American Lung Association, 1740 Broadway, New York, 10019.
17. Sosin A: Asthma camps: An up-to-date listing. Pediatr Asthma Allergy Immunol 5:39–50, 1991.
18. Strunk R, Mascia A, Lipkowitz M, Wolf S: Rehabilitation of a patient with asthma in the outpatient setting. J Allergy Clin Immunology 87:601–611, 1991.
19. Orenstein D, Reed M, Grogan F, Crawford L: Exercise conditioning in children with asthma. J Pediatr 106:556–560, 1985.
20. Fitch K: Sport, physical activity and the asthmatic. In Oseid S, Edwards A (eds): The Asthmatic Child in Play and Sport, pp. 246–258. London: Pitman, 1983.
21. Varray A, Mercier J, Terral C, Prefaut C: Individualized aerobic and high intensity training for asthmatic children in an exercise readaptation program. Chest 99:579–586, 1991.
22. Fireman P, Friday G, Gira C, et al: Teaching self-management skills to asthmatic children and their parents in an ambulatory care setting. Pediatrics 68:341–348, 1981.
23. Taggert V, Zucherman A, Lucas S, et al: Adapting a self-management education program for asthma for use in an outpatient clinic. Ann Allergy 58:173–178, 1987.
24. Parcel G, Nader P, Tiernan K: A health education program for children with asthma. J Dev Behav Pediatr 1:128–132, 1980.
25. Frankowski B, Foye H, Mainan L, et al: The effect of school absenteeism on an asthma education program using peer instructors [Abstract]. Am J Dis Child 140:298, 1986.
26. Whitman N, West D, Brough FK, Welch M: A study of a Self Care

Rehabilitation Program in pediatric asthma. Health Educ Q 12:333–342, 1985.

27. Platzker A: Chronic lung disease of infancy. *In* Ballard R (ed): Pediatric Care of the ICN Graduate, pp. 129–156. Philadelphia: WB Saunders, 1988.

28. Stocks J, Godfrey S: The role of artificial ventilation, oxygen, and CPAP in the pathogenesis of lung damage in neonates. Pediatr 57:352–362, 1976.

29. Desmond M, Thurber S: Historical perspectives. *In* Ballard R (ed): Pediatric Care of the ICN Graduate, pp. 3–11. Philadelphia: WB Saunders, 1988.

30. Lew C, Keens T: Outcome after neonatal intensive care with chronic lung disease. *In* Ballard R (ed): Pediatric Care of the ICN Graduate, pp. 317–321. Philadelphia: WB Saunders, 1988.

31. Bader ND, Ramos AD, Lea CD, et al: Persistent exercise and pulmonary dysfunction in late childhood following BPD [Abstract]. Clin Res 35(1):240A, 1987.

32. Balesy JE, Hancharik SM, Rivers A: Observations of a support group for parents of children with severe bronchopulmonary dysplasia. J Dev Behav Pediatr 9:19–24, 1988.

33. Shosenberg N, Minde K, Swyer PR, et al: The Premature Infant: A Handbook for Parents. Toronto: The Hospital for Sick Children, 1980.

34. Thurber SD, Armstrong LB: Developmental Support of the Low Birth Weight Infant: Parents' Guide, Nurses' Guide, 2nd ed. Houston: Office of Educational Resources, Texas Children's Hospital, 1982.

35. Meisels S, Plunkett JW, Roloff DI, et al: Growth and development of preterm infants with respiratory distress syndrome and bronchopulmonary dysplasia. Pediatrics 77:345–352, 1988.

36. Martin M, Seilheimer D: The development of performance objectives for the self management of CF. Pediatr Pulmonol 2(Suppl A172):141, 1988.

37. Spinelli S, Bartholomew K, Seilheimer D: A needs assessment approach to planning educational and psychosocial programs for CF families [Abstract]. CF Caregivers Report, p. 41, 1985.

38. Schwartz R, Ford E, Swender P, et al: Are patient support groups successful? CF Club Abstracts 23:113, 1982.

39. Lippincott C, Wery K: CF teen girls support group. Pediatr Pulmonol 2(Suppl A170): 141, 1988.

II Evaluation

6 CLINICAL ASSESSMENT OF PULMONARY DISEASE IN INFANTS AND CHILDREN

BETTINA C. HILMAN, M.D.

The clinical assessment of an infant or a child with a respiratory problem involves the application of problem-solving skills, including gathering information (history), examining the patient, obtaining pertinent laboratory studies, evaluating the collected data, formulating a presumptive diagnosis, and reevaluating the initial diagnostic assessment over time, excluding other diagnostic possibilities (differential diagnosis).

Respiratory problems can be evaluated by characterizing the predominant anatomic site of the clinical symptoms and signs or by the type of abnormalities in respiratory function. Classification by anatomic location distinguishes problems involving the airways (upper or lower) from problems of the lung parenchyma that involve either the alveolar airspaces or the pulmonary interstitium. Abnormalities in respiratory function are usually designated obstructive, restrictive, or mixed obstructive and restrictive lung disease. It is also possible to use information from clinical assessment for classifying presentation patterns of respiratory diseases into broad categories by identifying the site of maximal involvement:[1] (1) airway obstruction caused by obstruction of large intrathoracic airways, (2) airway obstruction caused by small intrathoracic obstruction, (3) airway obstruction caused by large extrathoracic airway obstruction, (4) reduced compliance of lung or chest wall with restrictive lung disease, and (5) disorders of respiratory control.

In addition to the qualitative and quantitative aspects of respiratory symptoms, it is important to determine the probable origins of the underlying respiratory problem (e.g., infectious, familial/inherited, metabolic, immunologic), the type of onset (acute, subacute, chronic), and the potential severity (immediately life-threatening, progressive, self-limited, recurrent, or indeterminant).

In this chapter, the history and physical examination are discussed in detail, and only a brief outline of some of the pertinent laboratory procedures used for clinical assessment of pediatric respiratory problems is presented. Diagnostic procedures are discussed in more detail in Chapters 8 to 13, 15, 16, and 89.

HISTORY

The history must be comprehensive and should include environmental, family, and psychosocial information, in addition to the medical history. In the past medical history, it is important to begin with an account of the perinatal events, including the occurrence of maternal infections, metabolic disorders, exposure to drugs or cigarette smoking, and any difficulties during labor and delivery. The birth weight, the Apgar score, special requirements for resuscitation, oxygen supplementation, mechanical ventilation, meconium aspiration, asphyxia, respiratory distress, apnea, infections, or difficulties with feedings should also be documented. For the period of infancy and childhood, it is important to review growth and development, immunizations, feeding problems, significant respiratory illnesses, pertinent abnormal laboratory studies, hospitalizations, and injuries. The review of organ systems should include specific inquiry with regard to appetite, activity level, exercise tolerance, sleep disturbances, skin rashes, and associated gastrointestinal, neuromuscular, and cardiovascular symptoms.

The focus of the history is on the respiratory system, beginning with a description of the chief complaints or reasons for referral. This description should include the duration of respiratory problems, followed by a chronological account of the history of the respiratory symptoms. The response to therapeutic interventions and the types and results of any diagnostic studies should also be reviewed.

The qualitative and quantitative characteristics of the predominant respiratory complaints should be described in detail, as should the timing of the symptom (time of day and relationship to phases of the respiratory cycle); triggering, aggravating, or alleviating factors; type of onset (sudden or gradual); and duration. The age at which onset of symptoms occurred is especially important; symptoms occurring soon after birth may be related to underlying congenital anomalies or may be a manifestation of an inherited disease. If an infectious etiologic agent is suspected, it is important to determine the sources of the patient's contacts with infectious agents.

In the evaluation of the duration of symptoms of respiratory disease, an arbitrary time frame is assigned to each of the three categories of acute ($<$3 weeks), subacute ($>$3 weeks and $<$3 months), and chronic ($>$3 months). In the last category, it is important to distinguish chronic or persistent symptoms from recurrent symptoms. If there is a well-defined, symptom-free period in between episodes of illness, the symptom or disease process is referred to as *recurrent*. (The problem of differentiating recurrent from persistent pneumonia is discussed in more detail in Chapter 18.) Clues leading to the distinction between recurrent and persistent pneumonia can be helpful in determining the underlying cause and management of the respiratory disease. The concept of inertia of the respiratory disease process may be helpful in assessing the type and duration of treatment. Disorders of low inertia are variable in severity and begin and end rapidly, whereas those of high inertia have a slower onset, are longer in duration, and are more difficult to improve.[2]

Environmental history should include evaluation of excessive exposure to infectious agents (e.g., crowded conditions in the home, in a babysitter's house, in a day-care center, or in school) and to noxious inhaled agents such as organic antigens, wood-burning stoves, or passive cigarette smoking (see Chapter 85). It is especially important to identify agents known to cause hypersensitivity pneumonitis and to remove the child from this environment before chronic interstitial pneumonitis and fibrosis develop. In children with allergic respiratory disease, a detailed assessment of the environment is essential in identifying inhalant allergens that can be eliminated or reduced by environmental control measures. A careful review of the social and environmental history may also help identify risk factors for human immunodeficiency virus (HIV) infection in parents or in older children.

Review of the family history can help in the evaluation for inherited or familial disorders. Inquiry should be made into the health status of any siblings, especially as it relates to respiratory illnesses.

Certain symptoms such as cough, wheezing, noisy breathing (e.g., stridor, grunting), dyspnea, chest pain, and cyanosis are often associated with respiratory disease. Each patient with respiratory complaints should be assessed for the presence of these symptoms; if documented, each symptom should be characterized in detail.

COUGH

Cough is one of the earliest and most common clinical manifestations of respiratory disease. Secretions from the larger airways are moved primarily by coughing. A cough can be characterized by its nature (dry or productive), its quality (brassy, croupy, paroxysmal, or staccato), the timing (nocturnal, intermittent, on arising, constant, or persistent), triggering factors (cold air; exercise or exertion such as feeding or positioning), alleviating factors (response to bronchodilators or antibiotics, change in

position), and the presence of associated symptoms (e.g., wheezing, vomiting).

A dry, nonproductive cough may be suggestive of inhaled irritants in the respiratory tract, the presence of allergens in an allergic child, or infections caused by viral, fungal, or mycobacterial agents. A brassy cough is suggestive of tracheal irritation, whereas a croupy or barking cough indicates glottic or subglottic involvement. A cough that sounds wet or productive implies either an increase in airway fluid (mucus, purulent secretions, blood, aspirated liquids) or abnormalities in the clearance of airway secretions. It is helpful to identify the pathophysiologic mechanisms of the increased airway fluid, such as increased production of normal respiratory secretions or abnormal airway clearance mechanisms. (Respiratory mucus is discussed in Chapter 3.) It may be difficult to document that a cough is productive because infants, young children, and many older children swallow rather than expectorate their respiratory secretions. A productive cough, often increased on arising in the morning, is suggestive of bronchiectasis or chronic inflammation of the airways (e.g., cystic fibrosis). It is important to document the color, consistency, volume, and odor of sputum, as well as the presence of any blood streaking or frank hemoptysis.

The timing and associated circumstances of a cough are also helpful in detecting the underlying etiologic process. A dry nocturnal cough may indicate subclinical or "cough-variant" asthma or postnasal drip caused by allergic respiratory disease or sinusitis. A recurrent cough associated with wheezing is suggestive of airway obstruction and can be caused by asthma, cystic fibrosis, aspiration syndromes (including foreign body in the bronchi), abnormalities in clearance of airway secretions, congenital anomalies, and mediastinal masses. A cough associated with alterations in phonation (dysphonia or aphonia) implies hypopharyngeal or laryngeal disorder (e.g., foreign body, papilloma of the larynx, infectious or allergic croup, or psychogenic causes). The evaluation of chronic cough is addressed in detail in Chapter 17.

Cough associated with feedings indicates (1) aspiration syndromes; (2) congenital anatomic or physiologic abnormalities of the airways, the hypopharynx, or the esophagus; or (3) incoordination of swallowing and breathing.

WHEEZING

Wheezing, a prolonged, high-pitched musical respiratory sound of varying intensity, is more commonly heard during expiration than during inspiration. Wheezing can be intermittent or persistent. Table 6-1 outlines the differential diagnosis of wheezing. Although the presence of wheezing implies respiratory disease or dysfunction, expiratory wheezing can be heard in normal persons as a result of flow limitation produced by a forced expiratory maneuver.

Paroxysmal or intermittent wheezing is suggestive of asthma. Persistent wheezing with sudden onset may indicate aspiration of a foreign body. Slowly progressive onset of wheezing may signify extraluminal bronchial obstruc-

Table 6–1. DIFFERENTIAL DIAGNOSIS OF WHEEZING IN INFANTS AND CHILDREN

Inflammatory
Retropharyngeal or peritonsillar abscess
Laryngitis: Diphtheritic and nondiphtheritic
Epiglottitis
Laryngotracheobronchitis
Acute spasmodic laryngitis (croup diathesis)
Bronchitis; "asthmatic bronchitis"*
Bronchiectasis
Pheumonitis
Cystic fibrosis*
Bronchiolitis*
Mechanical Obstruction
Enlarged adenoids; polyps of larynx
Mucus vibrating in respiratory passages
Extrinsic compression: Lymph nodes, tumor, foreign body in
  esophagus
Intraluminal obstruction: endobronchial foreign body*
Cardiovascular: vascular ring,*
  Anomalies of great vessels
  (double aortic arch)*
Congenital anomalies of the respiratory tract
  Choanal atresia
  Tracheal stenosis
  Bronchial stenosis
  Flaccid epiglottis
  Tracheomalacia
  Cysts (thyroglossal duct)
  Redundant folds of mucous membranes
  Subglottic hemangioma
  Congenital web larynx
  Lobar emphysema
  Bronchopulmonary sequestration
  Agenesis of lobe of lung
Metabolic
Stridor of tetany
Neurologic
Paralysis of recurrent laryngeal nerve
Stridor of cerebral palsy
Traumatic
Dislocation of fixation of cricoarytenoid joint
Other
Psychogenic (laryngeal wheezing or "factitious asthma")

*More commonly encountered disorder.

tion caused by enlarging lymph nodes (e.g., tuberculous adenitis or other intrathoracic mass).

In asthma, it is important to determine what triggers the wheezing (exercise, laughter, cold air, exposure to cigarette smoke, strong odors or perfume, specific allergens, infection). In some older children or adolescents with emotional disturbances or with vocal cord dysfunction, wheezing may be generated at the laryngeal level.

NOISY BREATHING

Various respiratory noises described as "noisy breathing" include snoring, stridor, and grunting.

Snoring. In snoring, a rough, snorting sound that may be present in both inspiration and expiration originates from the flutter of tissues in the oropharynx. It may be heard intermittently during sleep in normal children with upper respiratory infections or with seasonal allergic rhinitis. The snoring is heard more consistently in children with nasal polyps, adenoidal and tonsillar hypertrophy, or congenital anomalies such as Pierre Robin syndrome. Children with chronic nocturnal snoring should be evaluated for other signs of obstructive sleep apnea.

Stridor. Stridor is a high-pitched, harsh, loud musical sound of single pitch caused by oscillations of narrowed large extrathoracic airways. Obstructive lesions in the larynx cause inspiratory stridor. Obstructive lesions in the trachea can cause a combination of inspiratory and expiratory stridor, but more often the inspiratory stridor is predominant. The inspiratory stridor varies in intensity, being loudest during crying or with increased ventilatory rate. Stridor may be affected by changes in position. Stridor is worse when the infant is in the supine position with the neck flexed and better in the prone position with the neck extended.

Grunting. Grunting, a low-pitched expiratory noise usually with musical qualities, is caused by partial closure of the glottis. In infants with neonatal respiratory distress syndrome, grunting is produced by adduction of vocal cords and is used to generate end-expiratory pressures. It is often associated with chest pain in older children who have pneumonia and pleural involvement.

CHEST PAIN

Chest pain may be caused by respiratory as well as other causes. Pleural pain is frequently related to respiration; the respirations are often shallow and rapid and may be accompanied by an expiratory grunt. Parietal pleural pain is usually localized over the involved area. Pain from diaphragmatic pleural irritation can be referred to the base of the neck or to the abdomen.[2] It is important to obtain a detailed description of the type, location, frequency, and severity of the pain, as well as the relationship of the pain to sleep, exercise, or trauma (see Chapter 19).

DYSPNEA

Dyspnea is defined as difficulty in breathing or a subjective sensation of breathlessness. It is important to remember the subjective nature of this condition. Idiopathic hyperventilation is associated with extreme dyspnea, whereas serious conditions such as oversedation produce dangerous hypoventilation without any complaint of dyspnea.

CYANOSIS

Cyanosis refers to the blue color of the skin or mucous membranes when hemoglobin is desaturated: that is, when the concentration of reduced hemoglobin content of arterial blood is at least 3 g/100 ml, or 4 to 6 g/100 ml in capillary blood. Clinical cyanosis occurs at different levels of arterial oxygen saturation, varying with the amount of total hemoglobin present. It may be difficult to detect cyanosis early in anemic patients. Peripheral cyanosis (confined to the skin of the extremities) should be distinguished from central cyanosis, which includes the tongue and mucous membranes. Cyanosis can occur with normal arterial hemoglobin saturation if cardiac output is decreased or if peripheral perfusion is poor. Cyanosis is neither a reliable nor an early sign of hypoxemia. Central cyanosis indicates cardiorespiratory disease resulting from alveolar hypoventilation, ventilation/perfusion mismatching, alveolar-capillary diffusion abnormalities, or right-to-left shunts (cyanotic congenital heart disease, congenital pulmonary arteriovenous fistulae, or intrapulmonary shunting). With the exception of right-to-left shunts, cyanosis responds to small increases in supplemental oxygen in the inspired air.

PHYSICAL EXAMINATION

The importance of a careful, comprehensive physical examination cannot be overemphasized. The use of quantitative diagnostic techniques as a part of the physical examination is especially helpful for assessing younger or uncooperative patients, as well as in the longitudinal follow-up of patients with known respiratory disease. Four quantitative extensions of the physical examination are helpful in the assessment of the respiratory status of children and are discussed separately: clubbing index, chest depth/width ratios derived from thoracic anthropometric measurements, sleeping/resting respiratory rates, and differential segmental auscultation of the chest. The classical components of the physical examination (inspection, palpation, auscultation, and percussion) should also be an integral part of the comprehensive physical examination of any patient, although the order of these components varies with the age of the child, the degree of cooperativeness, and other circumstances particular to pediatric patients. The characteristics of breathing, including respiratory rate, depth, rhythm, and degree of effort, should be observed during inspection and further evaluated during auscultation of the chest.

INSPECTION

Respiratory rate, a noninvasive measurement of pulmonary and thoracic compliance, varies normally with age; with state of wakefulness, sleep, activity, or exercise; and with anxiety. Other nonrespiratory conditions or disorders that can affect the respiratory rate include acid-base status, fever, anemia, metabolic disorders, and central nervous system disturbances. The activity and behavioral status of the infant or child should be recorded when the respiratory rate is counted. The respiratory rate should be obtained while the child is resting or sleeping or whenever the child is as calm as possible. Monitoring of respiratory rate can be very helpful in infants and children with low-compliance disorders of the lungs and the thorax, such as pneumonia, interstitial lung disease, and pleural effusion.

The respiratory rate should be recorded over one full minute. It is preferable that the rate be counted for two or three separate determinations and that the average of the three determinations be recorded. It is difficult to obtain an accurate steady-state value for respiratory rate during

the physical examination in a clinic, an office, or a hospital setting. For children with chronic respiratory disorders, the parents are given instructions on how to measure sleep respiratory rates reliably and are asked to keep a respiratory rate log for longitudinal evaluation. Techniques that can assist in the accurate counting of respiratory rates in patients with shallow respiratory movements include evaluation of abdominal movements and the auscultation of breath sounds at the mouth or the nose.

Tachypnea, or an abnormally high respiratory rate, is associated with respiratory disease in patients with decreased compliance as well as other nonrespiratory disorders or conditions such as toxic drug ingestions (salicylate poisoning), hyperthyroidism, metabolic acidosis, fever, anemia, and anxiety. In contrast, *bradypnea,* or an abnormally low respiratory rate, occurs in patients with depression of the central nervous system or with metabolic alkalosis.

Terms used to describe the depth of respiration include *hyperpnea* (unusually deep respiration) and *hypopnea* (shallow breathing). Hyperpnea occurs in pulmonary disease with increased physiologic dead space associated with fever, severe anemia, metabolic acidosis, respiratory alkalosis, and intoxication by certain drugs (e.g., salicylates). Hypopnea can occur in metabolic alkalosis and respiratory acidosis associated with central nervous system depression. The depth of respiration is usually estimated by means of inspection of the amplitude of thoracic and abdominal excursions, but it may also be evaluated through auscultation of the chest or at the mouth and the nose.

Variations in the rhythm of breathing result in several recognizable breathing patterns, including apnea, periodic breathing, Kussmaul's breathing, Cheyne-Stokes breathing, and Biot's breathing. *Apnea* is described as cessation of respirations for more than 15 sec, or for less if accompanied by bradycardia or cyanosis. *Periodic breathing* is a respiratory pattern in which there are at least three respiratory pauses of 3- to 10-sec duration with less than 20 sec of respiration between pauses. This respiratory pattern is common in premature infants and is sometimes seen in normal full-term infants, usually under 3 months of age. *Kussmaul's breathing* is seen in ketoacidosis and is characterized by deep, slow, regular respirations with a prolonged expiratory phase.

In *Cheyne-Stokes breathing,* there are cycles of increasing and decreasing depths of tidal volumes (crescendo-decrescendo respiratory pattern) that are separated by periods of apnea; this pattern of breathing may be seen in children with increased intracranial pressure, cerebral trauma, and congestive heart failure. *Biot's breathing,* or cycles of irregular respiration at variable tidal volumes associated with periods of apnea of varying lengths, is usually seen in patients with severe brain damage.

Signs of distressed breathing or increased respiratory effort include retractions, use of accessory muscles of respiration, flaring of the alae nasi, head bobbing, grunting, wheezing, orthopnea, and increased pulsus paradoxus. In *dyspnea,* which is a physical sign as well as a symptom indicating difficult or labored breathing, there is increased work of breathing by the respiratory muscles and often the use of accessory muscles of respiration in an attempt to maintain adequate alveolar ventilation. It is difficult to quantitate dyspnea, especially in younger children; however, sternocleidomastoid muscle contractions have been shown to be correlated with severe abnormalities of pulmonary function in adults. *Retractions,* a sinking in or depression of the thoracic soft tissues in relation to the bony and cartilaginous thorax during inspiration, are produced by differences in pressure between the intrapleural space (intrathoracic pressure) and the pressure outside the thorax (atmospheric pressure). Mild intercostal retractions can be seen normally between the lower ribs in some children. With airway obstruction or increased lung stiffness, there are higher-than-normal increases of intrathoracic pressure during inspiration. Retractions of varying severity are often seen. In severe airway obstruction, retractions are more extensive and may involve the supraclavicular and infraclavicular areas. Retractions are best observed in the sixth and ninth intercostal spaces in the posterior axillary line with a light shining perpendicular to the plane of the middle ribs.[1] Subcostal retractions should be differentiated from other retractions because they are associated with flattening of the diaphragm seen in severe airway obstruction.

Bulging of Intercostal Interspaces

Inspection of the intercostal interspaces may also identify excessive expiratory effort (bulging of interspaces) as well as excessive inspiratory effort (retractions). In patients with diffuse bronchial obstruction, increased expiratory effort is required for emptying the lungs. Although intrathoracic pressure is normally subatmospheric during expiration, intrathoracic pressure in diffuse airway obstruction may exceed atmospheric pressure, causing the intercostal space to flatten or bulge outward during expiration (as in, e.g., cystic fibrosis, asthma, and bronchiolitis).

Bilateral *flaring* (enlargement) of alae nasi indicates that the accessory muscles of respiration are being recruited during inspiration. This is a sign of labored breathing or shortened inspiration time resulting from pain from pleuritis or thoracic trauma. The enlargement of the nares is caused by contraction of the anterior and posterior dilator muscles of naris (innervated by the facial nerves). Unilateral flaring is a sign of facial paralysis on the opposite side.

Head bobbing is the forward movement of the head as a result of neck flexion in an infant lying supine and unsupported (except for the suboccipital area). This sign is probably explained by contraction of the accessory muscles of respiration (scalene and sternocleidomastoid muscles), in which the counteraction from the extensor muscles of the neck is insufficient for fixing the cervical spine and head, resulting in flexion of the neck instead of raising of the sternum and the first two ribs.[2]

Grunting

Grunting, a low-pitched expiratory sound produced in the larynx, as mentioned earlier, is often found in infants with neonatal respiratory distress syndrome; the partial glottic closure helps to maintain a high expiratory pressure that keeps the alveoli open in the absence of normal amounts of surfactant. Other respiratory conditions associated with grunting include pulmonary edema and pneumonia with pleural involvement.

Clubbing

In digital clubbing, the nail bases of the fingers and toes are lifted by tissue proliferation on the dorsal surface of the terminal phalanx, which results in a focal enlargement of the soft tissues. Clubbing was first described by Hippocrates, and the pathogenesis is not clearly defined. Clubbing may be idiopathic, hereditary, or acquired. It has been associated with a wide spectrum of respiratory disorders, including bronchiectasis, pulmonary arteriovenous malformations, bronchiolitis obliterans, and pulmonary abscess (Table 6–2). There are various methods of determining clubbing; the one recommended by the author is the method of Waring and associates[3] in which the depth of a plaster cast of the index finger at the nail base is compared with the depth at the terminal interphalangeal fold. When this ratio exceeds 1.0, the finger is considered clubbed (Fig. 6–1). Serial measurements are helpful for monitoring the course of pulmonary diseases associated with clubbing.

Thoracic Configuration

It is extremely important to inspect the unclad thorax during quiet and forced breathing. Abnormalities of topography such as pectus excavatum (indrawing of the sternum), pectus carinatum (pigeon breast, or a bowing out of the sternal-costal border), or absence of one or both pectoral muscles are readily seen. Inspection also can

Table 6–2. CAUSES OF CLUBBING

Pulmonary
Bronchiectasis
    Cystic fibrosis
    Immotile cilia syndrome
    Bronchiolitis obliterans
Pulmonary abscess
Empyema
Interstitial infiltrates/fibrosis
    Hemosiderosis
    Immunodeficiency
        Congenital
        Acquired (including AIDS)
Malignancy (primary or secondary)
Sarcoidosis
Pulmonary arteriovenous fistulae
Cardiac
Congestive heart failure (chronic)
Congenital heart disease (cyanotic)
Subacute bacterial endocarditis
Other
Endocrine: thyrotoxicosis
Lymphomatoid granulomatosis
Hepatic cirrhosis (cystic fibrosis, alpha$_1$-antitrypsin deficiency)
Ulcerative colitis, Crohn's disease
Thalassemia

AIDS, acquired immunodeficiency syndrome.

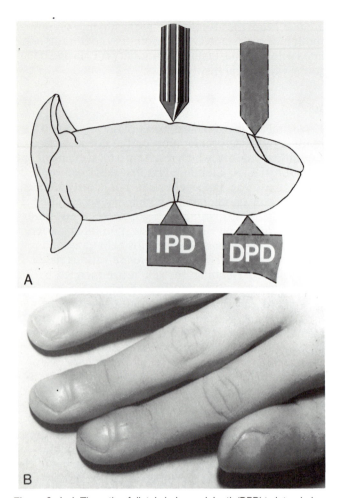

A

B

Figure 6–1. *A,* The ratio of distal phalangeal depth (DPD) to interphalangeal (IPD) is >1 in finger clubbing, in contrast to normal, which is <1. *B,* Photograph of digital clubbing in an 8-year-old white female with cystic fibrosis who previously was diagnosed with asthma.

reveal the use of accessory muscles of respiration with increased work of breathing. The sternocleidomastoid muscles are used as respiratory muscles to elevate the clavicles when lung capacity approaches 90% of vital capacity. The pectoral and lateral muscles also can be used as respiratory muscles when the arms are fixed in a tripod position so that these powerful muscles can expand the ribs. Symmetry of inspiration also should be confirmed.

Inspection of the chest reveals the presence of chronic air trapping, or the "barrel-shaped chest" that is characteristic of a number of disorders. The thorax of an infant is rounder than the chest of an older child. Although a subjective assessment of the anteroposterior diameter of the chest can be made on inspection, a more objective measurement of the anteroposterior and transverse diameters can be made with a conventional obstetric caliper. Serial measurements of anteroposterior and transverse diameters can be especially useful for following children with chronic obstructive lung disease. These diameters can be compared with diameters in normative tables and are used to compute the thoracic index, which is the anteroposterior diameter divided by the transverse diameter.[4] In severe lung disease, this value may be close to 1.0.

PALPATION

Tracheal Palpation

Tracheal palpation is important in the evaluation of an infant or a child for possible mediastinal shift. The trachea may be shifted when there are differences in thoracic pressure or in volume between the two sides of the thorax. Detection of the tracheal shift does not indicate in which hemithorax the volume or pressure change has occurred. For example, pneumothorax on the left adds to the volume of the left hemithorax; this is associated with increased negative intrathoracic pressure, causing the mediastinum and trachea to shift to the right. A foreign body completely obstructing the right main stem bronchus results in atelectasis distal to the site of obstruction. As air is absorbed from the collapsed alveoli, there is a decrease in the volume of the right hemithorax and a shift of the mediastinum to the right.

There are two methods of tracheal palpation: one for infants and small children (Fig. 6–2*A*) and the other for older children (Fig. 6–2*B*). The patient's neck should be slightly extended without any tilt or rotation from a midline position.

Pulsus Paradoxus

Pulsus paradoxus is an exaggeration of the normal decrease in systemic arterial pressure during inspiration. It is the result of a higher-than-normal increase in intrathoracic negative pressure as the patient inspires. This increase causes an exaggeration of the normal inspiratory-expiratory difference in left ventricular stroke volume. It is measured by determination of the difference in systolic pressure between inspiration and expiration. The highest pressure at which any systolic sound is heard is recorded. The pressure is then lowered until all systolic sounds are heard. The difference is normally less than 10 mm Hg. Values higher than this are believed to reflect bronchial obstruction. Although there is no accurate correlation of the magnitude of the pulsus paradoxus and the degree of airway obstruction, a change in the degree of pulsus during therapy for acute asthma is one reflection of the partial relief of the asthma.

AUSCULTATION

Auscultation of the chest with a stethoscope has been popular since the time of Laënnec (1781–1826). Waring described two basic rules for the successful assessment of breath sounds. The first is that the physician should rely on the stethoscope because it is an auditory instrument; the stethoscope diaphragm is generally used for most pulmonary auscultation because of its weighted frequency response toward higher frequencies.[2] Because breath sounds are higher pitched than heart sounds, they are better heard with the diaphragm. The second rule is that auscultation should be related to bronchopulmonary anatomy. (Figs. 6–3 to 6–6 show the surface projection of the bronchopulmonary segments on the anterior, right lateral, left lateral, and posterior chest wall.) It is important to correlate the auscultation of the chest with the topo-

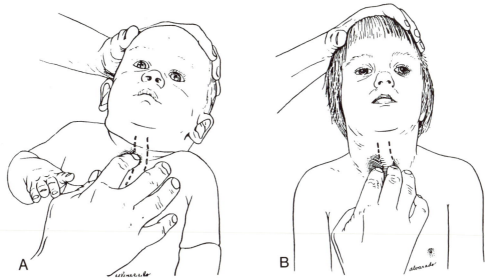

Figure 6-2. *A*, Technique of determining tracheal position in an infant. The index finger of the physician's palpating hand is placed in the suprasternal notch of the infant and gently slid inward in the midsagittal plane. It is essential that the infant's head be fixed in a neutral position and the neck be slightly extended. If the physician's finger consistently slides off one side of the infant's trachea, it can be concluded that the trachea is deviated in the opposite direction. In this illustration, the trachea is shifted to the left. *B*, Technique of determining tracheal position in an older child. Inspection of the suprasternal area may show asymmetry of the fossae bounded laterally by the sternocleidomastoid muscles and medially by the trachea. In this case, the fossa on the right is larger than that on the left, as indicated by its larger shadow. It is concluded that the trachea has been shifted to the left. The impression gained from inspection is then tested by two-finger palpation of the relative size of the two fossae. As shown, the physician's index finger fits easily between the right sternomastoid and the trachea of the patient, but the physician's middle finger is too large for the corresponding space on the left.

graphic anatomy and with the review of the chest radiographs (Figs. 6-7, 6-8). Careful differential auscultation of the chest, especially with a double stethoscope (double-headed, one earpiece for each ear) helps in the location of the disease. The correlation of the findings on physical examination with the chest radiographic findings can be useful in the recommendation for correct positioning for precise segmental bronchial drainage (Fig. 6-9).

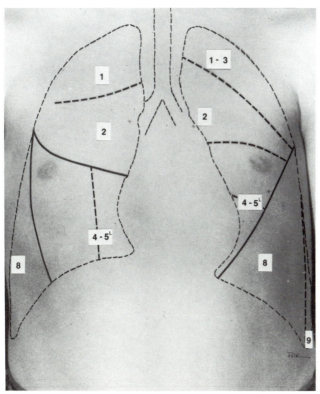

Figure 6-3. Topographic chest anatomy: anterior projection of bronchopulmonary segments.

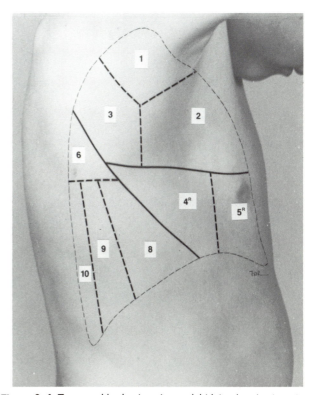

Figure 6-4. Topographic chest anatomy: right lateral projection of the bronchopulmonary segments.

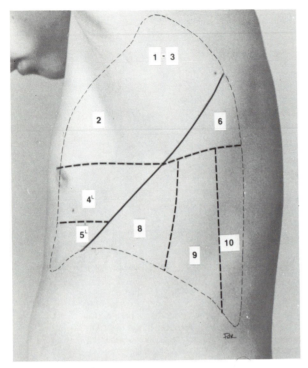

Figure 6–5. Topographic chest anatomy: left lateral projection of bronchopulmonary segments.

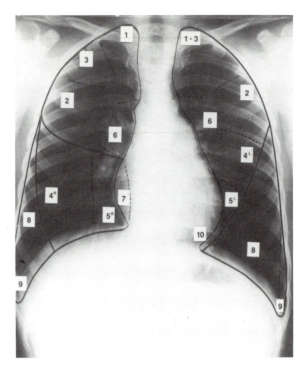

Figure 6–7. Radiographic chest anatomy: anterior view.

For complete assessment of the chest by auscultation, the physician should listen to one or two complete respirations in each of the bronchopulmonary segments listed in Figures 6–10A and 6–10B. The double stethoscope (Fig. 6–11) enables comparison of the sounds of homologous segments of the lung; the physician should be able to detect any significant difference in the breath sounds of the two segments (i.e., heterophony), which is usually a sign of pulmonary pathology.[5]

The sound transmitted to the diaphragm of the stethoscope through the chest wall is the sound of turbulent airflow in the conducting airways. The movement of air in

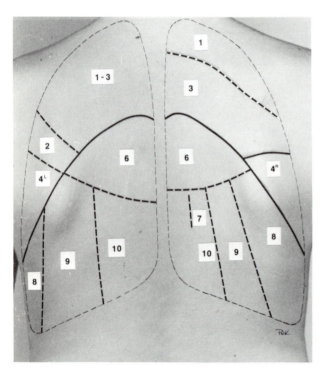

Figure 6–6. Topographic chest anatomy: posterior projection of bronchopulmonary segments.

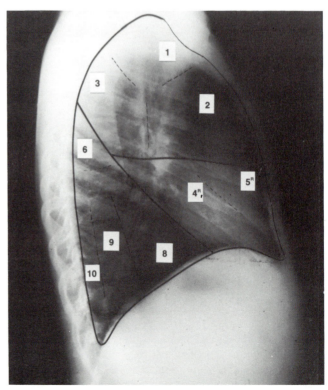

Figure 6–8. Radiographic chest anatomy: right lateral view.

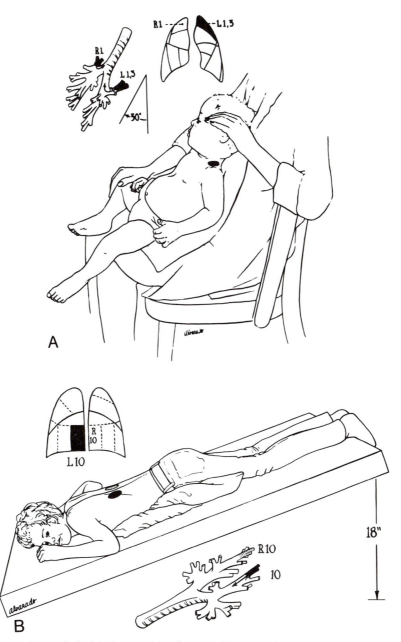

Figure 6–9. *A,* Left upper lobe. Segmental bronchial drainage. *B,* Left lower lobe, posterior basal segment.

large airways is more turbulent, and therefore more noisy, than that in more distal terminal airways. A simple clinical experiment can demonstrate this point. If the examiner places the diaphragm of the stethoscope over his or her own trachea, the harsh "tubular" sound in the expiratory phase is louder than in the inspiratory phase; this phenomenon is called *tracheal breathing.* A similar exercise in which the diaphragm is placed over the examiner's left axilla reveals a softer, lower-pitched sound in which inspiration is louder than expiration. This is the sound of air moving in the distal airways and is referred to as *vesicular breathing.* In a final exercise, the stethoscope is placed just below the center of the right clavicle. Sounds here are louder and more tubular than in vesicular breathing and are equal in loudness during inspiration and expiration. This is referred to as *bronchovesicular breathing.*

Bronchial breath sounds are a little louder during expiration than inspiration and are somewhat harsher but not as harsh as tracheal breathing. It is important that the clinician be familiar with the normal location of each of these sounds. Bronchial breathing heard in the axilla means either the interposition of a fluid medium that would transmit sound from a large airway or the presence of large bronchiectatic airways in the periphery of the lung.

Adventitious sounds in the lungs often are a source of confusion to the inexperienced clinician. These sounds are produced during the respiratory cycle by the presence of something abnormal in the conducting airway. Although there are a number of classifications, most of the pulmonary organizations have adopted common terminology. It is important to note loudness, pitch, and tim-

Lung Segments

Name/location	Number/key
RIGHT UPPER LOBE	
Apical	1
Anterior	2
Posterior	3
RIGHT MIDDLE LOBE	
Lateral	4
Medial	5
RIGHT LOWER LOBE	
Superior	6
Medial Basal	7
Anterior Basal	8
Lateral Basal	9
Posterior Basal	10
LEFT UPPER LOBE	
Apical—Posterior	1-3
Anterior	2
Lower-lingular	
Superior	4
Inferior	5
LEFT LOWER LOBE	
Superior	6
Anteriomedial Basal	7-8
Lateral Basal	9
Posterior Basal	10

A

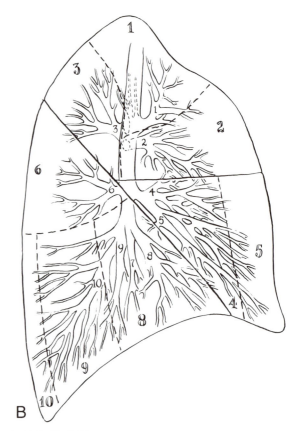

B

Figure 6–10. *A* and *B*, Bronchopulmonary segments.

ing during the cycle of these sounds in the various parts of the lung. It also is important to note the effect of respiratory maneuvers such as forced expiration or cough.

Crackles

A crackle is essentially an opening pop, the sound produced by the discontinuity of an air-fluid interface. During inspiration, a fluid meniscus is popped open as the airway dilates. This popping produces short, crackling

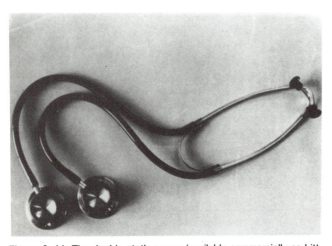

Figure 6–11. The double stethoscope (available commercially as Littman differential stethoscope). Each ear has its own bell-diaphragm chest piece; each of the chest pieces is equipped with spring-loaded on-off buttons so that the sound can be instantly cut off or restarted at any time.

sounds. The sounds may be low in pitch and may occur early in the respiratory cycle as fluid in a large airway is opened. This is referred to as a *coarse crackle* (also as a *coarse rale*), although this term is losing favor. Crackles that are heard later during inspiration and are higher in pitch are called *fine crackles.* Coarse crackles are usually indicative of fluid in the larger airways; fine crackles, of fluid in the smaller airways. Because the discontinuity of the meniscus of fluid happens only with dilatation of the airways, crackles are heard only during inspiration.

Another sound heard with breathing is caused by the production of turbulence resulting from the presence in the airway of a partial obstruction. The sounds are high-pitched, have a musical quality, and are referred to as "wheezes." *Wheezing* is a high-pitched, continuous (>200 msec), adventitious, musical lung sound that is associated with partial obstruction of one or more of the larger bronchi. The wheezes originate from an oscillation of the walls of narrowed airways. The frequency of the oscillations depends on type, airway size, elasticity, and the rate of airflow. The wheezing in asthma is usually generalized and polyphonic, in contrast to monophonic wheezing that accompanies obstruction of a single airway. Fixed monophonic wheezing is often associated with aspiration of a foreign body in the intrathoracic trachea or the lobar bronchi.

PERCUSSION

Although distinguishing percussive changes is not as useful in children as in older adults, many pediatricians are surprised to find that they can do so in a patient with an infiltrate or pleural effusion. Usually the third finger of the examiner's dominant hand strikes the terminal phalanx (not the joint) of the third finger of the other hand. The presence of consolidation is detected as much by feel as by sound.

CONCLUSION

Clinical assessment of pediatric pulmonary disease requires all five senses and time, patience, and common sense. Challenging and invigorating, the integration of the medical history and the data obtained in the clinical assessment forms a solid basis for conclusions about the nature and prognosis of pediatric pulmonary disease.

REFERENCES

1. Waring WW, Menendez R: General considerations in the management of respiratory diseases. *In* Shirkey HC (ed): Pediatric Therapy, 6th ed, pp. 621–635. St. Louis: CV Mosby, 1980.
2. Waring WW. The history and physical examination. *In* Chernick V (ed): Kendig's Disorders of the Respiratory Tract, 4th ed, pp. 56–76. Philadelphia: WB Saunders, 1983.
3. Waring WW, Wilkinson RW, Wiebe RA, et al: Quantitation of digital clubbing in children: Measurement of casts of the index finger. Amer Rev Respir Dis 104:166–174, 1971.
4. Waring WW, Golladay ES, Acker SE, et al: Shape and size of the thorax in children with chronic lung disease. South Med J 454:1582, 1965.
5. Waring WW: Physical examination of children: Quantitative extensions. *In* Sackner MA (ed): Diagnostic Techniques in Pulmonary Disease, pp. 49–85. New York: Marcel Dekker, 1981.

7 LUNG SOUNDS AND PHONOPNEUMOGRAPHY

WILLIAM W. WARING, M.D.

Unlike other organs (the liver, for example), the lung does not suffer insults silently. It is a noisy organ. Only in very slow, shallow breathing is it truly quiet. With increasingly deep breaths through an open mouth, the sounds of breathing can be heard across the room as a nonmusical, to-and-fro rustling. When diseased, the lung becomes downright vociferous: rattling, crackling, piping, snoring, and wheezing. All of these sounds are intrinsic to the lung. If the concept of "lung" is extended to include the trachea and the larynx, further sounds are derived from stridor and cough: *brassy, honking, croupy, barking, paroxysmal,* and *staccato* are common terms for these additional sounds.

The French 19th-century clinical investigator René Laënnec made the first major efforts to correlate lung sounds and disease. What he heard with his stethoscope from diseased lungs was correlated strongly with what he saw in them on the autopsy table. In the sense of relating sound to its pathologic source, it is disappointing that the science of lung sound recording and analysis (phonopneumography) and the ability to look inside the lungs by modern scanning and imaging have not been more productively developed. Nevertheless, there is a slowly growing wealth of information that relates sound to pulmonary function and disease. More details about these relationships than are contained in this short chapter are provided in the excellent series of articles on lung sounds in *Seminars in Respiratory Medicine.*[1]

Much of the problem with phonopneumography lies in the nature of the signal. It is easily contaminated by background noise and by artifacts related to equipment and movement by the patient. The site of recording varies widely (at the mouth, over the trachea, from the chest wall). Processing of artifact-free sound, once recorded, also presents many obstacles and raises many questions. Should the sample for analysis be limited in any way— inspiratory, expiratory, or mixed sound? If it is limited, should it contain a certain portion of inspiration or expiration? Is the patient required to take deeper-than-normal breaths or to perform some other special breathing maneuver? Should undesirable frequencies be removed by filtering before analysis? If so, which ones? What sort of signal within the sound is the examiner listening for: certain frequencies or certain amplitudes?

The answers to these questions depend on the goals of the phonopneumographic effort. In short, there is no standardized procedure. Indeed, if there is no conventional clinical application of this method, why should phonopneumography be mentioned in a clinical pulmonary text such as this? It should be included because its application has shed new light on pulmonary auscultation in general and on the physical nature of the sounds that people hear in particular.

EQUIPMENT

The equipment for phonopneumography can be extremely simple or extremely complex. Necessary in all

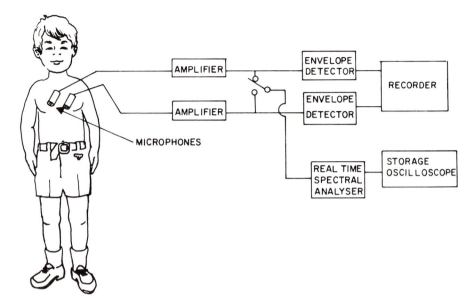

Figure 7–1. Block diagram of respiratory sound analysis system for differential phonopneumography. (From Wooten FT, Waring WW, Wegmann MJ, et al: Method for respiratory sound analysis. Med Instrum 12:254–257, 1978.)

systems are (1) a recording environment that minimizes contamination of the sound signal by background noise (quiet room, sound chamber); (2) at least one microphone that for most applications can be coupled to the chest wall in order to entrain sound from the lungs; (3) a recording device, usually an AM or FM tape recorder; and (4) signal processing equipment, which can include filters (to eliminate unwanted sound frequencies), a spectral analyzer or computer for fast Fourier transform (FFT), a video monitor, and strip chart recorder. Multichannel systems permit simultaneous recording of sound from more than one location along with other data, such as gas flow signals from a pneumotachograph at the mouth. The choice of equipment obviously depends on numerous factors, including the need for precision, the complexity of the observations, the magnitude of the anticipated signal, the sophistication of the analysis, and, always, the budget. Figure 7–1 depicts one such system that enables recording and analysis of breath sounds from two separate locations.

What has the use of equipment of this type revealed about lung sounds? This question is answered in the following sections (Breath Sounds and Adventitious Sounds).

BREATH SOUNDS

Present concepts hold that breath sounds, as monitored from the chest wall, are low in pitch (frequency), almost all less than 500 Hz. They are complexly attenuated and selectively filtered sounds that are generated in the central airways, including the trachea and the major bronchi, but not in the bronchioles or the alveoli. The sound is produced by air turbulence, which can occur only in large airways, wherein high requisite flows can be achieved. As monitored by auscultation of the trachea, this sound is loud, can be heard equally during inspiration and expiration, and has a high-pitched, tubular quality. Auscul-

tation over the lung apex and base in one normal subject reveals sounds with qualities markedly different from those of sounds in the trachea (Fig. 7–2). In a normal sub-

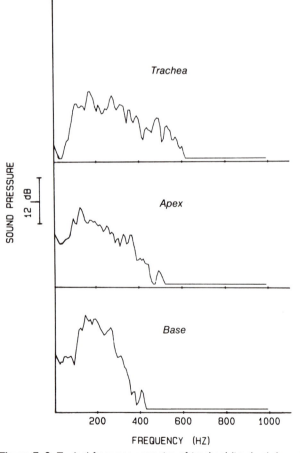

Figure 7–2. Typical frequency spectra of tracheal (trachea), bronchovesicular (apex), and vesicular (base) breath sounds. (From Kraman SS: Vesicular (normal) lung sounds: How are they made, where do they come from, and what do they mean? Sem Respir Med 6:186, 1985.)

ject, regardless of age, breath sounds auscultated over the upper lobes are generally higher pitched than those auscultated over the lower lobes. Although these peripheral lung sounds thus differ from each other, they are much softer and lower in pitch than those of the trachea. Also, unlike those heard over the trachea, they are heard exclusively or mainly during inspiration.

These differences are probably attributable to variations in effective filtering of large airway sounds. It is thought that unfiltered sounds, generated in the larger airways, are transmitted down the tracheobronchial tree, and at some point, the sound leaves the airways and travels more slowly through the lung parenchyma, finally reaching the chest wall. During the parenchymal portion of its journey, the sound is low-pass filtered; that is, low-frequency components pass through the lung, whereas those of higher frequency are reflected and absorbed and never reach the chest wall. The efficacy of this filtering process is thought to depend largely on two related factors: the distance of airways from the chest wall and the number of alveoli through which the sound must pass. The vesicular breath sounds at the lung bases in adults are lower pitched and softer than the bronchovesicular sounds in infants and young children, probably because there are many more filtering alveoli in adults. Thus the intensity and the pitch of breath sounds are related to age and undoubtedly reflect lung growth throughout childhood.

The efficacy of this filtering process can be quantified by phonopneumography and FFT, in which sound amplitude is displayed as a function of sound frequency. FFT has permitted a comparison of breath sounds recorded at various sites on the chest wall. Two spectral displays obtained by FFT from homologous bronchopulmonary segments are shown in Figure 7–3.

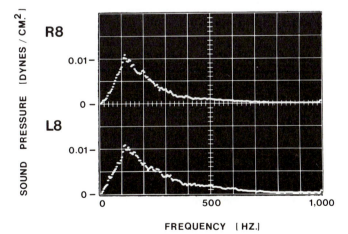

Figure 7–3. Frequency spectra of the same breaths recorded from the chest wall over the right (R8) and left (L8) anterior basal segments of the lower lobes in a 12-year-old child. On clinical auscultation, no difference in the pitch of breath sounds could be appreciated; this observation was confirmed in these spectra by the striking similarity of the breath sound frequencies of the two sides (equivalent to pitch homophony), although slightly more sound in frequencies above 500 Hz is observable on the left side. (From Waring WW: Physical examination of children. In Sackner MA [ed]: Diagnostic Techniques in Pulmonary Disease, Part I, p. 67. New York: Marcel Dekker, 1980.)

Pulmonary disease, especially consolidating diseases such as lobar pneumonia, may impair the sound-filtering function of the lung. The parenchyma filters sound by differentially reflecting higher frequency waves as they move from a gaseous medium in an alveolus to an aqueous medium in alveolar walls; this process is known as impedance mismatch. If gas within the alveoli is replaced by transudative or exudative fluid, the sound pathway no longer contains air-fluid interfaces. Impedance mismatch is reduced, and the bronchial breath sounds emerging from the chest wall more closely resemble tracheal than bronchovesicular breath sounds. They are loud, tubular, and well heard through expiration.

If the topographic distributions of the bronchopulmonary segments are projected onto the chest wall and auscultation is performed over the center of each such segment, the sounds that are heard reflect those that have been generated, transmitted, and filtered by the airways and parenchyma of that segment. They become evidence of the health or disease of that segment. A differential or double stethoscope contains two chest pieces; the sound from one chest piece goes only to the left ear, and sound from the other chest piece goes only to the right ear. If such an instrument is used for auscultation over equivalent (homologous) segments in the two lungs (e.g., the posterior basal segment of the right lower lobe and the same segment of the left lower lobe), the sounds in healthy people seem identical; that is, they begin, peak, and disappear at the same time and are equal in intensity and pitch. This state of phase, amplitude, and pitch likeness in the compared segments has been called *homophony* and is strong evidence that the lungs are normal (Figs. 7–3, 7–4). Differences in phasing, amplitude, or pitch between homologous segments constitute *heterophony* and thus suggest disease (Figs. 7–5, 7–6). Phonopneumography can be used to objectify and quantify both homophonous and heterophonous states.

ADVENTITIOUS SOUNDS

The term *adventitious* simply means "added on" and by itself does not imply a pathologic cause. However, most adventitious sounds indicate that the state of pulmonary health is less than perfect. Current practice decries the confusion that has evolved over the years in the various uses of the French word *râle* and the Latin word *rhonchus,* which were used as synonyms by Laënnec himself. Neither of these terms is now recommended; instead, the intrinsically descriptive terms *crackle* and *wheeze* have been advocated vigorously by Forgacs[2] and have been widely accepted.

The term *crackle* refers to soft or loud intermittent popping, snapping, frying, or crackling sounds, each of which is almost always less than 20 msec in duration. Although there may be more than one explanation for their production, the majority of crackles are thought to be caused by the sudden opening of an airway with accompanying noisy pressure equalization. They are often repetitive; that is, each crackle occurs at the same moment in the

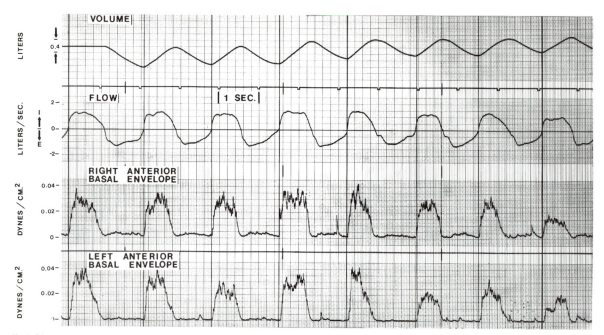

Figure 7-4. Phonopneumographic tracing of eight consecutive breaths in a normal 30-year-old man. Volume and flow signals, obtained at the mouth by a pneumotachograph, are used to analyze the corresponding sound amplitude envelopes as a function of time. Recordings were made simultaneously from the chest wall over right (R8) and left (L8) anterior basal segments of the lower lobes. The amplitudes and phasings of each set of paired breaths are very similar (equivalent to intensity and phase homophony). (From Waring WW: Physical examination of children. *In* Sackner MA [ed]: Diagnostic Techniques in Pulmonary Disease, Part I, p. 66. New York: Marcel Dekker, 1980.)

same phase of breathing with every breath. Crackles are thus frequently volume dependent.

Interstitial lung diseases typically are associated with end-inspiratory crackles, probably as a result of multiple small airways snapping open almost synchronously. Chil-

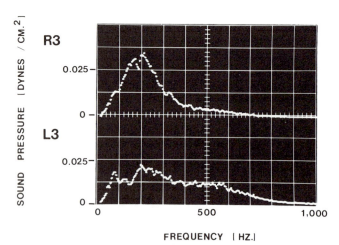

Figure 7-5. Frequency spectra of the same breaths recorded from the chest wall over the right (R3) and left (L3) posterior segments of the upper lobes in a 9-year-old child with a history of foreign body aspiration. Although peak frequencies are the same bilaterally (200 Hz), there is a striking difference between the two spectra: more sounds of higher frequencies (400 to 800 Hz) on the left than on the right. Clinical auscultation showed easily perceptible differences at these homologous sites with higher pitched breath sounds on the left (pitch heterophony). (From Waring WW: Physical examination of children. *In* Sackner MA [ed]: Diagnostic Techniques in Pulmonary Disease, Part I, p. 69. New York: Marcel Dekker, 1980.)

dren with bronchiectasis caused by cystic fibrosis, however, typically have paninspiratory crackles, which suggests that airways are opening throughout inspiration; the crackles may also be produced by the bubbling of air as it passes through bronchial secretions.

The different qualities of crackles have resulted in different descriptive terms. The crackles in interstitial lung disease are termed dry, fine, close to the ear, or "Velcro," whereas those in chronic obstructive lung disease are described as coarse or wet. Expanded waveform analysis, a variant of phonopneumography, has been used for studying crackles. A computer and analog-digital/digital-analog converters are used to slow down the recordings of crackles so that their waveforms can be precisely displayed. From such displays, crackle intensity over time can be measured. Two such measurements on each crackle have been suggested for use in discriminating between crackles that have been termed "fine" and those termed "coarse" by a competent auscultator: initial deflection width (IDW) and the two-cycle duration (2CD) (Fig. 7-7). Fine crackles have shorter IDWs (<1 msec) and 2CDs (<6 msec) than coarse crackles. Other methods of differentiating crackle types have been described. It is clear that computers enable the counting, displaying, and timing of discontinuous adventitious lung sounds with a precision that far exceeds that of the human ear.

Continuous adventitious lung sounds differ in many ways from discontinuous adventitious lung sounds, as exemplified by crackles. The continuous sounds are longer and are almost always phenomena of the large airways. They may be extrapulmonary (stridor) or intrapulmonary (wheeze) in origin. Regardless of the site of origin,

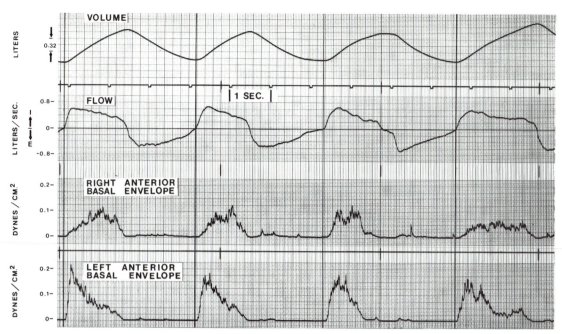

Figure 7–6. Phonopneumographic tracing of four consecutive breaths in a 9-year-old child (same patient as in Fig. 7–5) recorded from the chest wall over the right and left anterior basal segments. Volume and flow signals corresponding to the sound tracings are shown. Although breaths begin and end synchronously on the two sides, there is a striking lag in the buildup of sound on the right, resulting in a gap between peaking of inspiratory sound signals on the two sides. On the first breath, this gap is approximately 800 msec in duration. Only the left inspiratory sound envelope is in phase with the inspiratory flow signal at the mouth, whereas peak sound intensity on the right is usually reached considerably after maximal inspiratory flow has occurred at the mouth. These recorded breath sounds document a striking phase heterophony previously noted on auscultation with a differential (double) stethoscope. (From Waring WW: Physical examination of children. *In* Sackner MA [ed]: Diagnostic Techniques in Pulmonary Disease, Part I, p. 70. New York: Marcel Dekker, 1980.)

stridor and wheeze share many acoustic qualities and are probably produced by similar mechanisms. A wheeze may be low-pitched or high-pitched, may alter its pitch, and, to the ear, may resemble chirps, coos, groans, or squeaks. Most have a distinctly musical quality and must last long enough for a judgment of musicality to be made

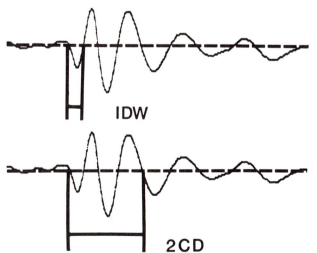

Figure 7–7. Expanded waveform analysis. Two measurements can be made for each crackle in order to separate fine from coarse crackles. The initial deflection width (IDW) shows the time (in milliseconds) of the first deflection of an identifiable crackle above or below the base line. The two cycle duration (2CD) is the time (in milliseconds) for two S-shaped waves, or cycles, to occur. (From Murphy RLH Jr: Discontinuous adventitious lung sounds. Sem Respir Med 6:212, 1985.)

(usually more than 20 msec). The pitch may range from 60 to >2000 Hz. Sound is probably produced by a resonating airway or glottis (in the case of stridor) that has been narrowed to near closure. The pitch of a wheeze is in theory set by airway size, tone, and structure, in addition to gas density and flow rate. Lower elasticity and higher airway mass, as well as lower flow rates, create lower pitched sounds. It is probable that continuous adventitious lung sounds require the faster gas flow rates that are characteristic of the large central airways and for that reason are not thought to originate in small airways, in which slow gas flows are the rule.

Phonopneumography has been used to visually display wheezes (Fig. 7–8) and to document the severity of asthma by automatically calculating the percentage of breaths containing the sustained frequencies that are characteristic of wheezing. Such methods should enable evaluation of triggers for acute episodes of asthma, as well as efficacy of therapy.

What is the future of phonopneumography? Murphy[3] speculated that "establishing standard ways of noting the presence of abnormal sounds over the chest at many sites (lung sound mapping) is likely to provide a method for following the course of some diffuse lung diseases. . . ." The key word here is *standard;* however, it is simply too early for standardization. Much more must be learned about lung sounds before phonopneumography equipment will roll off assembly lines. Although no uniform approach to lung sounds has yet been developed for this method, knowledge derived from unstandardized pho-

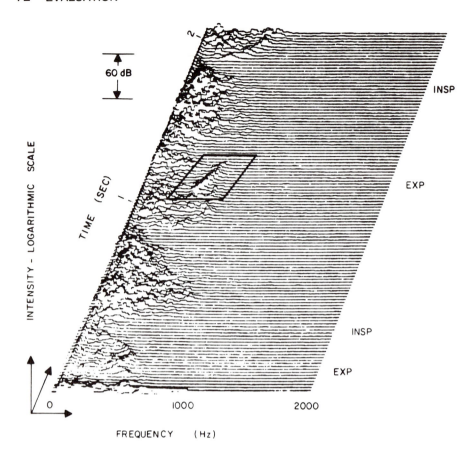

Figure 7–8. Phonopneumographic display with frequency (in Hertz) on the *x* axis, intensity (in decibels) on the *y* axis, and time (in seconds) on the *z* axis. The box marks an expiratory wheeze of about 250 msec that rises in pitch from 400 to 600 Hz over time. (From Wooten FT, Waring WW, Wegmann MJ, et al: Method for respiratory sound analysis. Med Instrum 12:254–257, 1978.)

nopneumographic techniques has both strengthened and improved the use of the conventional stethoscope (e.g., the timing of crackles during inspiration as a clue to the differentiation between restrictive and obstructive lung diseases). Modest as such advances individually may seem, collectively they greatly enhance auscultatory skills while the standardization of lung sound mapping is being developed.

REFERENCES

1. Kraman SS (ed): Lung Sounds [Special Issue]. Sem Respir Med 6:157–242, 1985.
2. Forgacs P: Lung Sounds, p. 2. London: Baillière Tindall, 1978.
3. Murphy RLH Jr: Future directions and potentials. Sem Respir Med 6:239–241, 1985.

8 APPLICATION OF DIAGNOSTIC IMAGING TECHNIQUES IN PEDIATRIC PULMONARY DISEASES

DENISE MULVIHILL, M.D.

The array of equipment and techniques available today in the field of diagnostic imaging is impressive and, at the same time, confusing. Engineering advances surpass the radiologist's ability to adequately evaluate the newer imaging devices and to formulate guidelines for efficient and cost-effective diagnostic evaluation. To date, no single modality adequately handles the wide spectrum of anatomy and disease presented to the pulmonologist. Applications formulated for adults may be inappropriate for pediatric diseases and usually fail to account for the small size and rapid respiratory rate of young children and infants. This chapter is an attempt to describe currently available techniques, and (in the second section) describe their strengths and weaknesses in delineating specific areas in relation to pulmonary disease. Detailed knowledge of each modality enables a diagnostic imaging approach to be tailored to each patient.

TYPES OF IMAGING TOOLS

Imaging methods can be categorized by the type of information provided: (1) anatomic studies, which include both plain radiographs and tomography; (2) dynamic examinations, such as fluoroscopy and ultrasonography; and (3) functional studies, which are basically nuclear medicine procedures.

With the development of each new piece of equipment, it has been the hope that the diagnostic information available would surpass simple anatomic description and would provide tissue characterization such as benign versus malignant or inflammatory versus neoplastic. To date, no imaging method—computed tomography (CT), ultrasonography, or magnetic resonance imaging—has been able to reliably fulfill this dream.

ANATOMIC STUDIES

Standard Radiographs

Despite all the new equipment, standard radiography remains the primary screening tool for evaluating pulmonary diseases and their complications. Anatomic information, with few exceptions, most appropriately begins with the global view provided by standard radiographs. In pulmonary disease, this view is most often provided by a frontal and a lateral chest film. Attempts at screening with only a single view have been unsuccessful.[1] Not only does the addition of a lateral view increase confidence and provide better localization of disease, but significant areas of the thorax are not adequately visualized on a frontal film. Although most examinations are ideally obtained at peak inspiration, an end-expiratory phase exposure is occasionally desired. Oblique projections further increase the ability to localize or confirm disease and are particularly helpful when ribs or mediastinal structures overlie a lesion. The information from oblique views may be important for determining which imaging procedure is most appropriate when further information is necessary.

On high-kilovoltage exposures, bone appears less dense radiographically, and thus the air-containing structures are accentuated and evaluation of the mediastinum and airway is easier. The addition of a filter aids in fading out the shadows produced by overlying bone. Similar enhancement can be obtained with the digitalization of standard radiographs. Digitalization has been extensively evaluated for the chest and will probably become the routine in all large diagnositc imaging departments. The decrease in resolution of some radiographic units to date has not affected significantly the detection of disease, and the advantages are many.[2] These advantages include the ability to manipulate the image, which enables the magnification of select areas as well as improving visualization of the mediastinum and retrocardiac areas through changing penetration and contrast. Comparable films for which the same technical factors are used can be reproduced, which makes the follow-up after disease easier.[3]

Another standard radiographic projection is the lateral decubitus examination, for which the patient lies on his or her side and the x-ray beam is parallel to the floor. In such films, gravity is used to demonstrate pathologic processes that may be obscured by overlapping shadows. In this way, free pleural effusion layers on the dependent side and free air rises. Because both air and fluid can be obscured by mediastinal structures, suspected air or fluid should be made to rise or fall to the periphery. In children, the restriction of motion in the dependent thorax can be used in decubitus radiographs to provide an expiratory view of the lung on the bottom (dependent lung) and an inspiratory view of the lung on top (nondependent lung). In this way, air trapping can be assessed[4] (Fig. 8–1). A forced expiratory film is another method of checking for focal air trapping. This is accomplished by manually compressing the abdomen during normal expiration in an attempt to obtain an end-expiratory exposure.[5] Both these techniques are used to obtain inspiratory and expiratory films in young children who cannot cooperate with radiographic procedures.

The cross-table lateral examination is less optimal for using gravity as an aid in diagnosis than the techniques described earlier. Cross-table lateral studies are obtained only for patients who cannot turn on their side, usually because of the presence of chest tubes or other apparatus. This technique can identify air that rises to the anterior thorax, but the findings are often difficult to interpret because of the superimposition of structures.

Standard radiographs of the extrathoracic areas associated with pulmonary disease focus on the head and neck. Routine sinus views usually consist of Waters, posteroanterior, lateral, and basal views. The basal projection is very difficult or impossible to obtain in all children except adolescents. If feasible, the examination should be obtained in the upright position in order to evaluate for air-fluid levels. A cross-table lateral exposure may be substituted, but, as with most cross-table examinations,

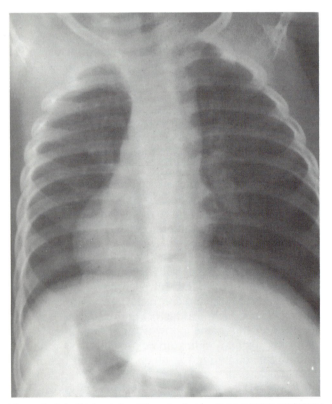

Figure 8–1. Left lateral decubitus chest view demonstrates expiratory changes in the dependent lung with diffuse increased opacity to the lung, narrowing of the rib interspaces, and elevated left hemidiaphragm, in comparison with the well inflated right lung.

superimposed structures makes interpretation of the findings difficult.

In the initial evaluation of the nasopharynx and the oropharynx, the lateral view is sufficient. Overlapping facial bones render the frontal image worthless. The hypopharynx, the larynx, and the extrathoracic trachea are best examined with frontal and lateral projections. It is technically difficult to obtain an adequate lateral neck view in a young child. The film must be obtained at full inspiration with the head extended. A filter and a high-kilovoltage technique improve airway visualization in the anteroposterior view.[6] Faulty interpretation of poor-quality studies is responsible for many of the misdiagnoses in this area.

Tomography

Tomography enables visualization of anatomic detail of a small area devoid of overlapping shadows and thereby increases delineation of structures. Plain tomography is no longer used in diagnosing pulmonary and neck disease. The long exposure time and increased scatter radiation render this modality useless for children. This form of tomography has been supplanted by CT and magnetic resonance imaging (MRI). Both types of imaging equipment display anatomic detail tomographically.

The superiority of CT over standard tomography is attributable in part to the greatly enhanced ability of CT to differentiate radiographic densities. This is in the order of a factor of 10.[7] The usual method of display is limited to axial projection; coronal imaging is available for the head and face in patients who can adequately extend the neck. Multiplanar reconstruction, such as that generated in coronal, sagittal, or oblique sections, can be generated from axial scans, although the resolution is significantly lower. Scans can be obtained with a slice thickness that varies between 1.5 mm and 10 mm. The choice of slice thickness is determined by the size and location of the suspected abnormality. Both radiation exposure and examination time are decreased with the use of wider slices, but information averaging can obscure pathologic processes, particularly in small children.

Other variables include slice spacing, which can vary from widely spaced cuts (slices) for diffuse lung disease to contiguous slicing necessary for viewing the hila and the mediastinum and when the suspected pathologic process could be smaller than the slice thickness. Scan time can also be selected. Short scan times of approximately 2 sec improve image quality because of the reduction in respiratory and cardiac motion but, at the same time, lose some resolution. This can be a problem with the rapid respiratory rate of infants. Breath holding by a patient who can cooperate is rewarding in terms of study quality.

Contrast enhancement is an attempt to increase the natural intrinsic contrast between adjacent structures. Injection of iodinated contrast material opacifies vascular structures and is often important for evaluating mediastinal disease in children, in whom little or no mediastinal fat is present to provide natural differentiation as in adults. Vascular masses can also be studied in this manner. Because the contrast agent passes into the extravascular compartment in a matter of seconds, interval doses may be needed. This procedure is difficult to accomplish in infants and children.

Finally, manipulation of the digitalized image enables the enhancement of specific areas. By adjusting the density and window width, maximal diagnostic information can be displayed for the mediastinum, bronchial anatomy, lung parenchyma, and bone. At this time, sagittal, coronal, and even oblique reconstruction can be obtained (Fig. 8–2).

Because of the number of variables in generating a diagnostic image, CT should not be considered a screening procedure, and specific information should be sought. This information may be the further delineation of an abnormality already detected on plain radiographs or a specific area suspected on clinical examination. The more information available, the better the examination can answer a particular diagnostic problem.

High-resolution CT scans are attempts to improve spatial resolution.[8] Methods for optimizing examinations of the lung parenchyma in adults are now available.[9] Such procedures require thin collimation on the order of 1.5 mm and the use of a special high–spatial-frequency algorithm. This may necessitate an increase in the radiation dose to the patient.

Machines capable of generating ultrafast CT were initially developed for evaluating the heart. The acquisition of data in ultrafast CT is different from that in conventional CT, and standard machines cannot be upgraded to this technology. Therefore, the number of units in use is low, and their availability in the future is uncertain. This equipment is capable of generating an image in less than 1 sec and as many as 20 slices can be obtained in 10 sec-

onds. Not only can most studies be done without sedation of the patient, but there is a reduction in radiation dose to the skin.[10] Most striking, however, is an ability to eliminate respiratory and cardiac as well as voluntary motion on the image in children.[11] Such motion artifacts significantly degrade the image quality and diagnostic information in conventional CT scans. Ultrafast scan times are obtained at the cost of spatial resolution and slice thickness, which is in the range of 8 mm. Some compromise can be obtained with newer software that operates at 100 msec. The speed of the examination markedly reduces the amount of intravenous contrast required and ensures adequate opacification of the vessels. High-quality examinations can be obtained with approximately half the usual contrast dose.[10]

The newest tomographic modality is MRI. It is difficult to discuss MRI adequately because it is still in its infancy as an imaging tool and technical advances are occurring rapidly. The lack of ionizing radiation is clearly a significant advantage. Other important parameters in comparison with CT are superior soft tissue contrast and the ability to image in multiple planes, such as coronal and sagittal in addition to axial.

MRI makes use of the magnetic property of the hydrogen nuclei. When a patient is placed in a magnetic field, the protons align either with or against the applied field, but there is a small difference in the two populations that results in a slight net magnetization. The presence of this applied magnetic field not only aligns the protons but causes a precessional motion that is analogous to a spinning top. In order to generate a signal, a second magnetic field induced by a radio frequency signal is applied perpendicular to the main magnetic field, causing the protons to rearrange. When the radio frequency field is discontinued, a signal is emitted as the protons realign to the main magnetic field. This process is known as *relaxation,* and the time required for realignment is labeled T_1. At the same time, the protons lose coherence, spinning in different directions, and a further loss in signal strength is observed. This further loss in detectable current is also called *relaxation,* and the time required for this loss is referred to as T_2.

The observed differences in relaxation times for different tissues is related largely to the total water content and the proton density of the tissue. An increase in water content increases both T_1 and T_2. These relaxation times determine the contrast between tissues and enable application of techniques that increase tissue differentiation.

In order to shorten the length of time necessary for acquiring sufficient information to generate an image, several fast-scanning techniques were developed. These scanning parameters are constantly changing in an effort to reduce motion artifact. Application to the chest is still limited in pediatric patients. Further difficulties in the thorax occur at soft tissue–air interfaces, where differences in magnetic susceptibility cause signal loss. Millisecond MRI units are being designed and may have value in imaging the chest.

At the present time, spatial resolution is poorer in MRI than in conventional CT because of the inherent cardiac and respiratory motion artifacts produced by the long data-acquisition times for conventional MRI. These

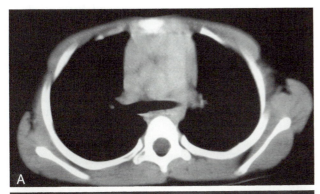
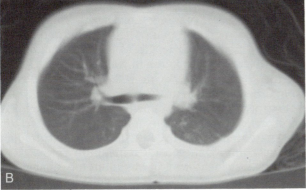

Figure 8–2. *A,* Computed tomographic (CT) scan of the chest obtained at the level of the carina with settings for evaluation of mediastinum. *B,* CT scan at same level but at settings chosen for parenchymal viewing.

times are in the span of several minutes, as opposed to several seconds for CT. The poorer resolution can cause a cluster of small nodes to appear as one enlarged node. Although cardiac gating is easily performed, respiratory gating is technically more difficult, and both techniques significantly prolong an examination.

A second significant problem in chest MRI is an inability to obtain a signal from calcifications on routine scans. The presence or absence of calcifications is important in the diagnosis of some chest diseases. In addition, MRI scans are technically more difficult to obtain. It is necessary to place the patient entirely within the magnet, which is encased in the 6-foot-long tube. Claustrophobia and difficulty in monitoring patients can present problems. Pulse oximeters that function reliably within the magnet are available.[12] Adaptations for oxygen and compressed air in the room can be made for most machines. Ventilators that run on compressed air have been used, but such apparatus is much more difficult to use during MRI than during the performance of a CT scan.

DYNAMIC IMAGING

Dynamic imaging procedures display chest anatomy over time, which enables observations to be made during a respiratory or cardiac cycle.

Fluoroscopy

Fluoroscopy has traditionally been the dynamic imaging technology most often used in chest diseases. The resolution is less than that observed with plain radiographs, but the information provided by real-time viewing is often significant and unique. Fluoroscopy still plays a useful role in localizing and confirming disease before more definitive studies. Digitalization of fluoroscopic images is currently being assessed, but it also creates further loss of spatial resolution. However, the significant decrease in radiation makes this a promising technique.

The addition of a barium esophogram aids in evaluation of the swallowing mechanism, which can be studied in only this way and helps in the identification of mediastinal disease.

The role of bronchography seems limited today. In most cases, the bronchi can be imaged with less invasive procedures. The examination, however, can be easily obtained in a patient already intubated.

Dynamic Computed Tomography

Dynamic CT involves rapid sequential scanning in one given area. This may involve a single slice or a few slices. This technique is usually used for the evaluation of suspected vascular lesions. With conventional scanners, this type of study requires breath holding for optimal results. The development of ultrafast scanners enables multiple images to be obtained during one respiratory cycle. This allows dynamic display of structures such as the trachea during inspiration and expiration.[11]

Ultrasonography

Ultrasound examination of the chest is severely limited by the inability of sound waves to penetrate air or bone. Both air-containing tissue and bone scatter the sound waves, thereby preventing any diagnostic assessment beyond these structures. Ultrasonography can accurately distinguish fluid from solid tissue and can readily visualize pleural and chest wall lesions. Intrathoracic masses that abut the chest wall can likewise be evaluated, as can fluid or a mass adjacent to the diaphragm, which is easily viewed from the abdomen (Fig. 8–3). The speed, the lack of radiation, and the portability of ultrasound equipment are important assets. Only very rarely is sedation needed for patients.

Angiography

Conventional angiography is rarely used for pulmonary disease because many vascular lesions can be identified by significantly less invasive means, specifically MRI. Digital subtraction angiography (DSA) can be performed through the venous route if fine vascular detail is not needed. DSA can also be performed as an arterial study, which allows the use of small catheters and small amounts of contrast. The difficulty with digital subtraction studies is the need for the patient to remain motionless during the filming in order for the subtraction of overlying structures to be achieved. Any motion results in significant degradation of the image.

Digital subtraction techniques have been used for structures other than vessels. Bones and soft tissues can be subtracted, which enables visualization of predictably moving structures such as the diaphragm and airway. Again, the patient must be motionless.

FUNCTIONAL IMAGING STUDIES

Functional imaging procedures rely on radionuclides to delineate specific structures or organs. A radioactive gas such as zenon or, more commonly, a radionuclide-tagged particle is used. Spatial resolution is generally quite poor, but the target organ is specific, and overlying structures do not interfere with the image. Anatomic detail has improved with the development of single photon emission computed tomography. This tomographic technique is applied to images of a functional agent. Three-dimensional reconstruction provides better delineation. Such procedures increase the length of the examination and increase the need for sedation in young children.[13]

Ventilation-perfusion scans remain the most commonly ordered functional study in pulmonary disease. The lung perfusion is determined through the injection of tagged particles that form microemboli within the perfused lung parenchyma. Because the particles are trapped by the lung, images are generated in multiple projections, which provides identification of various lobes, including segments. In ventilation techniques with xenon, the child must breathe the gas from a mask while remaining motionless. Images are obtained during inspiration, equi-

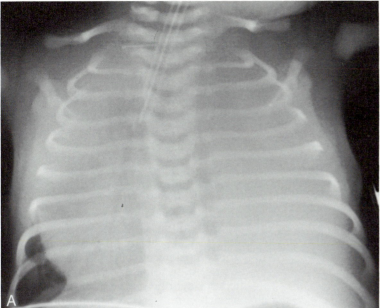

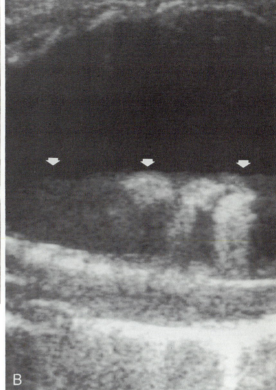

Figure 8–3. *A,* Anteroposterior chest view in a newborn reveals an opaque left hemithorax with shift of heart and mediastinum to the right. *B,* Ultrasound scan left hemithorax demonstrates collapsed lung *(arrows)* with very large fluid collection, which on examination proved to be chylous fluid.

librium, and washout phases. Because these phases are very short, the scans can be acquired in only one projection, usually the posterior. Thus segmental and subsegmental disease may be difficult to localize in only the posterior projection. Aerosol ventilation studies were developed for circumventing this problem. In this technique, aerosolized radionuclide particles are inhaled and deposited in ventilated lung. This enables different views to be obtained, although air trapping cannot be evaluated. This technique also requires some cooperation, but not to the degree that xenon ventilation studies demand. A newer agent, krypton 81m, has a very short half-life, resulting in low radiation doses and ease in use. Cooperation by patients is less critical; however, the agent is very expensive at the present time.

Aerosolized particles have likewise been used to evaluate mucus velocity (ciliary efficacy) in bronchi and trachea.[14] The location of precipitation can be controlled by the size of the labeled particles. These studies require the patient to remain motionless under a camera as the rate of the nuclide particle clearance is determined. Submicronic-sized labeled particles have been used in the evaluation of the integrity of the pulmonary epithelium after both acute and chronic insult.[15]

Ingestion of radionuclide-incorporated food or milk has been used to study gastric emptying, gastroesophageal reflux, and reflux-related aspiration. The evaluation of reflux by this method is cumbersome and mostly supplanted by pH probe monitoring. Aspiration, however, can be easily viewed with scanning of the lungs approximately 8 h after the ingestion of a radionuclide tracer.

This technique is specific in that any activity found in the lungs is abnormal, but the test may be insensitive. The rate of positive results in large series seems low, although the true incidence of disease is unknown.[16]

Both gallium 67 citrate– and indium-labeled white blood cells have been used to localize abscesses. These agents require up to 24-hr delay before imaging, and gallium 67 citrate cannot distinguish an abscess from a site of recent surgery.[17] The disadvantage of indium is that it does not localize in chronic infections. Both agents result in a higher radiation dose than do other labeled agents. Preliminary studies with technetium microaggregated albumin-labeled white blood cells, which require only a 30-min delay before imaging, are being evaluated.[13]

Radionuclide-tagged red blood cells have been used to study vascular lesions, particularly those that sequester red blood cells such as hemangiomas. For the best results, the patient's cells are removed and labeled. Other techniques involve the use of tagged red blood cells to identify bleeding sites.

APPLICATION OF IMAGING TOOLS

In this section, the application of different diagnostic modalities is discussed in relation to either specific anatomic areas or morbidity rates: (1) disease of the nasopharynx and sinuses, (2) abnormalities of the extrathoracic trachea, (3) obstruction of the intrathoracic trachea, (4) wheezing, (5) acute cough and fever, (6) chronic or recurrent lung disease, and (7) apnea and tachypnea.

NASOPHARYNX AND SINUSES

Anatomic Evaluation

Standard radiographs of the sinuses include Waters, frontal, and lateral views, which are obtained with the patient upright if at all possible. These views can provide limited anatomic detail in assessment of the maxillary sinuses and the frontal sinuses when they become aerated. Opacification or masses are signs of disease. The ethmoid air cells can not be accurately evaluated with standard radiographs. It is now believed that the ethmoid sinus is the space most commonly infected and is probably the focus from which infection spreads to the frontal and maxillary sinuses. Obstruction at the middle and superior meatal complex interferes with drainage of the frontal and maxillary sinuses, which is important in the pathogenesis of chronic sinusitis.[18]

Accurate anatomic detail can at present be obtained only from CT.[19] Mini-CT examinations consisting of five views in axial projection have been proposed as a form of initial screening.[20] This is followed by high-resolution scans if surgical intervention is contemplated. Direct coronal projection is preferred and, although somewhat uncomfortable, usually can be accomplished except in small children. Although high-resolution scans require a longer time, reasonable studies can be obtained because respiratory motion is not a problem (Fig. 8–4).

Other forms of obstruction, such as choanal atresia, require more specific anatomic detail than can be pro-vided by plain radiographs.[21] Bony atresia is clearly separated from membranous atresia, and coexisting anomalies can be identified. Bone defects, such as associated with tumor, are also readily demonstrated. CT is preferred to MRI in all cases in which accurate bone detail is needed. However, if lesions associated with the brain, such as encephaloceles, are being considered, MRI is superior because of better soft tissue discrimination and coronal projection.

Dynamic Evaluation

Fluoroscopy enables more precise positioning for a lateral view of the nasopharynx and for evaluation of the airway during inspiration and expiration. This is most helpful in infants and young children, in whom large adenoidal tissues can appear to fill the nasopharynx. Movement of the soft palate and lateral walls of the pharynx can also be studied. In some cases, a small amount of contrast instilled through the nose is necessary to delineate the airway. A barium swallow examination readily reveals reflux into the nasopharynx.

ABNORMALITIES OF THE EXTRATHORACIC TRACHEA

Obstruction of the airway is a common clinical problem. Children presenting with stridor can usually be des-

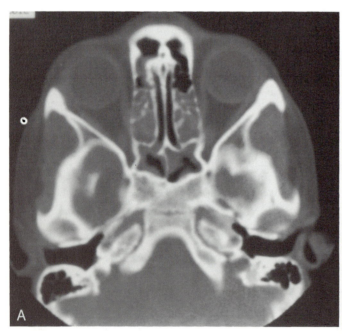

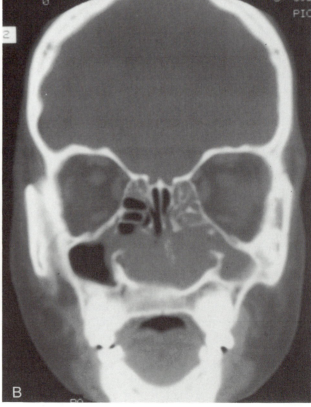

Figure 8–4. *A*, CT scan of the sinuses at the level of the ethmoids in the axial view shows opacification of posterior ethmoid air cells and sphenoid sinus. *B*, CT scan in the coronal projection reveals a large mass in the nasopharynx with opacification of left maxillary sinus and ethmoids. Clinical diagnosis was juvenile angiofibroma.

ignated by clinical examination as having findings suggestive of either extrathoracic or intrathoracic disease.

Anatomic Evaluation

In case of laryngeal and upper tracheal disease, anatomic evaluation of the airway begins with a soft tissue technique lateral radiograph of the neck. This view alone may be sufficient in cases of foreign body and epiglottitis, but when a more detailed display of this anatomy is needed, an anteroposterior view obtained with high kilovoltage and a copper-aluminum filter is indicated. The use of a filter and a high-kilovoltage technique changes the x-ray beam quality to allow the air column to stand out in comparison with the spine.[6] The added visualization is usually insufficient for complete characterization of pathologic processes but may suffice to confirm the presence of disease.

The radiographic anatomy can be most precisely delineated with CT and MRI. This delineation is most helpful when a mass is associated with an abnormal airway. The appearance and effect of the pathologic process are helpful for both diagnosis and therapy. The multidirectional imaging ability and the easy identification of major vessels render MRI theoretically superior for evaluating large masses, but CT is more sensitive in small intratracheal lesions. In both techniques, significant degradation of the images is caued by both voluntary and involuntary motion. Therefore, a higher quality examination is obtained in older, more cooperative children who are able to suspend respiration.

Like MRI, ultrasonography can clearly identify the major vessels of the neck and characterize an extraluminal mass, but it cannot depict the trachea itself or involvement of the spine. Ultrasonography is often used to describe and follow the extraluminal component of a hemangioma or a cystic hygroma.

Dynamic Evaluation

Dynamic evaluation of the upper trachea is easily accomplished by fluoroscopy. This technique often is helpful for distinguishing normal from abnormal airway caliber, particularly when the lateral view is suboptimal. The normal buckling of the trachea can be distinguished from displacement by mass simply and quickly at fluoroscopy. Video taping that includes audio recording is available and a worthwhile addition to the examination. Cine-CT, accomplished by means of an ultrafast CT unit, can demonstrate laryngomalacia and distinguish fixed from variable lesions by acquiring multiple images taken throughout one respiratory cycle.[22]

Functional Studies

A definite diagnosis of an ectopic thyroid can be made by a thyroid radionuclide scan. Gallium localizes at the sight of an abscess or lymphoma but is rarely necessary in such a superficial location. Tagged red blood cells are known to accumulate in hemangiomas, which thus distinguishes these lesions from lymphangiomas and may be a helpful consideration in the planning of therapy.

OBSTRUCTION OF THE INTRATHORACIC TRACHEA

Anatomic Studies

Anatomic evaluation of obstruction in this area begins with a frontal and a lateral chest film. Slight obliquity projects the tracheal air column away from the spine and improves visualization of the trachea and the carina. Oblique views are helpful for confirming and localizing a mediastinal mass but are not necessary if an obvious mass is to be studied by a more sensitive or specific modality. The CT characteristics of the normal trachea in children and infants have been studied over the years, and normal values for tracheal area and configuration have been determined.[23,24]

CT is particularly helpful for assessing intraluminal lesions and identifying or excluding associated masses. Small intraluminal lesions, however, may be missed, and image quality is, again, compromised by motion.

Although axial projections provide the most precise estimates of tracheal and bronchial narrowing, coronal and sagittal images are also helpful. Sagittal MRI sections are especially useful for localizing anteroposterior tracheal narrowing.[25] MRI, moreover, has a distinct advantage in an ability to demonstrate the mediastinal vessels clearly without contrast, which is extremely beneficial in view of the role of aberrant vessels in tracheal obstruction. The ability to obtain images along the long axis of the trachea in both coronal and sagittal projections also helps evaluate the extent of disease. Comparison of MRI with endoscopic evaluation of the trachea has shown close correlation of findings.[26]

Ultrafast CT, if available, may be the most appropriate examination for young infants. With only small amounts of contrast, mediastinal vessels are effectively demonstrated and consistently reveal vascular rings.

Dynamic Evaluation

Dynamic examination of the trachea helps distinguish fixed from variable lesions. This is readily accomplished with fluoroscopy. A slightly oblique projection, in which trachea appears separate from the spine, provides visualization of the entire trachea to the level of the carina. Video taping of the fluoroscopic study enables repeated observation. Fluoroscopy combined with a barium swallow study reveals most moderate-sized obstructing tracheal lesions.

Ultrafast CT has the advantage of obtaining optimal images at a predetermined site throughout one respiratory cycle. The exact role of dynamic CT in pediatric pulmonary disease is as yet unknown, although the information from one respiratory cycle may be useful for evaluating equivocal lesions. Because of the relatively thick slices, this technique is not helpful for identifying small, purely intraluminal lesions. However, tracheomalacia can be well demonstrated.[22]

Ultrasonography can image the mediastinum in infants under 6 months of age because of poor sternal ossification and a large thymus (Fig. 8–5). Cystic and solid masses are identifiable and can be easily distinguished from vascular

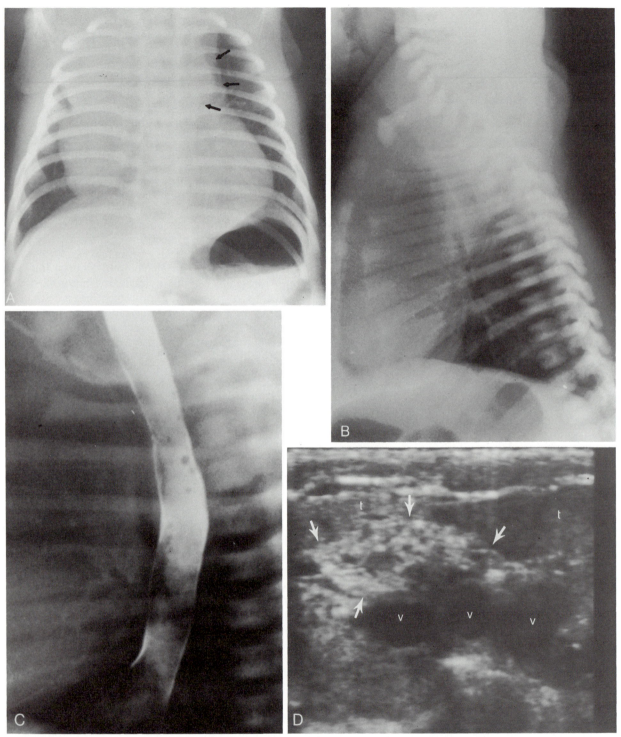

Figure 8–5. Posteroanterior (*A*) and lateral (*B*) chest views, in which a mass *(arrows, A)* is partially visualized through the thymic silhouette and mild posterior displacement of the trachea is shown on the lateral view. *C*, Lateral esophagram shows no displacement or mass effect. *D*, Ultrasound scan of the mediastinum localizes a mass *(arrows)* anterior to the major vessels (v) and behind the thymus (t).

structures by Doppler examination. The air column cannot be seen, and information about its caliber or configuration cannot be obtained.

Functional Studies

In the neck region, ectopic location of thyroid tissue is diagnosable by thyroid scan. Hemangiomas, which may be entirely in the thorax or may extend down from the neck, can be identified through the use of tagged red blood cells.

WHEEZING

Anatomic Evaluation

Radiographic assessment of obstruction at the level of the bronchi and smaller airways begins with a frontal and a lateral chest film. In cooperative children, such obstruction can be further studied by inspiratory and expiratory frontal views in order to detect air trapping. Deep inspiratory and expiratory radiographic exposures are difficult to obtain in small children, and so for this reason, right and left lateral decubitus projections are used. These films are sensitive to lobar obstruction, but segmental disease may be too subtle. A forced expiratory radiograph obtained by pressing the abdomen during expiration requires the help of additional radiography personnel, who are exposed to the primary x-ray beam. Although some investigators believe that this technique is more sensitive than the decubitus view,[5] it is not popular in many radiology departments.

CT scans performed with thin (1- to 2-mm) slices through the hilar areas can depict the major airways, even in young children. Respiratory motion resulting from the relatively long scanning time degrades images and almost eliminates the possibility of detecting small foreign bodies, such as food particles and small, purely intraluminal lesions. The disadvantage of ultrafast CT scanning, which can eliminate motion, is that scan slices are thick (approximately 7 mm) and thereby decrease resolution and average out small lesions.[10] Imaging of hilar masses, such as adenopathy, requires contrast in order to distinguish vessels from lymph nodes. Both conventional CT and ultrafast CT can demonstrate masses. However, the visualization of bronchial narrowing requires the spatial resolution of conventional CT, which is applicable in older children.

Spatial resolution is also decreased in MRI in comparison with conventional CT, but MRI can depict vessels without contrast. This facilitates the diagnosis of hilar masses and aberrant vasculature, such as a pulmonary artery sling. Although coronal images help confirm hilar masses, particularly when laterally placed, these accessory views do not add as much information when the trachea is imaged.

Dynamic Evaluation

Dynamic evaluation of the major bronchi by fluoroscopy provides limited information. The assessment of diaphragmatic movement or mediastinal shift secondary to air trapping is easily accomplished, but segmental disease is usually not perceived. Forced expiratory films can be obtained during fluoroscopy. Often the carina and the main stem bronchi are visualized, particularly in infants in whom the soft tissues of the thymus abut the major bronchi and are thus contrasted with the air column. Focal narrowing of the trachea may be visualized, but short stenotic segments may be missed. Dynamic CT can be used only indirectly to evaluate bronchial obstruction by depicting density differences in the lung throughout the respiratory cycle.[22] This technique should be sensitive even to segmental obstruction.

Functional Studies

Functional studies frequently reveal more widespread disease than is initially suspected. These studies include ventilation and perfusion scans and ciliary clearance studies. Xenon ventilation scans are sensitive to areas of decreased aeration and focal air trapping. Ventilation scans can be used to detect a suspected foreign body when chest radiographs are normal[27] or to confirm obstructive overinflation as opposed to compensatory hyperinflation.[28] Some degree of cooperation by the patient is needed, and the studies are usually unattainable in infants. Because only one projection is used, localization of disease is inexact. In aerosol ventilation studies, many projections ensure precise localization of the abnormality but do not demonstrate air trapping. Perfusion scans, which are easy to perform, generally match ventilation scans but may also give clues to congenital or developmental defects.

ACUTE COUGH AND FEVER

Anatomic Evaluation

Patients presenting with cough and fever usually require only a frontal and a lateral chest radiograph for initial diagnosis. It is the complications of acute infection, such as pleural effusion and abscess, that require further evaluation. Decubitus films are readily available and serve many purposes. Free fluid can be made to layer on the dependent side. Shifting free fluid to the side of the mediastinum enables the underlying lung parenchyma to be evaluated. Likewise, the use of gravity makes it possible to determine the extent of an abscess cavity containing air and fluid.

For further delineation, particularly in cases of pleural versus parenchymal disease, CT scanning is indicated. When a large, free pleural effusion is present, gravity can be used in prone and decubitus views to improve visualization of the parenchyma. In patients with both pleural and parenchymal disease, or for the localization of an abscess collection in the pleural space or parenchyma, CT examination is the preferred method. The shape of the lesion and the pleural-parenchymal interface facilitate assessment (Fig. 8–6), which usually requires contrast enhancement. Although CT can identify and localize focal fluid collections, the nature of the fluid cannot be

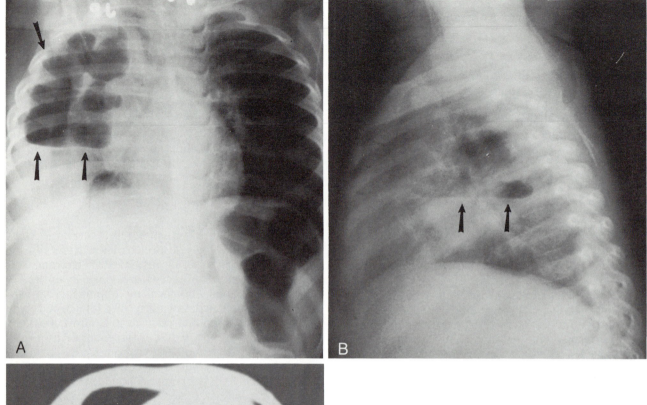

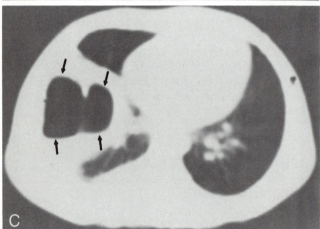

Figure 8–6. Posteroanterior (*A*) and lateral (*B*) chest views show large air fluid level in chest of a child with *Staphylococcus aureus* pneumonia. The exact location of the fluid was important for further therapy. *C*, CT scan localizes the loculated air and fluid collection to the pleural space.

determined, and empyemas appear similar to other fluid collections.

It was initially hoped that MRI would be able to characterize different fluids in the thorax. Intensity values from fluids vary, depending on protein content, but the complexity of biologic fluids have made categorization inconsistent.[29] Experimental models do show differences among various diseases, although these values have not been applied to the clinical situation. In one study, MRI distinguished fluid collections from masses with more certainty than did CT.[30] Also, pathologic processes near the apex and the diaphragm are better visualized with this modality[31] (Fig. 8–7). As of yet, MRI does not add sufficient additional information to the evaluation of the complications of acute inflammatory disease to justify its routine use.

Dynamic Studies

Ultrasound examination of the thorax provides a quick and easy assessment of pleural effusion, particularly loculated effusion. The area of maximal accumulation can be identified and marked for drainage. Deep collections located near the mediastinum are obscured by the lungs and are thus missed on ultrasound study; evaluation of such collections requires CT. The position of the diaphragm is easily determined, and subpulmonic fluid collection can be identified. Some characterization of fluid is possible when septations or floating debris are visualized.

The common uses of fluoroscopy are for checking diaphragmatic movement and for positioning or repositioning chest tubes for drainage of effusion or abscesses. In the presence of pleural effusion, diaphragmatic excursion is better judged through ultrasonography, in which the dia-

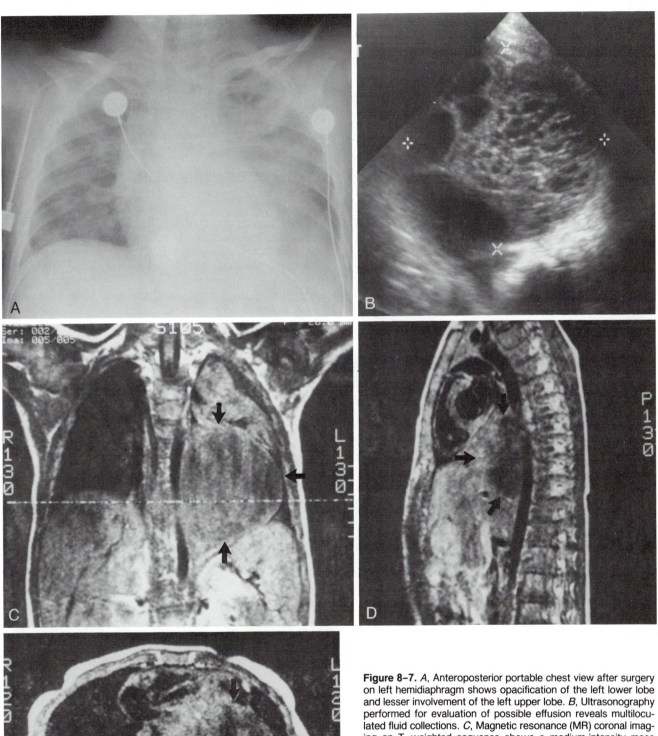

Figure 8–7. *A,* Anteroposterior portable chest view after surgery on left hemidiaphragm shows opacification of the left lower lobe and lesser involvement of the left upper lobe. *B,* Ultrasonography performed for evaluation of possible effusion reveals multiloculated fluid collections. *C,* Magnetic resonance (MR) coronal imaging on T_1-weighted sequence shows a medium-intensity mass *(arrows)* that is well defined and is causing atelectasis of left upper lobe and compression of aorta. *D,* MR sagittal midline image of same mass *(arrows)* compressing the aorta. *E,* MR axial view of mass *(arrows)* at the level of the right atrium. A loculated hematoma was found at surgery.

phragm is clearly visualized separately from the fluid in the chest. In the absence of thoracic disease adjacent to the diaphragm, fluoroscopy offers a larger field of viewing and an easier comparison of simultaneous movement of both hemidiaphragms than can be obtained with ultrasonography.

Functional Studies

Gallium 67 citrate scans play a significant role in the assessment of fluid collections and in excluding abscess when the anatomy is distorted. As of yet, indium-labeled leukocytes do not offer an advantage over gallium 67 citrate. Although gallium 67 citrate has been used to aid in the diagnosis of *Pneumocystis carinii* pneumonia in adults with acquired immunodeficiency syndrome, positive scans have been reported in cases of lymphoid interstitial pneumonitis; thus this test is sensitive but nonspecific.[32]

CHRONIC OR RECURRENT LUNG DISEASE

Anatomic Studies

Patients with chronic or recurrent lung disease usually have multiple chest radiographs, which are either nondiagnostic or inconclusive. Oblique views can help confirm or exclude an associated mass. When plain films show or suggest a mediastinal or hilar mass, CT or MRI is the next step for determining more precise anatomy. MRI is now generally undertaken for evaluation of posterior medias-

tinal masses because of its ability to evaluate the spine and easily depict vasculature, anomalies of which may be diagnostic in case of pulmonary sequestration.[33] Demonstration of enlarged bronchial vessels is an aid to the surgeon as well.

Middle mediastinal masses are well delineated by both CT and MRI procedures, and ultrafast CT, if available, is the technique of choice. The decrease in resolution, in comparison with conventional CT, would not significantly limit the evaluation of a mass recognized on plain film. The accurate identification of calcifications by CT generally renders conventional CT preferable to MRI if ultrafast CT is not available. An exception is in the evaluation of a vascular mediastinal mass or in mediastinitis for vascular compromise, in which case MRI is probably superior, particularly in young children (Fig. 8–8). Distinction among the mediastinal structures is often difficult even with contrast opacification. This is less of a problem in older children and teenagers.

Anterior and medial mediastinal masses in infants under 6 months of age can be studied with ultrasonography. This method clearly distinguishes cystic from solid structures and, in most cases, adequately delineates the extent of the lesion. Rapid respiratory rates and volume averaging by CT and MRI make for suboptimal study in infants.

In cases of chronic atelectasis, detailed demonstration of the hilum helps distinguish among the various causes. Anatomic assessment in children can be accomplished with ultrafast CT, if available, or, if not, with conventional CT. The ability to visualize calcifications and lobar bronchi by CT again outweighs the clearer identification of vascular structures by MRI.

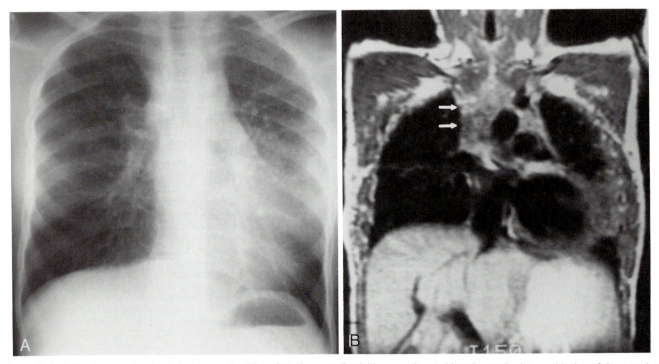

Figure 8–8. *A,* Posteroanterior chest view in a patient thought to have mediastinitis secondary to histoplasmosis shows widening of the superior mediastinum and loss of visibility of the left heart border. *B,* Magnetic resonance imaging (MRI) in coronal view shows loss of the expected signal void *(black areas)* from flowing blood in the region of the superior vena cava *(arrows).* This appearance is consistent with that of thrombus of the superior vena cava.

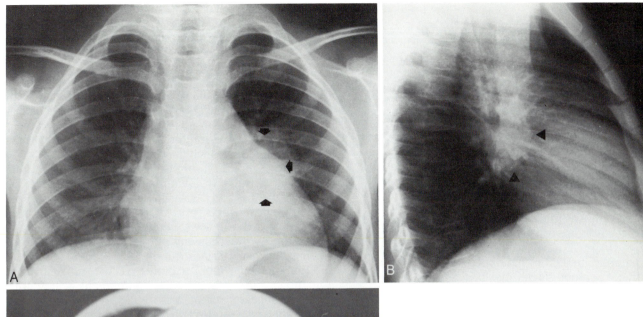

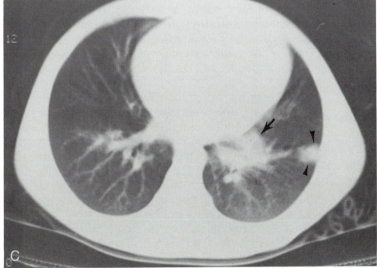

Figure 8–9. Posteroanterior (A) and lateral (B) chest views show a poorly defined left hilar mass *(arrows, A; arrowheads, B)*. *C*, CT scan reveals hilar mass *(arrows)*, an appearance consistent with that of adenopathy, as well as unsuspected lung nodule in the periphery *(arrowheads)*. Laboratory and clinical findings are consistent with histoplasmosis.

This area is also important in the recognition of bronchiectasis. Bronchiectatic changes have been clearly defined on high-resolution CT,[34] although initial reports with slices of 10 mm were disappointing for the detection of early disease.[35] Such scanning techniques as high-resolution CT increase the radiation exposure, prolong examination time, and are best directed to specific areas of disease rather than to the whole chest.

Parenchymal masses are in general still better imaged with CT than with MRI. The increase in resolution and the ability to identify landmarks such as fissures, as well as demonstration of calcifications, help localize and describe pathologic processes (Fig. 8–9). Much work has been done on characterization of interstitial lung disease in adults by CT and, more recently, by MRI. CT frequently shows involvement as being more extensive than as initially seen on plain films. This extent includes unsuspected involvement of remote areas and of locations difficult to evaluate, such as the retrocardiac space and the lung bases. Normal lung densities for children have been determined and make the detection of subtle disease easier.[36] Categorizing by localization (such as axial, middle,

and peripheral) and by configuration (such as reticular or nodular) has been attempted for some diffuse interstitial lung diseases in adults and has been suggested as a guide for lung biopsy. High-resolution CT scanning with 1.5-mm collimation is being used in adults to evaluate idiopathic pulmonary fibrosis, as well as in the categorization of fibrosing alveolitis, eosinophilic granuloma, and sarcoidosis.[37-39] Bullae, interstitial fibrosis with honeycombing, and small granulomas are clearly demonstrated when only uncertain or subtle findings are persistent on chest radiographs. In preliminary work on inflammatory disease, MRI showed differences in signal intensity for different pathologic processes.[40] As yet, these attempts at tissue characterization have not developed to a point of clinical significance.

One exception to the preferred evaluation of parenchymal disease with CT is in patients with cystic fibrosis. In these patients, it is difficult on chest radiographs to differentiate linear opacities from enlarged vessels, atelectasis, and bronchi with mucoid impaction. The ability of MRI to adequately evaluate mucoid impaction has proved helpful.[41]

Dynamic Studies

Dynamic studies in chronic and recurrent lung disease focus on the barium swallow examination. This method enables evaluation of the swallowing mechanism and the documentation of aspiration, tracheoesophageal fistula, dysmotility of the esophagus, obstruction, and reflux. Other methods are more sensitive to (and thus better indicators of) reflux, although it is important to look for causes of reflux such as partial gastric outlet or duodenal obstruction.

Some patients benefit from a contrast study of the tracheal and bronchial airways. This is usually limited to cases of multiple or diffuse narrowing that cannot be adequately studied by means of bronchoscopy.[42] This is possibly the only way in which the length, extent, and rigidity of a tight stricture can be determined in a young infant (Fig. 8–10).

Anatomic modalities have successfully demonstrated the site of hemoptysis but may be confusing in the presence of diffuse chronic lung disease.[43] Angiography is most helpful when there is active bleeding and when embolization of a large bronchial vessel is contemplated.

Functional Studies

Ventilation perfusion scans, like CT, often show more extensive disease than initially suspected from plain radiographs (Fig. 8–11). Abnormalities of perfusion give clues to congenital or developmental diseases because

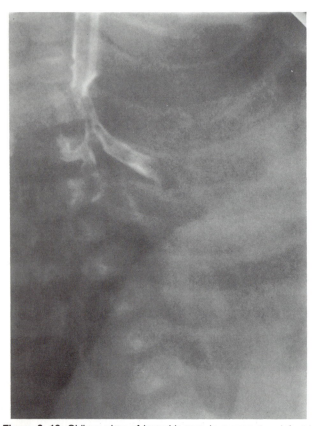

Figure 8–10. Oblique view of bronchiogram in a premature infant in whom bronchoscopy had been confusing. Severe narrowing of right main stem bronchus.

pulmonary emboli are rarely a diagnostic consideration in children. Overinflation can be categorized as compensatory or obstructive according to ventilation scans. Early changes of air trapping, particularly if diffuse, are difficult to detect on chest films.

Unlike indium-labeled white blood cells, gallium 67 citrate scans are useful in localizing chronic abscesses.[44] In the patient whose anatomy is distorted by previous disease, these functional studies may be helpful. However, in patients who have recently undergone surgery, results may be false, inasmuch as scans have remained positive for up to 18 months in adults.[17] Because gallium 67 citrate is highly sensitive to inflammatory processes, it can be used to identify and assess activity in interstitial lung disease, especially sarcoidosis.[44] More consistent results have been obtained with newer computerized methods of lung indexing.[45] Low specificity prevents this technique from being a primary diagnostic tool.

Radionuclide milk scanning is the only imaging method available for studying aspiration associated with gastroesophageal reflux. It is frequently performed with gastrointestinal scintigraphy for determination of reflux. These procedures require little cooperation. Quantification of reflux and of extent of reflux into the esophagus is readily available and is more accurate than barium swallow.

Tracheobronchial mucociliary clearance studies are performed in order to document and follow ciliary dysfunction.[45] In addition, pulmonary epithelial permeability studies have been performed with submicronic aerosol particles as a means of measuring the integrity of the pulmonary epithelium.[15] The role of these studies in diagnosis and follow-up is not yet clear, but they may be helpful for determining disease activity in patients with chronic interstitial pneumonitis.

Red blood cells tagged with technetium have been used to localize massive pulmonary hemorrhage when the anatomic modalities are nondiagnostic. Most reports have concerned patients with cystic fibrosis.[46] This technique has been shown to be effective if the patient is actively bleeding at the time. The sensitivity of this procedure is not known, and its chief role may be in patients who are not being considered for angiographic embolic therapy.

APNEA AND TACHYPNEA

Patients with apnea and tachypnea may have few clinical findings other than apnea of respiratory disease. Included in this group are patients with incidental findings noted on radiographs taken for other reasons, including preoperative chest films for nonpulmonary disease.

Anatomic Studies

Only occasionally are the pulmonary etiologic processes of apnea obvious on plain radiographs, but chest and neck films may demonstrate suspicious areas. Foreign bodies in the larynx and trachea rarely are sufficiently radiopaque to be diagnostic, but loss or irregularity of definition of the air column walls may warrant further evaluation. Many of the abnormalities causing tachypnea are

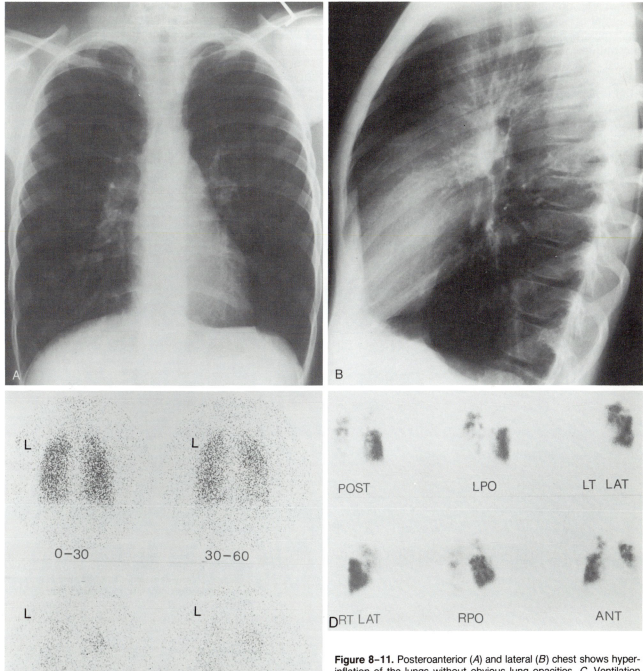

Figure 8–11. Posteroanterior (*A*) and lateral (*B*) chest shows hyperinflation of the lungs without obvious lung opacities. *C*, Ventilation scan reveals air trapping that is diffuse with the exception of the right lung base. *D*, Perfusion scan demonstrates severe, diffuse perfusion defects throughout the left lung and right upper and middle lobes. The right lower lobe is less involved.

present on chest films. These abnormalities include conditions that result in decreased anatomic or functional lung volume. In the patient with a spontaneous pneumothorax, an expiratory or decubitus chest film may be all that is needed to confirm a subtle finding on plain radiography. The air trapping in congenital lobar emphysema can be demonstrated with expiratory or lateral decubitus films.

More detailed anatomic imaging centers on the evalu-

ation of tracheal obstruction or mediastinal and parenchymal mass that replaces or compresses lung tissue. Further imaging of intratracheal obstruction for foreign body or soft tissue mass is best accomplished by CT, particularly by ultrafast scans. MRI is superior for determining the vascular nature of extratracheal masses, such as aberrant vessels causing rings or slings. Large mediastinal masses, such as bronchogenic cysts, can be defined by either CT or MRI. The advantage of MRI in defining the extent of a lesion is the ability to image in both coronal and sagittal projections. In the case of a posterior mediastinal mass, such as neurogenic tumor or extralobar sequestration, which is usually an incidental finding on chest radiograph, MRI is indicated and may be diagnostic.

MRI is also a technique of choice for small parenchymal lesions that cause respiratory disease through shunting of blood. The vascular nature of such arteriovenous malformations should be apparent on MRI, particularly with the newer techniques that give vessels a high-intensity signal.

Other Dynamic Studies

Although fluoroscopy has less resolution than do plain films, the dynamic imaging of the trachea may be suffi-

cient to confirm a tracheal intraluminal mass. Barium swallow is still the most rapid and inexpensive method of ruling out a vascular ring. However, the presence of an indentation on the esophagus is only indirect information and usually requires more definite imaging before surgery.

Both ultrasonography and fluoroscopy can be diagnostic aids in cases of diaphragmatic disorder, such as paralysis and hernia. The rocking motion visualized during fluoroscopy is diagnostic for diaphragmatic paralysis and distinguishes this entity from a right-sided diaphragmatic defect in which the liver has herniated into the chest. Similar findings are seen with ultrasonography. Likewise, an opaque hemithorax can be evaluated with ultrasonography which can accurately detect fluid in the pleural space or define mediastinal structures in the case of pulmonary agenesis. Left-sided diaphragmatic hernias in which

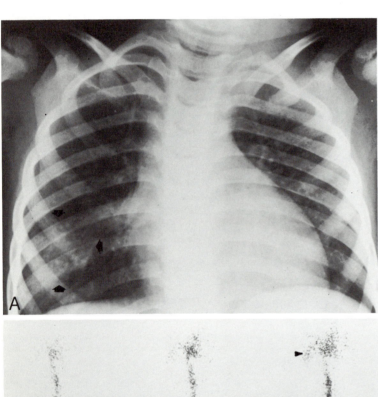

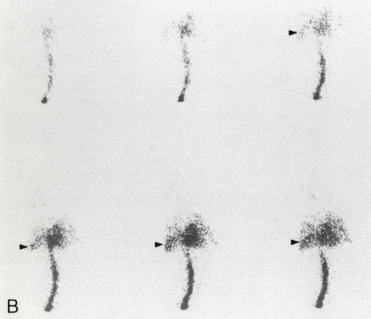

Figure 8–12. *A,* Posteroanterior chest view indicates an ill-defined opacity in the right lung *(arrows)* in a cyanotic patient. *B,* Radionuclide study with tagged red blood cells localizes a vascular malformation right lung base *(arrows).*

bowel loops are found in the thorax are more characteristic on plain chest. On occasion, this appearance may require differentiation from a cystadenomatoid malformation by means of a barium upper gastrointestinal study.

Functional Studies

The obstructive nature of congenital lobar emphysema and cystic adenomatoid malformation of the lung is best demonstrated on radionuclide lung scans. Either failure to ventilate or significant air trapping can distinguish the lesion from compensatory overinflation. Radionuclide-tagged red blood cells are another method for demonstrating vascular lesions in the lung such as arteriovenous malformations (Fig. 8–12).

REFERENCES

1. White H: Respiratory disease of later infancy. Semin Roentgenol 7:85–121, 1972.
2. Fraser RG, Breatnach E, Barnes GT: Digital radiography of the chest: Clinical experience with a prototype unit. Radiology 148:1–5, 1983.
3. Kogutt MS, Jones JP, Perkins, DD: Low-dose digital computed radiography in pediatric chest imaging. AJR 151:775–779, 1988.
4. Capitanio MA, Kirkpatrick JA: The lateral decubitus film: An aid in determining air-trapping in children. Radiology 103:460–462, 1972.
5. Wesenberg RL, Blumhagen JD: Assisted expiratory chest radiography. Radiology 130:538–539, 1979.
6. Joseph PM, Berdon WE, Baker DH, et al: Upper airway obstruction in infants and small children. Radiology 121:143–148, 1976.
7. Naidich DP, Zerhouni EA, Spiegelman SS: Computed Tomography of the Thorax. New York: Raven Press, 1984.
8. Webb WR, Stein MG, Finkbeiner WE, et al: Normal and diseased isolated lungs: High-resolution CT. Radiology 166:81–87, 1988.
9. Mayo JR, Webb WR, Gould R, et al: High-resolution CT of the lungs: An optimal approach. Radiology 163:507–510, 1987.
10. Frey EE, Sato Y, Smith WL, Franken EA: Cine CT of the mediastinum in pediatric patients. Radiology 165:19–23, 1987.
11. Brasch R: Ultrafast computed tomography for infants and children. Radiol Clin North Am 26:277–286, 1988.
12. McArdle C, Nicholas DA, Richardson CJ, Amparo EG: Monitoring of the neonate undergoing MR imaging: Technical considerations. Radiology 159:223–226, 1986.
13. Gainey MA, Capitanio MA: Recent advances in pediatric nuclear medicine. Radiol Clin North Am 26:409–418, 1988.
14. Zwas ST, Katz I, Belfer B, et al: Scintigraphic monitoring of mucociliary tracheo-bronchial clearance of technetium-99m macroaggregated albumin aerosol. J Nucl Med 28:161–167, 1987.
15. O'Brodovich H, Coates G: Pulmonary clearance of ^{99m}Tc-DTPA. A noninvasive assessment of epithelial integrity. Lung 165:1–16, 1987.
16. McVeagh P, Howman-Giles R, Kemp A: Pulmonary aspiration studied by radionuclide milk scanning and barium swallow roentgenography. Am J Dis Child 141:917–921, 1987.
17. Hatfield MK, MacMahon H, Martin WB, Ryan JW: The effects of previous thoracic surgery on gallium uptake in the chest. J Nucl Med 28:1831–1834, 1987.
18. Babbel RW, Harnsberger HR: A contemporary look at the imaging issues of sinusitis: Sinonasal anatomy, physiology, and computed tomography techniques. Semin Ultrasound CT MRI 12:526–540, 1991.
19. Zinreich SJ, Kennedy DW, Rosenbaum AE, et al: Paranasal sinuses: CT imaging requirements for endoscopic surgery. Radiology 163:769–775, 1987.
20. Arnold JP, Lee BCP, Seibert JA, McGahan JP: Mini CT of the paranasal sinuses: Replacement of the standard series on screening for benign sinus disease. Presented at the annual meeting of the Association of University Radiologists, New Orleans, 1988.
21. Slovis TL, Renfro B, Watts FB, et al: Choanal atresia: Precise CT evaluation. Radiology 155:345–348, 1985.
22. Brasch RC, Gould RG, Gooding CA, et al: Upper airway obstruction in infants and children: Evaluation with ultrafast CT. Radiology 165:459–466, 1987.
23. Griscom NT: Cross-sectional shape of the child's trachea by computed tomography. AJR 140:1103–1106, 1983.
24. Effmann EL, Fram EK, Vock P, Kirks DR: Tracheal cross-sectional area in children: CT determination. Radiology 149:137–140, 1983.
25. Fletcher BD, Dearborn DG, Mulopulos GP: MR imaging in infants with airway obstruction: Preliminary observations. Radiology 160:245–249, 1986.
26. Kangarloo H: Chest MRI in children. Radiol Clin North Am 26:263–275, 1988.
27. Samuel J, Houlder AE: Use of Xe-133 gas in the detection of foreign bodies in the lower respiratory tract. Clin Otolaryngol 12:115–117, 1987.
28. Loewy J, O'Brodovich H, Coates G: Ventilation scintigraphy with submicronic radioaerosol as an adjunct in the diagnosis of congenital lobar emphysema. J Nucl Med 28:1213–1217, 1987.
29. Moore EH, Webb WR, Muller N, Sollitto R: MRI of pulmonary airspace disease: Experimental model and preliminary clinical results. AJR 146:1123–1128, 1986.
30. von Schulthess GK, McMurdo K, Tscholakoff D, et al: Mediastinal masses: MR imaging. Radiology 158:289–296, 1986.
31. Epstein DM, Kressel H, Gefter W, et al: MR imaging of the mediastinum: A retrospective comparison with computed tomography. J Comput Assist Tomogr 8:670–676, 1984.
32. Schiff RG, Kabat L, Kamani N: Gallium scanning in lymphoid interstitial pneumonitis of children with AIDS. J Nucl Med 28:1915–1919, 1987.
33. Siegel MJ, Nadel SN, Glazer HS, Sagel SS: Mediastinal lesions in children: Comparison of CT and MRI. Radiology 160:241–244, 1986.
34. Grenier P, Maurice F, Musset D, et al: Bronchiectasis: Assessment by thin-section CT. Radiology 161:95–99, 1986.
35. Muller NL, Bergin CJ, Ostrow DN, Nichols DM: Role of computed tomography in recognition of bronchiectasis. AJR 143:971–976, 1984.
36. Vock P, Malanowski D, Tschaeppeler H, et al: Computed tomographic lung density in children. Invest Radiol 22:627–631, 1987.
37. Bergin CJ, Muller NL: CT of interstitial lung disease: A diagnostic approach. AJR 148:9–15, 1987.
38. Bergin CJ, Muller NL: CT in the diagnosis of interstitial lung disease. AJR 145:505–510, 1985.
39. Nakata H, Kimoto T, Nakayama T, et al: Diffuse peripheral lung disease: Evaluation by high-resolution computed tomography. Radiology 157:181–185, 1985.
40. Cohen MD, Eigen H, Scott PH, et al: Magnetic resonance imaging of inflammatory lung disorders: Preliminary studies in children. Pediatr Pulmonol 2:211–217, 1986.
41. Gooding CA, Lallemand DP, Brasch RC, et al: Magnetic resonance imaging in cystic fibrosis. J Pediatr 105:384–388, 1984.
42. Hauft SM, Perlman JM, Siegel MJ, Muntz HR: Tracheal stenosis in the sick premature infant. Am J Dis Child 142:206–209, 1988.
43. Haponik EF, Britt EJ, Smith PL, Bleecker ER: Computed chest tomography in the evaluation of hemoptysis. Chest 91:80–85, 1987.
44. Baughman RP, Shipley R, Eisentrout CE: Predictive value of gallium scan, angiotensin-converting enzyme level and bronchioadveolar lavage in two year follow-up of pulmonary sarcoidosis. Lung 165:371–377, 1987.
45. Specht HD, Brown PH, Haines JE, et al: Gallium-67 lung index computerization in interstitial pneumonitis. J Nucl Med 28:1826–1830, 1987.
46. Miller JH, Wang CI, Osher AB: The detection of sites of pulmonary hemorrhage in patients with cystic fibrosis utilizing technetium 99m red blood cells [Abstract]. J Nucl Med 27:923–924, 1986.

9 PULMONARY FUNCTION TESTING IN INFANTS

ROBERT TEPPER, M.D., Ph.D.

During the 1980s, there was an increase in interest in understanding the unique respiratory physiology of the infant and in the impact of respiratory illness during infancy on the subsequent growth and development of the lung. The motivation for being able to assess the pulmonary function of infants resulted in a reevaluation of some of the older methods that have been used to assess respiratory mechanics in infants, as well as a reevaluation of the development of some newer techniques. Pulmonary function testing of infants offers the same potential benefits that can be obtained from the testing of older children: (1) the assessment of respiratory physiology and the pathophysiologic processes associated with disease, (2) improving clinical assessment of respiratory disease, (3) assessing the efficacy of therapeutic interventions, and (4) understanding the natural history of acute and chronic respiratory disease.

Infants are usually evaluated while they are sleeping because they cannot actively cooperate with testing when they are awake. Sleep can be either spontaneous or aided by the oral administration of chloral hydrate (50 to 75 mg/kg). In this chapter, several methods for assessing pulmonary function in infants are reviewed. In addition, specific applications of some methods are presented.

METHODS

LUNG VOLUME

Functional Residual Capacity

The lung volume at the end of a passive tidal expiration is the functional residual capacity (FRC) and represents the lung volume that can most readily be measured in sleeping infants. The measurement of functional residual capacity allows for the assessment of lung growth with age. In addition, respiratory mechanics are related to lung volume, and therefore measurements are often referenced to the lung volume at which they are obtained.

Helium Dilution. In infants, FRC is most often measured by the helium dilution technique.[1, 2] The infant breathes into a closed circuit (Fig. 9–1) that contains a water-sealed spirometer, a helium analyzer, a blower for preventing rebreathing and for enhancing mixing in the

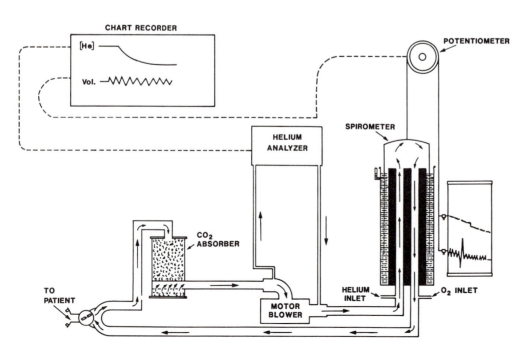

Figure 9–1. Closed-circuit helium dilution circuit for the measurement of functional residual capacity (FRC) in infants.

circuit, a CO_2 absorber, and an oxygen supply that can be regulated to compensate for the oxygen consumed during the measurement. While the infant breathes into the circuit, helium in the circuit equilibrates with the gas in the lungs.

The helium concentration decreases until it reaches a new steady state, and equilibration is considered to be complete when the helium concentration remains constant for 30 sec. From the known initial volume of the circuit (V_I), and the initial and final helium concentrations (He_I and He_F), the unknown lung volume (FRC) added to the circuit can be calculated as follows:

$$FRC = \frac{He_I - He_F}{He_F} V_I$$

In calculating FRC, the following volume changes need to be accounted for: (1) not accurately adjusting for oxygen consumption, (2) lung volume above FRC when an infant starts to equilibrate with helium, and (3) the dead space of the breathing valve and mask. Helium is an extremely insoluble gas, and no significant amount is absorbed from the lungs during the testing. The measurement of FRC is repeated in triplicate; most infants have three values that are within 10% of each other.

Nitrogen Washout. The nitrogen washout technique has also been used to measure FRC in infants. While 100% oxygen is inspired, the amount of nitrogen eliminated from the lung equals the lung volume at which oxygen breathing was initiated, divided by the initial nitrogen concentration in the lung. The amount of nitrogen expired can be quantified either by collecting the expired gas or by integrating the product of flow and nitrogen concentration.[3, 4] The latter method has been described for use in infants.

The infant breathes into a face mask attached to a T connector, which is supplied with a bias flow of gas at a precisely known flow rate. The bias flow rate is higher than the infant's peak inspiratory flow so as to prevent rebreathing. The infant exhales into the bias flow, which is directed through a mixing chamber in which the mixed exhaled nitrogen concentration is measured. While the bias flow is switched from room air to 100% oxygen, the mixed exhaled nitrogen concentration is measured continuously with a nitrogen analyzer, and the analog signal of the nitrogen concentration is integrated either electronically or digitally. The amount of nitrogen exhaled during the nitrogen washout equals the product of the integrated nitrogen signal, the known bias flow rate, and a calibration factor determined from a known volume of nitrogen. The concentration of the mixed exhaled nitrogen depends on the size of the infant, the bias flow rate, and the size of the mixing chamber. The amount of nitrogen washed out from stores in the body other than the lung is neglected in the calculation of FRC in infants.

Both the helium dilution and the nitrogen washout methods for measuring FRC reflect only the volume of gas that readily communicates with the central airways during tidal breathing. Airways that are either severely or totally obstructed do not equilibrate with either the helium or the oxygen. Therefore, these two methods for measuring FRC may underestimate the actual lung volume in infants with obstructive airway diseases such as bronchopulmonary dysplasia, bronchiolitis, cystic fibrosis, and congenital lobar emphysema.

Thoracic Gas Volume

The thoracic gas volume (TGV) represents the total amount of gas in the chest at end of expiration, regardless of whether the gas freely communicates with the central airways during tidal breathing or is trapped behind obstructed airways. TGV is most frequently measured in a constant-volume whole-body plethysmograph by the application of Boyle's law, as initially described by Dubois and associates[5] and applied to newborns by Auld and co-workers.[6] Respiratory efforts against an occluded airway produce changes in alveolar pressure (PA) and in box pressure (Pbox) secondary to movement of the chest wall. TGV can be calculated by assuming that during airway occlusion, the change in mouth pressure (Pm) reflects the change in PA and that the change in Pbox reflects the change in TGV:

$$TGV = (Pbar - 47) \times \frac{Pbox \times Bfact}{Pm \times Mfact},$$

where Bfact and Mfact are calibration factors and Pbar is barometric pressure.

The difference in the lung volume obtained by the gas dilution and the plethysmographic techniques is referred to as "trapped gas." This measurement has been used in older children and adults as an index of small airway obstruction in diseases such as asthma and cystic fibrosis. Although plethysmography has long been considered the gold standard for the assessment of lung volume, there has been increasing concern as to the accuracy of this method. Studies in adults have revealed that in the presence of airway obstruction, TGV can be an overestimate of lung volume secondary to the underestimation by Pm of the change in PA.[7, 8] In infants, the difference in the value of TGV measured at end of inspiration and end of expiration does not equal the volume measured during tidal expiration.[9, 10] This may result from airway closure at lower lung volumes and because Pm may not accurately reflect changes in PA. In addition, in comparison with a plethysmograph for an adult the box for infants has a high ratio of surface area to volume, which affects its thermal time constant. Sly and co-workers demonstrated that in the box for infants, gas compression is not adiabatic, and if it is not corrected, TGV will be overestimated.[11]

In contrast to these findings of overestimating TGV, Godfrey and collaborators found that TGVs were less than predicted in infants with bronchiolitis, which is contrary to the clinical and radiographic observations of hyperinflation in such patients.[12] In light of these results, the accuracy of the plethysmographic technique in measuring TGV in infants with obstructive airways disease remains uncertain.

COMPLIANCE

The elastic properties of the respiratory system are quantified by the measurement of compliance, which is defined as the change in volume that occurs for a given change in the applied pressure. Ideally, compliance should be measured under static conditions so that the measurement reflects the pressure required for overcoming the elastic forces of the respiratory system and not the additional pressure required for overcoming the resistive forces. In infants, compliance is generally measured at a lung volume in the range of tidal breathing. If the relationship between volume and pressure is nonlinear, then the measured value of compliance depends on the absolute lung volume at which the measurement is obtained.

Tidal volume in an infant can be measured directly by having the infant breathe into a spirometer or indirectly by integrating a flow signal measured by a pneumotachometer or by measuring pressure changes in a constant-volume plethysmograph. The volume change for the lung, the chest wall, and the total respiratory system (lung and chest wall) are the same; however, the applied pressures across each of their surfaces are different, which reflects the differences in their elastic properties. For pulmonary compliance, the applied pressure is measured as the difference in the airway and the pleural pressures. The chest wall compliance is measured from the difference in the pleural and ambient pressures, and the total respiratory system compliance is calculated from the difference in the airway and the ambient pressures.

Pulmonary Compliance

Changes in pleural pressure are estimated by measuring the esophageal pressure changes with a catheter passed through the nose or the mouth. Most often, the esophageal catheter is filled with air and has a small 1- to 2-cu cm balloon at its distal end to prevent secretions from occluding the catheter or dampening the pressure signal. The volume of air in the balloon needs to be adjusted so that the compliance of the air-filled balloon accurately transmits the changes in the applied pressure.[13] Water-filled catheters can also be used; however, it is necessary to ensure that the system has an adequate frequency response and that the signal is not dampened by air bubbles.[14] Compliance is calculated from the changes in pressure and volume between end of inspiration and expiration.[15] These two times are chosen because they are associated with zero airflow at the mouth and thus best approximate static conditions. This measurement, however, is referred to as *dynamic pulmonary compliance* (Cdyn) because the respiratory system is not truly under static conditions during spontaneous tidal breathing. In the presence of tachypnea or airway obstruction, Cdyn underestimates static compliance because there is inadequate time for the pressure and volume to equilibrate within the respiratory system.

Studies of premature infants and of infants with respiratory disease have raised concerns as to the validity of the assumption that changes in esophageal pressure accurately reflect changes in the pleural pressure.[16–19] In this age group, chest wall distortion during tidal breathing results in a pressure gradient along the esophagus, and therefore catheter position reflects only the local changes in pleural and esophageal pressures. Chest wall distortion changes with age, sleep state, body positioning, and res-

piratory disease. The airway occlusion test has been proposed as a method of evaluating the relationship between esophageal and pleural pressure.[20] Respiratory effort against an occluded airway should result in equal pressure changes at the mouth and in the esophagus, if esophageal pressure change accurately reflects changes in the pleural pressure. When these conditions are not met, the validity of the measurement must be questioned.

Total Respiratory System Compliance (Crs)

For measurement of Crs, mouth pressure is referenced to ambient pressure, and the need to estimate pleural pressure is eliminated. However, the relative contributions of the lung and the chest wall cannot be obtained, although in neonates the chest wall is very compliant and contributes relatively little to the compliance of the total respiratory system. Two different methods, the weighted spirometer and the airway occlusion technique, have been proposed for assessing total respiratory system compliance.

Weighted Spirometer Technique. In this method, the closed-circuit spirometer system described for the measurement of FRC is used.[21] While the infant breathes into the closed circuit, a weight is applied to the spirometer bell for 5 to 10 breaths. The weight produces a constant distending airway pressure (P) of approximately 3 cm H_2O within the circuit and results in an increase in the infant's end-expiratory lung volume (V) (Fig. 9–2). The Crs of the infant can be calculated by subtracting the volume change attributed to the circuit alone from the volume change measured with the infant's breathing into the circuit, and then dividing by the applied pressure (P). Different weights can be placed on the spirometer bell so that a pressure-volume curve can be constructed. This technique measures a quasi-static compliance. Although the infant continues to breathe during the measurement of Crs, the applied pressure is maintained over several breaths and therefore allows adequate time for equilibration of the pressure and volume changes in the lung. It is assumed that the positive end-expiratory pressure in the circuit does not produce respiratory effort at end of expiration, which would decrease chest wall compliance and Crs.

Airway Occlusion Technique. In neonates, airway occlusion elicits the Hering-Breuer reflex, a brief apnea with relaxation of the respiratory muscles. If the Hering-Breuer reflex is successfully obtained, mouth pressure increases and then plateaus for at least 200 msec, which reflects the recoil pressure of the respiratory system[22] (Fig. 9–3). By occluding the airways at different lung volumes within the tidal volume range, a pressure-volume curve can be constructed, and Crs can be calculated as the slope of the pressure-volume curve. In addition, the volume intercept of the pressure-volume curve reflects FRC (P = 0). In infants, end-expiratory lung volume can be higher than FRC, inasmuch as expiration may not be passive.[23] Compliance can also be calculated from a single end-expiratory airway occlusion. If the end-expiratory lung volume and FRC (P = 0) are the same, the inspiratory lung volume divided by the relaxation pressure at end of inspiration accurately reflects Crs. However, if the end-expiratory lung volume is above FRC, the pressure-volume

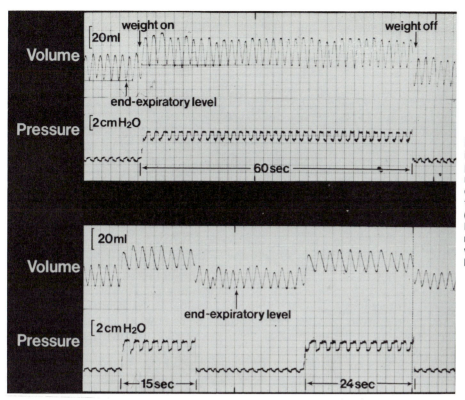

Figure 9–2. Volume-pressure tracings showing a constant end-expiratory level during a prolonged application of the weight to the spirometer bell *(top)* and reproducible changes in end-expiratory level during repetitive applications and removals of the weight *(bottom)*. (From Tepper RS, Pagtakhan RD, Taussig LM: Noninvasive determination of total respiratory system compliance in infants by the weighted-spirometer method. Am Rev Respir Dis 130:461–466, 1984).

curve does not have a zero intercept, and compliance is underestimated when calculated from the inspiratory volume. The actual volume above FRC can be measured by extrapolating to zero flow the linear pressure-volume curve that occurs when the airway is unoccluded after the Hering-Breuer reflex.[24, 25]

After the neonatal period and in the presence of an increased respiratory drive secondary to respiratory disease, the Hering-Breuer reflex becomes more difficult to elicit. The expiratory volume clamping (EVC) technique has been proposed as a method of enhancing the Hering-Breuer reflex by occluding the airway at elevated lung volumes.[26] Increased lung volumes are obtained by allowing

the infant to inhale through a nonrebreathing valve in which the expiratory port is occluded. After each tidal breath to an elevated lung volume, the Hering-Breuer reflex is more likely to be elicited before the next inspiration. After three inspiratory tidal volumes, the infant is then allowed to exhale. Crs can be calculated at a lung volume above FRC by measuring the slope of the measured inhaled volumes and recoil pressures.

AIRWAY FUNCTION

Distribution of Ventilation

The efficiency of the mixing of gas within the lung can be assessed from the equilibration of the helium in the closed circuit during the measurement of FRC.[1, 2] The mixing index is defined as the ratio of the predicted to the actual number of breaths required for the helium to reach 90% of its final concentration. The predicted number of breaths is calculated from an equation in which the measured FRC is considered a single, homogeneous lung volume ventilated with the measured tidal volume. In the presence of airways disease, the lung behaves as a multicompartment model with a heterogeneous distribution of ventilation. This heterogeneity results in an increase in the number of breaths required for the helium to equilibrate and therefore a lower mixing index. The mixing index is relatively sensitive to early stages of airway disease and can be low in the absence of overt clinical symptoms, as has been demonstrated in a group of asymptomatic infants with cystic fibrosis (CF) in whom chest radiographs were normal.[27] However, the mixing index is relatively insensitive to changes in respiratory status. A

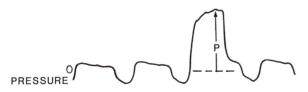
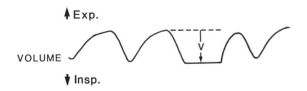

Figure 9–3. Tracings of tidal volume and mouth pressure. At end of inspiration, the airway is occluded, so that there is no change in volume. If the Hering-Breuer reflex is elicited, the mouth pressure rises rapidly to a plateau and represents the recoil pressure of the respiratory system. Exp., expirations; Insp., inspirations.

group of CF infants hospitalized for acute pulmonary exacerbation demonstrated improvement in their clinical status between admission and discharge, but the mixing index remained low with no significant change during hospitalization.[28]

Resistance

The resistance of the respiratory system can be measured either for the airway (Raw) or for the lung airways and the parenchyma combined (Rpulm). The difference in these two measurements relates to whether the driving pressure (P) producing the airflow is measured from mouth to alveoli (airway resistance) or from mouth to pleural space (pulmonary resistance).

Airways Resistance. The measurement of flow and alveolar pressure (PA) for the calculation of airways resistance can be performed in a constant-volume plethysmograph.[29] After thermal equilibrium has been attained within the plethysmographic box, the slope of airflow ($\dot{V}$) and box pressure (Pbox) is measured. In order to assess the relationship between Pbox and PA the infant's airway is occluded, and the slope of the mouth pressure (Pm) and Pbox is obtained. It is assumed that during airway occlusion, changes in Pm reflect changes in PA. Raw is calculated as follows:

$$\frac{Pm/Pbox}{\dot{V}/Pbox} = Pm/\dot{V} = PA/\dot{V} = Raw$$

Results are often expressed as airway conductance (Gaw), the reciprocal of resistance. Because there is a linear relationship between Gaw and lung volume, calculation of specific Gaw, $1/(Raw \times TGV)$, is an effective way of comparing differences in airway size that are caused by differences in lung volume.

Pulmonary Resistance. The measurement of pulmonary resistance requires the use of an esophageal catheter to estimate pleural pressure, which is similar to the method described for pulmonary compliance. Because resistance changes throughout tidal breathing, the measurement is most frequently standardized by calculating resistance at midinspiration and midexpiration.[30] Average respiratory resistance and average compliance over the respiratory cycle can be obtained through a least mean square analysis in which the driving pressure (P) is the sum of the elastic and resistive components:[31]

$$\Delta P_{pulm} = \frac{\Delta V}{C_{pulm}} + R_{pulm}\dot{V}$$

Total Respiratory System Resistance. The airway occlusion technique for the measurement of Crs can be used to measure total respiratory system resistance.[24] The product of resistance and compliance is in units of time (seconds) and is referred to as the time constant (τ), which reflects the time required for the respiratory system to empty. After an airway occlusion that elicits the Hering-Breuer reflex, unocclusion of the airway should result in a passive tidal exhalation.

The slope of the passive expiratory flow-volume curve is in units of 1/sec and represents the inverse of the time constant ($1/\tau$). If the flow-volume curve remains linear, it is assumed that the expiratory phase remained passive after the Hering-Breuer reflex. The total respiratory system resistance can be calculated by dividing τ by Crs, which is measured as described earlier.

The measurements of pulmonary and total respiratory system resistance include the combined resistances of the upper and lower airways. In infants, the nasal resistance alone can account for 40% of the total respiratory resistance.[32] Therefore, total airway resistance may be relatively insensitive to changes in the more peripheral airways. In addition, during a respiratory illness, upper respiratory symptoms can increase total resistance and further obscure the contribution of the lower airway.

Forced Expiratory Flow

The measurement of maximal expiratory flow-volume curves in infants represents a relatively new extension of infant pulmonary function testing methods that have routinely been used in older children and adults.[2, 33–36] At lower lung volumes, forced expiratory flow is limited by the mechanics of the lower airways and uninfluenced by the extrathoracic airways. Flow is measured by a pneumotachometer attached to a face mask. Care is taken to prevent upper airway obstruction either from compression of the nose and mandible with the face mask or from improper positioning of the head and neck. Volume is obtained by integration of the flow signal. The flow-volume curves can be displayed on a storage oscilloscope or a computer.

Forced expiratory flow is generated at end of inspiration by rapidly inflating (in <80 msec) a cuff that encircles the infant's chest and abdomen (Fig. 9–4). The cuff is inflated from a large-volume reservoir with an adjustable pressure. The partial expiratory flow-volume (PEFV) curves are quantified by measuring the flow at FRC. Forced expiratory flows are repeated at increasing compression pressures until a maximal expiratory flow at FRC, $\dot{V}_{max}$FRC, is obtained (Fig. 9–5A). It is important to continue to increase the applied pressures until a maximal flow is obtained because the actual pressure transmitted to the pleural space is not known. In addition, exceeding the optimal pressure for each infant can result in a decrease in the forced expiratory flow and the development of a concave shape to the PEFV curve. LeSouef and colleagues[37] suggested standardizing the transmitted pressure to the pleural space by measuring Pm generated during chest compression when the airway is occluded and with respiratory muscle relaxation produced by the Hering-Breuer reflex. This measurement, however, does not reflect the pleural pressure during the forced expiratory maneuver with the airway unoccluded and in the absence of the Hering-Breuer reflex. It is therefore most efficient to increase the applied pressure until a maximal flow-volume curve is obtained.

In normal, healthy infants, forced expiratory flow rises rapidly to a peak and then decreases: the PEFV curve has a linear or convex shape over the tidal volume range (Fig. 9–5A). In addition, there is a significant expiratory flow reserve between the tidal and the forced expiratory curves.

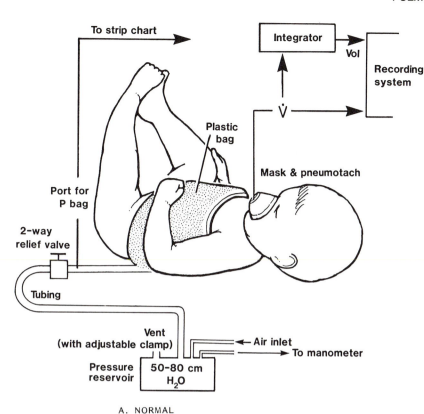

Figure 9–4. Schematic diagram of the rapid thoracic compression apparatus used to generate maximal expiratory flows in infants. (From Morgan WJ, Geller GE, Tepper RS, Taussig LM: Partial expiratory flow-volume curves in infants and young children. Pediatr Pulmonol 5:232–243, 1988.)

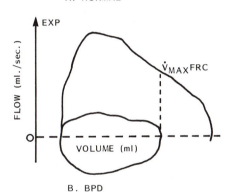

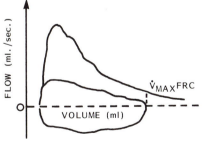

Figure 9–5. Partial expiratory flow-volume curves. Smaller inner curve represents tidal breathing, and larger curve represents maximal expiratory flow generated by rapid compression technique. Maximal expiratory flow at functional residual capacity ($\dot{V}_{max}FRC$) is indicated by dashed line. Difference between tidal breathing and maximal expiratory flow represents expiratory flow reserve. A, Convex to linear shape of maximal expiratory flow-volume curve, with large expiratory (EXP) flow reserve, in a normal control infant. B, Concave flow volume curve in an infant with bronchopulmonary dysplasia (BPD), with decreased expiratory flow reserve and decreased $\dot{V}_{max}FRC$, in comparison with the curve in A. (From Tepper RS, Morgan WJ, Cota K, Taussig LM: Expiratory flow limitation in infants with bronchopulmonary dysplasia. J Pediatr 109:1040–1046, 1986.)

In the presence of disease of the peripheral airways (bronchiolitis, cystic fibrosis, bronchopulmonary dysplasia), the flow-volume curve exhibits a rapid rise to a peak flow, the PEFV curve is concave, and the expiratory flow reserve decreases over the tidal volume range (Fig. 9–5B). In addition, $\dot{V}_{max}FRC$ is reduced. In infants with disease of the peripheral airways, the concavity of the PEFV curve reflects the rapid increase in airway resistance and the decrease of expiratory flow with decreasing lung volume.

The measurement of forced expiratory flows in infants has extended the ability to assess (1) respiratory physiology in infants, (2) the residual pulmonary dysfunction associated with bronchopulmonary dysplasia, (3) the impact of lower respiratory illness on the development of chronic lung disease, and (4) the effects of therapeutic interventions.[38–41] In addition, the forced expiratory maneuver has been effective in documenting and quantifying the presence of airway reactivity in infants.[42] The changes in the PEFV curves of a normal infant during a methacholine challenge are illustrated in Figure 9–6. After inhalation of normal saline and the lowest concentration of methacholine, there is no significant change in the PEFV curves. However, with increasing concentrations of methacholine, there is a decrease in $\dot{V}_{max}FRC$ and a change in the shape of the PEFV curve from convex to concave at the volume axis. Inhalation of metaproterenol results in bronchodilation and return of the PEFV curve to base line.

Airway obstruction in infants often produces wheezing, and the site of obstruction is sometimes difficult to localize clinically. In contrast to the concave shape of the flow-volume curve produced by peripheral airway obstruction, an obstruction in the central airways (vascular ring) pro-

METHACHOLINE BRONCHIAL CHALLENGE

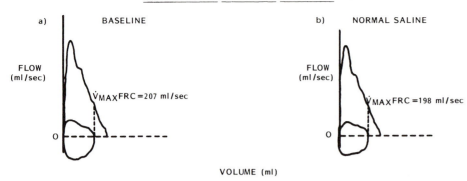

a) BASELINE

FLOW
(ml/sec)

$\dot{V}_{MAX}FRC = 207$ ml/sec

O

VOLUME (ml)

b) NORMAL SALINE

FLOW
(ml/sec)

$\dot{V}_{MAX}FRC = 198$ ml/sec

O

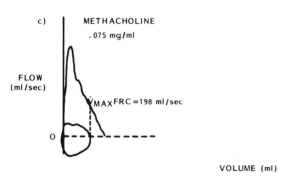

c) METHACHOLINE
.075 mg/ml

FLOW
(ml/sec)

$\dot{V}_{MAX}FRC = 198$ ml/sec

O

VOLUME (ml)

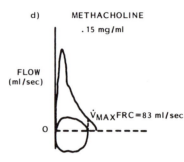

d) METHACHOLINE
.15 mg/ml

FLOW
(ml/sec)

$\dot{V}_{MAX}FRC = 83$ ml/sec

O

Figure 9–6. Partial expiratory flow-volume (PEFV) curves obtained during a methacholine challenge in a normal 5-month-old infant. There is no significant change in either the maximal expiratory flow at functional residual capacity ($\dot{V}_{max}FRC$) or the shape of the PEFV curve between base line and after inhalation of normal saline or the lowest concentration of methacholine (0.075 mg/ml). However, after inhalation of 0.15 mg/ml of methacholine, there is a significant decrease in $\dot{V}_{max}FRC$ and a concave shape to the PEFV curve. Inhalation of metaproterenol results in bronchodilation; $\dot{V}_{max}FRC$ returns to a level higher than base line, and the PEFV curve resumes a normal shape.

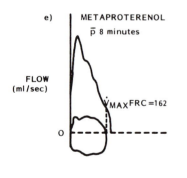

e) METAPROTERENOL
$\bar{p}$ 8 minutes

FLOW
(ml/sec)

$\dot{V}_{MAX}FRC = 162$

O

VOLUME (ml)

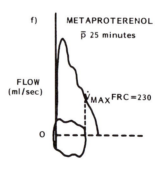

f) METAPROTERENOL
$\bar{p}$ 25 minutes

FLOW
(ml/sec)

$\dot{V}_{MAX}FRC = 230$

O

duces a flow-volume curve illustrated in Figure 9–7.[43] There is a poorly defined peak flow and a relatively constant reduced flow over the tidal volume range. This finding reflects the presence of flow limitation from a fixed lesion of the central airways in which resistance does not change with lung volume. After surgical correction of the vascular ring, the airway obstruction is relieved, and the PEFV curve appears normal.

CONCLUSIONS

In this chapter, several methods for assessing lung volume, compliance, and airway obstruction in infants have been reviewed. It is important to remember that in contrast to pulmonary function testing in older children and

VASCULAR RING

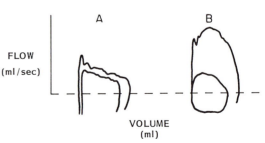

FLOW
(ml/sec)

A   B

VOLUME
(ml)

Figure 9–7. PEFV curves from an infant with a vascular ring (double aortic arch). *A*, Preoperative curve shows absence of a well-defined peak flow; the maximal expiratory flow remains relatively constant and low over the tidal volume range. *B*, One-year postoperative curve shows normal convex shape of PEFV curve with large expiratory flow reserve between the tidal and maximal flows. (From Tepper R, Eigen H, Brown J, Hurwitz R: Use of maximal expiratory flows to evaluate central airways obstruction in infants. Pediatr Pulmonol 6:272–274, 1989.)

adults, the methods used for infants have not been standardized with regard to technique, instrumentation, data acquisition, or how the results should be calculated. No single test can be applied universally to answer all questions related to respiratory function in infants. It is necessary to first ask a specific question and to then determine which method has the potential to answer that question. This choice depends on which measurement best reflects the physiology of interest and also on the intra- and intersubject variability of the measurement. Some pulmonary function tests are more sensitive for the early detection of pulmonary dysfunction, whereas others are better for assessing acute changes associated with respiratory disease and therapeutic interventions. Well-controlled clinical research studies will enable an assessment of the potential research and clinical applications of the many pulmonary function tests that are currently available for infants.

REFERENCES

1. Polgar G, Promadhat V: Pulmonary Function Testing in Children: Techniques and Standards. Philadelphia: WB Saunders, 1971.
2. Tepper RS, Morgan WJ, Cota K, et al: Physiologic growth and development of the lung during the first year of life. Am Rev Respir Dis 134:513–514, 1986.
3. Richardson P, Anderson M: Automated nitrogen-washout methods for infants: Evaluated using cats and a mechanical lung. J Appl Physiol 52:1378–1382, 1982.
4. Gerhardt T, Hehre D, Bancalari E, Watson H: A simple method for measuring functional residual capacity by N_2 washout in small animals and newborn infants. Pediatr Res 19:1165–1169, 1985.
5. Dubois A, Botelho S, Bedell G, et al: A rapid plethysmographic method for measuring functional residual capacity in normal subjects. J Clin Invest 35:322, 1956.
6. Auld P, Nelson N, Cherry R, et al: Measurement of thoracic gas volume in the newborn infant. J Clin Invest 42:476–483, 1963.
7. Shore S, Milic-Emili J, Martin JG: Reassessment of body plethysmographic technique for the measurement of thoracic gas volume in asthmatics. Am Rev Respir Dis 126:515–520, 1982.
8. Rodenstein D, Stanescu D, Francis C: Demonstration of failure of body plethysmography in airway obstruction. J Appl Physiol 52:949–954, 1982.
9. Beardsmore C, Stocks J, Silverman M: Problems in the measurement of thoracic gas volume in infancy. J Appl Physiol 52:995–999, 1982.
10. Helms P: Problems with plethysmographic estimation of lung volume in infants and young children. J Appl Physiol 53:698–702, 1982.
11. Sly P, Lanteri C, Bates J: Effect of the thermodynamics of an infant plethysmograph on the measurement of thoracic gas volume. Am Rev Respir Dis 139(Part 2):A382, 1989.
12. Godfrey S, Beardsmore CS, Maayan C, Bar-Yishay E: Can thoracic gas volume be measured in infants with airways obstruction? Am Rev Respir Dis 133:245–251, 1986.
13. Beardsmore CS, Helms P, Stocks J, et al: Improved esophageal balloon technique for use in infants. J Appl Physiol 49:735–742, 1980.
14. Asher M, Coates A, Collinge J, Milic-Emili J: Measurement of pleural pressure in neonates. J Appl Physiol 52:491–494, 1982.
15. Mead J, Whittenberger J: Physical properties of the human lungs measured during spontaneous respiration. J Appl Physiol 5:779, 1953.
16. Beardsmore CS, Stocks J, Silverman M: Esophageal pressure in infants at elevated lung volumes and positive airway pressure. J Appl Physiol 55:377–382, 1983.
17. LeSouef PN, Lopes JM, England SJ, et al: Influence of chest wall distortion on esophageal pressure. J Appl Physiol 55:353–358, 1983.
18. LeSouef PN, Loupes JM, England SJ, et al: Effect of chest wall distortion on occlusion pressure and the preterm diaphragm. J Appl Physiol 55:359–364, 1983.
19. Thomson A, Elliott J, Silverman M: Pulmonary compliance in sick low birthweight infants. Arch Dis Child 58:891–896, 1983.
20. Milic-Emili J, Mead J, Turner J, Glauser E: Improved techniques for estimating pleural pressures from esophageal balloons. J Appl Physiol 19:207–211, 1964.
21. Tepper RS, Pagtakhan RD, Taussig LM: Noninvasive determination of total respiratory system compliance in infants by the weighted-spirometer method. Am Rev Respir Dis 130:461–466, 1984.
22. Olinksy A, Bryan AC, Bryan MH: A simple method of measuring total respiratory system compliance in newborn infants. Afr Med J 50:128, 1976.
23. Mortola JP, Milic-Emili J, Noworaj A, et al: Muscle pressure and flow during expiration in infants. Am Rev Respir Dis 129:49–53, 1984.
24. LeSouef PN, England SJ, Bryan AC: Passive respiratory mechanics in newborns and children. Am Rev Respir Dis 129:552–556, 1984.
25. Guslets B, Wilkie R, England S, Bryan AC. Comparison of methods of measurement of compliance of the respiratory system in children. Am Rev Respir Dis 136:727–729, 1987.
26. Grunstein MM, Springer C, Godfrey S, et al: Expiratory volume clamping: a new method to assess respiratory mechanics in sedated infants. J Appl Physiol 62:2107–2114, 1987.
27. Tepper RS, Hiatt PW, Eigen H, Smith J: Total respiratory system compliance in asymptomatic infants with cystic fibrosis. Am Rev Respir Dis 135:1075–1079, 1987.
28. Tepper R, Ackerman V, Eigen H: Changes in lung function during hospitalization and at follow-up in CF infants. 2nd Annual North American CF Conference, Orlando, FL, 1988.
29. Stocks J, Levy NM, Godfrey S: A new apparatus for the accurate measurement of airway resistance in infancy. J Appl Physiol 43:155–159, 1977.
30. Kreiger I: Studies in mechanics of respiration in infancy. Am J Dis Child 150:439–448, 1963.
31. Bhutani V, Sivieri E, Abbasi S, Shaffer T: Evaluation of neonatal pulmonary mechanics and energetics: A two factor least mean square analysis. Pediatr Pulmonol 4:150–158, 1988.
32. Polgar G, King G: The nasal resistance of newborn infants. J Pediatr 67:557–567, 1965.
33. Hyatt R, Schilder D, Fry D: Relationship between maximum expiratory flow and degree of lung inflation. J Appl Physiol 13:331–336, 1958.
34. Adler SM, Wohl ME: Flow-volume relationship at low lung volumes in healthy term newborn infants. Pediatrics 61:636–640, 1978.
35. Taussig LM, Landau LI, Godfrey S, Arad I. Determinants of forced expiratory flows in newborn infants. J Appl Physiol 53:1220–1227, 1982.
36. Taussig LM: Maximal expiratory flows at functional residual capacity: A test of lung function for young children. Am Rev Respir Dis 116:1031–1038, 1977.
37. LeSouef P, Hughes D, Landau L: Shape of forced expiratory flow-volume curves in infants. Am Rev Respir Dis 138:590–597, 1988.
38. Tepper RS, Morgan WJ, Cota K, Taussig LM: Expiratory flow limitation in infants with bronchopulmonary dysplasia. J Pediatr 109:1040–1046, 1986.
39. Morgan WJ, Geller GE, Tepper RS, Taussig LM: Partial expiratory flow-volume curves in infants and young children. Pediatr Pulmonol 5:232–243, 1988.
40. Hiatt P, Eigen H, Yu P, Tepper RS: Bronchodilator responsiveness in infants and young children with cystic fibrosis. Am Rev Respir Dis 137:119–122, 1988.
41. Tepper R, Hiatt P, Eigen H, et al: Infants with cystic fibrosis: Pulmonary function at diagnosis. Pediatr Pulmonol 5:15–18, 1988.
42. Tepper RS: Airway reactivity in infants: A positive response to methacholine and metaproterenol. J Appl Physiol 62:1155–1159, 1987.
43. Tepper R, Eigen H, Brown J, Hurwitz R: Use of maximal expiratory flows to evaluate central airways obstruction in infants. Pediatr Pulmonol 6:272–274, 1989.

10 CLINICAL APPLICATIONS OF PULMONARY FUNCTION TESTING IN CHILDREN AND ADOLESCENTS

BETTINA C. HILMAN, M.D. / JULIAN L. ALLEN, M.D.

Pulmonary function tests enable clinicians to document normality or the degree of impairment of lung function and to monitor the effect of growth, disease, or treatment on lung function. When respiratory impairment is identified, pulmonary function tests enable physicians to characterize the type of dysfunction physiologically. Lung function testing also provides objective information for evaluating the risks of procedures or for assessing the prognosis of respiratory impairment. Some general clinical indications for pulmonary function studies in children and adolescents are outlined in Table 10–1.

Table 10–1. CLINICAL INDICATIONS OF PULMONARY FUNCTION STUDIES IN CHILDREN

To determine whether there is any objective evidence of significant impairment of lung function (e.g., to assess symptoms such as cough or dyspnea)

To quantify the degree of severity of impairment of lung function

To characterize any pulmonary dysfunction physiologically as obstructive, restrictive, or mixed obstructive and restrictive dysfunction

To assist in the identification of the site of airway obstruction (small versus large airway obstruction)

To differentiate fixed obstruction of central airway from variable obstruction of extra- or intrathoracic airway

To monitor the effect of growth on lung dysfunction

To follow the course of pulmonary disease (e.g., to determine evidence of persistent airflow obstruction in asthma)

To evaluate the risks of procedures on lung function (e.g., anesthesia during surgical procedures; side effects such as fibrosis from chemotherapy or radiation therapy)

To assess prognosis (e.g., scoliosis; muscular dystrophy)

To determine the response to therapy (e.g., response to bronchodilators; objective evaluation of bronchodilator inhalation techniques by metered dose inhaler)

To evaluate airway hyperreactivity and response to therapy after challenge with exercise, bronchial antigens, methacholine or histamine inhalation, hyperventilation with cold dry air, or ultrasonic nebulized distilled water

Anatomic and physiologic differences between the respiratory systems of children and adults must be considered in the performance and interpretation of pulmonary function studies. In children, changes in predicted "normal" reference standards are caused by growth and development. The ability to perform reproducible lung function tests varies with the child's age, the level of coordination, and the degree of cooperation in following instructions. By 6 years of age, most of the pulmonary function studies used to evaluate lung function in adults can be successfully performed in the majority of children.

Until the 1980s, lung function data in children under 6 years of age were limited because of the unavailability of noninvasive tests for infants and young children, who cannot perform voluntary forced expiratory maneuvers. During the 1980s, many procedures have been proposed to measure lung function in infants; the merits and limitations of the various methods of pulmonary function tests in infants have been the subjects of several reviews[1-3] and are discussed in Chapter 9.

EQUIPMENT AND PERFORMANCE OF PULMONARY FUNCTION TESTS

A variety of computerized lung function equipment has made pulmonary function testing available for children in most large hospitals and physicians' offices. Because these computerized devices automatically compare the measured pulmonary function parameters with reference values, it is important for clinicians to know what standards are being used in order to assess their appropriateness and to interpret the pulmonary function results.

In 1979, the American Thoracic Society (ATS) published standards for manufacturers of pulmonary function equipment; these standards were developed at the first ATS workshop on Standardization of Spirometry.[4] The ATS updated standards in 1987 to ensure quality performance of pulmonary functions for spirometry.[5] Because the initial ATS workshop (Snowbird Conference) was predominantly concerned with standards for pulmonary function testing in adults, Taussig and associates[6] later published specific guidelines for lung function studies in children. These guidelines included the recommendation that the results of the pulmonary function tests should be compared with reference standards obtained from the same race and gender.

Because volumes and flows tend to be lower in children, the pulmonary function equipment should be accurate at low volumes. Lemen and colleagues recommended that spirometers used to test children should have flat dynamic response up to 12 Hz for flow and 6 Hz for volume in order to obtain an accurate recording during a maximal expiratory vital capacity (VC) maneuver.[7] In addition to an initial calibration of the pulmonary function equipment, it is necessary to check the calibration of the equipment so as to ensure both accurate performance of lung function studies and that the equipment continues to meet the ATS standards.[8] It is important to have a graphic display of the lung function tests and to inspect the record for quality and reproducibility of the forced vital capacity (FVC) curves and the absence of artifacts resulting from coughing or from delayed onset or early termination of exhalation. Records of pulmonary function should also include a comment by the technologist as to whether expiratory effort was satisfactory; acceptable volume-time spi-

Table 10–2. GUIDELINES FOR SELECTION OF PEDIATRIC PULMONARY FUNCTION EQUIPMENT AND RECOMMENDATIONS FOR PEDIATRIC PULMONARY FUNCTION TESTING

Equipment should be responsive to small volumes and low flows, and meet the minimum specifications of American Thoracic Society[4, 5]

Equipment should be periodically calibrated and tested to insure continuing accuracy of function per American Thoracic Society guidelines[8]

Mouth piece size should be adjusted for size of the patient

Equipment should provide a printout of the test results

Testing area should be comfortable and pleasant, with few distractions

Procedures can be performed with the patient sitting or standing; the use of nose clips is encouraged

The technologist should have experience in testing children; the personality, as well as the technical skills, of the technologist are important in providing motivation to children for maximal performance in the effort-dependent pulmonary function tests

Adequate time for training and age-appropriate instructions; coaching during performance encourages maximal effort and correct performance in tests

Technologist should include comments on the degree of cooperation or effort and other factors that may affect performance in tests

The best of three attempts at a volume/time or MEFV curve (loop) used for evaluation; the curves are compared by using sums of FEV_1 and FVC in millimeters; the curve with the largest sum of FEV_1 and FVC must be used for calculation of $FEF_{25\%-75\%}$

Uniform method of selecting the "start part" of FVC maneuver studies such as the back extrapolation method.[13]

Exhaled values and airflow should be corrected to BTPS conditions.

MEFV, maximal expiratory flow-volume; FEV_1, forced expiratory volume in 1 sec; FRC, functional residual capacity; $FEF_{25\%-75\%}$, forced expiratory flow between 25% and 75% of vital capacity; BTPS, body temperature, saturated with water.

Table 10–3. PULMONARY VOLUMES AND CAPACITIES

Pulmonary Volumes

Tidal volume (TV)	Volume of air inspired and expired with each normal quiet breath
Inspiratory reserve volume (IRV)	Extra volume of air that can be inspired over and beyond the normal TV
Expiratory reserve volume (ERV)	Amount of air that can still be expired by forceful expiration after the end of a normal tidal (quiet) expiration or from resting respiratory position (RRP), the point in the respiratory cycle when there is an instantaneous balance of inspiratory and expiratory forces; in the nonobstructed lung, this coincides with FRC
Residual volume (RV)	Volume of air remaining in the lungs after the most forceful or maximal expiration: FRC − ERV

Pulmonary Capacities

Inspiratory capacity (IC)	Maximal amount of air that can be inspired beginning at the normal expiratory level (i.e., after a quiet expiration from RRP): TV + IRV
Functional residual capacity (FRC)	Amount of air remaining in the lungs at the end of a normal tidal volume expiration: ERV + RV
Vital capacity (VC)	Maximal amount of air that can be expelled from the lungs after first filling the lungs to the maximal extent (i.e., after the deepest inspiration): IRV + TV + ERV
Total lung capacity (TLC)	Amount of gas contained in the lung at the end of a maximal inspiration or the maximal volume to which the lungs can be expanded: VC + RV; IC + FRC; IRV + TV + ERV + RV

rograms should have an appropriate curve shape, should be sustained for at least 3 sec, and should be in agreement within 10% of the largest effort.[9] Guidelines for the selection of pulmonary function equipment and recommendations for performance of lung function tests in children are outlined in Table 10–2.

MEASUREMENTS OF LUNG FUNCTION

MEASUREMENT OF LUNG VOLUMES

The major subdivisions of lung volume are outlined in Table 10–3 and are depicted schematically in Figure 10–1. The two most commonly used methods of measuring lung volume are body plethysmography and gas dilution techniques.

Body Plethysmography. Functional residual capacity (FRC) is measured as total thoracic gas volume (TGV) in the body plethysmograph, according to the technique described by Dubois and co-authors[10] on the basis of Boyle's law. The routine use of body plethysmography is usually limited to children over 6 years of age. FRC can be tested in a younger child in a body plethysmograph if the child is held on an adult's lap and if the adult holds his or her breath at the time of the measurements in order to prevent distortion of the child's signal.[11]

The technique for measuring TGV in a constant-volume plethysmograph (pressure plethysmograph) is to

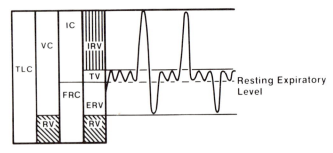

Subdivisions of the Lung

Figure 10-1. Subdivisions of lung volume. TLC, total lung capacity; VC, vital capacity; RV, residual volume; FRC, functional residual capacity; IRV, inspiratory reserve volume; ERV, expiratory reserve volume; TV, tidal volume; IC, inspiratory capacity.

occlude the airway of the patient by using a shutter at the end of tidal expiration. In this method, when there is no flow, it is assumed that the mouth pressure (Pm) is the same as the alveolar pressure (PA). When the child inhales against the shutter, the airway and alveolar pressures fall below atmospheric pressure, and TGV increases. The increase in TGV is associated with an increase in body box pressure.[12] During an expiratory effort against the shutter-occluded airway, alveolar and airway pressure rise above atmospheric pressure and TGV falls, resulting in a decrease in box pressure.[12]

TGV is calculated from Boyle's law, which states that at constant temperature, the product of pressure and volume in a closed system is constant:

$$P_1V_1 = P_2V_2.$$

During the expiratory portion of this maneuver,

P_1 = initial PA
   = atmospheric pressure − water vapor pressure;
V_1 = TGV;
P_2 = $P_1 + \Delta P$, where ΔP is the pressure change measured at the mouth;
V_2 = $V_1 - \Delta V$, where ΔV is the lung volume change derived from measuring the pressure change in the box (and prior knowledge of the pressure-volume curve of the box).

Assumptions implicit in this technique have been discussed in Chapter 1.

Helium Dilution. Functional residual capacity can also be measured by gas dilution techniques (helium dilution or nitrogen washout); details of these measurements are discussed in Chapter 1. These techniques are dependent on adequate mixing of the gases that are in free communication with the airways. The FRC measurement by body plethysmography, in contrast, includes both the obstructed and unobstructed gases (i.e., the total TGV). FRC measured by one of the gas dilution methods can be compared with FRC measured by body plethysmography in order to determine the volume of trapped air or the volume of gas that is not in free communication with the airways; this parameter is useful in the evaluation of airway obstruction and increases as the severity of airway obstruction increases.

MEASUREMENT OF AIRFLOWS

Spirometry, the measurement of certain pulmonary gas volumes and flow rates, is the pulmonary function measurement most commonly performed in children. In order to perform a spirogram, the child must be able to perform a forced expiratory maneuver, which consists of the following steps:

1. Taking a deep breath to total lung capacity (TLC).
2. Holding his or her breath 1 to 2 sec.
3. Exerting a maximal expiratory effort.
4. Completely emptying the lungs down to residual volume (RV).

There are two variants of spirometry: volume-time spirograms and maximal expiratory flow-volume curves (loops).

Volume-Time Spirogram. Figure 10-2 shows a normal volume-time spirogram. If there is no obstruction, the curve should reach a plateau within the first 3 sec. The pulmonary function parameters usually obtained from the volume-time spirogram are forced expiratory volume in 1 sec (FEV_1), forced vital capacity (FVC), FEV_1/FVC, and the forced expiratory flow at 25% to 75% of vital capacity ($FEF_{25\%-75\%}$). To determine $FEF_{25\%-75\%}$, a line is drawn connecting the points on the FVC curve that represent 25% and 75% of the expired volume. Once the slope of the line that connects these points is established, the two vertical lines at those points are connected, 1 sec apart (see Fig. 10-2). $FEF_{25\%-75\%}$ is the volume expired between the two intersections. $FEF_{25\%-75\%}$ is in the effort-independent portion of expiratory flow curve and is correlated with airflow in the peripheral airways. This parameter is thought to be more sensitive for detecting airflow limitation in the small airways than is FEV_1.

To ensure that the child has achieved the maximal effort in performing spirometry, triplicate testing is recommended. The best of the three values is selected for comparison with the reference standards. Observation of spirographic tracing helps identify poor effort (i.e., failure to achieve TLC or lack of complete deflation to RV). The spirogram should also be carefully reviewed to determine whether the child took an extra breath or coughed during

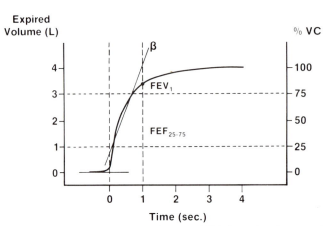

Figure 10-2. The volume-time spirogram. FEV_1, forced expiratory volume in 1 sec; $FEF_{25\%-75\%}$, forced expiratory flow at 25% to 75% of vital capacity.

the FVC maneuver. An appropriate expiratory curve starts with a steep slope.[9] The starting point (time 0) for expiration should be determined by extrapolating the steep initial part of the curve to the maximal inspiratory line.[9] One uniform method of selecting the zero point of the FVC maneuver is the back-extrapolation method.[13] Expired volume and airflows should be corrected to conditions of body temperature and saturated with water (BTPS) because the volume of gas expired from the lungs at BTPS may be higher than the volume of expired air at ambient temperature and pressure, saturated with water.

Maximal Expiratory Flow-Volume Curves/Loops. The maximal expiratory flow-volume (MEFV) curve/loop provides another method of displaying the forced vital capacity curve with flow ($\dot{V}$) on the vertical (y) axis and volume on the horizontal (x) axis (Fig. 10–3A). The expiratory flow is usually displayed on the upper part of the MEFV curve/loop and the inspiratory flow on the lower part of the loop; the point indicating RV is on the right of the MEFV curve, and the TLC point is on the left of the expiratory curve.

Flow rates are at least partially effort dependent; the effort-dependent flows are those measured at high lung volumes: that is, the first quarter of the expired FVC maneuver ($\dot{V}_{max}$ at 75% of VC). Flows at lower lung volumes are much less effort dependent[14] and more effort independent; the mechanism for the development of effort-independent flow is discussed in Chapter 1. Indeed, it is the fact that flows are effort independent that renders the MEFV curve a useful test of lung function; beyond modest efforts, flow rates within an individual are quite reproducible from day to day and are relatively independent of applied effort.

Flows at high lung volumes represent caliber of the central airways, whereas flows at low lung volumes represent

caliber of the peripheral airways. During forced expiration, resistive pressure losses within the airway from the alveoli to the mouth are more extensive at low lung volumes (smaller airway size and therefore higher airway resistance) than at high lung volumes. Thus the segment of the airway undergoing dynamic compression (which occurs because intra-airway pressure is low in relation to extra-airway or pleural pressure) migrates from the central to the peripheral airways during the course of a forced expiration; flow at high lung volumes therefore represents central airway events, whereas flow at low lung volumes represents peripheral airway events.

Partial Flow-Volume Curves. Partial expiratory flow-volume (PEFV) curves are obtained by means of a non-invasive technique for evaluating lung function and responses to various therapeutic interventions in infants and young children, who cannot perform voluntary MEFV maneuvers.[15-17] Taussig reported the successful measurement of maximal expiratory flows at end-tidal expiration (i.e., FRC) from partial expiratory flow volume curves in children aged 4 to 6 years (Fig. 10–4).[15] The intrasubject coefficient of variation for $\dot{V}_{max}$FRC was 16.9%, and intersubject coefficients of variation were 31% for girls and 36% for boys. These PEFV curves have subsequently been used in the assessment of children with cystic fibrosis and asthma and in 4- to 5-year-old children after cold air challenge. (A review of PEFV curves in infants and children by Morgan and colleagues[18] is suggested for additional reading.)

Peak Expiratory Flow Rate (PEFR). The peak flow rate as measured by a Wright peak flowmeter or a similar device is a simple pulmonary function test to perform in children and provides a measurement of the maximal flow attainable on forced expiration. This lung function study is both volume and effort dependent. The best of three, and preferably five, attempts is recorded as the observed PEFR. The PEFR is a measurement that lends itself to use in the patient's home for monitoring limitation of airflow or as an outpatient screening test for evaluating the degree of severity of airflow obstruction and response to therapy. Most children can perform a peak flow rate maneuver by 3 years of age. The Wright peak flowmeter (adult size) measures flow rates from 60 to 1000 l/min. PEFR can also be determined from the MEFV curve/loop or obtained from a variety of less complicated and less expensive flow rate measurement devices for home monitoring of pulmonary function.

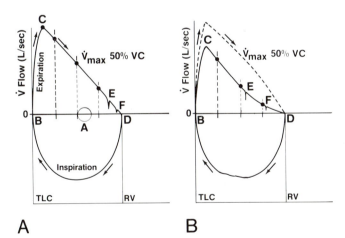

A   **B**

Figure 10–3. The maximal expiratory flow-volume curve. A, Schematic representation of a normal maximal expiratory flow-volume (MEFV) loop; for comparison, tidal volume ventilation is shown in point A. Point B represents the point of maximal inspiratory effort. The child is instructed to make a maximal expiratory effort and to exhale as fast and as completely as possible. The point of peak expiratory flow rate (designated by point C) represents an effort-dependent variable; shortly thereafter, flow becomes effort independent. Point D represents the RV. Point E corresponds to FEV$_1$. The forced expiratory volume at 3 sec (FEV$_3$) is identified by point F. $\dot{V}_{max}$ 50% VC is the flow rate at 50% vital capacity. B, MEFV curve in lower airway obstruction. $\dot{V}$, flow.

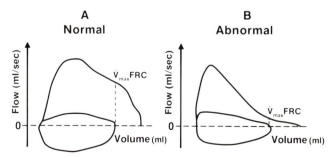

Figure 10–4. The partial expiratory flow-volume curve. Note that forced-flow starts at end-tidal inspiration, not at TLC. A, Normal curve; B, curve in lower airway obstruction.

AIRWAY RESISTANCE

An index of airway size that is more direct than flow is airway resistance (Raw). Raw and its reciprocal, airway conductance, can be measured in a body plethysmograph. Airway resistance is the ratio of the driving pressures (transairway pressure) to flow.[12] In the plethysmograph, Raw is the ratio of alveolar pressure (PA) divided by airflow. The relationship between plethysmographic pressure and PA can be calculated during airway occlusion. Thus airflow is measured by a pneumotachometer attached to the mouth piece of the body plethysmograph in two steps: first, the child pants through the flowmeter with the mouth shutter open and then continues to pant while the shutter is closed in order to measure TGV. Raw is measured at end-tidal expiration (FRC), the point when the airway is occluded in order to measure PA. When Raw is measured at a specific lung volume, it is referred to as specific airway resistance (SRaw). Raw is usually higher at smaller lung volumes and lower at larger lung volumes.

Airway conductance (Gaw), the reciprocal of Raw, is also useful in the assessment of airway size. Like Raw, Gaw is influenced by lung volume and should be corrected for volume or measured at a specific volume (SGaw). Gaw may be preferable to Raw for expressing airway caliber and to correct for volume change, inasmuch as the relationship of airway conductance to lung volume is linear. SGaw is useful in assessing response to bronchodilators, especially in children with extremely hyperresponsive airways in whom a forced expiratory maneuver can result in bronchoconstriction.[19]

INTERPRETATION OF PULMONARY FUNCTION TEST RESULTS

REFERENCE STANDARDS

The accuracy of interpretation of objective assessments of lung function in children depends on the availability of appropriate normal reference standards for comparison. Reference standards vary in children and adolescents because of growth, gender, and race.

Height, sex, and race are important predictors of lung function in children; height, rather than age, is used as a major predicting factor in regression equations for normal reference standards.[20] Reference normal standards are obtained by testing a group of children and adolescents of the same age, race, and sex who are, according to medical history, free of lung disease and who have not had a recent respiratory tract infection. It is crucial that a given laboratory's reference standards include the entire range of ages and heights of the population to be tested. Extrapolation beyond age or height ranges will lead to over- or underestimation of percent predicted values. Table 10–4 lists the sources of some of the published reference standards for the more commonly used lung volumes and flow rates in children.[20, 22-31] Flow rates and lung volumes increase with growth.[23] Several studies have confirmed the influence of race on pulmonary functions in children.[20, 21, 32, 33] Hsu and collaborators[20, 21] reported pulmonary function values for normal Mexican-American, black, and white children. VC was found to be significantly lower in black children than in white children of the same standing height. The lower VC values for black children are attributed to an average shorter upper body segment than in white children. The differences are greater with increasing height and during adolescence, which suggests that puberty influences the divergence in body habitus. FVC is slightly larger in Mexican-American children than in white children at the same standing height.[20] The influence of race on lung volume measurements has also been documented with Polynesian children.[33]

The need for more attention to standards for interpretation of pulmonary function tests in children was emphasized by Pattishell,[34] who reported on a survey of pulmonary function–testing laboratories. According to Pattishell's survey, 80% of the predicted value for three commonly used spirometric parameters (FVC, FEV$_1$, and FEF$_{25\%-75\%}$) was the standard most commonly used for

Table 10–4. PULMONARY FUNCTION STUDIES: NORMAL REFERENCE STANDARDS

Study	FEV$_1$	FVC	FEF$_{25\%-75\%}$	$\dot{V}_{max}$ FEF$_{50\%}$	$\dot{V}_{max}$ FEF$_{25\%}$	FRC (RV)	TLC
Dockery et al (1983)[23]	X	X		X			
Hsu et al (1979)[20]	X	X	X				
Knudson et al (1983)[24]	X	X	X	X	X		
Dickman et al (1971)[22]	X	X	X				
Polgar and Promadhat (1971)[25]	X	X	X			X	X
Godfrey et al (1970)[26]	X	X				X	X
Weng and Levison (1969)[27]	X	X	X			X	X
Zapletal et al (1969)[28]	X	X		X	X	X	X
DeMuth et al (1965)[29]		X				X	
Bjure (1963)[30]	X	X					
Cherniak (1962)[31]		X	X				

FEV$_1$, forced expiratory volume in 1 sec; FVC, forced vital capacity; FEF$_n$, forced expiratory flow at n% of vital capacity; $\dot{V}$, maximal flow; FRC, functional residual capacity; RV, residual volume; TLC, total lung capacity.

defining abnormality, although a 60% predicted cutoff value is probably more reasonable for $FEF_{25\%-75\%}$ because of its greater inherent variability.

Values exceeding 95% confidence limits (± 2 standard deviations) for any parameter of pulmonary function in comparison with predicted reference values from healthy age-, sex-, and race-matched controls should be used to define an abnormality of lung function and are considered preferable to a specific percentage cutoff value.[34] The expression of pulmonary function values as percentage of predicted normal reference values enables the evaluation of intersubject and intrasubject parameters of pulmonary functions with growth and permits assessment of the course of the pulmonary disease over time. Although pulmonary function values within two standard deviations of predicted reference standards are considered within the limits of normality, they may be associated with lung dysfunction in an individual patient. Serial testing can provide a better indication of normality of pulmonary function in any individual; a change of one standard deviation (or more than 10% change) is usually considered a significant intrasubject change in lung function. In a child with hyperreactive airway disease baseline flow rates that exceed the predicted normal range may drop significantly, whereas the absolute values still remain in the range of normal predicted values.

PHYSIOLOGIC CHARACTERIZATION OF PULMONARY DYSFUNCTION

Abnormalities of pulmonary function can be characterized physiologically and classified as (1) obstructive, (2) restrictive, and (3) mixed obstructive and restrictive dysfunction. Although pulmonary function studies do not provide a specific diagnosis, they do suggest possible diagnostic categories that are associated with each of these physiologic patterns of respiratory impairment. Table 10–5 outlines the physiologic classification of respiratory impairment and the more commonly used pulmonary function tests to identify obstructive and restrictive lung dysfunction.

Obstructive lung disease refers to a group of ventilatory disorders characterized by airflow impairment during expiration and can be identified by reduction in flow rates and alteration in some lung volumes. Flows such as FEV_1 are reduced in obstructive lung dysfunction. In contrast, the TLC is normal or moderately increased as a result of air trapping. With increasing airway obstruction, RV is increased and VC is decreased. These physiologic changes result primarily from a redistribution of the subdivisions of the lung (see Fig. 10–1). Although the FEV_1/FVC ratio may be reduced in obstructive dysfunction, it can be normal in mild disease. The average FEV_1/FVC ratio for children is 86%. Normal values are within two standard deviations (7%) of the predicted value. In obstructive lung dysfunction, flow-resistive properties of the airways, such as Raw or SRaw, are increased and Gaw or SGaw is decreased. The RV/TLC ratio is elevated with obstructive lung impairment. The $FEF_{25\%-75\%}$ is a more sensitive measure of obstruction in peripheral airways than is FEV_1.

Table 10–5. CLASSIFICATION OF LUNG FUNCTIONS BY PHYSIOLOGIC IMPAIRMENT

Obstructive Lung Dysfunction
Ventilatory disorder characterized by impairment during expiration identified by reduced maximal expiratory flow rates or airflow limitation ($\dot{V}_{max}$): FEV_1, $FEF_{25\%-75\%}$, PEFR, $\dot{V}_{max}$ at 50% VC, and $\dot{V}_{max}$ at 25% VC
- TLC: normal or moderately increased
- Increased RV/TLC
- Increased RV and decreased VC with increasing airway obstruction
- FEV_1/FVC reflects a disproportionate reduction in flow of FEV_1 to FVC
- Increased airway resistance (Raw, SRaw) or decreased airway conductance (Gaw, SGaw)

Restrictive Lung Dysfunction
Ventilatory disorder with reduction in lung volumes caused by decreased compliance of the lungs or chest wall, muscle weakness, or any combination, characterized by
- Symmetric reduction in lung volumes
- Vital capacity (FVC or VC) decreased; FVC < 80% predicted
- TLC decreased
- FEV_1/FVC ratio normal or slightly increased*
- RV/TLC normal, decreased, or increased (depends on whether TLC decreased more than RV)
- Flow rates normal or reduced in proportion to reduction in volumes
- Airway conductance (SGaw) normal

$\dot{V}_{max}$, maximal flow; FEV_1, forced expiratory volume in 1 sec; FEF_{25-75}, forced expiratory flow at 25% to 75% vital capacity; PEFR, peak expiratory flow rate; VC, vital capacity; TLC, total lung capacity; FVC, forced vital capacity; Raw, airway resistance; SRaw, specific airway resistance; Gaw, airway conductance; SGaw, specific airway conductance.
*Normal FEV_1/FVC for children is 86% (standard deviation, 7%).

Restrictive lung disease is characterized by decreased lung volumes. Decreased flow rates may be associated with decreased lung volumes because airflow is volume per unit of time; flows are decreased in proportion to volumes. Restrictive lung dysfunction can result from decreased compliance of the lungs or the chest wall, respiratory muscle weakness, or any combination of the three and is identified by symmetric reduction in lung volumes such as VC or FVC and TLC. The FEV_1/FVC ratio is normal or slightly increased. The RV/TLC ratio can be normal, decreased, or increased; an increase occurs more often in patients with expiratory muscle weakness. An increase in the RV/TLC ratio and a decrease in TLC differentiate restrictive lung dysfunction from obstructive lung disease. SGaw in restrictive lung dysfunction is normal. When a child has obstructive lung disease, it is difficult to confirm the presence of coexistent restrictive lung dysfunction by simple spirometry. With mixed obstructive and restrictive lung disease, spirometry most likely does not show an expiratory plateau before the child must curtail the breathing effort.

THE MEFV CURVE IN PERIPHERAL AND CENTRAL AIRFLOW OBSTRUCTION

Peripheral Airway Disease. Visual inspection of the shape of the MEFV curve can help to identify small airway dysfunction, which is characterized by a concavity in the expiratory curve that denotes low flows at lower lung volumes (Fig. 10–3*B*). Maximal expiratory flow is almost linearly related to expired volume in normal persons at all lung volumes more than 25% below full inflation. A curvilinearity score can be calculated by a ratio of the actual flow at 50% expired VC to the flow predicted from the straight line representing predicted maximal expiratory flow at all lung volumes more than 25% below full inflation.[9] Response to bronchodilators can also be noted by visual inspection of the MEFV curves (Fig. 10–5).

MEFV curves can be obtained when the child is breathing room air or a low-density gas mixture (80% helium and 20% oxygen), and the flow rates can be compared for estimates of the small peripheral airway contribution to expiratory flow resistance. Flows at $\dot{V}_{max50\%VC}$ can be compared, or the two curves can be superimposed and the lung volumes determined at the point where the expiratory flows are the same volume (Viso$\dot{V}$) or point of identical isoflow (PIF). During a forced expiration at high lung volumes, flow limitation occurs in large airways with turbulent airflow, and a low-density gas such as helium increases maximal flow (Fig. 10–6*A*). As the volume decreases, the flow-limiting segment moves into small (peripheral) airways, where flow is laminar and independent of density. At this lung volume (Viso$\dot{V}$), therefore, helium no longer increases maximal flow. In patients with obstructive lung disease, the major site of airflow resistance shifts from its normal location in the central airways to the more peripheral airways. Thus with the shift of the site of airflow resistance to peripheral airways with laminar flow, density dependence is decreased; flows do not increase as much with helium, and the Viso$\dot{V}$ occurs at higher lung volumes (Fig. 10–6*B*).

Central Airway Obstruction. The MEFV curve and the maximal inspiratory flow-volume curve (Fig. 10–7) can be useful in demonstrating fixed obstruction of the central airways (larynx, trachea, and main stem bronchi) and

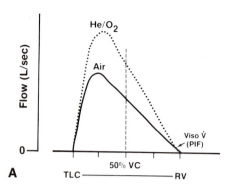

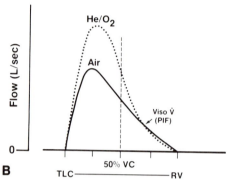

Figure 10–6. Maximal expiratory flow-volume curves while breathing air and an 80% helium/20% oxygen mixture. Viso$\dot{V}$, volume of isoflow; PIF, point of isoflow. *A*, Normal curve; *B*, lower airway obstruction. See text for explanation.

variable obstruction of the extrathoracic or intrathoracic airways. The relationship between reduced inspiratory flow to expiratory flow at mid-VC depends on the location of the airway obstruction (i.e., extrathoracic or intrathoracic central airway obstruction). Reduced expiratory flows at high lung volumes and reduced inspiratory flow rates are characteristic of mild obstruction of the central airways. With increasing degree of obstruction, expiratory flow is reduced at lower lung volumes. Because flow rates are effort dependent at higher lung volumes, it is important to encourage patients to use maximal effort in performing these studies.

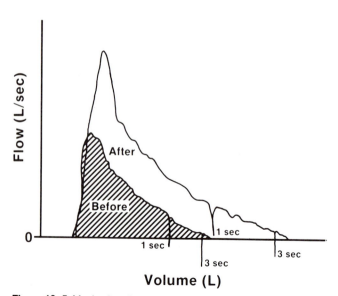

Figure 10–5. Maximal expiratory flow-volume curve in a patient with airflow obstruction: response to bronchodilators.

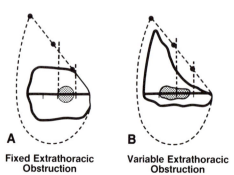

Figure 10–7. Maximal expiratory flow-volume curve in upper airway obstruction. Note decreased inspiratory flows and decreased expiratory flows at high lung volumes in fixed obstruction.

OTHER USES OF PULMONARY FUNCTION TESTS

Airway reactivity may be assessed by giving bronchodilators to patients with baseline airflow obstruction and reassessing lung function. In patients with normal baseline lung function, a variety of challenge tests can be used. The studies for airway hyperreactivity and hyperresponsiveness include physiologic tests (exercise testing, hyperventilation with cold air challenge, or ultrasonic nebulized distilled water challenge) and pharmacologic tests with methacholine or histamine, in addition to bronchoprovocation challenge with specific antigens. In cold air testing, one protocol is to have the patient hyperventilate at a rate of 25 times the baseline FEV_1 per minute; carbon dioxide is bled into the system to ensure that the patient does not become hypocapneic, and end-tidal CO_2 should be monitored. A decrease in FEV_1 of more than 10% is considered a positive challenge.[35]

In pharmacologic challenges, the assessment is somewhat different. Increasing doses of the testing agent (e.g., histamine or methacholine) are given, and the results are expressed as the dose of agent required to produce a percentage (e.g., 20%) decrease in FEV_1. Thus the lower this dose is, the more airway reactivity is present.

The effect of inhalation of normal saline should be determined before beginning either type of challenge study; if a fall in FEV_1 of $>10\%$ occurs, the validity of any challenge should be questioned, and testing should be deferred to another day. A variety of other circumstances can also make it difficult to interpret the challenge studies, such as presence of respiratory infections (especially viral infections and sinusitis), seasonal exposure to pollens, and drugs (e.g., cromolyn sodium, antihistamines, and beta-agonists). Studies for evaluation of airway hyperresponsiveness should be performed only in laboratories with experience in airway challenges and by appropriately trained personnel available for careful monitoring and interpretation of results. (For further discussions of these tests for airway hyperresponsiveness see Chapters 15 and 16.)

In preoperative assessment of respiratory function, peak expiratory flow rate can give a rough estimate of whether a child can generate flows adequate for raising secretions by coughing during the postoperative period. Froese[36] suggested that the inspiratory capacity is also helpful in predicting the patient's ability to breathe unaided postoperatively. In children with documented airway obstruction or a history of airway hyperresponsiveness, pulmonary function tests help evaluate the degree of airflow limitation and the extent of reversibility of the obstruction with bronchodilators. This documentation is useful in assessment of the need for bronchodilator therapy during the preoperative, intraoperative, and postoperative periods.

Inspiratory force measurements are helpful in the evaluation and monitoring of patients with muscular weakness and of patients who require mechanical ventilation and in whom extubation is being considered. The technique for measuring inspiratory force by an aneroid manometer is simple and enables objective evaluation of respiratory muscle strength.

NONINVASIVE ASSESSMENT OF GAS EXCHANGE

OXIMETRY

The measurement of arterial oxygen saturation by spectrophotoelectric oximetry is a noninvasive method of monitoring the deoxygenation status of infants and children. Pulse oximetry, a test of pulmonary gas exchange function, can be used continuously *in vivo* as well as intermittently. There are two important limitations of this method of which clinicians should be aware. First, pulse oximetry fails to function well in the presence of peripheral circulatory failure; the oximeter identifies poor perfusion as a poor pulse signal. Second, the amount of oxygen saturation displayed on the oximeter is inaccurate if heart rate from electrocardiogram does not agree with heart rate displayed on the pulse oximeter.

In the pulse oximeter, two wavelengths of light (660 and 940 nm) are used to calibrate oxygenated and deoxygenated hemoglobin, and the influx of arterial blood is identified by plethysmography. The "pulse added" absorbance signal exceeding diastolic tissue absorbance is measured at the two wavelengths, and the ratio is calculated by a microprocessor in the oximeter device. An increase in the light absorbance ratio at the two wavelengths is interpreted by the pulse oximeter as a fall in oxygen saturation because reduced hemoglobin gives off a different spectrophotometric wavelength than does oxygenated hemoglobin. The amplitude of the waveform depends on the size of the arterial pulse change, the wavelength of light used, and the oxygen saturation of arterial hemoglobin. Because the waveform results solely from arterial blood, it can be viewed as beat-to-beat arterial hemoglobin saturation.

A finger (usually the index), a toe, or a hand of an infant or a child, with its pulsating arterial vascular beds, can be placed between a two-wavelength light source and a detector. The expansion and contraction of the pulsating vascular bed creates a change in the length of the light path that modifies the amount of light detected, resulting in a plethysmograph waveform.

Some of the main disadvantages of pulse oximetry are that it does not reflect decreasing arterial saturation until the arterial oxygen pressure (Pa_{O_2}) is less than 80 mm Hg, this method cannot differentiate a Pa_{O_2} of 80 from one of 120 mm Hg, and all measures may read 100% saturation. The measurement of arterial saturations below 70% to 80% also have important and clinically significant limitations, and the possibility of erroneously high pulse oximetry values may fail to identify patients with serious desaturation. The two-wavelength system does not enable the oximeter to differentiate between more than two hemoglobins (i.e., reduced and oxygenated hemoglobin); thus in the presence of abnormal hemoglobins, oximetry readings are not reliable.

Another limitation of pulse oximetry is the fact that the accuracy of oximetry can be affected by movement of the patient,[37, 38] compression of the sensors,[37-39] severe desaturation,[39] low-perfusion states,[37, 38, 40] abnormal types of hemoglobin,[40-43] nail polish,[44] surgical electrocautery,[38, 40] and infrared heating lamps.[37, 40, 45] Because infrared heat lamps, fluorescent or high-intensity lighting, and sunlight may interfere with pulse oximetry, the photodetector should be protected from light in order to prevent these effects.

CAPNOGRAPHY

Capnography provides a breath-by-breath noninvasive analysis of expired CO_2. In this technique, gas is sampled from the airway and aspirated into a capnometer, in which the CO_2 is measured by an infrared absorption method. Rapid respiratory rates and pulmonary disease produce uneven mixing of expired gas and may cause severe limitations of this technique in critically ill infants or small children. McEvedy and co-workers[46] compared end-tidal CO_2 and arterial CO_2 tension (Pa_{CO_2}) in critically ill neonates and demonstrated the limitations of using end-tidal CO_2 as an estimate of Pa_{CO_2}. The coefficient of determinant for linear regression between end-tidal CO_2 and Pa_{CO_2} was 0.39, which increased to 0.72 when patients with respiratory rates >70/min or with O_2 requirements >70% O_2 were excluded. This technique should be helpful in monitoring patients with normal or minimally damaged lungs (e.g., monitoring degree of hyperventilation in children with increased intracranial pressure).[47] In children receiving assisted ventilation, there are sampling problems of the expired gas for end-tidal CO_2 measurements. Samples taken at the proximal end of the endotracheal tube are underestimates of the CO_2 because they contain a mixture of exhaled gas and fresh gas from the ventilator. The best sampling site is close to the end of the endotracheal tube.

REFERENCES

1. Wall M, Coates A, Buist S, et al: Controversies in pediatric pulmonary medicine: Infant pulmonary function tests. Am Rev Respir Dis 138:1069–1073, 1988.
2. England SJ: Current techniques for assessing pulmonary function in newborn and infant: Advantages and limitations. Pediatr Pulmonol 4:48–53, 1988.
3. Davis GM, Coates AL: Pulmonary function testing in infants and neonates. Sem Respir Med 2:185–196, 1990.
4. American Thoracic Society: ATS Statement—Snowbird workshop on standardization of spirometry. Am Rev Respir Dis 119:831–838, 1979.
5. American Thoracic Society: Standardization of Spirometry—1987 Update. Am Rev Respir Dis 136:1285–1293, 1987.
6. Taussig LM, Chernick V, Wood R, et al: Standardization of lung function testing in children. J Pediatr 97:668–676, 1980.
7. Lemen R, Gerdes C, Wegmann M, et al: Frequency spectra of flow and volume events for forced vital capacity. J Appl Physiol 53:977–984, 1982.
8. Quality assurance in pulmonary function laboratories: Proposed ATS recommended guidelines. ATS News 10(2):4–5, 1984.
9. Lemen RJ: Pulmonary function testing in the office and clinic. In Kendig EL, Chernick V (eds): Disorders of the Respiratory Tract in Children, 5th ed, pp. 147–154. Philadelphia: WB Saunders, 1990.
10. Dubois AB, Botelho SY, Bedell GN, et al: A rapid plethysmographic method for measuring thoracic gas volume. J Clin Invest 35:322–326, 1956.
11. Lindemann H: Body plethysmograph measurements in children with an accompanying adult. Respiration 37:278, 1979.
12. Fisher B: Pulmonary function testing in infants and small children. In Nussbaum E, Gallant SP (eds): Respiratory Disorders, pp. 233–249. Orlando, FL: Grune & Stratton, 1984.
13. Proceedings and Recommendations of the GAP Conference Committee, CF Foundation, Ashville, NC, September 18–20, 1978.
14. Allen JL, Castile RG, Mead J. Positive effort dependence of maximal expiratory flow. J Appl Physiol 62:718–724, 1987.
15. Taussig LM: Maximal expiratory flows at functional residual capacity: A test of lung function for young children. Am Rev Respir Dis 116:1031–1038, 1977.
16. Wall MA, Misley MC, Dickerson D: Partial expiratory flow-volumes curves in young children. Am Rev Respir Dis 129:557–562, 1984.
17. Buist AS, Adams BE, Sexton GJ, et al: Reference values for functional residual capacity and maximal expiratory flow in young children. Am Rev Respir Dis 122:983–988, 1980.
18. Morgan WJ, Geller DE, Tepper RS, Taussig LM: Partial expiratory flow-volume curves in infants and young children. Pediatr Pulmonol 5:232–243, 1988.
19. Gayrard P, Orehek J, Grimaud C, et al: Bronchoconstrictor effects of a deep inspiration in patients with asthma. Am Rev Respir Dis 3:433–439, 1975.
20. Hsu HK, Jenkins DE, Hsi BP, et al: Ventilatory functions of normal children and young adults: Mexican-American, white and black. I: Spirometry. J Pediatr 95:14–23, 1979.
21. Hsu HK, Jenkins DE, Hsi BP, et al: Ventilatory functions of normal children and young adults: Mexican-American, white and black. II: Wright Peak Flow Meter. J Pediatr 95:192–196, 1979.
22. Dickman ML, Schmidt CD, Gardner RM: Spirometric standards for normal children and adolescents (ages 5 years through 18 years). Am Rev Respir Dis 104:680–687, 1971.
23. Dockery DW, Berkey CS, Ware JH, et al: Distribution of forced vital capacity and forced expiratory volume in one second in children 6 to 11 years of age. Am Rev Respir Dis 128:405–412, 1983.
24. Knudson RJ, Lebowitz MD, Holberg C, Burrows K: Changes in the normal maximal expiratory flow-volume with growth and aging. Am Rev Respir Dis 127:725–734, 1983.
25. Polgar G, Promadhat V: Pulmonary Function Testing in Children: Techniques and Standards. Philadelphia: WB Saunders, 1971.
26. Godfrey S, Kamburoff PL, Nairn JR, et al: Spirometry, lung volumes and airway resistance in normal children aged 5–18 years. Br J Dis Chest 64:15–24, 1970.
27. Weng TR, Levison H: Standards of pulmonary function in children. Am Rev Respir Dis 99:879–894, 1969.
28. Zapletal A, Motoyama EK, Van De Woestijne KP, et al: Maximum expiratory flow-volume curves and airway conductance in children and adolescents. J Appl Physiol 26:308–316, 1969.
29. DeMuth GR, Howatt WF, Hill B: Growth of lung function. I: Lung volumes. Pediatrics 35:162, 1965.
30. Bjure J: Spirometric studies in normal subjects, IV: Ventilatory capacities in healthy children 7–17 years of age. Acta Paediatr 52:232–240, 1963.
31. Cherniack RM: Ventilatory function in normal children. Canad Med Assoc J 87:80–81, 1962.
32. Wall MA, Olson D, Bonn BA, et al: Lung function in North American Indian children: Reference standards for spirometry maximum expiratory flow volume curves and peak expiratory flow. Am Rev Respir Dis 125:158–162, 1982.
33. Asher MI, Douglas C, Stewart AW, et al: Lung volumes in Polynesian children. Am Rev Respir Dis 136:1360–1368, 1987.
34. Pattishell EN: Pulmonary function testing reference values and interpretations in pediatric training programs. Pediatrics 85:768–773, 1990.
35. McLaughlin FJ, Dozor AJ: Cold air inhalation challenge in the diagnosis of asthma in children. Pediatrics 72:503–509, 1983.
36. Froese AB: Preoperative evaluation of pulmonary function. Pediatr Clin North Am 26:645, 1979.
37. Yelderman M, New W: Evaluation of pulse oximetry. Anesthesiology 59:349–352, 1983.
38. Coté CJ, Goldstein EA, Coté MA, et al: A single blind study of pulse oximetry in children. Anesthesiology 68:184–188, 1988.
39. Mihm FG, Halperin BD: Noninvasive detection of profound arterial desaturation using a pulse oximetry device. Anesthesiology 62:85–87, 1985.
40. Mertzlufft F, Zander R: Noninvasive oximetry using the Biox III oximeter: Clinical evaluation and physiological aspects. In Payne

JP, Severinghaus JW (eds): Pulse Oximetry, pp. 76–77. New York: Springer-Verlag, 1986.

41. Barker SJ, Tremper KK: The effect of carbon monoxide inhalation on pulse oximetry and transcutaneous PO2. Anesthesiology 66:677–679, 1987.
42. Barker SJ, Tremper KK, Hyatt J, et al: Effects of methemoglobinemia on pulse oximetry and mixed venous oximetry. Anesthesiology 67(Suppl):A171, 1987.
43. Anderson ST, Hajduczek J, Barker SJ: Benzocaine-induced methemoglobinemia in an adult: Accuracy of pulse oximetry with methemoglobinemia. Anesth Analg 67:1099–1101, 1988.

44. Cotè CJ, Goldstein EA, Fuchsman WH, et al: The effects of nail polish on pulse oximetry. Anesth Analg 67:683–686, 1988.
45. Jennis MS, Peabody JL: Pulse oximetry: An alternative method for the assessment of oxygenation in newborn infants. Pediatrics 79:524–528, 1987.
46. McEvedy BAB, McLeod ME, Mulera M, et al: End-tidal, transcutaneous, and arterial pCO2 measurement in critically ill neonates: A comparative study. Anesthesiology 69:112–116, 1988.
47. Matthew DJ: The role of noninvasive techniques in the pediatric intensive care unit. Curr Opin Pediatr 2:519–521, 1990.

11 PEDIATRIC RIGID BRONCHOSCOPY

RICHARD BRYARLY, M.D. / RONALD HIROKAWA, M.D.

PEDIATRIC RIGID BRONCHOSCOPY

The first endoscope was developed in the 1890s by Adolf Kussmaul and consisted of an open-ended tube illuminated by the reflected light of a gasoline lamp.[1] The development of pediatric endoscopes lagged behind that of endoscopes for adults after visualization through telescopes was introduced in the 1880s, probably because the amount of light available at the area of visualization was small as a result of the enormous amount of absorption of light by the lens system. The smaller diameter tubes used at that time did not provide much illumination or visualization.

Modern pediatric endoscopy began with the development of the Hopkins rod lens system in the early 1950s. Professor H. H. Hopkins produced a telescope with rod-like lenses that provided more illumination; this angulated telescope was also able to visualize the upper lobes of the lungs. Further refinements included incorporation of fine fiberoptics to supply illumination with the fibers positioned to encircle the Hopkins lens in the telescope. A 2.7-mm–diameter telescope that offered excellent illumination and excellent visualization was developed. At about the same time, Karl Storz developed bronchoscope tubes made from a strong but thin-gauge metal (Fig. 11–1). These tubes enabled the use of small-diameter bronchoscopes to provide adequate ventilation even in small premature infants.

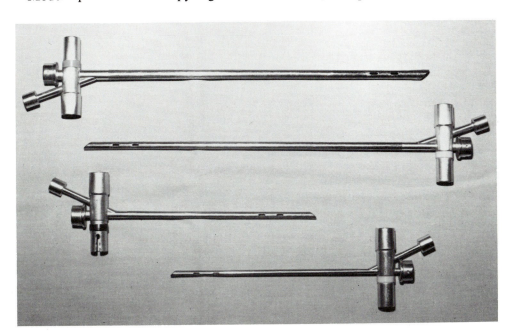

Figure 11–1. Storz bronchoscope tubes ranging from 2.5 mm *(bottom)* to 5 mm *(top)*.

INDICATIONS

In general, the indications for rigid bronchoscopy include diagnostic evaluation, removal of foreign bodies, removal of thick secretions, and the establishment of an airway. Although flexible endoscopes are useful for some of these problems, rigid bronchoscopes have several advantages.

In the diagnostic evaluation of stridor, recurrent aspiration, or persistent cough, the rigid bronchoscope enables easy access to the respiratory tract. Detailed examination of the respiratory mucosa is possible with the Hopkins telescope, enabling the detection of subtle changes such as laryngeal cleft or tracheoesophageal fistula. Vascular compressions can also be evaluated during rigid bronchoscopy. By applying pressure to the vessel, the examiner can obtain information about its anatomic source by noting changes in the radial and carotid pulses.

At present, rigid bronchoscopy is for several reasons the method of choice for removal of foreign bodies. First, the rigid bronchoscope offers the advantage of passing varied types of endoscopic forceps appropriate for the removal of foreign bodies. In addition, the instruments are larger, ensuring a better grip on the foreign body (Figs. 11–2, 11–3). During removal of a foreign body, ventilation may be better maintained with rigid bronchoscopy. The side vents on most rigid bronchoscopes allow visualization of one of the main bronchi while providing ventilation to the other patent bronchi (Fig. 11–4).

Rigid bronchoscopy can rapidly and effectively remove thick secretions from bronchi; this is helpful in inflammatory conditions in which the accumulation of thick, purulent debris results in atelectasis or airway obstruction. The larger caliber suction catheters available with rigid bronchoscopes enable effective evaluation of bleeding from the airway, even with brisk hemorrhage. Thick clots can be removed either with suction or with foreign body forceps.

In airway compromise secondary to edema or granulation tissue, the rigid bronchoscope enables dilatation of the airway. This feature can be useful in the emergency establishment of an airway. While the airway is maintained with the bronchoscope, a tracheostomy can be performed less hurriedly than usual. Although repeated dilatations with the rigid bronchoscope are of limited value today, enlargement of the airway is helpful in subglottic stenosis. Until the advent of the CO_2 laser and the development of open laryngotracheoplasty, such enlargement was the only effective method of treatment of this problem.

The CO_2 laser can be used with rigid bronchoscopes for resection of respiratory lesions. Because the emitted beam of the CO_2 lasers is absorbed by water, the effects are superficial and easily controlled. The adjacent tissue cells sustain little injury, and associated edema is minimal.[2, 3] This is particularly important when the lasers are used in the small pediatric airway. In vessels ranging from 0.2 to 0.5 mm, the CO_2 laser is capable of sealing openings in vascular walls, providing instantaneous hemostasis.[2]

The accessibility of the rigid bronchoscope to the smaller terminal airways is limited because it cannot deviate from a straight passage. The flexible bronchoscope is the instrument of choice for access to these areas.

In a child with airway compromise, the rigid bronchoscope offers a larger portal for ventilation and oxygenation than does the flexible bronchoscope. The presence of the flexible bronchoscope in the airway produces partial airway obstruction, and supplemental oxygen may not overcome this problem, depending on the bronchoscope size and airway size. Fiberoptic bronchoscopes that can pass through both 3.0- and 2.5-mm endotracheal tubes are available (see Chapter 12).

PREOPERATIVE CONSIDERATIONS

With either rigid or fiberoptic bronchoscopes, certain undesirable physiologic responses to bronchoscopy may

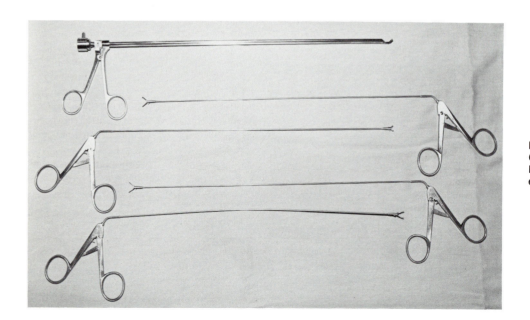

Figure 11–2. Endoscopic forceps. Optical forceps is used with Storz-Hopkins telescope to provide excellent visibility.

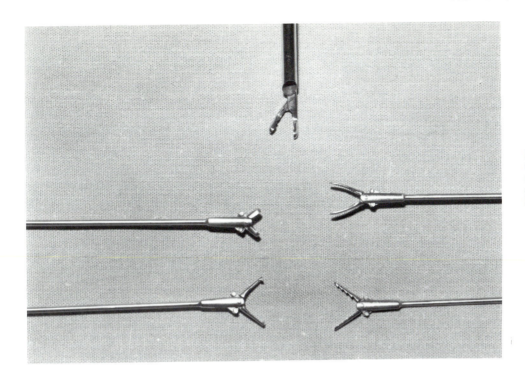

Figure 11-3. Close-up view of forceps. Optical forceps at top. The different types of jaws can be used according to the type of foreign body.

occur; in the pediatric patient, these may include bradycardia, anaphylaxis, and laryngospasm. To minimize bradycardia, an anticholinergic agent such as atropine or glycopyrrolate (Robinul) is administered 30 to 60 min before the procedure. Adequate doses are 0.01 to 0.03 mg/kg for atropine and 0.002 mg/lb for glycopyrrolate (0.004 mg/lb may be needed for children below two years of age). Glycopyrrolate has a somewhat longer duration of activity. In addition to their effects on heart rate, both agents

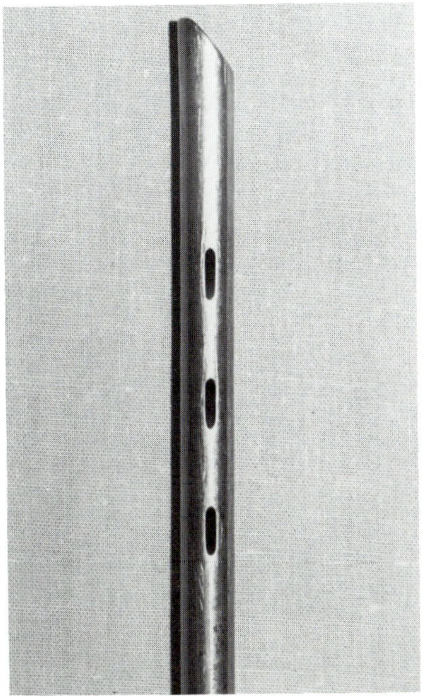

Figure 11-4. Close-up view of bronchoscopic tube reveals side vents for ventilation. Two other side vents, which are not visible, are located on opposite side.

provide other beneficial effects such as decreasing salivary and bronchial secretions.

Vagal stimulation and resultant bradycardia can be minimized by use of topical anesthesia to the pharynx and larynx. When thiopental is used in conjunction with general anesthesia, there is a tendency for laryngospasm to occur with tactile stimulation of the larynx.[4] The use of a topical anesthetic before instrumentation of the larynx may prevent this problem.

Anticholinergic agents tend to alleviate bronchospasm, which can result from instrumentation of the airway, especially when inflammation and hypoxia are present. Intraoperative and postoperative bronchospasm should be considered, especially in patients with hyperreactive airway disease. Intraoperative bronchospasm is somewhat less of a problem with general anesthesia than with local anesthesia when halothane (a bronchodilator) is used; these patients require bronchodilators postoperatively.

Bronchoscopy is associated with a certain amount of edema of the respiratory tissue caused by trauma of instrumentation. The frequency and the degree of this problem depend on the skill of the bronchoscopist. A careful, brief examination is the first step in prevention of postoperative respiratory tract edema. Preoperative use of steroids in a single large dose is advocated for reducing postinstrumentation edema.[5] Intravenous dexamethasone (Decadron) up to doses of 1.5 mg/kg (a maximum of 25 mg) is recommended just before the procedure.[6] In addition, selection of the proper-sized instrument is necessary for keeping postoperative edema, particularly subglottic, to a minimum. Table 11-1 lists the proper sizes of instrument for the ages of patients. Variables such as the presence of inflammatory airway disease and the size of the patient must be kept in mind.

The timing of the procedure is not always an easy deci-

Table 11–1. RECOMMENDED BRONCHOSCOPE SIZE IN RELATION TO AGE OF PATIENT

Bronchoscope Size	Age of Patient
2.5	Premature to neonate
3.0	Neonate to 6 months
3.5	6 to 18 months
4.0	18 to 36 months
5.0	3 to 8 years
6.0	Over 8 years

sion. The child with stridor and severe airway compromise should undergo immediate endoscopic examination. However, in the child with recurrent or persistent pneumonia, it is often difficult to determine the proper timing. Instrumentation of an inflamed airway can lead to increased edema and hemorrhage, and anesthesia can interfere with the ciliary clearance mechanisms. Conversely, conservative observation of the patient may delay removal of thick inspissated secretions, which would offer more rapid drainage of the infected area. The risks of anesthesia must be weighed against the expected benefits of the procedure.

The most important considerations in approaching a patient for bronchoscopy are probably the experience and the skill of the bronchoscopist. A skillful bronchoscopist is able to examine all areas of the airway in the shortest time, thereby decreasing the chance of complications. Postoperative complications such as bronchospasm or vocal cord edema are more likely to occur after a lengthy procedure and with traumatic intubation.

POSTOPERATIVE MANAGEMENT

Regardless of which anesthetic technique or which type of bronchoscope is used, certain postoperative considerations must be taken into account. Despite the skill of the bronchoscopist or the length of the procedure, the patient's vital signs should be carefully monitored. A croupy or barking cough within the first few hours after bronchoscopy is not uncommon in some pediatric patients; however, stridor and substernal retractions indicate progression of the subglottic edema.

Patients undergoing bronchoscopy may need supplemental oxygen and humidification. After rigid bronchoscopy, chest radiography should be performed. Pneumothorax can result from excessive positive pressure ventilation, especially in neonates. Foreign bodies can produce a ball-valve effect with resultant air trapping and pneumothorax, if excessive positive pressure ventilation is used.

A child undergoing bronchoscopy for persistent pneumonia or atelectasis should receive postural drainage postoperatively, especially when an obstructing lesion is removed. Postoperative postural drainage continues the process of removal started by bronchoscopic aspiration. In the removal of a foreign body from the bronchus, it is desirable to remove it in one piece; however, some objects are friable and fragment easily. When this occurs, postural drainage (concentrating on the area of the lung involved) may facilitate the removal of these fragments.

REFERENCES

1. Gans SL, Bersi G: Advances in endoscopy of infants and children. J Pediatr Surg 6:199–231, 1971.
2. Simpson GT, Healy GB, McGill T, Strong MS: Benign tumors and lesions of the larynx in children: Surgical excision by CO2 laser. Ann Otol Rhinol Laryngol 88:479–485, 1979.
3. Stellar S, Polanyi TG, Bredemeir HD: Lasers in surgery. In Wolbarsht ML (ed): Laser Applications in Medicine and Biology, Vol. 2, pp. 241–293. New York: Plenum Press, 1973.
4. Tucker GF: Anesthesia in peroral endoscopy. Oto Clin North Am 1:37–68, 1968.
5. Deming MV, Oech SR: Steroid and antihistaminic therapy for post intubation subglottic edema in infants and children. Anesthesiology 22:933–936, 1961.
6. Healy GB: Personal communication, 1985.

12 FLEXIBLE BRONCHOSCOPY IN CHILDREN

ROBERT E. WOOD, Ph.D., M.D.

In the past two decades, technical advances have made bronchoscopy a more reasonable and productive technique for obtaining information about the lower airways and the lungs. When the glass rod telescope is passed through a rigid (open-tube) bronchoscope, the view is superior to that obtained with standard open-tube bronchoscopes, and all the capabilities for instrumentation as well as ventilation of the patient are preserved during the procedure. The flexible fiberoptic bronchoscope, which revolutionized the approach to lung disease in adults, became available for pediatric use only as recently as 1981. It has some special advantages over the open-tube instruments and also has some major limitations. The primary advantages include the ability to examine the airways of infants and children in comfort and safety without the use of general anesthesia, the ability to examine the entire airway (from nares to segmental bronchi) without introducing major mechanical distortions that are encountered with the passage of open-tube instruments passed orally, and the capability of passage of flexible instruments (especially the ultrathin models) through endotracheal or tracheostomy tubes. The major limitations of the flexible instruments include the inability to pass instruments through the bronchoscope (thus precluding foreign body extraction except in special circumstances) and the fact that the patient must breathe around, rather than through, the flexible bronchoscope.

INSTRUMENTATION

The current standard flexible pediatric bronchoscope is 3.5 to 3.7 mm in outer diameter and has a 1.2-mm suction channel.[1] Smaller models are now available for special applications;[2] the most useful is the model with a 2.2-mm outer diameter and controlled angulation at the tip, but no suction channel (Olympus BF 22). This instrument passes through a 2.5-mm–diameter endotracheal tube. Adult-size flexible instruments have become smaller; new bronchoscopes 4.8 to 4.9 mm in diameter can be used in children as young as 3 to 4 years, whereas the older 5.8- to 6.0-mm–diameter instruments cannot be used safely in children younger than 8 to 10 years.[3]

Rigid (open-tube) bronchoscopes come in a variety of sizes, and a different nomenclature system is used to describe their sizes. Whereas flexible bronchoscopes are characterized by their outer diameter, open-tube instruments are classified by the size of the largest instrument that can pass through them. For example, the Olympus BF 3C20 (nominal outside diameter, 3.5 mm) passes easily through a Storz-Hopkins 3.5-mm rigid bronchoscope, which itself is 4.5 to 5.0 mm in outer diameter. This distinction has practical consequences, especially when the instruments are used to gauge the size of an airway.

SELECTION OF INSTRUMENTS FOR BRONCHOSCOPY IN PEDIATRIC PATIENTS

Since the development of pediatric flexible bronchoscopes, there has been some controversy over which instrument should be used and who should perform the procedure. If there is a choice, the procedure should be conducted with the most suitable instrument by the most skilled operator available. In the majority of cases, flexible bronchoscopes provide the necessary information (including specimens of secretions or washings from the lower airways) with minimal risk and minimal discomfort to the patient. Rigid instruments should always be used for the extraction of foreign bodies. Rigid instruments are also usually necessary for obtaining tissue specimens, although in older pediatric patients the flexible bronchoscopes for adults may be used for transbronchial biopsies. Other indications for use of the open-tube bronchoscope include the operative management of stenosis or obstruction by tissue masses, the detailed assessment of bilateral abductor vocal cord paralysis, and assessment of massive hemoptysis. Anatomic interarytenoid fixation cannot always be evaluated adequately with a flexible bronchoscope. In addition, the search for an H-type tracheoesophageal fistula is most readily facilitated by rigid, rather than flexible, bronchoscopy. The flexible bronchoscope may be suitable for virtually all other indications, provided that the bronchoscopist is skilled in its use and that a rigid bronchoscope is available if needed.

INDICATIONS FOR BRONCHOSCOPY

There is only one indication for bronchoscopy: the need to obtain information about the airways or pulmo-

Table 12–1. COMMON INDICATIONS FOR
BRONCHOSCOPY IN PEDIATRIC PATIENTS

Stridor
Atelectasis
Persistent wheezing (especially if patient is unresponsive to
    bronchodilators)
Suspected or known foreign body
Hemoptysis
Cough (persistent and unresponsive to therapy)
Evaluation of airway trauma (accident, prolonged intubation)
Localized air trapping
Abnormal cry, hoarseness
Suspected vocal cord paralysis
Unexplained upper airway obstruction
Recurrent aspiration
Pneumonia in a compromised host
Recurrent or persistent pneumonia
Suspected tuberculosis with radiographic abnormalities
Congenital anomalies (vascular ring, esophageal atresia,
    tracheoesophageal fistula, abnormal airway branching patterns, etc.)
Pulmonary hemosiderosis
Pulmonary parenchymal mass lesions, abscesses

nary parenchyma that can be obtained better by bronchoscopy than by other means. Chevalier Jackson once said, "When in doubt as to whether bronchoscopy should be performed, bronchoscopy should always be performed."[4] This statement, made in 1915, is still true, but the advice must be moderated by the availability of proper equipment and expertise in its use.

The specific indications for bronchoscopy vary somewhat with the age of the patient. In adults, the most common indications for bronchoscopy are malignancy or specific forms of infection. In children, congenital malformations, abnormal airway dynamics, and aspirated foreign body are more common indications for bronchoscopy than is malignancy. Specific frequent indications for bronchoscopy in pediatric patients are listed in Table 12–1. Many of these indications overlap: for example, in a child with persistent pneumonia, a foreign body should also be suspected.

In children, a negative bronchoscopic examination is often of equal importance to the management of the patient as a positive finding. This is especially true in the case of a suspected foreign body. A review of experience with the flexible bronchoscope in pediatric patients indicates that significant diagnostic information is obtained in a high percentage of patients.[5]

STRIDOR

The evaluation of infants with stridor is one of the major indications for endoscopic procedures in pediatric patients. In most cases, these procedures are most effectively performed with a flexible instrument, which enables the operator to examine the entire upper airway, including the nose and the palate. Also, it does not introduce distorting mechanical forces, inasmuch as the instrument passes through the nose into the posterior pharynx, while the head and neck are in a natural position, without displacing the tongue or laryngeal structures. Patients with acute, apparently infectious croup do not need endoscopic evaluation unless there are unusual

features of the patient's illness or history (e.g., prolonged or repeated stridor, history of prior intubation, onset at a very early age). It may be difficult to distinguish infectious laryngeal edema from subglottic stenosis complicated by acute infection; manipulation of the edematous larynx may produce more obstruction, thus precipitating the need for an artificial airway.

The majority of infants with persistent stridor have laryngomalacia, but there are other possibilities, such as foreign body, subglottic and supraglottic mass lesions (hemangiomas, cysts), congenital or acquired subglottic stenosis, hypotonia of the pharyngeal airway, enlarged adenoids or tonsils or both, and choanal stenosis. Stridor may be produced by lesions in the trachea, most notably tracheomalacia and extrinsic tracheal compression, or by an esophageal foreign body or an anomalous vessel (usually the innominate artery). In a significant percentage of patients with stridor caused by a laryngeal or supralaryngeal problem, there are also abnormalities in the lower airway,[6] and a complete endoscopic evaluation is usually indicated. The lower airway can be visualized endoscopically if there is no significant laryngeal edema or stenosis. If the patient has stridor at the time of the examination, the vibrating structures producing the stridor are always seen.

In patients with acute onset of stridor, a foreign body, which may be in the airway or the esophagus, must always be suspected. The younger the patient when the stridor develops, the more likely it is to be the result of a congenital anomaly.

ATELECTASIS

Atelectasis is another common indication for bronchoscopy in children. The more extensive the atelectasis and the younger the patient, the more likely it is to respond to bronchoscopic suctioning. Atelectasis that persists despite adequate medical therapy should be investigated with bronchoscopy, unless it is known to be caused by an underlying lung disease that predisposes the patient to atelectasis (e.g., cystic fibrosis). This diagnostic evaluation enables the clinician to rule out the presence of a foreign body and also provides specimens from the site for culture and microscopic examination. In the presence of established airway disease (as in cystic fibrosis), the probability of relieving atelectasis by bronchoscopy is relatively low. In small infants, atelectasis of the right upper lobe is relatively common and does not usually respond well to bronchoscopic suctioning. It is difficult to suction the right upper lobe of young infants without obstructing the rest of the airway.

FOREIGN BODY ASPIRATION

If a pulmonary foreign body is known to be present, it should be removed as soon as possible with an open-tube bronchoscope. Many special instruments for foreign body extraction are available, and patients should not be deprived of their benefit. Manipulation of foreign bodies with the flexible bronchoscopes currently available is extremely difficult and should not be attempted except under special circumstances. In the acute situation, it should not be too difficult to determine with reasonable accuracy (history, physical examination, radiography) which patients should undergo bronchoscopy for removal of a foreign body. On the other hand, in many patients the evidence of foreign body is equivocal, and the physician may be justifiably reluctant to send such patients for general anesthesia and rigid bronchoscopy. In addition, the presence of a foreign body is often not accompanied by a typical history or typical physical examination or radiographic findings. In these situations, the flexible bronchoscope may be most useful.[7] If a foreign body is found, it should not be manipulated, but the patient should promptly undergo rigid bronchoscopy. Consultation between the bronchoscopists using flexible and rigid instruments may be helpful for determining which procedure should be performed. The result of this practice is that some patients have to undergo two bronchoscopies, but the number of foreign bodies missed and the well-known consequences are reduced.

PERSISTENT WHEEZING

Persistent wheezing that is unresponsive or poorly responsive to bronchodilators may be the result of airway anomalies such as tracheomalacia, extrinsic compression of airways, endobronchial lesions such as granulation tissue, or foreign bodies.[1,6] In some patients, the source of the wheeze may be the upper airway. At the time of bronchoscopy, the esophagus may also be examined for evidence of esophagitis (which would raise suspicion of gastroesophageal reflux as a cause of the wheezing). However, the visual examination of the esophagus is not totally reliable, and biopsy may be required in order to verify the presence of inflammation in the lower esophagus.

HEMOPTYSIS

Hemoptysis is unusual in pediatric patients, and if there is no ready explanation on the basis of known disease, bronchoscopic evaluation may be required. To locate the source of the bleeding, the bronchoscopy must be performed during active bleeding, unless there is a visible endobronchial lesion. In some patients, it may be unclear whether blood is coming from the lungs or from another source, even when the airways are examined. Saline lavage may be helpful in this situation, as the washings may contain either frank blood or hemosiderin-laden macrophages. Hemosiderin appears in macrophages beginning 48 to 72 hours after acute intrapulmonary bleeding (or aspiration of blood, if it reaches the alveolar spaces).[8] In the diagnostic evaluation and management of massive hemoptysis, it is probably better to use rigid rather than flexible instruments because of their relatively greater capacity for suctioning large volumes of blood. Occasionally, after large bleeds, the airways may be filled with clots; these may be more readily removed through a rigid bronchoscope.

CHRONIC PERSISTENT COUGHING

Patients with persistent cough may require bronchoscopic investigation, especially if the cough is severe and persistent despite appropriate therapy. Children with abnormal airway dynamics (e.g., tracheomalacia) may develop a cough that persists after the resolution of an acute infectious illness, as a result of a cycle of mechanical stimulation of the airway walls with expiratory collapse, which in turn leads to more irritation and cough. In other patients, cough may be a manifestation of an occult infection or a foreign body. In an occasional patient, bronchoscopy can rule out the lungs as the source of a persistent cough and direct definitive investigation elsewhere.

AIRWAY TRAUMA

Bronchoscopy may be helpful in the management of patients with trauma to the airway, whether from external trauma or from prolonged or difficult intubation. Infants are particularly susceptible to airway damage from suction catheters and may develop granulation tissue and cicatricial stenosis, especially in the right main stem bronchus and the right lower lobe. It is not always possible to predict the subsequent course after trauma from the appearance of the subglottic space, although if the mucosa has been widely disrupted, subsequent subglottic stenosis is more likely.

LOCALIZED HYPERINFLATION

Radiographic evidence of localized air trapping may lead to suspicion of foreign body, bronchial obstruction, or other lesions. If there is an acute history of choking, the patient should undergo rigid bronchoscopy. Bronchography may be performed easily through flexible bronchoscopes; the additional visual examination leads to a much more informative procedure than do bronchograms performed through a catheter alone. In addition, the flexible bronchoscope may be directed much more selectively than a catheter, and the resulting bronchogram may be of higher quality with the use of less contrast material.

VOCAL ABNORMALITIES

The flexible bronchoscope is a useful tool for the evaluation of patients with abnormalities of the voice (e.g., persistent hoarseness, abnormal cry). Vocal cord movement may be observed easily in most cases, especially because general anesthesia is not used. In some cases, rigid laryngoscopy may be required, such as in patients with floppy supralaryngeal structures that obscure the view of the glottis or in patients with bilateral cord paralysis. In the latter case, it may be important to distinguish between neurogenic paralysis and interarytenoid fixation; this distinction may be accomplished with a rigid instrument.

UPPER AIRWAY OBSTRUCTION

Flexible endoscopy may be very useful for determining the causes of upper airway obstruction. The transnasal passage of a flexible bronchoscope may reveal anatomic findings or dynamics that are not apparent on physical or radiographic examination. In this setting, it may be of importance to examine the patient both awake and asleep, because the airway dynamics often change dramatically between the two states. The use of an ultrashort-acting barbiturate such as methohexital at doses sufficient to produce light sleep for 1 to 2 min (0.5 to 1.0 mg/kg intravenously) is often very helpful especially in patients who have sleep-associated obstruction. In some patients with anatomic obstruction, it may be necessary to examine the nasopharynx from the pharyngeal aspect, using a rigid telescope with a 120-degree prism after retracting the soft palate.

RECURRENT OR PERSISTENT PNEUMONIA

Recurrent or persistent pneumonia may be associated with a variety of causes, including occult tracheoesophageal fistula, foreign body, bronchial abnormalities, and recurrent aspiration. Bronchoscopy may be helpful in eliminating surgically correctable lesions, documenting the microbial flora of the lower respiratory tract, diagnosing immotile cilia syndrome and its variants, and defining aspiration on the basis of microscopic examination of bronchial washings (lipid-laden macrophages). Specimens of bronchial washings should always be sent for cytologic examination as well as for culture and other studies. The cytology laboratory should be informed of the specific nature of the questions being asked so that the appropriate staining can be performed.

SPECIAL TECHNIQUES AND APPLICATIONS

In many children with radiographic or physical evidence of lower airway disease, parenchymal disease, or both, adequate specimens of secretions for bacteriologic and cytologic study are difficult to obtain. This may be of special importance in immunocompromised patients. Direct lung puncture may be useful in selected cases, but is accompanied by a relatively high incidence of complications such as pneumothorax. In adults, specimens can be obtained through the flexible bronchoscope with the use of a special bronchial brush, which is protected from contamination by being enclosed in two outer catheters with the ends plugged. Unfortunately, the pediatric flexible bronchoscope is too small for use with a protected brush, and so specimens obtained through a bronchoscope either by direct aspiration or by saline lavage must to some degree be suspected of contamination with upper airway flora. Microscopic examination of the aspirate or washings can be helpful in identifying specimens with oral contamination. If the organism is a pathogen, no matter where found in the airway (e.g., *Pneumocystis carinii*), the specimen is of diagnostic benefit. Quantitative culture technique is of great value in assessing the validity of bronchial washings. With care and skill, adequate specimens can be obtained in the majority of pediatric patients, and bronchoscopy with localized saline lavage is a very useful diagnostic procedure.

The flexible bronchoscope is extremely useful for the facilitation of tracheal intubation in patients for whom inhalation would otherwise be very difficult.[9] Such patients include those with cervical or temporomandibular ankylosis and those with oral or pharyngeal mass lesions. The standard pediatric flexible bronchoscope can be used with an endotracheal tube as small as 4.5 mm in inside diameter; the 2.2-mm instrument can be used with a tube as small as 2.5 mm. Additional advantages of using the bronchoscope to facilitate intubation include the visual examination of the entire airway during the intubation and the ability to position the tip of the endotracheal tube without having to depend on a radiograph to verify tube position.

Questions are commonly raised with regard to the lower airways in patients already intubated. A flexible bronchoscope of appropriate size can be passed through the tube to examine the lower airways without extubating the patient. If the tube is small, the bronchoscope can be inserted and removed within a very short time (e.g., 30 to 45 sec) so as to minimally interrupt ventilation. When a bronchoscope is passed through an existing tube, it may be difficult to be certain of the anatomy, because the entire airway is not visualized. If the tip of the tube is below the carina or if there are anatomic variants (such as tracheal bronchus to the right upper lobe), considerable confusion may result. In patients with a tracheostomy, it may be helpful to pass the flexible bronchoscope through the glottis and then alongside the tracheostomy tube, thus leaving the airway unobstructed. A smaller tracheostomy tube may be placed temporarily to facilitate such examinations.

Patients with esophageal atresia and tracheoesophageal fistula should probably undergo bronchoscopy in preparation for surgical repair, in order to be certain that there are not two fistulas (i.e., an H-type fistula in addition to the distal fistula). The open-tube bronchoscope is superior to a flexible instrument in a search for a fistula because it enables the operator to probe the posterior tracheal wall with a catheter, which may then be passed through the fistula and left in place for easier localization of the fistula during the subsequent surgical repair. Furthermore, the open-tube instrument gives a better view of the posterior aspect of the upper trachea than can be obtained with the flexible instruments, and positive pressure can be applied in order to distend the trachea and thus more easily identify the fistula. It is also useful to examine the esophageal pouch for evidence of a second fistula if it is not seen from the tracheal side.

Bronchoscopy can be performed in even the smallest infants for either diagnostic or therapeutic reasons. Massive atelectasis is not uncommon in premature infants receiving ventilatory support, especially after extubation, and is often caused by large central mucus plugs. Bronchoscopy is suitable for relieving this condition and may be less traumatic to the airways and more effective than repeated reintubation and blind suctioning. With a bronchoscope, suctioning is more effective and can be directed to the proper area, and the results can be assessed visually. In addition, endobronchial abnormalities may be diagnosed. Either rigid or flexible bronchoscopes may be used for this purpose; with either, the small size and the clinical fragility of these patients mandates a very careful approach.

CONTRAINDICATIONS TO BRONCHOSCOPY

If bronchoscopy is the most effective and safest method of obtaining information that is vitally needed, there are no contraindications to bronchoscopy. In this statement, of course, it is assumed that suitable equipment and techniques are used and that all necessary measures are taken to reduce or eliminate risk factors. The specific risk factors present in a given situation may dictate the choice of technique. For example, in a patient with known airway obstruction, a rigid bronchoscope may be required in order to maintain ventilation during the procedure, or an ultrathin instrument may be required to pass through a narrowed area without producing further obstruction or edema. In general, bronchoscopes of either type should not be passed through a critically narrowed point in the airway. Patients with bleeding problems may be given platelet or clotting factor transfusions before bronchoscopy, and in these patients, flexible bronchoscopy is probably safer than rigid bronchoscopy. The only absolute contraindication to bronchoscopy is the lack of a rational indication.

ANESTHESIA FOR BRONCHOSCOPY

Because of the mechanical considerations inherent in the use of the open-tube bronchoscope, general anesthesia is preferred for almost all cases in which these instruments are used. In patients who are believed to be at serious risk with anesthesia, the procedure may be performed with topical anesthesia and extreme caution. With the flexible bronchoscope, general anesthesia is virtually never required. However, adequate topical anesthesia of the larynx is always necessary. Flexible bronchoscopy should be performed on a patient who is comfortable. Comfort may be ensured by chemical sedation or, in selected older patients, by relaxation facilitated by hypnotic techniques. Hypnoanalgesia is a useful adjunct to chemical sedation in patients of all ages.

Standard techniques for sedation in children may be used for flexible bronchoscopy, such as intramuscular meperidine/promethazine/chlorpromazine (or DPT: Demerol/Phenergan/Thorazine) or narcotics given intravenously. Intravenous sedation appears to be more satisfactory because the dose may be titrated to achieve the desired level of sedation, and most patients awaken more readily after the procedure is over. Whatever method is used, adequate sedation to maintain calm and comfort without reaching a level of general anesthesia makes the procedure safer and probably more successful, as well as reduces stress on the patient.

The author prefers to use intravenous meperidine (1 to 2 mg/kg) in combination with midazolam (0.05 to 0.1 mg/kg). If necessary, the effects of meperidine can be instantly reversed by the administration of naloxone (Narcan). The potential for respiratory depression exists if the patient is too deeply sedated. The usual dose of meperidine is 1 to 2 mg/kg, given as an intravenous infusion over 30 to 60 sec. In children aged 7 to 8 years and older, 0.5 to 1.0 mg/kg may be equally effective. The maximal effect should be apparent within 5 to 10 min, and the dose may be titrated upward to achieve the desired effect.

In some patients, especially those who are agitated upon entering the procedure room, rapid induction of sedation with an ultra–short-acting barbiturate may be very helpful. Agents such as methohexital in intravenous doses of 0.5 to 1.0 mg/kg produce deep sedation that lasts for 1 to 2 min; if necessary, administration of methohexital may be repeated once or twice during the procedure. Agents such as methohexital produce effects bordering on general anesthesia; therefore, extreme caution is needed in their use because respiratoy depression can be a major problem. Furthermore, if more than one dose is used, the combined effects of the barbiturate and the narcotic may last much longer. Therefore, when such drugs are used, the physician must be prepared to support the patient's ventilation in the immediate postprocedure period. In some patients, especially those with sleep-associated airway obstruction, intravenous short-acting barbiturate may be used alone if the total duration of the procedure is to be no more than 2 to 3 min. Patients undergoing sedation must be carefully monitored.[10]

As noted earlier, hypnoanalgesic techniques may substantially reduce the dose of drugs needed. Training in hypnosis is useful for a bronchoscopist. A few principles may be stated here: Control of the patient's expectation of the experience modifies to a major degree the perception of the experience, and the physician can manipulate the patient's expectation advantageously. Likewise, it is important to control the flow of information to the patient during the procedure. Patients under stress may be more receptive to suggestion than they would ordinarily be. Even though the patient may appear to be asleep, subtle (or not-so-subtle) comments or other sounds may have significant impact on the patient during the procedure. Positive suggestions of calm, comfort, and reassurance during the procedure are extremely helpful. At the end of the procedure, suggestions regarding feelings of well-being, hunger, and so forth may reduce postsedation nausea.

Topical anesthesia of the upper airway and larynx is always required, even in patients under general anesthesia. Lidocaine is probably the safest agent and may be used in 2% concentration in saline. Inadequacy of anesthesia is the most common cause of difficulty in getting a flexible bronchoscope through the glottis and may also result in serious complications (i.e., vagal stimulation with bradycardia or laryngospasm). Topical agents may also be used in the lower airways to control cough and to reduce the possibility of bronchospasm, which is especially important in patients with a history of asthma. The total dose of lidocaine necessary for topical anesthesia varies with the size of the patient, and should not in general exceed 5 to 7 mg/kg. In practice, much of the lidocaine instilled into the upper or lower airways may be removed immediately by suctioning, and so the absorbed dose is usually much lower than the administered dose.

Atropine may be optionally used before bronchoscopy in order to reduce airway secretions. In most patients undergoing general anesthesia, this is routinely done. For most pediatric patients undergoing fiberoptic bronchoscopy, atropine is not necessary because the duration of the procedure is short. The doses of atropine normally used for preoperative preparation are not vagolytic and thus do not afford additional protection against laryngospasm.

COMPLICATIONS OF BRONCHOSCOPY

The complications of bronchoscopic procedures depend on the instrument used and the clinical situation in which the procedure is done, as well as on the skill and experience of the bronchoscopist. The most common complication of rigid bronchoscopy is subglottic edema, which may develop within minutes to hours after the procedure. Subglottic edema is more common after prolonged procedures, especially those requiring extensive manipulation (such as extraction of foreign bodies). Other complications of rigid bronchoscopy include mechanical trauma to the airway (bleeding, air leakages), infection (from aspirated secretions or contamination of instruments from upper airway flora), arrhythmias, laryngospasm or bronchospasm, hypoxia, and anesthetic complications.

Because the flexible bronchoscope must be sufficiently small that the patient can breathe around it, it is more difficult to produce subglottic edema than with a rigid instrument. The most common complications with the flexible instruments include epistaxis (because the instrument is passed through the nose), hypoxia with bradycardia (especially in very small infants who cannot adequately ventilate around the instrument), and minor anesthetic problems (urticaria or other drug reactions). Bronchospasm or laryngospasm can occur (although the risk can be minimized by adequate topical anesthesia). All the other potential complications of rigid bronchoscopy can also occur with flexible bronchoscopy. Clinical experience indicates that the incidence of complications is lower with flexible bronchoscopes than with rigid instruments. However, the incidence of complications is influenced by the skill and judgment of the bronchoscopist and by the selection of patients for bronchoscopy.

REFERENCES

1. Wood RE, Postma D: Endoscopy of the airway in infants and children. J Pediatr 112:1–6, 1988.
2. Wood RE, Azizkhan RG, Lacey SR, et al: Surgical applications of ultrathin flexible bronchoscopes in infants. Ann Otol Rhinol Laryngol 100:116–119, 1991.
3. Sackner MA: Bronchofiberscopy. Am Rev Respir Dis, 111:62–88, 1975.
4. Jackson C: Peroral Endoscopy and Laryngeal Surgery, p. 201. St. Louis: The Laryngoscope Company, 1915.
5. Wood RE: The diagnostic effectiveness of flexible bronchoscopes in pediatric patients. Pediatr Pulmonol 1:188–192, 1985.
6. Wood RE, Spelunking in the pediatric airways: Explorations with the flexible bronchoscope. Pediatr Clin North Am 31:785–799, 1984.
7. Wood RE, Gauderer MWL: The flexible bronchoscope in the management of tracheobronchial foreign bodies in children: The value of a combined approach with open tube bronchoscopy. J Pediatr Surg 19:693–698, 1984.
8. Sherman JM, Winnie G, Thomassen MJ, et al: Time course of hemosiderin production and clearance by human pulmonary macrophages. Chest 86:409–411, 1984.
9. Rucker RW, Silva WJ, Worcester CC: Fiberoptic bronchoscopic nasotracheal intubation in children. Chest 76:56–58, 1979.
10. Guidelines for the elective use of conscious sedation, deep sedation, and general anesthesia in pediatric patients. Pediatrics 76:317–321, 1985.

13 BRONCHOALVEOLAR LAVAGE

WARREN E. REGELMANN, M.D. / GREG R. ELLIOTT, M.D.

The introduction of the pediatric bronchoscope (Olympus BF 3C4) made possible the exploration of the respiratory tract of infants and small children with sedation but without general anesthesia. The advantage of this bronchoscope over previous small fiberoptic bronchoscopes was that it enabled the passage of lavage material and small uncovered brushes through its 1.2-mm–inside diameter (ID) suction channel. By the mid-1980s, studies of bronchoalveolar lavage (BAL) in children with diffuse lung diseases were being conducted.[1-14] Reviews concerning the use of this technique in children soon followed.[15,][16] The indications for BAL and protocols for analysis of the resulting fluid in the children are still evolving. Nonetheless it is now clear that several diseases affecting children may be more efficiently and safely diagnosed through BAL than by previously available means.

EQUIPMENT

BAL is accomplished most reliably by a flexible fiberoptic bronchoscope because it can be directed to a specific area of the lung and gently wedged into a lobar, segmental, or subsegmental bronchus without significantly damaging the airway wall. The most experience with BAL in infants and small children so far has been gained with the use of a 3.5-mm–outside diameter (OD) bronchoscope. However, thinner bronchoscopes are available with small suction channels. These ultrathin bronchoscopes currently do not have directed distal flexion capabilities. Disposable thin bronchoscopes with external diameters of <2.5 mm may be useful for BAL, but wedging may be difficult because the distal tips may not be smooth; thus there exists the potential of traumatizing the bronchial wall. These disposable bronchoscopes also do not have directed distal flexion capability.

A limitation of the 3.5-mm–OD bronchoscopes is that the channel is too small for passing biopsy forceps or protected brushes. The 4.5-mm–OD bronchoscope is the smallest bronchoscope currently available that has a large enough working channel (2.0-mm ID) to permit the use of transbronchial biopsy forceps or protected brushes. The authors have successfully used the 4.5-mm–OD bronchoscope in children as young as 6 years of age when transbronchial biopsies or the use of covered brushes are indicated in addition to BAL.

TECHNIQUES OF FLEXIBLE BRONCHOSCOPY WITH BRONCHOALVEOLAR LAVAGE

Techniques for performing BAL vary according to status of the patient and facilities available. In many children, it is possible to perform BAL with light to moderate sedation and adequate amounts of topical anesthesia. The authors' practices generally include a short-acting narcotic with or without an intravenous benzodiazepine. The procedure begins with aerosolization of 2 to 4 ml of 4% lidocaine before sedation. Next, topical 4% lidocaine gel is used in the nasal passage and 1% lidocaine through the bronchoscope to anesthetize the glottic region. Small amounts of 1% lidocaine (without preservative) are used via the bronchoscope in the airway to improve the control of coughing. In order to obtain an adequate BAL sample, it is important to maintain firm wedging of the bronchoscope. This is difficult if the patient moves or coughs excessively. The risk of bleeding with such movement is also increased if there is thrombocytopenia or a coagulopathy. BAL is frequently performed in children who are immunocompromised, in whom these problems with hemostasis are more common. As a general rule, the authors make every effort to maintain the patient's plate-

let count at >50,000 and correct coagulopathies before BAL. If these precautions are taken, significant bleeding is rarely a problem. Because so many of these high-risk pediatric patients also have severe airway inflammation respiratory compromise with hypoxia, and excessive anxiety, the authors prefer to electively intubate such patients in whom BAL is to be done.

The 3.5-mm–OD bronchoscope passes easily through a 5.0-mm endotracheal tube and through some, but not all, 4.5-mm endotracheal tubes. For this reason, if general anesthesia is required, bronchoscopy is performed in small children while they are ventilated through a mask under general anesthesia. To accomplish this, adaptors that have adequate side ports to allow the entry of the bronchoscope through the mask are used.

All patients who undergo BAL should be monitored closely. The procedure should be done in the safest setting, in which resuscitative equipment is immediately available. Such settings include intensive care units, special procedures areas, and operating rooms. The authors recommend monitoring the cardiac rate and rhythm, continuous oxygen saturation by pulse oximetry, and monitoring blood pressure every 1 to 3 min at minimum. A trained clinician other than the bronchoscopist should monitor the patient. Airway obstruction is a significant problem in small children; hence BAL should be performed as quickly as possible. The authors generally evaluate the airway, remove excessive mucus, and then remove the bronchoscope for a few minutes before proceeding with the lavage.

In patients with diffuse disease, the authors' experience, as well as that of others, has been that the most suitable segments for lavage are in the right middle lobe or the lingula.[16-19] In these areas the wedge is accomplished more easily, and the volume of BAL return is generally much higher than that recovered from the lower or upper lobes. The volume of BAL return is generally between 50% to 75% of the volume of solution instilled but may be less in patients with obstructive airway disease.[17-19]

Physiologic sterile saline without preservatives is used as the standard solution for BAL. In adult patients, instilled volumes range from five aliquots of 20 ml each to three aliquots of 50 ml each per lobe lavaged. Lavage is occasionally repeated in another lobe. The total volume instilled generally should not exceed 300 ml.[18, 19] Total volumes used in children have ranged from 5% to 15% of the functional residual capacity (FRC), which is proportional to the total volume per FRC used in adults.[4, 5] The FRC can be estimated on the basis of the patient's height.[20] The relationship between volume instilled and diagnostic yield has not been adequately evaluated in children or adults. Because a higher proportion of lung may be obstructed and lavaged with the wedge located more centrally in infants and small children, the incidence of hypoxia caused by ventilation-perfusion mismatching may be increased in this age group.[21,22] However, using the lavage quantity of 5% to 10% of FRC and minimizing dwell time, the authors have not observed significant complications in more than 200 lavages in children. BAL procedures must be terminated immediately when arterial oxygen saturation (Sa_{O_2}) by continuous oximetry falls significantly.

After the bronchoscope is wedged, lavage solution is instilled through the suction channel. The fluid can be recovered by manual suction through a syringe; however, the authors have found it more efficient to use a series of traps in line-to-wall suction. In this setup, suction tubing is connected to the suction port of the bronchoscope. A three-way stopcock is connected in this line. Its side port is connected to a syringe containing the lavage material. Its main port is connected by suction tubing to sterile suction specimen collection traps connected in series. The exit port of the last trap is connected by suction tubing to a wall suction apparatus set at ≤120 mm Hg of negative pressure. Excessive negative pressure may cause the airways distal to the bronchoscope to collapse, preventing the aspiration of BAL fluid. Negative pressure of 120 mm Hg is adequate for obtaining sufficient return of the lavage fluid via the 1.2-mm–ID channel of the 3.5-mm pediatric bronchoscope. The suction is used minimally, and the sterile traps are bypassed until the time of the lavage so as to minimize contamination of the collected material with upper airway secretion. Lavage material is then collected in the traps, pooled, and distributed to the appropriate specimen containers for laboratory analysis. Data is insufficient for evaluating whether diagnostic yield is affected by inclusion of the initial lavage return. In general, it is included in diagnostic lavages.

RISKS OF FIBEROPTIC BRONCHOSCOPY WITH BRONCHOALVEOLAR LAVAGE

BAL has not been shown to cause major life-threatening complications in addition to those seen with bronchoscopy alone.[19, 23] BAL increases the time necessary for the bronchoscope to remain in the airway (dwell time), which may lead to significant hypercapnea, hypoxia, or both in certain high-risk patients, especially small children. BAL increases the likelihood of postbronchoscopy fever,[17, 23] and it may increase the risk of pulmonary infection or hemorrhage.[22] The authors have not observed documented infectious or hemorrhagic complications in BAL in more than 200 severely immunocompromised children. Special attention is paid to optimizing the platelet count to >50,000/cu mm and to correcting coagulation abnormalities. The authors usually infuse platelets simultaneously with BAL in patients in whom optimal counts cannot be achieved beforehand. Careful cleaning and sterilization of bronchoscopes minimizes the risk of nosocomial infection.[24]

DIAGNOSTIC APPLICATIONS OF FLEXIBLE BRONCHOSCOPY WITH BRONCHOALVEOLAR LAVAGE

THE IMMUNOCOMPROMISED CHILD AND THE DIAGNOSIS OF OPPORTUNISTIC INFECTIONS

Pediatric BAL is most commonly used for diagnosis of opportunistic infections in immunocompromised children when less invasive approaches have not yielded sat-

isfactory findings or when more invasive procedures are considered to entail too high a risk.[3, 4, 15, 25] The presence of *Pneumocystis carinii, Mycobacterium tuberculosis,* and *Legionella, Nocardia, Histoplasma, Cryptococcus, Blastomyces,* and *Coccidioides* organisms in the BAL of these patients provides etiologic diagnosis of the lung disease. In immunosuppressed patients with diffuse lung infiltrates, *P. carinii* can be identified in BAL with a sensitivity of ≥85%.[3, 25–27] Absence of *P. carinii* in BAL in immunosuppressed patients has a negative predictive value of >90%. These data are based on response to therapy or histologic findings on biopsy or autopsy.[26–28] These values are comparable with those obtained in the past from open-lung biopsy, and the incidence of morbidity from the procedure is significantly lower. In these patients, the sensitivity for detecting *M. tuberculosis* is ≥95%. The negative predictive value of absence of *M. tuberculosis* on BAL is ≥90%.[26, 27]

The recovery from BAL of microbes such as *Aspergillus, Candida,* atypical *Mycobacteria,* cytomegalovirus (CMV), and common flora of the upper respiratory tract does not necessarily imply that these organisms are causing the lung disease, even in immunocompromised hosts. Diagnosis of pulmonary infections caused by these organisms is often presumptive. The positive predictive value for CMV pneumonia associated with detection or culture of CMV in BAL in the absence of positive cytologic BAL findings is uncertain.[29] In one study,[30] the detection of CMV in BAL from immunocompromised children with pneumonitis was correlated with clinical improvement in respiratory status when the CMV was eliminated by gancyclovir. In bone marrow transplant patients who were in the postoperative period, the elimination of CMV from BAL was successfully accomplished by gancyclovir, but this was not associated with reversal of their respiratory disease. This suggests that non–CMV-related lung damage remained in these patients. Drug toxicity, graft-versus-host disease, adult respiratory distress syndrome, pulmonary edema, radiation injury, and oxygen toxicity may contribute to pulmonary disease in these patients.

Quantitative bacterial cultures of BAL have been used to diagnose pneumonia in immunocompromised and immunocompetent patients. When BAL with <1% squamous epithelial cells was analyzed, the finding of >10⁵ colony-forming units of a single bacterial species per milliliter of BAL was correlated with bacterial pneumonia in comparison with BAL from normal subjects.[31–33] BAL has also been useful for establishing the cause of acute pneumonia in patients on ventilators.[34]

THE CHILD WITH RECURRENT OR CHRONIC PULMONARY INFILTRATES

Eliciting sputum from children is frequently difficult. BAL is a rational alternative to more invasive pulmonary sampling procedures in children with persistent or recurrent pulmonary infiltrates of unknown cause. In an outpatient setting, it has enabled the recovery of mycobacterial species that were not recovered in multiple gastric aspirates or urine.[35–39] This recovery may be important in children living in areas of the world where multiple resistant *M. tuberculosis* strains are prevalent or where the infecting strain has not been recovered from the adult source.

Examination of the alveolar cells and fluid recovered in BAL may provide a definitive diagnosis of noninfectious causes of recurrent or persistent pulmonary infiltrates. In patients with pulmonary alveolar proteinosis, combined staining of BAL by Alcian blue and periodic acid–Schiff (PAS) demonstrates large amounts of PAS-positive material, scant Alcian blue staining, and relatively few alveolar macrophages.[14, 19, 40, 41] In diseases associated with pulmonary hemorrhage, such as idiopathic pulmonary hemosiderosis, Wegener's granulomatosis, and Goodpasture's disease, positive staining of a majority of alveolar macrophages for hemosiderin is strongly suggestive of chronic hemorrhage.[42, 43] The changes in BAL over time after pulmonary hemorrhage have been described and provide useful guidelines in interpreting the results of hemosiderin staining.[44] Lipid-laden macrophages have been associated with aspiration syndromes.[45, 46] However, studies suggest that in neonates, these macrophages may be present in other disorders as well.[47] The presence of Langerhans cells staining with the monoclonal antibody OKT-6 is highly suggestive of pulmonary histiocytosis X.[48] Increased generation of reactive oxygen species by alveolar macrophages was described in children with idiopathic interstitial lung disease; steroid treatment decreased this response.[5] It may be possible to evaluate the efficacy of steroid therapy by assessing its ability to reduce increased number of lymphocytes in BAL.[49] The decision to use other drugs in idiopathic interstitial lung disease may be supported by demonstrating the presence of eosinophils or neutrophils in BAL. This finding has been documented in adults,[49] but its applicability to children remains to be established. Reynolds[18] and Gibson and associates[19] reviewed the use of BAL in the diagnosis and management of adults with diffuse interstitial lung disease.

LABORATORY PROCESSING OF BRONCHOALVEOLAR LAVAGE

Because the primary clinical indication for BAL is for diagnostic purposes, quality-controlled transport and laboratory procedures should be in place at the time the BAL is obtained.

The authors' routine laboratory analysis in an immunocompromised patient is an attempt to confirm the presence of likely opportunistic microbes as soon as possible (Table 13–1). The techniques include rapid antigen detection, silver methenamine staining, Gram's stain, potassium hydroxide preparation, and acid-fast staining. In addition to routine aerobic cultures, special media for isolation of *Nocardia, Legionella,* and *Mycobacteria* species and of fungi are used. Cultures for respiratory and herpes group viruses are performed. Gluteraldehyde fixation for electron microscopy is performed as needed. Wright's staining of the cells recovered is used to determine a differential count of inflammatory cells. The results of the stains for bacteria, fungi, *P. carinii,* and rapid antigen detection for *Legionella* species, respiratory syncytial virus, and CMV should be available on the day of the procedure.

The authors' routine analysis for evaluation of a child with persistent or recurrent infiltrates is designed to detect likely microbes, to characterize any inflammatory cell response, to detect proteinosis, to quantify the proportion of lipid- and hemosiderin-laden macrophages, and to detect and characterize any abnormal cells, such as Langerhans cells. A number of other tests may be included for specific indications or research.

Normal cell differential analysis for children[5] is similar to that for adults[18, 19, 50–52] (Table 13–2). Two methods of determining the differential counts have been used. The most commonly used technique is cytocentrifugation, but this technique has been shown to underestimate the

Table 13–1. EVALUATION OF BRONCHOALVEOLAR LAVAGE IN IMMUNOCOMPROMISED PATIENTS

Stains	Cultures	Antigen Determinations	Cytology
KOH	Bacterial	*Legionella*	Cell count
Gram's	Routine aerobic	RSV	differential
Silver methenamine	*Legionella*	CMV	
Pneumocystis carinii	*Nocardia*		
Fungi	*Mycobacteria*		
Actinomyces	Viral		
Wright	CMV		
Chlamydial inclusions	Respiratory battery		
H&E	RSV		
Routine cytology	Influenza		
	Parainfluenza		
	Adenovirus		
	Enteroviruses		
	Fungal		
	Aspergillus		
	Candida		
	Chlamydia		

KOH, potassium hydroxide; CMV, cytomegalovirus; RSV, respiratory syncytial virus; H&E, hematoxylin and eosin.

Table 13-2. TOTAL AND DIFFERENTIAL CELL COUNTS IN BRONCHOALVEOLAR LAVAGE FROM CHILDREN AND ADULTS

Subjects	Alveolar Macrophages	Lymphocytes	Polymorphonuclear Neutrophils	Eosinophils	Other
Children*	89 ± 1.6	9 ± 1.4	1 ± 0.3	<1	<1
Adults†	85	10	—	<1	<1

*Mean ± standard deviation. Data from Clement et al. (1987).[5] †Data from Columbo and Hallberg (1987).[45]

number of lymphocytes in comparison with a filtration method.[53] Cell count per unit of BAL volume has not been standardized. It depends on the number of cells in the alveolar lining fluid, the volume of lung lavaged, and the percentage of lavage recovered. Because of variations in technique and the volume used as the denominator in the calculation of the cell count, comparisons of results from different studies are difficult to interpret. In one study in children aged 1 to 15 years, cell counts per milliliter of returned lavage fluid in patients with interstitial pneumonitis were compared with those of controls without lower respiratory disease. The control patients had mean cell counts (± standard error of the mean) of 255 (± 41) × 10^3 in comparison with 748 (± 81) × 10^3 cells per milliliter of returned lavage fluid in patients with diffuse lung disease.[5]

ADDITIONAL INTERPRETATION TECHNIQUES

Open (uncovered) brushes are available for obtaining cultures with 3.5-mm–OD fiberoptic bronchoscope (with a working channel of 1.2 mm). A significant limitation with the use of open brushes is the high probability of contamination by upper airway flora. Covered brushes can be used when the working channel is ≥2 mm. This type of brush consists of a series of telescoping plugged catheters. The covered catheter is extended beyond the bronchoscope tip, the plug is expelled, and a sample is taken by the brush. The brush is withdrawn into its protected catheter before it is pulled back into the bronchoscope. This technique has been shown to reduce, but not eliminate, the risk of upper tract contamination of the brush culture.[32, 54] Because of the limited number of sizes of bronchoscopes for younger children, covered brushing cannot be performed with the equipment currently available.

Pediatric transbronchial biopsy is at present limited to use in older children, in whom the airway enables safe passage of 4.5-mm–OD bronchoscopes, most of which have 2-mm–ID channels. The major advantage of biopsy is the ability to recover lung tissue that has not been exfoliated into the alveolar space or bronchial lumen. A biopsy specimen potentially adds information to the BAL results about tissue morphologic characteristics and invasion of tissue by inflammatory cells, tumor, or microbes. Caution must be exercised, in interpreting biopsy results. With current technology, the biopsy samples are small and hence may not contain pathologic processes that are actually present. The specimens are also prone to crush artifact. The risks of pneumothorax and bleeding are slightly increased. Nonetheless, transbronchial biopsy from multiple sites may prove to be a necessary addition to BAL in the diagnosis of interstitial lung diseases and of rejection after lung transplantation.

THERAPEUTIC USES OF FIBEROPTIC BRONCHOSCOPY WITH BRONCHOALVEOLAR LAVAGE

Therapeutic uses of fiberoptic bronchoscopy with BAL are not as yet defined. One generally accepted role of therapeutic lavage is in the treatment of pulmonary alveolar proteinosis. However, to ensure airway control and to obtain lavage of large volumes of the lung, therapeutic lavage in pulmonary alveolar proteinosis is performed with a cuffed double-lumen endotracheal catheter rather than with a fiberoptic bronchoscope.[55]

Multiple uncontrolled studies of therapeutic lavage in patients with cystic fibrosis who have severe mucus plugging of the airway or atelectasis have been reported. In the majority of these studies, a rigid bronchoscope was used. In some cases, bronchial washing with a rigid or fiberoptic bronchoscope has been associated with temporary improvement in pulmonary functions and a decrease in hypercapnea.[56–58] However, these techniques must be critically evaluated in comparison with current intensive antimicrobic, anti-inflammatory, and chest physiotherapeutic measures for relative risk and benefit.[59] The airway secretions found in the lungs of cystic fibrosis patients are invariably too thick to remove in quantity with the small working channel of the fiberoptic bronchoscope. However, stimulating the cough reflex and hydrating the mucus with lavage fluid may be of benefit. This remains to be proved in a controlled study.

The potential value of instilling high concentrations of antimicrobic or chemotherapeutic agents in local areas of the lung via the fiberoptic bronchoscope remains to be explored.

RESEARCH USES OF FLEXIBLE BRONCHOSCOPY WITH BRONCHOALVEOLAR LAVAGE

The role of BAL in the diagnosis, management, and therapy of pediatric lung diseases is emerging. At least three new areas of investigation involving the use of BAL in children seem particularly promising: (1) the study of cellular and biochemical correlates of the acute alveolar and bronchial injury that results in bronchopulmonary dysplasia and in pulmonary fibrosis following acute respiratory distress syndrome;[8, 60–66] (2) the study of pulmonary microbiology and cellular response, especially in cystic fibrosis;[67–69] and (3) the study of the cellular and biochemical changes in the airway contents that may aid in understanding the pathogenesis of asthma[70] (see Chapter 66).

In these diseases, it is currently known that many cells and biochemical mediators are capable of producing tissue injury. However, to assign causation and to develop a rationale for pharmacologic intervention, criteria similar to Robert Koch's postulates should ideally be fulfilled. The cell or mediator should be found at or near the site of the abnormal response. The amount of mediator detected should be sufficient to produce a biologic effect. The arrival of the cell or mediator should precede the pathologic event. Last, the inhibition of the cell influx or mediator release should reduce the intensity or duration of the pathologic response.[71] Bronchoscopy with BAL enables access close to the site of the pathologic response in selected lung diseases in children. The relatively low risk of complications permits sampling early and repeatedly during the evolution of these diseases. In patients defined to be at high risk for the development of pathologic changes, it may be performed before the development of these changes. During clinical trials of drug interventions, it can be used to document change in the cellular or mediator levels.

The major limitation in the research use of BAL is that it does not sample bronchoalveolar tissue or products that have not entered the bronchoalveolar lining fluid. Technical improvements that aid in the interpretation of BAL would be the development of biopsy equipment and covered brushes that can be used in pediatric flexible bronchoscopes.

REFERENCES

1. Antolini I, Miglioranzi P, Boner AL: Pulmonary fibrosis in children: Diagnosis and therapy. Pediatr Med Chir 8:675–682, 1986.
2. Ariole P, Bouquillard E, Barneon G, et al: Alveolar microlithiasis in children: Contribution of bronchoalveolar lavage. Arch Fr Pediatr 44:291–293, 1987.
3. Bye MR, Bernstein L, Shah K, et al: Diagnostic bronchoalveolar lavage in children with AIDS. Pediatr Pulmonol 3:425–428, 1987.
4. de Blic J, McKelvie P, Le Bourgeois M, et al: Value of bronchoalveolar lavage in the management of severe acute pneumonia and interstitial pneumonitis in the immunocompromised child. Thorax 42:759–765, 1987.
5. Clement A, Chadelat K, Masliah J, et al: A controlled study of oxygen metabolite release by alveolar macrophages from children with interstitial lung disease. Am Rev Respir Dis 136:1424–1428, 1987.
6. Clement A, Masliah J, Houssett B, et al: Decreased phosphatidyl choline content in bronchoalveolar lavage fluids of children with bronchopulmonary dysplasia: A preliminary investigation. Pediatr Pulmonol 3:67–70, 1987.
7. Clement A, Sardet A, Chadelat K, et al: Activation of alveolar macrophages from children with the acquired immunodeficiency syndrome–related complex. Pediatr Pulmonol 5:192–197, 1988.
8. Hallman M: Lung surfactant phospholipids in the foetus, newborn, and in the adult: Evidence of abnormality in respiratory failure. Ann Chir Gynaecol 71(Suppl) 19–23, 1982.
9. Leigh MW, Henshaw NG, Wood RE: Diagnosis of *Pneumocystis carinii* pneumonia in pediatric patients using bronchoscopic bronchoalveolar lavage. Pediatr Infect Dis 4:408–410, 1985.
10. Milburn HJ, Prentice HG, du Bois RM: Role of bronchoalveolar lavage in the evaluation of interstitial pneumonitis in recipients of bone marrow transplants. Thorax 42:766–772, 1987.
11. Nagy B, Marodi L, Jezerniczky J, Karmazsin L: Immunoglobulin levels in bronchoalveolar lavage fluid of children with recurrent obstructive bronchitis. Acta Paediatr Hung 27:205–210, 1986.
12. Nagy B, Marodi L, Karmazsin L: Characterization of cells in bronchoalveolar lavage fluid of children with recurrent obstructive bronchitis. Acta Paediatr Hung 27:211–219, 1986.
13. Postle AD, Hunt AN, Normand IC: The proteins of human lung surfactant. Biochim Biophys Acta 837:305–313, 1985.
14. Prakash UB, Barham SS, Carpenter HA, et al: Pulmonary alveolar phospholipoproteinosis: Experience with 34 cases and a review. Mayo Clin Proc 62:499–518, 1987.
15. Pattishall EN, Noyes BE, Orenstein DM: Use of bronchoalveolar lavage in immunocompromised children with pneumonia. Pediatr Pulmonol 5:1–5, 1988.
16. European Society of Pneumology Task Group: Technical recommendations and guidelines for bronchoalveolar lavage (BAL): Report of the European Society of Pneumology Task Group. Eur Respir J 2:561–585, 1989.
17. Pingelton SK, Harrison DJ, Stechschulte DJ, et al: Effect of location, pH, and temperature of instillate in bronchoalveolar lavage in normal volunteers. Am Rev Respir Dis 128:1035–1037, 1983.
18. Reynolds HY: State of the art: Bronchoalveolar lavage. Am Rev Respir Dis 135:250–263, 1987.
19. Gibson PG, Robinson BW, McLennan G, et al: The role of bronchoalveolar lavage in the assessment of diffuse lung diseases. Aust N Z J Med 19:281–291, 1989.
20. O'Brodovich HN, Chernick V: The functional basis of respiratory pathology. *In* Kendig EL, Chernick V (eds): Disorders of the Respiratory Tract in Children, 4th ed, pp. 3–46. Philadelphia: WB Saunders, 1983.
21. Leong AB: On risks of fiberoptic bronchoscopy and bronchoalveolar lavage (BAL) [Letter]. Pediatr Pulmonol 4:128, 1988.
22. Wagner JS: Fatality of fiberoptic bronchoscopy in a two-year-old child. Pediatr Pulmonol 3:197–199, 1987.
23. Crystal RG, Reynolds HY, Kalica AR: Bronchoalveolar lavage: The report of an international conference. Chest 90:122–131, 1986.
24. Elford B: Care and cleansing of the fiberoptic bronchoscopy. Chest 73:761–763, 1978.
25. Frankel LR, Smith DW, Lewiston NJ: Bronchoalveolar lavage for diagnosis of pneumonia in the immunocompromised child. Pediatrics 81:785–788, 1988.
26. Martin W II, Smith T, Brutinel W, et al.: Role of bronchoalveolar lavage in the assessment of opportunistic pulmonary infections: Utility and complications. Mayo Clin Proc 62:549–557, 1987.
27. Stover D, Zaman M, Hajdu S, et al.: Bronchoalveolar lavage in the diagnosis of diffuse pulmonary infiltrates in the immunosuppressed host. Ann Intern Med 101:1–7, 1984.
28. Williams D, Yungbluth M, Adams G, Glassroth J: The role of fiberoptic bronchoscopy in the evaluation of immunocompromised hosts with diffuse pulmonary infiltrates. Am Rev Respir Dis 131:880–885, 1985.
29. Cordonnier C, Escudier E, Nicolas JC, et al.: Evaluation of three assays on alveolar lavage fluid in the diagnosis of cytomegalovirus pneumonitis after bone marrow transplantation. J Infect Dis 155:495–500, 1987.
30. Gudnason T, Belani KK, Balfour HH Jr: Ganciclovir treatment of cytomegalovirus disease in immunocompromised children. Pediatr Infect Dis 8:436–440, 1989.
31. Kahn FW, Jones JM: Diagnosing bacterial respiratory infection by bronchoalveolar lavage. J Infect Dis 155:862–869, 1987.
32. Kirkpatrick MB, Bass JBJ: Quantitative bacterial cultures of bronchoalveolar lavage fluids and protected brush catheter specimens from normal subjects. Am Rev Respir Dis 139:546–548, 1989.
33. Thorpe JE, Baughman RP, Frame PT, et al: Bronchoalveolar lavage for diagnosing acute bacterial pneumonia. J Infect Dis 155:855–861, 1987.
34. Torres, A, Puig de la Bellacasa J, Xaubet A, et al: Diagnostic value of quantitative cultures of bronchoalveolar lavage and telescoping plugged catheters in mechanically ventilated patients with bacterial pneumonia. Am Rev Respir Dis 140:306–310, 1989.
35. Danek SJ, Bower JS: Diagnosis of pulmonary tuberculosis by fiberoptic flexible bronchoscopy. Am Rev Respir Dis 119:677–679, 1979.

36. de Gracia J, Curull V, Vidal R, et al: Diagnostic value of bronchoalveolar lavage in suspected pulmonary tuberculosis. Chest 93:329–332, 1988.
37. Jett JR, Cortese DA, Dines DE: The value of bronchoscopy in the diagnosis of mycobacterial disease. Chest 80:575–578, 1981.
38. Wallace JM, Deutsch AL, Harrell JH, Moser KM: Bronchoscopy and transbronchial biopsy in evaluation of patients with suspected active tuberculosis. Am J Med 70:1189–1194, 1981.
39. Wilcox PA, Benatar SR, Potgieter PD: Use of the flexible fiberoptic bronchoscope in diagnosis of sputum-negative pulmonary tuberculosis. Thorax 37:598–601, 1982.
40. Martin R, Coalson J, Rogers R, et al.: Pulmonary alveolar proteinosis: The diagnosis by segmental lavage. Am Rev Respir Dis 121:819–825, 1980.
41. Samuels MP, Warner JO: Pulmonary alveolar lipoproteinosis complicating juvenile dermatomyositis. Thorax 43:939–940, 1988.
42. Levy J, Wilmott RW: Pulmonary hemosiderosis. Pediatr Pulmonol 2:384–391, 1986.
43. Sanchez MJ, Ettensohn DB: Alveolar hemorrhage in Wegener's granulomatosis. Am J Med Sci 297:390–393, 1989.
44. Sherman JM, Winnie G, Thomassen MJ, et al: Time course of hemosiderin production and clearance by human pulmonary macrophages. Chest 86:409–411, 1984.
45. Columbo JL, Hallberg TK: Recurrent aspiration in children: Lipid-laden alveolar macrophage quantitation. Pediatr Pulmonol 3:86–89, 1987.
46. Corwin RW, Irwin RS: The lipid-laden alveolar macrophage as a marker of aspiration in parenchymal lung disease. Am Rev Respir Dis 132:576–581, 1985.
47. Moran JR, Block SM, Lyerly AD, et al: Lipid-laden alveolar macrophage and lactose assay as markers of aspiration in neonates with lung disease. J Pediatr 112:643–645, 1988.
48. Chollet S, Soler P, Dournovo P, et al: Diagnosis of pulmonary histiocytosis X by immunodetection of Langerhans cells in bronchoalveolar lavage fluid. Am J Pathol 115:225–232, 1984.
49. Turner-Warwick M, Haslam PL: The value of serial bronchoalveolar lavages in assessing the clinical progress of patients with cryptogenic fibrosing alveolitis. Am Rev Respir Dis 135:26–34, 1987.
50. Crystal R, Bitterman P, Rennard S, et al: Interstitial lung diseases of unknown cause: Disorders characterized by chronic inflammation of the lower repiratory tract (Part 1). New Engl J Med 310:154–166, 1984.
51. Crystal R, Bitterman P, Rennard S, et al: Interstitial lung diseases of unknown cause: Disorders characterized by chronic inflammation of the lower respiratory tract (Part 2). New Engl J Med 310:235–244, 1984.
52. Henderson R: Use of bronchoalveolar lavage to detect lung damage. In Gardner DE, Crapo JD, Massaro EJ (eds): Toxicology of the Lung, pp. 239–268. New York: Raven Press, 1988.
53. Saltini C, Hance A, Ferrans V, et al: Accurate quantification of cells recovered by bronchoalveolar lavage. Am Rev Respir Dis 130:650–658, 1984.
54. Halperin S, Suratt P, Gwaltney J Jr, et al: Bacterial cultures of the lower respiratory tract in normal volunteers with and without experimental rhinovirus infection using a plugged double catheter system. Am Rev Respir Dis 125:678–680, 1982.
55. Ramirez J: Bronchopulmonary lavage: New techniques and observations. Dis Chest 50:581–588, 1966.
56. Dahm L, Ewing C, Harrison G, Rucker R: Comparison of three techniques of lung lavage in patients with cystic fibrosis. Chest 72:593–596, 1977.
57. Kulczycki L: Experience with 632 bronchoscopic bronchial washings (BBW) done on 173 cystic fibrosis (CF) patients during a 16 year period (1965–1980). In Warwick W (ed): 1000 Years of Cystic Fibrosis, pp. 95–112. Minneapolis: University of Minnesota Press, 1981.
58. Quick C, Warwick W: Bronchoscopy and lavage in management of pulmonary complications of cystic fibrosis. Chest 73S:755S-758S, 1978.
59. Sherman JM: Bronchial lavage in patients with cystic fibrosis. Pediatr Pulmonol 2:244–246, 1986.
60. Hallman M, Maasilta P, Sipilä I, Tahvanainen J: Composition and function of pulmonary surfactant in adult respiratory distress syndrome. Eur Respir J [Suppl] 2:104s–108s, 1989.
61. Lachmann B, Hallman M, Bergmann KC: Respiratory failure following anti-lung serum: Study on mechanisms associated with surfactant system damage. Exp Lung Res 12:163–180, 1987.
62. Lilly CM, Sandhu JS, Ishizaka A, et al: Pentoxifylline prevents tumor necrosis factor–induced lung injury. Am Rev Respir Dis 139:1361–1368, 1989.
63. Modig J: Adult respiratory distress syndrome: Pathophysiology and inflammatory mediators in bronchoalveolar lavage. Prog Clin Biol Res 308:17–25, 1989.
64. Rich EA, Panuska JR, Wallis RS, et al: Dyscoordinate expression of tumor necrosis factor-alpha by human blood monocytes and alveolar macrophages. Am Rev Respir Dis 139:1010–1016, 1989.
65. Robertson B, Grossmann G, Jobe A, et al: Vascular to alveolar leak of iron dextran (120 kD) in the immature ventilated rabbit lung. Pediatr Res 25:130–135, 1989.
66. Warburton D, Parton L, Buckley S, et al: Combined effects of corticosteroid, thyroid hormones, and beta-agonist on surfactant, pulmonary mechanics, and beta-receptor binding in fetal lamb lung. Pediatr Res 24:166–170, 1988.
67. Garlich DJ, Clawson CC, Elliott GR: Ultrastructure and peroxidase active of alveolar macrophages in cystic fibrosis. In Bailey GW (ed): Proceedings of the Electron Microscopy Society of America, pp. 838–839. San Francisco: San Francisco Press, 1987.
68. Martin HG, Warren JR, Dunn MM: The pulmonary clearance of smooth and rough strains of Pseudomonas aeruginosa. Am Rev Respir Dis 140:206–210, 1989.
69. Woods RE: Treatment of CF lung disease in the first two years. Pediatr Pulmonol Suppl 4:68–70, 1989.
70. Wegner C, Gundel R, Reilly P, et al: Intercellular adhesion molecule-1 (ICAM-1) in the pathogenesis of asthma. Science 247:456–459, 1990.
71. Said SI: Peptides and lipids as mediators of acute lung injury. In Zapol W, Falke K (eds): Acute Respiratory Failure, pp. 435–462. New York: Marcel Dekker, 1985.

14 RAPID DIAGNOSIS OF VIRAL RESPIRATORY INFECTIONS

PENELOPE H. DENNEHY, M.D.

The laboratory diagnosis of viral infections has undergone major change since 1980. Viral diagnosis in the past consisted of either cell-culture isolation or serologic identification of the virus involved. Both methods are labor intensive and expensive and yield results days to weeks after onset of the viral infection. Today many viral infections can be diagnosed in hours because of the development of new viral diagnostic techniques. These techniques are rapid and inexpensive and can often be performed in a community hospital microbiology laboratory.

The rapid identification of virus contributes to the management of patients in a number of important ways. Probably the most important role of rapid viral diagnosis is in the use of antiviral agents. With the advent of drugs such as ribavirin for respiratory syncytial virus bronchiolitis and pneumonia, the rapid identification of respiratory viruses has become necessary if an antiviral drug is to be beneficial to the patient. Currently available antivirals and those under development are all likely to be most effective if initiated early in the course of infection and to be active against a narrow spectrum of respiratory viruses; thus prompt identification of the infecting virus is mandatory if antiviral therapy is to be beneficial.

Rapid viral diagnosis offers additional benefits. The availability of a specific viral diagnosis can eliminate the expense of unnecessary diagnostic tests and the additional expense and possibly harmful effects of inappropriate antibiotic therapy. Rapid identification of viral respiratory infections enables the prompt initiation of specific infection control measures in the hospital and also of specific public health measures in the community that are designed to control the spread of virus, such as vaccine campaigns or use of prophylactic drugs.

SPECIMEN REQUIREMENTS FOR THE RAPID DIAGNOSIS OF VIRAL INFECTIONS

Before the techniques available for rapid diagnosis of viral respiratory infections are reviewed, certain prerequisites for viral diagnosis should be outlined. No technique, regardless of how rapid, is useful unless the quality of the specimen—including the source, the means of collection, and the method of transport—is adequate.

SPECIMEN SELECTION

Viral respiratory tract infections involve the epithelium of the respiratory tract, and sampling should be performed from this site. Specimens may be taken from the throat or nasopharynx and obtained from coughed or aspirated sputum or by bronchial washings or bronchoalveolar lavage. Aspirates or washes are generally preferred to swabs because of increased isolation rates in comparison studies,[1-7] although a more recent study has found swabs to be comparable to aspirates.[8]

SPECIMEN COLLECTION

Specimens should be collected early in the acute phase of infection. The duration of shedding of respiratory viruses varies from a mean of 3 days in influenza to 7 days on the average in respiratory syncytial virus and parainfluenza infections; the exception is adenovirus, which may be shed asymptomatically for months after infection. Because virus is present in highest titer at the onset of illness, specimens should be obtained as early in the illness as possible.

Specimens may be collected from the upper respiratory tract by means of swabs, cytology brushes, plastic scrapers, washes, or aspiration.[9] Swab specimens are collected with cotton, rayon, or calcium alginate swabs. Throat specimens are collected by swabbing the posterior pharynx. To collect nasopharyngeal swab specimens, a flexible wire swab is inserted into the nose and gently pushed backward until resistance is felt; the swab is rotated and then removed. Throat and nasopharyngeal swabs are often combined.

Plastic scrapers and cytology brushes have been used on a limited basis to enhance recovery of nasal epithelial cells for immunofluorescence testing.[10-12] Excess secretions are removed by aspiration, and a plastic scraper designed specifically to sample the upper respiratory tract is gently scraped over the posterior nasal cavity. Scrapings are then transferred to transport media. Specimens may also be obtained by inserting a 2-mm cytology brush approximately 2 cm into the nasal cavity. The posterior respiratory epithelial surface is gently brushed, and the brush is agitated in transport media to loosen and suspend epithelial cells.

Samples of nasal mucus and exfoliated respiratory epithelial cells for culture or rapid testing may be obtained by a nasal wash or by aspiration of the nasopharynx. The nasal wash is performed by tilting the patient's head back at an angle of approximately 70 degrees. A rubber bulb syringe containing 3 to 7 ml of phosphate-buffered saline is inserted until it occludes the nostril. The specimen is collected with one complete squeeze and release of the bulb. The nasopharyngeal aspirate is obtained by inserting either a No. 6 or a No. 8 French catheter attached to a specimen trap into the nares and gently aspirating.

Sputum may also be used for viral culture or rapid testing. Specimens may be freshly expectorated sputum or may be obtained by tracheal aspiration through an endotracheal tube. Specimens obtained by either bronchial wash or bronchoalveolar lavage may be submitted for rapid viral testing.

SPECIMEN TRANSPORT AND STORAGE

Respiratory viruses vary in stability outside of the human host, but the majority survive poorly. Specimens should be transported as rapidly as possible to the laboratory for processing to maintain integrity of the virus and cells in the specimen. Because virus survival is optimal at 4°C, specimens should be kept cool during transport with cold packs or wet ice. Specimens should not be frozen because significant losses of virus titer occur after a freeze-thaw cycle. If specimens are held more than 5 days before processing, they should be frozen at −70°C and transported with dry ice.

TECHNIQUES USED IN THE RAPID DIAGNOSIS OF VIRAL INFECTIONS

The major emphasis in rapid viral diagnosis has been to develop tests capable of detecting virus or its components in clinical specimens. Because these techniques eliminate the need to cultivate virus in cell culture, they are faster and less expensive than traditional methods. They also have the advantage of detecting virus that may be non-cultivable in conventional cell culture systems or virus that is no longer infectious.

VIRAL CYTOPATHOLOGY AND ELECTRON MICROSCOPY

The analysis of viral cytopathology is the oldest form of rapid viral diagnosis. The respiratory tract may yield cytologic material for rapid diagnosis. Smears of cells obtained by nasal or throat swabs, tracheal aspirates, sputum, bronchial washings and brushings, and bronchoalveolar lavage may contain infected cells with cytologic changes that are diagnostic of viral infection. Rapid diagnosis of respiratory syncytial virus and parainfluenza bronchitis or pneumonia by cytologic changes in respiratory epithelial cells has been described by Naib and colleagues,[13] but this technique is not commonly used in the diagnosis of pediatric viral respiratory disease.

Electron microscopy for the rapid detection of virus in clinical specimens relies on the identification of viruses by their characteristic structure. Virus must be present in sufficient quantity (approximately 10^5 to 10^6 particles per milliliter) to be detected by direct electron microscopy. Procedures such as ultracentrifugation and immunoelectron microscopy may be used to increase the sensitivity. In general, there are too few virions in unconcentrated respiratory secretions to enable an electron microscopic diagnosis, and differentiation between the various orthomyxoviruses and paramyxoviruses cannot be made on direct electron microscopy.[14, 15] As a result, electron microscopy is not used in the routine diagnosis of viral respiratory infections.

IMMUNOFLUORESCENCE

The most frequently used method for detecting viral antigens in clinical specimens from the respiratory tract is immunofluorescence.[16, 17] This method is rapid, precise, and sensitive when high-quality reagents are used, when attention is paid to the technique of obtaining and processing the specimens, and when adequate technical help is available for the interpretation. Respiratory viral infections with respiratory syncytial virus, parainfluenza 1, 2, and 3 viruses, influenza A and B viruses, and adenovirus may be diagnosed by this technique. Nasal secretions are collected from the patient by aspiration or nasal wash. Virus-infected epithelial cells are washed and separated from nasal mucus by centrifugation and are then applied to a slide, dried, and fixed with acetone. Staining may be direct, with the use of a specific antiviral antibody with an attached fluorescein dye, or indirect, with the use of unlabeled specific antiviral antibody followed by fluorescein-labeled antibody directed against the initial antibody. The indirect test may be more sensitive than the direct test, although a study by Ray and Minnich[18] suggests that the sensitivity is comparable. The indirect test requires additional time and expensive reagents in comparison with direct assay. A fluorescence microscope is used to read the slides. Immunofluorescence has several advantages: a slide can be prepared and stained for a number of different viruses at a single time; the adequacy of the specimen can be determined; and slides may be made and sent to a reference laboratory for reading.[19] The disadvantages of immunofluorescence include the expertise required in the preparation of specimens and reading of slides as well as the expense of good-quality, high-titer antibody. Immunofluorescence testing for respiratory infections is often more sensitive than virus culture because it does not require intact viable virus; as a result a secretion may be positive by immunofluorescence after cultures are negative.[20, 21] Immunofluorescence is most suitable for a hospital with highly skilled and experienced virology technologists.

ENZYME IMMUNOASSAY

A second type of rapid viral test in wide clinical use is the enzyme immunoassay (EIA) or enzyme-linked immunosorbent assay, in which a double or multiple antigen-antibody reaction is used to amplify the presence of viral antigen and to increase the sensitivity. Antiviral antibody raised in an animal species is attached to a plastic plate or tube. The clinical specimen is added and incubated. If viral antigen is present, it will attach specifically to the antibody bonded to the solid phase. After washing, the bound antigen is detected by adding a second antiviral antibody, usually raised in a different animal species, that has been conjugated to an enzyme. Most often, peroxidase or alkaline phosphatase is used, although avidin and biotin are also employed. Antigen quantity is measured either visually or with a spectrophotometer after incubation with a substrate that changes from clear to colored in the presence of bound enzyme–labeled antibody. EIAs can measure quantities of antigen as small as a few nanograms and have a sensitivity that is usually comparable with that of virus culture or immunofluorescence.[22] Respiratory viral infections with respiratory syncytial virus, influenza A and B, parainfluenza, rhinovirus, and adenovirus may be diagnosed by means of EIA.

A further simplification of EIA, called a membrane EIA, takes minutes to perform and does not require specialized equipment or trained personnel. In the membrane EIA, a porous membrane is used as the capture phase, which is packaged in a single-use disposable plastic device filled with absorbent material for containment of waste liquids. Antiviral antibody is fixed to the membrane. The clinical specimen is poured into the device, and fluid is drawn by capillary action through the membrane directly into the reservoir below while viral antigens are bound by the antibody on the membrane. Alternatively, the clinical specimen may be initially incubated with antiviral antibody fixed to latex beads, which bind viral antigen present in the specimen. This mixture is then poured into the filtration device, and the latex beads are trapped directly on the membrane. A reagent containing enzyme-labeled antibody is then applied to the membrane and is followed by a substrate solution, which causes a color change on the membrane if viral antigen is present. Alternatively, membrane-bound viral antigen may be detected by the use of a particulate label consisting of liposomes with antiviral antibodies in the outer membrane and highly colored dyes in the interior. Sensitivity is comparable with that of standard EIAs. Membrane EIAs are currently available for respiratory syncytial virus and influenza A.

The major advantages of EIA are ease of interpretation, objectivity (because reading may be performed by spectrophotometer), and ability to detect viral antigen in specimens collected or handled in a manner that disrupts intact infected cells needed for immunofluorescence. Membrane EIAs have the further advantages of rapidity—most take 10 to 15 min to perform—and simplicity.

The disadvantages of EIA include the potential for nonspecific reactions, which may give false-positive results, and the ability of the test to identify the presence of only one virus; with immunofluorescence, in contrast, the presence of any one of several viruses can be determined on a single specimen by one procedure. EIAs are best suited for hospitals without virology laboratories or with virology laboratories that lack experience in immunofluorescence testing, where rapid respiratory viral testing would not otherwise be available.

RADIOIMMUNOASSAY

Radioimmunoassays are variations of the EIA technique that involve the use of antibody tagged with radioisotope, usually iodine 125 or iodine 131, in place of enzyme-labeled antibody. The binding of labeled antibody is detected in a gamma counter rather than a spectrophotometer. This technique is used primarily for hepatitis viruses but has been used experimentally for adenovirus,[23] respiratory syncytial virus, parainfluenza 1, 2, and 3 viruses, and influenza A and B viruses.[24–29]

TIME-RESOLVED FLUOROIMMUNOASSAY

The time-resolved fluoroimmunoassay is a detection system based on metal chelate chemistry and time-lapse fluorometry.[30–32] A fluorescent probe, a europium metal chelate attached to a detector antibody, is excited with a light pulse from a xenon lamp. The instrument then measures specific fluorescence after a delay time during which autofluorescence of the reagents and the background fluorescence in the plastic wells and specimens disappear. After a pause, the xenon lamp again excites the probe, and the cycle is repeated approximately 1000 times during the total counting time of 1 sec. The fluorescence is measured in a single-photon-counting fluorometer. This technique has been used experimentally for adenovirus, respiratory syncytial virus, parainfluenza 1, 2, and 3 viruses, and influenza A and B viruses.[30, 31, 33–38]

LATEX AGGLUTINATION ASSAYS

A fourth type of rapid viral test is the latex agglutination assay. In this method, a single antibody-antigen reaction occurs. Antiviral antibody is linked to a latex sphere, and visible agglutination is seen in the presence of a specimen containing viral antigen. This technique is simple and rapid but is less sensitive than the immunofluorescence and EIA tests. The latex agglutination tests have an advantage over the EIA tests in that they take only 5 to 10 min in comparison with several hours, require no special equipment, and can be easily performed in a doctor's office or in a small laboratory. Latex agglutination tests are not currently available for any of the respiratory viruses.

NUCLEIC ACID HYBRIDIZATION

A more recently developed technique for the detection of virus in clinical specimens is the use of nucleic acid probes to hybridize with viral nucleic acid in the specimen. Recent advances in molecular cloning have made hybridization possible by supplying large quantities of small segments of virus-specific nucleic acid to use as detectors or probes. A clinical specimen is treated to free DNA from proteins, RNA, and membranes. The DNA is then immobilized on nitrocellulose filters by filtration and baking. Probes of labeled virus-specific nucleic acid can then be hybridized to the DNA bound to the filter for detection of any viral DNA present. The probes may be labeled with enzyme or radioisotope. At present this technique has been used experimentally for adenovirus,[33, 39-42] influenza A,[43-46] rhinovirus,[47-50] and respiratory syncytial virus.[51] It is unlikely that nucleic acid hybridization will gain widespread use in the diagnosis of respiratory infections, for two reasons. First, the mucus in respiratory secretions often interferes with the preparation of DNA from the secretion. Second, the adaption of hybridization techniques to detect single-stranded RNA, such as the genomes of orthomyxoviruses and paramyxoviruses, in clinical specimens has been technically difficult.

Polymerase chain reaction (PCR), a powerful new technique developed in the early 1990s, also entails the use of reagents obtained by molecular cloning to amplify viral DNA in clinical specimens, allowing detection of small quantities of virus. The clinical specimen is initially treated to obtain viral DNA. The DNA is added to a reaction mixture that contains oligonucleotide primers designed to bind specifically to the viral DNA and to initiate new DNA chains, nucleotide precursors, and an enzyme, DNA polymerase, which catalyzes the production of new DNA by extension of the primers with the original viral DNA as a template. The reaction mixture is heated to denature the viral nucleic acid into single-stranded DNA, and the reaction is allowed to proceed. The reaction mixture is then heated to release new DNA chains from the original strand of viral DNA. Both the original DNA and the newly made copies may then serve as templates in a new round of DNA replication. This procedure is repeated 30 to 50 times, thus amplifying the nucleic acid from a few copies to as many as a million copies. After PCR, viral DNA is present in quantities sufficient to be detected by the probe technique described previously.

PCR has the sensitivity to detect as few as 10 infected cells in a clinical specimen. It has so far been used only experimentally to detect rhinovirus.[52] PCR is likely to come into widespread use but will probably be restricted to viral diagnostic laboratories because scrupulous care is required for avoiding contamination and misreading of specimens, and careful selection of primers is necessary to avoid amplification of related viruses.

CULTURE AMPLIFICATION TECHNIQUES

Because many specimens contain too little viral antigen to be detected directly from a clinical specimen, attempts have been made to use viral amplification in cell culture, followed by rapid detection of virus by antibody binding. Two approaches are now coming into widespread use in viral diagnostic laboratories.

The first approach is to inoculate the clinical specimens into cell culture and to screen the culture by EIA or immunofluorescence for the presence of virus 24 to 48 h after inoculation. This approach has been used experi-

mentally for respiratory syncytial virus,[53] rhinovirus,[54] and influenza.[55-57]

The second approach is called spin-amplification culture. This technique combines centrifugation of the clinical specimen onto cell culture on a coverglass in a small shell vial, which increases the efficacy of infection with screening of the culture for virus by immunofluorescence from 16 to 80 h after inoculation. Spin-amplified cultures have been used experimentally for adenovirus,[58-61] influenza A and B virus,[56, 62-64] and respiratory syncytial virus.[64-67]

The major advantage of both approaches is rapidity, in comparison with conventional cell culture. The spin-amplified culture may also be more sensitive than conventional viral culture for some viruses. As with all rapid tests, the major disadvantage is that screening is for a specific virus, thus, unsuspected viruses that may be present in the specimen may be missed. The culture plus early screening may be less sensitive than conventional culture, especially if the specimen contains very small amounts of virus that may still be below the levels of detection of the rapid test when the culture has incubated for a short period.

VIRAL SEROLOGY

Serology has been part of the traditional diagnostic approach to viral infection. As with conventional cell culture isolation of virus, the serologic response provides results too late in the course of the illness to be useful in the diagnosis and treatment of the patient. An exception is the immunoglobulin M (IgM) antibody assay, which may be used to detect active viral infections, because antibodies of this class appear early in the illness and seldom persist for extended periods. Virus-specific IgM antibodies in patient sera may be detected by either EIA or immunofluorescence in the same manner as described earlier for viral antigen. Results of IgM testing should be interpreted carefully with the following points in mind: (1) IgM may persist for long intervals, especially in the immunosuppressed patient, and (2) IgM responses may be cross-reactive for closely related viruses.[68] IgM detection has been used experimentally in the diagnosis of parainfluenza and respiratory syncytial virus infections but has not demonstrated sufficient sensitivity to be currently used in the diagnosis of viral respiratory infection.[69-72]

RAPID DIAGNOSIS OF THE RESPIRATORY VIRUSES

RESPIRATORY SYNCYTIAL VIRUS

With the availability of ribavirin for the treatment of serious respiratory syncytial virus infections, diagnostic tests for the detection of respiratory syncytial virus are increasingly important. Current methods for the diagnosis of respiratory syncytial virus include virus isolation from nasopharyngeal secretions in cell culture, immunofluorescence staining of exfoliated nasopharyngeal epithelial cells for detection of respiratory syncytial virus antigens, and EIA for the detection of respiratory syncytial virus antigens in nasopharyngeal secretions.

The choice of specimen submitted to the laboratory for diagnosis of respiratory syncytial virus is as important as the choice of test if accurate results are to be obtained. The preferred specimen is either a nasal wash or nasopharyngeal aspirate. The use of nasopharyngeal or throat swab specimens for diagnosis of respiratory syncytial virus has been associated with a decrease in virus recovery in culture[1, 4, 5, 7] and decreases in immunofluorescence[1] and EIA[1, 5] sensitivities.

Virus isolation is the most reliable method for detection of respiratory syncytial virus and is the gold standard against which the other detection methods are compared. Respiratory syncytial virus isolation requires being near a virology laboratory, because culture is most successful if specimens are transported on ice to the laboratory and inoculated within 3 h.[73, 74] A more serious drawback of culture is the fact that the majority of cultures require between 4 to 6 days for the appearance of respiratory syncytial virus.[4] Because results from culture are not often helpful in initial treatment decisions, more rapid techniques have been developed.

Immunofluorescence staining of nasopharyngeal epithelial cells is the technique most frequently used in virology laboratories to rapidly diagnose respiratory syncytial virus. Immunofluorescence is quite accurate compared with culture, with sensitivities ranging from 72% to 97% and specificities of 69% to 99% in published studies.[12, 18, 22, 53, 65, 75–87] Immunofluorescence produces results 2 to 5 h after receipt of the specimen and also detects nonviable virus, especially when transport from a distant hospital may have decreased the titer of virus in the specimen appreciably. The sensitivity of immunofluorescence testing, however, is dependent on the quality of the specimen, the antisera used, and the experience of the observer.

EIAs have also been adapted for detection of respiratory syncytial virus antigens in nasopharyngeal specimens. EIAs produce results in 15 min to 5 h, will detect nonviable virus, are easily automated, and require less technical skill than immunofluorescence. There are three commercially available EIAs and two membrane EIAs for the diagnosis of respiratory syncytial virus. In comparison with virus culture, the sensitivity of these tests has ranged from 53% to 100% in published studies, with specificities of 80% to 100%.[65, 77, 79, 81, 84, 86–100] A drawback of EIA testing is that only respiratory syncytial virus is identified, whereas culture will detect other viruses, if present.

Cell-culture amplification followed by immunofluorescence staining has been used for the diagnosis of respiratory syncytial virus. Meziere and associates[53] used an immunofluorescence staining method to detect virus in cell cultures, with a sensitivity of 80%. Shell vial culture with fluorescent antibody detection of respiratory syncytial virus has been developed and can be used to rapidly detect approximately 70% to 90% of these viruses 16 to 48 h after inoculation.[64–66]

INFLUENZA VIRUSES

Methods currently used for the diagnosis of influenza include virus isolation in cell culture or embryonated eggs

and immunofluorescence and EIA for the detection of influenza antigens in nasopharyngeal secretions. The preferred specimen for diagnosis is either a nasal wash or nasopharyngeal secretions obtained by suction catheter. The use of nasopharyngeal swab specimens for diagnosis of influenza has been associated with a 28% decrease in virus recovery in culture,[6] and the use of throat swabs resulted in a 40% decrease in sensitivity in either immunofluorescence or EIA results in comparison with nasal washes or swabs.[101]

Virus isolation is considered the reference method for detection of influenza viruses against which the all other detection methods are compared. Conventional recommendations suggested testing viral cultures for hemabsorption or hemagglutinating activities of influenza 3 to 7 days after inoculation with respiratory samples or when cytopathic effect is observed.[9] Because culture with such a schedule of hemabsorption is usually too slow to be helpful in initial treatment decisions, Minnich and Ray[102] studied daily hemabsorption from day 1 after inoculation and found that 38% of influenza isolates could be detected within 24 h, 69% within 48 h, and 100% of influenza A isolates within 3 days and influenza B isolates within 4 days.

Immunofluorescence staining of nasopharyngeal epithelial cells is the technique most frequently used in virology laboratories to rapidly diagnose influenza. Immunofluorescence with polyclonal antibodies has been disappointing in comparison with culture; sensitivities range from 43% to 86% for influenza A in published studies.[18, 22, 82, 103–107] The introduction of monoclonal antibodies directed against several epitopes on the influenza virus have increased the sensitivity of immunofluorescence to 56% to 100% for influenza A and 100% for influenza B.[6, 78, 107–109] One commercial membrane EIA is available for detection of influenza A. Sensitivity and specificity of this assay are 100% and 92%, respectively, in comparison with virus culture.[109] Experimental EIAs for influenza have had sensitivities ranging from 49% to 100%.[22, 28, 101, 104, 110–114]

Cell-culture amplification followed by immunofluorescence or immunoperoxidase staining have been used for the diagnosis of both influenza A and B viruses. Swenson and Kaplan[57] used an indirect immunoperoxidase staining method with type-specific monoclonal antibodies to influenza to detect virus in cell cultures with a sensitivity of 86%, whereas Evans and Olson[104] obtained a 93% sensitivity rate by using fluorescent antibodies directed against influenza to stain tissue culture at 24 to 48 h after inoculation. Shell vial culture with fluorescent antibody detection of influenza types A and B has been developed and can be used to rapidly detect approximately 70% to 80% of these viruses 24 h after inoculation.[6, 56, 62–64, 115]

PARAINFLUENZA VIRUSES

Current methods for the diagnosis of parainfluenza infections are isolation of virus from nasopharyngeal secretions in cell culture and immunofluorescence staining of exfoliated nasopharyngeal epithelial cells for detection of parainfluenza antigens. The preferred specimen for virus isolation or immunofluorescence is either a nasal wash or nasopharyngeal secretions obtained by suction catheter. The use of nasal swab specimens for diagnosis of parainfluenza has been associated with a 17% decrease in virus recovery in culture.[3]

Virus isolation is the most reliable method for detection of parainfluenza viruses and is the gold standard against which the other detection methods are compared. As with influenza, conventional recommendations suggested testing for hemabsorption or hemagglutinating activities of parainfluenza 3 to 7 days after inoculation with respiratory samples or when cytopathic effect is observed.[9] Minnich and Ray[102] studied daily hemabsorption from day 1 after inoculation, hoping to decrease the time to detection for parainfluenza viruses. However, they found that only 7% of parainfluenza isolates could be detected within 5 days. Results of immunofluorescence testing are quite variable, depending on the antisera used and the type of parainfluenza virus studied; sensitivities ranged from 31% to 99% in comparison with viral culture in published studies.[3, 18, 82, 116–119] EIAs are not available for parainfluenza viruses.

ADENOVIRUSES

Detection methods currently available for adenovirus are virus isolation from respiratory secretions in cell culture, immunofluorescence staining of exfoliated nasopharyngeal epithelial cells, and EIAs for the detection of adenovirus antigens in nasopharyngeal secretions.

Virus isolation is the most reliable method for detection of adenovirus and is the method against which the other detection methods are compared. A serious drawback is that cultures require an average of 10 days for the appearance of typical adenovirus cytopathic effect. Because results from culture are not often helpful in initial treatment decisions, more rapid techniques have been developed.

Immunofluorescence staining of nasopharyngeal epithelial cells has been used to rapidly diagnose adenovirus infections, but results have been disappointing. When compared with viral culture, sensitivities of immunofluorescence range from 11% to 66%.[18, 41, 82, 117, 120, 121] EIAs for the diagnosis of adenovirus respiratory infections offer more promise; reported sensitivities ranged from 50% to 98% compared with virus culture.[34, 41, 58, 122–125] An EIA kit containing monoclonal antibody is now available commercially. Cell-culture amplification followed by immunofluorescence or EIA has also been used for the diagnosis of adenovirus. Shell vial culture with fluorescent antibody detection of adenovirus has been developed and can be used to detect 70% to 87% of these viruses within 72 h of inoculation.[58, 60, 61]

REFERENCES

1. Ahluwalia G, Embree J, McNicol P, et al: Comparison of nasopharyngeal aspirate and nasopharyngeal swab specimens for respiratory syncytial virus diagnosis by cell culture, indirect immunofluorescence assay, and enzyme-linked immunosorbent assay. J Clin Microbiol 25:763–767, 1987.
2. Cruz JR, Quinonez E, de Fernandez A, et al: Isolation of viruses from nasopharyngeal secretions: Comparison of aspiration and swabbing as means of sample collection. J Infect Dis 156:415–416, 1987.
3. Downham MAPS, McQuillin J, Gardner PS: Diagnosis and clinical significance of parainfluenza virus infections in children. Arch Dis Child 49:8–14, 1974.
4. Hall CB, Douglas RG Jr: Clinically useful method for the isolation of respiratory syncytial virus. J Infect Dis 131:1–5, 1975.
5. McIntosh K, Hendry RM, Fahnestock ML, et al: Enzyme-linked immunosorbent assay for detection of RSV infection: Application to clinical samples. J Clin Microbiol 16:329–333, 1982.
6. McQuillin J, Madeley CR, Kendal AP: Monoclonal antibodies for the rapid diagnosis of influenza A and B virus infections by immunofluorescence. Lancet 2:911–914, 1985.
7. Treuhaft MW, Soukup JM, Sullivan BJ: Practical recommendations for the detection of pediatric respiratory syncytial virus infections. J Clin Microbiol 22:270–273, 1985.
8. Frayha H, Castriciano S, Mahony J, Chernesky M: Nasopharyngeal swabs and nasopharyngeal aspirates equally effective for the diagnosis of viral respiratory disease in hospitalized children. J Clin Microbiol 27:1387–1389, 1989.
9. Chernesky MA, Ray CG, Smith TF: Laboratory Diagnosis of Viral Infections. Washington, DC: American Society for Microbiology, 1982.
10. Barnes SD, LeClair JM, Forman MS, et al: Comparison of nasal brush and nasopharyngeal aspirate techniques in obtaining specimens for detection of respiratory syncytial viral antigen by immunofluorescence. Pediatr Infect Dis J 8:598–601, 1989.
11. Jalowayski AA, England BL, Temm CJ, et al: Peroxidase-antiperoxidase assay for rapid detection of respiratory syncytial virus in nasal epithelium specimens from infants and children. J Clin Microbiol 25:722–725, 1987.
12. Jalowayski AA, Walpita P, Puryear BA, Connor JD: Rapid detection of respiratory syncytial virus in nasopharyngeal specimens obtained with the Rhinoprobe scraper. J Clin Microbiol 28:738–741, 1990.
13. Naib Z, Stewart J, Dowdle W, et al: Cytologic features of viral respiratory tract infections. Acta Cytol 12:162–171, 1968.
14. Doane FW, Anderson N, Chatiyananda K, et al: Rapid laboratory diagnosis of paramyxovirus infections by electron microscopy. Lancet 2:751–753, 1967.
15. Joncas JH, Berthiaume L, Williams R, et al: Diagnosis of viral respiratory infections by electron microscopy. Lancet 1:956–959, 1969.
16. Almeida JD, Atanasiu P, Bradley DW, et al: Manual for Rapid Viral Diagnosis, WHO Offset Publication No. 47. Washington, DC: World Health Organization, 1979.
17. Gardner PS, McQuillin J: Rapid Virus Diagnosis: Application of Immunofluorescence, 2nd ed. London: Butterworth's, 1980.
18. Ray CG, Minnich LL: Efficiency of immunofluorescence for rapid detection of common respiratory viruses. J Clin Microbiol 25:355–357, 1987.
19. Downham MAPS, Elderkin FM, Platt JW, et al: Rapid virus diagnosis in paediatric units by a postal service. Respiratory syncytial viral infection in Cumberland. Arch Dis Child 49:467–471, 1974.
20. Gardner PS, McQuillin J, McGuckin R: The late detection of respiratory syncytial virus in cells of respiratory tract by immunofluorescence. J Hyg (Lond) 68:575–580, 1970.
21. Gardner PS, McQuillin J: The coating of RS virus infected cells in the respiratory tract by immunoglobulins. J Med Virol 2:77–87, 1978.
22. Takimoto S, Grandien M, Ishida MA, et al: Comparison of enzyme-linked immunosorbent assay, indirect immunofluorescence assay, and virus isolation for detection of respiratory viruses in nasopharyngeal secretions. J Clin Microbiol 29:470–474, 1991.
23. Meurman O, Ruuskanen O, Sarkkinen H: Immunoassay diagnosis of adenovirus infections in children. J Clin Microbiol 18:1190–1195, 1983.
24. Coonrod JD, Betts RF, Linnemann CC Jr, et al: Etiological diagnosis of influenza A virus by enzymatic radioimmunoassay. J Clin Microbiol 19:361–365, 1984.
25. Ehrlicher L, Hoffmann HG, Habermehl KO: Detection of respiratory virus antigens in nasopharyngeal secretions from patients with acute respiratory disease by radio-immunoassay and tissue culture isolation. Med Microbiol Immunol 173:37–44, 1984.

26. Ehrlicher L, Hoffmann HG, Habermehl KO: Detection of respiratory virus antigens in nasopharyngeal secretions from patients with acute respiratory disease by radio-immunoassay and tissue culture isolation. J Virol Methods 12:105–110, 1985.

27. Habermehl KO: Rapid diagnosis of respiratory virus infections in patients with acute respiratory disease. Diagn Microbiol Infect Dis 4:17S–22S, 1986.

28. Sarkkinen HK, Halonen PE, Salmi AA: Detection of influenza A virus by radioimmunoassay and enzyme immunoassay from nasopharyngeal specimens. J Med Virol 7:213–220, 1981.

29. Vesikari T, Kuusela A-L, Sarkkinen HK, et al: Clinical evaluation of radioimmunoassay of nasopharyngeal secretions and serology for diagnosis of viral infections in children hospitalized for respiratory infections. Pediatr Infect Dis 1:391–394, 1982.

30. Halonen P, Meurman O, Lovgren T, et al: Detection of viral antigens by time-resolved fluoroimmunoassay. Curr Top Microbiol Immunol 104:133–146, 1983.

31. Halonen P, Obert G, Hierholzer JC: Direct detection of viral antigens in respiratory infections by immunoassays: A four year experience and new developments. *In* de la Maza LM, Peterson EM (ed): Medical Virology IV, pp. 65–83. Hillsdale, NJ: Erlbaum, 1985.

32. Lovgren T, Hemmila I, Pettersson K, Halonen P: Time-resolved fluorometry in immunoassay. *In* Collins WP (ed): Alternative Immunoassays, pp. 203–217. New York: Wiley, 1985.

33. Dahlen P, Hurskainen P, Lovgren T, Hyypia T: Time-resolved fluorometry for the identification of viral DNA in clinical specimens. J Clin Microbiol 26:2434–2436, 1988.

34. Hierholzer JC, Johansson KH, Anderson LJ, et al: Comparison of monoclonal time-resolved fluoroimmunoassay with monoclonal capture-biotinylated detector enzyme immunoassay for adenovirus antigen detection. J Clin Microbiol 25:1662–1667, 1987.

35. Hierholzer JC, Bingham PG, Coombs RA, et al: Comparison of monoclonal antibody time-resolved fluoroimmunoassay with monoclonal antibody capture-biotinylated detector enzyme immunoassay for respiratory syncytial virus and parainfluenza virus antigen detection. J Clin Microbiol 27:1243–1249, 1989.

36. Nikkari S, Halonen P, Kharitonenkov I, et al: One incubation time-resolved fluoroimmunoassay based on monoclonal antibodies in detection of influenza A and B viruses directly in clinical specimens. J Virol Methods 23:29–40, 1989.

37. Walls HH, Johansson KH, Harmon MW, et al: Time-resolved fluoroimmunoassay with monoclonal antibodies for rapid diagnosis of influenza infections. J Clin Microbiol 24:907–912, 1986.

38. Waris M, Halonen P, Ziegler T, et al: Time-resolved fluoroimmunoassay compared with virus isolation for rapid detection of respiratory syncytial virus in nasopharyngeal aspirates. J Clin Microbiol 26:2581–2585, 1988.

39. Gomes SA, Nascimento JP, Siqueira MM, et al: In situ hybridization with biotinylated DNA probes: A rapid diagnostic test for adenovirus upper respiratory infections. J Med Virol 28:159–162, 1989.

40. Hyypia T: Detection of adenovirus in nasopharyngeal specimens by radioactive and nonradioactive DNA probes. J Clin Microbiol 21:730–733, 1985.

41. Lehtomaki K, Julkunen I, Sandelin K, et al: Rapid diagnosis of respiratory adenovirus infections in young adult men. J Clin Microbiol 24:265–268, 1986.

42. Virtanen M, Laaksonen M, Soderlund H, et al: Novel test for rapid viral diagnosis: Detection of adenovirus in nasopharyngeal mucus aspirates by means of nucleic-acid sandwich hybridization. Lancet 1:381–383, 1983.

43. Pliusnin AZ, Nolandt OV, Lipina NV, et al: The results of using the molecular hybridization of nucleic acids in the complex study of nasopharyngeal smears from patients with influenza and other acute respiratory diseases. Zh Mikrobiol Epidemiol Immunobiol (2):14–17, February 1990.

44. Pljusnin AZ, Rozhkova SA, Nolandt OV, et al: Molecular hybridization with DNA-probes as a laboratory diagnostic test for influenza viruses. Virologie 38(2):111–114, 1987.

45. Pljusnin AZ, Nolandt OV, Bryantseva EA, et al: Molecular hybridization with DNA probes as a laboratory diagnosis test for influenza viruses: Further investigations on the possibilities of the method. Virologie 40:39–42, 1989.

46. Richman DD, Cleveland PH, Redfield DC, et al: Rapid viral diagnosis. J Infect Dis 149:298–310, 1984.

47. al-Nakib W, Stanway G, Forsyth M, et al: Detection of human rhinoviruses and their molecular relationship using cDNA probes. J Med Virol 20:289–296, 1986.

48. Auvinen P, Ziegler T, Skern T, et al: Identification of rhinoviruses by cDNA probes. J Virol Methods 27:61–868, 1990.

49. Bruce CB, al-Nakib W, Almond JW, Tyrrell DA: Use of synthetic oligonucleotide probes to detect rhinovirus RNA. Arch Virol 105(3–4):179–187, 1989.

50. Forsyth M, al-Nakib W, Chadwick P, et al: Rhinovirus detection using probes from the 5′ and 3′ end of the genome. Arch Virol 107(1–2):55–63, 1989.

51. Van Dyke RB, Murphy-Corb M: Detection of respiratory syncytial virus in nasopharyngeal secretions by DNA-RNA hybridization. J Clin Microbiol 27:1739–1743, 1989.

52. Gama RE, Horsnell PR, Hughes PJ, et al: Amplification of rhinovirus specific nucleic acids from clinical samples using the polymerase chain reaction. J Med Virol 28:73–77, 1989.

53. Meziere A, Mollat C, Lapied R, et al: Detection of respiratory syncytial virus antigen after seventy-two hours of culture. J Med Virol 31:241–244, 1990.

54. Dearden CJ, al-Nakib W: Direct detection of rhinoviruses by an enzyme-linked immunosorbent assay. J Med Virol 23:179–189, 1987.

55. Phipps PH, McCulloch BG, Miller HR, Rossier E: Rapid detection of influenza virus infections in human fetal lung diploid cell cultures. J Infect 18:269–278, 1989.

56. Stokes CE, Bernstein JM, Kyger SA, Hayden FG: Rapid diagnosis of influenza A and B by 24-h fluorescent focus assays. J Clin Microbiol 26:1263–1266, 1988.

57. Swenson PD, Kaplan MH: Rapid detection of influenza virus in cell culture by indirect immunoperoxidase staining with type-specific monoclonal antibodies. Diagn Microbiol Infect Dis 7:265–268, 1987.

58. August MJ, Warford AL: Evaluation of a commercial monoclonal antibody for detection of adenovirus antigen. J Clin Microbiol 25:2233–2235, 1987.

59. Espy MJ, Hierholzer JC, Smith TF: The effect of centrifugation on the rapid detection of adenovirus in shell vials. Am J Clin Pathol 3:358–360, 1987.

60. Mahafzah AM, Landry ML: Evaluation of immunofluorescent reagents, centrifugation, and conventional cultures for the diagnosis of adenovirus infection. Diagn Microbiol Infect Dis 12:407–411, 1989.

61. Woods GL, Yamamoto M, Young A: Detection of adenovirus by rapid 24-well plate centrifugation and conventional cell culture with dexamethasone. J Virol Methods 20:109–114, 1988.

62. Espy MJ, Smith TF, Harmon MW, Kendal AP: Rapid detection of influenza virus by shell vial assay with monoclonal antibodies. J Clin Microbiol 24:677–679, 1986.

63. Mills RD, Cain KJ, Woods GL: Detection of influenza virus by centrifugal inoculation of MDCK cells and staining with monoclonal antibodies. J Clin Microbiol 27:2505–2508, 1989.

64. Waris M, Ziegler T, Kivivirta M, Ruuskanen O: Rapid detection of respiratory syncytial virus and influenza A virus in cell cultures by immunoperoxidase staining with monoclonal antibodies. J Clin Microbiol 28:1159–1162, 1990.

65. Johnston SL, Siegel CS: Evaluation of direct immunofluorescence, enzyme immunoassay, centrifugation culture, and conventional culture for the detection of respiratory syncytial virus. J Clin Microbiol 28:2394–2397, 1990.

66. Smith MC, Creutz C, Huang YT: Detection of respiratory syncytial virus in nasopharyngeal secretions by shell vial technique. J Clin Microbiol 29:463–465, 1991.

67. Woods GL, Johnson AM: Rapid 24-well plate centrifugation assay for detection of influenza A in clinical specimens. J Virol Methods 24:35–42, 1989.

68. Lennette EH, Jensen FW, Guenther RW, et al: Serologic responses to parainfluenza viruses in patients with mumps virus infection. J Lab Clin Med 61:780–788, 1963.

69. Hornsleth A, Friis B, Grauballe PC, et al: Detection by ELISA of IgA and IgM antibodies in secretion and IgM antibodies in serum in primary lower respiratory syncytial virus infection. J Med Virol 13:149–161, 1984.

70. Kadi Z, Dali S, Bakouri S, Bouguermouh A: Rapid diagnosis of respiratory syncytial virus infection by antigen immunofluorescence detection with monoclonal antibodies and immunoglobulin M immunofluorescence test. J Clin Microbiol 24:1038–1040, 1986.

71. Meddens MJ, Herbrink P, Lindeman J, van Dijk WC: Serodiagnosis of respiratory syncytial virus (RSV) infection in children as measured by detection of RSV-specific immunoglobulins G, M, and A with enzyme-linked immunosorbent assay. J Clin Microbiol 28:152–155, 1990.

72. van der Logt JTM, van Loon AM, van der Veen J: Detection of parainfluenza IgM antibody by hemadsorption immunosorbent technique. J Med Virol 10:213–221, 1982.

73. Bromberg K, Daidone B, Clarke L, et al: Comparison of immediate and delayed inoculation of HEp-2 cells for isolation of respiratory syncytial virus. J Clin Microbiol 20:123–124, 1984.

74. Hambling MH: Survival of the respiratory syncytial virus during storage under various conditions. Br J Exp Pathol 45:647–655, 1964.

75. Blanding JG, Hoshiko MG, Stutman HR: Routine viral culture for pediatric respiratory specimens submitted for direct immunofluorescence testing. J Clin Microbiol 27:1438–1440, 1989.

76. Cheeseman SH, Pierik LT, Leombruno D, et al: Evaluation of a commercially available direct immunofluorescent staining reagent for the detection of respiratory syncytial virus in respiratory secretions. J Clin Microbiol 23:155–156, 1986.

77. Halstead DC, Todd S, Fritch G: Evaluation of five methods for respiratory syncytial virus detection. J Clin Microbiol 28:1021–1025, 1990.

78. Hornsleth A, Jankowski M: Sensitive enzyme immunoassay for the rapid diagnosis of influenza A virus infections in clinical specimens. Res Virol 141:373–384, 1990.

79. Hughes JH, Mann DR, Hamparian VV: Detection of respiratory syncytial virus in clinical specimens by viral culture, direct and indirect immunofluorescence, and enzyme immunoassay. J Clin Microbiol 26:588–591, 1988.

80. Lauer BA: Comparison of virus culturing and immunofluorescence for rapid detection of respiratory syncytial virus in nasopharyngeal secretions: Sensitivity and specificity. J Clin Microbiol 16:411–412, 1982.

81. Masters HB, Weber KO, Groothuis JR, et al: Comparison of nasopharyngeal washings and swab specimens for diagnosis of respiratory syncytial virus by EIA, FAT, and cell culture. Diagn Microbiol Infect Dis 8:101–105, 1987.

82. Minnich LL, Ray CG: Comparison of direct immunofluorescent staining of clinical specimens for respiratory virus antigens with conventional isolation techniques. J Clin Microbiol 12:391–394, 1980.

83. Minnich LL, Shehab ZM, Ray CG: Application of pooled monoclonal antibodies for 1-hr detection of respiratory syncytial virus antigen in clinical specimens. Diagn Microbiol Infect Dis 7:137–141, 1987.

84. Thomas EE, Book LE: Comparison of two rapid methods for detection of respiratory syncytial virus (RSV) (TestPack RSV and Ortho RSV ELISA) with direct immunofluorescence and virus isolation for diagnosis of pediatric RSV infection. J Clin Microbiol 29:632–635, 1991.

85. Waner JL, Whitehurst NJ, Jonas S, et al: Isolation of viruses from specimens submitted for direct immunofluorescence test for respiratory syncytial virus. J Pediatr 108:249–250, 1986.

86. White JM, Poupard JA, Knight RA, Miller LA: Evaluation of two commercially available test methods to determine the feasibility of testing for respiratory syncytial virus in a community hospital laboratory. Am J Clin Pathol 90:175–180, 1988.

87. Woodin KA, Hall CB, Leibenguth KC, et al: Variables affecting the rapid diagnosis of respiratory syncytial virus [Abstract no. 1114]. Presented at the 28th Interscience Conference on Antimicrobial Agents and Chemotherapy, Los Angeles, 1988.

88. Ahluwalia GS, Hammond GW: Comparison of cell culture and three enzyme-linked immunosorbent assays for the rapid diagnosis of respiratory syncytial virus from nasopharyngeal aspirate and tracheal secretion specimens. Diagn Microbiol Infect Dis 9:187–192, 1988.

89. Chonmaitree T, Bessette-Henderson BJ, Hepler RE, et al: Comparison of three rapid diagnostic techniques for detection of respiratory syncytial virus from nasal wash specimens. J Clin Microbiol 25:746–747, 1987.

90. Christensen ML, Flanders R: Comparison of the Abbott and Ortho enzyme immunoassays and cell culture for the detection of respiratory syncytial virus in nasopharyngeal specimens. Diagn Microbiol Infect Dis 9:245–250, 1988.

91. Hornsleth A: A rapid test for detection of respiratory syncytial virus in nasopharyngeal secretion. Eur J Clin Microbiol Infect Dis 9(5):356–358, 1990.

92. Kok T, Barancek K, Burrell CJ. Evaluation of the Becton Dickinson Directigen test for respiratory syncytial virus in nasopharyngeal aspirates. J Clin Microbiol 28:1458–1459, 1990.

93. Kumar ML, Super DM, Lembo RM, et al: Diagnostic efficacy of two rapid tests for detection of respiratory syncytial virus antigen. J Clin Microbiol 25:873–875, 1987.

94. Masters HB, Bate BJ, Wren C, et al: Detection of respiratory syncytial virus antigen in nasopharyngeal secretions by Abbott Diagnostics enzyme immunoassay. J Clin Microbiol 26:1103–1105, 1988.

95. Rothbarth PH, Hermus M-C, Schrijnemakers P: Reliability of two new test kits for rapid diagnosis of respiratory syncytial virus infection. J Clin Microbiol 29:824–826, 1991.

96. Subbarao EK, Whitehurst NJ, Waner JL: Comparison of two enzyme-linked immunosorbent assay (EIA) kits with immunofluorescence and isolation in cell culture for detection of respiratory syncytial virus (RSV). Diagn Microbiol Infect Dis 8:229–234, 1987.

97. Subbarao EK, Dietrich MC, De Sierra TM, et al: Rapid detection of respiratory syncytial virus by a biotin-enhanced immunoassay: Test performance by laboratory technologists and housestaff. Pediatr Infect Dis J 8:865–869, 1989.

98. Swierkosz EM, Flanders R, Melvin L, et al: Evaluation of the Abbott TestPack RSV enzyme immunoassay for detection of respiratory syncytial virus in nasopharyngeal swab specimens. J Clin Microbiol 27:1151–1154, 1989.

99. Waner JL, Whitehurst NJ, Todd SJ, et al: Comparison of directigen RSV with viral isolation and direct immunofluorescence for the identification of respiratory syncytial virus. J Clin Microbiol 28:480–483, 1990.

100. Wren CG, Bate BJ, Masters HB, Lauer BA: Detection of respiratory syncytial virus antigen in nasal washings by Abbott TestPack enzyme immunoassay. J Clin Microbiol 28:1395–1397, 1990.

101. Greene WH, Betts RF, Menegus MA: Direct detection of influenza virus in different clinical specimens by histochemical enzyme immunoassay (HEIA), indirect fluoroimmunoassay (IFA) and direct fluoroimmunoassay (DFA) [Abstract no. 205]. Presented at the 28th Interscience Conference on Antimicrobial Agents and Chemotherapy, Los Angeles, 1988.

102. Minnich LL, Ray CG: Early testing of cell cultures for detection of hemabsorbing viruses. J Clin Microbiol 25:421–422, 1987.

103. Anestad G, Breivik N, Thoresen T: Rapid diagnosis of respiratory syncytial virus and influenza A virus infections by immunofluorescence: Experience with a simplified procedure for the preparation of cell smears from nasopharyngeal secretions. Acta Pathol Microbiol Immunol Scand 91:267–271, 1983.

104. Evans AS, Olson B: Rapid diagnostic methods for influenza virus in clinical specimens: A comparative study. Yale J Biol Med 55:391–403, 1982.

105. Liu C: Rapid diagnosis of human influenza infection from nasal smears by means of fluorescein-labelled antibody. Proc Soc Exp Biol Med 92:883–887, 1956.

106. McQuillin J, Gardner PS, McGuckin R: Rapid diagnosis of influenza by immunofluorescent techniques. Lancet 2:690–695, 1970.

107. Shalit I, McKee PA, Beauchamp H, et al: Comparison of polyclonal antiserum versus monoclonal antibodies for the rapid diagnosis of influenza A virus infections by immunofluorescence in clinical specimens. J Clin Microbiol 22:877–879, 1985.

108. Pothier P, Denoyel GA, Ghim S, et al: Use of monoclonal antibodies for rapid detection of influenza A virus in nasopharyngeal secretions. Eur J Clin Microbiol 5:336–339, 1986.

109. Waner JL, Todd SJ, Shalaby H, et al: Comparison of Directigen FLU-A with viral isolation and direct immunofluorescence for the rapid detection and identification of influenza A virus. J Clin Microbiol 29:479–482, 1991.

110. Chomel JJ, Thouvenot D, Onno M, et al: Rapid diagnosis of influ-

enza infection of NP antigen using an immunocapture ELISA test. J Virol Methods 25:81–91, 1989.

111. Grandian M, Pettersson CA, Gardner PS, et al: Rapid viral diagnosis of acute respiratory infections: Comparison of enzyme-linked immunosorbent assay and the immunofluorescence technique for detection of viral antigens in nasopharyngeal secretions. J Clin Microbiol 22:757–760, 1985.

112. Harmon MW, Pawlik KM: Enzyme immunoassay for direct detection of influenza type A and adenovirus in clinical specimens. J Clin Microbiol 15:5–11, 1982.

113. Harmon MW, Russo LL, Wilson SZ: Sensitive enzyme immunoassay with beta-D-galactosidase-Fab conjugate for detection of influenza A virus antigen in clinical specimens. J Clin Microbiol 17:305–311, 1983.

114. Yolken RH, Torsch VM, Berg R, et al: Fluorometric assay for measurement of viral neuraminidase—Application to the rapid detection of influenza virus in nasal wash specimens. J Infect Dis 142:516–523, 1980.

115. Seno M, Kanamoto Y, Takao S, et al: Enhancing effect of centrifugation on isolation of influenza virus from clinical specimens. J Clin Microbiol 28(7):1669–1670, 1990.

116. Gardner PS, McQuillin J, McGuckin R, et al: Observations on the clinical and immunofluorescent diagnosis of parainfluenza virus infections. Br Med J 2:7–12, 1971.

117. Salomon HE, Grandien M, Avila MM, et al: Comparison of three techniques for detection of respiratory viruses in nasopharyngeal aspirates from children with lower acute respiratory infections. J Med Virol 28:159–162, 1989.

118. Schneider S, Masters H, Lauer B: Rapid detection of respiratory viruses by immunofluorescence (Bartel's immunodiagnostics) [Abstract no. 207]. Presented at the 28th Interscience Conference on Antimicrobial Agents and Chemotherapy, Los Angeles, 1988.

119. Wong DT, Welliver RC, Riddlesberger KR, et al: Rapid diagnosis of parainfluenza virus infection in children. J Clin Microbiol 16:164–167, 1982.

120. Avila M, Salomon H, Carballal G, et al: Isolation and identification of viral agents in Argentinian children with acute lower respiratory tract infection. Rev Infect Dis 12:S974–S981, 1990.

121. Gardner PS, McGuckin R, McQuillin J: Adenovirus demonstrated by immunofluorescence. Br Med J 3:175, 1972.

122. Bruckova M, Grandien M, Pettersson C-A, Kunzova L: Use of nasal and pharyngeal swabs for rapid detection of respiratory syncytial virus and adenovirus antigens by enzyme-linked immunosorbent assay. J Clin Microbiol 27:1867–1869, 1989.

123. Harmon MW, Drake S, Kasel JA: Detection of adenovirus by enzyme-linked immunosorbent assay. J Clin Microbiol 9:342–346, 1979.

124. Roggendorf M, Wigand R, et al: Enzyme-linked immunosorbent assay for acute adenovirus infection. J Virol Methods 4:27–35, 1982.

125. Yolken RH: Enzyme immunoassays for the detection of infectious antigens in body fluids: Current limitations and future prospects. Rev Infect Dis 4:35–68, 1982.

15 BRONCHIAL CHALLENGE TECHNIQUES IN CHILDREN: METHACHOLINE, HISTAMINE, HYPERVENTILATION, AND OSMOLAR

RUSSELL JAMES HOPP, D.O./ ROBERT TOWNLEY, M.D. / BRIAN A. BRENNAN, M.D. / NIKHIL K. DAVE, M.D.

Airway hyperresponsiveness is essential to the definition and the understanding of the pathogenesis of asthma.[1-3] The severity of asthma also correlates with the degree of hyperresponsiveness.[1-3] In asthma, airway hyperresponsiveness likely arises from both genetic and acquired mechanisms.[4]

Bronchial challenges, using both physiologic and pharmacologic methods, are important tools to advance the understanding of airway reactivity and the pathogenesis of bronchial asthma. The purposes of such testing include diagnosis, research, epidemiology, and evaluation of pharmacologic agents for the treatment of asthma.[5-7] For further details of the mechanisms and management of asthma, the readers are referred to a review by Townley, Hopp, and colleagues[8] and Chapters 66 to 68.

Children are generally capable of performing inhalation challenges by 8 years of age, although many younger children are able to participate in bronchial challenges if properly instructed. Children younger than 5 years have difficulty performing reproducible and reliable forced expiratory maneuvers. There have been, however, reports of inhalation challenges in younger children through the use of both simple and sophisticated methods.[9-11]

The patient with known asthma shows hyperresponsiveness to a wide variety of physiologic and pharmacologic stimuli. There are, however, important differences in the mechanism responsible for bronchoconstriction. Methacholine and histamine induce direct smooth muscle constriction, whereas exercise, inhalation of cold, dry air, and inhalation of ultrasonically nebulized distilled water (UNDW) appear to do so by more indirect mechanisms, including mast cell mediator release.

The differences between the pharmacologic and physiologic bronchial challenges are both qualitative and quantitative. Tests with exercise, inhaled water, or hyperventilation of cold, dry air do not usually produce a 20% fall in the forced expiratory volume in 1 sec (FEV_1) in subjects without asthma, even with the maximal stimulus. In contrast, pharmacologic challenges with methacholine or histamine can produce significant airway narrowing in some subjects without asthma. This lack of specificity is most pronounced in the pediatric population.

INDICATIONS FOR TESTING

The primary clinical indication for performing a bronchial challenge is to identify the presence of bronchial hyperreactivity, an essential component of the asthmatic patient.[1, 6, 7, 12-15] Most patients with asthma have characteristic symptoms, and diagnostic bronchial challenges are not necessary. In pediatric patients, however, cough or dyspnea may be the only symptom, and physical findings and spirometry results may be normal. In these situations, a bronchial challenge may be useful. In addition, bronchial challenges have been used in children for epidemiologic research and as part of clinical trials of drug efficacy.

MEASUREMENT OF RESPONSE

The FEV_1 remains the most important measurement of airway responsiveness in adults and children.[16] It is both simple to perform and reproducible, and measurement is readily available. Other tests may be used, but it is important that an FEV_1 value also be included for comparison.

Other commonly used tests include airway resistance and specific airway conductance (SGaw), which can be measured by a body plethysmograph, and the peak expiratory flow rate (PEFR), which is often measured by using a hand-held peak flowmeter. These measurements provide sensitive measures of response, but they have the disadvantage of being more variable and less reproducible than the FEV_1.

FACTORS INFLUENCING RESPONSE

Factors that can influence the response to bronchial challenge should be taken into consideration when interpreting challenge results. These include acute viral respi-

Table 15–1. RECOMMENDED IDEAL TIME INTERVAL BETWEEN LAST MEDICATION AND BRONCHIAL CHALLENGE*

Drug	Time Interval (Hours)
Inhaled bronchodilators	
Isoproterenol	4
Isoetharine	6
Metaproterenol	8
Terbutaline	12
Salbutamol	12
Atropine and its analogs	10
Injected bronchodilators	
Epinephrine	4
Terbutaline	12
Oral bronchodilators	
Liquid theophylline preparations	12
Short-acting theophylline preparations	18
Aminophylline preparations	18
Intermediate-acting theophylline preparations	24
Long-acting theophylline preparations	48
Cromolyn sodium	48
Long-acting antihistamines	48
Hydroxyzine	96
Terfenadine	72

*Patients with a forced expiratory volume in 1 sec less than 70% of the predicted value should not be tested.

ratory infections and bacterial respiratory infections, such as sinusitis. Seasonal or sporadic exposure to naturally occurring antigens or recent antigen challenge may increase nonspecific airway hyperresponsiveness. This may be important when repeated bronchial challenges are performed for comparison. Children without asthma may have an exaggerated response to methacholine or histamine,[17, 18] as do many infants.[11] A variety of drugs can influence the results of a bronchial challenge. The recommended withdrawal times before challenge are listed in Table 15–1.

DELIVERY OF AEROSOL CHALLENGE

Aerosol with appropriate and reproducible properties must be delivered to the subject for valid airway responsiveness studies. Important aerosol properties include the electric charge, surface area, particle density, composition, volatility, and shape.[19]

The DeVilbiss Jet Nebulizer, model 646, is commonly used for methacholine and histamine. The other commonly used nebulizer is the Wright nebulizer, which generates an aerosol with a smaller mean mass diameter than does the DeVilbiss 646.[19] Similar histamine bronchoconstricting effects and dose-response curves have been produced with a DeVilbiss 646 (with dosimeter) and a Wright nebulizer with 2 min of tidal breathing.[20]

Tubing, mouthpieces, and other devices between the aerosol generator and the patient's mouth should remain the same for all measurements because particle size varies as a result of evaporation and impaction of the larger droplets within the tubing.

Ultrasonic nebulization is produced when high-frequency sound waves are focused onto an air-liquid inter-

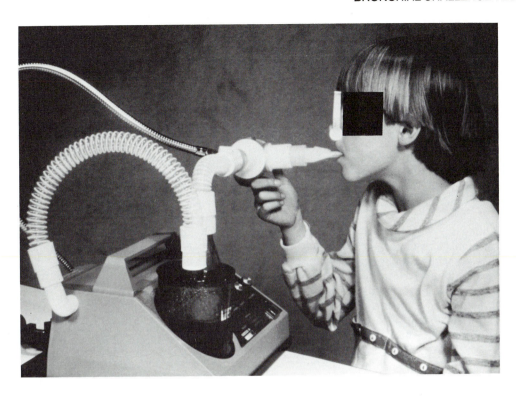

Figure 15–1. Typical setup for ultrasonic nebulized distilled water challenge.

face. The initial average particle diameter is a function of the crystal frequency used to generate the sound waves. The different ultrasonic nebulizers vary considerably in output and in ability to induce bronchoconstriction (see Fig. 15–1).

The effect of inhalation of normal saline must be determined before the dose-response relationship of any agent is obtained. If a fall in FEV_1 of 10% to 20% occurs after saline solution, the validity of any subsequent results is questionable, at least for that day. The time between inhalation and spirometry measurement should be constant. The responses should then be compared with the postsaline measurement. The inhaled agents are delivered in stepwise increasing doses. Concentrations of the broncho-provocation agent are increased until the FEV_1 has decreased by 20%, the airway conductance or resistance have changed by 35% to 40%, or the final dose is reached.

RESULTS

Several factors affect the interpretation of tests of airway responsiveness. These are the dose delivered, how the dose-response curve is plotted, the values used to express its position, the slope and shape of the dose-response curve, and the lung function test used.

The results are expressed as the provocation dose causing a 20% drop (PD_{20}) in FEV_1 or PD_{35} if SGaw is used. The degree of airway responsiveness to methacholine can be expressed as milligrams per milliliter for concentration (noncumulative), micromoles, and breath units (cumulative) for individuals with severe, moderate, and mild asthma as well as normal subjects.

The dose is expressed in breath units for methacholine or histamine. One breath unit is defined as one inhalation of a concentration of 1 mg/ml.[6, 7] It is also appropriate to express the dose in milligrams or micromoles and to specify whether the dose is cumulative or noncumulative.

The $PD_{20}FEV_1$ is the usual method of expressing results. When using methacholine or histamine, some nonasthmatic pediatric subjects and approximately 25% of subjects with allergic rhinitis may have a positive reaction and attain a $PD_{20}FEV_1$ but achieve a plateau phenomenon at higher doses.[2, 21, 22] In subjects with a plateau response, the further administration of methacholine or histamine fails to produce progressive airway narrowing. Woolcock[22] and Townley and co-workers[2, 21] showed that, when a $PD_{35}FEV_1$ is used, it is possible to differentiate patients with this plateau phenomenon from those with asthma. Beyond a $PD_{35}FEV_1$, the severity of airway narrowing makes further administration of the bronchoconstrictive agent too uncomfortable and dangerous.[21, 22]

In practical terms, the $PD_{20}FEV_1$ is the best measurement of changes in pulmonary function during histamine and methacholine challenges. If a pediatric subject has a 20% fall in FEV_1 by the end of the test, it is considered positive. A positive response to methacholine or histamine does *not*, however, indicate that the patient is asthmatic.

If the bronchial response to the inhaled bronchoconstrictor is monitored by changes in SGaw, a change in SGaw of 35% to 60% from base line is considered positive. A change in the PEFR of 10% is considered positive, although a fall of 20% or more is desirable, especially for research studies. Neither SGaw nor PEFR is as reproducible or reliable as FEV_1.

Challenges with physiologic agents are less likely to induce a significant response unless the patient is an asthmatic. Physiologic challenges can be performed with single doses (exercise, UNDW, cold air hyperventilation challenge [CAHC]) or with increasing doses (UNDW, CAHC).

METHODS FOR PHARMACOLOGIC CHALLENGES

Of the pharmacologic challenge agents, methacholine and histamine are most commonly used in children. Methacholine is a parasympathomimetic agent that stimulates the muscarinic receptors on bronchial smooth muscles. Histamine induces bronchoconstriction primarily by a direct bronchoconstrictive effect and partly by vagal reflex stimulation.[23] Selection of the agent to be used depends on the investigator's experience and familiarity with the agent. Histamine has a shorter duration of action and may cause headache, flushing, and hoarseness at higher doses.[24, 25]

Before testing, the patient should have a general physical examination and baseline pulmonary function testing. Unless the FEV_1 is at least 70% of the predicted value, testing should be postponed. Patients should receive a thorough explanation of tests, and their parents or legal guardian should be asked to sign an informed consent form. Because severe bronchospasm may result from the testing, a physician and emergency equipment should be present. Two methods of challenge with methacholine and histamine are widely used, and both require nebulization of the solution.[26] Serial dilutions of either methacholine or histamine solutions are prepared. The standard procedure is to use concentrations in a sequence of five inhalations of 0.075, 0.15, 0.31, 0.62, 1.25, 2.5, 5.0, 10, and 25 mg/ml for a total of 225 breath units.[6, 7] An abbreviated version of the American Academy of Allergy dose schedule has been suggested.[14] Two milliliters of the solution is placed in the DeVilbiss 646 nebulizer, and the tubing is attached to the compressed air reservoir. The aerosol is generated by the compressed air delivered at 20 psi through the nebulizer. Input is controlled by a valve triggered by inspiration and is kept open for 0.6 sec. The subjects use a nose clip and are instructed to inhale slowly from functional residual capacity to total lung capacity. During the inhalation, the vent of the nebulizer is kept open. Three minutes after the aerosol inhalation of each dilution, spirometric measurements are taken. The test is usually terminated if the FEV_1 drops by 20% or more of the control value or if the final dilution is reached. A decrease in FEV_1 of less than 20% is considered to be a negative challenge. The inhalation method and the continuous tidal breathing method was reviewed by Townley and Hopp in 1987.[26]

Throughout the challenge, spirometric measurements are taken in duplicate. Consistency is defined as two FEV_1 values within 5% of each other, and the best of the two values is taken for the challenge evaluation at each step. If the challenge is to be repeated in the same subject, the same nebulizer should be used to avoid internebulizer variation.[7]

METHODS FOR PHYSIOLOGIC CHALLENGES

Inhalation challenge studies with the use of graded exercise, CAHC, and UNDW can also produce bronchoconstriction in susceptible persons. These tests are used to assess latent asthma, to evaluate the severity of known exercise-induced bronchoconstriction, or to evaluate the effects of medications.[8, 13, 14] Although specificity for asthma approaches 100%, the sensitivity varies from 50% to 100%..

EXERCISE

Exercise studies can be performed with free running, treadmill running, or bicycle ergometer.[27] In free running, however, there are many uncontrollable factors that make the test less reliable.[27] As a result, treadmill running and bicycle ergometer studies in a controlled environment are more frequently performed in children.

With exercise challenges, the energy of each subject should be quantified by a measurement of the work rate[28] needed to increase the oxygen consumption by 30 to 40 ml/min/kg[29, 30] or to increase the heart rate by 80% to 90% of maximal heart rate based on the subject's age.[28] With subjects younger than 25 years, the target heart rate can be reached in the first 1 to 2 min of exercise.[27] The target heart rate should be sustained for 6 to 8 min for a maximal response. Exercise for longer periods does not increase the bronchoconstriction and may even promote bronchodilation.[27, 29–32]

Within the first 4 min of exericise, bronchodilation occurs and is thought to be caused by increased sympathetic drive.[27] This is followed by a progressive airway constriction that peaks 3 to 4 min after the completion of 8 min of exercise.[27, 28] Pulmonary function returns to normal an average of 20 to 30 min later.[27, 28]

Cold Air Hyperventilation Challenge

CAHC provides an alternative to exercise challenge, and a strong correlation exists between the two.[15, 28, 32] The cold air delivery system consists of compressed air entrained through a heat exchanger capable of generating a final temperature at the patient's mouth of at least $-10°C$.[15] It is necessary to measure and control minute ventilation ($\dot{V}_E$). End-tidal carbon dioxide (CO_2) levels need not be measured, but CO_2 needs to be added to the system. Hyperventilation produces hypocapnia, which itself causes bronchoconstriction.[28]

To initiate the test, the subject undergoes a baseline spirometry to determine the FEV_1. $\dot{V}_E$ is then set at (1) 20 to 30 times the baseline FEV_1, which is comparable with the $\dot{V}_E$ attained with moderately strenuous exercise[15, 33]; (2) maximal voluntary ventilation (MVV)[34]; or (3) a cumulative dose response of 20%, 40%, 60%, or 80% of predicted MVV or 7.5, 15, 30, 60 l/min and then MVV.[35, 36] Regardless of the method, each is maintained for 3 to 4 min.[15, 35, 36] Although a single $\dot{V}_E$ of 20 to 35 times the FEV_1 may produce good results, MVV alone or with a cumulative dose produces more consistent results.[36] A cumulative dose method also decreases the chance of marked bronchoconstriction and has the advantage of qualification by providing a dose-response curve.

As with exercise tests, the maximal bronchoconstrictive response peaks 4 to 8 min after the challenge, starts resolving within the next 5 min, and approaches base line after 15 to 60 min.[28, 35] Controversy exists as to what is considered a positive response. Most agree that a positive response is at least a 10% decrease in FEV_1; for SGaw a positive response is a change of 30% or more. Measurements are performed at 2- to 3-min intervals until maximal response is achieved and then at 5-min intervals until recovery begins.[37, 38] The results can be expressed in terms of $\dot{V}_E$, the respiratory heat exchange,[38] or the maximal drop in pulmonary function that was obtained.

Ultrasonically Nebulized Distilled Water Inhalation

UNDW is a relatively new addition to bronchial challenge procedures. Its use in children is limited at present.[39, 40] The positive test appears to be very specific for asthma, but the sensitivity ranges between 30% to 100%. The correlation of UNDW challenge to methacholine is variable; a better correlation to exercise and CAHC is found.[41]

Various methods of UNDW challenge are being used, and a standardized protocol has yet to be established. The three basic principles of UNDW challenges are as follows: (1) begin with a minimal dose of nebulized water; (2) increase the dose gradually; and (3) obtain a dose-response curve. Single-dose challenges have been used, however.[34] UNDW challenge is a safe, specific, moderately sensitive test for bronchial asthma, and it can be used as a valuable research tool in testing the pathophysiology of asthma. In 1990, Virant and associates demonstrated that hypertonic saline provides results similar to those of UNDW.[42]

REFERENCES

1. Townley RG, Dennis M, Itkin JM: Comparative action of acetyl-beta-methacholine, histamine and pollen antigens in subjects with hay fever and patients with bronchial asthma. J Allergy 36:121–137, 1965.
2. Townley RG, Bewtra AK, Nair NH, et al: Methacholine inhalation challenge studies. J Allergy Clin Immunol 64(2):569–574, 1979.
3. Cockcroft DW, Killian DN, Mellon JJA, Hargreave FE: Bronchial reactivity to inhaled histamine: A method and clinical survey. Clin Allergy 7:235–243, 1977.
4. Townley RG, Bewtra A, Wilson AF, et al: Segregation analysis of bronchial response to methacholine inhalation challenge in families with and without asthma. J Allergy Clin Immunol 77:101–107, 1986.
5. Boushey HA, Holtzman MJ, Sheller JR, Nadel JA: Bronchial hyperreactivity. Am Rev Respir Dis 121:389–413, 1980.
6. Chai H, Farr RS, Froehlich LA, et al: Standardization of bronchial inhalation challenge procedures. J Allergy Clin Immunol 56:323–327, 1975.
7. Cropp GJ, Bernstein IL, Boushey HA Jr, et al: Guidelines for bronchial inhalation challenges with pharmacologic and antigenic agents. ATS News, pp. 11–19, 1980.
8. Townley RG, Weiss S, Lang W, et al: Mechanisms and management of bronchial asthma. In Spittel JA Jr (ed): Clinical Medicine, pp. 1–29. Philadelphia: Harper & Row, 1986.
9. Adinoff AD, Schlosberg RT, Strunk RC: Methacholine inhalation challenge in young children: Results of testing and follow-up. Ann Allergy 61:282–286, 1988.
10. Mochizuki H, Mitsuhashi M, Tokuyama K, et al: Bronchial hyper-responsiveness in younger children with asthma. Ann Allergy 60:103–106, 1988.
11. Tepper RS: Airway reactivity in infants: A positive response to

12. Itkin IH: Bronchial hypersensitivity to mecholyl and histamine in asthma subjects. J Allergy 40:245–256, 1967.
13. Bewtra AK, Townley RG: Bronchoprovocative tests—Clinical usefulness and limitations. Arch Intern Med 144:925–926, 1984.
14. Rosenthal RR: Difference in response between hayfever and asthmatic patients. In Spector SL (ed): Provocative Challenge Procedures: Bronchial, Oral, Nasal, and Exercise, vol. 1, pp. 113–118. Boca Raton, FL: CRC Press, 1983.
15. Deal EC, McFadden ER, Ingram RH, et al: Airway responsiveness to cold air and hyperpnea in normal subjects and in those with hay fever and asthma. Am Rev Respir Dis 121:621–628, 1980.
16. Kanner RE, Schenker MB, Munoz A, Speizer FE: Spirometry in children. Methodology for obtaining optimal results for clinical and epidemiologic studies. Am Rev Respir Dis 127:720–724, 1983.
17. Riedel F, von der Hardt H: Bronchial sensitivity to inhaled histamine in healthy, nonatopic children. Pediatr Pulmonol 2:15–18, 1986.
18. Hopp RJ, Bewtra A, Nair N, Townley RG: The effect of age on methacholine response. J Allergy Clin Immunol 76:609–613, 1985.
19. Swift DL: Aerosol generation for inhalation challenge in airway responsiveness. In Hargreave FE, Woolcock AJ (eds): Airway Responsiveness: Measurement and Interpretation, pp. 1–8. Mississauga, Ontario, Canada: Astra Pharmaceuticals Canada, Ltd., 1985.
20. Ryan G, Dolovich MB, Roberts RS, et al: Standardization of inhalation provocation tests: Two techniques of aerosol generation and inhalation compared. Am Rev Respir Dis 123:195–199, 1981.
21. Townley RG, Ryo UY, Kolotkin BM, Kang B: Bronchial sensitivity to methacholine in current and former asthmatic and allergic rhinitis patients and control subjects. J Allergy Clin Immunol 56:429–442, 1975.
22. Woolcock AJ: Expression of results of airway hyperresponsiveness in airway responsiveness. In Hargreave FE, Woolcock AJ (eds): Airway Responsiveness: Measurement and Interpretation, pp. 80–85. Mississauga, Ontario, Canada: Astra Pharmaceuticals Canada, Ltd., 1985.
23. Simonsson BG, Jacobs FM, Nadel JA: Role of the autonomic nervous system and the cough reflex in the increased responsiveness of airways in patients with obstructive airway disease. J Clin Invest 46:1812–1818, 1967.
24. Hargreave FE, Ryan G, Thomson NC, et al: Bronchial responsiveness to histamine or methacholine in asthma: Measurement and clinical significance. J Allergy Clin Immunol 68:347–355, 1981.
25. Kang B, Townley RG, Lee CK, Kolotkin BM: Bronchial reactivity to histamine before and after sodium cromoglycate in bronchial asthma. Br Med J 1:867–870, 1976.
26. Townley RG, Hopp RJ: Inhalation methods for the study of airway responsiveness. J Allergy Clin Immunol 80:111–127, 1987.
27. Godfrey S: Exercise-induced asthma—Clinical, physiological, and therapeutic implications. J Allergy Clin Immunol 56:1–17, 1975.
28. Sourhrada JF, Kivity S: Exercise testing. In Spector SL (ed): Provocative Challenge Procedures: Bronchial, Oral, Nasal, and Exercise, vol. 2, pp. 75–102. Boca Raton, FL: CRC Press, 1983.
29. Cropp GJA: The exercise bronchoprovocation test: Standardization of procedures and evaluation of response. J Allergy Clin Immunol 64:627–633, 1979.
30. Eggleston PA, Rosenthal RR, Anderson SD, et al: Guidelines for the methodology of exercise testing of asthmatics. J Allergy Clin Immunol 64:642–645, 1979.
31. Anderson SD, Schoeffel RE: Standardization of exercise training in the asthmatic patient: A challenge in itself. In Hargreave FE, Woolcock AJ (eds): Airway Responsiveness: Measurement and Interpretation, pp. 51–59. Mississauga, Ontario, Canada: Astra Pharmaceuticals Canada, Ltd., 1985.
32. Anderson SD: Issues in exercise-induced asthma. J Allergy Clin Immunol 76:763–772, 1985.
33. McLaughlin FJ, Dozor AJ: Cold air inhalation challenge in the diagnosis of asthma in children. Pediatrics 72:503–509, 1983.
34. Fabbri LM, Mapp CE, Hendrick DJ: Comparison of ultrasonically nebulized distilled water and hyperventilation with cold air in asthma. Allergy 53:172–177, 1984.
35. Nair N, Hopp RJ, Alper BI, et al: Correlation of methacholine-induced non-specific bronchial reactivity and cold air hyperventilation challenge. Ann Allergy 56:226–228, 1986.

36. Malo JL, Cartier A, L'Archeveque J: Cold air inhalation has a cumulative bronchospastic effect when inhaled in consecutive doses for progressively increasing degrees of ventilation. Am Rev Respir Dis 134:990–993, 1986.
37. O'Bryne PM: Airway challenge using isocapnic hyperventilation. In Hargreave FE, Woolcock AJ (eds): Airway Responsiveness: Measurement and Interpretation, pp. 60–65. Mississauga, Ontario, Canada: Astra Pharmaceuticals Canada, Ltd., 1985.
38. Tessier P, Cartier A, L'Archeveque J, et al: Within and between day reproducibility of isocapnic cold air challenges in subjects with asthma. J Allergy Clin Immunol 78:379–387, 1986.
39. Galdes-Sebalt M, McLaughlin FJ, Levison H: Comparison of cold air, ultrasonic mist, and methacholine inhalations as tests of bronchial reactivity in normal and asthmatic children. J Pediatr 107:526–530, 1985.
40. Hopp RJ, Christy J, Bewtra AK, et al: Incorporation and analysis of ultrasonically nebulized distilled water challenges in an epidemiology study of asthma and bronchial reactivity. Ann Allergy 60:129–133, 1988.
41. Bascom B, Bleecker ER: Bronchoconstriction induced by distilled water. Am Rev Respir Dis 134:248–253, 1986.
42. Virant FS, Williams PV, Bierman CW, et al: Hyperosmolar saline challenge in children: Relationship to methacholine, exercise challenge and therapy. J Allergy Clin Immunol 85:259, 1990.

16 BRONCHOPROVOCATION BY INHALATION CHALLENGE WITH ANTIGEN IN CHILDREN

RICHARD R. ROSENTHAL, M.D.

Bronchoprovocation is an inhalation challenge method by which bronchospasm is deliberately induced. It is used in children as well as in adults to identify patients with hyperreactive airways, regardless of the cause and to measure the extent of the hyperreactivity. The methacholine challenge is commonly used today for this purpose and is now a standardized procedure: it is described elsewhere.[1,2]

Inhalation challenge with antigen is still primarily a research tool. It is used to characterize specifically the bronchomotor response to a particular antigen when it is given by inhalation. As in the case of methacholine, clinical indications for inhalation challenge with antigen have been established.[3,4] Inhalation challenge with antigen is used to clarify the role of specific allergens in asthma, especially when other diagnostic criteria are inadequate. A false-positive reaction, however, is possible; that is, allergic patients may show bronchoreactivity to allergens that are clinially unrelated to their asthma.

When the medical history is not clear, antigen challenge may be useful for diagnostic purposes if the results of cutaneous or serum tests are equivocal. Antigen provocation is particularly useful when there is a clinical decision to be made such as whether to initiate immunotherapy, or to indicate the need to avoid specific allergens. (This is especially important in treating children who are often reluctant to avoid asthma-provoking pets.)

Antigen challenge may be used to define the natural history of antigen sensitivity when there has been no immunologic intervention, and it may also be used to evaluate the therapeutic effect of immunotherapy.

Antigen challenge is not helpful in distinguishing the presence of airways hyperreactivity, because an allergic patient may have a reaction without having hyperreactive airways. Antigen sensitivity measured by inhalation challenge may compare favorably with that measured by skin sensitivity, but the results are not necessarily related to the presence of asthma.[5] Alternatively, a patient with a positive skin test may have a negative bronchial challenge with the same antigen.

Although allergen challenge testing cannot be used as an easy method of distinguishing between asthma and nonasthma, it is an adequate way of characterizing the atopic patient's bronchial sensitivity to a particular antigen, regardless of the disease process, and therefore may be used to rule out the causal role of a specific antigen in an asthmatic patient. It may be used to establish whether the lung is a target organ independently of whether the skin test has indicated the presence of immunoglobulin E (IgE) specific to the antigen. In some asthmatics, antigen challenge may be the only procedure available for defining the lung as a target organ.[6] In addition, there are a number of research applications of antigen challenge, especially in the field of new drug evaluation.

METHODOLOGY AND INTERPRETATION OF RESULTS

CONDUCT OF THE STUDY

A standard method for the inhalation challenge technique has been published under the aegis of the National Institutes of Health.[7] The fundamental concept underlying this method is that doses of inhaled agonists are given by intermittent aerosol in a stepwise incremental manner and that pulmonary function is measured by testing after each dose.

On the basis of these incremental doses and the response measurement, a reproducible dose-response curve is constructed. From this curve, the provocation dose causing a 20% drop in baseline forced expiratory volume in 1 sec ($PD_{20}FEV_1$) may be interpolated for any given agonist. The $PD_{20}FEV_1$ is an accepted index of airway sensitivity.

The first step after determining the patient's baseline pulmonary function and before inhalation challenge with the specific antigenic agonists (such as extract of cat dander or ragweed) is to determine pulmonary function after inhalation of a saline diluent control. (This is also the first step before bronchial challenge with the nonspecific agonists histamine and methacholine.) Also, anything that can influence the response to inhalation challenge may have to be taken into account at the time the test is conducted. The most important factor is the medication currently being used by the patient. Most bronchodilators, cromolyn sodium, and, possibly, antihistamines may inhibit antigenic challenges. See Hopp and colleagues' study[1] for a table of recommended time intervals between the last medication and bronchial challenge.

Inhalation of a saline diluent control is performed because all of the agonists are diluted in saline, and it is important to be able to subtract the bronchodilatory or bronchoconstrictor effects of aerosol inhalation itself from the effects of the agonist diluted in saline. In addition, if the saline control itself causes more than a 15% decrease in FEV_1, the inhalation challenge is generally not performed because the airways are too hyperreactive. This in itself may establish the diagnosis of airway hyperreactivity in the case of nonspecific airway irritability.

The nebulization dosimeter (Fig. 16–1) is often used to deliver consistent amounts of aerosol from breath to breath. This consistency enables the construction of fairly reproducible dose-response curves. In the configuration shown in Figure 16–1, the nebulization dosimeter regulates the interval of aerosol duration, and this is adequate for most clinical applications. If there is no breath holding at the end of the aerosol inflow, the length of time that the aerosol remains in the lungs and the amounts of aerosol in the lungs are relatively consistent from breath to breath.

The dosimeter may also be used in parallel with a spirometer from which the inspired air is drawn; this regulates the inspiratory flow rate, the lung volume at which aerosol is given, as well as the aerosol inflow interval.[8] This configuration may be used to enhance reproducibility of aerosol administration further and to enable calibration of the elements in order to regulate the delivery of specific target quantities of agonist. This may be useful for dose-range studies.

Antigen provocation is similar to methacholine challenge but is somewhat more critical. Before performing the antigen challenge, not only should the baseline and saline control pulmonary functions be established, but the patient's skin must also be tested with the antigen in question. If the skin test is negative, the patient is unlikely

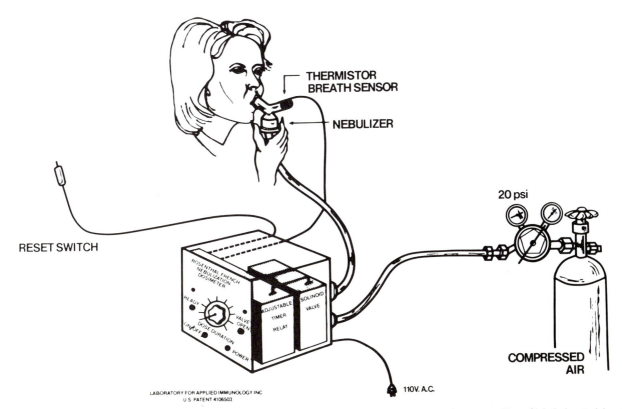

Figure 16–1. The nebulization dosimeter is an aerosol delivery device that can be used to measure consistent quantities of inhaled material such as antigen. It may be breath actuated or triggered manually. (Courtesy of the Laboratory for Applied Immunology, Inc., Fairfax, Virginia.)

to respond to an inhalation challenge with the antigen. If the skin test is positive, it can be used to establish the first dose of antigen to be used in the inhalation challenge because the magnitude of bronchial sensitivity is generally thought to relate to antigen skin test sensitivity in a quantitative manner. (This differs from the procedure used with methacholine challenges in which standard doses are used.)

The antigen concentration that causes a 2^+ skin test (10-mm wheal), expressed as protein nitrogen units (PNU), is usually the best concentration to use as the first dose given by inhalation; this is generally very conservative. In antigen challenge, inhalation units are conveniently described as one breath of a solution containing 1 PNU/ml or 1 μg of protein nitrogen per milliliter.

First, baseline pulmonary functions are established, and, under current standards, if the patient's FEV_1 is less than 80% of the predicted value, inhalation challenge is not performed. If the FEV_1 is 80% or more of the predicted value and the patient is a suitable subject for inhalation challenge, five inhalations of saline are then given, and the absolute value of the FEV_1, or any other airway parameter, is known as 100% of saline control.

From this control value, a 20% fall in FEV_1 to 80% saline control is computed and noted on the flow sheet (to be discussed). This computation enables the operator to determine when a fall of 20% or more in FEV_1 has occurred and to discontinue the challenge at that time. This is very important because patients may have a significant drop in airway function after administration of the initial doses of agonist, and this would contraindicate administration of any subsequent doses.

After the 100% saline control values are established and the target value of the patient's 20% fall in FEV_1 (80% of saline control) is computed, the actual challenge begins with the first dose of agonist. Inhalation should be taken from the normal resting level of lung inflation, or functional residual capacity. When the nebulization dosimeter is used, 0.6 sec is the customary interval of nebulization. This can, however, be varied between 0.1 and 3.0 sec. Because the effects of doses linger, inhalation units are cumulated.

A pulmonary function test is performed 10 min after each dose of five inhalations of antigen, unlike challenge with methacholine, in which pulmonary function testing is performed immediately after each dose. As discussed, the FEV_1 (or any other airway parameter) after inhalation challenge is computed in terms of percentage of the control values. If this FEV_1 is higher than 80% of the control, the next dose is given as scheduled.

When the postchallenge FEV_1 is between 15% and 20% less than the saline control value, it may be advisable to administer a subsequent dose that is either a repeat of the last dose or only a few of the five inhalations of the next concentration that normally would be given. This should be done to prevent an excessive decrease in pulmonary function.

A sample spirometry flow sheet for antigen challenge is shown in Figure 16–2. The cumulative dose schedule in inhalation units, which is the aggregate of breath time inhalations, varies with the concentration of the first dose used.

Recovery from methacholine and histamine inhalation challenge usually occurs spontaneously, and it is usually not necessary to administer a bronchodilator drug after this type of inhalation challenge. This is not the case in antigen challenge. After an antigen challenge, it is advisable to provide treatment with an inhaled beta-agonist, usually by means of a metered dose inhaler, unless the intention is to monitor for a delayed reaction.

In at least 25% of patients, a delayed reaction does occur, and this may be caused by either a late response to the antigen or the wearing off of the inhaled bronchodilator. In antigen challenge, some allowance should be made for these possibilities, such as giving the patient a metered dose inhaler to take home, prescribing other quick-acting bronchodilators to be taken orally, and advising the patient to call for assistance should respiratory distress occur.

Although inhalation challenge is often performed in outpatient settings, some provision for postchallenge care should be established if a delayed reaction occurs after the patient has left the clinical area.

FACTORS TO CONSIDER IN TESTING CHILDREN

In children, pulmonary function tests are performed for the same reasons as in adults. There are some tests of lung function that may be useful for children younger than 6 years,[9] but about 6 or 8 years[1] is generally the lower age limit for routine spirometry.

In children older than 6 to 8 years, spirometry, lung volume, maximal expiratory flow-volume curves, and diffusing capacity tests are performed in much the same way as in adults. There are, however, some technical factors and factors related to body and lung growth that should be taken into consideration in the pulmonary testing of children.

In testing of children, because of the lower volumes and flows, the instruments should be accurate at low volumes (± 3% of the reading or 30 ml, whichever is greater). A closed-circuit system or pneumotachygraph may be used to determine whether the inspiratory effort is adequate and to ensure that forced expiratory maneuvers start from total lung capacity. Also, mouthpiece size should be adjusted for the size of the child.

In general, regression equations that interpret adult lung function are not applicable to children. Computerized devices that measure lung function parameters and compare them with reference standards on the basis of sex, age, height, and race must have suitable pediatric reference, and if these standards are not used, the information may be misleading.

A child's body size is determined by height, which is the most significant predictor of lung function. Unlike the reference values for adults, age is usually not included in the determination of reference values for children's lung function.

Children's flow rates and lung volumes increase as a curvilinear function of height raised to a power between 2.5 and 3.0, and children track lung function percentiles in a manner similar to those of their height growth. Sig-

Name: Date:

Conditions	Cumulative units	Minutes	FVC	FEV$_1$	MMEF	FEV$_1$/FVC	FEV$_1$ Percent control	FEV$_1$ Percent baseline
Baseline								100%
Saline control							100%	
1 PNU/ml Ag	5	10						
2 PNU/ml Ag	15	10						
4 PNU/ml Ag	35	10						
8 PNU/ml Ag	75	10						
15 PNU/ml Ag	150	10						
30 PNU/ml Ag	300	10						
60 PNU/ml Ag	600	10						
120 PNU/ml Ag	1,200	10						
240 PNU/ml Ag	2,400	10						
480 PNU/ml Ag	4,800	10						
960 PNU/ml Ag	9,600	10						
2,000 PNU/ml Ag	19,600	10						
4,000 PNU/ml Ag	39,600	10						
8,000 PNU/ml Ag	79,600	10						
Post bronchodilator								

20% Fall in FEV$_1$:_____

Figure 16–2. A sample spirometry flow sheet for antigen inhalation challenge. This type of flow sheet can be used to track the response to an antigen inhalation sequence. Five inhalations of each concentration are administered. One inhalation unit is defined as one inhalation of antigen, 1 protein nitrogen unit per milliliter; the total dose is cumulated. It is helpful to compute a 20% fall in forced expiratory volume in 1 sec (FEV$_1$) from the saline control value as a target, although absolute values may be graphed as well. Cumulative units given may then be graphed against an airway parameter, such as FEV$_1$ or specific airway conductance (SGaw), and the provocation-dose causing a 20% drop (PD$_{20}$) in FEV$_1$ (or PD$_{35}$SGaw) may then be determined.

nificant deviation may indicate the presence of disease. There are also sex-related and race-related patterns of lung volumes and functions that must be taken into consideration in pulmonary tests for children.[9]

With adult patients, two or three spirograms are usually performed after each dose. If two FEV_1s are within 150 ml of each other, the third one need not be performed. The spirogram with the highest sum of the forced vital capacity and FEV_1 is usually taken as the patient's "best." The FEV_1 or other spirometric parameters are taken from this spirogram.[10]

In the case of children, age and previous experience in performing pulmonary function tests are the factors most important for obtaining the required three acceptable spirograms. Most children require eight or fewer forced expirations to achieve this; older children and adolescents may need as few as three tests.

For children, a minimum of five attempts is sometimes recommended, but with young children, because of boredom and fatigue, large numbers of spirograms may not improve the assessment of lung function. Spirometric tracings should be reviewed during the testing to determine when to discontinue further attempts and to use the available data.[9]

HOW TO GRAPH THE RESULTS

Figure 16–3 illustrates a method of graphing the data generated from inhalation challenges. Semilog paper is used and, with the log scale on the abscissa, cumulative antigen units are graphed against the percentage control on the ordinate. Thus all dose-response curves start from 100%. Usually, FEV_1 is used, but in the example shown, both FEV_1 and specific airway conductance (SGaw), determined by a whole-body plethysmograph, are graphed simultaneously.

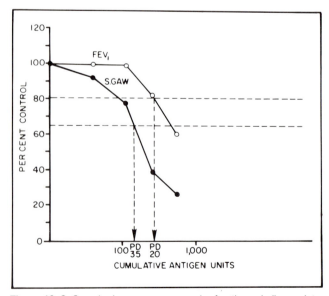

Figure 16–3. Sample dose-response graph of antigen challenge data. Cumulative doses of inhaled antigen agonist are plotted against airway functions such as forced expiratory volume in 1 sec or specific airway conductance in terms of percent saline control values to determine the provocative doses.

Table 16–1. MINIMUM ACCEPTABLE CHANGES IN PULMONARY FUNCTION TESTS AFTER BRONCHIAL PROVOCATION CHALLENGES

Test	Minimum Change From Base Line (%)
Vital capacity	−10
FEV_1	−20
MMEF (FEF_{25-75} or $\dot{V}max_{50}$)	−25
Peak expiratory flow rate	−25
Specific airway conductance	−35–40
Functional residual capacity	+25

From Guidelines for bronchial inhalation challenges with pharmacologic and antigenic agents. ATS News, 16, 1980.

FEV_1, forced expiratory volume in 1 sec; MMEF, maximal midexpiratory flow rate; FEF_{25-75}, forced expiratory flow between 25% and 75% of vital capacity; $\dot{V}max_{50}$, flow at 50% of vital capacity.

When the data illustrated in Figure 16–3 were obtained, SGaw tests were performed first, followed by a forced spirogram in which the FEV_1 was determined. The FEV_1 from the best spirogram at each dose was plotted, and a dose-response curve was constructed from this. The last data point should be at 80% of saline control or lower. The $PD_{20}FEV_1$ can then be interpolated from the dose-response curve. Table 16–1 lists the interpolated provocation doses used for other spirometric parameters.

The provocative dose (e.g., the $PD_{20}FEV_1$) is a measure of the patient's sensitivity to the inhaled agonist. Reactivity reflects the slope of the curve, but this assessment is not in general use. Still another method of analysis is to compute the area under the curve; this type of analysis is used primarily in research applications.[11]

In a comparison of the usefulness of several spirometric measurements in detecting asthmatic reactions after allergen bronchial challenge in asthmatic children, Murray and Ferguson[12] found that the ranking of tests from most sensitive to least sensitive in detecting the early asthmatic reaction was FEV_1, forced expiratory flow at 50% of vital capacity (FEF_{50}), FEF_{25-75}, peak expiratory flow rate (PEFR), and FVC. For the late reaction, the ranking was FEF_{50}, FEF_{25-75}, PEFR, and FVC.

In the same study it was found that although no one single test detected all the early or all the late reactions, a combination of FEV_1 and FEF_{25-75} (which is influenced by obstruction of small airways) detected all early and late asthmatic reactions. Although Murray and Ferguson found the FEV_1 to be the single most useful test, they recommended using it with the FEF_{25-75} test to ensure the detection of all asthmatic reactions induced by bronchial challenge with antigen.[12]

REPRODUCIBILITY OF RESULTS

Antigen challenges are fairly reproducible on a day-to-day basis but may be somewhat variable. Earlier studies demonstrated a tenfold day-to-day variation in the $PD_{35}SGaw$.[13] In one study of reproducibility of bronchial provocation with house dust in children, reproducibility was found in 80% of the tests performed. It was also found that reproducibility was better when lower doses were used.[14] The authors of another study of bronchial responsiveness, in testing asthmatic children with cat dander, found that sensitivity to antigen varied over time.[15]

PRECAUTIONS AND RISKS

The most obvious risk in conducting inhalation challenge with antigen in any age group is causing antigen overdosage by inhalation. A caveat that may be more relevant to the conduction of challenge in children, however, is that they may be less likely than adults to inform the challenge administrator that they are becoming uncomfortable. Accordingly, it is important that the baseline FEV_1 not be below 80% of the predicted value before challenge is initiated and that the 20% decrement from the saline control value be calculated and be exceeded only minimally during challenge.

It should be recognized that if an investigational protocol requires that antigen challenge be performed to evaluate the protective effects of an experimental drug, a particular risk may be introduced: the delivery of excessive doses of inhaled antigen under the protective influence of the study drug.

When the study drug wears off, the effects of the antigen may linger, causing more of an airway response than would have occurred without the protecting influence of the experimental drug. In addition, if higher doses of antigen are given, the risk of a severe delayed reaction may be greater than would have been possible without the protection from the immediate reaction by the drug under study.

Late asthmatic reactions may follow after recovery from the immediate response.[16-20] These characteristically occur 6 to 12 h after spontaneous recovery from the immediate response and may be more severe. The frequency of delayed or late reaction may be quite high. In one study, a 73% incidence of late reactions after antigen challenge was reported, and these late reactions often were more prolonged and severe than the immediate response to the challenge.[21] Similarly, in another study, an 86% incidence of late responses was reported.[22] These late reactions may be accompanied by an increase in nonspecific airway hyperreactivity, as measured by methacholine sensitivity, that may last days or weeks.[16, 18, 20, 23, 24]

A particularly significant risk factor is that the delayed reaction may occur in the absence of an immediate reaction[25] and that extent of the delayed reaction is not related to the extent of the immediate reaction when both do occur.[26] The mechanism of the delayed reaction is the subject of much speculation. This mechanism has been associated with the presence of antigen-specific IgG_4.[27]

A last caveat relates to the possibility of systemic symptoms after antigen challenge. Although these reactions are unusual, a study of eight patients who had a history of anaphylaxis revealed that six of them had at least some systemic symptoms after inhalation challenge with antigen to which they were allergic.[28] Accordingly, it is important to determine whether systemic symptoms other than bronchospasm have occurred in subjects before they are exposed to inhalation challenge, lest this risk factor not be taken into account for these patients.

Because the risk of late reaction cannot be predicted from the nature or even from the presence or absence of the immediate reaction, and because late reaction carries with it the further risk of sustained airway inflammation with enhanced nonspecific airway hyperreactivity, the relative value of conducting the challenge should always be weighed against the risks. Informed consent should be obtained, and a full explanation of the risks and benefits of the procedure should be given to the patient and parents. The challenge should be performed in a clinical setting that can accommodate the exigencies of unplanned untoward reactions and in which ancillary staff and patients are prepared accordingly.

APPLICATIONS

DIAGNOSIS OF ASTHMA

It is unusual for antigen challenge to be required for the routine diagnosis of allergic asthma, because positive skin tests or positive radioallergosorbent test (RAST) determinations and an indicative medical history are usually sufficient to indict a given antigen as the cause of the allergic asthma.

Strong correlations have been reported between skin testing and bronchoprovocation tests[29-31] and, in some studies, RAST testing as well.[32-34] Because the response to inhaled antigen so closely replicates the pathophysiologic processes of asthma (given the caveat of possible false-positive inhalation challenges), the bronchomotor response to such provocational agents has been considered to be the most reliable index of the "true diagnosis" of asthma.[35]

In one reported study, suspicion of asthma resulting from exposure to dog dander was confirmed with bronchoprovocation,[36] and in another the indication for immunotherapy with dog dander was predicated on the results of bronchoprovocation.[37] In the latter study, immunotherapy resulted in an increase in blocking IgG levels and decreased skin test sensitivity to dog dander antigen and was associated with short-term physical tolerance of exposure to dogs.

RESEARCH

Inhalation challenge with antigens may be suitable for a variety of research applications, ranging in scope from basic immunology and the physiology of immunologically mediated bronchospasm to clinical trials with investigational drugs. For example, a study that demonstrated the therapeutic effects of ketotifen in children with asthma required that the diagnosis of pollen asthma be verified with bronchoprovocation.[38]

Clinical trials with antigen inhalation challenge also may yield useful information regarding the nature of the response to allergen as well as information regarding the efficacy of the study drug for the treatment of allergic bronchospasm, thereby shedding even more light on pathophysiologic mechanisms. A study of the protective effects of cromolyn in children, for example, demonstrated that both the immediate and delayed responses to antigen inhalation were blocked by the study drug,[39] and a similar study by other investigators[24] confirmed those observations when the early and late responses to inhalation of house dust mite *(Dermatophagoides pteronyssimus)* were observed before and after cromolyn pretreatment. The latter investigation, moreover, showed that antigen challenge brought about an increase in nonspecific reactivity as measured by methacholine challenge, an observation with important clinical implications, and showed as well that this increase was also attenuated by cromolyn pretreatment.

REFERENCES

1. See Chapter 15 in this volume.
2. Rosenthal RR: Inhalation challenge. N Engl Reg Allergy Proc 9:113–119, 1988.
3. Spector S, Farr R: Bronchial challenge with antigens. J Allergy Clin Immunol 64(6, Pt. 2):580–586, 1979.
4. Rosenthal RR, Chai H, Mathison DA, et al: Indications for inhalation challenge. J Allergy Clin Immunol 64(6, Pt. 2):603, 1979.
5. Bruce CA, Rosenthal RR, Lichtenstein LM, Norman PS: Quantitative inhalation bronchial challenge in ragweed hay fever patients: A comparison with ragweed allergic asthmatics. J Allergy Clin Immunol 56:331–337, 1975.
6. Chai H: Antigen and methacholine challenge in children with asthma. J Allergy Clin Immunol 64(6, Pt. 2):575–579, 1979.
7. Chai H, Farr RS, Froehlich LA, et al: Standardization of bronchial inhalation challenge procedures. J Allergy Clin Immunol 56:323–327, 1975.
8. Laube BL, Adams GK III, Norman PS, Rosenthal RR: The effect of inspiratory flow rate regulation on nebulizer output and on human airways response to methacholine aerosol. J Allergy Clin Immunol 76:708–713, 1985.
9. Eisenberg JD, Wall MA: Pulmonary function testing in children. Clin Chest Med 8(4):661–667, 1987.
10. American Thoracic Society. Standardization of spirometry—1987 update. Am Rev Respir Dis 136:1285–1298, 1987.
11. Hopp RJ, Weiss SJ, Nair NM, et al: Interpretation of the results of methacholine inhalation challenge tests. J Allergy Clin Immunol 80:821–830, 1987.
12. Murray AB, Ferguson AC: A comparison of spirometric measurements in allergen bronchial challenge testing. Clin Allergy 11(1):87–93, 1981.
13. Rosenthal RR, Norman PS, Summer WR: Bronchoprovocation: Effect on priming and desensitization phenomenon in the lung. J Allergy Clin Immunol 56:338–346, 1975.
14. Rufin P, Benoist MR, Scheinman P, Paupe J: A study on the reproducibility of specific bronchial provocation testing in children. Clin Allergy 14(4):387–397, 1984.
15. Neijens HJ, Kerrebijn KF: Variation with time in bronchial responsiveness to histamine and to specific allergen provocation. Eur J Respir Dis 64(8):591–597, 1983.
16. Foresi A, Mattoli S, Corbo GM, et al: Late bronchial response and increase in methacholine hyperresponsiveness after exercise and distilled water challenge in atopic subjects with asthma with dual asthmatic response to allergen inhalation. J Allergy Clin Immunol 78(6):1130–1139, 1986.
17. Pepys J, Hargreave FE, Chan M, McCarthy DS: Inhibitory effects of disodium chromoglycate on allergen inhalation test. Lancet 2:134, 1968.
18. Cockcroft DW, Ruffin RE, Dolovich J, Hargreave FE: Allergen-induced increase in nonallergic bronchial reactivity. Clin Allergy 7:503, 1977.
19. Cartier A, Thomson NC, Frith PA, et al: Allergen-induced increase in bronchial responsiveness to histamine: Relationship to the late asthmatic response and change in airway caliber. J Allergy Clin Immunol 70:170, 1982.
20. Mormile F, Mattoli S, Rosati G, et al: Allergen-induced increase in nonallergic bronchial responsiveness to ultrasonic mist. Prog Respir Res 19:256, 1985.
21. Warner JO: Significance of late reactions after bronchial challenge with house dust mite. Arch Dis Child 51(12):905–911, 1976.
22. Price JF, Hey EN, Soothill JF: Antigen provocation to the skin, nose and lung, in children with asthma: Immediate and dual hypersensitivity reactions. Clin Exp Immunol 47(3):587–594, 1982.
23. Mattoli S, Foresi A, Corbo GM, et al: The protective effect of two doses of DSCG on allergen-induced increase in methacholine responsiveness [Abstract]. J Allergy Clin Immunol 77(Suppl.):123, 1986.
24. Mattoli S, Foresi A, Corbo GM, et al: Protective effect of disodium cromoglycate on allergen-induced bronchoconstriction and increased hyperresponsiveness: A double-blind placebo-controlled study. Ann Allergy 57(4):295–300, 1986.
25. Hill DJ: Inter-relation of immediate and late asthmatic reactions in childhood. Allergy 36(8):549–554, 1981.
26. Price JF, Turner MW, Warner JO, Soothill JF: Immunological studies in asthmatic children undergoing antigen provocation in the skin, lung and nose. Clin Allergy 13(5):419–426, 1983.
27. Gwynn CM, Ingram J, Almousawi T, Standworth DR: Bronchial provocation tests in atopic patients with allergen-specific IgE4 antibodies. Lancet 1(8266):254–256, 1982.
28. Broom BB, Fitzharris P: Life-threatening inhalant allergy: Typical anaphylaxis induced by inhalational allergen challenge in patients with idiopathic recurrent anaphylaxis. Clin Allergy 13(2):169–179, 1988.
29. Murray AB, Ferguson AC, Morrison BJ: Diagnosis of house dust mite allergy in asthmatic children: What constitutes a positive history? J Allergy Clin Immunol 71(1, pt. 1):21–28, 1983.
30. Kurimoto Y: Relationship among skin tests, bronchial challenge and serology in house dust and Candida albicans allergic asthma. Ann Allergy 35(3):131–141, 1975.
31. Lim DT, Ganju A: Reaginic sensitivity to Mus musculus extract in a group of Chicago urban asthmatics. Ann Allergy 44(5):267–272, 1980.
32. Pola J, Zapata C, Valdivieso R, et al: Cockroach asthma: Case report and literature review. Allergol Immunopathol (Madr) 16(1):61–65, 1988.
33. Wuthrich B, Guerin B, Hewitt B, Luggen-Brun H: House dust allergy: correlation between in vivo and in vitro diagnostic tests. Ann Allergy 46(2):100–104, 1981.
34. Businco L, Borsetto-Menghi AM, Lucarelli S, et al: Intradermal skin tests with Dermatophagoides pteronyssinus in asthmatic children: Correlation with specific IgE and bronchial provocation tests. Clin Allergy 9(5):459–463, 1979.
35. Stafanger G, Andersen JK, Koch C, et al: Specific diagnosis of exogenous bronchial asthma in children. Allergy 41(2):110–117, 1986.
36. Vanto T, Koivikko A: Dog hypersensitivity in asthmatic children. Acta Paediatr Scand 72(4):571–575, 1983.
37. Valovirta E, Viander M, Koivikko A, et al: Immunotherapy in allergy to dog. Immunologic and clinical findings of a double-blind study. Ann Allergy 57(3):173–179, 1986.
38. Broberger U, Graff-Lonnevig V, Lilja G, Rylander E: Ketotifen in pollen-induced asthma: A double blind placebo-controlled study. Clin Allergy 16(2):119–127, 1986.
39. Ryo UY, Kang B, Townley RG: Cromolyn therapy in patients with bronchial asthma. Effect on inhalation challenge with allergen, histamine, and methacholine. JAMA 236(8):927–931, 1976.

17 EVALUATION OF CHRONIC OR RECURRENT COUGH

PHILIP BLACK, M.D.

Cough may be voluntary or involuntary, infrequent and hardly noticeable, or painful, disruptive, and debilitating. Various aspects of cough, as well as the observers' beliefs, contribute to decisions to seek evaluation and treatment.

Cough serves at least two fundamental purposes: (1) the protection of the tracheobronchial tree from penetration by potentially injurious substances and (2) the removal of endogenous secretions and other materials, such as blood, pus, or necrotic tissue. Cough may be viewed as a continuum of health through disease and is a useful host defense mechanism.

Chronicity and recurrence are associated aspects of coughs that impress patients, parents, or other close observers as something abnormal. Chronic cough is present continuously for some period of time, at least 3 weeks and often 6 weeks or longer. Recurrent cough occurs, resolves for variable periods, and recurs in a repeating pattern.

Cough may be the initial or only sign of disease, such as a mediastinal tumor compressing the airway. A cough may be a component of reactive airway disease, such as asthma. In this and other contexts, cough may be somewhat maladaptive, either by failing to achieve its expected physiologic role or by imparting morbidity that outweighs the benefit.

There is limited information on the prevalence of chronic cough in children. The challenges of definition and variations in thresholds of awareness contribute to this gap. One survey reported a 7% to 10% prevalence of chronic cough in 7- to 15-year old urban children; a declining prevalence was seen in preadolescents.[1] These data were derived from questionnaires. Surveys of adults have found similar values but with a very wide range of and poor agreement between symptom reporting and more objective assessments.

Cough is an extremely common presenting complaint in pediatric medicine, commonly caused by irritation or inflammation of the respiratory tract. Most often, cough is a component of an upper respiratory infection (URI), which is usually self-limited. Preschool children have an average of seven or eight URIs per year. This number increases with the intensity of direct or indirect contact with the viral pool of their community. Direct contact may be through group day care,[2] play groups, and church nurseries or through shopping facilities or social gatherings. Indirect contact may be through siblings in school or other groups or through adult household members with a high degree of public contact. Even under very similar conditions, there is a wide range of frequency of infection in otherwise healthy, immunologically competent children.

PHYSIOLOGY

Cough physiology is important in the evaluation of chronic or recurrent cough for several reasons. First and most fundamental, knowledge of the anatomy and function of cough receptors forms a logical basis for the evaluation of cough. Second, some degree of cough ineffectiveness may be the underlying cause of chronicity; a working knowledge of cough physiology is fundamental to this concept. Finally, specific or nonspecific therapy has a basis of action at various points in the reflex pathway. The potential benefits and needed modifications of therapy may be anticipated in working within a physiologic framework.

Cough physiology is an integration of neurophysiology, respiratory and upper airway muscle function, lung mechanics, and fluid dynamics.[3,4] Any cough must begin with an input stimulus, either voluntary or arising from a "cough receptor." The stimulus is then carried over afferent nerves to the incompletely defined "cough center," which is probably in the pons. Complex efferent signals are then sent to various effectors, including inspiratory muscles, the larynx, and expiratory muscles. These effectors must then control lung volume, pleural pressure, and expiratory flow, all of which culminate in a single cough. To be effective, this process must somehow eliminate or lessen the original stimulus, expectorating the offending foreign material or accumulated mucus, expelling the irritant gas, or successfully preventing aspiration. Aspects of regional expiratory flow, velocity, turbulence, and anatomy interact with fluid mechanics to achieve or limit cough effectiveness.

COUGH RECEPTORS

Cough receptors are irritant nerve fibers located throughout the upper and lower airways as well as in the paranasal sinuses, pericardium, pleura, diaphragm, and external ear. They respond to mechanical, thermal, and a variety of chemical stimuli.[5] Their highest concentration is in the larger airways, especially at the carina and other bifurcations. These receptors probably function in respiratory defense mechanisms other than cough, such as laryngospasm, mucus secretion, and bronchoconstriction.

The observation that bronchodilators could relieve cough not accompanied by wheeze led to the hypothesis that cough "reception" is mediated by local bronchoconstriction that stimulates stretch receptors in airway walls. Experimentally induced cough and bronchoconstriction can be separated,[6] both by specificity of triggering agents[7, 8] and by differing response to drugs.[9] However, local bronchoconstriction may be very difficult to measure.

COUGH MECHANICS

Although cough may occur as a sudden glottic closure and subsequent expulsive exhalation, it most commonly begins with inhalation of a variable amount of air, generally one and one-half to three times tidal volume (Fig. 17–1).[10] This is followed by a compressive phase, consisting of, first, glottic closure and then a coordinated contraction of the expiratory muscles, including the thoracic cage and abdominal and pelvic muscles. This phase lasts about 200 msec and is followed by the opening of the glottis, resulting in explosive exhalation. There may be a single interval of expiratory flow, or there may be repeated glottic closure with continued expiratory muscle contraction, creating successive coughs at progressively lower lung volumes. There may also be repeated inspirations with a large degree of voluntary control; a person often chooses to take a deeper inspiration if the initial cough is not perceived to have been effective.

Higher lung volume contributes to cough effectiveness in several ways. The length-tension relationship of expiratory muscles has the greatest advantage at higher lung volumes, providing the best opportunity for the development of high pleural pressure. The proportion of poorly ventilated lung units is decreased, potentially providing the benefits of cough to areas in most need of clearance. Finally, at higher lung volumes, elastic recoil is at a peak, maximizing the effort-independent component of expiratory flow and providing more support and higher caliber to conducting airways.

Glottic closure is a usual but not always essential part of cough. Effective cough is possible without glottic closure[11] or even with tracheostomy; however, because of force-velocity relationships, the attainment of high pleural pressure is facilitated by glottic closure.[12] High pleural pressure increases expiratory flow as well as airway compression, both of which contribute to the increase in the velocity of expired gas. Glottic closure also more closely aligns peak pleural pressure with high lung volume, further enhancing peak expiratory flow. Finally, glottic opening allows the rapid exhalation of a bolus of air displaced from the central airways, producing the "spike," or "flow transient" (Fig. 17–2), that is characteristic of cough. Only the most proximal airways are exposed to flow from this spike; therefore, its contribution to cough effectiveness may be limited to the larynx and the trachea. However, its presence is a sign of central airway compression, and this may be the more essential contribution. Finally, repeated glottic closure and opening causes repeated central airway compression and re-expansion, thought to shake loose the secretions in these airways. Clinical observation of patients with tracheostomies suggests that the absence of glottic closure impairs cough effectiveness.

In the expiratory phase of cough, only the flow transient and a portion of flow from the peripheral lung are affected by expiratory effort. The physiologic basis of effort independence is the counterbalancing effect of increased driving pressure and increased airway resistance, secondary to

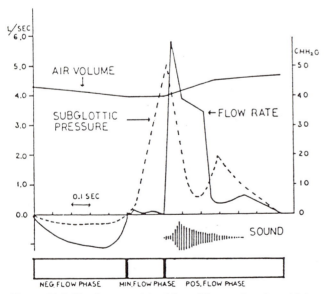

Figure 17–1. Simultaneous plots of flow at the mouth, spirometric lung volume change, subglottic pressure, and sound during a representative single cough. Negative flow is the inspiratory phase of cough, minimum flow is the compressive phase, and positive flow is the expiratory phase. (From Yanagihara N, von Leden H, Werner-Kukuk E: The physical parameters of cough: The larynx in a normal single cough. Acta Otolaryngol [Stockh] 61:495–510, 1966.)

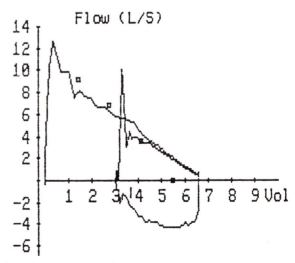

Figure 17–2. A flow transient produced by a cough superimposed on a maximal expiratory flow-volume loop; its presence demonstrates the ability to achieve the dynamic airway compression necessary for high linear velocity in coughing.

airway compression, that occurs with more expiratory effort. With expiratory flow preserved and airway cross-sectional area reduced, air velocity increases, raising shearing forces and kinetic energy.

During glottic closure, pleural and airway luminal pressures equalize, and airways achieve their sizes on the basis of the characteristics of the supporting anatomy and airway compliance. Once the glottis is opened, airway pressure falls to the greatest extent closest to the glottis (supraglottic pressure increases). Airway pressure rises peripherally. On the basis of expiratory effort (pleural pressure), local anatomy, and airway compliance, there is a point at which intraluminal and extraluminal pressures are equal (Fig. 17–3). This is the equal pressure point (EPP), or choke point.[13] Downstream, or mouthward, of this point, airways are compressed and velocity is increased. As lung volume decreases, this point moves peripherally, changing the selection of airways that experience high velocity. It is clear that some very changeable factors, such as bronchoconstriction, lung volume, accumulated secretions, strength, endurance, and even posture, may influence the distribution of airway compression and, consequently, cough effectiveness. Voluntary maneuvers, such as coughing through pursed lips or through a partially narrowed glottis, as in throat clearing, increase airway pressure and move the choke point downstream, possibling eliminating airway compression.

The level of the tracheobronchial tree at which cough is effective is not precisely known. Although it is generally believed that cough is most effective in the larger, more central airways, it does not follow that its contribution to clearance of smaller airways is unimportant. Theoretical considerations of fluid mechanics suggest that cough could augment mucociliary clearance down to at least the 12th airway generation in a normal adult.[14]

COUGH INEFFECTIVENESS

The cough reflex may be defective at any point, resulting in failure to adequately protect or cleanse the tracheobronchial tree.[15] Failure of cough receptors, afferent nerves, central processing of this input, or efferent nerves results in absence of appropriate cough and might manifest as lung disease, not cough. However, impairment of the musculoskeletal, airway, or mucociliary aspects of cough usually causes persistent, albeit ineffective, cough.

Inadequate inspiration predictably has negative influences on cough effectiveness, such as reducing flows and pressures, which result in incomplete or absent inflation of some lung units. Impaired inspiration may accompany many diseases, such as muscular dystrophy, cerebral palsy, scoliosis, and obesity; it may also be quasi-voluntary, limited by traumatic or postoperative pain or by the patient's attempts to suppress cough.

Similarly, weakness or thoracic deformity may limit expiratory effort. In one study, weakness induced by partial curarization of normal subjects produced a progressive loss of pleural pressure with little or no effect on expiratory flow. Diminution and loss of the flow transient closely followed the diminution of pleural pressure.[16] Similar findings have been reported in a number of muscle diseases.[17] In this study, all patients who were independently judged to have a weak, ineffective cough were also unable to produce a flow transient, although subjective assessment was able to identify only 75% of those without flow transients. Maximal expiratory pressure less than 60 cm H_2O was found to be an excellent indicator of absent flow transient.

Primary lung disease, however, is undoubtedly the most common cause of ineffective cough. This disease may result from abnormalities of airway structure and function; from characteristics of mucus production, rheology, and clearance; or from a combination of these factors.

Diseases with associated hyperinflation (measured functionally, not radiographically) cause a relative limitation of inspiration. Inspiratory capacity decreases as functional residual capacity approaches total lung capacity, thereby reducing the usable reserve that could be recruited when an increase in flow is needed. However, in spite of limited inspiratory capacity, the geometry of the expiratory muscles is still optimized, in contrast to the disadvantages of reduced inspiratory capacity resulting from

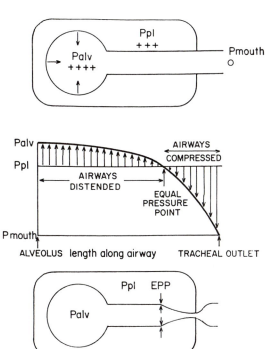

Figure 17–3. Upper panel: Model of lungs during cough. Pleural pressure (Ppl) is greater than atmospheric. Pressure in the alveoli (Palv) is greater than Ppl because of the elastic recoil of the lungs *(arrows)*. Mouth pressure is atmospheric. Because Ppl is approximately the pressure acting on the outer wall of the airways, the pressure in the airways at the alveolar end is greater than the pressure outside them. The opposite is true at the mouth end. Thus, there must be points along the airway where intraluminal pressures equal pleural pressure (equal pressure points [EPPs]). Compression of the airways occurs between EPP and the thoracic outlet (lower panel). The pressure interrelationships are shown diagrammatically in the middle panel, which plots a hypothetical pressure drop from the alveolus (Palv) to the tracheal outlet within the airways (curved line). The pressure outside the airways (Ppl) is given by the horizontal line. EPPs are shown where the two lines intersect. Between EPP and alveoli, the airways are distended *(upward-directed arrows)*. Between EPP and the tracheal outlet, airways are compressed *(downward-directed arrows)*. (From Macklem PT: Physiology of cough. Ann Otol 83:761–768, 1974.)

other causes. In addition, airway obstruction is the usual cause of hyperinflation. If the obstruction is caused by relatively widespread airway narrowing, an increase in velocity relative to flow is achieved, possibly offsetting some of the disadvantages of decreased flow. However, the inability to reach lower lung volumes may have additional disadvantages.[13]

Airways with minimal or no airflow, such as bronchiectatic sacs or occluded airways surrounded by atelectasis, may empty best by being squeezed at low lung volumes. The EPP must therefore shift to a point peripheral to the opening of such an airway in order for its contents to be emptied into the conducting airway.

Focal intrathoracic airway obstruction, either fixed or dynamic, may impair cough effectiveness in two ways. First, the obstructed airway may simply be too small to permit adequate flow of mucus, especially tenacious mucus, thereby increasing the degree of obstruction. Second, the progression of the EPP toward the smaller airways depends, in part, on lung emptying and decreasing elastic recoil. Therefore, a focal expiratory obstruction may keep the EPP stuck at the point of the obstruction. Such proximal lesions as tracheal stenosis, tracheomalacia, bronchomalacia, extrinsic compression, or foreign bodies may conceivably impair the airway-cleansing effectiveness of cough at points quite distant from the lesions, allowing accumulation of secretions and enhancing susceptibility to infection.

The characteristics of airway mucus and the mucociliary apparatus may also influence cough effectiveness or at least the effectiveness of mucus removal. In this capacity, cough is of greatest value under conditions of excess mucus accumulation, whether from increased production or from inadequate mucociliary function. In simulated cough, clearance of mucus is directly related to the depth of the mucus layer and inversely related to the viscosity and elasticity of mucus.[14, 18] The fluid dynamics of the airways include a liquid layer, called the periciliary fluid or serous layer, that underlies the mucus layer. The characteristics of this fluid may influence both the movement of the mucus layer and the function of the cilia. Other abnormalities affecting ciliary function, such as the ciliary dyskinesia syndrome or postinflammatory squamous metaplasia, may less directly limit cough effectiveness by failing to deliver mucus to the central airways. Finally, mucociliary transport may be slowed for hours after a moderate amount of coughing.[19, 20]

AGE-RELATED CHANGES IN PHYSIOLOGY

The development of cough is incompletely understood[21] both in health and in disease. In response to direct laryngoscopy without sedation, only half of term infants and a quarter of premature infants coughed.[22] This suggests that the absence of cough is not inherently dangerous. Likewise, the presence of cough does not indicate its effectiveness. There are major changes in respiratory mechanics from fetal life through adulthood.[23, 24] Some characteristics of the infant may be critical for the transition from intrauterine to extrauterine life but may

Table 17–1. INFANT DISADVANTAGES

High thoracic compliance
Respiratory muscle fatigability
Low elastic recoil of lung
High airway compliance
Poor collateral ventilation
High mucus gland density
Frequent regurgitation

become disadvantageous when challenged by respiratory disease (Table 17–1). The high compliance of the newborn thorax is evident with the dramatic sternal retraction that often accompanies the first breath. This compliance is believed to be useful in allowing the infant's passage through the birth canal and in partially emptying the lungs of amniotic fluid before the first breath of air. However, it subsequently limits inspiratory mechanics, both by consuming a portion of volume displacement accomplished by the diaphragm and by failing to provide rigid levers for the action of accessory muscles of inspiration.

The respiratory muscles of the newborn are of relatively low bulk and exhibit a fiber-type distribution that is sensitive to fatigue. Fatigue is probably not important in most episodic coughs but may occur as part of a respiratory illness, thus secondarily affecting cough performance and increasing the impact of the illness. Elastic recoil is also low in newborns and increases throughout childhood and adolescence. This allows airway closure at a higher relative lung volume. Airway compliance, as well, is higher in younger infants and children, at least partially because of incomplete development of cartilaginous support but probably also because of contributions of smooth muscle tone and the interaction of airway configuration with extrinsic supporting structures.[25, 26] This degree of compliance may result in a relative airway malacia, with influences on the positioning of the EPP as discussed previously here. Collateral ventilation is absent or very poorly developed in infancy and early childhood. During times of health, it is probably irrelevant. However, during times of increased airway secretions, this absence increases the likelihood of atelectasis in obstructed regions. The absence of air distal to airway obstruction severely impairs the ability of cough to clear that airway. Finally, there is in relation to healthy adults an increase in the density of mucus glands in younger children,[23, 27] which is comparable with the density in an adult with chronic bronchitis. This increase probably leads to more mucus production in response to infection, aspiration, or environmental irritants.

The mouth, the oropharynx, and the hypopharynx serve a dual function for passage of air and of fluids and solid matter, including endogenous secretions. The nasopharynx may also become involved in both roles, primarily as a reservoir of fluid after regurgitation of gastric contents or oropharyngeal reflux during feeding. As such, pharyngeal and esophageal function are critical adjuncts of cough in the role of airway protection.[27-29] Preterm infants swallow six times per minute, in comparison with six times per hour for adults. Regurgitation is very common in normal infants and very rare in normal adults. It is also common for infants to choke at the onset of feeding, but this is very rare beyond infancy. Infants and children with productive coughs are frequently observed to swallow, presumably respiratory secretions, after coughing. Thus it appears that insufficiency of the swallowing mechanism could pose a threat to airway protection that may be only partially accommodated by coughing. A portion of successful airway protection by coughing may be negated if the material removed from the airway remains in the pharynx to be aspirated.

CAUSES OF CHRONIC OR RECURRENT COUGH

The causes of chronic cough in children are innumerable. There are, however, a fairly manageable number of entities that underlie most chronic coughs. Many coughs may have overlapping causes, such as infection and reactive airway disease or cystic fibrosis and bronchial hyperreactivity.

ASPIRATION SYNDROMES

As discussed previously, pharyngeal and esophageal function are important components of airway protection. This is true for all ages but probably more often poses a challenge to the infant. Not only is the infant physiologically immature, but a large proportion of the day is spent sucking and swallowing, often supine and frequently in transition between wakefulness and sleep. Feeding may also be physically demanding, enhancing the risk of fatigue aspiration.[30]

Recurrent aspiration may accompany neurologic or neuromuscular disease, in which esophageal dysfunction may be a cardinal symptom. Laryngeal disorders, such as a laryngeal cleft or vocal cord paralysis, are also risk factors for aspiration. Adenoidal and tonsillar hypertrophy have been shown to greatly increase aspiration of contrast material from the hypopharynx during sleep.[31] This may occur because of impaired swallowing secondary to the mass effect of enlarged tonsils and also because of higher inspiratory gas velocity combined with upper airway narrowing, the corollary of an "inspiratory cough."

GASTROESOPHAGEAL REFLUX

A certain amount of gastroesophageal reflux (GER) is normal in all humans but is more common in infants. GER may contribute to cough in two ways. First, it may simply present gastric contents to the hypopharynx, thereby increasing the likelihood of aspiration and necessitating cough for its prevention. Second, there is probably a reflex pathway by which lower esophageal receptors cause cough or bronchoconstriction. This pathway may be augmented in the presence of esophagitis, but reflux may also increase with esophagitis.

The relationship of GER to respiratory disease is complex.[32, 33] A great deal of GER may be present without respiratory symptoms. Conversely, prominent respiratory symptoms may markedly improve after therapy for min-

imal reflux. In addition, respiratory disease may increase reflux. GER should be considered in children with chronic cough, especially if there is inadequately explained lung disease[34] (see Chapter 57).

ASTHMA

Cough-variant asthma has become well known in children[35] and adults.[36, 37] Modern asthma management includes close attention to cough as a prelude to bronchoconstriction. Patients with chronic cough may have mild to moderate obstructive lung disease evident on routine spirometry and often show improvement after inhaling a bronchodilator. Pulmonary function testing may demonstrate a normal base line, but obstructive disease may be apparent with provocation testing, such as exercise,[35, 38] methacholine inhalation,[39, 40] or histamine inhalation.[35, 38]

Airway hyperreactivity may be a component of other major diseases, notably cystic fibrosis or bronchopulmonary dysplasia. Other types of lung injury, such as hydrocarbon aspiration, near-drowning, and inhalation of noxious gases may predispose the patient to the development of clinical "asthma." In experimental animals, repeated aspiration of very small quanities of milk caused an increase in airway hyperresponsiveness.[41] Cough may not be a simple precursor to wheezing. As discussed in the section on cough receptors, cough and wheeze are probably distinct but interdependent phenomena[42] that possibly require different therapies.[43]

CHRONIC BRONCHITIS

Chronic bronchitis is an imprecise term. In a survey of physicians' use of this term, Taussig and colleagues[44] demonstrated differences between pediatricians and family physicians; the latter group's definition came closer to the definition used for adults: productive cough for more than 3 months of the year. However, operational descriptions were almost indistinguishable from those of asthma.

POSTNASAL DRIP

Drainage of nasal secretions into the oropharynx, the nasopharynx, and possibly the larynx is assumed to be the cause of cough that may improve with the use of antihistamines and decongestants. This is reported to be very common cause of chronic cough in adults[45–47] and is usually diagnosed by history taking and by physical examination. However, there is a reluctance to accept this explanation for children.[30] In both adults and children, the mechanism is more assumed than delineated. As with other entities, it is probably better for postnasal drip to be a diagnosis of relative exclusion.

SINUSITIS

Sinus disease is common in children with respiratory tract allergy[48] and is closely associated with nasal symptoms.[49] Sinusitis is an aggravating factor in asthma, such that asthma medication can often be reduced after treatment of sinusitis.[50] Mechanisms by which sinusitis may cause cough are not completely understood, but the presence of sinusitis should be considered in the evaluation of cough.

FOREIGN BODY ASPIRATION

Although more often considered a cause of sudden respiratory distress and wheezing, foreign body aspiration may also cause chronic cough that is remote in time from the aspiration episode. The local cough reflex from a foreign body wedged in the airway may be extinguished in a few hours. Cough can then re-emerge after a variable latent interval. Renewed symptoms are probably a result of atelectasis and overflow bronchorrhea. In one large series on inhaled foreign bodies, there was a close correlation between presentation with cough and the presence of atelectasis on the chest radiograph.[51] It must be kept in mind that a negative history of foreign body aspiration is common, especially in preschool children.[52] An esophageal foreign body can also cause cough, either by tracheal compression or by interfering with swallowing, resulting in aspiration.

CYSTIC FIBROSIS

A high prevalence of bronchial hyperreactivity can be demonstrated by nonspecific challenge[53, 54] or bronchodilator response.[55] Although there are distinct group differences between cystic fibrosis and asthma in terms of airway sensitivity to irritants or drugs, there is considerable overlap[56] and intrapatient variability.[57] There is a subset of patients who have both asthma and cystic fibrosis.[54, 57] Quantitative analysis of sweat chloride is necessary for ruling out cystic fibrosis.

TUBERCULOSIS

Tuberculosis must be considered in the differential diagnosis of chronic or recurrent cough in children. Complacency toward its detection may lead to resurgence, as occurred for pertussis and measles. Many infected children are asymptomatic, free of cough and other constitutional signs. However, cough may be the presenting sign or symptom. Endobronchial tuberculosis may be associated with a productive cough, whereas airway compression from enlarged peribronchial or mediastinal nodes can cause a dry cough. Mantoux's purified protein derivative (PPD) intradermal skin test is recommended whenever definitive diagnosis of tuberculosis infection is sought. The PPD tuberculin skin test may be falsely negative, especially early in the infection, with malnutrition or with overwhelming disease. Repeated tests 6 to 12 weeks later may be necessary for ruling out the diagnosis.[58]

DRUGS

Many drugs, including illegal drugs, can cause cough. The mechanism may be potentiation of underlying asthma, hypersensitivity reactions, or direct pulmonary toxicity. Beta blockers,[59] used for therapy of hypertension and some types of headache disorders, are well-known potentiators of asthma. Angiotensin-converting enzyme inhibitors may cause cough, probably by a similar mechanism.[60] Antineoplastic drugs can cause specific pulmonary toxicity,[61] including a nonproductive cough. This response can be fairly remote in time from their administration. Nitrofurantoin carries a moderate risk of acute or subacute pulmonary toxicity.[61] An extensive list of drugs can cause pulmonary infiltrates with eosinophilia (PIE), although a chest radiograph and a complete blood count may quickly shift the workup from cough to PIE.

INFECTION

Uncomplicated infection is rarely a cause of prolonged cough beyond early infancy, when chlamydial infection and pertussis are strong considerations. *Pneumocystis carinii* can cause cough in immunocompromised hosts, including poorly nourished infants, and may be the initial manifestation of acquired immunodeficiency syndrome. If immunization is incomplete, pertussis may cause cough lasting 4 to 6 weeks as a component of the primary infection at any age. As previously discussed, chronic infection is an important aspect of other disorders causing chronic cough, such as sinusitis, cystic fibrosis, other disorders with bronchiectasis, foreign body aspiration, or bronchogenic cyst.

POSTINFECTIOUS COUGH

This is a loosely defined concept that is usually applied to cough that begins with an acute respiratory infection but persists for weeks or even months beyond resolution of other aspects of the original illness. Cough is often a manifestation of asthma or transient increased bronchial hyperreactivity. Bronchial provocation testing is of questionable validity if performed within 2 months of a respiratory infection. However, most presentations of postinfectious cough are improving at the time of evaluation, although the rate of improvement is unacceptably slow. Bronchodilator therapy may be helpful if the underlying diagnosis of asthma is related to bronchial hyperreactivity.

IMMUNODEFICIENCY

Frequent, poorly resolving, or chronic respiratory infection can be caused by immunodeficiency. Cough can be a component of this disorder, but other signs of infection are usually present. Partial response to bronchodilators may be seen, but this does not mean that bronchial hyperreactivity or asthma is the primary disease.[62]

BRONCHIECTASIS

Cylindrical or saccular dilation of airways impairs mechanical clearance by cough and is usually associated with chronic or recurrent infection. Local mucus hypersecretion may participate in a vicious cycle with infection. Bronchiectasis is usually acquired, and chronic aspiration (with or without GER), pertussis, measles, and foreign body aspiration are important predisposing factors. Cystic fibrosis is a disease that includes bronchiectasis but should be considered in the evaluation of chronic cough. Bronchiectasis is a hallmark of advanced allergic bronchopulmonary aspergillosis. Anatomic lesions, such as tracheomalacia, bronchomalacia, granulomas, or extrinsic compression can impair local cough and mucociliary clearance, predisposing the patient to local infection and bronchiectasis. The diagnosis of bronchiectasis can be difficult and expensive. A tentative diagnosis may lead to very useful therapy while underlying causes are considered.

PSYCHOGENIC COUGH

The literature on psychogenic cough consists almost exclusively of case series and case reports with accompanying observation and opinion. The cough has several distinguishing characteristics. It is almost uniformly a very loud bark or honk, distinctly louder than most coughs observed in children with respiratory diseases. The coughs are usually single, as opposed to cough paroxysms, and absent during sleep. In the only pediatric series of appreciable size,[63] 29 of 33 subjects with psychogenic cough were 7 to 12 years old. It is often implied that the cough is essentially fake and that personal or family psychopathologic processes are present. These contentions are unsupported in children, although they may be valid for adults.[64] Limited long-term follow-up suggests that the symptom is not usually replaced by another after successful intervention and that the emergence of psychological disturbance is unusual. Management centers on powerful suggestion, convincing the subject that the cause of the cough is known and definitive cure is being administered. Results are more magical than medical, and the children often express gratitude.

CARDIOVASCULAR DISEASE

Cough can be a manifestion of congestive heart failure with pulmonary edema. This is probably most common in infants. Compensated chronic failure without pulmonary edema can also cause cough by way of left atrial enlargement compressing the left main stem bronchus. Whether this can cause bronchomalacia in infants is unclear but is primarily a semantic point (high airway compliance allows collapse with much less mechanical stress). Vascular malformations, such as a vascular ring or a pulmonary artery sling, can also cause airway compression and cough, although stridor or wheezing is more common.

CONGENITAL MALFORMATIONS

Congenital malformations, including H-type tracheoesophageal fistula, laryngeal cleft, cleft palate, or vocal cord paralysis, can permit aspiration and thereby cause cough, although other signs may predominate. Bronchogenic cysts, cystic adenomatoid malformation, or sequestered lobe can be associated with drainage of secretions, with or without infection, and cause cough. Cysts may cause cough by compressing the airways. Congenital lobar emphysema causes significant lung distortion, including compressive atelectasis of normal lung tissue, and can manifest with coughing.

MEDIASTINAL MASS

Malignant tumors, hamartomas, or mediastinal lymphadenopathy can cause cough by way of (1) airway compression without significant effects on ventilation or clearance or (2) airway obstruction with impaired clearance of distal airways, resulting in bronchorrhea with or without infection. There may be associated stridor.

PRIMARY CILIARY DYSKINESIA

Cough, otitis, sinusitis, and recurrent lower respiratory infections are the clinical hallmarks of primary ciliary dyskinesia,[65, 66] also known as immotile cilia syndrome. Approximately half of patients have situs inversus. Presentation is often in infancy or early childhood and may overlap with other diseases discussed here (see Chapter 60).

INEFFECTIVE COUGH

As pointed out previously, muscle weakness, tracheostomy, vocal cord paralysis, thoracic deformity, or tenacious secretions can all limit the effectiveness of cough and underlie its chronicity or recurrence, in such a way that the pathologic process is the act of coughing rather than the trigger. The physiologic disadvantages of newborns and older infants can enable persistence of cough in a similar manner, especially with any degree of debilitation.[67, 68] Diaphragm paralysis can occur without other muscle involvement and impairs the inspiratory limb of coughing.

TOBACCO SMOKE AND OTHER NONALLERGIC ENVIRONMENTAL IRRITANTS

Smoking is the major cause of chronic cough in adults[69] and causes a high prevalence of cough and phlegm production in secondary school students.[70] A smoking habit is often well established by the midteen years.[70, 71] Exposure to parental smoking has similar but less dramatic effects.[72] In addition, environmental tobacco smoke exposure reduces the incremental increase of forced expiratory volume in 1 sec[73] and can increase nonspecific bronchial reactivity[74] in children, which suggests a pivotal role in the development of asthma in some children.[75] Passive smoking is a well-established aggravating factor in chronic asthma,[76] which may be undiagnosed when the child is first evaluated for cough. A wood-burning stove is often another source of indoor air pollution that causes cough.[77] Outdoor air pollution, even at levels below current standards,[78] has been associated with increased cough in children.

ALPHA₁-ANTITRYPSIN DEFICIENCY

Alpha$_1$-antitrypsin deficiency[79, 80] is a genetic disorder; the onset of lung disease usually occurs in the third to fifth decades of life. There are a very few reported cases of lung disease in children. These children present with dyspnea and minimal or no cough.

MISCELLANEOUS

The ontogeny of the respiratory system scatters cough receptors to unusual places. Anecdotes of unusual causes of cough abound, including hair in the external ear,[81] a lima bean in the nose, and fiber wrapped around the uvula.

EVALUATION OF PATIENTS

Depending on age, severity, associated symptoms, and prior knowledge of a patient's general health, the evaluation of cough may range from a telephone consultation to open-lung biopsy. An exhaustive, hospital-based workup or more limited consideration of the likely possibilities may be indicated, followed by a therapeutic trial or period of observation. Limited evaluation should always include appropriate consideration and elimination of serious possibilities even when they are unlikely (e.g., tuberculosis or cystic fibrosis).

As is true with other organ systems, mild, subtle symptoms may signal serious respiratory disease in the neonate or young infant. Uncomplicated cough is not necessarily rare in this age group (younger than 6 months),[82–84] but life-threatening disorders such as congenital heart disease with congestive heart failure, aspiration syndromes, or lower respiratory tract infection should be seriously considered. Infections, which at a later age may pass with uncomplicated upper respiratory tract symptoms, may be accompanied by apnea or aspiration in very young infants. Conversely, frequent cough may be very common in school-age children and can be significantly increased by environmental tobacco smoke,[72] personal smoking habits,[70] or air pollution.[78] If the impact of a cough is mild and overall health is good, diagnostic restraint may be most appropriate.[85] Whenever specific workup is not pursued, this nonpursuit should be part of a diagnostic plan, including a threshold in time beyond which further evaluation will be reconsidered.

Evaluation of many of the specific causes of chronic or recurrent cough can be found in chapters devoted to these entities. Particular aspects of history, physical examination, and diagnostic studies that help to narrow the differential diagnosis are presented here.

HISTORY

AGE OF ONSET

Specific causes of cough may uniquely affect, or come to attention in, certain age ranges.[86, 87] Important considerations are listed in Table 17–2 and discussed next.

Congenital malformations, including most congenital heart diseases, are most often detected in infancy. Many malformations predispose patients to aspiration. As discussed previously, GER is common, although presenting features may vary widely. Certain infections are unique to this age (chlamydia, congenital viral infection, and *Pneumocystis*), whereas others are of greater impact later in life (pertussis, many viruses). Immunodeficiency may be seen, especially after maternal antibodies disappear. Passive smoking, especially by the primary caregiver, can have its greatest impact during infancy. Asthma is possible, although probably very uncommon before the age of 6 months and not as responsive to bronchodilators as it is later in childhood. Cystic fibrosis often manifests with cough in infancy. Tuberculosis can be congenital or acquired; miliary tuberculosis is a higher risk in infancy.

Atopic disorders may develop in toddlers and preschool children, and cough can result from asthma, rhinitis, or sinusitis. Asthma may also exist without a clearly atopic constitution. With increasing activity and decreasing observation, foreign body aspiration is more likely. Tonsillar and adenoidal hypertrophy develop during these years, possibly predisposing patients to aspiration or increased upper respiratory tract secretions. Cystic fibro-

Table 17–2. IMPORTANT CAUSES OF COUGH BY AGE GROUP

Infancy
  Aspiration/swallowing dysfunction
  Gastroesophageal reflux with or without aspiration
  Congenital malformations
  Cystic fibrosis
  Environmental tobacco smoke exposure
  Infection, especially chlamydia or pertussis
  Immunodeficiency
Toddlers and Preschoolers
  Asthma, usually with atopy
  Other atopic diseases: rhinitis, possibly sinusitis
  Cystic fibrosis
  Foreign body aspiration
  Community-acquired viral infections
Middle and Later Childhood
  Asthma
  Cystic fibrosis
  Infection, especially mycoplasma
  Psychogenic cough
  Smoking experimentation
Adolescence
  Asthma
  Cystic fibrosis
  Primary smoking

sis is diagnosed most frequently in infancy or early childhood. Tuberculosis is more likely to be confined to the lung when acquired after infancy. More contact with the outside world increases the frequency of URI, possibly exacerbating many underlying diseases.

In the early school years, at 5 to 12 years of age, the incidence of foreign body aspiration declines. Physical activity, especially sports, becomes more sustained and vigorous, possibly unmasking asthma or cystic fibrosis. Psychogenic cough is most prominent in the later part of this age range. Primary smoking may be tried or established.[71]

Adolescence is accompanied by an increased prevalence of primary smoking. Occupational exposure to irritants may begin. Psychogenic cough is probably uncommon. Asthma, cystic fibrosis, or tuberculosis may first become apparent in adolescence.

QUALITY AND TIMING

Whether a cough is productive (wet) or nonproductive (dry) is a major point in pursuing its cause. However, communication of these concepts may be difficult, especially when the history is taken from an observer, even a parent. Upper airway secretions may cause very wet sounds. A cough that a medically informed observer would consider productive may be reported as nonproductive if nothing is expectorated. These concepts are most useful if the patient can describe production of sputum. Chronic productive cough may be seen in asthma or suppurative lung disease and may often be more prominent after awakening. Sputum volume is generally minimal in asthma. A nonproductive cough may also be seen in asthma, often with a somewhat characteristic "tight" sound, and can be worse during the night or predawn hours. Paroxysms of cough may be present in many diseases but are suggestive of pertussis, chlamydial infection, or cystic fibrosis. Extremely loud coughs in the proper age group can, as mentioned earlier, be psychogenic.

MODERATING FACTORS

Activities or conditions that increase or decrease the frequency or severity of the cough are important. Exercise may aggravate many coughs, but prominent aggravation is suggestive of asthma or cystic fibrosis. The same is true for changes in the weather. Seasonal variation, especially during pollen seasons, is suggestive of asthma or rhinitis. Improvement while the patient is away from home brings household factors such as indoor allergens or smoke into question.

PREVIOUS THERAPY

It is uncommon to encounter a truly untreated cough. Some nonprescription medication may have been beneficial; whether this contained an antihistamine is helpful information. Often some form of bronchodilator has been tried with incomplete but suggestive success. Seven-

to 10-day antibiotic courses may be helpful in sinusitis, but the cough recurs shortly after discontinuation of the drugs.

MEDICAL HISTORY AND REVIEW OF SYSTEMS

Growth, development, appetite, activity level and habits, stool frequency and characteristics, and frequency and usual course of viral respiratory infections are essential points of history. A significant number of children with cystic fibrosis have normal growth, but they accomplish this by a very high food intake, or they do not have pancreatic insufficiency. Pneumonia can develop in children with asthma, aspiration, or cystic fibrosis. Cough that persists after resolution of more than one URI is suggestive of asthma, cystic fibrosis, foreign body aspiration, or bronchiectasis. Relative inactivity may be an adaptation to breathlessness with exertion. A history of recent travels is important in the evaluation of chronic cough.

FAMILY HISTORY

A family history of atopy is usually present in asthma, although this is not very specific. Tuberculosis in children is most often acquired through family contact. It is important to inquire about histories of cystic fibrosis in other family members.

HOUSEHOLD AND ENVIRONMENTAL FACTORS

The allergen and irritant loads of a household are important. Pets, potted plants, carpets, stuffed animals, and heating and cooling systems may be offending sources. Specific questioning should be directed toward exposure to passive smoking. Smokers in the household may not be mentioned if they do not smoke in the immediate presence of the child.

PHYSICAL EXAMINATION

Physical examination should include evaluation of height and weight on appropriate growth charts. Previous growth data increase the usefulness of this examination. Respiratory rate may vary widely with activity state and is potentially misleading most often in younger, awake children. Activity state should be noted with the recording. General nutrition and vigor should be noted. The fingers should be examined for clubbing. The nasal mucosa should be inspected and the gag reflex tested. An examination of the neck may reveal accessory respiratory muscle use; the scalenes cannot be seen, but their tensing with inspiration may be palpable. Tracheal deviation should be assessed. Retractions may be present at rest or may emerge with a voluntary deep and rapid inspiration. The shape of the thorax should be noted. Auscultation of the lungs should include all lung segments. Deep breathing and forced exhalation may bring out inspiratory crackles or wheezes and expiratory wheezes in patients without adventitious sounds at rest. Crying, exertion, or a thoracic squeeze may provide some of these findings in a patient unable to perform voluntarily. Inspiratory and expiratory timing should be noted, especially for forced expiratory prolongation. Every effort should be made to hear the cough in question, and any spontaneous coughing that occurs during this interview or the examination should be noted. Pressure over the trachea or a thoracic squeeze may induce a cough. Selected parts of the examination may be repeated after provocation by exercise or methacholine or after administration of an inhaled beta-agonist.

DIAGNOSTIC STUDIES

History and physical examination often yield a specific diagnosis. When they do not, additional studies may be considered. A chest radiograph is often the first test ordered. Although this does not usually provide a diagnosis, it gives a general view of lung health, especially for ruling out extensive lung injury, and reveals hidden processes such as lobar atelectasis or emphysema, cardiomegaly, or a radiopaque foreign body. Inspiratory and expiratory films or fluoroscopy may add information. Lateral neck or sinus radiographs may be ordered to investigate upper airway problems. A barium swallow and pH probe are used for investigating swallowing and GER as well as for delineating mediastinal anatomy.

For subjects able to participate, pulmonary function studies are among the most useful tests. Baseline studies showing obstructive lung disease may be checked for improvement after administration of an inhaled beta-agonist. Normal or mildly abnormal studies may be followed by bronchial provocation with exercise, an inhaled cholinergic drug or histamine, or cold, dry air challenge. Challenges with cholinergic drugs have been reported to be useful studies in adults[45] and children[39, 40] with chronic cough. Galvez and associates reported that a positive response to methacholine was a poor predictor of response to bronchodilator therapy.[40]

Sputum should always be grossly examined if available; vigorous efforts to obtain a sample may be immeasurably rewarded in some cases. In undiagnosed children with purulent sputum and in all children suspected of having asthma, quantitative sweat chloride should be measured after sweat is induced by pilocarpine iontophoresis. Many other studies may be considered for specific diagnoses.

MANAGEMENT

Cough does not always require therapy. Specific therapy, based on elucidation of the underlying disease, is often highly successful and almost uniformly recommended. Nonspecific therapy may be a useful adjunct to specific therapy, or it may be appropriate if used alone in selected circumstances. Cough suppressants are inherently dangerous both because of their direct pharmacologic effects and because of their influence on the perception and evaluation of the underlying illness. They should be used sparingly and only as a part of a therapeutic plan that includes reassessment at a defined point in time.

REFERENCES

1. Dockery DW, Gold DR, Rotnitsky A, et al: Effects of age, sex and race on prevalence of respiratory symptoms among children. Am Rev Respir Dis 139(4):A23, 1989.
2. Fleming DW, Cochi SL, Hightower AW, Broome CF: Childhood upper respiratory tract infections: To what degree is incidence affected by day-care attendance? Pediatrics 79:55–60, 1987.
3. Leith DE: Cough. In Brain JD, Proctor DF, Reid L (eds): Lung Biology in Health and Disease: Respiratory Disease Mechanisms, pp. 545–592. New York: Marcel Dekker, 1977.
4. Leith DE, Butler JP, Sneddon SL, Brain JD: Cough. In Macklem P, Mead J (eds): Handbook of Physiology. The Respiratory System, Section 3, vol. 3, pt. 1, pp. 315–336. New York: Oxford University Press, 1986.
5. Irwin RS, Rosen MJ, Braman SS: Cough: A comprehensive review. Arch Intern Med 137:1186–1191, 1977.
6. Pounsford J: Cough and bronchoconstriction. Bull Eur Physiopathol Respir 23(Suppl. 10):37s–40s, 1987.
7. Eschenbacher WL, Boushey HA, Sheppard D: Alteration in osmolarity of inhaled aerosols cause bronchoconstriction and cough, but absence of a permeant anion causes cough alone. Am Rev Respir Dis 129:211–215, 1984.
8. Mitsuhashi M, Mochizuki H, Tokuyama K, et al: Hyperresponsiveness of cough receptors in patients with bronchial asthma. Pediatrics 75:855–888, 1985.
9. Sheppard D, Rizk NW, Boushey HA, Bethel RA: Mechanism of cough and bronchoconstriction induced by distilled water aerosol. Am Rev Respir Dis 127:691–694, 1983.
10. Yanagihara N, von Leden H, Werner-Kukuk E: The physical parameters of cough: The larynx in a normal single cough. Acta Otolaryngol (Stockh) 61:495–510, 1966.
11. Young S, Abdul-Sattar N, Caric D: Glottic closure and high flows are not essential for productive cough. Bull Eur Physiopathol Respir 23(Suppl. 10): 11s–17s, 1987.
12. Gal TJ: Effects of endotracheal intubation on normal cough performance. Anesthesiology 52:324–329, 1980.
13. Macklem PT: Physiology of cough. Ann Otol 83:761–768, 1974.
14. Scherer PW, Burtz L: Fluid mechanical experiments relevant to coughing. J Biomech 11:183–187, 1978.
15. McCool FD, Leith DE: Pathophysiology of cough. Clin Chest Med 8:189–195, 1987.
16. Arora NS, Gal TJ: Cough dynamics during progressive expiratory muscle weakness in healthy curarized subjects. J Appl Physiol 51:494–498, 1981.
17. Szeinberg A, Tabachnik E, Rashed N, et al: Cough capacity in patients with muscular dystrophy. Chest 94:1232–1235, 1988.
18. King M, Brock G, Lundell C: Clearance of mucus by stimulated cough. J Appl Physiol 58:1776–1782, 1985.
19. Smaldone GC, Itoh H, Swift DL, Wagner HN Jr: Effect of flow-limiting segments and cough on particle deposition and mucociliary clearance in the lung. Am Rev Respir Dis 120:747–758, 1979.
20. Kamishima K, Yamamoto R, Shida A, et al: Effect of voluntary coughing on bronchial mucociliary clearance in smokers and the patients with chronic obstructive pulmonary disease. Am Rev Respir Dis 127(4, pt. 2):165, 1983.
21. Leith DE: The development of cough. Am Rev Respir Dis 131(Suppl.)S39–S42, 1985.
22. Miller HC, Proud GO, Behrle FC: Variations in the gag, cough, and swallow reflexes and tone of the vocal cords as determined by direct laryngoscopy in newborn infants. Yale J Biol Med 24:284–291, 1952.
23. Wohl MEB, Mead J: Age as a factor in respiratory disease. In Kendig EL, Chernick V (eds): Disorders of the Respiratory Tract in Children, 4th ed, pp. 135–141. Philadelphia: WB Saunders, 1983.
24. Bryan AC, Wohl MEB: Respiratory mechanics in children. In Macklem P, Mead J (eds): Handbook of Physiology: The Respira-

tory System, Section 3, vol. 3, pp. 179–191. New York: Oxford University Press, 1986.
25. Croteau JR, Cook CD: Volume-pressure and length-tension measurements in human tracheal and bronchial segments. J Appl Physiol 16:170–172, 1961.
26. Penn RB, Wolfson MR, Shaffer TH: Influence of smooth muscle tone and longitudinal tension on the collapsibility of immature airways. Pediatr Pulmonol 5:132–138, 1988.
27. Mellins RB: Pulmonary protective mechanisms. Am Rev Respir Dis 131(Suppl.):S62, 1985.
28. Thach BT, Menon A: Pulmonary protective mechanisms in human infants. Am Rev Respir Dis 131(Suppl.):S55–S58, 1985.
29. Mansell AL: Update: Signs and symptoms of pulmonary disease in children. Clin Chest Med 8:329–334, 1987.
30. Eigen H: The clinical evaluation of chronic cough. Pediatr Clin North Am 29:67–78, 1982.
31. Konno A, Hoshino T, Togawa K: Influence of upper airway obstruction by enlarged tonsils and adenoids upon recurrent infection of the lower airway in childhood. Laryngoscope 90:1708–1716, 1980.
32. Boyle JT, Tuchman DN, Altschuler SM, et al: Mechanisms for the association of gastroesophageal reflux and bronchospasm. Am Rev Respir Dis 131(Suppl.):S16–S20, 1985.
33. Orenstein SR, Orenstein DM: Gastroesophageal reflux and respiratory disease in children. J Pediatr 112:847–858, 1988.
34. Malfroot A, Vandenplas Y, Verlinden M, et al: Gastroesophageal reflux and unexplained chronic lung disease in infants and children. Pediatr Pulmonol 3:208–213, 1987.
35. Cloutier MM, Loughlin GM: Chronic cough in children: A manifestation of airway hyperreactivity. Pediatrics 67:6–12, 1981.
36. McFadden ER Jr: Exertional dyspnea and cough as preludes to acute attacks of bronchial asthma. N Engl J Med 292:555–559, 1975.
37. Carrao WM, Bramam SS, Irwin RS: Chronic cough as the sole presenting manifestation of bronchial asthma. N Engl J Med 300:633–637, 1979.
38. Konig P: Hidden asthma in childhood. Am J Dis Child 135:1053–1055, 1981.
39. de Benedictis FM, Canny GJ, Levison H: Methacholine inhalational challenge in the evaluation of chronic cough in children. Asthma 23(6):303–308, 1986.
40. Galvez RA, McLaughlin FJ, Levison H: The role of the methacholine challenge in children with chronic cough. J Allergy Clin Immunol 79:331–335, 1987.
41. Colombo JL, Hallberg TH: Airway hyperresponsiveness following repeated milk aspiration in rabbits. Am Rev Respir Dis 131(4):A249, 1985.
42. Anonymous: Cough and wheeze in asthma: Are they interdependent? Lancet 1:447–448, 1988.
43. Dolovich J, Ruhno J, O'Byrne P, Hargreave FE: Early/late response model: Implications for control of asthma and chronic cough in children. Pediatr Clin North Am 35:969–979, 1988.
44. Taussig LM, Smith SM, Blumenfeld R: Chronic bronchitis in childhood: What is it? Pediatrics 67:1–5, 1981.
45. Irwin RS, Corrao WM, Pratter MR: Chronic persistent cough in the adult: The spectrum and frequency of causes and successful outcome of specific therapy. Am Rev Respir Dis 123:413–417, 1981.
46. Irwin RS, Curley FJ, French CL: Chronic persistent cough: The spectrum of causes, key components of diagnostic evaluation, and outcome of specific therapy in 1987. Am Rev Respir Dis 137(4, pt. 2):330, 1988.
47. Poe RH, Harder RV, Israel RH, Kallay MC: Chronic persistent cough: Experience in diagnosis and outcome using an anatomic diagnostic protocol. Chest 95:723–728, 1989.
48. Rachelefsky GS, Goldberg M, Katz RM, et al: Sinus disease in children with respiratory allergy. J Allergy Clin Immunol 61:310–314, 1978.
49. Sacha RF, Tremblay NF, Jacobs RL: Chronic cough, sinusitis, and hyperreactive airways in children: An often overlooked association. Ann Allergy 54:195–198, 1985.
50. Rachelefsky GS, Katz RM, Siegel SC: Chronic sinus disease with associated reactive airway disease in children. Pediatrics 73:526–529, 1984.

51. Pyman C: Inhaled foreign bodies in childhood: A review of 230 cases. Med J Aust 1:62–68, 1971.
52. Davis CM: Inhaled foreign bodies in children: An analysis of 40 cases. Arch Dis Child 41:402–406, 1966.
53. Mellis CM, Levison H: Bronchial reactivity in cystic fibrosis. Pediatrics 61:446–450, 1978.
54. Van Asperen P, Mellis CM, South RT, Simpson SJ: Bronchial reactivity in cystic fibrosis with normal pulmonary function. Am J Dis Child 135:815–819, 1981.
55. Hordvik NL, Konig P, Morris D, et al: A longitudinal study of bronchodilator responsiveness in cystic fibrosis. Am Rev Respir Dis 131:889–893, 1985.
56. Mitchell I, Corey M, Woenne R, et al: Bronchial hyperreactivity in cystic fibrosis and asthma. J Pediatr 93:744–748, 1978.
57. Holzer FJ, Olinsky A, Phelan PD: Variability of airways hyperreactivity and allergy in cystic fibrosis. Arch Dis Child 56:455–459, 1981.
58. Starke JR: Modern approach to the diagnosis and treatment of tuberculosis in children. Pediatr Clin North Am 35:441–464, 1988.
59. Braman SS, Corrao WM: Cough: Differential diagnosis and treatment. Clin Chest Med 8:177–188, 1987.
60. Kaufman J, Casanova JE, Riendl P, Schlueter DP: Bronchial hyperreactivity and cough due to angiotensin-converting enzyme inhibitors. Chest 95:544–548, 1989.
61. Kercsmar CM, Boat TF: Lung diseases caused by chemotherapeutic agents. In Kendig EL, Chernick V (eds): Disorders of the Respiratory Tract in Children, 4th ed., pp. 916–922. Philadelphia: WB Saunders, 1983.
62. Sotomayor JL, Douglas SD, Wilmott RW: Pulmonary manifestations of immune deficiency diseases. Pediatr Pulmonol 6:275–292, 1989.
63. Cohlan SW, Stone SM: The cough and the bedsheet. Pediatrics 74:11–15, 1984.
64. Grumet GW: Psychogenic coughing: A review and case report. Compr Psychiatry 27:28–34, 1987.
65. Turner JAP, Corkey WB, Lee JYC, et al: Clinical expressions of immotile cilia syndrome. Pediatrics 67:805–810, 1981.
66. Rossman CM, Newhouse MT: Primary ciliary dyskinesia: Evaluation and management. Pediatr Pulmonol 5:36–50, 1988.
67. Williams HE: Chronic and recurrent cough. Aust Paediatr J 11:1–8, 1975.
68. Phelan PD, Landau LI, Olinsky A: Cough. In Respiratory Illness in Children, 2nd ed., pp. 204–220. St. Louis: CV Mosby, 1982.
69. Wynder EJ, Lemon FR, Mantel N: Epidemiology of persistent cough. Am Rev Respir Dis 91:679–700, 1965.
70. Adams L, Lonsdale D, Robinson M, et al: Respiratory impairment induced by smoking in children in secondary schools. Br Med J 288:891–895, 1984.
71. Baugh JG, Hunter SM, Webber lS, Berenson GS: Developmental trends of first cigarette smoking experience of children: The Bogalusa heart study. Am J Public Health 72:1161–1164, 1982.
72. Charlton A: Children's coughs related to parental smoking. Br Med J 288:1647–1649, 1984.
73. Tager IB, Weiss ST, Munoz A, et al: Longitudinal study of the effects of maternal smoking on pulmonary function in children. N Engl J Med 309:699–703, 1983.
74. Martinez FD, Antognoni G, Macri F, et al: Parental smoking enhances bronchial responsiveness in nine-year-old children. Am Rev Respir Dis 138:518–523, 1988.
75. Tager IB: Passive smoking—bronchial responsiveness and atopy. Am Rev Respir Dis 138:507–509, 1988.
76. Murray AB, Morrison BJ: Passive smoking and the seasonal difference of severity of asthma in children. Chest 94:701–708, 1988.
77. Honicky RE, Akpom CA, Osborne JS: Infant respiratory illness and indoor air pollution from a woodburning stove. Pediatrics 71:126–128, 1983.
78. Schwartz J, Dockery DW, Wypii D, et al: Acute effects of air pollution on respiratory symptom reporting in children. Am Rev Respir Dis 139(4, pt. 2):A27, 1989.
79. Talamo RC: Emphysema and alpha₁-antitrypsin deficiency. In Kendig EL, Chernick V (eds): Disorders of the Respiratory Tract in Children, 4th ed., pp. 475–483. Philadelphia: WB Saunders, 1983.
80. Idell S, Cohen AB: Alpha-1-antitrypsin deficiency. Clin Chest Med 4:359–375, 1983.

154

81. Wolff AP, May M, Nuelle D: The tympanic membrane: A source of the cough reflex. JAMA 223:1269, 1973.
82. Cloutier MM: The coughing child: Etiology and treatment of a common symptom. Postgrad Med 73(3):169–175, 1983.
83. Schneider AP II, Daws WR, Adams RD: The coughing child: A primary care perspective. Postgrad Med 74:253–260, 1983.
84. Cloutier MM: Commentary: Cough in children. Postgrad Med 73(4):260, 1983.
85. Cunningham AS: Beware of overtreating children! Am J Dis Child 143:786–788, 1989.
86. Cloutier MM: Finding the cause of chronic cough in children. J Respir Dis 1:20–28, 1980.
87. Mellis CM: Evaluation and treatment of chronic cough in children. Pediatr Clin North Am 26:553–564, 1979.

18 RECURRENT AND PERSISTENT PNEUMONIA

ELIZABETH CRAVEN, M.D. / BETTINA C. HILMAN, M.D.

Recurrent or persistent pneumonia is suggestive of deficiencies in local or systemic host defenses or of other underlying disorders that alter lung defenses. In the evaluation of a child with recurrent or persistent lower respiratory infections, a physician must determine whether the child has normal lung defenses and is just unfortunate or whether there is an underlying cause for the recurrent infections.[1] Underlying disorders can result from structural, functional, or environmental causes. When pneumonia recurs or persists in the same area, structural abnormalities of the respiratory tract or aspiration syndromes should be considered. Obstruction of the airways by abnormal respiratory secretions, foreign body, or extrinsic compression (e.g., enlarged lymph nodes, mediastinal tumors, cardiomegaly, vascular rings, or esophageal foreign bodies) can increase the risk of respiratory infections. Although many children have no underlying disorder, the assessment of each patient provides the physician a challenge in the timing and extent of the diagnostic evaluation. A careful history, physical examination, and review of chest radiographs enable the physician to decide which further diagnostic studies are indicated. This chapter focuses on the pathophysiologic processes, differential diagnosis, and evaluation of recurrent and persistent pneumonia in infants, children, and adolescents.

Because there is no universally accepted definition of either recurrent or persistent pneumonia, the true incidence of these clinical problems is not known. The term *persistent* implies chronicity; thus there arises the critical question of when a pneumonia should be considered chronic. Duration of symptoms or persistence of chest radiographic findings for three or more months is frequently used to define *chronic*. Other authors have arbitrarily defined chronic or persistent pneumonia as persistence of radiographic abnormalities beyond the expected time for resolution, a chronic cough that is present on most days for 3 months and is associated with a persistent abnormal chest radiograph, or both.

Fernald and associates,[2] in a 4-year review of 184 children (median age of 3.5 years) referred for evaluation with chronic or potentially chronic lung disease, found that 48% had recurrent pneumonia. Of this 48%, only 22% were found to have a specific underlying disorder, such as cystic fibrosis, bronchopulmonary dysplasia, immunodeficiency disorders, aspiration syndromes, or congenital anomalies. Eigen and colleagues[3] found an identifiable underlying cause in only 20 of 81 children with radiologic evidence of chest infiltrates that had recurred or had not resolved in the expected way.

It is often difficult to determine whether pneumonia is persistent or recurrent unless there has been a symptom-free interval during which chest radiographs have documented clearing of the pneumonic infiltrations. Bacterial pneumonias may appear to be recurrent infections if infection is persistent because therapy was inappropriate for the underlying pathogen or because the duration of appropriate therapy was inadequate as a result of noncompliance. Even when chest radiographs are available, there may be problems in distinguishing between persistent and recurrent pneumonia. Variability in the technical quality and positioning of chest radiographs may result in misinterpretation of resolution of the pulmonary pathologic process. Reappearance of radiologic densities in the same area on subsequent films may be attributed to recurrence, whereas the densities actually represent persistence of previous pulmonary lesions.

PATHOPHYSIOLOGY

The underlying disorders associated with recurrent or persistent pneumonia can be classified into several broad categories (Table 18–1): aspiration syndromes, congenital anomalies, abnormalities of clearance of airway secretions, other disorders associated with airway obstruction, and immunologic disorders (Table 18–2). In children with underlying immunologic disorders, the infections

Table 18-1. ETIOLOGIC FACTORS: RECURRENT/
PERSISTENT PNEUMONIA

Aspiration Syndromes
Respiratory Foreign Body
Airway Anomalies
Swallowing Dysfunction and Defects
Immaturity swallowing mechanism
Neurologic and neuromuscular disorders
Gastroesophageal Reflux
Poor Feeding Techniques and Practices

Congenital Anomalies
Airway Anomalies
Pierre Robin syndrome
Cleft palate
Laryngotracheal cleft
Tracheoesophageal fistulae
Bronchopulmonary
Bronchogenic cyst
Pulmonary
Pulmonary sequestration
Congenital adenomatoid malformation of lung
Pulmonary hypoplasia
Cardiovascular
Vascular rings
Congenital heart disease

Abnormalities of Clearance of Airway Secretions
Cystic Fibrosis
*Bronchopulmonary Dysplasia and Other NICU Survivors of
    Prolonged Mechanical Ventilation*
Defects in Ultrastructure of Cilia or Ciliary Dyskinesis
Immotile cilia syndromes
Physiologic Congenital Anomalies
Tracheomalacia
Bronchomalacia
Environmental
Pollutants/irritants
    (e.g., cigarette smoke, active or passive exposure)
Organic antigen exposure:
    hypersensitivity pneumonitis
Overcrowding/excessive exposure to infection
    (day care centers; nursery or play schools)
Other Altered Mucociliary Clearance
Sequelae to infections:
    Mycoplasma pneumoniae; viral infections (e.g., adenovirus)
Swallowing dysfunction defects
Repair of congenital anomalies
    (e.g., tracheoesophageal fistula; congenital diaphragmatic hernia)
Young's syndrome*

Other Disorders Associated with Airway Obstruction
Asthma
Acquired Airway Compression
Lymph nodes
Masses
Intraluminal secretions
Immunologic Disorders
Disorders of Systemic Immunity
Specific immune disorders (see Table 18-2)
Disorders/Diseases of Local Immunity

NICU, neonatal intensive care unit.
*Young's syndrome consists of male infertility, chronic sinopulmonary infections, normal electron microscopy of respiratory cilia, azoospermia caused by obstruction of epididymis by inspissated secretions, and normal sweat electrolytes.

Table 18-2. DISORDERS OF SYSTEMIC IMMUNITY

Specific Immune Disorders
Primary Immunodeficiency
Antibody-mediated immunodeficiency
    X-linked agammaglobulinemia
    Autosomal recessive agammaglobulinemia
    Immunodeficiency with hyper-IgM syndrome
    Common variable immunodeficiency
    IgG subclass deficiencies:
        Selective IgG_{2-4} deficiency
    Antibody deficiency with normal immunoglobulins:
        Poor response to polysaccharide antigens
    Selective IgA deficiency
Cellular immunodeficiency
    Congenital thymic aplasia (DiGeorge's syndrome)
    Chronic mucocutaneous candidiasis
    Cartilage-hair hypoplasia
    T lymphocyte deficiency with abnormal immunoglobulin synthesis
        (Nezelof's syndrome)
    Interleukin-2 deficiency
Combined immunodeficiency diseases
    Severe combined immunodeficiencies (SCID)
    Adenosine deaminase deficiency
Partial combined immunodeficiencies
    Wiskott-Aldrich syndrome
    Ataxia telangiectasia
Acquired Immunodeficiency
HIV infection
Neoplasms
Immunosuppressive agents
Malnutrition

Nonspecific Immune Disorders
Phagocyte Defects and Disorders
Neutropenia
    Cyclic
    Congenital
Motility defects
    Chemotactic defects
    "Lazy" leukocyte
    Hyper-IgE (Job's) syndrome
    Chediak-Higashi syndrome
    Shwachman's syndrome
Lethal defects
    Chronic granulomatous disease
    Myeloperoxidase deficiency
    Glucose-6-phosphate dehydrogenase deficiency
Generalized dysfunction
    Down's syndrome
Complement Disorders
Deficiencies of C3, C6, or C3b
Other Disorders of Respiratory Host Defenses
Hyposplenism
    Sickle cell disease
    Postsplenectomy

IgM, immunoglobulin M; IgG_{2-4}, immunoglobulins G_2 to G_4; IgA, immunoglobulin A; HIV, human immunodeficiency virus; IgE, immunoglobulin E.

this group of children, the rate of resolution of pulmonary infiltrates depends on the etiologic agent. Pulmonary infiltrates in bacterial infection with *Streptococcus pneumoniae* normally resolve in 6 to 7 weeks.[4] In contrast, resolution of radiologic findings in adenovirus pneumonia may take up to 12 months.[5] Many normal and otherwise healthy children may have from 6 to 10 respiratory infections per year, which are usually caused by viral agents.[6, 7] The number of respiratory infections is increased if there is exposure to other children in day-care settings[8-10] or to siblings in the home environment. When one or two bacterial respiratory infections also occur, there is concern

are more severe and more likely to be caused by unusual organisms. Children with no alteration of systemic immunity and no other causes of chronic illness are usually healthy between episodes of infection. However, even in

over possible immunodeficiency disorders or other underlying causes for the recurrent respiratory illnesses. Respiratory allergy can be confused with respiratory infections; a large percentage of children (up to 30% in some series) with recurrent pneumonia may have underlying respiratory allergic disease.[7]

Recurrent or persistent pneumonia can be caused by intrabronchial or extraluminal bronchial obstruction (Table 18–3). Conditions associated with abnormalities of respiratory mucus or alterations in the clearance of airway secretions, such as cystic fibrosis, bronchopulmonary dysplasia, tracheoesophageal fistula, and defects in the ultrastructure or function of cilia, may be the mechanism underlying recurrent pneumonia. Children recovering from viral or other infections such as *Mycoplasma pneumoniae* may exhibit altered mucociliary function for variable periods of time. Infants and children with disorders of swallowing, coughing, or other neuromuscular function may have problems in clearing the airways of secretions and thus impairment of respiratory host defenses. Congenital anomalies may be the underlying cause of recurrent or persistent pneumonia such as intralobar and extralobar sequestration (Figure 18–1), pulmonary hypoplasia associated with congenital diaphragmatic hernia, or congenital adenomatoid malformation of the lung. Obstruction of airways by secretions may be a result of extrinsic compression from lymph nodes, vascular rings, bronchogenic cysts, or cardiac chamber enlargement.

Other Alterations in Pulmonary Host Defenses. Ultrastructural abnormalities of cilia can result in ciliary dysfunction and contribute to recurrent respiratory infections. The syndrome of sinusitis, bronchiectasis, and situs inversus (Kartagener's syndrome) has been shown to include an associated congenital malformation of ciliary ultrastructure. There are a variety of genetically determined ultrastructural defects of the cilia: absence of outer, inner, or both dynein arms; radial spoke defects; and microtubular transposition. Electron microscopic examination of nasal scrapings and brushings or biopsy of nasal or airway mucosa can determine if ciliary ultrastructure is normal. In addition, there are instances of ciliary dyskinesis with normal ultrastructural organization but functional impairment associated with respiratory infections, such as sinobronchitis and bronchiectasis. Phase microscopy has been used to evaluate ciliary motility (see Chapter 60).

Recurrent or chronic aspiration alters pulmonary host defenses and may be associated with upper airway abnormalities, immature or abnormal swallowing function, gastroesophageal reflux, mental or motor retardation, cerebral palsy, seizures, and other neuromuscular disorders. Acute aspiration is usually recognized easily if extensive; however, chronic aspiration of small amounts of secretions or feedings may not be obvious and may be even more difficult to document. No available tests are both sensitive and specific for the diagnosis of chronic aspiration.[11] The presence of lipid-laden macrophages in respiratory secretions is highly suggestive of lipid aspiration into the respiratory tract[12] and is considered by some authors to be diagnostic evidence of aspiration pneumonia. Colombo and Hallberg[11] evaluated bronchial washings from 45 patients (mean age of 3.3 years) for lipid-laden macrophages and graded the amount of intracellular oil red O-positive material to derive a semiquantitative lipid-laden macrophage index. The studies by Colombo and Hallberg[11] suggested that simple identification of lipid-laden macrophage was nonspecific, but quantification of these cells was a fairly reliable test of food aspiration in children and more sensitive than radiographic studies to document aspiration.

Gastroesophageal reflux (GER) may also be difficult to document with the use of radiologic techniques. Demonstrating the relationship of GER to recurrent, persistent, or chronic pneumonia is even more difficult. GER can be documented by pH probe monitoring or modified Bernstein's test;[13] these studies, however, do not yield any information about aspiration into the lungs that may occur secondary to GER. Pulmonary aspiration often can be documented by barium esophagogram. Barium swallowing or cine-esophagogram is usually the first-line diagnostic test for determining whether aspiration occurs with swallowing or because of GER. Although the barium swallow procedure may be helpful in confirming the presence of a tracheoesophageal fistula, a laryngeal cleft, or a vascular ring, it is extremely insensitive in detecting chronic aspiration of small quantities of feedings, especially when it occurs intermittently. Another confounding factor in interpretation of the relationship of GER to recurrent, persistent, or chronic lower respiratory tract disease is the relationship of the role of GER without aspiration into the tracheobronchial tree; this may cause respiratory symptoms in some patients by means of reflex bronchospasm.

CLINICAL EVALUATION

HISTORY

One of the major objectives of the history is to identify evidence of any underlying cause. Both medical and environmental histories are essential components of the initial

Table 18–3. RECURRENT PNEUMONIA: TWO OUTCOMES OF BRONCHIAL OBSTRUCTION

Intraluminal	Extraluminal
Foreign body	Enlarged nodes
Tumor	Malignancy
Bronchiectasis	Sarcoidosis
Right middle lobe syndrome	Broncholithiasis
(RML atelectasis)	Fungus (e.g., *Histoplasma*)
Mucoid impaction	Tuberculosis
Bronchial stenosis	Cardiac disorders
Allergic bronchopulmonary	Vascular ring
aspergillosis	Congenital heart disease
	(enlarged cardiac chamber)
	Pulmonary sequestration
	Congenital lung cyst
	Repair of congenital anomalies
	Tracheoesophageal fistula
	Congenital diaphragmatic hernia
	Vascular ring

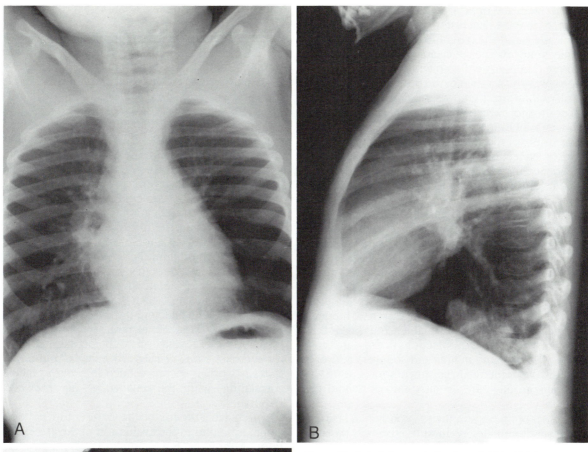

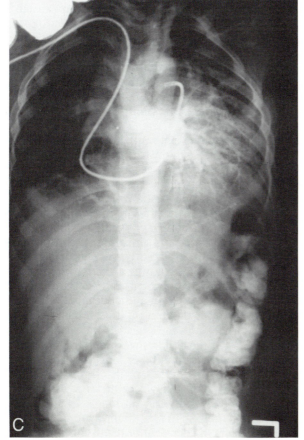

Figure 18–1. *A*, Anteroposterior view of child with lobar sequestration. *B*, Lateral view of child with lobar sequestration. *C*, Lobar sequestration demonstrated by pulmonary angiography.

evaluation for recurrent or persistent pneumonia. As with any comprehensive medical history, a detailed account of the family history and the perinatal events is important. For example, abnormalities in clearance of airway secretions are present in many children with a history of bronchopulmonary dysplasia or other exposure to prolonged mechanical ventilation. Inquiry should also be directed toward exposure to oxygen, maternal infections (virus, *Chlamydia,* human immunodeficiency virus [HIV]), and blood transfusions (especially those given from 1981 to 1985[7]). A detailed feeding history is important for detecting any evidence of swallowing dysfunction or defects, GER, or poor feeding techniques.

Environmental history should indicate the risk of exposure to respiratory tract infections, crowded conditions, exposure to pollutants and irritants, and potential respiratory inhalant allergies in a child with allergic diathesis or family history of allergy. Risk factors for sources of exposure to respiratory infections should be evaluated; these may include contact with school-age siblings, crowded conditions at home or in a baby sitter's house, day-care centers, church or synagogue nurseries, kindergarten, or school. Currently available data suggest a higher incidence of respiratory infections in day-care center attendees.[8-10] For many infants and younger children, the initial episode of the recurrent pneumonia coincides with placement in day care or entry into preschool or kindergarten.

Other significant findings in the environmental history include exposure to inhaled pollutants, especially passive tobacco smoke, which may depress normal respiratory defenses. The incidence and the severity of respiratory illnesses are increased with exposure to passive smoking.[14-20] The impact of passive smoking appears to be greatest in children under 1 year of age and is most closely related to maternal smoking.[21] A detailed history of smoke exposure helps assess the role of this risk factor in an individual patient. Among children chronically exposed to passive smoking, the degree of exposure varies widely, depending on the number of cigarettes smoked indoors, the proximity of exposure, and the amount of time that the child spends indoors (or riding in an automobile with closed windows) exposed to cigarette smoking, as well as to the adequacy of ventilation during exposure in closed areas. Numerous studies have shown a strong correlation between urinary cotinine (the major metabolite of nicotine that is specific for tobacco) and the level of exposure to environmental tobacco smoke in all age groups.[17-22]

A careful history of exposure to organic antigens is important for detecting hypersensitivity pneumonitis as a possible underlying cause of a recurrent pneumonia. In addition, exposure to fumes from wood-burning stoves or fireplaces or to other noxious fumes should be documented.

It is important to inquire about any family history of asthma, allergic disease, cystic fibrosis, congenital anomalies, or recurrent infections suggesting immunologic disorders. A history of maternal blood transfusion or a lifestyle suggestive of risk factors for acquired immunodeficiency syndrome (AIDS) should be carefully evaluated in order to rule out possible exposure to maternal HIV infection.[7]

The age of onset of the pneumonia is one of the key factors in the evaluation of underlying etiologic agents; the sooner after birth the symptoms and signs of respiratory disease occur, the greater is the possibility that there may be an associated congenital anomaly or hereditary disorder.

As detailed an account as possible of the first recognized episode of "pneumonia" should be obtained. Particular attention should be paid to the sequence of events leading to the diagnosis of the lower respiratory tract disease, such as the nature and duration of the cough, presence and duration of fever, documentation by a physician of rales or wheezing, chest radiographic findings (location of infiltrates, atelectasis), type and duration of antibiotic therapy (if any), response to antibiotics (if given), requirements for hospitalization, and the use of supplemental oxygen. Similar information about subsequent episodes of "pneumonia" should be obtained. A chronological account of the time sequence of each episode of lower respiratory tract disease and the symptom-free intervals, if any, in between episodes of respiratory disease should be reviewed. The acquisition of the actual medical records for documentation of rales, wheezing, or pulmonary infiltrates is strongly recommended in order to facilitate the correlation with the review of all previous chest radiographs.

A detailed account of the nature and pattern of the cough is helpful in the evaluation of the associated respiratory symptoms. For example, a brassy cough is suggestive of tracheal irritation, whereas a croupy cough implies involvement of the glottis or subglottis.[23] A paroxysmal cough may be associated with the presence of a foreign body in the respiratory tract. It is important to determine whether there is any relationship of the cough to feeding or swallowing, to positional changes, to time of day, or to exposure to irritating agents. If the cough is productive, the type and degree of productivity should be carefully described.

It is important to determine whether episodes of "pneumonia" are associated with wheezing and whether they occur at the same time each year. Evidence of seasonal cough or wheezing may suggest underlying allergic respiratory disease. Cough-variant asthma with wheezing can be triggered by viral respiratory infections. It is important to determine the pattern of events following or initiated by respiratory infections. In some patients, for instance, coughing may be initiated by exercise or laughter, or it may occur predominantly at night, which is suggestive of subclinical or cough-variant asthma. In the 81 children who, according to Eigen and colleagues,[3] showed radiographic evidence of chest infiltrates that had recurred or had not resolved in the expected way, 31% had a history of asthma. Of the children who had had abnormal chest radiographs for 3 months or longer, as reported by Fernald and associates,[2] 71% of the 143 children without a specific diagnosis had wheezing as a major symptom. Review of the history for other signs of allergic diathesis may also be helpful in identifying allergy as one of the etiologic factors in persistent or recurrent pneumonia.

PHYSICAL EXAMINATION

The goal of a complete physical examination with a focus on the respiratory system is the detection of any underlying etiologic factors and the documentation of any evidence of respiratory disease or dysfunction. In the evaluation of recurrent or persistent pneumonia, it is important to determine the location of the bronchopulmonary disease: that is, airways or lung parenchyma. Careful segmental auscultation of the chest helps localize involved bronchopulmonary segments. Quantitative recording of any abnormal auscultatory findings can help in the evaluation and management of persistent or recurrent pneumonia. The use of the double stethoscope can facilitate quantitative auscultation of the chest (Fig. 18–2).

An important part of the physical examination is inspection for clubbing of the fingers or toes, increased anteroposterior diameter of the chest, retractions, and the pattern of breathing, including use of any accessory muscles of respiration or flaring of the alae nasae. The presence of digital clubbing is important evidence of underlying bronchiectasis, although it has been reported in other pulmonary diseases, such as lung abscess, congenital heart disease, hepatic disease, certain intestinal disorders, and endocrine disorders (e.g., thyrotoxicosis).

Because of the association of malnutrition and poor host defenses against infection, it is important to assess the nutritional status of children with recurrent or persistent respiratory infections. Failure to thrive is a symptom or sign of many underlying conditions such as cystic fibrosis and some immunodeficiency syndromes, especially T cell defects.

Assessment of the patient for some of the characteristic physical signs of immunodeficiency syndromes includes such features as "fish mouth" with hypertelorism (DiGeorge's syndrome), associated periodontal disease (phagocytic dysfunction), telangiectasia of eyes or ears (ataxia telangiectasia), and sparse hair (adenosine deaminase deficiency). Each patient should be assessed for the presence of adenoidal or tonsillar tissue and age-appropriate lymphadenopathy.

Because of the association of atopic respiratory disease with recurrent or persistent respiratory symptoms, it is important to observe specifically for physical stigmata of the allergic diathesis such as the "allergic salute," transverse nasal crease, "allergic shiners," cobblestone appearance of posterior pharynx, and pale, boggy allergic turbinates. Many children referred with the diagnosis of recurrent "pneumonia" or chronic or recurrent "bronchitis" have asthma. Although not all asthma is atopic, the presence of other signs of the allergic diathesis may implicate allergic respiratory disease as one of the underlying factors contributing to asthma. This association may be helpful in younger children in whom hyperreactivity cannot be documented by pulmonary function studies.

RADIOGRAPHIC EVALUATION

Evaluation of chest radiographs (erect posteroanterior and lateral views) for the location and extent of infiltrates and the resolution over time is essential in the assessment of recurrent or persistent pneumonia. The use of other diagnostic imaging techniques such as computed tomography of the chest, magnetic resonance imaging, ventilation/perfusion scans, and selected bronchograms may be helpful in the more comprehensive evaluation of recurrent and persistent pneumonias.

It is important to document the specific area of pulmonary infiltrates on all chest radiographs. Recurrence of infiltrates in the same localized area is suggestive of obstruction (see Table 18–3) by a respiratory foreign body, a congenital anomaly, or a tumor. In contrast, recurrence of more diffuse infiltrates is suggestive of aspiration, especially if infiltrates are in the right middle lobe, the lingula, or the lower lobes. Infants lying supine may also aspirate into upper lobes. Infiltrates recurring in different lobes or segments are more likely to be associated with underlying generalized disorders such as cystic fibrosis or immunodeficiency syndromes. Pneumonia in the right middle lobe is frequently slow to resolve and may be associated with atelectasis caused by poorly developed collateral ventilation in that lobe. Children with asthma and allergic respiratory disease may develop recurrent right middle lobe pneumonia or atelectasis.

The misdiagnosis of pneumonia may be made when wheezing and airway obstruction result from airway inflammation rather than parenchymal involvement as the underlying cause of the abnormal auscultatory findings. If no chest radiographs are taken, it may be difficult to distinguish bronchitis from pneumonitis clinically, especially in an uncooperative child. In some children with asthma, however, the discovery of infiltrates on chest radiographs may precede the development of wheezing; these children may present with recurrent pneumonia.

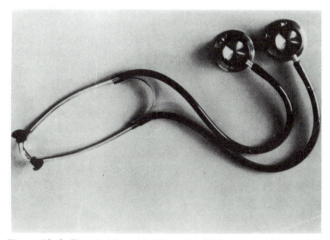

Figure 18–2. The double stethoscope (available commercially as Littmann differential stethoscope). Each ear has its own bell-diaphragm chest piece; each of the chest pieces is equipped with spring-loaded on-off buttons so that the sound can be instantly cut off or restarted at any time.

PULMONARY FUNCTION STUDIES

Pulmonary function studies offer an objective evaluation for the identification and quantification of lung dysfunction in children old enough to perform these studies reliably and consistently. Spirometry is the most commonly performed pulmonary function test in children over 6 years of age. In instances of airflow limitation, the response of the airway obstruction to bronchodilators should be objectively evaluated. In selected cases, airway challenge studies may be indicated.

A variety of studies are available for evaluating airway hyperreactivity in older children; they include challenge of methacholine or histamine, cold air hyperventilation ultrasonic nebulized distilled water, exercise, and bronchial antigen (see Chapters 15 and 16). Of the children without an underlying cause of their recurrent/persistent pneumonia as reported by Eigen and colleagues,[3] 92% had positive airway hyperreactivity, as demonstrated by inhalational challenge.

In addition to spirometry, older children can be evaluated for lung volumes (body plethysmography and gas dilution techniques), airway resistance and conductance (body plethysmography), diffusing capacity studies, and distribution of pulmonary gas (ventilation and perfusion studies, multiple-breath nitrogen washout studies, and helium dilution technique studies.)

In many medical centers, specialized equipment is now available for pulmonary function testing in infants and younger children who cannot perform standardized spirometric tests (see Chapter 9). Partial expiratory flow-volume curves, especially helpful in evaluating infants and young children, were reviewed by Morgan and collaborators.[24] Other objective tests of pulmonary function available for assessment of the patient with persistent or recurrent pneumonia include pulse oximetry, blood gas analysis, and assessment of respiratory rates. In addition, most larger medical centers have either capnography or end-tidal CO_2 measurements for noninvasive assessment of CO_2.

IMMUNOLOGIC EVALUATION

The majority of children referred because of a history of recurrent respiratory infections do not have a recognized specific immunologic defect, although there may be subtle or transient alterations in host defenses that cannot be currently identified.

For infants and children who are otherwise healthy except for recurrent or persistent pneumonia, only a limited laboratory workup may be necessary after a comprehensive history and physical examination. These children are more likely to have a period of freedom from symptoms or improvement of abnormalities on chest radiographs in between episodes of "pneumonia," and they exhibit normal growth and development before the onset of respiratory disease. For many children in this group, a temporal relationship between lifestyle change and the onset of recurrent or persistent respiratory infections is evident (e.g., entry into preschool, kindergarten, day care, or church or synagogue nursery). A large proportion of these apparently healthy children with persistent or recurrent pneumonia have associated wheezing. Although most of the respiratory infections in these children appear to have the characteristics of viral infections, the occurrence of two or more bacterial respiratory infections may be indicative of immunodeficiency disorders and warrants further evaluation.

The extent and severity of respiratory disease, as well as other clues in the history and physical examination that suggest possible underlying immunologic abnormalities, influence the urgency and intensity of the immunologic evaluation. In addition, the assessment of the chest radiograph may also suggest certain associated immunologic abnormalities. For example, if the predominant pattern on the chest radiograph is an interstitial pattern consistent with lymphoid interstitial pneumonitis and if possible risk factors for exposure to HIV are identified in the history, prompt immunologic evaluation to rule out AIDS is essential. If the predominant bronchopulmonary pathology is bronchiectasis, the immunologic evaluation may be delayed until after the results of quantitative sweat electrolyte tests and other additional diagnostic imaging studies are completed.

Alterations of respiratory host defenses that are not related to impairment of systemic immunity are discussed under the section "Other Alterations in Pulmonary Host Defenses" under Pathophysiology. Defects in systemic immunity include abnormalities of phagocytic cells (nonspecific immunity), specific cellular (T cell) immunity, antibody- (B cell–) mediated immunity, combined immunodeficiency (T and B cells), and complement defects (see Table 18–2). The presence of other features of the recognized specific immunodeficiency syndromes provides supportive evidence of disorders of specific immunity. Patients with defects in systemic immunity also have a propensity to develop infection in skin and gastrointestinal tract, in addition to the respiratory tract.

Screening immunologic evaluation includes quantitative serum immunoglobulins (IgG, IgM, IgA, and IgE), complete blood count and differential, and skin tests of delayed hypersensitivity to *Candida* and tetanus toxoid. Although normal total immunoglobulin findings do not ensure normal counts of IgG subclasses, there are wide ranges for normal values for each of the IgG subclasses. Interpretation of IgG subclass values necessitates assaying immunocompetence of the subclasses directed toward protein antigens (IgG_1 and IgG_3) and those responsive predominantly to polysaccharide antigens (IgG_2 and IgG_4). Measurement of specific pneumococcal antibodies before and after administration of polyvalent pneumococcal vaccine in children over 2 years of age enables functional evaluation of antibody responses to the polysaccharide antigens. Patients with deficiency of IgA in association with deficiency of IgG_2 are more prone to recurrent respiratory tract infections than are patients with IgA deficiency alone.

Additional studies include T and B cell subset quantification and response of T cells to mitogen stimulation. These studies may be necessary for evaluating further the immunologic status of patients with persistent pulmonary disease or recurrent pulmonary infiltrates.

Table 18–4. EVALUATION FOR RECURRENT OR PERSISTENT PNEUMONIA

Chest Radiograph
EPA and lateral views

Quantitative Sweat Electrolyte Analysis
After collection of sweat by pilocarpine iontophoresis

Pulmonary Function Studies
Pre- and postbronchodilation

Tests for Bronchial Hyperreactivity
If normal pulmonary function tests, methacholine challenge

Skin Tests (Delayed Hypersensitivity)
PPD 5TU
Candida
Diphtheria/Tetanus

Hematologic Studies
CBC with differential
Total eosinophil count
Sedimentation rate

Gram's Stain and Culture of Sputum (for Bacteria)
Sensitivity of bacterial pathogens identified

Nasal Smear for Eosinophils

Quantitative Serum Immunoglobulins
IgG, IgA, IgM, IgE
IgG subclasses

Serologic Studies
Pneumococcal antibodies (pre- and postvaccination with Pneumovax)
Haemophilus influenzae antibodies (if not protective, vaccination with
   H. influenzae vaccine and repeat antibody studies)
Tetanus/diphtheria antibodies (pre- and postimmunization)
HIV status (when risk factors or LIP present)
T and B cell quantifications: C4+, helper/inducer
T and B cell subsets: C8+, suppressor/cytotoxic

Serum Alpha₁-Antitrypsin

Nasal Cilia Scrapping/Biospy
For patients with bronchiectasis or chronic sinobronchial disease,
   electron microscopic morphologic studies

Neutrophil Function
NBT
Chemiluminescence
Hexose monophosphate shunt studies

Oxygen Saturation (Oximetry)
Arterial blood gases, if oximetry findings abnormal

Bronchoscopy
If abnormality of bronchial anatomy or foreign body suspected

Tests for Aspiration Pneumonia
Swallowing
   Barium swallow
   Cine-esophagogram
Gastroesophageal reflux
   Esophagogram
   pH Monitoring
   Esophagael manometry
   Lung scans to demonstrate aspiration (milk technetium scan)
Quantification of lipid-laden alveolar macrophages from tracheal
   aspiration or bronchial washings

Ventilation-Perfusion Scans

Computed Tomography of the Chest

EPA, erect posteroanterior; PPD 5TU, purified protein derivative, 5 tuberculin units; CBC, complete blood count; IgE, IgG, IgA, IgM, immunoglobulins E, G, A, M; HIV, human immunodeficiency virus; LIP, lymphoid interstitial pneumonitis; NBT, nitroblue tetrazolium.

Many laboratories now characterize lymphocyte subsets by means of flow cytometry and monoclonal antibodies. Monoclonal antibodies, through their definition of the surface characteristics, identify the stages of lymphocyte differentiation. Functional tests, in addition to indirect assessments, of T cell subsets are needed for more complete evaluation of T cell function. Proliferative responses to mitogens are little more than screening tests. The most relevant tests of T cell capacity are proliferative and cytolytic target responses to a particular antigen or response of cells to various cytokines.[6]

If phagocyte defects are suspected after screening tests for insufficient numbers of neutrophils, specific tests for ruling out lethal defects or motility defects are indicated. Findings that rule out chronic granulomatous disease include the inability of affected phagocytes to reduce the nitroblue tetrazolium dye *in vitro,* decreased neutrophil chemiluminescence, and abnormalities in hexose-monophosphate shunt.

Defects in complement are uncommon; patients with congenital absence of C3 are prone to recurrent infections with encapsulated bacteria, as are patients with deficiencies of C5, C6, or C3b. A defect in complement activation, such as that in sickle cell disease, also predisposes to infection with encapsulated bacteria.

Specific disorders of systemic immunity are described in detail in Chapter 75. The subject of most controversy is the evaluation and management of IgG subclass deficiency. This controversy is attributable in part to the variability in quantification of the IgG subclasses. It is important to evaluate response to specific antibodies in the evaluation of possible IgG subclass deficiency.

The evaluation of recurrent or persistent pneumonia can be difficult. Table 18–4 summarizes the laboratory studies useful in the search for an underlying cause, such as a congenital anomaly, a neuromuscular disorder, an abnormality in mucociliary function, an inherited disorder, an immunodeficiency, or the presence of a foreign body.

REFERENCES

1. Rubin BK: The evaluation of the child with recurrent chest infections. Pediatr Infect Dis 4:88–98, 1985.
2. Fernald GW, Denny FW, Fairclough DL, et al: Chronic lung disease in children referred to a teaching hospital. Pediatr Pulmonol 2:27–34, 1986.
3. Eigen H, Laughlin JJ, Homrighausen J: Recurrent pneumonia in children and its relationship to bronchial hyperreactivity. Pediatrics 70:698–704, 1982.
4. Jay SJ, Johanson WG, Pierce AK: The radiographic resolution of *Streptococcus pneumoniae* pneumonia. N Engl J Med 293:798–801, 1975.
5. Osborne D, White P: Radiology of epidemic adenovirus-21 infection of the lower respiratory tract in infants and young children. AJR 133:397–400, 1979.
6. Stiehm ER: Clinical and laboratory evaluation of the child with suspected immunodeficiency. Pediatr Rev 7(2):53–61, 1985.
7. Stiehm ER: They're back: Recurrent infections in pediatric practice. Contemporary Pediatr 7:20–40, 1990.
8. Denny FW, Clyde WA Jr: Acute lower respiratory tract infections in nonhospitalized children. J Pediatr 108:635–646, 1986.
9. Denny FW, Collier AM, Henderson FW: Acute respiratory infections in day care. Rev Infect Dis 8:527–532, 1986.
10. Loda FA, Glezen WP, Clyde WA Jr: Respiratory disease in group day care. Pediatrics 49:428–437, 1972.

11. Colombo JL, Hallberg TK: Recurrent aspiration in children: Lipid-laden alveolar macrophage quantitation. Pediatr Pulmonol 3:86–89, 1987.
12. Williams HE, Freeman M: Milk inhalation pneumonia, the significance of fat filled macrophages in tracheal secretions. Aust Pediatr 9:286–288, 1973.
13. Orenstein SR, Orenstein DM: Gastroesophageal reflux in children. J Pediatr 112:847–858, 1988.
14. Hasselblad V, Humble CG, Graham MG, et al: Indoor environmental determinants of lung function in children. Am Rev Respir Dis 123:479–485, 1981.
15. Ware JH, Dockery DW, Spiro A, et al: Passive smoking, gas cooking and respiratory health of children living in six cities. Am Rev Respir Dis 129:366–374, 1984.
16. Ekwo EE, Weinberger MM, Lachenbruch PA, et al: Relationship of parental smoking and gas cooking to respiratory disease in children. Chest 84:662–668, 1983.
17. Matsukura S, Taminato T, Kitano N, et al: Effects of environmental tobacco smoke on urinary cotinine excretion in nonsmokers: Evidence for passive smoking. N Engl J Med 311:828–832, 1984.
18. Greenberg RA, Bauman KE, Glover LH, et al: Ecology of passive smoking by infants. J Pediatr 114:774–780, 1989.
19. U.S. Department of Health and Human Services: Health effects of environmental tobacco smoke exposure. In The Health Consequences of Involuntary Smoking: A report of the Surgeon General, pp. 17–118. Rockville, MD: U.S. Public Health Service, 1986.
20. Committee on Passive Smoking, Board of Environmental Studies of Toxicology, National Research Council: Effects of Exposure to Environmental Tobacco Smoke on Lung Function and Respiratory Symptoms in Environmental Tobacco Smoke: Measuring Exposures and Assessing Health Effects, pp. 202–209. Washington, DC: National Academy Press, 1986.
21. Denny FW: Acute respiratory infections in children: Etiology and epidemiology. Pediatr Rev 9(5):135–146, 1987.
22. Wald NJ, Boreham J, Bailey A, et al: Urinary cotinine as marker of breathing other people's tobacco smoke. Lancet 1:230–231, 1984.
23. Waring WW: The history and physical examinations. In Kendig EL, Cherniak V (eds): Disorders of the Respiratory Tract in Children, 4th ed, pp. 57–78. Philadelphia: WB Saunders, 1983.
24. Morgan WJ, Geller DE, Tepper RS, et al: Partial expiratory flow-volume curves in infants and young children. Pediatr Pulmonol 5:232–243, 1988.
25. Hilman BC: How to work up recurrent or persistent pediatric pneumonia. J Respir Dis 12:315–332, 1991

19 EVALUATION OF CHEST PAIN IN CHILDHOOD AND ADOLESCENCE

MARTHA FRANZ, M.D.

Chest pain in children and adolescents has many possible causes. Media reports of sudden deaths of young athletes and medical emphasis on prevention and treatment of hypertension and atherosclerotic cardiovascular disease have focused the attention of children, adolescents, and their parents on chest pain. Although the majority of causes of chest pain in young patients are benign, it is essential to identify promptly the small group of patients whose chest pain is serious or life threatening.

The flow diagrams[1] presented as Figures 19–1 and 19–2 aid in developing a diagnostic plan for differentiating the various causes. Chest pain can occur in children of all ages. In several studies, the mean age of chest pain in children has been reported to be between 12 and 14 years.[2] The incidence of functional chest pain is higher in teenagers than in younger children. Chest pain frequently is chronic, lasting more than 6 months in as many as one third of the patients reported in some studies.[3–5]

CLINICAL MANIFESTATIONS

Chest wall pain is one of the most frequent causes of chest pain in adolescents and children. Irritation of the chest wall tissues causes a localized, superficial, sharp pain by stimulating the dermatomal intercostal nerve plexus in the area. This pain is reproducible by percussion or chest wall movement.

Chest pain arising from the thoracic or upper abdominal viscera is deep, is poorly localized, and may radiate from the visceral site. It usually cannot be reproduced by movement. In addition to the autonomic afferent fibers that accompany efferent autonomic fibers to the viscera and blood vessels, visceral pain fibers are believed to be present in these pathways. Excessive contraction of nonstriated smooth muscle, excessive tension on a viscus, or certain pathologic processes produce visceral pain. In these instances, vague pain may be felt in the region of the viscus itself (true visceral pain), or the pain may be experienced in a region of skin or other somatic tissue

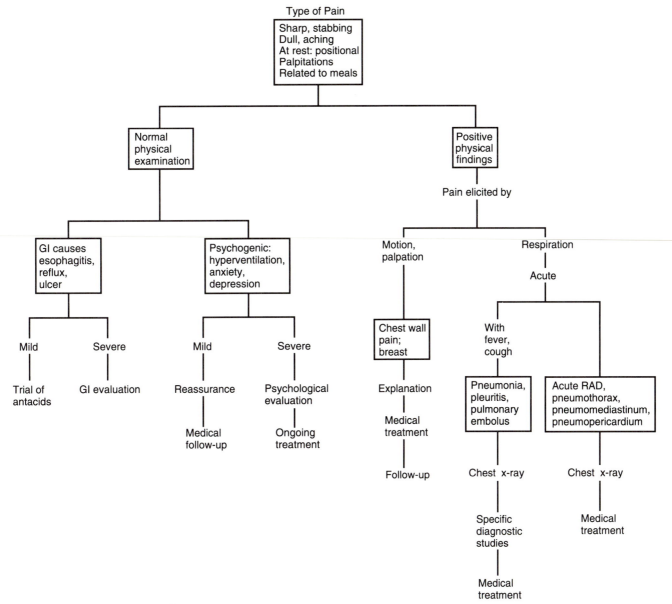

Figure 19–1. Flow chart for evaluating patients with nonanginal chest pain. If the physical examination findings are negative, gastrointestinal causes and psychogenic pain are important diagnostic considerations. When a positive physical finding of pain is elicited by motion or palpation, causes involving the chest wall are suggested. For chest pain with positive respiratory findings, chest radiography and other studies for specific diagnosis and treatment are required. GI, gastrointestinal; RAD, reactive airway disease. (Adapted from Brenner JI, Ringel RE, Berman MA: Cardiologic perspectives of chest pain in childhood: A referral problem? To whom? Pediatr Clin North Am 31:1241–1258, 1984.)

whose sensory nerve fibers enter the same segments of the spinal cord that receive afferent fibers from the involved viscus (referred pain). Referred pain may be associated with tenderness of the skin at the referred site[6] (Figure 19–3).

In general, the afferent sensory fibers that accompany the pre- and postganglion fibers of the sympathetic system have a segmental arrangement. Figure 19–4 shows the distribution of the dermatomal intercostal nerve complexes. Dermatomes T1 to T8 cover an area of the thorax from the clavicles to below the xyphoid process and also the anteromedial portions of the arms and forearms. Deep pain felt in this area may originate in any viscera whose afferent sensory fibers enter the spinal cord at these dermatomal levels. Pain at dermatome levels T1 to T4 may arise from most of the thoracic viscera (e.g., myocardium and esophagus). Pain at dermatome levels T5 to T8 may originate in the lower thoracic wall, the diaphragm, and the abdomen. The pain usually is maximal in the xyphoid region and in the back inferior to the scapula.[4]

Pain impulses from the heart enter the spinal cord through the first to fifth thoracic spinal nerves. They are carried mainly in the middle and inferior cardiac nerves. Peripherally, these fibers pass through the cardiac plexuses and along the coronary arteries. Anoxia of the cardiac muscle causes angina pectoris with deep, crushing presternal pain and referred pain over a large part of the

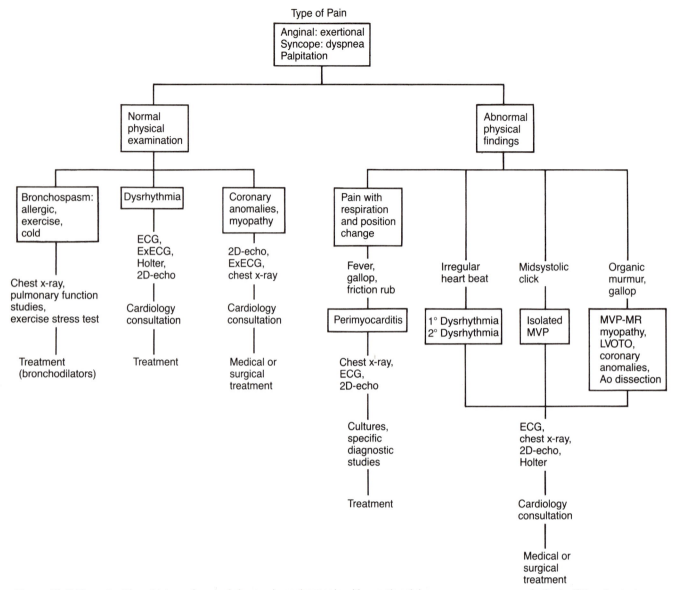

Type of Pain

Anginal: exertional
Syncope: dyspnea
Palpitation

Normal physical examination

Bronchospasm: allergic, exercise, cold

Chest x-ray, pulmonary function studies, exercise stress test

Treatment (bronchodilators)

Dysrhythmia

ECG, ExECG, Holter, 2D-echo

Cardiology consultation

Treatment

Coronary anomalies, myopathy

2D-echo, ExECG, chest x-ray

Cardiology consultation

Medical or surgical treatment

Abnormal physical findings

Pain with respiration and position change

Fever, gallop, friction rub

Perimyocarditis

Chest x-ray, ECG, 2D-echo

Cultures, specific diagnostic studies

Treatment

Irregular heart beat

1° Dysrhythmia
2° Dysrhythmia

Midsystolic click

Isolated MVP

Organic murmur, gallop

MVP-MR myopathy, LVOTO, coronary anomalies, Ao dissection

ECG, chest x-ray, 2D-echo, Holter

Cardiology consultation

Medical or surgical treatment

Figure 19–2. Flow chart for a history of anginal chest pain or chest pain with exertional dyspnea, syncope, or arrhythmia. If the physical examination findings are normal, exercise-induced bronchospasm, dysrhythmia, and coronary anomalies are diagnostic possibilities. Abnormal physical findings of fever with a gallop rhythm or pericardial friction rub mandate evaluation for perimyocarditis. Irregular heart beat, organic murmur, or midsystolic click requires further cardiac studies. ECG, electrocardiogram; ExECG, exercise electrocardiogram; Holter, 24-h ambulatory ECG monitor; 2D-Echo, two-dimensional echocardiogram; 1°, primary; 2°, secondary; Dys, dysrhythmia; MVP, mitral valve prolapse; MR, mitral regurgitation; LVOTO, left ventricular outflow tract obstruction; Ao, aortic). (Adapted from Brenner JI, Ringel RE, Berman MA: Cardiologic perspectives of chest pain in childhood: A referral problem? To whom? Pediatr Clin North Am 31:1241–1258, 1984.)

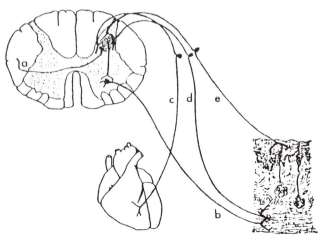

Figure 19–3. Diagram of possible neural path for referred chest pain of path *a* and path *b* as shown on diagram. Nerve impulses (c) from heart are transmitted to an "irritable area" in gray matter of cord. Nerve fibers from skin and muscle (d and e) enter the same region. Nerve fibers from this region carry impulses over path *a* to the spinothalamic tract and the cerebral cortex and over path *b* to the chest muscles, which contract in an exaggerated manner. (From Miller MA, Leavell LC: Sensation: Tactile sense, kinesthesia, temperature, pain, taste, smell, hearing, equilibrium, and vision: Structure components. *In* Kimber-Gray-Stockpole's Anatomy & Physiology, 16th ed, p. 234. New York: Macmillan, 1972.)

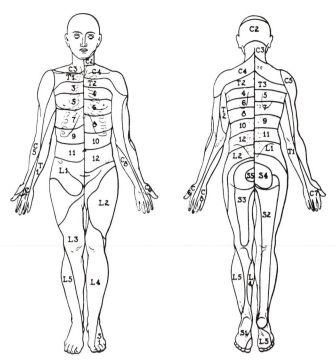

Figure 19–4. The distribution of the spinal dermatomes. The maximal extent of each dermatome is shown. (Modified from Ford FR: Diseases of the Nervous System in Infancy, Childhood, and Adolescence, 6th ed. Springfield, IL: Charles C Thomas, 1973.)

left chest, radiating to the left shoulder, to the inner side of the left arm, and upward along the neck or downward to the epigastrium.[6]

Disease of the lung itself may be extensive without producing chest pain because the lung tissue and visceral pleura have no sensory nerve fibers. The parietal pleural is supplied by sensory fibers from the intercostal nerves and the diaphragm. These sensory fibers are stimulated by inflammation or stretching of the membrane. Pleural pain usually underlies the area where the pain originates except when the diaphragmatic pleura is involved.

Diaphragmatic pain has different loci, depending on the area of pathologic processes. The posterior third and the lateral portions of the diaphragm are innervated by nerve segments T7 to T12 and produce pain in the lower chest, the upper abdomen, and the lumbar area. The anterior third and central portions of the diaphragm are innervated by the phrenic nerve, whose sensory afferent fibers enter the cervical cord mainly in the posterior nerve roots of C3 and C4. This pain is referred to the neck and the upper shoulders.[7]

HISTORY

A detailed history taken in a reassuring manner is the physician's most important diagnostic tool. First, an older child or an adolescent should describe the pain in his or her own words. Important considerations in the history include (1) the location, duration, and quality of the chest pain, (2) the activities that exacerbate or alleviate the pain, and (3) the descriptions of any associated signs and symptoms.

Pain that is sharp, superficial, and localized is most likely chest wall or pleuritic pain. Deep, gnawing, or burning pain is characteristic of visceral pain. This type of pain is poorly localized and radiates from the site. Brief recurrent episodes of chest pain are suggestive of chest wall or precordial pain. Gnawing pain lasting an hour or more that is substernal or epigastric may be associated with esophagitis or gastroesophageal reflux.

Chest pain that increases with breathing, movement, or cough frequently originates in the chest wall or pleura. Substernal pain that increases both with exercise and with lying down may be caused by gastroesophageal reflux and esophagitis. Pain that does not awaken the patient at night should lead the physician to suspect psychogenic pain. Conversely, chest pain that is worse or awakens the patient at night is strongly suggestive of organic causes.

In many children and adolescents with multiple somatic complaints, chest pain is often psychogenic in origin. In contrast, patients with other signs of illness such as fever, weight loss, or syncope require a thorough diagnostic workup for organic illness.[2, 3]

During history taking, the parents' and child's interactions and the parents' response to the child's pain should be assessed. If a psychogenic cause is suspected, tactful questions should be asked in order to determine whether a stressful school, social, or family situation exists.[8] A child with organic pain may also have compounding psychological problems.[8]

PHYSICAL EXAMINATION

It is important to evaluate the severity of the pain and the patient's anxiety regarding the pain at the time of the physical examination. Signs of impending cardiorespiratory embarrassment must be recognized immediately and prompt action taken. If the patient is stable, the child and parents should be reassured, and the child should be made as comfortable as possible during the examination.

CHEST WALL

Examination of the chest wall should include inspection for evidence of trauma, such as bruising or swelling. Shallow respiration with splinting caused by localized pain may be present. Palpation and percussion should be used to reproduce and localize chest wall pain. Tenderness of breast tissue to palpation may be described as "chest pain" by both boys and girls. Radicular pain, such as that associated with herpes zoster, can be reproduced by palpation over the involved nerve.

RESPIRATORY

The physician should evaluate the child for any evidence of acute or chronic respiratory disease. An abnormal breathing pattern (rate, depth, rhythm, and effort of breathing) may indicate respiratory disease. The child with chest pain may have rapid, shallow respirations. If deep breathing exacerbates the pain, an anxious or uncomfortable child or adolescent may hyperventilate; the dyspneic child, however, also shows signs of increased effort in breathing.

CARDIAC

Although cardiovascular causes of chest pain are reported in only 2% to 7% of cases of chest pain in children, a careful cardiac examination is essential in evaluating chest pain.[9] A hyperdynamic cardiac thrust extending over one or more interspaces may accompany hypertrophy and dilatation of the ventricles. On palpation, the apical impulse may be heaving in left ventricular hypertrophy. In right ventricular hypertrophy, a sternal and peristernal lift may be felt. Apical thrills are more easily palpated when the patient is in the left lateral position, whereas basal thrills are more easily palpated while the patient is sitting and leaning forward. Percussion of cardiac borders is more helpful for diagnosing pericardial effusion or mediastinal shift (secondary to pulmonary or pleural space disease) than for diagnosing cardiac disease. A third sound is a protodiastolic gallop, heard in myocarditis and in congestive heart failure. A fourth heart sound produced with atrial systole is generally associated with significant obstruction to ventricular filling or ejection. Aortic or pulmonic ejection sounds early in systole are heard frequently in aortic and pulmonic stenosis.[10]

Murmurs of congenital heart disease may be widely transmitted to both sides of the neck and back. It is crucial to auscultate the heart with the patient in both the supine and sitting positions and, if possible, after exercise. Mitral systolic and diastolic murmurs are more easily heard when the patient is in the left lateral position, especially after exercise. Basal murmurs may be more obvious when the patient is in the sitting position during breath holding.

Evaluation of the pulse for arrhythmia or persistent tachycardia is important. Persistent tachycardia is defined as a sustained pulse rate of >200/min in neonates, >150 in infants, and >120 in older children. If possible, the pulse rate should be obtained when the patient is quiet and relaxed. A water hammer pulse in the forearm or Corrigan's pulse in the carotid arteries signifies high pulse pressure, as is found in patent ductus arterosis, aortic insufficiency, or general vasodilation.

The presence of cervical venous distension or pulsations should be evaluated with the patient propped in bed at an angle of about 45 degrees and the neck muscles relaxed. Venous pulsations can occur in congestive heart failure, severe pulmonic stenosis, tricuspid insufficiency or stenosis, and constrictive pericarditis. Venous distension without pulsation is produced in obstruction of the superior vena cava.[10]

ABDOMINAL

Abdominal organs are a major source of pain referred to the chest. Tenderness in the epigastric or periumbilical area that may or may not radiate to the sternum or laterally into the chest is suggestive of esophagitis or gastroesophageal reflux. Abdominal masses or tenderness is often found with hepatic abscesses and tumors, peptic and duodenal ulcers, cholelithiasis, pancreatitis, and splenic infarction.

VERTEBRAL COLUMN

The spine should be examined routinely by percussion and inspection, including range of motion. Radicular pain may be referred to the chest by diseases or anatomic changes that impinge on the spinal cord or nerve roots. Kyphoscoliosis can cause severe restrictive lung disease and pain over the thoracic spine. Vertebral collapse from trauma, infiltrative processes, infections, abscess formation, and aseptic necrosis from prolonged steroid use also produces referred chest pain.[4]

EXTREMITIES

The joints should be examined for any evidence of arthritis that would be suggestive of a collagen disease. Bruising of the extremities may indicate trauma that had been previously overlooked. Examination of the skin may reveal a clue to underlying systemic disease or associated infection.

Skin rashes may manifest in collagen vascular diseases, Kawasaki's disease, and coxsackievirus and echovirus illnesses.

DIFFERENTIAL DIAGNOSIS

MUSCULOSKELETAL CHEST PAIN

Musculoskeletal sources are the most common specific causes of chest pain found. The spectrum of musculoskeletal causes include (1) muscle strain, spasm, and stress fractures, (2) costochondritis, (3) Tietze's syndrome, (4) direct trauma, (5) slipping rib syndrome, (6) chest wall tumors, (7) connective tissue disorders, and (8) breast pain. Muscle strain, spasm, and stress fractures are usually caused by strain or overuse of muscles. Often, no initiating factor is found; however, a history of participation in sports such as gymnastics or weight lifting is helpful in the diagnosis. Strain of the upper back muscles (latissimus dorsi or trapezius) can cause lateral or posterior chest pain. Stress fractures of ribs are seen in tennis, rowing, and repeated ball throwing. A stress fracture may be associated with evidence of soft tissue damage.[4]

Costochondritis has been reported to account for 10% to 22% of all pediatric chest pain. The pain usually is preceded by exercise or an upper respiratory infection. This condition is characterized by sharp pain in the anterior chest wall that is localized or radiates to the back or the abdomen. The pain tends to be unilateral, more commonly on the left, at the fourth to sixth costochondral junctions. It is diagnosed from the finding of tenderness on palpation over the affected rib cartilages where the ribs are attached to the sternum. Costochondritis is more common in girls and may persist for up to several months. Motion of the arm and shoulder on the affected side may produce the pain.[11]

In Tietze's syndrome, a spindle-shaped swelling is visible at the sternochondral junction. The swelling is usually localized at the right sternoclavicular or second sternochondral junction. It is believed to be caused by minor trauma. The pain is localized and may last up to several weeks. The swelling may persist for several months to years. In histologic reports of specimens, increased cartilage and lack of inflammatory changes have been described.[4]

Direct trauma to the chest wall may be incurred from sports, accidents, or child abuse. External signs such as bruising or swelling may not be present. Serious acute injuries that require immediate attention include pneumothorax, hemothorax, lung contusion, and vascular injuries. Incomplete rib fractures or pectoral muscle tears produce less serious injuries. Recurrent chest pain may be manifest long after the initiating musculoskeletal trauma.[2]

The patients with slipping rib syndrome report pain under the ribs or in the upper abdominal quadrants. A clicking or popping sound may be heard when the patient lifts objects or bends forward. The cause is believed to be the tip of the eight, ninth, or tenth rib (floating ribs) overriding the rib above. The onset of the pain is sudden, and the pain may last for several hours, with residual tenderness of several days' duration. The so-called hooking maneuver, in which the affected rib margin is grasped and pulled anteriorly, reproduces the pain. Surgical resection of the rib tip may be required in instances of severe pain.[4]

Primary malignant tumors of the chest wall are rare. Rhabdomyosarcomas originating in the chest wall musculature have been described; in one study, 50% of children with localized tumor were reported to be free of recurrence at a median time of more than 4 years after diagnosis.[12] Primary Ewing's sarcoma of the rib can occur. Leukemia can infiltrate the periosteum and the sternum.

Dermatomyositis and polymyositis can produce recurrent myalgias that involve the chest wall. Signs and symptoms of generalized disease are usually present. Electromyograms of affected muscles are abnormal. Arthritic involvement of the sternoclavicular joints and costochondral junctions may cause chest pain in juvenile rheumatoid arthritis.[13]

Breast-related chest pain is found in boys and girls; of the five adolescents with breast pain studied by Pantell and Goodman, four were male.[14] Fear of breast cancer can produce significant concern in either sex.

RESPIRATORY CAUSES OF CHEST PAIN

There are a variety of respiratory causes of chest pain, including (1) cough, (2) asthma, (3) pneumonia, (4) foreign bodies in the respiratory system, (5) pleuritis and pleural effusions, (6) pneumothorax, (7) pneumomediastinum and pneumopericardium, (8) pulmonary embolism, (9) sickle cell disease, and (10) idiopathic pulmonary hypertension.

Chronic and paroxysmal episodes of coughing were diagnosed as the cause of chest pain in 6% to 12% of pediatric and adolescent patients.[2] This pain usually is caused by overuse of the chest wall muscles. Tenderness may be elicited by pressure over the involved area, which is most often in the anterolateral lower intercostal muscles. This pain does not increase with deep inspiration, as is characteristic of pleural pain. It is aggravated by coughing but may persist between paroxysms of coughing. Severe paroxysmal coughing may produce rib fractures.[7]

Reactive airway disease is a leading respiratory cause of chest pain. Exacerbations of wheezing, hyperpnea, dyspnea, hyperinflation, cough, and muscle strain often lead to chest discomfort. Exercise-induced asthma was found to be the cause of chest pain on exertion in 9.5% of 147 children and adolescents tested with maximal exercise.[15] The majority of these patients did not have a history of asthma.

Pneumomediastinum has been reported to occur in 5% of patients during an acute, severe asthmatic attack. Pneumothorax is a less frequent cause of chest pain in asthma.[16]

Pneumonia that causes irritation of the parietal pleura may be the cause of pleural pain. Associated physical findings, such as rales, rapid shallow respirations, chest retractions, or fever, are suggestive of underlying pneumonia. Infectious etiologic agents are most common, but chemical pneumonitis (such as hydrocarbon aspiration) can also produce pleuritic pain.

Aspiration of respiratory foreign bodies can partially obstruct the airways, causing irritation, cough, and chest pain. Localized wheezing or rales, radiographic evidence of atelectasis, unilateral hyperinflation, or mediastinal shift with exhalation may confirm the diagnosis of foreign body aspiration.

Inflammation of the pleural membranes is usually the result of diseases of contiguous structures (e.g., adjacent pulmonary or subdiaphragmatic infectious foci) or of systemic diseases such as lymphoma and systemic lupus erythematosus. Rarely is pleuritis the result of disturbances primarily in the pleura.

Pneumonia is the most common cause of pleural effusion in children and adolescents. Pleural pain is sharp and is produced by inspiration or cough. As the effusion increases and separates the pleural membranes, pleuritic pain becomes a dull ache and may disappear. In the presence of any significant pleural effusions, thoracentesis is required for determining the character of the fluid and for diagnosing the specific cause. Children and adolescents often experience sudden pain in the chest or pain referred to the shoulder with pneumothorax; symptoms such as dyspnea, cyanosis, and rapid, shallow breathing may also occur. Early recognition of pneumothorax is required, especially in patients with clinical situations associated with this complication (see Chapter 62).

Protracted vomiting and drug abuse can produce pneumothorax and pneumomediastinum. Pneumomediastinum causes severe substernal pain that may radiate to the back, neck, and shoulders. Subcutaneous air may be palpated in the neck and chest wall. Pneumomediastinum rarely leads to severe cardiorespiratory distress; when it does, high mediastinal pressure can produce hypotension, and aspiration of mediastinal air is required. The mediastinal air usually dissects along the fascial planes into the subcutaneous tissues of the neck and the chest wall along the aorta to the peritoneum or into the pleural space and relieves mediastinal pressure.

Pneumopericardium can be managed conservatively unless it produces cardiac tamponade, in which case immediate pericardiocentesis is required.

Pneumomediastinum as well as pneumothorax has been reported after cocaine inhalation and marijuana smoking; both can cause acute chest pain and dyspnea.[17] Marijuana smoking and inhalation of crack cocaine is often accompanied by prolonged Valsalva maneuvers, use of positive pressure devices, or mouth-to-mouth blowing; these practices increase intrapleural pressure, leading to pneumomediastinum, pneumothorax, or pneumopericardium as a result of barotrauma. Free-basing cocaine has more frequently been described as producing severe chest pain by inducing cardiac arrhythmias, coronary artery spasm, and myocardial infarction. In view of the increasing rate of drug abuse in the United States, evaluation for cocaine or marijuana use must be considered in an adolescent who presents with acute chest pain. A careful history for drug use, chest radiographic evaluation, and electrocardiography are important tools in the diagnosis.

Pulmonary embolism is a rare occurrence in childhood and adolescence. The high-risk factors in adolescent girls include the use of oral contraceptives, pregnancy, and elective abortion. Recent trauma to a lower extremity, surgery (especially orthopedic surgery), central venous catheters, intravenous drug abuse, prolonged immobilization, systemic infection, and collagen vascular disease are potential predisposing factors for both sexes. The most common presenting complaint was pleuritic pain in 84% of the teenagers studied by Bernstein and associates.[18] Deep vein thrombosis of a lower extremity was found in 58% of the patients. Radionuclide perfusion scans and pulmonary arteriography when radionuclide scans are equivocal are necessary diagnostic tools.

Vaso-occlusive crises are responsible for severe chest pain in children and adolescents with sickle cell disease. Intravascular sickling leads to the formation of microthrombi, which occlude small arterioles and produce ischemia and multiple microinfarcts. Extensive pulmonary infarction may be difficult to differentiate from pneumonia because both are associated with fever.

Primary pulmonary hypertension is a rare cause of chest pain on exertion and is associated with dyspnea and often syncope. Chest radiographs demonstrate prominence of a pulmonary artery segment, moderate cardiac enlargement, and a decrease in pulmonary vascularity. Prognosis is poor. Intrapulmonary veno-occlusive disease represents another histologic class of primary pulmonary hypertension. Intimal proliferation and fibrosis of the intrapulmonary veins and venules occur. Chest radiographs show increased bronchovascular markings and Kerley B lines resulting from increased pulmonary capillary pressures. Survival after diagnosis is usually less than 2 years.[19]

CHEST PAIN OF GASTROINTESTINAL ORIGIN

Chest pain of gastrointestinal origin is caused by (1) esophagitis and gastroesophageal reflux, (2) hiatal hernia (partial thoracic stomach), (3) achalasia, (4) esophageal spasm, (5) presence of esophageal foreign bodies, (6) corrosive esophagitis, (7) esophageal perforations, (8) gastric and duodenal ulcer disease and pylorospasm, and (9) gastric distension.

A significant number of children and adolescents with chest pain in the retrosternal or substernal area demonstrate esophagitis and gastroesophageal reflux. Pain with gastroesophageal reflux is produced typically after eating and is increased with intra-abdominal pressure or in a reclining position. Because both the heart and the esophagus have similar neural pain pathways (the cardiac plexus and the esophageal plexus both arise from the vagus nerves and sympathetic trunks), it may be difficult to separate esophageal from cardiac chest pain.[20] In infancy and childhood, aspiration pneumonia, chronic cough, and wheezing may be prominent features.

Hiatal hernia, or partial thoracic stomach, may be a cause of chest pain in children. The most common type of herniation is the sliding hernia, in which the gastroesophageal junction and a portion of the stomach are within the chest. This condition usually is associated with gastroesophageal reflux and esophagitis. A feeling of excessive fullness with eating, epigastric pain, retrosternal pain, vomiting, and dysphagia are associated symptoms. In paraesophageal hernia, the gastroesophageal junction is positioned normally and a portion of the stomach is herniated through a patent esophageal hiatus. Infarction of the herniated stomach is a rare complication.[21]

Achalasia is the inability of the lower esophageal sphincter to relax, producing obstruction and esophagitis. Symptoms in addition to retrosternal or epigastric pain include difficulty in swallowing, vomiting, cough from overflow of fluids into the trachea, recurrent pneumonia, and failure to gain weight. The diagnosis is made radiographically by means of barium swallow, which demonstrates a persistently narrowed gastroesophageal junction and absence of propulsive peristaltic esophageal waves.[21]

Abnormalities of esophageal peristalsis, although more common in adults, can produce chest pain in children. Pressure type of pain, dysphagia, and symptoms of gastroesophageal reflux are the usual manifestations.[21]

Foreign bodies in the esophagus usually cause chest pain and difficulty in swallowing solid foods. Dyspnea may occur if the larynx is compressed. Patients may also have a history of an initial incident of coughing, choking, or retrosternal chest pain. If the presence of a foreign body is not promptly diagnosed, edema and inflammation may produce complete esophageal obstruction. Perforation of the esophagus, with severe chest pain, fever, mediastinitis, and shock, occasionally results.[21]

Ingestion of household cleaning products such as strong alkali preparations, hydrochloric acid, sulfuric acid, and bleaches can cause severe esophageal burns and pain from corrosive esophagitis. The clinical findings include inability to swallow, substernal or back pain, and excessive drooling.

Esophageal perforations may cause chest pain. Immediate recognition of this cause of chest pain is crucial because it can become a fatal condition rapidly, and aggressive treatment is required for a successful outcome. A mortality rate in excess of 20% has been reported.[22] Findings include vomiting followed by severe substernal pain, fever, leukocytosis, and mediastinal air in the majority of patients. Mediastinitis and septic shock must be immediately treated or prevented if possible. The most common causes of perforation are iatrogenic (instrumentation for pre-existing disease or accidental cutting of the esophagus during surgical procedures). The esophagus may perforate spontaneously as a result of a sudden increase of esophageal pressure, caused by violent vomiting, automobile accidents, or compression in the birth canal.[21] Diagnosis of perforation can be made by an esophagogram (always with the use of water-soluble contrast media), which shows extraluminal penetration of the contrast media.

Referred chest pain can originate in the stomach, the pylorus, and the duodenum from ulcers or pylorospasm. The pain tends to occur in the region of the xyphoid process and in the back, inferior to the scapula. Midepigastric pain, burning or gnawing in character, may also be present. Ingestion of food or antacids may relieve the pain. Tenderness in the midepigastric area may or may not be present.[23]

Gastric distension caused by swallowing air or delayed stomach emptying can produce spasm of the left hemidiaphragm with pain either in the lower left chest and the upper abdomen or referred to the left shoulder. Percussion over the stomach and relief with belching of air may help in the diagnosis.

CARDIAC CAUSES OF CHEST PAIN

Although a cardiac cause for chest pain is found in only a small percentage of children and adolescents evaluated with this complaint, chest pain has become a major source of referral to pediatric cardiologists. Chest pain raises anxiety in both the patient and the family about serious heart disease.

Cardiac disorders produce chest pain by causing myocardial ischemia or by irritation of pericardial or pleural serosa. Exertional chest pain associated with dizziness or syncope and sustained tachycardia are suggestive of myocardial ischemia. Pleural or pericardial inflammation leads to chest pain with positional changes or with respiration. Fever and respiratory distress are likely to be present with acute inflammatory processes (myopericarditis).

There are three categories of cardiac diseases that cause chest pain: (1) structural abnormalities, (2) acquired myopericardial or coronary disease, and (3) dysrhythmias.[1] Left ventricular outflow tract obstruction is the most frequent cause of ischemic myocardial dysfunction in children.[24] It comprises a small but significant group of diseases that have the potential to produce sudden death

from ventricular rhythm disturbance. All are likely to cause chest pain when the obstruction increases stress in the left ventricular wall, resulting in inadequate subendocardial perfusion and ischemic pain. Physical findings of a fixed left ventricular obstruction (valve or subvalve stenosis) include a loud, harsh systolic ejection murmur, caused by flow across the area of obstruction. The murmur is most clearly heard at the upper right sternal border radiating to the carotids.[1]

Because of the autosomal dominant inheritance pattern of hypertrophic cardiomyopathy, a family history of recurrent syncope or premature cardiac death is often found. In all lesions of left ventricular outflow tract obstruction, diagnosis is made by two-dimensional Doppler echocardiography.

Markiewicz and colleagues reported mitral prolapse in 5% to 22% of young women (aged 17 to 35 years).[26] Nonexertional chest pain was the chief complaint in 18% of children with mitral valve prolapse in one study.[25] The pain is presumed to be the result of papillary muscle ischemia or left ventricular endocardial ischemia. Cardiac examinations usually elicit the findings of a midsystolic click, a late systolic murmur, or both. The patient should be examined in the supine, sitting, and standing positions because the click and the murmur may vary greatly with position and from one examination to another.

Most children and adolescents with mitral valve prolapse remain asymptomatic. The association of mitral valve prolapse with supraventricular and ventricular dysrhythmias should be considered. Kavey and co-authors[27] reported serious rhythm disturbances in 18.5% of mitral prolapse patients during treadmill exercise and 24-h ambulatory electrocardiographic monitoring. Specific diagnosis is made by two-dimensional and M-mode echocardiography, which also rule out the presence of associated cardiac defects.[24] Follow-up clinical evaluations are important, as is reassurance of the patient and family when no associated cardiac defect or serious rhythm disturbance is found.

Coronary artery anomalies are rare causes of chest pain and myocardial ischemia, especially with exercise, with emotional distress, or after eating a large meal. This pain may be associated with syncope. Exercise electrocardiography and radionuclide perfusion scans should be obtained. Cardioangiography is diagnostic. Surgical repair may be necessary in order to prevent progressive disability or death.[1]

Marfan's syndrome, an autosomal dominant disorder of connective tissue, is characterized by skeletal, ocular, and cardiovascular abnormalities. The common cardiac lesion is dilation of the aorta, beginning at the aortic valve and usually limited to the ascending aorta. The valve ring is stretched, leading to aortic insufficiency. Cystic medial necrosis of the aorta may result in dissection of the aorta, a medical emergency requiring prompt angiographic diagnosis and surgical correction.[28]

Patients with Turner's syndrome have also been reported to develop aortic dissection and aortic aneurysmal rupture, in addition to the cardiac anomalies more commonly described (bicuspid aortic valve and aortic coarctation).[29] In instances of marked or rapidly progressive aortic dilatation, sudden onset of aortic regurgitation, unexplained episodes of chest pain, or progressive development of left ventricular enlargement, elective surgical therapy should be considered.[29]

One of the sinuses of Valsalva may be weakened by congenital or acquired disease, producing an aneurysm that ruptures, usually into the right atrium or ventricle. This can cause sudden, crushing substernal pain. A new "machinery" type of murmur similar to a ductus arteriosus murmur or a murmur of aortic insufficiency may be heard. A wide pulse pressure is present. If this diagnosis is suspected, immediate evaluation by two-dimensional echocardiography and angiography is necessary.[30]

Atrial septal defects, small ventricular septal defects, pulmonary valve stenosis, and mild aortic valve stenosis should not result in myocardial ischemia.

Acquired Myopericardial or Coronary Disease

Acute inflammatory myocarditis may manifest with chest pain resulting from inflammation, ischemia, or arrhythmia. The most common inflammatory agents causing myocarditis are viruses. Coxsackievirus B is found in almost half the cases of myocarditis with a known cause. Infected infants often present with a sudden illness and acute cardiorespiratory distress; older children and adolescents more often present with fever, dyspnea, precordial chest pain, and mild cardiac decompensation. Diagnosis depends on viral culture from the stools and an increasing coxsackievirus antibody titer.[31]

Acute myocarditis may be a complication of a number of acute processes. Acute myocarditis can be produced by many infectious pathogens, including viruses, bacterial toxins, bacteria, rickettsiae, parasites, and fungi. Physical and chemical agents such as radiation treatment, chemotherapy, lead ingestion, and poisonous bites can also cause myocarditis. Chronic myocarditis occurs with collagen disease, type II glycogen storage disease, progressive muscular dystrophy, and Hurler's syndrome.[31, 32]

Clinical findings of myocarditis, regardless of origin, include precordial chest pain, tachycardia, gallop rhythm, and cardiac enlargement. Heart murmurs or friction rubs are present in about one fourth of cases. Chest radiographs usually demonstrate globular cardiac enlargement. Electrocardiographic findings include S-T depression with or without T wave inversion. Both narrow and wide complex tachyarrhythmias occur.

Although the incidence of rheumatic fever is decreasing, the possibility of rheumatic pericarditis must be considered in children who are actually ill with fever, dyspnea, and pericardial pain. Systolic or diastolic murmurs or both are usually present, as is other evidence of rheumatic fever. Pericardial friction rub is common.[33]

Purulent (bacterial) pericarditis should be suspected in a young febrile child acutely ill with tachypnea, precordial pain, peripheral edema, and hepatomegaly. The heart is enlarged, and a friction rub may be present. Echocardiography confirms a pericardial effusion. The causative bacterium is identified by culture of the pericardiocentesis fluid. Pulsus paradoxus may be present. *Haemophilus influenzae* and *Staphylococcus aureus* are the most common etiologic agents. Intravenous therapy with appropriate antibiotics is required; however, surgical drainage of the pericardium is also usually necessary.

Pericarditis caused by tuberculosis is followed by a fibrotic reaction, which may lead to constrictive pericarditis. The effusion may clear more rapidly if corticosteroid therapy is added to the treatment regimen.[33]

Viral pericarditis may follow an upper respiratory tract infection, especially an enteroviral illness. The onset is usually acute and self-limited, but recurrences have been observed in up to 20% of the patients.[33]

The possibility of Kawasaki's mucocutaneous lymph node syndrome must be considered in an infant or a young child with heart failure and a prolonged, severe febrile illness. The disease is characterized by conjunctivitis, stomatitis, palmar and solar erythema with desquamation of the digits, lymphadenopathy, and erythema multiforme–type rashes. Platelet levels are commonly elevated. Myocarditis often begins early in the course of the disease. Pericarditis also may be present. Coronary artery vasculitis is a serious problem in Kawasaki's disease. Coronary artery aneurysms secondary to coronary vasculitis have been reported in 15% to 20% of children with Kawasaki's disease.[31, 34] Chest pain is a common complaint in children 4 years of age and older with Kawasaki's disease and myocardial infarction. One to two percent of children with the disease die of myocardial infarction secondary to obstruction of coronary arteries.[35]

Tumor involvement of the pericardium or the adjacent pleural space can occur in children and adolescents with Hodgkin's disease, acute lymphoblastic leukemia, non-Hodgkin's lymphoma, and metastatic osteogenic sarcoma. Radiation therapy to the mediastinum in patients with malignant tumors also produces pericarditis. Many children and adolescents with collagen diseases, especially lupus erythematosus and rheumatoid arthritis, develop pericarditis. Severe renal disease is a cause of uremic fibrous pericarditis.

Dysrhythmias

In children without associated cardiac diseases, prolonged supraventricular tachycardia may result in cardiac decompensation, insufficient myocardial oxygen supply, and ischemic chest pain. This pain must be differentiated from the sensation of chest discomfort caused by palpitation. Dizziness and syncope may be present. Resting electrocardiograms and Holter monitoring are diagnostic.

Isolated premature ventricular contractions or brief episodes of unsustained ventricular tachycardia rarely produce symptoms. Ventricular dysrhythmia associated with ventricular abnormality, dyspnea, and syncope, as well as demonstrated ventricular tachycardia during exercise, requires aggressive cardiac evaluation.[1]

PSYCHOGENIC CHEST PAIN

In most studies on chest pain in children authors have reported a significant number of cases in which no organic disease is found. Pantell and Goodman,[14] in a prospective study, found that of 100 adolescents with chest pain, 43 did not have a specific organic cause. Lababidi and

Wankum identified 36 of 98 children referred for chest pain as having idiopathic chest pain.[36] A diagnosis of psychogenic chest pain should be considered in children and adolescents when no organic etiologic agent is demonstrated and if a stressful situation, such as a recent death of or a separation from a significant family member or friend, is documented.[37] A family history of chest pain is often found in children with psychogenic chest pain. Children with recurrent or chronic organic disease often experience stress, anxiety, or depression associated with the illness and are at risk for developing psychogenic pain. Green emphasized that children with organic disease may have concomitant psychogenic symptoms.[38]

Psychogenic chest pain is real pain. It is responsible for significant restriction in physical activities and work or school absenteeism in children and adolescents.[4] The parents and the patient may distrust or deny initial suggestions of a psychogenic cause of the pain. The physician evaluating a child or an adolescent with psychogenic chest pain must carefully explain the findings to the patient and the parents, provide reassurance that no life-threatening illness exists, offer symptomatic relief of the pain, and schedule close clinical follow-up. In patients and families for whom serious psychological problems are diagnosed, a team approach with longitudinal follow-up, including evaluation and treatment by a psychiatrist, is needed in order to provide resolution of the emotional conflicts.

Hyperventilation is a common cause of psychogenic chest pain. The chest discomfort is presumed to result from (1) hypocapnic alkalosis, which causes coronary artery vasoconstriction; (2) aerophagia, which produces stomach distension and spasm of the left hemidiaphragm; or (3) transient arrhythmias.[14] Patients usually have associated paresthesias, dizziness, and weakness. Chest pain may occur in the subacute or chronic forms without obvious hyperventilation. In hyperventilation, the history usually reveals an underlying anxiety. Long-term treatment includes (1) reassurance by family and friends that hyperventilation can produce symptoms and (2) counseling to bring about resolution of the underlying stress.[4]

MISCELLANEOUS CAUSES OF CHEST PAIN

Pain attributed to so-called precordial catch syndrome occurs in some children aged 8 to 16 years. It is located at the left sternal border or apex and is described as a transient stabbing or knifelike pain that lasts less than 1 min. It is relieved by a forced inspiration and stretching from a slouched position. No cause has been identified. Reassuring the child and parents of its benign and self-limited nature is important.[39]

Chest pain from a stitch is believed to be caused during running by stress on the peritoneal ligaments, which are attached both to the rapidly moving diaphragm and to the heavy abdominal viscera. A sharp, cramping sensation is felt in the costal margin, and the pain can radiate to the right shoulder. It ceases with rest.[40]

Radicular pain may occur from vertebral column diseases or anatomic changes that impinge on the spinal cord or nerve roots. Examples include severe kyphoscoliosis

and vertebral collapse from infiltrative tumors, abscess formations, and aseptic necrosis from excessive and prolonged use of steroids.

Upper abdominal disease processes such as subdiaphragmatic abscess, hepatic tumor abscess, pancreatitis, splenic infarct, and cholelithiasis can produce pain referred to the chest.

REFERENCES

1. Brenner JI, Ringel RE, Berman MA: Cardiologic perspectives of chest pain in childhood: A referral problem? To whom? Pediatr Clin North Am 31:1241–1258, 1984.
2. Selbst SM: Evaluation of chest pain in children. Pediatr Rev 8(2):56–62, 1986.
3. Selbst SM: Chest pain in children. Pediatrics 75:1068–1070, 1985.
4. Coleman WL: Recurrent chest pain in children. Pediatr Clin North Am 31:1007–1026, 1984.
5. Selbst SM, Ruddy RM, Clark BJ, et al: Pediatric chest pain: A prospective study. Pediatrics 82:319–323, 1988.
6. Warwick R, Williams PL: Gray's Anatomy, 35th ed, pp. 1081–1083, 1194–1195. Philadelphia: WB Saunders, 1973.
7. Fraser RG, Paré JAP, Paré PD, et al: Methods in clinical, laboratory, and functional investigation. In Manke D (ed): Diagnosis of Diseases of the Chest, 3rd ed, vol. 1, pp. 393–394. Philadelphia: WB Saunders, 1988.
8. Green M: Sources of pain. In Levine M, Carey W, Crocker A, Gross R (eds): Developmental-Behavioral Pediatrics, pp. 512–518, Philadelphia: WB Saunders, 1983.
9. Fukushige J, Tsuchihashi K, Harada T, Ueda K: Chest pain in pediatric patients. Acta Paediatr Jpn 30:604–607, 1988.
10. Gersony WM: Evaluation of the cardiovascular system. In Behrman RE, Vaughan VC (eds): Nelson Textbook of Pediatrics, 12th ed, pp. 1100–1104. Philadelphia: WB Saunders, 1983.
11. Brown RT: Costochondritis in adolescents. J Adolesc Health Care 1:198–201, 1981.
12. Raney RB: Localized sarcoma of the chest wall. Med Pediatr Oncol 12:116–118, 1984.
13. Schaller JG, Wedgwood RJ: Rheumatic diseases of childhood. In Behrman RE, Vaughan VC (eds): Nelson Textbook of Pediatrics, 12th ed, pp. 579–582. Philadelphia: WB Saunders, 1983.
14. Pantell RH, Goodman BW: Adolescent chest pain: A prospective study. Pediatrics 71:881–887, 1983.
15. Nudel DB, Diamant S, Brady T, et al: Chest pain: Dyspnea on exertion, and exercise induced asthma in children and adolescents. Clin Pediatr 26:388–392, 1987.
16. Bierman CW, Pearlman DS: Asthma. In Kendig EL Jr, Chernick V (eds): Disorders of the Respiratory Tract in Children, pp. 497–538. Philadelphia: WB Saunders, 1983.
17. Luque MA, Cavallaro DL, Torres M, et al: Pneumomediastinum, pneumothorax, and subcutaneous emphysema after alternate cocaine inhalation and marijuana smoking. Pediatr Emerg Care 3:107–109, 1987.
18. Bernstein D, Coupey S, Schonberg SK: Pulmonary embolism in adolescents. J Dis Child 140:667–671, 1986.
19. Rich S: Primary pulmonary hypertension. Prog Cardiovasc Dis 31:205–238, 1988.
20. Berezin S, Medow MS, Glassman MS, Newman LJ: Chest pain of gastrointestinal origin. Arch Dis Child 63:1457–1460, 1988.
21. Herbst JJ: The esophagus: Development and function of the esophagus. In Behrman RE, Vaughan VC (eds): Nelson Textbook of Pediatrics, 12th ed, pp. 891–899. Philadelphia: WB Saunders, 1983.
22. Ajalat GM, Mulder DG: Esophageal perforations: The need for an individualized approach. Arch Surg 119:1318–1320, 1984.
23. Herbst JJ: The stomach and intestines: Ulcer disease. In Behrman RE, Vaughan VC (eds): Nelson Textbook of Pediatrics, 12th ed, pp. 901–904. Philadelphia: WB Saunders, 1983.
24. Brenner JI, Ringel RE, Berman MA: Chest pain in children: Identifying a source. Maryland Med J 34:481–487, 1985.
25. Markiewicz W, Stoner J, London E, et al: Mitral valve prolapse in one-hundred presumably healthy young females. Circulation 53:464–473, 1976.

26. Bissett GS, Schwartz DC, Meyer RA, et al: Clinical spectrum and long-term follow-up of isolated mitral valve prolapse in 119 children. Circulation 62:423–429, 1980.
27. Kavey RE, Sondheimer HM, Blackman MS: Ventricular arrhythmias and mitral valve prolapse in childhood. J Pediatr 105:885–890, 1984.
28. Gersony WM: Marfan syndrome: Cardiovascular manifestations. *In* Behrman RE, Vaughn VC (eds): Nelson Textbook of Pediatrics, 12th ed, p. 1167. Philadelphia: WB Saunders, 1983.
29. Lin AE, Lippe BM, Geffner ME, et al: Aortic dilation, dissection, and rupture in patients with Turner syndrome. J Pediatr 109:820–826, 1986.
30. Brenner JI, Berman MA: Chest pain in childhood and adolescence. J Adol Health Care 3:271–276, 1983.
31. Hohn AR, Stanton RE: Myocarditis in children. Pediatr Rev 9(3):83–87, 1987.
32. Gersony WM: Diseases of the myocardium: Conditions causing myocardial damage. *In* Behrman RE, Vaughan VC (eds): Nelson Textbook of Pediatrics, 12th ed, pp. 1183–1185. Philadelphia: WB Saunders, 1983.
33. Gersony WM: Diseases of the pericardium. *In* Behrman RE, Vaughan VC (eds): Nelson Textbook of Pediatrics, 12th ed, pp. 1191–1193. Philadelphia: WB Saunders, 1983.
34. Melish ME: Kawasaki syndrome (the mucocutaneous lymph node syndrome). Pediatr Ann 11:255–286, 1982.
35. Kato H, Schinose E, Kawasaki T: Myocardial infarction in Kawasaki disease: Clinical analyses in 195 cases. J Pediatr 108:923–927, 1986.
36. Lababidi Z, Wankum J: Pediatric idiopathic chest pain. Missouri Med 80:306–308, 1983.
37. Asnes RS, Santulli R, Benporad JR: Psychogenic chest pain in children. Clin Pediatr 20:788–791, 1981.
38. Green M: Psychogenic pain disorders. *In* Green M, Haggerty RJ (eds): Ambulatory Pediatrics III, pp. 245–249. Philadelphia: WB Saunders, 1984.
39. Diehl AM: Chest pain in children: Tip-offs to cause. Postgrad Med 73:335–342, 1983.
40. Feinstein RA, Daniel WA: Chronic chest pain in children and adolescents. Pediatr Ann 15:685–694, 1986.

20 CONTINUOUS NONINVASIVE MONITORING OF BLOOD GASES

ARUN K. PRAMANIK, M.D. / JAVIER DIAZ-BLANCO, M.D.

In critically ill, immature infants, oxygenation and ventilation may fluctuate widely, depending on the underlying pathologic entity and its management. Hypoxia may lead to injury of multiple organs, including brain damage, whereas hyperoxia may result in blindness from retinopathy of prematurity.

Until the 1980s repeated measurement of arterial blood gases was the mainstay in monitoring such infants, as it was for older patients with a variety of clinical disorders and during elective anesthesia or endoscopy. However, it is invasive and intermittent and requires replacement blood transfusion. Continuous measurement of cutaneous oxygen and carbon dioxide concentrations has been found to be an effective and valuable adjunct to the measurement of arterial blood gases in evaluating and managing critically ill patients regardless of age, in monitoring medical and surgical procedures, in studying sleep apnea, and in a variety of other situations.[1-4] Continuous monitoring of arterial oxygen saturation with a pulse oximeter is becoming standard practice in the care of these patients and in the care of healthy persons who require anesthesia or analgesia for diagnostic or surgical procedures.[5]

TRANSCUTANEOUS O_2 AND CO_2 MONITORS

The first record of measurement of gases through the skin is found in the 1851 experiments by P. Gerlach, a German veterinarian, who postulated a possible relationship between the measured values of transepidermal gas and skin blood flow.[6] After a dormant period of a century, research in blood gas measurement led to the development of the Clark O_2 electrode and the CO_2 electrode devised by R. W. Stowe and J. W. Severinghaus in the 1950s.[6-8] Finally, after several years of research in the 1970s, A. Huch, R. Huch, and M. Eberhard were the first scientists to independently report use of a heated Clark electrode to measure skin oxygen equivalent to the arterial oxygen tension.[9]

It is essential for physicians and others working with transcutaneous monitors to understand its principles. Thus in developing transcutaneous monitors, it was necessary to evolve a technique by which the skin (P_{O_2}) approximated the oxygen tension in the arterial blood (Pa_{O_2}). This was accomplished by heating the skin to

Skin Resistance To Oxygen Diffusion

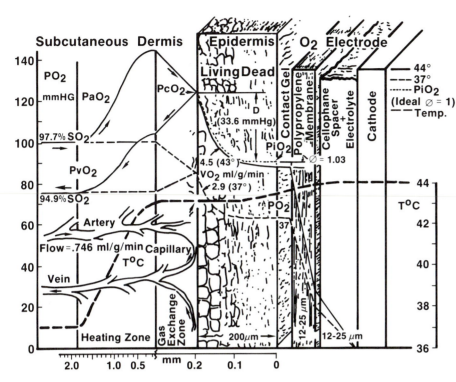

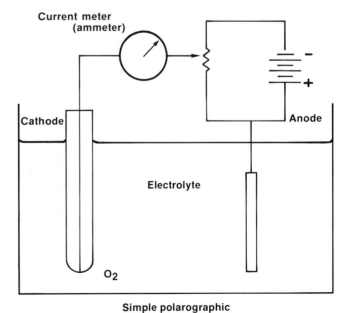

Figure 20–1. Schematic representation of the profiles of temperature and P_{O_2} within the normal adult skin and electrode membrane. The interrupted P_{O_2} line should be with a non-O_2-consuming electrode. (From Stow RW, Randall BF: Electrical measurements of the PCO_2 of blood. Am J Physiol 179:678, 1954.)

increase blood flow in the area under the sensor until it reached an independent flow state, consequently increasing the diffusion of oxygen to the epidermis. Heat increases the skin blood flow to levels above its metabolic needs, thereby increasing the amount of oxygen available to the sensor (Fig. 20–1).[10] Although concurrent increases in the metabolism of the living epidermis decrease oxygen availability, the shift in the hemoglobin-oxygen dissociation curve to the right increases oxygen release and thus the amount of oxygen available to the sensor. Heating also decreases oxygen solubility in the blood, further increasing P_{O_2}. This is again counterbalanced by oxygen consumption by the electrode and the diffusion gradients of the skin and membrane, all of which lower the measured P_{O_2}.[4,10] These opposing effects cancel each other, the net result being that the skin P_{O_2} approximates the Pa_{O_2}.

In order for oxygen to be available to the sensor, the hemoglobin saturation must be at least 50% to meet the oxygen demand for the increased skin metabolism with the higher temperature; conversely, at Pa_{O_2} levels above that necessary to maintain 100% saturation of hemoglobin, the excess oxygen is dissolved back into plasma faster than the molecules can be reduced in the oxygen sensor. Consequently, the best correlation with transcutaneous oxygen tension (tcP_{O_2}) occurs when the Pa_{O_2} is between 50 and 100 mm Hg. Subtle differences in sensor temperature, membrane properties, and electrode manufacture can affect the measured P_{O_2}, as can the patient's condition—for example, such factors as skin perfusion, skin thickness, edema, and drugs that affect blood flow.[4]

The tcP_{O_2} electrode is a modified Clark electrode,[6] wherein the oxygen sensor is a polarographic cell consisting of two electrodes (Fig. 20–2). In the working electrode,

or cathode, oxygen molecules are reduced (oxygen consumed) or measured and a new product is formed.[1,3,6,9,11] The cathode is made of a metal such as gold or platinum to prevent oxides from coating the surface of the electrode. The reference electrode, or anode, is where the measurement is standardized or compared. Both electrodes are dipped in an electrolyte bath and connected to

Figure 20–2. Diagramatic representation of the principle of an oxygen electrode.

a measuring instrument. The cathode is connected to an external circuit that produces a polarizing voltage that is measured in a current meter. When the cathode is made negative with regard to the anode, the oxygen molecules at the surface of the cathode are reduced, which results in a current that can be measured (see Fig. 20–2).

The transcutaneous carbon dioxide (tcP_{CO_2}) electrode is a modified glass pH electrode designed according to the principle that when two solutions are separated by glass, the potential difference from one side to the other is proportional to the difference in pH of the solutions.[1, 7, 12] Figure 20–3 shows that the tcP_{CO_2} electrode is housed behind a membrane that can be permeated by carbon dioxide molecules, with a bicarbonate layer placed between the pH electrode and the membrane. The pH electrode is the working electrode and is placed along with the reference electrode in a bicarbonate solution. When the bicarbonate solution is exposed to a study specimen, alterations in the pH change the baseline potential difference across the glass surface, and this difference is registered as a voltage change in the voltmeter. The glass pH electrode is separated from the specimen by a membrane permeable by carbon dioxide; thus, when the CO_2 molecules diffuse into the bicarbonate solution, its pH changes (Fig. 20–4). Because the relationship between CO_2 and voltage is curvilinear, the CO_2 electrode is calibrated with two carbon dioxide mixtures (usually 5% and 10%) and is thereafter checked for drift every four hours.[7, 8, 12–16]

The combined tcP_{O_2}/P_{CO_2} sensor is a single device in which a Clark polarographic electrode (platinum wire) is used with a Stowe-Severinghaus CO_2 electrode bulb of pH-sensitive glass and a common reference electrode, an electrolyte solution, a heating element, and a membrane.[2, 17–19] The electrode solution contains potassium chloride, sodium bicarbonate, and ethylene glycol.[2] The membrane is usually made of cellophane or polytef (Teflon). The combined sensor consistently overestimates the

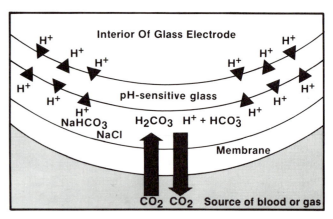

Principle Of The Practical Carbon Dioxide Electrode

Figure 20–4. Close-up view of the carbon dioxide electrode, demonstrating the exchange of carbon dioxide and H ion between the membrane and the glass.

tcP_{CO_2}. The reason for this overestimation is not clear; it has been attributed to heat-induced increase in metabolism, to anaerobic heating coefficient of blood, and to accumulated CO_2 not consumed by the skin or by the CO_2 sensor.[14, 16] The partial pressure of CO_2 at the level of the skin must be less than the arterial CO_2 tension (Pa_{CO_2}) in order for CO_2 to diffuse to the surface of the skin. Several studies have shown a strong correlation between tcP_{CO_2} and Pa_{CO_2} with the introduction of a correction factor.[2, 13–16] Some manufacturers have addressed this problem by a built-in correction mechanism. In one study in which two combined tcP_{O_2}/P_{CO_2} sensors were compared for neonates, infants, and children, the instruments were to be convenient to use, and even though the tcP_{O_2} was acceptable in both models (Kontron and Radiometer), the tcP_{CO_2} electrode had reduced performance in comparison with a single electrode.[20]

In the tcP_{CO_2} or tcP_{O_2}/P_{CO_2} electrode, in order to avoid drift, the membrane must not be exposed to air for long periods of time. These electrodes should be frequently used, and when not used, they should be kept exposed to a calibration gas or covered. Drift is presumed to be caused by the interaction of $H+$ and $OH-$ with the glass surface, which alters the electrolyte ionic composition.[13, 14, 19]

CLINICAL USES

During the 1980s, transcutaneous monitoring was found to be useful in preventing hyperoxia or hypoxia in newborns, particularly premature infants. Hyperoxia causes retinopathy of prematurity, which is the leading cause of blindness in early infancy. Several authors have suggested that the incidence of retinopathy of prematurity may be decreased by the use of transcutaneous oxygen monitoring.[4, 21] In a prospective study, in the group with continuous tcP_{O_2} monitoring, Bancalari and associates[22] did not observe a decrease in incidence of retinopathy of prematurity in infants with a birth weight less than 1000 g; however, in infants with a birth weight more than 1000

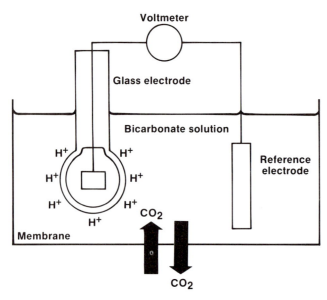

A carbon dioxide electrode system

Figure 20–3. Schema of the principle involved in a carbon dioxide electrode.

g, the incidence of retinopathy of prematurity decreased with continuous tcP_{O_2} monitoring. The tcP_{O_2} monitoring may also reduce the hyperoxia that occurs when assisted manual ventilation is administered to premature infants. The tcP_{O_2} sensor may underestimate Pa_{O_2} in infants with hyperoxemia ($Pa_{O_2} > 100$ mm Hg).[4, 23] Rome and colleagues[24] showed that the validity of tcP_{O_2} monitoring may be significantly improved in infants with bronchopulmonary dysplasia beyond 10 weeks of age when approximately 15 mm Hg is added to the resting tcP_{O_2} value.

The complications related to the manipulation of arterial catheters (e.g., thrombosis, infection) and the total number of blood gases and blood transfusions, along with laboratory costs per patient, may be decreased with the use of TcP_{O_2} monitors.[25] Because critically ill neonates are sensitive to external stimuli, even routine nursing procedures (such as endotracheal suctioning, nipple or gavage feeding, nasogastric tube placement, starting intravenous lines, and weighing), medical procedures (such as lumbar puncture, bladder catheterization, umbilical vessel catheterizations, intubation, and chest tube placement), and noise may lead to significant hypoxemia.[26]

Uses in Apnea of Prematurity

Apnea leading to sustained hypoxia and other complications can be prevented. The tcP_{O_2} monitor may also help to differentiate obstructive apnea from apnea of central origin. Conventional respiratory rate monitors are designed to detect only respiratory movements by perceiving a change in the impedance between the electrodes. In obstructive apnea, the chest movement persists in spite of lack of air movement, and the patient becomes hypoxic, which may be detected through the appropriate use of continuous tcP_{O_2} monitoring.[4]

Uses in Persistent Pulmonary Hypertension

The tcP_{O_2} monitors may also be helpful in the diagnosis and management of persistent pulmonary hypertension of the newborn (PPHN). When patients are suspected of having PPHN, a hyperoxia test is usually performed to rule out the possibility of cyanotic heart disease; tcP_{O_2} sensors can assist in determining the oxygenation response. Also, through the placement of tcP_{O_2} sensors pre- and postductally, the degree of right-to-left shunt through the patent ductus arteriosus can be estimated not only in patients with PPHN but also in patients with respiratory distress syndrome.[27]

Uses in Infants, Children, and Adults

Transcutaneous monitoring of P_{O_2} and P_{CO_2} has also been used successfully in some pediatric and adult patients and in animal experiments to detect early blood loss, shock, and venous diseases.[28–33] Furthermore, Fanconi and co-workers[34] found in a prospective study that tcP_{CO_2} monitoring was a reliable and objective tool for managing patients with upper airway obstruction, whereas croup scores were misleading.

LIMITATION OF TRANSCUTANEOUS MONITORS

The use of transcutaneous monitors, particularly tcP_{CO_2}, may not correlate with Pa_{CO_2} in patients with congenital heart disease and in cardiac patients after surgery, presumably because of a decrease in peripheral circulation.[35]

Certain pharmacologic agents altering cutaneous blood flow may affect transcutaneous O_2 and CO_2 values. Tolazoline (Priscoline), which causes peripheral vasodilation, may alter the tcP_{O_2}/Pa_{O_2} ratio.[36] Halothane and nitrous oxide may produce falsely high tcP_{O_2} values.[37] However, manufacturers have increased the negative potential difference of the electrodes in order to minimize this problem.

Some clinicians have found tcP_{O_2} monitors to be unreliable, particularly when the peripheral skin perfusion is decreased. The tcP_{O_2} electrodes are designed to measure oxygen tension at the level of the skin, and thus skin O_2 tension is equivalent to arterial O_2 tension only when certain prerequisite conditions are met, adequate skin perfusion being one of them (as described in the introduction to this section). Therefore, in patients with severe edema, acidosis, anemia, and shock or in those given an inhaled anesthetic, the tcP_{O_2} values are not equivalent to Pa_{O_2}.[3, 4, 36] In such conditions, the clinician, after ruling out technical reasons for poor correlation, should look for pathologic causes of poor skin perfusion and correct them rather than dismiss the tcP_{O_2} measurement as unreliable and useless. The earliest indicator of imminent shock may be a poor correlation between tcP_{O_2} and Pa_{O_2} values preceding tachycardia and decrease in blood pressure.[3, 4, 30, 31] This poor tcP_{O_2} reliability has been found to be helpful in the administration of parenteral fluids in clinical conditions with impending hypotension, shock, and necrotizing enterocolitis.[30, 31, 38]

Causes of High tcP_{O_2}

1. Hyperoxemia.
2. Technical reasons: air leak around the adhesive tape or in the electrolyte solution; faulty membrane preparation and calibration.
3. Physiological reasons: excessive sensor temperature ($>44°C$) for a very premature infant (even though the recommendation is 44°C for the premature baby, 43.5°C or less may be necessary when tcP_{O_2} is overestimating Pa_{O_2}).
4. Pharmacologic reasons: halothane, nitrous oxide.

Causes of Low tcP_{O_2}

1. Hypoxemia.
2. Technical reasons: temperature $>45°C$, skin burn, pressure on electrode (e.g., infant lying on it); positioning the electrode over bony prominence; lack of skin preparation; presence of meconium, vernix, or oily medications.
3. Physiologic reasons: shock, hypothermia, postcardiac surgery, congenital cyanotic heart disease, severe

edema, severe acidosis, severe anemia, postductal shunt position.

Side Effects Encountered with tcP_{O_2} Monitoring

All side effects are local. Transient erythema under the electrode site is present in all infants. Blisters occur in 0.1% of cases and can be avoided by changing the location of the tcP_{O_2} electrode every 4 h.[4, 13] However, patients with poor skin perfusion are more prone to blistering because the heating power of the electrode must increase in order to maintain the desired skin temperature.[13] Hyperpigmented skin craters have also been reported.[39]

Transcutaneous monitors are a valuable adjunct in the management of ill newborns. Not only does tcP_{O_2} give information about the infant's oxygenation status, but a fall in tcP_{O_2} may alert the clinician to an impending hypotension. Similarly, tcP_{O_2} readings may give a clue to a mechanical problem within the ventilator or the endotracheal tube or perhaps to an intrinsic problem caused by a change in the patient's clinical status.

Adequate performance of transcutaneous electrodes requires not only certain minimal benchmark standards but also a thorough understanding by the operator of the underlying physiology and technique.[1, 2, 4, 10, 11, 13, 14, 23, 24] Limitations of the apparatus are not widely understood, and marketing in some instances is misleading with regard to the simplicity of the method.[4] Before purchasing a device, the operator should evaluate the performance data obtained on the skin of human neonates throughout the range of Pa_{O_2} or P_{CO_2} values, or both, for which its use is recommended, by using the same device and specifying crucial details such as operating temperature.

PULSE OXIMETRY

The purposes of the rest of this chapter are (1) to familiarize the reader with the important milestones in the development of pulse oximetry, (2) to review the principles of pulse oximetry and their limitations, (3) to provide a background for evaluating the use of the pulse oximeter in a specific clinical situation, and (4) to discuss the advantages and disadvantages of some of the commonly marketed pulse oximeters.

HISTORICAL PERSPECTIVE IN THE MEASUREMENTS OF OXYGEN SATURATION AND PULSE OXIMETRY

The spectroscope, invented in 1860 by Robert Bunsen, first enabled analysis of the wavelength composition of light, but it was not until the selenium barrier-layer photocell became practical in the 1930s that spectra could be used for quantitative analysis of O_2 saturation. The reaction of oxygen with hemoglobin greatly increases the transmission of red light through hemoglobin solutions and blood; in the infrared wavelength, the effect is opposite, making blood more opaque.

Spectrophotometric analysis of O_2 saturation in tissue was introduced in 1932.[40] However, the first devices that could measure O_2 saturation through tissues were developed independently by K. Mathes and K. Kramer in 1935.[40, 41] Kramer showed that transmission of red light was dependent on oxygen saturation, but he used only a single wavelength of light, one that was dependent on oxygen saturation (and the other independent), thus compensating for hemoglobin content and tissue thickness. Mathes and others originally used green light as the saturation-independent wavelength. Because the filters that they used to produce green light were transparent to infrared light and because little green light penetrates the tissue, these pioneers actually were unknowingly using infrared light as the saturation-independent wavelength.

Stimulated by the needs of the aviation industry during World War II, research in this field progressed rapidly. In 1940, Squire reported that a tissue oximeter reading could be reduced to zero by compressing the tissue to squeeze out the blood. He was also the first scientist to equalize the light intensities of the red and infrared light when blood was flowing in the tissue.

These ideas contributed to modern pulse oximetry. Glen Millikan coined the term *oximetry* and in 1942 developed a small ear oximeter for aviation research. A few years later, two Mayo Clinic investigators, Earl Wood and J. Geraci, improved on Millikan's ear oximeter by incorporating an inflatable capsule for zeroing and by devising an electronic method of dividing the red signal by the infrared signal to display saturation continuously; this method became a standard technique for physiologic research.[5, 40, 41] In the 1960s, Robert Shaw developed a self-calibrating ear oximeter, manufactured by Hewlett-Packard Company, that was accurate but not widely used because it was cumbersome and expensive. In 1975, S. Nakajima and his associates introduced the pulse oximeter.[40] By analyzing the ratio of the pulse-added absorbances of red and infrared light, their device could accurately determine the hemoglobin saturation on various thickness and skin colors through the use of only two wavelengths of light. In this device, developed by Minolta, fiberoptics were used to transmit the light signals to and from a finger sensor. Because the device was cumbersome, it was quickly replaced in the early 1980s by BTI Biox (Boulder, Colorado), in which light-emitting diodes (LEDs) in a finger or ear sensor produced the red and infrared light. This innovation led to the manufacture of the modern light-weight, inexpensive monitors and sensors. Even disposable sensors have been devised.

Today, it is commonplace to use pulse oximeters to diagnose hypoxemia in the management of patients in intensive care units, in operating rooms, and in a variety of clinical settings.[5, 41, 42] For a more comprehensive history on the development of oximetry, the reader is referred to several excellent reviews.[40, 41, 43]

PRINCIPLES OF PULSE OXIMETRY

Noninvasive pulse oximeters estimate arterial hemoglobin saturation by measuring red and infrared light transmitted through a tissue bed at two different wave-

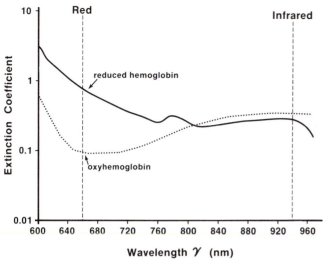

Figure 20-5. Light absorption (extinction) as a function of wavelength for the two hemoglobins measured by a pulse oximeter: oxyhemoglobin and deoxyhemoglobin.

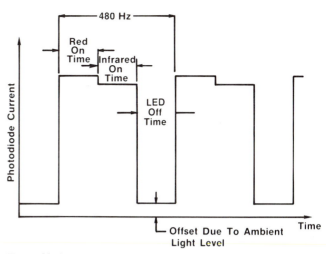

Figure 20-6. Light-emitting diode on-off cycle for a pulse oximeter. During a third phase, both the red and infrared diodes are off and are built in Ohmeda 3700 to compensate for ambient light. (Reproduced with permission from Ohmeda.)

lengths (Fig. 20–5) in order to effectively distinguish between the two commonly present hemoglobin species: oxyhemoglobin (HbO_2) and reduced hemoglobin, or deoxyhemoglobin.[5, 42–44] Most pulse oximeters in current use accomplish this by means of a light source that consists of two LEDs: one emitting red light (at 660 nm) and the other infrared light (at 940 nm). HbO_2 appears red because it absorbs less red light than does deoxyhemoglobin. At the infrared wavelength, the opposite is true, although to a lesser extent (Fig. 20–5). The instrument passes red and infrared light through pulsatile tissue at the sensor site and, many times each second, measures the amount of light that is transmitted through the tissue. Each LED is illuminated in turn at varying frequencies, which may be as high as several hundred Hertz. Some manufacturers of pulse oximeters have used a third phase in which both LEDs are off (Fig. 20–6), thus allowing the oximeter to compensate for extraneous light sources that may interfere with measurements by striking the photodetector.[43, 44] The photodetector is positioned on the opposite side of the tissue (e.g., finger, foot, ear, or nose) that is being monitored and cannot differentiate between different sources or wavelengths of light. Therefore, at any given time, the software of the oximeter assumes that the wavelength of the light reaching the photodetector corresponds to that of the concurrently illuminated LED.

During each cardiac cycle, the light absorption by the tissue beds varies cyclically (Fig. 20–7). During each diastole, the light is absorbed by venous and capillary blood, tissue, pigment (e.g., melanin, nail polish), and bone. During systole, light absorption increases, which is assumed to be the result of an influx of arterialized blood into the tissue bed. By subtracting the peak absorption during the systole from its background readings during diastole at both red and infrared wavelengths, the absorption computed by the oximeter is assumed to be that of arterialized blood. Oxygen saturation is calculated by the pulse oximeter (Sp_{O_2}) from the red infrared absorption ratio, which is an estimate of arterial oxygen saturation (Sa_{O_2}).[43, 44]

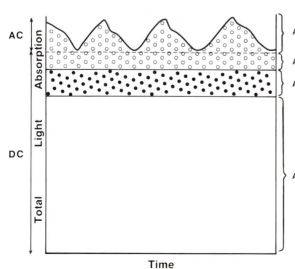

Figure 20-7. Schematic illustration of the light absorption through the various layers of tissue. The AC signal is triggered by the pulsatile component of the arterial blood; the DC signal is composed of all the nonpulsatile absorbers in the tissue, in nonpulsatile arterial blood, in venous and capillary blood, and in all other tissues.

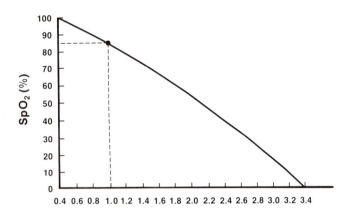

$$R = \frac{AC_{660}/DC_{660}}{AC_{940}/DC_{940}}$$

Figure 20–8. Typical empirically determined calibration curve showing oxygen saturation (Sp_{O_2}) as a function of red:infrared absorption ratio. Note that the Sp_{O_2} estimate is determined from the ratio (R) of the pulse-added red absorbance at 660 nanometers to pulse-added infrared absorbance at 940 nanometers. This ratio is one at a saturation of approximately 85%. (From Tremper KK, Barker SJ: Pulse oximetry. Anesthesiology 70:98–108, 1989.)

LIMITATIONS OF PULSE OXIMETERS

It is important to note not only that light is absorbed by the hemoglobin but also that refraction and scattering of this light beam occur within the tissue bed. Light scatter or reflection at the interphase of red blood cells and plasma may account for more than 50% of the absorption of whole blood at 660 nm,[43, 44] whereas at the tissue-bone interface, reflection may account for differences in calibration between the pulse oximeter probes used on the ear and those used on the finger or the feet, as in neonates.[44]

Because of reflection or light scattering, manufacturers have calibrated pulse oximeters by using empirical *in vivo* data from adult volunteers (Fig. 20–8). Because reliable human calibration data involving saturation levels of less than 70% and different forms of hemoglobin (e.g., fetal hemoglobin) are not available, the accuracy of pulse oximeters is decreased during extreme hypoxemia and hyperoxemia.[5, 43, 45–49] Hyperbilirubinemia, which is common in the neonatal period, does not interfere with pulse oximetry;[50] neither does skin pigmentation.[51] Table 20–1 outlines the advantages and disadvantages of pulse oximetry in comparison with transcutaneous P_{O_2} monitoring. Some of the intrinsic substances and extrinsic factors that interfere with the saturation readings of pulse oximeters are listed in Table 20–2.

Intrinsic Interference

Intrinsic interference is caused by substances within the patient's body that have an absorption at either a 660- or a 940-nm wavelength of light.[5, 43] Because only these two wavelengths are used in all currently manufactured pulse oximeters, these devices do not differentiate between more than two types of hemoglobin (i.e., HbO_2 and deoxyhemoglobin). If another form of hemoglobin is present, pulse oximetry readings may correlate poorly with co-oximetry values of HbO_2.[5, 43, 44, 52] Barker and Tremper reported that in carbon monoxide poisoning, pulse oximetry readings are higher than true HbO_2 levels by co-oximetry; consequently, the physician is not alerted to potentially lethal hypoxia.[52] Methemoglobin formation also affects pulse oximeter readings.[53] Methemoglobin is formed by converting the iron in the hemoglobin to ferric state, in which it cannot bind to oxygen. Methemoglobin absorbs more light at both 660 and 940 nm than does HbO_2 or deoxyhemoglobin but has disproportionately higher absorbance at 660 nm. The result, an increase in the 660-/940-nm absorbance ratio, is interpreted by the pulse oximeter as a reduction in oxygen saturation. It is estimated that when methemoglobin constitutes more than 65% of total hemoglobin, the 660-/940-nm light absorption ratio approaches 1.27, generating Sa_{O_2} readings of 75% to 80% even though the maximal possible HbO_2 value is 35%.[53] Therefore, with increasing methemoglobin concentrations, the pulse oximeter progres-

Table 20–1. ADVANTAGES AND DISADVANTAGES OF PULSE OXIMETRY AND OF TRANSCUTANEOUS PO_2 MONITORING

Pulse Oximetry	Transcutaneous PO_2 Monitoring
Advantages	***Advantages***
No skin heating	May be combined with a P_{CO_2} electrode
No calibration	Good correlation with Pa_{O_2} in younger neonates
No drift	If $tcP_{O_2} > 100$, possible hyperoxemia (if no air under electrode)
More reliable for detecting hypoxia	May detect early hypotension
Measures arterial pulse additionally (accurately with C-lock in Nelcor-200)	May diagnose right-to-left shunt through patent ductus arteriosus
Disadvantages	***Disadvantages***
Movement artifacts (minimized with Nelcor-200)	Skin burning and abrasion (minimized with skin temperature at 43°C and with site change every 4 h)
Poor circulation registered by low-quality signal	Requires calibration
Interference with phototherapy	Electrode drift
Pressure necrosis/infection in extremely small, critically ill neonates	Requires membrane change
Unreliable in diagnosing hyperoxia: because of the flat part of the HbO_2 dissociation curve, poor correlation with Pa_{O_2} at $Sa_{O_2} > 95\%$	Falls off patient easily
	Air may leak under electrode
	Interference with drugs (e.g., tolazoline [Priscoline], halothane, nitrous oxide)
	Poor circulation results in low values

Table 20–2. FACTORS INTERFERING WITH RELIABILITY OF PULSE OXIMETERS

Intrinsic Substances
Carboxyhemoglobin
Methemoglobin
Dyes (e.g., methylene blue, indigo carmine, indocyanine green)
Nail polish (other than red), footprint dye
Severe desaturation
Extrinsic Factors
Motion artifact
Compression of sensor or reuse of disposable sensor (adhesive)
Weak pulse signals
Electrocautery
Overhead xenon-arc surgical or infrared heating lamps

sively overestimates oxygen saturation, and the physician is unaware of the dangerous hypoxic state of the patient. A disparity between oxygen saturation calculated from Pa_{O_2} values and pulse oximetry readings can be an important clue to the presence of abnormal hemoglobins. Therapy in these instances should be guided by direct measurement of HbO_2 and of methemoglobin or carboxyhemoglobin and not by measurements by means of pulse oximetry or an estimate of calculated oxygen saturation.[54]

A number of dyes (e.g., methylene blue, indigo carmine, and indocyanine green) have a dose-dependent artifactual effect on HbO_2 and therefore on Sa_{O_2} readings.[5, 43, 55] These effects are transient, lasting for less than 10 min because of redistribution; when dye has redistributed to the nonpulsatile tissue compartment, there is no further effect on pulse oximetry readings.[5]

Opaque coatings of nail polish[43] or dyes[56] used to obtain footprints in neonates may significantly decrease light transmission, rendering oximeters inoperative. Certain shades of blue nail polish have strong absorption bands in the vicinity of 660 nm, resulting in falsely low pulse oximeter readings.

Extrinsic Interference

A patient's movement interferes with pulse oximeter readings. First, because of the shape and the bulk of the oximeter probe, the orientation of the probe with regard to the finger tends to change with motion. In evaluating several probes, Alexander and co-workers concluded that oximeters with large or massive probes (e.g., Physio-Control, Invivo) were more susceptible to artifactual reading caused by motion than were relatively light-weight probes (e.g., SensorMedics, Criticare).[43] A possible second source of motion interference is the current that is induced in the connecting cable when it moves in relation to the earth's magnetic field. In order to determine whether oximeters were able to update readings during motion rather than displaying previously obtained data, experiments were conducted on healthy volunteers who breathed a hypoxic gas mixture until Sp_{O_2} was 90% and who were then asked to wiggle their fingers while discontinuing the hypoxic gas mixture.[43] Most oximeters returned quickly to their pre-hypoxia level except the one by Physio-Control, which was unable to keep track of changes and continued to show readings of 0% Sa_{O_2} for approximately 15 sec before recovering.[43]

In conventional pulse oximeters, movement by the patient and poor peripheral pulses may interfere with performance because the oximeter is unable to distinguish between the true optical pulse signal and background noise. A novel approach to this problem was introduced by Nelcor with its C-lock electrocardiographic synchronization, wherein the pulse oximeter uses the electrocardiographic QRS complex as a timing indicator that optical pulse will soon appear at the sensor site; this technique theoretically improves the instrument's ability to distinguish a true pulse resulting from myocardial contractility from motion artifact and background noise, which normally are random with regard to the electrocardiogram. However, one group of investigators reported that readings by this oximeter may be synchronized with the electrocardiographic artifact caused by motion or shivering, thereby giving erroneous readings.[43] Furthermore, because of the synchronization, the pulse rates by the oximeter and the cardiac monitor are the same and should therefore not be used as an indicator that the displayed saturation data are valid.

Pulse oximeters differ considerably in ability to function in the presence of electrocautery. Because of special shielding and suppression circuiting, there is no interference by electrocautery in the Datascope oximeter.[43] In other monitors (Criticare, Nelcor-200, Physio-Control, and SARA) that were evaluated on patients with weak pulse signals, there appeared to be erroneous readings during electrocautery.[43, 57] The oximeter by Ohmeda stops acquiring data and gives an error message when interfered with by electrocautery.[43]

Xenon-arc surgical lamps and infrared lamps, because of their flicker frequencies, may interfere with pulse oximeters and produce erroneously high or low readings.[5, 43] This problem can be minimized by using a probe designed to prevent extraneous light from reaching the photodetector. Probes with this modification are oximeters by Criticare and SARA.[43] Other oximeters, such as Ohmeda and Invivo, that have a built-in mechanism to detect extrinsic light sources (i.e., not coming from LEDs) indicate interference with an error message or an abnormal waveform, in which case the problem can be corrected easily by covering the probe with an opaque sheet. In contrast, oximeters such as the Nelcor-200 that lack a waveform or diagnostic message display may give false readings even without interference and with no improvement from electrocardiographic synchronization, as discussed earlier.[43]

SIGNAL VERIFICATION[5, 43, 57]

As mentioned, a true pulse waveform ensures that valid pulses rather than interfering signals are being detected.[5, 43–44, 58] By increasing the amplitude of weak signals, some oximeters (e.g., Ohmeda, Invivo) enable signals to be easily visualized. Several devices (Catalyst, Datascope, Invivo, Ohmeda) show absolute signal strength, which indicates that the Sa_{O_2} readings are reliable and also serves as an indicator of relative peripheral perfusion (e.g., decrease in signal strength may indicate vasoconstriction or low cardiac output). The Ohmeda device has a real-time display of signal strength and pulse waveforms, which may be helpful for comparing other cardiovascular events and therapy in the patient. Some manufacturers (e.g., SARA, Datascope) enable the oximeter waveform to be displayed on other monitors, which may be cost effective in some circumstances.

STATUS MESSAGES, PULSE BEEPS, AND ALARMS[5, 43, 57, 58]

Several units warn the user about possible problems by displaying specific messages on the screen.[43] Some (e.g., Nelcor, Physio-Control) use "pulse search" for most abnormal situations, which is an undesirable system because it may pick up motion artifact.

All pulse oximeters emit a beep, which coincides with the detection of each systolic wave. In the optimal design present in most oximeters (except Catalyst, Criticare, and SARA), the pitch of the beep is proportional to the Sp_{O_2}. Thus any physician providing care for the patient can be made aware of changes in Sp_{O_2} before the alarm is triggered, even if the digital Sp_{O_2} reading is not in the direct field of vision.

A variety of alarms and their adjustability, acceptability, retention in memory, interferences, and accidental disabling are discussed in detail elsewhere.[5, 43, 57] Before purchasing an oximeter, the authors found it worthwhile to get the primary care providers to understand and evaluate these features so that they would be used to their full potential; for example, alarms would not be turned off because they were annoying or were confused with other alarms in the intensive care unit.

ACCURACY

A number of investigators and manufacturers have compared the Sp_{O_2} reading of oximeters with a gold standard: namely, *in vitro* Sa_{O_2} measurements.[5, 44, 47–49, 54, 58–61] Unfortunately, this comparison is misleading because the correlation coefficient does not measure agreement; instead, it measures association.[5] Pulse oximeter Sp_{O_2} and Sa_{O_2} values are highly associated, and so a significant correlation is to be expected. This form of analysis does not indicate whether one method is superior to the other or what degree of confidence an investigator can have in a new measurement. Therefore, it has been proposed that the means and the standard deviation of the difference between the two methods of measurement should be estimated. The mean of the difference is called *bias* and shows a systematic overestimate or underestimate of one method in relation to the other. The standard deviation, on the other hand, indicates precision and represents variability, or random error. If systematic random errors are clinically acceptable, one method can be replaced by the other.

Unfortunately, many investigators of pulse oximetry have used correlation coefficient and linear regression analysis, and thus it is difficult to compare their results for accuracy without bias and precision values.[5, 44, 47–49, 58–61] Most manufacturers contend that their pulse oximeters are accurate within $\pm 2\%$ from 70% to 100% saturation and within $\pm 3\%$ from 50% to 70% saturation, with no specified accuracy below 50% saturation. Thus for Sp_{O_2} values higher than 70%, approximately 68% of the data can be expected to fall within $\pm 2\%$ of a line of identity and 95% of the data to fall within $\pm 4\%$ (or 2 standard deviations).

In two reports, investigators compared data from various authors and discussed the limitations in accuracy and response of oximeters by different manufacturers.[5, 43] It is also important to consider whether the equipment was tested both on normal volunteers and on critically ill patients in different age groups and in a variety of settings.

OXIMETER AND PROBE DESIGN

The size, ease of use, and accessibility of controls in the monitor are also factors that should be considered before a new unit is obtained.[5, 43, 57] Most oximeters have internal batteries that enable the unit to operate for 0.5 to 12 h before recharging; this factor should be taken into consideration if oximeters are going to be used for transporting critically ill patients.[61] There are two types of display screens, which must also be considered: (1) liquid crystal displays, which have the advantage of low battery drain but may be difficult to read, particularly if the back is not lit,[43] and (2) LED displays, which are easier to read but may be invisible through the protective glasses used with CO_2 lasers in the operating room.[43]

Probes can be those with (1) Velcro or straps, which are designed to be placed around the finger or the palms and soles of infants, or (2) clips for the earlobe or the tongue.[43, 57] These probes may be disposable or reusable. A number of these devices have been tested.[43, 57] If probes are inaccessible because of drapes during surgery or a diagnostic procedure, they must be taped securely over the fingers, the palm, or the sole. However, caution must be exercised to avoid excessive pressure, which may cause pulsatile venous congestion and result in falsely low Sp_{O_2} readings. Tape-on probes are less susceptible to motion artifact. When disposable probes are reused, stray adhesive on the optical surface may produce erroneous readings.[43] Clip-on probes are used in adults and older children in whom the detection of rapid Sp_{O_2} response changes to inspired oxygen is critical, in patients with poor peripheral perfusion, or when the arm is not accessible. Rubbing the ear with alcohol or nitroglycerin ointment increases earlobe perfusion and, therefore, the performance of the oximeter.[43]

CHOICE OF OXIMETER

This question is often asked, but there is no simple answer. Each institution or user should evaluate several oximeters that meet the specific purpose, keeping in mind the principles and problems discussed earlier in this chapter. The cost of the oximeter and the probes (particularly the disposable ones) varies considerably and is not necessarily reflected in accuracy or reliability of the device. The reader is again referred to several excellent reviews that focused on this issue.[5, 43, 57] It must also be kept in mind that significant software and hardware changes are constantly being introduced in this rapidly expanding market.

CLINICAL APPLICATIONS

During Anesthesia

Pulse oximetry has been widely used by anesthesiologists. With the development of this new technology, it is important and ethically feasible for clinicians to undertake carefully controlled, randomized studies in order to evaluate its effectiveness. In such a carefully undertaken clinical study, Cote and colleagues established the necessity of continuous Sp_{O_2} monitoring during pediatric anesthesia.[62] They monitored Sp_{O_2} continuously in 152 anesthetized patients, for half of whom the anesthetic team was not given the Sp_{O_2} values. An Sp_{O_2} value of $\leq85\%$ for 30 sec or longer was defined as a major desaturation event. In the group for which the Sp_{O_2} data were unavailable to the anesthesia team, the incidence of such major desaturation events was twice as high (24 of 76 patients) as that in the group for which the data were available (11 of 76 patients).[62] In both groups, the majority of such events occurred in patients ≤2 years of age, possibly because infants have a greater tendency to desaturate as a result of relatively high oxygen consumption, lesser functional residual capacity, and proneness to revert to the fetal circulatory pattern.[62, 63] In another study in which Sp_{O_2} data were blindly collected from 108 patients undergoing outpatient gynecologic surgery, moderate desaturation ($Sp_{O_2} \leq 90\%$) was found in 10% of patients and severe hypoxemia ($Sp_{O_2} \leq 85\%$) in 5%.[64] These studies paved the way for the routine use of pulse oximeters during anesthesia, during transport, and in the recovery period.[5, 43, 61–63]

The status of Sp_{O_2} during transport to the recovery room has been studied in children and adults.[5, 62] In one such study, in which 71 children who were otherwise healthy were monitored, 28% were found to have Sp_{O_2} values $\leq90\%$; of these, 45% were cyanotic. In a comparable evaluation of adult patients, 35% had Sp_{O_2} values $\leq90\%$, and 12% of these values $\leq85\%$. In both studies, it was concluded that all patients should receive supplemental oxygen during transport from the operating room to the recovery room.[5]

Both pediatric and adult patients have been evaluated for adequacy of oxygenation through the use of pulse oximetry. Using a postanesthesia recovery (PAR) score based on motor activity, respiratory effort, blood pressure, and color in children, Soliman and collaborators found no correlation between Sp_{O_2} ($\geq95\%$ is considered adequate oxygenation) and the PAR score.[65] They inferred that infants and children should be monitored continuously with pulse oximetry or should be administered supplemental oxygen regardless of their apparent wakefulness and that an acceptable Sp_{O_2} value should be included among the recovery room discharge criteria.[65] Morris and coinvestigators evaluated Sp_{O_2} of 149 adult patients upon arrival in the recovery room, after 5 min,

after 30 min, and immediately before discharge (they excluded the personnel caring for the patients from their observations) and noted that 14% of the patients had Sa_{O_2} levels $<90\%$, in association with age, obesity, extensive surgery, and American Society of Anesthesiologists physical status; they were more desaturated at the time of discharge than at other times of Sa_{O_2} measurement. Further studies are in progress in this area.[5]

Uses in Infants and Children

Pulse oximetry has been used in the neonatal period in the delivery room to assess oxygenation status during resuscitation;[66, 67] during transport of critically ill neonates;[61] in the intensive care unit to monitor premature infants with respiratory distress syndrome,[48, 58–60, 68] repair of diaphragmatic hernia,[69] and cardiovascular surgery;[70] during monitoring children with cyanotic congenital heart disease;[71] in assessment of testicular torsion;[72] and in identifying children with wheezing.[73] Pulse oximetry is very helpful in diagnosing hypoxia and is therefore used in conjunction with tcP_{O_2} monitoring. Unlike the tcP_{O_2} monitoring, pulse oximetry has several advantages (Table 20–2): for example, ease in application and reliability. However, the authors urge caution in its use and in the interpretation of these data for patients with high Pa_{O_2}.[74] It should be obvious from the flat portion of the Hb_{O_2} dissociation curve that Sa_{O_2} levels should not be relied on for predicting "safe" high Pa_{O_2} levels in order to prevent oxygen damage to the retina. Currently, it is recommended that the steady-state Pa_{O_2} should be kept between 50 and 90 mm Hg so as to prevent retinopathy of prematurity.[21, 22] Bucker and associates designed a study to diagnose hyperoxemia during suctioning and bagging in newborns with various lung diseases who required oxygen and assisted ventilation.[74] Bucker and associates concluded that pulse oximeters may be sensitive to hyperoxemia if alarm limits are set (the two pulse oximeters studied were Nelcor N-100 and Ohmeda Biox 3700), and a low specificity is accepted.[74] However, because of the small sample size in this study and the reasons described earlier, the authors caution against using pulse oximeters to diagnose hyperoxemia, particularly in premature infants, until further studies are available.

In patients with bronchopulmonary dysplasia the Pa_{O_2} should be kept above 55 mm Hg to prevent further increase in pulmonary vascular resistance. Clinical status, capillary P_{O_2}, Pa_{O_2} with arterial puncture (crying), and tcP_{O_2} should not be relied on for monitoring oxygenation status in most patients with bronchopulmonary dysplasia, but several studies have shown that Sp_{O_2} by pulse oximetry is an effective method of monitoring the oxygenation status of these infants.[75–77] Pulse oximetry has also been used successfully in the pediatric intensive care unit[78, 79] and the pediatric ward[80] in patients with upper airway disorders (croup, epiglottitis, and retropharyngeal cellulitis),[81] asthma, pneumonia, adult respiratory distress syndrome, trauma, aspiration syndrome,[82] cardiothoracic diseases, or neurosurgical diseases.[83] Some hospitals use it to monitor oxygenation in all respiratory illnesses. It has also been used during diagnostic procedures such as bronchoscopy and esophagoscopy.[80] More recently, it has been used in the outpatient setting and has been accepted by children, their parents, and the staff.[80] Familiar and brightly painted objects on the probes (e.g., butterflies) have certainly improved acceptability by apprehensive children. Movement artifacts are minimized with sedation, with sucking (on a pacifier), and during sleep. There has been one report of a few minor side effects in three infants: one with a localized skin burn (under the probe) that turned into a blister, another one of mild skin erosion, and a third one with skin tanning under the probe.[84]

REFERENCES

1. Severinghaus JW: Transcutaneous blood gas analysis. Respir Care 27:152–159, 1982.
2. Bhat R, Diaz-Blanco J, Chaudhry U, et al: Transcutaneous oxygen and carbon dioxide monitoring in sick neonates using a combined sensor. Chest 88:890–894, 1985.
3. Tremper KK, Waxman K, Bowman R: Continuous transcutaneous oxygen monitoring during respiratory failure, cardiac decompensation, cardiac arrest and CPR. Crit Care Med 8:377–381, 1980.
4. Report of consensus meeting: Task Force on transcutaneous oxygen monitors, American Academy of Pediatrics, December 5 to 6, 1986. Pediatrics 83:122–126, 1989.
5. Tremper KK, Barker SJ: Pulse oximetry. Anesthesiology 70:98–108, 1989.
6. Clark LC, Wolf R, Granger D, et al: Continuous reading of blood oxygen tensions by polarography. J Appl Physiol 6:189–193, 1953.
7. Stow RW, Randall BF: Electrical measurements of the PCO_2 of blood. Am J Physiol 179:678, 1954.
8. Severinghaus JW, Bradley AF: Electrodes for blood PO_2 and PCO_2 determination. J Appl Physiol 13:515–520, 1958.
9. Lubbers DW: History of transcutaneous PO_2 measurement. Crit Care Med 9:693, 1981.
10. Thunstrom AM, Stafford MJ, Severinghaus JW: A two-temperature, two-PO_2 method of estimating the determinants of $tcPO_2$. In Huch A, Huch R, Lucey JF (eds): Continuous Transcutaneous Blood Gas Monitorings, pp. 167–182. New York: Liss, 1979.
11. Lubbers DW: Theoretical basis of the transcutaneous blood gas measurements. Crit Care Med 9:721–733, 1981.
12. Hansen TN, Tooley WH: Skin surface carbon dioxide tension in sick infants. Pediatrics 64:942–945, 1979.
13. Herrel N, Martin R, Pultusker M, et al: Optimal temperature for the measurement of transcutaneous carbon dioxide tension in neonate. J Pediatr 94:113–117, 1988.
14. Monaco F, McQuitty JC, Nickerson BG: Calibration of heated transcutaneous carbon dioxide electrode to reflect arterial carbon dioxide. Am Rev Respir Dis 127:322–324, 1983.
15. Laptook A, Oh W: Transcutaneous carbon dioxide monitoring in the newborn period. Crit Care Med 9:759–760, 1981.
16. Martin RJ, Beoglos A, Miller MJ, et al: Increasing arterial carbon dioxide tension: Influence on transcutaneous carbon dioxide tension measurements. Pediatrics 81:684–687, 1988.
17. Whitehead MD, Halsall D, Pollitzer MJ, et al: Transcutaneous estimation of arterial PO_2 and PCO_2 in newborns with a single electrochemical sensor. Lancet 1:111–114, 1980.
18. Messer J, Livolsi A, Willace D: Evaluation of a single transcutaneous measurement of PO_2 and PCO_2 in the neonate. In Huch A, Huch R, Rooth G (eds): Continuous Transcutaneous Monitoring, pp. 45–50. New York: Plenum Press, 1986.
19. Severinghaus JW: A combined transcutaneous PO_2-PCO_2 electrode with electrochemical HCO_3 stabilization. J Appl Physiol 51:1027–1032, 1981.
20. Lee HK, Broadhurst E, Helms P: Evaluation of two combined oxygen and carbon dioxide transcutaneous sensors. Arch Dis Child 64:279–282, 1989.
21. Yamanouchi I, Igarashi I, Ouchi E: Incidence and severity of retinopathy in low birth weight infants monitored by $tcPO_2$. In Huch A, Huch R, Rooth G (eds): Continuous Transcutaneous Monitoring, pp. 105–108. New York: Plenum Press, 1986.
22. Bancalari E, Flynn J, Goldbert RN, et al: Influence of transcutaneous oxygen monitoring on the incidence of retinopathy of prematurity. Pediatrics 79:663–669, 1987.
23. Anderson PK, Brinklov MM, Stokke DB, et al: Inaccuracy of oxygen electrodes at high blood oxygen tensions. Anesthesiology 49:61–62, 1978.
24. Rome ES, Stork EK, Carlo WA, et al: Limitations of transcutaneous PO_2 and PCO_2 monitoring in infants with bronchopulmonary dysplasia. Pediatrics 74:217–220, 1984.
25. Lucey JF, Dehner L: $tcPO_2$ monitoring reduces cost of blood gas monitoring. Pediatr Res 14:604, 1980.
26. Long JG, Lucey JF, Phillips AG: Noise and hypoxemia in the intensive care nursery. Pediatrics 65:143–145, 1980.
27. Pearlman SA, Maisels MJ: Preductal and postductal transcutaneous oxygen tension measurements in premature newborns with hyaline membrane disease. Pediatrics 83:98–100, 1989.
28. Ross-Russell RI, Helms PJ: Comparative accuracy of pulse oximetry and transcutaneous oxygen in assessing arterial saturation in pediatric intensive care. Crit Care Med 18:725–727, 1990.
29. Mahutte CK, Michiels TM, Hassell KT, et al: Evaluation of a single transcutaneous PO_2-PCO_2 sensor in adult patients. Crit Care Med 12:1063–1066, 1984.
30. Gottrup F, Gellett S, Kirkegaard L, et al: Effect of hemorrhage and resuscitation on subcutaneous, conjunctival, and transcutaneous oxygen tension in relation to hemodynamic variables. Crit Care Med 17:904–907, 1989.
31. Tremper KK, Shoemaker WC: Transcutaneous oxygen monitoring of critically ill adults, with and without low flow shock. Crit Care Med 9:706–709, 1981.
32. Tremper KK, Shoemaker WC, Shippy CR, et al: Transcutaneous PCO_2 monitoring on adult patients in the ICU and operating room. Crit Care Med 9:752–755, 1981.
33. Quigley FG, Faris IB: Transcutaneous oxygen potentials in venous diseases. Aust N Z J Surg 59:165–168, 1989.
34. Fanconi S, Burger R, Maurer H, et al: Transcutaneous carbon dioxide pressure for monitoring patients with severe croup. J Pediatr 117:701–705, 1990.
35. Venus B, Patel KC, Pratap KS, et al: Transcutaneous PO_2 monitoring during pediatric surgery. Crit Care Med 9:714–716, 1981.
36. Versmold HT, Linderkamp O, Holtzman H, et al: Transcutaneous monitoring of PO_2 in newborn infants. In Huch R, Huch A, Lucey J (eds): Continuous Transcutaneous Blood Gas Monitoring, pp. 285–294. New York: Liss, 1979.
37. Eberhard P, Mindt W: Interference of anesthetic gases at skin surface sensors for oxygen and carbon dioxide. Crit Care Med 9:717–720, 1981.
38. Butain WL, Conner E, Emrico J, et al: Transcutaneous oxygen ($tcPO_2$) measurement as an aid to fluid therapy in necrotizing enterocolitis. J Pediatr Surg 14:728–732, 1979.
39. Golden SM: Skin craters—A complication of transcutaneous oxygen monitoring. Pediatrics 67:514–516, 1981.
40. Severinghaus JW: History, status and future of pulse oximetry. Adv Exp Med Biol 220:3–8, 1987.
41. Barker SJ, Tremper KK: Pulse oximetry: Applications and limitations. Int Anesthesiol Clin 25:155–175, 1987.
42. Schratz WW: Pulse oximetry: A review with emphasis on applications in dentistry. Anesth Prog 34:100–101, 1987.
43. Alexander CM, Teller LE, Gross JB: Principles of pulse oximetry: Theoretical and practical considerations. Anesth Analg 68:368–376, 1989.
44. Pologe JA: Pulse oximetry: Technical aspects of machine design. Int Anesthesiol Clin 25:137–153, 1987.
45. Pologe JA, Raley DM: Effects of fetal hemoglobin on pulse oximetry. J Perinatol 7:324–326, 1987.
46. Harris AP, Sendak MJ, Donham RT, et al: Absorption characteristics of human fetal hemoglobin at wavelengths used in pulse oximetry. J Clin Monit 4:175–177, 1988.
47. Baeckert P, Bucher HU, Fallenstein F, et al: Is pulse oximetry reliable in detecting hyperoxemia in the neonate? Adv Exp Med Biol 220:165–169, 1987.
48. Durand M, Ramanathan R: Pulse oximetry for continuous oxygen monitoring in sick newborn infants. J Pediatr 109:1052–1056, 1986.
49. Ramanathan R, Durand M, Larrazabal C: Pulse oximetry in very low birth weight infants with acute and chronic lung disease. Pediatrics 79:612–617, 1987.

50. Veyckemans F, Baele P, Guillaume JE, et al: Hyperbilirubinemia does not interfere with hemoglobin saturation measured by pulse oximetry. Anesthesiology 70:118–122, 1989.

51. Emery JR: Skin pigmentation as an influence on the accuracy of pulse oximetry. J Perinatol 7:329–330, 1987.

52. Barker SJ, Tremper KK: The effect of carbon monoxide inhalation on pulse oximetry and transcutaneous PO_2. Anesthesiology 66:677–679, 1987.

53. Watcha MF, Connor MT, Hing AV: Pulse oximetry in methemoglobinemia. Am J Dis Child 143:845–847, 1989.

54. Hodgson AJ: Is co-oximetry a reliable standard for pulse oximetry in the neonate? J Perinatol 7:327–328, 1987.

55. Kessler MR, Eide T, Humayun B, et al: Spurious pulse oximeter desaturation with methylene blue injection. Anesthesiology 65:435–436, 1986.

56. Eide TR, Humayun-Scott B, Poppers PJ: More on dyes and pulse oximetry. Anesthesiology 67:148–149, 1987.

57. Kopotic RJ, Mannino FL, Colley CD, et al: Display variability, false alarms, probe cautions, and recorder use in neonatal pulse oximetry. J Perinatol 7:340–342, 1987.

58. Hay WW Jr: The uses, benefits, and limitations of pulse oximetry in neonatal medicine: Consensus on key issues. J Perinatol 7:347–349, 1987.

59. Walsh MC, Noble LM, Carlo WA, et al: Relationship of pulse oximetry to arterial oxygen tension in infants. Crit Care Med 15:1102–1105, 1987.

60. Henderson GW: Accuracy and reliability of pulse oximetry in premature neonates with respiratory distress. J Am Assoc Nurse Anesth 56:224–228, 1988.

61. Hankins CT: The use of pulse oximetry during infant transport from outside facilities. J Perinatol 7:346, 1987.

62. Cote CJ, Goldstein EA, Cote MA, et al: A single-blind study of pulse oximetry in children. Anesthesiology 68:184–188, 1988.

63. Miyasaka K, Katayama M, Kusakawa I, et al: Use of pulse oximetry in neonatal anesthesia. J Perinatol 7:343–345, 1987.

64. Raemer DB, Warren DL, Morris R, et al: Hypoxemia during ambulatory gynecologic surgery as evaluated by the pulse oximeter. J Clin Monit 3:244–248, 1987.

65. Soliman IE, Patel RI, Ehrenpreis MB, et al: Recovery scores do not correlate with post-operative hypoxemia in children. Anesth Analg 67:53–56, 1988.

66. House JT, Schultetus RR, Gravenstein N: Continuous neonatal evaluation in the delivery room by pulse oximetry. J Clin Monit 3:96–100, 1987.

67. Maxwell LG, Harris AP, Sendak MJ, et al: Monitoring the resuscitation of preterm infants in the delivery room using pulse oximetry. Clin Pediatr (Phila) 26:18–20, 1987.

68. Barrington KJ, Finer NN, Ryan CA: Evaluation of pulse oximetry as a continuous monitoring technique in the neonatal intensive care unit. Crit Care Med 16:1147–1153, 1988.

69. Norman EA: Pulse oximetry during repair of congenital diaphragmatic hernia (Letter). Br J Anaesth 58:934–935, 1986.

70. Friesen RH: Pulse oximetry during pulmonary artery surgery. Anesth Analg 64:376, 1985.

71. Boxer RA, Gottesfeld I, Singh S, et al: Noninvasive pulse oximetry in children with cyanotic congenital heart disease. Crit Care Med 15:1062–1064, 1987.

72. Kram HB, Miyamoto E, Rajfer J, et al: Testicular oximetry: A new method for the assessment of tissue perfusion and viability following torsion and detorsion. J Pediatr Surg 24:1297–1302, 1989.

73. Rosen LM, Yamamoto LG, Wiebe RA: Pulse oximetry to identify a high-risk group of children with wheezing. Am J Emerg Med 7:567–570, 1989.

74. Bucker HU, Fanconi S, Baeckert P, et al: Hyperoxemia in newborn infants: Detection by pulse oximetry. Pediatrics 84:226–230, 1989.

75. Eggert LD: The clinical use of pulse oximetry with bronchopulmonary dysplasia. J Perinatol 7:336, 1987.

76. White MP: Pulse oximetry in children with bronchopulmonary dysplasia (Letter). Lancet 1:652, 1988.

77. Solimano AJ, Smyth JA, Mann TK, et al: Pulse oximetry advantages in infants with bronchopulmonary dysplasia. Pediatrics 78:844–849, 1986.

78. Fanconi S, Doherty P, Edmonds JF, et al: Pulse oximetry in pediatric intensive care: Comparison with measured saturations and transcutaneous oxygen tension. J Pediatr 107:362–366, 1985.

79. Fanconi S: Pulse oximetry and transcutaneous oxygen tension for detection of hypoxemia in critically ill infants and children. Adv Exp Med Biol 220:159–164, 1987.

80. Levene S, McKenzie SA: Pulse oximetry in children (Letter). Lancet 1:415–416, 1988.

81. Gussack GS, Tacchi EJ: Pulse oximetry in the management of pediatric airway disorders. South Med J 80:1381–1384, 1987.

82. Fait CD, Wetzel RC, Dean JM, et al: Pulse oximetry in critically ill children. J Clin Monit 1:232–235, 1985.

83. Brooks TD, Gravenstein N: Pulse oximetry for early detection of hypoxemia in anesthetized infants. J Clin Monit 1:135–137, 1985.

84. Miyasaka K, Ohata J: Burn, erosion, and "sun" tan with the use of pulse oximetry in infants. Anesthesiology 67:1008–1009, 1987.

III Respiratory Infections

INFECTIOUS DISEASES

21 PEDIATRIC HUMAN IMMUNODEFICIENCY VIRUS INFECTION

LAURA S. INSELMAN, M.D.

Since 1979, when the acquired immunodeficiency syndrome (AIDS) was first recognized, the number of people with AIDS has risen exponentially; more than 500,000 cases occurred worldwide during the subsequent 9 years.[1] The disease now represents the most serious pandemic of the past 70 years and is comparable to the eras of poliomyelitis, tuberculosis, syphilis, and smallpox. It is estimated that at least 8 million people globally are infected with the virus and that, by the year 2000, the syndrome will develop in 8 million adults.[1-3] In the United States, as of December 1991, approximately 203,000 adults and 3500 children had AIDS, 133,000 had died, 1 million were infected with the virus, 1 out of every 30 men aged 20 to 50 years was a carrier of the virus, and 50% of those infected with the virus could develop AIDS within the ensuing 10 years.[3-5] As the months pass, these statistics are no longer valid.

ETIOLOGY

The human immunodeficiency virus (HIV-1), which was earlier described as human T cell lymphotropic virus (HTLV-III)/lymphadenopathy-associated virus, causes AIDS (Fig. 21–1).[6,7] This virus has been isolated from persons with HIV infection from cells (peripheral lymphocytes, mononuclear phagocytes, pulmonary alveolar macrophages, fibroblasts), fluid and secretions (cell-free plasma, cerebrospinal fluid, saliva, tears, semen, cervical secretions, urine, amniotic fluid, breast milk), and organs (lungs, lymph nodes, retina, thymus, bone marrow, liver, kidneys, heart, pancreas, brain, spinal cord, peripheral nerves).[7-13]

HIV-1 is part of a group of RNA lymphotropic retroviruses, which includes HTLV-I, II, IV, and V and HIV-2 (Table 21–1).[6,14-17] The HTLV-I, II, and V viruses cause leukemia and lymphoma. Like HIV-1, they are endemic in the Caribbean, southern Japan, and Africa but are now widespread throughout western and eastern Europe and North and South America. HTLV-IV and HIV-2 have been identified in Africa and the United States and may be associated with a less severe form of AIDS.[16,17] Infection with a retrovirus is lifelong, and multiple retroviral infections can occur simultaneously.[18,19]

Through the activity of reverse transcriptase (a retroviral enzyme that enables RNA to synthesize DNA), the genes of the retrovirus are integrated and duplicated with normal genes of an infected cell.[14,20] All newly produced cells contain the viral genes, which then govern the expressive actions of the cell. Retroviruses contain three structural genes: *gag* (group associated), which codes for viral core antigens; *pol* (polymerase), which is responsible for formation of reverse transcriptase; and *env* (envelope), which produces envelope proteins, the major serologic antigens in infected persons. Another gene, *tat* (transactivation of transcription), enhances viral replication.[10,19,20] On each end of this retroviral genome is a long terminal repeat (LTR) sequence, which controls transcription and expression of the viral genes. HIV-1 has five additional genes that regulate viral multiplication and infectivity: *rev* (regulator of expression of virion proteins), *nef* (negative regulatory factor), *vif* (virion infectivity factor), *vpu* (viral protein U), and *vpr* (viral protein R).[10,21,21a]

The HTLV viruses are distinguished serologically by their *gag, env, tat,* and LTR proteins.[10,15,19,20] All have a *gag* p24 protein. The major immunogenic antigens of HIV-1 identified serologically in humans are the *gag* p24 and the *env* gp160/120 and gp41 proteins.[19] Unlike HIV-1, HIV-2 lacks gp41, which is of major serologic importance in differentiating these viruses.[22] In addition, HIV-1 itself may represent a spectrum of different viruses with varying degrees of similarity in their genomes, particularly in the *env* gene, or, alternatively, HIV-1 may be one virus with differing viral genomes within one individual at different times.[6,10,23,24]

HIV-1 and some strains of HIV-2 are cytopathic to T4 lymphocytes (see Table 21–1) but not to monocytes.[6,10,14,23] The *env* gp120 gene may be responsible for cytopathogenicity.[25] In contrast, HTLV-I, II, IV, and V do not kill the cells that they infect but transform them to reproduce indefinitely and become "immortalized" (see Table 21–1).[6,15] Retroviruses induce the formation of syncytial, or multinucleated, virus-infected cells with intracellular flow of cations and water, resulting in cell membrane disruption.[6,10,23,25,26] The syncytium then spreads to neighboring normal cells.[23]

EPIDEMIOLOGY

HIV infection is transmitted in humans by exposure to the virus in body fluids through sexual contact, contami-

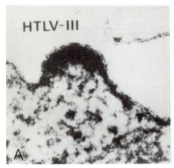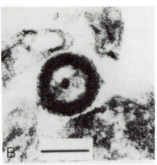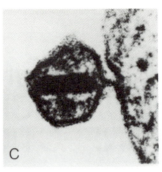

Figure 21–1. Electron microscopic views of budding (A), immature (B), and mature (C) forms of human immunodeficiency virus (HIV). The bar in (B) indicates 100 nm. (Reproduced with permission, from Gallo RC, Wong-Staal F: A human T lymphotropic retrovirus [HTLV-III] as the cause of the acquired immunodeficiency syndrome. Ann Intern Med 103:681, 1985.)

nated needles, and blood and blood products and by passage of the virus from an infected mother to the fetus across the placenta.[14, 22, 27, 28] Pediatric HIV infection can occur through any of these routes of transmission.

Eighty-one percent of pediatric HIV infections occur in children younger than age 5 years.[4, 27] Eighty-eight percent of these children acquire the virus perinatally, and in another 8%, HIV infection develops as a result of transfusions of blood and blood products.[4] Identifiable risk factors in the remaining pediatric infections are unknown.

AIDS develops in approximately one third of children born to HIV-1–infected mothers.[29] AIDS can also develop in children born to women with HIV-2 infection.[29] More than one fifth of all cases of AIDS in women in the United States are acquired during the teenage years.[2] Most of the reported adult and pediatric cases of HIV infection have occurred in New York, New Jersey, Florida, California, and Washington, D.C.[4]

DEFINITION

AIDS is defined by the Centers for Disease Control (CDC) as an illness characterized by the presence of an

Table 21–1. AIDS-RELATED VIRUSES

Virus	Associated Disease	Cellular Effect
HTLV-I	Adult T cell leukemia, lymphoma, neurodegenerative disease, polymyositis	Immortalizes and transforms T lymphocytes
HTLV-II	Hairy cell leukemia	Immortalizes and transforms T lymphocytes
HIV-1 (HTLV-III; LAV-1)	AIDS (HIV infection)	Cytopathic to T4 lymphocytes
HTLV-IV	Possible "slim" disease	Infects T4 lymphocytes without cytopathic effect
HTLV-V	Leukemia, mycosis, fungoides	Immortalizes and transforms T lymphocytes
HIV-2 (LAV-2)	AIDS (HIV infection)	Some strains cytopathic to T4 lymphocytes
STLV-I	Lymphoma in primates	
STLV-III	AIDS in primates	Cytopathic to T4 lymphocytes

AIDS, acquired immunodeficiency syndrome; HTLV, human T cell lymphotropic virus; HIV, human immunodeficiency virus; LAV, lymphadenopathy-associated virus; STLV, simian T lymphotropic virus.

indicator disease and by the status of laboratory documentation of HIV infection.[30, 30a] The continuum of HIV infection includes seroconversion, laboratory abnormalities, persistent generalized adenopathy, and AIDS itself.[7, 21, 30, 31]

Confirmation of AIDS in children is more difficult than in adults because of the occurrence of congenital immunodeficiencies in childhood, persistence of passively acquired maternal HIV antibody until age 15 months, and differing manifestations of the syndrome in children and adults.[30, 32, 33] Features unique to pediatric AIDS include the occurrence of lymphoid interstitial pneumonitis, parotid gland enlargement, low birth weight, failure to thrive, unexplained recurrent pyogenic bacterial infections, neurodevelopmental dysfunction, and a possible fetal AIDS syndrome manifested by craniofacial dysmorphism and growth failure.[31, 33–35] Children with HIV infection who are younger than age 13 years are considered to have pediatric HIV infection, whereas those who are 13 years of age or older are classified as adults infected with HIV.[30a, 33] Thus adolescents are excluded from the CDC definition of pediatric HIV infection.

Pediatric HIV infection can be classified according to the presence and type of symptoms and immune function (Table 21–2).[33] Indeterminate infection occurs in a child younger than age 15 months who has had perinatal exposure and has a positive HIV immunoglobulin G (IgG) antibody titer without other evidence of HIV infection.[33] However, this classification may eventually be revised as more information about this age group becomes available with new diagnostic techniques, such as the polymerase chain reaction (PCR).[12]

PATHOPHYSIOLOGY: IMMUNOLOGY

Normally, approximately 70% of circulating lymphocytes are thymus-derived T cells, which confer cell-mediated immunity, whereas 10% to 15% of circulating lymphocytes are bursa-derived B cells, which are responsible for humoral immunity (Fig. 21–2).[36, 37] The remaining 15% to 20% are null cells, which are composed of killer cells and natural killer cells and play a role in cellular cytotoxic defense mechanisms.[36, 38] T lymphocytes mature into helper, suppressor, inducer, and cytotoxic cells, and the helpers and suppressors regulate B lymphocyte differentiation and T lymphocyte proliferation and cytotoxicity (see Fig. 21–2).[36, 37] Helper T cells enable B lymphocytes to mature and synthesize specific immunoglob-

Table 21–2. CENTERS FOR DISEASE CONTROL CLASSIFICATION OF PEDIATRIC HIV INFECTION

Category	Findings
Class P-0	Indeterminate infection
Class P-1	Asymptomatic infection
Subclass A	Normal immune function
Subclass B	Abnormal immune function (humoral or cellular)
Subclass C	Immune function not tested
Class P-2	Symptomatic infection
Subclass A	Nonspecific (fever, failure to thrive, weight loss, generalized lymphadenopathy, hepatosplenomegaly, parotitis, diarrhea)
Subclass B	Progressive neurologic disease (loss of developmental milestones or intellectual ability, acquired microcephaly, brain atrophy, progressive symmetric motor deficits)
Subclass C	Lymphoid interstitial pneumonitis
Subclass D	Secondary infectious diseases (opportunistic infections, recurrent serious bacterial infections)
Subclass E	Secondary cancers (Kaposi's sarcoma, B cell non-Hodgkin's lymphoma, primary lymphoma of brain)
Subclass F	Hepatitis, cardiopathy, nephropathy, anemia, thrombocytopenia, dermatologic diseases associated with HIV

HIV, human immunodeficiency virus.
Modified from Centers for Disease Control: Classification system for human immunodeficiency virus (HIV) infection in children under 13 years of age. MMWR 36:225–236, 1987.

ulins.[36, 37, 39] Suppressor T cells inhibit this differentiation and also inhibit helper T cell function.[37, 40] As a result of deficient numbers and function of helper T cells in HIV infection, cell-mediated immunity is defective, and immunoglobulin synthesis is altered.[10, 14, 31] In addition, cytotoxicity mediated by T8 lymphocytes and natural killer cells is impaired, resulting in defective cytotoxicity against virus-infected cells.[14, 31, 38]

As T cell precursors mature, they acquire surface markers, or differentiation antigens, that specifically characterize these cells.[31, 36, 38, 40, 41] One T cell subset has the CD4 (T4, OKT4, Leu-3) antigen and is composed primarily of helpers and, to a lesser degree, inducers, suppressors, and cytotoxic cells. Another T cell subset has the CD8 (T8, OKT8, Leu-2) antigen and is composed mainly of suppressors, although it may also have inducers. Normally, 60% of T lymphocytes are T4 cells and 30% are T8 cells; hence the T4/T8 ratio is 2.0 in peripheral blood.[24, 38] In HIV infection, as a consequence of a selective reduction in the number of T4 cells, the T4/T8 ratio is reversed, with a value of less than 1.0.[24, 38]

Polyclonal hypergammaglobulinemia occurs as a result of augmented B lymphocyte activation, but the B lymphocytes are qualitatively dysfunctional in their ability to respond to new antigenic stimuli.[14, 31, 42–44] In addition, HIV-1 antibodies occur and reflect the hyperactivity of the B cells.[43]

Deficient monocyte chemotaxis, cytotoxicity, and secretion of lymphokine interleukin-1 (IL-1) also occur with HIV infection.[14, 31] Normally, IL-1 induces secretion of another lymphokine, interleukin-2 (IL-2), from T4 lymphocytes.[24, 39] IL-2 is a T cell growth factor that regulates helper and suppressor T lymphocyte proliferation, interferon production, and natural killer cell activation.[38] Deficiency in IL-2 secretion with HIV thus results in diminished numbers of T4 cells and decreased activity of natural killer cells. As with B lymphocytes, monocytes are activated and yet fail to respond to new antigens.[14] This predisposes to infection with cytomegalovirus, mycobacteria, *Pneumocystis carinii, Cryptococcus neoformans,* and *Toxoplasma gondii,* resistance to all of which requires properly functioning monocytes.[23]

Thus persons with HIV have dysfunction of cellular, humoral, and phagocytic components of the immune system. This is associated with functional hypogammaglobulinemia, despite quantitative polyclonal hypergammaglobulinemia; with defective cytotoxicity, chemotaxis, helper lymphocyte and monocyte activity; and with relative enhancement of suppressor T cell function. Possible

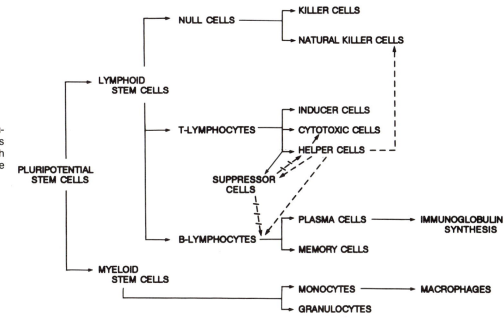

Figure 21–2. Differentiation of leukocytes. Arrows with dashed lines indicate activation. Arrows with dashed lines and slashes indicate inhibition.

causes of these alterations include a direct effect of HIV in its binding to the CD4 molecule of the T4 lymphocyte and monocyte, the actions of lymphokines secreted by the HIV-infected T4 cell and monocyte, a direct effect of HIV on the B lymphocyte, the formation of nonviable syncytial cells, autoimmune processes, and other viral infections.[9, 14, 42, 45] These immunologic abnormalities provide the setting for opportunistic infections and the development of malignancies.

PULMONARY SPECTRUM

The pulmonary spectrum of pediatric HIV infection includes infection with opportunistic organisms and lymphocytic interstitial pneumonitis.[27, 46, 47] This is in contrast with the pulmonary diseases in adult HIV infection, which are characterized primarily by opportunistic infections and Kaposi's sarcoma.[48, 49] The reasons for these differences are not clear. In addition, the types of opportunistic organisms in the lung differ, with an increased incidence of bacterial pneumonias in children and of mycobacterial disease in adults. Children may be more likely than adults to acquire serious pyogenic bacterial infections because of exposure to these organisms while they are immunodeficient.[43, 50] In contrast, many years of normal immunologic function precede immunodeficiency in adults, who have antibodies to these organisms and can respond more appropriately on re-exposure. In both pediatric and adult AIDS, several pulmonary infections can occur simultaneously.

OPPORTUNISTIC ORGANISMS

Pneumocystis carinii

P. carinii is the pulmonary opportunistic organism most frequently identified in both pediatric and adult AIDS, causing pneumonia in 55% of children with HIV.[27] It is a disease indicator used as a criterion for the diagnosis of AIDS.[30] *P. carinii* is usually localized to the lungs, even in fatal cases, although extrapulmonary infection in AIDS has also been identified.[51] This newly classified fungus,[51] which was previously considered a protozoan parasite, exists in two forms: as thick-walled cysts containing up to eight oval sporozoites (Fig. 21–3) and as thin-walled extracysts called trophozoites.[52, 53] In otherwise healthy persons, subclinical infection without histologic evidence of disease can occur, resulting in low titers of antibody to *P. carinii* during early childhood.[51–53] Clinical disease can develop later with reactivation of this latent infection by stress or immunodeficiency. Human-to-human airborne spread of *P. carinii* can also occur.[52, 53]

P. carinii causes primarily an intra-alveolar rather than interstitial inflammation.[49, 52] Initially, only isolated cysts with minimal changes are seen in alveolar septa, and clinical disease is absent.[52] Alveolar cells then desquamate, the cysts multiply within pulmonary alveolar macrophages in the alveolar lumen, and clinical symptoms can be present at this stage.[52] Eventually, a diffuse desquamative alveolitis ensues, and alveoli are filled with a

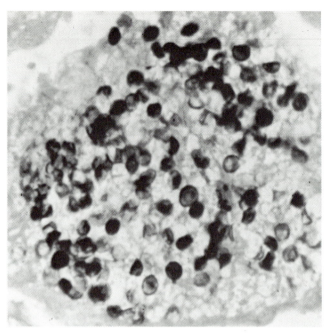

Figure 21–3. Thick cyst walls of *Pneumocystis carinii* in lung. Gomori's methenamine silver stain, magnification 1250×. (From Fishman JA: Protozoan infections of the lung. *In* Fishman AP [ed]: Pulmonary Diseases and Disorders, 2nd ed, p. 1660. New York: McGraw-Hill, 1988, with permission.)

foamy eosinophilic exudate of cysts, sporozoites, and macrophages. Interstitial inflammation occurs, pneumonia is evident clinically and radiographically, and mild interstitial fibrosis and focal alveolar hemorrhage may be present.[49, 52]

P. carinii pneumonia in pediatric AIDS has an acute onset of symptoms with rapid progression to respiratory failure.[46] It usually occurs in younger children, aged 4 to 8 months, and is often associated with failure to thrive and encephalopathy.[54] The infection is characterized initially by high fever, nonproductive cough, tachypnea, and crackles, with subsequent development of hypoxemia, cyanosis, retractions, and flaring of nasal alae.[46, 52] Chest radiographs reveal diffuse alveolar and interstitial infiltrates starting in the perihilar or basilar areas and spreading peripherally (Fig. 21–4).[52, 53] Hyperexpanded lungs, air bronchograms, lobar consolidation, hilar adenopathy, miliary and honeycomb patterns, spontaneous pneumothoraces, and endobronchial lesions can also occur.[52, 53, 55, 56] However, the chest radiograph can be normal despite the presence of severe clinical disease or a positive gallium lung scan.[53]

Lung function testing reveals restrictive lung disease, diminution in diffusing capacity, ventilation/perfusion imbalance, and arterial hypoxemia at rest.[51, 57, 58] In children with one episode of *P. carinii* pneumonia but without HIV, these abnormalities apparently resolve without clinical or histologic sequelae.[58]

Cytomegalovirus

Cytomegalovirus (CMV) is the second most frequent organism isolated in lungs of children with HIV.[27] To

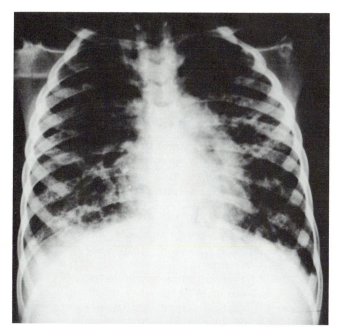

Figure 21–4. Bilateral interstitial infiltrates on an anteroposterior radiographic view of the chest of a 4½-year-old girl with acquired immunodeficiency syndrome. *Pneumocystis carinii* and parainfluenza type 3 virus were isolated from bronchoalveolar lavage fluid.

monic intranuclear and cytoplasmic inclusions in pulmonary alveolar macrophages, desquamated alveolar epithelial cells, and endothelial and interstitial cells.[62] The intranuclear inclusions are the viral particles, which are centrally located and surrounded by a lucent area, whereas the cytoplasmic inclusions are coarse, basophilic granules with a mucopolysaccharide envelope (Fig. 21–5).[62, 63] A diffuse or localized interstitial pneumonia results with minimal involvement of the intra-alveolar lumen,[62, 64] in contrast to *P. carinii* pneumonia. Proteinaceous alveolar exudates and alveolar hemorrhages can occur, but necrosis is rare.[62, 64] CMV can also be present without clinical or histologic evidence of lung disease.[48, 59]

Respiratory distress occurs gradually within 2 weeks of onset of the disease and includes fever, nonproductive cough, dyspnea, adventitious lung sounds, and hypoxemia.[60] Chest radiographs reveal diffuse interstitial infiltrates or lobar consolidation.[60, 65] CMV pneumonia can be fatal.

Bacteria, Viruses, Fungi, Protozoa

Patients, particularly children, with HIV infection are at increased risk for severe, life-threatening bacterial pulmonary infections.[43, 47, 48, 50] Although many of these bacteria are not normally considered opportunistic organisms, they are included in this discussion, along with certain viruses, fungi, and protozoa, because of their propensity for causing serious, recurrent, or unremitting pulmonary disease in HIV infection (Table 21–3). Several of these organisms are used as criteria for the diagnosis of HIV infection,[30, 33] and the presence of recurrent serious pyogenic bacterial infections, particularly with *Haemophilus influenzae* and *Streptococcus pneumoniae,* is considered a diagnostic criterion for pediatric HIV infection.[30, 33] Each organism listed causes nonspecific manifestations of respiratory distress, such as fever, dyspnea, adventitious lung sounds, hypoxemia, and cough, which may be productive in some infections in an older child. Other systemic manifestations associated with the specific

define its role in pediatric HIV infection more clearly and to rule out the presence of congenital CMV infection, the onset of CMV disease must occur after the age of 1 month for CMV to be considered an opportunistic organism with HIV.[30, 33] Acquired CMV infection, which occurs in AIDS, is transmitted by contact with virus-containing body fluids (saliva, urine, tears, stool, breast milk, cervical secretions, semen, leukocytes) and transplanted organs or tissues.[59–61] The virus may be secreted for years, may cause subclinical infection, and may be reactivated by stress or immunodeficiency, resulting in clinical disease.[59, 60]

This DNA virus belongs to the herpesvirus family[59–61] and characteristically causes cytomegaly with pathogno-

Figure 21–5. Intranuclear (N) and cytoplasmic (C) inclusions of cytomegalovirus in lung stained with hematoxylin-eosin (*A*) and Gomori's methenamine silver (*B*), magnification 600×. (From Gorelkin L, Chandler FW, Ewing EP Jr: Staining qualities of cytomegalovirus inclusions in the lungs of patients with the acquired immunodeficiency syndrome: A potential source of diagnostic misinterpretation. Hum Pathol 17:926, 1986.)

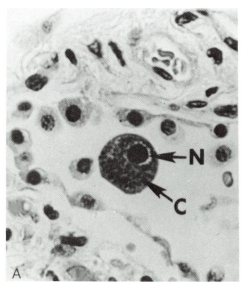

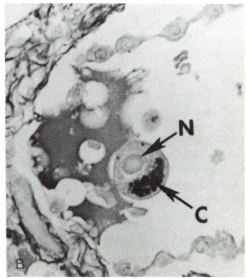

Table 21–3. PULMONARY OPPORTUNISTIC ORGANISMS
IN HIV INFECTION

Bacteria
*Bordetella pertussis**
*Branhamella catarrhalis**
Corynebacterium equi
*Enterobacter aerogenes**
*Escherichia coli**
Group B *Streptococcus**
Haemophilus influenzae type b*
Klebsiella pneumoniae
*Legionella pneumophila**
*Mycobacterium avium-intracellulare,** M. bovis,* M. gordonae,*
   M. kansasii, M scrofulaceum,* M. tuberculosis**
*Mycoplasma pneumoniae**
Nocardia asteroides
*Proteus mirabilis**
*Pseudomonas aeruginosa**
*Salmonella enteritidis, S. typhimurium**
Staphylococcus aureus, S. epidermidis**
Streptococcus pneumoniae, S. sanguis,* S. viridans**

Viruses
Adenovirus*
Cytomegalovirus*
Epstein-Barr virus*
Herpes simplex virus*
Influenza viruses*
Measles virus*
Respiratory syncytial virus*
Herpes zoster-varicella virus*

Fungi
*Aspergillus fumigatus, A. niger**
Candida albicans, C. (Torulopsis) glabrata**
Coccidioides immitis
*Cryptococcus neoformans**
Histoplasma capsulatum
Petriellidium boydii
*Pneumocystis carinii**

Protozoa
Cryptosporidium
Leishmania donovani
*Toxoplasma gondii**

HIV, human immunodeficiency virus.
*Reported in literature in pediatric HIV infection.

pathogen may also be present and include meningitis, encephalitis, diarrhea, skin lesions, and bone and joint involvement. Specific pulmonary radiographic changes occur with many of these organisms, and some of the pulmonary diseases, even if treated, can be fatal.

Mycobacteria

Pulmonary disease resulting from tuberculous and nontuberculous mycobacteria occurs with increased frequency in HIV infection,[48, 66] although infection with nontuberculous mycobacteria often occurs simultaneously with another opportunistic organism.[44, 46] The manifestations, the clinical course, and radiographic and histologic features of mycobacterial infections with HIV are atypical of lung disease caused by these organisms in non–HIV-infected persons.[48, 66-68] Extrapulmonary disease caused by tuberculous or nontuberculous mycobacteria is a criterion for the diagnosis of AIDS.[30]

Mycobacterium avium-intracellulare (MAI) is the mycobacterium most frequently isolated from patients with HIV.[66] It is ubiquitous in the environment and typically causes lymphadenitis in immunocompetent children.[66, 69] Serotypes 4, 6, and 8 are present with increased frequency in HIV infection.[66] The gastrointestinal tract is the likely portal of entry for MAI; airborne transmission has not been a documented mode of spread of the organism between people.[69]

Patients with both HIV and MAI initially have nonspecific systemic signs and symptoms, such as fever, weight loss, anorexia, malabsorption, and abdominal pain, which may be attributed initially to HIV instead of to MAI.[66] Respiratory manifestations develop later and include progressive dyspnea, productive or nonproductive cough, fevers, and night sweats.[70] Adventitious lung sounds and marked respiratory distress are unusual.[66, 70] Pulmonary symptoms may not be prominent, and identification of MAI in respiratory secretions may be the only initial manifestation of pulmonary infection with this organism.[66] Chest radiographs are usually normal[70] or indicate another concurrent pulmonary infection.[71] On histologic examination, atypical granulomas are present with macrophages that are filled with acid-fast bacilli but devoid of epithelioid cells, giant cells, and caseation necrosis.[66, 71] Histologic changes may also be minimal.[72] MAI disease is often diagnosed only at autopsy in AIDS, probably because of its insidious onset and the concomitant presence of other life-threatening illnesses.[66]

HIV infection is associated with an increased incidence of both pulmonary and extrapulmonary tuberculosis.[48, 66, 68] Tuberculosis frequently precedes the diagnosis of AIDS by years,[66, 68] and its onset may be predictive of the presence of infection with the retrovirus in a person in a group at high risk for HIV. The reversed sequence can also occur (i.e., AIDS is diagnosed before the development of tuberculosis).[48, 66, 68] Because *Mycobacterium tuberculosis* is more virulent than *P. carinii* or *T. gondii,* it is more likely to cause disease earlier in the course of HIV infection than are these other organisms.

Although spread of tuberculosis can occur among patients with active disease and HIV, the presence of tuberculosis in a person with HIV infection is usually a result of reactivation of latent tuberculosis.[73] Thus it is more likely to be recognized in adults than in children. However, tuberculosis has been diagnosed in children with HIV infection.[74, 75]

Pulmonary tuberculosis with HIV differs clinically, radiographically, and histologically from the disease in non–HIV-infected individuals.[48, 66-68] Mediastinal and hilar adenopathy and middle and lower lobe lesions are more likely to occur with HIV, in contrast to the apical, cavitary disease typical of tuberculosis in immunocompetent adults.[48, 66-68] The radiographic changes vary with the degree of T4 lymphocyte deficiency, with diffuse infiltrates occurring more frequently with low T4 cell counts, whereas upper and lower lesions, mediastinal adenopathy, and pleural effusion are more likely to be associated with a less severe diminution of T4 lymphocytes.[76]

HIV infection is also associated with an increased incidence of miliary and lymphatic tuberculosis, in contrast

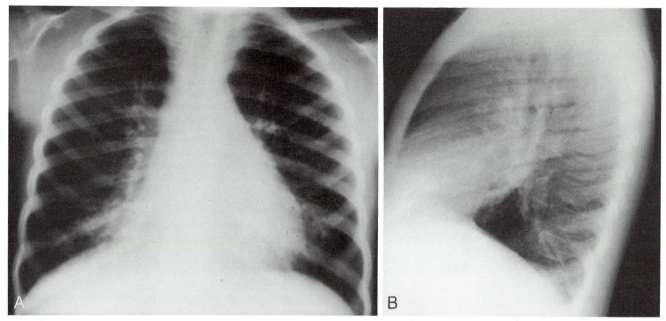

Figure 21–6. Lymphocytic interstitial pneumonitis on anteroposterior (*A*) and lateral (*B*) chest radiographs of a 6-year-old girl with acquired immunodeficiency syndrome. Diffuse infiltrates, which are more prominent in the lower lobes, are present bilaterally.

to tuberculosis without HIV infection.[66, 68, 77] In addition, extrapulmonary tuberculosis appears to be related to a more profound degree of T4 cell deficiency and has a graver prognosis than does pulmonary disease.[76] In general, children with tuberculosis are less likely than adults to have systemic manifestations, such as fever, night sweats, and weight loss.[69, 78]

On histologic examination, both well-formed and atypical granulomas can be identified in tuberculosis with HIV, in contrast to MAI with HIV.[48, 79] Tuberculosis may occur even if granulomas are absent and acid-fast bacilli are not visualized;[66, 68, 79] these features are unusual in tuberculosis without HIV infection.

LYMPHOCYTIC INTERSTITIAL PNEUMONITIS

Lymphocytic interstitial pneumonitis (LIP) is one of the two most frequently diagnosed lung lesions in pediatric HIV infection, the other being *P. carinii* pneumonia.[27, 46, 47, 80, 81] LIP is a unique feature of pediatric AIDS, is a criterion for its diagnosis,[30, 33] and occurs infrequently in adult AIDS.[48, 49] It is probably a response of the lung to an injury,[80, 82] such as could occur with the retrovirus itself, a component of the retrovirus, or another agent causing a currently unidentified opportunistic infection. No infectious microorganism has been histologically recognized in LIP,[80] although the Epstein-Barr virus genome[83, 84] and HIV-1 RNA[84] have been observed in lungs of children with LIP and AIDS.

LIP is characterized by markedly thickened alveolar septae filled with lymphocytes, histiocytes, plasma cells, immunoblasts, lymphoid nodules, and giant cells.[80–82, 85, 86] The lesion may be so severe as to completely alter normal lung morphology.[80] It can progress to interstitial fibrosis, a honeycomb lung, and respiratory failure.[86, 87] Although both B and T lymphocytes are present in the infiltrate, the majority are T8 cells.[83, 85, 88]

LIP is one of several pulmonary lymphocytic proliferative lesions occurring in pediatric AIDS. These lesions include pulmonary lymphoid hyperplasia (PLH), characterized by nodules of lymphocytes and plasma cells in the interstitium and near the bronchioles; bronchial-associated lymphoid tissue hyperplasia; and polyclonal polymorphic B cell lymphoproliferative disorder, consisting of aggregates of plasma cells and varying stages of lymphocytes in the lungs, the liver, the spleen, and the lymph nodes.[46, 81, 86, 89] LIP occurs in immune disorders other than AIDS, such as Sjögren's syndrome, autoimmune hemolytic anemia, pernicious anemia, myasthenia gravis, chronic active hepatitis, and alterations in levels or function of humoral immunoglobulins.[83, 86, 87]

LIP has an insidious course in pediatric AIDS; respiratory distress is milder than in the pneumonias associated with *P. carinii* or CMV, which cause a more rapid progression of pulmonary symptoms.[46, 87] In contrast to *P. carinii* pneumonia, LIP usually develops in older children.[54] Initial manifestations include cough and dyspnea.[87] Lymphadenopathy, clubbing of fingers and toes, parotid gland enlargement, and mild hypoxia occur more frequently in the LIP/PLH spectrum than with the opportunistic pneumonias, whereas fever, tachypnea, retractions, and adventitious lung sounds occur less often.[46] On chest radiographs, bilateral reticulonodular interstitial infiltrates, which are more prominent in the lower lobes, characterize LIP (Fig. 21–6),[46, 49, 86, 87] whereas PLH appears as scattered nodules that increase in size with progression of the disease and is associated with mediastinal and hilar adenopathy.[46] Pulmonary function testing

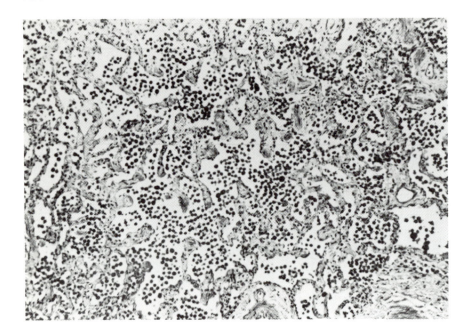

Figure 21–7. Desquamative interstitial pneumonitis with a sparse interstitial infiltrate of lymphocytes and plasma cells, alveoli filled with macrophages, and preservation of lung morphology. (From Katzenstein A-LA, Askin FB: Idiopathic interstitial pneumonia/idiopathic pulmonary fibrosis. *In* Bennington JL [ed]: Surgical Pathology of Non-Neoplastic Lung Disease, 2nd ed, p. 76. Philadelphia: WB Saunders, 1990.)

reveals restrictive lung disease, diminution of diffusing capacity, and arterial hypoxemia, which is more prominent with exercise.[86, 87]

DESQUAMATIVE INTERSTITIAL PNEUMONITIS

Desquamative interstitial pneumonitis (DIP) occurs in pediatric AIDS[80, 81] but has not been described in adult HIV infection.[48, 49, 72] It results from lung injury and can progress to interstitial fibrosis, a honeycomb lung, and respiratory failure.[80, 81, 87] It is characterized by a thin interstitial infiltrate of lymphocytes and plasma cells, cuboidal metaplasia of type II epithelial cells, intra-alveolar migration of monocytes and macrophages, and preservation of normal lung architecture (Fig. 21–7).[80, 81, 87, 90] Iron-containing inclusions within the intra-alveolar macrophages can be present but are also observed in other disorders.[90] Lymphocytic aggregates, hyaline membranes, viral inclusions, granulomas, and necrosis are not identified in DIP,[80, 90] although histologic evidence of an opportunistic infection or LIP may be present.[80, 81] DIP also occurs in pulmonary eosinophilic granuloma, in pneumoconiosis, in congenital rubella, after viral pneumonia, and in disorders involving the lymphoreticular system, such as acute lymphatic leukemia and chronic granulomatous disease.[80, 81, 90]

DIP has an insidious course, beginning with a dry-sounding cough, shortness of breath, and rapid respirations.[87] With progressive lung disease, crackles in the lower lobes, digital clubbing, and cyanosis can occur with DIP.[87] Chest radiographs reveal a triangular ground-glass pattern radiating from the hila to the lower lung fields but sparing the costophrenic angles.[87, 90] Radiographic changes are absent in 10% of patients with DIP.[87] Pulmonary function testing reveals restrictive lung disease, a reduced diffusing capacity, and arterial hypoxemia, which worsens with exercise.[87] These changes can be present in DIP despite normal results of a physical examination.[87]

DIFFUSE ALVEOLAR DAMAGE

Diffuse alveolar damage (DAD) occurs in both pediatric and adult HIV infection.[49, 72, 80, 81] Like LIP and DIP, DAD represents an interstitial inflammatory response of the lung to an injury, which, with DAD and AIDS, is probably a combination of positive-pressure ventilation, supplemental oxygen, and an infection with an opportunistic organism.[49, 72, 81, 91] DAD is also observed in other conditions, such as severe pulmonary infections with viruses and *Mycoplasma,* inhalation of toxic gases, exposure to chemotherapeutic agents or radiation, shock, near-drowning, uremia, and high altitude.[91, 92] Some of the pathologic abnormalities in bronchopulmonary dysplasia reflect the organizing state of DAD, and histologic changes in the acute respiratory distress syndrome are also a result of DAD.[91, 92]

An initial acute, or exudative, stage occurs within the first week of the lung injury and causes (1) damage to alveolar epithelial cells, the alveolar capillary membrane, and capillary endothelial cells; (2) thickening of the interstitium with fluid, plasma cells, lymphocytes, and histiocytes; (3) intra-alveolar hemorrhage and edema; (4) atelectasis; and (5) hyaline membrane formation (Fig. 21–8).[91, 92] Hyaline membranes are characteristic of DAD, are present throughout the acinus, and are composed of fibrin, protein, and necrotic epithelial cells.[92] Replication of alveolar epithelial type II cells begins during this stage in an attempt to repair the damage.[91]

One to 2 weeks after the lung injury, a proliferative, or organizing, stage occurs with interstitial inflammation, edema, and fibrosis. Fibroblasts multiply within the hyaline membranes, resulting in formation of organized fibrous tissue within the acinus. If the patient survives,

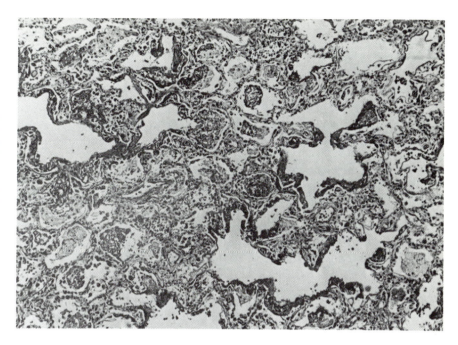

Figure 21–8. Acute diffuse alveolar damage with hyaline membranes, interstitial and alveolar edema, and alveolar hemorrhage. (From Katzenstein A-LA, Askin FB: Acute lung injury patterns: Diffuse alveolar damage, acute interstitial pneumonia, bronchiolitis obliterans-organizing pneumonia. *In* Bennington JL [ed]: Surgical Pathology of Non-Neoplastic Lung Disease, 2nd ed, p. 13. Philadelphia: WB Saunders, 1990.)

intra-alveolar fibrosis results with alveolar destruction, remodeling, and a honeycomb pattern.[91,92] The two stages of DAD may not be distinct, and recovery can occur in the exudative stage without further progression.[91]

DAD is characterized clinically by a rapid onset and severe respiratory distress that usually progresses to respiratory failure.[91,92] Interstitial pneumonitis, lung collapse, pulmonary edema, and a honeycomb lung may be present on chest radiographs.[91,92] The few children in whom DAD and HIV have been identified died of the lung disease.[80]

CHRONIC INTERSTITIAL PNEUMONITIS

A chronic interstitial pneumonitis occurs in pediatric HIV infection and is characterized by T8 and T11 lymphocytes in the infiltrate, with occasional T4 and B cells.[93] The infiltrate consists of lymphocytes, plasma cells, and pulmonary alveolar macrophages that invade and partially destroy bronchioles.[93] The macrophages fill alveoli, and interstitial fibrosis can occur.[93,94] Viral inclusions and evidence of an opportunistic infection are absent.[93] The clinical and radiographic features are similar to those in LIP.[93,94]

PULMONARY TUMORS

Approximately 4% of children with HIV infection have Kaposi's sarcoma,[27] but there are no reports to date of the tumor's occurring in the lungs in pediatric AIDS. Kaposi's sarcoma is described in children as a cutaneous lesion or a disseminated malignancy of the lymph nodes, the spleen, and the thymus, with proliferation of lymphocytes, plasma cells, and immunoblasts.[95,96] Children with nonpulmonary Kaposi's sarcoma have died of respiratory failure unrelated to the tumor.

Pulmonary Kaposi's sarcoma in adult AIDS has an acute onset and an aggressive clinical course and can result in respiratory failure.[97,98] The lesions have a characteristic red or violaceous color and consist of spindle-shaped cells with hyperchromatic nuclei, slitlike spaces filled with erythrocytes and hemosiderin, and intra-alveolar hemorrhage.[49,72,97–99] The tumor can occur as tracheobronchial or endobronchial lesions, nodular masses, interstitial infiltrates, pleural effusions, and mediastinal and hilar adenopathy.[49,72,98,99] Patients may be afebrile, and radiographs may reveal infiltrates for several months before the diagnosis is made.[98]

Other pulmonary tumors have been described in pediatric HIV infection. Pulmonary immunoblastic sarcoma consists of multiple tumor masses in the lungs, the liver, the spleen, the kidneys, and the adrenal glands.[94] The lung lesion is associated with hilar adenopathy and invasion of bronchial walls and pleura. Pulmonary leiomyomas can be associated with other smooth muscle tumors in the stomach and in the large and small intestines.[100] This primary pulmonary neoplasm can be parenchymal or endobronchial, and pulmonary metastases from the gastrointestinal lesions have been noted.

LABORATORY DIAGNOSIS

The pulmonary diseases in pediatric HIV infection are diagnosed from a history of respiratory difficulties (cough, tachypnea, dyspnea, fever), physical examination (nasal flaring, retractions, abnormal or adventitious lung sounds, cyanosis, clubbing of fingers and toes), and laboratory evaluation. Studies include anteroposterior and lateral radiographic views of the chest; cultures and stains for opportunistic organisms in respiratory secretions, bronchoalveolar lavage (BAL), pleural fluid, and lung tissue obtained by open-lung biopsy; serum antigen and antibody tests and immunofluorescent antibody determinations of respiratory secretions for viruses; DNA hybridization, including the PCR; and histologic examination of lung tissue. Arterial blood gas measurements and pulmonary function testing provide additional information.

PNEUMOCYSTIS CARINII

P. carinii pneumonia is diagnosed by stains of respiratory secretions in children by either induced sputum or BAL (with the use of 5- to 10-ml aliquots of sterile nonbacteriostatic saline).[48, 52] The thick cyst walls of *P. carinii* stain brown-black with Gomori's methenamine silver (see Fig. 21–3) and purple-violet with toluidine blue O stains, whereas the sporozoites and trophozoites are recognized with Giemsa, Wright's, and polychrome methylene blue stains.[51–53] Although BAL studies can detect *P. carinii* in more than 80% of cases,[101] microscopic examination of lung tissue provides more definitive identification of the organism in the remainder. Additional studies include serologic determination of a *P. carinii* IgG antibody, measured by enzyme-linked immunosorbent assay (ELISA), and of an antigen, analyzed by latex particle agglutination; indirect immunofluorescence for identifying monoclonal antibodies in respiratory secretions and tissue; and DNA hybridization techniques.[102–106]

P. carinii pneumonia in adults usually develops when peripheral T4 lymphocyte counts are ≤200 cells/cu mm, or 20% or fewer of the total lymphocytes.[107] Thus serial peripheral T4 counts can be used to evaluate the occurrence of *P. carinii* pneumonia in adults. However, the number of T4 cells may be higher in children with *P. carinii* pneumonia, and thus serial counts are less useful in this age group.[108]

Serial serum lactate dehydrogenase (LDH) levels can be used to follow the course of *P. carinii* pneumonia.[46, 109] Although both *P. carinii* pneumonia and LIP are associated with elevated serum LDH concentrations, the enzyme levels are higher with *P. carinii,* particularly during the acute infection. A decline in serum LDH levels occurs with clinical recovery, and relapse is preceded by a rise again in the enzyme level.[109]

CYTOMEGALOVIRUS

CMV pneumonia is diagnosed by examination of respiratory secretions, BAL, or lung tissue.[48, 62, 63, 65, 101] Gomori's methenamine silver and periodic acid–Schiff stains identify the cytoplasmic inclusions, whereas hematoxylin-eosin stains reveal both cytoplasmic and intranuclear inclusions (see Fig. 21–5).[63] The organism can be seen in lavage fluid in more than 80% of cases,[101] and histologic examination of lung tissue is required for the rest. Serologic antibody tests for diagnosis include complement fixation, indirect fluorescence, anticomplement and macroglobulin immunofluorescence, and ELISA.[59, 60] DNA probes and monoclonal antibodies to CMV proteins in the lung are also available.[61, 110, 111]

BACTERIA, VIRUSES, FUNGI, PROTOZOA

The diagnosis of bacterial pneumonia includes cultures and Gram's stain of respiratory secretions, sputum, BAL and pleural fluids, and lung tissue. Viral pneumonia is identified by cultures of nasopharyngeal or airway secretions and of lung tissue; microscopy of these secretions and tissue for viral inclusions; immunofluorescence, radioimmunoassay, and ELISA antigen studies of nasal secretions; a fourfold rise in antibody titers between acute and convalescent sera; and DNA probes of lung tissue for viruses.[83, 84] However, viral cultures are not always positive in acute respiratory infections proved to be viral by other methods, and CMV, Epstein-Barr virus, adenovirus, and herpes simplex virus can be identified in the lung without associated clinical or laboratory manifestations of respiratory illness that result from these organisms.[112]

Pulmonary fungal infections are evaluated with appropriate stains and cultures of respiratory secretions, pleural fluid, BAL, and lung tissue. Stains include silver, periodic acid-Schiff, and wet mount with India ink for *Cryptococcus;* Gomori's methenamine silver and wet mount with 10% potassium hydroxide for *Coccidioides;* and Gomori's methenamine silver and hematoxylin-eosin for *Histoplasma.*[113–115] Fungi can be cultured from lavage fluid in 80% of cases,[101] and histologic examination of lung tissue aids in confirming the diagnosis. Measurements of serum antibody titers and antigen are also available.[113–116]

Pulmonary protozoan infections are identified by stains of lung tissue.[117, 118] Additional studies for *Toxoplasma* include indirect fluorescence and ELISA testing for serum antibody, ELISA testing for serum antigen, and DNA probes of lung tissue.[119, 120] Protozoa cannot be grown *in vitro.*[118]

MYCOBACTERIA

Definitive diagnosis of pulmonary mycobacterial infections depends on identification of the organism in airway secretions, sputum, gastric washings, BAL and pleural fluids, and lung tissue.[68, 69, 79, 101, 121] Culture media include BACTEC-Middlebrook (which can also be used to isolate mycobacteria from blood), Lowenstein-Jensen, and Middlebrook.[69, 122] Acid-fast stains (such as Ziehl-Neelsen and Kinyoun) and fluorescence techniques of respiratory secretions and tissue help identify the presence of these organisms,[69, 121] but the sensitivity of this technique may be diminished as a result of the presence of nontuberculous mycobacteria in drinking water in some areas of the United States.[69, 123] Histologic identification of granulomas and caseation necrosis aids in the diagnosis,[69, 79, 121] but these findings are unusual in infection with MAI and HIV.[48, 66, 122] Other techniques that may be helpful in diagnosing active tuberculosis when cultures are negative include a radioactive-labeled gallium lung scan, ELISA testing for antibody to antigen 5 of *M. tuberculosis,* and DNA hybridization, which can rapidly identify mycobacteria in respiratory secretions if treatment has not been initiated.[123–125]

Mantoux's tuberculin skin testing with five tuberculin

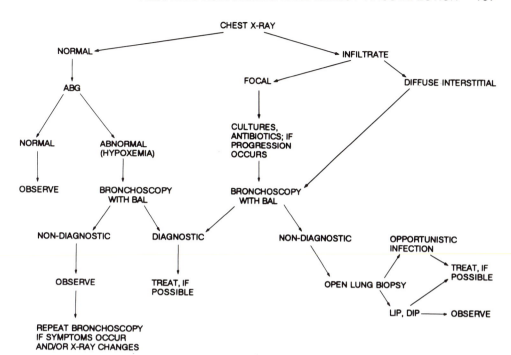

Figure 21–9. Diagnostic evaluation of pulmonary involvement in pediatric HIV infection. ABG, arterial blood gas; BAL, bronchoalveolar lavage; LIP, lymphocytic interstitial pneumonitis; DIP, desquamative interstitial pneumonitis.

units (TU) of purified protein derivative (PPD) identifies the presence of tuberculous infection and confirms exposure to *M. tuberculosis,* if positive (see Chapter 38).[66, 69, 123] A skin test reaction with ≥ 5 mm of induration after 48 to 72 h in HIV infection indicates tuberculous exposure or disease.[69, 76] Although tuberculin skin test reactions with HIV infection can be negative (≤4 mm of induration) as a result of anergy,[66, 68, 123, 126] the reaction is significant in at least two fifths of patients infected with both *M. tuberculosis* and HIV.[48, 76]

HIV-infected patients should be evaluated with a 5 TU PPD. A chest radiograph and examination for extrapulmonary tuberculosis are indicated if AIDS is present, regardless of the tuberculin skin test reaction.[66, 68, 126] If the PPD and/or the chest radiograph is positive, the possibility of tuberculous infection or disease must be investigated further.[66, 68, 123, 126] The presence of risk factors for HIV should be examined when infection or disease with *M. tuberculosis* occurs, particularly if tuberculosis is severe or unusual, and HIV testing should be considered if these risk factors are present.[66, 68, 76, 126]

The diagnosis of pulmonary tuberculosis is made more difficult in HIV infection because of false-negative tuberculin skin test reactions and radiographic findings that are unusual in tuberculosis without HIV infection.[77] Consequently, tuberculosis may be misdiagnosed as *P. carinii* pneumonia in this setting.[77] However, neither *P. carinii* pneumonia nor HIV itself is associated with the hilar or mediastinal adenopathy typical of pulmonary tuberculosis.[76, 77]

LIP, DIP, AND DAD

LIP, DIP, and DAD differ in radiographic patterns and clinical course. They are diagnosed definitively through microscopic examination of lung tissue obtained from open-lung biopsy (see Figs. 21–7, 21–8). The round or

oval iron-containing inclusions in macrophages in DIP react positively with periodic acid-Schiff and are blue-gray with hematoxylin-eosin stains.[90] Although polyclonal hypergammaglobulinemia characterizes HIV infection, the highest elevation in serum IgG levels occurs with LIP.[46] This finding can be used to help identify LIP clinically and to distinguish between LIP and *P. carinii* pneumonia.[46]

ALGORITHM

The algorithm in Figure 21–9 provides an overall plan for the evaluation of lung disease in pediatric HIV infection.[48, 127, 128] If both the chest radiograph and arterial blood gas measurements are normal, additional studies are usually postponed, particularly because respiratory symptoms are likely to be absent at this time. If the chest radiograph is normal but respiratory symptoms or arterial hypoxemia is present, bronchoscopy with BAL is performed to obtain secretions for cultures and stains in order to determine the presence of an infection. If these studies are nondiagnostic, the patient is observed, and, if respiratory symptoms or radiographic changes occur, bronchoscopy is repeated. If the BAL studies indicate an infection, therapy is initiated, if possible.

A focal infiltrate on a chest film most likely has a bacterial or viral etiology. Cultures, stains, and antigen studies of respiratory secretions and arterial blood gas measurements are obtained, and appropriate antimicrobial therapy is instituted, if possible. However, if the lung disease progresses radiographically or clinically, bronchoscopy with BAL is performed. If the BAL studies are nondiagnostic, an open-lung biopsy helps determine the type of infection present or whether LIP or DIP is the lesion.

Diffuse interstitial infiltrates usually occur with nonbacterial infections, LIP, and DIP. Bronchoscopy with BAL is performed initially. If findings are nondiagnostic, an open-lung biopsy is indicated, particularly if arterial hypoxemia or respiratory symptoms are present.

HUMAN IMMUNODEFICIENCY VIRUS

The possibility of HIV infection should be evaluated in children with an unexplained pulmonary opportunistic infection, interstitial pneumonitis, or any of the clinical features suggestive of HIV disease. The following laboratory abnormalities are used to diagnose pediatric HIV infection: growth of or histologic evidence of HIV-1 or HIV-2 in the patient's tissues; serum antigen, particularly p24, or antibody to HIV-1; polyclonal hypergammaglobulinemia, although hypogammaglobulinemia can also occur; diminished numbers of total and helper T lymphocytes; reversed helper/suppressor T lymphocyte ratio; absolute lymphopenia, which is defined as <1500 lymphocytes/cu mm and is present less frequently in HIV infection in children than in adults; and elevated levels of serum beta$_2$-microglobulin and neopterin and of urine neopterin.[30, 33, 47, 129, 130]

The presence of p24 antigen indicates active HIV multiplication. This antigen is more likely to be detected shortly after the initial infection with HIV, before antibody formation, and in the late stages of disease when the immune system is ineffective in suppressing HIV replication.[131] In addition, increasing concentrations of beta$_2$-microglobulin and neopterin indicate progression of HIV infection to AIDS.[130–132]

HIV-1 antibody is detected through an initial screening test, such as an enzyme immunoassay (EIA), in blood, BAL, cerebrospinal fluid, and urine.[106, 133–136] The EIA can be associated with false-positive results secondary to nonspecific serologic reactions and with false-negative studies as a result of testing before the development of measurable antibody.[134] If two EIA tests on the same specimen are reactive, the more specific Western blot test is then used; this test, if positive, indicates the presence of HIV-1 antibody.[134, 135] Other tests, such as isoelectric focusing and affinity immunoblotting, may be helpful in determining the presence of HIV-1 antigen-specific IgG antibody, particularly in congenital HIV infection.[137]

In addition, the PCR can detect HIV-1 DNA in peripheral blood monocytes and lymphocytes in persons who initially test negatively for HIV-1 antigen or antibody.[12, 106, 138] This technique amplifies DNA for hybridization in small quantities of cells, and the availability of results within 3 to 4 days makes it a potentially useful test clinically. The high specificity and moderate sensitivity of the current technique for the PCR allow identification of HIV-1 infection in children younger than age 15 months who could not be diagnosed previously because of the persistence of maternal IgG antibody to HIV. The PCR may eventually be used to detect the presence of other viruses when other tests are initially negative.[111]

Additional immunologic abnormalities in pediatric HIV infection include loss of *in vitro* T cell function with decreased lymphoproliferative responses to mitogens and antigens, cutaneous anergy, loss of *in vitro* B cell function, increased numbers of B lymphocytes, diminished plasma thymulin levels, and the presence of circulating immune complexes.[31, 42, 88, 139] Many children also have antibody titers to Epstein-Barr virus, CMV, hepatitis B virus, herpes simplex and zoster viruses, and *Toxoplasma*.[44, 83, 84, 140]

A reversed helper/suppressor T lymphocyte ratio is not pathognomonic of HIV infection, even in persons at risk for development of AIDS.[50, 140] A reversed ratio can occur in acute viral infections, such as infections with CMV, Epstein-Barr virus, or herpes zoster virus, or with hypersensitivity pneumonitis.[50, 140] However, the number of T4 cells is unaltered and the number of T8 cells is elevated in these diseases, unlike the changes seen with HIV.[50] Tuberculosis also results in a reversed T4/T8 ratio, which normalizes after a few months of antituberculous chemotherapy.[141] Persistent T cell depletion and dysfunction after initiation of therapy is likely to be indicative of infection with HIV.[141]

Transplacental passage of HIV-1 antigen is believed not to occur.[142] Therefore, its presence in a newborn most likely indicates active neonatal infection.[142] In addition, high maternal titers of antibody to gp120 of HIV-1 appear to protect full-term infants from the develpment of HIV infection.[143]

DIFFERENTIAL DIAGNOSIS

The differential diagnosis of the pulmonary diseases in pediatric HIV infection centers on the differential diagnosis of HIV infection itself. In general, the interstitial pneumonias have a more insidious clinical presentation with a milder course than do the opportunistic infections. However, they are diagnosed only through definitive histologic or microbiologic studies.

Other conditions that may mimic HIV infection are Nezelof's and Wiskott-Aldrich syndromes. These disorders are not associated with HIV antibodies and do not have an epidemiologic pattern of spread. In addition, low or normal serum immunoglobulin levels are characteristic of Nezelof's syndrome,[140, 144] and decreased platelet size is characteristic of Wiskott-Aldrich syndrome.[50]

THERAPY

The dosages and side effects of antimicrobial agents used in therapy for the pulmonary disorders in pediatric HIV infection are outlined in Table 21–4. Treatment of *P. carinii* pneumonia includes pentamidine isethionate and trimethoprim-sulfamethoxazole (TMP-SMX). The high incidence of adverse effects with TMP-SMX in HIV infection frequently prevents its use in these patients.[48, 52, 127, 128, 145] Despite the recommended 14 to 21 days of therapy with pentamidine or TMP-SMX, clinical and histologic recurrences of *P. carinii* pneumonia are frequent, and longer courses of therapy may be necessary.[127, 128, 145] In adults with moderate to severe *P. carinii* pneumonia, as defined by an arterial oxygen tension of <70 mm Hg or an alveolar-arterial oxygen gradient of >35 mm Hg, early use of corticosteroid therapy is advised in combination with an anti-*Pneumocystis* agent to reduce the progression of the disease.[146, 147] Guidelines for the use of corticosteroids in children with *P. carinii* pneumonia are not

Table 21–4. ANTIMICROBIAL THERAPY FOR PULMONARY DISORDERS IN PEDIATRIC HIV INFECTION

Pulmonary Disorder	Antimicrobial Therapy	Side Effects
Pneumocystis carinii	Pentamidine isethionate (Pentam 300): treatment: 4 mg/kg/dose IM or IV slowly once daily for 14–21 days; prophylaxis: 300 mg aerosolized via Respirgard II inhaler once monthly	Temporary hypotension, tachycardia, arrhythmias, hypoglycemia, hyperglycemia, hypocalcemia, pancreatitis, hepatotoxicity, reversible nephrotoxicity, megaloblastic anemia, granulocytopenia, gastrointestinal distress, increased incidence of side effects when given IV
	TMP-SMX (Bactrim, Septra): treatment: 20 mg/kg/day TMP or 100 mg/kg/day SMX po or IV in 4 divided doses for 14–21 days (maximum, 320 mg TMP/day and 1600 mg SMX/day); prophylaxis: 150 mg/sq m/day TMP and 750 mg/sq m/day SMX po in 2 divided doses 3 times weekly on consecutive days	Skin rashes, gastrointestinal distress, stomatitis, transient jaundice, headache, depression, hallucinations, irreversible nephrotoxicity, bone marrow suppression; increased incidence of fever, malaise, skin rash and pancytopenia with HIV; reduce dose in renal or liver disease or G6PD deficiency; contraindicated under age 2 months; potentiates oral anticoagulants and phenytoin
	Dapsone: prophylaxis: 1 mg/kg/day (maximum, 100 mg/day) po once daily	Agranulocytosis, hypersensitivity, peripheral neuropathy
	Leucovorin 1 mg/kg/day po, IM or IV as 1 dose (max. 10 mg/day)	Decreases actions of phenytoin, phenobarbital, primidone
Cytomegalovirus	DHPG (ganciclovir [Cytovene]) 6.0–7.5 mg/kg/day IV in 2–3 divided doses for 10–20 days	Reversible leukopenia, thrombocytopenia, gastrointestinal distress, skin rashes, nephrotoxicity, hepatotoxicity, neurotoxicity, phlebitis at IV site, increased toxicity with zidovudine
Respiratory syncytial virus	Ribavirin (Virazole) 6 g vial aerosolized for 12–20 h/day for 3–7 days	Bronchospasm, conjunctivitis, skin rashes, attenuated action with zidovudine
Influenza A virus	Amantadine hydrochloride (Symmetrel) 5–8 mg/kg/day po in 2 divided doses (max. 200 mg/day)	Insomnia, vertigo, fatigue, orthostatic hypotension, congestive heart failure, psychosis, urinary retention; increased toxicity with renal dysfunction, hydrochlorothiazide-triamterene, ipratropium; interacts with anticholinergics to cause confusion and hallucinations
Herpes simplex and zoster-varicella viruses	Acyclovir sodium (Zovirax) 45 mg/kg/day as 2-h IV infusion or po in 3 divided doses for 5–7 days	Phlebitis at IV site, skin rashes, nephrotoxicity, hepatotoxicity, neurotoxicity, bone marrow suppression, nausea; increased toxicity with zidovudine, interferon, probenecid
	Vidarabine (Vira-A) 10 mg/kg/day as 6-h IV infusion for 5 days	Gastrointestinal distress, phlebitis at IV site, neurotoxicity, increased toxicity with allopurinol, increases theophylline half-life
	DHPG (ganciclovir [Cytovene]) 6.0–7.5 mg/kg/day IV in 2–3 divided doses for 10–20 days	Reversible leukopenia, thrombocytopenia, gastrointestinal distress, skin rashes, nephrotoxicity, hepatotoxicity, neurotoxicity, phlebitis at IV site, increased toxicity with zidovudine
Toxoplasma	Pyrimethamine (Daraprim) 2 mg/kg/day for initial 3 days, then 1 mg/kg/day po in 2 divided doses (max. 25 mg/day)	Bone marrow suppression via folic acid antagonism
	Sulfadiazine, trisulfapyrimidine 120–150 mg/kg/day po in 4 divided doses (max. 4 g/day)	Bone marrow suppression, hemolytic anemia, hepatotoxicity, nephrotoxicity, skin rashes; potentiates actions of phenytoin, oral hypoglycemics, oral anticoagulants
	Leucovorin 1 mg/kg/day po, IM or IV as 1 dose (max. 10 mg/day)	Decreases actions of phenytoin, phenobarbital, primidone
Fungi	Amphotericin B (Fungizone) 0.25 mg/kg/day as 6-h IV infusion, increasing dose by 0.25 mg/kg/day every 2–3 days (max. 1 mg/kg/day, 30–35 mg/kg total dose)	Phlebitis at IV site, nephrotoxicity, gastrointestinal distress, hypokalemia, reversible anemia; chills, fever, vomiting during administration; increases nephrotoxicity of other drugs, attenuated action with miconazole, increased toxicity with flucytosine and corticosteroids
	Ketoconazole (Nizoral) 5–10 mg/kg/day po as 1–2 doses	Gastrointestinal distress, hepatotoxicity, photophobia, headache, decreased testosterone synthesis; decreases effects of antacids, isoniazid, rifampin; potentiates effects of oral anticoagulants
	Flucytosine (Ancobon) 150 mg/kg/day po in 4 divided doses	Gastrointestinal distress, skin rashes, hepatotoxicity, pancytopenia, increased toxicity with amphotericin B

Table 21–4. ANTIMICROBIAL THERAPY FOR PULMONARY DISORDERS IN PEDIATRIC HIV INFECTION *Continued*

Pulmonary Disorder	Antimicrobial Therapy	Side Effects
Mycobacterium tuberculosis	Isoniazid 10–15 mg/kg/day po or IM (max. 300 mg/day) plus rifampin (Rimactane, Rifadin) 10–20 mg/kg/day po (max. 600 mg/day) plus, for the initial 2 months, either pyrazinamide 20–30 mg/kg/day po in 3–4 divided doses (max. 2 g/day) or ethambutol (Myambutol) 15–25 mg/kg/day po (max. 1.5 g/day)	Isoniazid: hepatotoxicity, peripheral neuritis, arthritic symptoms, vasculitis, potentiates action of anticonvulsants, inhibits action of pyridoxine Rifampin: hepatotoxicity, red-orange color of secretions, bone marrow suppression; inhibits actions of oral contraceptives, digoxin, oral hypoglycemics, corticosteroids, methadone Ethambutol: reversible optic neuritis, impaired visual acuity Pyrazinamide: hepatotoxicity, hyperuricemia, arthralgia
Mycobacterium avium-intracellulare	Isoniazid 10–15 mg/kg/day po or IM (max. 300 mg/day) plus ethambutol (Myambutol) 15–25 mg/kg/day po (max. 1.5 g/day) plus ansamycin (Rifabutine) 5 mg/kg/day po in 1–2 divided doses (max. 300 mg/day) plus clofazimine (Lamprene) 2–5 mg/kg/day po in 1–3 divided doses (max. 300 mg/day) for 6–24 months	Clofazimine: gastrointestinal distress; red-brown color of urine, skin, cornea, retina, tears; anticholinergic effect Ansamycin: same as rifampin
Mycobacterium kansasii	Isoniazid 10–15 mg/kg/day po or IM (max. 300 mg/day) plus rifampin (Rimactane, Rifadin) 10–20 mg/kg/day po (max. 600 mg/day) plus ethambutol (Myambutol) 15–25 mg/kg/day po (max. 1.5 g/day) for 15 months; may add streptomycin 20–40 mg/kg/day IM twice weekly (max. 1 g/day) for the first 3 months	Streptomycin: nephrotoxicity, vestibular and auditory ototoxicity, inactivated by high concentrations of ticarcillin; potentiates actions of neuromuscular blocking agents, ethacrynic acid, cephalosporins, amphotericin B
Lymphocytic interstitial pneumonitis, desquamative interstitial pneumonitis, diffuse alveolar damage	Corticosteroids: prednisone 1–2 mg/kg/day po in 1–2 divided doses; hydrocortisone (Solu-Cortef) 10 mg/kg/day IV or IM in 4 divided doses; methylprednisolone (Solu-Medrol) 1–2 mg/kg/day IV or IM in 4–6 divided doses	Pituitary-adrenal inhibition, osteoporosis, growth suppression, hypokalemic alkalosis, edema, psychosis, myopathy, peptic ulcer; potentiates neuromuscular blocking agents; attenuated action with barbiturates, phenytoin, rifampin

IM, intramuscular; IV, intravenous; TMP, trimethoprim; SMX, sulfamethoxazole; po, oral; HIV, human immunodeficiency virus; G6PD, glucose-6-phosphate dehydrogenase; DHPG, 9-(1,3-dihydroxy-2-propoxymethyl)guanine.

currently established. Additional therapeutic modalities currently under consideration include dapsone, eflornithine, and the combination of trimetrexate and leucovorin.[51, 104, 148]

In adults, TMP-SMX or aerosolized pentamidine is prescribed to prevent clinical *P. carinii* pneumonia, particularly when the T4 lymphocyte count is <200/cu mm or <20% of the total lymphocytes.[48, 52, 53, 148, 149] A folate agent, leucovorin, is often prescribed to counteract the antifolate side effects of TMP-SMX.[145] In children, TMP-SMX prophylaxis is presently recommended for all HIV-infected children who are older than 1 month, have fewer than 1500 T4 cells/cu mm, or have had a previous episode of *P. carinii* pneumonia.[150] As the age of an HIV-infected child increases, the level of T4 cells used for determining the use of *P. carinii* prophylaxis decreases.[150] In HIV-infected children aged 5 years or older who cannot tolerate TMP-SMX, aerosolized pentamidine is recommended. Alternatively, dapsone may be used in children 1 month of age or older.

CMV pneumonia can be treated with ganciclovir, which results in only temporary improvement.[48, 61, 104, 151] CMV immune globulin administered in serial doses can prevent the development of CMV disease in certain clinical settings[61, 152] and may be applicable in HIV infection. Therapy of other viruses includes ribavirin for respiratory

syncytial virus, amantadine for influenza A virus, and acyclovir, vidarabine, and 9-(1,3-dihydroxy-2-propoxymethyl)guanine (DHPG) for herpes simplex and herpes zoster-varicella viruses.[112, 153, 154]

Pyrimethamine combined with either trisulfapyrimidine or sulfadiazine is used to treat *Toxoplasma* infections.[104, 118, 120] Leucovorin is also included so as to prevent bone marrow suppression caused by pyrimethamine.[120] Treatment is for a minimum of 3 to 4 weeks but may be prescribed indefinitely.

Amphotericin B or ketoconazole can be used to treat pulmonary disease resulting from infection with *Histoplasma* or *Coccidioides*.[114, 115] Disease with *Candida* or *Cryptococcus* is treated with both flucytosine and amphotericin B, although *Candida* infections can be treated with amphotericin B alone.[104, 113, 116] Antifungal drugs are usually prescribed for approximately 6 weeks.[113–116]

The duration of chemotherapy for patients infected with both *M. tuberculosis* and HIV is not known. Although antituberculous drug therapy should be prescribed for at least 9 months, which includes a minimum of 6 months after three cultures no longer grow *M. tuberculosis,* a longer regimen may be necessary.[66, 68, 126] If isoniazid or rifampin is not included because of drug resistance or toxicity, treatment should last for at least 18 months with a minimum of 12 months after culture conversion.[66, 68, 126] Alternatively, isoniazid therapy can be continued indefinitely.[66, 68] Patients with HIV infection and *M. tuberculosis* usually improve with antituberculous drugs.[66, 68, 126, 141]

Because HIV-infected patients with positive tuberculin skin test reactions have an increased chance of the development of tuberculosis, they should receive prophylactic isoniazid for at least 12 months.[66, 68, 126] In addition, patients whose specimens contain tubercle bacilli and who have HIV or high-risk factors for HIV should receive antituberculous chemotherapy.[68]

The administration of Calmette-Guérin bacillus (BCG) vaccine is recommended for asymptomatic HIV-infected children who are at increased risk for the development of tuberculosis.[155] However, BCG sepsis has occurred in this setting.[75] The BCG vaccine contains a live attenuated bacillus and is not administered to children with HIV infection who are symptomatic or who are unlikely to acquire tuberculosis.[155]

Drug therapy for nontuberculous mycobacteria is not standardized because most of these organisms respond poorly to chemotherapeutic agents. An exception is *M. kansasii,* which frequently responds to combined isoniazid, rifampin, and ethambutol therapy (see Table 21–4).[66, 69, 126] Ansamycin and clofazimine are investigational drugs at present.

Corticosteroids are often used in the treatment of LIP, DIP, and DAD.[87, 91, 156] In general, clinical, radiographic, and histologic features of DIP are more likely to respond to corticosteroids than are those of LIP.[87] However, LIP in pediatric AIDS appears to improve, even if transiently, with corticosteroids.[156]

Assisted ventilation, increased oxygen concentrations, positive end-expiratory pressure, and other supportive therapeutic modalities are used to treat respiratory failure secondary to these pulmonary diseases. In addition, children with HIV are frequently treated with serial intravenous gammaglobulin infusions in an attempt to enhance humoral immunity with new antigens.[50, 88, 104, 144, 156]

PROGNOSIS

The clinical course of the pulmonary diseases in pediatric HIV infection can be acute or chronic, waxing or waning. LIP appears to carry a relatively better short-term prognosis than does *P. carinii* pneumonia. Recurrent or low-grade persistence of *P. carinii* pneumonia occurs and eventually results in respiratory failure. The response of LIP and DIP to corticosteroids is variable.[87, 156] Although any of the opportunistic organisms can cause fatal pulmonary disease, bacteria and *M. tuberculosis* respond well to antimicrobial therapy, even with HIV. However, MAI and CMV infections are difficult to treat.

AIDS itself is fatal, and at present there is no cure. Several drugs, such as zidovudine (Retrovir) and dideoxyinosine, are available for treatment of HIV itself[104, 157-161] but they are not curative, and their use has resulted in reports of drug resistance. Although the time interval between the initial infection with the virus and clinical AIDS may be 10 to 12 years[104, 162] or even longer, the median age of survival for infants is 6 months and, for older children, 20 months.[27] The immunodeficiency is progressive, and pulmonary disease is the usual cause of death.

REFERENCES

1. Sato PA, Chin J, Mann JM: Review of AIDS and HIV infection: Global epidemiology and statistics. AIDS 3:S301–S307, 1989.
2. Centers for Disease Control: World AIDS Day 1990. AIDS in women—United States. MMWR 39:845–846, 1990.
3. Barnes DM: AIDS: Statistics but few answers. Science 236:1423–1425, 1987.
4. Centers for Disease Control: HIV/AIDS Surveillance Report, pp. 1–22, January 1992.
5. Centers for Disease Control: AIDS and human immunodeficiency virus infection in the Unites States: 1988 update. MMWR 38:1–38, 1989.
6. Wong-Staal F, Gallo RC: Human T-lymphotropic retroviruses. Nature 317:395–403, 1985.
7. Maynard EP, Frame B, Lewis CE, et al: Acquired immunodeficiency syndrome. Ann Intern Med 104:575–581, 1986.
8. Ho DD, Rota TR, Schooley RT, et al: Isolation of HTLV-III from cerebrospinal fluid and neural tissues of patients with neurologic syndromes related to the acquired immunodeficiency syndrome. N Eng J Med 313:1493–1497, 1985.
9. Gartner S, Markovits P, Markovitz DM, et al: The role of mononuclear phagocytes in HTLV-III/LAV infection. Science 233:215–219, 1986.
10. Levy JA: Human immunodeficiency viruses and the pathogenesis of AIDS. JAMA 261:2997–3006, 1989.
11. Ziegler JB, Cooper DA, Johnson RO, Gold J: Postnatal transmission of AIDS-associated retrovirus from mother to infant. Lancet 1:896–897, 1985.
12. Rogers MF, Ou C-Y, Rayfield M, et al: Use of the polymerase chain reaction for early detection of the proviral sequences of human immunodeficiency virus in infants born to seropositive mothers. N Engl J Med 320:1649–1654, 1989.
13. Salahuddin SA, Rose RM, Groopman JE, et al: Human T lymphotropic virus type III infection of human alveolar macrophages. Blood 68:281–284, 1986.
14. Fauci AS: The human immunodeficiency virus: Infectivity and mechanisms of pathogenesis. Science 239:617–622, 1988.
15. Manzari V, Gismondi A, Barillari G, et al: HTLV-V: A new human retrovirus isolated in a Tac-negative T cell lymphoma/leukemia. Science 238:1581–1583, 1987.
16. Molbak K, Lauritzen E, Fernandes D, et al: Antibodies to HTLV-IV associated with chronic, fatal illness resembling "slim" disease [Letter]. Lancet 2:1214–1215, 1986.
17. Clavel F, Mansinho K, Chamaret S, et al: Human immunodeficiency virus type 2 infection associated with AIDS in West Africa. N Engl J Med 316:1180–1185, 1987.
18. Harper ME, Kaplan MH, Marselle LM, et al: Concomitant infection with HTLV-I and HTLV-III in a patient with T8 lymphoproliferative disease. N Engl J Med 315:1073–1078, 1986.
19. Gallo RC, Wong-Staal F: A human T-lymphotropic retrovirus (HTLV-III) as the cause of the acquired immunodeficiency syndrome. Ann Intern Med 103:679–689, 1985.
20. Wong-Staal F, Gallo RC: The family of human T-lymphotropic leukemia viruses: HTLV-I as the cause of adult T cell leukemia and HTLV-III as the cause of acquired immunodeficiency syndrome. Blood 65:253–263, 1985.
21. Haseltine WA: Silent HIV infections. N Engl J Med 320:1487–1489, 1989.
21a. Cohen EA, Terwilliger EF, Jalinoos Y, et al: Identification of HIV-1 'vpr' product and function. J Acquired Immune Deficiency Syndromes 3:11–18, 1990.
22. Quinn TC, Mann JM, Curran JW, Piot P: AIDS in Africa: An epidemiologic paradigm. Science 234:955–963, 1986.
23. Ho DD, Pomerantz RJ, Kaplan JC: Pathogenesis of infection with human immunodeficiency virus. N Engl J Med 317:278–286, 1987.
24. Selwyn PA: AIDS—What is now known: I. History and immunovirology. Hosp Prac 21:67–82, 1986.

25. Levy JA: Changing concepts in HIV infection: Challenges for the 1990s. AIDS 4:1051–1058, 1990.
26. Resnick L, Novatt G: Human T-cell lymphotropic viruses: Syncytia formation. JAMA 255:3421, 1986.
27. Rogers MF, Thomas PA, Starcher ET, et al: Acquired immunodeficiency syndrome in children: Report of the Centers for Disease Control national surveillance, 1982 to 1985. Pediatrics 79:1008–1014, 1987.
28. Lapointe N, Michaud J, Pekovic D, et al: Transplacental transmission of HTLV-III virus [Letter]. N Engl J Med 312:1325–1326, 1985.
29. Morgan G, Wilkins HA, Pepin J, et al: AIDS following mother-to-child transmission of HIV-2. AIDS 4:879–882, 1990.
30. Centers for Disease Control: Revision of the CDC surveillance case definition for acquired immunodeficiency syndrome. MMWR 36:3S–15S, 1987.
30a. Chang SW, Katz MH, Hernandez SR: The new AIDS definitions. Implications for San Francisco. JAMA 267:973–975, 1992.
31. Seligmann M, Pinching AJ, Rosen FS, et al: Immunology of human immunodeficiency virus infection and the acquired immunodeficiency syndrome. An update. Ann Intern Med 107:234–242, 1987.
32. Centers for Disease Control: Update: Acquired immunodeficiency syndrome (AIDS)—United States. MMWR 32:688–691, 1984.
33. Centers for Disease Control: Classification system for human immunodeficiency virus (HIV) infection in children under 13 years of age. MMWR 36:225–236, 1987.
34. Marion RW, Wiznia AA, Hutcheon G, Rubinstein A: Fetal AIDS syndrome score: Correlation between severity of dysmorphism and age at diagnosis of immunodeficiency. Am J Dis Child 141:429–431, 1987.
35. Halsey NA, Boulos R, Holt E, et al: Transmission of HIV-1 infections from mothers to infants in Haiti. Impact on childhood mortality and malnutrition. JAMA 264:2088–2092, 1990.
36. Stiehm ER: Immunodeficiency. An overview. Chest 86:20S–23S, 1984.
37. Heinzel FP, Root RK: Antibodies. In Mandell GL, Douglas RG Jr, Bennett JE (eds): Principles and Practice of Infectious Diseases, 3rd ed, pp. 41–61. New York: Churchill Livingstone, 1990.
38. Wilson CB: The cellular immune system and its role in host defense. In Mandell GL, Douglas RG Jr, Bennett JE (eds): Principles and Practice of Infectious Diseases, 3rd ed, pp. 101–138. New York: Churchill Livingstone, 1990.
39. Waldmann TA, Tsudo M: Interleukin-2 receptors: Biology and therapeutic potentials. Hosp Prac 22:77–94, 1987.
40. Rosen FS, Cooper MD, Wedgwood RJP: The primary immunodeficiencies (first of two parts). N Engl J Med 311:235–242, 1984.
41. Nossal GJV: Current concepts: Immunology. The basic components of the immune system. N Engl J Med 316:1320–1325, 1987.
42. Pahwa S, Pahwa R, Saxinger C, et al: Influence of the human T-lymphotropic virus/lymphadenopathy-associated virus on functions of human lymphocytes: Evidence for immunosuppressive effects and polyclonal B-cell activation by banded viral preparations. Proc Natl Acad Sci 82:8198–8202, 1985.
43. Pahwa S, Fikrig S, Menez R, Pahwa R: Pediatric acquired immunodeficiency syndrome: Demonstration of B lymphocyte defects in vitro. Diagn Immunol 4:24–30, 1986.
44. Bernstein LJ, Ochs HD, Wedgwood RJ, Rubinstein A: Defective humoral immunity in pediatric acquired immune deficiency syndrome. J Pediatr 107:352–357, 1985.
45. Schnittman SM, Lane HC, Higgins SE, et al: Direct polyclonal activation of human B lymphocytes by the acquired immune deficiency syndrome virus. Science 233:1084–1086, 1986.
46. Rubinstein A, Morecki R, Silverman B, et al: Pulmonary disease in children with acquired immune deficiency syndrome and AIDS-related complex. J Pediatr 108:498–503, 1986.
47. Pahwa S, Kaplan M, Fikrig S, et al: Spectrum of human T-cell lymphotropic virus type III infection in children. Recognition of symptomatic, asymptomatic, and seronegative patients. JAMA 255:2299–2305, 1986.
48. Murray JF, Garay SM, Hopewell PC, et al: Pulmonary complications of the acquired immunodeficiency syndrome: An update. Report of the Second National Heart, Lung and Blood Institute Workshop. Am Rev Respir Dis 135:504–509, 1987.
49. Marchevsky A, Rosen MJ, Chrystal G, Kleinerman J: Pulmonary
complications of the acquired immunodeficiency syndrome: A clinicopathologic study of 70 cases. Hum Pathol 16:659–670, 1985.
50. Shannon KM, Ammann AJ: Acquired immune deficiency syndrome in childhood. J Pediatr 106:332–342, 1985.
51. Murray JF, Mills J: Pulmonary infectious complications of human immunodeficiency virus infection: Part II. Am Rev Respir Dis 141:1582–1598, 1990.
52. Walzer PD: Pneumocystis carinii. In Mandell GL, Douglas RG Jr, Bennett JE (eds): Principles and Practice of Infectious Diseases, 3rd ed, pp. 2103–2110. New York: Churchill Livingstone, 1990.
53. Young LS: Pneumocystis carinii. In Pennington JE (ed): Respiratory Infections: Diagnosis and Management, 2nd ed, pp. 570–582. New York: Raven Press, 1989.
54. Oxtoby MJ: Perinatally acquired human immunodeficiency virus infection. Pediatr Infect Dis J 9:609–619, 1990.
55. DeLorenzo LJ, Huang CT, Maguire GP, Stone DJ: Roentgenographic patterns of Pneumocystis carinii pneumonia in 104 patients with AIDS. Chest 91:323–327, 1987.
56. Gagliardi AJ, Stover DE, Zaman MK: Endobronchial Pneumocystis carinii infection in a patient with the acquired immune deficiency syndrome. Chest 91:463–464, 1987.
57. Sankary RM, Turner J, Lipavsky AJA, et al: Alveolar-capillary block in patients with AIDS and Pneumocystis carinii pneumonia. Am Rev Respir Dis 137:443–449, 1988.
58. Sanyal SS, Mariencheck WC, Hughes WT, et al: Course of pulmonary dysfunction in children surviving Pneumocystis carinii pneumonitis. A prospective study. Am Rev Respir Dis 124:161–166, 1981.
59. Hanshaw JB: Cytomegalovirus infections. In Feigin RD, Cherry JD (eds): Textbook of Pediatric Infectious Diseases, 2nd ed, pp. 1558–1566. Philadelphia: WB Saunders, 1987.
60. Ho M: Cytomegalovirus. In Mandell GL, Douglas RG Jr, Bennett JE (eds): Principles and Practice of Infectious Diseases, 3rd ed, pp. 1159–1172. New York: Churchill Livingstone,1990.
61. Sissons JGP, Borysiewicz LK: Human cytomegalovirus infection. Thorax 44:242–246, 1989.
62. Katzenstein A-LA, Askin FB: Infection: I. Unusual pneumonias. In Bennington JL (ed): Surgical Pathology of Non-Neoplastic Lung Disease, 2nd ed, pp. 323–326. Philadelphia: WB Saunders, 1990.
63. Gorelkin L, Chandler FW, Ewing EP Jr: Staining qualities of cytomegalovirus inclusions in the lungs of patients with the acquired immunodeficiency syndrome: A potential source of diagnostic misinterpretation. Hum Pathol 17:926–929, 1986.
64. Wallace JM, Hannah J: Cytomegalovirus pneumonitis in patients with AIDS: Findings in an autopsy series. Chest 92:198–203, 1987.
65. Schulman LL: Cytomegalovirus pneumonitis and lobar consolidation. Chest 91:558–561, 1987.
66. Snider DE Jr, Hopewell PC, Mills J, Reichman LB: Mycobacterioses and the acquired immunodeficiency syndrome. Am Rev Respir Dis 136:492–496, 1987.
67. Pitchenik AE, Robinson HA: The radiographic appearance of tuberculosis in patients with the acquired immune deficiency syndrome (AIDS) and pre-AIDS. Am Rev Respir Dis 131:393–396, 1985.
68. Centers for Disease Control: Tuberculosis and human immunodeficiency virus infection: Recommendations of the Advisory Committee for the Elimination of Tuberculosis (ACET). MMWR 38:236–250, 1989.
69. Smith MHD, Marquis JR: Tuberculosis and other mycobacterial infections. In Feigin RD, Cherry JD (eds): Textbook of Pediatric Infectious Diseases, 2nd ed, pp. 1342–1387. Philadelphia: WB Saunders, 1987.
70. Greene JB, Sidhu GS, Lewin S, et al: Mycobacterium avium-intracellulare: A cause of disseminated life-threatening infection in homosexuals and drug abusers. Ann Intern Med 97:539–546, 1982.
71. Sohn CC, Schroff RW, Kliewer KE, et al: Disseminated Mycobacterium avium-intracellulare infection in homosexual men with acquired cell-mediated immunodeficiency: A histologic and immunologic study of two cases. Am J Clin Pathol 79:247–252, 1983.
72. Nash G, Fligiel S: Pathologic features of the lung in the acquired

immune deficiency syndrome (AIDS): An autopsy study of seventeen homosexual males. Am J Clin Pathol 81:6–12, 1984.

73. Braun MM, Byers RH, Heyward WL, et al: Acquired immunodeficiency syndrome and extrapulmonary tuberculosis in the United States. Arch Intern Med 150:1913–1916, 1990.

74. Bye MR, Bernstein LJ: Identifying pulmonary sequelae in children with AIDS. J Respir Dis 10:27–39, 1989.

75. Houde C, Dery P: *Mycobacterium bovis* sepsis in an infant with human immunodeficiency virus infection. Pediatr Infect Dis J 7:810–812, 1988.

76. Chaisson RE, Slutkin G: Tuberculosis and human immunodeficiency virus infection. J Infect Dis 159:96–100, 1989.

77. Chaisson RE, Schecter GF, Theuer CP, et al: Tuberculosis in patients with the acquired immunodeficiency syndrome: Clinical features, response to therapy, and survival. Am Rev Respir Dis 136:570–574, 1987.

78. Inselman LS: Tuberculosis in children: Lessons in diagnosis. J Respir Dis 5:88–102, 1984.

79. Sunderam G, McDonald RJ, Maniatis T, et al: Tuberculosis as a manifestation of the acquired immunodeficiency syndrome (AIDS). JAMA 256:362–366, 1986.

80. Joshi VV, Oleske JM, Minnefor AB, et al: Pathologic pulmonary findings in children with the acquired immunodeficiency syndrome: A study of ten cases. Hum Pathol 16:241–246, 1985.

81. Joshi VV, Oleske JM: Pulmonary lesions in children with the acquired immunodeficiency syndrome: A reappraisal based on data in additional cases and follow-up study of previously reported cases [Letter]. Hum Pathol 17:641–642, 1986.

82. Joshi VV, Oleske JM, Minnefor AB, et al: Pathology of suspected acquired immune deficiency syndrome in children: A study of eight cases. Pediatr Pathol 2:71–87, 1984.

83. Fackler JC, Nagel JE, Adler WH, et al: Epstein-Barr virus infection in a child with acquired immunodeficiency syndrome. Am J Dis Child 139:1000–1004, 1985.

84. Andiman WA, Eastman R, Martin K, et al: Opportunistic lymphoproliferations associated with Epstein-Barr viral DNA in infants and children with AIDS. Lancet 2:1390–1393, 1985.

85. Chayt KJ, Harper ME, Marselle LM, et al: Detection of HTLV-III RNA in lungs of patients with AIDS and pulmonary involvement. JAMA 256:2356–2359, 1986.

86. Kradin RL, Mark EJ: Benign lymphoid disorders of the lung, with a theory regarding their development. Hum Pathol 14:857–867, 1983.

87. Fleetham JA, Thurlbeck WM: Desquamative interstitial pneumonia and other variants of interstitial pneumonia. *In* Chernick V (ed): Kendig's Disorders of the Respiratory Tract in Children, 5th ed, pp. 485–492. Philadelphia: WB Saunders, 1990.

88. Pahwa S, Fikrig S, Kaplan M, et al: Expressions of HTLV-III infection in a pediatric population. *In* Gupta S (ed): AIDS-Associated Syndromes, pp. 45–51. New York: Plenum Press, 1985.

89. Joshi VV, Kauffman S, Oleske JM, et al: Polyclonal polymorphic B-cell lymphoproliferative disorder with prominent pulmonary involvement in children with acquired immune deficiency syndrome. Cancer 59:1455–1462, 1987.

90. Katzenstein A-LA, Askin FB: Idiopathic interstitial pneumonia/idiopathic pulmonary fibrosis. *In* Bennington JL (ed): Surgical Pathology of Non-Neoplastic Lung Disease, 2nd ed, pp. 75–84. Philadelphia: WB Saunders, 1990.

91. Katzenstein A-LA, Askin FB: Acute lung injury patterns: Diffuse alveolar damage, acute interstitial pneumonia, bronchiolitis obliterans-organizing pneumonia. *In* Bennington JL (ed): Surgical Pathology of Non-Neoplastic Lung Disease, 2nd ed, pp. 10–34. Philadelphia: WB Saunders, 1990.

92. Mark EJ: Alveolar disease. *In* Lung Biopsy Interpretation, pp. 104–106. Baltimore: Williams & Wilkins, 1984.

93. Kornstein MJ, Pietra GG, Hoxie JA, Conley ME: The pathology and treatment of interstitial pneumonitis in two infants with AIDS. Am Rev Respir Dis 133:1196–1198, 1986.

94. Zimmerman BL, Haller JO, Price AP, et al: Children with AIDS—Is pathologic diagnosis possible based on chest radiographs? Pediatr Radiol 17:303–307, 1987.

95. Buck BE, Scott GB, Valdes-Dapena M, Parks WP: Kaposi sarcoma in two infants with acquired immune deficiency syndrome. J Pediatr 103:911–913, 1983.

96. Connor E, Boccon-Gibod L, Joshi V, et al: Cutaneous acquired immunodeficiency syndrome-associated Kaposi's sarcoma in pediatric patients. Arch Dermatol 126:791–793, 1990.

97. Bergfeld WF, Zemtsov A, Lang RS: Differentiation between AIDS-related and non-AIDS-related Kaposi's sarcoma. Clev Clin J Med 54:315–319, 1987.

98. Ognibene FP, Steis RG, Macher AM, et al: Kaposi's sarcoma causing pulmonary infiltrates and respiratory failure in the acquired immunodeficiency syndrome. Ann Intern Med 102:471–475, 1985.

99. Fouret PJ, Touboul JL, Mayaud CM, et al: Pulmonary Kaposi's sarcoma in patients with acquired immune deficiency syndrome: A clinicopathological study. Thorax 42:262–268, 1987.

100. Chadwick EG, Connor EJ, Hanson ICG, et al: Tumors of smooth-muscle origin in HIV-infected children. JAMA 263:3182–3184, 1990.

101. Stover DE, Zaman MB, Hajdu SI, et al: Bronchoalveolar lavage in the diagnosis of diffuse pulmonary infiltrates in the immunosuppressed host. Ann Intern Med 101:1–7, 1984.

102. Pifer LLW, Woods DR, Edwards CC, et al: *Pneumocystis carinii* serologic study in pediatric acquired immunodeficiency syndrome. Am J Dis Child 142:36–39, 1988.

103. Kovacs JA, Ng VL, Masur H, et al: Diagnosis of *Pneumocystis carinii* pneumonia: Improved detection in sputum with use of monoclonal antibodies. N Engl J Med 318:589–593, 1988.

104. Nicholas SW, Sondheimer DL, Willoughby AD, et al: Human immunodeficiency virus infection in childhood, adolescence, and pregnancy: A status report and national research agenda. Pediatrics 83:293–308, 1989.

105. Wakefield AE, Pixley FJ, Banerji S, et al: Detection of *Pneumocystis carinii* with DNA amplification. Lancet 336:451–453, 1990.

106. Husson RN, Comeau AM, Hoff R: Diagnosis of human immunodeficiency virus infection in infants and children. Pediatrics 86:1–10, 1990.

107. Phair J, Muñoz A, Detels R, et al: The risk of *Pneumocystis carinii* pneumonia among men infected with human immunodeficiency virus type 1. N Engl J Med 322:161–165, 1990.

108. Leibovitz E, Rigaud M, Pollack H, et al: *Pneumocystis carinii* pneumonia in infants infected with the human immunodeficiency virus with more than 450 CD4 T lymphocytes per cubic millimeter. N Engl J Med 323:531–533, 1990.

109. Silverman BA, Rubinstein A: Serum lactate dehydrogenase levels in adults and children with acquired immune deficiency syndrome (AIDS) and AIDS-related complex: Possible indicator of B cell lymphoproliferation and disease activity. Effect of intravenous gammaglobulin on enzyme levels. Am J Med 78:728–736, 1985.

110. Grody WW, Lewin KJ, Naeim F: Detection of cytomegalovirus DNA in classic and epidemic Kaposi's sarcoma by in situ hybridization. Hum Pathol 19:524–528, 1988.

111. Shibata D, Martin WJ, Appleman MD, et al: Detection of cytomegalovirus DNA in peripheral blood of patients infected with human immunodeficiency virus. J Infect Dis 158:1185–1192, 1988.

112. Kauffman RS: Viral pneumonia. *In* Pennington JE (ed): Respiratory Infections: Diagnosis and Management, 2nd ed, pp. 427–442. New York: Raven Press, 1989.

113. Diamond RD, Levitz SM: *Cryptococcus neoformans* pneumonia. *In* Pennington JE (ed): Respiratory Infections: Diagnosis and Management, 2nd ed, pp. 457–471. New York: Raven Press, 1989.

114. Drutz DJ: Coccidioidal pneumonia. *In* Pennington JE (ed): Respiratory Infections: Diagnosis and Management, 2nd ed, pp. 472–500. New York: Raven Press, 1989.

115. Sarosi GA, Davies SF: *Histoplasma capsulatum* pneumonia. *In* Pennington JE (ed): Respiratory Infections: Diagnosis and Management, 2nd ed, pp. 501–507, New York: Raven Press, 1989.

116. Jacobs RF, Bradsher RW: The mycoses other than histoplasmosis. *In* Chernick V (ed): Kendig's Disorders of the Respiratory Tract in Children, 5th ed, pp. 787–798. Philadelphia: WB Saunders, 1990.

117. Ma P, Villanueva TG, Kaufman D, Gillooley JF: Respiratory cryptosporidiosis in the acquired immune deficiency syndrome. Use of modified cold Kinyoun and Hemacolor stains for rapid diagnoses. JAMA 252:1298–1301, 1984.

118. Krugman S, Katz SL, Gershon AA, Wilfert CM: Toxoplasmosis. *In* Infectious Diseases of Children, 8th ed, pp. 388–397. St. Louis: CV Mosby, 1985.

119. Israelski DM, Skowron G, Leventhal JP, et al: Toxoplasma peri-

tonitis in a patient with acquired immunodeficiency syndrome. Arch Intern Med 148:1655–1657, 1988.

120. Koskiniemi M, Lappalainen M, Hedman K: Toxoplasmosis needs evaluation. An overview and proposals. Am J Dis Child 143:724–728, 1989.

121. Des Prez RM, Heim CR: *Mycobacterium tuberculosis. In* Mandell GL, Douglas RG Jr, Bennett JE (eds): Principles and Practice of Infectious Diseases, 3rd ed, pp. 1877–1906. New York: Churchill Livingstone, 1990.

122. Saltzman BR, Motyl MR, Friedland GH, et al: *Mycobacterium tuberculosis* bacteremia in the acquired immunodeficiency syndrome. JAMA 256:390–391, 1986.

123. Inselman LS: Tuberculosis in children: Update on diagnosis and therapy. J Respir Dis 4:11–25, 1983.

124. Daniel TM, Debanne SM: The serodiagnosis of tuberculosis and other mycobacterial diseases by enzyme-linked immunosorbent assay. Am Rev Respir Dis 135:1137–1151, 1987.

125. Brisson-Noel A, Gicquel B, Lecossier D, et al: Rapid diagnosis of tuberculosis by amplification of mycobacterial DNA in clinical samples. Lancet 2:1069–1071, 1989.

126. Centers for Disease Control: Diagnosis and management of mycobacterial infection and disease in persons with human immunodeficiency virus infection. Ann Intern Med 106:254–256, 1987.

127. Stover DE, White DA, Romano PA, et al: Spectrum of pulmonary diseases associated with the acquired immune deficiency syndrome. Am J Med 78:429–437, 1985.

128. Hopewell PC, Luce JM: Pulmonary involvement in the acquired immunodeficiency syndrome. Chest 87:104–112, 1985.

129. Le Tourneau A, Audouin J, Diebold J, et al: LAV-like viral particles in lymph node germinal centers in patients with the persistent lymphadenopathy syndrome and the acquired immunodeficiency syndrome-related complex: An ultrastructural study of 30 cases. Hum Pathol 17:1047–1053, 1986.

130. Lange JMA, de Wolf F, Goudsmit J: Markers for progression in HIV infection. AIDS 3:S153–S160, 1989.

131. Polis MA, Masur H: Predicting the progression to AIDS. Am J Med 89:701–705, 1990.

132. Ellaurie M, Rubinstein A: Beta-2-microglobulin concentrations in pediatric human immunodeficiency virus infection. Pediatr Infect Dis J 9:807–809, 1990.

133. Resnick L, Pitchenik AE, Fisher E, Croney R: Detection of HTLV-III/LAV-specific IgG and antigen in bronchoalveolar lavage fluid from two patients with lymphocytic interstitial pneumonitis associated with AIDS-related complex. Am J Med 82:553–556, 1987.

134. Centers for Disease Control: Update: Serologic testing for antibody to human immunodeficiency virus. MMWR 36:833–845, 1988.

135. Centers for Disease Control: Interpretation and use of the Western blot assay for serodiagnosis of human immunodeficiency virus type 1 infections. MMWR 38:1–7, 1989.

136. Connel JA, Parry JV, Mortimer PP, et al: Preliminary report: Accurate assays for anti-HIV in urine. Lancet 335:1366–1369, 1990.

137. Slade HB, Pica RV, Pahwa SG: Detection of HIV-specific antibodies in infancy by isoelectric focusing and affinity immunoblotting. J Infect Dis 160:126–130, 1989.

138. Katz SL, Wilfret CM: Human immunodeficiency virus infection of newborns. N Engl J Med 320:1687–1689, 1989.

139. Blanche S, Le Deist F, Fischer A, et al: Longitudinal study of 18 children with perinatal LAV/HTLV III infection: Attempt at prognostic evaluation. J Pediatr 109:965–970, 1986.

140. Rubinstein A, Sicklick M, Gupta A, et al: Acquired immunodeficiency with reversed T4/T8 ratios in infants born to promiscuous and drug-addicted mothers. JAMA 249:2350–2356, 1983.

141. Pitchenik AE, Burr J, Suarez M, et al: Human T-cell lymphotropic virus-III (HTLV-III) seropositivity and related disease among 71 consecutive patients in whom tuberculosis was diagnosed. A prospective study. Am Rev Respir Dis 135:875–879, 1987.

142. Epstein LG, Boucher CAB, Morrison SH, et al: Persistent human immunodeficiency virus type 1 antigenemia in children correlates with disease progression. Pediatrics 82:919–924, 1988.

143. Goedert JJ, Mendez H, Drummond JE, et al: Mother-to-infant transmission of human immunodeficiency virus type 1: Association with prematurity or low anti-gp120. Lancet 2:1351–1354, 1989.

144. Rubinstein A: Acquired immunodeficiency syndrome in infants. Am J Dis Child 137:825–827, 1983.

145. Fischl MA, Dickinson GM, LaVoie L: Safety and efficacy of sulfamethoxazole and trimethoprim chemoprophylaxis for *Pneumocystis carinii* pneumonia in AIDS. JAMA 259:1185–1189, 1988.

146. Masur H, Meier P, McCutchan JA, et al: Consensus statement on the use of corticosteroids as adjunctive therapy for *Pneumocystis* pneumonia in the acquired immunodeficiency syndrome. The National Institutes of Health-University of California Expert Panel for Corticosteroids as Adjunctive Therapy for *Pneumocystis* Pneumonia. N Engl J Med 323:1500–1504, 1990.

147. Bozzette SA, Sattler FR, Chiu J, et al: A controlled trial of early adjunctive treatment with corticosteroids for *Pneumocystis carinii* pneumonia in the acquired immunodeficiency syndrome. N Engl J Med 323:1451–1457, 1990.

148. Centers for Disease Control: Guidelines for prophylaxis against *Pneumocystis carinii* pneumonia for persons infected with human immunodeficiency virus. MMWR 38:1–9, 1989.

149. Montgomery AB, Debs RJ, Luce JM, et al: Aerosolised pentamidine as sole therapy for *Pneumocystis carinii* pneumonia in patients with acquired immunodeficiency syndrome. Lancet 2:480–483, 1987.

150. Centers for Disease Control: Guidelines for prophylaxis against *Pneumocystis carinii* pneumonia for children infected with human immunodeficiency virus. MMWR 40:1–13, 1991.

151. Collaborative DHPG Treatment Study Group: Treatment of serious cytomegalovirus infections with 9-(1,3-dihydroxy-2-propoxymethyl) guanine in patients with AIDS and other immunodeficiencies. N Engl J Med 314:801–805, 1986.

152. Snydman DR, Werner BG, Heinze-Lacey B, et al: Use of cytomegalovirus immune globulin to prevent cytomegalovirus disease in renal-transplant recipients. N Engl J Med 317:1049–1054, 1987.

153. Barnes DW, Whitley RJ: Antiviral therapy and pulmonary disease. Chest 91:246–251, 1987.

154. Dorsky DI, Crumpacker CS: Drugs five years later: Acyclovir. Ann Intern Med 107:859–874, 1987.

155. Centers for Disease Control: Use of BCG vaccines in the control of tuberculosis: A joint statement by the ACIP and the Advisory Committee for Elimination of Tuberculosis. MMWR 37:663–675, 1988.

156. Rubinstein A, Bernstein LJ, Charytan M, et al: Corticosteroid treatment for pulmonary lymphoid hyperplasia in children with the acquired immune deficiency syndrome. Pediatr Pulmonol 4:13–17, 1988.

157. McKinney RE Jr, Maha MA, Connor EM, et al: A multicenter trial of oral zidovudine in children with advanced human immunodeficiency virus disease. N Engl J Med 324:1018–1025, 1991.

158. Hirsch MS. Azidothymidine. J Infect Dis 157:427–431, 1988.

159. Yarchoan R, Mitsuya H, Myers CE, Broder S: Clinical pharmacology of 3′-azido-2′,3′-dideoxythymidine (zidovudine) and related dideoxynucleosides. N Engl J Med 321:726–738, 1989.

160. Balis FM, Pizzo PA, Murphy RF, et al: The pharmacokinetics of zidovudine administered by continuous infusion in children. Ann Intern Med 110:279–285, 1989.

161. Butler KM, Husson RN, Balis FM, et al: Dideoxyinosine in children with symptomatic human immunodeficiency virus infection. N Engl J Med 324:137–144, 1991.

162. Burger H, Belman AL, Grimson R, et al: Long HIV-1 incubation periods and dynamics of transmission within a family. Lancet 336:134–136, 1990.

22 BRONCHIOLITIS

CYNTHIA BLACK-PAYNE, M.D.

Bronchiolitis is a common, acute, contagious respiratory illness of infants and young children that involves the lower respiratory tract. It is the most significant respiratory illness of young children.[1] Bronchiolitis is a viral syndrome;[2, 3] respiratory syncytial virus (RSV) causes 50% to 90% of cases.[3-5] Initially named the *chimpanzee coryza agent,* RSV was first isolated in 1956 from chimpanzees, and the investigation for its role in human disease ensued.[6-8] It was subsequently established that RSV is the major respiratory pathogen in infancy and early childhood.[9]

When RSV is prevalent in a community, it is virtually the solitary cause of bronchiolitis.[10, 11] When bronchiolitis is sporadic, other infectious agents account for higher numbers of cases. The relative frequencies of etiologic agents causing bronchiolitis are summarized in Table 22–1. Parainfluenza viruses are the second most frequently isolated cause.[3, 12] At present, there exists no convincing proof that bacteria are primary etiologic agents of bronchiolitis.[3, 13]

There is evidence that the course of bronchiolitis may be atypical or unusually severe if there is simultaneous infection with other pathogens.[14, 15] Of 189 children hospitalized with documented RSV bronchiolitis, pneumonia, or both, 9 (4.8%) were found to have concomitant evidence of adenovirus, *Pneumocystis carinii,* cytomegalovirus, or *Streptococcus pneumoniae* infection.[14] Other investigators have likewise observed the co-occurrence of RSV-associated wheezing and *S. pneumoniae* bacteremia in young infants.[15] The potential role of coinfections (viral-viral, viral-bacterial) in bronchiolitis has been theorized.[16] In data collected in the 1950s, bronchiolitis was associated with laboratory evidence of typable *Haemophilus influenzae* infection.[17, 18] Sera from those patients also demonstrated evidence of RSV infection when subsequently analyzed.[1] In additional reports, RSV infection in infancy was associated with rhinovirus, influenza A, influenza B, parainfluenza, herpes simplex, enterovirus, and *Chlamydia trachomatis* infection.[19, 20] Bacterial complications after RSV infections of the lower respiratory tract in hospitalized patients probably occur infrequently.[19]

EPIDEMIOLOGY

The epidemiologic features of bronchiolitis closely parallel those of RSV, the predominant etiologic agent. This syndrome is a clinical continuum that incorporates viral lower respiratory tract infection and infection-induced airway hyperresponsiveness.

Bronchiolitis occurs worldwide and has typically been documented during RSV surveillance studies.[21-25] Seasonality of bronchiolitis caused by RSV is striking and predictable. The incidence peaks during winter and early spring and reaches near zero in late summer and autumn in both hemispheres (Fig. 22–1).[11, 23, 26, 27] In tropical climates, occurrence of RSV bronchiolitis tends to coincide with the rainy season.[25, 28] RSV outbreaks usually last about 5 months, and alternating short (7- to 12-month) and long (13- to 16-month) intervals between epidemics have been observed.[11] Bronchiolitis caused by other agents occurs throughout the year.[3, 29]

The age for peak incidence of RSV bronchiolitis is between 2 and 6 months; approximately 80% of all cases occur during the first year of life.[30, 31] The attack rate for bronchiolitis is believed to range from 11.4 to 19.6 cases per 100 children in the first year.[3, 32] Although the age for peak incidence in urban areas may be 2 to 3 months,[27, 31] bronchiolitis is seen in children as old as 2 years in more remote localities and in areas where risk of exposure is reduced.[29, 33] The rural or suburban (middle-income) setting has also been associated with a lower incidence of severe disease, as determined by the need for hospitalization.[13, 27, 29] Prematurity is a risk factor for severe lower respiratory tract illness (bronchiolitis, pneumonia) that necessitates hospitalization.[34] Bronchiolitis is not typically described in infants younger than 4 to 6 weeks of

Table 22–1. INFECTIOUS AGENTS ASSOCIATED WITH ACUTE BRONCHIOLITIS

Infectious Agent		Relative Frequency (%)
Respiratory syncytial virus		50
Parainfluenza viruses		25
Type 1	8	
Type 2	2	
Type 3	15	
Adenoviruses		5
Mycoplasma pneumoniae		5
Rhinoviruses		5
Influenza viruses		5
Type A	3	
Type B	2	
Enteroviruses		2
Herpes simplex viruses		2
Mumps virus		<1

From Welliver R, Cherry JD: Bronchiolitis and infectious asthma. *In* Feigin RD, Cherry JD (eds): Textbook of Pediatric Infectious Diseases, pp. 278–287. Philadelphia: WB Saunders, 1987.

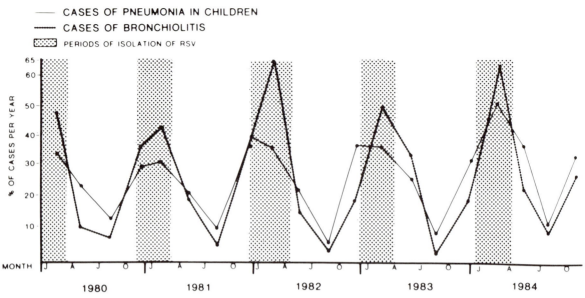

Figure 22–1. The proportion of cases of pediatric pneumonia and bronchiolitis reported in Rochester, New York, from 1980 to 1984 is shown in relation to the periods of isolation of respiratory syncytial virus (RSV). The major peaks of pneumonia and bronchiolitis occurred simultaneously and in association with the periods of RSV isolation. (From Hall CB: Respiratory syncytial virus. *In* Feigin RD, Cherry JD: Textbook of Pediatric Infectious Diseases, p. 1656. Philadelphia: WB Saunders, 1987.)

age,[3, 31, 35] although the same viral agents are known to infect and cause other manifestations, such as apnea, upper respiratory tract infections, and pneumonia, in neonates.[36]

Bronchiolitis is slightly more common in boys,[3, 27] and they appear to be more likely to experience severe disease.[33, 37] Wheezing-associated respiratory infections and lower respiratory tract illness continue to be more common in boys until the age of 6 to 9 years, at which time the incidence is equal in both sexes.[3] One study revealed no sex predilection for bronchiolitis in children under 1 year of age.[32]

Some observers have indicated that socioeconomic status may stratify the risk and severity of RSV bronchiolitis.[13] Estimations of rates of hospitalization for RSV diseases in infants under 1 year of age are higher (10 in 1000) in centers serving predominantly low-income families than in those serving middle-income populations (1 in 1000).[37] Several factors are presumed to influence disease frequency and severity in socioeconomically deprived families. The lower incidence of breast feeding among families in lower socioeconomic classes[38] may be one of these factors. Existing data suggest that breast feeding seems to protect against RSV and other wheezing respiratory illnesses in the first four months of life.[39, 40]

Poor immunization compliance in low-income areas[41] may be a contributing factor to the early age at which RSV disease occurs and its increased severity. There is evidence that the administration of oral polio vaccine, an attenuated viral vaccine, may stimulate production of endogenous interferon which leads to modification or prevention of other viral infections.[42, 43] In the Chapel Hill, North Carolina, studies, children from middle-income families had received three doses of oral polio

vaccine at monthly intervals beginning at 1 month of age, and 50% were breast fed for an average of 3 months. In this population, serious lower respiratory tract illnesses were infrequent. Fewer than 1% of the children required hospitalization, and RSV rarely produced disease of the lower respiratory tract in infants under 5 months of age. The investigators observed that infants from low-income families who were admitted to the hospital for RSV bronchiolitis or pneumonia were not breast fed, and virtually all were inadequately vaccinated.[29] In another study, it was noted that infants less than 2 years old who were hospitalized with bronchiolitis or pneumonia were more likely than control infants to have not been immunized the month before hospitalization.[34]

Infants who reside in crowded environments and have older siblings may be at risk by virtue of increased exposure frequency and large viral challenge doses.[27, 35, 40, 44] It has been shown that for healthy children under 2 years of age, regular attendance at a day-care center (with more than six children) may be a risk factor for illness of the lower respiratory tract (bronchiolitis, pneumonia).[34] Care received outside of the home in a day-care home (with six or fewer children) was not associated with the same incidence of illness.

Exposure to passive smoking, particularly maternal smoking, has been shown to be a risk factor for bronchiolitis in infancy.[44, 45] In a study that demonstrated a strong association between mild bronchiolitis in infancy and wheezing nearly 8 years later,[45] it was shown at 13-year follow-up that maternal smoking was a more powerful predictor of wheezing-associated morbidity than was the history of mild bronchiolitis.[46] Data from China indicate that there may be a synergistic effect of passive smoking and formula feeding on the risk of respiratory

Table 22–2. ESTIMATED RISK OF HOSPITALIZATION FOR BRONCHIOLITIS BY POPULATION AND AGE

Study	Manifestation	Population	Age	Hospitalization Rate
Washington, 1973[11]	Bronchiolitis	Low income	0–12 months	1/100
Seattle, 1973[51]	Bronchiolitis	Prepaid group	0–5 months 6–11 months 1–2 years	1/164 1/370 1/667
England, 1976[27]	LRD caused by RSV*	Urban Industrial Rural	0–2 months 0–2 months 0–2 months	1/38–1/62 1/60–1/76 1/102–1/135
Great Britain, 1978[22]	LRD caused by RSV*†	Urban Industrial Rural Total Total Urban Industrial Rural Total	1–3 months 1–3 months 1–3 months 1–3 months 0–12 months 1–5 years 1–5 years 1–5 years 1–5 years	1/60 1/40 1/80 1/56 1/114 1/588 1/227 1/714 1/476
North Carolina, 1979[3, 50]	Bronchiolitis	Middle income‡	78%, <5 years	<1/100
Houston, 1981[52]	LRD caused by RSV	Low income	<6 months	<1/100
Rochester, 1986[44]	Bronchiolitis	Middle income‡	Mean, 7.1 months	6/100
Tucson, 1989[32]	LRD*	Prepaid group	0–12 months	1/100

LRD, lower respiratory tract disease; RSV respiratory syncytial virus.
*Predominantly bronchiolitis. †Collaborative study at 10 centers. ‡Private pediatric practice, middle-income population.

illness that mandates hospitalization during the first 18 months of life.[47] It has also been observed that young American Indian children living in homes with wood-burning stoves are at higher risk of clinical bronchiolitis and pneumonia.[48]

In the majority of infants with bronchiolitis, the illness is mild, but approximately 1% to 5% require hospitalization.[45, 49] To estimate the rate of morbidity from virus-associated wheezing episodes, the rates of hospitalization from eight studies are summarized in Table 22–2.[3, 11, 22, 27, 32, 44, 50, 51, 52] Although definitions and study techniques varied, it is apparent that the infants at highest risk for hospitalization are those under 1 year of age, particularly those younger than 3 months. Environmental and socioeconomic conditions apparently contribute to this risk.

Nosocomial acquisition of bronchiolitis occurs primarily during seasons when RSV infection is prevalent.[27, 53] It has been shown that when RSV infection is epidemic, infants hospitalized for other problems have a 45% risk of acquiring the infection if they are inpatients for a week or more. The risk escalates with increasing length of stay to 100% for stays longer than 4 weeks.[54]

PATHOPHYSIOLOGY

RSV is transmitted primarily during close contact with infected persons by direct inoculation of large droplets or by self-inoculation (touching contaminated items or secretions).[55] Once RSV infects the eye or the nose, the incubation period is usually 2 to 8 days.[57] Involvement of the respiratory tract appears to occur principally by cell-to-cell transmission of infectious virus through fusion of cell membranes and formation of intracellular bridges, and, eventually, of syncytia (multinucleated cells).[58, 59] The respiratory tract may subsequently become infected throughout.

After viral invasion of the respiratory epithelium, replication occurs and is followed by cell death and ultimately necrosis.[60, 61] The host responds by mobilizing a peribronchiolar, predominantly mononuclear infiltrate. The submucosal and adventitial tissues become edematous, with apparent sparing of elastic fibers and muscle. Secretion of mucus is enhanced. Thick plugs composed of cellular debris, mucus, and fibrin form in the lumens of the small airways (Fig. 22–2). The alveoli are relatively spared unless immediately adjacent to an affected bronchiole. Hilar lymph nodes exhibit moderate reactive hyperplasia. Some investigators speculate that bronchiolitis with hypoxemia may produce pulmonary vasoconstriction, thereby altering gas-exchange structures.[62]

Infants with bronchiolitis are particularly vulnerable to airway obstruction from mucus because of small airway caliber and underdeveloped collateral ventilation. Ventilation in an affected infant may be compromised by several potential mechanisms:[60]

1. Airflow may be partially obstructed during both inspiration and expiration, which leads to impairment in ventilation with minimal air trapping or volume loss.
2. Bronchiolar obstruction may permit normal inspiratory volumes, but inadequate expiration results in air trapping and hyperinflation.
3. Peripheral airways can become completely obstructed, which leads to collapse of the distal respiratory unit.

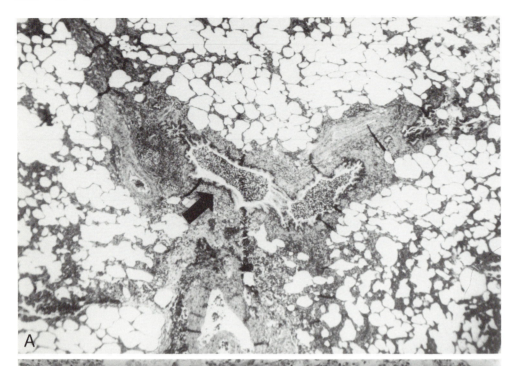

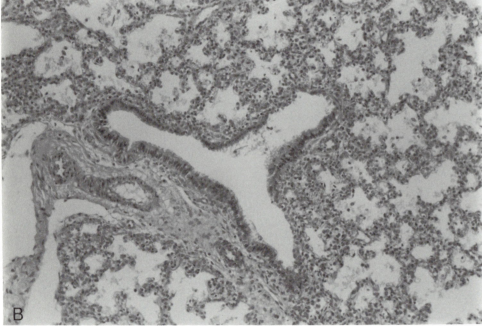

Figure 22–2. *A*, Histologic specimen from an 18-month-old infant dying of respiratory syncytial virus bronchiolitis. The arrow denotes a bronchiole filled with inflammatory exudate, with comparatively normal alveoli. (Courtesy of Caroline B. Hall, M.D., University Medical Center, Rochester, New York.) *B*, Histologic specimen from a 7-day-old infant dying of congenital heart disease, for comparison. Bronchiole is free of inflammation. (Courtesy of Marjorie Fowler, M.D., Louisiana State University Medical Center, Shreveport, Louisiana.)

4. A ball-valve mechanism may exist, allowing only the outflow of air; this leads to collapse of the distal airway that is more rapid than occurs with obstruction only.

It is apparent that any or all of these mechanisms may be operative and lead to the clinical continuum of air trapping, lobular collapse, or both.

Growth of the airways greatly alleviates the clinical consequences of mucus plugging that is characteristic of bronchiolitis, as illustrated by the tubes of different caliber in Figure 22–3. Scientific laws governing frictional resistance to flow of gases in tubes may be applied to gas flow within airways. Airflow can be either laminar

(streamlined) or turbulent. Resistance to airflow during laminar airflow, which predominates in the small airways, is governed by Poiseuille's law.[63] According to this law, the resistance to laminar flow is directly proportional to the viscosity of the fluid and the length of the tube and is inversely proportional to the fourth power of the radius of the tube:

$$R = \frac{8nl}{\pi r^4},$$

where R is the resistance to airflow, n is the viscosity of the gas, l is the length of the tube, and r is the radius.

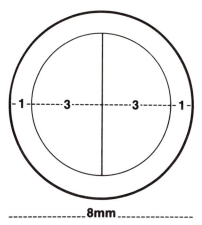
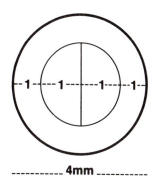
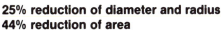

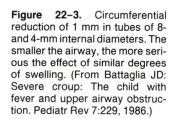

Figure 22–3. Circumferential reduction of 1 mm in tubes of 8- and 4-mm internal diameters. The smaller the airway, the more serious the effect of similar degrees of swelling. (From Battaglia JD: Severe croup: The child with fever and upper airway obstruction. Pediatr Rev 7:229, 1986.)

8mm

25% reduction of diameter and radius 44% reduction of area

4mm

50% reduction of diameter and radius 75% reduction of area

Because resistance to laminar airflow in small airways is inversely proportional to the radius to the fourth power, narrowing of the lumen in a small airway results in more obstruction of airflow than an equal narrowing in a larger airway.

During the repair phase of bronchiolitis, the respiratory epithelium regenerates in 3 to 4 days, but the process may not be complete for several weeks.[60, 62] Cilia reappear around the 15th day. Mucus plugs are eventually removed by macrophages. Additional evidence suggests that increase in gland size, increase in goblet cell population, and muscle hypertrophy may persist.[62] These anatomic sequelae are of unclear clinical and prognostic consequence.

Infected infants usually shed RSV for almost 7 days; some excrete virus for 3 to 4 weeks.[64, 65] Immunocompromised children may excrete the virus or viral antigen for prolonged or intermittent intervals.[66, 67]

The pathologic changes of bronchiolitis result in gas-exchange disturbances that are commensurate with the severity of disease. In a survey of infants requiring hospitalization for RSV disease, all had hypoxemia, which was prolonged and moderately severe.[68] The severity of hypoxemia was correlated significantly with duration of viral shedding in some children but not with clinical severity. The likely mechanism underlying the hypoxemia is mismatching of alveolar ventilation and capillary perfusion, which results from variable airway obstruction and atelectasis. Pulmonary arteriovenous shunting may contribute minimally to the hypoxemia associated with bronchiolitis, but the observation that most patients improve with supplemental oxygen further deemphasizes its clinical significance. In the majority of infants, hypercapnia does not occur because the alveoli that are functional can compensate for those that are not adequately aerated.[69] The potential contribution of bronchospasm to the hypoxemia associated with bronchiolitis remains obscure.[62]

In bronchiolitis, the work of breathing is increased because respiratory mechanics are altered.[70, 71] Infants with bronchiolitis breathe at high lung volumes, which contributes to a decrease in dynamic lung compliance. The compliance is further reduced by the variable distribution of intrathoracic resistances.[33] Some investigators have observed that the total work of breathing is increased an average of sixfold in bronchiolitis.[71] Previous pulmonary function tests in infants with broncolitis yielded variable results.[72, 73] More recently, newer techniques were used to measure pulmonary functions in 14 spontaneously breathing infants and two ventilated infants, all with acute RSV bronchiolitis.[74] During acute disease, there was a significant reduction in forced expiratory flow rates and an increase in respiratory resistance. Thoracic gas volume at functional residual capacity was increased. Of interest is that some infants did not compensate for airways narrowing with hyperinflation, and they exhibited severe expiratory flow limitation. The reasons for impaired compensatory mechanisms in these infants were unclear. Upon retesting 3 to 4 months later, lung function in the infants recovering from acute bronchiolitis showed improvement, but it remained significantly different from that of normal infants.[74]

The pathogenesis of bronchiolitis has been extensively studied, but the observations remain largely theoretical. It is apparent that the degree of bronchospasm and inflammation occurring during a viral illness is variable among patients, and thus the progression of disease and the response to therapy vary. It has been demonstrated that infants born with reduced lung function have an increased risk of experiencing illness of the lower respiratory tract with wheezing during the first 12 months.[75] This, coupled with the prior observation that adults may have lower levels of lung function years after an episode of lower respiratory tract illness in infancy,[76] suggests that some people are predisposed to wheezing in association with common viral respiratory infections from birth.[75]

There are several hypotheses about the pathogenesis of bronchiolitis, particularly bronchiolitis secondary to RSV infection. These theories concern the immune complex mechanisms, cell-mediated factors, developmental immunologic immaturity, immunoglobulin E– (IgE-) mediated hypersensitivity, and alternative mechanisms.

Immune Complex (Type III). This theory suggests that there is a type III hypersensitivity reaction (antigen-antibody, immune complex) injury in the bronchiole. According to this controversial explanation, RSV antigen reacts with maternally derived immunoglobulin G (IgG) antibody in the lungs of infants.[77] *In vitro* experiments have demonstrated that in RSV infection, immune complex activation of neutrophils results in release both of oxygen radicals and of products of arachidonic acid metabolism, potential effectors of tissue damage and bronchoconstriction.[78] Two groups of investigators working independently have demonstrated antibody-mediated enhancement of RSV infection in macrophagelike cell lines.[79, 80] The *in vivo* significance is unknown.

Cell-Mediated (Type IV). The exact role of cell-mediated (type IV) mechanisms in the pathogenesis of RSV bronchiolitis is not clear. Some authors have speculated that cell-mediated sensitization may contribute to the altered response to natural infection that occurred after the use of inactivated RSV vaccine and that transplacentally conferred lymphocyte sensitization to RSV might play a role in the pathogenesis of the first episode of RSV bronchiolitis in early infancy.[81]

Developmental Immunologic Immaturity. According to this theory, young infants become severely ill with RSV because of immunologic immaturity.[57, 82]

IgE-Mediated (Type I). Evidence implicating the possible adverse role of RSV-specific IgE in nasopharyngeal secretions has been refined.[83, 84] RSV-specific IgE is detectable in the exfoliated nasopharyngeal epithelial cells of acutely RSV-infected persons, but the persistence of RSV-specific IgE is more common in patients with wheezing than in those with upper respiratory tract illness or pneumonia. In a subsequent study, titers of RSV-specific IgE and histamine concentration of respiratory secretions were significantly higher in RSV-infected infants with wheezing.[84] Peak titers of RSV-specific IgE and concentrations of histamine correlated significantly with hypoxemia, which led the investigators to postulate that these phenomena may adversely affect the outcome of RSV infection.[84]

Other investigators, using different techniques, have demonstrated RSV-specific IgE and RSV-specific IgG$_4$ in sera of RSV-infected children. As in studies involving the use of nasopharyngeal secretions, RSV-specific IgE and RSV-specific IgG$_4$ serum levels were higher in children who had illnesses with wheezing.[85]

Severe RSV bronchiolitis may result from an IgE-mediated hypersensitivity reaction to viral antigens. This theory is further supported by the observation that concentrations of leukotrienes (mast cell mediators of bronchoconstriction and increased mucus secretion) are higher in the nasopharyngeal secretions of infants wheezing with RSV infection than in those of infants with only upper respiratory tract symptoms.[86] In another study, plasma levels of histamine and a prostaglandin metabolite, both bronchoconstrictive mediators of inflammation in bronchiolitis, were markedly elevated.[87]

Additional evidence for an IgE-mediated reaction in bronchiolitis is the allergic predisposition among affected infants, as determined by results of serum IgE testing, radioallergosorbent test scores, and nasal smears for eosinophils, mast cells, or both.[88]

Alternative Mechanisms. The anatomy of the developing lung may predispose an infant to severe impairment secondary to bronchiolitis because of immature compensatory mechanisms.[33, 62] Exposure of immature lungs to a large viral inoculum may predispose infants to severe disease. Postviral bronchoconstriction in adults may result from denudation of airway epithelium with exposure of irritant receptors.[89] These receptors become "sensitized" to inhaled irritants, which cause enhanced bronchoconstriction by way of a vagal reflex. The role that this mechanism plays in infantile bronchiolitis is unknown.

CLINICAL MANIFESTATIONS

The clinical definition of bronchiolitis is not completely refined; therefore, delineation among acute bronchiolitis, viral pneumonia, and infantile asthma remains indistinct. This dilemma is unlikely to reach a timely resolution because viral infections of the lower respiratory tract produce a continuum of disease dictated by the idiosyncrasy of an enigmatic interaction between host and pathogen. Most authorities agree that wheezing and hyperinflation of the lungs are features required for the diagnosis of bronchiolitis.[33, 45, 57] Other terms often used to describe bronchiolitis include wheezy bronchitis, asthmatic bronchitis, parainfectious bronchial hyperreactivity, and virus-associated wheezing.

The clinical course of bronchiolitis usually begins with symptoms of a viral infection of the upper respiratory tract for 2 to 4 days, typically with cough and profuse rhinorrhea, followed by dyspnea and wheezing.[90] The pattern of fever is variable (Table 22–3), depending on the viral etiologic agent and the severity of illness.[28, 30, 91] There may be signs of irritability, restlessness, decreased appetite, or vomiting. Most infants and children with bronchiolitis have mild disease and do not require medical attention. These "happy wheezers," despite mild breathlessness, continue near normal activity during illness.[92] In mild cases, symptoms usually last about a week. In infants with more severe disease, symptoms worsen over a period of 3 to 7 days. The common clinical signs and symptoms observed in 114 children (90 inpatients, 24 outpatients) with bronchiolitis are listed in Table 22–3.[28]

Initial physical examination typically reveals cough and fever with tachypnea. The cough is brief rather than severe and paroxysmal.[90] Breathing is labored and nasal flaring, grunting, thoracic retractions, or audible wheezes may be present. A prolonged expiratory phase and, infrequently, cyanosis may be apparent. Auscultation of the chest may reveal high-pitched expiratory wheezes, faint end-expiratory wheezes, or fine inconstant inspiratory crackles (rales, crepitations).[30, 69] Tachycardia is usually present. Additional abnormal features on physical examination may include conjunctivitis, pharyngitis, and otitis media. The liver and spleen may be easily palpable because of downward displacement by the hyperinflated chest.

Table 22–3. SYMPTOMS AND SIGNS IN 114 CHILDREN WITH ACUTE BRONCHIOLITIS

Symptom/Sign	Children with Symptom/Sign	
	No.	%
Symptoms		
Rapid breathing	105	92.1
Chest retraction	103	90.4
Refusal to feed	75	65.8
Fever	81	71.1
Vomiting with cough	39	34.2
Signs		
Respiratory rate >50/min	106	93.0
Retraction		
Subcostal	106	93.0
Intercostal	98	86.0
Suprasternal	21	18.4
Crepitations	89	78.1
Temperature		
>37°C	72	63.2
>38°C	24	21.1
>38.5°C	10	8.8
Hyperresonance on percussion	46	40.4
Flaring of alae nasi	38	33.3
Wheeze (audible without stethoscope)*	29	25.4
Grunting	21	18.4
Cyanosis	6	5.3

Reproduced with permission from Cherian T, Simoes EA, Steinhoff MC, et al: Bronchiolitis in tropical south India. Am J Dis Child 144:1027, 1990. Copyright 1990, American Medical Association.

*Wheeze, audible on auscultation, was present in all cases.

Features predictive of the severity of bronchiolitis are respiratory rates of 60 to 70 per minute, crackles, cyanosis, and an "ill" or "toxic" general appearance.[68, 93, 94] Decreased transcutaneous hemoglobin oxygen saturation (Sao_2 < 90% to 95%, measured by pulse oximetry) was the best single predictor of disease severity in several studies.[93, 94] Infants with these findings should be hospitalized. Before the use of specific antiviral therapy, hospital stays for bronchiolitis and viral pneumonia were typically 3 to 7 days, and clinical improvement was apparent by day 3 or 4.[64, 68] Despite clinical improvement, hypoxemia of some degree persisted for 3 to 7 weeks.[68] The usual natural course of bronchiolitis is remarkably constant. The duration of maximal respiratory distress is 1 to 2 days, followed by dramatic clinical improvement. During convalescence, some wheezing and prolongation of the expiratory phase during respiration may be observed for 7 to 10 days.[30]

It is estimated that 20% of children experience a protracted course as a result of bronchiolitis.[33] These children may have pulmonary function abnormalities and gas-exchange disturbances for weeks to months. An enlarging number of patients forming this group are infants who are immunocompromised or have pre-existing pulmonary impairment.[66, 67, 95, 96] Affected infants may experience more severe and prolonged RSV disease, and the risk may extend beyond infancy.[96] At-risk groups include infants with congenital heart disease; infants with bronchopulmonary dysplasia, reactive airway disease, or both; premature infants; infants with gastrointestinal disorders; infants with cystic fibrosis or other genetic disorders; and those with compromised immune function.

Adverse events during bronchiolitis and RSV infection that required intubation and mechanical ventilation occurred in approximately 7% to 15% of hospitalized patients before the availability of antiviral therapy.[97–99] Indications for ventilatory support were clinical deterioration (tachycardia of >200 beats per minute, advancing respiratory insufficiency, listlessness or lethargy, poor peripheral perfusion), hypoxia or clinical cyanosis, or hypercapnia.[97] Duration of mechanical ventilation averaged 4 to 5 days, the longest periods of ventilation being 16 to 18 days.[97, 100] In one study, infants who required ventilation for bronchiolitis were significantly smaller, younger, and more likely to have been born prematurely than were those who did not require ventilation (40% versus 16%).[100]

Prolonged hospitalization has been associated with decreased initial oxygen saturation in previously healthy infants with RSV infection.[99] In another study that included 56 healthy patients who did not require intubation, respiratory rate, presence or absence or fever on admission, hypoxemia, complete blood count changes and chest radiograph findings were not predictive of length of hospitalization.[98] After a review of the entire study group, the investigators concluded that only the presence of underlying cardiorespiratory disease or anomalies and the need for intubation and mechanical ventilation were useful predictors of prolonged hospitalization for children with RSV infection.[98]

Abrupt, unpredictable apnea may be associated with RSV infection.[35, 68, 97] The cause is unknown; however, a study of sleep apnea in infants with mild to moderate bronchiolitis indicated that the number of brief respiratory pauses (<15 sec) significantly increased during quiet sleep.[101]

DIAGNOSTIC APPROACHES

Bronchiolitis in pediatric practice is a clinical diagnosis. Supportive and confirmatory laboratory tests and chest radiography are helpful in the diagnosis as well as in the selection of therapy.

In a series of 207 infants with bronchiolitis who required hospital care, 74% had white blood cell counts less than 12,500 (only 12% with a neutrophil fraction greater than 60%). The investigator commented that "a normal leukocyte count was the most common finding."[30]

Because disease severity may be difficult to assess on clinical grounds alone, measurement of blood gas tensions and pH are useful in addressing supportive measures and specific therapy. At present, measurement of oxygen saturation by pulse oximetry is widely used.[93, 94, 99] In the hospitalized patient, a hemoglobin determination should be obtained in order to ensure adequate oxygen carrying capacity. Pre-existing diseases, prior therapy, and state of hydration dictate the need for additional laboratory testing.

A confirmatory diagnosis of the etiologic agent in

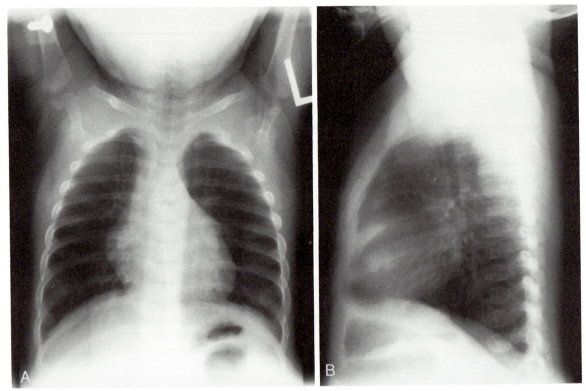

Figure 22–4. EPA (*A*) and lateral (*B*) chest radiographs of a 4-month-old infant with RSV bronchiolitis. Hyperinflation is apparent in both views.

bronchiolitis is possible through the use of rapid antigen detection, viral isolation in cell culture, or serologic analysis. An etiologic agent is usually sought in hospitalized infants. As specific antiviral therapy for RSV is available, rapid diagnosis is desirable. Respiratory secretions are tested directly for RSV antigen by enzyme-linked immunosorbent assay (EIA) or immunofluorescence.[102, 103] Interpretation of results requires a spectrophotometer for EIA and a fluorescence microscope for immunofluorescence. EIA and immunofluorescence are sensitive and specific for detection of RSV antigen in nasal secretions.[102, 103] The viral antigen is stable in transport, and test results are available within a few hours. Several specimen collection techniques are recommended.[103, 104] Rapid antigen detection tests for other respiratory viruses have been developed but are not widely available. Nucleic acid hybridization for detection of RSV in clinical specimens is being improved.[105]

Viral isolation in cell culture is becoming increasingly available to the clinician. In the patient with atypical or unusually severe pulmonary infection, respiratory secretions should be inoculated into cell culture for viral isolation in addition to rapid antigen testing. This maneuver may reveal dual viral pathogens or an unexpected viral agent. If adequate respiratory secretions are collected, transported, and inoculated promptly, RSV shows the characteristic cytopathic effect in an average of four days.[104] Maximal sensitivity is ensured by inoculation of tissue cultures at the patient's bedside. Isolation time for other respiratory viruses is variable, but most such viruses can be identified within a week.[106]

Serologic methods are available for retrospective detection of most viral agents.[106] In patients with severe bronchiolitis, serologic studies are indicated. Results of acute and convalescent serologic tests are delayed and of little help in acute management; however, a confirmatory test may be invaluable for prognosis if cultures and rapid antigen techniques are negative.

Chest radiographs provide nonspecific evidence of bronchiolitis in affected patients.[107, 108] Findings range from normal to an extensive spectrum, including hyperinflation, atelectasis, and consolidation. Typical findings are depressed diaphragms, bulging intercostal spaces and attenuated hilar structures (Fig. 22–4). Fullness of the retrosternal space may be apparent on lateral view. Some infants demonstrate interstitial pneumonia associated with diffuse hyperinflation. Others have areas of atelectasis that may be impossible to differentiate from lobar or segmental consolidation. Small pleural effusions and hilar enlargement are reported in rare instances.

There is generally strong correlation between radiograph appearance and clinical severity of illness,[94, 107] although patients sufficiently ill to require hospitalization may have normal films.[33] Interstitial changes usually clear in 7 to 10 days; regression of consolidated areas is slower.[107]

Differential Diagnosis. The causes of wheezing in infancy are numerous (Table 22–4).[69, 92] Initially, it must be established whether the respiratory distress originates from the upper or lower airways.[92] Obstructive processes in the upper airways tend to be characterized by inspiratory difficulty, which may be associated with stridor in addition to nasal flaring and retractions. Common examples include enlarged adenoids, croup, epiglottitis,

Table 22–4. DIFFERENTIAL DIAGNOSIS OF WHEEZING IN INFANCY

Causes of Acute Wheezing in Previously Healthy Infants*
Bronchiolitis
Pneumonia
Pertussis
Aspiration of a foreign body
Allergic reaction
Toxic inhalation
Parasite migration
Salicylate poisoning
Acidosis
Anemia
Hyperpyrexia
Extrinsic airway compression
   Mediastinal mass
   Enlarged lymph node
Viral myocarditis (congestive
   heart failure)

Predisposing Factors Associated With Wheezing in Infants†
Bronchopulmonary dysplasia
Cystic fibrosis
Neuromuscular disorders
Reactive airway disease
Gastroesophageal reflux
Bronchiectasis
Ciliary dyskinesia syndrome
Immune dysfunction
Anatomic defects
   Cardiovascular
      Congenital heart defects (congestive
         heart failure, pulmonary hypertension)
      Vascular rings
   Airway
      Tracheoesophageal fistula
      Bronchial stenosis
      Lung cysts
      Emphysema
      Chondromalacia

*Infants with silent underlying diseases may experience decompensation out of proportion to that expected from triggers of acute wheezing.
†All at-risk infants may have particularly severe wheezing precipitated by the acute events just listed, particularly bronchiolitis.

or aspiration of a foreign body. The predominant sign of lower respiratory tract obstruction is wheezing. Nasal flaring and thoracic retractions appear late in the course of obstructive processes in the lower respiratory tract.

MANAGEMENT

Trends in management of bronchiolitis follow, and at times, outpace the current understanding of the disease. Management includes supportive, specific, controversial, experimental, and preventive modalities.[109]

SUPPORTIVE

The comfort of the affected infant is of utmost importance in maximizing the desired benefit of specific therapies. Many infants with mild bronchiolitis may be managed in an outpatient setting. Caretakers should be advised of the contagiousness of the disease and should isolate the infant. Acceptable hydration and nourish-

ment techniques are emphasized. Infants with bronchiolitis may be more comfortable in the supine position with the head of the crib slightly elevated.[69] Infant seats are discouraged because in infants with poor head control the head may bob or lag and inadvertently compromise the upper airway. The caretaker should be aware of the signs and symptoms of clinical deterioration and the need for reevaluation. Infants with severe bronchiolitis may deteriorate unexpectedly.[35, 68, 97] For hospitalized infants, heart rate and respiratory or apnea monitors should be ordered.

Infants with bronchiolitis are at risk for dehydration from cough-induced vomiting, poor intake, or breathlessness. Intravenous fluids are frequently warranted because respiratory distress may preclude adequate nursing. Bronchiolitis of infancy may be associated with both increased antidiuretic hormone (ADH) secretion and hyperreninemia with secondary hyperaldosteronism, which leads to water retention.[110] This study suggested that the increased ADH secretion and plasma renin activity were not inappropriate but possibly indicated a response to the perception of hypovolemia by intrathoracic receptors. In certain cases, body weight and relationships between plasma osmolality and urinary osmolality should be monitored because serum sodium levels may be misleading.[110]

Mist therapy is not indicated in the treatment of bronchiolitis; it may act as an irritant, resulting in reflex bronchoconstriction.[111] Only humidification of oxygen and vehicles for delivery of aerosolized antivirals are recommended. Chest physiotherapy in previously healthy children has been shown to offer no benefit.[112] Overly zealous physiotherapy could potentially be harmful in small, dyspneic infants.

Body temperature of an infant should be monitored closely because temperature instability and the infant's effort to maintain it increase oxygen consumption.[33] Efforts to conserve heat in small infants should include the use of radiant heat as needed and close monitoring of ambient temperature in oxygen delivery systems. In infants with a significant febrile response, hydration should be adjusted accordingly.

Mechanical ventilation for respiratory failure is well tolerated and safe in acute bronchiolitis.[97, 100] Extracorporeal membrane oxygenation has been used successfully in a small number of infants with RSV bronchiolitis whose condition deteriorated despite maximal ventilator management.[113]

SPECIFIC

Hypoxemia is present in practically all infants hospitalized for bronchiolitis.[68] Oxygen administration in concentrations of 35% to 40% is adequate for most affected infants.[114, 115] A number of infants with bronchopulmonary dysplasia who contract bronchiolitis present additional concerns. Some have chronic compensated carbon dioxide retention, and hypoxemia is the major stimulus to breathe.[33] Oxygen administered to treat the bronchiolitis-induced hypoxemia should be monitored closely and restricted to the fractional inspired oxygen

Table 22–5. CANDIDATES FOR RIBAVIRIN TREATMENT

Infants at High Risk for Severe or Complicated Respiratory Syncytial Virus Infection
Congenital heart disease
Bronchopulmonary dysplasia
Other chronic lung conditions (cystic fibrosis)
Certain premature infants
Children with immunodeficiency (especially severe combined)
Recent transplant recipients
Children undergoing chemotherapy for malignancy

Infants Hospitalized With Respiratory Syncytial Virus Who Are Severely Ill
Pa_{O_2} less than 65 mm Hg
Increasing Pa_{CO_2}

Other Candidates for Treatment
Those who are hospitalized with lower respiratory tract disease that is not initially severe but who may be at some increased risk of progressing to a more complicated course by virtue of young age (less than 6 weeks) or in whom prolonged illness might be particularly detrimental to an underlying condition, such as multiple congenital anomalies or neurologic or metabolic diseases

Adapted from American Academy of Pediatrics, Committee on Infectious Diseases: Ribavirin therapy of respiratory syncytial virus. *In* Peter G (ed): Report of the Committee on Infectious Diseases, 22nd ed, pp. 581–587. Elk Grove Village, IL: American Academy of Pediatrics, 1991. Used with permission of the American Academy of Pediatrics.

(FI_{O_2}) that maintains arterial saturation in the range of 94% to 96%. Excessive inspired oxygen tensions remove the infant's drive to breathe; carbon dioxide retention may escalate, followed by apnea.

Empiric antibiotic therapy in bronchiolitis has been of no advantage.[116] Unfortunately, the clinical presentation, laboratory results, and chest radiograph may not sufficiently distinguish between viral and bacterial infection or eliminate the possibility of a dual infection.[14–20] In these instances, appropriate bacterial cultures should be obtained and empiric antibiotic therapy initiated on the basis of age-specific, community-acquired pathogens or, in the case of nosocomical acquisition, hospital-associated organisms.

Ribavirin is a synthetic nucleoside with anti-RSV properties. Ribavirin is dissolved in sterile water (20 mg/ml) and nebulized into an oxyhood, a tent, or a mask by a small-particle aerosol generator during 12 to 18 h each day for 3 to 7 days. The Committee on Infectious Diseases of the American Academy of Pediatrics issued a revised statement recommending criteria for therapy (Table 22–5).[117] Aerosolized ribavirin is not currently approved by the U. S. Food and Drug Administration for RSV-infected infants who require mechanical ventilation, but it has been used successfully in this group.[118, 119]

The six available investigations (four[120–123] in previously healthy children and two in children with predisposing risk factors[124, 125]) of the therapeutic role of ribavirin in RSV infections have engendered considerable controversy.[126–129] Although results of all six indicated that ribavirin-treated patients seemed to experience more rapid clinical resolution, numerous authors have questioned the actual impact on disease course and caution against its overuse in previously healthy children.

Additional potential benefits of ribavirin may be diminished viral shedding,[124] inhibition of other respiratory viruses that may be causing infection,[130] and favorable alteration of RSV-specific IgE response in respiratory secretions.[131] In one review on adverse reactions to ribavirin, it was concluded that the aerosolized drug appeared to be reasonably safe for patients and health care providers.[132] Women who are pregnant or may become pregnant should avoid ribavirin exposure pending development of more efficient delivery systems.[117]

CONTROVERSIAL

Empiric use of bronchodilators for therapy of bronchiolitis is a logical consideration if bronchiolitis and asthma actually share a common pathogenesis. Unfortunately, neither the approach nor the concept has been supported. Two studies of inhaled albuterol provide some evidence of benefit for infants with bronchiolitis.[133, 134] It seems reasonable to try an inhaled bronchodilator in infants with bronchiolitis; however, if no beneficial response is observed after several treatments, it should be discontinued. In a single retrospective study, theophylline showed no beneficial effects in the majority of infants with acute bronchiolitis.[135] A therapeutic trial of theophylline in infants with respiratory failure secondary to bronchiolitis is advocated by some investigators.[136]

Corticosteroids currently have no consistent role in the treatment of bronchiolitis. Sizable controlled studies have yielded no support for their use.[137]

EXPERIMENTAL

Investigators have used intramuscular injections of recombinant interferon-α_{2a}, postulating that benefit was derived from its antiviral properties.[138] Since an untreated control group was not included, beneficial effect was not ascertained. A trial of intravenous immunoglobulin containing high titers of RSV-neutralizing antibody was conducted and demonstrated decreased viral shedding and reduction in hypoxemia in infected infants, but this treatment failed to shorten hospitalization.[139]

PREVENTIVE

Attempts to develop an RSV vaccine have been largely unsuccessful; use of the inactivated vaccine in the 1960s resulted in enhanced disease severity in immunized participants.[140] A goal of current research is the development of an effective live RSV vaccine.[141] Infants at high risk for bronchiolitis should receive age-appropriate influenza immunization.[142]

PROGNOSIS

The prognosis for previously healthy infants with bronchiolitis is uniformly good; mortality rates are usually below 1%.[22] Infants with significant underlying diseases, particularly cardiorespiratory disease, are at a 30% risk of a fatal outcome.[66, 143] Another 1% of infants develop chronic bronchiolitis that may persist for weeks to months or may ultimately be fatal.[144] Clinically, these cases closely resemble those of obliterative bronchiolitis.

Immunity to RSV, the major cause of bronchiolitis, is imperfect. The disease recurs throughout life, although amelioration of symptoms with subsequent exposures is the general rule in otherwise healthy people.[145, 146] However, in previously healthy adults with documented RSV infection, total respiratory resistance has been shown to be significantly altered for weeks.[147]

A number of studies (with samples that included ambulatory patients but consisted predominantly of hospitalized patients) demonstrate a relationship between bronchiolitis and subsequent development of reactive airway disease or chronic abnormalities of pulmonary function.[45, 46, 148–151] The importance of atopy as a risk factor was variable in these studies. Welliver and colleagues, who studied RSV-specific IgE in nasal secretions of hospitalized infants with bronchiolitis, reported at follow-up several years later that subsequent wheezing developed in 20% of those without an RSV-specific IgE response at initial testing and in 70% of those with the highest responses. They suggested that the magnitude of RSV-specific IgE response at the onset of RSV bronchiolitis may be a useful predictor for recurrent wheezing.[152] Evidence based on follow-up studies of ambulatory populations with bronchiolitis indicates that children with milder disease are not at increased risk for long-term airway hyperreactivity or abnormalities in pulmonary function.[153, 154]

Pulmonary function abnormalities observed in symptom-free children 10 years after hospitalization for bronchiolitis have led other investigators to speculate that residual parenchymal or airways lesions may be permanent and could lead to chronic obstructive lung disease.[155] Studies of parainfluenza bronchiolitis and pneumonia in rodents indicate that when disease occurs in early life, it may induce abnormal alveolar development and bronchiolar hypoplasia, which are associated with abnormalities in pulmonary function.[156] Continued postnatal lung growth does not compensate for early virus-induced damage to alveolar and bronchiolar growth. Similar sequelae in virus-infected human infants have been postulated.[62]

The relationship of bronchiolitis in infancy and chronic obstructive pulmonary disease in later life remains an area of intense speculation.[157, 158] According to existing evidence, bronchiolitis may be the most important respiratory disease of infancy. Development of effective antiviral therapies and protective vaccines may alter the epidemiologic features of lower respiratory tract disease in all ages.

REFERENCES

1. Cherry JD: Newer respiratory viruses: Their role in respiratory illness in children. *In* Shulman I (ed): Advances in Pediatrics, vol. 20, pp. 225–290. Chicago: Year Book Medical Publishers, 1973.
2. Beem M, Wright FH, Fasan DM, et al: Observations on the etiology of acute bronchiolitis in infants. J Pediatr 61:864–869, 1962.
3. Henderson FM, Clyde WA, Collier AM, et al: The etiologic and epidemiologic spectrum of bronchiolitis in pediatric practice. J Pediatr 95:183–191, 1979.
4. Gardner PS: Respiratory syncytial virus infections. Postgrad Med J 49:788–791, 1973.
5. Urquhart GED, Walker GH: Immunofluorescence for routine diagnosis of respiratory syncytial virus infection. J Clin Path 25:843–845, 1972.
6. Morris JA, Blount RE Jr, Savage RE: Recovery of a cytopathogenic agent from chimpanzees with coryza. Proc Soc Exp Biol Med 92:544–549, 1956.
7. Chanock R, Roizman B, Myers R: Recovery from infants with respiratory illness of a virus related to the chimpanzee coryza agent (CCA): I. Isolation, properties and characterization. Am J Hyg 66:281–290, 1957.
8. Chanock R, Finberg L: Recovery from infants with respiratory illness of a virus related to chimpanzee coryza agent (CCA): II. Epidemiologic aspects of infection in infants and young children. Am J Hyg 66:291–300, 1957.
9. Parrott RH, Kim HW, Brandt CD, et al: Respiratory syncytial virus in infants and children. Prev Med 3:473–480, 1974.
10. Sandiford BR, Spencer B: Respiratory syncytial virus in epidemic bronchiolitis of infants. Br Med J 5309:881–882, 1962.
11. Kim HW, Arrobio JO, Brandt CD, et al: Epidemiology of respiratory syncytial virus infection in Washington, D.C.: I. Importance of the virus in different respiratory tract disease syndromes and temporal distribution of infection. Am J Epidemiol 98:216–225, 1973.
12. Welliver RC, Wong DT, Sun M, et al: Parainfluenza virus bronchiolitis: Epidemiology and pathogenesis. Am J Dis Child 140:34–40, 1986.
13. Loda FA, Clyde WA, Glezen WP, et al: Studies on the role of viruses, bacteria, and *M. pneumoniae* as causes of lower respiratory tract infections in children. J Pediatr 72:161–176, 1968.
14. Tristam DA, Miller RW, McMillan JA, et al: Simultaneous infection with respiratory syncytial virus and other respiratory pathogens. Am J Dis Child 142:834–836, 1988.
15. Timmons OD, Yamauchi T, Collins SR, et al: Association of respiratory syncytial virus and *Streptococcus pneumoniae* infection in young infants. Pediatr Infect Dis 6:1134–1135, 1987.
16. Nichol KP, Cherry JD: Bacterial-viral interrelations in respiratory infections in children. N Engl J Med 277:667–672, 1967.
17. Wood SH, Buddingh GJ, Abberger BF: An inquiry into the etiology of acute bronchiolitis of infants. Pediatrics 13:363–372, 1954.
18. Sell SHW: Some observations on acute bronchiolitis in infants. AM J Dis Child 100:31–39, 1960.
19. Hall CB, Powell KR, Schnabel KC, et al: Risk of secondary bacterial infection in infants hospitalized with respiratory syncytial virus infection. J Pediatr 113:266–271, 1988.
20. Waner JL, Whitehurst NJ, Jonas S, et al: Isolation of viruses from specimens submitted for direct immunofluorescence test for respiratory syncytial virus. J Pediatr 108:249–250, 1986.
21. Chanock RM, Kim HW, Vargosko AJ, et al: Respiratory syncytial virus: I. Virus recovery and other observations during 1960 outbreak of bronchiolitis, pneumonia, and minor respiratory diseases in children. JAMA 176:647–653, 1961.
22. Clarke SKR, Gardner PS, Poole PM, et al: Respiratory syncytial virus infection: Admissions to hospital in industrial, rural, and urban areas. Br Med J 2:796–798, 1978.
23. Lewis FA, Rae ML, Lehmann NI, et al: A syncytial virus associated with epidemic disease of the lower respiratory tract in infants and young children. Med J Aust 2:932–933, 1961.
24. Suto T, Yano N, Ikeda M, et al: Respiratory syncytial virus infection and its serologic epidemiology. J Epidemiol 82:211–224, 1965.
25. Spence L, Barratt N: Respiratory syncytial virus associated with acute respiratory infections in Trinidadian patients. Am J Epidemiol 88:257–266, 1968.
26. Hall CB, Douglas RG: Respiratory syncytial virus and influenza: Practical community surveillance. Am J Dis Child 130:615–620, 1976.
27. Sims DG, Downham MAPS, McQuillin J, et al: Respiratory syn-

cytial virus infection in northeast England. Br Med J 2:1095–1098, 1976.

28. Cherian T, Simoes EAF, Steinhoff MC, et al: Bronchiolitis in tropical south India. Am J Dis Child 144:1026–1030, 1990.

29. Glezen WP, Denny FW: Epidemiology of acute lower respiratory tract disease of children. N Engl J Med 288:498–505, 1973.

30. Ackerman BD: Acute bronchiolitis. Clin Pediatr 1:75–81, 1962.

31. Parrott RH, Kim HW, Arrobio JO, et al: Epidemiology of respiratory syncytial virus infection in Washington, DC: II. Infection and disease with respect to age, immunologic status, race, and sex. Am J Epidemiol 98:289–300, 1973.

32. Wright AL, Taussig LM, Ray CG, et al: The Tucson children's respiratory study: II. Lower respiratory tract illness in the first year of life. Am J Epidemiol 129:1232–1246, 1989.

33. Wohl MEB: Bronchiolitis. In Chernick V (ed): Kendig's Disorders of the Respiratory Tract in Children, 5th ed, pp. 360–370. Philadelphia: WB Saunders, 1990.

34. Anderson LJ, Parker RA, Strikas RA, et al: Day-care attendance and hospitalization for lower respiratory tract illness. Pediatrics 82:300–308, 1988.

35. Hall CB, Geiman JM, Biggar R, et al: Respiratory syncytial virus infections within families. N Engl J Med 294:414–419, 1976.

36. Bruhn FW, Mokrohisky ST, McIntosh K: Apnea associated with respiratory syncytial virus infection in young infants. J Pediatr 90:382–386, 1977.

37. Glezen WP: Pathogenesis of bronchiolitis-epidemiologic considerations. Pediatr Res 11:239–243, 1977.

38. Martinez GA, Kreiger FW: 1984 Milk-feeding patterns in the United States. Pediatrics 76:1004–1008, 1985.

39. Downham MAPS, Scott R, Sims DG, et al: Breast-feeding protects against respiratory syncytial virus infections. Br Med J 2:274–276, 1976.

40. Wright AL, Holberg CJ, Martinez FD, et al: Breast feeding and lower respiratory tract illness in the first year of life. Br Med J 299:946–949, 1989.

41. McMillan JA: What we must do for children in the 1990s. Contemp Pediatr 7:28–50, 1990.

42. Smorodintsev AA, Gvozdilova DA, Romanov YA, et al: Induction of endogenous interferon by use of standard live vaccines for prevention of respiratory viral infections. Ann N Y Acad Sci 173:811–822, 1970.

43. Voroshilova MK: Live enterovirus interferon inducers and their use for prevention of respiratory infections. In Proceedings of the International Conference on the Application of Vaccines Against Viral, Rickettsial, and Bacterial Diseases of Man, December 14–18, 1970, Scientific Publication #226, pp. 133–136. Washington, DC: Pan American Health Organization, 1971.

44. McConnochie KM, Roghmann KJ: Parental smoking, presence of older siblings, and family history of asthma increase risk of bronchiolitis. Am J Dis Child 140:806–817, 1986.

45. McConnochie KM, Roghmann KJ: Bronchiolitis as a possible cause of wheezing in childhood: New evidence. Pediatrics 74:1–10, 1984.

46. McConnochie KM, Roghmann KJ: Wheezing at 8 and 13 years: Changing importance of bronchiolitis and passive smoking. Pediatr Pulmonol 6:138–146, 1989.

47. Chen Y: Synergistic effect of passive smoking and artificial feeding on hospitalization for respiratory illness in childhood. Chest 95:1004–1007, 1989.

48. Morris K, Morganlander M, Coulehan JL, et al: Wood-burning stoves and lower respiratory tract infection in American Indian children. Am J Dis Child 144:105–108, 1990.

49. Glezen WP, Loda FA, Clyde WA, et al: Epidemiologic patterns of acute lower respiratory disease of children in a pediatric group practice. J Pediatr 78:397–406, 1971.

50. Denny FW, Clyde WA: Acute lower respiratory tract infections in nonhospitalized children. J Pediatr 108:635–646, 1986.

51. Foy HM, Cooney MK, Maletzky AJ, et al: Incidence and etiology of pneumonia, croup, and bronchiolitis in preschool children belonging to a prepaid medical care group over a four-year period. Am J Epidemiol 97:80–92, 1973.

52. Glezen WP, Paredes A, Allison JE, et al: Risk of respiratory syncytial virus infection for infants from low-income families in relation to age, sex, ethnic group, and maternal antibody level. J Pediatr 98:708–715, 1981.

53. Sims DG, Downham MAPS, Webb JKG, et al: Hospital cross-infection on children's wards with respiratory syncytial virus and the role of adult carriage. Acta Paediatr Scand 64:541–545, 1975.

54. Hall CB, Douglas RG, Geiman JM, et al: Nosocomial respiratory virus infections. New Engl J Med 293:1343–1346, 1975.

55. Hall CB, Douglas RG: Modes of transmission of respiratory syncytial virus. J Pediatr 99:100–103, 1981.

56. Hall CB, Douglas RG, Schnable KC, et al: Infectivity of respiratory syncytial virus by various roles of inoculation. Infect Immun 33:779–783, 1981.

57. Hall CB: Respiratory syncytial virus. In Mandell GL, Douglas RG, Bennett VE (eds): Principles and Practice of Infectious Diseases, 3rd ed, pp. 1265–1279. New York: Churchill Livingstone, 1990.

58. Taylor-Robinson D, Doggett JE: An assay method for respiratory syncytial virus. Br J Exp Pathol 44:473–480, 1963.

59. Shigeta S, Hinuma Y, Suto T, et al: The cell to cell infection of respiratory syncytial virus in HEp-2 monolayer cultures. J Gen Virol 3:129–131, 1968.

60. Aherne W, Bird T, Court SDM, et al: Pathological changes in virus infections of the lower respiratory tract in children. J Clin Pathol 23:7–18, 1970.

61. Ferris JAJ, Aherne WA, Locke WS, et al: Sudden and unexpected deaths in infants: Histology and virology. Br Med J 2:439–442, 1973.

62. Reid L: Anatomic and pathophysiologic factors in infections of the airways and pulmonary parenchyma in infants and children: Influence of the pattern of structural growth of lung susceptibility to specific infectious diseases in infants and children. Pediatr Res 11:210–215, 1977.

63. Levitzky MG: Mechanics of breathing: Airways resistance, laminar, turbulent and transitional flow. In Pulmonary Physiology, p. 35. New York: McGraw-Hill, 1990.

64. Hall CB, Douglas RG, Geiman JM: Quantitative shedding patterns of respiratory syncytial virus in infants. J Infect Dis 132:151–156, 1975.

65. Hall CB, Douglas RG, Geiman JM: Respiratory syncytial virus infections in infants: Quantitation and duration of shedding. J Pediatr 89:11–15, 1976.

66. Hall CB, Powell KR, MacDonald NE, et al: Respiratory syncytial viral infection in children with compromised immune function. N Engl J Med 315:77–81, 1986.

67. Chandwani S, Borkowski W, Krasinki K, et al: Respiratory syncytial virus infection in human immunodeficiency virus–infected children. J Pediatr 117:251–254, 1991.

68. Hall CB, Hall WJ, Seers DM: Clinical and physiological manifestations of bronchiolitis and pneumonia. Am J Dis Child 133:798–802, 1979.

69. Welliver R, Cherry JD: Bronchiolitis and infectious asthma. In Feigin RD, Cherry JD (eds): Textbook of Pediatric Infectious Diseases, 2nd ed, pp. 278–288. Philadelphia: WB Saunders, 1987.

70. Hall WJ, Hall CB: Clinical significance of pulmonary function tests: Alterations in pulmonary function following respiratory viral infection. Chest 76:458–465, 1979.

71. Stokes GM, Milner AD, Groggins RC: Work of breathing, intrathoracic pressure and clinical findings in a group of babies with bronchiolitis. Acta Paediatr Scand 70:689–694, 1981.

72. Godfrey S, Beardsmore CS, Maayan C, et al: Can thoracic gas volume be measured in infants with airways obstruction? Am Rev Respir Dis 133:245–251, 1986.

73. Mallol J, Hibbert ME, Robertson CF, et al: Inherent variability of pulmonary function tests in infants with bronchiolitis. Pediatr Pulmonol 5:152–157, 1988.

74. Seidenberg J, Masters IB, Hudson I, et al: Disturbance of respiratory mechanics in infants with bronchiolitis. Thorax 44:660–667, 1989.

75. Martinez FD, Morgan WJ, Wright AL, et al: Diminished lung function as a predisposing factor for wheezing respiratory illness in infants. N Engl J Med 319:1112–1117, 1988.

76. Samet JM, Tager IB, Speizer FE: The relationship between respiratory illness in childhood and chronic air flow obstruction in adulthood. Am Rev Respir Dis 127:508–523, 1983.

77. Chanock RM, Kapikian AZ, Mills J, et al: Influence of immunological factors in respiratory syncytial virus disease of the lower respiratory tract. Arch Environ Health 21:347–355, 1970.

78. Faden H, Kaul TN, Ogra PL: Activation of oxidative and arachidonic acid metabolism in neutrophils by respiratory syncytial

virus antibody complexes: Possible role in disease. J Infect Dis 148:110–116, 1983.
79. Krilov LR, Anderson LJ, Marcoux L, et al: Antibody-mediated enhancement of respiratory syncytial virus infection in two monocyte/macrophage cell lines. J Infect Dis 160:777–782, 1989.
80. Gimenez HB, Keir HM, Cash P: In vitro enhancement of respiratory syncytial virus infection of U937 cells by human sera. J Gen Virol 70:89–96, 1989.
81. Kim HW, Leikin SL, Arrobio J, et al: Cell-mediated immunity to respiratory syncytial virus induced by inactivated vaccine or by infection. Pediatr Res 10:75–78, 1976.
82. Bruhn FW, Yeager AS: Respiratory syncytial virus in early infancy. Am J Dis Child 131:145–148, 1977.
83. Welliver RC, Kaul TN, Ogra PL: The appearance of cell-bound IgE in respiratory-tract epithelium after respiratory-syncytial-virus infection. N Engl J Med 303:1198–1202, 1980.
84. Welliver RC, Wong DT, Sun M, et al: The development of respiratory syncytial virus–specific IgE and the release of histamine in nasopharyngeal secretions after infection. N Engl J Med 305:841–846, 1981.
85. Bui RHD, Molinaro GA, Kettering JD: Virus specific IgE and IgG$_4$ antibodies in serum of children infected with respiratory syncytial virus. J Pediatr 110:87–90, 1987.
86. Volovitz B, Welliver RC, DeCastro G, et al: The release of leukotrienes in the respiratory tract during infection with respiratory syncytial virus: Role in obstructive airway disease. Pediatr Res 24:504–507, 1988.
87. Skoner DP, Fireman P, Caliguiri L, et al: Plasma elevations of histamine and a prostaglandin metabolite in acute bronchiolitis. Am Rev Respir Dis 142:359–364, 1990.
88. Nagayama Y, Honda A, Sakurai N, et al: Allergic predisposition among infants with bronchiolitis. J Asthma 24:9–17, 1987.
89. Empey DW, Laitinen LA, Jacobs L, et al: Mechanisms of bronchial hyperreactivity in normal subjects after upper respiratory tract infection. Am Rev Respir Dis 113:131–139, 1976.
90. Wohl MEB, Chernick V: Bronchiolitis. Am Rev Respir Dis 118:759–781, 1978.
91. Putto A, Ruuskanen O, Meurman O: Fever in respiratory virus infections. Am J Dis Child 140:1159–1163, 1986.
92. Skoner D, Caliguiri L: The wheezing infant. Pediatr Clin North Am 35:1011–1030, 1988.
93. Mulholland EK, Olinsky A, Shann FA: Clinical findings and severity of acute bronchiolitis. Lancet 335:1259–1261, 1990.
94. Shaw KN, Bell LM, Sherman NH: Outpatient assessment of infants with bronchiolitis. 145:151–155, 1991.
95. Abman SH, Ogle JW, Butler-Simon N, et al: Role of respiratory syncytial virus in early hospitalizations for respiratory distress of young infants with cystic fibrosis. J Pediatr 113:826–830, 1988.
96. Groothuis JR, Salbenblatt CK, Lauer BA: Severe respiratory syncytial virus infection in older children. Am J Dis Child 144:346–348, 1990.
97. Outwater KM, Crone RK: Management of respiratory failure in infants with acute viral bronchiolitis. Am J Dis Child 138:1071–1075, 1984.
98. McMillan JA, Tristam DA, Weiner LB, et al: Prediction of the duration of hospitalization in patients with respiratory syncytial virus infection: Use of clinical parameters. Pediatrics 81:22–26, 1988.
99. Green M, Brayer AF, Schenkman KA, et al: Duration of hospitalization in previously well infants with respiratory syncytial virus infection. Pediatr Infect Dis J 8:601–605, 1989.
100. Lebel MH, Gauthier M, Lacroix J, et al: Respiratory failure and mechanical ventilation in severe bronchiolitis. Arch Dis Child 64:1431–1437, 1989.
101. Abreu e Silva FA, Brezinova V, Simpson H: Sleep apnoea in acute bronchiolitis. Arch Dis Child 57:467–472, 1982.
102. Halstead DC, Todd S, Fritch G: Evaluation of five methods for respiratory syncytial virus detection. J Clin Microbiol 28:1021–1025, 1990.
103. Ahluwalia G, Embree J, McNicol P, et al: Comparison of nasopharyngeal aspirate and nasopharyngeal swab specimens for respiratory syncytial virus diagnosis by cell culture, indirect immunoflurorescence assay, and enzyme-linked immunosorbent assay. J Clin Microbiol 25:763–767, 1987.
104. Hall CB, Douglas RG: Clinically useful method for the isolation of respiratory syncytial virus. J Infect Dis 131:1–5, 1975.
105. Van Dyke RB, Murphy-Cobb M: Detection of respiratory syncytial virus in nasopharyngeal secretions by DNA-RNA hybridization. J Clin Microbiol 27:1739–1743, 1989.
106. Drew WL: Controversies in viral diagnosis. Rev Infect Dis 8:814–824, 1986.
107. Rice RP, Loda F: A roentgenographic analysis of respiratory syncytial virus pneumonia in infants. Radiology 87:1021–1027, 1966.
108. Friis B, Eiken M, Hornsleth A, et al: Chest x-ray appearances in pneumonia and bronchiolitis: Correlation to virological diagnosis and secretory bacterial findings. Acta Paediatr Scand 79:219–225, 1990.
109. Milner AD, Murray M: Acute bronchiolitis in infancy: Treatment and prognosis. Thorax 44:1–5, 1989.
110. Gozal D, Colin AA, Jaffe M, et al: Water, electrolyte, and endocrine homeostasis in infants with bronchiolitis. Pediatr Res 27:204–209, 1990.
111. Taussig LM: Mists and aerosols: New studies, new thoughts. J Pediatr 84:619–622, 1974.
112. Webb MSC, Martin JA, Cartlidge PHT, et al: Chest physiotherapy in acute bronchiolitis. Arch Dis Child 60:1078–1079, 1985.
113. Steinhorn RH, Green TP: Use of extracorporeal membrane oxygenation in the treatment of respiratory syncytial virus bronchiolitis: The national experience, 1983 to 1988. J Pediatr 116:338–342, 1990.
114. Reynolds EDR: Arterial blood gas tensions in acute disease of lower respiratory tract in infancy. Br Med J 1:1192–1195, 1963.
115. Simpson H, Matthew DJ, Inglis JM, et al: Virological findings and blood gas tensions in acute lower respiratory tract infections in children. Br Med J 2:629–632, 1974.
116. Friis B, Anderson P, Brenoe E, et al: Antibiotic treatment of pneumonia and bronchiolitis: A prospective randomized study. Arch Dis Child 59:1038–1045, 1984.
117. Committee on Infectious Diseases: Ribavirin therapy of respiratory syncytial virus. In Peter G (ed): Report of the Committee on Infectious Diseases, 22nd ed, pp. 581–587. Elk Grove Village, IL: American Academy of Pediatrics, 1991.
118. Smith DW, Frankel LR, Mathers LH, et al: A controlled trial of aerosolized ribavirin in infants receiving mechanical ventilation for severe respiratory syncytial virus infection. N Engl J Med 325:24–29, 1991.
119. Outwater KM, Meissner HC, Peterson MB: Ribavirin administration to infants receiving mechanical ventilation. Am J Dis Child 142:512–515, 1988.
120. Hall CB, McBride JT, Walsh EE, et al: Aerosolized ribavirin treatment of infants with respiratory syncytial viral infection. N Engl J Med 308:1443–1447, 1983.
121. Taber LH, Knight V, Gilbert BE, et al: Ribavirin aerosol treatment of bronchiolitis associated with respiratory syncytial virus infection in infants. Pediatrics 72:613–618, 1983.
122. Barry W, Cockburn F, Cornall R, et al: Ribavirin aerosol for acute bronchiolitis. Arch Dis Child 61:593–597, 1986.
123. Rodriguez WJ, Kim HW, Brandt CD, et al: Aerosolized ribavirin in the treatment of patients with respiratory syncytial virus disease. Pediatr Infect Dis 6:159–163, 1987.
124. Hall CB, McBride JT, Gala CL, et al: Ribavirin therapy of respiratory syncytial viral infection in infants with underlying cardiopulmonary disease. JAMA 254:3047–3051, 1985.
125. Conrad DA, Christenson JC, Waner JL: Aerosolized ribavirin treatment of respiratory syncytial virus infection in infants hospitalized during an epidemic. Pediatr Infect Dis J 6:152–158, 1987.
126. Isaacs D: Ribavirin. Pediatrics 79:289–291, 1987.
127. Isaacs D, Moxon ER, Harney D, et al: Ribavirin in respiratory syncytial virus infection. Arch Dis Child 63:986–990, 1988.
128. Wald ER, Dashefsky D, Green M: In re ribavirin: A case of premature adjudication? J Pediatr 112:154–158, 1988.
129. Milner AD: Ribavirin and acute bronchiolitis in infancy. Br Med J 297:998–999, 1988.
130. Hall CB: Ribavirin: Beginning the blitz on respiratory viruses? Pediatr Infect Dis J 4:668–671, 1985.
131. Rosner IK, Welliver RC, Edelson PJ, et al: Effect of ribavirin therapy on respiratory syncytial virus–specific IgE and IgA responses after infection. J Infect Dis 155:1043–1047, 1987.
132. Janai HK, Marks MI, Zaleska M, et al: Ribavirin: Adverse drug reactions, 1986–1988. Pediatr Infect Dis J 9:209–211, 1990.

133. Soto ME, Sly PD, Uren E, et al: Bronchodilator response during acute viral bronchiolitis in infancy. Pediatr Pulmonol 2:85–90, 1985.
134. Schuh S, Canny G, Reisman JJ, et al: Nebulized albuterol in acute bronchiolitis. J Pediatr 117:633–637, 1990.
135. Brooks LJ, Cropp GJA: Theophylline therapy in bronchiolitis. Am J Dis Child 135:934–936, 1981.
136. Welliver RC: Today's approach to pediatric pneumonia and bronchiolitis. J Respir Dis 12:35–50, 1991.
137. Leer JA, Bloomfield NJ, Green JL, et al: Corticosteroid treatment in bronchiolitis. Am J Dis Child 117:495–503, 1969.
138. Portnoy J, Hicks K, Pacheo F, Olson L: Pilot study of recombinant interferon alpha-2a for treatment of infants with bronchiolitis induced by respiratory syncytial virus. Antimicrob Agents Chemother 32:589–591, 1988.
139. Hemming VG, Rodriguez W, Kim HW, et al: Intravenous immunoglobulin treatment of respiratory syncytial virus infections in infants and young children. Antimicrob Agents Chemother 31:1882–1886, 1987.
140. Kapikian AZ, Mitchell RH, Chanock RM, et al: An epidemiologic study of altered clinical reactivity to respiratory syncytial (RS) virus infection in children previously vaccinated with an inactivated RS virus vaccine. Am J Epidemiol 89:405–421, 1969.
141. McKay E, Higgins P, Tyrell P, et al: Immunogenicity and pathogenicity of temperature-sensitive modified respiratory syncytial virus in adult volunteers. J Med Virol 25:411–421, 1988.
142. CDC: Prevention and control of influenza. MMWR 39:1–15, 1990.
143. MacDonald NE, Hall CB, Suffin SC, et al: Respiratory syncytial viral infection in infants with congenital heart disease. N Engl J Med 307:397–400, 1982.
144. Hodges IGC, Milner AD, Groggins RC, et al: Causes and management of bronchiolitis with chronic obstructive features. Arch Dis Child 58:495–499, 1982.
145. Henderson FW, Collier AM, Clyde WA, et al: Respiratory-syncytial-virus infections, reinfections and immunity. N Engl J Med 300:530–534, 1979.
146. Hall CB, Walsh EE, Long CE, et al: Immunity to and frequency of reinfection with respiratory syncytial virus. J Infect Dis 163:693–698, 1991.
147. Hall WJ, Hall CB, Speers DM: Respiratory syncytial virus infection in adults. Ann Intern Med 88:203–205, 1978.
148. Hall CB, Hall WJ, Gala CL, et al: Long-term prospective study in children after respiratory syncytial virus infection. J Pediatr 105:358–364, 1984.
149. Weiss ST, Tager IB, Munoz A, et al: The relationship of respiratory infections in early childhood to the occurrence of increased levels of bronchial responsiveness and atopy. Am Rev Respir Dis 131:573–578, 1985.
150. Carlsen KH, Larsen S, Orstavik J: Acute bronchiolitis in infancy: The relationship to later recurrent obstructive airways disease. Eur J Respir Dis 70:86–92, 1987.
151. Sly PD, Hibbert ME: Childhood asthma following hospitalization with acute viral bronchiolitis in infancy. Pediatr Pulmonol 7:153–158, 1989.
152. Welliver RC, Sun M, Rinaldo D: Predictive value of respiratory syncytial virus–specific IgE responses for recurrent wheezing following bronchiolitis. J Pediatr 109:776–780, 1986.
153. Twiggs JT, Larson LA, O'Connell EJ, et al: Respiratory syncytial virus infection: Ten-year follow-up. Clin Pediatr 20:187–190, 1981.
154. McConnochie KM, Mark JD, McBride JT, et al: Normal pulmonary function measurements and airway reactivity in childhood after mild bronchiolitis. J Pediatr 107:54–58, 1985.
155. Kattan M, Keens TG, Lapierre JG, et al: Pulmonary function abnormalities in symptom-free children after bronchiolitis. Pediatrics 59:683–688, 1977.
156. Castleman WL, Sorkness RL, Lemanske RF, et al: Neonatal viral bronchiolitis and pneumonia induces bronchiolar hypoplasia and alveolar dysplasia in rats. Lab Invest 59:387–396, 1988.
157. Schroeckenstein DC, Busse WW: Viral "bronchitis" in childhood: Relationship to asthma and obstructive lung disease. Semin Respir Infect 3:40–48, 1988.
158. Ogra PL: Allergy, respiratory tract infections and bronchial hyperreactivity. Pediatr Infect Dis 8:347–352, 1989.

23 OBLITERATIVE BRONCHIOLITIS

KAREN HARDY, M.D.

Obliterative bronchiolitis (OB) is a potentially severe process of airway scarring in children after acute lower airway injury. It should be suspected in certain clinical situations, including (1) persistent coughing or wheezing after an acute pneumonia; (2) prolonged localized crackles or wheezing after severe acute respiratory failure; (3) prolonged exercise intolerance after an acute pulmonary injury; (4) respiratory symptoms that are severe in disproportion to the paucity of plain chest radiographic findings; (5) recurrent aspiration of gastric contents with persistent pulmonary symptoms; (6) the hyperlucent lung syndrome; and (7) severe lung disease with overinflation, difficulty in mechanical ventilation as a result of air leaks, and incomplete resolution of the process. Recognition and supportive treatment during the acute and chronic phases of this process may improve the functional status of these patients.

OB is a chronic lung disease that affects all age groups. Although it is infrequent, its prevalence was most recently described as 8 per 2987 autopsies in pediatric patients.[1] Initially noted in 1907 in adults who had inhaled noxious fumes, it has been reported more recently in patients of all ages.

OB is the result of an inflammatory process affecting mainly terminal bronchioles, respiratory bronchioles, and alveolar ducts. Patients may have documented obliteration of bronchi and of main stem bronchi. Many modes of epithelial damage can result in abnormal repair

Table 23–1. CONDITIONS ASSOCIATED WITH THE DEVELOPMENT OF OBLITERATIVE BRONCHIOLITIS

Inhalation of Toxins or Fumes
Ammonia chlorine
Chloropierin (trichloronitromethane)
Hydrochloric acid
Mustard gas (dichloroethyl sulfide)
Nitric acid
Nitrogen dioxide (silo-filler's disease)
Phosgene (carbonyl chloride)
Sulfuric acid
Talcum powder
Thermal injury
Zinc chloride

Infection
Viral
Adenovirus (types 1, 3, 7, 21)
Influenza
Measles (variable-zoster)
Bacterial
Bordetella pertussis
Staphylococcus aureus
Streptococcus Group B, beta-hemolytic
Other
Mycoplasma pneumoniae
Pneumocystis carinii

Connective Tissue Disease/Transplantation
Autoimmune hemolytic anemia
Bone marrow transplantation
Eosinophilic fasciitis
Heart-lung transplantation
Rheumatoid arthritis
Scleroderma
Sjögren's syndrome

Large Lesions
Alveolar proteinosis
Bronchopulmonary dysplasia
Congenital
Congestive heart failure
Cystic fibrosis
Lymphoma
Myasthenia gravis
Penicillamine therapy (rheumatoid arthritis)
Sulfasalazine therapy (ulcerative colitis)

Aspiration
Foreign bodies (prune pit, amniotic fluid)
Lipids (poppyseed oil)
Stomach contents (gastroesophageal reflux)

Idiopathic Conditions

that is characteristic of this disorder (Table 23–1). For example, OB is a typical finding in bronchopulmonary dysplasia, diffuse alveolar damage, and cystic fibrosis. It may also occur in patients who have had concomitant gastroesophageal reflux.

PATHOPHYSIOLOGY

The gross lesion consists of numerous small scars that fill airways and often have a pinpoint-sized lumen remaining when examined with a hand lens. These small nodules are easily palpable on the gross specimen. On microscopic examination, epithelial damage is associated with the invasion of a number of cells in the peribronchiolar space; fibroblasts begin to produce collagen. Polypoid cellular masses then fill the airway lumen and gradually become cicatrizing scars, obstructing airflow. Circumferential scarring occasionally occurs in the submucosal space, constricting the airway lumen and resulting in partial airway obstruction. In this form of OB, the diagnosis can be made only if the pathologist looks carefully and if elastic tissue stains are used to reveal remnants of airways. Complete or partial obstruction causes atelectasis or air trapping to develop. Poor mucociliary clearance and chronic inflammation can then lead to recurrent infection and bronchiectasis. The degree of compromise relates to the number of airways initially damaged and the degree of obliteration. Recanalization can occur and presumably accounts for slow improvement after the initial insult.

The descriptions of the pathologic changes were well summarized by Katzenstein and Askin.[2] Prior infection occurred in a majority of reported pediatric cases. Obliteration developed in a large number of children who had adenovirus pneumonia.[3–6] Other microbes known to cause necrotizing bronchiolitis that lead to the changes of obliteration include influenza A, *Mycoplasma,* and respiratory syncytial virus.[2, 7, 8] Obliteration developed in some patients after bacterial infection; however, most of these cases were reported before easy access of laboratory tests for viruses.[1] Gastroesophageal reflux is another problem that is associated with the development of obliteration reminiscent of animal models of this disease. Hydrochloric acid directly instilled into the trachea of dogs and rabbits reliably produces OB.[9] OB is also seen in association with collagen vascular disease. OB develops in approximately 50% of adult heart-lung transplant patients.[10] This growing number of affected patients provides the best opportunity to study the process of obliteration. Early detection via transbronchial biopsy and treatment with steroids have improved survival of patients.

CLINICAL MANIFESTATIONS AND DIAGNOSTIC APPROACHES

The clinical manifestation relates to the pathophysiologic process. Most children suffer from acute pneumonia, which can be quite ordinary in its original course. Cough, fever, and respiratory distress begin and may progress to warrant inpatient care, sometimes with mechanical ventilation. At other times, outpatient management alone is sufficient. Patients receive treatment appropriate to the degree of illness but do not fully recover. Those with symptoms severe enough initially to require mechanical ventilation may be particularly difficult to manage during the acute course, with severe air leaks as a result of pulmonary interstitial emphysema, pneumothorax, and pneumomediastinum. Most patients present to the subspecialist for persistent crackles and wheezing that lasts more than 6 weeks.[1] Some have poor tolerance for exercise.

Once the clinical setting arouses suspicion, multiple studies help to confirm the diagnosis of OB either radiographically or pathologically. Chest radiographs have been evaluated in large studies of pediatric and adult

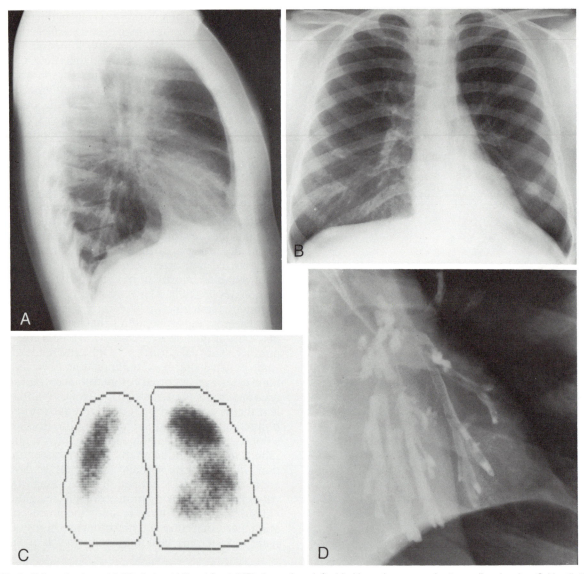

Figure 23–1. Obliterative bronchiolitis. Lateral (*A*) and frontal (*B*) views show left-sided hyperlucency and retrocardiac density. *C*, Ventilation scan shows moth-eaten appearance. *D*, Bronchogram with cutoff bronchiectasis.

patients.[11] Variable findings not specific to this problem are noted. It is remarkable that chest radiographs are often relatively normal in contrast to the physical examination. Occasionally, Swyer-James syndrome develops; obstruction causes air trapping, overdistension of the alveoli, and ultimately a decrease in pulmonary blood supply. Gradual atrophy of the affected tissue occurs, and a small, hyperlucent lung is visualized on plain film[6, 12] (Figs. 23–1*A*, 23–1*B*). This sequence of events occurred in 10% of Canadian children after adenovirus infection with OB.[3]

Other radiographic means of evaluating these children include the ventilation-perfusion scan, which shows a moth-eaten appearance of multiple matched defects in ventilation and perfusion (Fig. 23–1*C*).[13] Bronchiectasis is a complication of obliteration and can be diagnosed radiographically by bronchography and by high-resolution computed tomography (CT). For many years, bronchography has been the gold standard for displaying abnormally dilated airways but is associated with multiple complications (Fig. 23–1*D*).[14] Naidich and associ-

ates[15, 16] compared noninvasive recognition of bronchiectasis on CT with that on bronchograms and found 100% concordance in patients 14 years of age and older.[15] The most difficult problem is the recognition of bronchiectasis in young infants and children typically younger than 7 years. The high resolution possible with such advanced scanners as the GE 9800 in patients who are cooperative and who can hold their breath is now being approached by ultrafast high-resolution cine-CT. These studies have been helpful in documenting bronchiectasis in children as young as 4 months.[17]

Bronchoscopy has not been helpful in multiple studies.[1] Occasional mucosal abnormalities are seen, but typically findings are normal. Some authors proposed that with proper exclusions, the diagnosis of OB can be made from the clinical history, the abnormal ventilation-perfusion scan, and the documentation of bronchiectasis.

Pulmonary function testing has seldom been performed during the acute phase of an illness that ultimately led to OB. In the few patients who have undergone pulmonary function testing, it has shown decreased lung compliance as a result of parenchymal infiltration by interstitial fluid, as well as airflow obstruction. In the few reports of serial pulmonary function testing in pediatric patients, notable decreases in airflow with air trapping were present immediately and during the early chronic phase. As these patients are treated supportively and observed, pulmonary function can gradually improve, with an increase in airflow rates and a decrease in gas trapping. The condition of these patients continues to be quite labile, and repeated respiratory tract infections can cause rapid deterioration in pulmonary function.

The pathologic findings in pediatric patients can be demonstrated only after open-lung biopsy. This procedure entails definite risks of anesthetic and surgical nature, with increased cost and morbidity. In situations in which the sample contains few if any bronchioles, focal emphysema suggests more proximal airway obstruction and air trapping through collateral ventilation.[18] If patchy areas of interstitial fibrosis and organizing pneumonia are present, a careful examination of the airways for obliteration is needed.[19] In some cases, tissue destruction is so severe that bronchioles are not readily recognizable; elastic stains may reveal remnants of the airway wall.[2] During the acute phase, airway damage and necrosis may precede obliteration, and scarring may not yet be present. A biopsy early in the course of the cicatricial process may show bronchiolar necrosis and plugging with minimal fibroblastic response. Even major bronchi may be obliterated in children after infection,[20] although classically the bronchioles are involved.[21] Pathologic specimens from lobectomy have clearly demonstrated the intermittent obliteration of airways along the length of bronchi and bronchioles.[21] Transbronchial biopsy enables diagnosis in some adult patients, but it is not technically possible to perform this procedure in young pediatric patients.

MANAGEMENT

Once OB is diagnosed, the management of these patients is supportive. Most pediatric patients with this disorder who survive the initial insult gradually recover.[1] Some, however, remain severely intolerant of exercise because the total amount of functioning pulmonary tissue is severely decreased. Most patients exhibit chronic wheezing, which should be documented and assessed for bronchodilator responsivity. Because of the small numbers of patients with OB at any one center, random double-blind placebo control trials of corticosteroid therapy for prevention of obliteration have not been attempted. The case reports of series of children with OB who have received steroids have not demonstrated a clear benefit for the use of steroids given initially. The adult literature supports the use of steroids in patients in whom OB develops in many different settings. One summary suggests that steroids should be used in all patients but that the response is best in those in a postinfectious clinical setting.[22] Some patients in whom a localized discrete lesion has developed and who suffer from recurrent infections in that area of the lung respond very well to local resection. This procedure has been used in both adult and pediatric patients with minimally involved or normal areas of lung tissue.

REFERENCES

1. Hardy KA, Schidlow DV, Zaeri N: Obliterative bronchiolitis in children. Chest 93:460–466, 1988.
2. Katzenstein AL, Askin FB: Miscellaneous. I: Specific diseases of uncertain etiology. *In* Bennington JL (ed): Surgical Pathology of Non-Neoplastic Lung Disease, pp. 349–356. Philadelphia: WB Saunders, 1982.
3. Wenman WM, Pagtakhan RD, Reed MH, et al: Adenovirus bronchiolitis in Manitoba. Chest 81:605–609, 1982.
4. Gold R, Wilt JC, Adhikari PK, et al: Adenoviral pneumonia and its complications in infancy and childhood. J Can Assoc Radiol 20:218–224, 1969.
5. Cumming GR, MacPherson RI, Chernick V: Unilateral hyperlucent lung syndrome in children. J Pediatr 78:250–260, 1971.
6. Becroft DM: Bronchiolitis obliterans, bronchiectasis, and other sequelae of adenovirus type 21 infection in young children. J Clin Pathol 24:72–82, 1971.
7. Laraya-Cuasay LR, DeForest A, Huff D, et al: Chronic pulmonary complications of early influenza virus infection in children. Am Rev Respir Dis 116:617–625, 1977.
8. Stokes D, Sigler A, Khouri N, Talamo RC: Unilateral hyperlucent lung (Swyer-James syndrome) after severe *Mycoplasma pneumoniae* infection. Am Rev Respir Dis 117:145–152, 1978.
9. Moran TJ: Experimental aspiration pneumonia IV. Inflammatory and reparative changes produced by intratracheal injections of autologous gastric juice and hydrochloric acid. Arch Pathol 60:122–129, 1955.
10. McCarthy PM, Starnes VA, Theodore J, et al: Improved survival after heart-lung transplantation. J Thorac Cardiovasc Surg 99:54–59, 1990.
11. Gosink BB, Friedman PJ, Liebow AA: Bronchiolitis obliterans: Roentgenologic-pathologic correlation. AJR 117:816–832, 1973.
12. Swyer PR, James GCW: A case of unilateral pulmonary emphysema. Thorax 8:133–136, 1953.
13. Palmer J, Harke T, DeForest A, et al: Matched ventilation/perfusion defects in the lung scans of children with obliterative bronchiolitis and long term clinical followup. Am Rev Respir Dis 119:280, 1979.
14. Gregg I, Trapnell DH: The bronchographic appearances of early chronic bronchitis. Br J Radiol 42:132–139, 1969.
15. Naidich DP, McCauley DI, Khouri NF, et al: Computed tomography of bronchiectasis. J Comput Assist Tomogr 6:437–444, 1982.
16. Hansen TN: Bronchiolitis obliterans. Lung disease in children. Am Rev Respir Dis 1415–1416, 1990.
17. Hardy KA, Lynch DA, Brasch RC, Webb RW: Usefulness of high resolution cine computed tomography in infants and young children with cystic radiography. Am Rev Respir Dis, in press.
18. Blumgart HL, MacMahon HE: Bronchiolitis fibrosa obliterans: A clinical and pathologic study. Med Clin North Am 13:197–214, 1929.
19. Epler GR, Colby TV, McLoud TC, et al: Bronchiolitis obliterans organizing pneumonia. N Engl J Med 312:152–158, 1985.
20. Kargi HA, Kuhn C: Bronchiolitis obliterans: Unilateral fibrous obliteration of the lumen of bronchi with atelectasis. Chest 93:1107–1108, 1988.
21. Azizirad H, Polgar G, Borns PF, et al: Bronchiolitis obliterans. Clin Pediatr 14:572–584, 1975.
22. Epler G: The spectrum of bronchiolitis obliterans. Chest 83:161–162, 1983.

24 BRONCHIECTASIS

NORMAN J. LEWISTON, M.D.

Barker and Bardana[1] referred to bronchiectasis as an "orphan disease," implying that it is an uncommon disease that is neglected in research and treatment development. There is little argument with the progress of research in this area but much dispute about a lack of medical interest. A literature search of this topic for 1983 to 1989 revealed more than 700 articles on bronchiectasis. In a time when the incidence of this disease should be declining, evidence suggests that this is not the case: that the prevalence of bronchiectasis, although low, appears to be maintained. Fernald and co-workers[2] found that 9% of children referred to a teaching hospital for the workup of possible chronic lung disease had bronchiectasis. The severity of this disorder and the complicated approach to management should alert every pediatrician to the rightful place of bronchiectasis on the list of differential diagnoses.

PATHOGENESIS

The name *bronchiectasis* (Greek for "stretching of the windpipe") is appropriate for this disorder because it describes the pathologic process and suggests the pathogenesis. Bronchiectasis, the end result of a number of pulmonary conditions, causes permanent alteration in the structure and function of conducting airways. Bronchial walls derive rigidity from smooth muscle, elastic tissue, and cartilage. Pseudostratified ciliated columnar epithelium lines the bronchial walls; goblet cells and submucosal glands provide airway protection by means of the so-called mucus escalator, which serves to transport foreign matter out of the airway.

The bronchial dilation in bronchiectasis has been classified by Reid[3] into three types: (1) saccular, in which bronchi are dilated to form rounded blind sacs that usually do not communicate with the parenchyma; (2) cylindric, in which airways do not end blindly but communicate with more distal structures; and (3) varicose, in which local constrictions cause an irregularity of outline, occasionally causing the bronchi to terminate in a band of fibrous tissue, which may end distally as a nonpatent cord. The type of bronchiectasis is a result of the extent of airway damage. Saccular bronchiectasis causes destruction of the airway cartilage as well as damage to the elastic tissue and to the muscular coat. Retention of the supporting airway cartilage means that damage is probably limited to the cylindric stage. Whitwell[4] described changes in supportive structures and airway epithelium, the latter frequently resulting in squamous metaplasia interspersed with epithelial ulceration. Squamous metaplasia implies a discontinuity of the mucus escalator, necessitating clearing of the airways by gravity drainage or cough. Because of chronic inflammation, there is an increase in the size and activity of the bronchial and mucous glands. The presence of an increased amount of mucus that can be cleared only by cough explains, in large part, the symptoms and physical findings of this disease.

The pathophysiologic process of bronchiectasis is not well understood. A number of theories have been proposed, including traction on the airways caused by the collapse of surrounding structures, bulging of the airways caused by retention of secretions, weakening of the bronchial wall by infection or inflammation, and various combinations of these. Currently, the accumulation of secretions in an obstructed bronchus and damage to the bronchial walls by infection are believed to be the most important etiologic factors (Fig. 24–1).

Two classic animal studies are of importance in the understanding of bronchiectasis. Tannenberg and Pinner[5] ligated the bronchi of rabbits, allowing the bronchi to fill with secretions. Bronchiectasis did not occur unless the preparation inadvertently or intentionally became infected. The investigators found that the inflammation most likely to produce bronchiectasis was a purulent exudate within the bronchi and a desquamative pneumonic exudate within alveolar parenchyma. Cheng[6] ligated the bronchi of rats, which have a residual bronchial flora. All of these preparations became infected, and bronchiectasis developed in all rats, except for some in which the infection was controlled with chlortetracycline. This outcome led both groups of investigators to conclude that bronchiectasis was the result of the pressure of bronchial secretions on an inflamed bronchial wall. They believed that traction was not an important factor because surrounding structures were collapsed rather than stretched.

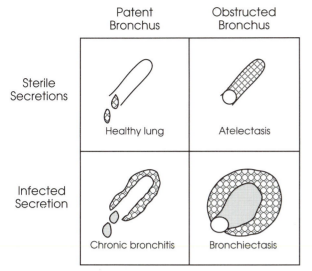

	Patent Bronchus	Obstructed Bronchus
Sterile Secretions	Healthy lung	Atelectasis
Infected Secretion	Chronic bronchitis	Bronchiectasis

Figure 24–1. The relationship between obstruction of the bronchus and infected secretions. An obstructed bronchus with sterile secretions becomes atelectatic. An obstructed bronchus with infected secretions probably will become bronchiectatic.

Similar findings have been noted in humans. Atelectasis resulting from a mucus plug or extrinsic compression can persist for months without damage to the bronchial wall or distal parenchyma if the material trapped in the bronchus is sterile. In disorders in which secretions are infected, the prevalence of bronchiectasis is very high. Hardy and colleagues[7] noted bronchiectasis as a sequela of obliterative bronchiolitis in children and urged that this disorder be suspected when persistent respiratory symptoms or signs follow acute pneumonia, when areas of hyperlucency are seen on chest radiographs, and when respiratory failure with overaeration is unresponsive to therapy. Kleinerman and Vauthy[8] found that the initial lesion in cystic fibrosis was bronchiolitis in airways distended with secretion. They predicted that this condition would progress to bronchiolitis obliterans and bronchiectasis as seen in more pronounced disease. Later work by Sobonya and Taussig[9] supported this theory of progression of cystic fibrosis, but they found that the degree of severity of disease varied greatly among patients of different ages.

Navaratnarajah[10] and Slavin and colleagues[11] reported a high incidence of bronchiolectasis in patients with respiratory failure who had been ventilated with positive end-expiratory pressure; this finding implied prolonged transmural pressure on bronchial walls that had been damaged by a number of factors. Bowen and coauthors[12] found that conditions leading to large bronchial casts ("plastic bronchitis") were associated with the development of bronchiectasis. There is a condition similar to bronchiectasis seen in respiratory bronchioles termed *diffuse panbronchiolitis*. This disease, described in reports from Japan, is characterized by thickening of the wall of the respiratory bronchiole with infiltration of lymphocytes, plasma cells, and histiocytes and extension of the inflammatory changes toward peribronchiolar tissue. In the advanced stage, large amounts of purulent sputum and dilation of the proximal terminal conducting bron-

chioli are seen, resembling bronchiectasis. The authors believed that this disease should be distinguished from bronchiectasis because there is often rapid progression with fatal outcome.[13]

The majority of bronchiectasis cases are diagnosed after severe lower respiratory infections. Glauser and associates[14] found that bronchiectasis was preceded by infection in 69% of patients, by aspiration in 16%, and by a genetic or congenital condition in 15%. Fernald[15] noted that a lower respiratory infection was the first known respiratory manifestation of the lung disease in two thirds of his patients. A similar association with infections has been noted in a number of studies (Table 24–1).

Certain infectious agents, among them adenovirus, seem to be highly associated with the development of bronchiectasis. Certain strains of adenovirus (especially strains 1, 3, 4, 7, and 21) can cause severe pneumonia. Simila and colleagues[16] reported a 10-year follow-up study on 22 Finnish children who had type 7 adenovirus pneumonia. Six of these subjects (27%) had bronchiectasis at 10-year follow-up. Among those who had the most lung disease, there was an increased prevalence of asthma and family histories of atopic disease. These results were compared with those of other long-term studies of adenovirus pneumonia. Of the 121 subjects, 28 (23%) had bronchiectasis and 59 (49%) had other residual changes. Sly and co-workers[17] found that young age at the time of viral pneumonia and the presence of a "measles-like" illness before its onset increases the chance of developing long-term pulmonary abnormalities.

Rubeola also is highly associated with the development of bronchiectasis. In the series reported by Fernald,[15] 17% of the patients had a history of measles. Measles pneumonia produces a profound inflammation of the bronchial wall as well as considerable exudate. Several authors[18–20] suggested an association between concurrent measles and another viral infection with the subsequent development of bronchiectasis. Although the numbers are small and the association is only tentative, acute infections with both viruses are known to have temporary but profound effects on the immune system.

Two diseases that generally are considered to have been largely eradicated by modern medicine are associated with the development of bronchiectasis. Both pertussis and tuberculosis produce a virulent necrotizing bronchi-

Table 24–1. PROBABLE CAUSES OF BRONCHIECTASIS IN CHILDREN

Variable	Fernald[15]	Landau et al.[60]	Glauser et al.[14]	Strang[43]
No. of patients	29*	29	187	209
Pneumonia (unspecified)	38%	21%	33%	35%
Measles	17%	23%	2%	10%
Pertussis	—	21%	12%	17%
Other infection	46%	—	4%	12%
Foreign body or aspiration	7%	—	7%	9%
Other or unknown	10%	35%	45%	35%

*Does not include nine children with congenital anomalies.

tis with a large amount of airway debris. Removal of pertussis antigen from routine childhood immunization has been associated with a predictable increase in the incidence of this disease.[21] Tuberculosis also has undergone a significant resurgence in association with the arrival of immigrants who had lived under poor health conditions. Adler[22] reported that the prevalence of tuberculosis among newborns and children up to 14 years of age in New York City is now 5%, more than five times that of the rest of the country.

Davis and associates[23] reviewed genetic factors that may predispose to bronchiectasis. She divided these into two main categories: those that predispose the carriers to the development of bronchial and pulmonary infections and those in which there is a congenital defect in the supporting structure of the bronchi. The former is more common and includes a constellation of immunodeficiencies as well as cystic fibrosis and the immotile cilia syndrome. Cystic fibrosis is the most common genetic cause of bronchiectasis and is discussed in detail in Chapters 69 to 72. Immotility of cilia is caused by abnormalities of ciliary ultrastructure, which result in lack of coordinated ciliary movement or absence of ciliary support of the mucus escalator important in bronchial hygiene. The incidence of ciliary ultrastructural abnormalities is 1 per 20,000. Another condition resulting in congenital bronchiectasis is the Williams-Campbell syndrome, a rare disorder of the bronchial wall cartilage.

Ciliary failure may be more common than generally is appreciated.[24] Corbeel and colleagues[25] described four patients who had morphologic abnormalities of respiratory cilia during acute or chronic respiratory infection. These abnormalities resolved after treatment of the respiratory illness. Wakefield and Waite studied ciliated epithelium in 13 patients with bronchiectasis.[26] All had morphologic abnormalities of bronchial and nasal cilia. Wakefield and Waite were interested in Polynesian bronchiectasis and suggested that there was a hereditary susceptibility of cilia to damage. A later study by those authors was unable to confirm a specific abnormality of nasal respiratory cilia specimens obtained by brushing.[27] Smith and Pearce noted that bronchiectasis was much more common in Maoris than in other New Zealanders.[28] Cornillie and associates analyzed bronchial cilia microstructure in 24 children with recurrent respiratory tract infections. They found a variety of nonspecific morphologic abnormalities in these patients, which suggest a pathogenic secondary influence from chronic infection.[29]

Allergic disease has been proposed as a causative factor in bronchiectasis. Field[30] and Varpela and co-authors[31] mentioned the presence of asthma in bronchiectasis as a negative prognostic factor. Plugging of airways with viscous asthmatic mucus can impair airway drainage, particularly if the poorly drained airway is bronchiectatic and chronically infected. O'Connor and collaborators concluded that there was no clear evidence that atopy was a risk factor for irreversible airflow obstruction in persons who did not have asthma.[32] Ostergaard[33] reported a series of patients who had non–immunoglobulin E–mediated asthma. He noted that among girls who had this disorder, there was a high incidence of declining lung function, pulmonary hyperinflation, and lung fibrosis. Of 67 patients, severe bronchiectasis developed in four girls and one boy. Patients who on repeated chest radiographs showed persistent hyperinflation of the lungs associated with fixed low forced expiratory volume in 1 sec to forced vital capacity ratio and a marked increase in total serum IgG were those at risk of the development of severe lung disease.[33]

Watts and colleagues[34] reviewed respiratory dysfunction in patients with common variable hypogammaglobulinemia (CVH). All 32 patients in their series had sinopulmonary symptoms and abnormal chest films suggestive of bronchiectasis.[34] Hausser and co-authors[35] agreed with this finding and noted that 9 of 30 children with CVH in their series had associated autoimmune diseases. Stanley and colleagues[36] found that patients with recurrent respiratory infections had significantly lower concentrations of serum IgG_2. IgG_4 was undetectable in 5 of 47 patients with chronic infection and in 4 of 53 patients with recurrent acute respiratory infections.[36] Heiner and associates described a familial bronchiectasis associated with IgG_4 deficiency.[37]

Bronchiectasis has been associated with a number of hypersensitivity diseases including allergic bronchopulmonary aspergillosis (ABPA). Hyphae of *Aspergillus* species grow in sputum plugs in the proximal bronchi. IgE against this antigen causes increased permeability of the respiratory mucosa, permitting IgG, complement, and neutrophils to flood into the airway. This flooding causes an intense localized inflammation, resulting in cylindric bronchiectasis at the site of the sputum plugs. Airways distal to the site of these plugs may be normal. Wang and colleagues reported ABPA in 13 children, 7 of whom had bronchiectasis.[38] Diagnosis of this disorder is important because the intense inflammation (and the lung damage) can be controlled with corticosteroids.

The concurrence of bronchiectasis and chronic sinusitis has been known for years. Although some of these cases may have been manifestations of the immotile cilia syndrome, Nemir proposed a reciprocal source of infection.[39] This suggests a "Ping-Pong" cycle in which infected sinus material drains into the trachea and infected sputum is coughed into the nasal passages and ultimately the sinuses. Efforts to clear the sinusitis with appropriate antimicrobial therapy or surgical drainage may be effective in breaking this cycle.

Finally, bronchiectasis has been associated with a number of other conditions, including Marfan's syndrome, rheumatoid arthritis, pulmonary sequestration, unilateral hyperlucent lung, tracheobronchomegaly, yellow nail syndrome, and peripheral neuropathy.[40] Although there is no immediate common denominator of these diseases, many of them are associated with poor bronchial drainage and disorders of immunity.

DIAGNOSIS

Certain signs and symptoms are useful in diagnosing bronchiectasis. Clark reported persistent cough in 81% of 116 patients and intermittent cough in an additional 12%.[41] Fifty-eight percent of the children had produced purulent sputum. Although the production of purulent

Table 24–2. LOBAR INVOLVEMENT IN CHILDHOOD BRONCHIECTASIS

Variable	Clark[41]	Glauser et al.[14]	Field[30]
No. of Patients	116	187	225
Right Lung			
Upper lobe	20%	21%	22%
Middle lobe	50%	41%	50%
Lower lobe	39%	71%	41%
Left Lung			
Upper lobe	10%	19%	13%
Lingula	73%	45%	55%
Lower lobe	77%	81%	61%

From Lewiston N: Bronchiectasis in childhood. Pediatr Clin North Am 31: 865–878, 1984.

sputum is an important clue, absence of sputum does not preclude bronchiectasis. Wilson and Decker found that 91% of children referred for bronchoscopy because of the production of more than 0.5 ml of sputum per day had evidence of bronchiectasis.[42] They also found that 32% of children who produced no sputum but who had other signs of bronchiectasis showed positive findings on bronchography. Hemoptysis and wheezing are rather uncommon presenting signs; they are seen in fewer than 10% of patients.[30, 41]

Physical examination may reveal two common findings in bronchiectasis. The first of these is the presence of bronchovesicular breath sounds over the affected area. This finding, frequently called "coarsening" of the breath sounds, means that the loudness of the expiratory phase of respiration is equal to that of the inspiratory phase when the diaphragm of the stethoscope is placed over the thorax in the vicinity of the bronchiectasis. The loudness of expiration denotes turbulent airflow in airways close to the chest wall, which are widened because of disease. This sound is heard in normal persons just above the clavicle at the apex of the right lung. The second finding is inspiratory crackles. Clark found these in 91% of his patients.[41] Crackles represent an "opening snap" or the discontinuity of a fluid-solid interface as the airway dilates during inspiration. This is a sign of fluid in the airways as a result of poor drainage or inflammation. Crackles usually are localized to one or more areas and are heard at the same site on re-examination, although they may clear transiently with coughing.

Bronchiectasis is found most commonly in the left lower lobe, the lingula, and the right middle lobe. Table 24–2 lists the locations of bronchiectasis found in three large series. The majority of the children studied had disease in more than one lobe. The most common combinations appear to be the left lower lobe and the lingula.

Clark reported an incidence of clubbed fingers in 3% of his pediatric patients with bronchiectasis, in comparison with 44% for Field and 51% for Strang.[30, 41, 43] Clark also reported that 43% of the children in his series measured below the 10th percentile for height and weight. It is now believed that the prevalence of both of these findings—clubbed fingers and growth failure—as presenting signs is lower than indicated in earlier series.

Findings characteristic of bronchiectasis may be seen on plain film radiographs. Felman[44] listed the following

criteria of the endobronchial-bronchiectasis pattern frequently seen in children: (1) ringlike densities with clear centers that represent thick-walled bronchi seen on end; (2) white, rounded densities produced when the bronchial lumina become plugged with mucopurulent material; (3) parallel lines (railroad tracks) that represent thick-walled bronchi seen from the side (these may branch and contain plugs of mucus); (4) irregular, ill-defined vascular markings that result from distortion of the normal vessels by adjacent diseased bronchi; and (5) unequal aeration that results from either partial or complete bronchial obstruction, which produces areas of focal atelectasis or hyperinflation. Bronchial walls, normally seen only in the central and perihilar regions on normal films, become apparent in the peripheral lung segments. Felman[44] recommended the study of serial films in order to appreciate some of the subtle changes just listed (Fig. 24–2).

Nadel and associates[45] reviewed the radiologic manifestations of immotile cilia syndrome. They found that the disease progresses from bronchial wall thickening with or without hyperinflation to increasing hyperinflation with parenchymal changes, including segmental atelectasis, consolidation, and bronchiectasis. There also was a predilection for anatomic middle-lobe abnormalities. The radiologic appearance and clinical symptoms were similar to those of cystic fibrosis, although they were less severe and less progressive.[45]

Naidich and collaborators[45] reviewed their experience with the use of computed tomography (CT) in the diagnosis of bronchiectasis. They noted four signs of this disorder: (1) air-fluid levels in distorted bronchi, (2) linear airways or cluster of cysts, (3) distended bronchi in the periphery of the lung, and (4) bronchial walls thickened by peribronchial fibrosis.[46] Joharjy and associates reported on the value of medium-thickness CT (4-mm–thickness cuts at 5-mm intervals) in the diagnosis of bronchiectasis.[47] CT scans correctly identified all cases of saccular and varicose bronchiectasis but missed the correct

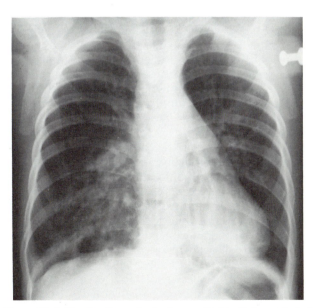

Figure 24–2. Chest radiograph of a 3-year-old girl with bronchiectasis of the left lower lobe. The film shows some of the thickened walls of the bronchiectatic lobe through the cardiac silhouette *(arrow)*.

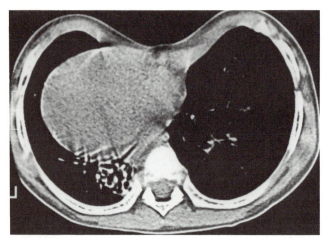

Figure 24–3. Computed tomographic view of the patient in Figure 24–2. The dilated bronchi and thickened bronchial walls are seen clearly in this view *(arrow).*

diagnosis in 3 of 52 segmental bronchi showing cylindric bronchiectasis; thus CT had 100% sensitivity for the two former types and 94% for cylindric bronchiectasis. Naidich and collaborators believed that the false-negative result was attributable to the presence of interstitial lung disease with hyperinflation and very localized mild disease in one case (Fig. 24–3).

Since about 1930, the standard means of confirming the diagnosis of bronchiectasis has been the bronchogram, which entails the instillation of radiocontrast media directly into the bronchus. Although this method produces clear radiographs, it has never been popular among pediatricians. Cameron and Holloway reported that the incidence of severe complications with this procedure in children was low but suggested that it be reserved for children who are thought to require surgical resection for bronchiectasis.[48]

Barker and Bardana identified three situations in which they believed that bronchoscopy might be of particular assistance: (1) when the history and laboratory information are nondiagnostic and other diseases such as a tumor or foreign body have been ruled out, but a strong suspicion of bronchiectasis remains; (2) when the diagnosis of bronchiectasis is clinically established, but it is suspected that a particular segment or lobe is the main contributor to massive secretions or bleeding; and (3) when bronchoscopy has not shown a discrete lesion in a patient with persistent hemoptysis.[1] Barker and Bardana believed that bronchoscopy and bronchography of both lungs are vital parts of the assessment of focal bronchiectasis for which surgical resection is contemplated.

As pediatricians gain experience with bronchoscopy, this modality assumes increased importance in the diagnostic plan of children with unexplained lung symptoms. Puhakka and colleagues reported the results of 1032 bronchoscopies performed in Finnish children; 2.5% of these children had bronchiectasis.[49] Godfrey and colleagues reported the results of bronchoscopy on 364 Israeli children; they found that the most common diagnoses in children younger than 1 year were related to congenital anomalies; in the 1- to 3-year-old group, to inhaled for-

eign bodies; and in children older than 3 years, to bronchiectasis.[50] Flower and Shneerson reviewed their experience with fiberoptic bronchoscopy in children. They agreed that bronchiectasis was the most common finding in older children and believed that the fiberoptic bronchoscope was the method of choice for obtaining segmental bronchograms.[51] Levy and co-workers found that the combined use of bronchoscopy and bronchography was a safe and sensitive means of obtaining a specific diagnosis in young children.[52]

A number of other procedures have been suggested as useful in the diagnosis of bronchiectasis. Gordon and associates[53] reviewed the results of radionuclide scintigraphy in 100 scans of children with a variety of cardiopulmonary disorders. The bronchiectatic segment retains the radionuclide, usually technetium 99m, during perfusion scan. These authors and Felman believed this to be a sensitive but not particularly specific means of diagnosing bronchiectasis or inhaled foreign body. They stated that the probability of bronchiectasis is small in the presence of a normal chest radiograph and a normal perfusion scan.[44, 53] Seibert and colleagues[54] found that chest ultrasonography was beneficial in the diagnostic workup of a child whose radiographs showed an opaque chest. They were able to locate the presence of bronchial foreign bodies and even see the bronchiectasis when the bronchi were filled with fluids.[54] Finally, Smith reviewed the value of nuclear magnetic resonance imaging. Smith indicated that this procedure would become the one of choice in the workup of children with chronic lung disease because of the high-resolution images that are possible without the use of ionizing radiation. As facilities become more readily available, time required per examination is decreased, and the cost of the procedure is reduced, this prediction will probably prove true.[55]

TREATMENT

The treatment plan for a child with bronchiectasis requires two phases. The first, or immediate, phase is directed at correcting as quickly as possible the factors that produce lung damage. Active infection should be treated with appropriate antimicrobial agents. Areas of atelectasis or mucus plugging should be cleared with bronchoscopy or vigorous chest physiotherapy. Bronchoscopy may be indicated to accomplish both culture of the inflamed site and lavage and suction of areas of mucus plugging. Most physicians believe that antimicrobial therapy should be as specific as possible and should be continued during acute exacerbations of infection.[56] There is no proven benefit of continuous antimicrobial therapy in bronchiectasis in patients who do not have a major underlying condition such as cystic fibrosis or immotile cilia syndrome. Maintenance of good bronchial hygiene is important. Because there has been disruption of the mucus escalator, the airways can be cleared only with vigorous coughing. Gravity drainage of affected lobes to permit the cough to be effective in clearing thick mucus is also important.

The second phase of treatment involves a long-term plan. Ultimately, the question of surgery must be considered. For this the primary physician's role as referring physician is important because guidelines for surgery in bronchiectasis are not well defined. Most surgeons believe that surgery may be necessary in the treatment of this disease. Pediatric pulmonary specialists, many of whom care for patients with cystic fibrosis, may opt for long-term conservative medical management.

Before the days of antibiotics and modern thoracic surgical techniques, bronchiectasis carried a poor prognosis. Improvement in anesthesia and surgical techniques after World War II offered hope to the population affected by it. By the late 1950s, however, lung disease specialists were beginning to question the advisability of surgery at all. An editorial in the *Lancet* in 1958 pointed out that the two most common causes of bronchiectasis in British children—obstruction of bronchi by enlarged tuberculous glands and persistent atelectasis after respiratory infections—were decreasing in frequency.[57] The authors stated, "Possibly by the time it has been finally settled when best to employ resection for bronchiectasis, there will be few opportunities to act on the knowledge." This prediction, like many others in medicine, has not been correct.

Field, in an elegant three-part study, reported a 20-year follow-up on 187 patients who acquired bronchiectasis in childhood.[30, 58, 59] In patients who did not undergo surgery, there was a tendency for symptoms to improve in the second decade of life and to remain unchanged during the third and fourth decades. Landau and associates[60] agreed with the tendency of bronchiectatic children to improve during adolescence. These conclusions have been quoted widely.

One of the major arguments for the surgical removal of diseased segments of lung is to prevent spread of infected sputum and debris to the unaffected lung. There has been disagreement on whether this actually occurs. Clark found new disease in 15 of 79 patients who were evaluated by repeated bronchography.[41] Wilson and Decker, however, found that only 2% of the patients in their series had extension of disease to healthy tissue.[42] They did, however, find progression of disease from ill-defined changes to bronchiectasis in 26% of young children. For this reason, they recommended delay of surgery until the extent of disease is defined, usually between 6 and 12 years of age.

Another argument for an attempt at complete alleviation of bronchiectatic symptoms deals with quality of life. Ellis and colleagues[61] reviewed the long-term social effects of the symptoms of bronchiectasis. Seventy-seven percent of the patients reported no social problems. Forty-six percent of the patients' spouses, however, found the cough annoying, and 29% of married patients reported difficulty with sexual relations. Ellis and colleagues concluded that although many of the severe effects of bronchiectasis have been mitigated by treatment, a significant percentage of patients still have severe physical and social problems as a result.

How likely is the possibility of a surgical cure? Zamir and co-workers reported complete relief of symptoms in 15 of 18 patients in their series.[62] The results of nine long-term follow-up studies of children with bronchiectasis are listed in Table 24–3. Criteria for evaluation vary with

Table 24–3. OUTCOME OF TREATMENT FOR BRONCHIECTASIS IN CHILDREN

Study	Mode†	No. Patients	Outcome Classification*			
			I	II	III	IV
Wilson and Decker[42]	Surg	96	39	45	22	0
	Med	87	0	0	9	91
Clark[41]	Surg	75	55	16	24	1
	Med	27	15	7	69	19
Field[30]	Surg	111	33	46	17	4
	Med	54	32	39	28	2
Strang[43]	Surg	155	31	37	12	40
Helm and Thompson[71]	Surg	32	46	19	28	6
Franklin[72]	Med	20	55	15	10	20
Fernald[15]	Surg	8	25	25	25	25
	Med	18	28	—	50	22
Voronov, et al.[70]	Surg	360	30	53	—	17
Lee and Conlan[69]	Surg	16	—	75	—	25
	Med	13	—	40	—	60

Adapted from Lewison, N: Bronchiectasis in childhood. Pediatr Clin North Am 31:865–878, 1984.
*Values are expressed in percentages. The outcome classification varies somewhat with each study but, in general, class I is "well or completely asymptomatic," class II is "mostly well with occasional symptoms or persisting abnormal bronchograms," class III is "improved over pretreatment condition," class IV is "unchanged or worse than pretreatment condition."
†Surg, surgery; Med, medicine.

each group, but a description of each study permitted categorization as follows: well, virtually asymptomatic with occasional exacerbations, improved over base line, and no change or worse. Patients treated by surgery seemed to fare better, although not all of the patients were carefully matched, and some of the patients managed medically would not have been surgical candidates. Probably the best comparison was by Wilson and Decker, who identified 87 children who were candidates for surgery but received only medical management. In this series, none of the 87 were well or much improved.[42] Ninety-one percent of these patients experienced no change in symptoms. This finding is consistent with those of Annest and colleagues[63] and Sanderson and associates,[64] who believed that patients with bronchiectasis who were candidates for surgery would have improved quality of life by decreasing symptoms and decreasing the need for medications after the operation. Laros and Westerman considered the late complications of major thoracic surgery in a large series. They found that in patients with bronchiectasis, the results were good with normal qualitative function; unsatisfactory results were found in patients with chronic obstructive pulmonary disease. The removal of nonfunctioning tissue apparently results in a compensatory increase in the vital capacity of the remaining segments.[65] Marmon and collaborators[66] and Steinkamp and co-workers[67] reported the results of pulmonary resection in a small number of patients with cystic fibrosis. They believed that resection was a satisfactory means of treating localized bronchiectasis and hemoptysis secondary to cystic fibrosis. One of the problems with this procedure is that patients who had even a limited thoracostomy may be disqualified as candidates for heart-lung transplantation (see Chapter 88).

In spite of these findings, most physicians caring for children with bronchiectasis at least consider a trial of conservative treatment. The reasons are varied but usually involve an unfavorable experience in which a child underwent resection of some bronchiectatic lung tissue, only to experience recurrence of the condition elsewhere. It is extremely important to realize that lung tissue can appear bronchiectatic after infection for several weeks (pseudobronchiectasis) and that surgery, if any, should be deferred until the status of the remaining lung tissue is well defined. With this in mind, it appears reasonable to consider surgery in a child with localized saccular bronchiectasis or with ongoing symptoms.

Wilson and Decker[42] provided the following indications for surgery:

1. Localized disease that produces severe symptoms such as sputum or cough that interfere with normal living.
2. Threatening hemorrhage from a demonstrated source.
3. Resectable disease associated with failure to thrive.
4. Resectable disease at a demonstrated site of recurrent acute infections of the lower respiratory tract.

The following additional indications may be appropriate:

1. Evidence of unstable disease associated with significant progression or extension of resectable disease.
2. Bronchiectasis not easily or totally resectable but associated with a failure to thrive.
3. Bronchiectasis not easily or totally resectable and associated with life-threatening or truly disabling symptoms such as hemorrhage or severe focal infections.
4. Localized disease producing minimal to moderate symptoms. Wilson and Decker stressed that patients in this category are not surgical candidates unless they are clearly symptomatic.

SUMMARY

Although bronchiectasis is uncommon in children, the prevalence of this disease remains relatively constant. It should be suspected in any child with an infiltrate on radiograph that fails to clear, persistent cough, purulent sputum, crackles or coarse breath sounds on auscultation of the chest, or hemoptysis.[68] Attempts should be made promptly to provide specific antimicrobial treatment of infected bronchial secretions and to establish normal bronchial drainage. Fiberoptic bronchoscopy may be particularly useful for this purpose. CT or nuclear magnetic resonance imaging of the chest may provide valuable information, particularly with repeated studies in an area of concern. Localized areas of bronchiectasis, particularly those producing symptoms, may be amenable to bronchographic evaluation and surgical resection.

REFERENCES

1. Barker A, Bardana E: Bronchiectasis: Update of an orphan disease. Am Rev Respir Dis 137:969–976, 1988.
2. Fernald G, Denny F, Fairclough K, et al: Chronic lung disease in children referred to a teaching hospital. Pediatr Pulmonol 2:27–34, 1986.
3. Reid L: Reduction in bronchial subdivision in bronchiectasis. Thorax 5:233–247, 1950.
4. Whitwell F: A study of the pathology and pathogenesis of bronchiectasis. Thorax 7:213–239, 1952.
5. Tannenberg J, Pinner MA: Atelectasis and bronchiectasis: An experimental study concerning their relationship. J Thorac Surg 11:571–616, 1942.
6. Cheng K-K: The experimental production of bronchiectasis in rats. J Pathol Bacteriol 67:89–98, 1954.
7. Hardy K, Schidlow K, Zaeri N: Obstructive bronchiolitis in children. Chest 93:460–466, 1988.
8. Kleinerman J, Vauthy P: Pathology of the Lung in Cystic Fibrosis. Rockville, MD: Cystic Fibrosis Foundation, 1976.
9. Sobonya R, Taussig L: Quantitative aspects of lung pathology in cystic fibrosis. Am Rev Respir Dis 134:290–295, 1986.
10. Navaratnarajah M, Nunn J, Lyons D, et al: Bronchiolectasis caused by positive end-expiratory pressure. Crit Care Med 12:1036–1038, 1984.
11. Slavin G, Nunn J, Crow J, et al: Bronchiolectasis, a complication of artificial ventilation. Br Med J [Clin Res] 285:931–934, 1982.
12. Bowen A, Oudjhane K, Odagiri K, et al: Plastic bronchitis: Large, branching, mucoid bronchial casts in children. AJR 144:371–375, 1985.
13. Homma H, Yamanaka A, Tanimoto S, et al: Diffuse panbronchiolitis: A disease of the transitional zone of the lung. Chest 83:63–69, 1983.
14. Glauser EM, Cook CD, Harris GBC: Bronchiectasis—A review of 187 cases in children with follow-up pulmonary functions studies in 58. Acta Pediatr Scand 165(Suppl):1–16, 1966.
15. Fernald GW: Bronchiectasis in childhood: A 10-year survey of cases treated at North Carolina Memorial Hospital. NC Med J 39:368–372, 1978.
16. Simila S, Linna O, Lanning P, et al: Chronic lung disease caused by adenovirus type 7: A ten-year follow-up study. Chest 80:127–131, 1981.
17. Sly PD, Soto-Quiros ME, Landau L, et al: Factors predisposing to abnormal pulmonary function after adenovirus type 7 pneumonia. Arch Dis Child 59:935–939, 1984.
18. Warner JO, Marshall WC: Crippling lung disease after measles and adenovirus infection. Br J Dis Chest 2:89–94, 1976.
19. Jean R, Benoist M, Rufin P, et al: Respiratory sequelae of severe measles. Rev Fr Mal Respir 9:45–53, 1981.
20. Kaschula R, Druker J, Kipps A: Late morphologic consequences of measles: A lethal and debilitating disease. Rev Infect Dis 5:395–404, 1983.
21. Johnstone T, Hull F: Whooping cough in the United States and Britain [Letter]. N Engl J Med 309:108–109, 1983.
22. Adler J: Tuberculosis test will be prerequisite to entering school in NYC. Pediatr News 23:17–21, 1989.
23. Davis PB, Hubbard VS, McCoy K, et al: Familial bronchiectasis. J Pediatr 102:177–185, 1983.
24. Turner J, Corkey C, Lee J: Clinical expressions of immotile cilia syndrome. Pediatrics 67:805–810, 1981.
25. Corbeel L, Cornillie F, Lauweryns J: Ultrastructural abnormalities of bronchial cilia in children with recurrent airway infections and bronchiectasis. Arch Dis Child 56:929–933, 1981.
26. Wakefield SJ, Waite D: Abnormal cilia in Polynesians with bronchiectasis. Am Rev Respir Dis 121:1003–1010, 1980.
27. Waite D, Wakefield S, Morairty K, et al: Polynesian bronchiectasis. Eur J Respir Dis [Suppl.] 127:31–36, 1983.
28. Smith A, Pearce N: Determinants of differences in mortality between New Zealand Maoris and non-Maoris aged 15–64. N Z Med J 97:101–108, 1984.
29. Cornillie F, Lauweryns J, Corbeel L: Atypical bronchial cilia in children with recurrent respiratory tract infections: A comparative ultrastructural study. Pathol Res Pract 178:595–604, 1984.
30. Field CE: Bronchiectasis, third report on a follow-up study of medical and surgical cases from childhood. Arch Dis Child 44:551–561, 1969.
31. Varpela E, Laitinen LA, Keskinen H, Korhola O: Asthma, allergy and bronchial hyper-reactivity to histamine in patients with bronchiectasis. Clin Allergy 8:273–280, 1978.
32. O'Connor G, Sparrow D, Weiss S: The role of allergy and non-specific airway hyperresponsiveness in the pathogenesis of chronic obstructive pulmonary disease. Am Rev Respir Dis 140:225–252, 1989.

33. Ostergaard PA: A prospective study on non–IgE-mediated asthma in children. Acta Paediatr Scand 77:112–117, 1988.
34. Watts W, Watts M, Dai W, et al: Respiratory dysfunction in patients with common variable hypogammaglobulinemia. Am Rev Respir Dis 134:699–703, 1986.
35. Hausser C, Virelizier J, Buriot D, Griscelli C: Common variable hypogammaglobulinemia in children: Clinical and immunologic observations in 30 patients. Am J Dis Child 137:833–837, 1983.
36. Stanley P, Corbo G, Cole P: Serum IgG subclasses in chronic and recurrent respiratory infections. Clin Exp Immunol 58:703–708, 1984.
37. Heiner D, Myers A, Beck C: Deficiency of IgG_4: A disorder associated with frequent infections and bronchiectasis that may be familiar. Clin Rev Allergy 1:259–266, 1983.
38. Wang J, Patterson R, Mintzer R, et al: Allergic bronchopulmonary aspergillosis in pediatric practice. J Pediatr 94:376–381, 1979.
39. Nemir R: Bronchiectasis. In Kendig E, Chernick V (ed): Disorders of the Respiratory Tract in Children, 4th ed, pp. 348–368. Philadelphia: WB Saunders, 1983.
40. Luce J: Bronchiectasis. In Murray J, Nadel J (eds): Textbook of Respiratory Medicine, pp. 1107–1125. Philadelphia: WB Saunders, 1988.
41. Clark NS: Bronchiectasis in childhood. Br Med J 1:80–88, 1963.
42. Wilson JF, Decker AM: The surgical management of childhood bronchiectasis. Ann Surg 195:354–363, 1982.
43. Strang C: The fate of children with bronchiectasis. Ann Intern Med 44:630–656, 1956.
44. Felman A: Radiology of the Pediatric Chest. New York: McGraw-Hill, 1987.
45. Nadel H, Stringer D, Levison H, et al: The immotile cilia syndrome: Radiological manifestations. Radiology 154:651–655, 1985.
46. Naidich DP, McCauley DI, Khouri NF, et al: Computed tomography of bronchiectasis. J Comput Assist Tomogr 6:437–444, 1982.
47. Joharjy I, Bashi S, Abdullah A: Value of medium thickness CT in the diagnosis of bronchiectasis. AJR 149:1133–1137, 1987.
48. Cameron EW, Holloway AM: Bronchography in children aged 3 years and under. Anesthetic techniques and results. S Afr Med J 54:271–275, 1978.
49. Puhakka H, Kero P, Erkinjuntti M: Pediatric bronchoscopy during a 17 year period. Int J Pediatr Otorhinolaryngol 13:171–180, 1987.
50. Godfrey S, Springer C, Maayen C, et al: Is there a place for rigid bronchoscopy in the management of pediatric lung disease? Pediatr Pulmonol 3:179–184, 1987.
51. Flower CD, Shneerson JM: Bronchography via the fiberoptic bronchoscope. Thorax 39:260–263, 1984.
52. Levy M, Glick B, Springer C, et al: Bronchoscopy and bronchography in children. Am J Dis Child 137:14–16, 1983.
53. Gordon I, Helms P, Fazio F: Clinical application of radionuclide lung scanning in infants and children. Br J Radiol 54:576–585, 1981.
54. Seibert R, Seibert J, Williamson S: The opaque chest: When to suspect a bronchial foreign body. Pediatr Radiol 16:193–196, 1986.
55. Smith F: The value of NMR imaging in pediatric practice: A preliminary report. Pediatr Radiol 13:141–147, 1983.
56. Dietesch H: Indications for antibiotic long-term treatment of chronic and recurring bronchitis. Kinderarztl Prax 47:175–178, 1979.
57. Surgery for bronchiectasis. Lancet 2:734–735, 1958.
58. Field C: Bronchiectasis in childhood. Pediatrics 4:21–45, 231–248, 355–372, 1949.
59. Field C: Bronchiectasis. A long-term follow-up of medical and surgical cases from childhood. Arch Dis Child 36:587–603, 1961.
60. Landau LI, Phelan PD, Williams HE: Ventilatory mechanics in patients with bronchiectasis starting in childhood. Thorax 29:304–312, 1974.
61. Ellis DA, Thornley PE, Wightman AJ, et al: Present outlook in bronchiectasis: Clinical and social study and review of factors influencing prognosis. Thorax 36:659–664, 1981.
62. Zamir I, Lernau O, Springer C: Lung resection for bronchiectasis in children. Kinderchir 42:282–285, 1987.
63. Annest L, Kratz J, Crawford F: Current results of treatment of bronchiectasis. J Thorac Cardiovasc Surg 83:546–550, 1982.
64. Sanderson JM, Kennedy MCS, Johnson MF, et al: Bronchiectasis, results of surgical and conservative management. A review of 393 cases. Thorax 29:407–416, 1974.
65. Laros C, Westerman C: Dilatation, compensatory growth, or both following pneumonectomy during childhood and adolescence. A 30-year follow-up. J Thorac Cardiovasc Surg 93:570–576, 1987.
66. Marmon L, Schilow D, Palmer J, et al: Pulmonary resection for complications of cystic fibrosis. J Pediatr Surg 18:811–815, 1983.
67. Steinkamp G, von der Hardt H, Zimmermann H: Pulmonary resection for localized bronchiectasis in cystic fibrosis. Report of three cases and review of the literature. Acta Paediatr Scand 77:565–575, 1988.
68. Lewiston N: Bronchiectasis in childhood. Pediatr Clin North Am 31:865–878, 1984.
69. Lee D, Conlan A: Bronchiectasis in urban black children. S Afr Med J 67:817–819, 1985.
70. Voronov A, Aleksandrov O, Kalechenkov M, et al: Immediate and long-term results of pulmonary resection in bronchiectasis. Vestnik Khir 137:3–6, 1986.
71. Helm WH, Thompson VC: The long term results of resection for bronchiectasis. Q J Med 27:353, 1958.
72. Franklin SW: The prognosis of bronchiectasis in childhood. Arch Dis Child 33:19, 1958.

25 DIAGNOSIS AND TREATMENT OF COCCIDIOIDOMYCOSIS

JOHN A. KAFKA, M.D. / ANTONINO CATANZARO, M.D.

Coccidioidomycosis is the infection caused by the fungus *Coccidioides immitis*. *C. immitis* is found naturally in a well-circumscribed geographic distribution consisting of desert areas of the southwestern United States and northern Mexico as well as certain limited areas of Central and South America. The fungus grows in the soil as a mycelium during the rainy season and forms highly friable arthrospores that easily become airborne during dry seasons. Infection is usually initiated by inhalation and proliferation of arthrospores in the airway or alveolar space. Infection with *C. immitis* is associated with a broad spectrum of clinical manifestations ranging from asymptomatic infection or mild flu-like illness to severe pneumonia with respiratory failure. Because the clinical findings are relatively nonspecific, the most important step in the diagnostic process is to suspect coccidioidomycosis. Historic information can be extraordinarily important. When coccidioidomycosis is suspected, the steps that must be taken to confirm or rule out the diagnosis are, in general, not difficult.

THE ORGANISM

C. immitis is a dimorphic fungus with two distinct life cycles.[1, 2] In the soil and under most laboratory conditions, it grows as a mold with septate hyphae that mature and may develop into small 2- to 5-μm thick-walled arthrospores. The organism grows well in the laboratory under a variety of culture conditions. Arthrospores can become readily detached and airborne. Laboratory-acquired infections may occur if cultures are not handled carefully.

When infection occurs in tissue, the arthrospore swells and forms a spherule. This is the characteristic form of the fungus that is seen in pathologic specimens (Fig. 25-1). Spherules vary from 10 to 80 μm in diameter. Endospores form within the cytoplasm of the spherule, which then bursts, releasing the endospores. The endospores grow into new spherules, continuing the life cycle.

Whereas arthrospores are highly infective, spherules and endospores are not; thus coccidioidomycosis is not transmissible from person to person, except, in rare instances, of vertical transmission from infected mother to the infant.

EPIDEMIOLOGY

Infection is usually initiated by inhalation of arthrospores into the respiratory tract. Activities that increase exposure to dust in endemic areas increase susceptibility to infection. Dust storms[3] and fomites[4] can result in infection outside the usual endemic area. Infections also occur in rare instances through vertical transmission or direct inoculation of the fungus in the skin.[5] Prospective studies in adults have shown that 60% of primary coccidioidal infections are asymptomatic and can be detected only through skin test conversion. Several factors can increase susceptibility to more severe infection. Increased intensity of exposure can result in development of symptoms in a higher proportion of patients, as demonstrated by outbreaks seen in archeology students[6] and in children digging in soil.[7, 8]

Although it has been stated that children are less likely to acquire severe or disseminated disease, available studies suggest that children and adults are similarly susceptible to severe infection.[9] Race is another factor that may affect susceptibility to serious infection. Blacks have been reported to have a twelvefold increase in the risk of dissemination;[10] other nonwhite patients have long been suspected to have higher rates of dissemination, but whether this represents differences in immunity or levels of exposure remains uncertain.[9, 11, 12] It is clear that conditions that impair immune function increase susceptibility to disseminated disease. This increase has been observed with neoplastic conditions, treated collagen vascular disease, and immunosuppression for transplantation or in association with acquired immunodeficiency syndrome.[13, 14] One report suggests that immunosuppression can trigger reactivation of an old healed primary lesion and dissemination years after the occurrence of primary infection.[15]

CLINICAL AND LABORATORY FINDINGS IN PRIMARY INFECTION

Symptoms of primary coccidioidomycosis occur after an incubation period of 5 to 20 days[16, 17] and may last from a few days to several weeks in uncomplicated cases. The most frequently observed symptoms in children[8, 16, 18] and

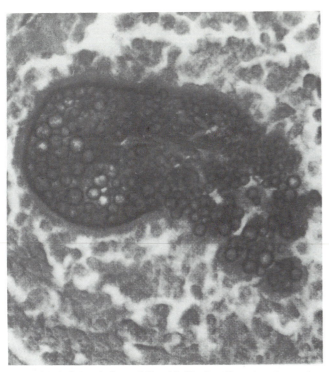

Figure 25–1. Spherule form of *Coccidioides immitis* undergoing rupture with release of endospores into surrounding tissue.

adolescents[6, 19, 20] are fever, sore throat, cough, skin rashes, and chest pain. Of these, chest pain and rash are the most suggestive of a possible diagnosis of coccidioidomycosis because, especially in combination, they occur rarely in other childhood illnesses.

Chest pain occurs in two thirds of cases and may be pleuritic or substernal in nature.[21] Skin rashes have also been reported in approximately two thirds of pediatric cases and are of two general types. The most common is a toxic erythema. It occurs in the first few days of illness, is usually a fine diffuse macular eruption on the trunk and extremities,[22, 23] and is occasionally associated with oral lesions.[18] This type of rash is indistinguishable from that of toxic erythema that commonly occurs with a variety of viral infections.

Hypersensitivity rashes include erythema multiforme and erythema nodosum. These eruptions, which occur in 5% to 20% of diagnosed primary coccidioidal infections, are associated with marked delayed-type hypersensitivity on skin testing to coccidioidal antigens. Erythema nodosum and erythema multiforme are markers of primary coccidioidal infection. Because the majority of primary cases have a favorable outcome, it is often said that erythema nodosum and erythema multiforme are associated with a favorable outcome. Unfortunately, patients with erythema nodosum and erythema multiforme have been observed to acquire more serious forms of coccidioidomycosis.[22, 23, 24]

Routine laboratory studies are rarely useful for confirming the correct diagnosis. Leukocyte counts are usually normal or mildly elevated, and eosinophilia is occasionally present.[22, 25] Eosinophilia may be associated with a poorer prognosis. The erythrocyte sedimentation rate may be elevated.[20]

Chest radiographs are abnormal in a majority of symptomatic patients.[26, 27] Unilateral parenchymal infiltrates typically are seen; these infiltrates may vary in appearance from patchy shadows to dense segmental infiltrates. Hilar adenopathy has been reported to occur in many cases (25%) (Fig. 25–2). Pleural reaction is seen in approximately 20% of patients and may range from mild pleural thickening to massive effusion.[25, 28]

Examination of pleural fluid is helpful. In one study of 28 pediatric and adult patients,[25] the pleural fluid contained a mean of 4600 leukocytes per cubic millimeter with a predominance of mononuclear cells. Pleural fluid cultures were positive in 20% of patients. Parietal pleural biopsy specimens yielded the organisms in all patients who underwent biopsy.

PULMONARY SEQUELAE OF PRIMARY INFECTION OR CHRONIC PULMONARY COCCIDIOIDOMYCOSIS

Spontaneous resolution of clinical and radiographic abnormalities is the outcome in the majority of patients.[25, 26] In approximately 30% of patients, coccidioidal pneumonia results in the formation of a focal residual lesion such as a cavity or a nodule.[18, 26, 29] Nodules typically evolve from infiltrates and are single without surrounding infiltrates. Depending on their size, they may resolve spontaneously over several months or become calcified.[18] Cavities may be thin or thick walled and single or multiple (Fig. 25–3). They are usually less than 3 cm in diameter and are centrally located. Although often benign, cavities may become obstructed and filled with necrotic material. Intermittent drainage may occur, which is suggestive of a lung abscess. In this stage, radio-

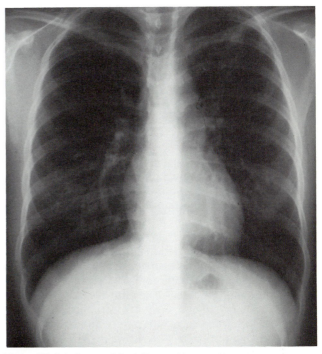

Figure 25–2. Left upper lobe infiltrate with central lucency in an 11-year-old girl. Hilar adenopathy is also present.

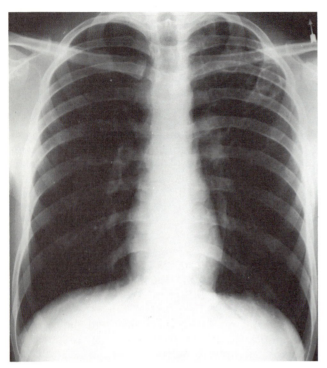

Figure 25–3. Multiple thin-walled cavities in the left upper lobe of a 14-year-old boy.

graphs may show lesions that resemble a mass or a nodule. If the forming cavity is close to the pleura, necrosis may cause collapse of the lung with hemoptysis, chest pain, and pyopneumothorax. In the absence of these complications, coccidioidal cavities may resolve spontaneously.

Miliary or progressive coccidioidal pneumonia has rarely been reported in the pediatric population.[30–32] Respiratory failure may develop in these patients. Coccidioidal skin tests are usually negative. The course of the illness may be relatively acute or may progress over an extended period of time. Aggressive antifungal and supportive treatment is required.

LARGE AIRWAY INFECTIONS

Laryngeal and tracheal infections with airway obstruction have been described in two settings. In several reported cases, large airway involvement has occurred without evidence of associated pulmonary parenchymal disease.[33–36] The patients were between 4 months and 2½ years of age and had symptoms of airway obstruction. Diagnosis was made through biopsy of endoscopically removed tissue. Treatment consisting of removal of infected tissue, temporary tracheostomy, and intravenous amphotericin B was reported to be successful.

Airway obstruction has also been reported during the course of coccidioidal pneumonia[37, 38] or in association with disseminated disease.[39] The clinical and pathologic findings in such patients suggest that infection can be spread into the airway from adjacent lymph nodes. Interestingly, this condition has been reported in children 5 years of age or older, in contrast with primary airway infections, which have occurred in infants and toddlers.

Treatment with a combination of endoscopic removal and intravenous amphotericin B has been reported to be successful in airway lesions secondary to coccidioidal pneumonia.

NEONATAL INFECTION

Coccidioidal infection in the first weeks of life is rare but potentially devastating. Infected infants usually have fever and exhibit poor feeding, with rapid progression to respiratory failure,[40–43] although extrapulmonary dissemination without severe pneumonia has also been reported.[44, 45] Death has occurred in most cases before the diagnosis could be established. Chest radiographs typically reveal diffuse bilateral nodular infiltrates without pleural effusion or hilar adenopathy.[46] Skin tests are invariably negative, and serologic tests are rarely diagnostic. The diagnosis can be established by identification of the organism in pulmonary secretions[43] or in lung biopsy specimens.

Pregnancy may be a significant risk factor for disseminated disease.[47, 48] Women who are newly infected with *C. immitis* during pregnancy are reported to be at increased risk of passing on these infections to the infant, particularly when the infection occurs in the last trimester of pregnancy. Furthermore, when the placenta is examined, it is often found to have granulomas and viable *C. immitis.* Under these circumstances, it is not surprising that a mother may infect her infant.[43, 49] There is some debate as to whether transplacental infection can occur, but most cases suggest transpartum aspiration of infected material as the source of neonatal infection.[49, 50] Infants may also become infected through the usual route of inhalation of arthrospores in endemic areas.[40, 42, 51]

DISSEMINATED COCCIDIOIDOMYCOSIS

Dissemination or extrapulmonary infection occurs in approximately 1% of symptomatic primary infections.[17] Manifestations of dissemination may appear simultaneously with the symptoms of pulmonary infection or may follow these by many months.[52] Dissemination can be to single or multiple sites. The most common sites of extrapulmonary dissemination are bones, joints, skin, subcutaneous tissue, and meninges. Disseminated coccidioidal diseases occur at other sites infrequently, including the eyes,[45] peritoneum,[53] and the uterus.[54] Trauma during the primary infection may result in later abscess formation and recovery of the organism from the site traumatized (*locus minoris resistentiae*). In some cases, there may be no clinical or radiographic evidence of preceding primary infection.

OSTEOMYELITIS AND SYNOVITIS

The most common sites of osteomyelitis are the vertebrae, the tibia, the skull, the metatarsus, and the metacarpus (Fig. 25–4).[55, 56] More than one bone is affected in 40% of patients. Radiographic findings vary with the site of

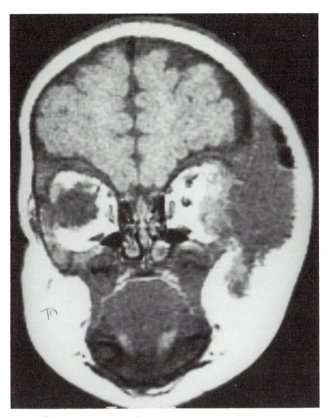

Figure 25–4. Large lesion of the temporal bone and retro-orbital space in a 6-month-old male infant.

involvement, but lytic lesions (Fig. 25–5) are typically followed by sclerosis, cortical thickening, or periosteal reaction.[57] Bone scans are more sensitive than skeletal radiographs in identifying the extent of involvement.[58] The diagnosis can be made through examination of surgical specimens. Joint infections may occur adjacent to bony lesions or through direct hematogenous spread.[22, 23] Isolated arthritis occurs most commonly in the knees or wrists.[56, 59] The organism can be identified by examination or culture of synovial membrane and, less commonly, from synovial fluid.[22, 23]

SKIN AND SUBCUTANEOUS ABSCESS

Subcutaneous abscesses are seen commonly in patients with disseminated disease. Lesions may be solitary or multiple, large or small. The most common locations are the back and the hips.[22, 23, 60] Subcutaneous abscesses also occur adjacent to foci of osteomyelitis or lymphadenitis.[52] In some patients, these abscesses may develop into chronic draining fistulae or ulcers.

Dermal infection may occur in two ways. Hematogenous dissemination may result in verrucous lesions, which appear most commonly on the face, the scalp, and the chest wall.[61] These lesions vary so much that in certain settings, it may be necessary to perform a biopsy on a chronic lesion to ensure that it is not coccidioidal. Biopsy reveals granulomatous inflammation with coccidioidal spherules. Cutaneous infection may also occur by primary inoculation of the skin.[5, 62]

MENINGITIS

The most serious manifestation of coccidioidomycosis is meningitis. Common symptoms include headache, vomiting, nuchal rigidity, and alterations in mental status. These symptoms develop over several weeks. In some children, a more insidious course may occur with symptoms such as malaise, weight loss, personality change, seizures, and disorientation.[52, 63] Because symptoms may be subtle, lumbar puncture should be performed in patients being evaluated for disseminated coccidioidomycosis.

Cerebrospinal fluid (CSF) findings include pleocytosis, elevated protein levels, and low glucose levels. White blood cell counts may range between 20 and 20,000 per cubic millimeter. Typically, there is a predominance of mononuclear cells; however, polymorphonuclear cells occasionally predominate during bursts of disease activity.[63] Eosinophils also may be seen. The diagnosis may be confirmed by serologic testing of CSF or serum. Serologic tests of CSF may be negative on initial examination. Additional examinations are necessary if cell count, protein levels, or glucose levels are abnormal.

DIAGNOSIS

Every effort must be made to recover the causative agent from the infected site. This is important because the manifestations of coccidioidal disease are the same as those of any granulomatous disease. Of course, immu-

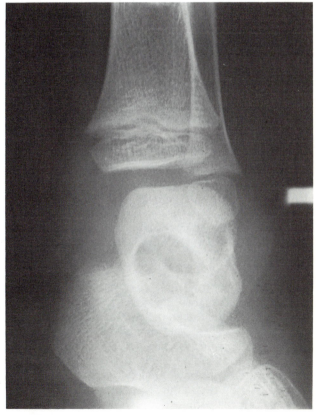

Figure 25–5. Lytic lesion of the talus and calcaneus in a 3-year-old boy.

nodiagnostic techniques are able to identify people who are producing an immune response to *C. immitis;* nevertheless, recovery of the organism is most reliable for diagnosis. Recovery of the organism is particularly important in determining the activity of the infection in severely affected patients. Techniques for collecting samples from infected tissues improved greatly during the 1980s. In pulmonary infections, sputum cultures are positive only rarely; however, bronchial lavage, brushing the airways, and transtracheal biopsies increase the yields dramatically. Skin lesions vary widely in their appearance; punch biopsies are simple, well tolerated, and definitive. The same can be said of thin-needle aspirations of lymph nodes, soft tissue, and bone.

IMMUNODIAGNOSIS

Immunodiagnosis of coccidioidomycosis is particularly useful because of the availability of specific antigens; however, there are pitfalls. Much of the data on the usefulness of immunodiagnosis was obtained before the widespread use of biopsy techniques referred to previously. Coccidioidin, an antigen developed from the mycelial phase of the fungus, is most commonly used, but spherulin (prepared from spherules) is also available now. Optimal interpretation of the skin test requires assessment of induration both 24 and 48 h after the intradermal injection of 0.1 ml of antigen. Reduced-strength (1:100) antigens should be used initially in patients with erythema nodosum or erythema multiforme because of the possibility of severe reactions. A positive skin test indicates the presence of cell-mediated immunity to coccidioidal antigen. This antigen could have been acquired any time before testing and does not necessarily mean that the illness being investigated is caused by *C. immitis.* In addition, patients with severe pulmonary or disseminated disease often have negative skin tests, and so a negative skin test cannot be used to rule out the diagnosis.

Serologic tests can be useful in diagnosis and in observing the course of the illness.[64, 65] They are best performed in experienced laboratories, and serial tests on the same patient should always be performed in the same laboratory. The tube precipitin test and the latex particle agglutination test measure an antibody that is present early in the illness. Eighty percent to 90% of symptomatic patients have positive tests in the first 4 weeks of illness.[17] After this, rates of positivity decrease rapidly. Results of the latex particle agglutination test must always be confirmed because false-negative (30%) and false-positive (10%) test results are common.

The complement fixation titer rises later in the illness. High titers (higher than 1:64) of complement-fixing antibodies are associated with more severe illness or disseminated disease. Whenever a patient's complement fixation titer is much higher than anticipated, it is prudent to review the history and physical findings and consider special tests such as lumbar puncture, gallium scan, bone scan, or computed tomographic scan. An elevated complement fixation titer alone, without an identified extrapulmonary focus of infection, is not sufficient for confirming the diagnosis of dissemination, and a low titer does not rule out dissemination or severe infection. Many patients with miliary disease manifest low complement fixation titers.

Immunodiffusion tests are sometimes used to measure the same antibody detected by the complement fixation test. If performed with appropriate controls, it may be as reliable as the complement fixation test performed in an experienced laboratory.

EVALUATION FOR THERAPY

After the diagnosis is established, it must be determined whether the disease is severe enough to warrant the risks associated with treatment. The considerations are clinical status, immune status, extent of disease, and site or sites of infection.

CLINICAL STATUS

Fever, anorexia, and weight loss or failure to grow all indicate that infection is active and progressive. At this stage, pulmonary lesions may cavitate, cavitary lesions may rupture, or dissemination may occur.

IMMUNE STATUS

The patient's immune response is of fundamental importance. Skin test and antibody responses obviously aid in establishing the diagnosis. In addition, however, it is known that cell-mediated immunity is necessary for controlling a coccidioidal infection, and high complement fixation titers are associated with T cell dysfunction. If the history reveals a concomitant illness associated with immune compromise or if immunosuppressive drugs are being administered, the prognosis is worse. In the assessment of delayed-type hypersensitivity, it is sometimes helpful to apply both coccidioidin and spherulin at low concentrations. If they are negative in the face of an established diagnosis, the test should be performed with higher concentrations. It is also informative to examine the response to other antigens such as *Candida* and diphtheria and tetanus toxoids that can be expected to yield a positive response in normal populations. After this procedure, the presence and extent of immunosuppression can be estimated. Although the antibody response is of obvious importance, these tests must not be overinterpreted. Serial complement fixation titers can be useful in observing the course of the illness. Titers fall as the patient improves.

EXTENT OF DISEASE

The extent of disease must be carefully assessed in the evaluation for treatment. There are two reasons: first, if extrapulmonary coccidioidal disease can be demonstrated, treatment is mandatory; second, new lesions that become clinically apparent after treatment has been started constitute prima facie evidence of drug failure unless it can be demonstrated that the lesion was present, although clinically occult, when treatment was started. Of course, any tissue can be infected by *C. immitis,* but the structures most commonly infected are the lymph nodes, skin, meninges, bone, and soft tissue. A careful physical examination identifies skin lesions and nearly all the lymph nodes. Coccidioidal meningitis can be totally asymptomatic, and so examination of CSF is necessary. Bone lesions may also be surprisingly asymptomatic, and so a bone scan is very helpful. Gallium scans occasionally reveal deep infections; the use of these tests can be restricted to only patients who manifest extremely high complement fixation titers. Positive cultures of the pulmonary secretions, urine, occasionally bone marrow, and any identified lesion provide definitive proof of the infection of that tissue.

TREATMENT

Treatment options include surgical excision and administration of amphotericin B, ketoconazole, itraconazole, and fluconazole. The role for surgery in the treatment of any infection is obviously limited to an adjunctive one. Specifically, surgery may be indicated for helping obtain the proper specimen for histologic examination and culture. Occasionally, the infection has caused so much tissue destruction or the reaction to the infection includes so much scar formation that removal of the distorted tissue results in an improved outcome, especially in osteomyelitis. As with other infections, chemotherapy is the mainstay of treatment.

Amphotericin B was introduced in 1950 and, despite the many problems associated with its use, remains the most effective, reliable treatment for nearly all manifestations of coccidioidomycosis.[22, 23] The drug is administered intravenously in doses of 1 mg/kg.[66] Frequently, lower doses are used during the first few days of treatment. Rapid infusion over 45 min is a safe alternative to traditional 4- to 6-h infusions and makes outpatient treatment possible. Symptoms such as fever, chills, generalized pain, and rashes may occur during the infusion. Renal toxicity, hypokalemia, and anemia occur in most patients undergoing amphotericin B treatment. Amphotericin B may also be administered intrathecally or intraventricularly in the treatment of meningitis.

Ketoconazole was the first orally absorbed antifungal agent to demonstrate efficacy in coccidioidal infections. Its use is limited by the relatively slow onset of antifungal effect and the high incidence of infection recurrence. Doses of 10 to 20 mg/kg/day have been used successfully in children. Adverse effects include gastrointestinal intolerance, hepatotoxicity, reduced serum testosterone levels, and a blunted adrenal response.[67] The triazoles fluconazole and itraconazole have become available as orally administered alternatives to amphotericin B and ketoconazole. Clinical studies in adults have revealed fluconazole to be an effective agent in coccidioidomycosis with much less toxicity than the older agents. A response rate of 58% to 90% was reported in adults with chronic pulmonary, soft tissue, or bone and joint disease treated for a mean of 18 months.[68] Experience with fluconazole in childhood coccidioidomycosis is limited at this time. Doses of 3 to 6 mg/kg/day have been suggested. Long courses of therapy are generally required. Itraconazole

has also been reported to be effective in adult patients, but drug intolerance and treatment failures have occurred more frequently than with fluconazole.[69] Again, experience with pediatric patients is lacking.

PRIMARY INFECTION

Early in the infection, the patient is usually not sick enough to warrant treatment with amphotericin B, and many patients recover with no treatment at all. Azoles have not been formally evaluated in primary infections. Many clinicians hoped that early treatment with an azole might forestall dissemination. Because no studies have been performed, the question is moot; however, patients have been observed to acquire disseminated disease while receiving ketoconazole treatment for pulmonary disease.

PROGRESSIVE PRIMARY PNEUMONIA

In patients with progressive primary pneumonia, necrotizing pneumonia may lead to empyema, or patients may acquire miliary disease, acute respiratory distress, meningitis, or widespread multifocal dissemination. These patients must be treated with amphotericin B.

MILIARY DISEASE

Miliary disease is the pulmonary manifestation of hematogenous disseminated disease. This manifestation is serious, and patients may deteriorate rapidly. Many of these patients have meningitis that is not readily apparent. Patients with miliary disease must be treated with amphotericin B.

PERSISTENT PULMONARY INFILTRATE

Patients with this condition typically have recovered from the pulmonary primary infection, but the infiltrate persists, often with a complement fixation titer in the range of 1:16 to 1:128. These patients can usually be managed with an azole treatment for 12 months. Serial clinical and serologic monitoring is needed on a monthly or bimonthly basis.

NEONATAL INFECTIONS

Because of the poor prognosis associated with neonatal infections, treatment with amphotericin B should be initiated as soon as the diagnosis is established.

RESIDUAL PULMONARY LESIONS

Solitary Pulmonary Nodule

The challenge in cases of solitary pulmonary nodules is to be certain of the diagnosis. If *C. immitis* or granuloma has been recovered from a nodule, no antifungal treatment is needed. Nodules may wax and wane in size. They may even empty their contents and become cavities. For these reasons, *C. immitis* may, on occasion, be recovered from airway secretions. If there are no symptoms, no treatment is needed.

Pulmonary Cavities

Pulmonary cavities may persist unchanged for many years. A few patients manifest cough, sputum production, small amounts of hemoptysis, and, in rare instances, systemic symptoms such as malaise, weakness, and fever. These symptoms are generally responsive to ketoconazole. Unfortunately, they are also likely to recur after the completion of therapy. In addition, pulmonary cavities may undergo development of complications such as superimposed infections, fungus balls, or hemoptysis, which at times can be significant in amount. These complications are usually treated with antibiotics such as ampicillin or trimethoprim-sulfamethoxazole. Patients who do not respond to that program usually respond to treatment with an azole. Fluconazole is particularly good in this situation because of improved tissue penetration in comparison with amphotericin B. Surgery may be used in patients refractory to medical treatment, but cavities may recur in some patients after surgery.

Pleural Effusion

Pleural effusion by itself does not change the outcome. If the effusion is symptomatic or persistent, an azole may be indicated.

Dissemination

Patients who have multifocal disease, have severe infection, or have rapidly developing disease must be treated with an antifungal agent.

Skin Lesions

If the patient has one or two skin lesions and no visceral disease, the likelihood of a satisfactory response to an azole is very high.

Osteomyelitis and Synovitis

Osteomyelitis and synovitis respond slowly and incompletely to any agent. Furthermore, recurrence after treatment with any agent is not unusual. Sometimes adjunctive surgery, with debridement and local administrations of amphotericin B, can be very useful. Some patients, particularly those with osteomyelitis, may receive amphotericin B initially followed by a long course (at least 12 months) of an azole.

Abscess

Abscess may involve lymph nodes, soft tissue, or any visceral organ. In general, if there is liquefaction, surgical drainage is useful. Local instillation of amphotericin B may be of value as an adjunct to systemic amphotericin B or to follow up an azole.

Meningitis

Meningitis is the most dreaded form of this infection. Untreated, this disease is 100% lethal. The blood-brain barrier prevents therapeutic amounts of amphotericin B. Treatment with systemic and intrathecal amphotericin B has been shown to be effective in this condition,[70-72] but this treatment is difficult to administer, and amphotericin B toxicity may occur. Promising results have been reported with fluconazole.[73]

REFERENCES

1. Fiese MJ: Coccidioidomycosis, pp. 23–52. Springfield, IL: Charles C Thomas, 1958.
2. Huppert M, Sun SH: Overview of mycology, and the mycology of *Coccidioidal immitis. In* Stevens DA (ed): Coccidioidomycosis, pp. 21–44. New York: Plenum Press, 1980.
3. Flynn NM, Hoeprich PD, Kawachi MM, et al: An unusual outbreak of windborne coccidioidomycosis. N Engl J Med 301:358–361, 1979.
4. Rothman PE, Graw RG, Harris JC, et al: Coccidioidomycosis—Possible fomite transmission. Am J Dis Child 118:792–801, 1969.
5. O'Brien JJ, Gilsdorf JR: Primary cutaneuous coccidioidomycosis in childhood. Pediatr Infect Dis J 5:485–486, 1986.
6. Werner SB, Pappagianis D: Coccidioidomycosis in northern California—An outbreak among archeology students near Red Bluff. Calif Med 119:10–20, 1973.
7. Winn WA, Levine HB, Broderick JE, et al: A localized epidemic of coccidioidal infection. N Engl J Med 268:867–870, 1963.
8. Ramras DG, Walch HA, Murray JP, et al: An epidemic of coccidioidomycosis in the Pacific Beach area of San Diego. Am Rev Respir Dis 101:975–978, 1970.
9. Pappagianis D: Epidemiology of coccidioidomycosis. Curr Top Med Mycol 2:199–238, 1988.
10. Smith CE, Beard RR, Whiting EG, et al: Varieties of coccidioidal infection in relation to the epidemiology and control of the diseases. Am J Public Health 36:1394–1402, 1946.
11. Johnson WM: Racial factors in coccidioidomycosis: Mortality experience in Arizona. Arizona Med 39:18–24, 1982.
12. Catanzaro A: Pulmonary mycosis in pregnant women. Chest 86:14S–18S, 1984.
13. MacDonald N, Steinhoff MC, Powell KR: Review of coccidioidomycosis in immunocompromised children. Am J Dis Child 135:553–556, 1981.
14. Bronnimann DA, Adam RD, Galgiani JN, et al: Coccidioidomycosis in the acquired immunodeficiency syndrome. Ann Intern Med 106:372–379, 1987.
15. Murphey SM, Drash AL, Donnelly WM: Disseminated coccidioidomycosis associated with immunosuppressive therapy following renal transplantation. Pediatrics 48:144–145, 1971.
16. Teel KW, Yow MD, Williams TW: A localized outbreak of coccidioidomycosis in southern Texas. J Pediatr 77:65–73, 1970.
17. Smith CE: Epidemiology of acute coccidioidomycosis with erythema nodosum. Am J Public Health 30:601–611, 1940.
18. Richardson HB, Anderson JA, McKay BM: Acute pulmonary coccidioidomycosis in children. J Pediatr 70:376–382, 1967.
19. Werner SB, Pappagianis D, Heindl I, et al: An epidemic of coccidioidomycosis among archeology students in northern California. N Engl J Med 286:507–512, 1972.
20. Yozwiak ML, Lundergan LL, Kerrick SS, et al: Symptoms and routine laboratory abnormalities associated with coccidioidomycosis. West J Med 149:419–421, 1988.
21. Tom PF, Long TJ, Fitzpatrick SB: Coccidioidomycosis in adolescents presenting as chest pain. J Adolesc Health Care 8:365–371, 1987.
22. Drutz DJ, Catanzaro A: Coccidioidomycosis: Part I. Am Rev Respir Dis 117:559–585, 1978.
23. Drutz DJ, Catanzaro A: Coccidioidomycosis: Part II. Am Rev Respir Dis 117:727–771, 1978.
24. Faber HK, Smith CE, Dickson EC: Acute coccidioidomycosis with erythema nodosum in children. J Pediatr 15:163–171, 1939.

25. Lonky SA, Catanzaro A, Moser KM, et al: Acute coccidioidal pleural effusion. Am Rev Respir Dis 114:681–688, 1976.
26. Salkin D, Birsner TW, Tarr AD, et al: Roentgen analysis of coccidioidomycosis pediatric cases in private practice. *In* Ajello L (ed): Coccidioidomycosis, pp. 63–67. Tucson: University of Arizona Press, 1967.
27. Lundergan LJ, Kernick SS, Galginni JN: Coccidioidomycosis at a university outpatient clinic: A clinical description. *In* Einstein HE, Catanzaro A (eds): *Coccidioidomycosis,* pp. 47–54. Washington, DC: National Foundation for Infectious Disease, 1985.
28. Pinckney L, Parker BR: Primary coccidioidomycosis in children presenting with massive pleural effusion. AJR 130:247–249, 1978.
29. McGahan JP, Graves DS, Palmer PE, et al: Classic and contemporary imaging of coccidioidomycosis. AJR 136:393–404, 1981.
30. Cohen R, Burnip R: Miliary coccidioidomycosis of the lungs—Report of a case in a child. Ann West Med Surg 3:413–414, 1949.
31. Gururaj VJ, Marsh WW, Aiyar SR: Fulminant pulmonary coccidioidomycosis in association with Coxsackie B$_4$ infection. Clin Pediatr 24:406–408, 1985.
32. Larsen RA, Jacobson JA, Morris AH, et al: Acute respiratory failure caused by primary pulmonary coccidioidomycosis—Two case reports and a review of the literature. Am Rev Respir Dis 131:797–799, 1985.
33. Winter B, Villaveces J, Spector M: Coccidioidomycosis accompanied by acute tracheal obstruction in a child. JAMA 195:1001–1004, 1966.
34. Ward PH, Berci G, Morledge D, et al: Coccidioidomycosis of the larynx in infants and adults. Otol Rhinol Laryngol 86:655–660, 1977.
35. Gardner S, Seilheimer D, Catlin F, et al: Subglottic coccidioidomycosis presenting with persistent stridor. Pediatrics 66:623–625, 1980.
36. Hajare S, Rakusan TA, Kalia A, et al: Laryngeal coccidioidomycosis causing airway obstruction. Pediatr Infect Dis J 8:54–56, 1989.
37. Moskowitz PS, Sue JY, Gooding CA: Tracheal coccidioidomycosis causing upper airway obstruction in children. AJR 139:596–600, 1982.
38. Benitz WE, Bradley JS, Fee WE Jr, et al: Upper airway obstruction due to laryngeal coccidioidomycosis in a 5-year-old child. Am J Otolaryngol 4:367–370, 1983.
39. Henley-Cohn J, Boles R, Weisberger E, et al: Upper airway obstruction due to coccidioidomycosis. Laryngoscope 89:355–360, 1979.
40. Christian JR, Sarre SG, Peers JH, et al: Pulmonary coccidioidomycosis in a twenty-one-day-old infant. Am J Dis Child 92:66–74, 1956.
41. Hyatt HW: Coccidioidomycosis in a 3-week-old infant. Am J Dis Child 105:93–98, 1963.
42. Westley CR, Haak W: Neonatal coccidioidomycosis in a southwestern Pima Indian. South Med J 67:855–857, 1974.
43. Bernstein DI, Tipton JR, Schott SF, et al: Coccidioidomycosis in a neonate: Maternal-infant transmission. J Pediatr 99:752–754, 1981.
44. Ziering WH, Rockas HR: Coccidioidomycosis—Long-term treatment with amphotericin B of disseminated disease in a three-month-old baby. Am J Dis Child 108:454–459, 1964.
45. Golden SE, Morgan CN, Bartley DL, et al: Disseminated coccidioidomycosis with chorioretinitis in early infancy. Pediatr Infect Dis J 8:45–56, 1989.
46. Child DD, Newell JD, Bjelland JC, et al: Radiographic findings of pulmonary coccidioidomycosis in neonates and infants. AJR 145:261–263, 1985.
47. Smale LE, Waechter KG: Dissemination of coccidioidomycosis in pregnancy. Am J Obstet Gynecol 107:356–361, 1970.
48. Wack EE, Ampel NM, Galgiani JN, et al: Coccidioidomycosis during pregnancy. Chest 94:376–379, 1988.
49. Spark R: Does transplacental spread of coccidioidomycosis occur? Arch Pathol Lab Med 105:347–350, 1981.
50. Cohen R: Placental coccidioides. Arch Pediatr 68:59–66, 1951.
51. Townsend TE, McKey RW: Coccidioidomycosis in infants. Am J Dis Child 86:51–53, 1953.
52. Kafka JA, Catanzaro A: Disseminated coccidioidomycosis in children. J Pediatr 98:355–361, 1981.
53. Chen KT: Coccidioidal peritonitis. Am J Clin Pathol 80:514–516, 1983.
54. Saw EC, Smale LE, Einstein H, et al: Female genital coccidioidomycosis. Obstet Gynecol 45:199–202, 1975.
55. Iger M, Larson J: Coccidioidal osteomyelitis. *In* Ajello L (ed): Coccidioidomycosis, pp. 89–92. Tucson: University of Arizona Press, 1967.
56. Iger M, Coppola AJ: Review of 135 cases of bone and joint coccidioidomycosis. *In* Einstein HE, Catanzaro A (eds): Coccidioidomycosis, pp. 379–389. Washington, DC: National Foundation for Infectious Diseases, 1985.
57. Deresinski S: Coccidioidomycosis of bones and joints. *In* Stevens DA (ed): Coccidioidomycosis, pp. 195–212. New York: Plenum Press, 1980.
58. Boddicker JH, Fong D, Walsh TE, et al: Bone and gallium scanning in the evaluation of disseminated coccidioidomycosis. Am Rev Respir Dis 122:279–287, 1980.
59. Bried JM, Galgiani JN: *Coccidioides immitis* infections in bones and joints. Clin Orthop 211:235–243, 1986.
60. Feigin RD, Shackelford PG, Lins RD, et al: Subcutaneous abscess due to *Coccidioides immitis*. Am J Dis Child 124:734–735, 1972.
61. Forbus WD, Bestebreurtje AM: Coccidioidomycosis: A study of 95 cases of the disseminated type with special reference to the pathogenesis of the disease. Milit Surgeons 654–713, 1946.
62. Winn WA: Primary cutaneous coccidioidomycosis. Arch Dermatol 92:221–228, 1965.
63. Caudill RG, Smith CE, Reinarz JA: Coccidioidal meningitis: A diagnostic challenge. Am J Med 49:360–365, 1970.
64. Smith CE, Saito MT, Simans SA: Pattern of 39,500 serologic tests in coccidioidomycosis. JAMA 160:546–552, 1956.
65. Pappagianis D: Serology and serodiagnosis of coccidioidomycosis. *In* Stevens DA (ed): Coccidioidomycosis, pp. 97–112. New York: Plenum Press, 1980.
66. Koren G, Lan A, Klein J, et al: Pharmacokinetics and adverse effects of amphotericin B in infants and children. J Pediatr 113:559–563, 1988.
67. Britton H, Shehab Z, Lightner E, et al: Adrenal response in children receiving high doses of ketoconazole for systemic coccidioidomycosis. J Pediatr 112:488–492, 1988.
68. Catanzaro A, Galgiani JN, Levine B, et al: Fluconazole in the treatment of chronic pulmonary or disseminated coccidioidomycosis. In preparation.
69. Graybill JR, Stevens DA, Galgiani JN, et al: Itraconazole treatment of coccidioidomycosis. Am J Med 89:282–290, 1990.
70. LeClerc M, Giammona ST: Coccidioidal meningitis: The use of amphotericin B intravenously and intrathecally by repeated lumbar punctures. West J Med 122:251–254, 1975.
71. Graybill JR: Current recommendations for treatment of coccidioidal meningitis. *In* Einstein HE, Catanzaro A (eds): Coccidioidomycosis, pp. 466–473. Washington, DC: National Foundation for Infectious Diseases, 1985.
72. Johnson RH, Brown JF, Haleman CM, et al: Coccidioidal meningitis: A 25 year experience with 194 patients. *In* Einstein HE, Catanzaro A (eds): Coccidioidomycosis, pp. 411–421. Washington, DC: National Foundation for Infectious Diseases, 1985.
73. Harrison HR, Galgiani JN, Reynolds AF, et al: Amphotericin B and imidazole therapy for coccidioidal meningitis in children. Pediatr Infect Dis 2:216–221, 1983.

26 CROUP AND EPIGLOTTITIS

STEPHEN D. LEVINE, M.D. / MARGARET ANN SPRINGER, M.D.

Croup and epiglottitis are two common pediatric manifestations of acute upper airway obstruction caused by infection. Anatomically contiguous, they share some common signs and symptoms; however, their causes, diagnostic workups, and management are quite different. Awareness of their similarities and differences facilitates prompt diagnosis and treatment, as well as the avoidance of severe and occasionally catastrophic consequences.

Both croup and epiglottitis are caused by infection in the upper airway, which leads to edema. The edema spreads throughout the supraglottis (or epiglottis), glottis, and subglottis because the mucosa is contiguous over all structures of oropharynx, nasopharynx, and trachea. The edema causes narrowing of the airway, which results in stridor, a common presenting sign in diseases causing upper airway obstruction. Epiglottitis usually connotes the area above the glottis, and croup, the subglottic area.

CROUP

Croup syndrome is a sometimes confusing collective term given to a range of symptoms that vary from minimal inspiratory stridor and occasional barking cough to dyspnea, hypoxia, and respiratory arrest.[1] In previous investigations, inconsistent nomenclature has caused problems with study design, data analysis, and interpretation. To avoid misunderstanding, the term *croup* in this chapter refers to an acute viral infection of the subglottic airway characterized by inspiratory stridor, barking cough, and low-grade fever. Allergic or spasmodic croup is a separate entity beyond the scope of this chapter.

Viral croup is the most common form of airway obstruction in children aged 6 months to 6 years and is responsible for 20,000 hospital admissions yearly in the United States; 1% to 5% of these children require intubation.[2] It is seasonal; most cases occur in the fall and winter.[3] The cause is overwhelmingly viral, usually parainfluenza I, II, or III. Other viruses, including respiratory syncytial virus, adenovirus, and influenza A and B, are implicated less often.[4]

Typically, the clinical manifestation of viral croup includes a prodrome of coryza, low-grade fever (less than 40°C), and general malaise. After 3 to 4 days, the characteristic barking cough begins, accompanied by inspiratory stridor. It is frequently the stridor that causes parents of patients to seek medical attention. Physical examination usually reveals some degree of respiratory distress, manifested by dyspnea, nasal flaring, and intercostal and suprasternal retractions. In extreme cases, there may also be air hunger, altered mental status, and cyanosis, all signs of impending respiratory arrest. Lungs are usually clear.

Laboratory data are usually not helpful in the diagnosis of viral croup: The white cell count may be normal or elevated.[2] Pulse oximetry is a noninvasive way to document oxygenation status. Radiographic diagnosis of viral croup is made on the basis of the steeple sign, seen on posteroanterior projections of the chest and neck as a narrowing of the trachea to a sharp point.[3]

The treatment of viral croup is as controversial as its definition. Many mild cases can be managed on an outpatient basis as long as the child is not dyspneic, hypoxic, or inadequately hydrated. Treatment consists of adequate oral hydration, antipyretics, and humidity. Although most evidence in support of humidification is anecdotal, some studies show that moist air softens secretions and makes the child more comfortable.[2, 3] Parents of these children should be thoroughly instructed in the signs and symptoms of worsening respiratory distress before taking their children home, and they should be aware of the waxing and waning nature of croup. All children observed on an outpatient basis should be reevaluated frequently.

Children who are hypoxic, dyspneic, or unable to hydrate themselves adequately should be admitted for observation and supportive care. Inpatient treatment may include humidity, oxygen supplementation, antipyretics, and intravenous fluids as needed. Antibiotics are usually not indicated. Some clinicians advocate the use of mist tents; others believe that cool-mist humidifiers are sufficient.[2] Supplemental oxygen, if required, should always be humidified. It may be administered by hood, mask, or nasal cannula, depending on the age of the child. Pulse oximetry is a convenient noninvasive means of monitoring for hypoxia. Children admitted with croup need close observation for signs of increasing ventilatory fatigue and impending respiratory arrest. Although most children do not require an artificial airway, it is an occasional necessity. In one study of 48 Australian children hospitalized for croup in 1981 and 1982, 81 required intensive care and 37 required intubation.[5] Tracheostomy, once the treatment of choice for respiratory failure in viral croup, is currently performed less often, probably

238

because of the increasing availability of mechanical ventilatory support and trained intensive care staff.[2, 6, 7]

Racemic epinephrine has been used in the treatment of croup since the early 1970s, although only since the late 1980s have controlled, double-blind studies documented its efficacy. Administered via nebulizer, the drug probably decreases airway edema by adrenergic stimulation and subsequent mucosal vasoconstriction.[2] Studies offer convincing evidence that racemic epinephrine decreases airway obstruction within 10 to 30 min of administration, waning over approximately 2 h. There is evidence of tachyphylaxis with "rebound" effects in some cases.[2] Most clinicians agree that administration of racemic epinephrine mandates hospital admission for this reason.

Adrenal corticosteroid therapy is another area of controversy in the management of viral croup. Used by many clinicians since the 1960s, corticosteroids supposedly decrease the local inflammatory reaction and reduce airway edema. Until the late 1980s, critics pointed out the lack of controlled, double-blind trials of steroid therapy in viral croup; however, as Skolnik[2] stated in his 1989 review, four of six prospectively randomized trials involving adequate doses of corticosteroids showed decreased length of severity of symptoms in comparison with placebo. Three studies showed decreased length of hospital stay.[2]

The prognosis of viral croup is good. Most patients recover without sequelae.

EPIGLOTTITIS

Epiglottitis (supraglottitis), in contrast to most cases of croup, is a true pediatric emergency. To parents and pediatricians, it is one of the most frightening experiences encountered in caring for children. Although epiglottitis is part of the spectrum of acute, infectious upper airway obstruction and although it must be considered in the diagnosis of stridor, its cause, manifestation, and management are all in stark contrast to those of laryngotracheobronchitis.

Epiglottitis is an infection of the epiglottis and supraglottic airway, usually caused by *Haemophilus influenzae* type B. *Streptococcus* and *Staphylococcus* species have also been implicated. The infection causes acute edema and inflammation, which lead to airway obstruction. The incidence is difficult to estimate. Studies have documented ranges from 11 to 70 per 100,000 each year in the most susceptible age group: children younger than 4 years.[8] Once considered only a pediatric disease, epiglottitis is now being reported as a disease of adults and of immunocompromised patients.[9]

The clinical manifestation of epiglottitis is remarkable for rapid onset of symptoms. The swollen epiglottis can cause complete airway obstruction, asphyxia, and death in a very short time from onset. It is not unusual for a child with epiglottitis to go to bed healthy and then awaken with a full-blown toxic illness. The temperature is high, usually more than 40°C. Many patients are flushed, often drooling, with the head thrust forward and the tongue protruding. "Tripod" posturing, in which the child leans forward on the hands and legs, forming a tripod, is common. When these patients arrive at the physician's office or at the emergency department, they appear acutely ill.

Management of acute epiglottitis requires prompt recognition, planning, preparation, and communication among personnel in emergency, pediatric, and otorhinolaryngology departments. A child with the clinical manifestation of acute epiglottitis should never be examined in the emergency room because increasing the child's distress might precipitate increased airway obstruction and sudden respiratory arrest. The child should be escorted calmly, preferably in a parent's arms, to a designated area (operating room or intensive care unit), accompanied by a pediatrician, an anesthesiologist, and an otorhinolaryngologist, with appropriate equipment and drugs at hand for emergency intubation or tracheostomy. Examination and visualization of the airway should be attempted only at the time of intubation, usually with sedation or general anesthesia. Under these conditions, the larynx can be visualized safely, an airway inserted, and the appropriate cultures obtained. Direct visualization usually reveals a grossly enlarged, cherry-red epiglottis.

Laboratory evaluation in epiglottitis is secondary to clinical evaluation. The white blood cell count is elevated, with a left shift, in most cases. In *H. influenzae* epiglottitis, the blood culture is positive in 50% to 70% of cases. Lateral neck radiographs (obtained in the operating room or intensive care unit with a physician present) show the characteristic "thumb sign" (the shape of the inflamed epiglottis on lateral neck radiographs).[10]

Management of epiglottitis requires, first, the stabilization of the airway. Most clinicians agree that this mandates the insertion of an artificial airway, although some advocate close observation and medical management. Although tracheostomy was the procedure of choice for decades, it has been superseded by nasotracheal intubation at many institutions. According to one report from The Children's Hospital in Boston, nasotracheal intubation with the patient under general anesthesia in the operating room and followed by supportive care in an intensive care setting is the optimal management for safe treatment of epiglottitis.[11] However, it was pointed out in that study that nasotracheal intubation in pediatric patients is difficult, particularly with acute obstruction, and personnel skilled in this procedure may not be available at smaller outlying hospitals. In these situations, and in hospitals without pediatric intensive care units, tracheostomy or transfer to another institution may be safer.[11]

All children with artificial airways should be observed closely in an intensive care unit. Besides maintaining a patent airway, supportive management may include mechanical ventilatory support, intravenous fluids, and sedation. The appropriate antibiotics should be instituted as soon as the airway is secured. Coverage for *H. influenzae* has historically included ampicillin and chloramphenicol. Today, a third-generation cephalosporin is also considered appropriate.[1, 11] Corticosteroid use is controversial, and there is disagreement concerning its efficacy.[11] Racemic epinephrine is of no benefit.[11]

After 2 to 3 days, most children are ready for extubation. Resolution of the edema can be detected by perception of an audible leak. At some centers, flexible fiberoptic bronchoscopy is used as a means of direct airway visualization at the time of extubation to document resolution of swelling.[11] After another 1 to 2 days of close observation, the child can be transferred to a ward service. Close observation for signs of recurrent airway obstruction is mandatory. At The Children's Hospital in Boston, a total of 7 days of intravenous antibiotics is completed and followed by 2 weeks of oral antibiotic therapy.[11] The child is discharged as soon as the clinical condition is stable and adequate outpatient follow-up is ensured.

REFERENCES

1. McLain LG: Croup syndrome. Am Fam Physician 36:207–214, 1987.
2. Skolnik NS: Treatment of croup: A critical review. Am J Dis Child 143:1045–1049, 1989.
3. Davis HW, Gartner JC, Galvis AG, et al: Acute upper airway obstruction: Croup and epiglottitis. Pediatr Clin North Am 28:859–880, 1981.
4. Couriel JM: Management of croup. Arch Dis Child 63:1305–1308, 1988.
5. Wagener JS, Landau LI, Olinsky A, et al: Management of children hospitalized for laryngotracheo-bronchitis. Pediatr Pulmonol 2:159–162, 1986.
6. Barku GA: Current management of croup and epiglottitis. Pediatr Clin North Am 26:565–579, 1979.
7. Fried MP: Controversies in the management of supraglottitis and croup. Pediatr Clin North Am 26:931–942, 1979.
8. Trollfars B, Nylen O, Strangert K, et al: Acute epiglottitis in children and adults in Sweden 1981–1983. Arch Dis Child 65:491–494, 1990.
9. Walsh TJ, Gray WC: Candida epiglottitis in the compromised host. Chest 91:482–485, 1987.
10. Hodge KM, Ganzel TM: Diagnostic and therapeutic efficiency in croup and epiglottitis. Laryngoscope 97:621–625, 1987.
11. Crockett DM, Mcgill TJ, Healy GB, et al: Airway management of acute supraglottitis at The Children's Hospital, Boston: 1980–1985. Ann Otol Rhinol Laryngol 97:114–119, 1988.

27 HISTOPLASMOSIS

JAMSHED KANGA, M.D. / H. DAVID WILSON, M.D.

Histoplasmosis was first described in 1906 by Darling.[1] He believed that the infection was caused by an encapsulated plasmodium that infected the reticuloendothelial system, hence the name *Histoplasma capsulatum*. In 1934, DeMonbreun[2] discovered that histoplasmosis was caused by a dimorphic fungus that exists in mycelial form at room temperature (22°C) and in yeast form at body temperature (37°C). In the United States, histoplasmosis is the most common systemic fungal infection. Although most infections are clinically insignificant, severe disease can occur in the immunocompromised host. Consequently, *H. capsulatum* infections are being seen with increasing frequency, especially in endemic areas.

Histoplasmosis has been reported worldwide. However, high rates of infection occur in certain endemic areas. Epidemiologic studies involving the use of histoplasmin skin reactivity in navy recruits have shown a high endemic rate of *H. capsulatum* infection in the central United States and, to a lesser extent, in surrounding states.[3] *H. capsulatum* grows on soil surfaces and especially well in areas where the soil contains bird and bat excreta.[4–6] Other factors known to enhance growth of the fungus are temperate climate (between 20°C and 30°C), high humidity, aerobic conditions, and acidic soil. These factors are present in abundance in the Ohio and Mississippi river valleys.

Small epidemics of histoplasmosis usually occur on the periphery of endemic areas (where there are more susceptible subjects) and are usually the result of dissemination from a highly contaminated source. Outbreaks of histoplasmosis have been reported after cleaning of chicken coops,[7,8] handling of bird nests, sawing of trees,[9] and working in bat-infested areas such as chimneys, bridges, and caves.[10, 11] Demolition and digging in areas close to blackbird roosts have resulted in outbreaks. *H. capsulatum* spores have been identified in roosts 10 years after birds have abandoned them.[12] Because the spores can be disseminated by the wind over great distances from construction sites, a history of exposure may not be elicited in many cases.

Persons living in areas endemic for histoplasmosis almost invariably are infected by *H. capsulatum*. In epidemiologic surveys with the histoplasmin skin tests, it has been estimated that approximately 30 to 40 million persons in the United States have been infected, at a rate of 0.5 million people per year.[13] Unlike tuberculosis, in which primary infection results in life-long tuberculin positivity, longitudinal studies of people living in endemic areas have shown a waxing and waning of histoplasmin skin test reactions, which is suggestive of reinfection.[14] Reinfection rather than reactivation of endogenous infection is more common in histoplasmosis.

PATHOPHYSIOLOGY

H. capsulatum exists in two forms. In soil and on culture medium, the organism is mycelial, with typical tuberculated chlamydospores (Fig. 27–1). Infections

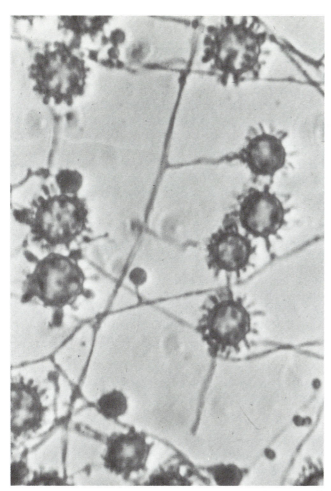

Figure 27–1. Mycelia of *Histoplasma capsulatum* in laboratory culture with the characteristic tuberculated spores.

usually occur as a result of inhalation of the spores. In the alveoli, the organisms convert to the yeast form, which is ingested by phagocytes. The organism multiplies in the macrophages. A primary focus of bronchopneumonia develops, varying in size from 1 mm to 2 cm.[15] Lesions may be single or multiple. The organisms are subsequently carried by the macrophages from the primary pulmonary focus to the regional lymph nodes. T cell immunity develops between 1 to 3 weeks after infection and enhances the activity of the macrophages, which results in control of the infection. The primary lesion involving the lung parenchyma and hilar nodes (similar to the Gohn complex in tuberculosis) becomes inactive and calcifies in most cases.[16, 17]

H. capsulatum occasionally disseminates outside the respiratory tract. Most often this dissemination is in the form of a self-limiting spread to the liver and spleen with development of tubercles, which become inactive and calcify.[18] Abnormalities of T cell function impair control of *H. capsulatum* infection, which results in other manifestations of the disease. Instead of the usual course of primary infection, inactivation, and calcification, the primary lesion may spread in the lung parenchyma, resulting in necrosis and cavitation. Hematogenous spread to the reticuloendothelial system and other organs may occur, especially in infants and in immuno-

compromised persons.[19, 20] Involvement of the bone marrow may result in anemia, leukopenia, or thrombocytopenia. Hematogenous dissemination to the lungs produces a miliary infection in the lungs and a "snowstorm" appearance on chest radiographs. Ulcerating lesions in the bowel, the skin, and the corneas may develop. *H. capsulatum* myocarditis, endocarditis, and meningitis have been reported.[21] Involvement of the adrenal glands, which produces caseous necrosis with adrenal failure, also occurs.

CLINICAL MANIFESTATIONS

The clinical spectrum of *H. capsulatum* infection is listed in Table 27–1. More than 50% of infections are asymptomatic and clinically insignificant (Fig. 27–2). Documentation of infection in these cases is either by conversion to a positive histoplasmin skin test or positive serologic tests. The primary lesion usually heals with calcifications in the lungs and hilar lymph nodes. In two studies of school-age children with positive histoplasmin skin tests, only 25% had chest radiographs suggestive of histoplasmosis infection.[22, 23] Adults living in endemic areas have a much higher incidence of pulmonary calcifications that, in the majority of cases, have been proved at autopsy to be attributable to histoplasmosis.[16, 17]

The incubation period for the development of symptoms after exposure to *H. capsulatum* appears to be dependent on the immune status of the patient. A short incubation period of 3 to 9 days is seen in persons who have immunity (live in endemic areas) and are exposed to a moderate-sized inoculum.[24, 25] In nonimmune adults and in children, the incubation period extends from 8 to 24 days, and the majority of such patients seek medical treatment between 12 and 16 days after exposure.[15]

The clinical spectrum of acute histoplasmosis varies from an extremely mild to an extremely severe infection (Table 27–1). The severity of the infection is dependent on the age and immune status of the individual and the magnitude of the exposure. In mild febrile illness, the usual duration of symptoms is 1 to 5 days[15] (Figs. 27–3*A*, 27–3*B*).

In moderate illness, the fever ranges from 38.3°C to 39.4°C and usually lasts 5 to 15 days. In addition, the

Table 27–1. CLINICAL SPECTRUM OF *HISTOPLASMA CAPSULATUM* INFECTION

Asymptomatic Infection
Acute Pulmonary Histoplasmosis
Mild febrile illness
Moderate flulike illness
Severe epidemic illness
Acute cavitary disease
Chronic Pulmonary Histoplasmosis
Noncavitary
Cavitary
Disseminated Histoplasmosis
Acute infantile type
Subacute type
Chronic adult type

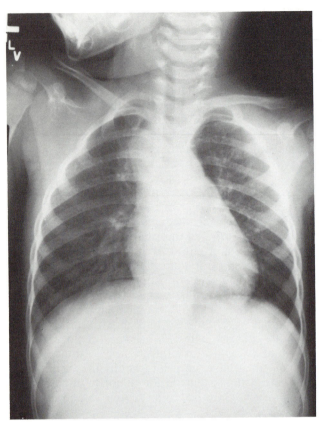

Figure 27–2. Asymptomatic histoplasmosis. Chest radiograph of a 2-year-old with a right suprahilar lymph node enlargement. The radiograph was taken after a neck injury. The diagnosis of histoplasmosis was confirmed by strongly positive serologic tests. The child remained asymptomatic, and a repeated chest radiograph 6 weeks later was normal.

subject complains of flulike symptoms with productive cough and chest pain. The chest pain is characteristically described as a substernal discomfort aggravated by deep breaths and may be related to mediastinal adenitis. Pleural effusion and pericarditis occasionally occur (Figs. 27–4A, 27–4B show esophageal obstruction).

In severe infection, usually after intensive exposure, bilateral pulmonary infiltration, high fever (38.9°C to 41.1°C), and dyspnea are prominent. Acute respiratory insufficiency secondary to the adult respiratory distress syndrome (ARDS) may also occur. The disease runs a protracted course of 10 to 20 days with slow recovery. Easy fatigability and malaise may last for months after a severe infection. Chronic pulmonary histoplasmosis is uncommon in children (Figs. 27–5A, 27–5B). However, a case of cavitary histoplasmosis in an immunocompetent child without underlying lung disease has been described.[26]

Disseminated disease occurs most often in children under 2 years of age and in immunocompromised persons (Figs. 27–6A, 27–6B). In the former category, no definite defect in cellular immunity can be demonstrated; however, evidence suggests that a transient T cell defect does exist.[20] The clinical spectrum of disseminated histoplasmosis can vary from an acute, fulminating disease resulting in death within a few weeks to a mild and protracted illness lasting many years. Goodwin and associates classified disseminated histoplasmosis on the basis of severity into acute, subacute, and chronic forms with some overlap between the three patterns.[20]

A severe, acute disease occurs most often in infants and in persons with immunodeficiency. The most characteristic features in infants are high fever, weight loss,

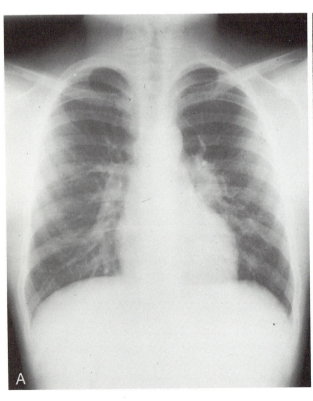

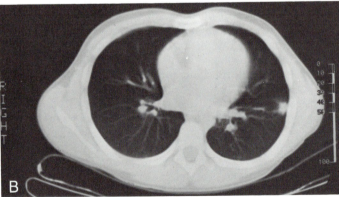

Figure 27–3. Acute pulmonary histoplasmosis. A, Chest radiograph of 13-year-old with a 1-week history of left pleuritic chest pain and cough. Left hilar adenopathy is noted. B, Computed tomographic (CT) scan shows a pulmonary parenchymal infiltrate and lymphangitis extending from the infiltrate to the enlarged hilar nodes. Histoplasma serologic tests were positive. The patient was treated with oral ketoconazole for 4 weeks and made an uneventful recovery. A follow-up chest radiograph 6 weeks later showed a decrease in size of the hilar adenopathy.

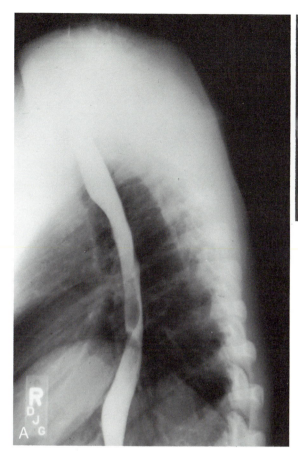

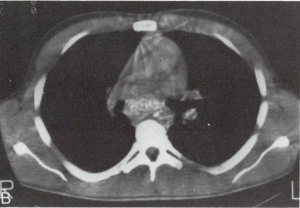

Figure 27–4. Esophageal compression. A 16-year-old patient presented with a history of fever, cough, chest pain, and dysphagia. The chest radiograph was normal; however, the barium eosphagogram (*A*) shows a large lymph node compressing the esophagus. The CT scan (*B*) shows a large subcarinal mass of matted lymph nodes compressing and displacing the barium-filled esophagus. Some calcification in the lesion is noted. Histoplasma serologic tests were all positive, and the patient recovered without antifungal therapy.

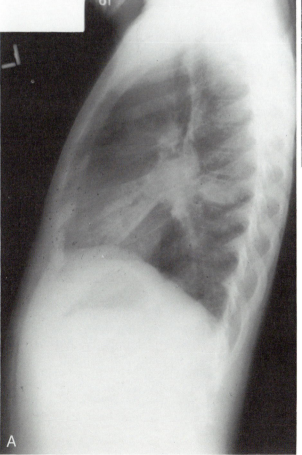

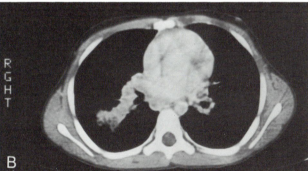

Figure 27–5. Chronic pulmonary histoplasmosis. *A*, Lateral chest radiograph with a right middle lobe infiltrate, atelectasis, and hilar adenopathy. *B*, CT scan findings of right hilar adenopathy and right middle lobe infiltrate. The 8-year-old patient had a 2-month history of cough, weakness, fever, and pneumonia that failed to respond to multiple courses of antibiotics. Serologic tests confirmed the diagnosis of histoplasmosis. He was treated with amphotericin B and corticosteroids for 4 weeks before he showed clinical and radiologic improvement. Clinical relapse occurred a few weeks after discontinuation of therapy, and a second course of amphotericin B therapy was required.

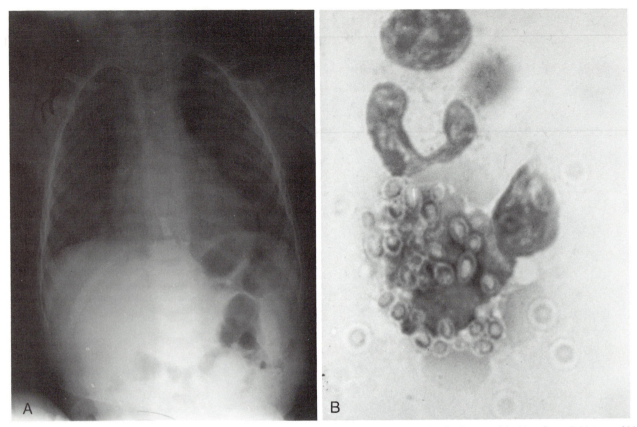

Figure 27–6. Acute disseminated histoplasmosis. *A,* Hilar adenopathy on the chest radiograph of a 2-year-old with a 6-week history of high fever, vomiting, abdominal pain, and anemia. *B,* The bone marrow smear shows a macrophage filled with histoplasma yeast and resulted in the diagnosis of disseminated histoplasmosis. Fungal serologic tests were negative; however, blood cultures grew *H. capsulatum.* The patient was treated with amphotericin B for 3 weeks with resolution of symptoms. He was subsequently found to have B and T cell immunodeficiency.

and irritability. A brassy cough and gastrointestinal symptoms are common. Hematologic abnormalities (anemia, leukopenia, thrombocytopenia) are seen in 80% of the patients. Hepatosplenomegaly (90%) with liver function abnormalities and peripheral lymphadenopathy are common features of this form of disseminated disease. Less common (70%) is the occurrence of endocarditis, meningitis, cerebritis, and ulceration of the skin and mucous membranes. Adrenal gland involvement has been demonstrated at autopsy or by computed tomographic (CT) scan in 80% to 100% of patients,[20, 27] and Addison's disease occurs in up to 15% of adult patients.[27-29] Renal involvement resulting in renal failure has been reported; the mechanism is unknown.[30-32] Untreated acute disseminated histoplasmosis is invariably fatal in a few weeks.

Acute disseminated histoplasmosis is seen with increasing frequency in patients with the acquired immunodeficiency syndrome (AIDS).[33-38] The acute form with fungemia, shock, ARDS, disseminated intravascular coagulation, and multiple organ involvement has been reported in one third of patients.[38] On the other hand, patients with AIDS may first present with mucocutaneous lesions of histoplasmosis.[39] Histologic features of histoplasmosis infection in AIDS patients are characterized by the paucity of granulomatous inflammatory reaction and giant cells in the lesion.[40] The majority of AIDS patients with disseminated histoplasmosis suffer relapse when treatment is discontinued.[34, 38]

Subacute disseminated disease is more common in adults but can also occur in infants and children. Goodwin and associates[20] reported six infants and one child among 19 patients with subacute disseminated disease. The subacute form is characterized by weight loss, weakness, and fever. Hepatosplenomegaly was present in all patients. Focal destructive lesions involving intestinal ulceration, oropharyngeal ulceration, Addison's disease, endocarditis, meningitis, cerebritis, or spinal cord compression were seen in 14 of 19 patients. Hematologic abnormalities occur less commonly than in the acute form. The duration of the illness varies from 2 months to 2 years, and death from general debility or a complication of the disease occurred in the majority of inadequately treated cases reported by Goodwin and associates.[20]

Chronic disseminated disease is characterized by low-grade infection, with few constitutional symptoms.[20] Ulceration in the mouth and pharynx is the most common finding. Hepatosplenomegaly and hematologic manifestations are less common than in the other two forms. Focal lesions such as meningitis, endocarditis, and adrenal gland involvement are seen as in the subacute form. Asymptomatic periods extending many years have been reported, and the disease course in the inadequately treated patient may last for 10 to 20 years.[41, 42] Of the patients reported by Goodwin and associates,[20] only one infant had chronic disseminated histoplasmosis. Disseminated disease covers a spectrum of disorders. In many cases, especially in infants, the initial primary infection may be followed by an asymptomatic period before acute disseminated disease occurs.

COMPLICATIONS

The thoracic complications of histoplasmosis infection are listed in Table 27–2. Respiratory distress caused by tracheal compression by large mediastinal lymph nodes is a common complication in children.[43–45] Atelectasis of the right middle lobe or the right lower lobe from external compression of the bronchus can occur, as in tuberculosis.[46] Prolonged obstruction and atelectasis may result in secondary bacterial infection and the development of bronchiectasis. Esophageal obstruction manifesting as dysphagia is not uncommon.[47, 48] The obstruction produced by acute lymphadenitis usually subsides within a few days to several weeks.

Mediastinal granuloma results from matting of lymph nodes and may vary in size from 3 to 10 cm. Central caseous necrosis and encapsulation of the mass occurs. On occasion, the central caseous material is expectorated, which results in a cystic mediastinal lesion. Mediastinal granulomas are usually asymptomatic but produce symptoms secondary to compression of adjacent structures in about one fourth of patients.[49, 50] Obstructive symptoms appear to be correlated with the thickness of the capsule surrounding the granuloma.[49]

Mediastinal fibrosis is a rare and serious complication of *H. capsulatum* infection. This extensive fibrosis is believed to be the result of an exaggerated host response to infection, resulting in excessive perihilar fibrosis that invades and encompasses mediastinal structures.[49, 50] Constriction of the airway, the pulmonary vessels, and the superior vena cava may occur and result in bronchial stenosis, pulmonary congestion and edema, cor pulmonale, and the superior vena caval syndrome.[49–51] Mediastinal fibrosis is a late complication of histoplasmosis; diagnosis is difficult because serologic tests may revert to negative by the time this complication occurs. Diagnosis is usually made by excluding other causes of fibrosing mediastinitis, such as tuberculosis.[52] The course may be benign or may result in death from pulmonary hypertension and cor pulmonale.[52]

Table 27–2. COMPLICATIONS OF HISTOPLASMOSIS INFECTION

Airway and esophageal obstruction
Mediastinal granuloma
Fibrosing mediastinitis
Broncholithiasis
Sinusitis and fistulae
Histoplasmomas
Pericarditis

Broncholithiasis caused by the erosion of caseous and calcified material from a lymph node into the bronchi usually results in bronchial inflammation and hemoptysis. The broncholith may produce significant airway obstruction and may cause wheezing, atelectasis, or pneumonitis. Relief of symptoms occurs after removal of the obstruction, either spontaneously by coughing or by bronchoscopy. In endemic areas, histoplasmosis is the most common cause of broncholithiasis and pulmonary calcifications. Infection by *H. capsulatum* can be demonstrated histologically within the broncholiths.[53–55]

Sinuses and fistulae probably result from the same process that produces broncholithiasis (i.e., invasion of caseous material from lymph nodes into adjacent structures such as bronchi, the esophagus, the aorta, or the pericardium). Bronchoesophageal fistulae, pneumopericardium, and cutaneous sinuses have been reported as complications of histoplasmosis.

A histoplasmoma results from central caseous necrosis of a large pulmonary infiltrate. The lesion becomes encapsulated and may appear as a single coin lesion. Calcification in concentric rings resulting from extension of the fibrosis around the capsule is a typical finding seen on chest radiographs. This exaggerated fibrous response is similar to that seen in mediastinal fibrosis. Gradual enlargement of the histoplasmoma occurs until the entire lesion is calcified.[56] Histoplasmomas are usually single; other causes of a single pulmonary nodule should be ruled out.

Pericarditis that follows active pulmonary histoplasmosis is probably the result of an inflammatory reaction to adjacent infected mediastinal nodes.[57, 58] Culture of pericardial fluid in such cases is sterile, and treatment with anti-inflammatory agents alone is effective in treating the pericarditis. Less often the pericarditis results from direct extension of the pulmonary infiltrate or erosion of a caseous node into the pericardium. Goodwin and associates[15] reviewed 37 reports of histoplasma pericarditis and found positive pericardial fluid culture in only three cases. This uncommon complication is usually seen in older children. Symptoms are similar to those of pericarditis from other causes and may result in cardiac tamponade requiring pericardiocentesis. Pericardial constriction and obstruction of blood vessels may develop, necessitating pericardectomy.

RADIOGRAPHIC FINDINGS

Radiographic manifestations of a primary infection caused by *H. capsulatum* vary with the clinical spectrum and severity of the infection. In 75% of cases of asymptomatic or mild infection, the chest radiograph is normal;[23] in the other 25%, there are one or more areas of pulmonary infiltrates, usually in the lower lobes, with hilar and mediastinal lymphadenopathy. In infants and young children, these infiltrates may coalesce into one large infiltrate. Calcification of healed parenchymal and hilar lesions is a common finding in persons living in endemic areas.[16, 17] Calcified nodules in the liver and spleen, seen on chest radiographs, are highly suggestive of histoplasmosis.

Intensive exposure resulting in widespread acute pulmonary infection may manifest as multiple small nodular or miliary infiltrates. Miliary infiltrates are believed to result from intensive exposure in persons who are already immune, and the presence of this radiographic pattern of infiltrates is usually not associated with hilar lymphadenopathy.[15] Calcification of the miliary infiltrates results in the typical "buckshot" appearance of chest radiographs. Isolated coin lesions may occur and are difficult to differentiate from pulmonary metastasis. Cavitary lesions involving the upper lobes occur in the chronic form of the disease.

Radiographic abnormalities are seen in two thirds of patients with disseminated disease. These abnormalities usually consist of multiple areas of pneumonitis and hilar adenopathy. Interstitial pneumonitis has also been reported in disseminated disease.[20] Computed tomography (CT scans) has been helpful in defining the extensive hilar and mediastinal lymphadenopathy. Early small parenchymal infiltrates that may not be seen on routine chest films are identified on chest CT scans. Bronchograms, although rarely necessary, may help identify bronchial obstruction from lymph node enlargement or mediastinal fibrosis. Esophagograms and cardiac catheterization are helpful in the diagnosis of obstruction of the esophagus and major blood vessels from granulomas or mediastinal fibrosis. Histoplasmosis may be the cause of acquired hyperlucent lung (Swyer-James syndrome), and radionuclide imaging is useful in demonstrating decreased perfusion and ventilation in the affected area.[59] Gallium scanning was helpful in identifying pericarditis caused by histoplasmosis and tuberculosis in a patient with fever of unknown origin.[29] In a report by Cohen and associates, magnetic resonance images of diffuse pulmonary diseases were different for histoplasmosis, tuberculosis, and allergic alveolitis and may in the future be the most specific imaging technique for the diagnosis of histoplasmosis.[60]

DIAGNOSIS

Although the histoplasmin skin test is used extensively in epidemiologic studies, it is not helpful in the diagnosis of active infection. In endemic areas (e.g., the Bluegrass region of Kentucky), 80% of the population have a positive reaction by age 20 years.[3, 5, 13] A positive reaction in nonendemic areas and in young children may be more suggestive of a recent infection. Cross reactions to histoplasmin may occur with other fungal infections such as coccidioidomycosis and blastomycosis, reducing its specificity as a diagnostic tool. Reaction to a histoplasmin skin test may also cause an increase in serologic histoplasmin titers.

The complement fixation test is the most widely available and sensitive serologic test used in the diagnosis of histoplasmosis. Both the yeast and mycelial antigens are used for testing, although yeast antigen is more sensitive for acute infection. After infection with *H. capsulatum*, it takes 3 to 4 weeks before antibodies can be detected by the complement fixation test. A complement fixation titer of 1:32 or higher, or a fourfold rise in titer, is diagnostic of active histoplasmosis.[61] In endemic areas, 5% to 24% of the population may have titers of up to 1:16 without evidence of active infection. In a study of 104 healthy blood donors tested for complement fixation titers, 24% had complement fixation antibody titers of 1:8 or 1:16 for one or both of the antigens, but none had titers above 1:16.[62] Unlike the histoplasmin skin test, which may remain positive for 10 years or more after infection, serologic titers decrease with time and may become negative in 2 to 5 years.[63] Elevated complement fixation titers are demonstrated in more than 90% of patients with symptomatic histoplasmosis and, to a lesser extent, in patients with asymptomatic infection. These titers, may however, be negative in severe disseminated disease and in immunosuppressed hosts. The height of complement fixation titer is not correlated with the severity of infection; however, the more severe the infection, the higher the yield of positive complement fixation titers.[64]

Precipitating antibodies, detected by immunodiffusion tests, may be helpful in the diagnosis of histoplasmosis. These tests have the advantage of being simple and require less time to perform than the complement fixation tests. Two major precipitin bands are designated the H and M bands. The presence of an M band is less specific for active infection and may persist after recovery or may be demonstrated after histoplasmin skin testing. The H band has higher diagnostic value because it disappears after the acute infection. The presence of both H and M bands is highly specific for active histoplasmosis, but the diagnosis should be confirmed by the more definitive complement fixation test. A negative immunodiffusion test does not rule out active infection, and the complement fixation test should be performed if histoplasmosis is suspected.

Detection of *H. capsulatum* antigen has been reported in the blood and urine of patients with histoplasmosis.[65] In disseminated disease, the antigen was detected in the urine of up to 90% of patients and in the blood of 50% of patients. The yield was lower (50%) in the acute form of the disease. Antigen detection is helpful as a rapid diagnostic test of histoplasmosis; it is also useful in following the response to treatment and predicting relapse. Wheat and colleagues[65] reported clearance of the urine and serum antigen in patients with disseminated histoplasmosis when amphotericin B treatment was instituted and reappearance of the antigen with relapse.

Direct microscopic examination of sputum using the standard potassium hydroxide preparation is not helpful in the diagnosis of histoplasmosis because of the small size and the intracellular location of the organism. Giemsa or Wright's stain of blood or bone marrow smears may reveal the small (2- to 5-μm–diameter) oval yeast cells of *H. capsulatum*. Similarly, histologic examination of caseous lymph nodes and smears from oropharyngeal or cutaneous ulcers may be diagnostic.

Culture of *H. capsulatum* from body tissue or secretions confirms the diagnosis. The site for acquisition of appropriate culture material depends on the form of the disease. The organism may be cultured from sputum, bronchial washings, blood, bone marrow aspirate, urine, and cerebrospinal fluid; from material obtained from lymph nodes, skin, and mucous membrane ulcers; and from liver and spleen biopsy specimens. Proper collection and rapid transport of material to the laboratory is essential. Freezing of specimens should be avoided because it is injurious to dimorphic fungi. Sabouraud's dextrose agar, which contains peptone, glucose, and antibiotics, is the commonly used culture medium.

H. capsulatum is generally a slow-growing organism. The rate of growth is dependent on the medium used and on the number of organisms present in the specimen. The lysis-centrifugation blood culture technique (Isolator) has been found to be a rapid and sensitive method for the diagnosis of fungemia, especially in immunosuppressed patients with disseminated histoplasmosis.[66, 67] The diagnosis of *H. capsulatum* infection is made by means of macroscopic and microscopic identification of the morphologic characteristics of the fungal growth.

Differential Diagnosis. Histoplasmosis can mimic a variety of conditions. The diagnosis of unusual manifestations of histoplasmosis such as parotitis, arthritis, interstitial nephritis, cutaneous lesions, and meningitis may be easily overlooked.[68] Probably the most common differential diagnosis is a mediastinal mass. Woods and collaborators[69] reported that of 68 children who presented with a mediastinal mass, six were found to have histoplasmosis; all six cases were originally believed to be lymphomas involving the mediastinal nodes.

Gaebler and co-workers[70] confirmed histoplasmosis in 21 (57%) of 37 children being evaluated for anterior and middle mediastinal masses. In only one case of histoplasmosis did the mass involve the anterior mediastinum. Most histoplasma-infected lymph nodes are in the middle mediastinum; anterior mediastinal masses secondary to histoplasmosis are uncommon.[71]

Disseminated histoplasmosis may mimic leukemia, especially when associated with bone marrow suppression. Histoplasmosis must be considered in all children with unexplained fevers, especially in endemic areas. Tuberculosis and histoplasmosis have many similar clinical and radiologic features. Other rare conditions such as reticuloendotheliosis usually require biopsy of the involved lymph nodes in order to establish the diagnosis.

TREATMENT

Amphotericin B remains the gold standard for comparison of antifungal agents. The mechanism of action is believed to be disruption of the cell membrane and autooxidation, which cause fungal cell damage. Amphotericin B is not absorbed from the gastrointestinal tract and must be given intravenously or intrathecally. Topical use in the form of mouth washes, bladder washes, or direct irrigation of wounds is also effective. Toxicity of amphotericin B is caused by binding of the drug to the cholesterol in cell membranes.

The major side effects of amphotericin B are bone marrow suppression and nephrotoxicity with potassium loss, especially with sodium depletion. Sodium loading improves renal function despite continued amphotericin administration.[72] Hematocrit, creatinine, and potassium levels should be determined before treatment is started and should be followed two to three times per week thereafter. Renal toxicity, manifested by an increase in serum creatinine levels, is frequently seen and may be minimized by decreasing the dosage or increasing the intervals between amphotericin B infusions. When the serum potassium level falls below 3.5 mEq/l, potassium replacement should be given. Anemia from bone marrow suppression usually resolves when the drug is stopped.

Ketoconazole is less toxic than amphotericin B, but it is also less effective in treating serious mycotic infections.[73, 74] It has the advantage of good absorption from the gastrointestinal tract. An acidic gastric pH is necessary for optimal drug absorption; thus the drug should not be given along with antacids[75] or to patients receiving cimetidine. Ketoconazole is metabolized by the liver and excreted in the bile. Because levels of active drug are low in the urine, ketoconazole is not recommended for genitourinary infections. Ketoconazole is not recommended for infections of the central nervous system because it penetrates the system poorly.[75] The most common adverse effects of ketoconazole are nausea, vomiting, and anorexia. Mild hepatic toxicity is fairly common. Symptomatic hepatic dysfunction is rarely seen and resolves with discontinuation of the drug.[73, 74] However, fatal hepatic necrosis has been reported.[76] Endocrine dysfunction secondary to blockage of synthesis of testosterone and adrenocorticosteroids is seen with high doses.[73, 74]

After infection with *H. capsulatum,* the majority of healthy persons are asymptomatic or have mild illness and require no treatment. Treatment of children with moderate illness (characterized by several weeks of fever, moderate anemia, lethargy, nonproductive cough, and splenomegaly) is controversial. Some physicians treat with a short course (2 weeks) of amphotericin B; others use no treatment. Evidence supporting use of an alternative treatment with ketoconazole in systemic histoplasmosis is accumulating.[73, 74]

A severe "epidemic"-type illness that results in respiratory insufficiency may be either a reinfection in partially immune persons or a severe primary infection. Some investigators believe that no intervention is indicated in such patients. In the authors' experience, a 2-week course of amphotericin B therapy alone or followed by treatment with ketoconazole results in prompt and full recovery in these cases.

Chronic pulmonary histoplasmosis with or without cavitary disease is rare in children. Intravenous amphotericin B for 2 to 4 weeks or 10 mg/kg/day (maximal dose of 400 mg/day) of ketoconazole for 3 to 6 months has been successful in these cases.

Although ketoconazole has been recommended as the drug of choice in non–life-threatening histoplasmosis,[74] amphotericin B remains the mainstay for the treatment of disseminated disease. Clinical response with amphotericin B is quicker than that with ketoconazole and is usually seen within 1 or 2 weeks. The mortality rate in untreated disseminated disease is higher than 90%; with treatment, it decreases to between 5% and 23%[69] among the immunocompetent hosts and as high as 73% among immunodeficient patients.[77] A total dose of 35 to 40 mg/kg is recommended for preventing relapses.[72] Young infants generally respond to a course of 2 to 3 weeks of therapy.[78] Patients with congenital immunologic diseases and immunosuppressed patients should receive treatment with amphotericin B for 6 to 10 weeks, perhaps followed by therapy with ketoconazole. Among patients with AIDS, there is a high incidence of relapse after discontinuation of amphotericin treatment.[37, 38] It has been recommended that a 6- to 8-week course of amphotericin B (1.0 to 1.5 g) followed by indefinite maintenance therapy with ketoconazole (400 mg/day) or amphotericin B (50 to 100 mg/week) be undertaken by adult patients with AIDS.[36, 63] Development of adrenal insufficiency appears to be associated with a higher incidence of relapses; thus diagnosis of adrenal insufficiency should be made, and adrenal hormone substitution therapy should be instituted. In relapses, treatment may be repeated with either amphotericin B or ketoconazole, dependent on the susceptibility of the fungus.[72]

Treatment for the various complications of histoplasmosis must be individualized. Patients with severe stridor or esophageal dysfunction may improve after a short course of steroid therapy along with amphotericin B treatment. The authors favor 2 mg/kg/day of intravenous methylprednisolone divided into four equal doses, one dose given every 6 h, for approximately 1 week. Amphotericin B is given in full doses (0.75 to 1.00 mg/kg/day) for 2 to 4 weeks.

Mediastinal granuloma may or not be symptomatic and may resolve without complications. For mild symptoms, the authors favor instituting ketoconazole treatment for several months with close follow-up by plain radiographs or CT scans.

Mediastinal fibrosis is believed to be caused by an exaggerated immune response to mediastinal histoplasmosis. Whether early treatment prevents this complication is unknown. Steroids and amphotericin B treatment may be useful at the earliest suggestion of mediastinal fibrosis; however, no data to substantiate this possibility are available. Surgical intervention for constricted vessels and airways has been disappointing.

Bronchiolithiasis secondary to histoplasmosis is rare, and the resulting complications are usually obstruction of airways or bacterial pneumonias. Treatment consists of removal of the broncholith and administration of antibiotics as indicated. The histoplasma infection is usually inactive at the time of this complication, and no therapy for histoplasmosis is indicated. Sinus and fistula penetration into adjacent organs from caseous lymph nodes are rarely seen in children. Surgical intervention and treatment with either ketoconazole or amphotericin B are usually required.

Treatment of histoplasmoma depends on the size and location of the lesion. Surgical removal is generally curative for large lesions. Smaller lesions could be followed clinically while ketoconazole treatment is undertaken.

Active pericarditis caused by histoplasmosis is another situation in which the authors favor a short course of treatment with methylprednisolone along with amphotericin B.[79] Oral treatment with ketoconazole after the amphotericin B might also be beneficial.

In the future, itraconazole,[72, 80–82] which is less toxic and has a longer half-life than ketoconazole, may well replace ketoconazole as the oral agent of choice for the treatment of histoplasmosis. Liposome-encapsulated amphotericin B may replace the current formulation for intravenous use because it can be given in higher doses, produces fewer systemic side effects and less nephrotoxicity, and at the same time attains higher blood levels.[83]

REFERENCES

1. Darling ST: Histoplasmosis: A fatal infectious disease resembling kala-azar found among natives of tropical America. Arch Intern Med 2:107–123, 1908.
2. DeMonbreun WA: The cultivation and characteristics of Darling's *H. capsulatum.* Am J Trop Med 14:93–137, 1934.
3. Edwards LB, Acquaviva FA, Livesay VT, et al: An atlas of sensitivity to tuberculin, PPD-B, and histoplasmin in the United States. Am Rev Respir Dis 99(Suppl):1–132, 1969.
4. Ajello L: Relationship of *Histoplasma capsulatum* to avian habitats. Pub Health Rep 79:266–270, 1964.
5. Campbell CC: The epidemiology of histoplasmosis. Ann Intern Med 62:1333–1336, 1965.
6. Emmons CW, Klite PD, Baer GM, et al: Isolation of *Histoplasma capsulatum* from bats in the United States. Am J Epidemiol 84:103–109, 1966.
7. Beatty OA, Zwick LS, Paisley CG: Epidemic histoplasmosis in Ohio with source in Kentucky. Ohio State Med J 63:1470–1472, 1967.
8. Furcolow ML, Menges RW, Larsh HW: An epidemic of histoplasmosis involving man and animals. Ann Intern Med 43:173–181, 1955.
9. Ward JI, Weeks M, Allen D, et al: Acute histoplasmosis: Clinical, epidemiologic and serologic findings of an outbreak associated with exposure to a fallen tree. Am J Med 66:587–595, 1979.
10. Englert E Jr, Phillips AW: Acute diffuse pulmonary granulomatosis in bridge workers. Am J Med 15:733–740, 1953.
11. Lottenberg R, Waldman RH, Ajello L, et al: Pulmonary histoplasmosis associated with exploration of a bat cave. Am J Epidemiol 110:156–161, 1979.
12. Vandiviere HM, Goodman NL, Melvin IG, et al: Histoplasmosis in Kentucky—Can it be prevented? J Ky Med Assoc 79:719–726, 1981.
13. Ajello L: Distribution of *Histoplasma capsulatum* in the United States. *In* Ajello L, Chick EW, Furcolow ML (eds): Histoplasmosis, pp. 103–122. Springfield, IL: Charles C Thomas, 1971.
14. Zeidberg LD, Dillon A, Grass RS: Some factors in the epidemiology of histoplasmin sensitivity in Williamson County, Tennessee. Am J Public Health 41:80–89, 1951.
15. Goodwin RA, Loyd JE, Des Prez RM: Histoplasmosis in normal hosts. Medicine (Baltimore) 60:231–266, 1981.
16. Mashburn JD, Dawson DF, Young JM: Pulmonary calcifications and histoplasmosis. Am Rev Respir Dis 84:208–216, 1961.
17. Straub M, Schwarz J: Healed primary complex in histoplasmosis. Am J Clin Pathol 25:727–741, 1955.
18. Okudaira M, Straub M, Schwarz J: The etiology of discrete splenic and hepatic calcifications in an endemic area of histoplasmosis. Am J Pathol 39:599–611, 1961.
19. Dismukes WE, Royal SA, Tynes BS: Disseminated histoplasmosis in corticosteroid-treated patients: Report of five cases. JAMA 240:1495–1498, 1978.
20. Goodwin RA, Shapiro JL, Thurman GH, et al: Disseminated histoplasmosis: Clinical and pathologic correlations. Medicine (Baltimore) 59:1–33, 1980.
21. Couch JR, Abdou NI, Sagawa A: Histoplasma meningitis with hyperactive suppressor T cells in cerebrospinal fluid. Neurology 28:119–123, 1978.
22. Smith RT: Histoplasmosis: A review with an epidemiological and clinical study of an outbreak occurring in Minnesota. Lancet 75:83–100, 1955.

23. Whitehouse WM, Davey WM, Engelke OK, et al: Roentgen findings in histoplasmin-positive school children. J Mich Med Soc 58:1266–1269, 1959.
24. Furcolow ML, Tosh FE, Larsh HW, et al: The emerging pattern of urban histoplasmosis. N Engl J Med 264:1226–1230, 1961.
25. Parrott T, Taylor G, Poston MA, et al: An epidemic of histoplasmosis in Warrenton, North Carolina. South Med J 48:1147–1150, 1955.
26. Chick EW, Dillon ML, Tahanasab A: Acute cavitary histoplasmosis. Chest 71:674–676, 1977.
27. Wilson DA, Muchmore HG, Tisdal RG, et al: Histoplasmosis of the adrenal glands studied by CT. Radiology 150:779–783, 1984.
28. Smith JW, Utz JP: Progressive disseminated histoplasmosis: A prospective study of twenty-six patients. Ann Intern Med 76:557–565, 1972.
29. Taillefer R, Lemieux RJ, Picard D, et al: Gallium-67 imaging in pericarditis secondary to tuberculosis and histoplasmosis. Clin Nucl Med 6:413–415, 1981.
30. Bullock WE, Artz RP, Bhathena D, et al: Histplasmosis: Association with circulating immune complexes, eosinophilia, and mesangiopathic glomerulonephritis. Arch Intern Med 139:700–702, 1979.
31. Murray JJ, Heim CR: Hypercalcemia in disseminated histoplasmosis: Aggravation by vitamin D. Am J Med 78:881–884, 1985.
32. Walker JV, Baran D, Yakub N, et al: Histoplasmosis with hypercalcemia, renal failure, and papillary necrosis: Confusion with sarcoidosis. JAMA 237:1350–1352, 1977.
33. Bonner JR, Alexander WJ, Dismukes WE, et al: Disseminated histoplasmosis in patients with the acquired immune deficiency syndrome. Arch Intern Med 144:2178–2181, 1984.
34. Johnson PC, Sarosi GA, Septimus EJ, et al: Progressive disseminated histoplasmosis in patients with the acquired immune deficiency syndrome: A report of 12 cases and a literature review. Semin Respir Infect 1:1–8, 1986.
35. Macher AM, De Vinatea ML, Tuur SM, et al: AIDS and the mycoses. Infect Dis Clin North Am 2:827–839, 1988.
36. Mandell W, Goldberg D, Neu H: Histoplasmosis in patients with the acquired immune deficiency syndrome. Am J Med 81:974–978, 1986.
37. Wheat LJ, Small CB: Disseminated histoplasmosis in the acquired immune deficiency syndrome. Arch Intern Med 144:2147–2149, 1984.
38. Wheat LJ, Slama TG, Zeckel ML: Histoplasmosis in the acquired immune deficiency syndrome. Am J Med 78:203–210, 1985.
39. Hazelhurst JA, Vismer HF: Histoplasmosis presenting with unusual skin lesions in acquired immunodeficiency syndrome (AIDS). Br J Dermatol 113:345–348, 1985.
40. De Vinatea M, Macher A, Sbaschnig R, et al: AIDS case for diagnosis series: Disseminated infection by *Histoplasma capsulatum* mimicking *Pneumocystis carinii* pneumonia and disseminated candidiasis. Milit Med 152:M57–M64, 1987.
41. Gelfand JA, Bennett JE: Active histoplasma meningitis of 22 years' duration. JAMA 233:1294–1295, 1975.
42. Morris RJ, Betts RF, Douglas RG, et al: Recurrent disseminated histoplasmosis. South Med J 71:621–623, 1978.
43. Greenwood MF, Holland P: Tracheal obstruction secondary to histoplasma mediastinal granuloma. Chest 62:642–645, 1972.
44. Friedman JL, Baum GL, Schwarz J: Primary pulmonary histoplasmosis. Am J Dis Child 109:298–303, 1965.
45. Woods LP: Mediastinal histoplasma granuloma causing tracheal compression in a 4 year old child. Surgery 58:448–452, 1965.
46. Riggs W, Nelson P: The roentgenographic findings in infantile and childhood histoplasmosis. AJR 97:181–185, 1966.
47. Dukes RJ, Strimlan CV, Dines DE, et al: Esophageal involvement with mediastinal granuloma. JAMA 236:2313–2315, 1976.
48. Jenkins DW, Fisk DE, Byrd RB: Mediastinal histoplasmosis with esophageal abscess: Two case reports. Gastroenterology 70:109–111, 1976.
49. Goodwin RA, Nickell JA, Des Prez RM: Mediastinal fibrosis complicating healed primary histoplasmosis and tuberculosis. Medicine (Baltimore) 51:227–246, 1972.
50. Schowengerdt CG, Suyemoto R, Main FB: Granulomatous and fibrous mediastinitis: A review and analysis of 180 cases. J Thorac Cardiovasc Surg 57:365–379, 1969.
51. Pate JW, Hammon J: Superior vena cava syndrome due to histoplasmosis in children. Ann Surg 161:778–787, 1965.
52. Dines DE, Payne WS, Bernatz PE, et al: Mediastinal granuloma and fibrosing mediastinitis. Chest 75:320–324, 1979.
53. Baum GL, Berstein IL, Schwarz J: Broncholithiasis produced by histoplasmosis. Am Rev Tuberc 77:162–167, 1958.
54. Kelly WA: Broncholithiasis, current concepts of an ancient disease. Postgrad Med 66:81–88, 1979.
55. Felson B, Klatte EC: Complications of the arrested primary histoplasmic complex. JAMA 236:1157–1161, 1976.
56. Goodwin RA, Snell JD: The enlarging histoplasmoma. Concept of a tumor-like phenomenon encompassing the tuberculoma and coccidioidoma. Am Rev Respir Dis 100:1–12, 1969.
57. Picardi JL, Kauffman CA, Schwarz J, et al: Pericarditis caused by *Histoplasma capsulatum*. Am J Cardiol 37:82–88, 1976.
58. Wheat LJ, Stein L, Corya BC, et al: Pericarditis as a manifestation of histoplasmosis during two large urban outbreaks. Medicine (Baltimore) 62:110–119, 1983.
59. Wieder S, White TJ, Salazar J, et al: Pulmonary artery occlusion due to histoplasmosis. Am J Radiol 138:243–251, 1982.
60. Cohen MD, Eigen H, Scott PH, et al: Magnetic resonance imaging of inflammatory lung disorders: Preliminary studies in children. Pediatr Pulmonol 2:211–217, 1986.
61. Chick EW, Baum GL, Furcolow ML, et al: The use of skin tests and serologic tests in histoplasmosis, coccidioidomycosis, and blastomycosis. Am Rev Respir Dis 108:156–159, 1973.
62. George RB, Lambert RS: Significance of serum antibodies to *Histoplasma capsulatum* in endemic areas. South Med J 77:161–163, 1984.
63. Wheat LJ: Systemic fungal infections: Diagnosis and treatment: I. Histoplasmosis. Infect Dis Clin North Am 2:841–859, 1988.
64. Larrabee WF, Ajello L, Kaufman L: An epidemic of histoplasmosis on the Isthmus of Panama. Am J Trop Med Hyg 27:281–285, 1978.
65. Wheat LJ, Kohler RB, Tewari RP: Diagnosis of disseminated histoplasmosis by detection of *Histoplasma capsulatum* antigen in serum and urine specimens. N Engl J Med 314:83–88, 1986.
66. Bille J, Stockman L, Roberts GD, et al: Evaluation of a lysis-centrifugation system for recovery of yeasts and filamentous fungi from blood. J Clin Microbiol 18:469–471, 1983.
67. Paya CV, Roberts GD, Cockerill FR: Laboratory methods for the diagnosis of disseminated histoplasmosis: Clinical importance of the lysis-centrifugation blood culture technique. Mayo Clin Proc 62:480–485, 1987.
68. Weinberg GA, Kleiman MB, Grosfeld JL, et al: Unusual manifestations of histoplasmosis in childhood. Pediatrics 72:99–105, 1983.
69. Woods WG, Singher LJ, Krivit W, et al: Histoplasmosis simulating lymphoma in children. J Pediatr Surg 14:423–425, 1979.
70. Gaebler JW, Kleiman MB, Cohen M, et al: Differentiation of lymphoma from histoplasmosis in children with mediastinal masses. J Pediatr 104:706–709, 1984.
71. Zeanah CH, Zusman J; Mediastinal and cervical histoplasmosis simulating malignancy. Am J Dis Child 133:47–49, 1979.
72. Sarosi GA, Bates JH, Bradsher RW, et al: Chemotherapy of the pulmonary mycoses. Am Rev Respir Dis 138:1078–1081, 1988.
73. Dismukes WE, Stamm AM, Graybill JR, et al: Treatment of systemic mycoses with ketoconazole: Emphasis on toxicity and clinical response in 52 patients. Ann Intern Med 98:13–20, 1983.
74. Dismukes WE, Cloud G, Bowles C, et al: Treatment of blastomycosis and histoplasmosis with ketoconazole. Ann Intern Med 103:861–872, 1985.
75. Nizoral [Product information]. *In* Physician's Desk Reference, 45th ed, pp. 1118–1119. Oradell, NJ: Medical Economics, 1991.
76. Duarte PA, Chow CC, Simmons F, et al: Fatal hepatitis associated with ketoconazole therapy. Arch Intern Med 144:1069–1070, 1984.
77. Kauffman CA, Israel KS, Smith JW, et al: Histoplasmosis in immunosuppressed patients. Am J Med 64:923–932, 1978.
78. Fosson AR, Wheeler WE: Short-term amphotericin B treatment of severe childhood histoplasmosis. J Pediatr 86:32–36, 1975.
79. Wilson HD: Histoplasmosis. *In* Nelson JD (ed): Current Therapy in Pediatric Infectious Disease—2, pp. 174–177. Toronto: BC Decker, 1988.
80. Dupont B, Drouhet E: Early experience with itraconazole in vitro and in patients: Pharmacokinetic studies and clinical results. Rev Infect Dis 9(Suppl):71–76, 1987.
81. Ganer A, Arathoon E, Stevens DA: Initial experience in therapy

for progressive mycoses with itraconazole, the first clinically studied triazole. Rev Infect Dis 9(Suppl):77–86, 1987.
82. Phillips P, Fetchick R, Weisman I, et al: Tolerance to and efficacy
of itraconazole in treatment of systemic mycoses: Preliminary
results. Rev Infect Dis 9(Suppl):87–93, 1987.

83. Meunier F, Sculier JP, Coune A, et al: Amphotericin B encapsulated in liposomes administered to cancer patients. Ann N Y Acad
Sci 544:598–610, 1988.

28 INFLUENZA

STEPHEN MARKER, M.D.

In 1933, Wilson Smith and Sir Christopher Andrew
first grew the influenza A virus from human tissue. The
original infected specimen came from Andrew's throat.[1]
Smith used these washings to inoculate a variety of experimental animals by several routes. Although Smith and
Andrew described the influenza virus in 1933, other records indicate that epidemics of influenza occurred as early
as 1173. The term influenza entered the English language
in 1743 from the Italian term *influence*. What becomes
clear from the many monographs dealing with these epidemics is that worldwide epidemics and pandemics in
which morbidity and mortality rates are substantially
high have occurred at irregular intervals. In the 20th century, pandemics occurred in 1918, 1957, 1968, and 1977.

Human influenza virus isolates have been available
since the experiments of Smith and Andrew in the early
1930s, and these isolates have been subjected to intense
scrutiny, as have the isolates from diverse animal species.
These investigations have provided insight into the nature
of the virus and the molecular basis of antigenic variation,
while at the same time suggesting the origin of these variations. Each yearly epidemic is associated with significant
morbidity but low mortality rates. Although death from
the influenza virus is uncommon in otherwise healthy
populations, the mortality rate does rise with increasing
age. Epidemics that are easily handled by healthy children
are devastating to the elderly. A microbiologic perspective
on the annual epidemics in children has been obtained
since 1960 by monitoring acute respiratory illness as
shown in Figure 28–1.[2–6]

Influenza B was recovered from humans in 1940.[7,8] Differences in the antigenicity of the nucleocapsid are the
basis of the classification of influenza into types A, B, and
C; in addition, there are substantial differences in biologic
activity and molecular structure.[9] Influenza B occurs in
yearly epidemics of smaller magnitude and severity than
those of influenza A. The influenza B virus seems to be
under less severe genetic selection. Although mutations
produce variations in the antigenic structure of influenza
B, the major changes associated with influenza A pandemics do not occur. Immunity acquired by natural influ-

enza B infection is not as protective as the natural immunity from influenza A.[4] Other biologic differences include
the stronger association of influenza B than of influenza
A with Reye's syndrome and acute myositis.[10,11] The hemagglutinin gene in influenza B contains a second reading
frame; thus the hemagglutinin in this virus is a pair of
proteins.

In 1949, influenza C was discovered.[12] This virus causes
a lesser illness than either influenza A or B because immunity in children is high, but the frequency of recognized
illness is low. As with influenza B, structural differences
are also seen; the influenza C virus has only a single surface glycoprotein and does not have neuraminidase
activity.[9]

PATHOPHYSIOLOGY

The influenza virion is about 0.1 μm in diameter and
contains 11 proteins (4690 copies), eight segments of neg-
ative-strand RNA (13,600 nucleotides and 11 genes), and
a lipid bilayer.[9,13] Interaction of this >5000-component,
self-assembling, self-replicating molecular collection with
the host tissues and defense mechanisms results in influenza. The hemagglutinin protein contains four important
antigenic regions. It also contains regions responsible for
cell attachment and virulence. The sequence and tertiary
structure of this glycoprotein trimer is known, and a schematic representation of the hemagglutinin is shown in
Figure 28–2. Antigenic site A on the hemagglutinin (a
loop of seven amino acids near the outer surface) seems
particularly important in that site A variations are seen
between strains of different yearly epidemics. This year-
to-year variation in antigenic structure seems to occur by
mutation of the RNA sequence and is termed *antigenic
drift*. Changes in a single epitope may prevent antibody
neutralization.

The major antigenic variants of the human influenza
hemagglutinin are called H1, H2, and H3; H4 to H13 are
found in other species. Pandemics are associated with the
appearance of influenza strains with a major antigenic

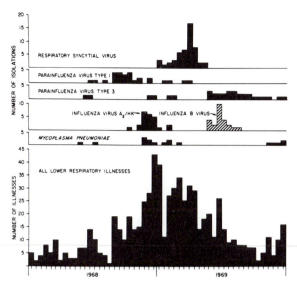

Figure 28–1. Weekly virus isolation of four major respiratory pathogens from children with lower respiratory disease. (From Glezen WP, Denny FW: Epidemiology of acute lower respiratory disease in children. N Engl J Med 288:498–505, 1973. Reprinted with permission from the *New England Journal of Medicine,* vol. 288, pp. 498–505, 1973.)

shift in the hemagglutinin or with the reappearance of a pre-existing hemagglutinin in an unimmunized population. This occurred in 1889 with H2, in 1899 with H3, in 1918 with H1, in 1957 with H2 (Asian influenza), in 1968 with H3 (Hong Kong influenza), and in 1977 with H1. For instance, in 1957 the Asian influenza (H2N2) contained four new genes: the hemagglutinin, neuraminidase, and two components of the RNA polymerase.[14] In 1968, the Hong Kong influenza H3N2 contained only a new hemagglutinin.[14, 15]

Among the 11 influenza proteins, the neuraminidase is the only protein other than hemagglutinin that is exposed on the surface of the virus. In this surface position, four neuraminadase antigenic sites are exposed.[16, 17] The sequence and tertiary structure of this tetrameric glycoprotein is known. N1 and N2 are the designations for the two major antigenic subtypes of human origin; N3 to N9 are found in other species. In 1957, N2 was among the four new gene products along with H2 that appeared for the first time, resulting in the Asian influenza pandemic.[14]

Nomenclature for influenza virus was revised in 1980 and contains the following elements: (1) antigenic type of nucleocapsid protein (A, B, or C); (2) host of origin (e.g., swine, horse, duck); (3) geographic origin; (4) strain number; and (5) year of isolation. For example, A/swine/Iowa/15/30 is one reference strain of H1N1 influenza A and was isolated from pigs in Iowa in 1930.

Influenza virus infects the epithelial cells of the respiratory tract. The subsequent cytopathic effects of viral replication, perhaps direct toxicity of viral proteins, and the host's inflammatory response result in the symptoms and complications of influenza. Indeed, the cytokines from interleukin-1 (IL-1) to IL-6 and at least a dozen other white blood cell mediators may be responsible for the sudden onset of fever, myalgia, headaches, poor appetite, and prolonged fatigue so typical of influenza.[18] Some effects of these cytokines are mediated by increases of arachidonic acid metabolites. For instance, the IL-1 from

stimulated monocytes causes prostaglandin E2 synthesis, resulting in its inflammatory properties.[19] Influenza and other viruses *in vitro* can stimulate the production of IL-6 (tumor necrosis factor, or cachectin).[20] Elevated levels of circulating IL-6 in influenza have not actually been demonstrated. However, the technologic capability for such a demonstration is available and has been used in acquired immunodeficiency syndrome (AIDS).[21]

The biologic characteristics of these cytokines are rapidly being elucidated. Tumor necrosis factor (TNF) α is a 157–amino acid protein encoded by a three-kilobase gene on human chromosome six, 200 kilobase pairs centromeric of human leukocyte antigen (HLA) B, and is derived from myeloid cells.[22] This protein has profound biologic effects on the host; production may be stimulated by interferon, and in turn the protein may exhibit direct antiviral effects.[23, 24] The complexities of these inflammatory responses and their specific involvement in influenza are yet to be fully elucidated, but progress has been made toward understanding and recognizing the symptoms of this disease.

In 1957, an Asian influenza pandemic led to many pathologic studies of human influenza.[25–30] A bronchoscopic study of this epidemic showed the early edema and redness of laryngotracheobronchial mucosa.[30] Histologic examination showed that the epithelial cellular swelling is quickly followed by all degrees of ciliary and cellular loss down to the basement membrane. The limited cellular infiltration is out of proportion to the marked extent of epithelial involvement. More lymphocytic infiltrates and a histiocytic infiltrate are seen with lesser numbers of neu-

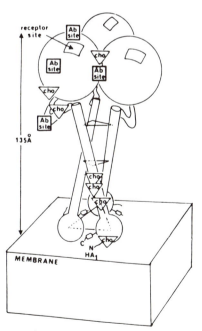

Figure 28–2. Schematic diagram of the trimer of the hemagglutinin of influenza A. Four antibody-binding sites are shown. The receptor site for the host oligosaccharide is also shown. CHO, carbohydrate attachment sites. (From Wiley DC, Wilson IA, Skehel JJ: Structural identification of the antibody-binding sites of Hong Kong influenza haemagglutinin and their involvement in antigenic variation. Reprinted by permission from Nature, vol 289, pp. 373–378; copyright © 1981 Macmillan Magazines Limited.)

trophils, eosinophils, and plasma cells. The degree of thickening of the basement membrane is extremely high. Histologic improvement begins, as early as the third day, with mitoses in the surviving basal cells. A new epithelium six to eight cells thick is present after 9 to 15 days. After 2 weeks, new cilia begin to appear.[31]

In fatal cases, respiratory mucosal ulceration or replacement by inflammatory granulation tissue may occur. Mucociliary flow is disrupted with the obvious consequences of bronchiolar plugging, atelectasis, and the stasis necessary for rapid local bacterial proliferation. In fatal Asian influenza-mediated pneumonia, the changes extend down to the respiratory bronchioles and alveolar ducts. There are cytopathogenic changes in the fixed alveolar cells, capillary thrombosis, and necrosis with focal leukocytic exudates. After 3 to 4 days, alveolar hyaline membranes form, and after 5 to 7 days, the epithelium begins regenerating to form a stratified metaplastic layer. The changes are focally distributed and not diffuse. A complicating bacterial pneumonia may be seen, but fatal cases of viral pneumonia without superinfection are not uncommon.

Virus shedding from the nasal mucosa peaks on the second day of infection and is usually ended after the fifth day, although children with a primary infection may shed virus for up to 3 weeks. It is unusual to detect viremia. In ferrets, as in humans, upper respiratory disease predominates. In this model, virus titers are more than 100 times higher in nasal turbinate tissue than in the lower respiratory tract.[32] In the lungs, infection is primarily in bronchial epithelium rather than in alveolar cells. This effect is not a result of diminished inoculum to the lower respiratory tissue. If alveolar cells are infected, little progeny virus is released. The absence of viremia in influenza may be explained by at least two mechanisms. First, virus does enter the local respiratory lymphatic tissue but is rapidly removed from the blood by the reticuloendothelial system. Many extra respiratory tissues grow influenza virus to high titers, but the barrier between blood and susceptible tissue seems impenetrable. Second, physiologic impairment parallels the pathologic state. Lung volumes are restricted, and alveolar-arterial (A-a) oxygen gradients increase. Increased bronchial reactivity occurs. Of 39 influenza A infected college students, 80% showed increased total pulmonary resistance and decreased helium-oxygen flow rates. Inhalation of carbachol aerosol resulted in airway hyperreactivity that was still measurable but substantially improved 3 weeks after infection.[33–35]

Bacterial superinfection, in addition to the disordered mucociliary clearance and accumulation of tracheobronchial debris, can occur through several mechanisms during influenza infection. Mononuclear and polymorphonuclear leukocyte metabolic and chemotactic functions are impaired by influenza virus.[36] These effects may be partially explained by a low level of viral component synthesis in polymorphonuclear leukocytes.[37] Influenza virus may induce staphylococcal receptors on epithelial cell surfaces.

Transplacental passage of influenza antibody provides protection to neonates.[38] Higher titers of this passively transferred antibody seem to exert a longer duration of protection. After the primary infection in children, symptomatic reinfections in subsequent years with antigenically similar viruses are uncommon.[4, 39] Some protection from prior infection may last up to 20 years, as seen during the reappearance of the H1 virus in 1977 after an absence of 20 years; its reappearance was primarily in persons less than 25 years old.[40]

CLINICAL MANIFESTATIONS

Within 24 h of the first sign of illness, coryza, fever, myalgia, sore throat, headache, and malaise ensue. Cough occurs in the second 24 h. Three to 5 days later, the fever subsides along with the sore throat and headache. Malaise may persist for an extended period.

Infants may manifest signs indistinguishable from those of neonatal sepsis. Many hospitalized older children have pneumonia, bronchiolitis, croup, seizures, or abdominal pain with vomiting and, less common, encephalitis, myocarditis, or myositis.[3, 7, 10, 41–44] During an influenza epidemic, infected children may have rectal temperatures higher than 39.5°C and appear acutely ill with clear rhinorrhea. Erythematous pharyngitis and enlarged, boggy, and inflamed tonsils accompany the coryza, cough, and irritability. Office visits often are prompted by accompanying otitis media.[5]

In utero infection has been described. In one case, maternal fever, chills, and uterine tenderness occurred, and the virus was grown from amniotic fluid. Mother and fetus recovered; no cesarean section was required.[45] During the 1918 and 1957 influenza epidemics, the risk of death from influenza in women was substantially increased by pregnancy. However, fetal infection was uncommon.[46]

Fatal disease of the lower respiratory tract is not common in influenza but certainly occurs both as primary viral pneumonia and as secondary bacterial pneumonia.[28, 29] Primary viral pneumonia progresses rapidly, and respiratory distress may occur within 36 h of the initial onset of illness. Associated cardiac illness is common. A fanning perihilar infiltrate of a diffuse, nodular appearance is present, and pleural effusions may occur. Secondary bacterial pneumonia follows a slightly different clinical pattern. Most patients have typical influenza followed by a period of improvement and then, 2 to 14 days later, shaking chills, pleuritic pain, or productive bloody or purulent sputum accompanying secondary pneumonia. Death may occur after another 2 to 4 days in both primary viral pneumonia and secondary bacterial pneumonia. These two illnesses may not be distinguishable on clinical grounds.

Toxic shock syndrome in association with influenza virus infection was described in 1987.[47, 48] Six of the first 10 patients described died of the illness. Hypotension and fever in the absence of bacterial sepsis were common to all patients. Renal and hepatic dysfunction, thrombocytopenia, and desquamation were common. Erythroderma and mucous membrane hyperemia were seen in several patients. *Staphylococcus aureus* was grown from cultures of the respiratory secretions in most patients. Although pulmonary infiltrates and laryngotracheitis were seen, they were not the causes of death. Toxic shock syndrome toxin-1 was found in all *Staphylococcus aureus* isolates.

Influenza is one of the causes of acute infectious bronchiolitis with wheezing; it may also provoke wheezing in children with established asthma. Respiratory syncytial virus is the most common cause of bronchiolitis and other acute lower respiratory illnesses in infants that result in hospitalization; however, influenza is another etiologic agent. Among 49 asthmatic children with 128 episodes of respiratory infection, 71 (55%) of those infections were associated with asthma attacks, seven of 15 rhinovirus infections caused asthma, and four of five influenza A infections were accompanied by wheezing.[49]

The role of salicylates in the development of Reye's syndrome has now overshadowed the well-known antecedent role of influenza B and, to a lesser extent, influenza A and other viruses. Since its description in 1963, this often fatal illness has been recognized to affect children a few days after the onset of viral infection.[11] Repetitive vomiting heralds the onset of the disease. Lethargy may be followed shortly by delirium and coma. Elevated levels of plasma ammonia and serum glutamic-oxaloacetic transaminase (and, to a lesser extent, hypoglycemia) accompany the potentially lethal increase in intracranial pressure. Warnings against the use of aspirin in children with influenza and varicella infections resulted in a reduction in the incidence of this disease.

Bacterial tracheitis is a life-threatening complication of influenza infection.[50] Influenza causes croup with some regularity, and the recognition of the rapid progression of respiratory insufficiency requiring airway intervention is life-saving.[51] Unexpectedly high fever with rapidly progressive croup may help clinically differentiate viral croup from bacterial tracheitis. The discovery of an extensive pseudomembrane or extensive tracheal inflammation at the time of intubation confirms the diagnosis. *Staphylococcus aureus* is perhaps the most common etiologic agent of this complication, although *Streptococcus pyogenes* and *Haemophilus influenzae* also may be causative.

Nosocomial influenza in children may complicate the course of the illness during influenza epidemics.[42] During April 1974, 12 of 17 infants (all less than 21 months old) in one hospital ward for more than 7 days acquired nosocomial influenza A; one half of these patients shed virus for 7 to 21 days.

DIAGNOSTIC APPROACHES

The diagnosis of influenza A can be confirmed by a rise in convalescent antibody, isolation of the virus, or direct detection of virus antigens from clinical specimens. Detection of virus antigen is the most rapid method, and with high-quality reagents, the specificity of these assays has become excellent.

Humans produce antibodies reactive against several viral proteins after influenza infection or vaccination. Antibody against the hemagglutinin is typically measured in the hemagglutination inhibition assay. Levels of hemagglutinin inhibition antibody are detectable 2 weeks after infection and peak in the third week, and presence of the antibody seems to last for a lifetime, as shown in Figure 28–3. Hemagglutinin inhibition antibody is specific for hemagglutinin types (i.e., antibody to H1 does not react to H2 hemagglutinin). After a primary infection with influenza virus, each subsequent infection produces a booster antibody to the initial hemagglutinin.[52] Antibody against the nucleocapside protein, a group-specific antigen, is often measured by complement fixation assay. This complement fixing antibody specificity to nucleocapsid antigens distinguishes among influenza groups A, B, and C.

Identification of influenza virus or antigen from respiratory secretions can be accomplished by several methods, including egg inoculation, cell monolayer culture, radioimmunoassay,[53] immunofluorescence, enzyme-linked immunoassay, and time-resolved fluoroimmunoassay.

The sensitivity of cultures of virus on cell monolayers is much improved by the use of trypsin in the medium. This *in vitro* use of trypsin mimics the *in vivo* posttranslational cleavage of the hemagglutinin leaving the two-disulfide–linked subunits. Proteolytic cleavage at amino acid 328 of the hemagglutinin at the cell membrane enables a conformational change necessary for infection to occur.[54] During standard virus isolation in cell monolayers, the cells are checked for cytopathogenic effect by light microscopy and for hemabsorption every few days. With cell monolayer culture methods, most isolates are found in the first 5 days after cultures are taken. Hemabsorption for detecting virus in these cultures after only 24 h results in the early detection of only 38% of isolates.

Several techniques are being used to speed the results of

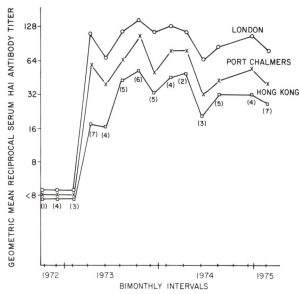

Figure 28–3. Persistence of hemagglutination inhibitory antibody after natural influenza infection (probably caused by A/London strain, January to March, 1973). Hemagglutination inhibitory antibody was tested with three strains of influenza: A/London, A/Hong Kong, and A/Port Chalmers. (From Wright PF, Ross KB, Thompson J, Karzon DT: Influenza A infections in young children: Primary natural infection and protective efficacy of live-vaccine–induced or naturally acquired immunity. N Engl J Med 296:829–834, 1977. Reprinted with permission from the *New England Journal of Medicine*, vol. 296, pp. 829–834, 1977.)

virus culture. In chamber slide assays, the inoculated cell layer on a slide is fixed at 24 h and infected cells are detected by immunofluorescent microscopy (75% as sensitive as cell culture).[55] In shell vial assays, the inoculated media and cells are centrifuged for 45 min before incubation. This step increases sensitivity; after 16 to 18 h, the cell layer is fixed, and infected cells are detected by immunofluorescent microscopy (84% as sensitive). Direct immunofluorescent microscopy of nasopharyngeal cells is a rapid method but is only 37% sensitive.[55] Enzyme-linked immunosorbent assay of nasal secretions requires less technical experience and may be more sensitive than direct immunofluorescence (53% sensitivity).[56] Time-resolved fluoroimmunoassay may detect antigen in nasopharyngeal aspirates with more (85%) sensitivity.[57] The use of pooled monoclonal mouse antisera broadly reactive to influenza A and B (prepared by the Centers for Disease Control and available since 1986) has improved the specificity of all these procedures.[58]

MANAGEMENT

In the United States, influenza is prevented by inactivated vaccine and amantidine and can be treated with amantidine. Live attenuated vaccines are used in other countries. Rimantadine, ribavirin, and interferon have not been approved for use in the treatment of influenza.

Vaccination against influenza in humans has been used since 1943. Sixty-four World Health Organization collaborating laboratories monitor influenza activity worldwide; thus antigenic changes are detected and can be incorporated into vaccines in a timely manner.[59] In 1986 and 1987, most isolates were closely related to A/Taiwan/1/86 (H1N1). Thirteen of 315 isolates were H3N2 variants. Since 1977, two influenza A strains (H1N1 and H3N2) and their antigenic variants have continued to circulate together. Both antigens are incorporated into the currently used vaccine along with influenza B antigen.

The rate of mortality from influenza is highest among the elderly. About 85% of the excess deaths from pneumonia and influenza are in persons over 65 years of age.[60] Approximately 10,000 excess deaths occur in the United States during the yearly influenza epidemic. There also is a high-risk group of children in whom influenza may further compromise respiratory status to the point of requiring hospitalization. This high-risk group includes patients with bronchopulmonary dysplasia, cystic fibrosis, severe asthma, congenital heart disease with high pulmonary flow or pressure, AIDS, and other immunodeficiency disorders with chronic pulmonary diseases. Each year the Immunization Practices Advisory Committee of the United States Public Health Service makes recommendations regarding influenza vaccine use for children, including (1) children with chronic disorders of the pulmonary or cardiovascular system (including asthma) who require regular medical follow-up or hospitalization during the preceding year; (2) children with chronic metabolic diseases (including diabetes mellitus), renal dysfunction, hemaglobinopathies, or immunosuppression; and (3) children who are receiving long-term aspirin therapy. The recommendations also pertain to health care personnel: (1) physicians, nurses, and other personnel who have extensive contact with high-risk patients (e.g., primary care and certain specialty clinicians and staff of chronic care facilities and intensive care units, particularly neonatal intensive care units) and (2) providers of home care to high-risk persons.

The efficacy of influenza vaccine in protection against clinical disease is less than that of other childhood vaccines, but it still should be given because it undoubtedly provides some measure of protection against severe or fatal disease. Children between the ages of 6 months and 3 years should be given 0.25 ml of vaccine repeated at 4 weeks. For children aged 3 to 12 years, the vaccine should be given in one dose of 0.5 ml. Older children and adults should receive the standard dose of 0.5 ml of vaccine. In subsequent years, patients should be given one dose of the appropriate vaccine. Although the vaccine is grown in egg culture, most patients who can tolerate ice cream or other egg-containing foods are able to receive the vaccine without difficulty. When there is concern about egg sensitivity, the vaccine can be used for an intradermal skin test if positive special protocols are followed.[61] It is important to give the vaccine to all family members of a child who is at high risk for the complications of influenza.

In patients with human immunodeficiency virus (HIV) infection, antibody response to influenza vaccination may not be adequately protective.[62] Only 13% to 50% (the percentage varies with the strain tested) of patients with AIDS or AIDS-related complex develop protective antibody responses. Even among asymptomatic HIV-seropositive patients, only 52% to 89% develop protective antibodies, in contrast to 94% to 100% of normal persons. Thus other measures are needed to protect these patients, such as the use of amantadine and the vaccination of health care personnel. The poor antibody response seen in patients with symptomatic AIDS and AIDS-related complex may reflect the known dependence of influenza antibody production on T cells and the decreased levels of helper (CD4) lymphocytes seen in these patients.

Live attenuated influenza vaccine holds promise of speedy production, ease in administration, and longer lasting mucosal and systemic immunity than that provided by inactivated vaccines.[63, 64] Live influenza vaccine is widely used in other countries. A unique live, cold-adapted vaccine has been tested extensively in the United States.[64] The vaccine contains a reassortment of genes between a cold-adapted strain and the wild-type virus of vaccine interest. The wild-type virus donates the genes for the two surface proteins, hemagglutinin and neuraminidase. The cold-adapted strain donates the remaining six genes for internal proteins, replicase, transcriptase, and nonstructural genes. This vaccine is immunogenic, genetically stable, and nonreactogenic in children and adults.

Intranasal interferon α, although theoretically appealing, has been less successful in the prevention of influenza A than of rhinovirus infections.[65-68] Dosages of 2 to 7 million units/day have reduced illness caused by challenge with influenza A/Eng/40/83. Four of 13 interferon users, in comparison with 10 of 17 placebo users, developed influenza symptoms.[68] Dosages of 5 million units/day for 7 days seems to be well tolerated and effective in reducing rhinovirus infections by about 85% and colds by 40%. Previously used dosages of 10 million units had resulted in unacceptable nasal irritation, and dosages of 2 million units were ineffective.[65] But at dosages of 5 million units, nasal symptoms were generally tolerable; nasal stuffiness, dryness, and tinging of nasal mucus with blood occurred in 13% of interferon users and 7% of placebo users.[67]

Amantadine has been licensed for use or approved by the Food and Drug Administration since 1966 in the United States for the prophylaxis of influenza A infections. Both amantadine and rimantadine are effective.[69, 70] When 452 volunteers received 100 mg of amantadine twice a day for 6 weeks during a natural outbreak of influenza A, laboratory-documented infection occurred in 21% of placebo users, 3% of rimantadine recipients, and 2% of amantadine recipients. Central nervous system side effects that included insomnia, jitteriness, and difficulty in concentrating occurred in 4% of placebo users, 13% of amantadine recipients, and 6% of rimantadine recipients. Both drugs have also been shown to be effective prophylactics against influenza in children.[69] Among 267 boys (aged 13 to 19 years) given amantadine (100 mg/day), only three had laboratory-proven influenza A, whereas among 269 who received no treatment, 29 had laboratory-proven infection. The low dosage of amantadine used in this study was associated with virtually no side effects.[70]

Although there is little information about the use of amantadine for preventing influenza A in children, this drug certainly should be considered for patients with severe chronic respiratory disease or disorders of the immune system. The recommended prophylactic doses are 4.4 to 8.8 mg/kg/24 h divided into two daily doses for children aged 1 to 9 years and 200 mg/24 h divided into two daily doses for children aged 9 years and older.

Amantadine is also more effective therapy for symptoms of influenza A than is aspirin.[71] During a natural outbreak of influenza B/Brazil/78 (H1N1), patients with illness of less than 2 days' duration experienced more symptomatic relief with 100 or 200 mg of amantadine than did aspirin recipients.

Amantadine seems to interfere at least in part with the low-pH membrane-fusion ability of influenza. The early events in influenza infection start with the attraction and binding of the hemagglutinin receptor site with clathrin (a 17,000-D membrane protein) coated pits on the cell surface.[15] The bound virus and membrane are rounded up into an endocytotic vesicle. This first cytoplasmic vesicle then fuses with a lysosome.[72] In the low-pH environment of the lysosome, the influenza membrane and the lysosomal membrane undergo a conformational change that enables fusion of the two membranes and eventual release of the virus internal components into the cytoplasm. A low-pH–induced conformational change in the hemagglutinin causes the fusion amino acid sequence to move outward from its usual interior location to at least the 3.5 nm needed for this sequence to be exposed to the exterior.[73, 74]

SUMMARY

Influenza is a major respiratory pathogen in children as well as in adults. Each year, an epidemic is caused by an influenza A virus whose antigenicity is different from that of the strain of the previous year. Molecular biologists have delineated the exact structures responsible for this change in antigenicity and perhaps even their origins. Children experience the primary infection with this virus during the first few years of life after a short period of protection provided by maternal antibody. A self-limited febrile respiratory illness occurs in the majority of children. The cytokines produced as part of the host response may also be responsible for many of the obvious disease symptoms (fever, myalgia, and fatigue). Some patients sustain serious respiratory injury with bronchiolitis, croup, pneumonia, bacterial tracheitis, and bacterial pneumonia. Children with already compromised respiratory status (such as patients with bronchopulmonary dysplasia, severe asthma, cystic fibrosis, immunodeficiency, or cardiac disease) may develop acute respiratory failure. Other organ systems may also be attacked with resultant encephalitis, Reye's syndrome, myocarditis, and myositis. This first experience with influenza results in significant immunity until the virus undergoes the next major shift in antigenic structure.

Inactivated vaccine and amantadine are readily available and effective in the prevention of influenza. Treatment with amantadine is also effective. These treatment and prevention methods are largely underused. Perhaps this underusage is attributable in part to lack of specific, rapid methods for confirming the exact identity of the virus responsible for the patients' symptoms. Timely identification of influenza virus as a cause of illness may result in more widespread use of the influenza vaccine during childhood.

REFERENCES

1. Stuart-Harris CH, Potter CW: The Molecular Virology and Epidemiology of Influenza, p. 1. London: Academic Press, 1984.
2. Glezen WP, Denny FW: Epidemiology of acute lower respiratory disease in children. N Engl J Med 288:498–505, 1973.
3. Glezen WP, Paredes A, Taber LH: Influenza in children: Relationship to other respiratory agents. JAMA 243:1345–1349, 1980.
4. Hall CE, Cooney MK, Fox JP: The Seattle virus watch study: IV. Comparative epidemiologic observations of infections with influenza A and B viruses in 1965–69 in families with young children. Am J Epidemiol 98:365–380, 1973.
5. Henderson RW, Collier AM, Sanyal MA, et al: A longitudinal study of respiratory viruses and bacteria in the etiology of acute otitis media with effusion. N Engl J Med 306:1377–1383, 1982.
6. Kim HW, Brandt CD, Arrobio JO, et al: Influenza A and B virus infection in infants and young children during the years 1957–1976. Am J Epidemiol 109:464–479, 1979.
7. Francis T Jr: A new type of virus from epidemic influenza. Science 92:405–408, 1940.
8. Magill TP: A virus from cases of influenza-like upper respiratory infection. Proc Soc Exp Biol Med 45:162–164, 1940.
9. Stuart-Harris CH, Schild GC, Oxford JS: Influenza, the Viruses and the Disease, 2nd ed, pp. 7–40. London: Arnold, 1985.
10. Middleton PJ, Alexander RM, Szymanski MT: Severe myositis during recovery from influenza. Lancet 2:533–535, 1970.
11. Ruben FL, Michaels RH: Reye syndrome with associated influenza A and B infection. JAMA 234:410–412, 1975.
12. Taylor RM: Studies on survival of influenza virus between epidemics and antigenic variants of the virus. Am J Public Health 39:171–178, 1949.
13. Kilbourne ED: Viral structure and composition. In Kilbourne ED (ed): Influenza, pp. 33–56. New York: Plenum Press, 1987.
14. Scholtissek C, Rohde W, Von Hoyningen V, Rott R: On the origin of the human influenza virus subtypes H2N2 and H3N2. Virology 87:13–20, 1978.

15. Lazarovits J, Roth M: A single amino acid change in the cytoplasmic domain allows the influenza virus hemagglutinin to be endocytosed through coated pits. Cell 53:743–752, 1988.

16. Colman PM, Varghese JN, Laver WG: Structure of the catalytic and antigenic sites in influenza virus neuraminidase. Nature 303:41–44, 1983.

17. Varghese JN, Laver WG, Colman PM: Structure of the influenza virus glycoprotein antigen neuraminidase at 2.9 A resolution. Nature 303:35–40, 1983.

18. Beutler B: The presence of chachectin/tumor necrosis factor in human disease states. Am J Med 85:287–288, 1988.

19. Dinarello CA: The biology of interleukin 1 and comparison to tumor necrosis factor. Immunol Lett 16:227–231, 1987.

20. Beutler B, Krochin N, Milsark IW, et al: Induction of cachetin (tumor necrosis factor) synthesis by influenza virus: Deficient production by endotoxin-resistant (C3H/HeJ) macrophages (abstr). Clin Res 34:491a, 1986.

21. Lahdevirta J, Maury CPJ, Teppo A, Repo H: Elevated levels of circulating cachectin/tumor necrosis factor in patients with acquired immunodeficiency syndrome. Am J Med 85:289–291, 1988.

22. Carroll MC, Katzman P, Alicot EM, et al: Linkage map of the human major histocompatibility complex including the tumor necrosis factor genes. Proc Natl Acad Sci USA 84:8535–8539, 1987.

23. Mestan J, Digel W, Mittnacht S, et al: Antiviral effects of recombinant tumor necrosis factor in vitro. Nature 323:816–819, 1986.

24. Wong GHW, Goeddel DV: Tumor necrosis factors alpha and beta inhibit virus replication and synergize with interferons. Nature 323:819–822, 1986.

25. Giles C, Shuttleworth EM: Post-mortem findings in 46 influenza deaths. Lancet 2:1224–1225, 1957.

26. Hers JF Ph, Goslings WRO, Masurel N, Mulder J: Death from Asiatic influenza in the Netherlands. Lancet 2:1164–1165, 1957.

27. Hers JF Ph, Masurel N, Mulder J: Bacteriology and histopathology of the respiratory tract and lungs in fatal Asian influenza. Lancet 2:1141–1143, 1958.

28. Louria DB, Blumenfeld HL, Ellis JT, et al: Studies on influenza in the pandemic of 1957–1958: II. Pulmonary complications of influenza. J Clin Invest 38:213–265, 1959.

29. Martin CM, Kunin CM, Gottlieb LS, et al: Asian influenza A in Boston, 1957–1958. Arch Int Med 103:515–531, 1959.

30. Walsh JJ, Dietlein LF, Low FN, et al: Bronchotracheal response in human influenza. Arch Intern Med 108:376–388, 1961.

31. Hers JF: The Histopathology of the Respiratory Tract in Human Influenza. Leiden, The Netherlands: Stenfert Kroese, 1955.

32. Smith H, Sweet C: Lessons for human influenza from pathogenicity studies with ferrets. Rev Infect Dis 10:56–75, 1988.

33. Empey DW, Laitinen LW, Jacobs L, et al: Mechanisms of bronchial hyperreactivity in normal subjects after upper respiratory tract infection. Am Rev Respir Dis 113:131–139, 1976.

34. Hall WJ, Douglas RG Jr, Hyde RW: Pulmonary mechanics after uncomplicated influenza A infection. Am Rev Respir Dis 113:141–148, 1976.

35. Little JW, Hall WJ, Douglas RG Jr, et al: Airway hyperreactivity and peripheral airway dysfunction in influenza A infection. Am Rev Respir Dis 118:295–303, 1978.

36. Abramson JS, Mills EL, Giebink GS, Quie PG: Depression of monocyte and polymorphonuclear leukocyte oxidative metabolism and bactericidal capacity by influenza A virus. Infect Immun 35:350–355, 1982.

37. Cassidy LF, Lyles DS, Abramson JS: Synthesis of viral proteins in polymorphonuclear leukocytes infected with influenza A virus. J Clin Microbiol 26:1267–1270, 1988.

38. Puck JM, Glezen WP, Frank AL, Six HR: Protection of infants from infection with influenza A virus by transplacentally acquired antibody. J Infect Dis 142:844–849, 1980.

39. Hoskins TW, Davies JR, Smith AJ, et al: Assessment of inactivated influenza-A vaccine after three outbreaks of influenza A at Christ's Hospital. Lancet 1:33–35, 1979.

40. Chakraverty P, Cunningham P, Pereira MS: The return of the historic influenza A H1N1 virus and its impact on the population of the United Kingdom. J Hyg (Lond) 89:89–100, 1982.

41. Brocklebank JT, Court SD, McQuillin J, Gardner PS: Influenza A infection in children. Lancet 2:497–500, 1972.

42. Hall CB, Douglas RG Jr: Nosocomial influenza infection as a cause of intercurrent fevers in infants. Pediatrics 55:673–677, 1975.

43. Paisley JW, Bruhn FW, Lauer BA, et al: Type A2 influenza viral infections in children. Am J Dis Child 132:34–36, 1978.

44. Price DA, Postlethwaite RJ, Longson M: Influenzavirus A2 infections presenting with febrile convulsions and gastrointestinal symptoms in young children. Clin Pediatr 15:361–367, 1976.

45. McGregor JA, Burns JC, Levin MJ, et al: Transplacental passage of influenza A/Bangkok (H3N2) mimicking amniotic fluid infection syndrome. Am J Obstet Gynecol 149:856–859, 1984.

46. Kort BA, Cefalo RC, Baker VV: Fatal influenza A pneumonia in pregnancy. Am J Perinatol 3:179–182, 1986.

47. MacDonald KL, Osterholm MT, Hedberg CW, et al: Toxic shock syndrome. A newly recognized complication of influenza and influenzalike illness. JAMA 257:1053–1058, 1987.

48. Sperber SJ, Francis JB: Toxic shock syndrome during an influenza outbreak. JAMA 257:1086–1087, 1987.

49. Minor TE, Dick EC, Baker JW, et al: Rhinovirus and influenza type A infections as precipitants of asthma. Am Rev Respir Dis 113:149–153, 1976.

50. Edwards KM, Dundon MC, Altemeier WA: Bacterial tracheitis as a complication of viral croup. Pediatr Infect Dis 2:390–391, 1983.

51. Howard JB, McCracken GH Jr, Luby JP: Influenza A2 virus as a cause of croup requiring tracheostomy. J Pediatr 81:1148–1150, 1972.

52. Wright PF, Ross KB, Thompson J, Karzon DT: Influenza A infections in young children: Primary natural infection and protective efficacy of live-vaccine–induced or naturally acquired immunity. N Engl J Med 296:829–834, 1977.

53. Sarkkinen HK, Halonen PE, Salmi AA: Detection of influenza A virus by radioimmunoassay and enzyme immunoassay from nasopharyngeal specimens. J Med Virol 7:213–220, 1981.

54. Lazarowitz SG, Goldberg AR, Choppin PW: Proteolytic cleavage by plasmin of the HA polypeptide of influenza virus: Host cell activation of serum plasminogen. Virology 56:172–180, 1973.

55. Stokes CE, Bernstein JM, Kyger SA, Hayden FG: Rapid diagnosis of influenza A and B by 24-h fluorescent focus assays. J Clin Microbiol 26:1263–1266, 1988.

56. Harmon MW, Pawlik KM: Enzyme immunoassay for direct detection of influenza type A and adenovirus antigens in clinical specimens. J Clin Microbiol 15:5–11, 1982.

57. Walls HH, Johansson KH, Harmon MW, et al: Time-resolved fluoroimmunoassay with monoclonal antibodies for rapid diagnosis of influenza infections. J Clin Microbiol 24:907–912, 1986.

58. Walls HH, Harmon MW, Slagle JJ, et al: Characterization and evaluation of monoclonal antibodies developed for typing influenza A and influenza B viruses. J Clin Microbiol 23:240–245, 1986.

59. Centers for Disease Control: Influenza—United States, 1986–87 season. MMWR 37:466–470, 475, 1988.

60. Immunization practices advisory committee: Prevention and control of influenza. MMWR 37:361–364, 1988.

61. Herman JJ, Radin R, Schneiderman R: Allergic reactions to measles (rubeola) vaccine in patients hypersensitive to egg protein. J Pediatr 102:196–199, 1983.

62. Nelson KE, Clements ML, Miotti P, et al: The influence of human immunodeficiency virus (HIV) infection on antibody responses to influenza vaccines. Ann Intern Med 109:383–388, 1988.

63. Clements ML, Betts RF, Murphy BR: Advantage of live attenuated cold-adapted influenza A virus over inactivated vaccine for A/Washington/80 (H3N2) wild-type virus infection. Lancet 1:705–708, 1984.

64. Johnson PR, Feldman S, Thompson JM, et al: Immunity to influenza A virus infection in young children: A comparison of natural infection, live cold-adapted vaccine, and inactivated vaccine. J Infect Dis 154:121–127, 1986.

65. Douglas RM, Albrecht JK, Miles HB, et al: Intranasal interferon alpha 2 prophylaxis of natural respiratory virus infection. J Infect Dis 151:731–736, 1985.

66. Douglas RM, Moore BW, Miles HB, et al: Prophylactic efficacy of intranasal alpha2-interferon against rhinovirus infections in the family setting. N Engl J Med 314:65–70, 1986.

67. Hayden FG, Albrecht JK, Kaiser DL, Gwaltney JM: Prevention of natural colds by contact prophylaxis with intranasal alpha2-interferon. N Engl J Med 314:71–75, 1986.

68. Phillpotts RJ, Higgins PG, Willman JS, et al: Intranasal lymphoblastoid interferon ("Wellferon") prophylaxis against rhinovirus and influenza virus in volunteers. J Interferon Res 4:535–541, 1984.

69. Dolin R, Reichman RC, Madore HP, et al: A controlled trial of amantadine and rimantadine in the prophylaxis of influenza A infection. N Engl J Med 307:580–584, 1982.
70. Payler DK, Purdham PA: Influenza A prophylaxis with amantadine in a boarding school. Lancet 1:502–504, 1984.
71. Younkin SW, Betts RF, Roth FK, Douglas RG Jr: Reduction in fever and symptoms in young adults with influenza A/Brazil/78 H1N1 infection after treatment with aspirin or amantadine. Antimicrob Agents Chemother 23:577–582, 1983.
72. Yoshimura A, Ohnishi SI: Uncoating of influenza virus in endosomes. J Virol 51:497–504, 1984.
73. Daniels RS, Downie JC, Hay AJ, et al: Fusion mutants of the influenza virus hemagglutinin glycoprotein. Cell 40:431–439, 1985.
74. Skehel JJ, Bayley PM, Brown EB, et al: Changes in the conformation of influenza virus hemagglutinin at the pH optimum of virus-mediated membrane fusion. Proc Natl Acad Sci USA 79:968–972, 1982.

29 LUNG ABSCESS

PRESTON W. CAMPBELL III, M.D.

A lung abscess is a circumscribed, thick-walled cavity containing purulent material. It is the result of complex interaction between an overwhelmed or impaired pulmonary host defense system and pyogenic organisms that cause pulmonary suppuration and parenchymal necrosis. Before the advent of antibiotics, lung abscess was relatively common, but its incidence subsequently decreased.[1] This is a result not only of appropriate antibiotic use, but also of a better understanding of the need to protect the airways of normal persons during procedures involving anesthesia, during dental procedures, and during episodes of altered consciousness. Lung abscess is less common in children than in adults. Chart reviews of children from Toronto (83 cases in 19 years),[2] Dallas (20 cases in 20 years),[3] and Montreal (31 cases in 18 years),[4] who had lung abscesses give an indication of its incidence in children since the advent of antibiotics.

Lung abscesses have traditionally been classified as either primary or secondary.[2] A primary abscess is one occurring in an otherwise healthy child. Lung abscesses occurring in children with pre-existing conditions such as cystic fibrosis, endocarditis, nephrotic syndrome, immunosuppression and in children after surgery are defined as secondary.

Although lung abscess in adults has been extensively reviewed,[5-10] there have been few studies in infants and children.[2, 4, 11, 12] The limited number of pediatric patients available for controlled studies has precluded definitive studies.

PATHOGENESIS AND ETIOLOGY

Microbes have access to the lung by at least four routes (Table 29–1): postpneumonic, hematogenous spread, direct extension or contamination, and aspiration. The list of organisms causing pneumonia with lung abscess spans the microbiologic spectrum, but *Staphylococcus aureus* has been the most common. In staphylococcal pneumonia, a segmental or lobar pneumonia is initially seen, and pleural effusions develop in a large percentage of patients.[13] Pulmonary pneumatoceles are seen after the early stages of pneumonia in as many as 85% of patients.[14] Pneumatoceles are usually small and thin walled with multiple cystic, air-filled cavities that result from alveolar and bronchiolar necrosis. Pyopneumothorax can also occur, and its presence is suggestive of staphylococcal disease.[2] Unlike pneumatoceles, lung abscesses are large (more than 2 cm in diameter) areas of necrosis with suppuration manifested by a ragged, thick-walled, fluid-filled cavity. Multiple abscesses can occur. It is unknown whether viral infections predispose the lung to lung abscess, but abscesses caused by *S. aureus* occur frequently during influenza epidemics.[15]

The more common pediatric bacterial pneumonias rarely cause lung abscesses.[2, 3, 16, 17] For example, pneumococcal pneumonia is a rare cause of lung abscess, although cases continue to be described.[18] Before routine *Haemophilus influenzae* vaccination, reports suggested that the prevalence of pneumonia caused by *H. influenzae* (almost always type B) was increasing among young children,[19-21] but lung abscesses remain a rare complication of infection with this organism.[18, 22]

Pneumonia caused by gram-negative enteric bacteria occurs mainly in newborns and older children who are immunosuppressed, but it rarely occurs in older normal children. Of these, *Klebsiella pneumoniae* causes particularly severe disease, and necrosis of lung parenchyma with abscess formation is common. *Pseudomonas aeruginosa* pneumonia occurs primarily in children with cystic fibrosis and rarely causes lung abscess.[23] Uncommon infections, including histoplasmosis, tuberculosis, coccidioidomycosis, aspergillosis, glanders, and *Legionella pneumophila*[24] pneumonia, may also result in lung abscess. Immunocompromised patients are more likely than normal persons to harbor unusual organisms.[25]

Table 29–1. ORIGINS OF LUNG ABSCESS IN CHILDREN

Postpneumonic
Pyogenic organisms (*Staphylococcus aureus, Klebsiella pneumoniae, Pseudomonas* species, others)
Tuberculosis
Fungal (*Histoplasma capsulatum, Coccidioides immitis, Aspergillus fumigatus*)
Actinomycetes
Hematogenous Spread
Bacteremia with seeding of lungs (*S. aureus*, gram-negative organisms, salmonellosis, *Yersinia*)
Emboli from phlebitis
Embolic septic thrombosis from an indwelling central catheter (coagulase-positive and coagulase-negative staphylococci and gram-negative organisms)
Endocarditis of the right side of the heart with septic embolization gram negative aerobic bacilli (*Streptococcus viridans, S. aureus, Staphylococcus epidermidis*)
Direct Extension or Contamination
Liver abscess (pyogenic and amebic)
Osteomyelitis of ribs or vertebrae
Penetrating injuries of the chest
Pulmonary surgery
Aspiration
Acute or chronic aspiration of oropharyngeal secretions (see Table 29–2)
Aspiration of foreign body
Other Associated Predisposing Conditions
Secondary infection of congenital lung cyst, lobar emphysema, bronchial stenosis, or sequestrated lobe
Immunodeficiency or immunosuppression
Benign pulmonary neoplasm (rare)

Hematogenous dissemination of microorganisms may cause lung abscess. Specific conditions place the lung at risk for septic emboli from infected peripheral systemic veins or septic thromboses from indwelling central catheters. Coagulase-positive and coagulase-negative staphylococci and the gram-negative enteric organisms are the organisms usually isolated in these cases. Endocarditis involving the right side of the heart may also result in septic emboli to the lung. Almost all affected children have some structural abnormality of the heart. Streptococci, staphylococci, gram-negative organisms, and fungi (in decreasing order of frequency) are the responsible microorganisms in children with endocarditis. Lung abscess may occur many weeks after an episode of clinical salmonellosis. In rare instances, lung abscess caused by *Yersinia enterocolitica* has been described in children.[26] Whatever their source, abscesses resulting from hematogenous spread are usually small, are often multiple, and are located in the subpleural zones of the lungs.[17]

In rare cases, organisms gain access to the lung parenchyma by direct extension, as with a liver abscess, in which the transmission occurs across the diaphragm or by way of the lymphatic vessels. *S. aureus* (33%) and gram-negative organisms (32%) have been the predominant isolates in children with liver abscesses,[27] although anaerobes are common as well. Amebic liver abscesses may also rupture into the lung. In the latter case, the sputum is reddish brown, has no foul odor, and contains trophozoites of *Entamoeba histolytica*. Finally, additional causes of lung abscess from extension or contamination include infections of the bony thorax and penetrating injuries of the chest.

Aspiration of oropharyngeal contents is the most common cause of lung abscess in adults and certainly plays a significant role in predisposed children as well (Table 29–2). This is understandable in view of the enormous bacterial load contained even in minute amounts of oropharyngeal secretions. For example, saliva contains about 10^6 to 10^9 bacteria per milliliter; 1000 times that amount of bacteria is found in the gingival crevices.[28] In contrast, inhalation of air, containing 15 organisms per cubic meter, for 1 h introduces approximately 10 organisms into the lungs.[29] Therefore, children who aspirate are at increased risk of lung abscess, and the involved organisms are those colonizing the oropharynx. Although most people occasionally aspirate scant amounts of oropharyngeal secretions, the aspirated pathogens are usually cleared by cough, mucociliary transport, and alveolar macrophages. In a few children, the bacterial load is overwhelming, resulting in pneumonia and subsequent lung abscess.

Brock[30] demonstrated that aspirated material flows by gravity into the dependent areas of the lung. Thus which lobe is affected depends on the patient's position at the time of aspiration. In the supine position, the posterior segments of the upper lobes and the apical segments of the lower lobes are those most severely affected. Abscesses are more common in the right lung, probably because of the less acute angle of the right main stem bronchus. Because most patients are supine when aspiration occurs, the most commonly affected lobes are the right and left upper lobes and the apical segments of both lower lobes.[8, 31, 32]

The organisms involved in aspiration pneumonia are those colonizing the oropharynx. Various studies have shown that anaerobic bacteria play a role in lung abscess.[11, 33, 34] Brook and Finegold,[11] using percutaneous transtracheal aspirates in children with lung abscesses, demonstrated the polymicrobial nature of these infections, including both aerobic and anaerobic organisms. The most common anaerobic isolates were *Peptostreptococcus, Bacteroides melaninogenicus, Peptococcus, Veillonella,* and *Fusobacterium nucleatum*. These organisms are remarkably similar to anaerobic isolates previously described in adults.[32] A number of aerobic and facultative organisms were also isolated including α-hemolytic streptococci, group A β-hemolytic streptococci, Group D streptococci, *S. aureus, Escherichia coli, K. pneumoniae, P. aeruginosa, Serratia marcescens,* and *Eikenella corrodens*. There is an important difference in bacterial etiology, depending on whether the patient aspirates in the hospital or in the community environment.[28, 35, 36] Aspiration occurring in the community yields primarily

Table 29–2. CONDITIONS PREDISPOSING TO ASPIRATION LUNG ABSCESS

Coma
Seizures
Mental retardation
Swallowing dysfunction
Absent epiglottic reflex
General anesthesia
Oropharyngeal or dental surgery
Tracheoesophageal fistula
Gastroesophageal reflux
Drowning

anaerobic disease, whereas various aerobic and facultative nosocomial pathogens such as *S. aureus, Klebsiella, Pseudomonas,* and *Proteus* species are more likely to be isolated from aspiration occurring in the hospital.

PATHOLOGY

Regardless of the route of infection, the initial event in the development of lung abscess is pneumonitis. In an attempt to control the infection, inflammatory cells, predominantly polymorphonuclear cells, migrate to the infection area; this migration eventually leads to tissue destruction. Studies in experimental animals indicate that 7 to 14 days elapse between bacterial challenge and the pathologic appearance of pulmonary abscess.[37] The extension of infection continues until the abscess is walled off by fibrous and granulation tissue and drainage into the bronchi or pleural space occurs.[17] Bronchial collateral vessels form a dense vascular plexus around the cavity, aiding in resolution and repair.[16] As healing progresses, the lining granulation tissue is replaced by ciliated epithelial cells, which grow in from the bronchi draining the cavity.

CLINICAL MANIFESTATION

The clinical manifestation of a lung abscess varies, depending on the patient's condition and the etiologic agent. Table 29–3 summarizes symptoms.[2, 4, 38] In most cases, the early manifestations are those of pneumonia, characterized by fever, anorexia, and cough. The course can be acute, subacute, or chronic. Lung abscess is often not suspected until sequential chest radiographs document its development. When the course has been indolent and treatment is delayed, weight loss is usual. Pleuritic chest pain is relatively common, and pleural thickening over the abscess is seen in most patients. With the communication of the abscess with the bronchial tree, the cough in older children becomes productive, with bloody or purulent sputum. The child may report the sensation of a bad taste or have foul breath. Although not always present, a putrid odor is diagnostic of an anaerobic infection.[32, 39] Occasionally, the course is fulminant.

Physical examination of the chest early in the course yields findings identical to those seen in consolidating pneumonia, including decreased breath sounds and ipsilateral crackles. Although 50% of adults develop empyema, it is less common in children.[3, 4, 38] Laboratory tests

Table 29–3. CLINICAL MANIFESTATIONS

Symptom	Percentage of Patients	No. of Patients/ Total
Fever	98%	46/47
Anorexia	84%	33/39
Cough	74%	35/47
Sputum production	50%	11/22
Chest pain	40%	19/47
Weight loss	30%	14/47

Compiled from data of Asher et al.,[4] Kosloske et al.,[38] and Mark and Turner.[2]

are usually nonspecific, but an elevated erythrocyte sedimentation rate and leukocytosis are often found.

DIAGNOSIS AND DIFFERENTIAL DIAGNOSIS

The typical lung abscess is diagnosed by means of chest radiograph, which reveals the classic thick-walled, fluid-filled cavity larger than 2 cm in diameter (Fig. 29–1*A*). Computed tomography (CT) of the chest with contrast and magnetic resonance imaging can localize abscesses and distinguish them from similar-appearing lesions such as congenital lung cysts (Fig. 29–1*B*). According to Mayer and co-authors,[40] features on CT that characterize lung abscess are (1) the well-marginated nature of the mass; (2) a sharp angle between the mass and the pleura, suggestive of the parenchymal nature of the lesion; (3) a density higher than that of water or simple pleural fluid; and (4) contrast enhancement that displays increased density in the tissues around the mass without a change in density centrally. Lesions that can be confused with a lung abscess include pneumatoceles, bronchogenic cysts, congenital pulmonary cysts, loculated empyema, and congenital lobar emphysema. On occasion, the physical findings and imaging studies are suggestive of a primary malignancy.[41]

MANAGEMENT

BACTERIAL DIAGNOSIS

Extended, appropriate antimicrobial therapy is recommended for abscess therapy. The choice of antibiotics depends on the source of infection and is guided by stains and cultures from uncontaminated specimens. These cultures are particularly helpful in aspiration pneumonia, in which the infection is likely to be polymicrobial, and in immunocompromised patients, in whom unusual organisms are seen. Unfortunately, sputum is an unsatisfactory guide for antibiotic therapy because of contamination by oropharyngeal microorganisms. In cultures of anaerobes, the only valid specimens are blood, pleural fluid, transtracheal aspirates, transthoracic pulmonary aspirates, specimens obtained at thoracotomy, and fiberoptic bronchoscopic aspirates obtained through the use of the protected brush.[31]

Although not particularly sensitive, blood cultures should be obtained routinely in all cases of lung abscess. Pleural fluid is the obvious culture source in patients with empyema. Endotracheal aspirates, like expectorated sputum, are contaminated by oropharyngeal organisms but occasionally yield valuable information. Another technique, percutaneous transtracheal aspiration, has been used by Finegold and others.[11, 42–45] It is safe and reliable when used by experienced clinicians. Transthoracic pulmonary aspirates (lung puncture) have been used primarily for diagnosis in peripherally located, consolidated pneumonias, but the benefit of this procedure for lung abscess is unclear. Potential complications include pulmonary hemorrhage or pneumonothorax. Bronchoscopic techniques with the use of protected brushes in

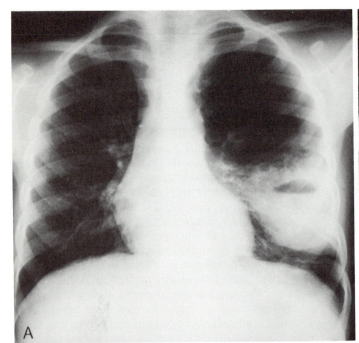

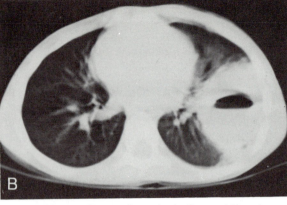

Figure 29–1. *A,* Chest radiograph of a 6-year-old boy demonstrates a thick-walled cavity in the left lower lobe with an air-fluid level. *B,* Computed tomogram of the chest demonstrates the same lesion and gives additional information regarding the amount of lung involved. *C,* Same lesion 5 weeks later, demonstrating significant resolution.

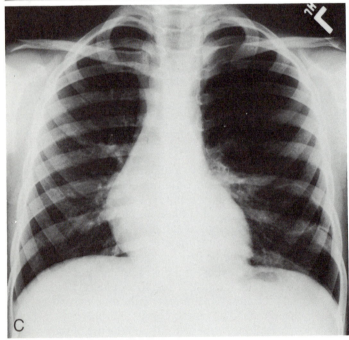

older children to prevent upper airway contamination have been described.[46,47] Specimens should be transported to the laboratory immediately under oxygen-free conditions for aerobic and anaerobic cultures.

ANTIMICROBIAL THERAPY

When *S. aureus* is involved, the treatment of choice is a penicillinase-resistant penicillin: a first- or second-generation cephalosporin or clindamycin. Methicillin-resistant *S. aureus* should be treated with vancomycin. If gram-negative coliforms are involved, aminoglycosides or cephalosporins are preferred.

The first large-scale prospective comparison of antibiotic regimens for the treatment of anaerobic lung abscess was reported in 1983 by Levison and co-workers,[48] who evaluated intravenous penicillin G and clindamycin. Patients treated with clindamycin had a shorter febrile period and produced fetid sputum on fewer days than did patients treated with penicillin G. Five of 11 penicillin-treated patients failed treatment, whereas none of the 10 clindamycin-treated patients failed treatment ($p < 0.01$). This study cast doubt on the position of penicillin G as the drug of choice for anaerobic pulmonary infections. Increasing resistance to penicillin among *Bacteroides* species may explain these results. Clindamycin (30 mg/kg/day given every 6 to 8 h intravenously, intramuscularly, or orally) is appropriate coverage both for anaerobes and for *S. aureus.* Nonetheless, some authorities still prefer penicillin on the basis of its historical pivotal position and its reduced cost and side effects. Penicillin given in 150,000 to 250,000 units/kg/day in equally divided doses every 4 h must be given in order to cover the anaerobic streptococci. Whenever penicillin is used in the presence of *Bacteroides* species, chloramphenicol or metronidazole must be added. Although metronidazole has excellent activity against all anaerobes, its use as a single agent has been associated with a high failure rate, probably because of its lack of activity against contributing aerobic and microaerophilic streptococci.

Antibiotics are usually given for extended periods of at least 2 to 4 weeks. Therapy must be tailored to clinical and radiographic improvement. Although oral antibiotics have been shown to be effective,[49] parenteral antibiotics are recommended until defervescence occurs, which usually follows 7 to 10 days of treatment.[30, 31] Prolonged fever suggests inadequate microbial coverage or inadequate drainage of the abscess.

ANCILLARY TREATMENT MODALITIES

Drainage of the abscess usually occurs through bronchial connections and may be maximized by using postural drainage. Positioning of the patient depends on the location of the cavity. If possible, the patient is taught to sleep in a position that facilitates drainage. Coughing is encouraged. More invasive modalities for draining the abscess are controversial[4] and should be reserved for atypical cases that are unresponsive to conservative treatment.

Bronchoscopy is indicated when aspiration of a foreign body is suspected, but convincing support of its routine use in facilitating drainage is lacking. Mark and Turner,[2] in their series of lung abscess in 83 children, noted that bronchoscopy did not alter the course. In some cases, bronchoscopic access to the cavity and, therefore, drainage of the cavity are precluded by inflammation and edema of the bronchus. In these circumstances, the passage of angiographic catheters through the bronchoscope into the abscess under fluoroscopic control can establish drainage and be used to obtain material for culture.[50-52] The catheter can be left in place for irrigation and drainage over extended periods if necessary.[53] Bronchoscopy is not without risks, however, and massive intrabronchial aspiration of the abscess contents has been described.[54] To prevent this complication, Hammer and co-authors[54] suggested the following precautions: (1) minimal prebronchoscopic sedation; (2) judicious use of topical lidocaine (Xylocaine) anesthesia in an effort to maintain some degree of the gag-and-cough reflex; (3) avoidance of manipulation of the abscess by the catheter or the forceps for biopsy; (4) observation in an intensive care unit for a period of up to 6 h after the bronchoscopic procedures; and (5) placement of the patient in the lateral position (with the affected lung dependent) until complete return of the gag-and-cough reflex, in an effort to prevent intrabronchial aspiration of infected material.

Surgery is rarely needed, but it may be life-saving in special circumstances. Transthoracic drainage by percu-taneous tube drainage may avoid thoracotomy and resection in acute illness that has been refractory to medical treatment.[55-58] Potential complications of transthoracic drainage include empyema and bronchopleural fistula,[7, 38] but with proper precautions, these are infrequent. Most children demonstrate clinical improvement after this approach, and thoracotomy is unnecessary. Thoracotomy should be reserved for children unresponsive to medical treatment and drainage by other means, for chronic abscess lasting longer than 3 months, for life-threatening hemoptysis, for bronchial stenosis, for significant bronchiectasis, and for massive pulmonary necrosis.[8, 56, 59, 60]

The experience of Bartlett and associates[61] and of Asher and colleagues[4] suggests that a conservative approach in primary lung abscess is warranted. Welch[60] suggested that earlier intervention is required in patients who are immunocompromised or have chronic medical conditions (i.e., transplant patients, oncology patients, and patients with inflammatory bowel disease) because the mortality rate is close to 20% in this already vulnerable group of patients.[62] Finally, Siegel and McCracken[53] suggested that surgical intervention is usually required in infants 8 weeks of age or younger because of the more virulent organisms that cause disease, because of diminished host resistance in this age group, and because of the possibility of anatomic malformations that may require surgical attention.

PROGNOSIS

An excellent outcome should be expected in children with primary lung abscess. The mortality rate, according to data compiled from pediatric reviews,[2-4, 11] is 3%. Most children are asymptomatic within several weeks, although the cavity resolves slowly. After effective treatment is begun, 13% of cavities disappear by 2 weeks, 44% by 4 weeks, 59% by 6 weeks, and 70% by 3 months.[63] Larger cavities and cavities in the right upper lobe resolve more slowly. The incidence of residual focal fibrocystic or bronchiectatic changes is about 80% when the diameter of the abscess is more than 4 cm.[64] In an evaluation of clinical status, lung volumes, and expiratory flow rates in children 9 years after treatment for primary lung abscess, Asher and colleagues[4] concluded that changes are probably insignificant; they found no abnormalities related to the disease.

The prognosis of secondary abscesses is variable and depends on the underlying condition. In a Toronto series, 54 of 58 patients with secondary lung abscess died, but the diagnosis of lung abscess was made post mortem in most cases.[2] In a Dallas series, 5 of 17 died.[3] In both series, fatalities were related to the underlying disease.

REFERENCES

1. Schweppe H, Knowles J, Kane L: Lung abscess: An analysis of the Massachusetts General Hospital cures from 1943 through 1956. N Engl J Med 265:1039–1043, 1961.
2. Mark PH, Turner JA: Lung abscess in childhood. Thorax 23:216–220, 1968.

3. McCracken GH Jr: Lung abscess in childhood. Hosp Pract 13(8):35–36, 1978.
4. Asher M, Spier S, Beland M, et al: Primary lung abscess in childhood: The long-term outcome of conservative management. Am J Dis Child 136:491–494, 1982.
5. Bartlett J: Anaerobic bacterial infections of the lung. Chest 91:901–909, 1987.
6. Bartlett JG: Lung abscess. In Baum GL, Wolinsky E (eds): Textbook of Pulmonary Disease, pp. 595–604. Boston: Little Brown, 1983.
7. Estrera A, Platt M, Mills L, et al: Primary lung abscess. J Thorac Cardiovasc Surg 79:275–282, 1980.
8. Gopalakrishna K, Lerner P: Primary lung abscess: Analysis of 66 cases. Cleve Clin Q 42:3–13, 1975.
9. Perlman L, Lerner E, D'Esopo N: Clinical classification and analysis of 97 cases of lung abscess. Am Rev Respir Dis 99:390–398, 1969.
10. Pohlson E, McNamara J, Char C, et al: Lung abscess: A changing pattern of the disease. Am J Surg 150:97–101, 1985.
11. Brook I, Finegold S: Bacteriology and therapy of lung abscess in children. J Pediatr 94:10–12, 1979.
12. Levine M, Ashman R, Heald F: Anaerobic (putrid) lung abscess in adolescence. Am J Dis Child 130:77–81, 1976.
13. Rebhan AW, Edwards HE: Staphylococcal pneumonia: A review of 329 cases. Canad Med Assoc J 82:513–517, 1960.
14. Hendren WH, Haggerty RJ: Staphylococcic pneumonia in infancy and childhood: Analysis of 75 cases. JAMA 168:6–16, 1958.
15. Asher M, Beaudry P: Lung abscess. In Kendig G, Chernick V (eds): Diseases of the Respiratory Tract in Children, 4th ed, pp. 369–375. Philadelphia: WB Saunders, 1983.
16. Charan N, Turk M, Dhand R: The role of bronchial circulation in lung abscess. Am Rev Respir Dis 131:121–124, 1985.
17. Spencer H: Lung abscesses. In Spencer H (ed): Pathology of the Lung, pp. 317–326. Philadelphia: WB Saunders, 1986.
18. Yangco B, Deresinski S: Necrotizing or cavitating pneumonia due to Streptococcus pneumoniae: Report of four cases and review of the literature. Medicine (Baltimore) 59:449–457, 1980.
19. Asmar BI, Slovis TL, Reed JO, et al: Haemophilus influenzae type B pneumonia 43 children. J Pediatr 93:389–393, 1978.
20. Jacobs NM, Harris VJ: Acute Haemophilus pneumonia in childhood. Am J Dis Child 133:603–605, 1979.
21. Potter AR, Fischer GW: Haemophilus influenzae, the predominant cause of bacterial pneumonia in Hawaii. Pediatr Res 11:504, 1977.
22. Kitagawa S, Kaplan S, Seilheimer D: Lung abscess due to Haemophilus influenzae type C. Am J Dis Child 133:650–651, 1979.
23. Canny G, Marcotte J, Levison H: Lung abscess in cystic fibrosis. Thorax 41:221–222, 1986.
24. Lewin S, Brettman LR, Goldstein EJC, et al: Legionnaires' disease: A cause of severe abscess forming pneumonia. Am J Med 67:339–342, 1979.
25. Williams D, Krick J, Remington J: Pulmonary infection in the compromised host: Part I. Am Rev Respir Dis 114:359–394, 1976.
26. Sebes JI, Mabry EH Jr, Rabinowitz JG: Lung abscess and osteomyelitis of rib due to Yersinia enterocolitica. Chest 69:546–548, 1976.
27. Dehner LP, Kissane JM: Pyogenic hepatic abscesses in infancy and childhood. J Pediatr 74:763–773, 1969.
28. Finegold SM: Anaerobic Bacteria and Human Disease. New York: Academic Press, 1977.
29. Mancinelli R, Shulls WA: Airborne bacteria in an urban environment. Appl Environ Microbiol 35:1095–1101, 1978.
30. Brock RC: Lung Abscess. Springfield, IL: Charles C Thomas, 1952.
31. Barnett T, Herring C: Lung abscess, initial and late results of medical therapy. Arch Intern Med 127:217–227, 1971.
32. Bartlett J, Finegold S: Anaerobic infections of the lung and pleural space. Am Rev Respir Dis 110:56–77, 1974.
33. Guillemot L, Halle J, Rist E: Recherches bacteriologigues et experimentales sur les pleuresies putrides. Arch Med Exper P d'Anat Pathol 16:571, 1904.
34. Bartlett JG, Finegold SM: Anaerobic pleuropulmonary infections. Medicine (Baltimore) 51:413–450, 1972.
35. Bartlett JG, Gorbach SL, Finegold SM: The bacteriology of aspiration pneumonia. Am J Med 56:202–207, 1974.
36. Lorber B, Swenson RM: Bacteriology of aspiration pneumonia: A prospective study of community and hospital acquired cases. Ann Intern Med 81:329–331, 1974.
37. Smith DT: Experimental aspiratory abscess. Arch Surg 14:231–239, 1927.
38. Kosloske A, Ball W, Butler C, et al: Drainage of pediatric lung abscess by cough, catheter, or complete resection. J Pediatr Surg 21:596–600, 1986.
39. Altemeier WA: The cause of the putrid odor of perforated appendicitis with peritonitis. Ann Surg 107:634–636, 1938.
40. Mayer T, Matlak M, Condon V, et al: Computed tomographic findings of neonatal lung abscess. Am J Dis Child 136:39–41, 1982.
41. Dehner L: Tumors and tumor-like lesions of the lung and chest wall in childhood: Chemical and pathological review. In Stocker JT (ed): Pediatric Pulmonary Disease, pp. 207–267. Washington, DC: Hemisphere, 1989.
42. Bartlett J: Diagnostic accuracy of transtracheal aspiration bacteriologic studies. Am Rev Respir Dis 115:777–782, 1977.
43. Bartlett J, Rosenblatt J, Finegold S: Percutaneous transtracheal aspiration in the diagnosis of anaerobic pulmonary infection. Ann Intern Med 79:535–540, 1973.
44. Kalinske RW, Parker RH, Brandt D, et al: Diagnostic usefulness and safety of transtracheal aspiration. N Engl J Med 276:604–608, 1967.
45. Pecora DV, Brook R: A method of securing uncontaminated tracheal secretions for bacterial examination. J Thorac Surg 37:653–654, 1959.
46. Wimberley N, Faling L, Bartlett J: A fiberoptic bronchoscopy technique to obtain uncontaminated lower airway secretions for bacterial culture. Am Rev Respir Dis 119:337–343, 1979.
47. Marquette CH, Ramon P, Courcol R, et al: Bronchoscopic protected catheter brush for the diagnosis of pulmonary infections. Chest 93:746–750, 1988.
48. Levison M, Mangura C, Lorber B, et al: Clindamycin compared with penicillin for the treatment of anaerobic lung abscess. Ann Intern Med 98:466–471, 1983.
49. Weiss W, Cherniack NS: Acute non-specific lung abscess: A controlled study comparing orally and parenterally administered penicillin G. Chest 66:348–351, 1974.
50. Connors J, Roper C, Ferguson T: Transbronchial catheterization of pulmonary abscesses. Ann Thorac Surg 19:254–260, 1975.
51. Groff D, Marquis J: Transtracheal drainage of lung abscesses in children. J Pediatr Surg 12:303–307, 1977.
52. Rowe L, Keane W, Jafek B, et al: Transbronchial drainage of pulmonary abscesses with the flexible fiberoptic bronchoscope. Laryngoscope 89:122–128, 1979.
53. Siegel J, McCracken G: Neonatal lung abscess: A report of six cases. Am J Dis Child 133:947–949, 1979.
54. Hammer D, Aranda C, Galati V, et al: Massive intrabronchial aspiration of contents of pulmonary abscess after fiberscopic bronchoscopy. Chest 74:306–307, 1978.
55. Lacey SR, Kosloske AM: Pneumonostomy in the management of pediatric lung abscess. J Pediatr Surg 18:625–627, 1983.
56. Weissberg D: Percutaneous drainage of lung abscess. J Thorac Cardiovasc Surg 87:308–312, 1984.
57. Yellin A, Yellin E, Lieberman Y: Percutaneous tube drainage: The treatment of choice for refractory lung abscess. Ann Thorac Surg 39:266–270, 1985.
58. Snow N, Lucas A, Horrigan T: Utility of pneumonotomy in the treatment of cavitary lung disease. Chest 87:731–734, 1985.
59. Nonoyama A, Tanaka K, Osako T, et al: Surgical treatment of pulmonary abscess in children under ten years of age. Chest 85:358–362, 1984.
60. Welch KJ: Lung abscess. In Ravitch MM, Welch KJ, Benson CD, et al (eds): Pediatric Surgery, 3rd ed, pp. 557–563. Chicago: Year Book Medical, 1979.
61. Bartlett J, Gorbach S, Tally F, et al: Bacteriology and treatment of primary lung abscess. Am Rev Respir Dis 109:510–518, 1974.
62. Schmitt G, Ohar J, Kanter K, et al: Indwelling transbronchial catheter drainage of pulmonary abscess. Ann Thorac Surg 45:43–47, 1988.
63. Weiss W: Cavity behavior in acute, primary, nonspecific lung abscess. Am Rev Respir Dis 108:1273–1275, 1973.
64. Kaplan K, Weinstein L: Abscess of the lung. In Feigin RD, Cherry JD (eds): Textbook of Pediatric Infectious Diseases, pp. 352–358. Philadelphia: WB Saunders, 1987.

30 PNEUMONIA OF INFANCY

RICHARD J. BONFORTE, M.D.

Respiratory diseases are a major cause of morbidity and mortality in the pediatric age group. A common approach to the diagnosis and treatment of childhood pneumonia involves grouping patients by age. Knowledge of the causative organisms that are most prevalent in each age group forms the basis of selection of appropriate antibiotic treatment. These age categories have traditionally been neonates, infants, toddlers, school-age children, and adolescents. The period of infancy is usually further subdivided to include a special category for infants less than 6 months of age. Pneumonia in that age group is the focus of this chapter.

Certain bacterial organisms are considered to be of specific concern in the origins of pneumonia in infants less than 6 months of age (Table 30–1). However, respiratory viruses are more frequent causes of pneumonia in the first several months of life and thus should be considered important pathogens (Table 30–2). Techniques for identifying viral agents are being used increasingly often, and specific antiviral therapy is available for some viruses (e.g., respiratory syncytial virus). (See Chapter 83.)

Pneumonia in the early months of infancy requires special attention because many of the etiologic agents may be acquired perinatally. Many of these organisms are commonly present in the female genitourinary tract, and primary infection in adults usually is asymptomatic. A variety of incomplete immune responses result in colonization of these organisms in infants, and in certain settings, infection and disease result.

HOST FACTORS

Evaluation of a patient with any infectious disease requires an assessment not only of causative agents but also of host factors. In the ideal setting, a host with intact defense mechanisms would be able to deal with an invading pathogen and prevent development of disease. Diseases, however, occur as a result of an imbalance in this ideal scheme. If the invading organism is highly pathogenic or the inoculum is large or, conversely, if the host's defenses are subnormal, disease develops. Any evaluation of infectious processes in general and of pneumonia in this age group in particular warrants an assessment of the host.

If a pneumonia is confined to a certain anatomic location—for example, the right middle lobe—questions must always be raised as to whether something is extrinsically or intrinsically obstructing the right main stem bronchus and may predispose the patient to infection. Infection in the right upper lobe caused by *Staphylococcus aureus* or *Pseudomonas aeruginosa* is suggestive of cystic fibrosis. Recurrent pneumonia is suggestive of aspiration resulting from a tracheoesophageal fistula or from gastroesophageal reflux.[1]

Questions should also be raised as to whether the host can mount an appropriate inflammatory response.[2] Infants with defective chemotaxis, with an inadequate number of white cells, or whose granulocytes are unable to phagocytose or kill organisms (e.g., as in chronic granulomatous disease) experience recurrent infections. Defects in the humoral or cell-mediated immune systems also place the host at risk.[3]

DIAGNOSIS

The question "Can one decide on a clinical basis whether a pneumonia has a bacterial or a viral etiology?" is often asked. Some clinical patterns (Table 30–2) may be more suggestive of one etiologic category than of another. Clinical signs are often a poor indicator of the extent of the pneumonic process, but certain signs are more frequently associated with abnormal chest radiographs (Table 30–3).

Although viruses are more common as etiologic agents of pneumonia in almost all age groups,[4–7] bacteria remain a very real concern because of their potential to significantly affect morbidity and mortality. The possibility that agents such as *S. aureus, Haemophilus influenzae,* and group B *Streptococcus* may cause lung damage and even death, if left untreated, often prompts the physician to use antibiotics prophylactically until either a definitive causative organism can be identified or the patient clinically improves. With more rapid and efficient diagnostic techniques available, the ability to diagnose specific infection has improved. Nevertheless, most clinicians still prescribe antibiotics until the results of further diagnostic studies can be confirmed or more specific therapy is introduced.

CHLAMYDIA

Beem and Saxon first described this distinctive pneumonia syndrome due to *Chlamydia trachomatis* in 1977.[8]

Table 30–1. BACTERIAL CAUSES OF PNEUMONIA

Staphylococcus aureus
Streptococcus pneumoniae
Haemophilus influenzae
Streptococcus hemolyticus, group A
Klebsiella pneumoniae and other gram-negative organisms
Chlamydia trachomatis

Chlamydia has long been known as a group of microorganisms associated with a variety of clinical entities.[9]

Chlamydial pneumonia manifests in infants between 2 and 12 weeks of age. The clinical features of this distinctive pneumonia syndrome include a gradual onset, fever, and initial nasopharyngitis or secretory otitis media or both followed by cough, tachypnea, and characteristic chest radiographic findings of hyperinflation with interstitial infiltrates. A history of conjunctivitis is present in some infants. The cough is characteristically staccato. Serum immunoglobulin M (IgM) levels are elevated, and in most cases, the concentration of immunoglobulin G (IgG) is also increased.[10] Peripheral eosinophilia is often found. Some children may also have hypoxemia. (This is discussed in detail in Chapter 31.)

MYCOPLASMAL INFECTIONS

Mycoplasma pneumoniae was initially isolated by M. D. Eaton and is often referred to as the atypical pneumonia agent of Eaton. *M. pneumoniae* is a well-recognized cause of pneumonia in school-age children. The data on age-specific attack rates of *M. pneumoniae* reported by Denny and Clyde[11] showed no isolates from children younger than 3 months of age, and the peak rates occurred in school-age children.[12] *M. pneumoniae* is discussed in detail in Chapter 33.

The role of genital *Mycoplasma* infections in pneumonia in infants has not been clearly defined. Two major genital mycoplasmal organisms, *Mycoplasma hominis* and *Ureaplasma urealyticum,* are frequently isolated from the female genitourinary tract, and colonization by these organisms may occur in neonates. The prevalence of *M. hominis* in the genital tract during normal pregnancy varies from 12% to 50%, depending on the population under study. There is a high rate of colonization in infants exposed to these organisms. They have been implicated in a variety of neonatal infections, including pneumonia. *U. urealyticum* was originally known as the *t* strain of *Mycoplasma,* in reference to the tiny form of colonies that these organisms form on agar culture. These organisms contain urease and hydrolyze urea, which distinguishes them from other *Mycoplasma* microbes. There appears to be an association between this organism and perinatal infections, prematurity, and, on occasion, pneumonia.

ADENOVIRUS

Adenoviral infections are particularly common in the pediatric population and cause a wide spectrum of illness, from upper respiratory infections and bronchitis to bronchiolitis and pneumonia. The former tend to occur most commonly in childhood and adolescence; the latter tend to occur more commonly in younger infants. Conjunctivitis is common, and adenoviruses frequently cause a pertussis-like syndrome.

Severe forms of disease cause problems such as bronchiolitis obliterans and acute respiratory distress syndrome. For infants who survive, respiratory sequelae include bronchiectasis and bronchiolitis obliterans. Bilateral disease is commonly present, as is multilobar involvement.

Adenoviruses are commonplace; more than 40 distinct types cause human infection. Certain hosts such as small infants and malnourished infants appear to be more susceptible to the more severe forms of pneumonia. Treatment is primarily supportive. For additional details, see Chapter 34.

CYTOMEGALOVIRUS

Cytomegalovirus is a ubiquitous organism, present in 10% to 30% of pregnant women at term and in 10% to 20% of nursing women. However, there is a definite inverse link between infection rate and socioeconomic factors.[13] The presence of the organism in the female genitourinary tract, in breast secretions, and in isolates from the respiratory tract is strongly associated with the transmission of this agent to neonates with resulting illness. About 1% of all infants are infected in utero and excrete the virus at birth; severe disease with manifestations at birth occurs in about 5% of these infants. Maternal cervical infections are common and over 50% of infants who are exposed perinatally become infected. Most of these infants will remain asymptomatic, but some neonates develop symptomatic infection. Features include fatigue, loss of appetite, fever, malaise and thrombocytopenia. Interstitial pneumonia may develop in patients in the early months of life. This organism is one of the common opportunistic infections associated with the human immunodeficiency virus (HIV) and may make this infection one of the presenting manifestations of pediatric AIDS. CMV infection in immunocompromised infants is discussed further in Chapter 36.

Table 30–2. VIRUSES CAUSING PNEUMONIA

Common
Respiratory syncytial virus
Parainfluenza viruses 1, 2, and 3
Adenoviruses
Influenza viruses A and B

Uncommon
Rhinoviruses
Enteroviruses
Coronaviruses
Rubeola virus
Varicella virus
Cytomegalovirus
Herpesvirus hominis
Rubella virus

Table 30–3. CLINICAL SIGNS WITH OR WITHOUT RADIOGRAPHIC FINDINGS

Sign	Percentage of Patients	
	With Radiographs	Without Radiographs
Appears ill	21	11
Cough	21	9
Nasal flaring	31	16
Grunting	42	17
Tachypnea	32	7
Rales	33	14
Pallor	39	15

$p < 0.05$.

PNEUMOCYSTIS CARINII

Pneumocystis carinii is an opportunistic organism and is often associated with human immunodeficiency virus (HIV) infections. Currently, the *P. carinii* infection is considered a manifestation of acquired immunodeficiency syndrome (AIDS) until proved otherwise. This organism causes acute, diffuse pneumonitis associated with fever, hypoxia, cough, and a deteriorating clinical course. The chest radiograph often shows bilateral interstitial infiltrates with hyperaeration and linear and segmental atelectasis. Decreased oxygen saturation, elevated serum levels of immunoglobulins (particularly IgM) and peripheral eosinophilia are common. The organism is readily obtained from bronchoalveolar lavage, from bronchoscopic biopsy specimens, and from closed- and open-lung biopsies. Toluidine blue and methenamine silver nitrate are the stains most commonly used to identify the organism. Pneumonia caused by this organism is discussed in Chapter 36.

RESPIRATORY SYNCYTIAL VIRUS

Respiratory syncytial virus may cause acute respiratory illness in patients at any age, but it is the most common cause of bronchiolitis and pneumonia in infants and young children.[14] The disease tends to occur in yearly outbreaks in winter and spring, and virtually all children are infected in the first few years of life. The number of infants requiring hospitalization is estimated to vary from one in 50 to one in 1000. The mortality rate among hospitalized infants is less than 1%. It is estimated that bronchiolitis develops in two thirds of infected persons and pneumonia in one third. In infants with underlying diseases such as immunodeficiency and cardiopulmonary disease, the mortality rate may be higher.

The virus is easily isolated from nasopharyngeal secretions; however, rapid diagnostic procedures with enzyme-linked immunosorbent assay and immunofluorescent staining techniques are readily available and have a high rate of sensitivity.

Interest in this particular disease has increased as a result of the availability of specific antiviral therapy.[15] Most previously normal infants improve solely with supportive care. There is strong evidence that in some children, hyperreactive airway disease and recurrent infections of the lower respiratory tract occur later in life. Ribavirin, an antiviral drug, is available as an aerosolized form of treatment for serious respiratory syncytial virus infections. Recommendations for use of the drug have been suggested by the AAP-Committee on Infectious Diseases.[16] This drug is expensive, and there is continuing concern about its cost/benefit analysis, although morbidity and mortality rates appear to be reduced in high-risk patients undergoing treatment.

HIV (AIDS)

No discussion of infant pneumonia would be complete without some consideration of HIV infection. Pneumonia in an infant warrants special consideration of the socioeconomic factors that place the patient under consideration at risk for infection with HIV.[17]

Pediatric AIDS is acquired primarily as a result of maternal infection transmitted prenatally or perinatally. The association of pediatric AIDS in lower socioeconomic groups and its relationship to the epidemic of substance abuse warrant strong consideration. Thus infants with pneumonia in most urban settings, particularly in the first few months of life, should be assessed for the presence of risk factors for AIDS. This is especially true if either or both parents are known substance abusers. AIDS is discussed in detail in Chapter 75.

REFERENCES

1. Bonforte RJ: Evaluation of the child with repeated infections. Pediatr Ann 5:432–447, 1977.
2. Murphy S, Florman AL: Lung defenses against infection: A clinical correlation. Pediatrics 72:1–15, 1983.
3. Josephs SH: Immunologic mechanisms in pulmonary disease. Pediatr Clin North Am 31:919–936, 1984.
4. Maletzky AJ, Cooney MK, Luce R, et al: Epidemiology of viral and mycoplasmal agents associated with childhood lower respiratory illness in a civilian population. J Pediatr 78:407–414, 1971.
5. Glezen WP, Loda FA, Clyde WA, et al: Epidemiologic patterns of acute lower respiratory disease of children in a pediatric group practice. J Pediatr 78:397–406, 1971.
6. Glezen WP, Denny FW: Epidemiology of acute lower respiratory disease in children. N Engl J Med 288:498–505, 1973.
7. Murphy TF, Henderson FW, Clyde WA, et al: Pneumonia: An eleven-year study in a pediatric practice. Am J Epidemiol 113:12–21, 1981.
8. Beem MO, Saxon EM: Respiratory-tract colonization and a distinctive pneumonia syndrome in infants infected with *Chlamydia trachomatis*. N Engl J Med 296:306–310, 1977.
9. Schachter J: Chlamydial infections (first of three parts). N Engl J Med 298:428–435, 1978.
10. Hammerschlag MR, Anderka M, Semine DZ, et al: Prospective study of maternal and infantile infection with *Chlamydia trachomatis*. Pediatrics 64:142–148, 1979.
11. Denny FW, Clyde WA Jr: Acute lower respiratory tract infections in nonhospitalized children. J Pediatr 108:635–646, 1986.
12. Foy HM, Kenny GE, Cooney MK, et al: Naturally acquired immunity to pneumonia due to *Mycoplasma pneumoniae*. J Infect Dis 147:967–973, 1983.
13. Stagno S, Dworsky ME, Torres J, et al: Prevalence and importance of congenital cytomegalovirus infection in three different populations. J Pediatr 101:897–900, 1982.

14. Parrott RH, Kim HW, Brandt CD, et al: Respiratory syncytial virus in infants and children. Prev Med 3:473–480, 1974.
15. Hall CB, McBride JT, Walsh EE, et al: Aerosolized ribavirin treatment of infants with respiratory syncytial viral infection. N Engl J Med 308:1443–1447, 1983.
16. Committee on Infectious Diseases: Ribavirin therapy of respiratory syncytial virus. Pediatrics 79:475–478, 1987.
17. Falloon J, Eddy J, Wiener L, et al: Human immunodeficiency virus infection in children. J Pediatr 114:1–30, 1989.

31 THE CHLAMYDIAE

JOSEPH A. BOCCHINI, Jr., M.D.

The chlamydiae are a group of widely distributed organisms that are responsible for a number of infections in humans, other mammals, and birds.[1,2,3] Since the early 1970s, advances in culture techniques and serologic tests have rapidly expanded our knowledge of these organisms and the diseases that they cause. It is now clear that chlamydial species are common causes of respiratory diseases in infants, children, and adults. The role of *Chlamydia trachomatis* in respiratory disease in infants was first recognized in 1975.[4] In subsequent studies, *C. trachomatis* has been identified as a common pathogen in the upper and lower respiratory tracts of infants under 6 months of age.[5] In addition, a newly identified species of *Chlamydia, C. pneumoniae,* appears to be a frequent cause of respiratory disease in older children and adults.[6] Human infections from *Chlamydia psittaci,* which is a pathogen primarily among birds, are uncommon in the United States.

C. trachomatis is the most common sexually transmitted disease in the United States. The incidence of cervical infection in pregnant women varies from 2% to 36% in different populations,[2,7,8] and the overall incidence is 6% to 8%. Chlamydial infection rates are highest in poor, nonwhite, and adolescent populations.[9] *C. trachomatis* is most likely to be acquired by infants during the perinatal period. Infection of most infants probably occurs during vaginal delivery through the infected cervix.[9,10] Ascending infection after rupture of the amniotic membranes can also occur, as shown by the fact that some infants delivered by cesarean section acquire *C. trachomatis.*[11,12]

The rate of transmission of *C. trachomatis* to newborns is high; 60% to 70% of infants born to mothers with cervical infection develop an antibody response to the organism.[5,8] The most common clinical manifestation of *C. trachomatis* infection in infants is inclusion conjunctivitis, which is seen in 33% to 50% of infants born to infected mothers.[2,3,7,8] Infection of the upper respiratory tract commonly accompanies inclusion conjunctivitis and can be present in the absence of clinically apparent eye disease. Pneumonia is seen in 10% to 20% of infants of infected women.[2,3,6–8] If the overall chlamydial infection rate during pregnancy is assumed to be 5%, the rate of

pneumonia caused by *Chlamydia* is 5 to 10 per 1000 live births.[8] Using a figure of 3 million live births a year in the United States, Hammerschlag[13] estimated that 15,000 to 30,000 infants contract chlamydial pneumonia annually.

Prevalence studies indicate that *C. trachomatis* is the most common cause of pneumonia in children under 6 months of age, accounting for 25% to 45% of pneumonias in this age group.[10,14–16] In one study, 30% of 30 consecutive infants under 6 months of age hospitalized with pneumonia were infected with *C. trachomatis.*[14] In another prospective study of 193 hospitalized infants (1 to 3 months of age), 36% were found to be infected with *C. trachomatis.*[15] Seventy-three percent of afebrile pneumonias in infants under 6 months of age are caused by *C. trachomatis.*[10]

C. pneumoniae was originally labeled "TWAR" after the designation of the first two laboratory isolates.[17] The epidemiologic features, the clinical manifestations, the mode of transmission, and the spectrum of diseases caused by this agent are under investigation. In studies to date this agent has been identified as the cause of 6% to 12% of cases of community-acquired pneumonia in adults and in approximately 10% of patients hospitalized for pneumonia.[6,18]

Antibody prevalence studies indicate that approximately 50% of adults from different areas of the world have an antibody against *C. pneumoniae.*[6,18] Antibody begins to appear in children at 5 years of age; the prevalence of the antibody increases rapidly during adolescence, and seropositivity rates increase more slowly thereafter.[6,18] Reinfection is common. Endemic[19] and epidemic[20] diseases have been described.

PATHOPHYSIOLOGY AND PATHOLOGY

The genus *Chlamydia* has been divided into three species: *C. psittaci, C. trachomatis,* and *C. pneumoniae. C. psittaci* is an avian pathogen that can infect humans. *C. trachomatis* and *C. pneumoniae* primarily infect humans. *C. trachomatis* strains include at least 15 human serotypes:[2] the 12 serotypes associated with trachoma or sexually transmitted infections and the three serotypes associated with lymphogranuloma venereum. Only a single strain of *C. pneumoniae* has been identified.[18]

The chlamydiae are unique organisms.[1, 2, 7] They are small, coccus-shaped bacteria that have a complex cell wall similar to that of gram-negative agents. They contain both DNA and RNA. Although they possess ribosomes and metabolic enzymes, they are not capable of energy production; hence they are obligatory intracellular parasites.

The chlamydiae primarily infect columnar epithelial cells in the mucous membranes of the respiratory, genitourinary, and gastrointestinal tracts and the conjunctivae. The life cycle of the organism consists of an extracellular phase and an intracellular phase. The organism exists extracellularly as the elementary body, a 300- to 350-nm particle, which is the infectious form of the organism. Elementary bodies are relatively stable in the extracellular environment. There appear to be specific receptor sites on the host cell for elementary body attachment. After the elementary body attaches to the host cell, it enters the cell by an organism-induced, host cell–directed phagocytic process. The elementary body remains within the invaginated host cell membrane and inhibits the fusion of the phagosome with cell lysosomes.

Once inside the phagosome, the elementary body undergoes a reorganization to form the larger (700- to 1000-nm), metabolically active reticulate body (initial body). The reticulate body divides by binary fission. Later, some reticulate bodies undergo reorganization to form elementary bodies and then are released from the host cell to begin another infectious cycle.

Because most infants with *C. trachomatis* experience a self-limited illness even without antibiotic therapy, little has been reported about the pathologic changes associated with the disease. Griffin and associates[21] reviewed previously published results of lung biopsies and autopsies and a more recent biopsy. The histologic findings included a diffuse intra-alveolar infiltrate of histiocytes, lymphocytes, plasma cells, eosinophils and neutrophils; necrotizing bronchiolitis and alveolitis; and emphysema, airway plugging, and atelectasis. Also, they identified by electron microscopy an elementary body in an alveolar macrophage and reticulate bodies in alveolar epithelial cells.

The first open-lung biopsies of two infants with *C. trachomatis* pneumonia were described by Beem and Saxon[22] in 1977 and revealed an interstitial pneumonia. Light, immunofluorescence, and electron microscopy studies were negative. In an open-lung biopsy from a patient from whom both *C. trachomatis* and cytomegalovirus were grown, diffuse interstitial and alveolar infiltrates of monocytes and neutrophils were found.[23]

Arth and colleagues[24] found bronchoalveolar involvement in a patient with *C. trachomatis*, which was characterized by near obliteration of the involved alveoli (primarily with mononuclear cells) and a widespread necrotizing bronchiolitis. They postulated that the biopsy may have been performed at an earlier stage of the infection, before interstitial involvement occurred.

Mardh and co-authors[25] in 1984 described a premature infant who died 52 h after birth. Lung tissue studies showed collapsed alveoli, dilated bronchioles with eosinophilic membranes, and advanced interstitial edema. Numazaki and co-workers[26] described interstitial bleeding, atelectasis, and emphysema in autopsy tissue from a premature infant. Intracytoplasmic inclusions of *C. trachomatis* were found through the use of fluorescence-labeled monoclonal antibodies.

CLINICAL MANIFESTATIONS

Beem and Saxon[22] in 1977 were the first to describe a distinctive pneumonia syndrome in a group of patients from whom *C. trachomatis* was isolated and in whom elevated levels of antibodies were found. *C. trachomatis* was isolated from secretions obtained at bronchoscopy but not from the lung biopsies of two infants. Later, the successful isolation of *C. trachomatis* from lung tissue of a patient with pneumonia confirmed the association of *C. trachomatis* with pneumonia in young infants.[23]

More recent studies have further defined the clinical characteristics and laboratory findings of the chlamydial pneumonia syndrome. Table 31–1 lists selected clinical findings from two studies[10, 27] of infants with documented *C. trachomatis* pneumonia. Most infants with *C. trachomatis* are under 8 weeks of age at the onset of symptoms; however, infections occur in infants up to 6 months of age. The initial symptoms of respiratory infection from *C. trachomatis* are usually those of nasopharyngitis. Rhinitis with a mucoid nasal discharge is frequently found. Some degree of nasal obstruction is common, and severe

Table 31–1. SELECTED CLINICAL AND LABORATORY FEATURES OF INFANTS WITH *CHLAMYDIA TRACHOMATIS* PNEUMONIA

Clinical Feature	% With Feature	
	Tipple et al.[10] (N = 41)	Schaad and Rossi[27] (N = 115)*
Age and Mode of Onset		
Presentation at 4–11 weeks	98	88
Onset <7 weeks†	93	87
Prodrome >1 week	78	83
Apnea	—‡	5
Physical Findings		
Afebrile	100	99
Conjunctivitis	46	47
Ear abnormalities	59	39
Staccato cough	59	77
Expiratory wheeze	12	18
Laboratory Values		
Eosinophils >300/cu mm	71	69
↓Pa$_{O_2}$; Pa$_{CO_2}$ normal	NR	76
Elevated levels		
IgA	83	NR
IgG	93	84
IgM	100	93
IgG and IgM	93	NR
IgA, IgG, and IgM	76	NR

N, number of subjects studied; NR, not reported.
*Not all patients evaluable for each finding (range, 59–115).
† <8 weeks in Schaad and Rossi.[27]
‡Occurred; number not documented.

nasal obstruction resulting in apnea with cyanosis has been described.[28] Apnea can occur abruptly.[29] Middle ear abnormalities are found in more than 50% of infants with nasopharyngeal involvement.

In early studies, approximately 50% of infants with pneumonia were noted to have a history of inclusion conjunctivitis or evidence of conjunctivitis at the time of presentation.[10] Because many hospitals now use erythromycin or tetracycline for ophthalmologic prophylaxis, the occurrence of inclusion conjunctivitis in *Chlamydia*-infected infants has been reduced but not eliminated.[30]

Within a week of onset of respiratory symptoms, patients develop cough and tachypnea. These symptoms worsen gradually over the next week or two. Patients may have a history of poor oral intake and failure to thrive if nasal obstruction or tachypnea is severe enough. Some infants present abruptly with respiratory distress, respiratory failure, or apnea. The cough in chlamydial pneumonia is often distinctive. It was initially described as a paroxysm of closely spaced staccato coughs, each separated by a brief inspiration. This characteristic cough is present in more than 50% of the infants. In severe cases, the cough can be pertussislike, but the coughing spell does not usually result in cyanosis, emesis, or an inspiratory whoop.

Children with *C. trachomatis* pneumonia are typically afebrile. On physical examination, there is usually rhinitis with a mucoid nasal discharge, an elevated respiratory rate (usually 50 to 60 breaths per minute), and rales widely distributed throughout the lung fields. In addition, mild expiratory wheezing can be present with an expiratory phase that is normal or only slightly prolonged.

The course of chlamydial pneumonia is frequently prolonged. Beem and collaborators[31] reported worsening of pneumonia or lack of improvement over a period ranging from 24 to 61 days, with a mean of 43 days, in a group of hospitalized infants treated with supportive care only. All infants continued to shed *C. trachomatis* throughout this period.

C. trachomatis pneumonia has also been described in premature infants.[32, 33] Case reports suggest the possibility of a more severe illness in this group of patients, especially those requiring ventilator therapy for respiratory distress syndrome.[32]

The frequency of symptomatic infection and the clinical manifestations of *C. pneumoniae* infection in young children are not yet known. Preliminary data indicate that the infection in normal adolescents and young adults is usually mild or asymptomatic. *C. pneumoniae* infection typically begins with a sore throat that is often severe and, in many cases, accompanied by hoarseness.[6, 18] A cough develops about a week later, often giving the appearance of a biphasic illness. Fever may be present in the early stages of illness but is absent in many patients with lower respiratory tract involvement. Pneumonia and bronchitis are the common manifestations. Most patients have a mild prolonged course with cough that lasts up to 2 months. Some patients have more severe respiratory symptoms and require hospitalization.

C. psittaci produces an acute respiratory illness commonly associated with chills and high fever. Severe headache is a frequent finding.

Table 31–2. INITIAL RADIOGRAPHIC FINDINGS IN *CHLAMYDIA TRACHOMATIS* PNEUMONIA IN 125 INFANTS

Feature	Severity of Radiographic Findings (N = 125)*				
	Absent	1+	2+	3+	4+
Bilateral lung involvement	0	0	0	0	125
Interstitial infiltrates	10	27	23	39	26
"Alveolar" infiltrates†	23	36	38	25	3
Atelectasis	0	26	39	45	15
Hyperexpanded lungs	11	19	31	44	20
Presence of thymus	10	39	37	27	12
Lobar consolidation	120	0	5‡	0	0
Pleural effusion	125	0	0	0	0
Cardiomegaly	125	0	0	0	0
Congestive heart failure	125	0	0	0	0

From Radkowski MA, Kranzler JK, Beem MO, et al: Chlamydia pneumonia in infants: Radiography in 125 cases. AJR 137:703–706, 1981.
*1+, mild; 2+, moderate hyperexpansion and moderate infiltrates; 3+, moderate hyperexpansion and marked infiltrates; 4+, severe hyperinflation and marked infiltrates.
†More confluent densities considered to be mainly atelectasis.
‡Probably atelectasis; cleared rapidly.

DIAGNOSTIC APPROACHES

The chest radiographic pattern of *C. trachomatis* pneumonia is not diagnostic. Most infants show bilateral and symmetric interstitial pulmonary infiltrates along with bilateral hyperexpansion. Table 31–2 shows the findings in a series of 125 patients from Chicago.[34]

Infants with *C. trachomatis* pneumonia are frequently mildly to moderately hypoxic. Although arterial oxygen levels are low, arterial carbon dioxide levels are usually normal. The total white blood cell count is usually normal; however, the absolute eosinophil count is elevated (>400/cu mm) in approximately 69% of patients. Quantitative studies of immunoglobulins G (IgG) and M (IgM) show that IgG and IgM levels are more than two standard deviations above normal in 93% and 100% of patients, respectively.[10] Although the elevated eosinophil count and the elevated immunoglobulin levels occur more frequently in patients with chlamydial infection, other pathogens can also be associated with similar elevations of values. In one study, elevated values were not predictive of *C. trachomatis* infection.[15] Thus although elevations in absolute eosinophil count and in IgG and IgM levels in the presence of the characteristic clinical syndrome are suggestive of *C. trachomatis* infection, they cannot be relied on alone to establish the diagnosis.

The presence of *C. trachomatis* can be documented in most patients with pneumonia by tests of nasopharyngeal secretions with culture or with antigen detection. In most patients with pneumonia, nasopharyngeal culture for *C. trachomatis* is positive. Isolation, however, requires tissue culture techniques that are not routinely available in most hospital and office settings. The organisms are labile and can be lost during transport in spite of the availability of special transport media. The chlamydiae are also sensitive to freeze-thaw cycles. If sent to a reference laboratory for culture, specimens must be immediately inoculated into transport media and frozen at −60°C to maximize viability. The involved mucous membrane must be vigorously swabbed or scraped in order to obtain an adequate specimen.

Cyclohexamide-treated McCoy's cells are used for isolation of *C. trachomatis*.[35] The cell monolayer is grown on 13-mm coverglass. The specimen is centrifuged onto the coverglass in a glass vial at approximately 2800 g for 1 h and then incubated for 2 to 3 days. The coverglass is then stained, and the cells are examined for the presence of inclusions. Staining can be performed with either iodine or fluorescein-conjugated monoclonal antibody. A single blind passage of negative material can be expected to increase the isolation rate by as much as 10%. Flat-bottom microtiter plates can be used for coverglass. This technique allows for the processing of large numbers of specimens but is less sensitive than the vial procedure.

C. trachomatis antigen detection techniques that have proved to be reliable and practical in comparsion with tissue culture diagnosis have also been developed.[36, 37] Two types of assays for detection of *C. trachomatis* antigen are available. The first is a direct fluorescent antibody assay in which monoclonal antibody that reacts with all 15 known serotypes of *C. trachomatis* is used. The antibody enables staining of elementary bodies in specimens. The second technique is an enzyme immunoassay in which a polyclonal antibody to *C. trachomatis* is used to detect chlamydial antigens in specimens. Both assays have been licensed for use on respiratory secretions of infants with pneumonia. Because tissue culture is not readily available in most hospitals, antigen detection methods are the most practical means available for determining *C. trachomatis* infection in infants.

Multiple investigators have reported that other respiratory pathogens can be isolated along with *Chlamydia* in 25% to 50% of patients.[10, 14-16] Thus the search of *C. trachomatis* in culture or through antigen detection should be supplemented by specific antibody titers when an absolute diagnosis is required. For most cases, however, establishment of *C. trachomatis* infection by culture or antigen testing enables the decision to begin specific antibiotic therapy. The patient can then be monitored for appropriate clinical response.

Serologic techniques are also available for detecting infections caused by the chlamydiae.[35] The complement fixation antibody test measures antibody to all chlamydiae and thus cannot be used for specific diagnosis. In 1970 a microimmunofluorescence test was devised for the identification of both IgG and IgM antibody responses to *C. trachomatis*. This test has proved to be sensitive and specific.[35]

Although microimmunofluorescent *C. trachomatis* antibody titers are a reliable method for diagnosing infection, IgG titers must be interpreted with caution in young infants. Many infants born to infected mothers have transplacentally transmitted antichlamydial IgG, which can be present for up to 6 to 9 months. Patients with pneumonia but not with conjunctivitis often manifest a diagnostic titer rise of IgG (fourfold or higher rise in titer).[38] In addition, many infants with pneumonia exhibit high titers of IgM antibody.[38] This IgM response does not occur in patients with conjunctivitis and only occasionally develops (usually with low titers) in patients with nasopharyngitis. Microimmunofluorescent antibody tests are

not readily available. If desired, they can be performed at reference laboratories.

The radiographic findings in patients with *C. pneumoniae* pneumonia are also nonspecific.[6, 18] The chest radiographic abnormalities can range from a single subsegmental infiltrate in milder cases to extensive bilateral pneumonitis in more severe cases.

C. pneumoniae can be isolated from the throat of a patient with pneumonia or bronchitis caused by this organism; however, it is more difficult to grow *C. pneumoniae* than *C. trachomatis*.[6, 18] Currently, HeLa 229 cells and the yolk sacs of embryonated chicken eggs are used for isolation of this agent. Identification of this organism is enhanced by fluorescent staining of cultures with monoclonal antibody directed against a *C. pneumoniae* elementary body antigen. Currently, the HeLa cells and the embryonated eggs necessary for the growth of this organism are not usually available to the clinician. IgG and IgM microimmunofluorescent tests with the use of *C. pneumoniae*–specific elementary body antigen have also been developed. Because there is no significant cross reaction between *C. trachomatis* and *C. pneumoniae* in these tests, antibody responses to these two species can be readily distinguished. Currently, *C. pneumoniae* microimmunofluorescent antibody titers are not commercially available. Thus the diagnosis of *C. pneumoniae* infection cannot be established routinely at the present time.

C. psittaci produces an interstitial pneumonia that is often extensive. There are no characteristic findings on radiographs. The chlamydial complement fixation test has been used in the past to document psittacosis. Because infection with *C. pneumoniae* also produces a rise in complement fixation titer, the use of the complement fixation test to document infection with *C. psittaci* must be reevaluated.

DIFFERENTIAL DIAGNOSIS

Many other respiratory pathogens can produce an afebrile pneumonia in infants under 6 months of age and must be considered in the differential diagnosis of *C. trachomatis* pneumonia. Respiratory viruses, such as respiratory syncytial virus (RSV), adenovirus, parainfluenza and influenza, and the enteroviruses can cause pneumonia in young infants. Pertussis may also need to be considered. The course of *C. trachomatis* is usually more gradual than that seen in respiratory viral infections. In addition, patients with respiratory viral infections are more likely to have fever, and other household members may have a history of respiratory symptoms. Wheezing can occur with any viral pneumonia but is very common in RSV infections in young children. RSV pneumonia with bronchiolitis can be difficult to distinguish from *C. trachomatis* infection of the lower respiratory tract. Cytomegalovirus, *Pneumocystis carinii*, and *Ureaplasma urealyticum* each can produce an afebrile pneumonia syndrome that is clinically indistinguishable from *C. trachomatis* pneumonia unless specific diagnostic tests are performed.

Another factor complicating diagnosis is the fact that

approximately 25% to 50% of infants with *C. trachomatis* pneumonia have mixed infections. In one study there was no evidence of increased severity of disease when another pathogen was found along with *C. trachomatis.*[10] Another study of a small number of patients indicated that infants with mixed infections had more severe disease, as manifested by increased need for oxygen, incidence of apnea, and requirement for mechanical ventilation.[15]

C. pneumoniae pneumonia most often resembles infections caused by *Mycoplasma pneumoniae.* Viral respiratory pathogens such as influenza A and B, adenovirus, parainfluenza, and RSV also need to be considered. *C. psittaci* likewise must be differentiated from other causes of atypical pneumonia. Recent exposure to imported birds or wild birds, such as turkeys, even if the birds are asymptomatic, should lead to evaluation for psittacosis in any patient with pneumonia.

MANAGEMENT

No prospective placebo-controlled studies have been performed to evaluate the effect of antibiotic therapy in infants with *C. trachomatis* pneumonia. Beem and collaborators[31] in 1979 compared the clinical course and the quantity and duration of nasopharyngeal shedding of *C. trachomatis* in 11 patients who received supportive care with those of 32 patients who were treated with either erythromycin ethylsuccinate (40 mg/kg/day) or sulfisoxazole (150 mg/kg/day). The 11 patients treated with supportive care continued to worsen or failed to improve for weeks and continued to shed *C. trachomatis* for the entire time that they were followed. The mean duration of unimproved or worsening pneumonia was 43 days. In the treated patients, the two antibiotic regimens proved equally effective. There was a rapid decrease in the number of inclusions noted per coverglass in cultures after the start of either antibiotic. Cultures became negative in all treated patients by the 6th day of therapy. Clinical improvement was documented by the end of 1 week of therapy in 83% of patients. Improvement with erythromycin was seen at a mean time of 5.8 days and with sulfisoxazole at a mean of 5.5 days.

No subsequent large series of patients with *C. trachomatis* pneumonia have been reported; however, 14 days of oral erythromycin has become the accepted course of therapy. The recommended dose of erythromycin is 50 mg/kg/day in four divided doses. Parents should also be treated.

Most patients with *C. trachomatis* pneumonia can be treated as outpatients. Those with significant hypoxia or poor feeding initially require inpatient management. Oxygen supplementation and intravenous fluids may be needed for a short period of time. The patients who present abruptly with apnea need intensive care management. Some, in addition to those with respiratory failure, require a period of ventilator support.

After successful antibiotic therapy, radiographic abnormalities can persist for a prolonged period of time.[16] Recurrent episodes of wheezing can also be expected. Although more information is required for determining the long-term outcome after *C. trachomatis* infection, two studies raise the possibility of significant sequelae.

Weiss and associates[39] evaluated 18 children 7 to 8 years after hospitalization with documented *C. trachomatis* pneumonia and compared them with 19 control children from the same community. Risk factors for obstructive pulmonary disease were the same in the two groups. Patients with *C. trachomatis* pneumonia had significant limitations of expiratory airflow and signs of abnormally elevated volumes of trapped air in comparison with control children. The obstruction was responsive to inhalation of isoproterenol. Six of the 18 patients had been diagnosed as having asthma, a significantly higher number than that of the matched controls.

In a retrospective analysis of banked serum that was collected in a study to evaluate the long-term sequelae of acute infection of the lower respiratory tract in infants, *C. trachomatis* was found to be the cause of such infection in 10 patients.[40] These children, in comparison with patients who had lower respiratory tract infections caused by other respiratory pathogens, had more severe chronic cough and were more likely to exhibit abnormalities on pulmonary function tests. They also experienced more wheezing and coughing than did age-matched normal infants.

No prospective trials of antibiotic therapy have been performed in patients with *C. pneumoniae* infections. Because the organism is susceptible to tetracycline and erythromycin in tissue culture, both drugs have been used empirically. Experience suggests that antibiotic therapy may alter the clinical course.[6, 18] The recommended adult regimens include 500 mg of tetracycline every 6 h for 14 days; 100 mg of doxycycline every 12 h for 14 days; and 500 mg of erythromycin every 6 h for 14 days or 250 mg every 6 h for 21 days. Even with antibiotic therapy, recovery is slow, and cough and malaise may persist for weeks.

C. psittaci infections are treated with tetracycline for at least 10 to 14 days after defervescence. Erythromycin is recommended for children under 9 years of age.

REFERENCES

1. Schachter J: Chlamydial infections. N Engl J Med 298:428–435, 490–495, 540–549, 1978.
2. Schachter J, Caldwell HD: Chlamydiae. Annu Rev Microbiol 34:285–309, 1980.
3. Schachter J, Grossman M: Chlamydial infections. Annu Rev Med 32:45–61, 1981.
4. Schachter J, Lum L, Gooding CA, et al: Pneumonitis following inclusion blennorrhea. J Pediatr 87:779–780, 1975.
5. Schachter J, Grossman M, Holt J, et al: Prospective study of chlamydial infection in neonates. Lancet 2:377–380, 1979.
6. Grayston JT, Campbell LA, Kuo CC, et al: A new respiratory tract pathogen: *Chlamydia pneumoniae* strain TWAR. J Infect Dis 161:618–625, 1990.
7. Hammerschlag MR: Medical progress: Chlamydial infections. J Pediatr 114:727–734, 1989.
8. Wilfert CM, Gutman LT. *Chlamydia trachomatis* infections of infants and children. Adv Pediatr 33:49–75, 1986.
9. Frommell GT, Rothenberg R, Wang S, McIntosh K: Chlamydial infection of mothers and their infants. J Pediatr 95:28–32, 1979.
10. Tipple MA, Beem MO, Saxon EM: Clinical characteristics of the afebrile pneumonia associated with *Chlamydia trachomatis* infection in infants less than 6 months of age. Pediatrics 63:192–197, 1979.
11. Givner LB, Rennels MB, Woodward CL, et al: *Chlamydia tracho-*

matis infection in infant delivered by cesarean section. Pediatrics 68:420–421, 1981.

12. La Scolea LJ Jr, Paroski JS, Burzynski L, et al: *Chlamydia trachomatis* infection in infants delivered by cesarean section. Clin Pediatr 23:118–120, 1984.

13. Hammerschlag MR, Chlamydial pneumonia in infants [editorial]. N Engl J Med 298:1083–1084, 1978.

14. Harrison HR, English MG, Lee CK, et al: *Chlamydia trachomatis* infant pneumonitis: Comparison with matched controls and other infant pneumonitis. N Engl J Med 298:702–708, 1978.

15. Stagno S, Brasfield DM, Brown MB, et al: Infant pneumonitis associated with cytomegalovirus, *Chlamydia, Pneumocystis,* and *Ureaplasma:* A prospective study. Pediatrics 68:322–329, 1981.

16. Brasfield DM, Stagno S, Whitley RJ, et al: Infant pneumonitis associated with cytomegalovirus, *Chlamydia, Pneumocystis,* and *Ureaplasma:* Follow-up. Pediatrics 79:76–83, 1987.

17. Grayston JT, Kuo CC, Wang SP, et al: A new *Chlamydia psittaci* strain, TWAR, isolated in acute respiratory tract infections. N Engl J Med 315:161–168, 1986.

18. Grayston JT, Wang SP, Kuo CC, Campbell LA: Current knowledge on *Chlamydia pneumoniae,* strain TWAR, an important cause of pneumonia and other acute respiratory diseases. Eur J Clin Microbiol Infect Dis 8:191–202, 1989.

19. Marrie TJ, Grayston JT, Wang SP, et al: Pneumonia associated with TWAR strain of *Chlamydia.* Ann Intern Med 106:507–511, 1987.

20. Kleemola M, Saikku P, Visakorpi R, et al: Epidemics of pneumonia caused by TWAR, a new *Chlamydia* organism, in military trainees in Finland. J Infect Dis 157:230–236, 1988.

21. Griffin M, Pushpanathan C, Andrews W: *Chlamydia trachomatis* pneumonitis: A case study and literature review. Pediatr Pathol 10:843–852, 1990.

22. Beem MO, Saxon EM: Respiratory-tract colonization and a distinctive pneumonia syndrome in infants infected with *Chlamydia trachomatis.* N Engl J Med 296:306–310, 1977.

23. Frommell GT, Bruhn FW, Schwartzman JD: Isolation of *Chlamydia trachomatis* from infant lung tissue. N Engl J Med 296:1150–1152, 1977.

24. Arth C, Von Schmidt B, Grossman M, et al: Chlamydial pneumonitis. J Pediatr 93:447–449, 1978.

25. Mardh PA, Johansson PJ, Svenningsen N: Intrauterine lung infection with *Chlamydia trachomatis* in a premature infant. Acta Paediatr Scand 73:569–572, 1984.

26. Numazaki K, Chiba S, Kogawa K, et al: Chronic respiratory disease in premature infants caused by *Chlamydia trachomatis.* J Clin Pathol 39:84–88, 1986.

27. Schaad UB, Rossi E: Infantile chlamydial pneumonia—A review based on 115 cases. Eur J Pediatr 138:105–109, 1982.

28. Cohen SD, Azimi PH, Schachter J: *Chlamydia trachomatis* associated with severe rhinitis and apneic episodes in one-month-old infant. Clin Pediatr 21:498–499, 1982.

29. Brayden RM, Paisley JW, Lauer BA: Apnea in infants with *Chlamydia trachomatis* pneumonia. Pediatr Infect Dis J 6:423–425, 1987.

30. Black-Payne C, Bocchini JA, Cedotal C: Failure of erythromycin ointment for postnasal ocular prophylaxis of chlamydial conjunctivitis. Pediatr Infect Dis J 8:491–495, 1989.

31. Beem MO, Saxon E, Tipple MA: Treatment of chlamydial pneumonia of infancy. Pediatrics 63:198–203, 1979.

32. Attenburrow AA, Barker CM: Chlamydial pneumonia in the low birthweight neonate. Arch Dis Child 60:1169–1172, 1985.

33. Amato M, Inaebnit D: Perinatal *Chlamydia trachomatis* infection in a low birth weight infant. J Perinat Med 16:487–489, 1988.

34. Radkowski MA, Kranzler JK, Beem MO, et al: Chlamydia pneumonia in infants: Radiography in 125 cases. AJR 137:703–706, 1981.

35. Schachter J: Chlamydia. *In* Balows A, Hausler WJ Jr, Isenberg HD, et al (eds): Clinical Microbiology, 5th ed, pp. 1045–1053. Washington, DC: American Society for Microbiology, 1991.

36. Paisley JW, Lauer BA, Melinkovich P, et al: Rapid diagnosis of *Chlamydia trachomatis* pneumonia in infants by direct immunofluorescence microscopy of nasopharyngeal secretions. J Pediatr 109:653–655, 1986.

37. Hammerschlag MR, Roblin PM, Cummings C, et al: Comparison of enzyme immunoassay and culture for diagnosis of chlamydial conjunctivitis and respiratory infections in infants. J Clin Microbiol 25:2306–2308, 1987.

38. Schachter J, Grossman M, Azimi PH: Serology of *Chlamydia trachomatis* in infants. J Infect Dis 146:530–535, 1982.

39. Weiss SG, Newcomb RW, Beem MO: Pulmonary assessment of children after chlamydial pneumonia of infancy. J Pediatr 108:659–664, 1986.

40. Harrison HR, Taussig LM, Fulginiti VA: *Chlamydia trachomatis* and chronic respiratory disease in childhood. Pediatr Infect Dis 1:29–33, 1982.

32 BACTERIAL PNEUMONIA

TERRY W. CHIN, M.D. / ELIEZER NUSSBAUM, M.D. / MELVIN MARKS, M.D.

Infection of the lower respiratory tract is one of the most common reasons for hospital admissions, especially during the winter months. It has been estimated that 0.4% of all infants under 1 year of age are hospitalized for pneumonia.[1] It has further been estimated that the frequency of mortality among hospitalized infants is between 1% and 10%. In a study of outpatient cases, Denny[2] found the frequency of pneumonia to be between 1.0 and 4.5 per 100 children per year, the highest frequency occurring in children between 2 and 3 years of age. Another survey of patients in a clinic setting indicated that pneumonia accounted for 13% of infectious illnesses during the first 2 years of life.[3]

Bacterial infections account for 10% to 50% of lower respiratory infections, depending on the population of patients, the age range, and the type of diagnostic procedures used. Treatment of pneumonia is straightforward when an etiologic agent is identified. However, management of the patient must be initiated before definitive identification is available. Although the majority of infections of the lower respiratory tract are viral, bacterial infections are common, can be severe and life-threatening, and require prompt antibiotic therapy. There is considerable overlap in signs and symptoms of pneumonia caused by viral and bacterial pathogens, often making a specific diagnosis difficult.

PATHOPHYSIOLOGY

Infectious agents enter the lower respiratory tract by hematogenous spread or by inhalation or aspiration into the tracheobronchial tree. It is thought that large clumps of organisms, with or without other blood components that are too large to pass through the pulmonary circulation, lodge there and subsequently invade lung parenchyma. Metastatic pneumonias from endocarditis (right-sided) or from septic thrombophlebitis are also well documented. Pulmonary staphylococcal infections may result from a primary infection elsewhere in the body in 15% to 20% of cases and are especially invasive, frequently causing abscesses and pneumatoceles. Hematogenous spread appears to be an important mechanism for *Escherichia coli* pneumonia. Although primary meningococcal pneumonia is common in adults, it is usually secondary to meningococcemia in children.[4] However, because only about 10% to 15% of children with pneumonia have bacteremia,[5] most cases of pediatric pneumonia probably occur by nonhematogenous mechanisms.

Inhalation of bacteria can occur in several ways. Unlike viruses, airborne transmission of bacteria is uncommon, except in the acquisition of pulmonary tuberculosis. Aspiration of potentially pathogenic bacteria from the oropharynx is the most frequently implicated mechanism of bacterial pneumonia.[6] Indeed, most bacteria that cause pneumonia normally inhabit the upper respiratory tract. These include *Streptococcus pyogenes, Neisseria* species, *Branhamella catarrhalis,* and anaerobic bacteria. Antibiotics, prolonged hospitalization, or manipulation of the upper respiratory tract by endotracheal intubation or tracheostomy can result in colonization of the upper airways by other potential pathogens (e.g., gram-negative bacilli), which may then cause pneumonia. Usually, the mucociliary clearance system is able to remove aspirated bacteria. However, if the inoculum is massive, if the pathogen is especially virulent, or if the pulmonary defenses are compromised or overwhelmed, pneumonia can develop.

Several host defense mechanisms account for pulmonary protection from various infectious agents. The upper airway passages are capable of filtering and trapping pathogens; the mucociliary defense system, including the cough reflex, eliminates organisms that escape the upper airway barriers. Potential pathogens are caught on a layer of mucus and expelled after transport by the ciliary escalator and by coughing. Alveolar macrophages eliminate organisms that reach the alveoli. The alveolar macrophages have high phagocytic activity and can recruit other inflammatory cells that help eliminate the bacterial pathogens. Elimination of infectious organisms is enhanced by immunoglobulins G and A (IgG and IgA) and other factors such as complement, antiproteases, lysozyme, and fibronectin.[7]

Any process that impairs these defense mechanisms increases the likelihood of pulmonary infection. Endotracheal and tracheostomy tubes, which bypass the upper airways, are examples of conditions under which nosocomial infections commonly occur. Administration of drugs that impair mucociliary clearance or that may suppress the cough reflex may also increase the risk of pulmonary infection. Similarly, conditions that adversely affect ciliary action, such as the inhalation of noxious gases or the sequelae of viral or mycoplasmal infections, also predispose the patient to the development of pneumonia. In the presence of pulmonary edema, from congestive heart failure, nephrotic syndrome, or other causes, fluid accumulation in the alveoli decreases the effectiveness of pulmonary clearance mechanisms and may increase the risk of pneumonia. Patients with altered host defenses may have respiratory infections that are caused by unusual or opportunistic organisms; they may also have recurrent pneumonias that are caused by the usual bacterial pathogens. Chapter 2 provides a detailed discussion of lung defenses. The ability of antipolysaccharide antibodies to facilitate phagocytosis and opsonization enables the immune system to fight *Streptococcus pneumoniae* and *Haemophilus influenzae* infections. Therefore, deficiencies in these antibody responses (such as hypogammaglobulinemia) or, specifically, in IgG subclass 2 and 4 activity have resulted in recurrent pneumonias and subsequent chronic pulmonary disease[8] (see Chapter 18).

As many as half of pediatric outpatients and 25% to 75% of hospitalized patients with bacterial pneumonia have concurrent viral infections.[9-14] Therefore, differentiation of viral and bacterial pneumonia may not be as important as identifying the patient in whom viral infections may play a role in the subsequent development of bacterial infection. Ciliary action is impaired by viral infection of ciliated cells and subsequent cell destruction, either by virus-induced cytopathologic processes or by host immune mechanisms of lysis of virus-infected cells. In addition, changes in nasal epithelial water and electrolyte balance with hypersecretion of mucus may increase aspiration of upper airway bacteria and decrease the efficiency of ciliary clearance. Thus it is not surprising that both pneumococcal and staphylococcal pneumonias have been documented to follow infection by influenza virus.

CLINICAL PRESENTATION

The signs and symptoms of pneumonia are dependent on the age of the patient, the severity of the disease, and the organism responsible for the infection. Young children may be difficult to evaluate because of uncooperativeness and the fact that the thin chest wall may transmit upper airway sounds, adding confusion to the auscultatory findings. It is not unusual to see extensive infiltrates on chest radiograph with only minimal auscultatory findings and, conversely, a normal radiograph with much auscultatory noise.

Neonates with pneumonia may have nonspecific symptoms such as fever, irritability or lethargy, and decreased appetite or activity. Tachypnea, nasal flaring, chest retrac-

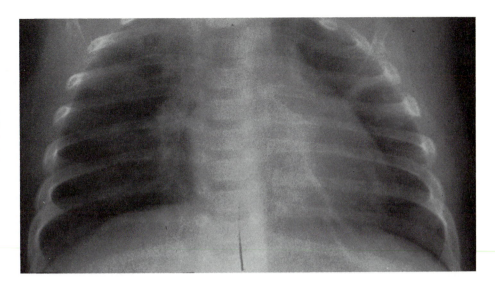

Figure 32–1. Small infiltrates seen radiographically in the right upper, left upper, and left lower lobes in a 2-month-old with group B streptococcus meningitis who had tachypnea in the absence of fever.

tions, or grunting further supports a possible pulmonary source. A chest radiograph should be obtained in any neonate with suspected infection who exhibits these findings. Neonates with a history of prolonged rupture of membranes and acute respiratory distress syndrome should be suspected of being infected by group B *Streptococcus*. Apnea and septic shock may rapidly develop in such patients. In older neonates, meningitis and pneumonia may occur concurrently (Fig. 32–1).

In infants beyond the neonatal period, the presence of tachypnea is a good predictor of an abnormal chest radiograph, especially if it is accompanied by rales or pallor.[15] An infant under 1 year of age with a respiratory rate of less than 50 is highly unlikely to have pneumonia.[16] Wheezes or rhonchi and decreased breath sounds may also be found, but these are not specific for pneumonia. Other symptoms such as cough and coryza may indicate upper

respiratory tract infection. Afebrile infants with tachypnea and cough with a history of rhinitis or conjunctivitis (in about half of cases) should be evaluated for *Chlamydia* pneumonitis.

Children from a few months to about 5 years of age with sudden onset of high fever and respiratory distress may have bacterial rather than viral pneumonia. In a cooperative child, rales, bronchial breathing, or diminished breath sounds can be auscultated. In one study, respiratory rates of higher than 40 per minute and chest retractions were reliable indicators in children between 1 and 3 years of age.[16] Percussion may be performed in some patients; dullness indicates either consolidation or pleural fluid (Fig. 32–2). Upper respiratory tract infection with otitis media may also be present. The peak ages for children hospitalized with pneumococcal pneumonia are 13 to 18 months of age.[17] In contrast, 30% of cases of staph-

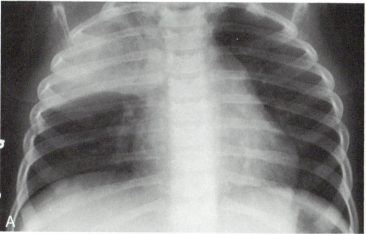
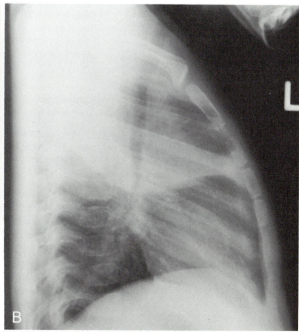

Figure 32–2. *A* and *B*, Right upper lobe consolidation attributed to *Haemophilus influenzae* in a 7-month-old. Patient was successfully treated as an outpatient with amoxicillin for 10 days.

ylococcal pneumonia occur in infants under 3 months of age and two thirds in children under 12 months of age.[18] The mean age for *H. influenzae* pneumonia is 9½ months.[19] A predominance of males has been noted among patients with pneumococcal[17] and those with *H. influenzae* pneumonias.[20, 21]

Older children and adolescents are more likely to exhibit the classical features of pneumococcal pneumonia: namely, acute onset, high fever, chills, cough, and marked toxicity. Finally, involvement of the right lower lobe may be manifested by symptoms of acute abdominal pain. Pleural effusions may develop with pleuritic pain that may result in referred meningismus. The peak incidence of pneumonias caused by *Mycoplasma pneumoniae* is between the ages of 5 and 18 years, and they are characterized by a prodromal stage of malaise, upper respiratory tract symptoms, sore throat, and headache. Persistent cough and fever are common.

Extrapulmonary involvement may be present and aids in the identification of the suspected pathogen. Epiglottitis may be associated with pneumonia caused by *H. influenzae*. Exanthems, hemolysis, and neurologic disease may be seen in *Mycoplasma* infection. The presence of skin abscesses or extrapulmonary abscesses may indicate secondary staphylococcal pneumonia. Finally, skin petechiae or arthritis in a teenager with pneumonia indicates possible involvement by *Neisseria meningitidis*.

DIAGNOSIS

Demonstration of pathogenic bacteria in the lung can be considered evidence of bacterial pneumonia. The difficulty lies in obtaining a specimen that is not contaminated with the flora of the upper airways. Therefore, cultures from sputum, nasopharyngeal aspirates, and even bronchoscopic aspirates contain, in decreasing probability, contaminated flora that may either reflect normal flora colonization or result in overgrowth of fastidious pathogens by the usual flora. Specimens in which this problem does not occur include transtracheal aspirates, transthoracic needle aspirates, pleural fluid, blood cultures, and a specimen from bronchial lavage obtained by a specially designed double-lumen catheter. For example, bacterial pathogens were identified in 13% of pediatric pneumonias documented by lung puncture.[22]

Identification of some agents, however, regardless of the source of specimen, is indicative of lower respiratory tract infection, if the chest radiograph shows changes. These agents include *Legionella, Mycobacterium tuberculosis, M. pneumoniae,* certain fungi, and viruses.

The approach in establishing the diagnosis depends upon the index of suspicion of a particular pathogen. This, in turn, reflects the age of the patient (Table 32–1)[58] and the clinical setting (Table 32–2). Nonspecific laboratory findings of a high white blood cell count (>15,000),

Table 32–1. ETIOLOGIC PATHOGENS IN PEDIATRIC PULMONARY INFECTIONS

Age	Bacteria	Other
Neonate (under 1 month)	Group B streptococci Gram-negative bacilli (especially *E. coli*, occ. *Klebsiella*) Occ. anaerobes Occ. *Haemophilus influenzae* Occ. *Streptococcus pneumoniae* Occ. group A streptococci Occ. *Staphylococcus aureus* Rarely *Chlamydia*	Respiratory viruses Enteroviruses Occ. herpes simplex virus Occ. cytomegalovirus Occ. varicella Rarely *Mycobacterium* Rarely *Listeria*
Infant (1–3 months)	*Chlamydia* Occ. *S. aureus* Occ. group B streptococci Occ. *H. influenzae* Occ. *S. pneumoniae* Occ. *S. aureus* Occ. group A streptococci	Respiratory viruses Enteroviruses Occ. *Bordetella pertussis* Occ. cytomegalovirus Occ. *Ureaplasma* Occ. *Pneumocystis carinii*
Young child (3 months to 5 years)	*H. influenzae* *S. pneumoniae* Occ. *S. aureus* Occ. group A streptococci Occ. *Mycoplasma*	Respiratory viruses (esp. RSV, occ. parainfluenza, adenovirus, influenza; rarely rhinovirus) Rarely *Mycobacterium*
Older child (5–10 years)	*S. pneumoniae* *Mycoplasma* Occ. *S. aureus* Occ. group A streptococci Rarely *H. influenzae*	Respiratory viruses (influenza, adenovirus) Occ. *Mycobacterium*
Teenager (>10 years)	*S. pneumoniae* *Mycoplasma* Occ. *S. aureus* Occ. group A streptococci Occ. *Klebsiella* Rarely *Neisseria meningitidis* Rarely *H. influenzae* Rarely *Legionella*	Respiratory viruses Occ. *Mycobacterium*

Adapted from Gilsdorf JR: Community-acquired pneumonia in children. Semin Respir Infect 2:146–151, 1987.
Occ., occasionally; RSV, respiratory syncytial virus.

Table 32–2. SPECIAL SITUATIONS AND POSSIBLE ORIGINS OF PNEUMONIC INFILTRATES

Clinical Setting	Bacterial	Other
Aspiration pneumonitis	Anaerobic bacteria (*Peptostreptococcus, Fusobacterium, Bacteroides melaninogenicus,* etc.)	Chemical
Hospital acquired pneumonia	Gram-negative bacilli (*Klebsiella, Escherichia coli, Proteus, Pseudomonas*) *Staphylococcus*	
Cystic fibrosis	*Staphylococcus aureus* *Haemophilus influenzae* *Pseudomonas*	Viruses *Aspergillus*
Immunocompromised Hypogammaglobulinemia	*Streptococcus pneumoniae* *H. influenzae*	
Neutropenia or WBC dysfunction	*S. pneumoniae* *S. aureus* Gram-negative bacilli (e.g., *Serratia*)	*Aspergillus* *Legionella*
Lymphocyte dysfunction	*Mycobacterium tuberculosis* *Mycobacterium avium-intracellulare* *Legionella*	Fungi Viruses *Nocardia* *Toxoplasma* *Pneumocystis carinii*
Hyper-IgE	*S. aureus* *Neisseria meningitidis*	
Sickle cell disease	*S. pneumoniae* *Chlamydia*	Pulmonary infarction

WBC, White blood cell count; IgE, immunoglobulin E.

elevated erythrocyte sedimentation rate, or presence of C-reactive protein suggest the diagnosis of pneumonia.[23, 24] However, the overall clinical impression, which is based on the physical examination that is suggestive of respiratory involvement, remains the most useful in terms of cost effectiveness. When this clinical suspicion is supported by a chest radiograph indicating pneumonitis, therapy is usually initiated on the basis of the likely pathogens.

Certain radiographic findings can be incorporated into the initial impression of which etiologic agent is respon-sible for the pneumonia.[25] If pleural effusion is present, a viral process is less likely. Lobar or segmental consolidation with fever and tachypnea is suggestive of infection with either *S. pneumoniae* or *H. influenzae* (Fig. 32–3). A diffuse, patchy bronchopneumonia or perihilar infiltrate is often associated with viral or *Mycoplasma* pneumonia; hyperaeration is usually present. Finally, the presence of pneumatocele or abscess suggests involvement of *Staphylococcus aureus* or, on occasion, gram-negative bacteria. However, these generalities are not invariably true. Hence pleural fluid can be present with infections by *S. aureus*,

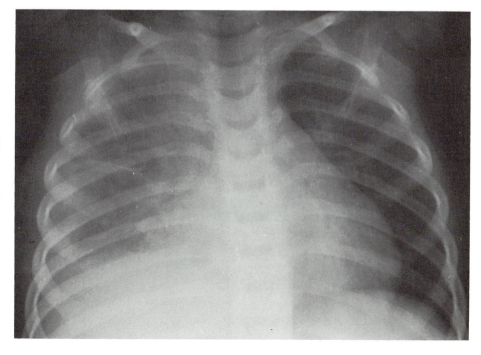

Figure 32–3. Right lower lobe pneumonia and effusion, from which *S. pneumoniae* was isolated, in a 27-month-old with a 1-week history of coughing, tachypnea, decreased appetite, and low-grade fever. Increased lethargy and abdominal pain prompted medical attention.

H. influenzae, M. tuberculosis, M. pneumoniae, or respiratory viruses.

Several points must be kept in mind in consideration of the diagnosis of pneumonia and radiography. First, clinical pneumonia may be present despite a normal chest radiograph, especially very early in the course of the illness. Second, although lobar consolidation is most often associated with bacterial infection, there are exceptions. At times, lobar or segmental infiltrates may represent atelectasis secondary to aspiration of a foreign body or development of a mucus plug, rather than infection. Similarly, the presence of pleural effusion usually, but not always, occurs with a bacterial process. Diffuse patchy or perihilar infiltrates do not invariably indicate that the pneumonia is caused by a virus or *Mycoplasma.* A major problem in the interpretation of chest radiographs is the prevalence of atelectasis, which may be caused by inefficient collateral air circulation through the pores of Kohn (particularly in the right middle lobe) and the ducts of Lambert, especially in infants and young children. Although some authors contend that radiographic differentiation between viral and bacterial pneumonia is possible,[26] clinical correlation and appropriate laboratory studies are the mainstay of diagnosis.[27, 28] Indeed, the question is the appropriateness of chest radiographs in children with acute disease of the lower respiratory tract. In the setting of presumed viral pneumonia, a chest radiograph may indicate bacterial involvement and a change of therapy to include antibiotics.[29]

In patients with underlying factors that predispose to involvement by unusual organisms (such as malignancy or immunodeficiency), the etiologic agent responsible for the pneumonia should be identified as early as possible. As mentioned, nasopharyngeal and sputum cultures may be contaminated by flora in the upper respiratory tract or may be difficult to obtain in younger children. Blood cultures are positive in only a small percentage of patients (10% to 20%). Indeed, the results of bacterial and viral cultures are usually not available when therapy is initiated. However, advances in technology have speeded the processing of results. Urine, serum, pleural fluid, and respiratory washes may be tested for antigens (*S. pneumoniae, H. influenzae,* group B *Streptococcus,* and *N. meningitidis*) by counterimmunoelectrophoresis,[30] latex particle agglutination or enzyme-linked immunosorbent assay (ELISA) techniques. Further development of polymerase chain reaction tests for pneumonia in early diagnosis looks promising. These tests are valuable especially when prior antimicrobial treatment has inhibited bacterial growth and isolation. However, positive detection alone may not indicate bacterial involvement in the lungs; one study indicated that 16% of patients with otitis media had antigenemia (caused by *S. pneumoniae* and *H. influezae*).[31] If the tests are not conclusive, invasive procedures such as bronchial brush biopsy and lavage, transtracheal and lung aspiration, and open-lung biopsy may be necessary for obtaining appropriate and adequate specimens for identification of the etiologic agent.

Development of respiratory distress in patients who use humidification equipment suggests that contaminated solutions may be responsible. Infection by gram-negative bacilli and molds should be suspected and evaluated by appropriate tests such as special microbiologic media and delayed hypersensitivity assays. The presence of anaerobic and gram-negative bacteria should be suspected in situations in which aspiration of stomach contents is likely, such as in comatose or neurologically impaired patients, in children with nasogastric tube feedings, in patients who have undergone seizure activity or apnea, and in children with gastroesophageal reflux. This suspicion is based on the fact that such aspiration causes the high incidence of colonization of the upper respiratory tract by gram-negative bacilli in hospitalized patients. Indeed, up to 60% of nosocomial pneumonias may be caused by gram-negative bacilli, and a significant percentage is also attributed to anaerobic organisms.[32]

Documentation of certain bacterial infections may also indicate underlying disease.[33] Infection of the lower respiratory tract by *Legionella* is not common in the normal pediatric population. Involvement may indicate underlying neutrophil deficiency, such as chronic granulomatous disease[34] and leukemia.[35] Repeated bouts of infection with polysaccharide-encapsulated bacteria may indicate immunoglobulin subclass deficiency; IgG subclass levels should be evaluated, and production of specific antibody toward the bacteria (usually *H. influenzae* or *S. pneumoniae*) should be measured. Similarly, repeated *Neisseria* infections are suggestive of complement component deficiency.

DIFFERENTIAL DIAGNOSIS

In patients with pulmonary infiltrates on chest radiography or with other clinical evidence suggestive of pneumonia, there is always the possibility of atelectasis, especially in patients who may be prone to mucus plugs, such as those with cystic fibrosis or asthma. The difficulty in differentiating between bacterial and other infectious causes of pneumonia has already been discussed. Neonates are susceptible to bacterial infections caused by group B *Streptococcus,* gram-negative coliforms, and occasionally *S. aureus.* Viral pneumonia, on the other hand, is more frequent in infants and preschoolers. Rapid immunofluorescent tests of nasal washings may detect involvement of respiratory syncytial virus or influenza viruses. Other viruses such as cytomegalovirus or pathogens such as *Ureaplasma* and *Chlamydia* may also be involved.

Mycoplasma infection is common among school-age children. Bacterial (e.g., pneumococcal) pneumonia may occur at any age after the neonatal period. Other infectious causes of pneumonia should be evaluated in certain patients at high risk, such as those with tuberculosis. History of travel to endemic areas, such as desert areas of California, Arizona, or New Mexico, is suggestive of coccidioidomycosis, whereas travel to the Missouri, Mississippi, and Ohio river valleys adds histoplasmosis to the differential diagnosis. Exposure to pets and wild animals should be assessed. Every patient should be questioned about underlying illness, chest trauma, and aspiration or inhalation of foreign material, gases, and so forth.

Age of the patient is also considered in the determination of noninfectious causes of pulmonary infiltrates (Table 32–3). In neonates with respiratory distress, struc-

Table 32–3. NONINFECTIOUS DIFFERENTIAL DIAGNOSIS OF PNEUMONIA RELATED TO THE AGE GROUP

Neonatal Pneumonia

Respiratory distress syndrome (hyaline membrane disease)
Transient tachypnea of the newborn
Meconium aspiration
Pneumothorax
Congenital heart disease
Thymic shadow
Congenital anomalies (e.g., diaphragmatic hernia)
Cystic adenomatoid malformation
Segmental bronchiectasis
Bronchogenic cyst with secondary compression

Childhood Pneumonia

Hyperreactive airway disease with segmental atelectasis
Aspiration:
    Foreign body
    Gastric content
    Drowning
Cystic fibrosis
Immotile cilia syndrome
Congenital pulmonary anomalies (e.g., sequestration)
Hypersensitivity pneumonitis (or disorders)
Drug-induced pneumonitis
Neoplastic (leukemia, histiocytosis, neuroblastoma, etc.)
Leukoagglutinin reactions
Pulmonary embolus and infarction
Sarcoidosis
Pulmonary edema
Pulmonary hemosiderosis
Adult respiratory distress syndrome
Congestive heart failure
Allergic bronchopulmonary aspergillosis
Acquired immunodeficiency syndrome
Desquamative interstitial pneumonitis or fibrosing alveolitis
Pulmonary collagen-vascular disease

tural abnormalities must be suspected. Sterile or septic aspiration may also have occurred. Respiratory distress syndrome and hyaline membrane disease must be considered with any neonatal infection caused by group B *Streptococcus.* The presence of pleural effusion is uncommon in the former but may occur with the latter. In older populations, mechanical or chemical insults to the lungs are usually suggested by the history.

The possibility of foreign bodies and structural anomalies must be evaluated if the pulmonary infiltrates persist in the same location. Fiberoptic bronchoscopy, when performed by experienced clinicians, is a relatively safe and effective procedure for evaluating persistent atelectasis.[36, 37] Recurrent pneumonias also may indicate immunodeficiency, cystic fibrosis, or aspiration. Therefore, serum quantitative immunoglobulin concentrations and a sweat chloride test are mandatory in such patients. Barium swallow and upper gastrointestinal radiographic studies may help in diagnosing structural abnormalities as well as the presence of gastroesophageal reflux. However, to actually document aspiration in the airways, bronchoalveolar washings showing lipid-laden macrophages may be very helpful.[38]

Drug-induced pneumonitis should be considered, especially in patients with cancer.[39] If the chest has been exposed to radiation, a clinical spectrum of effects are possible in the differential diagnosis, ranging from subclinical pneumonitis to chronic pulmonary fibrosis. Transfusion reactions and pulmonary infiltration by neoplastic cells are other possible causes of pneumonitis.

The presence of chest infiltrates can create a difficult diagnostic dilemma in patients with sickle cell disease. Because these patients are at increased risks for vaso-occlusive phenomena as well as for pneumococcal pneumonia, differentiation between bacterial pneumonia and pulmonary emboli or infarction should be made. Abnormal arterial blood gases and abnormal lung scans may occur in both. Bacterial pathogens in the blood are detected in only about 8% of patients,[40] but this rate can approach 50% if detection is vigorously sought. The general impression is that the pulmonary events in young children with sickle cell disease are predominantly pneumonia,[41] especially *Chlamydia,*[42] however, in adults these events are mainly pulmonary infarction.[43]

Pulmonary function tests (PFTs) in children older than 6 years of age may assist in establishing the diagnosis as well as differentiating obstructive from restrictive pulmonary disease (see Chapter 10). In addition, pre- and post-bronchodilator PFTs may elucidate the presence of reversible hyperreactive airway disease, as may the magnitude of response to aerosolized bronchodilators such as specific beta$_2$-agonists. Primary diffusion abnormalities, although rare in children, may be detected by the single-breath carbon monoxide diffusing capacity method.

MANAGEMENT

As reviewed earlier, the clinical symptoms and signs, laboratory data, and radiography indicate infection of the lower respiratory tract. However, the management plan depends on the patient's age because this factor also determines which pathogens are most likely involved and, indeed, which appropriate laboratory tests should be conducted (see Table 32–1). Identification of the etiologic agent is established by culture or antigen detection in blood, urine, or pleural effusion in fewer than 25% of hospitalized children with pneumonia and in a smaller percentage of ambulatory patients. Thus, definitive etiologic identification of pneumonia can be difficult and time consuming, and empiric therapy is often required.

Neonates. Neonates may be considered immunologically compromised and, as such, should be vigorously treated. Infection with group B *Streptococcus* carries a mortality rate of up to 50%. The clinical and radiographic features may resemble those of hyaline membrane disease. Grunting, nasal flaring, and chest retractions occur. Cyanosis, apnea, and hypotension may also be present and require management. Colonization of the mother's birth canal with gram-negative bacteria (*Escherichia coli, Klebsiella,* and *Pseudomonas*) indicates possible infection of the neonate with these organisms. Systemic or meningeal involvement must also be evaluated. Consequently, initial antimicrobial therapy must be structured to reflect these concerns. Therefore, a penicillin (usually ampicillin) is prescribed together with an aminoglycoside or a third-generation cephalosporin (Table 32–4). Intravenous immunoglobulin studies or white blood cell transfusions are encouraging but remain experimental.[44, 45]

Table 32–4. CLINICAL PICTURE, COMPLICATIONS, AND TREATMENT OF BACTERIAL PNEUMONIA

Organism	Clinical Features	Complications	Treatment
Group B *Streptococcus*	Early onset, similar to respiratory distress syndrome; late onset may be associated with meningitis	Mortality high; apnea, hypotension common	Penicillin with aminoglycoside until meningitis is excluded; minimum of 14 days
Streptococcus pneumoniae[59]	Accounts for 25% of pediatric bacterial pneumonia Infants: sudden fever, occasionally febrile convulsions, respiratory distress Classically acute onset, high fever, chills, cough, toxicity Usually winter-spring seasons	Quick resolution with antibiotic; excellent prognosis with no sequelae; SIADH common Empyema (20%); abscess (rarely)	Penicillin, 50–100 mg/kg/day for 7–10 days; organisms resistant to pencillin are rare
Group A *Streptococcus*[60, 61]	Accounts for 1% of pediatric bacterial pneumonia Patients appear extremely ill with respiratory distress, anemia Peak incidence winter Common URI symptoms ⅓ of patients have pharyngitis Usual age, 5–6 years	Slow resolution with antibiotic; SIADH and empyema common; pericarditis (1%–10%); occasionally pneumatocele, pneumothorax	Penicillin, 50–100 mg/kg/day for 10–14 days
Staphylococcus aureus[18, 62, 63]	Primary pneumonia: accounts for 25% of infantile bacterial pneumonia; usually high fever and respiratory distress; Median age is 6 months, 70% less than 1 year of age; peak incidence, winter; 50% with URI symptoms Secondary pneumonia: fever, generalized toxicity; median age, 5½ years; 67% over 3 years of age; 11% with URI symptoms	Empyema (70%), pneumothorax (30%), pneumatocele (23%), occasionally abscess (6.3%)	Penicillinase-resistant penicillin (nafcillin, 150 mg/kg/day, or vancomycin, 40 mg/kg/day) for 3–6 weeks, depending on complications; surgical treatment of empyema or abscess may be required
Haemophilus influenzae[19–21]	Neonatal involvement similar to group B *Streptococcus* In children similar to *S. pneumoniae* 73% under 2 years of age 80% in winter-spring seasons 65% had URI symptoms, 98% with fever, 75% with cough	Good if no other organ involved; pleural fluid (49%), pericarditis (4%), epiglottitis (6%), meningitis (18%), pneumothorax (11%), and rarely pneumatocele	Amoxicillin, 25–50 mg/kg/day; Augmentin, 40–80 mg/kg/day; cefaclor, 40–60 mg/kg/day; 7–10 days in mild disease, 2–3 weeks if severe or complication; may require parenteral therapy with cefuroxime (100–150 mg/kg/day), or ampicillin plus chloramphenicol initially
Gram-negative bacilli[32]	Copious, thick mucous secretions in immunocompromised patients	Necrotizing process with high mortality; empyema, occasionally cystic changes; lung abscess may occur with associated anaerobes	Penicillin G (50,000–250,000 units/kg/day or clindamycin (15–40 mg/kg/day)
Chlamydia[64]	Afebrile, persistent tachypnea, and staccato cough Otitis (50%) Conjunctivitis (50%) Wheezing (70%) Occasionally apnea Patients are usually between 3–12 weeks of age	Usually good prognosis, but hyperactive airway disease may be present	Erythromycin, 25–40 mg/kg/day for 7–10 days; tetracycline, 25–50 mg/kg/day if patient older than 7 years
Mycoplasma[65, 66]	Infants: cough, tachypnea, retraction Wheezing common; mild but protracted course of fever and cough Only 3% require hospitalization	May have associated neurologic and joint disease May result in hyperreactive airway disease after 4–6 weeks and abnormal PFT up to 3 years later	Erythromycin, 30–50 mg/kg/day for 7–10 days
Legionella[67, 68]	Infrequently documented despite seroconversion; usually with fever, chills, nonproductive cough	Diarrhea, confusion, hepatic involvement common	Erythromycin, 30–50 mg/kg/day for 7–10 days

SIADH, syndrome of inappropriate antidiuretic hormone; URI, upper respiratory infection; PFT, pulmonary function test.

Infants. Beyond the perinatal period, bacterial pneumonia is usually caused by *S. pneumoniae* and *H. influenzae,* and *S. aureus* is a frequent pathogen in undernourished infants. Infants are also exposed to respiratory viruses and *Chlamydia*. In addition, studies by Stagno and colleagues indicate a significant involvement by cytomegalovirus.[46] However, the roles of *Ureaplasma* and *Pneumocystis carinii* remain unknown. Ribavirin therapy for respiratory syncytial virus infection may need to be supplemented by cefotaxime or a third-generation cephalosporin in this age group.

Young Children. In children from 3 months to 5 years

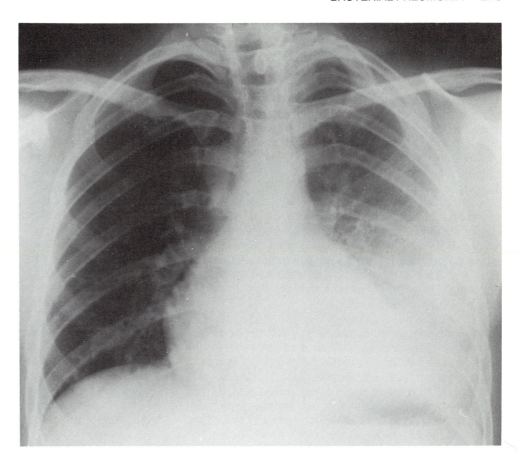

Figure 32–4. Significant left lower lobe pneumonia and empyema in a 14-year-old with fever, left lower chest pain, and dyspnea. A four-fold rise in *M. pneumoniae* CF titers was observed. No virus or bacterial pathogens were isolated from pleural fluid.

of age, the predominant bacteria are *S. pneumoniae* and *H. influenzae.* If there is a significant incidence of lactamase-positive *H. influenzae* in the community, the use of erythromycin-sulfisoxazole, trimethoprim-sulfamethoxazole, clavulanic acid/amoxicillin, or cefaclor is appropriate. When the risk of ampicillin-resistant *H. influenzae* is low, therapy with an aminopenicillin (amoxicillin or cyclacillin) is usually initiated.[47] However, viral pneumonias occur more frequently than bacterial pneumonias. There appears to be no increased morbidity or mortality in withholding antibiotics pending the results of cultures or antigen detection tests if nonbacterial pneumonia is strongly suspected.[48] Whatever the therapeutic choice, it is essential that adequate follow-up occurs, either by telephone conversation or by clinical examination within 24 to 48 h. If a child does not improve or the child's condition deteriorates, further evaluation is necessary. Teaching the parents to measure the respiratory rate during sleep or when the child is at rest enables objective information to be relayed. The chest radiograph may also be repeated. If initial treatment fails, depending on the reevaluation, possible hospitalization and additional diagnostic studies should be considered, in addition to alterations in therapy.

Older Children. *S. pneumoniae* remains a major bacterial cause of pneumonia in this age group; however, involvement with *Mycoplasma* must be considered (Fig. 32–4). Because of this, most physicians initiate therapy with erythromycin. Uncommon treatment failures with erythromycin may occur with resistance of some strains

of group A streptococci, *S. pneumoniae,* and staphylococci. In ambulatory practice, some physicians prefer a therapeutic trial over testing for cold agglutinins when *Mycoplasma* pneumonia is strongly suspected.[49] In hospitalized patients, however, cold agglutinins, *Mycoplasma* cultures, and serologic studies should be considered.

Special Host. Special situations (see Table 32–2) in which the patient's bacterial flora are altered or host defenses are depressed affect the selection of antibiotics (see Table 32–4). As mentioned previously, major predisposing conditions for aspiration pneumonia include seizure disorders, severe cerebral palsy, profound mental retardation, myopathies and neuromyopathies, general anesthesia, esophageal anomalies (tracheoesophageal fistulae, achalasia, anomalies of oral structures), and nasogastric tube feeding. Radiographic evidence of pneumonia in the posterior segments of the upper and lower right lobes is common in aspiration pneumonia. Abscess formation or empyema are also frequent in such cases and may require surgical intervention. Because anaerobic bacteria are part of the normal oral flora, outnumbering aerobes in a ratio of 10:1, documentation of their role in pneumonia may be difficult when there is no pleural fluid to extract for culture. Therefore, empiric antibiotic therapy is usually instituted in patients with clinical or radiographic evidence of aspiration pneumonia with antibiotics such as penicillin or clindamycin, which are active against anaerobic bacteria. Some physicians prefer clindamycin because of the increasing numbers of lactamase-producing strains of anaerobic bacteria and clinical treatment failures with penicillin therapy.[50]

Another special setting is the development of pulmonary infiltrates and respiratory distress with fever in a hospitalized patient. Organisms not normally found in the upper airways may appear at this stage and spread to the lower respiratory tract as a result of colonization from prior antimicrobial use or serious illness. In addition, colonization of the lower airways occurs within 24 h after a tracheostomy. The predominant organisms are gram-negative coliforms as well as potential pathogens such as *S. pneumoniae* and nontypable *H. influenzae*.[51] *Klebsiella* is the most frequent coliform, followed by *Pseudomonas*. Infection by *E. coli*, *Enterobacter*, and *Acinetobacter* can also occur.[32] In rare instances, *Proteus* and *Serratia* are involved. Because of the difficulty of establishing an etiologic pathogen, treatment is usually instituted empirically with a lactam antibiotic combined with an aminoglycoside. If aspiration pneumonia also appears likely, clindamycin may be added.

Cystic fibrosis represents a pediatric equivalent of chronic obstructive pulmonary disease in adult patients; however, the microbiologic flora of children and young adults with this disease is unique.[52] It consists of persistent colonization of the lower respiratory tract secretions with *S. aureus* in the earliest stages of the disease; a mixture of *S. aureus*, nontypable *H. influenzae*, and rough strains of *Pseudomonas aeruginosa* in the intermediate phase; and persistent colonization with mucoid *P. aeruginosa* in late stages. Because of this flora, antibiotic therapy is often tailored specifically to combat these microbes, even in episodes of viral infection, in which the objective of treatment is suppression of bacterial superinfection.

GENERAL MANAGEMENT AND FOLLOW-UP

Supportive care should never be overlooked in any pneumonia. Monitoring of arterial blood gases may be necessary when cyanosis, severe dyspnea, or tachypnea occurs. Normal arterial oxygen pressure should be maintained with supplemental oxygen. A rising arterial carbon dioxide pressure is suggestive of pulmonary hypoventilation, which may require ventilatory support. Although mist treatment may not influence the duration of hospitalization, it is generally believed that humidification of the airways aids in clearing secretions by pulmonary toilet (postural drainage and percussion). Adequate hydration and nutrition must be provided. Development of hyponatremia may be present in almost half of hospitalized children with pneumonia.[53] Therefore, dehydration caused by anorexia and increased respiratory rate must be prevented, but the syndrome of inappropriate secretion of antidiuretic hormone, which requires limitation of fluid intake, must also be considered. Electrolyte and blood urea nitrogen levels may need to be followed.

A chest radiograph obtained at the conclusion of treatment may not show resolution. Grossman and associates[54] showed that 80% of patients show complete clearing of the infiltrate after 3 to 4 weeks and 100% by 3 months. Documentation of resolution is essential in patients with recurrent pneumonias because it is evidence against pulmonary sequestration. Some authors recommend a chest radiograph in all patients after 3 months.[55] However, whether this is needed after treatment of uncomplicated, first-time pneumonia is controversial.

Lack of a response after 2 to 3 days should result in investigation of complicating factors (see Table 32-4). Drainage of pleural effusions may be needed. Patients with staphylococcal empyema require chest tube drainage for a median of 7 days as opposed to those with pneumococcal or *H. influenzae* infection, who require only 3 or 4 days of drainage.[56] It has been estimated that 60% to 80% of patients with empyema or effusion eventually require tube thoracostomy. Development of abscess and pneumatocele requires longer antibiotic treatment (up to 3 weeks). In repeated episodes and whenever the clinical course has been prolonged, bronchoscopy is important not only for obtaining diagnostic specimens but also for searching for a foreign body, evaluating anatomic defects, and in certain cases aiding in clearance of secretions and removal of mucus plugs. Superinfection with new bacterial pathogens such as aerobic gram-negative rods, *Aspergillus*, *Candida*, or the phycomycetes is a concern in immunocompromised patients.[57] Typically, after a week into the course of treatment, fever returns with increased sputum production, new infiltrates on chest radiographs, and new organisms that appear to be morphologically different on Gram's stain of the sputum.

REFERENCES

1. Glezen WP, Denny FW: Epidemiology of acute lower respiratory disease in children. New Engl J Med 288:498–505, 1973.
2. Denny FW: Acute lower respiratory tract infections in nonhospitalized children. J Pediatr 108:635–646, 1986.
3. Klein JO, Schlesinger PC, Karasic RB: Management of the febrile infant three months of age or younger. Pediatr Infect Dis 3:75–79, 1984.
4. Llorens-Terol J, Martínez-Roig A, Mur A: Pneumonia associated with meningococcal bacteremia and/or meningitis. Helv Pediatr Acta 39:189–192, 1984.
5. Davidson M, Tempest B, Palmer DL: Bacteriologic diagnosis of acute pneumonia. JAMA 235:158–163, 1976.
*6. Stratton CW: Bacterial pneumonias: An overview with emphasis on pathogenesis, diagnosis and treatment. Heart Lung 15:226–244, 1986.
*7. Murphy S, Florman AL: Lung defenses against infection: A clinical correlation. Pediatrics 72:1–15, 1983.
8. Umetsu DT, Ambrosino DM, Quinti I, et al: Recurrent sino-pulmonary infection and impaired antigen in children with selective IgG subclass deficiency. New Engl J Med 313:1247–1251, 1985.
9. Turner RB, Lande AE, Chase P, et al: Pneumonia in pediatric outpatients: Cause and clinical manifestations. J Pediatr 111:194–200, 1987.
10. Hughes JR, Sinha DP, Cooper MR, et al: Lung tap in childhood: Bacteria, viruses and mycoplasmas in acute lower respiratory tract infections. Pediatrics 44:477–485, 1969.
11. Mufson MA, Krause HE, Mocega HE, et al: Viruses, *Mycoplasma pneumoniae*, and bacteria associated with lower respiratory tract disease among infants. Am J Epidemiol 91:192–202, 1970.
12. Zollar LM, Krause HE, Mufson MA: Microbiologic studies on young infants with lower respiratory tract disease. Am J Dis Child 126:56–60, 1973.

*Recommended reading.

13. Escobar JA, Dover AS, Duenas A, et al: Etiology of respiratory tract infections in children in Cali, Colombia. Pediatrics 57:123–130, 1976.
14. Paisley JW, Lauer BA, McIntosh K, et al: Pathogens associated with acute lower respiratory tract infection in young children. Pediatr Infect Dis 3:14–19, 1984.
15. Leventhal JM: Clinical predictors of pneumonia as a guide to ordering chest roentgenograms. Clin Pediatr 21:730–734, 1982.
16. Chenian T, John TJ, Simoes E, et al: Evaluation of simple clinical signs for the diagnosis of acute lower respiratory tract infection. Lancet 2:125–128, 1988.
17. Klein JO: The epidemiology of pneumococcal disease in infants and children. Rev Infect Dis 3:246–253, 1981.
18. Chartraud SA, McCracken GH: Staphylococcal pneumonia in infants and children. Pediatr Infect Dis 1:19–23, 1982.
19. Ginsburg CM, Howard JB, Nelson JD: Report of 65 cases of *Haemophilus influenzae* B pneumonia. Pediatrics 64:283–286, 1979.
20. Asmar BI, Slovis TL, Reed JO, Dajani AS: *Haemophilus influenzae* type B pneumonia in 43 children. J Pediatr 93:389–393, 1978.
21. Jacobs NM, Harris VJ: Acute *Haemophilus* pneumonia in childhood. Am J Dis Child 133:603–605, 1979.
22. Silverman M, Stratton D, Diallo A: Diagnosis of acute bacterial pneumonia in Nigerian children. Arch Dis Child 52:925–931, 1977.
23. McCarthy PL, Lembo RM, Fink UD, et al: Observation, history and physical examination is diagnostic of serious illnesses in febrile children less than 24 months. J Pediatr 110:26–30, 1987.
24. McCarthy PL, Spiesel SZ, Stashwick CA: Radiographic findings and etiologic diagnosis in ambulatory childhood pneumonias. Clin Pediatr 20:686–691, 1981.
25. Eichenwald HF: Pneumonia syndromes in children. Hosp Pract 11:89–93, 1976.
26. Swischuk LE, Hayden CK: Viral vs bacterial pulmonary infections in children. Pediatr Radiol 16:278–284, 1986.
27. Zukin DD, Hoffman JR, Cleveland RH, et al: Correlation of pulmonary signs and symptoms with chest radiographs in the pediatric age group. Ann Emerg Med 15:792–796, 1986.
28. Isaacs D: Problems in determining the etiology of community-acquired childhood pneumonia. Pediatr Infect Dis J 8:143–148, 1989.
29. Alario AJ, McCarthy PL, Markowitz R, et al: Usefulness of chest radiographs in children with acute lower respiratory tract disease. J Pediatr 111:187–193, 1987.
30. Turner RB, Hayden FG, Hendley JO: Etiologic diagnosis of pneumonia in pediatrics outpatients by counterimmunoelectrophoresis of urine. Pediatrics 71:780–783, 1983.
31. Ramsey BW, Marcuse EK, Foy HM: Use of bacterial antigen in the diagnosis of pediatric lower respiratory tract infections. Pediatrics 78:1–9, 1986.
*32. Levison ME, Kaye D: Pneumonia caused by gram-negative bacilli: An overview. Rev Infect Dis 7(Suppl 4):S656–S665, 1985.
*33. Stiehm ER, Chin TW, Haas A, Peerless AG: Infectious complications of the primary immunodeficiencies. Clin Immunol Immunopathol 40:69–86, 1986.
34. Peerless AG, Liebhaber M, Anderson S, et al: *Legionella* pneumonia in chronic granulomatous disease. J Pediatr 106:783–785, 1985.
35. Kovatch AL, Jardine DS, Dowling JN, et al: Legionellosis in children with leukemia in relapse. Pediatrics 73:811–815, 1984.
36. Nussbaum E: Flexible fiberoptic bronchoscopy and laryngoscopy in infants and children. Laryngoscopy 93:1073–1075, 1983.
37. Nussbaum E: Pediatric flexible bronchoscopy and its application in infantile atelectasis. Clin Pediatr 24:379–382, 1985.
38. Nussbaum E, Maggi JC, Mathis R, Galant SP: Association of lipid-laden alveolar macrophages and gastroesophageal reflux in children. J Pediatr 110:190–194, 1987.
*39. Ries F, Sculier JP, Klastersky J: Diffuse bilateral pneumopathies in patients with cancer. Cancer Treat Rev 14:119–130, 1987.
40. Ceulaer K, McMullen KW, Mande GU, et al: Pneumonia in young children with homozygous sickle cell disease: Risk and clinical features. Eur J Pediatr 144:255–258, 1985.
41. Barrett-Connor E: Bacterial infection and sickle cell anemia. Medicine 50:97–112, 1971.
42. Miller ST, Hammerschlag MR, Chirgwin K, et al: Role of *Chlamydia pneumoniae* in acute chest syndrome of sickle cell disease. J Pediatr 118:30–33, 1991.
43. Davies SC, Luce PJ, Win AA, et al: Acute chest syndrome in sickle-cell disease. Lancet 1:36–38, 1984.
44. Stiehm ER: Intravenous immunoglobulins in neonates and infants: An overview. Pediatr Infect Dis 5:S217–S219, 1986.
45. Christensen RD, Anstall HB, Rothstein G: Review: Deficiencies in the neutrophil system of newborn infants and the use of leukocyte transfusions in the treatment of neonatal sepsis. J Clin Apheresis 1:33–41, 1982.
46. Stagno S, Brasfield DM, Brown MB, et al: Infant pneumonitis associated with cytomegalovirus, *Chlamydia, Pneumocystitis* and *Ureaplasma:* A prospective study. Pediatrics 68:322–329, 1981.
*47. Grossman M, Kline JO, McCarthy DL, et al: Consensus: Management of presumed bacterial pneumonia in ambulatory children. Pediatr Infect Dis 3:497–500, 1984.
48. Friis A, Andersen FH, Krasilnikoff PA, et al: Antibiotic treatment of pneumonia and bronchitis: A prospective randomized study. Arch Dis Child 59:1038–1045, 1984.
*49. Gooch WM: Bronchitis and pneumonia in ambulatory patients. Pediatr Infect Dis 6:137–140, 1987.
*50. Brook I: Direct and induced pathogenicity of anaerobic bacteria in respiratory tract infections in children. Adv Pediatr 34:357–377, 1987.
51. Johanson WG, Pierce AK, Sanford JP: Changing pharyngeal bacterial flora of hospitalized patients: Emergence of gram-negative bacilli. New Engl J Med 281:1137–1140, 1969.
52. Stutman HR, Marks MI: Pulmonary infections in children with cystic fibrosis. Semin Respir Infect 2:166–176, 1987.
53. Shawn F, Germer S: Hyponatremia associated with pneumonia or bacterial meningitis. Arch Dis Child 60:963–966, 1985.
54. Grossman LK, Wald ER, Nair P, Dapiez J: Roentgenographic follow-up of acute pneumonia in children. Pediatrics 63:30–31, 1979.
*55. Marks MI: Pediatric pneumonia: Viral or bacterial? J Respir Dis 3:108–126, 1982.
56. Barrett FF: Bacterial pneumonia of infants and children. *In* Laraya-Cuasay LR, Highes WT (eds): Interstitial Lung Disease in Children, pp. 165–173. Boca Raton, FL: CRC Press, 1988.
57. Parrino TA, Stollerman GH: The management of pneumonia. Adv Intern Med 30:113–151, 1984.
*58. Gilsdorf JR: Community-acquired pneumonia in children. Semin Respir Infect 2:146–151, 1987.
59. Finland M: Conference on the pneumococcus, summary and comments. Rev Infect Dis 3:358–371, 1981.
60. Molteni R: Group A β-hemolytic streptococcal pneumonia. Am J Dis Child 131:1366–1371, 1977.
61. Burech DL, Koranyi KI, Haynes RE: Serious group A streptococcal diseases in children. J Pediatr 88:972–974, 1976.
62. Hieber JP, Nelson AJ, McCracken GH: Acute disseminated staphylococcal disease in childhood. Am J Dis Child 131:181–185, 1977.
63. Shulman ST, Ayoub EM: Severe staphylococcal sepsis in adolescents. Pediatrics 58:59–66, 1976.
*64. Wilfert CM, Gutman LT: *Chlamydia trachomatis* infections of infants and children. Adv Pediatr 33:49–75, 1986.
65. Azimi PH, Chace PA, Petru AM: Mycoplasmas: Their role in pediatric disease. Curr Probl Pediatr 14:1–46, 1984.
66. Sabato AR, Martin AJ, Marmion BP, et al: *Mycoplasma pneumoniae:* Acute illness, antibiotics and subsequent pulmonary infection. Arch Dis Child 59:1034–1037, 1984.
67. Millunchick EW, Floyd J, Banks J: Legionnaires' disease in an immunologically normal child. Am J Dis Child 135:1065–1066, 1981.
68. Muldoon RL, Jaecker DL, Kiefer HK: Legionnaires' disease in children. Pediatrics 67:329–332, 1981.

33 *MYCOPLASMA PNEUMONIAE* INFECTIONS

HAILEN MAK, M.D., M.P.H.

Mycoplasmas have been recognized as pathogenic agents in diseases of humans, animals, and plants. In humans, the organism has been isolated from the respiratory tract, the urogenital tract, and synovial fluid. Among the 100 or more recognized species, three have been associated with disease in humans: *Mycoplasma pneumoniae,* which has been associated with respiratory diseases; *Mycoplasma hominis,* which has been shown to be a cause of postpartum fever and pelvic inflammatory disease; and *Ureaplasma urealyticum,* which causes nongonococcal urethritis, infertility, chorioamnionitis, and spontaneous abortion. Studies[1,2,3] indicate that there is a significant association between *U. urealyticum* colonization of the respiratory tract and development of chronic lung disease in infants of very low birth weight. In this chapter, the clinical spectrum of *M. pneumoniae* in respiratory diseases is discussed, with emphasis on epidemiology, clinical manifestations, diagnosis, and treatment.

BACTERIOLOGY

Mycoplasma pneumoniae, initially called the Eaton agent, was isolated by Eaton and co-workers in 1944 as the cause of primary atypical pneumonia.[4] This febrile respiratory disease did not respond to sulfonamide or penicillin therapy and was associated with the development of cold hemagglutinins. The Eaton agent was originally believed to be a virus until B. P. Marmion and A. M. Goodburn in 1961 showed that it was identical to pleuropneumonia-like organisms initially isolated from cattle with contagious pleuropneumonia.

Myocplasmas are the smallest free-living microorganisms known to survive outside of host cells. Lacking cell walls, they are pleomorphic and thus resistant to penicillin and other cell wall–active antimicrobials.[5] Adherence to and penetration of the respiratory epithelium are necessary for the initiation of infection.[6] When confined to the epithelium of the respiratory tract, the organism causes submucosal and peribronchial lesions. Cellular damage leads to ciliostasis, which accounts for the prolonged paroxysmal coughing.[7]

EPIDEMIOLOGY

M. pneumoniae infections are endemic throughout the year, but they occur in epidemics every several years. The organism is transmitted in droplets from the respiratory tract of one person to that of another and may take several weeks to spread among people in close contacts, such as in family members, children and workers in day-care centers, and military personnel. In close contacts, the infection rate may be as high as 90%. The incubation period is 10 to 14 days.

In a long-term epidemiologic study of *M. pneumoniae* infections in a prepaid medical plan, Foy and associates[8] found that the rates of infection, as determined by four-fold or higher rise in complement fixation titer, in cohorts of school-aged children and young adults varied from 2% in endemic years to 35% during epidemic periods. However, the rate of clinically recognized pneumonia was only 10% among those infected. The age-specific rate of pneumonia was highest among 5- to 9-year-olds and second highest among 10- to 14-year-olds. In children under 5 years of age, the rate of mycoplasma pneumonia was half that of children aged 5 to 9 years, but this (the youngest) age group had the highest total rate of pneumonias, caused mainly by viral etiologic agents.

Primary infection, mostly asymptomatic, commonly occurs in the youngest age group. In monitoring infants and children aged 2 months to 8 years who attended a day-care center, Fernald and co-workers[9] found that the annual infection rate was approximately 12%. Primary infection may sensitize young children to more severe infections at an older age when reinfection occurs. The mild nature of the disease in young children and the increasing severity of the disease with age suggest that pulmonary involvement and extrapulmonary complications are the result of immunologic response to reinfection.

CLINICAL MANIFESTATIONS

The spectrum of *M. pneumoniae* infections ranges from asymptomatic or mild upper respiratory illnesses to severe pneumonia and extrapulmonary complications. The illness usually begins with malaise, fever, cough, pharyngitis, and headache. The cough may be quite severe and is frequently paroxysmal. It starts several days after onset of the illness and is initially nonproductive, but may become productive of mucoid sputum that contains polymorphonuclear leukocytes on Gram's stain. Skin rashes, tenderness of cervical lymph nodes, otitis, bullous myringitis, chest pain, nausea, vomiting, myalgias, and arthralgias may occur. Sinus involvement is frequent but usually asymptomatic.[10] In Stevens and co-authors' review of 44 children referred to the hospital for lower respiratory tract infection with *M. pneumoniae,*[11] cough, malaise, and fever were the most common findings. Among patients with chronic lung diseases such as asthma and chronic bronchitis, *M. pneumoniae* may precipitate an acute exacerbation.[12] For patients with subclinical asthma or undiagnosed reactive airway diseases, wheezing, dyspnea, and intractable coughing may become unexpectedly prominent.

Pneumonia occurs in 3% to 10% of infected persons, and physical findings include scattered rales, rhonchi, wheezing, and bronchial breath sounds. Radiographic manifestations are variable; reticular and interstitial patterns are seen early in the course of the disease, and segmental or patchy consolidation develops later. Pleural effusion is found in 20% of pneumonias for which decubitus films are taken.[13] Effusions are typically small, unilateral, and transient. Pleural fluid usually shows an exudative characteristic, with a normal glucose, and variable numbers of polymorphonuclear and mononuclear cells. Transient enlargement of the hilar lymph nodes is a characteristic of *M. pneumoniae* respiratory infections in children, as observed in 34% of Niitu's pediatric patients.[14] In *Mycoplasma* infections there is a poor correlation between the degree of patient's symptoms and the clinical findings on both physical examination and chest radiographs.

Without serologic determinations or cultural identification, routine laboratory studies are not diagnostic of *Mycoplasma* infection. The leukocyte count is usually normal, but the sedimentation rate may be elevated during the acute phase of the illness. Positive Coombs' test and reticulocytosis suggest that clinically inapparent anemia is present, although the red blood cell count is normal. Serum immunoglobulin M (IgM) is frequently elevated, whereas levels of immunoglobulins G and A (IgG and IgA) are normal.

Although severe pulmonary complications of *Mycoplasma* infections are rare in children, the few long-term sequelae reported are significant. Stokes and associates[15] described the development of unilateral hyperlucent lung (Swyer-James syndrome) after severe *Mycoplasma* pneumonia in an 11-year-old girl. Another 11-year-old girl developed obliterative bronchiolitis 5 years after the initial *M. pneumoniae* infection.[16] Persistent abnormalities of the small airways, demonstrated by helium flow-volume loops, were found in children 1 to 9 years after *M. pneumoniae* respiratory tract infections.[17] Like many viral infections that result in subsequent abnormalities of pulmonary functions, *Mycoplasma* infections in early childhood may predispose the patient to reactive airway disease later in life.

Extrapulmonary manifestations of *M. pneumoniae* infection involve multiple organ systems, including the skin and the musculoskeletal, cardiovascular, gastrointestinal, neurologic, and hematologic systems (Table 33–1). Sequelae from the central nervous system and the heart are the most serious complications.

A variety of nonspecific rashes have been reported to accompany *M. pneumoniae* infections in 11% to 25% of patients.[18] Erythematous maculopapular and vesicular

Table 33–1. CLINICAL MANIFESTATIONS OF *MYCOPLASMA PNEUMONIAE* INFECTION

Respiratory	Nonrespiratory
Upper Respiratory Tract	***Dermatologic***
Pharyngitis	Erythematous maculopapular and vesicular exanthems
Bronchitis	Erythema multiforme
Myringitis	Stevens-Johnson syndrome
Otitis media	***Musculoskeletal***
Otitis externa	Myalgia
Pulmonary	Arthralgia
Pneumonia	Polyarthritis
Pleural effusion	Rheumatic fever–like syndrome
Lung abscess	***Cardiovascular***
Pneumatoceles	Myopericarditis
Swyer-James syndrome	Hemopericardium
Bronchiolitis obliterans	Congestive heart failure
Bronchiectasis	Heart block
	Gastrointestinal
	Gastroenteritis
	Elevation of liver enzymes
	Hepatitis
	Splenomegaly
	Pancreatitis
	Neurologic
	Convulsion
	Meningitis
	Encephalitis
	Cerebral infarction
	Cerebellar ataxia
	Guillain-Barré syndrome
	Transverse myelitis
	Hematologic
	Hemolytic anemia
	Thrombocytopenia
	Intravascular coagulation

eruptions are most common, but bullous, urticarial, and petechial lesions have been observed, particularly in males. Stevens-Johnson syndrome is an uncommon but serious dermatologic manifestation. Recurrent erythema multiforme caused by *M. pneumoniae* was described in a 15-year-old boy.[19]

The most common manifestations of the musculoskeletal system are arthralgias and myalgias. The pattern of joint involvement is usually polyarticular and migratory, and the large joints are most often affected. Illnesses resembling rheumatic fever have been described.[20]

Cardiac complications occur in 4% to 8% of hospitalized patients; the majority of such patients are adults and are seriously ill. Myopericarditis, hemopericardium, complete heart block, and congestive heart failure may occur.

Gastroenteritis symptoms, including anorexia, nausea, vomiting, and diarrhea, are seen in 12% to 44% of cases. Transient elevation of liver enzymes, hepatitis, splenomegaly, and pancreatitis have been observed.

Various central nervous system manifestations of mycoplasma infection include convulsions, Guillain-Barré syndrome, cerebellar ataxia, transverse myelitis, aseptic meningitis, encephalitis, and cerebral infarction.[21] In one study, the median age of patients with neurologic diseases was 10 years, which indicates that the pediatric age group was most prone to complications of the central nervous system. The overall mortality rate was 10%, and one third of the patients had significant neurologic deficits. The neurologic syndromes are believed to be immunologically mediated, and circulating immune complexes and autoantibodies have been detected.

Significant hematologic complications are rare, but hemolytic anemia, diffuse intravascular coagulation, and thrombocytopenia have been reported.[18] Hemolytic anemia is seen in patients with severe pulmonary disease and high titers of cold agglutinins.

DIAGNOSIS

Although *Mycoplasma* organisms may be isolated from secretions of the respiratory tract, the slow growth of the organism renders cultures impractical in most clinical settings. Therefore, serologic methods are usually used in diagnosis. However, the immune response may not be evident until the second week of illness. *M. pneumoniae* evokes the formation of several distinct antibodies. Cold agglutinins for human O erythroyctes develop in about 50% of patients with pneumonia. Some patients develop agglutinins for the MG strain of nonhemolytic *Streptococcus*. Antibody to species-specific surface antigen of *Mycoplasma* may be detected by complement fixation, immunofluorescence, metabolic inhibition, and radioimmunoprecipitation tests.

Cold hemagglutinins are IgM autoantibodies that agglutinate human erythrocytes at 4°C. The presence of cold hemagglutinins is nonspecific, and they may be present in patients with infectious mononucleosis, rubella, influenza, adenovirus infections, malaria, psittacosis, and conditions associated with dysproteinemias and peripheral vascular disorders. A rapid screening test for cold agglutinins may be performed by collecting four drops of blood in a tube containing 0.2 ml of 3.8% sodium citrate solution. The tube is placed in ice water for 0.5 min and then is examined for agglutination by tilting it on its side.[22] Cold hemagglutinins begin to appear at 7 days, rise sharply in titer to peak at 4 weeks, and disappear by 3 months. Being the antibody first detected and first to disappear, its presence is correlated directly to the severity of the respiratory illness. In children, cold agglutinins do not appear frequently, but when present they are likely to occur with pneumonia.

The complement fixation test is the most commonly used method to detect antibodies against *M. pneumoniae*. A fourfold or higher rise in titers between acute- and convalescent-phase specimens is diagnostic. A single titer of at least 1:64 is also highly suggestive. The glycolipid antigen used in the complement fixation test cross-reacts with a variety of microorganisms, particularly those causing *Legionnaires'* disease, which has similar clinical features as mycoplasma pneumonia.

The enzyme-linked immunosorbent assay (ELISA) has been introduced for the detection of mycoplasma antibodies. In comparison with complement fixation testing, ELISA offers several advantages: increased sensitivity, simplicity, rapidity, and low cost. Since 1988, the MYCO-PLASMELISA II test kit (BioWhittaker, Inc., Walkersville, Maryland) has been available as a commercial

ELISA system designed to detect *M. pneumoniae* IgG antibody. Agreement between the MYCOPLASMELISA and the complement fixation tests was 96.6% for antibody detection and 93.9% for evaluation of paired sera.[23] The MYCOPLASMA STAT test, also developed by Bio-Whittaker, is a modified version of the MYCOPLAS-MELISA II test in which the total test time has been shortened from 3 to 1 h. Therefore, the MYCOPLASMA STAT test may be used is smaller laboratories as a rapid and convenient tool in the diagnosis of mycoplasma infections. The IgM-Mp TEST (Instar Corporation, Stillwater, Minnesota) is a solid-phase reverse ELISA test for the detection of specific IgM antibodies to *M. pneumoniae*. The determination of specific IgM antibodies, which characteristically appear early in most infections and rapidly decline over time, enables the early diagnosis of current infection in a single serum specimen. In contrast, the determination of specific IgG antibodies, which typically remain elevated for a prolonged period of time after a microbial infection, generally require acute and convalescent serum titers for clinical diagnosis.

The MERISTAR-MP latex agglutination test (Meridian Diagnostics, Inc., Cincinnati, Ohio) was developed in 1991 for the rapid detection of IgG and IgM antibodies to *M. pneumoniae*. In comparison with the standard complement fixation test, with positive tests defined by complement fixation titers of 64 or higher, the sensitivity and specificity of the latex agglutination test was 82% and 91%.[24] The total test time required for the latex agglutination test is approximately 10 min. Therefore, the latex agglutination test can serve as a simple and rapid screen for *M. pneumoniae* in a small medical clinic or office setting.

TREATMENT

Because mycoplasmas lack cell walls and penicillin-binding proteins, penicillin and other beta-lactam compounds are ineffective antimicrobial agents. Erythromycin is the most active drug in inhibiting the growth of *M. pneumoniae*.[25] Mardh[26] found that of the tetracyclines, doxycycline and minocycline were the most active. Because of the adverse effects of tetracycline on dentition, erythromycin is the drug of choice in children. Early administration of antibiotics delays but does not prevent infection or development of pneumonia. In one study, children given erythromycin during the first 7 days of illness experienced a shorter duration of fever than did patients treated with inappropriate medicine.[27] Organisms have been recovered from throat cultures and sputum during and after therapy.

Mycoplasma carrier status is not affected by antibiotic therapy; this explains the high infection rate among family members. The benefit of early treatment is unknown, because most cases involving complications are not diagnosed until late in the course of the disease. However, in clinical settings of young children with nontoxic but severe respiratory illness and debilitating cough, the judicious use of erythromycin to shorten the duration of symptoms of *Mycoplasma* infection and to eradicate other susceptible respiratory pathogens such as *Chla-mydia trachomatis* and *Bordetella pertussis* may be beneficial.

Finally, supportive therapeutic modalities, consisting of adequate rest, nutritional support, bronchodilators, and administration of oxygen, should be included as adjuncts to antimicrobial treatment. In severe cases of pneumonia, erythema multiforme, hemolytic anemia, and neurologic complications, corticosteroids have been found to be beneficial, but their clinical efficacy needs to be assessed in controlled, prospective studies. There is no effective method of preventing *Mycoplasma* infections. Therefore, attempts at limiting close contacts with infectious persons should be made.

REFERENCES

1. Sanchez PJ, Regan JA: *Ureaplasma urealyticum* colonization and chronic lung diseases in low birth weight infants. Pediatr Infect Dis J 7:542–546, 1988.
2. Wang EE, Frayha H, Watts J, et al: Role of *Ureaplasma urealyticum* and other pathogens in the development of chronic lung disease of prematurity. Pediatr Infect Dis J 7:547–551, 1988.
3. Cassell GH, Waites KB, Crouse DT, et al: Association of *Ureaplasma urealyticum* infection of the lower respiratory tract with chronic lung disease and death in very low birth weight infants. Lancet 2:240–245, 1988.
4. Eaton MD, Meiklejohn G, van Herick W: Studies on the etiology of primary atypical pneumonia; a filterable agent transmissible to cotton rats, hamsters, and chicken embryos. J Exp Med 79:649–668, 1944.
5. Hayflick L, Chanock R: *Mycoplasma* species of man. Bacteriol Rev 29:185–221, 1965.
6. Powell DA, Hu PC, Wilson M, et al: Attachment of *Mycoplasma pneumoniae* to respiratory epithelim. Infect Immun 13:959–966, 1976.
7. Broughton RA: Infections due to *Mycoplasma pneumoniae* in childhood. Pediatr Infect Dis 5:71–85, 1986.
8. Foy HM, Kenny GE, Cooney MK, et al: Long-term epidemiology of infections with *Mycoplasma pneumoniae*. J Infect Dis 139:681–687, 1979.
9. Fernald GW, Collier AM, Clyde WA: Respiratory infections due to *Mycoplasma pneumoniae* in infants and children. Pediatrics 55:327–335, 1975.
10. Griffin JP, Klein EW: Role of sinusitis in primary atypical pneumonia. Clin Med 78:23–27, 1971.
11. Stevens D, Swift PG, Johnston PG, et al: *Mycoplasma pneumoniae* infections in children. Arch Dis Child 53:38–42, 1978.
12. McNamara MJ, Phillips IA, Williams OB: Viral and *Mycoplasma pneumoniae* infections in exacerbations of chronic lung disease. Am Rev Respir Dis 100:19–24, 1969.
13. Fine NL, Smith LR, Sheedy PF: Frequency of pleural effusions in mycoplasma and viral pneumonias. N Engl J Med 283:790–793, 1970.
14. Niitu Y: *M. pneumoniae* respiratory diseases, clinical features—children. Yale J Biol Med 56:493–503, 1983.
15. Stokes D, Sigler A, Khouri NF, et al: Unilateral hyperlucent lung (Swyer-James syndrome) after severe *Mycoplasma pneumoniae* infection. Am Rev Respir Dis 117:145–152, 1978.
16. Isles AF, Masel J, O'Duffy J: Obliterative bronchiolitis due to *Mycoplasma pneumoniae* infection in a child. Pediatr Radiol 17:109–111, 1987.
17. Mok JY, Waugh P, Simpson H: *Mycoplasma pneumoniae* infection, a follow-up study of 50 children with respiratory illness. Arch Dis Child 54:506–511, 1979.
18. Murray HW, Masur M, Senterfit LB, et al: The protean manifestations of *Mycoplasma pneumoniae* infections in adults. Am J Med 58:229–242, 1975.
19. Welch KJ, Burke WA, Irons TG: Recurrent erythema multiforme due to *Mycoplasma penumoniae*. J Am Acad Dermatol 17:839–840, 1987.
20. Lambert HP: Syndrome with joint manifestations in association with *Mycoplasma pneumoniae* infection. Br Med J 3:156–157, 1968.
21. Behan PO, Feldman RG, Segerra JM, et al: Neurological aspects of mycoplasmal infection. Acta Neurol Scand 74:314–322, 1986.
22. Griffin JP: Rapid screening for cold agglutinins in pneumonia. Ann Intern Med 70:701–705, 1969.
23. Fischer GS, Sweimler WI, Kleger B: Comparison of MYCOPLAS-MELISA with complement fixation test for measurement of antibodies to *Mycoplasma pneumoniae*. Diagn Mycobiol Infect Dis 4:139–145, 1986.
24. Harvey SM, Tom S, Nikaido M: Mycoplasma pneumonia latex agglutination and complement fixation: Comparative serology. Am Clin Lab 11:16–18, 1992
25. McCracken GH Jr: Current status of antibiotic treatment for *Mycoplasma pneumoniae* infections. Pediatr Infect Dis 5:167–171, 1986.
26. Mardh PA: Human respiratory tract infections with mycoplasma and their *in vitro* susceptibility to tetracyclines and some other antibiotics. Chemotherapy 21(Suppl 1):47–57, 1975.
27. Sabato AR, Martin AJ, Marmion BP, et al: *Mycoplasma pneumoniae:* Acute illness, antibiotics, and subsequent pulmonary function. Arch Dis Child 59:1034–1037, 1984.

34 VIRAL PNEUMONIA

DANA G. KETCHUM, M.D., M.P.H. / RUSSELL B. VAN DYKE, M.D.

Viral pneumonia—inflammation of the lung due to infection with a virus—is the most common acute infectious disease of the lower respiratory tract in childen.[1] Most cases of viral pneumonia are mild and are treated on an outpatient basis, resolving without complications. Nevertheless, this disease entity is a major cause of serious (and potentially life-threatening) illness in infants and immunocompromised patients. Research has helped better define the epidemiologic characteristics of viral pneumonia and clarify which viruses are its most common causes. In addition, improvements in rapid diagnostic testing for respiratory viruses have enabled a specific viral diagnosis to be made with higher frequency. Although treatment remains mainly supportive, antiviral therapy is now available for some agents, enhancing the need for accurate, rapid diagnosis. Prevention still depends principally on strong infection control measures until specific effective vaccines are developed. Despite these advances, however, additional studies are needed in order to clarify the pathophysiologic processes of viral pneumonia and its relation to the development of chronic pulmonary disease.

Childhood pneumonia occurs most often in infants under 1 year of age, and decreases in frequency through school age to adolescence. Pneumonia caused by respiratory viruses usually spreads in an epidemic manner because of the contagiousness of the agents that are its most common causes (and because of their short incubation periods): respiratory syncytial virus (RSV), parainfluenza and influenza viruses, and adenoviruses. These viral agents are not usually found endemically except for parainfluenza virus type 3 and adenovirus. Outbreaks tend to be caused by only one virus at a time: an "interference phenomenon" whereby the widespread presence of one virus tends to exclude others may thus operate during epidemics.[2] Epidemic patterns are different for each viral agent. RSV occurs in midwinter epidemics, as do influenzae A and B. Parainfluenza viruses types 1 and 2 cause biannual fall outbreaks. Adenoviruses occur endemically but with seasonality, being most common from October to May. Children in day-care centers are easily exposed to respiratory viruses and provide an experimental model for the spread of these agents. For example, a group of healthy children in day care who were exposed to others with symptomatic adenovirus infection was studied over a 2-week period. Two thirds of the exposed children became ill and shed virus of the same serotype (a secondary attack rate of 67%).[3]

ETIOLOGY AND PATHOPHYSIOLOGY

Table 34–1 lists the viral agents that have been associated with pneumonia in children. In addition to the res-

piratory viruses just mentioned, rhinoviruses may infrequently cause pneumonia.[4] Enteroviruses (principally coxsackievirus A9 and B1[5, 6]) and coronaviruses[7] also appear to spread to the lungs by the respiratory route, occasionally causing disease.

The viruses of the herpes group (herpes simplex, varicella, cytomegalovirus, and Epstein-Barr virus) gain access to the lungs primarily by hematogenous dissemination as part of a systemic illness. The normal host immune response usually contains such spread, so these viruses produce pneumonia most often in immunocompromised patients and newborns. Rubella virus also spreads hematogenously to the lungs in infected neonates. Measles virus can gain access to the lungs by either the respiratory or the hematogenous route, and pneumonia often complicates infection with this agent.

The most common viral agents of pneumonia are transmitted by aerosol when close contact occurs with an infected person. RSV, parainfluenza, influenza, adenoviruses, rhinoviruses, enteroviruses, and coronaviruses are all spread by this respiratory route. The virus gains access to the upper respiratory tract and then spreads contiguously to the lower respiratory tract, invading the terminal bronchioles and the alveoli. In the small airways, the virus attacks the respiratory epithelium, resulting in loss of ciliary function and obstruction of the airways with mucus and mononuclear inflammatory cells. Incomplete airway obstruction may lead to air trapping distally with consequent hyperinflation of the lungs. Complete airway obstruction can cause adjacent alveoli to collapse in infants and young children, which leads to atelectasis because of lack of collateral ventilation via the pores of Kohn. Overwhelming infections (e.g., with influenza) may destroy the respiratory epithelium and cause a hemorrhagic exudate with both mononuclear and polymorphonuclear cells. In healthy children, the immune response (specific antibody, cytotoxic cells, and interferon) halts the spread of the virus and allows regeneration of the respiratory epithelium. An animal model of these pathologic processes has been described in hamsters infected intranasally with parainfluenza virus type 3.[8, 9]

CLINICAL MANIFESTATIONS

Viral pneumonia caused by respiratory viruses is usually preceded by several days of mild upper respiratory and constitutional symptoms. Patients may have a history of nasal congestion, decreased activity and appetite, and gradual development of fever, cough, and respiratory distress. The hallmark signs and symptoms of viral pneumonia are tachypnea with tachycardia, chest retractions (intercostal, subcostal, and suprasternal), and nasal flaring and grunting, all indicative of respiratory distress. Patients suffering apneic episodes or recurrent bouts of coughing and patients with significant ventilation-perfusion mismatch may be cyanotic, with dusky oral mucous membranes and nailbeds. Apneic episodes occur in young infants, especially with respiratory syncytial virus, and can be life-threatening.[23] Infants with pneumonia may also tend to become dehydrated as a result of tachypnea, increased temperature, and decreased oral intake.

Table 34–1. CAUSES OF VIRAL PNEUMONIA

Causative Agents	Primary Route of Spread to the Lung
Respiratory Viruses	
Respiratory syncytial virus	Respiratory
Parainfluenza viruses (types 1, 2, 3)	Respiratory
Influenza viruses (types A, B)	Respiratory
Adenoviruses (types 1–5, 7, 14, 21)	Respiratory
Rhinoviruses	Respiratory
Enteroviruses	Respiratory
Coronaviruses	Respiratory
Herpes Viruses	
Herpes simplex	Hematogenous
Varicella-zoster	Hematogenous
Epstein-Barr	Hematogenous
Cytomegalovirus	Hematogenous
Other Viral Agents	
Measles	Respiratory
Rubella	Hematogenous

On auscultation, children with viral pneumonia may exhibit crackles (rales), diminished breath sounds or dullness to percussion (indicative of consolidation or atelectasis), increased resonance with percussion (characteristic of air trapping), and wheezing. These physical findings are usually more easily detectable in older children and adolescents; infants and younger children may have only symptoms that are consistent with respiratory distress. Newborns with pneumonia may not even have specific respiratory symptoms (except for apnea) but may exhibit only decreased activity and difficulty with or reluctance in feeding.

Bacterial pneumonia classically presents with high fever, signs and symptoms of respiratory distress, and physical findings (dullness to percussion and decreased breath sounds over the affected area) that are characteristic of a lobar infiltrate. This clinical picture may also be consistent with viral pneumonia, however, and the two entities cannot be distinguished on the basis of physical examination alone. Children (especially those of school age) with pneumonia who are not in respiratory distress can be treated on an outpatient basis if they undergo close follow-up. Patients with respiratory distress, particularly infants, need to be hospitalized, and those who are in respiratory failure may need intensive care.

RSV is the leading cause of lower respiratory tract infection in children, especially in those under 2 years of age. Bronchiolitis is the most common disease caused by RSV, but this entity often coexists with pneumonitis (bronchiolitis is discussed in depth in Chapter 22). RSV disease of the lower respiratory tract in children begins with upper respiratory symptoms and low-grade fever, progressing to worsening cough, wheezing, and rales. Most infants recover in about a week, but reinfections are frequent. A small number of infants develop more serious disease with signs and symptoms of respiratory failure.

Parainfluenza viruses produce disease of the lower respiratory tract almost as frequently as RSV, also most commonly in children under 2 years of age. Parainfluenza types 1 and 2 usually cause croup (laryngotracheobronchitis), but pneumonia caused by these agents is also common and may accompany croup. Parainfluenza type 3 infection in infants can result in severe pneumonia analogous to RSV pneumonia.[10]

Influenza viruses A and B are the third most common cause of pneumonia in infants and toddlers and a leading cause of viral pneumonia in school-age children. Influenza pneumonia in children often manifests with a more rapid and severe onset than lower respiratory tract disease caused by other respiratory viruses. Symptoms initially include high fever, cough, pharyngitis, headache, and myalgia and progress to physical manifestations consistent with pneumonia. Influenza virus destroys the respiratory epithelium, and secondary infection with upper respiratory tract bacteria (pneumococci, *Streptococcus pyogenes, Haemophilus influenzae,* and staphylococci) may result from the consequent impairment of ciliary function.[11]

In most children, adenovirus infection is restricted to the upper respiratory tract, although it is often accompanied by high fever. In a large prospective series of children with acute respiratory illnesses, however, almost 7% of those with a clinical diagnosis of pneumonia produced nasal washings that tested positive for adenoviruses.[3] Adenovirus types 3, 7, 11, and 21 can cause life-threatening pneumonia in infants, producing an obliterative bronchiolitis. Chronic lung changes are common in patients who recover.[12-14] Adenoviruses of these types generally produce less serious illness in older children and adolescents, although types 4, 7, and 21 can cause fatal pneumonia.[15]

Pneumonia caused by the measles virus can resemble severe adenovirus infection and is a source of considerable mortality in developing countries. Immunocompromised patients, particularly those infected with human immunodeficiency virus (HIV), may develop severe primary measles pneumonia.[16] Herpes simplex virus most commonly causes pneumonia as part of disseminated herpes infection in newborns, but it sometimes produces lower respiratory tract disease in HIV-infected and transplant patients.[17] Cytomegalovirus is a more frequent cause of overwhelming pneumonia in immunosuppressed patients, and cytomegalovirus pneumonia can also occur in newborns after transfusion with unscreened blood.[18-20] Varicella-zoster virus is another cause of serious lower respiratory tract disease in immunocompromised children and may occasionally be a complication of chickenpox in normal patients.[21] Epstein-Barr virus infection can also lead to pneumonia in immunocompetent persons.[22]

DIAGNOSIS

Pneumonia can be conclusively diagnosed only by demonstrating infiltrates on chest radiographs. Chest radiographs of patients with viral pneumonia have characteristic features that help distinguish them from patients with bacterial disease. These radiologic features include bilateral scattered interstitial, peribronchial, and perihilar infiltrates. Multiple subsegmental areas of atelectasis are also seen in viral pneumonia, as is atelectasis of the right upper and middle lobes. In contrast, chest radiographs of bacterial pneumonia patients more often show better defined unilobular or unilateral infiltrates in the mid- to peripheral lung fields. Pleural effusions, abscesses, and pneumatoceles are also associated primarily with bacterial infections but occur with viral pneumonia on rare occasions.[24, 25] Adenovirus pneumonia may manifest with lobar infiltrates and pleural reaction. Chlamydial pneumonia in young infants yields radiographic findings (bilateral interstitial infiltrates) that are indistinguishable from those of viral pneumonia, as does mycoplasmal pneumonia.

In a child who is in severe respiratory distress or is in respiratory failure as a result of viral pneumonia, blood gases should be measured in order to assess blood pH and degree of hypercapnia and hypoxemia. For the child who is less ill but still appears cyanotic or in mild respiratory distress, noninvasive monitoring by pulse oximetry is useful.

White blood cell counts (WBCs) in viral pneumonia vary widely and may be in the normal range, and so they are of limited diagnostic value. An elevated WBC with viral pneumonia has been reported to occur most often with influenza and parainfluenza virus infections.[26] Other authors, however, have reported that the WBC is usually below normal with influenza. Increased white blood counts with an increase in the number of neutrophils and band forms are characteristic of bacterial pneumonia but cannot be used to conclusively rule out viral disease.

Tests that can be useful for differentiating viral pneumonia from other infectious causes of lower respiratory tract disease include a purified protein derivative (PPD) of 5 tuberculin units (TU) for tuberculosis (accompanied by a *Candida* skin test to rule out anergy); cold agglutinin tests or specific serologic tests for *Mycoplasma;* and, in young infants, a rapid screening test or culture on nasopharyngeal secretions for *Chlamydia.*

Children are not usually asymptomatic carriers of viruses in the respiratory tract (adenoviruses, although they can persist in tonsillar tissue, appear to be carried predominantly in the gastrointestinal tract).[3, 27] Detection of a specific virus in respiratory secretions of a patient with pneumonia is thus accepted as evidence that this particular agent is the cause of pulmonary infection (in contrast to suspected bacterial pneumonia, for which results of upper respiratory tract cultures are not useful for determining the causes of lower respiratory tract disease). Viruses in respiratory secretions can be identified by culture (which takes several days) and also by several rapid diagnostic procedures, including fluorescent antibody testing (FA), enzyme-linked immunosorbent assay (ELISA), and DNA probes. These rapid diagnostic tests for viral infections are described in detail in Chapter 14. Presumptive serologic diagnosis of viral pneumonia is also possible if a rise in antibody titer can be demonstrated between acute and convalescent serum specimens. Such testing is by nature retrospective, however, and of limited utility in clinical practice. If cytomegalovirus is present, it can be isolated from cultures of the throat, the urine, and the buffy coat of the blood. Tracheal aspirate and thoracentesis or open-lung biopsy to obtain lung tissue itself for direct examination and culture should be reserved for immunocompromised patients and severely ill immunocompetent patients whose lives may be saved by making a definitive diagnosis. Health care providers may find that obtaining surveillance cultures on a number of patients with suspected viral pneumonia may be useful during the respiratory virus season as a way of determining which viruses are most prevalent in their community.

DIFFERENTIAL DIAGNOSIS

The most common causes of bacterial pneumonia in preschool children over 1 month of age are the pneumococcus and *Haemophilus influenzae* type b. *Mycoplasma* is probably the principal cause of lower respiratory tract disease in school-age children.[1] Pulmonary infection caused by tuberculosis always needs to be considered, however, especially in children infected with HIV, indigent children, and migrants and refugees from developing countries. Pertussis should also be included in the differential diagnosis of bacterial pneumonia, particularly in unimmunized and incompletely immunized infants. Other infectious causes of pneumonia include *Chla-*

mydia, environmental (atypical) mycobacteria, fungal agents (blastomycosis, coccidioidomycosis, histoplasmosis) and parasites (*Pneumocystis carinii* in immunosuppressed patients and *Paragonimus westermani* in Southeast Asian refugees).

A variety of noninfectious conditions can produce a clinical picture similar to that of viral pneumonia. Reactive airway disease, especially with atelectasis, is probably the most common of these conditions in an outpatient setting. Other considerations include congestive heart failure, pulmonary infarction (especially in children with hemoglobinopathies), chronic lung disease, recurrent foreign body aspiration, underlying anatomic abnormalities of the lung, and pulmonary damage by physical agents (e.g., hydrocarbons).

MANAGEMENT

Supportive therapy is the primary form of treatment for viral pneumonia. Such therapy consists principally of ensuring that patients are well hydrated and well oxygenated with adequate humidity. Close monitoring of vital signs and of intake and output is essential, especially in infants at risk for apnea, who should be placed on a cardiorespiratory monitor. Chest physical therapy, suctioning of secretions, and fever control (with acetaminophen) are also important. The use of dextromethorphan or codeine to suppress cough is contraindicated and should be limited to older normal children with persistent cough that interrupts sleep.[28] Patients in respiratory failure may need mechanical ventilation in order to correct hypoxemia and hypercapnia.

ANTIBIOTICS

Antibiotics have no role in the treatment of patients with a diagnosis of viral pneumonia. Because the diagnostic evaluation of most pneumonia patients is limited, however, and a cause cannot be definitely established in many cases, empiric antibiotic treatment is often prescribed to cover the possibility of bacterial infection. Antibiotics effective against the pneumococcus and *H. influenzae* (and against *Mycoplasma pneumoniae* in older children and sickle cell patients) are usually employed. A broader range of bacterial agents must be considered in hospitalized patients with possible secondary bacterial infections and in immunocompromised children. Therapy for bacterial pneumonia is discussed in more detail in Chapter 32.

SPECIFIC ANTIVIRAL THERAPY

Specific antiviral therapy is usually reserved for seriously ill infants and immunocompromised children. Ribavirin administered by inhalation has been used to treat patients with severe pneumonia caused by RSV, especially infants with congenital heart disease[29] and bronchopulmonary dysplasia. Amantadine is most useful for preventing influenza A infection, but it may have a role in the treatment of critically ill children with influenza A, especially those with underlying risk factors. This agent has no efficacy against influenza B. Acyclovir has been used as specific therapy for varicella and herpes simplex pneumonia in immunocompromised patients. These antiviral agents are described in full in Chapter 83.

COMPLICATIONS

Most children with viral pneumonia recover rapidly without complications. Patients with bronchopulmonary dysplasia, congenital heart disease, and cystic fibrosis[30] are more likely to develop severe infections, however. Infants with bronchopulmonary dysplasia and congenital heart disease (particularly those with pulmonary hypertension) are especially at risk of potentially life-threatening pneumonia caused by RSV.[31]

By contrast, most immunosuppressed patients and children with hematologic malignancies are not usually at increased risk of infection with the common respiratory viruses that cause pneumonia. Such children are, however, at risk of severe infection with viruses capable of latency that spread hematogenously: cytomegalovirus and varicella. Patients with severe combined immunodeficiency disease are an exception; they are at high risk of serious respiratory infection with the more frequent agents of viral pneumonia, particularly parainfluenza type 3.[32] The relationship of viral pneumonia to longer term complications is unclear, but an association between chronic pulmonary disease and pneumonias caused by adenoviruses, influenza, and measles has been suggested.[33–35]

PROGNOSIS

Viral pneumonia in children is usually a self-limited illness and is rarely fatal except in young infants (especially those with underlying disease) and immunodeficient patients. Most practitioners schedule children treated on an outpatient basis for a follow-up visit 1 to several weeks after the diagnosis has been made. As long as the patient is clinically healthy at that time (and the majority are), repeating a chest radiograph is not necessary. One fifth of children with acute pneumonia diagnosed radiographically continue to have infiltrates on follow-up radiographs 3 to 4 weeks later, but almost all of these infiltrates have resolved 3 months afterwards. Chest radiographs should be repeated in children who continue to have symptoms and in those with a history of recurrent pneumonia or other forms of chronic lung disease.[36]

PREVENTION

Prevention of viral pneumonia in family, community, school, and day-care settings is extremely difficult, especially during acute outbreaks. Day-care centers should request that children with viral pneumonia remain at home or should restrict them to isolation rooms with separate caretakers. Prevention is equally difficult in the hospital setting, where health care personnel can act as intermediate hosts, carrying respiratory viruses in their upper respiratory tracts or, more likely, on their hands. The nosocomial spread of RSV is common, and patients with RSV pneumonia or bronchiolitis should be restricted to separate isolation rooms or wards.[37] Hospital personnel should avoid being contaminated with respiratory secretions and should practice efficient hand-washing technique. RSV is generally spread, not by aerosol, but by contact with respiratory secretions either directly by handling infected infants or indirectly via fomites. Control of nosocomial spread thus depends on thorough hand washing between patients and on fomite control. With infection control practices in addition to isolating infants and utilizing the cohort arrangement for the staff, the nosocomial infection rate dropped from 45% to 19% in one study.[38] In a subsequent study, use of eye-nose goggles reduced the nosocomial infection rate to 9%.[39]

Vaccines have been developed for influenza and adenoviruses, but only the influenza vaccine is recommended for use in children. The Committee on Infectious Diseases of the American Academy of Pediatrics currently recommends yearly influenza immunization for children over 6 months old with chronic lung disease, hemodynamically significant heart disease, sickle cell disease (and other hemoglobinopathies), and symptomatic HIV infection and for children receiving immunosuppressive therapy. Consideration should also be given to immunizing other children at increased risk of severe influenza infection, including those with diabetes, those with chronic kidney and metabolic disease, and patients receiving long-term aspirin treatment for arthritis or Kawasaki's disease (who are at increased risk of developing Reye's syndrome after an influenza infection). Immunization of family members of high-risk children, of children living with high-risk adults (e.g., those with symptomatic HIV infection), and of hospital personnel caring for high-risk pediatric patients is also encouraged. Influenza vaccination should be given in the autumn before the beginning of the influenza season.[40] Amantadine prophylaxis against influenza A may also be useful, especially in nonvaccinated persons and in immunosuppressed patients who do not respond adequately to the influenza vaccine (amantadine prophylaxis is discussed more fully in Chapter 83).

REFERENCES

1. Murphy TF, Henderson FW, Clyde WA Jr, et al: Pneumonia: An eleven-year study in a pediatric practice. Am J Epidemiol 113:12–21, 1981.
2. Glezen WP, Denny FW: Epidemiology of acute lower respiratory disease in children. N Engl J Med 288:498–505, 1973.
3. Edwards KM, Thompson J, Paolini J, et al: Adenovirus infections in young children. Pediatrics 76:420–424, 1985.
4. George RB, Mogabgab WJ: Atypical pneumonia in young men with rhinovirus infections. Ann Intern Med 71:1073–1078, 1969.
5. Eckert HL, Portnoy B, Salvatore MA, et al: Group B Coxsackie virus infection in infants with acute lower respiratory disease. Pediatrics 39:526–531, 1967.

6. Lerner AM, Klein JO, Levin HS, et al: Infections due to Coxsackie virus group A, type 9, in Boston, 1959, with special reference to exanthems and pneumonia. N Engl J Med 263:1265–1272, 1960.
7. McIntosh K, Chao RK, Krause HE, et al: Coronavirus infection in acute lower respiratory tract disease of infants. J Infect Dis 130:502–507, 1974.
8. Harmon AT, Harmon MW, Glezen WP: Evidence of interferon production in the hamster lung after primary or secondary exposure to parainfluenzae virus type 3. Am Rev Respir Dis 125:706–711, 1982.
9. Kimmel KA, Wyde PR, Glezen WP: Evidence of a T-cell-mediated cytotoxic response to parainfluenza virus type 3 pneumonia in hamsters. J Reticuloendothel Soc 31:71–83, 1982.
10. Glezen WP, Frank AL, Taber LH, et al: Parainfluenza virus type 3: Seasonality and risk of infection and reinfection in young children. J Infect Dis 150:851–857, 1984.
11. Glezen WP, Paredes A, Taber LH: Influenza in children: Relationship to other respiratory agents. JAMA 243:1345–1349, 1980.
12. Becroft DMO: Histopathology of fatal adenovirus of the respiratory tract in young children. J Clin Pathol 20:561–569, 1967.
13. Herbert FA, Wilkinson D, Burchak E, et al: Adenovirus type 3 pneumonia causing lung damage in childhood. Can Med Assoc J 116:274–276, 1977.
14. Zahradnik JM: Adenovirus pneumonia. Semin Respir Infect 2:104–111, 1987.
15. Dingle J, Langmuir AD: Epidemiology of acute respiratory disease in military recruits. Am Rev Respir Dis 97:1–65, 1968.
16. Siegel MM, Walter TK, Ablin AR: Measles pneumonia in childhood leukemia. Pediatrics 60:38–40, 1977.
17. Ramsey, PG, Fife KH, Hackman RC, et al: Herpes simplex virus pneumonia: Clinical, virologic, and pathologic features in 20 patients. Ann Intern Med 97:813–820, 1982.
18. Ballard RA, Drew WL, Hufnagle KG, et al: Acquired cytomegalovirus infection in preterm infants. Am J Dis Child 133:482–485, 1979.
19. Yeager AS: Transfusion-acquired cytomegalovirus infection in newborn infants. Am J Dis Child 128:478–483, 1974.
20. Yeager AS, Grumet FC, Hafleigh EB, et al: Prevention of transfusion-acquired cytomegalovirus infections in newborn infants. J Pediatr 98:281–287, 1981.
21. Feldman S, Hughes WT, Daniel CB: Varicella in children with cancer: Seventy-seven cases. Pediatrics 56:388–397, 1975.
22. Andiman WA, McCarthy P, Markowitz RI, et al: Clinical, virologic, and serologic evidence of Epstein-Barr virus infection in association with childhood pneumonia. J Pediatr 99:880–886, 1981.
23. Bruhn FW, Mokrohisky ST, McIntosh K: Apnea associated with respiratory syncytial virus infections in young infants. J Pediatr 90:382–386, 1977.
24. Khamapirad T, Glezen WP: Clinical and radiographic assessment of acute lower respiratory tract disease in infants and children. Semin Respir Infect 2:130–144, 1987.
25. McCarthy PL, Spiesel SZ, Stashwick CA, et al: Radiographic findings and etiologic diagnosis in ambulatory childhood pneumonias. Clin Pediatr (Phila) 20:686–691, 1981.
26. Foy HM, Cooney MK, McMahan R, et al: Viral and mycoplasmal pneumonia in a prepaid medical care group during an eight-year period. Am J Epidemiol 97:93–102, 1973.
27. Fox JP, Hall CE, Cooney MK: The Seattle Virus Watch: VII. Observations of adenovirus infection. Am J Epidemiol 105:362–386, 1977.
28. Committee on Drugs, American Academy of Pediatrics: Use of codeine- and dextromethorphan-containing cough syrups in pediatrics. Pediatrics 62:118–122, 1978.
29. Hall CB, McBride JT, Gala CL, et al: Ribavirin treatment of respiratory syncytial viral infection in infants with underlying cardiopulmonary disease. JAMA 254:3047–3051, 1985.
30. Wang EE, Prober CG, Manson B, et al: Association of respiratory viral infections with pulmonary deterioration in patients with cystic fibrosis. N Engl J Med 311:1653–1658, 1984.
31. MacDonald NE, Hall CB, Suffin SC, et al: Respiratory syncytial viral infection in infants with congenital heart disease. N Engl J Med 307:397–400, 1982.
32. Jarvis WR, Middleton PJ, Gelfand EW: Significance of viral infections in severe combined immunodeficiency disease. Pediatr Infect Dis 2:187–192, 1983.
33. Lang WR, Howden CW, Laws J, et al: Bronchopneumonia with serious sequelae in children with evidence of adenovirus type 21 infection. Br Med J 1:73–79, 1969.
34. Laraya-Cuasay LR, Deforest A, Huff D, et al: Chronic pulmonary complicatons of early influenza virus infection in children. Am Rev Respir Dis 116:617–625, 1977.
35. MacPherson RI, Cumming G, Chernick V: Unilateral hyperlucent lung: A complication of viral pneumonia. J Can Assoc Radiol 20:225–231, 1969.
36. Grossman LK, Wald ER, Nair P, et al: Roentgenographic follow-up of acute pneumonia in children. Pediatrics 63:30–31, 1979.
37. Hall CB: The shedding and spreading of respiratory syncytial virus. Pediatr Res 11:236–239, 1977.
38. Hall CB, Geiman JM, Douglas RG, et al: Control of nosocomial respiratory syncytial viral infections. Pediatrics 62:728–732, 1978.
39. Gala CL, Hall CB, Schnabel KC, et al: The use of eye-nose goggles to control nosocomial respiratory syncytial virus infection. JAMA 256:2706–2708, 1986.
40. Committee on Infectious Diseases, American Academy of Pediatrics: Report of the Committee on Infectious Diseases, 21st ed. Elk Grove Village, IL: American Academy of Pediatrics, 1988.

35 RESPIRATORY SEQUELAE OF VIRAL INFECTIONS

LOURDES R. LARAYA-CUASAY, M.D.

Almost 64 million people who live in the United States today are children under 17 years of age. In this group, respiratory disease is responsible for about 20% of all hospitalizations.[1] Pneumonia, influenza, and chronic obstructive pulmonary disease ranked as the fourth leading causes of death in the United States in 1986.[2] Among the pediatric population, viral respiratory illnesses and their sequelae account for a significant number of visits to physicians and school absenteeism. This chapter addresses some of sequelae of viral respiratory illnesses among the pediatric population. Figure 35–1 diagrammatically depicts the pathogenesis of the respiratory sequelae of viral infections.

APNEA

After respiratory syncytial virus (RSV) infections, prolonged apnea has been observed in young infants, especially those with low birth weights. Ten percent of infants with RSV bronchiolitis had one or more episodes of apnea, which was more frequent in preterm infants and those under 2 months of age.[3] RSV was the virus most often identified at autopsy in infants dying unexpectedly at home or when crib death was diagnosed.[4]

Apnea in bronchiolitis occurs mostly with RSV, but it also occurs with adenovirus. In one report, sleep apnea was mainly central in type and shorter than 15 sec.[5] Apneic episodes occur in quiet sleep during the index illness and are accompanied by a sigh or body movement. Transcutaneous oxygen tension is significantly reduced during apneic periods. The mechanism for central apnea is still undefined. Apnea is not more common in infants with hypoxia or hypercapnia. Apnea can also occur during severe bronchiolitis as fatigue sets in from the increased work of breathing.[6]

PNEUMOTHORAX

Although uncommon, spontaneous bilateral pneumothorax has been reported in RSV bronchiolitis[7] and unilateral pneumothorax in systemic adenovirus type 3 infection.[8] Airflow obstruction occurs as a result of mucus and cellular debris from the necrotizing process, bronchiolar wall edema, and even muscular spasm. Overdistended alveoli rupture and cause pneumothorax or pneumomediastinum. Partial obstruction to expiratory airflow results in hyperinflation of the lungs. With air trapping, the infant breathes at high lung volume, compromising inspiratory muscles function and limiting ventilation.

ATELECTASIS

Lobar collapse or segmental atelectasis may follow mucus plugging or mucus hypersecretion cells. Consolidation interspersed with zones of hyperinflation results from partial obstruction of small airways by inflammatory edema of the walls or by intraluminal cellular debris. Radiologic distinction between atelectasis and consolidation is a major problem without clinical correlation.[9] Atelectasis is common in children because of the paucity of collateral ventilation; the pores of Kohn and the canals of Lambert are deficient in number and size in infants and young children.[10]

PLEURAL EFFUSION

Pleural effusion occurring in viral infections is fibrinopurulent, serous, or fibrinous. The effusion may be small or massive and unilateral or bilateral and may lead to respiratory failure or resolve within a few weeks without specific treatment.

Pleural effusions have been reported with rubeola virus infection after immunization with killed measles vaccine,[11] Epstein-Barr virus (EBV),[12] cytomegalovirus (CMV), adenovirus, and influenza.[13] Lobar or segmental consolidation may also be present. The author observed minimal pleural effusion on a chest radiograph of an 8-month-old boy with CMV pneumonia who then had persistent interstitial pneumonia for 2 years.[14] The effusion resolved spontaneously after 2 months. A fatal case of EBV pneumonia with massive pleural effusion 4 weeks after the initial symptoms without a definable immunologic disorder has been reported.[15]

BRONCHIAL HYPERREACTIVITY

Children under 5 years of age are more susceptible to the development of a wheeze with viral upper respiratory infection.[16] Wheezing is most commonly observed in those with a family history of atopy and allergic disease.[17] Boys are more susceptible to bronchial hyperreactivity during viral respiratory infection.[18]

Bronchial hyperreactivity is not a universal response to the viral infection, and there is great variability in its response to treatment. The viral infection itself and interferon can enhance mediator release.[19] Histamine release produces airway obstruction directly or increases bronchial hyperreactivity by producing airway inflammation.

Acute airway injury leads to exfoliation of epithelial cells. The protective barrier is lost, enhancing presentation of antigen to antibody-producing cell and increasing immunoglobulin E (IgE) synthesis.[20] RSV-specific IgE, parainfluenza virus–specific IgE, and high levels of histamine in nasopharyngeal secretions support the hypothesis that respiratory viral infections may predispose patients to allergic sensitization.[21]

CHRONIC INTERSTITIAL PNEUMONITIS

In 1978, in a series of 90 cases of interstitial pneumonitis in infants and young children observed over a 7-year period, the author reported that most cases presented as acute onset of upper respiratory infection with or without accompanying rhinitis or fever.[14] Within a few days, the patients had dry cough, which gradually became loose and productive. Tachypnea was prominent. Crackles were heard over the lung fields. Diffuse interstitial densities running parallel to the bronchial tree were found in most chest radiographs. Overaeration was commonly seen in young infants. Patchy areas of atelectasis were often seen on radiographs, and some confluent bilateral densities were predominant in one or more lobes. Alveolar and interstitial densities were present together with interstitial densities, and differentiating them was difficult. Nonspecific interstitial pneumonitis was diagnosed histologically in most patients who underwent open-lung biopsy. There were thickened alveolar septae with cellular

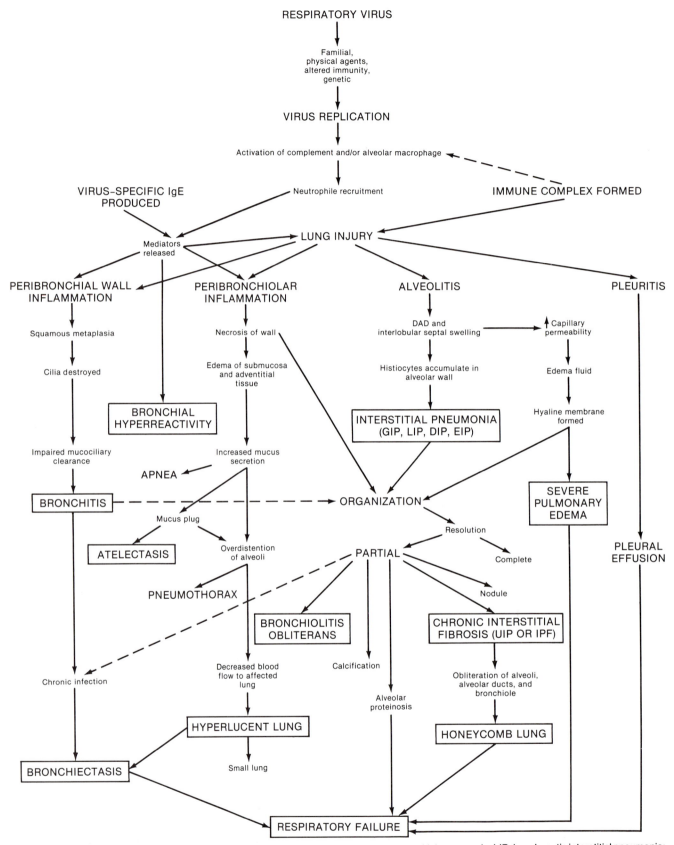

Figure 35–1. Pathogenesis of the sequelae of respiratory viral infections. GIP, giant cell interstitial pneumonia; LIP, lymphocytic interstitial pneumonia; DIP, desquamative interstitial pneumonia; DAD, diffuse alveolar damage; EIP, eosinophilic interstitial pneumonia; UIP, usual interstitial pneumonia; IPF, idiopathic pulmonary fibrosis. (Modified with permission from Laraya-Cuasay LR: The interstitial pneumonias. *In* Laraya-Cuasay LR, Hughes WT [eds]: Interstitial Lung Diseases in Children, vol. 3, p. 123. Boca Raton, FL: CRC Press, 1988.)

proliferation containing lymphocytes and plasma cells.[22] Similar diffuse interstitial infiltrates persisting long after symptoms and signs of acute lower respiratory tract disease have abated have been observed in respiratory viral infections secondary to influenza, rubeola, CMV, EBV, and adenovirus. Usual interstitial pneumonia after Texas A influenza infection in two adult patients was reported.[23]

PULMONARY FIBROSIS

Pulmonary fibrosis is the end result of unresolved interstitial pneumonitis. With progressive deposition of collagen in the interstitium, alveolectasia occurs, resulting in the honeycomb lung appearance on radiographs. Hypoxemia is a prominent feature with accompanying symptoms of gradually increasing exercise intolerance, dyspnea, tachypnea, cyanosis, and development of digital clubbing. Hemoptysis may be present. Gallium 67 scans are positive in about 70% of all patients with idiopathic pulmonary fibrosis.[24] Bronchoalveolar lavage may exhibit a pattern dominated by neutrophils and macrophages with smaller numbers of eosinophils and lymphocytes.[25]

OBLITERATIVE BRONCHITIS AND BRONCHIOLITIS

Obliterative bronchitis and bronchiolitis may complicate pneumonia, bronchitis, and bronchiolitis secondary to measles,[26] influenza,[27] adenovirus infection,[28] and RSV infection.[28] Prominent interstitial mononuclear infiltrate, interstitial fibrosis, honeycombing, and microcyst formation have been found in 10% of cases of bronchiolitis obliterans on histologic examination. Intrabronchiolar and intra-alveolar ductal exudate that undergoes organization in varying degrees has also been shown. The exudate is mainly lymphocytic in the early stages with some polymorphonuclear leukocytes. The damaged bronchiole is surrounded by lymphocytes and other chronic inflammatory cells that may occupy the adjacent peribronchiolar alveoli. Fibroplastic granulation tissue may appear as a polypoid mass, leaving a narrow crescentic slit in the intrabronchiolar lumen.[27] A honeycomb appearance results from the air trapping distal to the obstructed bronchioles.

When respiratory symptoms persist beyond the usual duration of the clinical course of bronchiolitis or pneumonia, obliterative bronchiolitis has probably complicated the clinical picture. Localized wheezing may be present. Diffuse interstitial and alveolar infiltrates may appear on radiographs. Hypoxemia may be present. Pulmonary function tests may document mixed restrictive and obstructive patterns. A period of relative lack of symptoms or signs may occur for several weeks or months after a lower respiratory tract disease, followed by progressive dyspnea, cyanosis, and nonproductive cough in some patients. For more information, see Chapter 23.

HYPERLUCENT LUNG

Unilateral hyperlucency of a lung develops with progressive air trapping after obliterative bronchiolitis.

Because obliterative endarteritis occurs together with obliterative bronchiolitis changes, one lung or a major portion of a lung can appear hyperlucent.[28] This phenomenon is more commonly recognized as Swyer-James or Macleod's syndrome. This has to be differentiated from unilateral bronchial obstruction by a foreign body or ball-valve mechanism or rarely from congenital absence of the pulmonary artery or branch stenosis of the pulmonary arteries. Congenital lobar hyperinflation, staphylococcal pneumatoceles, and pneumothorax are other differential diagnostic considerations in infants.

As a consequence of this hyperlucency, smallness of the lung results, with a decrease in volume of a whole lung or individual lobes. Air trapping is documented by fluoroscopy and prolonged helium time on lung volume measurements. Ventilation/perfusion lung scan is a noninvasive method of confirming poor perfusion or absence of perfusion and ventilation of a particular lobe or an entire lung. Even in noncooperative infants, this technique can be performed through the use of radionuclide-labeled microsonic particles.

BRONCHIECTASIS

Childhood bronchiectasis may be the sequela of pertussis, measles, primary influenza, and adenoviral pneumonia. Episodic obstruction by retained secretions and secondary bacterial infection account for fluctuation in the clinical course. Bronchiolar obliteration may contribute to bronchiectasis by leading to absorption atelectasis and fibrosis and by predisposing the patient anatomically and physiologically to stagnation of secretions, which results in inflammation. This is discussed in more detail in Chapter 24.

PULMONARY NODULES

Pulmonary nodules form in areas of organizing pneumonia. They may be present for months or years after viral lower respiratory tract illness. The postviral nodule should be considered in the differential diagnosis of solitary pulmonary nodules in younger patients, which includes cysts, arteriovenous malformation, metastasis, hamartoma, granuloma, lymphoma, sequestration, mucoid impaction, and xanthomatous postinflammatory pseudotumor. In older children, adolescents, and young adults, it is important to identify residual pulmonary nodules as postviral in cause so as to obviate the need for further invasive diagnostic tests to rule out metastatic lung disease. In a patient previously immunized with killed measles virus vaccine, the occurrence of a febrile illness accompanied by a rash should alert the clinician to the possibility of a benign postinflammatory condition.

PULMONARY CALCIFICATIONS

Scattered nodular opacities that may resolve within 2 months or slowly calcify after 3 to 5 years have been reported with varicella pneumonia. Nodular residua in a case of atypical measles pneumonia exhibited calcification in the nodules 6 years after the pneumonia. Leukemic patients in whom varicella developed did not exhibit calcification on follow-up.[29] Differentiation from tuberculosis and fungal diseases has to be made, but the history of previous varicella infection is most important.

PULMONARY ALVEOLAR PROTEINOSIS

Childhood pulmonary alveolar proteinosis (PAP) may simulate *Pneumocystis carinii* infection clinically and radiographically. This acquired syndrome produces symptoms referable to hypoxemia secondary to accumulation of lipid-rich granular material in the alveolar spaces. A proteinaceous substance that stains positively with periodic acid Schiff stain fills the alveoli. The chemical properties of this material resemble surfactant. It is possible that CMV infection is causal in some cases of PAP.[30] Characteristic nuclear and cytoplasmic inclusions of CMV were seen in the alveolar pneumocyte. Because CMV is able to replicate within granular pneumocytes without producing cytopathic effects and because the synthesis of host proteins and glycoproteins continues after infection, it is possible that CMV may cause infected granular pneumocytes to produce an excess of phospholipids.[31] An alteration in surfactant release by granular pneumocytes from causes other than CMV infection cannot be entirely ruled out.

When the diagnosis of PAP is made, it is important to rule out infection with CMV and *P. carinii*. Both infections can coexist in an immunocompromised host.[32] Specific therapy is available for either one so that early diagnosis is crucial. Bronchoalveolar lavage can be very useful both for diagnosis and for treatment in PAP.

CHRONIC OBSTRUCTIVE LUNG DISEASE IN ADULTHOOD

Among adults who have experienced previous acute respiratory illnesses, there is a significantly higher prevalence of physician-confirmed chronic respiratory disease. Some data suggest that viral respiratory infections predispose toward transient episodes of wheezing in children and may also contribute to the pathogenesis of obstructive lung disease in adulthood.[33-35]

In follow-up studies of symptomatic and asymptomatic children after bronchiolitis, measurements of airflow, lung volume, or blood gases and bronchial provocation challenge tests with exercise, cold air, or histamine have documented reduced airflow, air trapping, hypoxemia, and bronchial hyperreactivity. A male patient with postmeasles obliterative bronchiolitis and bronchiectasis acquired at 5 years of age continued to have small airway dysfunction 24 years after infection. He had an increased anteroposterior chest diameter and had recurrent episodes of wheezing that responded to bronchodilator therapy.

MANAGEMENT

Prevention is crucial for decreased rates of mortality and morbidity from respiratory viral infections. Measures

to control the spread of respiratory infections, such as habitual and hardy hand washing, have the greatest value in infection control. Prevention of virus transmission among siblings, restriction of parental cigarette smoking, and avoidance of the use of wood-burning stoves and other environmental pollutants reduce the morbidity associated with bronchiolitis and pneumonia.

Measles, mumps, and rubella and influenza vaccines are available. Children with underlying pulmonary diseases, such as cystic fibrosis and bronchopulmonary dysplasia, are candidates for influenza vaccination. For detailed instructions on the use of these vaccines, readers are referred to the American Academy of Pediatrics publication.[36] No effective vaccine is available for RSV, rhinovirus, or parainfluenza. Extensive research has been performed with killed and intranasally administered live, attenuated RSV vaccine. Immunity acquired after RSV infection is not permanent and has no demonstrable effect on the severity of RSV illness associated with reinfection 1 year later. Modification of illness severity rather than immunoprophylaxis is a more realistic goal.

Amantadine and rimantadine are orally administered in patients at high risk for serious influenza infection who have not been vaccinated or who have been vaccinated within 2 weeks of the onset of the influenza epidemic. Both amantadine and rimantadine have been used safely in children. Amantadine may be useful for close household or hospital ward contacts of patients with index cases, immunocompromised patients, and health care and community services personnel and when influenza vaccine is contraindicated (see Chapter 28).

Antiviral drugs have been used safely in RSV infection and in pneumonia and tracheobronchitis resulting from herpes simplex virus (HSV) and varicella zoster virus (VZV). See Table 35–1 for antiviral drugs, indications, dosage, and side effects. Ribavirin has antiviral properties against both RNA and DNA viruses *in vitro*. It also has mast cell–release inhibitory properties.[37] No toxic effects have been reported with ribavirin aerosol therapy, and drug-resistant viral strains have not emerged. Acyclovir triphosphate, used in HSV and VZV infections, interferes with HSV DNA polymerase and inhibits viral DNA replication. It is excreted through the urinary system, and so dosage has to be adjusted in accordance with the creatinine clearance rate.

CMV pneumonia in immunosuppressed hosts has been treated with the new nucleoside ganciclovir (9-[1,3-dihydroxy-2-propoxymethyl] guanine) with encouraging results.[38]

Bronchodilators with or without sodium cromoglycate have been useful when bronchial hyperreactivity is present and when pulmonary function testing shows significant improvement in airway obstruction with its use. Early use of selected antibiotics during exacerbation of chronic bronchitis or bronchiectasis has decreased the need for hospitalization because bacterial superinfection of stagnant secretions in the lower airways occurs frequently. The role of corticosteroids is not definitive in obliterative bronchiolitis with pulmonary fibrosis, although they have been used for their anti-inflammatory and antihypersensitivity effects. In obliterative bronchiolitis, Gosink and associates found considerable benefit

Table 35–1. ANTIVIRAL DRUGS USED IN LOWER RESPIRATORY TRACT INFECTIONS

Drug	Indication	Usual Dosage/Form	Duration	Side Effects
Acyclovir (Zovirax), 9-[(2-hydroxy ethoxy)methyl] guanine sodium	Pneumonia and tracheobronchitis from HSV or VZV in immunocompromised host	Oral: 200 mg 5 times a day; IV: 30 mg/kg/day in 3 divided doses; adjust dosage if renal function is abnormal; Form: 200-mg cap, 10-ml sterile vials containing 500 mg acyclovir	5–10 days	Nausea or vomiting, headache, diarrhea, skin rash, insomnia, fatigue, irritability, coarse tremor, clonus, phlebitis at injection site after infiltration of IV fluid, elevated serum creatinine, thrombocytopenia, jitters
Vidarabine (Vira-A), D-arabino-furanosyladenine-monohydrate	Varicella or zoster in immunocompromised host with pneumonia or tracheobronchitis	IV: 10 mg/kg/day in 1 dose over 12–24 h; dose adjusted when renal function is impaired; form: 5-ml vial contains 1 g of vidarabine (200 mg/ml)	5–10 days	GI: anorexia, nausea, vomiting, diarrhea; CNS: disturbance usually in patients with impaired hepatic or renal function; hematologic: anemia, leukopenia, thrombocytopenia; pain at injection site
Amantadine (Symmetrel), 1-adamantanamine hydrochloride	Prevention and treatment of influenza A infection	With normal renal function, oral: 1–9 years of age, 4.4–8.8 μg/kg/day in 2 doses up to 150 mg maximum; age 9 years: 200 mg/day in 2 doses. Form: 50 mg/5 ml syrup, 100 mg capsules	Prophylactic: use for entire winter season; treatment use: continue for 48 h after disappearance of symptoms for maximum of 5 days	Nausea, lightheadedness, dizziness, insomnia, euphoria, dysphoria, constipation, pruritus, depression, anxiety, irritability, hallucinations, confusion, anorexia, dry mouth, ataxia, slurred speech, visual disturbance; rarely leukopenia, neutropenia, oculogyric episodes
Rimantadine, methyl-1-adamantane methylamine hydrochloride	Prevention and treatment of influenza A infection	Oral 6.6 mg/kg/day, 150 mg/day for age 1–9 years; 200 mg/day divided into 2 doses	3–5 days	Nausea, vomiting, diarrhea, dry mouth, headache, dizziness, fatigue, anorexia, rash
Ribavirin (Virazole), 1-B-D-riba-furanosyl-1,2,4 triazole-3-carboxamide	Treatment of carefully selected hospitalized infants and young children with severe RSV bronchiolitis and pneumonia	Small-particle aerosol, 20 mg/2 ml for inhalation for 12–18 h each day via SPAG-2; form: 100-ml glass vials with 6 g of sterile water for injection with no preservatives added	3–7 days	Mild conjunctival edema, headache, dyspnea, chest soreness, significant deterioration of lung function, reticulocytosis, anemia

HSV, herpes simplex virus; VZV, varicella zoster virus; IV, intravenous; GI, gastrointestinal; CNS, central nervous system; RSV, respiratory syncytial virus; SPAG-2, small-particle aerosol generator-2.

from steroids even in the absence of hypersensitivity.[39] A controlled study of the use of steroids in children with obliterative bronchiolitis and pulmonary fibrosis is not available because of the rarity of such patients.

Chest physiotherapy and postural drainage are indicated for atelectasis and recurrent mucus plugging and to assist in evacuation of secretions. Endobronchial lavage has been tried for persistent atelectasis and for removal of mucus plugs. Lobectomy for localized obliterative bronchiolitis and bronchiectasis has been performed. The clinical decision of treatment is based on the predicted residual lung function postlobectomy.

Supportive therapy includes oxygen therapy at home or in the hospital. Diligent nutritional care improves the host's response to disease. Increased caloric intake is mandatory in anticipation of increased work of breathing as pulmonary fibrosis progresses.

Therapy in the future depends on the discovery of newer and safer antifibrotic, anti-inflammatory, and antiviral agents. Heart-lung and lung transplantations have shown early promise for end-stage pulmonary fibrosis (see Chapter 88).

The chronicity and unpredictability of some of the sequelae of respiratory viral infection support the holistic approach to management that necessarily includes the emotional and psychosocial support of the patients and their family members. For those with chronic respiratory insufficiency, adequate preparation and support throughout the dying process must be provided.

REFERENCES

1. Glezen WP: Viral pneumonia as a cause and result of hospitalization. J Infect Dis 147:765–770, 1983.
2. National Center for Health Statistics: Vital Statistics of the United States 1986, vol. 11: Mortality, Part A. DHHS Pub. No. (PHS) 88-1122, Public Health Service. Washington, DC: U.S. Government Printing Office, 1988.
3. Bruhn FW, Mokrohisky ST, McIntosh K: Apnea associated with respiratory syncytial virus infection in young infants. J Pediatr 90:382–386, 1977.
4. Scott DJ, Gardner PS, McQuillin J, et al: Respiratory viruses and cot death. Br Med J 2:12–13, 1978.
5. Abreu e Silva, FA, Brezinova V, Simpson H: Sleep apnea in acute bronchiolitis. Arch Dis Child 57:467–472, 1982.
6. Wohl ME, Chernick V: State of the art: Bronchiolitis, Am Rev Respir Dis 118:759–781, 1978.
7. Pollack J: Spontaneous bilateral pneumothorax in an infant with bronchiolitis. Pediatr Emerg Care 3:33–35, 1987.

8. Levy Y, Nitzan M, Beharab A, et al: Adenovirus type 3 infection with systemic manifestation in apparently normal children. Israel J Med Sci 22:774–778, 1986.
9. Swischuk LE, Hayden CK, Jr: Viral vs. bacterial pulmonary infections in children (is roentgenographic differentiation possible?). Pediatr Radiol 16:278–284, 1986.
10. Griscom NT, Wohl ME, Kirkpatrick JA Jr: Lower respiratory infections: How infants differ from adults. Radiol Clin North Am 16:367–387, 1978.
11. Margolin FR, Gandy TK: Pneumonia of atypical measles. Pediatr Radiol 131:653–655, 1979.
12. Young LW, Smith DI, Glasgow LA: Pneumonia of atypical measles: Residual nodular lesions. AJR 110:439–448, 1970.
13. Fine NL, Smith LR, Sheedy PF: Frequency of pleural effusions in mycoplasma and viral pneumonias. N Engl J Med 283:790–793, 1970.
14. Laraya-Cuasay LR: Pulmonary sequelae of acute respiratory viral infection. Pediatr Ann 7:42–53, 1978.
15. Offit PA, Fleisher GR, Koven NL, et al: Severe Epstein-Barr virus pulmonary involvement. J Adolesc Health Care 2:121–125, 1981.
16. McIntosh K, Ellis EF, Hoffman LS, et al: The association of viral and bacterial respiratory infections with exacerbations of wheezing in young asthmatic children. J Pediatr 82:578–590, 1973.
17. Laing I, Reidel F, Yap PL, et al: Atopy predisposing to acute bronchiolitis during an epidemic of respiratory syncytial virus. Br Med J 284:1070–1072, 1982.
18. Henderson FW, Collier AM, Clyde WA, et al: Respiratory syncytial virus infections, reinfections and immunity: A prospective, longitudinal study in young children. N Engl J Med 300:530–534, 1979.
19. Fitzpatrick FA, Stringfellow DA: Virus and interferon effects on cellular prostaglandin biosynthesis. J Immunol 125:431–437, 1980.
20. Welliver RC, Kaul A, Ogra PL: Cell-mediated immune response to respiratory syncytial virus infection: Relationship to the development of reactive airway disease. J Pediatr 94:370–375, 1979.
21. Welliver RC, Wong DT, Sun M, et al: The development of respiratory syncytial virus-specific IgE and the release of histamine in nasopharyngeal secretions after infection. N Engl J Med 305:841–846, 1981.
22. Niguidula FN, Balsara RK, Cuasay RS: The role of lung biopsy in interstitial lung diseases in children. In Laraya-Cuasay LR, Hughes WT (eds): Interstitial Lung Diseases in Children, vol. 1, pp. 101–109. Boca Raton, FL: CRC Press, 1988.
23. Pinsker KL, Schneyer B, Becker N, et al: Usual interstitial pneumonia following Texas A₂ influenza infection. Chest 80:123–126, 1981.
24. Line BR, Fulmer JD, Reynolds HY, et al: Gallium-67 citrate scanning in the staging of idiopathic pulmonary fibrosis: Correlation with physiologic and morphologic features and bronchoalveolar lavage. Am Rev Respir Dis 118:355–365, 1978.
25. Murphy S: The role of bronchoalveolar lavage in interstitial lung disease. In Laraya-Cuasay LR, Hughes WT (eds): Interstitial Lung Diseases in Children, vol. 1, pp. 111–128. Boca Raton, FL: CRC Press, 1988.
26. Laraya-Cuasay LR: Longitudinal follow-up of postmeasles obliterative bronchitis and bronchiolitis. Pediatr Res 25:368A, 1989.
27. Laraya-Cuasay LR, Deforest A, Huff D, et al: Chronic pulmonary complications of early influenza virus infection in children. Am Rev Respir Dis 116:617–625, 1977.
28. Becroft DM: Bronchiolitis obliterans, bronchiectasis, and other sequelae of adenovirus type 21 infection in young children. J Clin Pathol 24:72–82, 1971.
29. Stokes DC, Feldman S, Sanyal SK, et al: Pulmonary function following varicella-zoster pneumonia in children with leukemia. Pediatr Pulmonol 3:236–241, 1982.
30. Tirnoveanu G, Dobresco G, Gheorghiu C: Alveolar proteinosis in infants coexisting with viral (cytomegalovirus and measles virus) and microbial infections. Rev Med Chir Soc Med Nat Iasi 76:187–193, 1972.
31. Ranchod M, Bissell M: Pulmonary alveolar proteinosis and cytomegalovirus infection. Arch Pathol Lab Med 103:139–142, 1979.
32. Volpi A, Whitley RJ, Ceballos R, et al: Rapid diagnosis of pneumonia due to cytomegalovirus with specific monoclonal antibodies. J Infect Dis 147:1119–1120, 1983.
33. Burrows B, Knudson RJ, Lebowitz MD: The relationship of childhood respiratory illness to adult obstructive airway disease. Am Rev Respir Dis 115:751–760, 1977.
34. Carlsen KH, Larsen S, Orstavik I: Acute bronchiolitis in infancy: The relationship to later recurrent obstructive airways disease. Eur J Respir Dis 70:86–92, 1987.
35. Phelan PD: Does adult chronic obstructive lung disease really begin in childhood? Br J Dis Chest 78:1–9, 1984.
36. American Academy of Pediatrics: Report of the Committee on Infectious Diseases, 22nd ed. Elk Grove Village, IL: American Academy of Pediatrics, 1991.
37. Hall CB, McBride JT, Gala CL, et al: Ribavirin treatment of respiratory syncytial viral infection in infants with underlying cardiopulmonary disease. JAMA 254:3047–3051, 1985.
38. Collaborative DHPG Treatment Study Group: Treatment of serious cytomegalovirus infections with 9-(1,3-dihydroxy-2-propoxymethyl) guanine in patients with AIDS and other immunodeficiencies. N Engl J Med 314:801–805, 1986.
39. Gosink B, Friedman P, Liebow A: Bronchiolitis obliterans: Roentgenologic-pathologic correlation. AJR 117:816–832, 1973.

36 PNEUMONIA IN THE IMMUNOSUPPRESSED HOST

WALTER T. HUGHES, M.D.

In a sense, infections in the immunocompromised host begin with breaching of the skin or mucosal surfaces by microbial organisms. The type and extent of the infection are influenced by the number, virulence, and tropism of the organism, as well as the competence of the host's immune responses both at the port of entry and systemically. Although the skin and mucosal surfaces of the alimentary tract provide large surfaces for adherence and colonization of opportunistic organisms, the lungs offer the largest surface of the body exposed to environmental agents. The total pulmonary surface area is estimated to be about 200 sq m.[1,2] Considering the density of bacteria,

Table 36–1. LOCAL DEFENSE MECHANISMS TO PROTECT THE LUNG AGAINST INFECTION

Nasal hair
Aerodynamic airway filtration
Mucociliary clearance
Lymphohematogenous clearance
Alveolar macrophage
Polymorphonuclear leukocytes
Eosinophils
Lymphocytes
   Extrapulmonary lymph nodes
   Bronchus-associated lymphoid tissue
   Interstitial lymphocyte nodules
   Free lymphocytes in parenchyma and alveoli (immunoglobulins
     G, A, E)
   T lymphocyte system (macrophage and blood monocytes)
Mast cells
Complement
Lysozyme
Fibronectin
Antiproteases

Table 36–2. CAUSES OF PNEUMONITIS IN IMMUNOSUPPRESSED PATIENTS

Most Common
  Pneumocystis carinii
  Cytomegalovirus
  Varicella-zoster virus
  Candida species
  Aspergillus species
  Lymphoid interstitial pneumonia (cause unknown)
Less Common
  Toxoplasma gondii
  Cryptosporidium
  Epstein-Barr virus
  Herpes simplex virus
  Respiratory syncytial virus
  Adenovirus
  Legionella pneumophila
  Pseudomonas aeruginosa
  Escherichia coli
  Klebsiella pneumoniae
  Nocardia species
  Mycobacterium species
  Zygomycetes
  Cryptococcus neoformans

viruses, and fungi in the air and that the average person inspires between 10,000 and 20,000 l of air daily,[3] it is understandable why patients whose resistance is impaired are prone to serious pulmonary infections. The major components of the lung defense mechanisms are listed in Table 36–1. In this chapter, attention is given to severely immunocompromised patients such as those with cancer, organ transplantation, congenital immunodeficiency disorders, and acquired immunodeficiency disorders and those receiving immunosuppressive therapy for other diseases.

The frequently encountered causes of pneumonitis in compromised patients are listed in Table 36–2. In the discussions that follow, most of these causes are considered in some detail.

PNEUMOCYSTIS CARINII PNEUMONIA

Pneumonia resulting from *Pneumocystis carinii* occurs almost exclusively in immunocompromised hosts. Because most normal persons become asymptomatically infected early in life with *P. carinii,* the pneumonitis that occurs with immunocompromise is believed to represent activation of latent infection.

PATHOPHYSIOLOGY

The natural habitat seems to be limited to the lungs of humans and lower mammals. Transmission has been demonstrated only from animal to animal and by the airborne route.[4,5] It is not known whether animal-to-human or human-to-human transmission occurs. *P. carinii,* previously considered to be a protozoan, is now considered a fungus (see Chapter 21). The organism is found in the alveoli as a thick-walled cyst about 5 to 6 μm in diameter that contains up to eight intracystic daughter cells termed *sporozoites.* Extracystic forms are also found in abundance in the alveoli of patients with the pneumonitis. These are termed *trophozoites* and measure 1 to 5 μm in

diameter. *In vitro* culture studies with embryonic chick epithelial lung cells suggest that the trophozoite attaches to the alveolar cell surface and increases in size as the intracystic daughter cells develop, progressing to the cystic stage.[6] The cyst detaches from the host cell, never having reached an intracytoplasmic stage. Breaks occur in the cyst wall, and the sporozoites are expelled. Once excysted, the sporozoite becomes a trophozoite. In the infantile form of *P. carinii* pneumonitis, the interstitial septae are thickened because of lymphocyte and plasma cell infiltration. The alveolar epithelium is hyperplastic. The alveolar lumen contains desquamated epithelial cells, *P. carinii* organisms, a few neutrophils, many alveolar macrophages, and edema fluid. *P. carinii* organisms may be found in both the alveolar lumen and the interstitium.[7-9]

In children and adults with immunodeficiency disorders, the interstitial component and plasma cell infiltration may be absent or present only to a limited extent. The pattern in these patients is an extensive diffuse alveolitis.[10] The extensive alveolar infiltrates and foamy exudate of the lumen interfere with oxygenation, resulting in severe hypoxemia. Carbon dioxide retention does not become significant until the patient reaches near-terminal status.[11]

CLINICAL MANIFESTATIONS

The clinical features of *P. carinii* pneumonitis have been categorized into two general types. The infantile endemic interstitial plasma cell pneumonitis is seen in outbreaks in European nurseries; the child-adult type occurs in immunocompromised hosts with cancer, organ transplants, and congenital and acquired immunodeficiency disorders and in those undergoing iatrogenic immunosuppressive therapy. The infantile type is seen in debilitated infants 2 to 6 months of age. The onset of this type is subtle, with progression of tachypnea, cough, and intercostal retractions over a 1-week to 1-month interval. Rales are heard bilaterally, and fever is usually absent.

In the child-adult type of *P. carinii* pneumonitis, the onset is abrupt with fever, tachypnea, flaring of the nasal alae, and intercostal retractions. No rales are heard on auscultation. In some patients, especially those with acquired immunodeficiency syndrome (AIDS), the clinical manifestations may vary between the child-adult and the infantile types.

DIAGNOSTIC APPROACHES

The chest radiograph characteristically reveals diffuse, bilateral pneumonitis with an alveolar pattern. Air may be visible on bronchograms. In unusual cases, the pneumonitis may manifest as a lobar infiltrate or nodular lesions. Pleural effusion, pneumomediastinum, and pneumothorax are not uncommon.

To establish firmly the diagnosis of *P. carinii* pneumonitis, there must be clinical and radiographic evidence of pneumonitis in an immunocompromised host, and *P. carinii* must be demonstrated in lung tissue or secretions from the lower respiratory tract. Invasive procedures such as bronchoscopy with bronchoalveolar lavage and transbronchial biopsy, percutaneous transthoracic needle aspiration, and open-lung biopsy are highly successful in providing specimens for diagnostic purposes. A biopsy of the lung parenchyma is the most dependable and informative procedure. Pneumothorax is the most frequent complication of the invasive procedures. The organism may also be found in sputum; however, the pneumonitis is not often associated with sputum production, and spontaneously expectorated specimens are usually not available. Saline-induced sputum production has been used successfully in AIDS patients to obtain diagnostic specimens. If sputum specimens do not contain *P. carinii,* the diagnosis cannot be excluded. However, if the organism is found in sputum from an immunocompromised patient with pneumonitis, it may be considered diagnostic in the absence of other causes. Specimens are stained with Gomori-Grocott methenamine silver nitrate, Giemsa stain, or toluidine O stains. An immunofluorescent monoclonal antibody test has become commercially available for diagnostic use.[12]

Serologic tests for antibody and antigen are not diagnostic.

MANAGEMENT

Trimethoprim-sulfamethoxazole is the drug of choice for the treatment of *P. carinii* pneumonitis. The dosage is 15 mg of trimethoprim and 75 mg of sulfamethoxazole per kilogram per day intravenously or 20 mg of trimethoprim and 100 mg of sulfamethoxazole per kilogram per day orally in four divided doses. Usually a 2-week course of treatment is adequate, but patients with AIDS may require longer courses.

Patients who have adverse reactions to trimethoprim-sulfamethoxazole or who do not respond to this drug should be given pentamidine isethionate intravenously as a single daily dose of 4.0 mg/kg. This drug can also be given intramuscularly, but severe injection site reactions may occur. The duration of treatment is the same as for trimethoprim-sulfamethoxazole. Trimethoprim-sulfamethoxazole and pentamidine are equally effective, but the latter is associated with a higher adverse reaction rate.

For unknown reasons, the adverse reaction rates to trimethoprim-sulfamethoxazole and pentamidine are strikingly higher in AIDS patients than in non-AIDS patients. For patients who cannot tolerate either drug, experimental drugs are available through investigators or pharmaceutical companies for use in certain patients. These include dapsone,[13, 14] aerosolized pentamidine,[15] trimetrexate,[16] and pyrimethamine-sulfadiazine.[17]

Results of some studies of adults with AIDS suggest that the administration of corticosteroid drugs may improve oxygenation in certain cases of *P. carinii* pneumonitis,[18] but this therapy has not been studied in children.

P. carinii pneumonitis can be prevented in high-risk patients by the regular administration of trimethoprim-sulfamethoxazole in the dosage of 5.0 mg of trimethoprim and 25.0 mg of sulfamethoxazole per kilogram per day orally in two divided doses. The prophylaxis is effective when given daily[19] or only 3 consecutive days per week.[20] Aerosolized pentamidine has been used successfully in adults,[21] but no studies in children have been reported.

TOXOPLASMOSIS

Infection with the ubiquitous protozoan *Toxoplasma gondii* occurs frequently in many parts of the world. Most infections in otherwise healthy people are asymptomatic. In severely immunocompromised hosts, toxoplasmosis may be a serious, life-threatening infection. In most such infections, the disease is that of a necrotizing encephalopathy. However, other organs may be involved with disseminated toxoplasmosis. It is remarkable that pulmonary infection from *T. gondii* is unusual, even in immunocompromised hosts. In a review of the literature,[22] 20 cases of pulmonary toxoplasmosis described between 1941 and 1986 were tabulated. These were often associated with infection in other organs.

PATHOPHYSIOLOGY

Most cases of pulmonary toxoplasmosis are believed to be caused by recrudescence of a latent infection. Little is known of the histopathologic features of the pulmonary infection, usually acquired by ingestion of cysts or oocysts from inadequately cooked meats. The released organisms invade the intestinal epithelium and are spread by hematogenous or lymphatic distribution to various organs, where cysts are formed.

CLINICAL MANIFESTATION

There are no unique clinical manifestations of pulmonary toxoplasmosis. The symptoms are not specific. Cough, fever, and shortness of breath are the most frequent presenting symptoms. Generalized lymphadenopathy, rash, and neurologic signs of encephalitis may coexist with pulmonary lesions.

DIAGNOSTIC APPROACHES

The chest radiograph usually reveals diffuse bilateral infiltrates, but lesions may be limited to single lobes.[23] The demonstration of specific immunoglobulin M (IgM) antibodies by the indirect fluorescent antibody test is useful for diagnosing acute infection. A single high titer or a serial two-tube rise in IgM antibody titer is diagnostic of acute infection.[24] The absence of IgM antibodies does not rule out active infection. A search for *T. gondii* in tissues or secretions stained with hematoxylin and eosin augmented by Giemsa stain may reveal the organism in specimens obtained by bronchoalveolar lavage or open-lung biopsy. The trophozoite is an arc-shaped or oval cell 5 to 7 μm in maximal width.

MANAGEMENT

If pulmonary toxoplasmosis is discovered in an immunocompromised host, a search should be made to find infection in other organs, especially the brain. A computed tomographic (CT) scan of the head is warranted in such cases. The drug combination of pyrimethamine and a sulfonamide is the treatment of choice. The combination of clindamycin and pyrimethamine has also shown some promise for therapeutic efficacy but needs further study.[25] Unfortunately, the outcome is usually fatal.

LEGIONELLA PNEUMONIA

Pulmonary infection with *Legionella* species may occur in either immunocompromised or immunocompetent individuals, especially those in hospitals receiving cancer chemotherapy, undergoing organ transplantation, or receiving immunosuppressive drugs.[26–29] *Legionella* pneumonia has been reported most frequently in older adults but is also less frequently a cause of infection in immunocompromised children.[30]

PATHOPHYSIOLOGY

Legionella species may be found in potable water, air-conditioning cooling towers, evaporative condensers' nebulizers, shower baths, and whirlpools. Of the 11 species, *L. pneumophila* is the most frequently encountered. Bacteria are acquired by the airborne route. Hospitalized patients receiving renal or bone marrow transplants are at high risk for *Legionella* pneumonitis. After colonization of the nasopharynx, the lungs are believed to become infected through aspiration of nasopharyngeal secretions. A lobular or multilobular infiltrate develops and often progresses to lobar pneumonia with or without pleural effusion. The disease is predominantly alveolar, with an exudate of polymorphonuclear leukocytes and alveolar macrophages. The activated macrophage can inhibit growth of but cannot kill phagocytosed *Legionella* organisms.[31]

CLINICAL MANIFESTATIONS

Because the number of cases of *Legionella* pneumonitis in children is small, information on the clinical features in this age group is limited. The manifestations of fever, cough, and tachypnea are usual. In older persons, neurologic signs and symptoms may occur. These include disorientation, hallucinations, depression, delirium, and amnesia. Some patients may have diarrhea.

DIAGNOSTIC APPROACHES

The chest radiograph reveals one or more pneumonic infiltrates with no characteristic features. The diagnosis requires the identification of *Legionella* species by culture, stained smear, and serologic tests. Sputum or bronchoalveolar lavage specimens or biopsy tissue should be cultured with a modification of blood–charcoal-yeast extract (BCYE) agar supplemented with alpha-ketoglutarate. Smears, imprints, and tissue preparations may be stained with a direct fluorescent antibody method and Dieterle's stain. *Legionella* antigen can be detected by enzyme-linked immunosorbent assay (ELISA), radioimmunoassay (RIA), and latex agglutination methods. An indirect immunofluorescence test for serum antibodies is considered diagnostic if a fourfold or higher increase is found from a reciprocal titer of 128 or higher. New methods to identify specific *Legionella* species with DNA probes will likely come into general use in the near future.

MANAGEMENT

The recommended therapy is erythromycin. Rifampin may be added if the response to erythromycin is poor. An alternative therapy is trimethoprim-sulfamethoxazole.

LYMPHOID INTERSTITIAL PNEUMONITIS

A severe pulmonary parenchymal disease, referred to as lymphoid interstitial pneumonitis (LIP), has been associated with human immunodeficiency virus (HIV) infection in infants and children. It is the most frequent form of diffuse pneumonitis in pediatric patients with AIDS.

PATHOPHYSIOLOGY

The cause of LIP is not known, and there is no conclusive proof that it is an infectious process. However, a causative relationship among HIV, the Epstein-Barr virus (EBV), or other opportunistic organisms seems very likely. In a study by Rubinstein and colleagues,[32] four of five children with AIDS and LIP were found to have EBV-specific DNA in lung specimens, whereas in a comparative group of children with AIDS and *P. carinii* pneumonitis, no EBV-specific DNA was found. The usual histopathologic appearance is of nodules formed by clusters of mononuclear cells, including lymphocytes and plasma cells. These lesions are located around the bronchiolar epithelium and in the adjacent intra-alveolar septa. In addition, a diffuse lymphocytic interstitial infiltrate is present. (See Chapter 42.)

CLINICAL MANIFESTATIONS

The onset is often subtle with a slow progressive course and mild hypoxemia. The patients are usually afebrile and have generalized lymphadenopathy and enlargement of the salivary glands. Digital clubbing may be evident. Tachypnea, cough, and chest retractions may or may not be present.

DIAGNOSTIC APPROACHES

The chest radiograph shows bilateral, diffuse, fine nodular infiltrates, and hilar nodes may be enlarged. A definitive diagnosis requires histologic examination of a biopsy specimen.

MANAGEMENT

No specific therapy has been established. The treatment of AIDS with azidothymidine has been associated with improvement of LIP. Some uncontrolled studies suggest that corticosteroid therapy may evoke resolution of LIP.

CYTOMEGALOVIRUS PNEUMONIA

Although cytomegalovirus (CMV) pneumonia can occur in almost any category of disease or therapy causing extreme immunodeficiency, it occurs most commonly in patients receiving allogeneic bone marrow transplants for leukemia or other malignancies; the incidence rate is 15%. Once CMV pneumonia is clinically evident, the fatality rate is about 85%.[33] This pneumonitis occurs only rarely in syngeneic transplant patients and never in autologous transplant recipients.

PATHOPHYSIOLOGY

CMV pneumonitis may occur as a part of a systemic infection from the virus. Studies on the molecular epidemiologic characteristics of CMV infections suggest that at least some of the infections that occur after bone marrow transplantation may be caused by strains present before transplantation.[34] Also, the virus may be transmitted via transfusion of blood products to seronegative transplant recipients. CMV often causes enlargement of infected cells with intranuclear inclusions similar to those of other herpesvirus infections.

CLINICAL MANIFESTATIONS

The systemic CMV infection often presents with an infectious syndrome like mononucleosis, with fever, subclinical hepatitis, splenomegaly, and lymphocytosis with atypical lymphocytes. Tachypnea and signs of respiratory distress emerge as pneumonitis occurs. In some cases, the clinical features of pneumonitis may be the sole evidence of CMV infection.

DIAGNOSTIC APPROACHES

As with many other pneumonias of immunocompromised hosts, the chest radiograph shows bilateral diffuse interstitial infiltrates with no unique features. Although CMV can be isolated from sputum, pharynx, blood, or urine and the demonstration of CMV antibody serologically establishes the diagnosis of CMV infection, these findings do not prove that a concomitant pneumonitis is caused by CMV. The diagnosis of CMV pneumonitis is often difficult because subclinical CMV infection is present in most immunocompromised patients. To establish the diagnosis definitively, it is necessary to perform a biopsy of the lung parenchyma.

MANAGEMENT

No specific antiviral drug has been found to be highly effective against CMV infection. However, an acyclovir analog, ganciclovir, has activity against CMV.[35] Some clinical studies indicate efficacy for CMV retinitis in AIDS patients, but studies on the treatment of CMV pneumonitis are not conclusive at present. The drug has been effective in preventing CMV pneumonitis in bone marrow transplant recipients under controlled conditions.[36]

Attempts should be made to prevent CMV infection in transplant recipients if possible.[37] When transfusions of blood or blood products are needed, CMV antibody–negative blood or freezing and thawing of deglycerolized red blood cells aid in the prevention of transmission.

VARICELLA-ZOSTER VIRUS PNEUMONITIS

The most feared complication of varicella or herpes zoster is pneumonitis resulting from disseminated varicella-zoster virus infection. Although other organs may be affected with the systemic form of this disease, the fatality rate is highest with the pneumonitis. For example, of children with cancer who acquire varicella, approximately one third will progress to disseminated systemic varicella, with an overall mortality rate of 7%. In Feldman and coworkers' study,[38] all the deaths were related to varicella pneumonitis. In herpes zoster infection in cancer patients, systemic dissemination occurs in about 10%, and the overall mortality rate is 1% to 2% without treatment.[39]

PATHOPHYSIOLOGY

Airborne droplets with varicella-zoster virus reach the upper respiratory tract and conjunctiva. The virus invades and viremia occurs. During viremia, the virus is disseminated throughout the body. Virus replication may occur in the columnar epithelium of the respiratory tract, the alveolar epithelial cells, and the endothelial lining of the blood vessels. The virus then exits the capillaries and reaches the epidermis, causing the characteristic vesicular lesion. Affected cells enlarge and may exhibit eosinophilic inclusions in the nuclei causing the so-called ballooning degeneration. Pulmonary lesions resemble the poxlike lesions of the skin. There are scattered areas of necrosis and hemorrhage. The infection involves the alveolar walls, blood vessels, and small bronchioles.[40] There is usually extensive involvement of the trachea and larger bronchi.

CLINICAL MANIFESTATIONS

Usually the pneumonitis occurs while the rash of varicella or zoster is erupting. Rarely, if ever, does the pneumonitis occur before or without the rash. Cough and tachypnea are early signs, but eventually respiratory distress becomes more accentuated with intercostal retractions and cyanosis. Varicella in the immunosuppressed host is often complicated with secondary bacterial infection, and *Staphylococcus aureus* is the most frequent cause.

DIAGNOSTIC APPROACHES

The chest radiograph shows bilateral diffuse infiltrates. This finding, plus the typical skin lesions of varicella or zoster, is usually sufficient to establish the diagnosis of varicella pneumonitis. Efforts should be made to exclude other causes of pneumonitis because additional organisms may also cause pulmonary infection concomitantly with varicella, but this is unusual in the absence of varicella pneumonia.

MANAGEMENT

Acyclovir is the drug of choice for the treatment of varicella and zoster. It is believed that all immunosuppressed patients with these infections should be treated as soon as possible. Pneumonitis rarely occurs in patients who have started treatment before there is evidence of lung involvement. Acyclovir is administered in the dosage of 30 mg/kg as a 1-h infusion divided into three equal doses at 8-h intervals.[41, 42] The treatment should be given for 7 days or

for 2 days after no new skin lesions appear, whichever is longer. Immunosuppressed patients who are susceptible to varicella infection should be given varicella-zoster immunoglobulin within 3 days after exposure. This prophylaxis either prevents or modifies the varicella infection.[43]

A live, attenuated varicella-zoster virus vaccine is currently under study but is not yet available for general use.[44]

RESPIRATORY SYNCYTIAL VIRUS

Respiratory syncytial virus (RSV) is a frequent cause of nonfatal infections of the respiratory tract in normal infants and children. In the immunocompromised host, an exaggerated course of the infection may occur.

PATHOPHYSIOLOGY

In the normal host, RSV causes a mild acute upper respiratory tract illness or lower respiratory tract bronchiolitis, pneumonia, or croup starting 3 to 4 days after exposure to the virus; immunocompromised patients have a more severe disease of the lung and more prolonged virus excretion. Patients with T lymphocyte deficiencies seem to be especially prone to this infection. In reports of severe RSV infections, authors have described extensive pulmonary disease or giant cell pneumonia with prolonged virus shedding for as long as 100 days.[45] Underlying diseases have included AIDS resulting from HIV-1, severe combined immunodeficiency syndromes, malignancy, and graft-versus-host reactions.

CLINICAL MANIFESTATIONS

The clinical manifestations vary, and none is unique to RSV infection. Fever, dyspnea, wheezing, cough, or tachypnea may occur during the course of the disease.

DIAGNOSTIC APPROACHES

The virus is usually isolated from a nasal wash. Material may be inoculated onto HEp-2 cells. Typical cytopathic effects may be seen in 4 days. An earlier diagnosis may be made by immunofluorescent antibody techniques to identify viral antigen. ELISA and RIA methods are also useful.

MANAGEMENT

Only one drug, ribavirin, is available for specific anti-RSV treatment. The drug must be administered by aerosol in the same manner as for RSV bronchiolitis.[46] Serum immunoglobulin has been used to a limited extent,[47] but further controlled studies are needed for definitive recommendations. Nosocomial transmission of RSV occurs early, and infected patients should be placed in isolation during the infectious period; the use of gloves and gowns by hospital personnel must be emphasized.

PULMONARY CANDIDIASIS

The most frequent systemic fungal infection in immunocompromised hosts is candidiasis. *Candida albicans* and other species of *Candida* are components of the usual microbial flora of the oral cavity and intestinal tract and may become invasive with impairment of host defenses.

PATHOPHYSIOLOGY

Pulmonary candidiasis may result from systemic infection and disseminated infection by the hematogenous route or from direct invasion by bronchopulmonary infection.[47] The patients are often neutropenic and recipients of broad-spectrum antibiotics. Also concomitant bacterial and viral infection may be present. Histologically, pseudohyphae forms of *Candida* species invade alveoli and capillaries and may progress by direct invasion.

CLINICAL MANIFESTATIONS

The majority of patients with pulmonary candidiasis are febrile with or without respiratory symptoms. No single clinical pattern applies. Tachypnea and cough may occur in patients with extensive pneumonitis.[48]

DIAGNOSTIC APPROACHES

The most suggestive radiographic lesions of pulmonary candidiasis are rounded cotton boll–like infiltrates, either single or multiple. However, lobar, miliary, and other configurative lesions are common. The finding of *Candida* in the sputum is not diagnostic because this may occur in patients without pneumonitis. Blood cultures rarely yield the organism. The diagnosis requires a biopsy of the lesion to demonstrate yeast and pseudohyphal forms of the organism. Isolation in culture is necessary for confirming *Candida* as the agent. Serologic tests for antigen and antibody are not sufficiently sensitive and specific for firmly establishing the diagnosis.

MANAGEMENT

The combination of amphotericin B and flucytosine is probably the most effective treatment for pulmonary candidiasis. However, amphotericin B alone is the essential component of therapy. Doses of 0.5 mg/kg of amphotericin B intravenously daily and 150 mg/kg of flucytosine per day orally are usual. An alternative, although less effective, treatment is the administration of ketoconazole. A new drug, fluconazole, has anti-*Candida* activity but has not been adequately evaluated in pulmonary candi-

diasis. Some patients with systemic candidiasis have been treated successfully with this drug.[49]

PULMONARY ASPERGILLOSIS

The second most frequent mycotic pulmonary infection in immunocompromised hosts is aspergillosis. *Aspergillus* species, such as *A. fumigatus, A. flavus,* and *A. niger,* are ubiquitous in hospital environments as well as many extramural sites, and spores are often airborne.

PATHOPHYSIOLOGY

Most cases of pulmonary aspergillosis in immunocompetent patients originate from inhalation of airborne spores. Infection of the pulmonary parenchyma may be associated with direct invasion from the respiratory airway or from hematogenous dissemination to alveolar capillaries. The septate hyphae invade the alveolus and initiate a necrotizing or hemorrhagic pneumonic infiltrate.

CLINICAL MANIFESTATIONS

Fever is usually present and may be the only sign or symptom of pulmonary aspergillosis in the immunocompromised patient. Cough, tachypnea, chest pain, and hemoptysis may also occur but with no characteristic pattern. Severe neutropenia (less than 500/cu mm) is often present as a predisposing factor.

DIAGNOSTIC APPROACHES

The chest radiograph may reveal a fairly typical aspergilloma, which represents an area of consolidation with a central clearing bearing a "half-moon" sign. More common than this typical lesion is a nonspecific nodular or lobar lesion. For firmly establishing the diagnosis, an open-lung biopsy is the most dependable approach. However, isolation of *Aspergillus* species from the tracheobronchial airway or nares provides strong evidence for the cause if the clinical features are compatible with aspergillosis. Finding the organism in bronchoalveolar lavage specimens is even more convincing evidence. Serologic tests for antibodies of antigenic components of *Aspergillus* species are under study, but no test has proved adequate to confirm the diagnosis.

MANAGEMENT

Pulmonary aspergillosis is treated with amphotericin B. Starting with a daily intravenous dosage of 0.25 mg/kg/day, the dose is increased daily to a maintenance dose of 1.0 mg/kg/day. The minimal course is 4 to 6 weeks. When the lesion is well localized to an area of the lung away from the vital structures of the hilum, surgical excision of the lesion should be considered. The prognosis is poor in

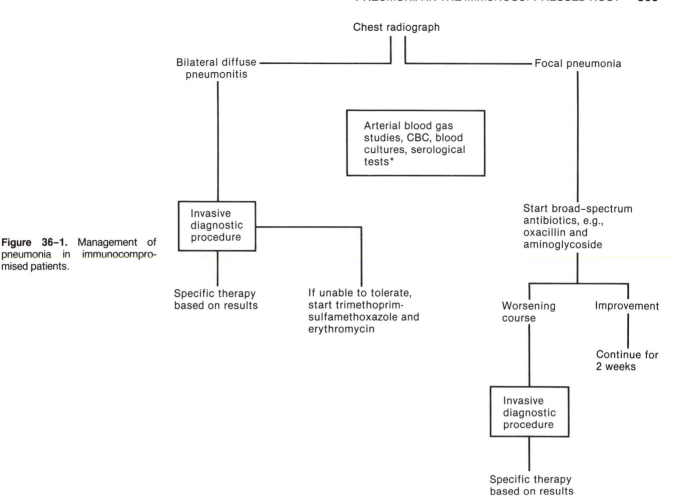

Figure 36–1. Management of pneumonia in immunocompromised patients.

patients who remain severely neutropenic. The role for granulocyte transfusions has not been established.

MANAGEMENT PLAN FOR PNEUMONIA IN THE IMMUNOCOMPROMISED HOST

No single straightforward scheme applies to all immunocompromised patients with pneumonia. In most instances, the etiologic diagnosis cannot be definitively established without an invasive procedure to identify the causative agent in pulmonary tissue. This does not necessarily mean that this approach is the best management for all patients. The approach in Figure 36–1 serves as a skeletal scheme to be modified as needed for the comprehensive management of these patients. For example, in a patient with terminal malignancy for whom no further anticancer therapy is available and whose primary disease will prove fatal in a few days or weeks, an open-lung biopsy is not in the best interest of the patient. Also some patients, because of bleeding tendency, may not tolerate an invasive pulmonary procedure. In these situations, empiric antibiotic therapy may be given. With bilateral diffuse pneumonia, erythromycin and trimethoprim-sulfamethoxazole is a combination that is effective against the majority of causes such as *P. carinii, Legionella, Chlamydia trachomatis,* and many gram-positive and gram-

negative bacterial infections. If the pneumonia is focal or lobar, broad-spectrum antibiotics such as an aminoglycoside plus a penicillinase-resistant penicillin may be used. If fungal infection is suspected, amphotericin B may be added.

REFERENCES

1. Huber GL, First MW: Perspectives: Pulmonary host defense. The host and the development of lung disease. Semin Respir Med 1:87, 1980.
2. Kersarwala HH, Fischer TJ: Pulmonary immunology. *In* Laraya-Cuasay LR, Hughes WT (eds): Interstitial Lung Diseases of Children, vol. 1, pp. 43–55. Boca Raton, FL: CRC Press, 1988.
3. Hinds WC: The drug and the environment. Semin Respir Med 1:197, 1980.
4. Hendley JO, Weller TH: Activation and transmission in rats of infection with *Pneumocystis.* Proc Soc Exp Biol Med 137:1401–1404, 1971.
5. Hughes WT: Systemic candidiasis: A study of 109 fatal cases. Pediatr Infect Dis J 1:11–18, 1982.
6. Pifer LL, Hughes WT, Murphy MJ: Propagation of *Pneumocystis carinii in vitro.* Pediatr Res 11:305–313, 1977.
7. Bommer W: *Pneumocystis carinii* in interstitial plasma-cell pneumonia. Am J Dis Child 102:121–126, 1961.
8. Post C, Dutz W, Nasarian F: Endemic *Pneumocystis carinii* pneumonia in south Iran. Arch Dis Child 39:35–45, 1964.
9. Sheldon WH: Pulmonary *Pneumocystis carinii* infection. J Pediatr 61:780–789, 1962.

10. Price RA, Hughes WT: Histopathology of *Pneumocystis carinii* infestation and infection in malignant disease in childhood. Hematol Pathol 5:737–744, 1974.

11. Hughes, WT, Sanyal SK, Price RA: Signs, symptoms and pathophysiology of *Pneumocystis carinii* pneumonitis. Natl Cancer Inst Monogr 43:77–83, 1976.

12. Kovacs JA, Ng V, Masur H, et al: Diagnosis of *P. carinii:* Improved detection in sputum using monoclonal antibodies. N Engl J Med 318:589–593, 1988.

13. Hughes WT, Smith BL: Efficacy of diaminodiphenylsulfone and other drugs in murine *Pneumocystis carinii* pneumonitis. Antimicrob Agents Chemother 26:436–440, 1984.

14. Leoung GS, Mills J, Hopewell PC, et al: Dapsone-trimethoprim for *Pneumocystis carinii* pneumonia in acquired immunodeficiency syndrome. Ann Intern Med 105:45–48, 1986.

15. Debs RJ, Blumenfeld W, Brunette EN, et al: Successful treatment with aerosolized pentamidine of *Pneumocystis carinii* pneumonia in rats. Antimicrob Agents Chemother 31:37–41, 1987.

16. Allegra CJ, Chabner B, Tuazon C, Kovacs J: Preliminary results of a phase I-II trial of trimetrexate therapy for Pneumocystis pneumonia in AIDS patients [Abstract no. TH 4.1]. Presented at the Third International Conference on AIDS, Washington, DC, June 1987.

17. Frenkel JK, Good JT, Schultz JA: Latent pneumocystis infection of rats: Relapse and chemotherapy. Lab Invest 15:1559–1577, 1966.

18. National Institutes of Health, University of California Expert Panel for Corticosteroids as Adjunctive Therapy for *Pneumocystis carinii* Pneumonia: Consensus statement on the use of adjunctive therapy for *Pneumocystis carinii* pneumonia in AIDS. N Engl J Med 323:1500–1504, 1990.

19. Hughes WT, Kuhn S, Chaudhary S, et al: Successful chemoprophylaxis for *Pneumocystis carinii* pneumonitis. N Engl J Med 297:1419–1426, 1977.

20. Hughes WT, Rivera G, Schell M, et al: Successful intermittent chemoprophylaxis for *Pneumocystis carinii* pneumonitis. N Engl J Med, 316:1627–1632, 1987.

21. Leoung GS, Feigal DW, Montgomery AB, et al: Aerosolized pentamidine for prophylaxis against *P. carinii* pneumonia. N Engl J Med 323:669–675, 1990.

22. Golden H, Gallicano W, Brandstetter RD: Pulmonary toxoplasmosis. Infect Surg 2:337–345, 1988.

23. Vietzke WM, Gelderman AH, Grimley PM, Vasamis MP: Toxoplasmosis complicating malignancy. Cancer 21:816–827, 1968.

24. Krick JA, Remington JS: Toxoplasmosis in the adult: An overview. N Engl J Med 298:550–553, 1978.

25. Navia BA, Petito CK, Gold JW, et al: Cerebral toxoplasmosis complicating the acquired immune deficiency syndrome: Clinical and neurological findings in 27 patients. Ann Neurol 19:224–238, 1986.

26. Gump DW, Keegan M: Pulmonary infection due to Legionella in immunocompromised patients. Semin Respir Infect 1:151–159, 1986.

27. Taylor RJ, Schwentker FN, Kakala TR: Opportunistic lung infections in renal transplant patients: A comparison of Pittsburgh pneumonia agent and Legionnaires' disease. J Urol 125:289–292, 1980.

28. Kugler JW, Armitage JO, Helms CM, et al: Nosocomial Legionnaires' disease: Occurrence of bone marrow transplants. Am J Med 74:281–288, 1983.

29. Tobin JO, Beare J, Dunnill MS, et al: Legionnaires' disease in a transplant unit: Isolation of the causative agent from shower baths. Lancet 2:118–121, 1980.

30. Ryan ME, Feldman S, Pruitt B, Fraser DW: Legionnaire's disease in a child with cancer. Pediatrics 64:951–953, 1979.

31. Horwitz MA, Silverstien SC: Activated human monocytes. J Clin Invest 66:441–450, 1980.

32. Rubinstein A, Morechi R, Silverman B, et al: Pulmonary disease in children with acquired immune deficiency syndrome and AIDS-related complex. J Pediatr 108:498–504, 1986.

33. Meyers JD, Flournoy H, Wade JC, et al: Biology of interstitial pneumonia after marrow transplantation. *In* Gale RP (ed): Recent Advances in Bone Marrow Transplantation, pp. 405–423. New York: Alan R. Liss, 1983.

34. Winston DU, Huang ES, Miller MJ, et al: Molecular epidemiology of cytomegalovirus infections associated with bone marrow transplantation. Ann Intern Med 102:16–20, 1985.

35. Cheng YC, Huang ES, Lin JC, et al: Unique spectrum of 9-(1,3-dihydroxy-2-propoxy) methyl-guanine against herpes viruses in vitro and its mode of action against herpes simplex virus type. Proc Natl Acad Sci USA 80:2770, 1983.

36. Schmidt GM, Horak DA, Niland JC, et al: A randomized, controlled trial of prophylactic ganciclovir for cytomegalovirus pulmonary infection in recipients of allogeneic bone marrow transplants. N Engl J Med 324:1005–1011, 1991.

37. Meyers JD, Flournoy H, Thomas ED: Risk factors for cytomegalovirus infection after human marrow transplantation. J Infect Dis 153:478–488, 1986.

38. Feldman S, Hughes WT, Daniel CB: Varicella in children with cancer: Seventy-seven cases. Pediatrics 56:388–397, 1975.

39. Feldman S, Hughes WT, Kim HY: Herpes zoster in children with cancer. Am J Dis Child 126:178–184, 1973.

40. Feldman S, Stokes DC: Varicella zoster and herpes simplex virus pneumonias. Semin Respir Infect 2:84–94, 1987.

41. Balfour HH Jr: Intravenous acyclovir therapy for varicella in immunosuppressed children. J Pediatr 104:134–136, 1984.

42. Balfour HH Jr, Brown B, Laskin OL, et al: Acyclovir halts progression of herpes zoster in immunocompromised patients. N Engl J Med 308:1448–1453, 1983.

43. Centers for Disease Control: Varicella-zoster immune globulin for the prevention of chicken pox. Ann Intern Med 100:859–865, 1984.

44. Gershon AA, Steinberg SP, Gelb L: Live attenuated varicella vaccine use in immunocompromised children and adults. Pediatrics 78(Suppl):757–763, 1986.

45. Ogra PL, Patel J: Respiratory syncytial virus infection and the immunocompromised host. Pediatr Infect Dis 7:246–249, 1988.

46. Hall CB, McBride JT, Walsh EE, et al: Aerosolized ribavirin treatment of infants with respiratory syncytial virus infection: A randomized double-blind study. N Engl J Med 314:20–26, 1986.

47. Hemming VG, Rodriquez W, Kim HW, et al: Intravenous immunoglobulin treatment of respiratory syncytial virus infection in infants and young children. Antimicrob Agents Chemother 31:1882–1886, 1987.

48. Hughes WT: Natural mode of acquisition for de novo infection with *Pneumocystis carinii.* J Infect Dis 145:842–847, 1982.

49. Kauffman CA, Bradley SF, Ross SC, Weber DR: Successful treatment of hepatic candidiasis with fluconazole [Abstract no. 577]. Presented at the Interscience Conference on Antimicrobial Agents and Chemotherapy, Atlanta, 1990.

37 SARCOIDOSIS

ROSALIND S. ABERNATHY, M.D.

Sarcoidosis, a systemic granulomatous disease of unknown cause, was originally described as a dermatologic curiosity by J. Hutchinson and E. Besnier. In 1899, Boeck, a Norwegian dermatologist, described granulomatous skin changes that he thought resembled sarcoma. He labeled this *sarcoid,* hence the term *sarcoidosis.* The systemic nature of the disease was described by J. Schaumann in 1916, when he noted involvement of the lungs, lymph nodes, bone, liver, and spleen. It was necessary for the incidence of tuberculosis to decline before the frequency of this granulomatous disease could be fully recognized, as it has been since the first international sarcoidosis conference in 1934.[1]

INCIDENCE AND EPIDEMIOLOGY

The incidence of sarcoidosis varies widely with race, age, and geographic location. White patients in northern Europe were originally described with the disease, but blacks have been most frequently affected in the United States. It is most commonly seen in young adults, between 20 and 40 years of age, with an increased incidence in women, and is rare in children 15 years of age or younger. McGovern and Merritt reported 104 cases of childhood disease described in the literature in their survey published in 1956.[2] Since 1964, nine series of seven to 60 patients each have added 242 cases of childhood sarcoidosis to the literature. Eighty-three percent of these cases were found in Virginia, North Carolina, South Carolina, and Arkansas, which suggests that the southeastern and south central states are an area endemic for childhood sarcoidosis.[3–11]

In most series of childhood sarcoidosis, the majority of the cases are reported to be in the age range of 13 to 15 years and with an equal sex ratio. The Arkansas patients were somewhat younger, with a median age of 11 years, and 60% were male. The percentage of black children in the series reported from the endemic areas ranged from 69% to 97%.[3–5] The exception was a study from Duke University, involving a largely referral population, in which 66% of the patients were reported to be male and 33% black.[6]

ETIOLOGY, PATHOGENESIS, AND PATHOLOGY

Although the cause of sarcoidosis is unknown, it appears to be an immunologic response to an unknown antigenic stimulus that gains access to the body via the lungs. The initial response to the antigen is alveolitis, characterized by infiltration of the alveolar septae by increased numbers of mononuclear cells, T lymphocytes, and macrophages. Macrophages interact with the antigen, are activated, and produce interleukin-1 (IL-1). This process activates the T cells, which develop receptors for interleukin-2 (IL-2) and also secrete IL-2, interferon γ, and lymphokines. Monocyte chemotactic factor attracts monocytes, and migratory inhibitory factor holds them in the lung. Activated T cells also stimulate the growth and differentiation of B lymphocytes, which secrete immunoglobulins. This secretion probably accounts for the characteristic hyperglobulinemia found in active sarcoidosis.

The immunologic reaction in the lung in sarcoidosis is compartmentalized. In contrast with the excess numbers of helper T cells in the lung, the peripheral blood shows a decreased number of T cells. This probably explains the paradoxical finding of relative anergy to skin test antigens found in patients with active sarcoidosis.

Interferon γ, produced by the activated T lymphocytes and acting on the accumulated mononuclear cells, induces macrophage differentiation and stimulates the formulation of the noncaseous granuloma, which is the characteristic pathologic lesion in sarcoidosis. Granulomas are found in tissues throughout the body. They may eventually resolve spontaneously or under the influence of corticosteroid therapy, leaving no residua, or they may progress to fibrosis (Fig. 37–1).[12, 13]

The constitutional symptoms in early sarcoidosis such as fever, weight loss, and muscle weakness could be induced by IL-1, which is identical to leukocyte pyrogen. The epithelioid cells of the granulomas have secretory functions, releasing lysozyme and angiotensin-converting enzyme (ACE).[13]

The puzzling finding of hypercalcemia and hypercalciuria in sarcoidosis was explained by the finding of elevated serum levels of 1,25-dihydroxyvitamin D_3 in sarcoidosis patients with hypercalcemia.[14] In sarcoidosis, this compound is not produced in its usual site (the kidney) inasmuch as it was found in elevated levels in the serum of an anephric patient with sarcoidosis and hypercalcemia.[15] Pulmonary alveolar macrophages from patients with sarcoidosis with normal calcium levels can be shown to convert 25-hydroxyvitamin D to the active 1,25-dihydroxyvitamin D form.[16] Studies have shown that 1,25-dihydroxyvitamin D inhibits the synthesis of IL-2, interferon γ, and immunoglobulins by activated lymphocytes. This suggests that the vitamin is part of a down-regulation response to the chronic granulomatous inflammation.[17]

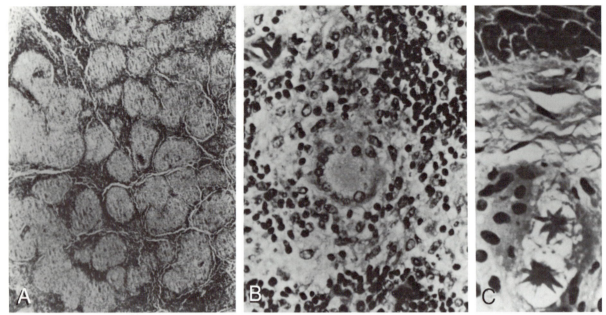

Figure 37-1. (*A*) Lymph node showing extensive infiltration with noncaseating granulomas (hematoxylin and eosin stain, ×100). (*B*) Multinucleated giant cell, epithelioid cells, and lymphocytes in lung tissue (×750). (*C*) Skin with a large giant cell containing two asteroid bodies, characteristic but not diagnostic inclusions sometimes seen in sarcoidosis (×1000). (Reprinted with permission from Abernathy RS: Sarcoidosis. *In* Laraya-Cuasay L, Hughes WT [eds]: Interstitial Lung Disease in Children, Vol. 3, pp. 51–61. Boca Raton, FL: CRC Press, 1988. Copyright by CRC Press, Boca Raton, FL.)

The diagnosis of sarcoidosis rests on (1) compatible clinical or radiographic findings, (2) histologic evidence of noncaseating granulomas, and (3) proof by means of special stains and cultures that these lesions are not produced by fungi, mycobacteria, or other organisms that can cause similar pathologic findings.

CLINICAL MANIFESTATIONS

Sarcoidosis may be asymptomatic, detected from characteristic chest radiographic findings on routine films. Up to 45% of adult patients may be initially diagnosed in this manner.[18] Because children rarely have routine radiographs, sarcoidosis in children is more likely to be symptomatic. In the endemic area, 90% of the children in several series were symptomatic.[3-6, 9] Symptoms are of two varieties. Generalized constitutional symptoms, which include weight loss, fatigue or lethargy, malaise, and occasionally fever, were present in more than half of the children in these series. Other symptoms are caused by the infiltration of granulomas into various organs. The most commonly affected are the lungs. Dyspnea, cough, and, to a lesser extent, chest pain were the complaints in nearly half of the children.[3-6] Other complaints include enlargement of peripheral lymph nodes in 15% to 45% and ophthalmologic symptoms such as redness or pain in the eyes and decreased visual acuity in 12% to 40%.[3-6, 9]

ORGAN SYSTEM INVOLVEMENT AND RADIOGRAPHIC FINDINGS

As in adults, the pulmonary system is almost universally involved in children with sarcoidosis. Physical findings of the chest are usually absent, except for tachypnea in the very severely affected. Abnormalities are detected on the chest radiograph. Since the 1950s, the radiographic appearance has conventionally been classified into three categories: stage I shows bilateral hilar and paratracheal adenopathy with normal-appearing lung parenchyma; stage II shows both bilateral adenopathy and parenchymal abnormalities; and stage III shows parenchymal disease without any hilar adenopathy. A normal radiograph can be designated stage 0. Figure 37–2 shows a stage II film with prominent adenopathy.

Parenchymal abnormalities may include a diffuse reticulonodular pattern or, less commonly, an acinar pattern, which may coalesce into areas of consolidation. Findings of linear strands extending out from the hilum or asymmetric bullae are suggestive of pulmonary fibrosis. Observations by early students of the disease over many years demonstrated sequential evolution from stage I to stage III. Parenchymal infiltrates often appear when hilar adenopathy is diminishing. After hilar nodes disappear, they never reappear. The prognosis for remission decreases as the stage increases.[19, 20]

The stage classification is strictly on the basis of the appearance of the standard radiograph. Alveolitis and granulomas may be demonstrated on lung biopsy specimens in patients with stage I films. Despite this, as long as the radiographic classification remains stage I, the prognosis is good.[19]

Granulomatous infiltration of peripheral lymph nodes is the second most common manifestation of sarcoidosis in children, occurring in 60% to 70%.[3-5] The nodes are nontender, rubbery, and freely movable and may be large enough to see from a distance. Table 37–1 shows the incidence of organ system involvement in three large series of childhood sarcoidosis from the endemic area in comparison with a worldwide adult group.[3-5, 18]

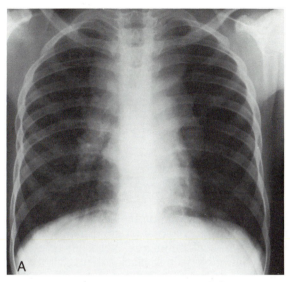
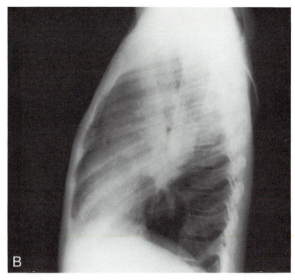

Figure 37–2. A 12-year-old black male presented in 1978 with large cervical lymph nodes, skin rash, follicular conjunctivitis, and mild iritis. Both skin and conjunctival biopsy specimens were positive. Anteroposterior (*A*) and lateral (*B*) radiographs show large hilar and paratracheal lymph nodes and typical reticulonodular infiltrate of stage II sarcoidosis. (Reprinted with permission from Abernathy RS: Sarcoidosis. *In* Laraya-Cuasay L, Hughes WT [eds]: Interstitial Lung Disease in Children, Vol. 3, pp. 51–61. Boca Raton, FL: CRC Press, 1988. Copyright by CRC Press, Boca Raton, FL.)

Ocular involvement is the second most dangerous manifestation, after involvement of the lungs, with the potential for serious residua. Granulomatous uveitis, which may be asymptomatic, is very characteristic of sarcoidosis. A complete ophthalmologic examination, including evaluation with the slit lamp, is mandatory in any patient suspected of having sarcoidosis. The presence of characteristic findings can help establish the diagnosis, and the patient can be offered the meticulous ophthalmologic care required to help ensure preservation of vision. Nodules can be found on the conjunctiva; lacrimal glands can be infiltrated. Cataracts or glaucoma may complicate uveitis both as part of the disease and as complications of topical steroid treatment. Loss of vision is the most severe complication.[3, 21]

A moderate degree of splenomegaly is a characteristic finding, but massive enlargement is occasionally seen. Complications include the possibility of traumatic rupture and hypersplenism.[22] Hepatomegaly may be present. Although the liver nearly always contains granulomas at postmortem examination, liver function abnormality is rarely noted. A syndrome of febrile hepatic granulomatosis, characterized by extreme enlargement of the liver and high fever, has been described as a form of sarcoidosis and was present in two children and two 19-year-old patients seen at the University of Arkansas.[3, 23]

Erythema nodosum has been seen as part of Lofgren's syndrome, along with fever, fatigue, polyarthralgia, and a stage I chest film. Spontaneous resolution without therapy occurs within 6 months in 80% of patients. This is most commonly seen in young adult white women and is rare in children and black patients.[1]

Children do have cutaneous lesions that contain noncaseating granulomas on biopsy. The most characteristic forms are small, flat-topped papules on the face and round, pigmented plaques, 2 to 3 cm in diameter, on the trunk. Subcutaneous nodules may also be seen. Skin lesions often appear first with a systemic exacerbation of the disease.[3]

Parotid gland enlargement may be seen either as an initial finding or developing during the course of the illness (see Table 37–1).

Table 37–1. ORGAN SYSTEM INVOLVEMENT IN SARCOIDOSIS

| | Children 15 Years of Age and Younger | | | | | | Adults (Worldwide)[38] (N = 1609) | |
| | North Carolina[29] (N = 60) | | Virginia[18] (N = 33) | | Arkansas[2] (N = 30) | | | |
Variable	No.	%	No.	%	No.	%	No.	%
Chest abnormality	56/59	95%	33	100%	30	100%	1416	88%
Peripheral lymphadenopathy	37	62%	23	70%	19	63%	451	28%
Splenomegaly	17	28%	9	27%	12	40%	161	10%
Hepatomegaly	22	37%	11	33%	9	30%	—	—
Eyes	31	52%	8	24%	12	40%	354	22%
Uveitis	—	—	7	21%	8	27%	—	—
Skin	24	40%	9	27%	9	30%	290	18%
Parotid	8	13%	4	12%	7	23%	97	6%
Seventh nerve palsy	1	2%	—	—	2	7%	—	—

Arthralgias without physical findings occur in some patients. Arthritis with nonpainful effusions and boggy synovial thickening in the large joints is characteristic of a small group of pediatric patients in whom the onset of sarcoidosis occurs during the preschool years. Other characteristic findings are diffuse dermatitis and granulomatous uveitis but no pulmonary involvement. The dermatitis, uveitis, and arthritis tend to be extremely chronic. Of 40 patients so far reported, 84% were white and 16% were black.[24, 25]

Involvement of the bones is nearly always asymptomatic and detectable only on radiographs. The characteristic finding is small, round lytic lesions in the small bones of the hands or feet. These lesions may remain unchanged for years. Larger, irregular lytic lesions in the long bones are occasionally seen and may heal without therapy.[3]

Renal disease in children is primarily the result of hypercalciuria, which causes the development of kidney stones and sometimes ureteral obstruction and secondary infection. Nephrocalcinosis may also develop.[1] In rare instances, there is granulomatous infiltration of the kidney and renal failure.[26]

The single most common neurologic abnormality in sarcoidosis is facial (seventh) nerve palsy (see Table 37–1). Other manifestations include aseptic meningitis, hydrocephalus, parenchymal disease of the central nervous system, other cranial or peripheral neuropathy, and myopathy. Intracranial or intraspinous mass lesions from sarcoidosis are highly responsive to steroid therapy.[27]

Cardiac involvement is uncommon in children. Among the 200 patients reported from the endemic area, only four had cardiac disease. The severity ranged from an electrocardiographic abnormality[4] to presumably transient myocarditis in two cases[6] to fatal cor pulmonale in a girl whose pulmonary sarcoidosis had been diagnosed 2½ years previously.[9] Moffat and colleagues reported a fatal case of cor pulmonale in a 14-year-old girl whose symptoms of dyspnea, cough, and weight loss over 1½ years had been incorrectly attributed to cystic fibrosis.[28]

Burton and associates reported a 15-year-old healthy boy hospitalized after experiencing 4 days of dyspnea, tachycardia, and cardiomegaly who died 5 days later of fulminating myocarditis.[29] The more characteristic finding is electrocardiographic abnormalities, of which premature ventricular contractions are the most common. Some adult patients have died suddenly. Steroids are the treatment of choice for cardiac sarcoidosis.[1]

DIAGNOSTIC APPROACHES

PULMONARY FUNCTION TESTING

Pulmonary function abnormalities are also approximately correlated with radiographic stage. Stage I findings are associated with normal forced vital capacity (FVC) and normal diffusing capacity (DL_{COsb}) in 80% and 70% of patients, respectively. In the presence of parenchymal disease, stages II and III, these values are normal in only 35% of patients. Restrictive abnormality with a decreased FVC is the classic pulmonary function abnormality, but rarely does it fall below 50% predicted. Changes in DL_{COsb} usu-

ally mirror those in the FVC. A small number of children show mild obstructive findings. Children usually have nearly normal functions on follow-up, but a small number may have severe restrictive abnormalities secondary to pulmonary fibrosis.[30, 31]

Observing pulmonary function changes is an important part of the ongoing evaluation of children with sarcoidosis. Because nearly all pediatric patients are 6 years of age or older, they are capable of undergoing pulmonary function tests.

LABORATORY STUDIES

Hyperglobulinemia, present in two thirds of cases, is the most common laboratory abnormality in sarcoidosis. Hyperimmunoglobulinemia is usually present and is most commonly seen in black patients.[3–5] A white blood cell count of less than 5000 and a moderate degree of eosinophilia are common findings but are, by no means, evidence of sarcoidosis. Hypercalcemia, with serum calcium levels higher than 11 mg/dl, is present in about one third of childhood cases.[3, 5] Hypercalciuria is seen almost twice as frequently as hypercalcemia but is difficult to document. It can be detected by measuring creatinine and calcium levels in a single, fasting, voided specimen. A calcium/creatinine ratio of more than 0.20 is indicative of hypercalciuria.[32] This technique, which has not been widely used in evaluating pediatric sarcoidosis patients, deserves more attention.

Delayed hypersensitivity skin testing with purified protein derivative (PPD), *Candida,* and tetanus helps to complete the evaluation. A negative PPD test is less of an indicator of sarcoidosis than a reassurance that the granulomatous disease is not tuberculosis. The combination of elevated levels of immunoglobulins with negative results of skin tests for *Candida* and tetanus is certainly supportive of the diagnosis of sarcoidosis.

NEW DIAGNOSTIC TECHNIQUES

In the 1980s, three new diagnostic procedures were described as appearing to be much more sensitive measures of the inflammatory response in sarcoidosis and to allow more accurate diagnosis and prognosis than the traditional means of evaluation. Bronchoalveolar lavage has been the tool by which much of the pathophysiologic processes of pulmonary sarcoidosis have been understood.[26] However, it is too invasive to use routinely in children. Gallium 67 scans of the lungs appear to reflect the presence of granulomas accurately.[33] A negative gallium 67 scan suggests a very small likelihood that pulmonary sarcoidosis will become active during the following 2 years.[34] Unfortunately, the high radiation exposure from this procedure makes it undesirable for children.

The serum ACE level can be determined in children. Normal values for children, higher than those for adults, have been established. It was demonstrated that children with sarcoidosis had significantly higher values than did normal children.[35, 36] Unfortunately, false-negative serum ACE test results are found in both stage I and stage III patients.

Regrettably, none of the new tests are specific for sarcoidosis, and they offer less diagnostic aid than originally expected. They also have failed to predict the long-term prognosis in pulmonary sarcoidosis and to identify patients in whom pulmonary fibrosis will develop. The chest radiograph and pulmonary functions remain the best predictors of progression of the disease.[12, 37]

DIAGNOSTIC BIOPSY SPECIMENS

The diagnosis of sarcoidosis rests on finding noncaseating granuloma in a biopsy specimen and proving that it is not the result of a known granuloma-producing infection. Less invasive biopsy procedures should be performed whenever possible. Results of biopsies of skin lesions and subcutaneous nodules are nearly always positive. Specimens from less obviously diseased tissue such as the lower lip for minor salivary glands often have a significant yield.[38] The conjunctival biopsy result is nearly always positive if a small millet-seed nodule can be sampled for biopsy, but even in the absence of such a nodule, granulomas can be obtained in 70% of patients if bilateral biopsy specimens are taken.[39] All of these procedures can be performed on an ambulatory basis. The site most frequently chosen for biopsy in children has been a peripheral lymph node, including the scalene fat pad biopsy. This entails a low-risk procedure, but anesthesia and hospitalization or ambulatory surgery are usually required. Other biopsy sites in children have been the liver, lung parenchyma, the parotid gland, bone, striated muscle, and the testes.[3–5]

Transbronchial biopsy with a flexible bronchoscope has become the procedure of choice for adults because it is simple and safe and may be performed without general anesthesia. Roethe and co-workers showed that multiple specimens are needed—five for stage II disease and 10 for stage I disease—in order to ensure a positive biopsy result.[40] Mediastinoscopy provides a very high yield of positive specimens in any patient with hilar adenopathy. It is safe, but anesthesia is required.[41] Either of these procedures could be performed in a cooperative teenage patient.

DIFFERENTIAL DIAGNOSIS

The noncaseous granuloma is the characteristic pathologic finding in sarcoidosis, but this finding on biopsy does not automatically establish the diagnosis. Caseous granulomas are characteristically seen in tuberculosis, histoplasmosis, coccidioidomycosis, syphilis, brucellosis, leishmaniasis, leprosy, and Crohn's disease. However, noncaseous granulomas are occasionally seen in all these diseases. They can be differentiated from sarcoidosis by serologic studies, skin tests, cultures from the biopsy material, and the clinical course. Noncaseous granulomas may be seen in regional lymph nodes draining a malignancy such as carcinoma of the breast, melanoma, or lymphoma. Other characteristics differentiate these malignancies from sarcoidosis.[42]

Lymphoma is often suspected from the appearance on the chest radiograph of very large hilar nodes. It was stated in 1973, and reconfirmed more recently, that young adult patients with only asymptomatic bilateral hilar adenopathy can be considered to have sarcoidosis without confirmation by biopsy. Unilateral hilar adenopathy should certainly be examined in diagnostic biopsy because the patients, especially if symptomatic, are more likely to have lymphoma or Hodgkin's disease.[41]

The diagnosis of sarcoidosis rests on finding the characteristic clinical picture, noncaseous granuloma on biopsy, failure to identify other causes of granuloma, and the course of the disease. If adolescent patients are considered to have sarcoidosis on the basis of being asymptomatic and of a characteristic chest radiograph, they must be observed until the lymphadenopathy disappears. If the radiograph shows progression to stage II, a biopsy should be performed at that time for confirmation.

MANAGEMENT

The indications for treatment of pulmonary sarcoidosis vary with the radiographic appearance at diagnosis. About 70% of patients with stage I disease experience a spontaneous remission. Spontaneous remission rates with stage II and stage III chest radiographs are 50% and 30%, respectively. Patients with parenchymal disease (stage II or stage III) should be treated if they are symptomatic or if abnormalities appear to be progressing. The response is good if granulomatous inflammation is present, but fibrosis does not respond. Because there is no way to determine whether fibrosis is present, all patients should have the benefit of a trial of treatment. Some authorities believe that early treatment with corticosteroids may suppress inflammation and decrease the possibility of progression to fibrosis.[42] Extrapulmonary sarcoidosis often requires treatment. Indications for treatment include persistent hypercalcemia and hypercalciuria, massive splenomegaly with hypersplenism, infiltration into vital structures such as the myocardium and the central nervous system, uveitis uncontrolled by topical steroids, disfiguring skin disease, severe hepatic involvement, and progressive constitutional symptoms such as fever and weight loss.

The drug of choice for treatment is oral prednisone, beginning with 1 mg/kg daily and changing to an alternative-day schedule once improvement has occurred. Medication is given once daily in the morning. The duration of therapy depends on the rapidity of clearing of signs and symptoms but often is many months or even years.

Among children with generalized sarcoidosis, there is a 50% incidence of systemic exacerbation after initial improvement, either spontaneous or induced by prednisone treatment. Exacerbation is usually heralded by weight loss. Other manifestations are the appearance of skin lesions, the onset or recurrence of hypercalcemia or hypercalciuria, splenomegaly, and parotid swelling. Granulomatous uveitis may progress, or abnormality of the chest radiograph or pulmonary functions may worsen. Exacerbations are usually equally responsive to prednisone treatment.[3]

The overall prognosis for children is similar to that for

adults and is less favorable for blacks and for patients with generalized disease. Most children belong to both of these categories. According to worldwide statistics, the mortality rate is 5% in London and New York but only 1.8% in Paris, where 84% of the patients are white.[18] Kataria and co-authors reported a mortality rate of 5.5% among black patients but only 1.4% among white patients.[43] Pediatric reports include one death in 43 cases,[44] 1 in 60,[5] 1 in 18,[9] and 2 in 30.[3] Four of these five deaths were from pulmonary causes; all constitute a death rate of 5 of 151, or 3%, which is comparable with the rates reported in adults from largely black populations.

REFERENCES

1. Kerdel FA, Moschella SL: Sarcoidosis: An updated review. J Am Acad Dermatol 11:1–19, 1984.
2. McGovern JP, Merritt DH: Sarcoidosis in childhood. Adv Pediatr 8:97–135, 1956.
3. Abernathy RS: Childhood sarcoidosis in Arkansas. South Med J 78:435–439, 1985.
4. Kendig EL Jr: The clinical picture of sarcoidosis in children. Pediatrics 54:289–292, 1974.
5. Pattishall EN, Strope GL, Spinola SM, Denny FW: Childhood sarcoidosis. J Pediatr 108:169–177, 1986.
6. Grossman H, Merten DF, Spock A, Kirks DR: Radiographic features of sarcoidosis in pediatric patients. Semin Roentgenol 20:393–399, 1985.
7. Beier FR, Lahey ME: Sarcoidosis among children in Utah and Idaho. J Pediatr 65:350–359, 1964.
8. Reed WG: Sarcoidosis: A review and report of eight cases in children. J Tenn Med Assoc 62:27–36, 1969.
9. Schabel SI, Stanley JH, Shelley BE Jr: Pediatric sarcoidosis. J SC Med Assoc 76:419–422, 1980.
10. Schmitt E, Appelman H, Threatt B: Sarcoidosis in children. Radiology 106:621–625, 1973.
11. Siltzbach LE, Greenberg GM: Childhood sarcoidosis—A study of 18 patients. N Engl J Med 279:1239–1245, 1968.
12. Soskel NT, Fox R: Sarcoidosis . . . or something like it. South Med J 83:1190–1204, 1990.
13. Thomas PD, Hunninghake GW: Current concepts of the pathogenesis of sarcoidosis. Am Rev Respir Dis 135:747–760, 1987.
14. Chesney RW, Hamstra AJ, DeLuca HF, et al: Elevated serum 1,25-dihydroxyvitamin D concentrations in the hypercalcemia of sarcoidosis: Correction by glucocorticoid therapy. J Pediatr 98:919–922, 1981.
15. Barbour GL, Coburn JW, Slatopolsky E, et al: Hypercalcemia in an anephric patient with sarcoidosis: Evidence for extrarenal generation of 1,25-dihydroxyvitamin D. N Engl J Med 305:440–443, 1981.
16. Singer FR, Adams JS: Abnormal calcium homeostasis in sarcoidosis. N Engl J Med 315:755–757, 1986.
17. Reichel H, Koeffler HP, Barbers R, Norman AW: Regulation of 1,25-dihydroxyvitamin D₃ production by cultured alveolar macrophages from normal human donors and from patients with pulmonary sarcoidosis. J Clin Endocrinol Metab 65:1201–1209, 1987.
18. Siltzbach LE, James DG, Neville E, et al: Course and prognosis of sarcoidosis around the world. Am J Med 57:847–852, 1974.
19. DeRemee RA: The roentgenographic staging of sarcoidosis. Historic and contemporary perspectives. Chest 83:128–133, 1983.
20. Pare JAP, Fraser RG: Synopsis of Diseases of the Chest, chap. 14. Philadelphia: WB Saunders, 1983.
21. Hoover DL, Khan JA, Giangiacomo J: Pediatric ocular sarcoidosis. Surv Ophthalmol 30:215–228, 1986.
22. Kataria YP, Whitcomb ME: Splenomegaly in sarcoidosis. Arch Intern Med 140:35–37, 1980.
23. Israel HL, Margolis ML, Rose LJ: Hepatic granulomatosis and sarcoidosis. Dig Dis Sci 29:353–356, 1984.
24. Mallory SB, Paller AS, Ginsburg BC, et al: Sarcoidosis in children: Differentiation from juvenile rheumatoid arthritis. Pediatr Dermatol 4:313–319, 1987.
25. Sahn EE, Hampton MT, Garen PD, et al: Preschool sarcoidosis masquerading as juvenile rheumatoid arthritis: Two case reports and a review of the literature. Pediatr Dermatol 7:208–213, 1990.
26. Turner MC, Shin ML, Ruley EJ: Renal failure as a presenting sign of diffuse sarcoidosis in an adolescent girl. Am J Dis Child 131:997–1000, 1977.
27. Stern BJ, Krumholz A, Johns C, et al: Sarcoidosis and its neurological manifestations. Arch Neurol 42:909–917, 1985.
28. Moffat RE, Sobonya RE, Chang CH: Childhood sarcoidosis with fatal cor pulmonale. Pediatr Radiol 7:180–182, 1978.
29. Burton DA, Kapur S, Shapiro SR, et al: Fulminant cardiac sarcoidosis in childhood. Am J Cardiol 58:177–178, 1986.
30. Pattishall EN, Strope GL, Denny FW: Pulmonary function in children with sarcoidosis. Am Rev Respir Dis 133:94–96, 1986.
31. Winterbauer RH, Hutchinson JF: Use of pulmonary function tests in the management of sarcoidosis. Chest 78:640–647, 1980.
32. Roy S III, Stapleton FB, Noe HN, Jerkins G: Hematuria preceding renal calculus formation in children with hypercalciuria. J Pediatr 99:712–715, 1981.
33. Abe S, Munakata M, Nishimura M, et al: Gallium-67 scintigraphy, bronchoalveolar lavage, and pathologic changes in patients with pulmonary sarcoidosis. Chest 85:650–655, 1984.
34. Baughman RP, Shipley R, Eisentrout CE: Predictive value of gallium scan, angiotensin-converting enzyme level and bronchoalveolar lavage in two-year follow-up of pulmonary sarcoidosis. Lung 165:371–377, 1987.
35. Beneteau-Burnat B, Baudin B, Morgant G, et al: Serum angiotensin-converting enzyme in healthy and sarcoidotic children: Comparison with the reference interval for adults. Clin Chem 36:344–346, 1990.
36. Rodriguez GE, Shin BC, Abernathy RS, Kendig EL Jr: Serum angiotensin-converting enzyme activity in normal children and in those with sarcoidosis. J Pediatr 99:68–72, 1981.
37. Rubinstein I, Baum GL: The persistent need to improve our approach to sarcoidosis [editorial]. Chest 87:710–711, 1985.
38. Nessan VJ, Jacoway JR: Biopsy of minor salivary glands in the diagnosis of sarcoidosis. N Engl J Med 301:922–924, 1979.
39. Karcioglu ZA, Brear R: Conjunctival biopsy in sarcoidosis. Am J Ophthalmol 99:68–73, 1985.
40. Roethe RA, Fuller PB, Byrd RB, Hafermann DR: Transbronchoscopic lung biopsy in sarcoidosis. Optimal number and sites for diagnosis. Chest 77:400–402, 1980.
41. Munkgaard S, Neukirch F: Comparison of biopsy procedures in intrathoracic sarcoidosis. Acta Med Scand 205:179–184, 1979.
42. DeRemee RA: Sarcoidosis. Current perspectives on diagnosis and treatment. Postgrad Med 76:167–172, 1984.
43. Kataria YP, Shaw RA, Campbell PB: Sarcoidosis: An overview II. Clin Notes Respir Dis 20:3–16, 1982.
44. Kendig EL Jr: Sarcoidosis. Am J Dis Child 136:11–12, 1982.

Suggested Reading
1. Lieberman J (ed): Sarcoidosis. Orlando, FL: Grune & Stratton, 1985.
2. Scadding JG, Mitchell DN: Sarcoidosis, 2nd ed. London: Chapman & Hall, 1985.

38 PULMONARY TUBERCULOSIS AND TUBERCULOUS INFECTION IN INFANTS, CHILDREN, AND ADOLESCENTS

BETTINA C. HILMAN, M.D.

Unlike smallpox and poliomyelitis, tuberculosis is not a disease of the past. Significant progress has been made in the control of tuberculosis in the United States, but this communicable disease has not yet been eradicated. From 1953 to 1984, the number of reported cases of tuberculosis in the United States decreased by 73.6%, but the decline in the number of reported cases essentially stopped in 1985.[1] The downward trend was reversed in 1986, with the first increase in the number of indigenous cases since national reporting began in 1953.[1-4] The increased numbers of cases of tuberculosis reported in the United States are in populations with certain racial and ethnic minorities, predominantly blacks, native American Indians, native Alaskans, and immigrants from Latin America, Asia, and the Pacific Islands. In 1989 Rieder and colleagues[4] reported the relative risks of tuberculosis in different segments of the U.S. population and documented that the overall risk of tuberculosis was, in comparison with that of non-Hispanic whites, 4.3 times higher for Hispanics, 4.7 times higher for native American Indians and native Alaskans, 6.4 times higher for non-Hispanic blacks, and 11.2 times higher for Asians and Pacific Islanders. The number of cases of childhood tuberculosis in the United States has changed little in recent years, and cases tend to cluster in some racial and ethnic groups and in certain geographic locations.[5]

The development of specific chemotherapy for tuberculosis revolutionized the prognosis of tuberculosis and offers the potential for eradication.[6] Tuberculosis is now potentially curable and preventable, but the full potential of antituberculous chemotherapy has not yet been achieved because of a variety of factors, including patients' compliance and problems of access to care.[6] Clinical trials of specific chemotherapy for tuberculosis have emphasized two basic principles: (1) treatment regimens must include multiple drugs to which the organisms are susceptible, and (2) drug therapy must continue for a sufficient period of time.[6]

The American Thoracic Society and the Centers for Disease Control (CDC) provide guidelines for the treatment of tuberculosis and tuberculous infections in both adults and children and periodically revise their joint statements on treatment.[6] Major changes in antituberculous chemotherapy in the 1970s and 1980s have included the demonstrated efficacy of short-term chemotherapy for pulmonary tuberculosis in adults.[6-10] The shorter courses of chemotherapy in adults have improved compliance with drug therapy and are more cost effective.[6] The rationale for the short-term chemotherapy is the rapid sterilization of lesions to reduce acquired resistance to the tubercle bacilli. Abernathy and associates[11] in 1983 reported that treatment with isoniazid and rifampin for 9 months was effective therapy for tuberculosis in children.[11] At least nine additional studies demonstrated the efficacy of short-term chemotherapy regimens in children.[12-20] The shorter drug regimens are not recommended when drug intolerance or toxicity occurs, in drug-resistant tubercle bacilli, or when there is systemic disease such as human immunodeficiency virus (HIV) infections, malignancies, or diabetes mellitus.

The Committee on Infectious Diseases for the American Academy of Pediatrics (AAP) published revised guidelines for chemotherapy in infants and children.[21] These recommendations are included later in this chapter.

This chapter focuses on the recognition of tuberculous infection in infants, children, and adolescents; the diagnosis and management of intrathoracic tuberculosis; the management of children in contact with cases of active tuberculosis; and infants exposed to mothers with tuberculous infection.

PATHOGENESIS AND PATHOPHYSIOLOGY

Mycobacterium tuberculosis, the etiologic agent of human tuberculosis, is almost exclusively transmitted from person to person through inhalation of airborne droplet nuclei (1 to 10 μm in diameter) containing viable tubercle bacilli. The rate of transmission of tuberculous infection varies with the number of viable tubercle bacilli

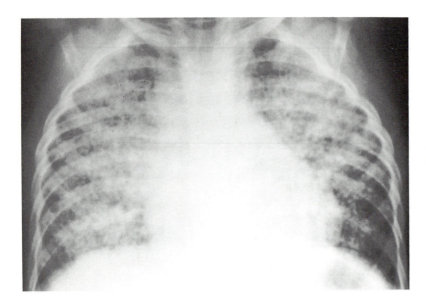

Figure 38–1. Posteroanterior chest radiograph of pulmonary miliary tuberculosis.

in sputum of patients with active tuberculosis, the exposure to infected aerosolized droplet nuclei (especially with coughing, sneezing, or laughing), the concentration of bacilli in the air, the degree of infectiousness of the active case, and the length of time that the susceptible host breathes the infected air.[22]

With the exception of older children and adolescents with "reactivation" tuberculosis, children rarely infect other children.[23] Most adults with pulmonary tuberculosis are no longer infectious after 2 to 3 weeks of chemotherapy, but patients with advanced cavitary disease who continue to cough and those with resistant mycobacterial organisms may remain infectious for longer periods of time.[24]

The primary lesion of tuberculosis occurs in the lung parenchyma in more than 95% of patients because the usual mode of tuberculous infection is by inhalation. When inhaled tubercle bacilli reach the alveoli, the organisms are engulfed by phagocytes but remain viable and continue to multiply. The tubercle bacilli are then carried from the primary focus in the lung parenchyma to the regional lymph nodes (hilar lymph nodes or paratracheal lymph nodes). The primary focus is usually single but may be multiple. Tubercle bacilli may also spread through the blood stream to generalized areas in the lungs or to more distant sites. Acute miliary tuberculosis is a generalized hematogenously spread disease that occurs as a complication of tuberculous infection and is more common in infants and younger children than in older children and adults (Fig. 38–1).

Acquired immunity develops over a period of several weeks after primary infection and is usually adequate for limiting further multiplication and spread of bacilli. The infected host may remain asymptomatic, and the initial lesion or lesions heal. The immune response can be demonstrated by a positive tuberculin skin test (delayed cutaneous hypersensitivity), which develops over a 2- to 10-week period after infection. The primary complex forms during this period and consists of the initial lung parenchymal focus, the involved regional lymph nodes, and the lymphatic vessels in between.

While hypersensitivity of the body tissue to the tubercle bacilli is developing, the primary focus may grow larger, but it is not encapsulated. The primary focus may become caseous; the caseous material is gradually inspissated and later calcifies or may completely disappear. In most cases of primary pulmonary tuberculosis, the initial parenchymal focus heals. However, the initial lesions may progress, pneumonitis may develop in the surrounding tissue, and the overlying pleura may thicken. In the stage of caseation, the caseous material may empty into one or more bronchi to form primary cavitary tuberculosis. Hematogenous dissemination is also more likely to occur during caseation. The regional lymph nodes also have a tendency to heal but often not as completely as the primary parenchymal focus. Even though partial healing has occurred, tubercle bacilli may persist in lymph nodes for years, as evidenced by the areas of calcification. Calcification develops over a period of 6 months, and evidence of calcification on chest radiographs suggests that the infection has been present for at least 6 months.

Infected regional lymph nodes may encroach on bronchi, causing extraluminal obstruction; atelectasis of the lung may develop distal to the obstruction if the bronchial obstruction is complete. Air trapping and hyperinflation result from partial airway obstruction. A caseous node may erode into the bronchial lumen and cause extrusion of its caseous contents, producing atelectasis or a combination of pneumonia (consolidation) and collapse. Figure 38–2 shows a collapse-consolidation pattern on the chest radiograph of a patient with primary pulmonary tuberculosis.

Most of the complications of primary tuberculosis occur within the first year after the initial infection. In some patients, however, complications and clinical illness develop after an interval of several years, when the tubercle bacilli that have persisted in the body begin to replicate and produce disease. The lung is one of the sites where foci of infection most commonly result in delayed disease. Tuberculous infection provides immunity against tubercle bacilli that may be subsequently inhaled, but the price is persistence of viable bacilli from the initial infection. In

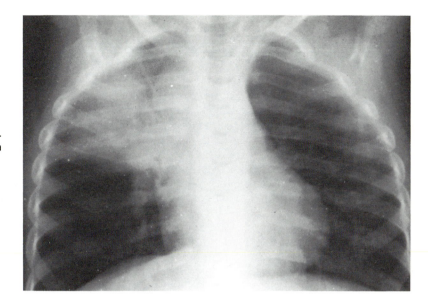

Figure 38–2. Endobronchial tuberculosis with a collapse-consolidation pattern on chest radiograph in an 11-month-old black female.

some patients, the persistence of viable tubercle bacilli leads to reactivation of infection and progressive disease. Resistance may be lowered by several factors such as chronic fatigue, malnutrition, stress (e.g., from surgery), hormonal changes (puberty, pregnancy), certain infections (measles, varicella, pertussis, HIV, and possibly other severe viral illnesses), corticosteroids, and other immunosuppressive therapy. Reactivation tuberculosis, or the adult type of tuberculosis, can occur in older children and adolescents. This type of tuberculosis is more common in females around the time of puberty (Fig. 38–3). In contrast to primary tuberculosis in children, reactivation tuberculosis is highly contagious.

DIAGNOSIS AND DIAGNOSTIC APPROACHES

A high index of suspicion is necessary for identifying either tuberculous infection or disease (tuberculosis) in

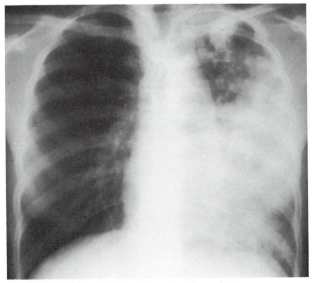

Figure 38–3. Reactivation tuberculosis in an adolescent female.

infants and children, because primary tuberculosis is often occult.[25] Even with pulmonary tuberculosis, children rarely cough and seldom produce sputum. In most cases, tuberculous infection is associated with a few organisms of *M. tuberculosis*. Unlike adults, children exhibit few clinical signs or symptoms of tuberculosis, and the diagnosis is not easily documented by microbiologic confirmation of the presence of *M. tuberculosis* on culture of sputum or gastric washings. The classic symptoms and signs of active tuberculosis (such as fever, weight loss or failure to thrive, cough, night sweats, anorexia, or malaise) are usually absent in most children. A positive tuberculin skin test result may be the initial and only indication of tuberculous infection in infants and children.

Tuberculous infection should always be considered whenever an infant, a child, or an adolescent is in contact with adults with active tuberculosis. The risk of tuberculous infection is highest among household or close contacts, and younger children are at higher risk of infection than are older children and adolescents. The risk of the development of clinically active disease among recent tuberculin skin test convertors has been estimated as one in every 30 cases exposed. Thus, prompt investigation of all children in contact with adults with active tuberculosis is important for preventing disease resulting from *M. tuberculosis* and its complications. It is important to determine the sensitivity of the infecting *M. tuberculosis* from the adult source case to ensure that the organisms are not resistant to isoniazid. There are at least three factors contributing to the increase in isoniazid-resistant mycobacteria in the United States: (1) concentration of active tuberculosis in noncompliant adults and adolescents, (2) the increase in refugees from populations with a high incidence of isoniazid-resistant organisms, and (3) failure to use adequate antituberculous chemotherapy in the initial treatment.

Bacteriologic confirmation from sputum cultures in pediatric patients is seldom feasible. Infants and young children seldom produce adequate samples of sputum for cultures, even when methods such as ultrasonic nebulization are used to induce sputum production. Results of cultures of *M. tuberculosis* in sputum from the source case, when known, provide indirect evidence to support the diagnosis in children in close contact with adolescents or adults who have active tuberculosis. Even gastric aspirates may result in a low yield of positive mycobacterial cultures. Of the 18,578 gastric lavages obtained over an 8-year period in 4251 patients reported by Gerbeaux,[26] only 4% yielded positive cultures (i.e., only 16.8% of the patients had positive cultures). In contrast, Wallgren[27] reported a higher percentage of positive cultures from gastric aspirates: more than 44% positive cultures in patients in his series with positive chest radiographic findings. In a review by Fox[25] of 350 children with occult tuberculosis, calcification developed in 20.8% with normal initial chest radiographs over 2 to 5 years; of the cultures obtained in 340 of these children from three gastric washings, only 8.5% were positive. Starke and Taylor-Watts,[5] in a review of 110 children (median age of 24 months), with active tuberculosis, reported gastric aspirate cultures positive for *M. tuberculosis* in 39% of children with pulmonary disease.

The low yield of positive cultures from gastric aspirates in children is a result of the small number of organisms in primary tuberculosis and possible inadequate techniques for collection of gastric aspirates. Gastric washings should be obtained early in the morning after an overnight fast. The contents of the stomach should be aspirated and placed in a sterile container for culture. Lavage of the stomach should then be performed with 20 to 60 ml of sterile (not tap) water and the lavage contents added to the sterile container with the fluid obtained by the initial gastric aspiration.

Satisfactory evidence of tuberculous infection in children includes two or more of the following findings: (1) positive result of intradermal tuberculin skin test (purified protein derivative [PPD] 5 tuberculin units [TU]) of ≥ 10 mm induration read at 48 to 72 h (occasionally, a recent conversion from negative to 5 to 8 mm in an infant or a young child in contact with active cases of tuberculosis may be read as positive); (2) abnormal chest radiograph that is compatible with tuberculous infection (e.g., hilar adenopathy with or without parenchymal infiltrate, pleural effusion, collapse-consolidation, or miliary lesions); (3) positive culture for *M. tuberculosis* in gastric aspirate, tissue, or sputum; (4) positive biopsy results that are consistent with a diagnosis of *M. tuberculosis* infection; and (5) household or close contact with an adult or an adolescent with proven active tuberculosis.

Because a skin test indicates the presence of tuberculous infection, it is essential to ensure that the skin test is properly applied (with the use of standardized solutions) and correctly interpreted. The tuberculin solution recommended for testing is the PPD because of its specificity. It is injected intracutaneously (i.e., Mantoux's intracutaneous test). The World Health Organization has used one lot number of PPD (no. 49608) as the international standard tuberculin PPD-S. Because it is adsorbed in variable amounts by glass and by plastic, a small amount (5 parts per million) of polysorbate 80 (Tween 80) is added to reduce this adsorption. It should be administered promptly intracutaneously. Exactly 0.1 ml of the PPD solution is injected intracutaneously on the volar surface

Table 38–1. FACTORS INFLUENCING FALSE-NEGATIVE OR FALSE-POSITIVE RESULTS FOR TUBERCULIN SKIN TESTS

False-Negative Results
Overwhelming infection with *Mycobacterium tuberculosis*
Early *M. tuberculosis* infection (before development of delayed hypersensitivity)
Deficiencies of immunity (congenital or acquired including corticosteroids and other immunosuppressive drugs)
Active infections (measles, rubella, mumps, varicella, influenza, infectious mononucleosis, mycoplasma, HIV)
Recent live virus vaccination
Diseases of the lymphoid system
Stressful conditions (e.g., burns, malnutrition)
Sarcoidosis
Problems with the tuberculin solution
  Improper handling (dilutional errors; storage in light, heat, or excessive cold; contamination)
  Adsorption to container walls
Errors in technique of skin test administration
  Incorrect administration
  Wrong amount given
  Injection subcutaneous (not intradermal)
  Adsorption to syringe walls because of delayed administration
Incorrect interpretation of skin test results
  Inexperience in detecting induration
  Mismeasurement of erythema
  Errors in recording
False-Positive Results
Cross-reactions to nontuberculous myobacteria
Reactions to impurities in the tuberculin solution
Incorrect technique of administration
Incorrect interpretation
Previous vaccination with BCG

HIV, human immunodeficiency virus; BCG, bacillus Calmette-Guérin.

of the forearm through a short-bevel 26- or 27-gauge needle. If any area of ecchymosis develops at the site of the skin test, the test should be repeated at another site.

The tuberculin skin test is read at 48 to 72 h, and the area of induration is measured at the widest transverse diameter. A positive test result is ≥ 10 mm induration; a doubtful result is 5 to 9 mm; and a negative result is less than 5 mm. Additional details of tuberculin skin testing are available from a variety of sources.[28, 29] It is important to be aware of causes of false-negative and false-positive reactions to tuberculin skin tests (Table 38–1). If the skin test results are doubtful, tests should be repeated at the same dose at a different site. Skin test readings in the doubtful range may indicate cross-reactivity with antigens of the nontuberculous mycobacteria. These antigens are not commercially available and are not standardized but have been available for investigative epidemiologic studies from the CDC in Atlanta, Georgia.

After the diagnosis of tuberculous infection is established or accepted, the next critical diagnostic consideration is the evaluation of the evidence for mycobacterial disease. With the lack of bacteriologic confirmation of tuberculous infection and the absence of diagnostic biopsy findings, the decision of presence or absence of disease may rest on the interpretation of the chest radiograph. Hilar adenopathy may be the only positive chest radiographic finding suggestive of the diagnosis of tuberculosis. Both anteroposterior and lateral views of the chest are indicated to evaluate hilar adenopathy. Figure 38–4 demonstrates hilar adenopathy in both anteroposterior

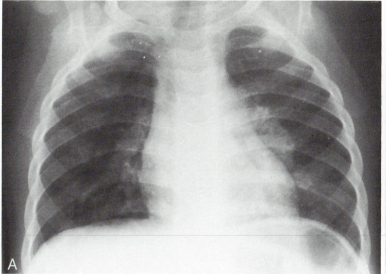

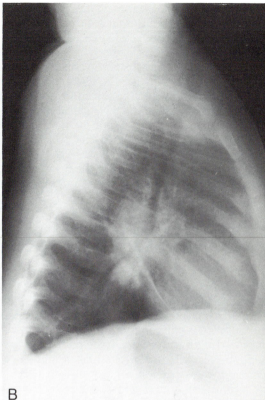

Figure 38–4. Hilar adenopathy in primary tuberculosis in both anteroposterior (*A*) and lateral (*B*) views. The child was in contact with his father, who had active tuberculosis.

and lateral views in a child in contact with an adult with active tuberculosis. Children should be carefully positioned for the chest radiographs because rotation can distort the hilar structures. Ideally, chest radiographs should be taken during maximal inspiration with the diaphragm at the eighth rib posteriorly. With expiratory chest radiographs, mediastinal widening can occur.

Special radiographic views such as apical lordotic views

can be helpful to demonstrate lesions or cavities in the apical regions of the lung. Figure 38–5*A* shows a plain chest radiograph of an adolescent with reactivation tuberculosis. Tomograms or computed tomographic (CT) examinations of the chest can more precisely define the extent of the cavitation or suspected cavities in reactivation tuberculosis (Fig. 38–5*B*). Lateral decubitus chest films may demonstrate the presence of pleural effusion.

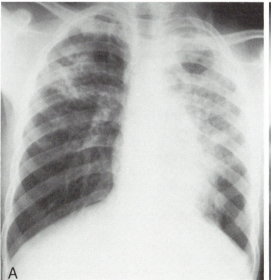

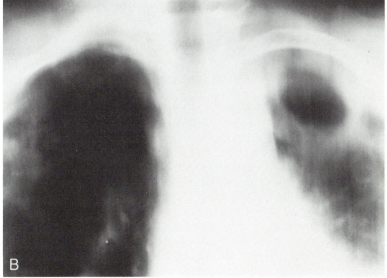

Figure 38–5. *A*, Plain chest radiograph of reactivation tuberculosis with cavity in adolescent black male. *B*, Tomogram of chest demonstrates cavitary lesion in the left upper lobe of an adolescent male with reactivation tuberculosis.

Other diagnostic imaging techniques for confirming pleural effusion include ultrasonograms or CT scans of the chest.

The primary complex is more likely to be seen on the chest radiograph in infants and younger children than in older children and adolescents. The majority (up to 75%) of children with tuberculous infection have normal chest radiographs; an additional 17% usually have an area of increased density in the region of the hilus without a demonstrable primary parenchymal focus.

In view of the increasing incidence of HIV infection in infants and children, HIV testing (with informed consent) is recommended when the diagnosis of tuberculosis is made in patients at risk for HIV infection.[21]

MANAGEMENT

Early recognition and adequate treatment of primary tuberculosis are necessary for minimizing the risk of complications from the lymphohematogenous spread of the tubercle bacilli, such as miliary tuberculosis, meningitis, and other extrapulmonary tuberculous lesions. Available since 1945, antituberculosis chemotherapy is aimed at sterilizing *M. tuberculosis* lesions promptly and completely, avoiding treatment failures caused by bacterial resistance, and preventing reactivation of tuberculous infection during adolescence and adulthood. Because there is no objective measurement that would indicate complete sterilization of lesions resulting from tubercle bacilli, it is difficult to determine when the primary goal has been reached. Compliance with prescribed drug therapy is the major problem with antituberculous chemotherapy. Other problems related to chemotherapy for *M. tuberculosis* include the variability in susceptibility of different bacterial populations because of pH of the environment and metabolic activity of the organisms. Tubercle bacilli multiply in spurts; drugs kill the tubercle bacilli but only at certain times (i.e., at the time of replication when the DNA is organized for dividing).

Various laboratory observations and experience from clinical drug trials have suggested a background for mycobacterial chemotherapy in relation to different bacterial populations.[30-33] There are different bacterial populations in cavitary lesions, in closed caseous lesions, and within macrophages. The tubercle bacilli in each site have different metabolic activities and different rates of replication; the frequency of replication varies with the available oxygen supply. The susceptibility of the tubercle bacilli depends on the pH of the environment as well as the metabolic activity of the organisms.

The population size of the tubercle bacilli also varies with each site. Open cavities have the largest number of mycobacteria. Naturally occurring drug-resistant mutants of *M. tuberculosis* occur within large bacterial populations even before tuberculous chemotherapy is started.[21] The frequency of drug-resistant mutants of the tubercle bacilli is proportional to the size of the mycobacterial population; resistant mutants are less frequent in caseous lesions and within macrophages than in open cavities.[21]

Mitchison[30, 31] described four populations of tubercle bacilli. Group I includes the metabolically active bacilli found in areas of neutral pH, which are rapidly and continuously growing. Isoniazid has bactericidal action, which is greatest for fast-growing organisms, whereas rifampin kills less quickly than isoniazid. Group II population includes tubercle bacilli in acid environments such as those found inside pulmonary macrophages. The drug that is most active against the small number of tubercle bacilli that multiply slowly inside macrophages is pyrazinamide (PZA). Pyrazinamide has sterilizing activity second only to that of rifampin. Group III tubercle bacilli have occasional spurts of active growth. Only rifampin is bactericidal for all three populations and against the tubercle bacilli that multiply intermittently. Group IV consists of dormant tubercle bacilli that are difficult to eradicate with current drugs; host defenses probably play a major role in their eradication. Isoniazid and rifampin are bactericidal against all populations of mycobacteria and are essential components in all treatment regimens for children. Isoniazid is the most potent and least toxic bactericidal drug. Streptomycin is most active against *M. tuberculosis* growing extracellularly in open cavities. Other drugs such as ethambutol and ethionamide prevent replication of mycobacteria but are not bactericidal.

Current chemotherapy entails the use of at least two bactericidal drugs to which *M. tuberculosis* is susceptible and can usually effect a cure in 6 to 9 months if the patient is compliant with the drug therapy.[21]

Three antituberculous drugs—isoniazid, rifampin, and pyrazinamide—can achieve tissue and body fluid levels adequate for killing *M. tuberculosis* in all body sites (Table 38–2). Infection with *M. tuberculosis* in most sites can be adequately treated by a 9-month course of isoniazid and rifampin[34, 35] or by 6-month chemotherapy regimens consisting of isoniazid, rifampin, and pyrazinamide for 2 months followed by isoniazid and rifampin for an additional 4 months.[12, 19, 20] Treatment of extrapulmonary tuberculosis (e.g., bone and joint tuberculosis) can require longer durations of therapy.[21] The treatment for tuberculous meningitis with isoniazid and rifampin has been generally accepted.[36] The Committee on Infectious Diseases of the AAP recommends a 12-month drug regimen, with initial therapy of isoniazid, rifampin, pyrazinamide, and streptomycin for 2 months followed by isoniazid and rifampin for 10 additional months.[21] The optimal therapy of tuberculosis in HIV-infected children has not yet been firmly established,[21] but it is anticipated that therapy would always include at least three drugs initially and would be continued for at least 9 months.

The specific treatment of tuberculous infection and tuberculosis in infants and children changed dramatically over the 1980s. The AAP Committee on Infectious Disease has developed a consensus statement on treatment,[21] and recommendations given in this chapter conform to most of these recommendations. The Committee recommends as standard therapy for drug-susceptible pulmonary tuberculosis a 6-month drug regimen consisting of isoniazid, rifampin, and pyrazinamide daily for 2 months, followed by isoniazid and rifampin for 4 additional months given daily to twice weekly. The twice-

Table 38–2. RECOMMENDED TREATMENT FOR PULMONARY (INTRATHORACIC) TUBERCULOSIS

Classification	Treatment Regimens	Comments
Asymptomatic Infection (Positive Skin Test Only)		
INH susceptible	INH, 9 months	A minimum of 6 consecutive months with good compliance and susceptible organisms
INH resistant	RIF, 9 months	If daily therapy not possible, give twice weekly; this should be continued at least 9 months
Pulmonary Infection (Manifest Intrathoracic Disease), Pulmonary or Hilar Adenopathy Only		
Predominant regimen	INH, RIF, and PZA daily initially for 2 months, followed by 4 months of INH and RIF daily INH, RIF, and PZA daily initially for 2 months, followed by 4 months of INH and RIF twice weekly (if directly observed)	With hilar adenopathy, 6-month regimen of INH and RIF has been successful when drug resistance is rare. If noncompliance is likely, regimens with direct observation offer a rational alternative; when drug resistance is highly likely, ethambutol or streptomycin should be considered for addition to initial therapy while drug susceptibility determined
Alternative regimen	INH and RIF daily 9 months, or INH and RIF daily for 1 month followed by 8 months of INH and RIF twice weekly (if directly observed)	

Modified from American Academy of Pediatrics, Committee on Infectious Diseases: Chemotherapy for Tuberculosis in Infants and Children. Elk Grove Village, IL: American Academy of Pediatrics, 1991.
INH, isoniazid; RIF, rifampin; PZA, pyrazinamide.

weekly drug regimen should be directly observed by a health care worker; the optimal duration of twice-weekly therapy is controversial, but durations of 6 to 9 months are usually successful for treating pulmonary disease and hilar adenopathy.[21] Additional alternative antituberculous drug regimens are given in detail in Table 38–3. The treatment of hilar adenopathy is usually the same as for pulmonary tuberculosis in infants and children when drug resistance is unlikely. A normal chest radiograph is not a criterion for discontinuation of antituberculosis chemotherapy in children because radiologic resolution may take as long as 2 or 3 years. With disseminated disease such as miliary tuberculosis, information is inadequate for recommending 6-month chemotherapy at this time.[21] The AAP Committee on Infectious Diseases also recommends a chemotherapy regimen of 9 months of isoniazid for infants and children with asymptomatic tuberculous infection as evidenced by only a positive tuberculin skin test result (PPD 5 TU) and no evidence of disease

clinically or by chest radiographs. Rifampin given for 9 months is recommended for children with isoniazid-resistant infection.[21]

Isoniazid can inhibit pyridoxine metabolism and can result in peripheral neuritis or convulsions. The administration of pyridoxine is not usually necessary for children taking isoniazid, except for those who are malnourished, breast-fed infants, adolescents on meat- and milk-deficient diets, and pregnant patients.[21]

Recommendations for the addition of corticosteroids to antituberculous chemotherapy is suggested for tuberculous meningitis,[37] for pleural[38] and pericardial effusions,[39] in endobronchial disease,[40] and in acute miliary disease.[21] When used, the corticosteroids are given daily for 4 to 6 weeks and then tapered for varying periods, usually over 2 to 3 weeks.

The potential chemotherapy for tuberculosis in children with HIV infection has not yet been firmly established. It is anticipated that longer duration of therapy will

Table 38–3. DRUGS FOR ANTITUBERCULOUS CHEMOTHERAPY IN INFANTS, CHILDREN, AND ADOLESCENTS

Variable	INH*†	RIF*‡	PZA	ETH	EMB§	STM
Form	Tablets, 100 and 300 mg (scored)	Capsules, 150 and 300 mg	Tablets, 500 mg	Tablets, 250 mg	Tablets, 100 and 400 mg	Vials, 1 and 5 g
Dose	10–15 mg/kg/day (po)	10–20 mg/kg/day (po)	20–40 mg/kg/day (po)	15–25 mg/kg/day (po)	15–25 mg/kg/day (po)	20–30 mg/kg/day‖ (im)
Maximum dose	300 mg/day, 900 mg twice/week	600 mg twice/week	2000 mg	1000 mg	2500 mg, 50–70 mg/kg twice/day	1000 mg/dose, 20–40 mg/kg, both twice/week

INH, isoniazid; RIF, rifampin; PZA, pyrazinamide; ETH, ethionamide; EMB, ethambutol; STM, streptomycin; po, orally; im, intramuscular.
*Rifamate capsules containing 150 mg INH and 300 mg RIF are available for older children and adolescents.
†A syrup of 10 mg/ml is available. Many experts do not recommend the use of INH syrup because it may be unstable and can be associated with frequent gastrointestinal complaints, including diarrhea. I do not recommend use of INH or RIF syrups.
‡A syrup of RIF can be formulated from the capsules; however, it is unstable. Many experts do not recommend this syrup because of its instability and possible error in dosage of various strengths of the active drug in these liquid preparations.
§EMB is bacteriostatic and should be used with caution, because monitoring of toxicity in infants or young children by visual acuity and color discrimination is difficult.
‖In one or two doses.

be necessary and should be continued for at least 9 months.[21] Therapy should include at least three drugs initially.[21] Culture confirmation with sensitivities of organisms is highly desirable.

DRUG RESISTANCE

Drug resistance to antibacterial agents is genetically coded in the genomes of the microorganisms; in the case of tubercle bacilli, resistance occurs as a result of a mutation, and the mutation rates to different drugs apparently are independent of one another.[41] The likelihood that a mutant organism is resistant to two drugs is extremely low; resistance to three drugs is almost nonexistent.

The treatment of drug-resistant tuberculosis should include at least two bactericidal drugs to which the *M. tuberculosis* isolated from the child or the source case is susceptible. Resistance to isoniazid and streptomycin is commonly encountered, whereas primary resistance to rifampin and pyrazinamide is rare.[21] It is important to obtain drug susceptibility information about the adult source case or the child in order to determine the risk of infection by drug-resistant mycobacterial organisms. Certain populations are more likely to have drug-resistant tuberculosis; these populations include people from high-risk areas (Asia, Africa, and Latin America), the homeless, and persons previously treated or who have a history of noncompliance with chemotherapy. Powell and associates[42] reported that one third of Indochinese refugees in the United States have tubercle bacilli resistant to at least one antituberculous drug.

Usually a fourth drug, such as ethambutol, is added to the initial chemotherapy regimen when there is primary resistance to isoniazid. Ethambutol is a bacteriostatic drug that delays the multiplication of both intracellular and extracellular organisms through interference with RNA synthesis.[29] Adverse side effects include retrobulbar optic neuritis with a decrease in visual acuity (diminished red-green color perception and loss of peripheral vision). These toxic effects usually subside when the drug is discontinued, but the retrobulbar neuritis may be irreversible. The drug should be discontinued when there is a two-line loss of visual acuity on the Snellen chart, loss of color vision, or loss of visual fields.[29]

MONITORING PATIENTS ON CHEMOTHERAPY

Frequent evaluation of infants, children, and adolescents receiving antituberculous chemotherapy is essential for assessing the effectiveness of treatment, for encouraging compliance with treatment, and for observation for possible adverse drug effects.

Adverse reactions to antituberculous chemotherapy are infrequent in infants and children; routine laboratory monitoring of complete blood count, liver function studies, and serum uric acid measurements are usually not necessary. However, with several hepatotoxic drugs used in combination or with severe disease, monitoring of liver function tests is advised, especially in the initial months or treatment.[21]

PREVENTION

Additional management issues in infants, children, and adolescents involve prevention of tuberculosis. These issues include

1. management of an infant born to a mother with tuberculosis;
2. treatment of infants, children, and adolescents exposed to active cases of tuberculosis in which the tuberculin skin test is negative; and
3. treatment of tuberculin skin test–positive patients receiving corticosteroids or other immunosuppressive therapy or patients with positive tuberculin skin tests who are undergoing the stress of surgery.

INFANTS BORN TO MOTHERS WITH TUBERCULOSIS

An infant born to a mother with tuberculosis should have a chest radiograph and a tuberculin skin test (PPD 5 TU) and begin treatment with isoniazid at 10 mg/kg/day for a minimum of 3 months. A second tuberculin skin test should be performed in 2 to 3 months. If the result is positive, the infant should be evaluated for tuberculosis. If the result is negative, maternal compliance is good, and the chest radiograph is negative, isoniazid can then be stopped. If maternal compliance is questionable or poor, isoniazid should be continued for 9 to 12 months,[29] or bacillus Calmette-Guérin (BCG) vaccine for the infant should be considered.[43] If BCG administration to the infant is chosen, the infant should be separated from the mother until the Mantoux tuberculin skin test reaction becomes positive from the BCG vaccine (usually about 6 to 8 weeks).[29] If isoniazid is selected, the infant can be returned to the mother's care as soon as the isoniazid therapy is instituted. In Kendig's study,[44] 38 of 73 infants born to mothers considered to have "inactive" tuberculosis became infected; three of the infected infants died of tuberculosis.

If the infant of a mother with tuberculosis has a positive skin test result, two drugs (usually isoniazid or rifampin unless there is drug resistance) should be used for 12 months. Short-course chemotherapy has not been evaluated extensively in the treatment of the newborn with tuberculosis.

Although rare, congenital tuberculosis can occur. It is anticipated that the incidence may rise in the future with increasing numbers of women in the childbearing age range with HIV infection. Congenital tuberculosis results from hematogenous dissemination of the tubercle bacilli transplacentally or from aspiration of infected amniotic fluid in utero or during delivery. Prompt recognition and treatment of this form of tuberculosis are essential. It is mandatory to examine the cerebrospinal fluid for evidence of tubercle bacilli and to search for organisms of *M. tuberculosis* in the respiratory secretions, gastric washings, urine, bone marrow, and liver.

CONTACTS OF ACTIVE CASES OF TUBERCULOSIS

All infants, children, and adolescents in close contact (e.g., household or extended household) with adults with active tuberculosis, as well as older children and adolescents with reactivation tuberculosis who have a negative tuberculin skin test result (PPD 5 TU) and no clinical or chest radiographic evidence of disease, should receive isoniazid for 3 months at 10 to 15 mg/kg/day. If the tuberculin skin test reaction remains negative after 3 months and contact with the active case is broken, or if the case is known to be smear negative and the source case is considered to be compliant with antituberculous chemotherapy, prophylactic isoniazid therapy can be discontinued. If the child remains in contact with an adult with active tuberculosis for longer than 3 months and there is concern about the compliance of the source case with antituberculous chemotherapy, tuberculin skin test reactivity should be monitored at 3-month intervals. If the smear of the source case remains positive, the tuberculin skin test reactivity of the close contacts should also be monitored at 3-month intervals.

TUBERCULIN-POSITIVE PATIENTS RECEIVING IMMUNOSUPPRESSIVE THERAPY

Patients who are tuberculin positive and who have been previously treated for tuberculous infection or disease should receive antituberculous chemotherapy simultaneously with immunosuppressive treatment (i.e., corticosteroids) for the duration of the immunosuppressive therapy.[45]

REFERENCES

1. Tuberculosis—United States, 1985—and the possible impact of human T-lymphotropic virus type III/lymphadenopathy-associated virus infection. MMWR 35:74–76, 1986.
2. Tuberculosis, final data—United States, 1986. MMWR 36:817–820, 1988.
3. Centers for Disease Control: Tuberculosis in the United States 1985–1986, publication no. CDC 88-8322. Washington, DC: U.S. Department of Health and Human Services, 1987.
4. Rieder HL, Cauthen GM, Kelly GD, et al: Tuberculosis in the United States. JAMA 262(3):385–389, 1989.
5. Starke JR, Taylor-Watts KT: Tuberculosis in the pediatric population of Houston, Texas. Pediatrics 84:28–35, 1989.
6. American Thoracic Society: Treatment of tuberculosis and tuberculosis infection in adults and children. Am Rev Respir Dis 134:355–363, 1986.
7. Dutt AK, Jones L, Stead WW: Short-course chemotherapy for tuberculosis with largely twice-weekly isoniazid-rifampin. Chest 75:441–447, 1979.
8. D'Esopo ND: Clinical trials in pulmonary tuberculosis. Am Rev Respir Dis 125(Suppl):85–93, 1981.
9. Snider DE Jr, Graczyk J, Bek E, et al: Supervised six-months treatment of newly diagnosed pulmonary tuberculosis using isoniazid, rifampin and pyrazinamide with and without streptomycin. Am Rev Respir Dis 130:1091–1094, 1984.
10. Coombs DL, O'Brien RJ, Geiter LS: USPHS tuberculosis short-course chemotherapy trial 21: Effectiveness, toxicity and acceptability. Ann Intern Med 112:397–406, 1990.
11. Abernathy RS, Dutt AK, Stead WW, et al: Short-course chemotherapy for tuberculosis in children. Pediatrics 72:801–806, 1983.
12. Anane T, Cernay J, Bensenovci A: Resultats compares des regimens et des regimens long dans la chimiotherapie de la tuberculose de l'enfant en Algerie. Presented at the African regional meeting, International Union Against Tuberculosis, Tunis, Tunisia, October 1984.
13. Pelosi F, Budani H, Rubinstein C, et al: Isoniazid, rifampin and pyrazinamide in the treatment of childhood tuberculosis with duration adjusted to the clinical status. Am Rev Respir Dis 131(Suppl):A229, 1985.
14. Starke JR, Taylor-Watts KT: Six-month chemotherapy of intrathoracic tuberculosis in children. Am Rev Respir Dis 139(Suppl):A314, 1989.
15. Khubchandani RP, Kumta NB, Bharucha NB, et al: Short-course chemotherapy in childhood pulmonary tuberculosis. Am Rev Respir Dis 141(Suppl):A338, 1990.
16. Ibanez S, Ross G: Quimioterapia abreviada de 6 meses en tuberculosis pulmonar infantil. Rev Chil Pediatr 51:249–252, 1980.
17. Varudkar BL: Short-course chemotherapy for tuberculosis in children. Indian J Pediatr 52:593–597, 1985.
18. Medical Research Council Tuberculosis and Chest Disease Unit: Management and outcome of chemotherapy for childhood tuberculosis. Arch Dis Child 64:1004–1012, 1989.
19. Biddulph J: Short-course chemotherapy for childhood tuberculosis. Pediatr Infect Dis J 9:794–801, 1990.
20. Kumar L, Ohand R, Singhi PD, et al: A randomized trial of fully intermittent and daily followed by intermittent short-course chemotherapy for childhood tuberculosis. Pediatr Infect Dis J 9:802–806, 1990.
21. American Academy of Pediatrics Committee on Infectious Diseases: Chemotherapy for tuberculosis in infants and children. Pediatrics 89:161–165, 1992.
22. Farer LS: Infectiousness of tuberculous patients. Am Rev Respir Dis 108:152–156, 1973.
23. Starke JR: Modern approach to the diagnosis and treatment of tuberculosis in children. Pediatr Clin North Am 35:441–464, 1988.
24. Nobel RC: Infectiousness of pulmonary tuberculosis after starting chemotherapy. Review of the available data on an unresolved question. Am J Infect Control 9:6–10, 1981.
25. Fox TG: Occult tuberculous infection in children. Tubercle 58:91–96, 1977.
26. Gerbeaux J: Primary Tuberculosis in Childhood. Springfield, IL: Charles C Thomas, 1970.
27. Wallgren A: Pulmonary Tuberculosis in Adults and Children. New York: Thomas Nelson, 1939.
28. Childs WH, Bass JB Jr: Using and interpreting tuberculin skin tests. J Respir Dis 4(12):18–26, 1983.
29. Inselman LS, Kendig EL Jr: Tuberculosis. In Chernik V (ed): Kendig's Disorders of the Respiratory Tract in Children, 5th ed, pp. 730–769. Philadelphia: WB Saunders, 1990.
30. Mitchison DA: Basic mechanisms of chemotherapy. Chest 76:771–781, 1979.
31. Mitchison DA: Treatment of tuberculosis. The Mitchell Lecture 1979. J R Coll Physicians Lond 14:91–99, 1979.
32. Dutt AK, Stead WW: Present chemotherapy for tuberculosis. J Infect Dis 146:698–704, 1982.
33. Starke JR: Multidrug chemotherapy for tuberculosis in children. Pediatr Infect Dis J 9:785–793, 1990.
34. Jacobs RF, Abernathy RS: The treatment of tuberculosis in children. Pediatr Infect Dis J 4:513–517, 1985.
35. Dutt AK, Moers D, Stead WW: Short-course chemotherapy for extrapulmonary tuberculosis. Ann Intern Med 107:7–12, 1986.
36. Jacobs RF, Sunakorn P: Tuberculous meningitis in children: An evaluation of chemotherapeutic regimens. Am Rev Respir Dis 141(Suppl):A337, 1990.
37. Escobar JA, Belsey MA, Ovenas A, et al: Mortality from tuberculous meningitis reduced by steroid therapy. Pediatrics 56:1050–1055, 1975.
38. Smith MHD, Matsaniotis N: Treatment of tuberculous pleural effusions with particular reference to adrenal corticosteroids. Pediatrics 22:1074–1087, 1958.
39. Strang JIG, Kakaza HHS, Gibson DG, et al: Controlled trial of prednisolone as adjunct in treatment of tuberculous contrictive pericarditis in Transkei. Lancet 2:1418–1422, 1987.
40. Nemir RL, Cordona J, Vaziri F, et al: Prednisone as an adjunct in the chemotherapy of lymph node-bronchial tuberculosis in child-

hood: A double-blind study. II. Further term observation. Am Rev Respir Dis 95:402–410, 1967.

41. Donath J, Chitkara RK: Drug-resistant tuberculosis: Principles of management. J Respir Dis 9(10):61–77, 1988.

42. Powell KE, Brown D, Farer LS: Tuberculosis among Indochinese refugees in the United States. JAMA 249:1455–1460, 1983.

43. Kendig EL Jr: BCG vaccination in Virginia. J Pediatr 51:54, 1957.

44. Kendig EL Jr: Prognosis of infants born of tuberculous mothers. Pediatrics 26:97, 1960.

45. Smith MHD: Tuberculosis in children and adolescents. Clin Chest Med 10:381–395, 1989.

DISEASES WITH A RESPIRATORY COMPONENT

39 CARDIOVASCULAR-RELATED RESPIRATORY DISEASE

SUNG MIN PARK, M.D. / JAMES W. MATHEWSON, M.D.

The close relationship between the respiratory and circulatory systems is well recognized. For example, the pulmonary hypertension of cor pulmonale may result in right ventricular hypertrophy and right ventricular failure. Not as well recognized is respiratory dysfunction resulting from congenital cardiovascular diseases. Because this dysfunction may be similar to that encountered in primary respiratory diseases, significant underlying and contributory cardiac abnormalities may be overlooked.

The lungs receive the entire output from the right side of the heart and must return the same volume to the left side. The lungs surround the heart, and the large airways and the great arteries are close to each other. This dual-organ system is enclosed within the rigid bony rib cage. Respiratory function may thus be altered by a variety of cardiac lesions. These lesions include those that (1) increase pulmonary blood flow and pressure, (2) impede return of pulmonary flow to the left heart, (3) result in compression of large airways by abnormally positioned or dilated blood vessels, and (4) result in decreased pulmonary blood flow and systemic hypoxemia. Table 39–1 lists several examples of each type of lesions.

RESPIRATORY DYSFUNCTION FROM INCREASED PULMONARY BLOOD FLOW AND PRESSURE

Patients with atrial septal defects (ASDs) are usually asymptomatic throughout childhood in spite of increased pulmonary blood flow. Pulmonary artery and venous pressure is not elevated because resistance in the lungs is low and the left atrium is decompressed by virtue of the atrial defect.

If the left-to-right shunt is large and in the absence of ASD or anomalous pulmonary venous return, the left side of the heart dilates, its end-diastolic pressure rises, and there is a concomitant rise in left atrial and pulmonary venous pressure, as seen in congestive cardiac failure.[1] Increased pulmonary venous capillary pressure follows. As pulmonary capillary pressure rises, fluid accumulates in the peribronchovascular and interstitial spaces. This fluid is initially removed by pulmonary lymphatic channels, but as left ventricular failure continues, the lymphatic channels are overwhelmed and can no longer remove fluid in proportion to the rate of its production. Alveolar flooding results. At this stage, congestive heart failure occurs.

Patients with increased pulmonary blood flow and pressure, as in a large ventricular septal defect (VSD), experience respiratory dysfunction even when there is no overt congestive heart failure (Figs. 39–1, 39–2). The respiratory dysfunction associated with large left-to-right shunt can be caused by the compression of large or small airways by the distended left atrium, distended pulmonary arteries, and arterioles. In severe cases of VSD, the pulmonary artery can dilate and compress the left lateral aspect of distal trachea, left main stem bronchus, and right lower lobe bronchus. A distended left atrium can compress the inferior aspect of main stem bronchi.[2]

Small airways can also be narrowed. It has been speculated that the involvement of small airways may be a result of compression by small, distended pulmonary arteries, formation of peribronchiolar edema, or stiffening of lung tissue by pulmonary vasculature, which is distended by increased flow and pressure.

Table 39–1. RESPIRATORY DYSFUNCTION FROM VARIOUS CONGENITAL CARDIOVASCULAR DISEASES

Increased Pulmonary Blood Flow and Pressure
Ventricular septal defect
Patent ductus arteriosus
Complete atrioventricular canal
Systemic-to-pulmonary shunt
Obstruction to Pulmonary Venous Return
Pulmonary venous stenosis
Mitral stenosis
Cor triatriatum
Total anomalous pulmonary venous return below the diaphragm
Compression of Large Airways
Vascular Anomalies
Vascular ring
Anomalous innominate artery
Pulmonary artery sling
Dilatation of Pulmonary Artery
Tetralogy of Fallot with absent pulmonic valve
Enlarged Left Atrium
Mitral valve disease
Large left-to-right shunt
Chronic Hypoxemia and Reduced Pulmonary Blood Flow
Tetralogy of Fallot
Tricuspid atresia

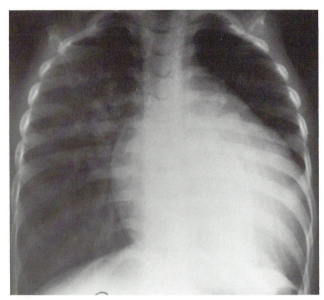

Figure 39–1. Anteroposterior chest view in a 3-year-old boy with a marked cardiomegaly resulting from ventral septal defect (VSD) and aortic insufficiency. Note left lower lobe atelectasis caused by compression to the left lower lobe bronchus.

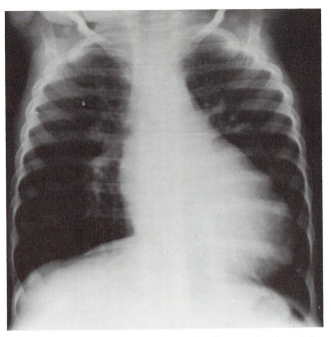

Figure 39–2. A frontal view of the chest, showing a marked hyperinflation of the chest in a 15-month-old male with VSD and truncus arteriosus. Note the hyperinflation resulting from compression of small airways by distended pulmonary arteries under high pressure.

Bancalari and colleagues[3] determined lung compliance in infants with increased pulmonary blood flow. These infants had significantly lower lung compliance than infants with decreased pulmonary blood flow. Specific lung compliance was inversely related to mean pulmonary artery pressure. In infants, lesions causing a large left-to-right shunt can produce significant respiratory morbidity without concomitant respiratory infections. Hordof and co-authors[4] studied the clinical course of 10 infants with VSD and large left-to-right shunts. The manifestations of airway obstruction included ronchi, wheezing, diffuse hyperinflation, lobar emphysema, atelectasis, and hypercapnia, all of which regressed rapidly after surgical repair of the defect. Radiographic studies by Oh and Markowitz and their associates[5, 6] showed that patients with left-ro-right shunts exhibited hyperinflation of the chest, which subsided after repair.

Children with increased blood flow may be at increased risk for complications of viral illness. MacDonald and co-workers[7] reported 27 patients with both congenital heart disease and respiratory syncytial virus (RSV) infection. These patients had a significantly higher rate of morbidity than did a control group. In addition, the degree of pulmonary artery hypertension was correlated positively with the severity of RSV illness. Eight of 11 infants with severe pulmonary artery hypertension and large VSD died during RSV illness.

The treatment is surgical, even in young infants. Those children who manifest persistent and frequent respiratory difficulties resulting from cardiovascular disease in spite of maximal medical management should undergo operation as soon as possible.

In infants weighing less than 2.5 kg, pulmonary artery banding may be an attractive alternative to total repair. The objective is to reduce pulmonary artery pressure and flow to tolerable levels. In heavier infants, total surgical repair is preferable. In either case, surgical morbidity and mortality rates are low when such patients are cared for in advanced pediatric intensive care units.

Pulmonary hypertension may make surgical repair of the heart lesion more difficult. Heard and colleagues[8] reported that preoperative pulmonary artery pressure and resistance were correlated positively with the duration of mechanical ventilation in patients recovering from surgical repair of congenital heart diseases. Bush and co-authors[9] reported 14 children with pulmonary artery hypertension and congenital heart disease in whom increased medial muscle thickness was correlated positively with an increased probability of perioperative death.

RESPIRATORY DYSFUNCTION FROM OBSTRUCTION OF PULMONARY VENOUS RETURN TO THE LEFT SIDE OF THE HEART

The lungs must accept the output from the right side of the heart. Although pulmonary vascular resistance is normally low, capacitance is limited. If the right ventricular stroke volume cannot make its way unimpeded back to the left side of the heart, pulmonary arterial and venous pressures must rise. Such patients clinically manifest symptoms similar to those of patients with large left-to-right shunts, including dyspnea and tachypnea. The volume of blood pumped by the heart, however, is less than that seen with a large left-to-right shunt; thus the caloric expenditure can maintain both cardiac output and the work of breathing. Many affected infants do not manifest rales, even in the presence of severe pulmonary edema. In contrast to the pulmonary arterial and venous pressure elevation seen with large left-to-right shunt, chest radiographs in pulmonary venous obstruction demonstrate pulmonary edema and engorged pulmonary veins without concomitant enlargement of the pulmonary arteries.

When the obstruction is at the level of the pulmonary veins in the neonate, the heart remains small. Long-standing pulmonary venous obstruction results in progressive enlargement of the right side of the heart and secondary cardiomegaly. When the level of obstruction is at the mitral valve, the left atrium may be huge. Pulmonary dysfunction is inevitable because of elevated pulmonary venous pressure and compression of the main stem bronchi with varying degrees of atelectasis, especially of the left lower lobe. Other lesions causing obstruction to pulmonary venous return to the left side of the heart include cor triatriatum and total anomalous pulmonary venous return (TAPVR) below the diaphragm with obstruction at the level of the sinus venosus. TAPVR to the right atrium may include obstruction to left ventricular inflow resulting from a small patent foramen ovale or ASD.

The neonate with TAPVR plus obstruction may exhibit clinical signs and symptoms that are essentially identical to those seen in severe respiratory distress syndrome. When such patients are evaluated for the possibility of patent ductus arteriosus, the differential diagnosis should always include obstructed anomalous pulmonary venous return.

Diagnosis starts with a chest radiograph and two-dimensional echocardiograms. Most obstructive congenital cardiac lesions that manifest in the neonatal period are amenable to either total corrective repair or palliation.

Pulmonary venous return to the left side of the heart may be impeded by the lesions such as mitral or aortic insufficiency. In either case, left atrial or left ventricular end-diastolic pressure is elevated, resulting in pulmonary venous hypertension and passive congestion of the lungs.

A similar mechanism for pulmonary dysfunction may be seen in patients who have primary myocardial dysfunction involving the left ventricular free wall or septal muscle. Such diseases include congestive or restrictive forms of cardiomyopathy. In each instance, left ventricular compliance is reduced, resulting in an elevation in left ventricular end-diastolic pressure. Left atrial and pulmonary venous pressures obligatorily rise, producing inevitable pulmonary dysfunction.

RESPIRATORY DYSFUNCTION FROM COMPRESSION OF LARGE AIRWAYS

Three types of cardiovascular lesions may result in compression of large airways: (1) vascular anomalies, (2) dilatation of the pulmonary arteries, and (3) enlarged left atrium.

VASCULAR ANOMALIES

Vascular anomalies include (1) vascular ring, (2) anomalous innominate artery, and (3) pulmonary artery sling (Table 39–2).

Vascular Ring

A vascular ring consists of a ring of vascular structures that surround the trachea and esophagus. These structures include the aorta, the main pulmonary artery, and a patent ductus arteriosis or ligamentum arteriosum. A double aortic arch may also produce a vascular ring. Desnos and associates[10] reviewed 680 cases of vascular strictures of the respiratory tract in children. The incidence of vascular ring was 54%. Interestingly, in their own series of 41 cases, the incidence was 29%. In a report by Waldman

Table 39–2. VASCULAR ANOMALIES THAT CAUSE AIRWAY COMPRESSION AND ABERRANT RIGHT SUBCLAVIAN ARTERY

Anomaly	Symptoms	Esophagogram	Bronchoscopy	Angiography	Treatment
Vascular ring	Stridor, respiratory distress, occasional swallowing difficulty, apnea	Bilateral indentation of esophagus on anteroposterior view, posterior indentation on lateral view	Bilateral tracheal compression, pulsatile, not essential in diagnosis	Diagnostic but not essential in diagnosis	Surgery
Anomalous innominate artery	Stridor, recurrent bronchitis, apnea	Normal	Pulsatile anterior tracheal compression, essential in diagnosis	Not necessary	Surgery for apnea and severe respiratory difficulties
Pulmonary artery sling	Stridor, respiratory distress, recurrent bronchitis	Anterior indentation of esophagus	Tracheobronchial compression or complete ring trachea and other anomalies	Diagnostic and essential in diagnosis	Surgery, postoperative respiratory management can be very difficult; preoperative bronchography recommended
Aberrant right subclavian artery	Asymptomatic	Oblique defect upward to the right on anteroposterior view, posterior indentation on lateral view	Usually normal	Diagnostic but not necessary	Usually no treatment from respiratory point of view

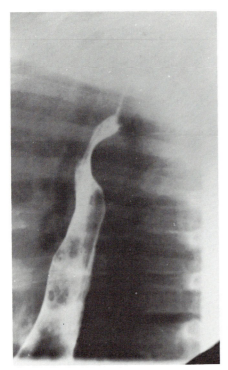

Figure 39–3. Esophagogram (lateral view) in a 14-month-old male with double aortic arch. Note the posterior indentation of the esophagus.

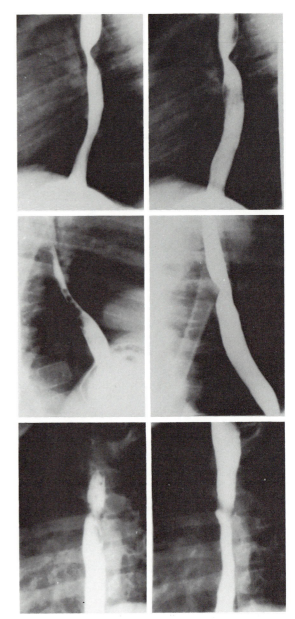

Figure 39–4. Esophagogram taken in various positions in a 5-year-old boy who has a vascular ring with right aortic arch and ligamentum arteriosum. Note the posterior indentation of the esophagus.

and colleagues[11] of 10 children with vascular compression of the upper airway, 4 patients had a vascular ring. The primary symptoms are stridor, dyspnea, and wheezing, which may be mistaken for asthma or persistent bronchitis. Some patients may exhibit dysphasia, although the primary manifestation of a vascular ring is usually respiratory. When wheezing in a child does not respond to appropriate bronchodilator therapy, a vascular ring should be included in the differential diagnosis. Apnea has also been reported as a presenting symptom.[12]

The diagnosis may be suggested in a standard frontal chest radiograph. Infants who are acyanotic and have a right aortic arch are highly likely to have a vascular ring. Infants with right aortic arch and cyanotic congenital heart disease usually do not have a vascular ring, because the ductus arteriosus or ligamentum arteriosum inserts anteriorly into the left subclavian artery. Additional confirmatory evidence may be obtained from an esophagogram (Fig. 39–3, 39–4). In the frontal view, bilateral indentation is evident, whereas in the lateral view, the posterior aspect of the esophagus appears to be indented. Invasive studies, such as bronchoscopy and angiography, usually are not required. Digital subtraction angiography and magnetic resonance imaging (MRI) scanning are relatively noninvasive and effective modalities for demonstrating right aortic arch with or without aberrant origin of the left subclavian artery. In cases in which noninvasive studies do not produce a clear diagnosis, cardiac catheterization and cineangiocardiography should be performed.

The treatment is surgical, and symptoms of severe respiratory distress improve immediately after surgery. Stridor, although diminished, may continue for several months or years until the tracheal deformation regresses completely. It is essential that parents be told of the time lag from surgery to the resolution of stridor.

Aberrant right subclavian artery with left aortic arch should be considered in this category because it can produce abnormal esophagographic findings similar to those seen in vascular ring. It occurs in 0.5% of the normal population.[13] These patients are usually asymptomatic. The esophagogram may show posterior indentation on the lateral view. In the frontal view, there is an oblique filling defect that extends upward and to the right. Such patients demonstrate a normal left aortic arch on frontal chest radiographs. If the indentation is caused by a vascular ring, a right aortic arch is likely to be present. Dysphasia occurs occasionally. Surgical repair is rarely indicated.

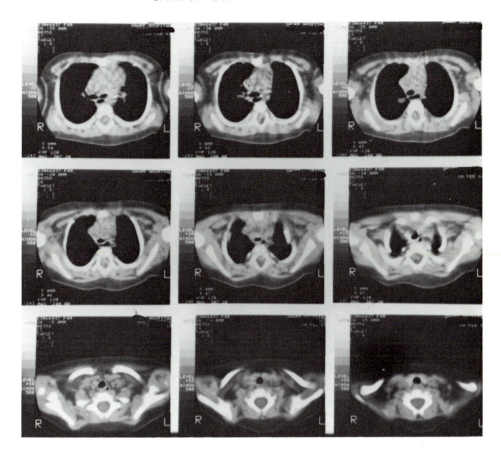

Figure 39–5. Computed tomographic scan of the chest in a 3-month-old female with innominate artery compression syndrome. Note tracheal compression at the midtracheal level. In this disease, the esophagogram is normal.

Anomalous Innominate Artery

In this lesion, the innominate artery arises from the aortic arch far to the left, courses in front of the trachea, and compresses it (Fig. 39–5). In a review of 680 cases of vascular compression of the airway by Desnos and colleagues,[10] the incidence of anomalous innominate artery was 20%. Presenting symptoms may include cough, stridor, and apnea.[12, 14] Of the 10 patients with vascular anomalies reported by Waldman and colleagues,[11] only one patient had apnea as a presenting symptom. Both the chest radiograph and esophagogram are normal. The diagnosis is made by bronchoscopy. An anterior pulsatile compression is demonstrated, and when the pulsatile area is compressed anteriorly by a rigid bronchoscope, the right radial pulse is abolished. Such findings are pathognomonic of this lesion. Three-dimensional MRI scanning is also useful for demonstrating compression of the trachea by the anomalous artery. Surgical treatment consists of aortopexy (tacking the aortic arch and the innominate artery forward to the sternum) and is indicated only in patients with severe symptoms and in those in whom apnea has been demonstrated. Supportive treatment is reserved for patients with mild to moderate symptoms without apnea.

Pulmonary Artery Sling

In this condition, the left pulmonary artery arises aberrantly from the right pulmonary artery, courses around and behind the trachea, and passes in front of the esophagus to enter the left lung[15] (Figs. 39–6 to 39–8). Clinical manifestations include stridor, recurrent respiratory infection, dyspnea, and wheezing. Important diagnostic modalities include esophagography, echocardiography, and bronchography. On esophagograms, an anterior indentation of the esophagus above the carina is visible, whereas on echocardiograms, the left pulmonary artery is seen to arise from the right pulmonary artery. The diagnosis should be confirmed by cineangiocardiography.

Severe respiratory symptoms are the result both of tracheal compression by the anomalously originating left pulmonary artery and of associated tracheobronchial malformations.[16, 17] The most common such malformation is stenotic complete tracheal ring rather than the normal horseshoe-shaped cartilage. Prognosis for this lesion is thus guarded if there are significant associated tracheobronchial abnormalities. Bronchography should be performed preoperatively in order to delineate these malformations. Postoperative respiratory management can be extremely difficult if they are present.

Prognosis

The prognosis for survivors of surgery for vascular ring, anomalous innominate artery, and pulmonary sling is generally good. All 54 patients reported by Marmon and associates[18] had immediate relief of respiratory symptoms after surgical repair of their lesions. Mild respiratory symptoms, however, persisted postoperatively from 3

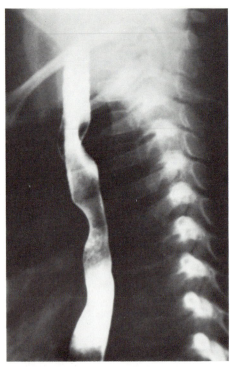

Figure 39–6. Esophagogram in an 11-month-old female with pulmonary artery sling. She also had aberrant subclavian artery *(lateral view)*. Note the anterior indentation of esophagus by pulmonary artery sling and posterior indentation by aberrant subclavian artery. The tracheobronchogram and the pulmonary angiogram are shown in Figures 39–7 and 39–8.

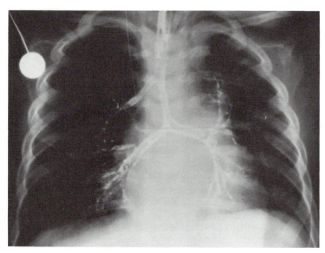

Figure 39–7. Tracheobronchogram in an 11-month-old female who had pulmonary artery sling and moderate tracheal bronchial stenosis. Note the severe narrowing of the distal trachea; the right upper lobe has a separate bronchus coming directly off the trachea. The bronchus that supplies right middle lobe and right lower lobe is also narrowed. The esophagogram and the pulmonary angiogram are shown in Figures 39–6 and 39–8.

months to 4 years. In 47 of 48 patients observed from 6 months to 14 years,[18] all respiratory symptoms completely resolved. Interestingly, nine of 17 patients who underwent pulmonary function testing demonstrated abnormal flow-volume loops, suggesting significant central airway obstruction.

DILATATION OF PULMONARY ARTERY

Massive dilatation of the main or branch pulmonary arteries may compress the distal trachea and right and left main stem bronchi.[2] For such dilatation to occur, there must be a high driving force (pressure) together with significant pulmonic insufficiency. If a connective tissue abnormality involves the main or branch pulmonary arteries, the degree of dilatation may be massive. Such massively dilated branch pulmonary arteries are commonly seen in tetralogy of Fallot with absent pulmonary valve[19, 20] (Fig. 39–9). The clinical picture consists of wheezing, air trapping, chest retractions, and dyspnea, which may be indistinguishable from the clinical picture of primary obstructive lung disease such as bronchiolitis and bronchial asthma. The presence of central cyanosis, overactive precordium, and a characteristic to-and-fro murmur that sounds like sawing wood suggest the diagnosis. Two-dimensional echocardiography may be used to make the definitive diagnosis both noninvasively and rapidly.

When patients first exhibit severe airway obstruction in early infancy, the pulmonary arteries are already markedly dilated and the prognosis is guarded. Those who present initially in later childhood usually can be managed medically. If respiratory failure cannot be managed, total surgical repair with the use of a valve prosthesis in the pulmonic position should be attempted. The presence of a pulmonary valve may halt further distention of the pulmonary arteries by limiting the stroke volume ejected into the pulmonary bed. Valve replacement in very small infants may be technically difficult because of the absence of readily available small-diameter valves. In older patients with massive dilatation of the branch pulmonary arteries, internal plication of the proximal pulmonary

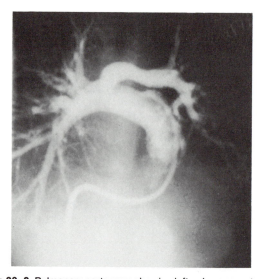

Figure 39–8. Pulmonary aortogram showing left pulmonary artery originating abnormally from far to the right and going behind trachea and in front of esophagus in an 11-month-old female with pulmonary artery sling. The esophagogram and the tracheobronchogram are shown in Figures 39–6 and 39–7.

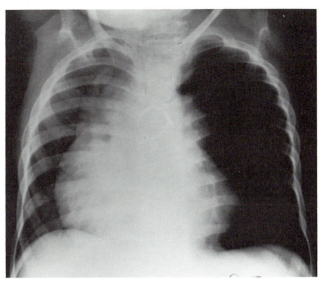

Figure 39–9. A frontal view of a chest showing hyperinflation of the left lung as a result of a distended pulmonary artery's compressing the left main stem bronchus in a 4-year-old female with tetralogy of Fallot and absent pulmonic valve. The left lung is very hyperinflated, and an artificial cardiac valve is visible.

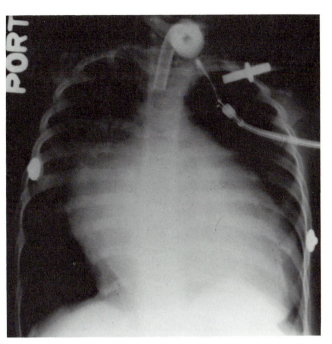

Figure 39–10. Anteroposterior chest radiographic view showing a gigantic left atrium in a 22-month-old female with congenital mitral regurgitation that is compressing main stem bronchi. Right lower lobe is hyperinflated, and right upper lobe is atelectatic. Left upper lobe is also hyperinflated. The patient could not be weaned off a ventilator.

arterial system has been successfully performed with the use of conduit material sewn inside the pulmonary arteries in association with a homograft pulmonary valve.

In the postoperative period, it is essential to maintain normal or increased systemic arterial oxygen tension and normal or low carbon dioxide tension. This prevents pulmonary arterial constriction and subsequent hypertension, which will in turn augment the pulmonary artery distension and result in further obstruction to the airways.

ENLARGED LEFT ATRIUM

Any cardiac lesion that results in a volume-pressure load on the left atrium will result in left atrium enlargement. Because the left atrium sits close to the inferior aspect of the main stem bronchi, variable degrees of compression of the structure result.[2] Cardiac lesions resulting in left atrium enlargement are mitral valve disease (Fig. 39–10) and large left-to-right shunt.

RESPIRATORY DYSFUNCTION FROM CHRONIC HYPOXEMIA AND REDUCED PULMONARY BLOOD FLOW

Children with cyanotic congenital heart disease associated with reduced pulmonary blood flow may have a blunted hypoxic respiratory drive. Blesa and co-workers[21] studied eight children aged 7 to 16 years with cyanotic congenital heart disease and with arterial oxygen saturation varying from 55% to 80%. The ventilatory response to acute hypoxia was subnormal. Such patients may not show the usual clinical findings such as tachypnea and chest retractions when their oxygenation is worsened by respiratory infections or other causes. They therefore need to be closely monitored during such events.

SUMMARY

In summary, the heart and lungs are intimately related both anatomically and physiologically. Blood must enter the lungs under low pressure and exit unimpeded for pulmonary function to be normal. Significant respiratory distress results from (1) lesions that produce increased pulmonary blood flow associated with increased driving pressure, (2) lesions that impede pulmonary venous return to the left side of the heart, (3) lesions that compress the large airways, and (4) lesions that are associated with reduced pulmonary blood flow and chronic systemic hypoxemia. The clinician should be aware of these mechanisms when attempting to treat patients who exhibit significant respiratory dysfunction if they have a history or physical findings of congenital heart disease. Most of the cardiac conditions discussed here either are curable or can be palliated surgically if the correct diagnosis is made in a timely manner.

REFERENCES

1. Murray J: The lungs and heart failure. Hosp Pract, pp. 55–68, May 1985.
2. Stanger P, Lucas R, Edwards J: Anatomic factors causing respiratory distress in acyanotic congenital cardiac disease. Pediatrics 43:760–768, 1969.
3. Bancalari E, Jesse M, Gelband H, Garcia O: Lung mechanics in congenital heart disease with increased and decreased pulmonary blood flow. J Pediatr 90:192–195, 1977.
4. Hordof A, Mellins R, Gersony W, Steeg C: Reversibility of chronic obstructive lung disease in infants following repair of ventricular septal defect. J Pediatr 90:187–191, 1977.
5. Oh SK, Park SC, Galvis AG, et al: Pulmonary hyperinflation in ventricular septal defect. J Thorac Cardiovasc Surg 76:706–709, 1978.

6. Markowitz R, Johnson K, Weinstein E: Hyperinflation of the lungs in infants with large left-to-right shunts. Invest Radiol 23:354–358, 1988.
7. MacDonald N, Hall C, Suffin S, et al: Respiratory syncytial viral infection in infants with congenital heart disease. N Engl J Med 307:397–400, 1982.
8. Heard G, Lamberti J, Park S, et al: Early extubation after surgical repair of congenital heart disease. Crit Care Med 13:830–832, 1985.
9. Bush A, Busst C, Haworth S, et al: Correlations of lung morphology, pulmonary vascular resistance, and outcome in children with congenital heart disease. Br Heart J 59:480–485, 1988.
10. Desnos J, Andrieu-Guitrancourt J, Dehesdin D, Dubin J: Vascular strictures of the respiratory tract in children. Int J Pediatr Otorhinolaryngol 2:269–285, 1980.
11. Waldman JD, Meltzer E, Miller K, et al: Vascular compression of the upper airway in children. West J Med 132:209–218, 1980.
12. Fearon B, Shortreed R: Tracheobronchial compression by congenital cardiovascular anomalies in children. Ann Otolaryngol 72:949–969, 1963.
13. Klenkhaimer SC: Esophagography in Anomalies of the Aortic Arch System. Baltimore: Williams & Wilkins, 1969.
14. Ardito J, Tucker G, Ossoff R, DeLeon S: Innominate artery compression of the trachea in infants with reflex apnea. Ann Otolaryngol 89:401–405, 1980.
15. Sade R, Rosenthal A, Fellows K, Castaneda A: Pulmonary artery sling. J Thorac Cardiovasc Surg 69:333–346, 1975.
16. Cohen S, Landing B: Tracheostenosis and bronchial abnormalities associated with pulmonary artery sling. Ann Otolaryngol 85:582–590, 1976.
17. Berdon W, Baker D, Wung JT, et al: Complete cartilage-ring tracheal stenosis associated with anomalous left pulmonary artery: The ring-sling complex. Pediatr Radiol 152:57–64, 1984.
18. Marmon L, Bye M, Haas J, et al: Vascular rings and slings: Long-term follow-up of pulmonary functions. J Pediatr Surg 19:683–692, 1984.
19. Lakier J, Stanger P, Heymann M, et al: Tetralogy of Fallot with absent pulmonary valve. Circulation 50:167–174, 1974.
20. Pinsky W, Nihill M, Mullins C, et al: The absent pulmonary valve syndrome. Circulation 57:159–162, 1978.
21. Blesa M, Lahiri S, Rashkind W, Fishman A: Normalization of the blunted ventilatory response to acute hypoxia in congenital cyanotic heart disease. J Med 296:237–296, 1977.

40 PULMONARY INVOLVEMENT IN COLLAGEN VASCULAR DISORDERS

SUSAN MILLARD, M.D. / LAIRTON VALENTIM, M.D. / RONI GRAD, M.D. / RICHARD J. LEMEN, M.D.

Collagen vascular diseases are chronic inflammatory disorders of unknown etiology. The inflammatory processes are similar to the normal response to foreign material; however, the specific antigenic triggers and the factors responsible for the ongoing response amplification are not known. Classification of these disorders is often difficult because many of these diseases share common features. Current hypotheses suggest that unknown antigens stimulate immune responses similar to the classic Coombs and Gell types I, II, III, and IV inflammatory responses.[1] Tissue damage during inflammatory processes results from the release of degradative lysosomal enzymes by inflammatory cells. These enzymes include the hydrolases, collagenases, neutral proteases, elastase, and cathepsin B. Degradative enzymes play an important role in the tissue-destructive changes observed in collagen vascular disorders and in the amplification of the inflammatory response. Tissue fibrosis results from the repair process after acute tissue inflammation.

In this chapter, the pulmonary complications of collagen vascular disorders are reviewed. The lung seems, at least in theory, to be vulnerable to the effects of the collagen vascular diseases. This vulnerability may result from the rich vascular supply of the lung and exposure of the lung to the entire cardiac output, with all of its circulating mediators. Very little is known about the lung involvement in childhood collagen vascular diseases. Pulmonary involvement appears to differ among specific syndromes; however, sporadic evidence from the literature suggests that all types of lung involvement may be seen in adults.

JUVENILE RHEUMATOID ARTHRITIS

Juvenile rheumatoid arthritis (JRA) is a common pediatric collagen vascular disorder. Three major varieties of this disorder are seen: Still's disease (a systemic disorder), polyarticular disease, and pauciarticular disease. Patients may have a genetic predisposition to JRA. The pathologic processes may be mediated by immune complexes. Unknown triggers stimulate the production of immunoglobulin G (IgG) and immunoglobulin M (IgM) directed against IgG (rheumatoid factor), forming immune complexes. These immune complexes activate synovial fluid complement, resulting in the chemotaxis of inflammatory cells. Rheumatoid arthritis cells develop, and various mediators (hydrolases, histamine, and fibrinogen) are released, amplifying the inflammatory response and leading to tissue damage.

Pleuropulmonary involvement is uncommon in children with JRA. If present, it is usually diagnosed in patients with systemic-onset JRA. Pneumonitis and pleuritis may be the presenting manifestations of this form of JRA. Pleural disease is occasionally noted as an incidental finding on chest radiographs in patients without respiratory symptoms. Cough, chest pain, dyspnea, and tachypnea are frequently experienced by children with pulmonary or pleural involvement.[2] Occasionally patients present with or acquire interstitial lung disease, pulmonary amyloidosis, recurrent pneumonitis, and pulmonary hemosiderosis. Evidence of airway involvement may be present. Patients with carditis may experience respiratory distress secondary to congestive heart failure. Sternoclavicular joint disease and thoracolumbar spine disease may contribute to the development of restrictive disease.

Radiographic findings are variable. Normal radiographs are frequently seen, even in the presence of abnormal pulmonary function studies. Abnormal findings may include solitary nodules, focal pneumonitis, diffuse interstitial disease, and pleural or pericardial effusions. In addition, pleural granulomas may be present.

Pulmonary function tests (PFTs) indicate restrictive and obstructive disease, as illustrated in Figure 40–1. Wagener and co-workers studied 18 children (ages 6–18 years) with JRA.[3] Six patients had normal PFT results. Two thirds of patients with polyarticular disease and one half of those with pauciarticular disease had abnormal pulmonary function. Seven of 15 patients had low carbon monoxide–diffusing lung capacity. Only one patient had an abnormal resting oxygen saturation, and only one had a significant change in diffusing capacity after exercise. Instead of the typical increase in oxygen saturation with exercise, two patients had a decreased arterial oxygen saturation (Sa_{O_2}) after adequate exercise. Results of physiologic tests are not correlated with clinical well-being or with radiographic findings.

Laboratory findings may be difficult to use in the definitive diagnosis of JRA. Leukocytosis and left shifts are present, and total white blood cell counts are usually between 15,000 and 35,000. The white blood cell count is made up primarily of neutrophils. The erythrocyte sedimentation rate is nonspecifically elevated. Rheumatoid factor is rarely found in JRA children, except in the polyarticular form. If present, systemic lupus erythematosus (SLE) should be suspected. Similarly, high titers of antinuclear antibody (ANA) and anti-DNA antibody should raise suspicion of SLE.

Treatment is aimed at suppression of the underlying inflammatory disease and includes acetylsalicylic acid and other nonsteroidal anti-inflammatory agents, corticosteroids, methotrexate, gold, and penicillamine. Fever in a patient with JRA may be suggestive of infection, especially if it occurs in conjunction with new pulmonary findings. The evaluation of fever should include cultures of sputum or bronchoalveolar lavage fluid. If a pleural

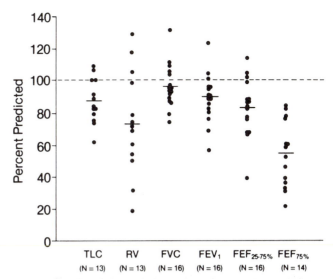

Figure 40–1. Restrictive and obstructive pulmonary disease indicated by pulmonary function tests. TLC, total lung capacity; RV, residual volume; FVC, forced vital capacity; FEV_1, forced expiratory volume in 1 sec; FEF_{25-75}, maximum midexpiratory flow; FEF_{75}, forced expiratory flow at 75% in patients with juvenile rheumatoid arthritis (JRA). Bars designate the mean for patients with JRA. (From Wagener JS, Taussig LM, Debenedetti C, et al: Pulmonary function in juvenile rheumatoid arthritis. J Pediatr 99:108–110, 1981.)

effusion is present, the pleural fluid should also be examined before the institution of, or increase in, anti-inflammatory therapy.

POLYARTERITIS NODOSA AND OTHER VASCULITIDES

Vasculitic syndromes are seen in childhood and include polyarteritis nodosa, Wegener's granulomatosis, Takayasu's arteritis, Churg-Strauss syndrome, and Henoch-Schönlein purpura. Inflammation and necrosis of the blood vessels are features of vasculitic syndromes. The cause of these disorders is unknown. This section focuses on polyarteritis nodosa, Wegener's granulomatosis, and Churg-Strauss syndrome.

Polyarteritis Nodosa. Polyarteritis nodosa is a vasculitic syndrome that involves the muscular arteries of multiple organs.[4] Thrombosis and segmental necrosis of blood vessels are seen most commonly in the kidneys, heart, and lungs. The gastrointestinal tract, liver, pancreas, muscles, epididymal ducts, skin, and brain may also be involved. A hypersensitivity response to an unknown antigenic trigger may be the basis of the pathophysiologic processes. Remote infections and drug exposures have been implicated in the pathogenesis of this disease.

Polyarteritis nodosa is uncommon in infants and children. There are two manifestations of the disease: the infantile form and the adult form. The infantile disease usually manifests with signs and symptoms suggestive of viral illness with fever, maculopapular erythema, erythema multiforme, or urticaria. Pulmonary disease is rare in infantile polyarteritis; there have been only scattered, isolated case reports. In the adult variety, many patients show evidence of pulmonary disease. Pulmonary edema of cardiac or renal origin is frequently seen in the adult population.

Wegener's Granulomatosis. Wegener's granulomatosis is characterized by a widespread necrotizing granulomatous vasculitis involving arteries and veins.[5] Wegener's granulomatosis may be present in infants as young as 3 months but is most commonly seen in young adults. Common findings are nasal and sinus discomfort; clear rhinorrhea progressing to brownish, purulent, and foul-smelling nasal discharge; epistaxis; and nasal mucosal ulceration. Fever, anorexia, malaise, and weight loss also are frequently seen. Other presenting signs include arthritis, skin ulcerations, serous otitis, conjunctivitis, corneal ulcerations, and hepatitis. The majority of patients exhibit renal involvement and hypertension.

Pulmonary involvement is commonly seen in Wegener's granulomatosis.[6] Patients may have fever, cough, chest pain, or hemoptysis. Subglottic and upper tracheal narrowing occur and are associated with nasal disease. These findings may be evident as a fixed extrathoracic or intrathoracic obstructive appearance on a flow-volume loop. Multiple or solitary nodular densities or infiltrates, varying in size from 0.5 to 10 cm and with vaguely or sharply demarcated borders, are seen on chest radiographs. The lesions may be bilateral and cavitary, with atelectasis, alveolar hemorrhage and hemoptysis, pleural effusions, mediastinal lymph node enlargement, and calcification of the lesion.

Churg-Strauss Syndrome. Churg-Strauss syndrome is actually a variant of polyarteritis nodosa. In this disease, small arteries are affected, and vascular and extravascular necrotizing granulomas are found.[7] The patient exhibits marked eosinophilia and reactive airway disease. Large doses of corticosteroids are used in the treatment, but cytotoxic agents may be necessary.

Prognosis. The long-term prognosis for children with polyarteritis nodosa and Wegener's granulomatosis is poor. Death is caused by renal failure, cardiac failure, or severe gastrointestinal or central nervous system disease. Corticosteroids and immunosuppressive agents may improve prognosis in polyarteritis nodosa, but in Wegener's granulomatosis, corticosteroid therapy is usually unsuccessful. Cytotoxic agents such as cyclophosphamide and chlorambucil are often chosen in the treatment of Wegener's granulomatosis.

SYSTEMIC LUPUS ERYTHEMATOSUS

SLE is a multisystem, chronic inflammatory disease of unknown cause. Multiple autoantibodies that participate in tissue damage are present. Genetic and immune defects, cell-surface antigenic abnormalities, and hormonal influences may also be involved. Patients may acquire this disease at any age. The most common problems are a skin rash, often located on the face in a butterfly conformation, and arthritis. Multiple organs are usually affected. For example, the patient may exhibit thrombocytopenia, conjunctivitis, ascites, pericarditis, and seizures.

Fifty to seventy percent of adults and children with SLE

Table 40–1. PULMONARY LESIONS IN SYSTEMIC LUPUS ERYTHEMATOSUS

Interstitial pneumonitis
Acute pneumonia
Vascular lesions (e.g., thromboemboli)
Pleural effusion
Pleural fibrosis
Hemorrhage
Pulmonary edema
Hyaline membranes
Alveolitis obliterans
Bronchiolitis obliterans
Pulmonary interstitial fibrosis
Alveolar overinflation
Alveolar septal calcinosis
Diaphragmatic lesions

have pulmonary involvement.[8] Pulmonary lesions are numerous in SLE, as shown in Table 40–1. Interstitial pneumonitis, atelectasis, pleuritis with effusions, bronchopneumonia, pulmonary edema, hemosiderosis, and alveolar hemorrhage are examples of pulmonary abnormalities.[9]

It is often difficult to establish the diagnosis of a specific pulmonary disease in patients with SLE because of the many potential causes. In addition, patients without clinical or radiographic evidence may have pulmonary function abnormalities. The diffusing capacity for carbon monoxide may be abnormal, and restrictive or obstructive disease is also seen on pulmonary function testing.[10] About 50% of the patients have distal airway disease, including obliterative bronchiolitis, bronchiolar dilatation, and focal panacinar emphysema.

Figure 40–2 is a chest radiograph of a patient with SLE and pulmonary disease. Four types of clinical patterns may have associated radiographic findings: (1) episodic pleurisy with effusions but normal lung fields; (2) pleuropericarditis with an elevated or thickened hemidiaphragm; (3) frequent attacks of either episodic, recurrent pleurisy or pleuropericarditis (as previously described) with persistent or progressive dyspnea; and (4) fibrosing alveolitis.

The pulmonary involvement in childhood may follow any of three patterns: (1) mild to moderate progressive impairment in pulmonary function without clinical symptoms or significant radiographic changes; (2) slow progression of pulmonary symptoms with radiographic changes; and (3) rapid onset of severe pulmonary distress and chronic interstitial pneumonitis.

Pulmonary failure is a common cause of death. Secondary infections may occur because of bacteria, fungi, or viruses. Examples are *Candida albicans, Aspergillus* species, cytomegalovirus, *Pneumocystis carinii, Klebsiella/Aerobacter* species, *Escherichia coli,* alpha-hemolytic streptococcus, and *Staphylococcus epidermidis.* Diagnostic workup for infectious diseases is indicated in patients with SLE and pulmonary infiltrates.

Management depends on the pulmonary diagnosis. For example, lupus pneumonitis develops when SLE is not under control; the symptoms are dyspnea and chest pain. These symptoms may also occur, however, in a patient with an infected pleural effusion or an opportunistic

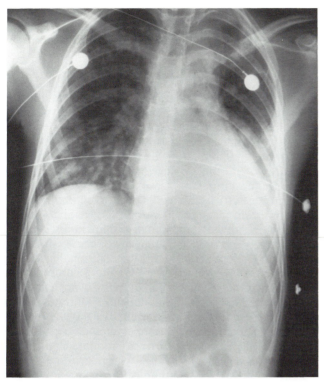

Figure 40-2. Chest radiograph showing a diffuse opacity in the left base, indicative of a pleural effusion. The pulmonary vascular pattern is mildly prominent. A pericardial drainage catheter is in place on the left side; it had been used to drain a pericardial effusion.

pneumonia. Serum complement levels and ANA titers are used to observe change in the disease activity. Sputum culture, thoracentesis, bronchoalveolar lavage, and lung biopsy may be performed to look for an infectious cause. Therapy is then based on the results and the clinical course of the patient. Treatment of SLE, in general, involves the use of corticosteroids and immunosuppressive agents such as cyclophosphamide, azathioprine, and chlorambucil.

MIXED CONNECTIVE TISSUE DISEASE

Mixed connective tissue disease (MCTD) has features of many collagen vascular disorders but is now considered a separate entity. The cause is unknown, although antibody and complement deposition in affected organs may play a role. MCTD manifests with nonspecific symptoms such as fever, lymphadenopathy, and hepatosplenomegaly. Polyarteritis, skin rashes, Raynaud's phenomenon, dysphagia, and muscle weakness may also occur. Cardiac, neurologic, and renal involvement may be present as well.

Antibodies for DNA and extractable nuclear antigen are seen in MCTD. Other abnormal laboratory findings include the presence of rheumatoid factor, leukopenia, lymphopenia, thrombocytopenia, anemia, and elevated muscle enzymes.

Pulmonary involvement is more common in adults than in children with MCTD. Common pulmonary abnormalities are diffuse interstitial lung disease, pleural effusions, and pulmonary hypertension.[11] A restrictive

pattern is a common pulmonary function finding. A decreased carbon monoxide–diffusing capacity, hypoxemia, and respiratory alkalosis are also seen. Several different chest radiographic findings may be observed and include a normal lung field with a prominent hilum, pleural effusions, bibasilar infiltrates, and a diffuse reticular nodular pattern. Pulmonary hypertension is frequently present and is associated with proliferative changes and thrombus formation in the pulmonary vascular bed. In addition, esophageal dysfunction may lead to the development of aspiration pneumonitis. Myocarditis and congestive heart failure lead to the development of pulmonary edema.

Arthritis is treated with nonsteroidal anti-inflammatory agents, and corticosteroids are used for treatment of dermal lesions. The systemic efficacy of corticosteroids has not been established, but steroids may be effective for the lung involvement.

DERMATOMYOSITIS

Polymyositis is characterized by inflammation and degeneration of skeletal muscle. A subgroup of patients with polymyositis have evidence of dermal and systemic involvement, a syndrome called *dermatomyositis.* Abnormalities in antibody production and cell-mediated immunity may be present; antimyosin antibodies, as well as vascular deposition of IgG, IgM, and C3 and sensitization of peripheral blood lymphocytes to muscle tissue, have been demonstrated in some affected patients. A viral cause has been suggested by the demonstration of Coxsackie virus in some patients.

The onset is insidious; proximal muscle weakness is the usual chief complaint in all age groups. Dermatologic manifestations are peripheral edema, a heliotrope rash, and a scaly dermatitis over the joints. Subcutaneous or periarticular calcification occurs as an end result of active disease. Palatal weakness, dysphagia, abdominal pain, small bowel hypomotility, cardiac arrythmias, and heart block have been reported. Generalized edema and ascites have been observed in the absence of renal involvement.

Diffuse pulmonary fibrosis is a well-documented complication, especially among adult patients.[12] The clinical onset of pulmonary disease may be acute with fever, dyspnea, and cough. Lower lobe crackles are commonly found on physical examination. Interstitial lung disease is another problem that is more frequent than previously reported.[13] Patients have dyspnea and cough. Bilateral diffuse nodular, reticulonodular, or irregularly shaped shadows are present on chest radiographs. Response to corticosteroid therapy is poor.

Other radiographic findings in dermatomyositis include patchy alveolar infiltrates, spontaneous pneumothorax, pneumomediastinum, and diminished lung volumes. PFTs typically reveal a restrictive defect. Lung disease also is caused by thoracic muscle weakness and poor mucociliary clearance, resulting in aspiration pneumonitis and hypoventilation.

Patients with active muscle disease usually improve with aggressive corticosteroid therapy. During this acute phase, many have respiratory and swallowing difficulties;

close observation for the development of pneumonia and respiratory failure is warranted.

KAWASAKI'S DISEASE

Kawasaki's disease, or mucocutaneous lymph node syndrome, is an acute febrile illness usually occurring in children younger than 4 years.[14] There are six principal symptoms: fever lasting at least 5 days; reddening of the palms and soles, followed by fingertip desquamation; rash; bilateral conjunctival congestion; cervical lymphadenopathy; and a strawberry tongue with reddened lips. Patients may have other problems such as arthralgias, encephalopathy, abdominal pain, and jaundice. Cardiac involvement is the most worrisome potential problem in children with Kawasaki's disease. The coronary arteries may dilate acutely, and aneurysms may develop. Valvular regurgitation, pericarditis, myocarditis, and myocardial infarction also occur in these patients. The most common cause of death is acute myocardial infarction, but pneumonia, respiratory failure, and lung hemorrhage are other reported causes of death. Pulmonary disease is not a commonly reported problem in Kawasaki's disease. Umezawa and colleagues reported that abnormal chest radiographs were found in 14.7% of the 129 patients they studied.[15] Reticulogranular patterns were the most frequent finding. Peribronchial cuffing, pleural effusion, atelectasis, and air trapping were also seen. It is possible that lower respiratory tract inflammation and pulmonary arteritis are the causes of respiratory disease.

Aspirin and intravenous gammaglobulin are therapies for Kawasaki's disease. Research protocols are under way for minimizing morbidity and mortality through the development of the most effective regimen.

BEHÇET'S SYNDROME

Behçet's syndrome is a multisystem disease but is typically diagnosed because of three problems: relapsing iridocyclitis, recurrent genital ulcerations, and recurrent oral ulcerations. Arthritis, thrombophlebitis migrans, and arterial aneurysms are examples of systemic complications. Adults are most commonly affected, but a minority of patients may have evidence of the disease before 18 years of age.[16] Pulmonary disease is not a prevalent problem. Raz and associates studied 72 patients with Behçet's syndrome, and only seven had pulmonary vascular involvement.[17] Massive hemoptysis and pulmonary hemorrhage are potential life-threatening events. Diffuse infiltration is the most common finding on chest radiographs. There is no specific therapy for these rare pulmonary complications.

SJÖGREN'S SYNDROME

Sjögren's syndrome is a chronic inflammatory disease resulting in decreased lacrimal and salivary gland secretion. Keratoconjunctivitis sicca and xerostomia result from the diminished secretions. Sjögren's syndrome is rare in childhood. Middle-aged women are most frequently affected.

Histologic features consist primarily of infiltrations of the parotid and lacrimal glands by mature-appearing T and B lymphocytes. Acinar atrophy develops with lymphoid replacement. A similar process involves glands in the gastrointestinal and respiratory tracts, and glandular hyposecretion in the tracheobronchial tree results in poor mucociliary drainage and secondary infection.

Salivary insufficiency results in difficulty chewing, swallowing, and phonating. Ulcers of the mucous membranes, lips, and tongue develop, as does dental caries. Dryness of the nasopharynx leads to epistaxis, hoarseness, and recurrent otitis. Raynaud's phenomenon is present, and nonthrombocytopenic purpura develops, usually accompanied by hypergammaglobulinemia. Hepatosplenomegaly, chronic active hepatitis, acute pancreatic disease, and gastric achlorhydria are additional findings.

Cough, dyspnea, and pleuritic pain are common primary complaints.[18] Chest radiographs do not exhibit a particular pattern, but diffuse interstitial infiltrates are the most common feature. Pleural effusions are also seen. Pulmonary function abnormalities include a restrictive defect and a diminished carbon monoxide–diffusing capacity. On pathologic studies, lymphocytic interstitial pneumonitis, pseudolymphoma, bronchopneumonia, malignant lymphoma, and diffuse interstitial pulmonary fibrosis may be diagnosed.

Treatment is symptomatic. Humidifying agents, such as 0.5% methylcellulose, are used to moisten mucous membranes. Steroids and immunosuppressive agents may be helpful.

PROGRESSIVE SYSTEMIC SCLEROSIS (SCLERODERMA)

Progressive systemic sclerosis is a generalized connective tissue disease with vascular lesions in the internal organs. Presenting symptoms include gradual swelling of the distal portions of the extremities, joint pain or stiffness, and thickening of the skin. The disease may begin at any time during childhood, and the clinical course is similar to that in adulthood. There is slow but progressive internal organ involvement. The heart, intestines, kidneys, and lungs are involved. Extensive fibrosis with connective tissue hyperplasia is the typical histologic finding.

The respiratory system is frequently affected by this disease. Lung disease is also a common cause of death.[19] Dyspnea is the most common respiratory complaint. Cough is not a typical complaint. Impairment of carbon monoxide–diffusing capacity is the earliest pulmonary function abnormality, even without evidence of clinical pulmonary disease.[20] The vital capacity is usually reduced. Obstructive lung disease may be seen late in the course of the disease. Chest radiographs reveal linear or nodular densities, which are usually more prominent in the lower lung fields. A diffuse fibrosis is seen in about one fourth of patients. Three scenarios are described when the pulmonary involvement of this disease is discussed: (1) lung fibrosis with obliteration of the vascular bed and cor pulmonale, (2) a combination of pulmonary parenchymal and vascular lesions, and (3) predominant vascular disease with right ventricular failure.

Many therapeutic regimens have been used for this disease without obvious benefit. The pulmonary involvement also has no specific treatment. D-penicillamine may be a potential drug for the pulmonary and skin disorders, but more studies need to be performed.

CONCLUSION

Overall, collagen vascular diseases in children are not common. When pulmonary involvement is present, restrictive lung disease and a lowered carbon monoxide-diffusing capacity are usually present. Often the patient may not have pulmonary symptoms or abnormal chest radiographs but may have abnormal responses on PFTs. Pulmonary complications are severe in some patients, and morbidity and mortality rates may be high. Because of the scarcity of patients at single medical centers and the absence of animal models, very little research (focusing on effective therapies, causes, and mechanisms of injury) has been performed. It is hoped that clinicians and researchers will provide new insights into these diseases in the near future.

REFERENCES

1. Coombs RR, Gell PG: The classification of allergic reactions of underlying disease. *In* Gell RG, Coombs RR (eds): Clinical Aspects of Immunology, pp. 317–337. Philadelphia: FA Davis 1968.
2. Athreya BH, Doughty RA, Bookspan M, et al: Pulmonary manifestations of juvenile rheumatoid arthritis: A report of eight cases and review. Clin Chest Med 1:361–374, 1980.
3. Wagener JS, Taussig LM, Debenedetti C, et al: Pulmonary function in juvenile rheumatoid arthritis. J Pediatr 99:108–110, 1981.
4. Amman AJ, Wara DW: Collagen vascular diseases (rheumatic diseases). *In* Rudolph AM, Hoffman JIE (eds): Pediatrics, 18th ed, p. 423. Norwalk, CT: Appleton & Lange, 1987.
5. Warren J, Pitchenik AE, Saldana MJ: Granulomatous vasculitides of the lung: A clinicopathologic approach to diagnosis and treatment. South Med J 82:481–491, 1989.
6. Cordier JF, Valeyre D, Guillevin L, et al: Pulmonary Wegener's granulomatosis: A clinical and imaging study of 77 cases. Chest 97:906–912, 1990.
7. Carrol JC, Taussig LM: Pulmonary disorders. *In* Stiehm ER (ed): Immunologic Disorders in Infants and Children, 3rd ed, p. 483. Philadelphia: WB Saunders, 1989.
8. Carrol JC, Taussig LM: Pulmonary disorders. *In* Stiehm ER (ed): Immunologic Disorders in Infants and Children, 3rd ed, pp. 488–489. Philadelphia: WB Saunders, 1989.
9. Eichacker PQ, Pinsker K, Epstein A, et al: Serial pulmonary function testing in patients with systemic lupus erythematosus. Chest 94:129–132, 1988.
10. Singsen BM, Platzker ACG: Pulmonary involvement in the rheumatic disorders of childhood. *In* Chernick V, Kendig EL (eds): Disorders of the respiratory tract in children, 5th ed, pp. 892–894. Philadelphia: WB Saunders, 1990.
11. Prakash UBS: Pulmonary manifestations in mixed connective tissue disease. Semin Respir Med 9:318–324, 1988.
12. Singsen BM, Platzker ACG: Pulmonary involvement in the rheumatic disorders of childhood. *In* Chernick V, Kendig EL (eds): Disorders of the Respiratory Tract in Children, 5th ed, pp. 901–903. Philadelphia: WB Saunders, 1990.
13. Takizawa H, Shiga J, Moroi Y, et al: Interstitial lung disease in dermatomyositis: Clinicopathological study. J Rheumatol 14:102–107, 1987.
14. Kato H, Inoue O, Akagi T: Kawasaki disease: Cardiac problems and management. Pediatr Rev 9:209–217, 1988.
15. Umezawa T, Saji T, Matsuo N, Odagiri K: Chest x-ray findings in the acute phase of Kawasaki disease. Pediatr Radiol 20:48–51, 1989.
16. Singsen BM, Platzker ACG: Pulmonary involvement in the rheumatic disorders of childhood. *In* Chernick V (ed): Kendig's Disorders of the Respiratory Tract in Children, 5th ed, p. 907. Philadelphia: WB Saunders, 1990.
17. Raz I, Okon E, Chajek-Shaul T: Pulmonary manifestations in Behçet's syndrome. Chest 95:585–589, 1989.
18. Strimlan CV, Rosenow EC, Divertie MB, Harrison EG: Pulmonary manifestations of Sjögren's syndrome. Chest 70:354–361, 1976.
19. Singsen BM, Platzker ACG: Pulmonary involvement in the rheumatic disorders of childhood. *In* Chernick V, Kendig EL (eds): Disorders of the Respiratory Tract in Children, 5th ed, pp. 898–901. Philadelphia: WB Saunders, 1990.
20. DeMuth GR, Furstenberg NA, Dabich L, et al: Pulmonary manifestations of progressive systemic sclerosis. Am J Med Sci 255:94–104, 1968.

41 PULMONARY HYPERTENSION AND COR PULMONALE IN CHILDREN

GREGORY J. REDDING, M.D.

Pulmonary hypertension is a condition resulting from altered mechanical properties of the pulmonary vascular bed that increase pulmonary vascular resistance and impedance to blood flow through the lungs. The major consequence of this condition is increased afterload on the right ventricle and increased right ventricular work, leading to the structural and functional changes that characterize cor pulmonale. Although the cardiac features of cor pulmonale are associated with certain congenital right heart diseases, the term *cor pulmonale* refers only to car-

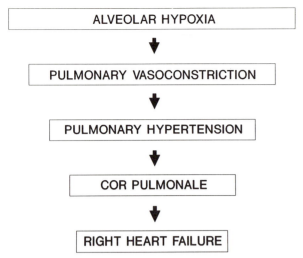

Figure 41–1. A small proportion of patients acquire pulmonary hypertension, and an even smaller proportion acquire right heart failure in comparison with patients with alveolar hypoxia.

diac changes resulting from pulmonary conditions. Causes of pulmonary hypertension that result from primary right or left heart abnormalities are, therefore, not discussed in detail.

The incidence of pulmonary hypertension among children is not known. Hemodynamic measurements have been made in few normal children invasively by right heart catheterization techniques. In contrast, investigators in multiple studies have measured pulmonary hemodynamic indexes within populations of children with various cardiopulmonary diseases. Examples of diseases in childhood in which pulmonary hypertension is likely to occur include congenital heart diseases with left-to-right shunts, chronic obstructive lung diseases such as cystic fibrosis and bronchopulmonary dysplasia, and interstitial lung diseases.[1-5]

The correlations among abnormal lung function, the severity of pulmonary hypertension, and cor pulmonale are only approximate and are not necessarily predictive of an individual's hemodynamic response to lung disease. For example, patients with primary pulmonary vasculitis have mild hypoxemia and minimal spirometric abnormalities despite significant pulmonary hypertension. Conversely, not everyone with alveolar hypoxia acquires pulmonary vasoconstriction, nor does everyone with pulmonary hypertension acquire cor pulmonale. Figure 41–1 illustrates this schematically for hypoxia-induced pulmonary hypertension. Experimental studies suggest that 10% or more of infant and adult animals have a minimal vasoconstrictive response to 12% inspired oxygen.[6] Whether this tendency is genetically determined in humans is unknown. Not all children whose pulmonary vessels vasoconstrict vigorously in response to hypoxia acquire the cardiac compensatory characteristics of cor pulmonale. Finally, not all children with cor pulmonale have clinical signs of right heart failure.

This chapter focuses on the pathogenic mechanisms producing pulmonary hypertension, its clinical and diagnostic features, and its treatment in children. When pediatric information is scant, literature involving pulmonary vascular features of adult humans or young animals is addressed in an effort to extrapolate data for the pediatric patients.

PATHOGENESIS AND PATHOPHYSIOLOGY OF PULMONARY HYPERTENSION

Multiple pathophysiologic mechanisms produce pulmonary hypertension at different sites in the pulmonary vascular bed. For conceptual purposes, the pulmonary vasculature can be divided into precapillary, capillary, and postcapillary compartments (Fig. 41–2). The arteries and arterioles, representing the precapillary compartment, can constrict, remodel into thick indistensible conduits, or become compressed. All of these processes lead to narrowing of the vessel lumen and, hence, increased resistance to blood flow. Compression by alveolar overdistension, atelectasis, or perivascular edema is the most common mechanism affecting pulmonary capillaries, which in turn increases pulmonary arterial pressure (Ppa). The postcapillary compartment, made up of venules and veins, may remodel, constrict, or become compressed as ways of producing pulmonary hypertension in the pulmonary arteries. Precapillary, capillary, and postcapillary compartments can all become occluded by emboli or thrombi as a result of coagulation activation, endothelial cell injury, polycythemia, or locally reduced pulmonary blood flow. Vessel obliteration resulting from progressive narrowing, perivascular inflammation, and pulmonary fibrosis can also involve all of these compartments, thereby producing pulmonary hypertension.

Acute pulmonary hypertension results from vasoconstriction, embolism, intravascular thrombosis, or alveolar overdistension. Pulmonary vasoconstriction occurs in response to a host of alveolar, neural, and humoral stimuli, as listed in Table 41–1. Some of these substances are made locally in the lung (e.g., thromboxane A2), whereas others circulate into the lung from distant organ sites (e.g., adrenal catecholamines). The pulmonary vessels with the greatest ability to constrict and therefore dictate pulmonary vascular resistance are muscular pulmonary arteri-

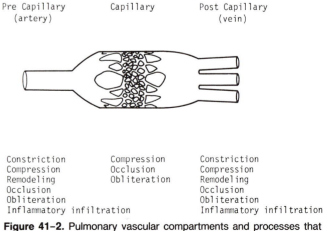

Figure 41–2. Pulmonary vascular compartments and processes that increase resistance to blood flow.

Table 41–1. ALVEOLAR, HUMORAL, AND NEURAL STIMULI PRODUCING PULMONARY VASOCONSTRICTION

Alveolar hypoxia
Acidosis
Thromboxane A_2
Prostaglandin H_2, D_2, $F_{2\alpha}$
Platelet activating factor
Complement fragments C_{5a}, C_{3a}
Norepinephrine
Acetylcholine
Substance P
Angiotensin II
Histamine
Leukotriene C_4, D_4

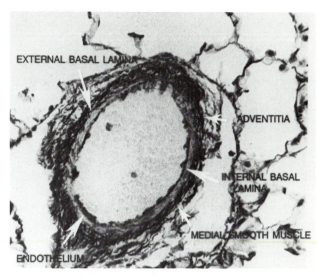

Figure 41–3. Micrograph of a normal pulmonary arteriole of 150-μm diameter. Anatomic components of the vessel wall include endothelium, internal and external basal laminae, medial smooth muscle, and surrounding adventitia.

oles, often referred to as pulmonary resistance vessels. Vasoconstriction is often reversible if the stimulus can be eliminated (e.g., treatment of alveolar hypoxia with supplemental oxygen). In contrast, acute pulmonary hypertension resulting from vascular obstruction is not readily reversible and carries with it a significant mortality rate.[7] Pulmonary hypertension associated with alveolar overdistension occurs in patients receiving positive-pressure mechanical ventilation and in those whose obstructive airway disease leads to hyperinflation and self-imposed positive end-expiratory pressure.[8] Relief of the airway disease and reduction in respirator pressures alleviate this mechanism of acute pulmonary hypertension.

Chronic pulmonary hypertension may result from long-term exposure of pulmonary vessels to a vasoconstrictive stimulus (i.e., hypoxia) but can also result from conditions that stress vessels independently of vasoconstriction.[9] For example, children with large ventricular septal cardiac defects experience increased pulmonary blood flow, which does not per se produce vasoconstriction. Instead, increased blood flow may produce shear stress on pulmonary endothelial cells, which in turn leads to structural changes in arterioles that produce clinical pulmonary hypertension. It is important to note that a "chronic" stimulus for pulmonary hypertension does not necessarily connote that the stimulus is continuously present. Nighttime sleep-related alveolar hypoxia in children and adults with lung disease and sleep apnea syndromes produces sustained pulmonary hypertension despite the presence of normal arterial oxygen tensions when these patients are awake.[10] As yet, the critical duration and severity of recurrent stimuli (such as hypoxia) necessary to produce chronic pulmonary hypertension in infants and children are unknown.

The pulmonary vascular response to intermittent and continuous long-term pathogenic stimuli is a structural alteration in vessel architecture known broadly as remodeling. The cellular processes that produce vascular remodeling and the reversal of the remodeling process are currently under active study by a number of investigators.[11,12] Large precapillary pulmonary vessels normally contain endothelium, an internal basal lamina, a smooth medial muscle layer peripheral to the internal elastic lamina, an external basal lamina, and outside adventitial tissue (Fig. 41–3). Elastic pulmonary arteries are preacinar vessels larger than 1000 μm in diameter that contain multiple

layers of medial smooth muscle separated by elastic laminae. Muscular pulmonary arteries are preacinar vessels that range from 150 to 1000 μm in diameter and contain discrete intimal, medial, and adventitial regions.

In vessels larger than 150 μm in diameter, smooth muscle completely encircles the vessel. As the vessel proceeds into the acinar region, the medial muscle thins and spirals around the vessel in such a way that the lumen of a particular arteriole may be only partially surrounded by smooth muscle. These small vessels are known as partially muscularized arterioles. These vessels also contribute to active control of pulmonary vascular resistance.[13] Partially muscularized arterioles then connect to nonmuscularized vessels, which in turn connect to pulmonary capillaries. Postnatal age influences the distribution of smooth muscle around pulmonary vessels 150 μm or less in diameter. The extension of medial musculature into smaller precapillary vessels and the increase in thickness of muscle walls in pulmonary vessels of different caliber normally occur in infancy, but both of these features can be modified by alveolar hypoxia and other pathogenic mechanisms at any age.[14] All portions of the pulmonary blood vessel wall are responsive to injury or mechanical stress and can remodel.[15]

Specific morphologic features of remodeled pulmonary vessels bear mention because they result from common pathogenic mechanisms and are encountered on lung biopsy and autopsy tissue examination.

HYPOXIA-INDUCED PULMONARY HYPERTENSION

Alveolar hypoxia leads to immediate vasoconstriction of the pulmonary arterioles and, to a lesser extent, venules in both humans and animals. The cellular mechanism accounting for hypoxic pulmonary vasoconstriction remains unclear despite extensive study by multiple

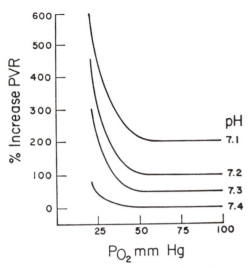

Figure 41–4. Changes in pulmonary vascular resistance (PVR) in response to changes in inspired oxygen pressure/tension under conditions of different blood pH for newborn calves. (From Rudolph AM, Yuan S: Response of the pulmonary vasculature to hypoxia and H+ ion concentration changes. J Clin Invest 45:399–411, 1966. Reproduced from the *Journal of Clinical Investigation*, 1966, vol. 45, pp. 399–411 by copyright permission of the American Society for Clinical Investigation.)

investigators.[16] Arteriolar vasoconstriction in response to hypoxia is important as a means of distributing regional pulmonary blood flow to the best ventilated, least hypoxic areas of lung, thereby maintaining optimal ventilation/perfusion matching and arterial oxygenation. Diffuse alveolar hypoxia, such as occurs during apnea, in hypoventilation syndromes, or at high altitude, leads to diffuse vasoconstriction and hence pulmonary hypertension. The classic relationship between oxygen tension and pulmonary vascular resistance is illustrated in Figure 41–4. The nonlinear changes in pulmonary vascular resistance at lower oxygen tensions is particularly important and has led to the use of oxygen therapy to minimize vasoconstriction by maintaining arterial oxygen pressure/tension (Pa_{O_2}) > 55 mm Hg and arterial oxygen saturation > 90%. Figure 41–4 also illustrates the additional influences of pH on the potency of hypoxic pulmonary vasoconstriction. Acidosis augments vasoconstrictive response, whereas alkalosis, particularly pH values greater than 7.50, attenuates hypoxic pulmonary vasoconstriction.[17]

The primary site of remodeling in the pulmonary vascular bed in response to chronic hypoxia is the precapillary compartment. All forms of lung disease that produce alveolar hypoxia, whether the result of abnormal ventilatory drive, primary lung parenchymal disease, airway obstruction, chest wall restriction, or respiratory muscle weakness, produce similar features of pulmonary vascular remodeling. Within 3 days of the onset of experimental alveolar hypoxia, rats begin to acquire sustained pulmonary hypertension.[18] By 10 days of exposure to hypoxia, pulmonary hypertension is more dramatic and is associated with the extension of medial smooth muscle into smaller arterioles. This occurs in part as a result of cellular proliferation, differentiation, and hypertrophy of two cell types: the intermediate cell within partially muscularized pulmonary arterioles and the pericyte within nonmuscularized arterioles. Both cells are surrounded by basement membrane and appear internal to the elastic

lamina in pulmonary vessels. Both also contain smooth muscle actin and myosin, which suggests that these cell types are capable of contracting and contributing to local vascular tone. By 14 days of exposure to hypoxia, both medial hypertrophy and hyperplasia of smooth muscle cells in muscular pulmonary arteries develop in rats.[18] Later the arterial number relative to alveolar structures declines, which is suggestive of vessel dropout and reduction in cross-sectional surface area of arteriolar conduits. Cellular and acellular elements in the adventitial tissue surrounding large pulmonary vessels also increase. Production of elastin and collagen increases, as does the number of fibroblasts within the adventitial part of the vessel.[19] Although endothelial swelling is present, little intimal proliferation occurs in response to hypoxia. The mechanical effect of these structural changes is to reduce the distensibility of the vessel and to reduce the caliber of the vessel lumen. This effect manifests functionally as an increase in pulmonary vascular resistance and also a disproportionate increase in Ppa in response to conditions of increased pulmonary blood flow (i.e., exercise). If vessel obliteration is significant, measurements of diffusing capacity may also be reduced in response to a reduction in alveolar-capillary surface area.

Although the mechanisms that promote these structural changes are not known, the prevailing concept is that increased tension across the vessel wall resulting from increased intraluminal distending pressure leads to structural changes that strengthen the vessel wall and minimize its distensibility.

With relief from alveolar hypoxia, these vascular features can regress coincidentally with a reduction in Ppa.[20] Smooth muscle hypertrophy regresses toward normal appearance; however, increased deposition of elastin and collagen in the adventitial region of the vessel persists. Obliteration of vessels and reduction in arteriolar number are also irreversible. The mechanical characteristics of the re-remodeled pulmonary vasculature have not been described, but hemodynamic measurements after definitive treatment (e.g., tonsillectomy for children with pulmonary hypertension resulting from upper airway obstruction) often revert toward normal values over a period of months.[21]

PULMONARY HYPERTENSION ASSOCIATED WITH INCREASED PULMONARY BLOOD FLOW

Another major cause of pulmonary hypertension is persistently increased pulmonary blood flow as occurs with congenital heart lesions associated with increased or decreased pulmonary blood flow. Some cardiac lesions produce pulmonary hypertension in adulthood, whereas others are associated with severe pulmonary vascular remodeling in infancy. Atrial septal defects, for example, lead to pulmonary hypertension primarily in adults and less often in children, which suggests that increased pulmonary blood flow per se is not a mechanism that promotes rapid structural change of the pulmonary vasculature. Vessel wall distension may accelerate vascular remodeling in the presence of increased blood flow. The distension produced by elevated systolic Ppa and right ventricular systolic pressures in patients with ventricular septal defects (VSDs) presumably promotes these structural changes in pulmonary vessels. As a result, 20% of infants with large VSDs acquire pulmonary hypertension as early as the first year of life.[3] Similarly, children with atrioventricular canal defects frequently acquire severe pulmonary hypertension in infancy. The incompetent mitral valve produces mitral regurgitation, pulmonary venous distension and hypertension, and, consequently, pulmonary artery hypertension. The triad of increased blood flow, increased pulmonary artery distension from an increased right ventricular systolic pressure, and pulmonary venous distension from mitral regurgitation may act collectively to accelerate vascular remodeling and pulmonary hypertension in these patients.

The structural changes in pulmonary arteries and arterioles in patients with increased pulmonary blood flow are similar to those encountered in patients with pulmonary hypertension resulting from chronic hypoxia.[22] Extension of smooth muscle into smaller precapillary vessels and the differentiation of intermediate cells and pericytes occur in the lungs of both types of patients, as do vascular medial smooth muscle hypertrophy and hyperplasia. In contrast to patients with chronic hypoxic pulmonary hypertension, increased pulmonary blood flow also injures endothelial cells and alters the intimal layer of the vessel. This occurs in response to endothelial shear stress resulting from the rapid velocity of blood elements streaming through individual vessels. Rabinovitch and others, using scanning and transmission electromicrographic techniques, demonstrated changes in the endothelial luminal surface contours from lung biopsies of children with high-flow congenital heart lesions.[23] Associated structural changes include degradation and repair of the internal elastic membrane and increased synthesis of connective tissue in the subendothelial layer of the vessel. These events lead to intimal layer thickening, which further reduces internal vessel caliber. When the lumen is narrowed sufficiently to reduce blood flow, thrombosis occurs, leading to vascular occlusion, loss of vessel number, and reduced precapillary cross-sectional vascular surface area throughout the lung.

The vascular morphologic features associated with cardiac lesions producing increased pulmonary blood flow and pulmonary hypertension were classified in 1958 by Heath and Edwards.[24] These categories, summarized in Table 41–2, were developed to predict which patients could survive surgical correction of the cardiac defect and which would die of progressive pulmonary hypertension and right heart failure despite surgical therapy. The classification has also been useful for describing the progressive vascular features in severe pulmonary hypertension. Late, irreversible changes include accumulation of collagenous material within the intimal layer, plexiform lesions, and fibrinoid necrosis of pulmonary arteries. Plexiform lesions are characterized by aneurysmal dilation of the vessel and thinning of the vessel wall with disruption of the elastic laminae. The lumen is filled with cells that connect to form septa, further reducing intraluminal caliber. Fibrinoid necrosis is necrosis of the vessel wall with accumulation of fibrin; the vessel therefore loses its integrity.

Table 41–2. HISTOLOGIC CLASSIFICATION OF PULMONARY VENULES IN PATIENTS WITH PULMONARY HYPERTENSION

Class	Description
I	Medial hypertrophy of small muscular arteries, medial muscle extension into nonmuscular arteries
II	Grade I changes plus cellular intimal proliferation in arterioles
III	Intimal fibrosis; conversion of intimal hypercellularity to acellular elements with "onion-skin" appearance; fragmentation of internal elastic laminae; extension of intimal changes into large pulmonary arteries
IV	Grade III changes plus "dilatation" lesions (plexiform lesions, angiomatoid lesions, veinlike branches of occluded pulmonary arteries)
V	More "dilatation" lesions plus extensive fibrosis of intima and media of small pulmonary arteries
VI	Fibrinoid necrosis of media, generalized pulmonary arteritis

Heath and Edwards' classification has been subsequently modified by several investigators in order to predict postoperative outcomes in patients with pulmonary hypertension but only mild to moderate (Heath and Edwards' grades I to III) pulmonary vascular changes on lung biopsy.[25, 26] They have also been used to correlate biopsy vessel morphologic features preoperatively with long-term hemodynamic function in children surviving cardiac repair.

OTHER MECHANISMS AND PATTERNS OF PULMONARY VESSEL REMODELING

Acute pulmonary vascular obstruction resulting from large thromboemboli does not produce structural remodeling of the pulmonary vasculature. However, chronic vascular obstruction resulting from incomplete recanalization and organization of extensive thrombi and emboli is associated with chronic pulmonary hypertension and cor pulmonale.[27] Chronic intravascular obstruction leads to medial smooth muscle hypertrophy, intimal proliferation, and plexiform lesions in the unoccluded portions of the pulmonary vascular bed. These regions receive a relatively increased pulmonary blood flow chronically in response to vascular occlusion elsewhere in the pulmonary bed. These features of remodeling mimic those of children with increased pulmonary blood flow resulting from cardiac lesions with left-to-right shunts. Intravascular thrombosis is also a common event in the lungs when a vessel's caliber is critically narrowed enough to slow blood flow through it. Consequently, thrombosis is a late but frequent pathologic finding, regardless of how the vasculature becomes narrowed. Chronic vascular obstruction resulting from thromboembolic events is uncommon, however, and accounts for less than 2% of cases of pulmonary thromboembolic disease among adults.[28] Its incidence in infants and children has not been addressed, nor have the pulmonary structural changes caused by this process been described in children.

An additional pattern of structural change in pulmonary vessels resulting in pulmonary hypertension is vascular obliteration. This results from inflammation and fibrosis in surrounding lung tissue that extends to involve or entrap adjacent pulmonary precapillary, capillary, and postcapillary vessels. As an example, idiopathic pulmonary fibrosis and other interstitial inflammatory lung diseases produce diffuse fibrosis of lung tissue and blood vessels within the fibrosed region. An alternative form of vascular obliteration results from pulmonary vasculitis with infiltration of the vessel wall with monocytes, eosinophils, and neutrophils, depending on the underlying disease. The end result is narrowing of the vessel lumen as a result of cellular infiltration and edema as well as intravascular fibrosis. This occurs with collagen vascular diseases such as polyarteritis nodosa, systemic lupus erythematosus, and dermatomyositis. Granulomatous arteritis and obliteration occurs with Wegener's granulomatosis, Churg-Strauss allergic granulomatosis, and sarcoidosis.[29] When the lung is diffusely involved by these diseases, widespread vascular obliteration leads to pulmonary hypertension. When the process is multifocal, as occurs with tuberculous granulomatous arteritis, individual vessels are obliterated, but there is no significant hemodynamic change as a result of the patchy distribution of vessel involvement.

Pulmonary veins can also be obstructed or obliterated, thereby producing pulmonary hypertension. When these processes primarily affect the small pulmonary veins, patients are diagnosed with pulmonary veno-occlusive disease. In cases of veno-occlusive disease, pulmonary arteries are also remodeled but to a lesser degree. Pathologic findings demonstrate intimal thickening, fibrosis, and thrombosis in both pulmonary veins and venules. Medial smooth muscle hypertrophy of pulmonary veins and venules also occurs with both veno-occlusive disease and left heart lesions (e.g., mitral stenosis) when wall tension within both pulmonary veins and arteries is increased.

The last process modifying the structure of pulmonary vessels is hypoplasia. This is not truly remodeling but abnormal growth and deviation from the normal developmental characteristics of the pulmonary vasculature at the time of birth. Intrauterine factors that influence structural characteristics of the pulmonary vessels include degree of lung underdevelopment (including vascular structures within the parenchyma), amount of fetal pulmonary blood flow, timing of prenatal events that lead to hypoplasia, site of vascular hypoplasia, and other factors as yet unidentified. Pulmonary vascular hypoplasia accompanies hypoplasia of airways and alveolar structures associated with in utero chest wall restriction, abdominal distension, phrenic nerve agenesis, diaphragmatic hernia, and primary pulmonary hypoplasia. Both size and number of precapillary, capillary, and postcapillary vessels are reduced in these conditions. In patients with normal lung parenchymal development but reduced intrauterine pulmonary blood flow (i.e., pulmonic valve atresia), the pulmonary vessels are also reduced in size and number with thin-walled arteries that contain reduced medial smooth muscle.[30] When it is less severe, reduced fetal pulmonary blood flow (as occurs in some patients with tetralogy of Fallot), precapillary vascular wall distension, and compensatory medial smooth muscle hypertrophy develop in the presence of reduced vessel size and number.[31]

When pulmonary venous outflow is obstructed in utero (as occurs with total anomalous pulmonary venous return and interrupted aortic arch), intravascular distension throughout the fetal pulmonary vascular bed produces medial hypertrophy and smooth muscle extension into very small vessels in both the precapillary and postcapillary compartments. Similar excessive smooth muscle hypertrophy and extension occurs in some children with persistent pulmonary hypertension of the newborn (PPHN) but does so in the absence of venous outflow obstruction.[32] Intrauterine ductal closure by ligation or prostaglandin inhibitor administration, fetal systemic hypertension in the presence of a patent ductus arteriosus (produced by ligation of a renal artery or an umbilical artery), and short periods of fetal hypoxia all lead to pulmonary vascular structural changes and postnatal pulmonary hypertension similar to that found in infants with PPHN.[33, 34] It is unclear how closely these experimental pathogenic mechanisms reflect the cause of PPHN in human newborns.

The pathogenic mechanisms that lead to vessel remodeling often act in concert with one another. This is illustrated in children with trisomy 21 and atrioventricular canals. These children have small upper airways, mildly hypoplastic lungs, and respiratory muscle weakness, all of which lead to chronic or recurrent hypoventilation and alveolar hypoxia.[35] This combination of hypoxic pulmonary remodeling and remodeling from high pulmonary blood flow associated with cardiac disease explains why these children acquire severe pulmonary hypertension early in life.

FUNCTIONAL FEATURES OF THE REMODELED PULMONARY VASCULATURE

Global remodeling of the pulmonary vascular bed and reduced vessel caliber increase pulmonary vascular resistance. The resistance is "fixed" in the sense that reversal of these structural changes may be slow, particularly when advanced stages of remodeling (e.g., plexiform lesions) are present. There is less information regarding the ability of such vessels to constrict or relax in comparison with the normal pulmonary vasculature. Stenmark and colleagues exposed calves immediately after birth to hypobaric hypoxia and produced dramatic remodeling and suprasystemic Ppa.[36] Further study of the vessels in vitro demonstrated a reduced ability to synthesize vasodilator compounds such as prostacyclin and a reduced ability to relax when exposed to pharmacologic vasodilators. Other investigators found that remodeled pulmonary vessels in adult rats exposed to chronic hypoxia were unable to vasoconstrict further in response to acute alveolar hypoxia.[37] These new findings provide initial insights into the alterations in synthesis and metabolism of vasoactive products by different cell populations within vessel walls. How metabolic functions and cell-cell interactions within remodeled pulmonary vessels specifically influence vascular reactivity awaits further study.

Such findings will, ideally, relate to clinical observations of enhanced vasoreactivity noted in infants recovering from surgical repair of diaphragmatic hernias and in children who experience pulmonary hypertensive crises in the immediate postoperative period after cardiopulmonary bypass and hypothermia. They may also help predict which pediatric populations are susceptible to reduced vasoreactivity, aside from the few patients with advanced pulmonary hypertension who are unresponsive to vasodilator drugs. Further clinical investigation must determine the role of vasomotor tone in right heart disease in children with remodeled pulmonary vessels associated with various chronic lung diseases. Such information will ultimately provide a more rational basis for therapeutic interventions.

FUNCTIONAL CONSEQUENCES OF PULMONARY HYPERTENSION

HEMODYNAMIC CHANGES

Pulmonary hypertension is present when mean Ppa is greater than 20 mm Hg. Normal mean Ppa is 10 to 16 mm Hg, and normal pulmonary artery systolic pressure is 15 to 25 mm Hg in older children.[38] Normal Ppa is therefore approximately one fifth of normal systemic artery pressure. Determinants of Ppa are cardiac output, pulmonary venous pressure (Pv), and altered vessel lumen caliber and wall characteristics that dictate pulmonary vascular resistance (PVR). Ppa is related to these variables by the formula

$$Ppa = cardiac\ output \times PVR + Pv$$

From this equation, it is apparent that increased cardiac output increases Ppa. Because a number of variables (e.g., intravascular volume, stress, and anesthetics) influence cardiac output when pulmonary hemodynamics are clinically assessed during cardiac catheterization, characterization of the pulmonary vascular bed is often made through the use of PVR to normalize Ppa for variability in pulmonary blood flow. PVR is expressed as resistance units (millimeters of mercury/liter/minute) or as dynes/second/cubic centimeter. Because cardiac output varies with body size in growing children, PVR is further transformed by normalizing cardiac output by body surface area to obtain a cardiac index for use in calculation of PVR. This enables comparison of an individual patient's hemodynamic data with normal values. Normal PVR values for older children and adults are 1 to 3 units/sq m.

These values are not applicable to the normal newborn during the immediate postnatal period. Ppa is approximately half of systemic pressure by 24 h of age and normally falls to adult values within 6 to 8 weeks after birth.[39] Similarly, PVR falls by 80% immediately after birth and continues to decrease more gradually over the next 10 to 15 days. Adult values for PVR are also reached by 6 to 8 weeks of age.[40]

Included indirectly in the equation are the influences of blood viscosity and intrathoracic pressure. Both influence PVR but do not reflect the condition of the pulmonary vasculature per se. In children with severe hypoxemia from chronic lung disease, the erythropoietin-induced increase in red blood cell mass can lead to an elevated hematocrit. A change in hematocrit depends on whether an increase in plasma volume develops in conjunction with changes in red blood cell mass. When hematocrit levels are higher than 55%, blood viscosity increases. The increased resistance to flow from increased blood viscosity can further elevate Ppa without additional changes in vessel caliber or cross-sectional area.

Positive intrathoracic pressure as occurs in patients on mechanical ventilation is transmitted across vessel walls and contributes to intravascular Ppa values. This may also occur in children with pulmonary hyperinflation in response to severe airway obstruction. In adults with chronic obstructive pulmonary disease (COPD), cardiac catheterization studies suggest that lower lobe overdistension increases pressure around the heart and extraparenchymal pulmonary veins, increasing PV and hence Ppa.[8]

The abnormal mechanical characteristics of remodeled vessels are accentuated by exercise. The normal lung is capable of receiving two- to threefold increases in pulmonary blood flow; minimal increases in Ppa result from the distensibility of the vessels and the recruitment of pulmonary vessels that are normally collapsed.[41] Pulmonary vascular resistance falls during exercise as a result of the large increase in flow relative to the small increase in Ppa. In contrast, increased pulmonary blood flow within indistensible and maximally recruited pulmonary vessels during exercise in patients with pulmonary hypertension produces dramatic increases in Ppa.[42] In contrast to normal persons, PVR in patients with pulmonary hypertension may stay the same or increase during exercise. Most patients with mild pulmonary hypertension associated with obstructive lung disease have normal hemodynamic measurements at rest but abnormal right ventricular pressure and Ppa during exercise.[43] In children with severe pulmonary hypertension, resistance to blood flow may be fixed and so great that the normal increase in cardiac output during exercise does not occur, so the increase in Ppa is not much greater than at rest.

Because of the distensibility of normal pulmonary vessels, it is estimated that at least 60% of the lung vasculature must be occluded acutely before pulmonary hypertension develops in response to acute pulmonary thromboembolism.[44] In contrast, patients with pulmonary hypertension who have remodeled vessels as a result of recurrent or chronic extensive thromboembolic disease experience significant increases in pulmonary pressure when small emboli recur.

All of the pathologic changes in vessel structure mentioned previously and all forms of vasoconstriction directly increase PVR independently of flow. Pulmonary venous obstruction increases Ppa because of passive vessel distension throughout the lung independently of resistance characteristics of precapillary and capillary vessels.

Increased mean and systolic Ppas impede emptying into the right ventricle. When the rise in pulmonary pressures is abrupt, the compliant thin-walled right ventricle in older children dilates to move into a more mechanically effective position of the Frank-Starling curve, and right ventricular end-diastolic volume increases. The right heart is unable to maintain normal stroke volume when Ppa of 50 mm Hg or more develops acutely, and

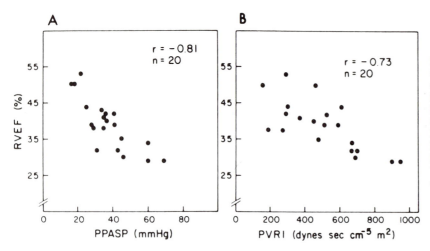

Figure 41–5. Relation of right ventricular ejection fracture (RVEF) to (*A*) peak pulmonary artery systolic pressure (PPASP) and (*B*) pulmonary vascular resistance index (PVRI) in 20 adults with chronic obstructive pulmonary disease. The greater the index of right ventricular afterload produces a lower RVEF. (From Berger HJ, Matthay RA, Loke J, et al: Assessment of cardiac performance with quantitative radionuclide angiography: Right ventricular ejection fraction with reference to findings in chronic obstructive pulmonary disease. Am J Cardiol 41:897–905, 1978.)

right heart failure develops.[45] This may be caused in part by a reduction in right coronary artery perfusion when the oxygen requirements of the right ventricle are increased in response to increased right ventricular work. Normally, perfusion of the right ventricle by the right coronary artery occurs during both systole and diastole. When right ventricular pressures increase in response to pulmonary hypertension, coronary perfusion of the right heart occurs only during diastole. If right ventricular pressures approximate aortic pressures, coronary perfusion pressure approaches zero. If diastole filling time is reduced, as can occur with tachyarrhythmias, right ventricular perfusion is further reduced. Subendocardial ischemia and infarction have been found at autopsy in patients with acute pulmonary hypertension.[46] This suggests that poor perfusion of the right myocardium occurs as a consequence of severe pulmonary hypertension.

The response to acute pulmonary hypertension is somewhat different in neonates in whom the right ventricle is hypertrophied as a result of fetal life. Although the critical Ppa at which the right heart fails in a newborn is not known, suprasystemic pressures have been achieved in the right hearts of infants with PPHN concomitantly with adequate if not optimal cardiac outputs. The condition of newborns with hypertrophic right ventricle is more analogous to that of older children with cor pulmonale from chronic pulmonary hypertension. Unlike acute pulmonary hypertension, the right heart compensates to chronically elevated afterload with hypertrophy more than dilation. However, before the onset of electrocardiographic changes that are suggestive of right ventricular hypertrophy, right ventricular ejection fraction falls below normal levels in inverse proportion to the severity of pulmonary hypertension.[47] This is illustrated in Figure 41–5, in which ejection fraction is compared with pulmonary arterial systolic pressure and PVR in 20 adult patients with COPD.[48]

Once hypertrophy develops in the right heart, the ventricle becomes less compliant, producing increased end-diastolic pressures, increased right atrial pressures, and systemic venous distension. The relationship between cardiac output and right atrial pressure, illustrated in Figure 41–6, suggests that right ventricular stroke volume is significantly reduced when right atrial pressures exceed 10

mm Hg in adult patients with pulmonary hypertension.[49] Similar relations have not been studied in infants and children. When Ppa is further increased, as during superimposed viral respiratory infections, the right heart fails. As with left-sided heart failure, right-sided heart failure leads to decreased cardiac output and a compensatory increase in circulating plasma volume. The increased preload may not further improve right heart function. Increased right atrial and systemic venous pressures then produce clinical signs of neck vein distension, hepatic congestion and enlargement, and edema of limbs and dependent tissues.

The left heart functions normally in most patients with pulmonary hypertension despite suboptimal right heart function.[50] A minority of patients, consistently described in clinical studies, have poor left ventricular function, which aggravates lung mechanics, gas exchange, and hence pulmonary hypertension. Controversy exists as to how much cor pulmonale per se contributes to left ventricular dysfunction in these patients.[51, 52] Hypoxia and respiratory acidosis associated with severe lung disease affect left ventricular function independently of changes

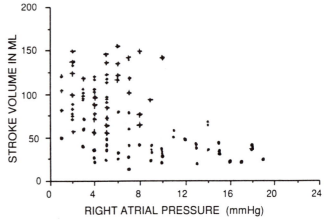

Figure 41–6. Relation of stroke volume to right atrial pressure at rest and during exercise in normal subjects (+) and patients with pulmonary hypertension. (From Reeves JT, Groves BM, Morrison DA, et al: Right ventricular function in pulmonary hypertension. *In* Weir EK, Reeves JT (eds): Pulmonary Vascular Physiology and Pathophysiology, pp. 325–351. New York: Marcel Dekker, 1985. Reprinted by courtesy of Marcel Dekker, Inc.)

in right ventricular geometry or pressures. Similarly, large negative intrathoracic pressures occurring with accentuated inspiratory efforts increase venous return to the right heart, further distending the ventricle in the presence of increased right ventricular afterload resulting from pulmonary hypertension. Such distension changes left ventricular configuration and decreases left ventricular compliance. Left ventricular end-diastolic pressure therefore increases, reducing pulmonary venous return and left ventricular stroke volume. Several authors have shown that poor left ventricular function is more frequently identified in patients with pulmonary hypertension when the cardiopulmonary system is stressed (i.e., during exercise).[53, 54]

CHANGES IN LUNG MECHANICS

In patients with primary pulmonary hypertension and infants with PPHN, measurements of lung mechanics demonstrate restrictive lung disease, on the basis of reduced lung compliance and reduced lung volumes.[55] These changes in lung mechanics are mild in relation to the pulmonary hemodynamic abnormalities. Restrictive lung disease in patients with pulmonary hypertension is not surprising conceptually, inasmuch as the vascular tree extends throughout lung tissue and becomes stiffer as a result of structural remodeling. Whether pulmonary vasoconstriction in the absence of remodeling produces equally significant restrictive lung mechanics is unclear. Obstructive changes in lung mechanics resulting directly from pulmonary hypertension have been reported less frequently.[56] Such changes presumably occur as a result of small airway compression by distended thick pulmonary arteries and encroachment by increased perivascular adventitial tissue. In lung diseases, which produce restrictive or obstructive changes themselves, the restrictive element resulting from vascular remodeling associated with pulmonary hypertension may add to the abnormal lung mechanics produced by the underlying disease.

CHANGES IN GAS EXCHANGE

Hypoxemia is the characteristic feature of primary pulmonary hypertension. It is associated with tachypnea, which results in part from both low arterial oxygen tension and increased physiologic dead space. These characteristics have been documented both at rest and during exercise in patients with pulmonary hypertension. The tachypnea in turn leads to increased minute ventilation and hypocapnia. The mechanism for hypoxemia may depend somewhat on the cause of pulmonary hypertension. In adults with primary pulmonary hypertension studied by inert gas analysis, Dantzker and co-workers found that ventilation/perfusion matching remained largely intact despite severe pulmonary hemodynamic abnormalities.[57] The patients were hypoxemic, but there was no increase in shunt fraction or increased perfusion to low ventilation/perfusion ratio regions. Instead, mixed venous oxygen tension was lower than normal because of increased tissue extraction as a result of limited cardiac output. Poor cardiac output in these patients resulted from poor left ventricular filling, high fixed PVR, and suboptimal right ventricular function. Hypoxemia in patients with pulmonary hypertension is also accentuated during exercise when increased tissue demands for oxygen cannot be met because of limited cardiac reserve.[58]

In neonates and older children with a patent foramen ovale, hypoxemia resulting from pulmonary hypertension can be severe and life-threatening. When Ppa reaches suprasystemic levels in newborns, blood flows right to left through the patent ductus arteriosus; this process leads to large extrapulmonary shunt. Ductal-dependent shunt is detected when oxygen tension is measured from the preductal ascending aorta and an artery emanating from the postductal descending aorta. Oxygen tension differences in blood taken from the right radial (preductal) artery and the umbilical artery (postductal source) of more than 10 mm Hg are suggestive of this condition.[59] Preductal versus postductal oxygen tension differences may be obscured by right-to-left interatrial shunts across the foramen ovale. The patent foramen allows desaturated venous blood to enter first the left atrium and ventricle and then the ascending (preductal) aorta. Addition of desaturated blood to the ascending aorta reduces the differences between preductal and postductal oxygen tensions, which are used to diagnose ductal right-to-left shunting. The presence of either of these persistent fetal channels predisposes a patient with pulmonary hypertension to much more profound hypoxemia.

Pulmonary hypertension associated with primary pulmonary parenchymal or airway disease leads to abnormalities in both oxygen and carbon dioxide tensions, depending on the severity of lung mechanics and the diffuse nature of the pulmonary process. As with most pulmonary diseases, these gas exchange abnormalities and pulmonary hypertension are worsened by reduced tidal volume, functional residual capacity, and reduced minute ventilation associated with sleep.[60]

CLINICAL FEATURES

SYMPTOMS AND SIGNS

Common symptoms and clinical signs associated with primary pulmonary hypertension in the absence of additional airway or parenchymal disease are listed in Table 41–3. The earliest complaint among 187 adults and chil-

Table 41–3. CLINICAL SYMPTOMS ASSOCIATED WITH PULMONARY HYPERTENSION (INDEPENDENT OF UNDERLYING LUNG DISEASE)

Dyspnea
Fatigue
Exercise intolerance (including feeding intolerance)
Failure to thrive in infancy
Excessive napping
Diaphoresis
Chest pain
Syncope
Palpitations

Table 41–4. PHYSICAL SIGNS ASSOCIATED WITH PULMONARY HYPERTENSION AND RIGHT HEART FAILURE

Tachypnea
Arrhythmias
Increased P_2 heart sound
Narrowed splitting of S_2 heart sound
Tachycardia
Diaphoresis
S_3 or S_4 heart sounds
Tricuspid insufficiency murmur
Pulmonic insufficiency murmur
Hepatic enlargement and pain
Pedal edema
Jugular venous distension (large "a" waves)

dren registered during the national multicenter pulmonary hypertension registry was dyspnea (60% of patients).[61] More than half (74%) also experienced fatigue after the onset of dyspnea. In young children, dyspnea and fatigability may be manifested by poor feeding (short duration of feeding despite apparent hunger), sweating during feeding, frequent rests during play, and excessive daytime napping. Orthopnea is unusual except when postcapillary pulmonary hypertension occurs and produces pulmonary edema. Symptoms of peripheral edema and palpitations reflect heart failure and are late manifestations of disease. None of these findings is specific for pulmonary vascular disease, especially in the presence of chronic or severe lung disease, which can produce many of the same findings in the absence of pulmonary hypertension. Consequently, a high index of suspicion is necessary in order to survey for pulmonary hypertension in children with various lung and airway disorders.

Physical findings of pulmonary hypertension are often obscured by similar signs associated with underlying lung disease until signs of right heart failure develop. Typical findings for pulmonary hypertension resulting from primarily vascular changes are listed in Table 41–4.[62,63] They reflect altered right heart function in response to increased right ventricular afterload. Giant "a" waves producing jugular venous distension occur as a result of increased right atrial force generated to pump blood into a poorly compliant right ventricle. A fourth heart sound (S_4) reflects a diastolic atrial gallop. Narrowing of the normal split between the pulmonic and aortic components of the second heart sound reflects earlier-than-normal closure of the pulmonic valve leaflets as a result of rapid falloff in right ventricular systolic pressure at the end of systole in the presence of increased right ventricular afterload. The diastolic murmur of pulmonic valve regurgitation is three times more common than the holosystolic murmur of tricuspid regurgitation. Tricuspid regurgitation and the presence of a third heart sound (S_3) are signs of advanced disease associated with right heart failure.

Clinical findings associated with signs and symptoms of pulmonary hypertension often help to identify the underlying process producing pulmonary hypertension. For example, snoring and obstructive sleep apnea result in central airway obstruction and nighttime alveolar hypoxia as a result of hypoventilation. Alternatively, a child may have a chronic productive cough associated with the bronchiectasis and lower airway obstruction that are characteristic of cystic fibrosis. Physical findings such as hyperinflation produced by lower airway disease can also obscure the detection of signs of pulmonary hypertension. Hyperinflation of the lungs overlying the heart reduces transmission of heart sounds to the examiner. Adventitial breath sounds resulting from underlying lung disease can also obscure the auscultatory cardiac features associated with pulmonary hypertension. Hence the apparent absence of these findings in the presence of severe lung disease should not dissuade the clinician from documenting the presence of pulmonary hypertension by using laboratory techniques.

IMAGING STUDIES

Imaging techniques are used to discern the underlying pathogenic mechanisms and the locations of disease within the thorax in patients with pulmonary hypertension. These techniques include chest radiographs, ventilation and perfusion scans, and pulmonary angiography. The images may indirectly reflect the functional status of the heart and lungs, but the appearance of the lungs and heart correlates poorly with hemodynamic function. The latter is measured more specifically and directly with right heart catheterization, electrocardiography, and echocardiography.

Chest radiographs of children with pulmonary hypertension are variable in appearance, depending on the cause and the severity of the disease. Radiographic features of pulmonary hypertension unobscured by parenchymal or lower airway diseases depend on whether the site of vascular narrowing is localized (e.g., pulmonary emboli) or diffuse and whether precapillary or postcapillary vessels are primarily involved.

Radiographic features of primary pulmonary hypertension range from normal appearance to cardiac and central pulmonary vessel enlargement, with "pruning" of intrapulmonary arteries so that peripheral lung tissue seems underperfused. In contrast, thromboembolic disease produces radiographic appearances ranging from normal to asymmetric central pulmonary vessel size and heterogeneous distribution of perfusion, depending on the locations of large-vessel occlusion. The most common findings associated with acute pulmonary embolism are localized infiltrates and volume loss in the thrombosed lung region. Veno-occlusive disease produces a radiographic pattern of diffuse reticular nodularity and Kerley B lines, which are indicative of pulmonary edema.

Underlying lung disease may alter the radiographic appearance of the chest so that features suggesting pulmonary hypertension are difficult to discern. Hyperinflation tends to lengthen the mediastinum, reducing the visual impact of cardiac enlargement. Interstitial infiltrates and bronchiectatic changes obscure the appearance of both central and peripheral pulmonary vessels. As in the case of physical findings, the lack of diagnostic radiographic features should not deter further investigation of pulmonary hypertension in the presence of chronic or severe cardiopulmonary disease.

Ventilation scintigraphic scans with radiolabeled xenon or diethylenetriamine penta-acetic acid (DTPA) and pulmonary perfusion scans with radiolabeled albumin are most useful in identifying lung regions that are not functioning normally. Ventilation/perfusion scans are most helpful in the diagnosis of thromboembolic disease, which affects regions of the lung heterogeneously. They are most diagnostic when the chest radiograph appears normal despite clinical signs of cardiopulmonary distress. One finding on the perfusion scan that may reflect generalized pulmonary vascular disease is the loss of normal gravity-dependent preferential blood flow to the bases of the lung in upright patients. A finding of homogeneous distribution of perfusion equally to upper and lower lobes suggests a generalized increase in PVR but does not distinguish vasoconstriction from vessel remodeling.

Pulmonary angiography is a more precise way of identifying the sites of vascular disease, especially vascular obstruction. Alteration in pulmonary vessel size and appearance is more apparent in angiography than in plain chest films. The more select the vascular area that receives the dye, the more precisely the process altering the vessel is described. Injection of contrast material into the main pulmonary artery results in dilution of dye, loss of visual detail because of generalized enhancement of overlapping vessels, and diversion of dye into the most normal vessels, which receive the highest amount of blood flow. Wedge pulmonary angiography is also used to evaluate the extent of the capillary "blush" resulting from dye transit through the pulmonary capillary network.[64] Reduction in the blush suggests reduced precapillary and capillary vessel number. In most cases, pulmonary angiography is combined with pulmonary hemodynamic assessment to determine the functional significance of angiographic findings.

FUNCTIONAL ASSESSMENT OF PULMONARY VESSELS AND THE HEART

Functional assessment of pulmonary hypertension can be accomplished to determine severity of the pathologic vascular process. It can also be used repeatedly to assess the impact of a therapeutic intervention or to observe the clinical course of the disease. The clinical tools most commonly used to assess pulmonary and right heart hemodynamic function in patients with pulmonary hypertension are electrocardiography, echocardiography, thallium scans, and right heart and pulmonary catheterization. Echocardiography and pulmonary catheterization are used to assess the interaction between pulmonary vascular mechanics and cardiac performance. Electrocardiography is used to evaluate only the cardiac response to increased right heart afterload. Thallium 201 (^{201}T) scans are used to image the septum and right ventricular free wall. Thallium uptake is dependent on both myocardial blood flow and myocardial mass; the sensitivity of this technique is greatest when blood flow to the heart is enhanced, as occurs during exericse.[65] None of these methods can be used to evaluate the extravascular pulmonary components, such as alveolar hypoxia and hyper-

Table 41–5. ELECTROCARDIOGRAPHIC FEATURES OF COR PULMONALE IN CHILDHOOD

Right QRS Axis Deviation (Associated with Right Ventricular Hypertrophy and Right Bundle Branch Block)
> +180 degrees in newborns
> +120 degrees in infants
> 90 degrees in children older than 3 years
Right Ventricular Hypertrophy in Infants and Children
R/S ratio:
    >1.5 in V_1, V_2 in infants 0–6 months old*
    >0.8 in V_1, V_2 in children >1 year old
    <1.0 in V_6 in infants >1 month old
Increased R voltage:
    V_1 (>20 mm in infants older than 1 month)
    V_2 (>30 mm 0–8 years; >25 mm in children older than 8 years)
Increased S voltage: V_6 (>10 mm in infants older than 1 month)
Upright T wave: V_1 (children older than 3 days and younger than 6 years)
q wave: V_1 (qR or qRs patterns: suggestive evidence)
Right Ventricular Hypertrophy in the Neonate
Pure R wave with no S wave in V_1 (>10 mm)
R wave in V_1 >25 mm
R wave in aVR >8 mm
qR pattern in V_1
Right Atrial Hypertrophy (P Pulmonale)
P wave >3 mm in II, V_1, V_2

---

*Especially when R wave is >5 mm.

capnia, that contribute to the severity of pulmonary hypertension.

Electrocardiography is a useful diagnostic tool for patients with pulmonary hypertension when its pattern reflects right ventricular strain, right ventricular hypertrophy, right atrial hypertrophy, and right bundle branch block. Unfortunately, significant alterations in right ventricular structure and function may develop before electrocardiographic patterns become diagnostic. The sensitivity of electrocardiograms for detecting cor pulmonale ranges from 28% to 75% in surveys in which other diagnostic techniques are compared with electrocardiograms.[66–69] Thallium 201 scans, vectorcardiography, and echocardiography are more sensitive for detecting right ventricular hypertrophy, particularly when pulmonary hypertension is only mild to moderate in severity. The advantage of the electrocardiogram is its availability and the ease of use by physicians and ancillary staff.

Specific electrocardiographic features that reflect acute or chronic cor pulmonale are listed in Table 41–5.[70] These findings must be interpreted in light of age-specific electrocardiographic features in normal children. Kilcoyne and associates identified an additional set of features that tend to reflect fluctuations in cardiopulmonary status in patients with pulmonary hypertension.[71] The four dynamic electrocardiographic features include (1) a right shift of the QRS of 30 degrees or more, (2) T wave abnormalities in the precordial leads, (3) ST depression in leads 2, 3, and aVF, and (4) transitory right bundle branch block. Such patterns appeared with mean Ppa rose to 25 mm Hg or more and when oxyhemoglobin saturation fell to less than 85% in adults with known pulmonary hypertension and cor pulmonale. The usefulness of this dynamic electrocardiographic assessment in children with pulmonary hypertension has not yet been demonstrated.

Echocardiographic evaluation of patients with suspected pulmonary hypertension and cor pulmonale includes assessment of right ventricular wall thickness and chamber size as well as motion of the interventricular septum and tricuspid and pulmonic valves. Evaluation of left ventricular dimensions and contraction is also important for ruling out left heart disease as a cause of pulmonary hypertension and for identifying poor left heart function as a complication of cor pulmonale. Right ventricular end-diastolic volume reflects the degree of ventricular dilation in response to intravascular preload and ventricular afterload produced by the pulmonary vasculature. Increased right ventricular anterior wall thickness and, to a lesser extent, interventricular septal wall thickness reflect right ventricular hypertrophy. Paradoxical septal wall motion is a sign of impending right ventricular strain and failure. Tricuspid valve regurgitation is also associated with limited right heart functional reserve in the presence of cor pulmonale.

Echocardiography in conjunction with an on-line electrocardiogram enables measurement of the right heart pre-ejection period (RPEP) and right ventricular ejection time (RVET). Pre-ejection period (PEP) is the duration of time after electrical activation of the ventricle as noted by the QRS complex to the onset of ejection during systole. RVET is measured from the time of opening to closure of the pulmonic valve during systole. In contrast to that of adults, the anatomy of children permits echocardiographic observation of pulmonic valve motion throughout the entire cardiac cycle, making these measurements of right heart function clinically feasible.[72] Increased right ventricular afterload resulting from pulmonary hypertension delays pulmonic valve opening until right ventricular systolic pressure exceeds Ppa. This delay lengthens RPEP. In contrast, increased Ppa shortens the duration of time the pulmonic valve is open after peak right ventricular systolic pressure has been reached, thus shortening RVET. The RPEP/RVET ratio accentuates these opposing influences of pulmonary hypertension on each time index, thus increasing the sensitivity of the ratio to elevated Ppa. This ratio is not specific for pulmonary hypertension. For example, reduced right ventricular contractility and compliance resulting from primary heart disease influence PEP and RVET similarly in the presence of normal Ppa. However, PEP/RVET, in conjunction with the other echocardiographic features of cor pulmonale, is specific for pulmonary hypertension and amenable to serial noninvasive assessments of its severity.

A major problem with this technique is the technical difficulty of obtaining interpretable information in children with obstructive lung diseases such as cystic fibrosis or bronchopulmonary dysplasia. Echocardiographic interference from overinflated lungs in front of the heart reduces the windows and angles through which the right ventricle and pulmonic valve can be assessed. Excessive body motion, especially in infants, also compounds the technical challenge of obtaining useful results.

Right heart catheterization is the most precise clinical method for measuring hemodynamic abnormalities associated with pulmonary hypertension and cor pulmonale. Individual measurements during the procedure include Ppa, pulmonary capillary wedge or arterial occlusion

Table 41–6. CLINICALLY USED PULMONARY VASODILATOR AGENTS

Isoproterenol
Hydralazine
Nitroprusside, nitroglycerin
Nifedipine, diltiazem, nitrendipine
Prostacyclin, prostaglandin E_1
Tolazoline
Diazoxide
Aminophylline
Captropril
Terbutaline
Amrinone

pressure, cardiac output, and arteriovenous oxygen difference. Catheterization techniques in conjunction with indicator dilution techniques (e.g., indocyanine green or thermodilution) also provide the means to document intracardiac shunts quantitatively. The foramen ovale is probe-patent in 50% of children under 5 years of age and in 25% of adults older than 20 years.[73] Angiographic documentation of right-to-left shunts through the foramen ovale helps to explain arterial hypoxemia in some patients with pulmonary hypertension.

A complete right heart catheterization depends on the clinical stability of the patient. Arrhythmias, hypotension, and acute pulmonary vasoconstriction with right heart failure have all been reported in children with severe pulmonary hypertension who are undergoing catheterization.[74] If the patient is stable, assessment of vasomotor tone and its reversibility are important for determining short-term therapy. This is accomplished by administering 100% inspired oxygen or vasodilator drugs such as those listed in Table 41–6. In Reeves and colleagues' retrospective review of multiple acute pulmonary vasodilator trials in adults, 45% of patients experienced a reduction in PVR of 30% or more.[75] Clinical improvement 3 to 6 months after catheterization occurred in 62% of patients with a significant response to acute vasodilator treatment, in contrast to only 6% of patients in whom PVR fell by less than 30% in response to the same drugs. The lack of hemodynamic response to vasodilating agents suggests that the high PVR is fixed as a result of structural changes in the vessels and is unlikely to respond to chronic vasodilator treatment. However, a significant response to vasodilators during an initial catheterization does not necessarily portend the same hemodynamic response in the future. Indeed, many patients in serial catheterization studies are found to become unresponsive to pulmonary vasodilator agents as pulmonary hypertension progresses.[76]

The acute hemodynamic response to supplemental oxygen is different from that to vasodilator drugs. Oxygen does not influence systemic artery pressure. It is, therefore, a relatively specific pulmonary vasodilator. In contrast, vasodilator agents reduce both pulmonary and systemic artery pressures to variable extents. Several hemodynamic patterns occur in response to vasodilator trials. The beneficial response is a reduction in Ppa more than systemic artery pressure and an increase in cardiac output with either no change or improvement in arterial oxygen tension. Such a response reflects reduction in right heart work and improved oxygen delivery to tissues. This response is relatively infrequent. A second pattern is a reduction in systemic artery pressure to a much greater degree than Ppa. This arises when PVR is fixed and cardiac output cannot increase to compensate for systemic hypotension. Coronary perfusion pressure to the right heart is reduced, and myocardial ischemia is more likely. The third pattern is an increase in cardiac output in response to reduced systemic artery pressure, but an increase in Ppa in response to increased pulmonary blood flow (i.e., the afterload to the right ventricle) has not been reduced despite an adequate cardiac compensatory response to hypotension.

These patterns reflect the hemodynamic responses in patients who have primary pulmonary vascular disease such as primary pulmonary hypertension. They do not take into account the adverse effects on gas exchange that occur when hypoxic pulmonary vasoconstriction in regions of poor ventilation is attenuated pharmacologically. One goal of therapy is to improve oxygen delivery to tissues. In patients with significant parenchymal or airway disease, oxygen is the optimal therapy insofar as it reduces Ppa and improves cardiac output and arterial oxygen tension. The benefit of vasodilators may be mixed as a result of favorable or adverse effects on gas exchange. Vasodilators can reduce arterial oxygen tension resulting from increased ventilation/perfusion mismatch. They can also increase arterial oxygen tension by improving cardiac output and increasing mixed venous oxygen tension as a result of reduced oxygen extraction from blood by peripheral tissues.

The rationale underlying the use of vasodilator trials is to assess the degree to which vasoconstriction contributes to right ventricular afterload and to the increased vascular wall tension that promotes remodeling of pulmonary vessels. Vasodilator trials are designed to prognosticate survival and the likely response to chronic vasodilator treatment. Retrospective data suggest that responders live longer than nonresponders, but this may reflect the state of the pulmonary vascular bed at the time of the vasodilator trial rather than the efficacy of chronic vasodilator agents. In addition, it is not known quantitatively how much of a "beneficial" vascular response to vasodilators or oxygen is necessary to influence prognosis regarding survival or response to other therapies. Furthermore, the samples in most studies have consisted of adult patients; the importance of vasomotor tone in the course of pulmonary hypertension of various causes in infants and children is even less clear.

CLINICAL APPROACHES TO PULMONARY HYPERTENSION IN CHILDREN

There are two situations in which the problem of pulmonary hypertension is considered in pediatrics. The first situation exists when a child with a known respiratory disorder that produces pulmonary hypertension is managed for the long term by the clinician. In this scenario, pulmonary hypertension is expected to occur, and manage-

ment is geared toward surveying for the development of cor pulmonale and subsequently monitoring its progression and response to therapy. Patients with cystic fibrosis, interstitial lung disease, upper airway obstruction, respiratory muscle weakness, and bronchopulmonary dysplasia are all at risk for acquiring pulmonary hypertension during the course of their disease. In children with these diseases, cor pulmonale represents a marker of severity of the underlying respiratory disorder. Later, cor pulmonale in these patients becomes a complication when right heart failure develops and contributes to death. Diagnostic methods are focused on early detection, monitoring of severity and progression, and treatment of both the vascular component and the underlying disease.

The second situation that confronts the clinician exists when a child presents with unexplained right heart failure and pulmonary hypertension. The clinician must ascertain the cause of the pulmonary hypertension and determine whether it is the result of underlying heart disease, lung disease, systemic disease, or isolated pulmonary vascular disease. Simultaneously, the patient must receive appropriate supportive care to reverse heart failure and coincidental hypoxemia, hypercapnia, and acidosis and prevent death. A useful algorithm for identifying the cause of unexplained right heart failure in children is outlined in Figure 41–7. Initial measures include assessment of left heart function and right heart structural lesions distinct from cor pulmonale. Once cor pulmonale has been diagnosed, arterial blood gas tension measurements identify patients with hypoventilation, patients with hypoxemia in the absence of carbon dioxide retention, and those with normal gas exchange when awake. The subsequent use of a chest radiograph and a complete physical examination helps identify respiratory disorders other than primary pulmonary vascular disease. When cor pulmonale is present in the absence of overt lung disease, sleep-related disorders of breathing must be considered in addition to pulmonary vasculitis, thromboembolic disease, and primary pulmonary hypertension. Evaluation of breathing during sleep is necessary when everything except the right heart seems to function normally during wakefulness. Lung perfusion scans and selective angiography are then appropriate for identifying vascular obstruction. When these studies are also negative, lung biopsy is appropriate for evaluating the nature of vessel structural alterations. However, lung biopsies may be of limited value insofar as the histologic findings may not reflect the cause of the disease as much as the degree of vascular remodeling. Clinical entities that produce pulmonary hypertension in children are listed in Table 41–7.

THERAPY AND OUTCOME

Therapy for patients with pulmonary hypertension is designed to prevent its progression, if not completely reverse the condition. The degree to which reversal is possible may depend on the severity of pulmonary remodeling at the time when treatment is initiated. Treatment of cor pulmonale and pulmonary hypertension includes therapies that improve the underlying pulmonary disor-

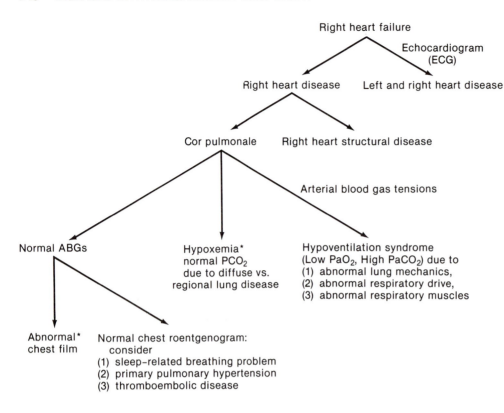

Figure 41–7. Diagnostic approach to unexplained right heart failure.

*Abnormal chest roentgenogram will lead to further diagnostic evaluation, depending on radiographic appearance of the chest (airway disease, interstitial lung disease, etc.)

der and those that modify the pulmonary vasculature directly. Examples of the former include tonsillectomy and adenoidectomy for upper airway obstruction resulting from tonsillar and adenoidal hypertrophy and anti-

Table 41–7. PEDIATRIC CONDITIONS CAUSING PULMONARY HYPERTENSION

Hypoxia
Bronchopulmonary dysplasia
Cystic fibrosis
Interstitial lung disease
Hypoventilation syndromes (central nervous system disorders)
Respiratory muscle weakness (e.g., Duchenne's muscular dystrophy)
Chest wall disorders (kyphoscoliosis, thoracic dystrophies)
Upper airway obstructions (tonsil and adenoid enlargement, macroglossia, obesity)
High Pulmonary Blood Flow
Left-to-right congenital heart lesions (e.g., ventricular septal defect)
Occlusion Disorders
Thromboembolism (acute, chronic)
Veno-occlusive disease
Sickle cell disease
Pulmonary Vasculitis
Collagen vascular disease (systemic lupus erythematosus, polyarteritis, scleroderma)
Granulomatous vascular disease (e.g., Wegener's granulomatosis)
Tuberculosis
Schistosomiasis
Vascular Obstructive Disease
Left ventricular failure
Obstructive anomalous pulmonary veins
Mitral valve stenosis
Cor triatriatum
Idiopathic
Primary pulmonary hypertension

biotics for children with bronchiectasis and cystic fibrosis. Figure 41–8 illustrates the immediate hemodynamic improvement in response to acute oxygen therapy and the long-term hemodynamic response 3 months after adenoidectomy in a child with upper airway obstruction. Mechanical ventilation is another form of therapy that reverses cor pulmonale associated with hypoventilation syndromes resulting from brainstem lesions and disorders producing respiratory muscular weakness.

Specific vascular treatment of pulmonary hypertension is best considered under three circumstances: (1) the immediate treatment of right heart failure associated with cor pulmonale, (2) the immediate treatment of suprasystemic pulmonary hypertension as occurs in PPHN, and (3) treatment of chronic pulmonary hypertension.

Treatment of right heart failure associated with cor pulmonale is designed to maintain cardiac output, maintain coronary perfusion to the right ventricle, and ensure adequate tissue oxygenation. These goals are accomplished by ensuring adequate right ventricular preload, maintaining systemic blood pressure to keep up adequate right coronary artery perfusion pressure, and reducing right ventricular work with judicious use of vasodilating agents in addition to oxygen. Intravascular fluid administration is important when inadequate preload is adversely affecting cardiac output. However, too much fluid leads to overdistension of the already dilated right ventricle, producing tricuspid insufficiency and perhaps reduced left ventricular diastolic filling volume. In such cases, quantitative monitoring of cardiac output directly, as with a thermodilution pulmonary artery catheter, provides immediate feedback as to how much intravascular fluid is needed.

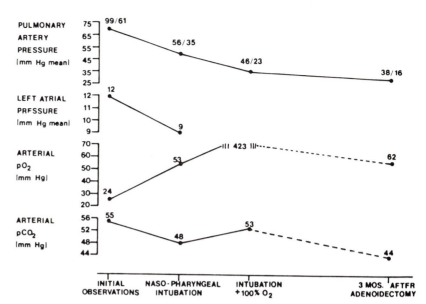

Figure 41–8. Short-term and long-term hemodynamic response of a child with adenoidal hypertrophy and pulmonary hypertension acutely to oxygen and long term after adenoidectomy. (From Levy AM, Tabakin BS, Hanson JS, et al: Hypertrophied adenoids causing pulmonary hypertension and severe congestive heart failure. N Engl J Med 277:506–511, 1967. Reprinted with permission from *The New England Journal of Medicine,* vol. 277, pp. 506–511, 1967.)

Maintaining systemic blood pressure with alpha-adrenergic agents such as phenylephrine or norepinephrine or, alternatively, with inotropic agents such as dopamine or dobutamine ensures adequate right coronary artery perfusion, and hence right ventricular perfusion, despite the increase in right ventricular work.[77] An alternative treatment in adults for maintaining systemic blood pressure has been aortic balloon counterpulsation.[78] This treatment has not been used for right heart failure in children. Diuretic therapy is used to reduce hepatic congestion and pedal edema in patients with right heart failure. This palliative approach is designed to increase the comfort of the child in right heart failure. In contrast, the effectiveness of diuretics in reducing right ventricular dilation in the presence of right heart failure is unclear and at times counterproductive to administration of intravascular fluids used for maintaining cardiac output.

The effectiveness of digitalis as treatment of right heart failure in patients with cor pulmonale remains unsubstantiated. Digitalis may improve myocardial contractility and cardiac output, particularly when left ventricular function is poor. However, digitalis also produces pulmonary vasoconstriction and can therefore increase right ventricular afterload.[79] Like diuretics, digitalis can also reduce systemic venous return and decrease cardiac output when right ventricular functional compensation exists in the presence of pulmonary hypertension.[80]

The use of vasodilators has been unpredictably beneficial because of the nonspecificity of vasodilating agents. Table 41–6 lists such agents used in both adults and children. As with fluid administration, the effectiveness of these agents in the presence of right heart failure is best monitored directly in the intensive care setting.

The treatment of PPHN is designed to improve pulmonary blood flow into the lungs and minimize blood flow bypassing the lungs via the ductus arteriosus and the foramen ovale. Such measures directly improve preductal arterial oxygenation by reducing Ppa to values less than systemic artery pressures and right atrial pressures to values lower than left atrial pressures. Therapies that have improved clinical outcome include assurance of optimal ventilation and alveolar oxygen tension with mechanical ventilation and supplemental inspired oxygen. They have also included measures to increase arterial pH to values above 7.55, both by hyperventilation to arterial carbon dioxide pressure/tension values of 20 to 30 mm Hg and by intravenous bicarbonate and tromethamine (THAM) administation, in order to further reduce pulmonary vasospasm.[81, 82] Sedation, paralysis, and minimizing episodic hypoxia, as occurs with endotracheal tube suctioning, have also been used as adjunctive forms of therapy. In addition, intravascular volume and systemic pressors such as dopamine are used, as in cases of right heart failure from cor pulmonale, in order to maintain cardiac output, right ventricular perfusion, and hence right ventricular function. Pulmonary vasodilators such as tolazoline (Priscoline) and prostacyclin were previously considered important components of treatment.[83, 84] However, the incidence of systemic hypotension and the unpredictable response to such agents by the pulmonary vasculature to dilate more than the systemic arterial bed have made this form of therapy uncommon.

The latest maneuver to reduce mortality from PPHN has been the use of extracorporeal membrane oxygenation (ECMO) in newborns. The use of the membrane oxygenator to increase venous oxygen pressure/tension and deliver it mechanically to the systemic circulation has improved survival rates among neonates with PPHN to more than 80%.[81] Although criteria for initiation of ECMO continue to evolve, the patient who fails the aforementioned approaches to treatment should be considered a candidate, and the regional neonatal ECMO program should be consulted to ensure safe transport and initiation of ECMO therapy.

The pulmonary vascular treatment of chronic pulmonary hypertension is based on the idea that processes leading to vascular remodeling must be reversed.[85] Despite dramatic histologic changes in pulmonary arterial architecture, the premise exists that ongoing vessel wall tension resulting from ongoing or recurrent vasoconstriction can be reduced, thereby reversing some of the structural features of remodeled vessels with narrow intraluminal dimensions. It is clear that in some patients with primary pulmonary hypertension, bronchopulmonary dysplasia, pulmonary veno-occlusive disease, and cystic fibrosis, the administration of oxygen reverses hypoxic pulmonary vasoconstriction and acutely reduces increased pulmonary vascular resistance despite the existence of pulmonary vascular remodeling.[86, 87] Animal studies suggest that a further benefit of longer term oxygen therapy of 20 weeks' duration is chronic reduction in vascular wall tension and actual reversal of medial muscle hypertrophy associated with chronic alveolar hypoxia.[88] Oxygen therapy may therefore have acute and chronic therapeutic effects that are distinct.

The amount and duration of supplemental oxygen necessary to provide maximal therapeutic benefit to a child with pulmonary hypertension are unknown. Two large-scale prospective studies involving adults with COPD and evaluating the effects of long-term oxygen therapy on survival provide the most cogent evidence for continuous oxygen therapy as a means of prolonging life in the presence of chronic lung disease and pulmonary hypertension. The British Medical Research Council (MRC) study compared survival among patients with COPD who received no oxygen therapy and a group that received 2 l/min of oxygen for 15 h/day.[89] Patients were observed for a period of 36 to 60 months. Both groups had carbon dioxide retention and moderate pulmonary hypertension at the time of enrollment. The mortality rate among patients receiving no oxygen therapy was approximately 67% over 5 years, in comparison with the group receiving part-time oxygen, among whom the mortality rate was 45% over the same duration. In a similar study, the National Institutes of Health–sponsored Nocturnal Oxygen Therapy Trial (NOTT) compared use of oxygen that maintained $Pa_{O_2} > 65$ mm Hg for 12 h/day with use of oxygen for more than 19 h/day in patients comparable with those studied in England.[90] The survival rate among patients using oxygen 12 h/day was 41% over 2 years, similar to the rate among British subjects using oxygen for 15 h/day. The mortality rate among subjects using oxygen 19 to 24 h/day was only 22% over the first 2 years of the study. These results are shown in Figure 41–9. The conclusion reached after a review of both studies is that some oxygen is good, and more continuous use of supplemental oxygen in patients with chronic lung disease and pulmonary hypertension improves survival even more. In both studies, oxygen tensions were maintained above 55 mm Hg. Results from an evaluation of the improvement in survival of children with Eisenmenger's syndrome who received home oxygen therapy confirm that these conclusions also apply to children with chronic pulmonary hypertension.[91]

Pulmonary hemodynamic changes associated with oxygen therapy in both the MRC and NOTT studies were not dramatic. Over the duration of the study, British subjects receiving oxygen for 15 h/day experienced no change in mean Ppa or PVR. In the NOTT study, continuous oxygen therapy resulted in greater reductions in pulmonary vascular resistance than in patients receiving oxygen for 12 h/day. However, the absolute amount of hemodynamic improvement in both groups was only modest, which suggests that reduction in pulmonary hypertension

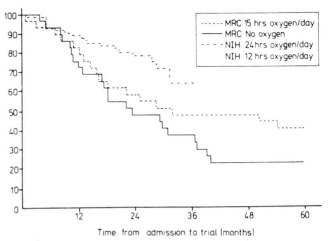

Figure 41–9. Survival curves from the British Medical Research Council and Nocturnal Oxygen Therapy Trial long-term oxygen therapy studies of adults with chronic obstructive pulmonary disease and pulmonary hypertension. Survival was greatest among patients who had used supplemental oxygen continuously.[62, 66]

and the prevention of the progression of pulmonary hypertension may not be the only explanation for improved survival in patients with COPD. The reduction in polycythemia and the improvement in tissue oxygen delivery in response to supplemental oxygen may also have influenced survival.

An exception to the strategy of continuous oxygen therapy applies to patients who clearly have sleep-related breathing disorders and sleep-exacerbated hypoxemia. When arterial blood gas tensions or oxyhemoglobin saturations are normal in conscious patients with pulmonary hypertension and sleep-related respiratory problems, nighttime oxygen treatment may be all that is necessary to reverse cor pulmonale and pulmonary hypertension. Along these lines, it is clear that patients with chronic airway obstruction, such as bronchopulmonary dysplasia, experience more hypoxemia when asleep than when awake and quiet.[92] Such patients may require more supplemental oxygen when asleep in order to maintain acceptable blood oxygen values. In this setting, a strategy for oxygen administration that separates sleep from awake oxygen requirements may provide the most rational and cost-effective form of chronic oxygen therapy in the hospital or at home.

Additional long-term therapies for chronic pulmonary hypertension for which the benefits are less well documented include pulmonary vasodilators, anticoagulants, and lung transplantation.

The effectiveness of long-term vasodilator therapy depends on the cause for pulmonary hypertension in each individual. Patients with chronic lung disease and hypoxemia may benefit more because of reversal of ongoing degree of pulmonary vasoconstriction resulting from alveolar hypoxia by vasodilator drugs. In contrast, children with primary pulmonary hypertension and advanced plexiform lesions are unlikely to derive much benefit from such agents. Furthermore, there are fewer pulmonary vasodilators available for long-term use because fewer oral preparations exist. The long-term vasodilators most commonly used to treat chronic pulmonary hypertension are calcium-channel blockers, nitroglycerin, and hydralazine. In studies of patients with COPD, hydralazine appeared to be superior to nitrates because it increased oxygen tissue delivery and cardiac index more predictably.[93] In young adults with cystic fibrosis, nifedipine reduced pulmonary vascular resistance, increased cardiac output, and improved exercise tolerance.[94] However, in a similar study, both nifedipine and hydralazine reduced pulmonary vascular resistance in adults with cystic fibrosis, but only hydralazine increased oxygen tissue delivery.[95]

The influence of vasodilators on survival of patients with chronic pulmonary hypertension remains unclear. Dosages of these drugs must be low enough to minimize systemic hypotension and its clinical consequences. In addition, pulmonary vasodilators may reduce efficient ventilation/perfusion matching because of loss of hypoxic pulmonary vasoconstriction and may lead to arterial hypoxemia. Current recommendations include the use of vasodilators in conjunction with supplemental oxygen to minimize arterial hypoxemia while minimizing the pulmonary vasoconstriction component of chronic pulmonary hypertension. Long-term collaborative studies are necessary to determine whether pulmonary vasodilators with or without concomitant oxygen therapy further improve survival in pediatric patients.

Anticoagulation therapy is the hallmark of chronic treatment for recurrent pulmonary thromboembolic disease. However, it may have an additional role in the treatment of chronic pulmonary hypertension regardless of cause. If thrombosis within narrowed, remodeled pulmonary vessels is a common late pathophysiologic event, anticoagulant therapy may delay final obliteration of such vessels and prolong survival. Results from a study conducted at the Mayo Clinic suggest that this may be the case. The clinical courses of 120 adult patients with nonembolic pulmonary hypertension were reviewed over a 3-year period. Survival in groups that received warfarin (Coumadin) was almost twice that of patients who did not receive anticoagulants.[96] Prospective therapeutic trials in both pediatric and adult patients must be performed to confirm these findings.

A final consideration in the future may be lung transplantation. Adults with Eisenmenger's syndrome and with primary pulmonary hypertension have successfully received single-lung, double-lung, and heart-lung transplants.[97] This is not currently a widespread clinical option for children with pulmonary hypertension. Its value will depend on the continued development of the transplantation expertise and availability.

REFERENCES

1. Allen H, Taussig LM, Gaines JA, et al: Echocardiograph profiles of the long-term cardiac changes in cystic fibrosis. Chest 75:428–433, 1979.
2. Goodman G, Perkin, R, Anas N, et al: Pulmonary hypertension in infants with bronchopulmonary dysplasia. J Pediatr 112:67–72, 1988.
3. Hoffman JIE, Rudolph AM: The natural history of ventricular septal defects in infancy. Am J Cardiol 16:634–653, 1965.
4. Reid JM, Stevenson JG, Coleman EN, et al: Moderate to severe pulmonary hypertension accompanying patent ductus arteriosus. Br Heart J 26:600–605, 1964.
5. Stack BHR, Choo-Kang YF, Heard BE: The prognosis of cryptogenic fibrosing alveolitis. Thorax 27:535–542, 1972.
6. Ahmed T, Oliver W, Wanner A: Variability of hypoxic pulmonary vasoconstriction in sheep. Am Rev Respir Dis 127:59–62, 1983.
7. Benotti JR, Dalen JE: The natural history of pulmonary embolism. Clin Chest Med 5:403–410, 1984.
8. Butler J, Schrijen F, Henriquez A, et al: Cause of increased right and left atrial pressures in patients with obstructed airflow disease. Chest 93:171S–172S, 1988.
9. Barer GR, Emery CJ, Bee D, et al: Mechanisms of pulmonary hypertension: An overview. In Wills JA (ed): The Pulmonary Circulation in Health and Disease, pp. 405–423. Orlando, FL: Academic Press, 1987.
10. Flenley DC: Sleep in chronic obstructive lung disease. Clin Chest Med 6:651–661, 1985.
11. Badesch DB, Orton EC, Zapp L, et al: Decreased arterial wall prostaglandin production in neonatal calves with severe chronic pulmonary hypertension, Am J Respir Cell Mol Biol 1:489–498, 1989.
12. Todorovich-Hunter L, Johnson D, Ranger P, et al: Altered elastin and collagen synthesis associated with progressive pulmonary hypertension induced by monocrotaline: A biochemical and ultrastructural study. Lab Invest 58:184–195, 1988.
13. Reid L: Vascular remodeling. In Fischman A (ed): The Pulmonary Circulation: Normal and Abnormal, pp. 343–352. Philadelphia: University of Pennsylvania Press, 1990.
14. Hislop A, Reid L: Pulmonary arterial development during childhood: Branching pattern and structure. Thorax 28:129–135, 1973.
15. Wagonvoort CA: Pulmonary veno-occlusive disease. In Fischman A (ed): The Pulmonary Circulation: Normal and Abnormal, pp. 343–352. Philadelphia: University of Pennsylvania Press, 1990.
16. Voelkel N: Mechanisms of hypoxic pulmonary vasoconstriction. Am Rev Respir Dis 133:1186–1195, 1986.
17. Rudolph AM, Yuan S: Response of the pulmonary vasculature to hypoxia and H$^+$ ion concentration changes. J Clin Invest 45:399–411, 1966.
18. Rabinovitch M, Gamble W, Nadas AS, et al: Rat pulmonary circulation after chronic hypoxia: Hemodynamic and structural features. Am J Physiol 236:H818–H827, 1979.
19. Yohn SE, Polan GJ, Tozzi CA, et al: Elastin synthesis in the hypertensive pulmonary artery of the rat. Am Rev Respir Dis 135:A130, 1987.
20. Fried R, Reid LM: Early recovery from hypoxic pulmonary hypertension: A structural and functional study. J Appl Physiol 57:1247–1253, 1984.
21. Levy AM, Tabakin BS, Hanson JS, et al: Hypertrophied adenoids causing pulmonary hypertension and severe congestive heart failure. N Engl J Med 277:506–511, 1967.
22. Rabinovitch M: Pulmonary hypertension in the presence of high blood flow. In Will J (ed): The Pulmonary Circulation in Health and Disease, pp. 423–442. Orlando, FL: Academic Press, 1987.
23. Rabinovitch M, Bothwell T, Hayakawa BN, et al: Pulmonary artery endothelial abnormalities in patients with congenital heart defects and pulmonary hypertension: A correlation of light with scanning electron microscopy and transmission electron microscopy. Lab Invest 55:632–653, 1986.
24. Heath D, Edwards JE: The pathway of hypertensive pulmonary vascular disease: A description of six grades of structural changes in the pulmonary arteries with special reference to congenital cardiac defects. Circulation 18:533–547, 1958.
25. Juaneda E, Haworth SG: Pulmonary vascular structure in patients dying after a Fontan procedure: The lung as a risk factor. Br Heart J 52:575–580, 1984.
26. Rabinovitch M, Keane JF, Norwood W, et al: Vascular structure in lung tissue obtained at biopsy correlated with pulmonary hemodynamic findings after repair of congenital heart defects. Circulation 69:655–667, 1984.
27. Moser K: Pulmonary vascular obstruction due to embolism and thrombosis. In Moser K (ed): Pulmonary Vascular Diseases, pp. 365–366. New York: Marcel Dekker, 1979.
28. Paraskos JA, Adelstein SJ, Smith RE, et al: Late prognosis of acute pulmonary embolism. N Engl J Med 289:55–58, 1973.
29. Dreisin RB: Pulmonary vasculitis. Clin Chest Med 3:607–618, 1982.

30. Haworth SG, Reid L: Quantitative structural study of pulmonary circulation in the newborn with pulmonary atresia. Thorax 32:129–133, 1977.

31. Hislop A, Reid L: Structural changes in the pulmonary arteries and veins in tetrology of Fallot. Br Heart J 35:1178–1183, 1973.

32. Murphy JD, Rabinovitch M, Goldstein JD, et al: The structural basis of persistent pulmonary hypertension of the newborn infant. J Pediatr 98:962–967, 1981.

33. Abman SH, Accurso FJ, Wilkening RB, et al: Persistent fetal pulmonary hypoperfusion after acute hypoxia. Am J Physiol 253:H941–H948, 1987.

34. Levin DL, Mills LJ, Parkey M, et al: Constriction of the fetal ductus arteriosus after administration of indomethacin to the pregnant ewe. J Pediatr 94:647–650, 1979.

35. Greenwood RD, Nadas AS: The clinical course of cardiac disease in Down's syndrome. Pediatrics 58:893–897, 1976.

36. Stenmark KR, Fasules J, Hyde DM, et al: Severe pulmonary hypertension and arterial adventitial changes in newborn calves at 4300 m. J Appl Physiol 62:821–830, 1987.

37. McMurtry IF, Petrun MD, Reeves JT, et al: Lungs from chronically hypoxic rats have decreased pressor response to acute hypoxia. Am J Physiol 235:H104–H109, 1978.

38. Cournand A, Bloomfield RA, Lauson HD: Double lumen catheter for intravenous and intracardiac blood sampling and pressure recording. Proc Soc Exp Biol Med 60:73–78, 1945.

39. Moss AJ, Emmanouilides G, Duffie ER: Closure of the ductus arteriosus in the newborn infant. Pediatrics 32:25–30, 1963.

40. Krovetz LJ, Goldbloom S: Normal standards for cardiovascular data. II: Pressure and vascular resistances. Johns Hopkins Med J 130:187–195, 1972.

41. Reeves JT, Dempsey JA, Grover RF: Pulmonary circulation during exercise. In Weir EK, Reeves JT (eds): Pulmonary Vascular Physiology and Pathophysiology, pp. 107–135. New York: Marcel Dekker, 1985.

42. Robin ED, Gaudia R: Cor pulmonale. Dis Mon May:3–38, 1970.

43. Jezek V, Schrijen F, Sadoul P: Right ventricular function and pulmonary hemodynamics during exercise in patients with COPD. Cardiology 58:20–31, 1973.

44. Brandfonbrener M, Turino G, Himmelstein A, et al: Effects of occlusion of one pulmonary artery on pulmonary circulation in man. Fed Proc 17:19, 1958.

45. Ohkuda K, Nakahara K, Weidner WJ, et al: Lung fluid exchange after uneven pulmonary artery obstruction in sheep. Circ Res 43:152–161, 1978.

46. Vlahakes GJ, Turley K, Hoffman JI: The pathophysiology of failure in acute right ventricular hypertension: Hemodynamic and biochemical correlations. Circulation 63:87–95, 1981.

47. Berger HJ, Matthay RA, Loke J, et al: Assessment of cardiac performance with quantitative radionuclide angiography: Right ventricular ejection fraction with reference to findings in chronic obstructive pulmonary disease. Am J Cardiol 41:897–905, 1978.

48. Brent BN, Berger HJ, Matthay RA, et al: Physiologic correlates of right ventricular ejection fraction in COPD: A combined radionuclide and hemodynamic study. Am J Cardiol 50:255–262, 1982.

49. Reeves JT, Groves BM, Morrison DA, et al: Right ventricular function in pulmonary hypertension. In Weir EK, Reeves JT (eds): Pulmonary Vascular Physiology and Pathophysiology, pp. 325–351. New York: Marcel Dekker, 1985.

50. Davies H, Overy HR: Left ventricular function in cor pulmonale. Chest 58:8–14, 1970.

51. Fishman AP: Chronic cor pulmonale. Am Rev Respir Dis 114:775–794, 1976.

52. Stool EW, Mullins CB, Leshin SJ, et al: Dimensional changes of the left ventricle during acute pulmonary arterial hypertension in dogs. Am J Cardiol 33:868–875, 1974.

53. Khaja F, Parker JO: Right and left ventricular performance in chronic obstructive lung disease. Am Heart J 82:319–327, 1971.

54. Matthay RA, Berger HJ, Davies R, et al: Right and left ventricular exercise performance in COPD: Radionuclide assessment. Ann Intern Med 93:234–239, 1980.

55. McIlroy MB, Apthorp GH: Pulmonary function in pulmonary hypertension. Br Heart J 20:397–402, 1958.

56. Fernandez-Bonetti P, Lupi-Herrera E, Martinez-Guerra ML, et al: Peripheral airways obstruction in idiopathic pulmonary artery hypertension. Chest 83:732–738, 1983.

57. Dantzker DR, Bower JS: Mechanisms of gas exchange abnormality in patients with chronic obliterative pulmonary vascular disease. J Clin Invest 64:1050–1055, 1979.

58. Dantzker DR: The influence of cardiovascular function on gas exchange. Clin Chest Med 4:149–159, 1983.

59. Heymann MA, Soifer SJ: Persistent pulmonary hypertension of the newborn. In Fishman A (ed): The Pulmonary Circulation: Normal and Abnormal, pp. 371–384. Philadelphia: University of Pennsylvania Press, 1990.

60. Krieger J: Breathing during sleep in normal subjects. Clin Chest Med 6:577–594, 1985.

61. Rich S, Dantzker DR, Ayres SM, et al: Primary pulmonary hypertension: A national prospective study. Ann Intern Med 107:216–223, 1987.

62. Gregaratos G, Karliner JS, Moser KM: Mechanisms of disease and methods of assessment. In Moser KM (ed): Pulmonary Vascular Disease, pp. 282–292. New York: Marcel Dekker, 1975.

63. Hill N: The cardiac exam in lung disease. Clin Chest Med 8:273–285, 1987.

64. Schrijen F, Jezek V: Haemodynamics and pulmonary wedge angiography findings in chronic bronchopulmonary disease. Scand J Respir Dis 58:151–158, 1977.

65. Newth CJ, Corey M, Fowler RS, et al: Thallium myocardial perfusion scans for the assessment of right ventricular hypertrophy in patients with cystic fibrosis. Am Rev Respir Dis 124:463–468, 1981.

66. Berger HJ, Matthay RA, Pytlik LM, et al: First pass radionuclide assessment of right and left ventricular performance in patients with cardiac and pulmonary disease. Semin Nucl Med 9:275–295, 1975.

67. Chipps BE, Alderson PO, Roland JM, et al: Non-invasive evaluation of ventricular function in cystic fibrosis. J Pediatr 95:379–384, 1979.

68. Chou TC, Masangkay MP, Young R, et al: Simple quantitative vectorcardiograph criteria for the diagnosis of right ventricular hypertrophy. Circulation 48:1262–1267, 1973.

69. Liebman J, Krause DA, Doershuk CF, et al: Orthogonal vectorcardiogram in cystic fibrosis: Diagnostic significance and correlation with pulmonary function tests. A four year follow-up. Chest 63:218–226, 1973.

70. Park MK, Guntheroth WG: How to Read Pediatric ECGs. Chicago: Yearbook Medical Publishers, 1987.

71. Kilcoyne MM, Davis AL, Ferrer MI: A dynamic electrocardiographic concept useful in the diagnosis of cor pulmonale. Circulation 52:903–924, 1970.

72. Nanda NC, Gramiak R, Robinson TI, et al: Electrocardiographic evaluation of pulmonary hypertension. Circulation 50:575–581, 1974.

73. Moss AJ, Adams FH, Emmanouilides GC: Heart Disease in Infants, Children and Adolescents, 2nd ed. Baltimore, MD: Williams & Wilkins, 1977.

74. Keane JF, Fyler DC: Hazards of cardiac catheterization in children with primary pulmonary vascular obstruction. Lancet 1:863, 1977.

75. Reeves JT, Groves BM, Turkevich D: The case for the treatment of selected patients with primary pulmonary hypertension. Am Rev Respir Dis 134:342–346, 1986.

76. Baughman R, Inkley SR: Letter to the editor. N Engl J Med 296:631–632, 1977.

77. Prewitt RM, Ghignone M: Treatment of right ventricular dysfunction in acute respiratory failure. Crit Care Med 11:346–352, 1983.

78. Spotnitz HM, Berman MA, Epstein SE: Pathophysiology and experimental treatment of acute pulmonary embolism. Am Heart J 82:511–520, 1971.

79. Kim YS, Aviado DM: Digitalis and the pulmonary circulation. Am Heart J 62:680–686, 1961.

80. Sylvester JT, Goldberg HS, Permutt S: The role of the vasculature in the regulation of cardiac output. Clin Chest Med 4:111–126, 1983.

81. Clarke WR: The transitional circulation: Physiology and anesthetic implications. J Clin Anesthesiol 2:192–211, 1990.

82. Drummond W, Gregory G, Heymann M, et al: The independent effects of hyperventilation, tolazoline and dopamine on infants with persistent pulmonary hypertension. J Pediatr 98:603–611, 1981.

83. Peckham GJ: The risk-benefit relationships of current therapeutic approaches. In Peckham GJ, Heymann MA (eds): Cardiovascular Sequelae of Asphyxia in the Newborn, 83rd Ross Conference on Pediatric Research, pp. 110–116. Columbus, OH: 1982.

84. Peckham G, Fox W: Physiologic factors affecting pulmonary artery pressure in infants with persistent pulmonary hypertension. J Pediatr 93:1005–1010, 1978.
85. Weir K: Acute vasodilator testing and pharmacologic treatment of primary pulmonary hypertension. In Fishman A (ed): The Pulmonary Circulation: Normal and Abnormal, pp. 485–500. Philadelphia: University of Pennsylvania Press, 1990.
86. Abman SH, Wolfe RR, Accurso FJ, et al: Pulmonary vascular response to oxygen in infants with severe bronchopulmonary dysplasia. Pediatrics 75:80–84, 1985.
87. Palevsky HI, Pietra GG, Fishman AP: Pulmonary veno-occlusive disease and its response to vasodilator agents. Am Rev Respir Dis 142:426–429, 1990.
88. Herget J, Suggett AJ, Leach E, et al: Resolution of pulmonary hypertension and other features induced by chronic hypoxia in rats during complete and intermittent normoxia. Thorax 33:468–473, 1978.
89. MRC Working Party: Long-term domiciliary oxygen therapy in chronic hypoxic cor pulmonale complicating chronic bronchitis and emphysema. Lancet 1:681–686, 1981.
90. Nocturnal Oxygen Therapy Trial Group: Continuous or nocturnal oxygen therapy in hypoxemic chronic obstructive lung disease: A clinical trial. Ann Intern Med 93:391–398, 1980.
91. Bowyer JJ, Busst CM, Denison DM, et al: Effect of long term oxygen treatment at home in children with pulmonary vascular disease. Br Heart J 55:385–390, 1986.
92. Garg M, Kurzner SI, Bautista DB, et al: Clinically unsuspected hypoxia during sleep and feeding in infants with bronchopulmonary dysplasia. Pediatrics 81:635–642, 1988.
93. Brent BN, Berger HJ, Matthay RA, et al: Contrasting acute effects of vasodilators on right ventricular performance in patients with COPD and pulmonary hypertension: A combined radionuclide-hemodynamic study. Am J Cardiol 51:1682–1689, 1983.
94. Michael JR, Kennedy TP, Fitzpatrick S, et al: Nifedipine inhibits hypoxic pulmonary vasoconstriction during rest and exercise in patients with cystic fibrosis and cor pulmonale. Am Rev Respir Dis 130:516–519, 1984.
95. Geggel RL, Dozor AJ, Fyler DC, et al: Effect of vasodilators at rest and during exercise in young adults with cystic fibrosis and cor pulmonale. Am Rev Respir Dis 131:531–536, 1985.
96. Foster V, Steele PM, Edwards WD, et al: Primary pulmonary hypertension: Natural history and the importance of thrombosis. Circulation 70:580–587, 1984.
97. Morrison D, Maurer JR, Grossman RF: Preoperative assessment for lung transplantation. Clin Chest Med 11:207–215, 1990.

42 INTERSTITIAL LUNG DISEASE IN CHILDREN

BETTINA C. HILMAN, M.D.

Interstitial lung disease (ILD) includes a heterogeneous group of disorders of both known and unknown causes that share a common finding—inflammation of the pulmonary interstitium (i.e., the alveolar walls and perialveolar tissues)—but differ in the type of inflammatory response and the degree of progression to interstitial fibrosis. Since 1970, considerable progress has been made in the understanding of ILD in adults; however, little information about ILD in pediatric patients is available. It is also not certain as to what extent the knowledge of ILD in adults[1-23] and in experimental animal models[24-27] can be applied to ILD in children. Currently, there is increased interest in ILD in children because of the expanding number of pediatric patients with acquired immunodeficiency syndrome (AIDS) who have lymphoid interstitial pneumonitis (LIP).

There are considerable differences in opinion about the exact definition of ILD in children. The author defines pediatric ILD (PILD) as a group of disorders characterized by inflammation of the pulmonary interstitium that can resolve completely or partially or progress to derangement of the alveolar structures with varying degrees of fibrosis and loss of functional alveolar units. Like ILD in adults, PILD includes a heterogeneous group of pulmonary disorders in which there is primary inflammation of the lung (primary lung disease) or the inflammatory disease in the lung is secondary to other underlying condi-

tions. Both ILD and PILD imply some degree of chronicity with a potential for progression to pulmonary fibrosis.

One of the underlying problems limiting the knowledge and understanding of PILD is the lack of a significant number of well-documented cases in any one medical center for critical scientific evaluation. Thus PILD could qualify as one of the pediatric "orphan lung diseases." To address this problem, a national cooperative effort has been initiated to improve the understanding of PILD and to formulate a mechanism for review of appropriate cases of PILD so that prospective multicenter studies can be conducted in the future. This chapter includes some of the information from this national working group.

The term *interstitial* is considered a misnomer because ILD histologically involves alveolar epithelial cells, endothelial cells, and perialveolar tissues of the small airways (bronchioles), as well as the small arteries and veins of the pulmonary parenchyma in some cases. The pulmonary interstitium is anatomically bounded by the alveolar epithelial and endothelial basement membranes and normally contains connective tissue components, mesenchymal cells, and inflammatory immune effector cells (monocytes, macrophages, and lymphocytes). Some authors object to the use of the word *disease* to refer to such a spectrum of clinical histologic findings that share a common pathogenic mechanism and pathophysiologic sequelae. The substitution of the term *disorder* for *disease* should dispel this semantic dispute.

There are no pathognomonic clinical or laboratory criteria for the diagnosis of PILD other than the characteristic histologic findings on lung biopsy. Thus a lung biopsy is the gold standard for determining whether the infant or child suspected of having PILD (either by clinical signs and symptoms or characteristic chest radiographic findings) meets the histologic criteria of ILD. The incidence of PILD is uncertain. However, if histologic criteria used to describe ILD in adults are applied, PILD would include disorders characterized by inflammation of the pulmonary interstitium and would require histologic confirmation by lung biopsy.

Because of the invasive nature of open-lung biopsy, children with persistent or chronic forms of ILD and children who are immunocompromised would be more likely to undergo histologic studies to confirm the diagnosis of ILD. Infants and children with acute forms of ILD or chronic forms that resolve completely or with few sequelae are usually not evaluated histologically. In this chapter, only the chronic forms of interstitial pneumonitis with and without fibrosis are discussed.

CLASSIFICATION

PILD can be classified by various criteria, including status of the lung disease (i.e., primary ILD or ILD associated with other conditions), type of onset, etiology, immune status, clinical course, and histologic appearance. Because histologic criteria are essential for the diagnosis, as well as for understanding the pathogenesis and clinical variants of this heterogeneous disorder, histologic findings are often used as the basis for classification (Table 42–1). Liebow[2] proposed six histologic classifications based on the predominant inflammatory cell type: lymphoid interstitial pneumonitis (LIP), giant cell interstitial pneumonitis (GIP), plasma cell interstitial pneumonitis (PIP), desquamative interstitial pneumonitis (DIP), usual interstitial pneumonitis (UIP), and bronchiolitis obliterans associated with interstitial pneumonitis (BIP). The inclusion of bronchiolitis obliterans or bronchiolitis obliterans with organizing pneumonia under ILD in a Liebow classification is not accepted by many pathologists because the clinical spectrum and prognosis of patients with these disorders are usually better than with UIP and many of the other types of ILD. Bronchiolitis obliterans is discussed in Chapter 23.

The term UIP refers to a nonspecific type of ILD of unknown cause associated with a progressive interstitial inflammatory process and fibrosis. Clinicians often use this term indiscriminantly with idiopathic pulmonary fibrosis or cryptogenic fibrosing alveolitis.

PATHOPHYSIOLOGY

If the pathogenesis of PILD is the same as that of ILD in adults, the common mechanism of this heterogeneous group of disorders is alveolitis. Alveolitis results from injury to the alveolar wall (i.e., to the alveolar epithelium

Table 42–1. CLASSIFICATION OF INTERSTITIAL LUNG DISEASE IN CHILDREN

Status of Pulmonary Disease
Primary pulmonary disease
Secondary to or associated with other conditions
Type of Onset
Acute
Chronic
Etiology
Known causes
Unknown causes
Associated with other conditions
Type of Host
Immunocompetent
Immunocompromised
Primary immunodeficiency
Acquired immunodeficiency (e.g., acquired immunodeficiency syndrome [AIDS])
Clinical Course
Asymptomatic (subclinical)
Symptomatic (stabilized or progressive)
Histologic Findings
Predominant Cell Type (e.g., LIP)
Granulomatous-Nongranulomatous
Pulmonary Fibrosis (Focal or Diffuse)
Clinical Histologic Diagnostic Categories
Nonspecific or usual interstitial pneumonitis (UIP)
Interstitial pneumonitis with sarcoidosis
Interstitial pneumonitis with pulmonary hemosiderosis (e.g., idiopathic pulmonary hemosiderosis)
Pulmonary alveolar proteinosis
Desquamative interstitial pneumonitis
Lymphoid interstitial pneumonitis
Idiopathic pulmonary fibrosis or interstitial pneumonitis with fibrosis
Associated Findings
Bronchiolitis obliterans*
Bronchiolitis obliterans with organizing pneumonia (BOOP)*
Alveolar proteinosis
Interstitial pneumonitis with giant cells
Pulmonary infiltrates with eosinophilia
Liebow's[2] Classification
Giant cell interstitial pneumonitis (GIP)
Plasma cell interstitial pneumonitis (PIP)
Bronchiolitis obliterans with interstitial pneumonitis (BIP)
Lymphoid interstitial pneumonitis (LIP)
Desquamative interstitial pneumonitis (DIP)

*Not accepted by many pathologists because the clinical spectrum and prognosis of patients with these disorders differ from those of the other types of interstitial pneumonitis.

or to the endothelium of the alveolar wall or to both) from known or unknown causes associated with a variable influx of inflammatory cells and immune effector cell responses.[10] The inflammatory responses in the alveolar walls and perialveolar tissues cause a thickening of the alveolar septum and distortion by inflammatory cells or fibrosis. The initial lesion is potentially reversible. However, if the alveolitis does not resolve completely, inflammatory changes may persist with variable stages of resolution and degrees of fibrosis before stabilization or progression to extensive fibrosis and irreversible lung disease. The cells involved in the alveolitis have a diverse armamentarium of inflammatory and immune mediators with the potential to cause derangement of alveolar structures,[10] or an alteration in the number, form, and location of the cellular and noncellular constituents of the normal alveolar structures.[5, 9, 10, 28] The rate, form, and extent of the derangement caused by the alveolitis appear to be related to the number, type, and state of activation of the effector cells involved.[10] The reversibility of the lesions in ILD seems to be controlled by the persistence of the derangement of the alveolar structures that is caused by the alveolitis.[5] Inflammatory cells vary in their potential to injure the alveolar wall. Neutrophils cause the most damage and lymphocytes the least damage; alveolar macrophages and eosinophils have intermediate potential to injure the alveolar wall. The derangement may be permanent when it is predominantly fibrosis resulting from injury by neutrophils, the most potent oxidant producers. If the derangement is caused by increased number of lymphocytes, the alveolar wall may be only temporarily distorted but may resolve without significant fibrosis as a sequela. The fate of the alveolar derangement depends in part on the relative integrity of the epithelial and endothelial basement membranes.[11] It is currently thought that alveolar structures have the potential to be restored to normal as long as the basement membrane is present to serve as a scaffolding to direct the repair process of new parenchymal cells.[10]

In ILD from known causes, the etiologic agent is thought to activate the inflammatory cells that are normally present in the lung, which then cause the alveolitis to propagate. Alternatively, the causative agent may directly injure the alveolar walls, and the damaged tissues subsequently initiate the inflammatory response. It is not well understood what initiates the inflammation in ILD of unknown cause; however, many of the mechanisms that maintain the inflammatory responses, once they have been initiated are understood and have been described in studies of ILD in adults and in animal models. The inflammatory process in ILD is driven, in part, by immune complexes. The immune complexes interact with alveolar macrophages and maintain the chronic state of activation of the inflammatory process.

With the development of techniques for bronchoalveolar lavage (BAL), it is possible to recover cells from patients with a spectrum of interstitial lung diseases and compare these findings with those obtained in the lavage fluid from normal persons.[3, 7, 13, 28] It is postulated from studies in adults that the alveolitis appears to be maintained by the local production of specific cell-derived chemotactic factors that recruit inflammatory cells from the blood into the interstitium of the lung, which results in a derangement of alveolar structures.[10] The histologic sequelae to the alveolitis include a change in the pulmonary parenchymal cell populations, lung parenchymal cell injury, granuloma formation, interstitial fibrosis, and a variable degree of distortion of the alveolar architecture.

In adults with ILD, the rate, form, and extent of the alveolar derangement appear to be a function of the number, type, and state of activation of the effector cell constituents and immune mediators.[10] Some of the overall changes in the inflammatory cell populations in ILD include an increase in the number of inflammatory cells, an increase in the number of effector cells present, an increase in the number of "activated" effector cells, and the accumulation of effector cells such as neutrophils that are not normally present in the alveolar structures in any significant amounts.[3, 18] Two types of alveolitis commonly found in interstitial lung disorders in adults are the mac-

rophage-lymphocyte type seen in sarcoidosis[6–8] and the macrophage-neutrophil type seen in idiopathic pulmonary fibrosis.[4, 7, 8, 10]

To understand the pathogenic mechanisms involved in ILD, it is necessary to understand the anatomy of the normal alveolar structures and pulmonary interstitium. The normal pulmonary interstitium of the lung is composed of connective tissue components (supporting connective tissue matrix of collagen, elastic fibers, proteoglycans, and various glycoproteins), mesenchymal cells (fibroblasts, pericytes, and rare smooth muscle cells), and inflammatory and immune effector cells (macrophages, monocytes, and lymphocytes) with the pulmonary capillaries interwoven through the interstitium.[29]

The lining of normal alveoli consists of a single layer of epithelial cells that rests on a thin, continuous basement membrane: the epithelial basement membrane. About 95% of the cells lining the normal alveoli are type I cells, the remainder being type II cells; it is the type II cells that proliferate when there is injury to the alveolar epithelium. The alveolar interstitium is normally just beneath the epithelial basement membrane. The capillary endothelium is composed predominantly of a cytoplasmic extension of endothelial cells, which also rests on a basement membrane: the endothelial basement membrane. These two basement membranes are in very close approximation and appear fused over the thin portions of the alveolar septum, where the pulmonary gas exchange occurs.[29] In the thicker portions of the alveolar septum, the basement membranes of the epithelial and endothelial cells are separated by the interstitial cellular and noncellular components.

Alveolar macrophages are the predominant inflammatory cell in the normal lung (up to 90%),[3, 4, 7, 28] T lymphocytes being the next most common type of inflammatory cell; only small numbers of B lymphocytes and monocytes and a tiny number of neutrophils (less than 1% to 2%) are present in the normal lung.[7, 10] The alveolar macrophages and lymphocytes are usually not activated in the normal lung. The presence of an increased number of inflammatory cells in ILD distorts the alveolar walls but may not damage the alveolar walls or perialveolar tissues, depending on the state of activation of these inflammatory cells. When the inflammatory cells are activated, there can be injury to the alveolar walls, especially to the type I epithelial cells and the capillary endothelial cells. If the alveolar wall inflammation is self-limited or suppressed with therapy, the pulmonary architecture can be preserved before injury is too severe, and alveolar capillary units may be spared. Alternatively, when extensive injury to the alveolar walls has occurred, the normal alveolar architecture cannot be fully reestablished. According to the studies in adults, the reversibility of ILD seems to be modulated in part by the integrity of the epithelial and endothelial basement membranes.[10, 11] The integrity of the basement membranes is presumably a critical determining factor in the reversibility of PILD; however, little information is available to confirm this hypothesis in children.

The normal alveolar wall is very thin (about 5 to 10 μm wide), and the width of the alveolar space is about 200 to 300 μm.[29] In ILD, there is a proliferation of the alveolar lining cells and thickening of the alveolar walls because of the influx of inflammatory cells or fibrosis. A wide spectrum of derangement of alveolar structures accompanies the inflammation of the alveolar walls and perialveolar tissues in ILD in adults.[10] These alveolar derangements can result in either temporary distortion or persistent distortion from fibrosis of the pulmonary interstitium. In sarcoidosis or early stages of hypersensitivity pneumonitis in adults, T lymphocytes, macrophages, and granulomas may distort the normal alveolar walls; however, there may be little injury to normal alveolar structures, and the inflammatory process can be reversible.[17, 22] In sarcoidosis, activated T lymphocytes release a monocyte-specific chemotactic factor that modulates the accumulation of blood monocytes in the alveolar structures.[17, 22] In contrast, in idiopathic pulmonary fibrosis in adults, alveolar macrophages are activated and release neutrophil-specific chemotactic factors that attract blood neutrophils to the lung.[12, 21] Very little information is available in children with ILD not related to AIDS. Bitterman and colleagues[30] reported on BAL in the children of patients with familial pulmonary fibrosis and demonstrated that they had mild alveolitis, even though they had no symptoms and no evidence of lung disease.

DIAGNOSIS AND DIAGNOSTIC APPROACHES

There are no pathognomonic clinical criteria for the diagnosis of PILD. This diagnosis is a challenge because of the wide spectrum of clinical manifestations and the extreme variability in symptoms and signs. Physicians should have a high index of suspicion of PILD in an infant or a child with tachypnea or dyspnea. Cough may also be present. Patients may exhibit radiologic evidence of ILD and no reportable symptoms. In contrast, some patients have clinical symptoms and signs of ILD but have normal chest radiographs. In the latter cases, the clinician institutes a diligent search for evidence of systemic disease that can be manifested by respiratory symptoms. It is well recognized that the plain chest radiograph is insensitive in detecting the earlier changes of ILD, manifested only by alveolar thickening. Some of the newer methods of diagnostic imaging, such as thin-cut computed tomographic (CT) scans of the chest, may be more sensitive in detecting the earlier stages of PILD.

An important goal in the clinical evaluation of any infant or child with tachypnea or dyspnea is to detect evidence of primary ILD or systemic disorders with an ILD component. Patients with suspected ILD should be assessed for evidence of hypoxemia, both at rest and with exercise. Chest radiographs of infants and children with any of the clinical manifestations suggestive of ILD should be reviewed for the presence of reticulonodular or nodular involvement.

CLINICAL MANIFESTATIONS

Clinical symptoms or signs of ILD are variable and may include cough, tachypnea, dyspnea, orthopnea, exercise intolerance, retractions, dry crackles, failure to thrive or weight loss, cyanosis, and other manifestations that can be attributed to the presence of underlying systemic or associated diseases. Chest pain may also occur and may be pleuritic. With the complication of a pneumothorax, the chest pain may be acute in onset and accompanied by sudden onset or exacerbation of dyspnea. Fever is uncommon and is usually caused by superimposed infection. Anorexia, weight loss, or failure to thrive may be seen with persistent or progressive disease. Failure to thrive or weight loss occurs when the increased caloric requirements from increased work of breathing are not being met. The cough is nonproductive, is usually inconsequential, and does not disturb sleep.

The onset of PILD is insidious; tachypnea or dyspnea is usually the earliest clinical sign or symptom. Dyspnea may appear first on exertion and later at rest, unaffected by position. With advanced disease, orthopnea may be present and can occur even with the use of supplementary oxygen. Sudden onset of dyspnea or orthopnea may be caused by a pneumothorax, an occasional complication of advanced PILD. Retractions (intercostal or subcostal) may be associated with tachypnea.

Exercise intolerance or easy fatigability may be another presenting symptom but may be difficult to document. Objective assessment of exercise tolerance and the documentation of hypoxemia or desaturation by oximetry with exercise or feeding in infants provides supporting evidence for the diagnosis of ILD. Oximetry is one of the important tools for monitoring the oxygenation status of patients with PILD.

The physical examination is often unimpressive. On auscultation, dry "Velcro" rales or crackles, which are short (<5 m/sec), low-pitched, discontinuous sounds heard late in inspiration, are characteristic of PILD. Digital clubbing may be one of the signs of significant pulmonary disease. Cyanosis can also occur with advanced or progressive lung disease. Cyanosis with digital clubbing may be present with DIP, LIP, and UIP; however, cyanotic heart disease must be considered and ruled out in the differential diagnosis. In addition to tachypnea, retractions (intercostal or subcostal) may be present. Both the measurement of the respiratory rate and the assessment for retractions should be performed when the patient is resting or at least when the patient is quiet and comfortable. The triad of tachypnea, intercostal retractions, and dry crackles in an infant or a child with a normal birth history is strongly suggestive of ILD, especially when other causes such as cystic fibrosis and aspiration syndromes are ruled out.

RADIOLOGIC EVALUATION

The plain chest radiograph should be assessed for lung volume, presence and pattern of lung opacities, and other associated findings such as lymphadenopathy, pleural abnormality, or cardiac enlargement. A reticular or reticulonodular pattern of lung opacities is the characteristic pattern in ILD. The distribution (homogeneous, lobar, segmental, central, or peripheral) and severity (degree of obstruction of normal structures) of the lung opacities should also be evaluated.

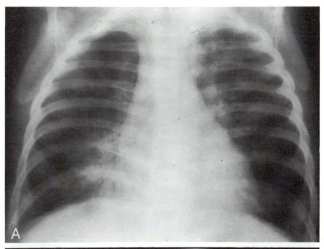

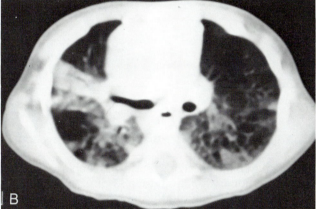

Figure 42–1. *A,* Chest radiograph (posteroanterior view) of a child with interstitial lung disease (ILD) of unknown cause, requiring prolonged oxygen; the child had persistent "Velcro" rales. *B,* Computed tomographic scan of chest of a child with unknown type of ILD, demonstrating the extensive interstitial involvement.

CT scans of the chest, expecially thin-cut sections, are sensitive for demonstrating the lesions of interstitial lung disease (Fig. 42–1). Nuclear scintigraphy (e.g., gallium scanning) has been proposed as a method of assessing alveolitis; it is more likely to be positive with active interstitial disease. This procedure exposes the infant or child to a considerable amount of radiation and is often not helpful in the diagnosis. Technetium scanning is another imaging technique that measures the intactness of the epithelial membrane with timed clearance from the lung of the inhaled tracer. This study may be useful but is not available in all medical centers, and its usefulness in the diagnosis has not been evaluated in prospective studies in children.

HISTOLOGIC FINDINGS

Because the histologic features are the basis for confirmation of the diagnosis as well as prognosis, the physician should be aware of the characteristic pathologic findings in PILD and its histologic variants. The histologic variants of three of the more common variants of PILD are discussed in the Differential Diagnosis section. Thickening of the alveolar wall is the hallmark for the diagnosis of

ILD. Involvement of the pulmonary interstitium, evidenced by thickening of the alveolar wall, can be documented, and the type of inflammation can be characterized by histologic examination of lung tissue. The thickening of the alveolar wall in ILD can be a result of edema, inflammation, and proliferation of immune effector cells.

For the optimal information from an open-lung biopsy, certain general guidelines are helpful in the selection of the biopsy site and in the handling of the tissue. Whenever possible, the site of the lung biopsy should be the area of predominant involvement on radiograph or thin-cut CT scan of the chest. The advantage of multiple over single sites for lung biopsy is controversial; however, experience in a few centers suggests that the use of multiple sites does not offer additional diagnostic advantages. The size of the lung biopsy tissue should be sufficient to provide at least three portions of tissue: one for formalin fixation, another for fixation in glutaraldehyde for electron microscopy studies, and a third for freezing without fixation in cryobath or liquid nitrogen or for touch preparations. It is preferable to have inflated tissue for formalin fixation. At a minimum, the tissue for review by consulting pathologists (e.g., those at the Armed Forces Institute for Pathology or the National Working Group for PILD) should include (1) a slide of biopsy tissue stained with hematoxylin-eosin, (2) a slide of lung tissue stained with a connective tissue stain (e.g., Masson's stain), and (3) a block of tissue that is unstained.

In the review of the biopsy, assessments should be made to determine (1) the predominant location and the extent of the pathologic process (i.e., alveolar, peribronchiolar, and so on); (2) the quantification of the alveolar wall thickness; (3) the evaluation of any changes in the alveolar lining cells; (4) the predominant type of inflammatory cell involved; (5) the presence of macrophages within the alveoli; (6) the type and extent of the derangement of the alveolar structures with a quantification of the type and degree of fibrosis (i.e., collagen deposition, fibroblast response); (7) the presence of associated findings such as viral inclusions, giant cells, alveolar proteinosis, bronchiolitis obliterans, diffuse alveolar damage, pleural reaction, and pulmonary lymphoid hyperplasia; and (8) a tentative or definitive diagnostic category that is consistent with the histologic findings (e.g., UIP, DIP, LIP). Figures 42–2 and 42–3 show thickening of the alveolar wall with fibrosis. In Figure 42–2, the tissue is stained with Masson's stain. Figure 42–3 shows fibrosis in biopsy stained with hematoxylin-eosin.

EVALUATION OF PULMONARY FUNCTION

Because tachypnea is one of the more characteristic clinical findings in ILD, the documentation of elevated respiratory rate in the infant or child at rest or during sleep is important in the confirmation of the diagnosis. The respiratory rate should be counted for a full minute. Assessment of oxygenation by pulse oximetry is a noninvasive technique used in the diagnosis and monitoring of infants and children with ILD; the fraction of inspired oxygen

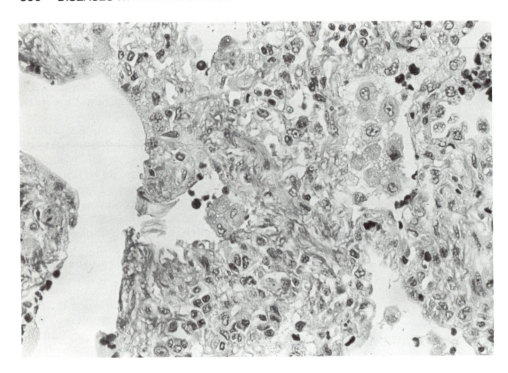

Figure 42–2. Thickening of the alveolar wall by fibrosis demonstrated by Masson's connective tissue stain of lung biopsy specimen; the patient was a 10-year-old female with ILD of unknown cause.

(F_{IO_2}) must be recorded when the oximetry readings are obtained. Oxygen saturation should be determined at rest and with exercise to observe for desaturation. The limitations of oximetry must be appreciated when this technique is used to monitor oxygenation (see Chapters 6 and 10). Arterial blood gases are the gold standard for the assessment of oxygenation; again, the F_{IO_2} must be recorded to calculate the alveolar-arterial gradient. If supplemental oxygen is required, it is important that the oxygen be delivered with a hood or a Venturi mask while the

blood gases are drawn so that F_{IO_2} can be accurately determined.

For children old enough to perform reliable and reproducible pulmonary function studies, spirometry and lung volumes by either helium dilution or body plethysmography should be part of the workup and monitoring of children with ILD. Diffusing capacity for carbon monoxide by the single-breath method is also useful in the diagnosis but is usually limited to children over 10 years of age. The values for diffusing capacity should be

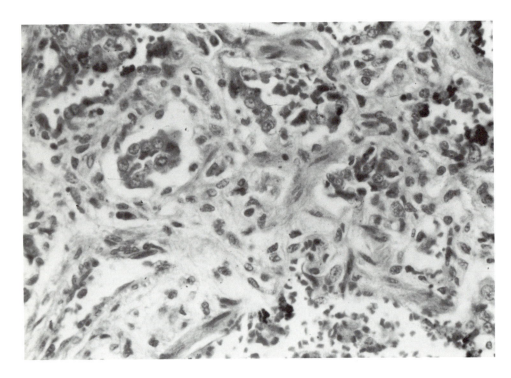

Figure 42–3. Thickening of alveolar wall by extensive fibrosis. Hematoxylin-eosin stain of lung biopsy tissue.

reported as D_L/V_A. A hemoglobin test should be conducted simultaneously with the diffusing capacity study.

For those children who do not demonstrate hypoxemia at rest, exercise challenge studies should be performed while oxygen saturation is monitored during modified submaximal exercise.

EVALUATION OF BRONCHOALVEOLAR LAVAGE FLUID

Although the use of BAL in adults has enabled investigation of the cells and mediators that may contribute to ILD, more studies are needed to determine the usefulness of this technique in the diagnosis and monitoring of disease activity in infants and children. Most of the experience with diagnostic microbiologic and cytologic examinations of BAL in PILD have been in immunocompromised infants and children,[31-34] and the data have been obtained from flexible fiberoptic bronchoscopy. BAL by means of a fiberoptic bronchoscope with local anesthesia has been reported to be safe and reduces the necessity of open-lung biopsy in the management of immunocompromised infants and children with interstitial pneumonitis associated with the human immunodeficiency virus (HIV).[35]

De Blic and associates demonstrated the value of microbiologic and cytologic studies in BAL in acute and chronic interstitial pneumonitis in HIV-infected children (3 months to 16 years).[35] They found the overall microbiologic yield was 75% in their series, *Pneumocystis carinii* being the predominant infective organisms in 63% of patients, but viral agents such as adenovirus and cytomegalovirus were also isolated. On cytologic studies, the *P. carinii* pneumonitis was associated with clumps of cel-lular debris, lymphocytosis, and an increase in neutrophils; this differed from the finding on BAL of pulmonary lymphoid hyperplasia without opportunistic infection. In the latter case, BAL provides supplementary evidence for diagnosis and offers a means of ruling out an opportunistic infection.[35, 36] The mean percentages of lymphoctyes and neutrophils were also found to be significantly different in children with *P. carinii* pneumonia. De Blic and associates proposed that the presence of lymphocytosis alone, in the absence of *P. carinii* and of neutrophils, offered support to the clinical and radiologic diagnosis of pulmonary lymphoid hyperplasia in pediatric patients with AIDS.[36] The mechanism for the development of the lymphocytosis is not clearly defined and may be linked to the HIV itself[37] or may be the result of a co-infection with Epstein-Barr virus.[38]

Standards for analysis of BAL need to be developed for its use in the diagnosis and monitoring of disease activity of non-AIDS forms of PILD. BAL is technically more difficult to obtain in small children than in adults. The smaller flexible bronchoscopes do not have a suction channel; the 3.5- to 3.7-mm flexible bronchoscopes have a suction channel, but it may easily become obstructed with mucus. For older children in whom the 4.9-mm bronchoscope can be used, BAL studies should be accomplished as easily as those performed in adults. The first aliquot of BAL should be used for culture for viruses, bacteria, fungi, mycobacteria, and mycoplasma. In addition, this specimen should include Gram's stain, acid-fast stain, and silver stain for *Pneumocystis*; fluorescent antibodies for *Chlamydia*, *Bordetella pertussis*, and *Legionella*; and enzyme-linked immunosorbent assay for respiratory syncytial virus. Figure 42–4 shows *Pneumocystis* organisms identified by BAL. The next aliquot is used for routine cytologic studies in order to look for hemosiderin-

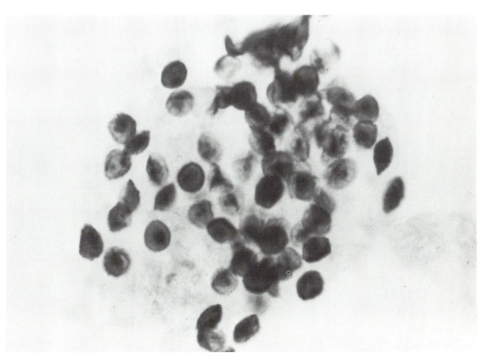

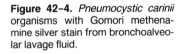
Figure 42–4. *Pneumocystic carinii* organisms with Gomori methenamine silver stain from bronchoalveolar lavage fluid.

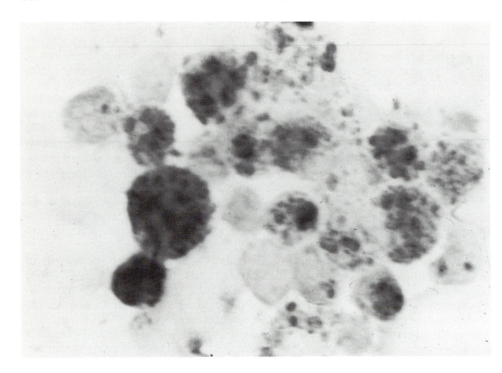

Figure 42–5. Hemosiderin-laden macrophages obtained from bronchoalveolar lavage in a patient with idiopathic pulmonary hemosiderosis.

laden macrophages (Fig. 42–5) or lipid-laden macrophages (Fig. 42–6). The third aliquot can be frozen or used for other specific studies, including immunofluorescence studies.

OTHER LABORATORY STUDIES

Because pediatric AIDS may become the most common cause of ILD in children in this country in the next several years, it is important to determine possible risk factors for each patient and to evaluate all infants and children with suspected ILD for HIV infection when any of the risk factors are present.

DIFFERENTIAL DIAGNOSIS

The differential diagnosis of ILD in infants and children is listed in Table 42–2. In the case of hypersensitivity pneumonitis, clinical manifestations and histologic responses are self-limited if the patient is removed from

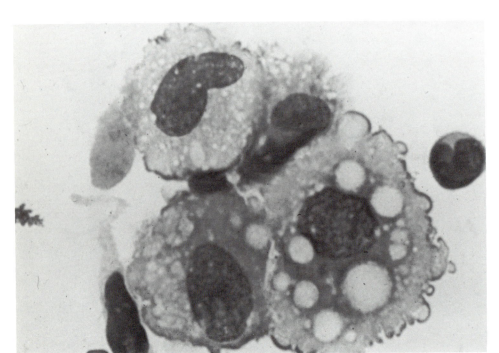

Figure 42–6. Lipid-laden macrophages in bronchoalveolar lavage fluid in a child with chronic aspiration of formula.

Table 42–2. DIFFERENTIAL DIAGNOSIS OF INTERSTITIAL LUNG DISEASE IN CHILDREN

Pediatric Acquired Immunodeficiency Syndrome (AIDS)
Testing for HIV antibodies or antigen
   ELISA or Western blot for HIV antibodies
   Polymerase chain reaction (PCR) for HIV antigen
Cystic Fibrosis
Quantitative analysis of sweat electrolytes
Gastroesophageal Reflux/Chronic Aspiration
Barium swallow
pH probe
Evaluation of gastric/tracheal aspiration or BAL for lipid-laden
   macrophages
Immunodeficiency
Quantitative immunoglobulins
Immunoglobulin G subclasses
Assay of antibody response to tetanus, diphtheria, Pneumovax,
   Haemophilus influenzae type b
T and B lymphocyte subset quantitation
Ciliary Disorders
Electron microscopy of nasal scrapings or
   tracheal biopsy for ciliary morphology
Collagen-Vascular Disorders
Antinuclear antibody (ANA)
Rheumatoid factor (RF)
Infectious Disease
Viral cultures/serology/viral probe studies, ELISA for respiratory
   syncytial virus
Cultures/serology tests for *Mycoplasma*
Culture for bacterial pathogens/Gram's stains
Fungal cultures/smears
Mycobacterial cultures/smear for acid-fast bacilli
Silver stains *(Pneumocystis carinii)*
Fluorescent antibodies for *Chlamydia, Legionella*
Immunofluorescense for *Pneumocystis carinii*
Hypersensitivity Pneumonitis
Serum precipitins
Pulmonary Hemosiderosis
Cytology (BAL fluid, lung biopsy)
   for hemosiderin-laden macrophages

HIV, human immunodeficiency virus; ELISA, enzyme-linked immunosorbent assay; BAL, bronchoalveolar lavage.

exposure to the offending organic antigens before irreversible inflammatory changes occur in the lung. If hypersensitivity pneumonitis can be documented by history, a lung biopsy may not be necessary. Assay for serum precipitins may also help to document the history of exposure to organic antigens such as pigeon or dove antigens. Pulmonary hemosiderosis is a special type of ILD. The use of BAL may confirm the presence of hemosiderin-laden macrophages. Infectious or postinfectious disease is currently the most common type of PILD. It is important to attempt to document an infectious cause in ILD whenever possible.

Because of the heterogeneity of the disorders that can cause PILD, it is important to consider the differential diagnosis from two approaches. The first is to differentiate ILD from other respiratory disorders that cause similar clinical signs or symptoms and laboratory findings. The second approach is to differentiate the various disorders that cause primary ILD from those of ILD with associated conditions. Table 42–3 is a classification of PILDs resulting from known or identified causes and includes both primary ILD and some types of ILD that are secondary to other conditions. Table 42–4 is a classification of PILDs

resulting from unknown causes and in which the lung disease is the predominant disease. Because the causes of this group of disorders are unknown, it is difficult to attribute these disorders to primary or secondary ILD. Table 42–5 is a classification of a group of disorders in which ILDs may be present at some time and are associated with other underlying conditions. The scope of this chapter does not allow a discussion of each of these disorders; for additional details, the reader is referred to the three-volume reviews of ILD by Laraya-Cuasay and Hughes.[39] Only three of the specific disorders that can be characterized histologically are discussed separately in this chapter (i.e., UIP, DIP, and LIP).

Usual Interstitial Pneumonitis

This term was proposed to describe pulmonary interstitial inflammatory disease associated with fibrosis, and the disorder is often referred to as Hamman-Rich syndrome[40] in children and as cryptogenic or idiopathic fibrosing alveolitis in adults. This type of ILD is characterized histologically by a spectrum of interstitial fibrosis ranging from scattered focal areas interspersed with mainly normal alveoli to a predominant fibrotic lung with marked derangement of alveolar structures. Variable degrees of proliferation of smooth muscle and inflammatory responses are seen in the alveolar walls with interstitial fibrosis. The exact pathogenetic mechanisms of the lesions in UIP are uncertain; however, it is thought to be initiated by injury to the alveolar wall that results in alveolitis. This alveolitis from a known or unknown agent is thought to damage the epithelium or endothelium of the alveolar wall and is associated with a variable influx of inflammatory and immune effector cells. The inflammatory responses result in a thickening of the alveolar septum by inflammatory cells and fibrosis (Fig. 42–7).

The cause of UIP or cryptogenic fibrosing alveolitis is unknown (idiopathic fibrosing alveolitis). A familial autosomal dominant form of this clinical and histologic entity, with age at onset ranging from infancy to adulthood, has been reported.[41, 42] Several human leukocyte antigen (HLA) types (HLA-B12, HLA-B7, HLA-B8) have been reported to be associated with UIP.[43] A viral cause has been suggested as another possible agent associated with the initial alveolitis. The original cases of UIP reported in the Hamman-Rich syndrome were noted to occur after a severe viral infection.

The role of immunologically mediated lung injury in UIP has received much support.[10] Identical histologic lung lesions are found in adults with a variety of collagen vascular diseases such as rheumatoid arthritis, scleroderma, dermatomyositis, and systemic lupus erythematosis. Deposition of immunoglobin in the lungs, in additon to circulating immune complexes, has been reported in these patients.[44] Rheumatoid factor and antinuclear factors have also been found in these patients in the absence of clinical rheumatoid arthritis and systemic lupus erythematosis.[45]

The clinical picture of UIP is usually one of insidious onset of dyspnea, which first appears on exertion but is progressive and, later in the course of the disease, is present at rest. Cough, when present, is nonproductive unless

Table 42–3. KNOWN CAUSES OF INTERSTITIAL LUNG DISEASE IN CHILDREN

Infections or Postinfections
Viral
Cytomegalic virus
Human immunodeficiency virus (HIV)
Respiratory syncytial virus
Adenovirus
Influenza virus
Parainfluenza viruses
Mycoplasma
Measles
Mycobacterial
Fungal
*Pneumocytis carinii**
Aspergillus species
Bacterial
Legionella pneumophila
Bordetella pertussis

Environmental Inhalants, Toxic Substances, Foreign Materials, or Antigenic Dusts
Inorganic Dusts
Silica
Asbestos
Talcum powder
Zinc stearate
Organic Dusts
Hypersensitivity pneumonitis
Fumes
Sulfuric acid
Hydrochloric acid
Gases
Chlorine
Nitrogen dioxide
Ammonia
Aerosols

Drug-Induced Disorders
Antineoplastic Drugs
Cyclophosphamide
Nitrosoureas (carmustine, lomustine)
Azothioprine
Cytosine arabinoside
6-Mercaptopurine
Vinblastine
Bleomycin
Methotrexate

Miscellaneous Drugs
Nitrofurantoin
Penicillamine
Gold salts

Radiation-Induced Neoplastic Diseases
Leukemia
Hodgkin's disease
Non-Hodgkin's disease lymphoma
Histiocytosis X
Letterer-Siwe disease
Hand-Schüller-Christian disease
Eosinophilic granuloma

Lymphoproliferative Disorders
Familial erythrophagocytic lymphohistiocytosis
Angioimmunoblastic lymphadenopathy
Lymphoid interstitial pneumonitis
Pseudolymphomas of the lung

Metabolic
Storage Disorders
Hermansky-Pudlak syndrome
Pulmonary Lipidosis
Gaucher's disease
Niemann-Pick disease
Disorders of Ion transport
Cystic fibrosis
Other
Cardiac failure
Renal disease

Degenerative Disorders
Idiopathic pulmonary alveolar microlithiasis

Neurocutaneous Syndromes With Interstitial Lung Disease
Tuberous sclerosis
Neurofibromatosis
Ataxia-telangiectasia

* P. carinii, previously considered a protozoan parasite, is now classified as a fungus.

there is a coexistent respiratory infection. Nonspecific findings are anorexia, failure to thrive, easy fatigability, and occasional chest pain (pleuritic or substernal).

Physical examination may not be conclusive early in the course of the lung disease; the most common finding is tachypnea with rapid shallow breathing. Fine ("Velcro") end-inspiratory rales or crackles may also be found on chest auscultation. Digital clubbing is usually seen in later stages of the lung disease. Physical findings consistent with pulmonary hypertension or cor pulmonale may also be noted, in association with extensive lung disease. Chest radiographs may also vary from normal to showing end-stage lung disease. The characteristic radiographic findings are diffuse reticulonodular lesions. As the lung disease progresses, there is a diminution of lung volume and the appearance of cystic lesions. There is currently

considerable interest in CT of the chest, specifically thin-cut CT, to better define the radiographic lesions.

UIP is characteristically progressive; complete and permanent arrest of the pulmonary pathology is unusual. Most children die of respiratory failure; often UIP is exacerbated or precipitated by an acute respiratory infection.

Desquamative Interstitial Pneumonitis

DIP, first described by Liebow and colleagues in 1965,[2] is the most common histologic variant of interstitial pneumonitis in infants and children. It was initially considered to be a distinct entity with a better prognosis than UIP; however, it is usually viewed as a part of the clinical and histologic spectrum of interstitial pneumonitis, with

Table 42-4. INTERSTITIAL LUNG DISEASE IN CHILDREN RESULTING FROM UNKNOWN CAUSES

Usual interstitial pneumonitis
    Diffuse idiopathic pulmonary fibrosis (cryptogenic fibrosing alveolitis)
Sarcoidoisis
Pulmonary hemosiderosis
    Idiopathic pulmonary hemosiderosis
Pulmonary alveolar proteinosis
Pulmonary infiltrates with eosinophilia
    Chronic eosinophilic pneumonia

Table 42-5. INTERSTITIAL LUNG DISEASE IN CHILDREN ASSOCIATED WITH OTHER CONDITIONS

Interstitial Lung Disease Associated With Collagen Vascular Disorder
Juvenile rheumatoid arthritis
Dermatomyositis/polymyositis
Scleroderma
Progressive systemic sclerosis
Ankylosing spondylitis
Sjögren's syndrome
Behçet's syndrome
Interstitial Lung Disease Associated With Pulmonary Vasculitides
Polyarteritis nodosa
Wegener's granulomatosis
Churg-Strauss syndrome
Lymphomatoid granulomatosis
Hypersensitivity vasculitis
Systemic necrotizing vasculitides
    "Overlap" vasculitis
Interstitial Lung Disease Associated With Liver Disease
Chronic active hepatitis
Primary biliary cirrhosis
Interstitial Lung Disease Associated With Bowel Disease
Ulcerative colitis
Crohn's disease
Interstitial Lung Disease Caused by Failure of Other Organs
Chronic left ventricular failure
Chronic left-to-right intracardiac shunt
Chronic renal disease with uremia
Amyloidosis
Graft-Versus-Host Disease
Recovering Phase of Adult Respiratory Distress Syndrome
Goodpasture's Syndrome
Hypereosinophilic Syndrome
Pulmonary Veno-Occlusive Disease

DIP the more cellular phase of UIP. DIP may progress to fibrosis and end-stage lung disease with honeycombing. The prognosis in response to corticosteroid therapy has been proposed to be more favorable with DIP than with UIP; however, a progressive clinical course has been reported in a 3-month-old infant with DIP who died despite corticosteroid therapy.[46] In addition to a more favorable response to corticosteroids, the diagnosis of DIP was based on the difference in histologic appearance and prognosis.[47] The mortality rate is reported to be significant.[46, 48-51] Hewitt and co-authors reported 31 cases of PILD, with a mean survival period of 4.7 months.[52] Kerem and colleagues reported response to high doses (pulses) of methylprednisolone and daily oral doses of hydroxychloroquine in children with chronic interstitial pneumonitis with a histologic appearance of DIP.[53] These authors used 10 mg/kg/day of methylprednisolone for 3 days in addition to 10 mg/kg/day of oral hydroxychloroquine, followed by other immunosuppressive agents.

The cause of DIP is unknown, although various causes have been proposed, including a response to foreign body, an autoimmune phenomenon, or a sequela to infection. DIP is not seen in collagen vascular disease with the same frequency as UIP, although antinuclear antibody and rheumatoid factor have been reported in DIP as well as in UIP. In some cases, DIP is associated with alveolar proteinosis.[52]

The main diagnostic criterion of DIP is the presence of a large number of macrophages within the alveolae (Fig.

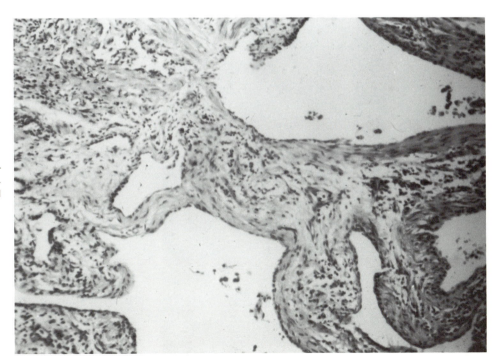

Figure 42-7. Thickening of alveolar wall as a result of marked septal fibrosis in a child with usual interstitial pneumonitis.

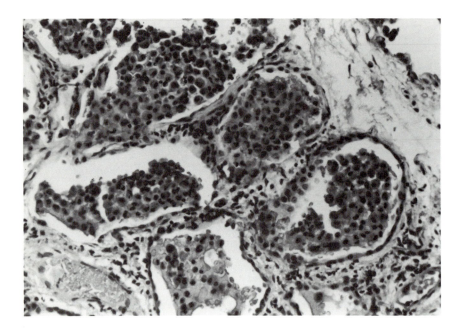

Figure 42-8. Open-lung biopsy specimen showing desquamative interstitial pneumonitis.

42-8). In addition, DIP is characterized histologically by (1) proliferation of cells lining the alveolar spaces (type II pneumocytes), (2) the presence of accumulation of periodic acid-Schiff– (PAS-) positive, diastase-resistant cytoplasmic granules free in alveolar spaces, and (3) the infiltration of lymphocytes, monocytes, plasma cells, and eosinophils into the interstitium (Fig. 42-9).[54–59] Eosinophilic intranuclear inclusions in both the alveolar lining cells and the desquamated cells have been described by Liebow (1965)[1] and may appear as "virus" type particles.[60,61] On electron microscopy, the inclusions consist of myelin figures. In contrast to UIP, there is no alveolar wall necrosis and no hyaline membrane lining the alveoli in DIP. Occasionally, macrophages fuse to form multinucleated cells that can resemble giant cells.

There is generally a mild degree of fibrosis; however,

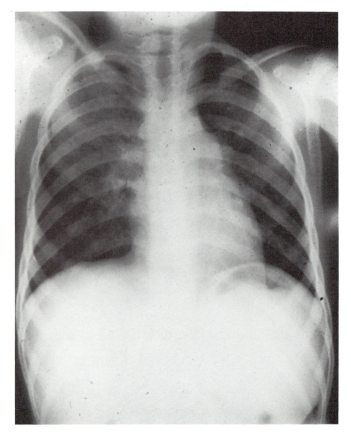

Figure 42-9. Posteroanterior chest radiograph of a child with desquamative interstitial pneumonitis.

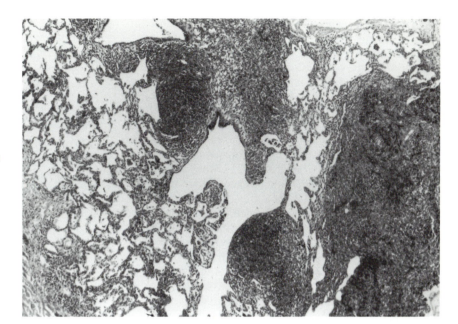

Figure 42–10. Lymphoid interstitial pneumonitis seen on open-lung biopsy specimen.

this varies with the stage of the ILD at the time of lung biopsy. Patients documented to have mild fibrosis initially in infancy may show extensive fibrosis; this has been confirmed on a second lung biopsy in some of our patients (Fig. 42–6).

Lymphoid Interstitial Pneumonitis

In LIP, the thickening of the alveolar wall is caused predominantly by the infiltration of lymphocytes, although occasionally plasma cells and histiocytes can be present and contribute to the alveolar wall thickening (Fig. 42–10).[62, 63] This type of ILD is one of the most frequent lung lesions seen in AIDS and as part of the spectrum of lymphoid lesions and is one of the criteria for the diagnosis of pediatric AIDS.[64] LIP should be differentiated from pulmonary lymphoid hyperplasia in pediatric patients with AIDs and also must be distinguished from opportunistic infection with *P. carinii*. LIP has an insidious onset (see Chapter 21 for more detail discussion). LIP can also be associated with other immunodeficiency disorders other than AIDS such as Sjögren's syndrome and chronic active hepatitis.

MANAGEMENT

The precise recommendations for drug therapy in PILD have not been determined by randomized, controlled clinical trials and remain controversial. No one medical center has enough of these cases to conduct prospective, randomized trials of adequate sample size. The efforts of the national working group are to establish a data registry for patients and to plan for multicenter prospective trials in the future. Until these goals can be accomplished, treatment is on an individualized basis. The use of corticosteroids initially is usually in the range of 1 to 2 mg/kg/day for variable periods of time, often with conversion to alternate-day therapy if there is

response to therapy and if the patient can be stabilized on this regimen. Bursts of corticosteroids are given with exacerbations, and intermittent pulses of high doses of corticosteroids have been proposed by some authors.[53] A variety of other immunosuppressive agents directed toward the suppression or control of the inflammatory process in the pulmonary interstitium have been tried in individual cases with varying degrees of success.

In general, managment includes both supportive and symptomatic treatment in addition to corticosteroid and immunosuppressive drugs. Symptomatic treatment includes the use of supplemental oxygen with the goal of maintaining the arterial blood oxygen tension at more than 60 mm Hg or the oxygen saturation at more than 90%. Supportive management is similar to that of infants and children with bronchopulmonary dysplasia (i.e., adequate nutritional support to provide extra calories for the increased work of breathing, growth, and basal metabolic needs). It is also important to minimize exposure of the child with ILD to respiratory infections and environmental respiratory irritants (e.g., cigarette smoking) whenever possible.

Heart and lung or bilateral lung transplantation is another option in selected cases for the definitive treatment for PILD when all other treatments offered appear to be failing and the ILD is progressing.

Honeycomb lung is a nonspecific description of end-stage lung disease, represents the outcome of a wide variety of lung injuries, and should not be confused with UIP, which has specific diagnostic characteristics.

HISTOLOGIC EVALUATION

The timing of the lung biopsy is one of the most critical diagnostic issues in the evaluation of ILD in children. The decision to perform a biopsy should be individualized and depends on the severity and rate of progression of the clinical and radiographic findings. In immunocompromised hosts with PILD, an aggressive approach is warranted in order to identify specific opportunistic infections or drug-induced causes. Because ILD is best confirmed by histologic criteria, the open-lung biopsy is considered the gold standard for the diagnosis of ILD in children. Transtracheal biopsies of the lung in infants and young children have not usually been feasible because of technical limitations such as airway size and development. Because physicians and parents are reluctant to subject children to invasive procedures, there is a need for a consensus on the clinical criteria for the diagnosis of ILD that would suggest indications for an open-lung biopsy. There is no consensus at this time for specific indications for open-lung biopsies in the diagnosis of ILD in children. Some of the criteria considered for the clinical diagnosis of PILD should include (1) compatible clinical symptoms or signs, (2) radiographic changes consistent with ILD, (3) normal birth history, and (4) the exclusion of other disorders in an infant or child in whom other causes of the clinical or radiologic findings have been ruled out (e.g., cystic fibrosis, ciliary disorders, and aspiration syndromes). It is important to determine the possibility of any underlying collagen vascular disorder or systemic vasculitides.

REFERENCES

1. Liebow AA, Steer A, Billingsley JG: Desquamative interstitial pneumonia. Am J Med 39:369–404, 1965.
2. Liebow AA: Definitions and classification of interstitial pneumonias in human pathology: Alveolar interstitium of the lung. International Symposium. Paris, 1974. Prog Respir Res 8:1–33, 1975.
3. Reynolds HY, Newball HH: Analysis of proteins and respiratory cells obtained from human lungs by bronchial lavage. J Lab Clin Med 84:559–573, 1974.
4. Crystal RG, Fulmer JD, Roberts WC, et al: Idiopathic pulmonary fibrosis: Clinical, histologic, radiographic, physiologic, scintigraphic, cytologic, and biochemical aspects. Ann Intern Med 85:769–788, 1976.
5. Weinberger SE, Crystal RG: Reactions of the interstitial space to injury. In Fishman AP (ed): Pulmonary Diseases. New York: McGraw-Hill, 1979.
6. Hunninghake GW, Fulmer JD, Young RC, et al: Localization of the immune response in sarcoidosis. Am Rev Respir Dis 120:49–57, 1979.
7. Hunninghake GW, Gadek JE, Kawanami O, et al: Inflammatory and immune processes in the human lung in health and disease: Evaluation by bronchoalveolar lavage. Am J Pathol 97:149–206, 1979.
8. Reynolds HY, Fulmer JD, Kazmierowski JA, et al: Analysis of cellular and protein content of bronchoalveolar lavage fluid from patients with idiopathic pulmonary fibrosis and chronic hypersensitivity pneumonitis. J Clin Invest 59:165–175, 1977.
9. Fulmer JD, Crystal RG: Interstitial lung disease. In Simmons DH (ed): Current Pulmonology, vol. 1, pp. 1–65. Boston: Houghton Mifflin, 1979.
10. Crystal RG, Gadek JE, Ferrans VJ, et al: Interstitial lung disease: Current concepts of pathogenesis, staging and therapy. Am J Med 70:542–568, 1981.
11. Vracko R: Significance of basal lamina for regeneration of injured lung. Virchows Arch [A] 355:264–274, 1972.
12. Hunninghake GW, Gadek JE, Fales HM, et al: Human alveolar macrophage-derived chemotactic factor for neutrophils: Stimuli and partial characterization. J Clin Invest 66:473–483, 1980.
13. Hunninghake GW, Gadek JE, Szapiel SV, et al: The human alveolar macrophage. In Harris CC, Trump BF, Stoner GD (eds): Methods and Perspectives in Cell Biology: Cultured Human Cells and Tissues in Biomedical Research, vol. 21, pp. 95–112. New York: Academic Press, 1980.
14. Gadek JE, Hunninghake GW, Zimmerman RL, et al: Regulation of the release of alveolar macrophage-derived neutrophil chemotactic factor. Am Rev Respir Dis 121:723–733, 1980.
15. Merrill WW, Naegel GP, Matthay RA, et al: Alveolar macrophage-derived chemotactic factor: Kinetics of in vitro production and partial characterization. J Clin Invest 65:268–276, 1980.
16. Crystal RG, Bitterman PB, Rennard SI, et al: Interstitial lung diseases of unknown cause: Disorders characterized by chronic inflammation of the lower respiratory tract. First of two parts. N Engl J Med 310:154–166, 1984.
17. Crystal RG, Bitterman PB, Rennard SI, et al: Interstitial lung diseases of unknown cause: Disorders characterized by chronic inflammation of the lower respiratory tract (second of two parts). N Engl J Med 310:235–244, 1984.
18. Hunninghake GW, Bedell GN: Interstitial lung disease, concepts of pathogenesis. Semin Respir Med 6:31–39, 1984.
19. Hunninghake GW, Garrett KC, Richerson HB, et al: State of art: Pathogenesis of the granulomatous lung diseases. Am Rev Respir Dis 130:476–496, 1984.
20. Gadek JE, Kelman JA, Fells GA, et al: Collagenase in the lower respiratory tract in patients with idiopathic pulmonary fibrosis. N Engl J Med 301:737–742, 1979.
21. Reynolds HY: Idiopathic interstitial pulmonary fibrosis: Contribution of bronchoalveolar lavage analysis. Chest 89:139S,–144S, 1986.
22. Daniele RP, Rossman MD, Kern JA, et al: Pathogenesis of sarcoidosis, state of the art. Chest 89:174S–177S, 1986.
23. Hunninghake GW, Gadek JE, Lawley TJ, et al: Mechanisms of neutrophil accumulation in the lungs of patients with idiopathic pulmonary fibrosis. J Clin Invest 68:259–269, 1981.
24. van Toorn DW: Experimental interstitial pulmonary fibrosis. Pathol Eur 5:97–104, 1970.
25. Ryan SF: Experimental fibrosing alveolitis. Am Rev Respir Dis 105:776–791, 1972.
26. Adamson IYR, Bowden DH: The pathogenesis of bleomycin-induced pulmonary fibrosis in mice. Am J Pathol 77:185–190, 1974.
27. Jennings FL, Arden A: Development of experimental radiation pneumonitis. Arch Pathol 71:437–446, 1961.
28. Barry BE, Crapo JD, Gehr P, et al: Population characteristics of the cells of the normal lung. Am Rev Respir Dis 119:287A, 1979.
29. Murray JF: The Normal Lung, 2nd ed. Philadelphia: WB Saunders, 1986.
30. Bitterman P, Hunninghake G, Keogh B, et al: Evidence for a focus regulating immune processes causing familial pulmonary fibrosis. Clin Res 29:314A, 1981.
31. Bye MR, Bernstein L, Shah K, et al: Diagnostic bronchoalveolar lavage in children with AIDS. Pediatr Pulmonol 3:425–428, 1987.
32. de Blic J, McKelvie P, Le Bourgeois M: Bronchoalveolar lavage in children with acquired immunodeficiency syndrome. Am Rev Respir Dis 135:A72, 1987.
33. Frankel LR, Smith DW, Lewiston NJ: Bronchoalveolar lavage for diagnosis of pneumonia in the immunocompromised child. Pediatrics 81:785–788, 1988.
34. Pattishall EN, Noyes BE, Orenstein DM: Use of bronchoalveolar lavage in immunocompromised children with pneumonia. Pediatr Pulmonol 5:1–5, 1988.
35. de Blic J, Blanche S, Danel C, et al: Bronchoaveolar lavage in HIV infected patients with interstitial pneumonitis. Arch Dis Child 64:1246–1250, 1989.
36. Couderc LJ, Herve P, Solal-Celigny P, et al: Pneumonie lymphoide interstitielle et polyadenopathies chez des sujets infectes par le virus LAV/HTLV III. Presse Med 15:1127–1130, 1986.
37. Plata F, Autran B, Martins LP, et al: AIDS virus-specific cytotoxic T lymphocytes in lung disorders. Nature 328:348–351, 1987.
38. Ho DD, Pomerantz RJ, Kaplan JC: Pathogenesis of infection with immunodeficiency virus. N Engl J Med 317:278–286, 1987.
39. Laraya-Cuasay LR, Hughes WT: Interstitial Lung Diseases in Children, vols. I, II, III. Boca Raton, FL: CRC Press, 1988.
40. Hamman L, Rich A: Acute diffuse interstitial fibrosis of the lung. Bull Johns Hopkins Hosp 74:177–204, 1944.
41. Swaye P, Van Ordstrand HS, McCormack LJ, et al: Familial Hamman-Rich syndrome. Report of eight cases. Dis Chest 55:7–12, 1969.
42. Solliday NH, Williams JA, Gaensler EA, et al: Familial chronic interstitial pneumonia. Am Rev Respir Dis 108:193–204, 1973.

43. Turton CWG, Morris LM, Lawler SD, et al: HLA in cryptogenic fibrosing alveolitis. Lancet 1:507–508, 1978.
44. Dreisin RB, Schwarz MI, Theofilopoulos AN: Circulating immune complexes in the idiopathic interstitial pneumonias. N Engl J Med 298:353–357, 1978.
45. Turner-Warwick M, Haslam P: Antibodies in some chronic fibrosing lung diseases. I. Non organ-specific autoantibodies. Clin Allergy 1:83, 1971.
46. Wiggers HJ, Berdon WE, Ores CN: Fatal desquamative interstitial pneumonia in an infant: Case report with transmission and scanning electron microscopical studies. Arch Pathol Lab Med 101:129–132, 1977.
47. Carrington CB, Gaensler EA, Coutu RE, et al: Natural history and treated course of usual and desquamative pneumonia. N Engl J Med 298:801–809, 1978.
48. Howatt WF, Heidelberger KP, LeGlovan DP, et al: Desquamative interstitial pneumonia: Case report of an infant unresponsive to treatment. Am J Dis Child 126:346–348, 1973.
49. Barnes SE, Godfrey S, Milward-Sadler GH, et al: Desquamative fibrosing alveolitis unresponsive to steroid or cytotoxic therapy. Arch Dis Child 50:324–327, 1975.
50. Tal A, Maor E, Bar-Ziv J, Gorodischer R: Fatal desquamative interstitial pneumonia in three infant siblings. J Pediatr 104:873–876, 1984.
51. Buchta RM, Park S, Giammona ST: Desquamative interstitial pneumonia in a 7 week old infant. Am J Dis Child 120:341–343, 1970.
52. Hewitt CJ, Hull D, Keeling JW: Fibrosing alveolitis in infancy and childhood. Arch Dis Child 52:22–37, 1977.
53. Kerem E, Bentur L, England S, et al: Sequential pulmonary function measurements during treatment of infantile chronic interstitial pneumonitis. J Pediatr 116:61–67, 1990.
54. Bhagwat AG, Wentworth P, Conen PE: Observations on the relationship of desquamative interstitial pneumonia and pulmonary alveolar proteinosis in childhood: A pathologic and experimental study. Chest 58:326–332, 1970.
55. Patchefsky AS, Fraimow W, Hoch WS: Desquamative interstitial pneumonia: Pathological findings and follow-up in 13 patients. Arch Intern Med 132:222–225, 1973.
56. McCann BG, Brewer DB: A case of desquamative interstitial pneumonia progressing to "honeycomb lung." J Pathol 112:199–202, 1974.
57. Valdivia E, Hensley G, Leory EP, et al: Morphology and pathogenesis of desquamative interstitial pneumonitis. Thorax 32:7–18, 1977.
58. Stillwell PC, Norris DG, O'Connell EJ, et al: Desquamative interstitial pneumonitis in children. Chest 77:165–171, 1980.
59. Hilman BC: Interstitial and hypersensitivity pneumonitis and their variants. Pediatr Rev 1(8):229–238, 1980.
60. Patchefsky AS, Banner M, Freundlich IM: Desquamative interstitial pneumonia: Significance of intranuclear viral-like inclusion bodies. Ann Intern Med 74:322–327, 1971.
61. McNary WF, Gaensler EA: Intranuclear inclusion bodies in desquamative interstitial pneumonia: Electron microscopic observations. Ann Intern Med 74:404–407, 1971.
62. O'Brodovich HM, Moser MM, Lu L: Familial lymphoid interstitial pneumonia: A long-term follow-up. Pediatrics 65:523–528, 1980.
63. Church JA, Isaacs H, Saxon A, et al: Lymphoid interstitial pneumonitis and hypogammaglobulinemia in children. Am Rev Respir Dis 124:491, 1981.
64. Joshi VV, Oleske JM, Minnefor AB, et al: Pathologic findings in children with the acquired immunodeficiency syndrome: A study of ten cases. Hum Pathol 16:241–246, 1985.

43 PULMONARY MANIFESTATIONS OF NEUROLOGIC DISEASE

MARGARET M. SULLIVAN, M.D.

The pediatric pulmonologist is often consulted to evaluate the respiratory status of a child with a neurologic disease. A variety of neurologic disorders ranging from central nervous system (CNS) dysfunction to peripheral neuropathies can result in significant respiratory compromise. The evaluation and management of patients with respiratory problems that develop as a consequence of disorders of the central and peripheral nervous system are discussed.

DISORDERS OF THE CEREBRUM AND BRAINSTEM

Abnormalities involving the cerebral hemispheres and the brainstem often have an impact on the respiratory status of a person. This is usually a result of adverse effects on the brainstem respiratory control centers, the pons, and the medulla. The pons and the medulla each have two regions concerned primarily with acid-base balance and oxygen homeostasis.[1] The pons contains the pneumotaxic center, which functions to modulate respiratory frequency and depth. The apneustic center in the pons produces atonic inspiratory spasm that is modulated by feedback mechanisms from the pneumotaxic center, the medulla, and afferent vagal impulses. Injury or ablation of the pons can result in gasping and uncoordinated respiratory pattern.[2]

The medulla contains the inspiratory and the expiratory centers, which are intrinsically rhythmic and modulated by pontine and vagal input. Medullary chemoreceptors monitor the acid-base status of the cerebral spinal fluid and alter ventilation, depending on the pH of the fluid (a lower pH increases ventilation and a higher pH slows ventilation). The medullary reticular system aids in maintaining the ability of the respiratory neurons to discharge spontaneously. This may be an important mechanism in initiating spontaneous respirations in the newborn.[2] These control centers of respiration, also labeled the central pattern generator, are modulated by feedback mechanisms that include input from central and peripheral chemoreceptors and afferent stimuli from lung stretch receptors and intercostal muscle and tendon propioceptors. The interaction of the central control centers and these feedback mechanisms creates an effective respiratory rate and rhythm.[2, 3]

Congenital malformations, disorders of the CNS, and various insults to the CNS can affect these respiratory centers and compromise ventilation. The more common disorders seen in children are discussed as follows.

SEIZURES

Seizures represent one of the most common neurologic disorders that can adversely affect respiratory status. Approximately 5% of children have one or more seizures.[3, 4] Seizures may be precipitated by prenatal or perinatal complications, meningitis, head trauma, fever, tumors, vascular lesions, metabolic disturbances, lead intoxication, drug ingestion, and idiopathic causes. There are various types of seizure disorders, each with its own electrophysiologic and clinical characteristics. Generalized seizures are discussed here because they have the most adverse effects on respiratory status.

In a generalized or tonic-clonic seizure, there is abnormal electrical activity in the neurons of both cerebral hemispheres. A large number of neurons discharge simultaneously and at high frequency in all areas of the cortex. Clinical manifestation of this type of seizure is an initial sustained contraction of the skeletal muscles (tonic phase) followed by intermittent, rapid muscle contractions and ocular movements (clonic phase). Ventilation is impaired in both phases. During the tonic phase, there is no gas exchange while all the skeletal muscles, including the diaphragm and the intercostal muscles, are in tonic contraction. During this phase, there may also be excessive salivation and emesis, which may result in aspiration. In the clonic phase, ventilation is characterized by a rapid panting pattern, which is ineffective. If the seizure is prolonged or recurrent, the condition of the patient may deteriorate to status epilepticus, in which the patient is usually unconscious. In status epilepticus, ventilation is impaired and complications of hypoxemia, respiratory, and lactic acidosis develop.

After a seizure (postictal phase), the brain function is diffusely impaired and the patient is lethargic and at risk for hypoventilation or apnea.[3, 4]

Management during a generalized seizure focuses on keeping the airway open and clear of secretions, protecting the patient from bodily injury, and stopping the seizure activity. The patient's clothes should be loosened, the airway cleared, and, if possible, an artificial oral airway created. Turning the patient onto the side may prevent aspiration. Oropharyngeal suctioning can be performed gently to avoid overstimulation and a possible increase in seizure activity. Oxygen should be given by

mask, intravenous access achieved, and anticonvulsants administered, if the seizure persists. The anticonvulsant drugs can depress ventilatory function, and the dosage and the patient must be carefully monitored. If the seizure is refractory to drug therapy, intubation and general anesthesia may be required.[5] After the seizure, the patient should continue to receive supplemental oxygen and be observed for apnea or hypoventilation. Once the patient is stable, the cause of the seizure should be investigated and appropriate diagnostic procedures completed.

COMA

Coma refers to an altered state of consciousness and can be classified into four stages. In stage I, there is stupor, but the patient may be aroused for a brief period of time and may exhibit some simple responses to pain. In stage II (light coma), the patient cannot be aroused even with painful stimuli but may be able to make some spontaneous verbal sounds or movements. Stage III is deep coma with no movement or response except possibly decerebrate posturing. In stage IV, the patient is flaccid and has no spontaneous respiration or pupillary reflexes, and all brainstem functions are absent.[4, 6]

The causes of coma include trauma, infection, metabolic encephalopathy, drug intoxication, tumor, vascular disease, postictal state, and hydrocephalus. The evaluation of a comatose patient should include a complete history from the family or caretakers, a thorough physical examination, and appropriate diagnostic tests.

The respiratory status of a comatose patient is guarded and requires constant monitoring for hypoventilation or apnea, which can progress to respiratory failure. In coma stages I to III, a child is usually able to maintain spontaneous respiration, but the adequacy needs to be assessed by tests of blood gases or oximetry. Intervention with supplemental oxygen or mechanical ventilation should be instituted when indicated. In stage IV coma, mechanical ventilation is needed.

In addition to monitoring arterial oxygen and carbon dioxide levels, the pulmonary management of a comatose child must include frequent physical examinations to detect deepening levels of coma, evidence of increased intracranial pressure, and further disruption of central respiratory control. Close observation of the respiratory pattern alerts the physician to respiratory center compromise. Hyperventilation may be caused by metabolic acidosis or may occur in respiratory alkalosis because of abnormal stimulaton of the medullary respiratory center (e.g., as in Reye's syndrome or hepatic coma). The onset of periodic or irregular breathing can indicate medullary dysfunction and may precede apnea. Observing pupillary responses provides information on brainstem status. Fixed and dilated pupils signal a brainstem insult; pinpoint pupils are seen in opiate or barbiturate ingestion and also with pontine lesions. Funduscopic examination gives information on the presence of increased intracranial pressure. If present, increased intracranial pressure should be treated with measures such as hyperventilation, osmotic diuresis, or ventricular taps. These measures lessen the disruption of the central respiratory control centers.

In addition to the monitoring for changes in central respiratory control, the respiratory management of a comatose child must include protecting the upper airway and preventing pulmonary infection from aspiration of saliva or vomitus. The patient should be placed semiprone or in a lateral position and should also undergo frequent suctioning of oropharyngeal secretions. If enteral nutrition is given, it should be administered via a nasogastric or, ideally, a nasojejunal tube in order to prevent aspiration.

Atelectasis may be a problem, particularly if the coma is prolonged. If the intracranial pressure is not elevated and there are no other contraindications, chest physiotherapy may be beneficial.

CENTRAL APNEA

In central apnea, there is a cessation of diaphragmatic and accessory muscle respiratory effort secondary to CNS disorder that results in a respiratory pause lasting more than 15 to 20 sec. In a number of congenital and acquired neurologic conditions in the pediatric population, apnea is a significant component. In infants, these conditions include apnea of prematurity, seizures, infection, cardiac arrhythmias, and gastroesophageal reflux. In older children central apnea may be a symptom of brainstem disease such as encephalitis, trauma, surgery, congenital malformation, metabolic abnormalities, infarction, and central depression. The severity of acquired apnea depends on the extent of medullary disruption.[3]

The diagnosis of central apnea can be made by polysomnography, which monitors chest wall movements, nasal airflow, and oral airflow; electrocardiogram (ECG) and electroencephalogram (EEG) recordings; and oxygen saturation levels while the patient is both awake and asleep. In patients with central apnea, chest wall movements and nasal and oral airflow cease during apneic episodes. Also oxygen desaturation and bradycardia may occur. Evaluation of the ECG and EEG recordings helps rule out any cardiac or seizure component. Once central apnea is diagnosed, computed tomography (CT) or magnetic resonance imaging (MRI) of the head should be performed to identify any anatomic disorder. Further evaluation of the apnea should include a thorough history, physical examination, and diagnostic testing to identify the various causes of central respiratory control dysfunction.

Management of patients with central apnea focuses on treating the underlying cause, if possible, and on preventing the apneic episodes and decreasing the risk of respiratory arrest or development of pulmonary hypertension and cor pulmonale. Many patients with acquired central apnea syndromes have a static condition resulting from the initial CNS insult. However, apnea from progressive systemic disease may advance to frank respiratory failure if the underlying disease process is not halted.[3]

Apnea of prematurity is a relatively common event, often during the non–rapid eye movement (REM) sleep stage, in up to 50% of infants who are less than 35 weeks of gestation. These apneic events are thought to be a result of the immaturity of the central respiratory center.[7, 8] These episodes ultimately resolve with maturity for the majority of infants.

In the evaluation of the premature infant with apnea it must first be determined whether the apneic events are precipitated by any of the causes listed previously. If the apnea is judged to be a result of prematurity, the use of theophylline therapy and an oscillating bed for continuous stimulation may be beneficial. The use of sleep-apnea monitors is essential for these patients. For patients who are discharged home from the neonatal nursery, their parents or caretakers should be trained in cardiopulmonary resuscitation and have the equipment at home for this (e.g., Ambubag).

Congenital central alveolar hypoventilation syndrome (CCHS), also called Ondine's curse, is a rare condition characterized by a marked depression of respiratory drive during sleep. In this condition, no other abnormalities of cardiac, lung, or neuromuscular disease can account for the apnea. Ventilation when the patient is awake is usually normal except during episodes of respiratory infection, when apnea and hypoventilation can be a problem in both the awake and asleep states. Guilleminault and coauthors demonstrated apnea, with evidence of hypoxia and hypercapnia, in infants with CCHS during stages 3 and 4 of the non-REM delta slow-wave sleep state.[9] This type of sleep develops progressively during the first few months of life, so that infants with this disorder are at increasing risk of respiratory failure and sudden death as they grow older.

The cause of CCHS is not well defined. Pathologic and radiologic studies to date seem to suggest a diffuse CNS process rather than a discrete lesion.[3, 10, 11] Some researchers believe that it is caused by a defect of the central chemoreceptors located in the medulla, and this accounts for the apnea during non-REM sleep when ventilation is maximally under chemical control.[9, 12] Others postulate that an autonomic nervous system defect may be operative because there is an association of CCHS and Hirschsprung's disease and also a higher incidence of ganglioblastoma in these patients. It is speculated that central chemoreception may be normal, but the integration of central information and autonomic central input may be defective.[9, 13, 14] There may be a genetic or familial component.[15]

Older children with evidence of central alveolar hypoventilation may have brainstem disease resulting from the various causes listed earlier. Evaluation includes polysomnography, MRI, or CT scan. Tests for evaluating the ventilatory response to hypoxia and hypercapnia can also demonstrate a blunted response in these patients. Voluntary control of ventilation is usually intact, and these patients can hyperventilate and normalize their arterial blood gases.[3]

Many of the patients with either congenital or acquired central alveolar hypoventilation syndrome require a tracheostomy with nighttime mechanical ventilation.[9] The patients must be evaluated regularly for correct ventilator settings and tracheostomy tube size to ensure adequate ventilation and the absence of air leaks. Use of a fenestrated tracheostomy tube allows for crying and the development of normal speech during the daytime. A non-fenestrated inner cannula can be placed at night for ventilatory support. Nocturnal monitoring is mandatory.

Phrenic nerve pacing has been performed in children with CCHS. In one study, seven infants with CCHS underwent bilateral phrenic nerve pacing. In the follow-up period, ranging from 6 months to 8 years postoperatively, six patients were adequately ventilated by pacing during sleep, and an additional patient was paced during the day and mechanically ventilated during the night. The pacing interval was either 12 continuous h or a total of 16 to 18 h in a 24-h period.[16] Some studies have shown that prolonged low-voltage electrophrenic pacing can be performed without damaging the phrenic curve.[17] Other studies have shown histologic changes in the phrenic nerve with prolonged pacing.[18] Obviously, more investigation is needed in this area; until then, continuous 24-h pacing is not recommended.

When these infants are paced, bilateral phrenic nerve pacers must be implanted because unilateral pacing does not sustain adequate ventilation.[16] A tracheostomy is also required during pacing because of problems with upper airway obstruction. There is an inability to synchronize laryngeal and upper airway muscle activity with diaphragmatic contraction.[16] When electrophrenic pacing is performed, the adequacy of ventilation is assessed via arterial blood gas sampling and oximetry. These patients can be managed at home, but such care does require close attention to detail by both the parents or caretakers and the medical team.

Arnold-Chiari malformation (ACM) is another CNS disorder in which apnea and hypoventilation may occur. In this condition, there is protrusion of the medulla oblongata and the cerebellum through the foramen magnum into the spinal canal. There is often associated hydrocephalus as well as a variety of neurologic abnormalities resulting from central and peripheral nervous system dysfunction.[19, 20] Oren and colleagues reported four patients with ACM and myelodysplasia who had abnormal ventilation characterized by hypoventilation, prolonged sleep apnea, and prolonged breath-holding spells. It is postulated that these events result from structural derangements in the pontomedullary respiratory control centers and in its afferent and efferent pathways (e.g., dysplastic development of vagal nuclei structures).[19] Hypoventilation may also result from compression of the brainstem respiratory centers. Herniation of the hindbrain into the spinal canal can displace the vascular supply and result in ischemia to the brainstem.[21]

The evaluation for apnea in ACM is as described for the other previously mentioned apnea disorders (polysomnography, MRI, and so on). These patients also must be evaluated for evidence of increased intracranial pressure and brainstem compression.

Management of the apnea in ACM often includes relief of the increased pressure or brainstem compression. Apnea has been alleviated in some of these patients after shunting procedures or decompression of the posterior fossa.[22] Also, in some of these patients who have apneic episodes associated with crying or painful stimuli, the apnea is controlled with atropine.[19] It is speculated that these episodes are secondary to disordered vagal activity resulting from dysplastic nuclei development or the stretching of vagal fibers when there is displacement of the posterior fossa structures into the spinal canal.[19]

Patients with ACM who do not respond to the therapies just described and who have significant apnea require tracheostomy with mechanical ventilation and oxygen supplementation.

CEREBRAL PALSY

Cerebral palsy is a CNS disorder that may lead to recurrent pneumonias and chronic upper airway problems. It is a chronic nonprogressive static encephalopathy. The primary insult involves the motor areas of the brain, including the pyramidal and extrapyramidal systems.

Histologic examination of the brains of these patients has revealed cerebral atrophy with cavity formation in the subcortical white matter and cystic degeneration of the white matter, as well as atrophy of the basal ganglia. In mild cases, the brain may appear normal but is decreased in weight.[4, 23–25]

Two major risk factors associated with the development of cerebral palsy are prematurity with low birth weight and intraventricular hemorrhage and asphyxiation.[4, 23, 26] Before the development of exchange transfusion and phototherapy, kernicterus secondary to hyperbilirubinemia was another significant etiologic factor in cerebral palsy. Bacterial meningitis and viral encephalitis in the early neonatal period can also result in motor deficits with signs and symptoms of cerebral palsy.

Clinically, the patient with cerebral palsy has abnormalities in posture, muscle tone, and motor coordination. The predominant neurologic signs are spasticity with hyperreflexia, tight fist clenching, extensor posturing, and scissoring of the legs. Patients with spastic quadriplegia are most often referred to the pulmonologist. These patients have severe limitations, many are mentally retarded, and they have pseudobulbar palsy, which entails paresis of the facial, lingual, and laryngeal muscles. This makes feeding and the handling of secretions very difficult, and recurrent aspiration is a problem. Some patients may have abnormal dyskinetic movements of the facial muscles, the tongue, and the palate. This is manifested by grimacing, swallowing, and feeding and speech abnormalities. There can also be a lack of coordination of the respiratory muscles with an erratic breathing pattern.[26] This feature exacerbates the chronic aspiration problems. Because of the musculoskeletal problem that exists, deformity of the thoracic cage develops, particularly scoliosis, which further compromises the respiratory status of these patients. Pediatric pulmonologists who evaluate patients with cerebral palsy must address three issues: (1) gastroesophageal reflux with pulmonary aspiration; (2) oropharyngeal muscular incoordination with subsequent aspiration of oral secretions and food, and (3) thoracic cage deformities (e.g., scoliosis).

Patients with severe cerebral palsy invariably have gastroesophageal reflux with frequent episodes of aspiration pneumonia. The cause of the reflux centers on the generalized muscular incoordination and spasticity, which does not allow for normal esophageal motility and gastric emptying. Also problems with positioning and a limited ability to flex the trunk and elevate the upper body can exacerbate the reflux and aspiration. The recurrent aspiration leads to life-threatening respiratory compromise, bacterial infection, and chronic lung disease. Reflux therapy is directed toward preventing aspiration. Positioning and nasogastric or nasojejunal tube feeding may be initially tried. Agents such as metoclopramide or bethanechol may also be tried with caution. Many of these patients require a gastric fundoplication with gastrostomy or gastrojejunal tube placement, which often helps in alleviating the reflux problem. However, a fair number of patients still aspirate chronically, and the surgical results may not be long-lasting. For these patients, placement of a percutaneous jejunal tube may be the best intervention.

Patients with pseudobulbar palsy have excessive pooling of oral secretions, resulting in obstruction of the upper airway and chronic aspiration of these secretions. Also there is aspiration of oral feedings as a result of dysfunctional oropharyngeal muscles. Treatment for this is directed at preventing aspiration. Therapy in young infants is initiated with the aid of a speech therapist and is aimed at inhibiting abnormal oral reflexes and encouraging more normal sucking and swallowing mechanisms. Included in this therapy are appropriate positioning of the head and manual facilitation of jaw control. The focus is on developing muscle control by normalizing the feeding patterns.[27] This therapy may help in the handling of secretions and may enable oral feedings in some patients.

If the oropharyngeal dysfunction does not allow for bulbar muscle training, therapy is directed toward keeping the upper airway free of secretions and food. This entails tube feeding, suctioning of the oropharynx, and chest physiotherapy to promote the drainage of aspirated secretions. A trial of atropine or glycopyrrolate may help these patients by decreasing the production of oral secretions.[28] These patients often need tracheostomy placement because of upper airway obstruction secondary to secretions and poor pharyngeal muscle tone. The tracheostomy maintains the airway, but secretion control and feeding must continue to be monitored.

For patients who have intractable pulmonary aspiration, Eisele and co-workers[29] proposed a tracheoesophageal diversion procedure for draining secretions into the esophagus. In this procedure, the upper respiratory tract is surgically separated from the digestive tract. The trachea is divided between the fourth and fifth rings, and the proximal segment is anastomosed to an anterior esophagotomy in an end-to-side manner. The distal tracheal segment is brought out to the skin as a tracheostoma. Eisele and colleagues reported successfully preventing aspiration in adult patients who underwent this procedure. These patients were also able to tolerate oral feeding.[29] For children with cerebral palsy, such a procedure might be considered only after failure of all of the other modalities for preventing the aspiration of upper airway secretions and gastric contents.

Another area of concern for children with severe cerebral palsy is the development of scoliosis. Thoracic cage deformity and scoliosis lead to problems of atelectasis, with subsequent complications of pneumonia, compromised ventilation, and restrictive lung disease. Medical management is directed at minimizing the development of thoracic cage deformity. The use of specially fitted chairs with proper support and positioning of the back and chest is indicated. Chest wall support through the use of custom-made vests also helps in promoting good pos-

ture. These modalities must be instituted early in growing and developing children. Physical therapy is important in helping develop upper body muscle strength. When problems with atelectasis do exist, chest physiotherapy and bronchial drainage are indicated. Also early recognition of pulmonary infection and prompt treatment with antibiotics are advised.

CRANIAL NERVE DYSFUNCTION

The ability to chew, swallow, and coordinate swallowing and breathing involves the interaction of branches of cranial nerves 5, 7, 9, 10, 11, and 12. Dysfunction in any of these nerves can result in problems with handling oral secretions and in swallowing, ultimately placing the patient at high risk for aspiration. Problems with these cranial nerves can also lead to obstructive apnea secondary to poor pharyngeal muscle tone and collapse of the pharyngeal airway during sleep when the tone of these muscles is decreased. Isolated cranial nerve disorders are not very common in the pediatric population, but a few syndromes that may require consultation by the pediatric pulmonologist do exist.

MÖBIUS'S SYNDROME

Möbius's syndrome is a nonprogressive condition in which there is a deterioration or a lack of development of the cranial nerve motor nuclei. Cranial nerves 6 and 7 are most often involved, but cranial nerves 5, 9, 10, 11, and 12 can be involved as well.[4, 30] Affected patients typically have bilateral facial palsy and ophthalmoplegia. When other cranial nerve nuclei are involved, there is difficulty with chewing and swallowing, and there are problems with aspiration pneumonia. Other associated congenital anomalies may include hearing loss, pectoral muscle defects, micrognathia, and hand and foot anomalies.

FAZIO-LONDE DISEASE

Fazio-Londe disease, or progressive bulbar paralysis of childhood, involves a decrease in the number of motor cells in the cranial nerve nuclei as well as degenerative changes in the brainstem and anterior horn cells. The cause is unknown, and it may be hereditary. Cranial nerve 7 is most often involved; however, cranial nerves 3, 4, 6, 10, and 12 can also be affected.[30] As in Möbius's syndrome, problems with chewing, swallowing, and aspiration of oral contents can occur. The symptoms tend to begin around the age of 3 years.

ARNOLD-CHIARI MALFORMATION

Children with myelodysplasia and Arnold-Chiari malformation can also have cranial nerve dysfunction as a result of structural derangement and compression of nerve structures.[19] These patients may have no gag or cough reflexes and may have oropharyngeal incoordination; these deficits lead to repeated episodes of aspiration pneumonia. Also, some patients with faulty innervation of the posterior cricoarytenoid muscles have bilateral abductor vocal cord paralysis and are at risk for aspiration. The presence of thoracolumbar myelodysplasia in these patients is associated with abdominal muscle weakness, which leads to an ineffective cough, obstruction of airway from secretions, and further respiratory compromise.[22]

The respiratory medical management of patients with Möbius's syndrome, Fazio-Londe disease, and ACM with cranial nerve dysfunction is similar to the treatment discussed for patients with pseudobulbar cerebral palsy. Management includes the prevention of aspiration pneumonia by the institution of tube feeding; frequent suctioning of oral secretions; chest physiotherapy and bronchial drainage; and speech therapy aimed at promoting the coordination of oropharyngeal movements.

SPINAL CORD PATHOLOGY

Lesions of the spinal cord from the level of C-1 to T-6 can impair ventilatory function. The most dramatic cases involve patients with quadriplegia. Quadriparesis can be secondary to an intrinsic spinal cord tumor, trauma, infection (e.g., poliomyelitis), or external compression of the cervical cord (e.g., a dislocated vertebra, tumor, or vascular anomaly). The degree of impairment depends on the level of the lesion.

High cervical cord lesions at the level of C-1 and C-2 and midcervical cord lesions at the level of C-3 to C-5 result in paralysis of the diaphragm, intercostal muscles, scalene muscles, and abdominal muscles. With these lesions, ventilation is seriously compromised and respiratory failure is inevitable, especially in infants and young children. Older children may attempt to use inspiratory neck muscles to breathe, and this results in pulling the sternum upward and expanding the upper rib cage in a lateral and anteroposterior direction with alteration of the rib cage contour. There is also paradoxical motion of the lateral wall of the lower rib cage, which may be related to a decrease in pleural pressures with inspiratory effort.[31] This chest wall motion, in addition to the fact that chest wall compliance is decreased, results in increased work of breathing. Also, with these cervical lesions, cough is ineffective, and bronchial secretions accumulate and lead to recurrent pneumonia and atelectasis.

The medical management of patients with high or midcervical cord lesions is aimed at identifying and treating the cause of the paralysis if possible (i.e., spinal cord tumor decompression, radiation, antibiotic therapy, chemotherapy). In cases in which the quadriplegia is permanent, the treatment must center on preventing respiratory failure, chronic pneumonia, and atelectasis. These patients usually require tracheostomy with either full-time or part-time mechanical ventilatory support. Older children may be trained to breathe on their own for hours by using their sternomastoid, trapezius, platysmus, myelohyoid, and sternohyoid muscles or by glossopharyngeal breathing.[3, 32] Hypertrophy of the sternomastoid and trapezius muscles has been noted in adult patients as well as electromyographic activity in the other muscles mentioned.[31, 33] In patients with high cervical lesions, the phrenic nerve nuclei are spared, and phrenic nerve pacing is possible. In patients with midcervical cord lesions, the motor nuclei of the phrenic nerve are lost, and so they are unresponsive to phrenic nerve pacing. These patients can be evaluated by percutaneous stimulation of the phrenic nerve in the neck and observed for abdominal movement or monitored for electrical activity of the diaphragm.[18] For patients with sparing of the phrenic nerve motor nuclei, successful pacing with the use of a very low-frequency electrical stimulus has been accomplished.[18, 34-36] Pacing enables increased mobility of the patient. The person being paced must be routinely evaluated through arterial blood gas measurements to ensure that adequate ventilation is being achieved. Ventilatory monitors with alarms should be attached to the patient, and a back-up portable mechanical ventilation system should be available. This is especially important if the patient is discharged home or to an institution. Most patients use the ventilator for a portion of the time (nights) and the pacers the rest of the time. Good tracheostomy care is necessary, as is the removal of secretions. Chest physiotherapy on a routine basis might help avoid atelectasis and secretion accumulation. A fenestrated tracheal tube can be used to enable speech while the patient is using the pacer.

Reports on the use of noninvasive means of ventilatory assistance in quadriplegic patients have been published.[37] These respiratory support techniques include direct positive airway pressure methods such as intermittent positive-pressure ventilation via the mouth or nose and the use of negative-pressure body ventilators and glossopharyngeal breathing techniques. In one report, the authors described the conversion of a large number of patients from mechanical ventilatory support via tracheostomy or endotracheal tube to positive-pressure ventilation by mouth.[37] This technique can be used during sleep as long as the chemotaxis centers have not been altered.

The advantages of using noninvasive means of ventilation are that a tracheostomy, with its inherent complications, and fear of disconnection from the ventilator are eliminated and effective speech can be allowed.

For positive-pressure ventilation by mouth, the patient must be alert and cooperative. Small children, infants, and mentally impaired persons are not candidates. Intact functional oropharyngeal musculature is also required.

Patients with spinal cord lesions between the levels of C-6 and T-6 have paralysis of the intercostal and abdominal muscles. Innervation to the diaphragm and neck muscles is intact, and mechanical ventilation is usually not needed. Pulmonary function testing can be performed on older children with these lesions. A restrictive pattern with a decrease in vital capacity and in total lung capacity is evident.[38] Positioning can affect the pulmonary function test results in these patients. When the position of a patient is changed from erect to supine, there is an increase in the vital capacity and a decrease in residual volume and total lung capacity.[39] It is postulated that the change in vital capacity is secondary to the change in the residual volume. The residual volume change is caused by changes in the position of the abdominal contents (i.e., in the upright position, there is bulging of the abdomen secondary to abdominal muscle paralysis, and in the supine position there is an upward displacement of the viscera because of gravity, resulting in the upward movement of the diaphragm). The use of an abdominal binder when the patient is sitting can prevent the abdominal bulging and can reduce residual volume (air trapping).[39]

Because function of the respiratory muscles is impaired and chest wall compliance is decreased, the work of breathing is increased. This can be a significant problem if pneumonia is present because the patient may not be able to meet the increased ventilatory requirements during an acute illness. Mechanical ventilation may be needed at these times.

Cough and secretion clearance are impaired in these patients, and the risk of pneumonia, chronic bronchial infection, and atelectasis is increased.

Therapy is focused on identifying and treating the cause of the paralysis if feasible and on maximizing the function of the neck and unaffected intercostal muscles. Intensive rehabilitation training is needed. Also routine chest physiotherapy to help clear secretions is beneficial. Mechanical ventilation (negative or positive) should be initiated if the patient shows evidence of hypoventilation (e.g., during acute illness or during sleep).

PERIPHERAL NERVE DYSFUNCTION

Disorders of the peripheral nervous system that can result in respiratory compromise include the neural components involved in diaphragmatic, intercostal, and accessory muscle innervation. Respiratory problems can be similar to those seen with upper spinal cord lesions, although in many cases they are not as severe. Two of the more common conditions in this category are phrenic nerve dysfunction and Guillain-Barré syndrome.

The phrenic nerve is composed of neural fibers originating from C-3, C-4, and C-5 nerve roots. Injury to this nerve results in flaccidity, loss of muscle tone, and elevation and eventual disuse atrophy of the diaphragmatic muscles. Isolated phrenic nerve dysfunction in pediatric patients can be caused by trauma (e.g., during the birth delivery process) or a consequence of a thoracic surgical complication. Phrenic nerve dysfunction can result with infection or malignancy (which is rare in children), or often it is idiopathic.[33, 40]

The clinical manifestation can range from severe respiratory distress with respiratory arrest to mild tachypnea or no respiratory symptoms at all. Neonates and older infants are particularly compromised whether there is unilateral or bilateral phrenic nerve dysfunction. This is because of the pliability of the chest wall and poor respiratory accessory muscle function. Infants may have cyanosis, dyspnea, and respiratory failure requiring mechanical ventilation. Lung atelectasis is present, and there is a high risk of pulmonary infection.[41]

Older children with unilateral phrenic nerve dysfunction may have tachypnea or evidence of accessory muscle use. They may be asymptomatic unless an infection develops in the atelectatic lung. On physical examination, when a patient with unilateral diaphragm paralysis inspires, there is an inward movement of the abdominal

wall instead of the expected outward movement. On auscultation, no change in diaphragm position is noted with inspiration, and decreased breath sounds or rales may be heard on the affected side. Dullness with percussion may be noted if atelectasis exists. The chest radiograph shows elevation of the hemidiaphragm on the affected side. This elevation must be differentiated from pleural and subpulmonic effusion and from eventration of the diaphragm.

Older children with bilateral phrenic nerve dysfunction have dyspnea, and respiratory failure develops. These patients use intercostal and accessory muscles to breathe, but during sleep these muscles are not active enough, and hypoventilation results.[33] Physical examination reveals tachypnea, dyspnea, and auscultative findings similar to those in unilateral dysfunction except that the abnormalities are bilateral. Chest radiographs show bilateral elevation of the diaphragm with probable atelectasis.

Fluoroscopy should be performed in patients with suspected diaphragm paralysis. In unilateral diaphragmatic paralysis, there is very little or no motion of the affected hemidiaphragm. A deep inspiration reveals an upward displacement of the affected hemidiaphragm instead of a downward shift; this is secondary to the increase in intraabdominal pressure occurring with the sudden downward motion of the contralateral functional hemidiaphragm.[42] In bilateral phrenic nerve injury, the lack of diaphragm motion is bilateral.

For older children who are able to perform pulmonary function testing, a restrictive pattern is observed. The vital capacity and the total lung capacity may be decreased, and the functional residual capacity may be normal.[33] Pulmonary function testing with the patient in the supine position reveals a further reduction in vital capacity in comparison with the upright position. This is caused by the gravitational effect of the upward displacement of the diaphragm when supine. Gas exchange may also be affected when the patient is supine, and there can be a decrease in arterial oxygen pressure/tension and a rise in the arterial carbon dioxide pressure/tension.

Further evaluation of phrenic nerve function is possible. Nerve conduction time can be measured by percutaneous stimulation of the phrenic nerve in the neck. This helps define whether the injury is in the peripheral nerve fibers or close to or at the spinal cord level. Evaluation of diaphragm function can be performed by recording pressures, simultaneously in the esophagus and in the stomach, with the use of a balloon-tipped catheter. The pressure difference, recorded during inspiration, between the esophagus and the stomach reflects the force generated by the diaphragm. With diaphragm paralysis, the pressure change is very small or zero.[18, 33]

The management of patients with phrenic nerve disorders must include identifying and treating the cause, if possible, and preventing respiratory compromise. For infants with unilateral or bilateral nerve dysfunction, intensive care with mechanical ventilation is required. In the case of Erb's palsy, phrenic nerve dysfunction is often temporary, and diaphragmatic function is recovered. If there has been avulsion of the anterior nerve roots (C-3, C-4, and C-5), recovery is unlikely.[43] In these cases, long-term mechanical ventilation is necessary, and surgical plication of the diaphragm is usually performed. Electrophrenic pacing has been attempted on infants with diaphragmatic paralysis and can be performed when the injury to the nerve is very close to the nerve root and most of the lower motor neuron is intact. Radecki and Tomatis reported using continuous bilateral phrenic nerve pacing in an infant.[40] As in CCHS, the use of low-frequency electrical pulses can avoid diaphragmatic fatigue and nerve injury. Because a surgical procedure is required and a tracheostomy is needed, the risks and benefits must be carefully considered. If the nerve injury is proximal and likely to be permanent, pacing is a viable alternative to continuous mechanical ventilation. If recovery of phrenic nerve function is a possibility, the implantation of pacers should be postponed and only mechanical ventilation used. In addition to mechanical ventilation, diaphragm plication, or electrophrenic pacing, therapy to prevent problems of atelectasis, secretion accumulation, and infection must be performed. The ventilatory status must be monitored carefully and routinely either by oximetry or by measurement of arterial blood gases; otherwise, there is the risk of acute respiratory arrest or chronic respiratory failure with the development of cor pulmonale.

In many older children with unilateral phrenic nerve dysfunction, no intervention is needed if ventilation is not compromised. However, these children are at risk for chronic infection of atelectatic lung segments on the affected side. Care in this situation consists of chest physiotherapy to minimize the atelectasis and of treatment with antibiotics. Older children can be trained to maximize the use of the intercostal and accessory muscles of respiration. The use of incentive spirometry can be an effective pulmonary rehabilitation method.[3] If ventilation is a serious problem, the use of a pacer can be considered if adequate lower motor neuron exists.

Older children with bilateral phrenic nerve dysfunction can also be trained to use the intercostal and accessory muscles to help improve ventilation. Most likely, however, mechanical ventilation is required, especially during sleep. If the phrenic nerve is permanently damaged, electrophrenic pacing may be considered. As indicated, routine monitoring of the ventilatory status, chest physiotherapy, and antibiotics should be part of the medical regimen.

Guillain-Barré syndrome affects the peripheral nervous system, and the major clinical features are areflexia and muscle weakness. It is a disease in which approximately 30% of the patients are under 20 years of age; two thirds are younger than 8 years, and boys tend to be affected more than girls.[44] It seems to be more prevalent in the fall and winter. The cause is unknown, but in more than half the patients, there is an antecedent upper respiratory or gastrointestinal illness.

Clinically, the patient may present with pain and paresthesias in the legs and feet. There is muscle weakness, which is progressive and symmetric, and there may be sensory deficits with respect to position and vibration. Most of the deficits are motor rather than sensory. Over time, weakness progresses, beginning in the legs and moving upward to include the arms, trunk, and facial muscles. There is a loss or diminution of the deep tendon reflexes. Findings in nerve conduction studies are abnormal in 80% of the patients.[45] The cranial nerves are involved in

50% of the cases; cranial nerve 7 is most commonly affected, followed by cranial nerves 9 and 10.[30, 44, 45] Many patients have gait disturbance, ataxia, and areflexia. The majority of symptoms evolve over 7 to 14 days. Autonomic imbalance, manifested as cardiac arrhythmias or blood pressure lability, may be observed, although not very commonly, in children. Respiratory compromise is a significant complication in at least 18% of pediatric cases.[44] The child loses the function of the intercostal and diaphragmatic muscles, and respiratory failure ensues. Compromise of oropharyngeal muscles makes handling secretions difficult and causes pulmonary aspiration. Progression to quadriplegia is possible, and the mortality rate in children is about 3% to 4%.[44]

The care of pediatric patients with Guillain-Barré syndrome is primarily supportive, but they should be placed in an intensive care unit setting. There must be continuous monitoring of the disease progression by neurologic examination. Plasmapheresis has shown some possible effectiveness in this group of patients and may be an alternative in a child whose condition is rapidly deteriorating.[46]

With regard to respiratory monitoring, signs of dyspnea, fatigue, agitation, deteriorating blood gases, and oximetry must be noted. Evidence of dysphagia or shoulder paresis mandates elective intubation. In older patients, the pulmonary function is a good indicator of pulmonary reserve. The first evidence of decline in respiratory muscle function is a decrease in the maximal inspiratory and expiratory pressures generated by the patient. These measurements may be more sensitive than monitoring of the vital capacity.[3] Vital capacity can be measured, and if it decreases to less than half the predicted value elective intubation should be performed. Ideally, intubation and mechanical ventilation should be performed under elective, controlled conditions rather than after respiratory failure occurs. Tracheostomy may be considered if mechanical ventilation is needed for more than 2 weeks. In addition to mechanical ventilation, these children need a pulmonary toilet regimen similar to that of patients with quadriplegia: chest physiotherapy and keeping the airway free of secretions and avoiding aspiration. Antibiotic therapy should be initiated if any evidence of infection exists. These patients ideally should not be fed; hyperalimentation is indicated.

The prognosis for these patients is generally good. At least 50% of patients recover within 6 months and 70% by 1 year. Some patients may be left with permanent neural deficits, particularly if they have a very prolonged course.[47]

REFERENCES

1. Phillipson EA: Control of breathing during sleep. Am Rev Respir Dis 118:909–939, 1978.
2. O'Brodovich H, Haddad G: The functional basis of respiratory pathology. *In* Chernick V, Kendig EL (eds): Disorders of the Respiratory Tract in Children, 5th ed, pp. 3–47. Philadelphia: WB Saunders, 1990.
3. Colice GL, Bernat JL: Neurologic disorders and respiration. Clin Chest Med 10:521–543, 1989.

4. Huttenlocher PR: The nervous system. *In* Behrman RE,Vaughan VC, Nelson WE (eds): Nelson Textbook of Pediatrics, 13th ed, pp. 1274–1328. Philadelphia: WB Saunders, 1987.
5. Dreiffuss FE: Focal and multifocal cortical seizures. *In* Swaiman KF (ed): Pediatric Neurology—Principles and Practice, pp. 393–411. St. Louis: CV Mosby, 1989.
6. Lockman L: Impairment of consciousness. *In* Swaiman KF (ed): Pediatric Neurology—Principles and Practice, pp. 157–167. St. Louis: CV Mosby, 1989.
7. Smith SA: Sleep disorders in children. *In* Swaiman KF (ed): Pediatric Neurlogoy—Principles and Practice, pp. 149–156. St. Louis: CV Mosby, 1989.
8. Gabriel M, Albani M, Schulte FJ: Apneic spells and sleep states in preterm infants. Pediatrics 57:142–147, 1976.
9. Guilleminault C, McQuitty J, Ariagno R, et al: Congenital central alveolar hypoventilation syndrome in six infants. Pediatrics 70:684–694, 1982.
10. Weese-Mayer DE, Brouillette RT, Naidich TP, et al: Magnetic resonance imaging and computerized tomography in central hypoventilation. Am Rev Respir Dis 137:393–398, 1988.
11. Liu HM, Loew JM, Hunt CE: Congenital central hypoventilation syndrome: A pathologic study of the neuromuscular system. Neurology 28:1013–1019, 1978.
12. Severinghaus JW, Mitchell RA: Ondine's curse: Failure of respiratory center automaticity while awake. Clin Res 10:122, 1962.
13. Haddad GG, Mazza NM, Defendini R, et al: Congenital failure of automatic control of ventilation, gastrointestinal motility and heart rate. Medicine (Baltimore) 57:517–526, 1978.
14. Korobkin R, Guilleminault C: Neurologic abnormalities in near miss for sudden infant death syndrome infants. Pediatrics 64:369–374, 1979.
15. Khalifa MM, Flavin MA, Wherrett BA: Congenital central hypoventilation syndrome in monozygotic twins. J Pediatr 113:853–855, 1988.
16. Ilbawi MN, Idress FS, Hunt CE, et al: Diaphragmatic pacing in infants: Techniques and results. Ann Thorac Surg 40:323–329, 1985.
17. Kim JH, Manuelidis EE, Glenn WW, et al: Light and electron microscopic studies of phrenic nerves after long-term electrical stimulation. J Neurosurg 58:84–91, 1983.
18. Nochomovitz ML, Petersen DK, Stellato T: Electrical activation of the diaphragm. Clin Chest Med 9:349–358, 1988.
19. Oren J, Kelly D, Todres ID, et al: Respiratory complications in patients with myelodysplasia and Arnold-Chiari malformation. Am J Dis Child 140:221–224, 1986.
20. Balk RA, Hiller FC, Lucas EA, et al: Sleep apnea and the Arnold-Chiari malformation. Am Rev Respir Dis 132:929–930, 1985.
21. Morley AR: Laryngeal stridor, Arnold-Chiari malformation and medullary haemorrhages. Dev Med Child Neurol 11:471–474, 1969.
22. Hoffman HJ, Hendrick EB, Humphres RP: Manifestations and management of Arnold-Chiari malformation in patients with myelomeningocele. Childs Brain 1:255–259, 1975.
23. Paneth N: Etiologic factors in cerebral palsy. Pediatr Ann 15:191–201, 1986.
24. Paneth N, Kiely JL: The frequency of cerebral palsy: A review of population studies from industrialized nations since 1950. Clin Dev Med 87:46–56, 1984.
25. Denhoff E: Medical aspects. *In* Cruickshank W (ed): Cerebral Palsy: A Development Disability, 3rd ed, pp. 29–71. Syracuse, NY: Syracuse University Press, 1976.
26. Barabas G, Taft LT: The early signs and differential diagnosis of cerebral palsy. Pediatr Ann 15:203–214, 1986.
27. Diamond M: Rehabilitation strategies for the child with cerebral palsy. Pediatr Ann 15:230–236, 1986.
28. Dickison AE: The normal and abnormal pediatric upper airway-recognition and management of obstruction. Clin Chest Med 8:583–597, 1986.
29. Eisele DW, Yarington CT, Lindeman RC: Indications for the tracheoesophageal diversion procedure and the laryngotracheal separation procedure. Ann Otol Rhinol Laryngol 97:471–475, 1988.
30. Swaiman KF: Anterior horn cell and cranial motor neuron disease. *In* Swaiman KF (ed): Pediatric Neurology—Principles and Practice, pp. 1083–1103. St. Louis, CV Mosby, 1989.
31. DeTroyer A, Estenne M, Vincken W: Rib cage motion and muscle use in high tetraplegics. Am Rev Respir Dis 133:1115–1119, 1986.
32. Dail CW, Affeldt JE, Collier CR: Clinical aspects of glossopharyngeal breathing. JAMA 158:445–449, 1955.
33. Tobin MJ: Respiratory muscles in disease. Clin Chest Med 9:263–286, 1988.
34. Danon J, Druz WS, Goldberg NB, et al: Function of the isolated paced diaphragm and the cervical accessory muscles in C-1 quadriplegics. Am Rev Respir Dis 119:909–919, 1979.
35. Garrido H, Mazaira J, Gutierrez P, et al: Continuous respiratory support in quadriplegic children by bilateral phrenic nerve stimulation. Thorax 42:573–577, 1987.
36. Glenn WW, Phelps ML, Elefteriades JA, et al: Twenty years of experience in phrenic nerve stimulation to pace the diaphragm. Pace 9:780–784, 1986.
37. Bach JR, Alba AS: Noninvasive options for ventilatory support of the traumatic high level quadriplegic patient. Chest 98:613–619, 1990.
38. DeTroyer A, Borenstein S, Cordier R: Analysis of lung volume restriction in patients with respiratory muscle weakness. Thorax 35:603–610, 1980.
39. Estenne M, DeTroyer A: Mechanisms of the postural dependence of vital capacity in tetraplegia subjects. Am Rev Respir Dis 135:367–371, 1987.
40. Radecki LL, Tomatis LA: Continuous bilateral electrophrenic pacing in an infant with total diaphragmatic paralysis. J Pediatr 88:969–971, 1976.
41. Canet E, Bureau MA: Chest wall diseases and dysfunction in children. *In* Chernick V, Kendig EL (eds): Disorders of the Respiratory Tract in Children, 5th ed, pp. 648–672. Philadelphia: WB Saunders, 1990.
42. Riley EA: Idiopathic diaphragmatic paralysis. Am J Med 32:404–416, 1962.
43. Mangurten HH: Birth injuries. *In* Faranoff AA, Martin RJ, Merkatz IR (eds): Behrman's Neonatal-Perinatal Medicine—Diseases of the Fetus and Infant, 3rd ed, pp. 216–239. St. Louis: CV Mosby, 1983.
44. Evans OB: Guillain-Barré syndrome in children. Pediatr Rev 8:69–74, 1986.
45. Asbury AK: Diagnostic considerations in Guillain-Barré syndrome. Ann Neurol 9:1–5, 1981.
46. Guillain-Barré Syndrome Study Group. Plasmapheresis and acute Guillain-Barré syndrome. Neurology 35:1096–1104, 1985.
47. Low N, Schneider J, Carter S: Polyneuritis in children. Pediatrics 22:972–990, 1958.

44 RESPIRATORY MUSCLE DISEASE AND DYSFUNCTION

GEORGE B. MALLORY, JR., M.D.

The traditional focus of pulmonary medicine has been the study of the lungs. However, basic and clinical research has broadened the focus of respiratory disease to include the thorax and its movers, the respiratory muscles. For children with serious respiratory disorders—from infants with slowly progressive respiratory insufficiency to asthmatic children in acute respiratory failure—physicians must use a diagnostic and therapeutic framework that recognizes the central role of the respiratory muscles in the maintenance of gas exchange. This chapter covers the spectrum of pediatric disorders that are associated with dysfunction of the respiratory muscles.

ANATOMY AND PHYSIOLOGY

The respiratory pump consists of the thorax, the respiratory muscles, and the central and peripheral nervous systems. Although this chapter focuses primarily on the respiratory muscles, pertinent aspects of the anatomy and physiology of the entire respiratory pump are briefly presented.

The thorax consists of the vertebral column, the ribs, the sternum, and the muscles and soft tissues that interconnect these bony structures. The function of the thorax (chest wall) is to provide the physical integrity that enables the bellows function of the respiratory pump. Early in postnatal human development, several anatomic and physiologic characteristics of the thorax predispose infants to respiratory compromise. In infants, the ribs and sternum contain a high ratio of cartilage to bone, and the bone itself is minimally mineralized, which renders the chest wall highly compliant, in comparison with that of older children and adults.[1] This compliance is a distinct advantage as the normal infant travels through the narrow straits of the birth canal. However, in the presence of respiratory load, this exaggerated compliance leads to a significant deformation of the infant's rib cage during forceful diaphragmatic contractions, leading to dissipation of work and an inefficient coupling of respiratory muscles and thorax.

In premature infants, the thorax is even more compliant and the inefficiency more significant. From empiric measurements of chest wall and diaphragm displacement in premature infants, it has been estimated that paradox-ical chest wall movements result in diaphragmatic volume changes approximately two times greater than the resultant lung volume changes.[2] In newborns, the ribs also extend from the vertebrae at a nearly right angle in the horizontal plane, contributing to a more circular configuration of the rib cage (Fig. 44–1A. This angulation results in a relatively elevated or rostral position of the

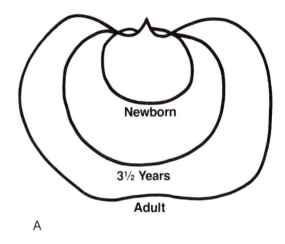

A

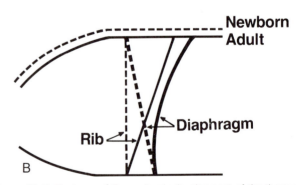

B

Figure 44–1. Features of the anatomic development of the thorax. *A,* Changes in the configuration of the thorax in the horizontal. (Adapted from Krahl VE: Anatomy of the mammalian lung. *In* Fenn WO, Rahn H (eds): Handbook of Physiology, Section 3, Vol. 1, p. 229. Bethesda, MD: American Physiological Society, 1964.) *B,* Orientation of the ribs and diaphragm in both newborn and adult in the sagittal plane. (Adapted from Muller NL, Bryan AC: Chest wall mechanics and respiratory muscles in infants. Pediatr Clin North Am 26:507, 1979.)

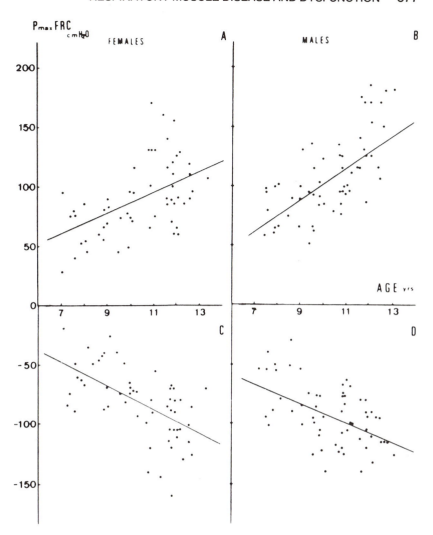

Figure 44–2. Maximal expiratory and inspiratory pressures in females and males from ages 7 to 13 years. Parts *A* and *B* represent maximal expiratory pressures; parts *C* and *D* represent maximal inspiratory pressures. (Adapted from Gaultier C, Zinman R: Maximal static pressures in normal children. Respir Physiol 51:52, 1983.)

sternum and anterior chest wall. The diaphragm is more horizontally oriented in infants than in adults (Fig. 44–1B); there is diminished movement with intercostal or accessory muscle contraction and a tendency for posterior movement of the anterior chest wall with diaphragmatic contraction.[3]

Total respiratory compliance progressively decreases during development; this decrease has been attributed to changes in chest wall compliance,[4] leading to increased chest wall stability and enhanced respiratory muscle efficiency. As young children grow and spend more time in the upright position, the anterior chest wall gradually descends, and the ribs become more caudally oriented (Fig. 44–1B). Thus the mechanical disadvantages of the thorax in early life decrease with age and somatic development.

Because of high chest wall compliance and the suboptimal configuration of the rib cage, the respiratory muscles of infants operate at a mechanical disadvantage. The mature diaphragm is designed for stamina and stress. Its muscle fiber composition reflects its requirement for power and fatigue resistance. Of the fibers in the mature diaphragm, 50% to 60% are slow-twitch, high-oxidative type I fibers, which are highly resistant to fatigue. In the diaphragm of a premature infant, the proportion of type

I fibers may be as low as 10%, and in full-term infants, the average is 30%.[5] By the age of 1 year, the proportions of fiber types reach adult levels in normal infants. Muscle mass also increases with age. Empiric measurement of respiratory muscle strength by maximal inspiratory and expiratory pressures also demonstrates relatively low values in infancy,[6] followed by a progressive increase that continues through somatic development[7] (Fig. 44–2). Thus in conjunction with anatomic changes within the thorax, developmental changes in respiratory muscle fiber type and mass lead to increased strength, efficiency, and probably stamina over the first several years of life in normal children.

The central and peripheral nervous systems control the pattern and coordination of respiratory muscle function. There are unique aspects of brainstem respiratory center function in premature and young infants. Because of the high compliance of the thorax in infants, functional residual capacity (FRC) tends to be particularly low in relation to total lung capacity except for the active role of respiratory muscles. Studies have demonstrated that healthy infants maintain FRC above relaxation volume by means of expiratory braking mechanisms.[8] These mechanisms involve a coordinated activation of the diaphragm and posterior cricoarytenoid muscles during the expiratory phase of breathing.[9] During rapid eye movement (REM) sleep, expiratory braking is markedly diminished, causing a significant fall in FRC,[10] which may result in desaturation or apnea.[11] Immature respiratory control contributes to apnea in young infants, as do chest wall compliance and the instability of FRC between sleep states. The need for newborns to depend on diaphragmatic function during both inspiration and expiration further increases the demands on the neonatal diaphragm.

PATHOPHYSIOLOGY

The normal infantile respiratory pump, because of its developmental deficiencies, has reduced reserve, which leads to early decompensation with pulmonary disease. Respiratory muscle fatigue is frequent in infancy. The majority of patients in acute or chronic respiratory failure in a typical pediatric center are infants. Respiratory failure, except when of central origin, usually involves respiratory muscle fatigue in combination with a respiratory load. The frequency of respiratory failure early in life can certainly be attributed in part to the frequency of severe intrinsic pulmonary disease such as hyaline membrane disease, bronchopulmonary dysplasia, respiratory syncytial virus–associated bronchiolitis, and the respiratory failure associated with congenital heart defects. In addition, the threshold of infants for respiratory muscle fatigue is particularly low. As stated before, the diaphragm of the normal infant must overwork to compensate for the chest wall distortion and paradoxical movement. Indeed, normal infants may show evidence of diaphragmatic fatigue during REM sleep, as manifested by an abnormal diaphragmatic electromyograph (EMG) frequency spectrum.[12] Diaphragmatic strength and endurance are diminished in very young rabbits in comparison with older rabbits.[13] Clinical and research data support the notion that the diaphragm in human newborns is markedly susceptible to fatigue.

Respiratory muscle fatigue has been defined as an inability of the inspiratory muscles to continue to generate sufficient pressure for adequate alveolar ventilation.[14] In general, muscle fatigue at the cellular level is manifested by impaired excitation-contraction coupling and depletion of adenosine triphosphate (ATP). The pathogenesis of muscle fatigue involves an imbalance between energy supply and expenditure. Energy supply depends primarily on blood flow to the diaphragm, blood oxygen content, and serum glucose level. Energy expenditure depends on work of breathing. In infants, energy expenditure of the respiratory muscles is high, and the demand becomes greater during respiratory disease. Energy supply may also be compromised with disease. In addition, the immaturity of the muscle itself contributes to an intrinsic predilection to fatigue.

Respiratory loads or metabolic stress place demands on the respiratory pump. The unique aspect of pediatric disease is the interaction of respiratory load, intrinsic muscle disease, and the metabolic stress of systemic disease with the vulnerable respiratory pumps of infants and young children. Hypoxia, acidosis, malnutrition, and respiratory loads all predispose infants without intrinsic respiratory muscle disease to diminished force generation.[14] In patients with primary neuromuscular disease, secondary changes subsequent to weakness of respiratory muscles play a central role in the ongoing pathophysiologic process. These secondary changes are described along with physiologic measurements of lung function.

DIAGNOSTIC APPROACHES

In pediatric patients with primary neuromuscular disease, respiratory symptoms may or may not be a prominent presenting complaint. Weakness and hypotonia are the most common general findings in infants and children with neuromuscular disease. The age at onset of weakness is markedly variable among the many neuromuscular disorders that commonly involve the respiratory musculature (Table 44–1). Myelomeningocele in infants is diagnosed in the delivery room, but respiratory complications, if they occur, manifest months to years later. Type I spinal muscular atrophy in infants can be identified in the early days or weeks after birth from marked hypotonia, bright eyes, and forceful diaphragmatic contractions, which are accentuated on visual inspection by weak intercostal and abdominal musculature. In young boys who have difficulty walking up stairs and standing up from a squat (Gowers' sign) because of Duchenne-type muscular dystrophy, respiratory symptoms may be more subtle. A description of the broad picture of signs and symptoms associated with even the most common neuromuscular disorders in pediatrics is beyond the scope of this chapter.

In patients with neuromuscular disease, it is appropriate to highlight the respiratory manifestations because of the high morbidity and mortality rates associated with respiratory complications.[15] Respiratory failure is the usual cause of death in infants and children who die of underlying neuromuscular disease. Thus in assessing an infant or child with weakness, it is important to elicit a detailed respiratory history. Muscle strength can be assessed from a description of the child's general activity level and the strength of the cry. The seriousness and frequency of lower respiratory infections and the presence and vigor of cough during infections should be discerned. The patient's feeding history is important, especially if there has been frequent vomiting, choking, or gagging. Questioning parents about a child's breathing during sleep with attention to snoring, restlessness, frequency of awakening, and daytime hypersomnolence is also helpful.

Visual inspection is the most fruitful aspect of the physical examination of the respiratory system in a patient with respiratory muscle dysfunction. The patient should be observed at length in a position of comfort, preferably while not wearing a shirt. Respiratory rate and the presence of retractions should be noted and recorded. Thoracic and abdominal wall movements should be carefully assessed for symmetry and pattern. Observation of the patient while awake and while asleep is ideal. An infant with spinal muscular atrophy lying in the supine position exhibits paradoxical inward movement of the anterior chest wall in concert with exaggerated abdominal wall movements, which reflect both the relative strength of the

Table 44–1. COMMON PEDIATRIC DISORDERS ASSOCIATED WITH SIGNIFICANT RESPIRATORY MUSCLE DYSFUNCTION

Site of Primary Pathology	Clinical Entity	Age of Onset	Respiratory Failure	Characteristics
Spinal cord	Spinal muscular atrophy type 1	Early infancy	Always	
	Spinal muscular atrophy type 2	Infancy	Always	Diaphragmatic "sparing"
	Spinal muscular atrophy type 3	Childhood	Common	
	Myelomeningocele	Birth	Uncommon	Depends on vertebral level and degree of kyphoscoliosis
	Cervical cord injury	Any age	Common	Depends on level of injury complications
Peripheral nerve	Guillain-Barré syndrome	Any age	Common	Recovery generally expected
Neuromuscular junction	Myasthenia gravis	Any age	Uncommon	Highly variable expression and outcome
	Botulism	Any age	Common	High fatality rate; recovery without residue
	Tick paralysis	Any age	Common	Variable depending on timing of intervention
Muscle	Myotonic dystrophy	Variable	Common	Diaphragm involvement common
	Congenital fiber type disproportion	Infancy	Uncommon	Variability; often improves with age
	Nemaline rod myopathy	Infancy	Common	Severe diaphragm involvement
	Infantile fascioscapulohumeral dystrophy	Infancy	Common	Respiratory involvement variable
	Congenital dystrophy	Infancy	Common	Respiratory involvement variable
	Myotubular myopathy	Infancy	Uncommon	Respiratory involvement variable
	Duchenne-type muscular dystrophy	Childhood	Always	Cardiomyopathy often present
	Metabolic myopathies	Variable	Variable	Commonly associated with central nervous system dysfunction
	Dermatomyositis	Childhood	Uncommon	Variable course
Diaphragm	Congenital eventration	Birth	Uncommon	Respiratory failure common if bilateral
	Paralysis	Any age	Uncommon	Respiratory difficulty common in infants
	Hyperinflation	Any age	Common if severe	Reflects underlying airway obstruction
Thorax	Scoliosis	Adolescence (usually)	Uncommon	Degree of angulation correlates with degree of respiratory compromise
Systemic conditions	Hypocalcemia	Any age	Uncommon	In a sick patient of any age, these conditions may reduce strength and stamina of respiratory muscles and contribute to respiratory failure
	Hypophosphatemia	Any age	Uncommon	
	Hypokalemia	Any age	Uncommon	
	Hypoxemia	Any age	Common	
	Acidosis	Any age	Common	
	Sepsis	Any age	Common	

diaphragm and the weakness of the abdominal and intercostal muscles. Adolescents with significant thoracic scoliosis exhibit reduced movement of the asymmetrically distorted thorax even with strong respiratory efforts. Children with severe cystic fibrosis may exhibit increased anterior-posterior diameter as a result of hyperinflation of the lungs and a variable degree of tachypnea and retractions. During sleep, the child with a myopathy, which includes significant involvement of the pharyngeal musculature, may exhibit exaggerated respiratory efforts and snoring, which reflect the presence of sleep-disordered breathing as a result of pharyngeal airflow obstruction. In patients with or without neuromuscular disease, bedside observation of chest and abdominal compartments may reveal the dyssynchronous movements that signify respiratory muscle fatigue and respiratory failure.[16]

RADIOGRAPHY

Plain chest radiographs can be helpful in the diagnosis of respiratory compromise in patients with respiratory muscle dysfunction. The position and configuration of the diaphragm can be suggestive of eventration, paresis, or paralysis. In a patient with bronchopulmonary dysplasia who is not being mechanically ventilated, the degree of hyperinflation is correlated with the degree of respiratory reserve (Fig. 44–3). The bell-shaped configuration of the

chest in patients with spinal muscular atrophy reflects the weakness of the intercostal muscles (Fig. 44–4).

If diaphragmatic paralysis or marked paresis is suspected, fluoroscopy or ultrasonography can assess diaphragm function in a qualitative manner. Ultrasonography has the distinct advantages of avoiding ionizing radiation and movement of unstable patients (the equipment can be brought to the bedside). The publication of normative data for axial movement of the right hemidiaphragm may enable the use of ultrasonography as a quantitative measure of diaphragm function in sick infants.[17]

HISTOPATHOLOGY

In patients with suspected muscle disease, an elective muscle biopsy has been a standard diagnostic tool for decades. Specimens are examined for histochemical and morphometric data by light microscopy and for ultrastructural abnormalities by electron microscopy. Although some disorders produce characteristic findings on muscle biopsy, others do not. Particularly confusing may be the muscle biopsy performed in early infancy that shows a relative predominance of type I muscle fibers, a finding that may be seen in myotonic dystrophy, nemaline rod myopathy, congenital muscular dystrophy, and congenital fiber-type disproportion.[18] Repeated biopsies after the age of 1 year may be necessary in many of these

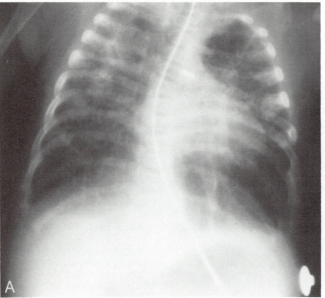

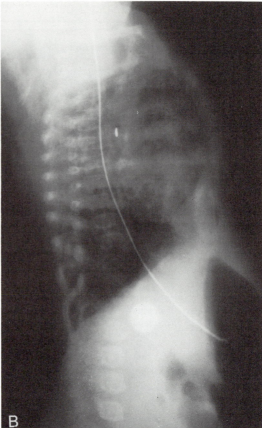

Figure 44–3. Anterior-posterior (A) and lateral (B) chest radiographs from a 1-year-old with bronchopulmonary dysplasia demonstrating marked hyperinflation and bilateral patchy infiltrates.

patients in order to pinpoint the correct diagnosis and thereby offer a more accurate prognosis to the family.

OTHER LABORATORY EVALUATIONS

Serum creatine kinase (CK) evaluation is easily performed on infants and children. Very high levels of CK ($>10,000$) are commonly found in the first 5 years of life in Duchenne-type muscular dystrophy. CK levels may also be a useful index of disease activity in dermatomyositis. In many other myopathies, there are modest elevations in CK, but test results do not differentiate one form of muscle disease from another.

EMG is a mildly invasive diagnostic tool that is often useful when performed by an experienced neurologist. There are distinct differences in EMG pattern between a primary myopathy and spinal muscular atrophy or other more proximal disorders. Within the myopathies, there may be subtle differences in EMG pattern and in the distribution of muscle involvement. One exception to the general similarity among myopathies is myotonic dystrophy, in which a pattern of waxing and waning of amplitude and frequency is found.[19]

MEASUREMENTS OF LUNG FUNCTION

In children and adolescents who can cooperate, pulmonary function testing can enable physicians to objectively measure respiratory strength, relative physiologic reserve, and serial changes in lung volumes. Maximal inspiratory and expiratory pressures are the most easily obtained measurements of respiratory muscle strength. In general, a decrement in maximal inspiratory pressure (MIP) precedes changes in lung volumes in slowly pro-

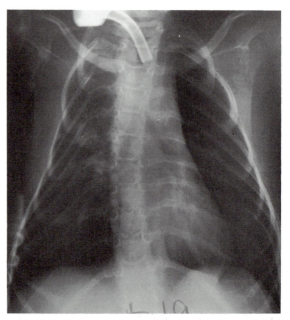

Figure 44–4. Anterior-posterior chest radiograph demonstrating the bell-shaped thorax of a child with spinal muscular atrophy who requires nocturnal mechanical ventilation.

gressive myopathies.[20] In congenital myopathies, MIP is reduced from birth. Maximal expiratory pressure (MEP) seems to be disporportionately reduced in patients with Duchenne-type muscular dystrophy.[21] MEP is correlated clinically with cough efficacy and is therefore a useful measure. Maximal voluntary ventilation (MVV) reflects respiratory muscle strength and stamina and is reduced in patients with primary muscle disease and related disorders. Measurement of transdiaphragmatic pressure and diaphragmatic electromyograms are more invasive but more sophisticated techniques that are usually used in the research setting and give more precise information on diaphragmatic function.[14]

Chest wall and lung compliance is usually reduced in chronic neuromuscular disorders, even in the absence of scoliosis. Chest wall compliance is reduced probably as a result of a variety of factors, including stiffening of thoracic tendons and ligaments as well as ankylosis of the costovertebral and costosternal joints.[22] Lung compliance also tends to become decreased as inspiratory capacity decreases, which probably reflects widespread microatelectasis.[23]

Spirometry is probably the most accessible measure of pulmonary function for cooperative children aged 6 years or older. There is a close clinical correlation between serial measures of forced vital capacity (FVC) and progression of respiratory muscle weakness, either in acutely ill patients with Guillain-Barré syndrome or in school-age children with Duchenne-type muscular dystrophy. The measurement of lung volumes, especially the partition of FVC into inspiratory capacity and expiratory reserve volume, has been recommended as the most helpful measure of respiratory function in chronic neuromuscular disease.[15] Airflow is usually normal, although obstructive changes may develop in patients with recurrent episodes of aspiration and infection. Attention to the contour of the flow-volume curve may provide evidence of upper airway obstruction (Fig. 44–5). Because bulbar involvement is common in many disorders and is often associated with serious complications, spirometry is probably indicated in all cooperative pediatric patients with significant neuromuscular disease, as well as in adults.[24]

In most patients with chronic neuromuscular disease, the partial pressure of arterial or capillary carbon dioxide is normal until life-threatening respiratory insufficiency has developed. An exception is myotonic dystrophy, in which stable hypercapnia may occur over an extended period.[25] In acute illnesses, blood gas analysis may be helpful, especially if there are previous data with which to compare. Pulse oximetry is a useful and noninvasive method of assessing oxygenation. In most patients with neuromuscular disease, there is no significant impairment of oxygenation (arterial oxygen saturation <90%) unless there is an acute respiratory illness or an end-stage respiratory insufficiency or except during sleep in selected patients.

POLYSOMNOGRAPHY

In all patients with respiratory insufficiency, sleep represents an especially vulnerable period of the day. Sleep-

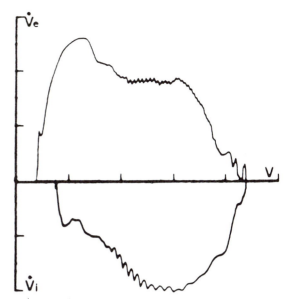

Figure 44–5. Maximum expiratory and inspiratory flow-volume curve in a patient with motor neuron disease and clinically significant bulbar weakness. (From Vincken W, Elleker G, Cosco MG: Detection of upper airway muscle involvement in neuromuscular disorders using the flow-volume loop. Chest 90:52–57, 1986.)

associated breathing disorders, including hypoventilation and apnea, should be considered in certain subgroups of neuromuscular disease: patients with myotonic dystrophy; patients with severe diaphragmatic weakness; and patients with known or suspected cor pulmonale. Polysomnography is an expensive but precise diagnostic tool that can identify potentially preventable complications of neuromuscular disease. It also enables the physician, the patient, and the family to choose among treatment modalities. Patients with myotonic dystrophy may have central sleep apnea that leads to daytime hypersomnolence.[26] Nemaline rod myopathy is often associated with severe weakness of the diaphragm and hypoventilation during sleep.[27] In Duchenne-type muscular dystrophy, significant hypoxemia during sleep may cause pulmonary hypertension and an increased load on an intrinsically abnormal right ventricle. Among patients with REM-associated oxygen desaturations similar to those demonstrated in Figure 44–6, administration of oxygen during sleep may have a significant impact on morbidity and mortality.[28] Overnight oximetry as a screening tool and polysomnography as a definitive study are important aids in the management of pediatric patients with respiratory muscle dysfunction. The degree of sleep-disordered breathing, however, is not always well correlated with daytime pulmonary function testing.[29]

DIFFERENTIAL DIAGNOSIS

The most common pediatric disorders associated with respiratory muscle dysfunction are listed by site of the pathologic process in Table 44–1. These disorders are heterogeneous in cause, mode of onset, and clinical manifestations and are briefly discussed by category according to the anatomic site of the primary pathologic process.

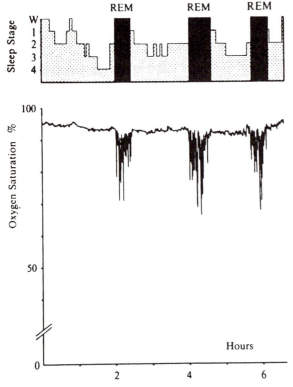

Figure 44–6. Overnight record of oxygen saturation and sleep staging in a 17-year-old with Duchenne-type muscular dystrophy. Stages 1 to 4 of non–rapid eye movement (REM) sleep are shown in the stippled area. REM sleep (in solid bars) is associated with persistent desaturation <90%. (Adapted from Smith PEM, Calverly PMA, Edwards RHT, et al: Practical problems in the respiratory care of patients with muscular dystrophy. N Engl J Med 316:1197–1207, 1987.)

SPINAL CORD

Patients with spinal muscular atrophy have generalized muscle weakness much like that of patients with intrinsic muscle disease. Spinal muscular atrophy is a unique form of diffuse anterior horn cell disease. Its three types differ in timing of onset. Acute Werdnig-Hoffmann disease, or type 1 infantile spinal muscular atrophy, manifests at birth or in the first days after birth and progresses to respiratory failure in the first months. Gastroesophageal reflux and recurrent aspiration of gastric contents or formula during feeding are common and contribute to respiratory complications.[30] Type 2, or chronic Werdnig-Hoffmann disease, may manifest later in infancy and progress more slowly. Respiratory insufficiency occurs in most patients but may not evolve to a terminal stage until the patient is of school age. The slow progression of this form of the disease may allow for kyphoscoliosis to develop and contribute to the pathophysiologic processes of respiratory insufficiency. Type 3, or Kugelberg-Welander disease, is typically noted between 5 and 15 years of age. Patients with this variant commonly acquire kyphoscoliosis, and respiratory insufficiency may develop in early adulthood. In all three types of spinal muscular atrophy, the diaphragm is relatively spared. The chest radiograph (see Fig. 44–4) shows a normal diaphragmatic configuration but a bell-shaped thorax and may demonstrate progressive collapse of the upper chest wall as intercostal muscle weakness increases.

Respiratory muscle involvement is markedly variable in infants with myelomeningocele, depending largely on the size and level of spinal involvement. In patients with lumbar myelomeningoceles, there may be weakness of the abdominal musculature, which may compromise the effectiveness of cough. Weakness of cough predisposes a patient to atelectasis and lower respiratory infection. If the level of the defect is thoracic, the intercostal muscles are likely to be involved; this may decrease inspiratory muscle strength. In addition, thoracic myelomeningoceles are commonly associated with severe kyphoscoliosis and associated respiratory complications (see discussion of the thorax). Brainstem respiratory center dysfunction, manifested by hypoventilation that is most severe during sleep, may also have a significant impact on respiratory function, especially in patients with spina bifida and Arnold-Chiari malformation; many of these patients have bulbar dysfunction and are at risk for recurrent aspiration, sleep apnea, and cor pulmonale.[31]

Injuries to the cervical spinal cord may occur at any age but peak in number in adolescence and the early adult years. The degree of interference with gas exchange depends on the level and completeness of injury. In general, if diaphragm function is intact, chronic ventilator dependence does not result. Injuries at the C-3 level and above result in paralysis or severe paresis of the diaphragm and in chronic respiratory failure. Patients with intact diaphragms (injury at the C-4 level and below) usually breathe most efficiently when supine.

PERIPHERAL NERVOUS SYSTEM

Guillain-Barré syndrome is an acute disease of the peripheral nerves with a variable involvement of the spinal cord and the autonomic nervous system. Respiratory muscles are often involved, and respiratory failure occurs in about 25% of patients. Once the diagnosis is made, expectant observation for ascending paralysis with particular attention to the respiratory system is imperative. Respiratory complications are treated with supportive measures, including mechanical ventilator support, oxygen supplementation, and antibiotics, because specific treatment is not available and reversibility is expected. Mechanical ventilator support for days or even weeks may be required.

NEUROMUSCULAR JUNCTION

Myasthenia gravis is a rare condition affecting infants and children. Its signs and symptoms reflect the characteristic predilection of the patient's muscles to fatigue. Bulbar involvement is the rule, and ptosis is frequently, although not always, present. On occasion, significant respiratory muscle involvement may be out of proportion to degree of involvement of other muscles.[32] Careful attention to respiratory status is necessary, especially in infants and young children, and occasionally may be life-saving.

Botulism is most prevalent among infants at present in the United States. Respiratory involvement is common, and mechanical ventilator support may be necessary. The manifestation of botulism, which may be similar to that of Guillain-Barré syndrome, may be fulminant.

Tick paralysis is rare but occurs more often in children than in adults. In its full-blown form, it may involve the respiratory musculature as part of a progressive, ascending paralysis and flaccidity. The key to diagnosis is the detection of a tick bite at history taking or physical examination. Treatment entails the removal of the tick and supportive therapy. Recovery, which usually occurs in 1 to 5 days, is complete.

MUSCLE

Several childhood myopathies are typically associated with significant respiratory muscle dysfunction. Many uncommon myopathies are typically associated with significant respiratory muscle dysfunction. Some entities manifest in early infancy and can be grouped under the rubric of congenital myopathies, even though there is considerable variability within and among these entities. Diffuse muscle weakness often associated with respiratory symptoms is the hallmark of congenital fiber-type disproportion, infantile muscular dystrophy, nemaline rod myopathy, congenital dystrophy, and myotubular myopathy. Myotonic dystrophy is highly variable in degree of severity and in time of manifestation. When symptomatic in infancy, it is similar to the other congenital myopathies in clinical manifestation. Neonatal myotonic dystrophy most commonly occurs when the mother is similarly affected.

In several inherited metabolic disorders, there is associated muscle involvement. Although respiratory failure resulting in part from respiratory muscle involvement may occur in these metabolic myopathies, the major pathologic process is often in other organs. Examples include Pompe's disease (infantile acid maltase deficiency), which features a severe form of cardiomyopathy and cytochrome c oxidase deficiency associated with severe lactic acidosis, hepatomegaly, and macroglossia.[19]

Duchenne-type muscular dystrophy is the most common myopathy and is inherited as an X-linked disorder. Its prevalence in the United States and western Europe is approximately 3 per 100,000. Clinical manifestations may begin in the second year of life. Weakness is generally mild during ther first several years of life. Ambulation becomes difficult near the end of the first decade of life. The child then requires a wheelchair, and it becomes increasingly difficult to prevent contractures. Progressive kyphoscoliosis is common during the second decade. Respiratory complications become frequent and more severe. Respiratory failure is the usual cause of death, although significant complications from cardiomyopathy may also contribute in some instances.

Dermatomyositis is most common in childhood; onset is usually during the second decade and is usually acute or subacute. Skin manifestations are often the presenting complaint. Weakness is more common than muscle pain, and dyspnea is rare in early stages. Pulmonary parenchymal involvement may sometimes occur as interstitial lung disease. The disease runs a variable course but occasionally progresses to respiratory failure in childhood. Severe pulmonary complications seem to be more common in adults with polymyositis.[33] Corticosteroids are the mainstay of therapy.

DIAPHRAGM

Because the diaphragm is the major inspiratory muscle of the body, some disorders of the diaphragm are worthy of consideration in this chapter. Congenital diaphragmatic hernia is a relatively common and serious respiratory disease in infancy and childhood. However, the primary pathophysiologic process relates to the associated pulmonary hypoplasia, not to any important interference with diaphragmatic function, and thus is not further discussed.

Congenital eventration of the diaphragm is relatively common and often of trivial significance to pediatric patients because of a lack of functional impairment. Eventration represents a region of the diaphragm in which normal muscle fails to develop, leaving an attenuated and often highly compliant region of the diaphragm. When eventration is large, significant elevation of the diaphragm is seen on radiographs with a relatively ineffective movement of the affected hemidiaphragm. If eventration is bilateral and extensive, significant pulmonary hypoplasia and respiratory failure may occur.[34, 35]

Paralysis of the diaphragm occurs most commonly in infants and children as a consequence of nerve root injury during traumatic delivery or as a complication of thoracic surgery. The phrenic nerve may recover in either clinical setting. The degree of impairment of respiration is variable; ventilatory assistance or surgical plication may be necessary because of inadequate ventilation of the associated lung and mediastinal swing that compromises ventilation of the contralateral lung.

Hyperinflation of the lungs is a common finding in diseases associated with intrathoracic airways obstruction. Hyperinflation appears to be partially caused by air trapping from frank airway closure or by a prolonged time constant of a given airway or airways. A major factor in asthma appears to be that many patients use their inspiratory muscles to brake expiration and maintain lung ventilation at high lung volumes.[36] In either case of hyperinflation, diaphragmatic length is shortened, which limits both force generation and length of potential contraction. The near-continuous contraction of the diaphragm adds to the risk of diaphragmatic fatigue in this clinical scenario.[14]

THORAX

The high compliance of the infantile thorax has already been discussed. An efficient thoracic cage requires relative rigidity, normal dimensions, and uninhibited range of motion of the costovertebral joints.

Secondary changes of the thorax occur in disease asso-

Table 44–2. TREATMENT OF ACUTE RESPIRATORY FAILURE ASSOCIATED WITH RESPIRATORY MUSCLE FATIGUE

Modality	Effect on Respiratory Muscles
Mechanical ventilatory support	Reduced work = reduced energy demand
Normalization of serum calcium, phosphorus, glucose, pH, and arterial oxygen pressure/tension	Increased energy supply or utilization
Correction of nutritional deficit	Increased energy supply
Improve cardiac output if abnormal	Increased energy supply
Treatment of underlying pulmonary disease	Reduced work
Gradual weaning of mechanical ventilatory support	Retraining muscles

ical impact on their function. Chemical imbalances such as hypocalcemia and hypophosphatemia are common in the modern hospital and may cause respiratory muscle dysfunction.[37, 38] Hypoxemia is a condition that has been treated aggressively. It is only since 1980 that the decrement in respiratory muscle contraction in the hypoxic state provided an additional imperative for adequate oxygenation to acutely and chronically ill patients.[39] Acidosis tends to cause organ dysfunction, including diaphragmatic contraction.[40]

Sepsis in a rat model and viral respiratory infection in humans have been shown to be associated with significant reductions in respiratory muscle strength that are independent of any detectable metabolic abnormality.[41, 42] Respiratory muscle function may be affected by many systemic conditions, and careful assessment of respiratory status in ill patients without intrinsic pulmonary disease is mandatory.

ciated with respiratory muscle dysfunction. The bell-shaped chest seen with intercostal muscle weakness has been mentioned in the discussion of infantile spinal muscular atrophy. The increased anteroposterior diameter of the chest seen in conjunction with chronic hyperinflation of the lungs, most typically in bronchopulmonary dysplasia or severe cystic fibrosis, involves a kyphosis of the thoracic vertebrae, anterior bowing of the sternum, and presumed remodeling of the ribs.

A common and potentially serious complication of neuromuscular disorders is kyphoscoliosis. Children without significant neuromuscular disease sometimes experience rapid angulation of the spine during the adolescent growth spurt. As the vertebral curvature progresses, costovertebral joint motion is limited and rib configuration is distorted, resulting in progressive inefficiency of intercostal muscle function. Chest wall compliance may fall dramatically. Even in patients without neuromuscular disease, maximal respiratory pressures fall, often before significant changes in lung volume. In patients with intrinsic neuromuscular dysfunction, further impairment of muscle function and concomitant reduction in regional ventilation of the lung may rapidly lead to respiratory insufficiency. In general, there is a direct relationship between the degree of scoliosis and the degree of respiratory impairment; milder degrees of scoliosis have more clinical import in patients with chronic neuromuscular disease than in normal patients.

SYSTEMIC CONDITIONS

Interest in respiratory muscle function has spawned a variety of methods for measuring respiratory muscle strength at the patient's bedside. It is now appreciated that a variety of clinical conditions predispose patients to respiratory muscle fatigue. The astute clinician considers this phenomenon in ill patients, especially in those with intrinsic neuromuscular disorders or severe intrinsic pulmonary disease.

The metabolic milieu in which muscles work has a log-

MANAGEMENT

RESPIRATORY MUSCLE FATIGUE WITHOUT UNDERLYING NEUROMUSCULAR PATHOLOGY

Acute respiratory failure is a common clinical problem in pediatric tertiary care centers. Pulmonary disease causing increased airway resistance or reduced lung compliance is the usual cause of interference with gas exchange. Respiratory muscle fatigue, however, is usually an interrelated phenomenon and should be considered in the therapeutic approach to respiratory failure. From a physiologic perspective, muscle fatigue is caused by a demand on energy output that exceeds energy supply. Therapy must therefore be aimed at restoring a balance between energy supply and demand (Table 44–2).

The mainstay of therapy for acute respiratory failure is mechanical ventilatory support with oxygen supplementation. The effects of such therapy on the respiratory muscles are (1) to reduce energy demand by decreasing the work of breathing, (2) to enhance energy supply or utilization by correcting serum pH and by increasing blood oxygen content, and (3) to improve cardiac output. Correction of other metabolic abnormalities (hypokalemia, hypocalcemia, hypophosphatemia) and the administration of intravenous or enteral nutrition may permit restoration of intracellular energy metabolism, including repletion of ATP and phosphocreatine. Therapy may be directed at the underlying pulmonary disease to improve lung compliance, as in adult respiratory distress syndrome, congestive heart failure, hyaline membrane disease, or severe pneumonia. Therapy may reduce airway resistance as in asthma, bronchiolitis, or acute epiglottitis. Both modalities result in more efficient gas exchange and reductions in energy demand on the respiratory muscles. Successful weaning of mechanical ventilatory support requires the reduction of respiratory load and the optimal reconditioning of respiratory muscles by allowing for appropriate exercise while avoiding fatigue.

RESPIRATORY MUSCLE FATIGUE ASSOCIATED WITH UNDERLYING NEUROMUSCULAR DISEASE

There is a broad spectrum of neuromuscular disorders. Acute disorders such as botulism, tick paralysis, and Guillain-Barré syndrome must be identified accurately and treated vigorously because their pathologic processes are reversible. Other disorders such as cervical cord injuries resulting in quadriplegia, spina bifida, and some myopathies are static disorders, and the prognosis for long-term survival is often good. Careful observation, especially during childhood development, is important in these patients for detecting complications and for offering timely intervention. Other disorders such as spinal muscular atrophy and Duchenne-type muscular dystrophy are progressive. Observing these patients with a comprehensive approach and educating their families may enable choices in therapy that benefit the patient in the short run; this approach may also allow the patient's inevitable death to occur within the context of a sensitive and caring relationship between physician and family.

For most of the disorders listed in Table 44–1, corrective or curative treatment is not available at present. Nevertheless, it remains an appropriate goal to treat the primary disease if possible. One traditional goal of the continuing basic research in intrinsic muscle disease is the understanding of basic muscle cell biologic processes. In the meantime, physicians involved in the care of neuromuscular disorders in childhood continue treating the complications of primary disease.

COMPLICATIONS AND THEIR TREATMENT

The most common complications of neuromuscular disease that have an impact on pulmonary function are listed in Table 44–3. In the absence of primary treatment, medical therapy should be aimed at prevention and treatment of these problems as long as the patient is likely to benefit.

Malnutrition is a common problem among infants with congenital myopathies who often have bulbar involvement that causes swallowing dysfunction. Severe malnutrition leads to skeletal muscle breakdown.[43] Gluconeogenesis is a secondary energy pathway for use when glycogen in the liver and skeletal muscle is depleted, and it involves the mobilization of alanine and other amino acids from skeletal muscle to generate glucose as an essential fuel for the brain. An inevitable effect is skeletal muscle protein degradation. It is logical that severe malnutrition affects the respiratory muscles. A study of malnutrition in hamsters showed that severe dietary restriction led to a decrease in muscle mass, a selective decrease in fast-twitch fibers, and reduction in force generation.[44] Undernourished adults without underlying pulmonary disease show reduced MIP, MEP, and MVV.[45] Pediatric patients and patients with underlying neuromuscular disease are particularly at risk for the detrimental effects of undernutrition. Assessment of nutritional

Table 44–3. COMMON RESPIRATORY COMPLICATIONS OF NEUROMUSCULAR DISEASE

Malnutrition
   Undernutrition
   Obesity
Gastroesophageal reflux
Scoliosis
Respiratory infection
Atelectasis
Sleep-disordered breathing
Cardiomyopathy
Respiratory insufficiency

status in patients with neuromuscular disease, however, requires more than plotting growth on standard curves. Because of reduced muscle bulk in most disorders, weight percentile should be expected to be lower than height percentile on standard growth curves. Serum albumin and prealbumin and triceps skin-fold measurements enable accurate assessment of sufficiency of dietary energy intake. Nutritional programs for patients with neuromuscular disease must be individually tailored and should embrace modest caloric restriction, adequate vitamin and mineral content, adjustment of volume and texture according to the patient's bulbar function, and modifications based on serial measurements of height, weight, and triceps skin fold.

Obesity may be a significant threat to a child with neuromuscular disease. It imposes an elastic load on the thorax and is often associated with an increase in pharyngeal resistance, which can predispose patients to obstructive sleep apnea.[46] With a preventive nutritional approach as outlined previously, obesity will likely be avoided. If obesity does develop, calorie restriction is recommended but must be instituted with care.[47]

Gastroesophageal reflux appears to be more common among patients with neuromuscular disease, particularly among those with spinal muscular atrophy and myopathies. Weak infants with bulbar dysfunction may often be unable to protect the larynx and thereby experience frequent "silent" aspiration.[30] Repeated aspiration episodes predispose patients to pneumonia, airway inflammation, and respiratory failure. Careful assessment of individual patients by radiography, endoscopy, and pH probe enables diagnosis of clinically significant dysfunction of swallowing and of the gastroesophageal sphincter. Metoclopramide or bethanechol may be of therapeutic aid, but a Nissen fundoplication with gastrostomy tube is often required for protecting patients with moderate to severe muscle weakness from recurrent aspiration. Improved nutrition can also more easily be delivered after surgical intervention.

Scoliosis itself may cause significant respiratory muscle dysfunction. Scoliosis, when associated with intrinsic neuromuscular disease, leads to an additive impairment of pulmonary function.[48] The advent of surgical approaches that obviate the prolonged immobilization of patients in cases has increased the safety of scoliosis repair for patients with neuromuscular disease.[49] Careful, frequent regular back examinations in conjunction with measurement of lung function should lead to precisely timed decisions for therapy. Bracing, a nonsurgical alternative to surgery, slows progression of scoliosis but does not seem to prevent the ultimate need for surgery in many patients[50] and is often associated with a reduction in vital capacity.[51] Surgery is often associated with improvement in sitting, overall comfort, and FVC.[52]

Respiratory infections, especially those involving the lower respiratory tract, are no more common in patients with than in those without neuromuscular disease, but complications occur more often. Vigorous and early treatment of respiratory infections is indicated. Immunization, including influenza vaccine and pneumococcal vaccine, should be offered to each patient at risk for pulmonary complications.

Atelectasis is a common pulmonary complication of neuromuscular disease.[53] Right upper lobe atelectasis is suggestive aspiration in the patient who lies in the supine position for feedings. Although atelectasis may be widespread and involve subsegments of any lobe, the left lower lobe seems to be the most common site of atelectasis, even in the absence of cardiomegaly. Patients at greatest risk for atelectasis are those with significant expiratory muscle weakness, those who are nonambulatory and relatively immobile, infants in whom airways are small in absolute caliber, and patients with a history of atelectasis or pneumonia. Chest physical therapy and postural therapy may be of particular benefit to patients with respiratory muscle weakness.

The use of intermittent positive-pressure breathing devices appears to be a logical method of expanding poorly ventilated regions of the lungs in patients with impaired inspiratory capacity. However, it has been difficult to demonstrate objective improvement in patients with quadriplegia or muscular dystrophy.[54] Incentive spirometry may be useful and less costly for patients with less severe muscle weakness.[55] Respiratory muscle training is an attractive option for patients with chronic neuromuscular disease affecting the respiratory muscles. Skeletal muscles can be trained for endurance in normal patients by alternating periods of exhausting exertion with rest. Inspiratory-resistive training has been used in adults and children with neuromuscular disease with modest success.[55-57] In general, muscle training appears to be an excellent method of involving the patient and family in a therapeutic program that highlights the significance of respiratory complications. Careful monitoring of the program is recommended.

Ventilation during sleep is often compromised in patients with neuromuscular disease. Central apnea and hypopnea have been documented in a variety of myopathies.[26, 29] Pharyngeal collapse causing frank upper airway obstruction may also cause obstructive hypopnea during sleep. Patients with significant respiratory muscle weakness may experience significant hypoventilation with hypoxemia during REM sleep when tonic inhibition of intercostal muscle function occurs (see Fig. 44–6). Treatment depends on the underlying mechanism of interference with gas exchange. Elective tonsillectomy and adenoidectomy may help some young patients with obstructive sleep apnea. Oxygen supplementation may

aid patients with mild degrees of sleep-disordered breathing. Mechanical ventilatory support by positive-pressure or negative-pressure devices can prevent abnormal gas exchange during sleep and may improve daytime function.[55, 58]

Cardiomyopathy is associated with Duchenne-type muscular dystrophy and, more rarely, with other myopathies. Medical treatment of congestive heart failure with digitalis and diuretics can prevent respiratory complications. Cor pulmonale resulting from sleep-associated hypoxemia may also indicate treatment of hypoventilation during sleep, especially in patients with associated cardiomyopathy.

Respiratory insufficiency may occur with a variety of neuromuscular disorders. The use of mechanical ventilatory support for acute, potentially reversible disorders requires anticipation and timely institution. The use of ventilators for severe static myopathies or progressive conditions is more controversial and is not always clearly in the patient's best interests. In a survey of muscular dystrophy clinics in the United States, there was no consensus about the use of ventilators in patients with progressive neuromuscular disease: 24% of clinics never prescribed, 33% routinely prescribed, and 42% selectively prescribed ventilatory assist devices.[59] Published experience of long-term ventilation of patients in chronic respiratory failure from static or progressive neuromuscular disease suggests that selection of patients may be the key to the adjudged success of the program.

Infants with severe congenital myopathies appear to have a poor outcome,[60] patients with Duchenne-type muscular dystrophy have a less predictable outcome,[61, 62] patients with spinal muscular atrophy often do well,[63] and patients with quadriplegia and other stable conditions may have the longest survival, albeit with a highly dependent lifestyle.[64]

The potential benefits for a given child and family depend on a variety of factors other than the underlying diagnosis, including the presence of other complications, the temperament and resources of the child and family, the attitude of third-party payers, and the support of the child's home community. The ideal management scheme of a patient with severe neuromuscular disease involves a comprehensive program.[65] The development of a deep sense of trust between family and caregivers is crucial. Good communication among the various health care specialists (neurologist, psychiatrist, and pulmonologist) is highly desirable. The child and family must be educated about prognosis and apprised of the progression of the underlying condition and associated complications as they relate to quality of life. Particular attention to pulmonary function and respiratory care in all patients with significant neuromuscular disease seems obvious in view of the morbidity and mortality rates associated with respiratory insufficiency.[15] A graduated program of therapeutic respiratory intervention should be developed and implemented in conjunction with education of patient and family.[55] Sensitivity to family goals, fiscal issues, and ethical concerns is critical for correct decision making.

If mechanical ventilatory support is chosen, a choice between positive-pressure and negative-pressure ventilatory support is required. Patients who require ventilatory support only during sleep or during portions of the day may be candidates for negative-pressure ventilation.[58] A major advantage is the avoidance of a tracheostomy. Disadvantages include the lack of access to airway secretions in the event of a lower respiratory tract infection and the possibility of inducing upper airway obstruction and sleep disruption.[66] Positive-pressure ventilation traditionally requires a tracheostomy. However, the use of a mouthpiece with positive-pressure ventilation has been surprisingly effective in some patients, both awake and asleep.[55] Nasal masks may be an even more practical route, and experience has shown this to be effective in patients with neuromuscular disease.[67, 68] Progressive respiratory muscle weakness inevitably requires a decision to proceed to tracheostomy and continuous mechanical ventilatory support or to withhold further therapy in favor of allowing the patient to die. It is imperative that the patient and family be given maximal moral support in order to minimize guilt if they decide against aggressive therapy. The patient's best interests must always be the central focus of ethical decision making. No single medical intervention program is applicable for all patients and families.

REFERENCES

1. Gerhardt T, Bancalari E: Chest wall compliance in full term and premature infants. Acta Paediatr Scand 69:359–364, 1980.
2. Heldt GP, McIlroy MB: Dynamics of chest wall in preterm infants. J Appl Physiol 62:170–174, 1987.
3. Muller NL, Bryan AC: Chest wall mechanics and respiratory muscles in infants. Pediatr Clin North Am 26:503–516, 1979.
4. Sharp JT, Druz WS, Balagot RC, et al: Total respiratory compliance in infants and children. J Appl Physiol 29:775–779, 1970.
5. Keens JG, Bryan AC, Levison H, Ianuzzo CD: Developmental pattern of muscle fiber types in human ventilatory muscles. J Appl Physiol 44:909–913, 1978.
6. Malsch E: Maximal inspiratory force in infants and children. South Med J 71:428–429, 1978.
7. Gaultier C, Zinman R: Maximum static pressures in healthy children. Respir Physiol 51:45–61, 1983.
8. Kosch PC, Stark AR: Dynamic maintenance of end-expiratory lung volume in full-term infants. J Appl Physiol 57:1126–1133, 1984.
9. Kosch PC, Hutchison AA, Wozniak JA, et al: Posterior cricoarytenoid and diaphragm activities during tidal breathing in neonates. J Appl Physiol 64:1968–1978, 1988.
10. Henderson-Smart DJ, Read DJ: Reduced lung volume during behavioral active sleep in the newborn. J Appl Physiol 46:1081–1085, 1979.
11. Gabriel M, Albani M, Schulte FJ: Apneic spells and sleep states in preterm infants. Pediatrics 57:142–147, 1976.
12. Muller N, Gulston G, Cade D, et al: Diaphragmatic muscle fatigue in the newborn. J Appl Physiol 46:688–695, 1979.
13. Le Souef PN, England SJ, Stogryn HA, Bryan AC: Comparison of diaphragmatic fatigue in newborn and older rabbits. J Appl Physiol 65:1040–1044, 1988.
14. Roussos C, Macklem PT: Inspiratory muscle fatigue. In Macklem PT, Mead J (eds): Handbook of Physiology, Section 3: The Respiratory System, Vol. 3, pp. 511–527. Bethesda, MD: American Physiological Society, 1986.
15. Macklem PT: Muscular weakness and respiratory function. N Engl J Med 314:775–776, 1986.
16. Pardee NE, Winterbauer RH, Allen JD: Bedside evaluation of respiratory distress. Chest 85:203–206, 1984.
17. Laing IA, Teele RL, Stark AR: Diaphragmatic movement in newborn infants. J Pediatr 112:638–643, 1988.
18. Iannaccone ST, Bove KE, Vogler CA, Buchino JJ: Type I fiber size disproportion: Morphometric data from 37 children with myopathic, neuropathic, or idopathic hypotonia. Pediatr Pathol, 7:395–419, 1987.
19. Brooke, MH: A Clinician's View of Neuromuscular Diseases. Baltimore: Williams & Wilkins, 1986.
20. Black LF, Hyatt RE: Maximal static pressure in generalized neuromuscular disease. Am Rev Respir Dis 103:641–650, 1971.
21. Inkley SR, Oldenburg FC, Vignos PJ: Pulmonary function in Duchenne muscular dystrophy related to stage of disease. Am J Med 56:297–306, 1974.
22. Estenne M, Heilporn A, Delhez L, et al: Chest wall stiffness in patients with chronic respiratory muscle weakness. Am Rev Respir Dis 128:1002–1007, 1983.
23. Gibson GJ, Pride NB, Davis JN, Loh LC. Pulmonary mechanics in patients with respiratory muscle weakness. Am Rev Respir Dis 115:389–395, 1977.
24. Vincken W, Elleker G, Cosio MG: Detection of upper airway muscle involvement in neuromuscular disorders using the flow-volume loop. Chest 90:52–57, 1986.
25. Gillam PMS, Heaf PJD, Kaufman L, Lucas BGB: Respiration in dystrophia myotonica. Thorax 19:112–120, 1964.
26. Cummiskey J, Lynn Davies P, Guilleminault C: Sleep study and respiratory function in myotonic dystrophy. In Guilleminault C, Dement WC (eds): Sleep Apnea Syndromes, pp. 295–308. New York: Alan R. Liss, 1978.
27. Maayan C, Springer C, Armon Y, et al: Nemaline myopathy as a cause of sleep hypoventilation. Pediatrics 77:390–395, 1986.
28. Smith PE, Calverley PM, Edwards RH, et al: Practical problems in the respiratory care of patients with muscular dystrophy. N Engl J Med 316:1197–1205, 1987.
29. Smith PE, Calverley PM, Edwards RH: Hypoxema during sleep in Duchenne muscular dystrophy. Am Rev Respir Dis 137:884–888, 1988.
30. Grunebaum M, Nutman J, Nitzan M: The pharyngo-laryngeal deficit in the acute form of infantile spinal muscular atrophy (Wernig-Hoffman disease). Pediatr Radiol 11:67–70, 1981.
31. Oren J, Kelly DH, Todres ID, Shannon DC: Respiratory complications in patients with myelodysplasia and Arnold-Chiari malformation. Am J Dis Child 140:221–224, 1986.
32. Mier-Jedrzejowicz AK, Brophy C, Green M: Respiratory muscle function in myasthenia gravis. Am Rev Respir Dis 138:867–873, 1988.
33. Dickey BF, Myers AR: Pulmonary disease in polymyositis/dermatomyositis. Semin Arthritis Rheum 14:60–76, 1984.
34. Rodgers BM, Hawks P: Bilateral congenital eventration of the diaphragms: Successful surgical management. J Pediatr Surg 21:858–864, 1986.
35. Moerman P, Fryns J, Devlieger H, et al: Congenital eventration of the diaphragm: An unusual cause of intractable neonatal respiratory distress with variable etiology. Am J Med Genet 27:213–218, 1987.
36. Martin J, Powell E, Shore S, et al: The role of respiratory muscles in the hyperinflation of bronchial asthma. Am Rev Respir Dis 121:441–447, 1980.
37. Aubier M, Viires N, Piquet J, et al: Effects of hypocalcemia on diaphragmatic strength generation. J Appl Physiol 58:2054–2061, 1985.
38. Aubier M, Murciano D, Lecocguic Y, et al: Effect of hypophosphatemia on diaphragmatic contractility in patients with acute respiratory failure. N Engl J Med 313:420–424, 1985.
39. Jardim J, Farkas G, Prefaut C, et al: The failing inspiratory muscles under normoxic and hypoxic conditions. Am Rev Respir Dis 124:274–279, 1981.
40. Howell S, Fitzgerald RS, Roussos C: Effects of uncompensated and compensated metabolic acidosis on canine diaphragm. J Appl Physiol 59:1376–1382, 1985.
41. Boczkowski J, Dureuil B, Branger C, et al: Effects of sepsis on diaphragmatic function in rats. Am Rev Respir Dis 138:260–265, 1988.
42. Nier-Jedrzejowicz A, Brophy C, Green M: Respiratory muscle weakness during upper respiratory tract infections. Am Rev Respir Dis 138:5–7, 1988.
43. Goldberg AL, Chang TW: Regulation and significance of amino acid metabolism in skeletal muscle. Fed Proc 37:2301–2307, 1978.
44. Kelsen SG, Ference M, Kapoor S: Effects of prolonged undernutri-

tion on structure and function of the diaphragm. J Appl Physiol 58:1354–1359, 1985.

45. Arora NS, Rochester DF: Respiratory muscle strength and maximal voluntary ventilation in undernourished patients. Am Rev Respir Dis 126:5–8, 1982.

46. Luce JM: Respiratory complications of obesity. Chest 78:626–631, 1980.

47. Edwards RHT, Round JM, Jackson MJ, et al: Weight reduction in boys with muscular dystrophy. Dev Med Child Neurol 26:384–390, 1984.

48. Kurz LT, Mubarak SJ, Schultz P, et al: Correlation of scoliosis and pulmonary function in Duchenne muscular dystrophy. J Pediatr Orthop 3:347–353, 1983.

49. Luque ER: Segmental spinal instrumentation for correction of scoliosis. Clin Orthop 163:192–198, 1982.

50. Colbert AP, Craig C: Scoliosis management in Duchenne muscular dystrophy: Prospective study of modified Jewett hyperextension brace. Arch Phys Med Rehabil 68:302–304, 1987.

51. Noble-Jamieson CM, Heckmatt JZ, Dubowitz V, Silverman M: Effects of posture and spine bracing on respiratory function in neuromuscular disease. Arch Dis Child 61:178–181, 1986.

52. Piasecki JO, Mahinpour SL, Levine DB: Long-term follow-up of spinal fusion in spinal muscular atrophy. Clin Orthop 30:177–182, 1986.

53. Schmidt-Nowara WW, Altman AR: Atelectasis and neuromuscular respiratory failure. Chest 85:792–795, 1984.

54. McCool FD, Mayewski RF, Shayne DS, et al: Intermittent positive pressure breathing in patients with respiratory muscle weakness. Chest 90:546–552, 1986.

55. Bach JR, O'Brien J, Krotenberg R, Alba AS: Management of end stage respiratory failure in Duchenne muscular dystrophy. Muscle Nerve 10:177–182, 1987.

56. Estrup C, Lyager S, Noeraa N, Olsen C: Effect of respiratory muscle training in patients with neuromuscular diseases and in normals. Respiration 50:36–43, 1986.

57. Martin AJ, Stern L, Yeates J, et al: Respiratory muscle training in Duchenne muscular dystrophy. Dev Med Child Neurol 28:314–318, 1986.

58. Curran FJ: Night ventilation by body respirators for patients in chronic respiratory failure due to late stage Duchenne muscular dystrophy. Arch Phys Med Rehabil 62:270–274, 1981.

59. Colbert AP, Schock NC: Respirator use in progressive neurmuscular diseases. Arch Phys Med Rehabil 66:760–762, 1985.

60. Iannaccone ST, Guilfoile T: Long-term mechanical ventilation in infants with neuromuscular disease. J Child Neurol 3:30–32, 1988.

61. Alexander MA, Johnson EW, Petty J, Stauch D: Mechanical ventilation of patients with late stage Duchenne muscular dystrophy: Management in the home. Arch Phys Med Rehabil 60:289–292, 1979.

62. Rideau Y, Gatin G, Bach J, Gines G: Prolongation of life in Duchenne muscular dystrophy. Acta Neurol 5:118–124, 1983.

63. Gilgoff IS, Kahlstrom E, MacLaughlin E, Keens TG: Long-term ventilatory support in spinal muscular atrophy. J Pediatr 115:904–909, 1989.

64. Splaingard ML, Frates RC, Harrison GM, et al: Home positive pressure ventilation: Twenty years' experience. Chest 84:376–382, 1983.

65. Mallory GB, Stillwell PC: The ventilator-dependent child: Issues in diagnosis and management. Arch Phys Med Rehabil 72:43–55, 1991.

66. Levy RD, Bradley TD, Newman SL, et al: Negative pressure ventilation: Effects on ventilation during sleep in normal subjects. Chest 95:95–99, 1989.

67. Kerby GR, Mayer LS, Pingleton SK: Noctural positive pressure ventilation via nasal mask. Am Rev Respir Dis 135:738–740, 1987.

68. Leger P, Jennequin J, Gerard M, Robert D: Home positive pressure ventilation via nasal mask for patients with neuromuscular weakness or restrictive lung or chest-wall disease. Respir Care 34:73–79, 1989.

45 PULMONARY COMPLICATIONS OF SICKLE CELL DISEASE

JUDY PALMER, M.D. / J. LAWRENCE NAIMAN, M.D.

Sickle cell disease is a genetic disorder in which a small DNA substitution results in the production of hemoglobin S rather than hemoglobin A. This product, under certain conditions of oxygen desaturation, forms a viscous gel within the red blood cell, distorting it into the characteristic rigid sickle shape. It is believed that this property in a person who is heterozygous for hemoglobin A and for hemoglobin S confers a degree of resistance to malaria. A person who is homozygous for hemoglobin S (about 1 in 500 black Americans) has sickle cell disease, which is characterized by recurrent episodes of anemia, hemolysis, and vascular occlusion.

Because the sickling process is a function of deoxygenation, the lung has an important role in the manifestations of sickle cell disease. In the first case report of a patient with sickle cell disease, respiratory infections were responsible for three of five hospitalizations.[1] In 1950, Henderson[2] reported pneumonia as the presenting manifestation in 25% of 54 patients with sickle cell disease. Among patients dying from sickle cell disease, acute chest conditions (pneumonia, embolism, or both) were the most common causes reported by Thomas and colleagues.[3] Pulmonary lesions occur but are less common in persons with the milder sickle hemoglobin variants such as sickle hemoglobin C, sickle cell–thalassemia, sickle cell–hemoglobin D disease, and possibly sickle cell trait.[4–6]

Acute pulmonary disease (abacteremic febrile episode with a pulmonary infiltrate) has been reported to be the single most common reason for hospitalization of patients with sickle cell disease.[7]

Because of the difficulty in distinguishing infection and

infarction, the term *acute chest syndrome* was coined to describe the occurrence of fever, chest pain, increased leukocytosis, and pulmonary infiltrate.[8] In a report from the Cooperative Study of Sickle Cell Disease by the Sickle Cell Branch of the National Institutes of Health, 73 deaths occurred among 2824 patients under 20 years of age. Six of the 73 deaths were attributed to acute chest syndrome.[9]

Acute chest syndrome commonly occurs in patients hospitalized for narcotic treatment of painful crises involving the trunk. The presence of pain and shallow breathing may prompt a chest radiograph, which is usually found to be normal initially (Fig. 45–1*A*). Two or 3 days later, fever and tachypnea develop, and a chest radiograph at this time may show new infiltrates[10–12] (Fig. 45–1*B*). In spite of antibiotic administration, the fever and respiratory distress may persist for several days.

Overhydration was suggested as a possible cause.[8] However, the observation of prolonged fever and tendency to recurrences led to speculation that inflammatory reaction and regional hypoxia might promote sickling and stasis, delaying the resolution of the inflammatory process.[13] In published reports on acute chest syndrome, infection has been uncommon except among the sicker patients.[8, 12, 14–16]

In addition, coexistent infection and arterial occlusion may be pathogenically interrelated and produce similar clinical manifestations.[17, 18] Alveolar wall necrosis, apparently secondary to sickling in association with intravascular infiltrates, was seen at autopsy in 17% of 72 patients with sickle cell disease and may help explain the protracted clinical course of pulmonary disease seen in some patients.[19]

Narcotic administration for the treatment of painful crisis has been linked in several reports to the development of acute chest syndrome.[11, 12, 20] In at least three cases, inadvertent overdose of morphine has occurred.[20] Acute chest syndrome developing during painful crisis (especially involving the trunk) may be caused in part by the hypoventilation produced by the chest wall splinting as a result of the truncal pain, by respiratory depression caused by the narcotic agents, or by both.[11, 12]

Multiple pulmonary microinfarctions may be another cause of this syndrome.[21] Postmortem examination of a young adult who died during an episode of acute chest syndrome showed multiple scattered recent pulmonary infarcts without morphologic evidence of thrombosis; these findings suggest that intravascular sickling may be a major factor in the pathogenesis of this disorder.[22] The authors proposed that the lung could be a favorable site for intravascular sickling because of the low mixed venous pH and oxygen tension, which could be lowered further by superimposed bronchospasm accompanying viral infections of the upper respiratory tract.[22]

DIFFERENTIAL DIAGNOSIS OF ACUTE CHEST SYMPTOMS IN SICKLE CELL DISEASE

PNEUMONIA

In Barrett-Connor's review of 166 patients with sickle cell anemia who required hospitalization over a 10-year period, 67 were hospitalized 152 times for episodes of acute respiratory disease.[23] Although bacteriologic confirmation was possible in only 50%, it was believed that most of these episodes represented pneumonia because of the young average age of the patients affected, lack of association with clinical crisis, and clinical characteristics of the illness.[23] In a large, prospective, controlled study in Jamaica, pneumonia was found to be equally common among children with sickle cell disease and normal controls until the age of 8 months. After 8 months, there was an increase in the occurrence of pneumonia among the children with sickle cell disease, so that by the age of 4 years, the relative risk exceeds a factor of four.[24]

Children with sickle cell disease are more prone to pneumococcal bacteremia because of impaired splenic function, defects in alternate complement pathway, and lack of type-specific pneumococcal antibodies.[25] In established pneumonia, hypoxia may also impair pulmonary defenses against infection and hinder recovery.[18]

Pneumonia should be considered in patients with symptoms of infection (coryza, cough, or purulent spu-

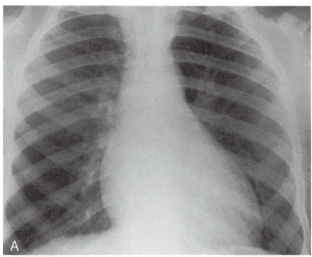
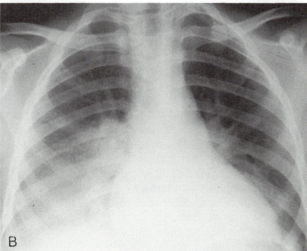

Figure 45–1. *A*, Chest radiograph on admission of a child with acute chest syndrome, showing no evidence of acute disease. *B*, Chest radiograph of same child 48 h later, showing bibasilar infiltration.

tum). Prior administration of cough suppressants could hinder clearance of secretions and promote the development of infection. The physical and radiographic findings in pneumonia resemble those of acute chest syndrome so closely that clinical differentiation between the two conditions is generally not possible.

In patients with sickle cell disease and sickle C hemoglobinopathies, mycoplasma infections have been reported to be more severe, with prolonged fever, pleural effusion, and serious respiratory distress with slow resolution.[26-29] In one patient with sickle hemoglobin C and *Mycoplasma pneumoniae,* a prominent vesicular rash was noted.[27] Failure of these patients to respond to initial antibiotic therapy may be a clue to the presence of *Mycoplasma* infection.[26]

Neither the frequency nor the severity of tuberculosis in patients with sickle cell disease differs from those in patients without hemoglobinopathy.[23]

In patients with pneumonia who underwent transfusion between 1977 and 1985, the possibility of *Pneumocystis carinii* secondary to acquired immunodeficiency syndrome (AIDS) should be considered.

INFARCTION

Emboli and infarcts are seen frequently at autopsy in adults with sickle cell disease but are rare in children.[30] Probable pulmonary infarction has been reported in infants as young as 7 months[31] and in a 6-year-old girl with sickle cell disease.[32] Fat embolism resulting from marrow infarct has been reported in an adult patient with sickle cell C disease.[33] Emboli may consist of tangled masses of sickled erythrocytes, fat, and particles of bone and marrow.[30] Hemoptysis may occur in major infarctions but is an uncommon sign.

CARDIAC DISEASE

In older patients, acute chest syndrome may be confused with myocardial ischemia.[10] Acute pericarditis is another condition that may also manifest with chest pain.[34]

ABDOMINAL PATHOLOGY

Cholecystitis and splenic infarction may manifest with pain referred to the chest.[34] Ultrasonography of the gallbladder and splenic scanning may be useful in distinguishing these conditions.

PULMONARY EDEMA

Pulmonary edema, which is less commonly seen, has been reported in young adults with sickle cell disease during treatment of painful crisis with intravenous fluids and narcotic analgesics.[35] The incidence of pulmonary edema among patients with sickle cell disease has been found at autopsy to be higher than among controls.[19]

INFARCT OF STERNUM OR RIB

Infarct of the sternum or rib cage with superficial tenderness may be a cause of chest pain in the patient with sickle cell disease.[34, 36]

OTHER PULMONARY DISEASES

Other pulmonary diseases have been reported in patients with sickle cell disease, including asthma,[37] cystic fibrosis,[38] and sarcoidosis.[39] Therefore, when clinical findings are suspicious, appropriate studies are warranted.

DIAGNOSTIC APPROACHES TO ACUTE CHEST SYMPTOMS IN SICKLE CELL DISEASE

Acute episodes are often diagnostic dilemmas that require thorough evaluation. Acute pulmonary complications of sickle cell disease are contrasted in Table 45-1.

The diagnostic approach to the patient with sickle cell disease and acute chest syndrome is greatly facilitated when previous pulmonary studies on the patient are available as a base line for comparison with findings during the acute episode. This was demonstrated in 16 asymptomatic adult patients[40] in whom baseline chest radiographs, measurements of arterial blood gases, spirometric findings, and radioisotopic lung scans were obtained. Of the four patients in whom acute chest disease later developed, three experienced the occurrence of new abnormalities, which were suggestive of vascular occlusion; in the other patient, the knowledge of pre-existing abnormalities avoided unnecessary therapy for the patient[40] (Figs. 45-2A, 45-2B).

HISTORY

A history of cough and fever in association with painful truncal crisis should raise the suspicion of acute chest syndrome.[11] Medication usage should be carefully reviewed because excessive narcotic administration may provide a clue to the presence of respiratory depression.

PHYSICAL EXAMINATION

Smallness of the chest with decreased lateral diameter has been observed in patients with sickle cell disease.[41] Other investigators have noted decreased rib expansion and diminished movement of the diaphragm.[42] These physical features may inhibit ventilation and facilitate the development of chronic changes.

During episodes of acute lung disease, physical examination may reveal tachypnea, signs of consolidation, pleural friction rub, or effusion.[10] Signs of upper respiratory infection (otitis, rhinitis, and pharyngitis) may be present. Patients with truncal pain may exhibit splinting of respirations.

Table 45–1. ACUTE PULMONARY COMPLICATIONS OF SICKLE CELL DISEASE

Feature	Infection	Infarction	Acute Chest Syndrome
Cause	Encapsulated bacteria *Mycoplasma*	Emboli: fat and marrow or in situ thrombi	Intravascular sickling
Age	Especially < 6 years	Older, especially <12 years	Any age
Concurrent crisis	+	+++	++
Fever	+++	+	+
Preceding upper respiratory infection	+++	+	++
Chest pain	+	++	++
Leukocytosis	+++	+++	+++
Blister cells	−	+++	?
Normal initial chest radiography	+	+++	+++
Lobes usually affected	Upper/middle	Lower lobes	Lower lobes
Perfusion scan	Normal/increased/decreased	Decreased or absent	?
Ventilation scan	Decreased	Normal	?
Gallium scan	Negative	Positive	?

−, absent; +, occasionally present; ++, commonly present; +++, usually present; ?, unknown.

HEMATOLOGIC EXAMINATION

Leukocyte counts are often elevated in children with sickle cell anemia who are not sick. Increased leukocytosis and initial thrombocytopenia were observed in children with acute chest syndrome studied by Poncz and co-workers.[43] In patients with pneumococcal infections, the white blood cell count exceeded the usual values for sickle cell disease; leukocytosis and large numbers of mature and immature granulocytes were present.[17] *M. pneumoniae* in patients with sickle cell disease is associated with leukocytosis in contrast to the same infection in patients without hemoglobinopathies.[26]

The finding of Howell-Jolly bodies in the erythrocytes on peripheral smear indicates splenic hypofunction, with an increased risk of serious bacteremia.[17] "Blister cells" (red cells that have presumably been damaged during passage through narrowed arterial channels) have been reported in patients with sickle cell disease and pulmonary embolism.[30, 44]

CHEST IMAGING

In acute chest syndrome, chest radiographs may be initially normal or may show infiltrates, especially in the lower lobes.[8, 11, 14, 45] In patients without hemoglobinopathy, *M. pneumoniae* is usually limited to one of the lower lobes. However, patients with sickle cell disease typically have involvement of more than one lobe, occasionally accompanied by pleural effusion.[26, 46] Pleural effusion in those patients may be associated with a variety of pulmonary and extrapulmonary conditions including infection, infarction, or intra-abdominal disorders.[47]

Isotopic lung scan may not be useful unless a previous study has been performed recently while a patient is well[34, 40] (Fig. 45–2). Angiography has a theoretical risk of increasing sickling because of the hypertonic contrast solutions.[10, 48] Although this procedure is rarely indicated, a prior partial exchange transfusion may reduce the risk.

PULMONARY FUNCTION TESTING

Pulmonary function tests are probably not useful during an episode of acute pulmonary disease, but serial studies should be performed in patients with recurrent episodes of acute chest syndrome.[34] Because of the high frequency of acute pulmonary problems in patients with sickle cell disease, it is useful to obtain baseline pulmonary function tests and repeat them at least annually in all such patients after the age of 6 or 7 years.

ARTERIAL BLOOD GAS

Although hypoxemia may be acutely present, the occurrence of mild to moderate degrees of hypoxemia in some asymptomatic patients points to the importance of obtaining baseline studies for comparison with findings during acute respiratory illness.[10, 40]

BACTERIOLOGY AND SEROLOGY

Pneumonia in patients with sickle cell disease is difficult to distinguish from noninfectious causes of acute lung disease.[10] Therefore, appropriate cultures and studies for the rapid identification of bacterial and viral antigens are useful.

In those children with proven pneumonia, pneumococcus is the most common organism isolated. Other organ-

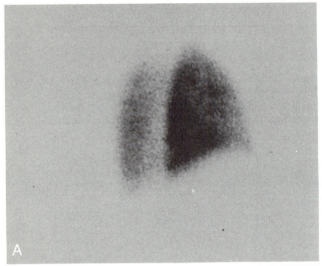

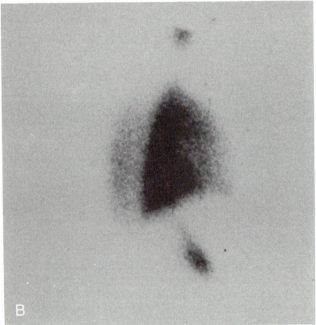

Figure 45-2. Ventilation (*A*) and perfusion (*B*) scans of patient with sickle cell disease performed during an asymptomatic period, showing matched ventilation and perfusion defects in the right upper lobe.

isms, including *Haemophilus influenzae,* *Mycoplasma,*[26, 49] and *Chlamydia,*[45] are occasionally present. In the case of *Mycoplasma,* cultures, cold agglutinins, and complement-fixation titers may help establish the diagnosis.[15, 26] Opportunistic organisms such as cytomegalovirus, *Cryptococcus,* and *Legionella pneumophila* have been reported.[50–52] Obvious alternative predisposing conditions were not observed in these cases.

OTHER TESTS

Sputum smears stained for fat may occasionally be positive in patients with pulmonary emboli from bone marrow infarcts.[34] An electrocardiogram showed progressive

right heart strain and pulmonary hypertension that preceded fatal pulmonary infarction in one young adult.[34]

MANAGEMENT OF ACUTE EPISODES OF LUNG DISEASE

ANTIBIOTICS

Patients with fever and respiratory symptoms should receive antibiotics such as ampicillin or a cephalosporin. If *Mycoplasma* or *Chlamydia* infection is suspected, erythromycin should be added pending the results of microbial studies, especially in the autumn or if cold agglutinins are positive.[10, 15, 34, 45] In patients with sickle cell disease who have infections with *M. pneumoniae,* the response to erythromycin may be suboptimal.[26]

ANALGESIA

Uncontrolled truncal pain can cause splinting of respiratory movements and hypoventilation. Analgesics should be administered cautiously in amounts sufficient to ease the pain but not completely eradicate the pain, in order to avoid respiratory depression. Respiratory status must be closely monitored by observing the frequency and depth of breathing and by obtaining arterial blood gas studies.

OXYGEN

Oxygen administration should be undertaken only to correct hypoxemia; arterial blood gases should be carefully monitored.[10] Continuous nasal oxygen administration in clinically stable patients has been associated with a decrease in the number of sickled cells; however, when oxygen is discontinued, there may be a rebound increase in sickling, which has been associated with clinical crisis.[53]

MECHANICAL VENTILATION

If mechanical ventilation is required, arterial blood gases should be carefully monitored. Hyperventilation and hypocapnia should be avoided; cerebellar infarction (possibly secondary to sickling from focal cerebral hypoxia resulting from hypocapnia-induced carotid artery constriction) has been reported.[54, 55] In one child with pulmonary infarction, positive end-expiratory pressure was helpful in restoring functional residual capacity and in improving ventilation/perfusion mismatch and shunting.[56]

BLOOD TRANSFUSION

In one report, 23 children who underwent transfusion at the time of admission for acute chest syndrome had clinical improvement within 24 h, whereas in nine children who did not undergo transfusion, recoveries were significantly more prolonged.[16] Transfusion may also be necessary for improving oxygen delivery in patients with severe anemia and acute pulmonary disease.[10] Exchange transfusion was thought to be helpful in cases of severe pulmonary involvement,[10, 57] and a hypertransfusion program has been helpful in a few patients with recurrent episodes.[34, 58, 59] An episode of life-threatening acute chest syndrome in a young woman was successfully treated with extracorporeal membrane oxygenation.[60]

ANTICOAGULANT THERAPY

In the absence of other risk factors (i.e., ingestion of oral contraceptive pills, postoperative immobilization), arterial occlusion in sickle cell disease is usually caused by intravascular sickling; therefore, anticoagulant therapy is not indicated. It has been suggested that anticoagulant therapy be reserved for patients with documented deep venous thrombosis; however, this is a very rare occurrence.[34]

PREVENTIVE MEASURES FOR SICKLE CELL LUNG DISEASE

PNEUMOCOCCAL AND HAEMOPHILUS INFLUENZAE TYPE B VACCINE

Pneumococcal vaccine, although useful, is not totally effective in children with sickle cell disease because it contains only 80% of the strains causing disease, and children with sickle cell disease may show a weaker-than-normal antibody response to some of the vaccine strains.[61] Deaths from pneumococcal infections in previously vaccinated sickle cell patients have been reported.[61, 62] However, good immunologic and clinical response to vaccine has been observed in children with sickle cell disease, and it is generally recommended that pneumococcal vaccine be given at the age of 2 years,[61, 63] with booster injection 3 to 5 years later.[64] Some authors have recommended giving the vaccine at the age of 6 to 12 months and a booster at 2 years because the antibody response to injections before the age of 2 years, although suboptimal, may confer some protection.

Although poorly immunogenic in young children with sickle cell disease, *H. influenzae* type b polysaccharide vaccine has been recommended for children older than 5 years.[65] Preliminary evidence suggests that polysaccharide protein–conjugated *H. influenzae* vaccine might prove useful in children even younger than 5 years of age.[66]

ANTIBIOTIC PROPHYLAXIS

Antibiotic prophylaxis has been shown to decrease the incidence of death and serious infection in patients with sickle cell disease.[67] It should be started at 4 months of age and continued at least to 6 years of age. After this age, acute febrile illnesses (temperature >38°C) should con-

tinue to be treated aggressively with antibiotics in therapeutic doses.[61]

SMOKING CESSATION

Smoking cessation and the avoidance of second-hand smoke are essential because cigarette smoke compromises lung defenses, and the presence of carbon monoxide might further compromise oxygen delivery to tissues.[39]

PHYSIOLOGY AND LONG-TERM COURSE OF SICKLE CELL LUNG DISEASE

LUNG FUNCTION IN SICKLE CELL DISEASE

In early reports of patients with sickle cell disease, spirometric studies showed that the majority of patients had reduced vital capacity[42, 68–71] and reduced total lung capacity,[69–71] usually without evidence of airway obstruction[42, 70] or air trapping,[72] in comparison to predicted values for normal subjects (most of whom are white). Because equations used to predict normal values for pulmonary function are based on height, age, and weight, the relatively long limbs and narrow chest in patients with sickle cell disease may cause underestimation of values relative to the actual body requirements.[41] Prediction equations that take into account this growth disorder and anemia have been developed for use in adults with sickle cell disease in order to assess lung volumes and single-breath carbon monoxide–diffusing capacity.[73]

During a quiescent phase of sickle cell disease, affected children have lung volumes comparable with those of height-matched and race-matched control subjects.[74] Black children, both those with sickle cell disease and healthy controls, have values lower than those of white children of the same height.

In adults with sickle cell disease, the carbon monoxide–diffusing capacity is lower than normal.[41, 70, 71] However, the diffusion capacity is disproportionately high in relation to the hemoglobin level, possibly because of the expanded pulmonary capillary bed.[70, 71] Membrane-diffusing capacity is lower in patients with a history of previous acute pulmonary complications.[41] In children, the diffusing capacity is above normal when corrected for anemia and in comparison with subjects with similar total lung capacity (Table 45–2).[74]

GAS EXCHANGE IN SICKLE CELL LUNG DISEASE

Arterial desaturation is common in patients with sickle cell disease.[42, 68, 69, 75] Arterial oxygen tension is often below normal, and the arterial-alveolar gradient is increased.[69] More pronounced abnormalities are seen in patients with evidence of underlying lung disease.[69] Hypocapnia has also been reported in stable adult patients.[68]

The most important mechanism of hypoxemia appears

Table 45–2. FEATURES OF CHRONIC LUNG DISEASE IN PATIENTS WITH SICKLE CELL DISEASE

Restrictive Lung Disease in Older Patients
Small chest
Repeated episodes of infection or infarction
Hypoxemia and Arterial Desaturation
Low diffusing capacity (high for degree of anemia possibly because of expanded pulmonary capillary bed)
Intrapulmonary shunt
Ventilation/perfusion imbalance in some patients (especially those with history of recurrent chest episodes)
Right-Shifted Oxygen Dissociation Curve
Increased 2,3-diphosphoglyceric acid
Increased oxygen affinity of hemoglobin S
Increased Susceptibility to Infection
Hyposplenism
Impaired opsonization and phagocytosis as a result of a defect in alternate pathway of complement activation
Deficiency in opsonization of encapsulated bacteria
Pulmonary Hypertension and Chronic Cor Pulmonale in Advanced Stages

to be left-to-right shunting within the lungs. Studies in adults[42, 69, 76] and children[74] with sickle cell disease demonstrated above-normal shunt fraction during breathing of 100% oxygen in all those studied ($>7\%$ in children and a mean of 12% in adults). Low levels of inspired oxygen (less than 15%) exaggerate the effects of impaired diffusion and minimize the effect of venous admixture.[76] Therefore, the increased alveolar-arterial oxygen tension gradient that lessened during breathing of 9% to 15% oxygen suggests admixture of unsaturated blood as a cause of arterial desaturation in patients with sickle cell disease.[68, 76] Damage from repeated bouts of infection or infarction may allow blood to traverse unaerated segments of lung parenchyma.[76] In some patients, increased ratio of dead space volume to tidal volume (V_D/V_T) suggestive of ventilation/perfusion imbalance, is present.[42]

Nocturnal oxygen desaturation in patients with sickle cell disease has been reported; in one 10-year-old patient, oxygen saturations fell from 98% and 87% while awake to 55% and less than 50%, respectively, while asleep.[77] In another case, a six-year-old girl with sickle cell disease and multiple strokes had obstructive sleep apnea with severe desaturation (47%).[78] This was not related to painful crisis and was relieved by removal of the tonsils and adenoids.[78]

OXYHEMOGLOBIN DISSOCIATION IN SICKLE CELL DISEASE

Oxygen affinity falls with increasing anemia.[79, 80] This is a normal response to anemia for improving release of oxygen to tissues. A right-shifted oxyhemoglobin dissociation curve has been observed in patients with sickle cell disease.[68, 79, 81, 82] This phenomenon results in lower arterial saturation[82] but promotes the unloading of oxygen to the tissues[82] and is partially a result of increased levels of 2,3-diphosphoglyceric acid (2,3-DPG) in red blood cells.[82, 83] However, the lowered oxygen affinity appears to be more closely associated with hemoglobin S concentrations than

with 2,3-DPG content.[80, 84] This is true in spite of the finding that isolated hemoglobin S has a dissociation curve similar to that of hemoglobin A[85] and that increasing concentrations of hemoglobin F are associated with only modest decreases in oxygen affinity.[79, 80]

EXERCISE STUDIES IN SICKLE CELL LUNG DISEASE

Exertional dyspnea is commonly reported by adults with sickle cell disease and may be related to anemia, hypoxemia, and lung volumes that are small in proportion to body size.[86] The symptoms may include intermittent chest pain and cough with later development of more severe and prolonged chest pain, chronic cough, fatigue, decreased exercise tolerance, dyspnea at rest, unexplained syncopal attacks, and eventually total disability.[42, 87] The presence of ischemic pain on awakening is suggestive of nocturnal oxygen desaturation sufficient to cause increased sickling, which leads to vaso-occlusion.[77]

Exercise studies in adults with sickle cell disease have shown that severe anemia (hemoglobin levels of >8 g/dl) is associated with increased anaerobic metabolism, presumably resulting at least in part from failure of increased tissue extraction to compensate for the decreased oxygen delivery.[86] Blood transfusion improves exercise capacity in patients with sickle cell disease, enabling them to perform increased amounts of work at lower heart rates. Increased hemoglobin concentration[88] and improved flow properties of hemoglobin A–containing cells[89] have been thought to be the major benefits of transfusion.

CHRONIC LUNG DISEASE IN SICKLE CELL DISEASE

The incidence of chronic pulmonary disease increases with age. This increase is believed to be the result of recurrent acute lung disease[87, 90] or progressive obliteration of small pulmonary vessels caused by obstruction by sickled cells.[91] It has been reported in less than 10% of adults with sickle cell disease and often is not very severe, although it can be a cause of pulmonary hypertension, cor pulmonale, and death.[91, 92]

Early diagnosis of chronic lung disease in sickle cell disease is difficult because chest radiographs, electrocardiograms, and echocardiograms may be normal in the initial phases of the process.[92] Chest radiographs in the early stages of chronic lung disease in sickle cell disease may be normal or may show decreased distal pulmonary vascularity, hyperexpansion, and increased interstitial markings, which progress to severe pulmonary fibrosis in the later stages.[87] Arterial oxygen tension falls progressively during the course of this disease.[87] The mortality rate is high, and most patients die within 30 months of onset of fixed dyspnea.[92]

The progression of chronic lung disease in sickle cell disease through four stages has been described.[87] In stage 1 disease, the patient has recurrent chest pain with mild pulmonary function and chest radiograph abnormalities but normal oxygen saturation and electrocardiogram. As the disease progresses to stage 4, the severe disability develops with fixed dyspnea, severe arterial desaturation, and pulmonary hypertension.[87]

Therapy is not established but has included anticoagulative agents, continuous oxygen, phlebotomy, and partial exchange transfusion.[87] A program of regular red blood cell transfusions may be necessary for maintaining physiologic levels of hemoglobin and seems to accelerate recovery.[87]

REFERENCES

1. Herrick JB: Peculiar elongated and sickle-shaped red blood corpuscles in a case of severe anemia. Arch Intern Med 6:517–521, 1910.
2. Henderson AB: Sickle cell anemia. Clinical study of fifty-four cases. Am J Med 9:757–765, 1950.
3. Thomas AN, Pattison C, Serjeant GR: Causes of death in sickle-cell disease in Jamaica. Br Med J 285:633–635, 1982.
4. Smith EW, Conley CL: Clinical features of the genetic variants of sickle cell disease. Bull Johns Hopkins Hosp 94:289–318, 1954.
5. Topley JM, Cupidore L, Vaidya S, et al: Pneumococcal and other infections in children with sickle cell-hemoglobin C (SC) disease. J Pediatr 101:176–179, 1982.
6. Buchanan GR, Smith SJ, Holtkamp CA, Fuseler JP: Bacterial infection and splenic reticuloendothelial function in children with hemoglobin SC disease. Pediatrics 72:93–98, 1983.
7. Barrett-Connor E: Pneumonia and pulmonary infarction in sickle cell anemia. JAMA 224:997–1000, 1973.
8. Charache S, Scott JC, Charache P: Acute chest syndrome in adults with sickle cell anemia. Arch Intern Med 139:67–69, 1979.
9. Leikin SL, Gallagher D, Kinney TR, et al: Mortality in children and adolescents with sickle cell disease. Pediatrics 84:500–508, 1989.
10. Charache S, Lubin B, Reid CD: Management and Therapy of Sickle Cell Disease. U.S. Department of Health and Human Services PHS NIH Publication No. 84-2117, pp. 20–21. Washington, DC: U.S. Government Printing Office, 1984.
11. Palmer J, Broderick KA, Naiman JL: Acute lung syndrome during painful sickle crisis—Relation to site of pain and narcotic requirement. Blood 62(Suppl. 1):59a, 1983.
12. Sprinkle RH, Cole T, Smith S, Buchanan GR: Acute chest syndrome in children with sickle cell disease: A retrospective analysis of 100 hospitalized cases. Am J Pediatr Hematol Oncol 8:105–110, 1986.
13. Petch MC, Serjeant GR: Clinical features of pulmonary lesions in sickle-cell anaemia. Br Med J 3:31, 1970.
14. Davies SC, Luce PJ, Win AA, et al: Acute chest syndrome in sickle cell disease. Lancet 1:36–38, 1984.
15. Poncz M, Kane E, Gill FM: Acute chest syndrome in sickle cell disease: Etiology and clinical correlates. J Pediatr 107:861–866, 1985.
16. Mallouh AA, Asha M: Beneficial effect of blood transfusion in children with sickle cell chest syndrome. Am J Dis Child 142:178–182, 1988.
17. Seeler RA, Metzger W, Mufson MA: Diplococcus pneumoniae infections in children with sickle cell anemia. Am J Dis Child 123:8–10, 1972.
18. Bromberg PA: Pulmonary aspects of sickle cell disease. Arch Intern Med 133:652–657, 1974.
19. Haupt HM, Moore GW, Bauer TW, Hutchins GM: The lung in sickle cell disease. Chest 81:332–337, 1982.
20. Cole TB, Sprinkle RH, Smith SJ, Buchanan GR: Intravenous narcotic therapy for children with severe sickle cell pain crisis. Am J Dis Child 140:1255–1259, 1986.
21. Onwubalili JK: Sickle cell disease and infection. J Infect 7:2–20, 1983.
22. Athanasou NA, Hatton C, McGee JO, Weatherall DJ: Vascular occlusion and infarction in sickle cell crisis and the sickle chest syndrome. J Clin Pathol 38:659–664, 1985.
23. Barrett-Connor E: Bacterial infection and sickle cell anemia: An analysis of 250 infections in 166 patients and a review of the literature. Medicine 50:97–112, 1971.
24. DeCeulaer K, McMullen KW, Maude GH, et al: Pneumonia in young children with homozygous sickle cell disease: Risk and clinical features. Eur J Pediatr 144:255–258, 1985.
25. Landesman SH, Rao SP, Ahonkhai VI: Infections in children with sickle cell anemia: Special reference to pneumococcal and salmonella infections. Am J Pediatr Hematol Oncol 4:407–418, 1982.
26. Shulman ST, Bartlett J, Clyde WA, Ayoub EM: The unusual severity of Mycoplasma pneumonia in children with sickle-cell disease. N Engl J Med 287:164–167, 1972.
27. Chusid MJ, Lachman BS, Lazerson J: Severe Mycoplasma pneumonia and vesicular eruption in SC hemoglobinopathy. J Pediatr 93:449–451, 1978.
28. Solanki DL, Berdoff RL: Severe Mycoplasma pneumonia with pleural effusions in a patient with sickle-cell hemoglobin C (SC) disease. Am J Med 66:707–710, 1979.
29. Lobel JS, Sturm R, Carroll WL, Limouze SC: Mycoplasma pneumonia in a 15-month-old girl with hemoglobin SC disease. Am J Pediatr Hematol Oncol 3:444–446, 1981.
30. Diggs LW: Pulmonary lesions in sickle cell anemia. Blood 34:734, 1969.
31. Victor AB, Imperiale LE: The pulmonary and small bone changes in infants with sickle cell anemia. N Y State J Med 57:1403–1408, 1957.
32. Babiker MA, Obeid HA, Ashong EF: Acute reversible pulmonary ischemia: A cause of the acute chest syndrome in sickle cell disease. Clin Pediatr (Phila) 24:716–718, 1985.
33. Ober WB, Bruno MS, Simon RM, Weiner L: Hemoglobin S-C disease with fat embolism: Report of a patient dying in crisis; autopsy findings. Am J Med 27:647–658, 1959.
34. Davis JR: Curr Probl Pediatr 20:26–29, 1980.
35. Haynes J Jr, Allison RC: Pulmonary edema: Complication in the management of sickle cell pain crisis. Am J Med 80:833–840, 1986.
36. Harcke HT, Capitanio MA, Naiman JL: Sternal infarction in sickle-cell anemia: Concise communication. J Nucl Med 22:322–324, 1981.
37. Perin RJ, McGeady SJ, Travis SF, Mansmann HC: Sickle cell disease and bronchial asthma. Ann Allergy 50:320–322, 1983.
38. Porter RC, Cloutier MM, Brasfield DM, et al: Cystic fibrosis in two black children with sickle cell anemia. J Pediatr 94:239–240, 1979.
39. Young RC Jr, Castro O, Baxter RP, et al: The lung in sickle cell disease: A clinical overview of common vascular, infectious, and other problems. J Natl Med Assoc 73:19–26, 1981.
40. Walker BK, Ballas SK, Burka ER: The diagnosis of pulmonary thromboembolism in sickle cell disease. Am J Hematol 7:219–232, 1979.
41. Miller GJ, Serjeant GR: An assessment of lung volumes and gas transfer in sickle-cell anaemia. Thorax 26:309–315, 1971.
42. Lemle A, Hazan EM, Mandel MB, Pinto JC: The defect in pulmonary gas transfer in patients with sickle cell disease. Rev Bras Pesqui Med Biol 9:279–291, 1976.
43. Poncz M, Greenberg J, Gill FM, Cohen A: Hematologic changes during acute chest syndrome in sickle cell disease. Am J Pediatr Hematol Oncol 7:96–99, 1985.
44. Barreras L, Diggs LW, Bell A: Erythrocyte morphology in patients with sickle cell anemia and pulmonary emboli. JAMA 203:569–573, 1968.
45. Miller ST, Hammerschlag MR, Chirgwin K, et al: Role of chlamydia pneumoniae in acute chest syndrome in sickle cell disease. J Pediatr 118:30–33, 1991.
46. Smith JA: Cardiopulmonary manifestations of sickle cell disease in childhood. Semin Roentgenol 22:160–167, 1987.
47. Oestreich AE: Pleural effusion in sickle cell disease. J Natl Med Assoc 69:579–580, 1977.
48. Cheatham ML, Brackett CE: Problems in management of subarachnoid hemorrhage in sickle cell anemia. J Neurosurg 23:488–493, 1965.
49. Barrett-Connor E: Acute pulmonary disease and sickle cell anemia. Am Rev Respir Dis 104:159–165, 1971.
50. Haddad JD, John JF, Pappas AA: Cytomegalovirus pneumonia in sickle cell disease. Chest 86:265–266, 1984.
51. Hardy RE, Cummings C, Thomas F, Harrison D: Cryptococcal pneumonia in a patient with sickle cell disease. Chest 89:892–894, 1986.
52. Woronow DI, Tenney JH: Legionnaires' disease in a patient with sickle cell anemia. Md State Med J 30:53–54, 1981.

53. Embury SH, Garcia JF, Mohandas N, et al: Effects of oxygen inhalation on endogenous erythropoietin kinetics, erythropoiesis, and properties of blood cells in sickle-cell anemia. N Engl J Med 311:291–295, 1984.
54. Protass LM: Possible precipitation of cerebral thrombosis in sickle-cell anemia by hyperventilation. Ann Intern Med 79:451, 1973.
55. Arnow PM, Panwalker A, Garvin JS, Rodriguez-Erdmann F: Aspirin, hyperventilation, and cerebellar infarction in sickle cell disease. Arch Intern Med 138:148–149, 1978.
56. Maggi JC, Nussbaum E: Massive pulmonary infarction in sickle cell anemia. Pediatr Emerg Care 3:30–32, 1987.
57. Kleinman S, Thompson-Breton D, Breen D, et al: Exchange red blood cell pheresis in a pediatric patient with severe complications of sickle cell anemia. Transfusion 21:443–446, 1981.
58. Warrier RP, Ducos R, Yu LC: Acute chest syndrome in sickle cell disease [Letter]. J Pediatr 109:731, 1986.
59. Poncz M, Gill FM: Acute chest syndrome in sickle cell disease [Letter]. J Pediatr 109:731, 1986.
60. Gillett DS, Gunning KE, Sawicka EH, et al: Life threatening sickle chest syndrome treated with extracorporeal membrane oxygenation. Br Med J 294:81–82, 1987.
61. Ahonkhai VI, Landesman SH, Fikrig AM, et al: Failure of pneumococcal vaccine in children with sickle-cell disease. N Engl J Med 301:26–27, 1979.
62. Castro R, DelDuca V: Pneumococcal vaccine failure in a child with sickle-cell disease: A case report. Del Med J 59:21–22, 1987.
63. Ammann AJ, Addiego J, Wara DW, et al: Polyvalent pneumococcal-polysaccharide immunization of patients with sickle-cell anemia and patients with splenectomy. N Engl J Med 297:897–900, 1977.
64. Weintrub PS, Schiffman G, Addiego JE, et al: Long term follow-up and booster immunization with polyvalent pneumococcal polysaccharide in patients with sickle cell anemia. J Pediatr 105:261–263, 1984.
65. Rubin LG, Voulalas D, Carmody L: Immunization of children with sickle cell disease with *Haemophilus influenzae* type b polysaccharide vaccine. Pediatrics 84:509–513, 1989.
66. Frank AL, Labotka RJ, Frisone LR, et al: *H. influenzae* b immunization of children with sickle cell diseases. Pediatr Res 21:324A, 1987.
67. Gaston MH, Verter JI, Woods G, et al: Prophylaxis with oral penicillin in children with sickle cell anemia. New Engl J Med 314:1593–1599, 1986.
68. Fowler NO, Smith O, Greenfield JC: Arterial blood oxygenation in sickle cell anemia. Am J Med Sci 234:449–458, 1957.
69. Bromberg PA, Jensen WN: Arterial oxygen unsaturation in sickle cell disease. Am Rev Respir Dis 96:400–407, 1967.
70. Femi-Pearse D, Gazioglu KM, Yu PN: Pulmonary function studies in sickle cell disease. J Appl Physiol 28:574–577, 1970.
71. Elegbeleye OO: Pulmonary function studies in sickle cell anaemia. Trop Geogr Med 30:473–476, 1978.
72. Young RC Jr, Wright P III, Banks DD: Lung function abnormalities occurring in sickle cell hemoglobinopathies. A preliminary report. J Natl Med Assoc 68:201–205, 1976.
73. Miller GJ, Serjeant GR, Saunders MJ, et al: Interpretation of lung function tests in the sickle-cell haemoglobinopathies. Thorax 33:85–88, 1978.
74. Wall MA, Platt OS, Strieder DJ: Lung function in children with sickle cell anemia. Am Rev Respir Dis 120:210–214, 1979.
75. Leight L, Snider TH, Clifford GO, Hellems HK: Hemodynamic studies in sickle cell anemia. Circulation 10:653–662, 1954.
76. Sproule BJ, Halden ER, Miller WF: A study of cardiopulmonary alterations in patients with sickle cell disease and its variants. J Clin Invest 37:486–495, 1958.
77. Scharf MB, Lobel JS, Caldwell E, et al: Nocturnal oxygen desaturation in patients with sickle cell anemia. JAMA 249:1753–1755, 1983.
78. Robertson PL, Aldrich MS, Hanash SM, Goldstein GW: Stroke associated with obstructive sleep apnea in a child with sickle cell anemia. Ann Neurol 23:614–616, 1988.
79. Bromberg PA, Jensen WN: Blood oxygen dissociation curves in sickle cell disease. J Lab Clin Med 70:480–488, 1967.
80. May A, Huehns ER: The concentration dependence of the oxygen affinity of haemoglobin S. Br J Haematol 30:317–335, 1975.
81. Becklake MR, Griffiths SB, McGregor M, et al: Oxygen dissociation curves in sickle cell anemia and in subjects with sickle cell trait. J Clin Invest 34:751–755, 1955.
82. Milner PF: Oxygen transport in sickle cell anemia. Arch Intern Med 133:565–572, 1974.
83. Charache S, Grisolia S, Fiedler AJ, Hellegers AE: Effect of 2,3,-diphosphoglycerate on oxygen affinity of blood in sickle cell anemia. J Clin Invest 49:806–812, 1970.
84. Seakins M, Gibbs WN, Milner PF, Bertles JF: Erythrocyte Hb-S concentration: An important factor in the low oxygen affinity of blood in sickle anemia. J Clin Invest 52:422–432, 1973.
85. Allen DW, Wyman J Jr: Equilibre de l'hemoglobine de drepanocytose avec l'oxygene. Rev D'Hematol 9:155–157, 1954.
86. Miller GJ, Serjeant GR, Silvapragasam S, Petch MC: Cardio-pulmonary responses and gas exchange during exercise in adults with homozygous sickle-cell disease (sickle-cell anaemia). Clin Sci 44:113–128, 1973.
87. Powars D, Weidman JA, Odom-Maryon T, et al: Sickle cell chronic lung disease: Prior morbidity and the risk of pulmonary failure. Medicine (Baltimore) 67:66–76, 1988.
88. Charache S, Bleecker ER, Bross DS: Effects of blood transfusion on exercise capacity in patients with sickle-cell anemia. Am J Med 74:757–764, 1983.
89. Miller DM, Winslow RM, Klein HG, et al: Improved exercise performance after exchange transfusion in subjects with sickle cell anemia. Blood 56:1127–1131, 1980.
90. Oppenheimer EH, Esterly JR: Pulmonary changes in sickle cell anemia. Am Rev Respir Dis 103:858–859, 1971.
91. Reynolds J: The Roentgenological Features of Sickle Cell Disease and Related Hemoglobinopathies, pp. 183–218. Springfield, IL: Charles C Thomas, 1965.
92. Collins FS, Orringer EP: Pulmonary hypertension and cor pulmonale in the sickle hemoglobinopathies. Am J Med 73:814–821, 1982.

IV Noninfectious Disorders of the Respiratory Tract

46 ALPHA₁-ANTITRYPSIN DEFICIENCY

ROBERT H. SCHWARTZ, M.D.

Alpha₁-antitrypsin (α1AT) deficiency is a prime example of how the interaction of certain heredity risk factors and environmental risk factors can accelerate inflammation and influence the early appearance of disease. The management of α1AT deficiency is an example of how health behavior modification and gene product replacement therapy potentially can slow and halt these processes.

Alpha₁-antitrypsin deficiency was first described by Laurell and Eriksson[1] in 1963. In 1965, Eriksson[2, 3] established an association of α1AT deficiency with an inherited form of panacinar emphysema. In 1969, Sharp and associates[4] reported the association of familial juvenile cirrhosis with the homozygous deficiency. These early important clinical observations were followed by epidemiologic efforts to define the prevalence of the deficiency and the incidences of pulmonary and hepatic diseases in adult and pediatric populations. It then became possible to appreciate the natural history of α1AT deficiency. None of this could have occurred without the development of newer technologies in genetics and molecular biology. Since the 1970s, these multidisciplinary investigative efforts have enabled an understanding of the genetic and molecular pathophysiologic basis for the conditions associated with α1AT deficiency. Today, investigators are on the threshold of a rational approach to prevention, early diagnosis, and innovative therapy.

The pulmonary disease associated with α1AT deficiency clinically begins in adulthood. It is rarely diagnosed in children. Treatment occurs mainly in specialty clinics serving adults.[5] It is likely that tests of pulmonary dysfunction, more sensitive than those that exist now, will be developed. Therefore, in the future, preventive and potentially curative therapies may have to be offered to younger patients.

PATHOPHYSIOLOGY

THE PROTEASE-ANTIPROTEASE IMBALANCE THEORY

Alpha₁-antitrypsin is a plasma glycoprotein that accounts for 90% of the area under the alpha₁ peak in serum protein electrophoresis (Fig. 46–1), and is responsible for 80% to 90% of serum trypsin inhibitory capacity. Its historical name is derived from these two properties. However, α1AT has a broader spectrum of protease inhibitor (Pi) activity, including elastase, other leukocyte and bacterial proteases, collagenase, chymotrypsin, plasmin, and thrombin. It shares a common molecular structure and

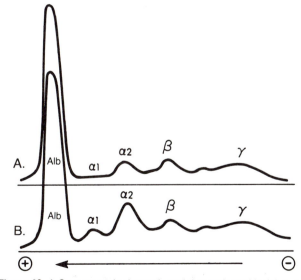

Figure 46–1. Serum protein electrophoresis in a patient with alpha₁-antitrypsin deficiency (Pi ZZ) (A) and in a normal subject (Pi MM) (B).

mechanism with other members of the serpin (serine proteinase inhibitor) family, which includes antithrombin, antiplasmin, and C_1-esterase inhibitor.[6] The serpins probably arose by gene duplication of an ancestral gene.[7] They control the balance of inflammatory cascades such as coagulation, kinin release, fibrinolysis, and complement activation. The main biologic targets of α1AT are proteases released by stimulated leukocytes, particularly human neutrophil elastase.[6, 7] Alpha$_1$-antitrypsin is synthesized and secreted predominantly by hepatocytes. Because of its relatively small molecular size (52,000 D), it readily diffuses throughout the interstitial fluids after entering the plasma.[6, 7] In the lung, it crosses the endothelial-interstitial-epithelial barrier to bathe the alveolar walls.[6, 7] The antineutrophil elastase activity of α1AT is thought to serve a homeostatic function in lungs. It protects elastin fibers of alveolar septa and bronchiole walls from the esterolytic action of endogenous elastaselike enzymes, which are released from neutrophil leukocytes and alveolar macrophages. A deficiency or relative deficiency of α1AT-Pi activity results in *protease-antiprotease imbalance* and impairment of the local screen that inhibits neutrophil elastase that is released normally by a chronic low-level burden of inflammatory cells or by increased levels in response to infectious or inflammatory stimuli. The *protease-antiprotease imbalance theory* not only explains the loss of lung elasticity normally accompanying aging but also explains the accelerated loss of lung elasticity in premature emphysema in smokers and in persons with α1AT deficiency.

Heavy tobacco smoking contributes to proteolysis imbalance in a number of ways.[6] It increases migration of polymorphonuclear neutrophils into large airways. It also increases the number of alveolar macrophages and their elastolytic activity while suppressing their endocytotic function.[6] Cadmium, contained in tobacco smoke, is capable of inactivating α1AT.[6] An important part of the reactive center of the α1AT molecule is methionine, which fits neatly into the active center of elastase.[6] Both oxygen radicals contained in tobacco smoke and oxygen radicals released by stimulated neutrophils are capable of oxidizing methionine to methionine sulfoxide, inactivating α1AT by making the reactive center too large to fit in the active center of elastase.[6] Antielastase activity of α1AT can also be reduced by the enzymatic action of free elastase on α1AT, which could occur at local sites of inflammation and infection, where enzyme activity would be in excess. Parenchymal and endobronchial infection with *Pseudomonas aeruginosa,* known to elaborate elastase, may also contribute to elastase excess.

In severe α1AT deficiency states (PiZZ, PiSZ), the lung bases are the predominant areas of emphysematous change, presumably because these areas have the most pulmonary blood flow and are thought to be one of the "graveyards" of aging neutrophils.[6]

The possibility that other exogenous and endogenous disease determinant risk factors may be operative is suggested by the following observations: (1) pulmonary disease associated with α1AT deficiency usually becomes clinically evident during adulthood (third and fourth decades); (2) sometimes pulmonary symptoms begin in childhood; and (3) not all α1AT-deficient persons acquire pulmonary disease. These additional risk factors are not completely understood.[6]

THE PROTEASE INHIBITOR (Pi) SYSTEM AND DEFICIENCY

The serologic expression (phenotype) of α1AT is determined by two autosomal codominant alleles (genotype). The α1AT gene has been localized to the long arm of chromosome 14 at q31-32.[8] The gene locus is highly polymorphic. More than 60 allelic protease inhibitor (Pi) variants have been identified at the protein level.[9] These variants are characterized by their electrophoretic mobility in starch and polyacrylamide gels. The most common alleles are designated Pi*M (midrange mobility), Pi*S (slow mobility), Pi*F (fast mobility), and Pi*Z (slowest mobility). In the homozygous state, there is a double dose (one copy per parental genome) of the same allelic product. Homozygous phenotypes are PiMM, PiSS, PiFF, and PiZZ. Heterozygous combinations include PiMS, PiMZ, PiSZ, PiFM, PiFS, and PiFZ. In electrophoretic analysis, both allelic phenotypes appear as a mixture (codominant alleles). Almost all of the electrophoretic variants have no pathophysiologic significance. Deficiency alleles that are considered clinically significant are those that result in the production of 20% or less of the normal amount of plasma α1AT. This designation is based on epidemiologic studies showing that α1AT levels less than 50 mg/dl were associated with a high risk of emphysema; levels above 80 mg/dl conferred no increased risk.[10, 11]

In some cases of α1AT deficiency, no α1AT can be detected at all. Neither of the two parental α1AT genes is expressed. This rare form is called the null-null state.[12] A study of one of these (null bellingham–null bellingham) demonstrated that a patient with emphysema had α1AT genes that were grossly intact, but the cells that normally expressed these genes contained no detectable α1AT messenger RNA (mRNA) transcripts.[13] Cloning and sequencing the null bellingham gene demonstrated that the promoter region, the coding exons, and all exon-intron junctions were normal except for a single base substitution in exon III, which caused the normal lys217 (AAG) to become a stop codon (TAG).[13] Other varieties of the null (QO) allele include: QObolton, QOludwigshafen, QOgranitefalls, QOhongKong, QOmattawa, QOrouen, and QOboston. QOgranitefalls and QOhongKong are also known to be nonproductive because of stop codons.[14]

The genetic basis of common homozygous Z mutation (PiZZ) is very different from that of the null (QO) forms. Alpha$_1$-antitrypsin mRNA levels are normal, and there is normal translation of the mRNA. A mutation, involving an amino acid substitution, Glu342→Lys, results in the production of a Z protein with a high mannose-type carbohydrate side chain that tends to aggregate in the rough endoplasmic reticulum of the hepatocyte and cannot be translocated to the Golgi secretion system.[14] Investigative evidence indicates that the Z mutation causes the loss of a normal salt bridge (i.e., negatively charged Glu342 adjacent to positively charged Lys290 changed to positively charged Lys342 adjacent to positively charged Lys290).[14] Final processing of approximately 85% of the carbohy-

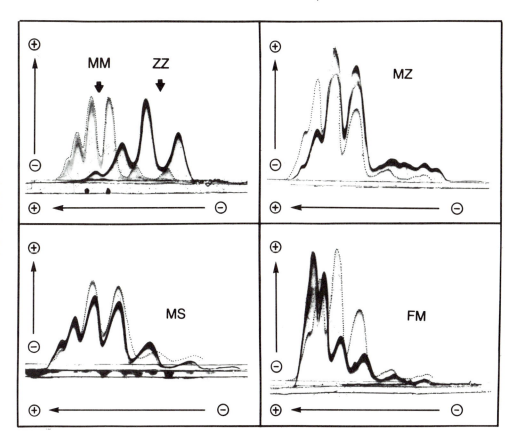

Figure 46-2. Alpha₁-antitrypsin Pi types by starch gel electrophoresis (horizontal migration) followed by crossed immunoelectrophoresis (vertical migration). Pi ZZ (upper left), Pi MZ (upper right), Pi MS (lower left), and Pi FM (lower right) are each superimposed on the common Pi MM type.

drate side chains of α1AT appears to be blocked, which results in a serum level of 15% of normal. Repair of the secretion defect has been accomplished in an *in vitro* eukaryotic expression system by addition of a second mutation, reestablishing the salt bridge (i.e., Lys290→Glu290).[14] Aggregation of α1AT and failure in transport of the Z protein results in microscopically visible periodic acid-Schiff–positive inclusions, most apparent in the rough endoplasmic reticulum of the periportal hepatocytes where there is active synthesis.

Several other alleles can produce a deficiency similar to the Pi*Z allele (3% to 15% of normal): Mmalton, Mduarte, Mheerlen, Mprocida, and Mcobalt. Mduarte and Mmalton produce a defect in secretion and are associated with liver inclusions. Mmalton also tends to aggregate.[14] Another rare deficient α1AT phenotype (PiP), associated with only 25% to 30% of the normal serum concentration, was reported in a 41-year-old woman with chronic obstructive pulmonary disease.[15] The entire protein has been sequenced; an amino acid substitution, Asp256→Val, has been found. This substitution is the result of an A-to-T transversion in exon III of the gene.

SEROLOGIC DIAGNOSIS

ELECTROPHORETIC ANALYSIS OF ALPHA₁-ANTITRYPSIN

Electrophoretic analysis alone cannot distinguish PiMM from PiMnull, PiSS from PiSnull, or PiZZ from PiZnull because their serologic expression (phenotypes) are similar. Therefore, by convention, persons are designated PiM, PiS, PiZ, and so forth, unless family studies establish that they are true homozygotes. Figure 46-2 illustrates the serologic phenotypic expression of established Pi types ZZ, MZ, MS, and FM superimposed upon the common MM type. This method of Pi typing, called acid starch gel electrophoresis (horizontal axis) followed by crossed immunoelectrophoresis (vertical axis), was developed by Fagerhol and colleagues.[16, 17] Heterogeneity reflected by a number of high and low peaks for each Pi type depends on different numbers of negatively charged terminal sialic acid residues on the sugar moieties of the glycoproteins. The slower migrations of some PiMS, PiMZ, and PiZZ components to the left (toward the anode) reflect fewer net negative charges as a result of amino acid content that is different from the common MM type. For PiMS, valine has replaced glutamic acid (264glu→val) in the PiS allelic product; for PiMZ, lysine has replaced glutamic acid (342glu→lys) in one PiZ allelic product; and for PiZZ, substitution has occurred in both PiZZ allelic products.[9] Thus there are electrophoretic heterogeneity within Pi types and electrophoretic differences between Pi types. Newer methods of Pi typing include isoelectric focusing in polyacrylamide gels (PIEF) and PIEF followed by immunofixation with the use of specific α1AT antibody. Agarose gel electrophoresis may be necessary to distinguish deficiency variants that are not readily differentiated by PIEF.[14] DNA haplotypes may be useful for distinguishing rare deficiency alleles and for tracing their evolution from precursor alleles.[9] In the future, it is likely that specific oligonucleotide probes—for deficiency variants that have been sequenced—will be

Table 46–1. ALPHA$_1$-ANTITRYPSIN PROTEASE INHIBITOR (Pi) TYPES: PREVALENCE AND QUANTITY, MONROE COUNTY, NEW YORK

Pi Type	Prevalence No.	Prevalence Percentage	EID Mean	EID Range	TIC Mean	TIC Range
MM	839	90.4	223	114–500	1.26	0.53–2.77
MS	55	5.9	178	130–340	1.15	0.73–2.02
MZ	21	2.3	125	90–151	0.88	0.67–1.53
IM	7	0.8	262	262–298	1.61	1.07–2.08
SZ	4	0.4	90	80–100	ND	ND
SS	2	0.2	150	140–160	ND	ND
Total	928	99.9				

Total, 464 parent pairs (mothers and fathers); random sample of parents. EID, Electroimmunodiffusion quantitation (mg/dl); TIC, Trypsin inhibitory capacity (mg trypsin inhibited/ml serum); ND, no data available.

used to identify the variant gene in a few cells from which DNA has been amplified by the polymerase chain reaction (PCR).

QUANTIFICATION OF ALPHA$_1$-ANTITRYPSIN

The quantity of α1AT in serum and biologic fluids can be determined by electroimmunodiffusion (EID: "rocket" technique), radial immunodiffusion (Mancini's method), enzyme-linked immunosorbent assay (ELISA), and laser nephelometry. These methods are used to measure immunoreactive protein and depend on specific antiserum to α1AT (all Pi types give reactions of identity) and a standard reference serum pool that represents adult normality. Results are expressed in milligrams per milliliter or in milligrams per 100 milliliters of serum. Because of the questionable accuracy of absolute levels in reference pools, it has been recommended that results be expressed as a percentage of standard pool. This convention enables comparisons between laboratories. Table 46–1 illustrates the α1AT serum levels (1 mg/100 ml serum − reference pool = 195 mg/100 ml serum) of various established Pi types from a random sample of adults (both mothers and fathers of children under 17 years of age) in Monroe County, New York. Mean serum levels for PiMS, PiMZ, and PiSZ are progressively lower than the most common PiMM type. PiZZ levels are only 10% to 20% of the common PiMM type. Thus serum α1AT levels are under genetic control, as determined by the Pi genotype. Profound deficiency as occurs in PiZZ, PiSZ, and Pi-null is the least prevalent (1:2000, 1:500, and very rare), but

these are the types most commonly associated with lung and liver disease. A relative quantitative deficiency occurs with PiMS (80% of PiMM) and, to a greater extent, with PiMZ (60% of PiMM). There is evidence, still controversial, that PiMZ persons also are at risk of developing pulmonary disease:[18–26] when (1) they are exposed over time to exogenous factors (tobacco, infections, pollutants, irritants) that are conducive to pulmonary inflammation; (2) they have another deficient endogenous host defense mechanism (IgA deficiency) accounting for recurrent infection; or (3) they have an overabundance of metabolic cellular enzymatic elements (leukocytic elastase) that, in the presence of partial α1AT deficiency, works to the disadvantage of the host. Theoretically, protease-antiprotease balance may be interrupted in numerous ways, resulting in disease that can be conceived of only as being multifactorial.

Clinically significant α1AT deficiency should be suspected when there is a flat α1 region on simple serum protein electrophoresis or when low serum levels in the range of 20% or less of the common PiMM are found. A similar pattern exists for Pi-null. When these findings are observed, more definitive testing and family studies should be pursued.

Alpha$_1$-antitrypsin is an acute-phase reactant. Serum concentrations rise three- to fourfold in response to infection, inflammation, and stress.[27] It is likely that cytokines such as interleukin-6 regulate production in hepatocytes.[7] Serum levels are also influenced by hormones, especially estrogens. Levels are higher in females than in males, and they rise during pregnancy and in females taking birth control pills (Table 46–2). With these stimuli, the percentage rises in serum level and in absolute levels achieved are less with PiZZ, PiSZ, and PiMZ than with PiMM, thus accentuating the relative deficiencies under dynamic conditions. Glucocorticosteroids, which are used to reduce inflammation in chronic pulmonary conditions, indirectly lower raised levels. Danazol, an "impeded" androgen, is able to augment the release of α1AT from the liver in some but not all persons with PiZ;[28] stanazolol, another testosterone analog, does not.[28]

PREVALENCE, INCIDENCE, RISKS, AND SURVIVAL

Most epidemiologic studies have found the prevalence of PiZ homozygotes to be between 1/1670 and 1/3500; thus α1AT deficiency is as common as cystic fibrosis.[5] Approximately 100,000 persons in the United States pop-

Table 46–2. NORMAL ADULT SERUM ALPHA$_1$-ANTITRYPSIN CONCENTRATIONS: INFLUENCE OF SEX AND BIRTH CONTROL PILLS

Pi Type	Males	Females	Females + B.C.	Females − B.C.
MM	207 ± 38	238 ± 55	284 ± 50	223 ± 48
MS	178 ± 31	204 ± 41	231 ± 49	193 ± 31
MZ	138 ± 27	147 ± 22	175 ± 14	137 ± 15

Concentration: mg/dl ± standard deviation. Method of determination: electroimmunodiffusion. Standard serum reference pool: 195 mg/dl + B.C., on birth control pills; − B.C., off birth control pills. Normal adults: random sample of parents (mothers and fathers), Monroe County, New York (Rochester, New York).

ulation are affected.[5] However, it has been estimated that approximately 5% of affected persons escape clinical sequelae, and normal life spans (up to 87 years) have been reported.[29] PiZ is rare among Asian and black populations. PiS is more common among people in southern Europe. In Monroe County, New York (see Table 46–2), the most common Pi-type is PiMM. Approximately 10% of the population are the common heterozygotes PiMS (6.0%) and PiMZ (3.6%). This percentage is similar to prevalences found in other studies.[30] It is now generally believed that the common heterozygote PiMZ, with serum α1AT levels of approximately 60% of normal, is not usually at increased risk for the development of clinically detectable emphysema.[10, 11] If a PiMZ person does develop lung disease, it is because the risk potential has been highly influenced or modified by other environmental and genetic factors.

Tobacco smoking accelerates the loss of lung elasticity in the normally aging lung. The effect is even more profound in the presence of α1AT deficiency.[31] In New Zealand, Janus and co-workers[32] studied 69 PiZ subjects. The forced expiratory volume in 1 sec (FEV₁) of nonsmoking controls decreased at the rate of 36 ml/year, in comparison with 80 ml/year for nonsmoking PiZ subjects. The FEV₁ of smoking controls decreased at a rate of 45 to 90 ml/year, depending on whether significant airflow obstruction was developing. In the PiZ smokers, the average FEV₁ loss was 300 ml/year. In a 14-year follow-up of 246 PiZ adults in Sweden, Larsson[29] found that 47% of 95 nonsmokers developed emphysema, in comparison with 85% of 151 smokers. PiZ smokers developed dyspnea at an earlier age (40 years) than did nonsmokers (50 years).

In a New Zealand 13-year follow-up study of 69 PiZ homozygotes, Janus and co-workers[32] reported that 14 of 19 deaths were from emphysema, the mean ages at death being 67 years in nonsmokers and 48 years in smokers. Brantly and co-authors[33] offered another perspective by comparing the cumulative probability of survival of the total U.S. population with 120 PiZ adults (smokers and nonsmokers) evaluated at the National Institutes of Health (NIH). At age 50 years, the survival rates were 93% for the total population and 52% for the PiZ subjects; at age 60 years, the respective survival rates were 85% and 16%.

Larsson[29] reported the cause of death for 91 PiZ patients. Fifty-six patients died of chronic obstructive pulmonary disease (COPD); 54 died of respiratory insufficiency and two of pneumothorax. Twelve died of liver cirrhosis with or without hepatoma; nine died of hepatic failure and three of bleeding esophageal varices.

DISEASES ASSOCIATED WITH ALPHA₁-ANTITRYPSIN DEFICIENCY IN ADULTS

PULMONARY DISEASE

Approximately 12% of adult patients with emphysema have α1AT deficiency. Emphysema in general is more common in men. Emphysema associated with α1AT deficiency occurs with equal frequency in men and women. Most (80%) but not all patients develop overt symptom-atic disease. Progressive dyspnea, without cough or sputum production, may begin in the third decade of life, significantly earlier than does emphysema in general. Panacinar emphysema may be evident from increased basilar lucency on chest radiographs at this stage. As the disease progresses, chronic cough, chronic bronchitis, and bronchiectasis may add to the clinical picture. The variability of the clinical course in α1AT (PiZ) deficiency is stressed. Smoking definitely contributes to earlier onset of symptoms and more severe disease. In smokers, dyspnea begins soon after age 30 and usually before age 40; death is likely by age 50. In nonsmokers, dyspnea begins after age 50, and handicapping emphysema begins later.[29]

HEPATIC DISEASE

Almost all adult PiZZ homozygotes show histologic evidence of liver damage, and about 12% eventually develop cirrhosis.[34] The risk is higher for males. Cox and Smyth[35] found that the frequency of liver disease in 115 adults with α1AT deficiency was 15% in men between 50 and 60 years of age. Reports on the association of α1AT deficiency with cirrhosis and malignant hepatoma in adults began to appear in the 1970s.[36] Eriksson and collaborators[36] assessed the risk of these complications in a retrospective study based on 17 autopsies of patients with α1AT deficiency identified during the period 1963 to 1982 in the city of Malmö, Sweden. From studies of population prevalence and autopsy rates, it is thought that 21 cases have existed. Of the 17 patients who died, one was a 1½-year-old boy who died of complications of cirrhosis. Of the remaining 16, who were adults, 6 presented with decompensated cirrhosis, 1 with rheumatoid arthritis, and 1 with gastric carcinoma; both of the latter two had had cirrhosis at autopsy. None of these patients had clinical signs of COPD, but all had emphysema that had been histologically verified at the time of autopsy. The remaining patients had presented primarily with pulmonary symptoms and had been found to have severe emphysema; some also had mild liver disease. After each case was matched with four control autopsies, calculation of the Mantel-Haenszel odds ratio indicated a strong relation between α1AT deficiency and both cirrhosis and primary liver cancer. When the data were stratified for sex, these associations were statistically significant only for male patients. The possible pathogenetic mechanism leading to cirrhosis has been discussed; the one leading to primary liver cancer remains unknown.

Like the association of α1AT heterozygosity and pulmonary disease, the notion of susceptibility of PiMZ persons to liver disease is controversial.[37] Because liver disease may be accompanied by other inflammatory processes that can increase PiMZ α1AT serum concentrations into the normal PiMM range, it is important to verify phenotypes by Pi typing with starch gel electrophoresis, isoelectric focusing, or PiZ-specific antibodies. In a study of 857 consecutive patients with liver disease, plasma α1AT levels were subnormal in only 50% of 64 (7.5% of the total number of patients) identified heterozygotes. Malignant hepatoma occurred in 9.4%, in comparison with 1.6% of non-PiZ patients.[37] Eriksson believed that these findings supported the idea that intermediate deficiency predisposes affected persons to chronic liver disease and hepatoma.[34, 36] The risk is thought to be 10% to 15%.

DISEASE ASSOCIATED WITH ALPHA₁-ANTITRYPSIN DEFICIENCY IN CHILDREN

PULMONARY DISEASE

In children with severe α1AT deficiency, chronic progressive respiratory disease may develop, but this is uncommon.[38] Buist and associates[39] studied 19 children aged 3 to 7 years with α1AT deficiency (PiZZ or PiSZ). Using a case control design, the investigators were unable to find significant differences in functional residual capacity or maximal expiratory flow at functional residual capacity. They concluded that through age 7 years, there is no gross impairment of pulmonary function. However, Wagener and colleagues[40] found mild diffuse airspace and bronchial gland enlargement and slight dilation of small airways in postmortem studies of two adolescents with α1AT deficiency who died of hepatic cirrhosis. They concluded that pulmonary anatomic changes may occur before the onset of clinically and pathologically significant emphysema. There have been other reports of α1AT deficiency disease in children.[41, 42] Chronic cough, progressive dyspnea, and wheezing may begin early in infancy or any time thereafter. Digital clubbing occurs when respiratory disease is severe or with the juvenile cirrhosis that also is a manifestation of α1AT (PiZZ and PiSZ) deficiency in childhood. Both panacinar emphysema alone and emphysema complicated by chronic bronchitis, bronchiectasis, or localized pulmonary cavitation may occur. Liver and lung disease may coexist in children, mimicking a similar combination that occurs in some children with cystic fibrosis (Fig. 46–3). Thus α1AT deficiency should be considered in the differential diagnosis of recurrent and chronic pulmonary disease and can be confused with cystic fibrosis, immunodeficiency disorders, and asthma.

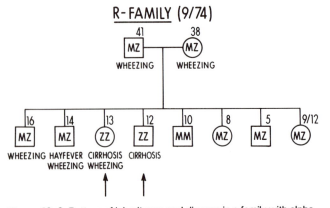

Figure 46–3. Pattern of inheritance and disease in a family with alpha₁-antitrypsin deficiency. Hepatic (*arrows*) as well as pulmonary disease is present. (From Schwartz RH: Nonallergic chronic pulmonary disease. *In* Bierman CW, Pearlman DS [eds]: Allergic Diseases of Infancy, Childhood and Adolescence, pp. 622–641. Philadelphia: WB Saunders, 1980.)

HEPATIC DISEASE

Before the description of the association of familial juvenile cirrhosis with α1AT deficiency by Sharp and associates[4] in 1969, many newborns with cholestatic jaundice received a diagnosis of idiopathic neonatal hepatitis with giant cell transformation. Since then, 13% to 40% of children with neonatal cholestatic jaundice have been found to have either PiZ or PiSZ α1AT deficiency.[34, 35, 43] In one study of 100 patients with neonatal hepatitis, 21 had biliary atresia, 13 had α1AT deficiency, 6 had other metabolic or chromosomal abnormalities, and 14 tested positively for hepatitis B virus.[44] In a prospective study of 200,000 Swedish newborns screened for α1AT deficiency between 1972 and 1974, Sveger[30] identified 127 children with α1AT deficiency. Eighty-three percent appeared healthy at birth; 11% had neonatal cholestasis, and 6% showed other signs of liver dysfunction.

Alpha₁-antitrypsin–deficient newborns with liver disease and cholestatic jaundice in the first month of life present with pale stools, failure to thrive, and hepatosplenomegaly. The jaundice may persist as long as 8 months. Most patients recover, but 2% to 3% acquire juvenile cirrhosis. The course of hepatic disease, although originally described as relentlessly progressive and fatal, is now known to be variable, with periods of quiescence interspersed with periods of hepatocellular damage. Persistent elevation of serum glutamic-oxaloacetic transaminase levels through the third year of life is associated with a poor prognosis. The chances for complete recovery remain uncertain. Of the 127 PiZ children identified by Sveger[30] and observed from infancy to 12 years of age, four with neonatal liver disease died: two of liver cirrhosis at age 7 years, one of aplastic anemia at age 4 years (but who was found at autopsy to have cirrhosis), and a fourth as the result of an accident and who was found to have mild periportal fibrosis. Another PiZ child died of anaphylactic shock, and one PiSZ child died of sudden infant death syndrome. None of the remaining children had any clinical symptoms of liver disease. In PiZ children, the incidence of abnormal results of liver enzyme tests decreased from 50% and 70% to 3% to 6% and about 15% by the age of 12 years. Abnormal S-GT and S-ALAT levels were found in about 20% of PiSZ infants; this rate decreased to 2% by the age of 12 years.

The pathogenetic mechanisms responsible for liver disease in α1AT-deficient persons are still unknown. Protease-antiprotease imbalance, a result of the deficiency of plasma protein, could render the hepatocyte more susceptible to proteolytic damage by extracellular enzymes. Alternatively, liver damage could be the result of the intracellular accumulation of aggregated protein Z. Experiments in surrogate cell systems indicate that the build-up of protein Z causes a switch from intracellular metabolism to proteolysis. Presumably, cell death occurs in the periportal hepatocytes, in which the accumulation of material is greatest.[7, 34, 45] The latter theory explains both why liver disease may also occur more frequently in PiMZ persons, in whom some protein Z accumulates in hepatocytes, and why hepatocellular damage has not been observed in Pi-null persons, who have a block in the production of α1AT at the transcription level. If this explanation is correct, the augmentation of hepatic synthesis of

Table 46–3. MEAN POPULATION CHARACTERISTICS AND PULMONARY
FUNCTION STUDIES: COMPARISON OF PiMM CONTROLS WITH MATCHED
PiMZ AND PiMS HETEROZYGOTE SUBJECTS

Characteristic	PiMZ	PiMM	PiMS	PiMM
No. subjects	16	16	27	27
Age (years)	15.4 ± 6	14.6 ± 4	15.2 ± 5	15.4 ± 5
Height (cm)	158 ± 13	158 ± 12	154 ± 12	154 ± 11
No. smokers	1	1	2	2
Function studies				
FVC (% of predicted)*	81.4 ± 8	86.6 ± 9	84.8 ± 9	81.4 ± 7
FEV₁ (% of predicted)†	83.8 ± 6	91.3 ± 5	86.2 ± 5	86.8 ± 5
FEV₁/FVC (% of predicted)‡	95.2 ± 8	101 ± 6	98.3 ± 7	97.6 ± 7
R3 − R9 (frequency dependency index)	1.83 ± 0.56	1.24 ± 0.57	1.7 ± 0.55	1.5 ± 7
V$_{max\,40}$	30 ± 6	34 ± 8	30 ± 8	29 ± 8
VisoV	12.5 ± 7	7.3 ± 6	5.3 ± 4	6.3 ± 4

From Vance JC, Hall WJ, Schwartz RH, et al: Heterozygous alpha-1-antitrypsin deficiency and respiratory function in children. Pediatrics 60:263–272, 1977.
FVC, forced vital capacity; FEV₁, forced expiratory volume in 1 sec; V$_{max\,40}$, maximal flow in 40 sec; VisoV, volume of isoflow.
*$p < .02$. †$p < .01$. ‡$p < .20$.

α1AT with danazol in PiZ, PiSZ, and PiMZ persons could potentially be dangerous.

The possibility that other genetic and hormonal factors play a role in determining the severity of hepatic disease is suggested by the observations that progression to cirrhosis is more likely to occur in males or if another sibling has been affected.[42] Also, not all PiZ α1AT-deficient patients treated with danazol respond with increased serum concentrations of α1AT; this occurred in 66% of men and only 25% of women studied.[28]

Breast-feeding may offer some protection against both severe liver disease and death in infants with α1AT deficiency. Udall and co-workers[46, 47] investigated the early feeding histories of 32 full-term children who had been identified as having α1AT deficiency in Boston between 1969 and 1983. Severe liver disease was observed in eight (40%) bottle-fed infants and in one (8%) breast-fed infant. Of the 32 infants, 24 were still alive at the end of the study; the 8 who had died had been bottle-fed. It has been postulated that until gut closure occurs, intestinal luminal enzymes in the neonate are transported into the systemic circulation and reach the liver, where they may cause inflammation and, eventually, fibrosis. Breast milk contains protease inhibitors that bind these enzymes.[46, 47]

The risk to a PiZZ fetus of developing severe liver disease has been estimated at 13% when a previous PiZZ sibling had no liver disease or liver disease that resolved during early childhood and at 40% when a previous PiZZ sibling had developed severe liver disease.[42] This is one instance in which prenatal diagnosis may be desired.

THE HETEROZYGOTE CONTROVERSY

Functional abnormalities of peripheral airways have been described in partially α1AT-deficient, asymptomatic, nonasthmatic PiMZ children. Vance and collaborators[22] evaluated 224 children from Rochester, New York, families in which at least one parent was heterozy-

gous for α1AT. No differences were found in respiratory symptoms or physical findings between 75 PiMS and 37 PiMZ children and 104 PiMM children. However, when pulmonary function tests were evaluated by a matched-pair analysis designed to minimize other genetic and environmental risk factors, PiMZ subjects demonstrated statistically significant differences in forced expiratory flow rates and in an increased number of frequency-dependent characteristics of total pulmonary resistance (Table 46–3). These abnormalities were similar to those previously described in adult PiMZ subjects. Whether these children were predisposed to the development of lung disease is still not known.

Some investigators[19, 23] have found that PiMZ adults may have an increased risk for the development of COPD, whereas other investigators[48] have found no evidence for such an association. Abnormal arterial oxygen tension, lung elastic recoil, maximal expiratory flows, and closing capacity have been observed in groups of PiMZ adults in comparison with PiMM adults; pulmonary function abnormalities were consistent with those of emphysema, and cigarette smoking was a significant additive risk factor. Horne and associates[23] studied 28 PiMZ grain elevator workers and 28 PiM matched controls in Saskatchewan. The PiMZ grain elevator workers had significantly lower mean values for FEV₁, ratio of FEV₁ to forced vital capacity, maximal midexpiratory flow rate, and maximal flow at 50% of vital capacity (V$_{max50\%VC}$). These observations reinforce the concept that genetic and environmental factors together may produce obstructive lung disease. Prospective studies of PiZZ, PiSZ, and PiMZ children are obviously needed in order to fully appreciate the natural history of their health or disease and to place various other genetic and environmental risk factors in proper quantitative perspective. Until this is done, routine screening of the general population and of newborns and attempts at prenatal diagnosis for α1AT deficiency are not warranted. Testing is, of course, indicated in children and adolescents with chronic lung disease and hepatic disease of undetermined cause and families in which α1AT deficiency is found to be associated with disease in any one member.

Results of several studies have implicated an association of partially deficient α1AT variants (PiMZ and PiMS) in adults and children with asthma.[49, 50] The prevalence of Pi variants has been reported to be increased among nonallergic asthmatic children in comparison with normal children.[51] Such an association has not been found in non–steroid-dependent, mildly atopic asthmatic children living in Rochester, New York, or in a mostly steroid-dependent group of more severely atopic asthmatic children living at an asthma residential treatment center in Denver, Colorado.[52] Because wheezing is a manifestation of symptomatic α1AT deficiency in children, α1AT deficiency should be suspected in any symptomatic child in whom bronchial obstruction cannot be relieved with bronchodilators, corticosteroids, or both.

OTHER DISEASE RELATIONSHIPS

Because α1AT plays a central role in modulating and containing the enzymatic effects of inflammation, more fulminant forms of various inflammatory diseases are expected to be associated with α1AT deficiency. The importance of this consideration is that adjunctive therapies may be available in these situations.

A variety of diseases and physical factors can cause cutaneous panniculitis. Neutrophils are the principal type of cells participating in fat necrosis and ulceration. Some cases of this disease have been reported as "Weber-Christian Disease," or relapsing febrile nodular nonsuppurative panniculitis.[53] Pittelkow and co-authors[54] reviewed 18 cases, associated with α1AT deficiency, reported since 1972. Twelve patients had the PiZ phenotype, and the others had the PiMZ or an unknown phenotype. Two PiZ patients with severe cutaneous panniculitis were treated with parenteral α1AT infusions. There were marked clinical improvement and eventual healing of extensive cutaneous ulceration. The heterozygote controversy exists for this condition also. The author has observed one PiMZ female with mild but troublesome panniculitis provoked mainly by trauma. Her condition did not warrant expensive treatment with α1AT.

TREATMENT

The first step in the prevention and treatment of pulmonary disease is encouraging smokers to stop smoking and nonsmokers not to start. The epidemiologic data overwhelmingly support the prediction that smoking precipitates both the early appearance of disease and early death in persons with α1AT deficiency. Avoidance of atmospheric conditions with respiratory irritants should also be encouraged. Immunization against current respiratory pathogens such as influenza A and B, *Pneumococcus,* and *Haemophilus influenzae* B should be kept current. Infections of the lower respiratory tract should be treated early and aggressively with appropriate antibiotics.

Alpha$_1$-proteinase inhibitor (human), prepared from human immunodeficiency virus antibody–negative and hepatitis B surface antigen–negative plasma pooled from normal human donors, is now being used in a multicenter, National Institutes of Health–sponsored clinical trial to evaluate the effect of chronic replacement (augmentation) on the development of emphysema in adult patients with early symptomatic α1AT deficiency of the PiZ type.[5] It has been estimated that 300 patients in the treated group and 300 in the untreated control group, observed for three years, are needed in order to show efficacy by a decrease of 50% in the rate of decline in the FEV_1.[55] The rationale for weekly intravenous infusions of 60 mg/kg body weight is based on epidemiologic and experimental data. Patients with α1AT serum levels <50 mg/dl have a risk of more than 80% of developing emphysema over the lifetime.[10, 11] Those with serum levels >80 mg/dl do not seem to have an increased risk. This observation is the basis both for selection of patients and for trying to achieve serum "threshold" levels higher than 80 mg/dl.

Weekly infusions for 4 weeks to a 35-year-old emphysema patient with the P-null-null phenotype provided an opportunity to examine the contribution of α1AT antineutrophil elastase protection to the lower respiratory tract.[56] His serum antineutrophil elastase capacity was <5% of normal, and that of the epithelial lining fluid of the lower respiratory tract was 13% of normal. The serum α1AT level peaked at >300 mg/dl, and trough levels were 81 ± 2 mg/dl. Both α1AT and antineutrophil elastase activity in the epithelial lining fluid rose to values within the lower range of normal. These observations indicated that infusions of α1AT at weekly intervals can raise and maintain blood levels at and above the "protective threshold" level despite a half-life in the blood of 5.2 days and that infused α1AT crosses the endothelial-interstitial-epithelial barrier to bathe alveolar walls. A second study of 21 patients with the PiZZ form of α1AT and emphysema demonstrated that infusions of α1AT derived from plasma are safe and can reverse the biochemical abnormalities in serum and lung fluid.[55] Steady-state serum α1AT rose from 30 mg/dl to 126 mg/dl when weekly infusions were given for up to 6 months. Serum antineutrophil elastase rose from 5.4 to 13.3 μmol. When measured 6 days after infusion, epithelial lining fluid α1AT had increased significantly ($p < .0001$) from 0.46 ± 0.16 to 1.89 ± 0.17 μmol, and antineutrophil elastase capacity had risen from 0.81 ± 0.13 to 1.65 ± 0.13 μmol. The only adverse reaction in 507 infusions was four episodes of self-limited fever, which resolved within 24 h. The serum half-life of the preparation did not decrease over 6 months of therapy; this indicates the probable absence of development of anti-α1AT antibody that could interfere with α1AT metabolism. During this long-term controlled clinical trial of replacement therapy, alternative treatment strategies are being considered.

The α1AT gene has been successfully cloned. It can be genetically engineered by a technique called site-directed mutagenesis. By changing the genetic code, Rosenberg and colleagues[57] were able to substitute a valine for the methionine at the 358 residue of the protein. Alpha$_1$-antitrypsin is normally inactivated by oxidation of methionine. Substitution of another amino acid circumvents this event and prolongs the biologic half-life of α1AT. Further experimental and clinical trials are necessary for proving the effectiveness and safety of this type of preparation.

Hubbard and co-workers[58] administered aerosolized recombinant α1AT by compressed air-driven nebulizer to 14 patients with emphysema secondary to α1AT deficiency. There was a significant increase in its concentration in pulmonary epithelial lining fluid, and some α1AT was detectable even in the serum, which demonstrates its permeability of lower respiratory epithelium.

The mechanism of liver disease seems to be quite distinct from that of the pulmonary disease; there is no reason to believe that plasma therapy would be beneficial. Prenatal diagnosis may be considered for the fetus at risk because of a family history of a child with α1AT deficiency who has developed severe cirrhosis. Liver transplantation is the only known therapy. Perhaps other therapies will be developed when the pathogenesis of the liver disease becomes more completely understood. A useful model for studying this aspect of the disease has been developed in transgenic mouse lineages carrying the human normal (M) or human mutant (Z) alleles.[45] Those with the M allele produced and secreted protein M normally into the serum. Those with the Z allele had serum concentrations of the Z allele protein one tenth the serum concentration of the M allele protein. Protein Z accumulated in hepatocytes in diastase-resistant cytoplasmic granules that could be revealed in the periodic acid-Schiff reaction. Irregular foci of liver cell necrosis also occurred. These findings, along with runting in the neonatal period, resemble those observed with α1AT deficiency–associated neonatal hepatitis.

REFERENCES

1. Laurell CB, Eriksson S: The electrophoretic alpha₁-globulin pattern of serum in alpha₁-antitrypsin deficiency. Scand J Clin Lab Invest 15:132–140, 1963.
2. Eriksson S: Pulmonary emphysema and alpha₁-antitrypsin deficiency. Acta Med Scand 175:197–205, 1964.
3. Eriksson S: Studies in alpha₁-antitrypsin deficiency. Acta Med Scand Suppl 432:1–85, 1965.
4. Sharp HL, Bridges RA, Krivit W, et al: Cirrhosis associated with alpha-1-antitrypsin deficiency: A previously unrecognized inherited disorder. J Lab Clin Med 73:934–939, 1969.
5. Buist AS: α1-Antitrypsin deficiency in lung and liver disease. Hosp Pract (Off Ed) 24:51–59, 1989.
6. Carrell RW: α1-Antitrypsin: Molecular pathology, leukocytes, and tissue damage. J Clin Invest 78:1427–1431, 1986.
7. Kalsheker N: Alpha₁-antitrypsin: Structure, function and molecular biology of the gene. Biosci Rep 9:129–138, 1989.
8. Long GL, Chandra T, Woo SL, et al: Complete sequence of the cDNA for human α1-antitrypsin and the gene for the S variant. Biochemistry 23:4828–4837, 1984.
9. Nukiwa T, Brantly ML, Ogushi F, et al: Characterization of the gene and protein of the common α1-antitrypsin normal M2 allele. Am J Hum Genet 43:322–330, 1988.
10. Gadek JE, Fells GA, Zimmerman RL, et al: Antielastases of the human alveolar structures: Implications for the protease-antiprotease theory of emphysema. J Clin Invest 68:889–898, 1981.
11. Gadek JE, Klein HG, Holland PV, et al: Replacement therapy of alpha₁-antitrypsin deficiency: Reversal of protease-antiprotease imbalance within the alveolar structures of PiZ subjects. J Clin Invest 68:1158–1165, 1981.
12. Talamo RC, Langley CE, Reed CE, et al: α1-Antitrypsin deficiency: A variant with no detectable α1-antitrypsin. Science 181:70–71, 1973.
13. Satoh K, Nukiwa T, Brantly M, et al.: Emphysema associated with complete absence of α1-antitrypsin in serum and the homozygous inheritance (corrected) of a stop codon in an α1-antitrypsin-coding exon. Am J Hum Genet 42:77–83, 1988.
14. Cox DW, Billingsley GD: Rare deficiency types of α1-antitrypsin: Electrophoretic variation and DNA haplotypes. Am J Hum Genet 44:844–854, 1989.
15. Faber J, Weidinger S, Goedde H, et al: The deficient alpha-1-antitrypsin phenotype Pi P is associated with an A-to-T transversion in exon III of the gene. Am J Hum Genet 45:161–163, 1989.
16. Fagerhol MK, Laurell CB: The polymorphism of "prealbumins" and alpha-1-antitrypsin in human sera. Clin Chim Acta 16:199–203, 1967.
17. Fagerhol MK, Hauge HE: Serum Pi types in patients with pulmonary diseases. Acta Allergol 24:107–114, 1969.
18. Klasen EC, Biemond I, Laros CD: α1-Antitrypsin deficiency and the flaccid lung syndrome: The heterozygote controversy. Clin Genet 29:211–215, 1986.
19. Mittman C, Lieberman J, Rumsfeld J: Prevalence of abnormal protease inhibitor phenotypes in patients with chronic obstructive lung disease. Am Rev Respir Dis 109:295–296, 1974.
20. Schwartz RH, Johnstone DE, Talamo RC, et al: Alpha-1-antitrypsin (AAT) protease inhibitor (Pi) types in recurrent and chronic lung disease of childhood. J Allergy Clin Immunol 51:85, 1973.
21. Hall WJ, Hyde RW, Schwartz RH, et al: Pulmonary abnormalities in intermediate alpha-1-antitrypsin deficiency. J Clin Invest 58:1069–1077, 1976.
22. Vance JC, Hall WJ, Schwartz RH, et al: Heterozygous alpha-1-antitrypsin deficiency and respiratory function in children. Pediatrics 60:263–272, 1977.
23. Horne SL, Tennent RK, Cockcroft DW, et al: Pulmonary function in Pi M and MZ grainworkers. Chest 89:795–799, 1986.
24. Ostrow DN, Cherniack RM: The mechanical properties of the lungs in intermediate deficiency of alpha-1-antitrypsin. Am Rev Respir Dis 106:377–383, 1972.
25. Shigeoka JW, Hall WJ, Hyde RW, et al: The prevalence of alpha-1-antitrypsin heterozygotes (PiMZ) in patients with obstructive pulmonary disease. Am Rev Respir Dis 114:1077–1084, 1976.
26. Bruce RM, Cohen BH, Diamond EL, et al: Collaborative study to assess risk of lung disease in PiMZ phenotype subjects. Am Rev Respir Dis 130:386–390, 1984.
27. Talamo RC: Basic and clinical aspects of the alpha-1-antitrypsin. Pediatrics 56:91–99, 1975.
28. Wewers MD, Gadek JE, Keogh BA, et al: Evaluation of danazol therapy for patients with PiZZ alpha-1-antitrypsin deficiency. Am Rev Respir Dis 134:476–480, 1986.
29. Larsson C: Natural history and life expectancy in severe alpha₁-antitrypsin deficiency, PiZ. Acta Med Scand 204:345–351, 1978.
30. Sveger T: Liver disease in alpha₁-antitrypsin deficiency detected by screening of 200,000 infants. N Engl J Med 294:1316–1321, 1976.
31. Harris JO, Olsen GN, Castle JR, et al: Comparison of proteolytic enzyme activity in pulmonary alveolar macrophages and blood leukocytes in smokers and nonsmokers. Am Rev Respir Dis 111:579–586, 1975.
32. Janus ED, Phillips NT, Carrell RW: Smoking, lung function, and α1-antitrypsin deficiency. Lancet 1:152–154, 1985.
33. Brantly M, Courtney M, Crystal RG: Repair of the secretion defect in the Z form of α1-antitrypsin by addition of a second mutation. Science 242:1700–1702, 1988.
34. Eriksson SG: Liver disease in α1-antitrypsin deficiency. Scand J Gastroenterol 20:907–911, 1985.
35. Cox DW, Smyth S: Risk of liver disease in adults with alpha₁-antitrypsin deficiency. Am J Med 74:221–227, 1983.
36. Eriksson S, Carlson J, Velez R: Risk of cirrhosis and primary liver cancer in alpha₁-antitrypsin deficiency. N Engl J Med 314:736–739, 1986.
37. Carlson J, Eriksson S: Chronic 'cryptogenic' liver disease and malignant hepatoma in intermediate alpha₁-antitrypsin deficiency identified by a PiZ-specific monoclonal antibody. Scand J Gastroenterol 20:835–842, 1985.
38. Talamo RC, Levison H, Lynch MJ, et al: Symptomatic pulmonary emphysema in childhood associated with hereditary alpha-1-antitrypsin and elastase inhibitor deficiency. J Pediatr 79:20–26, 1971.

39. Buist AS, Adams BE, Azzam AH, et al: Pulmonary function in young children with alpha-1-antitrypsin deficiency: Comparison with matched control subjects. Am Rev Respir Dis 122:817–822, 1980.
40. Wagener JS, Sobonya RE, Taussig LM, et al: Unusual abnormalities in adolescent siblings with alpha-1-antitrypsin deficiency. Chest 83:464–468, 1983.
41. Dunand P, Cropp GA, Middleton E: Severe obstructive lung disease in a 14-year old girl with alpha-1-antitrypsin deficiency. J Allergy Clin Immunol 57:615–622, 1976.
42. Langley CE, Berninger RW, Wolfson SL, Talamo RC: An unusual type of α1-antitrypsin deficiency in a child. Johns Hopkins Med J 144:161–165, 1979.
43. Cox DW, Mansfield T: Prenatal diagnosis of α1-antitrypsin deficiency and estimates of fetal risk for disease. J Med Genet 24:52–59, 1987.
44. Porter CA, Mowat AP, Cook PJ, et al: 1-Antitrypsin deficiency and neonatal hepatitis. Br Med J 3:435–439, 1972.
45. Dycaico MJ, Grant SG, Felts K, et al.: Neonatal hepatitis induced by α1-antitrypsin: A transgenic mouse model. Science 242:1409–1412, 1988.
46. Udall JN, Bloch KJ, Walker WA: Transport of proteases across neonatal intestine and development of liver disease in infants with alpha-1-antitrypsin deficiency. Lancet 1:1441–1443, 1982.
47. Udall JN, Dixon M, Newman AP, et al: Liver disease in alpha-1-antitrypsin deficiency: A retrospective analysis of the influence of early breast- vs. bottle-feeding. JAMA 253:2679–2682, 1985.
48. Cooper DM, Hoeppner V, Cox D, et al: Lung function in alpha$_1$-antitrypsin heterozygotes (Pi type MZ). Am Rev Respir Dis 110:708–715, 1974.
49. Szczeklik A, Turowska B, Czerniawska-Mysik G, et al: Serum alpha 1-antitrypsin in bronchial asthma. Am Rev Respir Dis 109:487–490, 1974.
50. Katz RM, Lieberman J, Siegel SC: Alpha-1-antitrypsin levels and prevalence of Pi variant phenotypes in asthmatic children. J Allergy Clin Immunol 57:41–45, 1976.
51. Arnaud P, Chapuis-Cellier C, Souillet G, et al: High frequency of deficient Pi phenotypes of alpha-1-antitrypsin in nonatopic asthma of children. Clin Res 24:488A, 1976.
52. Schwartz RH, Van Ess JD, Johnstone DE, et al: Alpha-1-antitrypsin in childhood asthma. J Allergy Clin Immunol 59:31–34, 1977.
53. Hendrick SJ, Silverman AK, Solomon AR, Headington JT: α1-Antitrypsin deficiency associated with panniculitis. J Am Acad Dermatol 18:684–692, 1988.
54. Pittelkow MR, Smith KC, Su WP: Alpha-1-antitrypsin deficiency and panniculitis: Perspectives on disease relationship and replacement therapy. Am J Med 84(Suppl 6A):80–86, 1988.
55. Wewers MD, Casolaro A, Sellers SE, et al: Replacement therapy for alpha$_1$-antitrypsin deficiency associated with emphysema. N Engl J Med 316:1055–1062, 1987.
56. Wewers MD, Casolaro MA, Crystal RG: Comparison of alpha-1-antitrypsin levels and antineutrophil elastase capacity of blood and lung in a patient with alpha-1-antitrypsin phenotype null-null before and during alpha-1-antitrypsin augmentation therapy. Am Rev Respir Dis 135:539–543, 1987.
57. Rosenberg S, Barr PJ, Najarian RC, et al: Synthesis in yeast of a functional oxidation-resistant mutant of human alpha-1-antitrypsin. Nature 312:77–80, 1984.
58. Hubbard R, Stephans L, Crystal RG: Delivery of α1-antitrypsin by aerosol: Direct augmentation of lung anti-elastase defenses in α1-antitrypsin deficiency. Clin Res 36:625A, 1988.

47 ADAPTATION TO HIGH ALTITUDE

GEOFFREY KURLAND, M.D.

THE CHALLENGE OF ALTITUDE

Approximately 20 to 30 million people live year-round at an altitude of at least 3000 meters (9842 feet) above sea level,[1] and additional millions of low-altitude residents travel to areas of high elevation. The ability to adapt to the stresses of altitude determines a person's ability to survive and thrive at high altitude. In this chapter, some of the stresses involved, as well as several of the physiologic adaptations to these stresses, are discussed.

ACUTE MOUNTAIN SICKNESS

Acute mountain sickness (AMS) is a clinical syndrome that occurs in healthy persons who ascend rapidly to high altitude. Because acclimatization to high altitude takes time, it is commonly believed that the rapidity of ascent is a major factor in the development of AMS. However, the altitude attained is also important; this syndrome is rare under 2500 m. The amount of time at altitude is also important; brief exposures (<24 h) to altitude may lead to the development of important but not life-threatening symptoms of AMS. Although susceptibility to AMS is not related to sex or physical stress, children over 2 years of age are particularly susceptible. With modern air travel, people may rapidly move to high-altitude areas. Ski areas in Colorado, for example, are often 2400 to 2800 m at base altitudes; maximal altitudes at mountain summits are 3500 m. AMS is therefore possible in a fairly large population, including children.

CLINICAL FEATURES OF AMS

The most common symptom of AMS is headache, which occurs in the majority of persons in whom AMS develops according to an incidence study by Hackett and co-workers.[2] Other symptoms, in descending order as reported by those authors, include insomnia, anorexia, nausea, dizziness, excessive dyspnea on exertion or at rest, oliguria, lassitude, vomiting, and incoordination.

The headache of AMS typically is frontal in location and occurs within a few hours of ascent to altitude or on awakening after spending a first (often restless) night at altitude. As noted by Hackett and Hornbein, the early symptoms of AMS are "remarkably similar to those of alcohol hangover."[3]

Life-threatening complications of AMS include high-altitude pulmonary edema (HAPE) and high-altitude cerebral edema (HACE). Because of the morbidity and mortality rates associated with these, they are discussed as separate entities, although it is likely that they are extremes of a pathophysiologic spectrum in AMS rather than entities totally separate from AMS.

INCIDENCE OF AMS

Hackett and colleagues[2, 3] studied, interviewed, and examined 278 trekkers to Pheriche in the Everest region of Nepal (elevation, 4243 m). They reported that the overall incidence of AMS was 53%. AMS was more prevalent among trekkers who flew rather than trekked from Kathmandu (1370 m) to Lukla (2800 m), rapidly ascended, and spent fewer nights acclimatizing. The incidence was equal in males and females and was unrelated to previous experience at altitude or to load carried. Younger trekkers tended to be more severely affected with AMS. Singh and associates,[4] studying Indian troops moved from lowlands to 3350 to 5490 m by truck or airplane, reported the incidence of AMS to vary from 0.1% to 8.3%. Airplane travel to altitude was associated with more severe symptoms, and they reported that allowing 1 week for acclimatization at 2400 m (8000 feet), 3350 m (11,000 feet), and 4270 m (14,000 feet) was adequate for preventing severe symptoms at higher altitudes.

PATHOPHYSIOLOGY OF AMS

In a review of AMS, Johnson and Rock[5] summarized the current concepts of the pathogenesis of AMS. Although the sojourner at high altitude encounters numerous stresses, it is likely that alveolar hypoxia and resistant tissue hypoxia are the major causes of AMS. With hypoxia secondary to low ambient barometric pressure, there are numerous physiologic changes, which include increased minute ventilation, peripheral alkalosis, changes in cerebrospinal fluid (CSF) pH and hydrogen ion concentration, and an increase in cerebral blood flow (CBF). This latter change appears to be central in the appearance of HACE and is discussed. Fluid shifts that occur in AMS and its complications may be augmented by alterations in volume regulation. Indeed, diuresis during ascent is more commonly seen in persons in whom severe AMS did not develop.[4] Hackett and others[6] also documented weight loss, as well as diuresis, in high-altitude sojourners who did not acquire AMS, whereas those who acquired symptoms of AMS had weight gain, which is consistent with fluid retention. Hypocapnia, which is secondary to the increased minute ventilation on ascent

to altitude, has been implicated as another important facet in the pathogenesis of AMS. Studies by Grubb and co-workers[7] reported a linear relationship of CBF to arterial carbon dioxide pressure/tension (Pa_{CO_2}). Hansen and Evans,[8] however, suggested that hypocapnic hypoxia is protective against an increased CSF pressure and that hyperventilation is protective against AMS. Several studies showed that a relatively decreased hypoxic ventilatory response, measured at either sea level or high altitude, is related to the development of symptoms of AMS.[9, 10] Paradoxically, the inhalation of 3% carbon dioxide at altitude has been suggested as a treatment for moderate AMS by Harvey and co-authors.[11]

Hackett and Rennie,[12] in their review of AMS, pointed out that the major initial clinical manifestations of AMS are neurologic (e.g., headache, insomnia, lassitude, anorexia, and so on). They argued that AMS is basically a "cerebral disorder" and that a basic underlying pathologic feature is probably cerebral vasodilation. There is evidence for an increase in CBF on exposure to altitude,[4, 13, 14] and this increase temporally matches the normal course of AMS, with an increased CBF over 6 to 36 h after ascent and a gradual decrease to normal after 5 to 6 days.

HAPE, another severe complication of AMS, is probably a permeability-type edema in that left ventricular failure is not present,[15] although changes in pulmonary vascular resistance, pulmonary artery pressure, and physical features such as shear stress on the pulmonary capillary endothelium all are believed to play some role in its development. Maher and co-workers[16] reported, as an alternative, that hypocapnia was protective in subjects exposed to simulated altitude. It is difficult to reconcile the conclusions of these two studies, although the small numbers of subjects, as well as varying conditions of study, suggest that further investigation of the relationship of arterial carbon dioxide pressure/tension (Pa_{CO_2}) to AMS may be fruitful. It is likely that hypocapnia or eucapnia affects people differently because there appears to be a wide intersubject variability in susceptibility to the symptoms of AMS.

AMS, however, is probably not simply the result of hypoxia per se but rather the combination of hypoxia and a lack of normal acclimatization by a slow ascent to altitude in susceptible persons. Some persons have reproducible symptoms if the altitude achieved and rate of ascent are similar. The fact that there is a lag phase of several hours between attainment of altitude and appearance of the first symptoms of AMS suggests that factors other than alveolar hypoxia are involved in its pathogenesis.

HIGH-ALTITUDE PULMONARY EDEMA

HAPE is a clinical entity usually occurring within the first 3 days of ascent to altitude. Rapidity of ascent is believed to contribute to the development of HAPE. Persons affected tend to be relatively young, physically fit, and free of underlying cardiac or respiratory disease. Males are more commonly affected by HAPE than are females. There have been cases of HAPE that have developed in the absence of other symptoms of AMS.

Several epidemiologic studies of HAPE confirm its high incidence among children. Hultgren and Marticorena[17] studied residents of an Andean mining village (altitude, 3750 m) who had experienced HAPE after initial exposure or on re-exposure to high altitude after a sojourn to sea level. The incidence of HAPE was 6.5% in 402 exposures to altitude by residents 1 to 19 years of age, as opposed to 0.45% in older persons. Hultgren and Marticorena stated that HAPE was rare before the age of 2 years. In a larger study of the same population,[18] the incidence of HAPE overall was 6.1%, but among persons 2 to 12 years old, it was 10%, and among those 13 to 20 years old, it was 17%. These younger persons also tended to have more severe episodes of HAPE.

Other reviews of AMS (and the severe complication HAPE) refer to the increased incidence in younger adults and children.[3, 19, 20] Scoggin and colleagues[21] reported on 39 episodes of HAPE requiring hospitalization of 32 residents of Leadville, Colorado (elevation, 3100 m), who had returned after a sojourn to a lower altitude (<2200 m). The mean age of those affected was 11.9 years; only two cases occurred in persons older than 21 years. In contrast to other studies, many of the low-altitude sojourns preceding HAPE in this study were less than 7 days in length; 3 of the 39 episodes followed a 1-day sojourn.

CLINICAL FEATURES

Numerous descriptions of HAPE exist in the literature[2, 22-25] and are summarized briefly here. Early manifestations of HAPE are dyspnea on exertion, fatigue, and weakness. Dry cough develops, and peripheral cyanosis may be seen. Orthopnea and sleep difficulty are common. Dyspnea, tachypnea, tachycardia, production of pink sputum, central cyanosis, and occasionally hemoptysis are seen in severe disease. In children, restlessness, anorexia, and vomiting may be prominent symptoms. Fever up to 38.5°C is common and is one reason why HAPE may be confused with bacterial or viral pneumonia. Crackles are commonly heard on auscultation of the chest; these may first appear in the right middle lung field. The chest radiographs in HAPE often show patchy, fluffy densities that may be unilateral (more often on the right) or bilateral. Pleural effusion and cardiomegaly are rare, although the pulmonary outflow tract or central branches of the pulmonary artery may be prominent. Chest radiographic findings often improve rapidly with treatment, and the chest radiographs often return to normal over 48 h.

Mild leukocytosis (13,000 to 15,000/cu mm) with "left shift" may be seen, but often the white blood cell count is normal. Arterial blood gas measurements show hypoxemia and respiratory alkalosis with a widened alveolar-arterial oxygen gradient. Electrocardiograms during HAPE have evidence of acute right ventricular and right atrial overload: peaked P waves, R waves in the right precordial leads, prominent S waves in leads V_5 and V_6, and right-axis deviation in severe cases.

Several reports of lung lavage fluid from patients with HAPE have appeared. Schoene and colleagues[26] performed bronchoalveolar lavage (BAL) on three climbers with HAPE and three controls. BAL fluid from HAPE victims contained more erythrocytes and neutrophils, although alveolar macrophages remained the predominant cell type. The HAPE fluid also contained much higher amounts of total protein, albumin, and immunoglobulins. Hackett and coworkers[27] simultaneously reported that the amount of total protein in direct secretions from the lung of a patient with HAPE was essentially equal to serum concentrations. Both these reports suggested that HAPE is the result of an increased pulmonary capillary permeability.

PATHOGENESIS OF HAPE

As pointed out by Wagner,[19] pathophysiologic changes leading to HAPE are still unclear. A variety of potential mechanisms have been reviewed by Hultgren and associates[18, 25] and include antidiuresis and fluid retention, increased capillary permeability transarterial leakage, "neurogenic" pulmonary edema, lung shifts into the pulmonary vasculature, cardiac left ventricular failure, and overperfusion. The last mechanism is indicative of nonhomogeneous hypoxic pulmonary vasoconstriction, which would lead to relative overperfusion of nonconstricted precapillary arterioles, with transmission of high pressure to the capillary bed and resulting interstitial and alveolar edema.

Evidence of pulmonary hypertension on exposure to hypoxia is abundant and has been extensively reviewed by Wagner.[19] Wagner also suggested that shear forces from increased local blood flow in the pulmonary vascular bed may play a role in the development of HAPE by injuring the capillary endothelium.

HIGH-ALTITUDE CEREBRAL EDEMA

HACE is rare, generally affecting less than 2% of persons at risk. Dickinson[28] in 1983 and Hackett and Hornbein[3] in 1988 reviewed HACE. HACE is a severe form of AMS with cerebral dysfunction, and yet it is difficult to establish the exact definition and diagnosis because the few cases that occur usually are in remote areas where sophisticated medical care is unavailable. Few cases of HACE have come to autopsy, but cerebral edema is an important feature in most of these.

The symptoms of HACE overlap with those of AMS in that both have neurologic features. In HACE, however, disturbance of consciousness, ataxia, papilledema, and retinal hemorrhage are more significant. Some patients are comatose in the absence of papilledema. HACE, like AMS and HAPE, has wide intersubject variability; some persons become severely affected at an altitude at which others do not.

The pathophysiologic mechanisms of HACE are believed to be similar to those of AMS and HAPE. Sutton and Lassen[29] suggested that cerebral vasodilation and increased CBF secondary to hypoxia lead to increased pressure in the microvasculature, resulting in cerebral edema. Other proposed mechanisms were reviewed by Dickinson.[28]

TREATMENT OF AMS, HAPE, HACE

The most important aspect of treating AMS and its severe complications is their early recognition. AMS, HAPE, or HACE should be suspected when neurologic, pulmonary, or, in the case of children, certain nonspecific symptoms such as restlessness, lassitude, or anorexia appear in a person who has ascended rapidly to high altitude.

The definitive treatment for AMS is descent to lower altitude. Although a small drop in altitude may markedly improve the condition of the person with mild AMS or HAPE, more descent is usually needed in the presence of HACE. Oxygen may be life-saving in HAPE,[30] but its usefulness as therapy in HACE is not as well established.[31]

Various medications have been used in the treatment of AMS, but few have been evaluated in a double-blind, placebo-controlled manner. Aspirin may relieve headache associated with AMS, although side effects including dyspnea have been noted after its administration.[12] Diuretics have been advocated for preventing or treating symptoms of AMS. Singh and colleagues[4] reported that furosemide relieved symptoms of AMS within 6 to 48 h, although data on placebo control–treated subjects are lacking. Gray and associates[32] reported that furosemide given regularly from the time of arrival at altitude caused dehydration, with evidence of vascular collapse in some patients.

Acetazolamide may be useful in treating AMS and is commonly taken as a preventive medication. Controlled studies of its effectiveness are lacking. Its mechanisms of action in treating AMS are controversial. As a carbonic anhydrase inhibitor, it leads to renal bicarbonate loss (metabolic acidosis) and inhibition of red blood cell carbonic anhydrase and decreased respiratory loss of carbon dioxide (respiratory acidosis). Both conditions increase ventilation and increase the arterial oxygen tension/pressure (Pa_{O_2}). It is not clear whether the most important mechanism is the carbonic anhydrase inhibition in the kidney or in the red blood cell.[33] Plasma bicarbonate levels are lowered and ventilation is increased, increasing the Pa_{O_2} and speeding the process of acclimatization.[34]

Corticosteroids, particularly dexamethasone and betamethasone, have been used in treating AMS and HACE.[5] At least one clinical trial demonstrated the efficacy of dexamethasone in reducing symptoms of AMS, although objective physiologic abnormalities associated with AMS were not improved.[35] The authors concluded that dexamethasone should be used to treat AMS only when descent is impossible.

Because experimental hypoxic pulmonary hypertension is responsive to calcium-channel blockers[36, 37], Oelz and co-workers[38] administered nifedipine to six subjects with HAPE after their ascent to 4559 m. All subjects exhibited both a decrease in subjective complaints such as shortness of breath and improvement in the alveolar-arterial oxygen gradient, pulmonary artery pressure, and radiographic evidence of pulmonary edema. Because of the small number of subjects, Oelz and co-workers[38] cautioned against the regular use of nifedipine in lieu of descent in cases of HAPE; nifedipine, however, may prove to be beneficial in those instances in which descent is impossible or delayed.

PREVENTION OF AMS, HAPE, HACE

The most important preventive measure is slow ascent to altitude. Hackett and co-workers[2] noted that slow ascent to altitude was associated with decreased incidence of AMS. Their study also suggested some effectiveness of acetazolamide when taken before symptoms developed. Other studies also suggested a useful role for acetazolamide as a preventive medication.[22, 34, 39, 40]

Two double-blind crossover trials of dexamethasone in young, healthy male subjects exposed to a simulated altitude of 4575 m suggested that it may be useful in preventing symptoms of AMS.[41, 42] The investigators, however, cautioned against extrapolation of their results to travelers to high altitude. Further study of both dexamethasone and acetazolamide is needed in order to better decide who will benefit from each drug and to optimize dosing schedule and duration of treatment.

The use of narcotics, alcohol, sedative-hypnotics, or any other medications that depress ventilatory drive should be avoided in patients with AMS. Digoxin, previously suggested in the treatment of HAPE, is also not recommended because left ventricular dysfunction is not a common problem in this setting. Medical management in the treatment of established severe AMS (including HAPE and HACE) is probably less effective than descent to lower altitude, which remains the treatment of choice for this disorder.

EFFECTS OF ALTITUDE ON GROWTH AND LUNG MECHANICS

FETAL GROWTH AND BIRTH WEIGHT

When socioeconomic and nutritional factors are controlled for, high-altitude gestation is associated with a decreased birth weight.[43–45] Studies by Kruger and Arias-Stella[43] suggest that placental weight increases and placental septation decreases at high altitude. The latter change would bring about an increase in the proportion of functioning parenchyma in the placenta. Jackson and co-workers, although unable to confirm placental weight differences at high altitude,[46] documented histologic changes interpreted as adaptations that optimize placental gas exchange.[47, 48] Thus there appears to be a direct relationship among maternal ventilation, arterial oxygenation, and infant birth weight at high altitude.[49, 50]

THORACIC SIZE, LUNG VOLUMES, AND LUNG MECHANICS

Living in high-altitude areas leads to a reduction in linear growth of children.[51–54] In addition, thoracic size and forced vital capacity in such children are increased.

Brody and co-workers[55] compared forced vital capacity, static lung pressure-volume characteristics, and expiratory flow-volume curves in native-born young adult Peruvian males. The results suggested that conducting airways, which form in fetal life, are not involved in adaptation to altitude. Therefore, the increase in the size of the lungs of highland dwellers is most likely the result of post-

Table 47–1. ADAPTIVE RESPONSES TO ALTITUDE: CHANGES RELATIVE TO SEA LEVEL CONTROL VALUES

Variable	Immediate Change	Early Adaptation	Chronic Acclimatization
Ventilation Parameters			
Minute ventilation	↑	↑	↑
Respiratory rate	V	V/↑	V
Tidal volume	↑	↑	↑
Arterial oxygen pressure/tension	↓	↓	↓
Arterial carbon dioxide pressure/tension	↓	↓	↓
Arterial pH	↑	↑/NC	↑/NC
Pulmonary Function Tests			
Vital capacity	↓	↓	NC
Total lung capacity	↑	↓/NC	↑
Residual volume	↑	↑	↑
Functional residual capacity	↑	↑	↑
Diffusing capacity	↑	↑	↑
Cardiopulmonary			
Cardiac output	↑	NC	NC/↓
Pulmonary vascular resistance	↑	↑	↑
Hematologic Parameters			
Hemoglobin	NC	↑	↑
Erythropoietin	↑	↑	NC
P_{50}	↑	↑	↑
2, 3-diphosphoglycerate	NC/↑	↑	↑

Modified from Guenter CA, Welch MH (eds): *Pulmonary Medicine,* 2nd ed, p. 11. Philadelphia: JB Lippincott, 1982.
↑, increased; ↓, decreased; V, variable response; NC, no change, or equivalent to sea-level value.

natal hypoxic stimulation of more peripheral lung growth. This concept of "dysynaptic" lung growth (i.e., disproportionate growth patterns in different constituent parts of the lung) was first proposed by Green and co-workers[56] and has been shown to originate in childhood.[57]

Cruz, studying airway mechanics in adults moved from sea level to Cerro de Pasco, Peru (4350 m), noted a decrease in airway resistance of 6% and a modest but statistically significant increase in forced expiratory volume in 1 sec.[58] However, because of the decreased density of air at that elevation, airway resistance was expected to fall further. Cruz suggested that some degree of bronchoconstriction at high altitude may have explained the observed results.

Mansell and co-workers, however, offered an alternative mechanism to explain changes in airway resistance at altitude.[59] They reported an increase in residual volume and a decrease in lung compliance, with a loss of elastic recoil at 60% total lung capacity after at least 9 days at altitude. These changes, they argued, could be best explained by an increase in fluid in the lung interstitium and a non-homogeneous loss of lung recoil. Evidence for such an increase in lung fluid has been documented through use of the technique of transthoracic electrical impedance. Jaeger and co-workers[60] postulated an initial increase in thoracic intravascular fluid volume at high altitude, followed by an increase in extravascular (interstitial) fluid, especially in dependent portions of the lungs. Hoon and colleagues,[61] studying lowlanders taken to areas of high altitude, noted that subjects who were symptomatic with signs of altitude sickness or pulmonary edema exhibited a progressive drop in transthoracic electrical impedance, whereas the impedance values of other asymptomatic or less symptomatic subjects decreased only transiently.

In summary, most studies have confirmed a negative effect of high altitude on both birth weight and linear growth. Above the altitude of at least 2500 m, there appears to be an adaptive increase in chest size (depth, width, and circumference) along with parameters of lung volumes, including the forced vital capacity. Migration from a low altitude to a high altitude during infancy or childhood leads to these changes. Flow rates and lung elastic recoil do not appear to be affected by increasing altitude, but a fall in vital capacity and an increase in residual volume and functional residual capacity are seen. Several of these changes are summarized in Table 47–1.

THE EFFECTS OF ALTITUDE ON RESPIRATORY PHYSIOLOGY

VENTILATION, GAS EXCHANGE, AND DIFFUSION AT ALTITUDE

Ventilation and Ventilatory Control

There are three phases of respiratory adaptation to high altitude. The first phase is an immediate response (within minutes to hours) to hypoxia and is best elicited in persons who are exposed to high-altitude conditions either in a decompression chamber or after rapid ascent in aircraft or motorized vehicle. Such exposure leads to an increase in minute ventilation, which, in turn, leads to hypocapnia and respiratory alkalosis.[62] In unacclimatized persons, this ventilatory increase does not occur until the Pa_{O_2} is 50 to 60 mm Hg at an elevation of approximately 3650 m (12,000 feet) if the respiratory quotient is assumed to be 0.85. The increase in ventilation is accomplished mainly by an increase in tidal volume, with a variable increase in respiratory frequency.[63] Mouth occlusion pressure, an

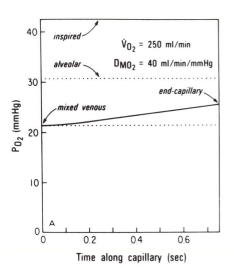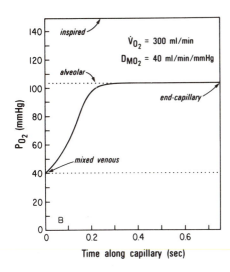

Figure 47–1. *Left,* calculated time course of the oxygen pressure/tension (P_{O_2}) in the pulmonary capillary of a climber at rest on the summit of Everest. Note the slow rate of rise of P_{O_2} and the marked alveolar–end capillary P_{O_2} difference. *Right,* normal time course at sea level for comparison. V_{O_2} is oxygen uptake; D_{MO_2} is the diffusing capacity of the alveolar-capillary membrane. (From West JB, Wagner PD: Predicted gas exchange on the summit of Mt. Everest. Respir Physiol 42:1–16, 1980.)

index of neuromuscular inspiratory drive, is also increased at altitude, reflecting an increase in central nervous system drive brought on by hypoxia[64] (Fig. 47–1).

With rapid ascent, blunting of this initial hyperventilatory response may occur after a few minutes, leading to a lower but still elevated respiratory rate. This down-regulation is thought to be secondary to the inhibitory effect of respiratory alkalosis on the respiratory drive of central and peripheral chemoreceptors.[65]

Results of studies by Weil and colleagues and others[66-68] suggested that the hypocapnic inhibition of the hypoxic drive is dependent on ventilatory responsiveness to carbon dioxide (CO_2). This CO_2 responsiveness is mediated by brainstem receptors, which are, in turn, sensitive to changes in H^+.[66-68]

It might be expected that hypoxemia would adversely affect the central nervous system, leading to a blunting of the acute hypoxic ventilatory response. However, Morrill and co-workers[69] found that any blunting of the central hypoxic drive by central nervous system hypoxia takes effect only when the resultant alveolar oxygen tension/pressure (PA_{O_2}) is much lower than that expected at all but the most extreme altitudes.[69]

In the late 1920s and 1930s, Heymans and co-workers[70] showed that the carotid bodies are the primary respiratory peripheral chemoreceptors. They increase their neural output in response to a decrease in Pa_{O_2} and an increase in P_{CO_2} and H^+. The carotid bodies appear to be more sensitive to oxygen pressure/tension (P_{O_2}) changes, with a hyperbolic relationship between the number of impulses generated and the P_{O_2}. A decrease in Pa_{O_2} from 500 to 75 mm Hg under normocapnic conditions results in a minimal increase in carotid body output, whereas further decreases in P_{O_2} lead to a marked increase in output, correlating with an increase in minute ventilation.[70-72]

The second phase in the ventilatory response to altitude takes place over the ensuing hours to days after exposure and is called *ventilatory acclimatization.* This acclimatization is characterized by a further increase in ventilation through an increase in tidal volume and some increase in respiratory frequency (Fig. 47–2). Rahn and Otis[62] pointed out that in comparison with values obtained on acute exposure to hypoxia (the unacclimatized state),

"the alveolar P_{CO_2} is always lower and the O_2 higher" in acclimatized persons.

The precise mechanism for ventilatory acclimatization remains unknown, although several factors are involved, which results in different explanatory theories for this acclimatization. Initially, it was believed that renal bicarbonate loss and H^+ conservation compensated for the acute respiratory alkalosis at altitude, increasing the sensitivity of the central respiratory drive to the effects of hypoxia. However, arterial alkalosis persists during the first several days of acclimatization, which argues against this explanation.

Ventilatory Adaptation to Chronic Hypoxia

The third phase of respiratory adaptation to high altitude occurs over months to years of exposure. Successful

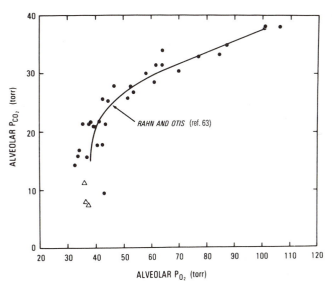

Figure 47–2. Oxygen-carbon dioxide diagram showing alveolar gas composition in acclimatized subjects at high altitude. At extreme altitudes (open triangles), marked hyperventilation maintains alveolar oxygen pressure/tension at approximately 35 mm Hg. The data fall on the curve first described by Rahn and Otis.[63] (From West JB, Hackett PH, Maret KH, et al: Pulmonary gas exchange on the summit of Mt. Everest. J Appl Physiol 55:678–687, 1983.)

prolonged residence at high altitude requires several changes in respiratory control as well as alterations in other systems such as the cardiovascular or hematopoietic systems. Most investigators documenting the adaptive mechanisms have studied the respiratory physiology of lifelong inhabitants of high-altitude regions.[73–81]

As pointed out by Rahn and Otis,[62] acclimatization to altitude is accompanied by an increase in ventilation, which results in a decrease in alveolar carbon dioxide pressure/tension (PA_{CO_2}) and an increase in PA_{O_2}. Lifelong residency at altitude by Andean Indians or Sherpas in the Himalayas, however, leads to an intermediate level of ventilation. This results in intermediate values for PA_{CO_2} and PA_{O_2} for highland natives.[82] Several studies have shown that lifelong adult residents at high altitude have a blunted hypoxic ventilatory response, which is not reversed on return to sea level.[74–76, 83, 84] Limited studies in Tibetan highland natives, however, have suggested that their minute ventilation is similar to that of acclimatized sojourners; hypoxic ventilatory control, however, has not been studied.[85]

Data from children living at high altitude suggest that this blunted hypoxic ventilatory response is acquired rather than genetically determined.[79] For example, Lahiri and co-workers[79] reported that 41 of 43 Andean children under 12 years of age had a normal hypoxic ventilatory response. Of 58 high-altitude natives between the ages of 13 and 22 years studied, 16 had an intermediate and 10 a blunted response to hypoxia. The remainder had a normal increase in ventilation. Forty high-altitude natives over 22 years of age were also studied, and all had blunted hypoxic responses. Newborn infants under 5 days of age also showed normal responses to hypoxia. Thus the abnormal response to hypoxia in high-altitude dwellers appears to be environmentally rather than genetically determined.

The progressive loss of the hypoxic ventilatory response, seen in high-altitude natives, is paralleled by a slow return of the normal response when a long-time high-altitude resident migrates to sea level. Although the lack of hyperventilation on exposure to hypoxia is present initially in these people, a normal response is seen after several years at sea level.[79] The mechanism for the blunted hypoxic ventilatory response at altitude is not clear. The enlargement of the carotid body, with chief cell hyperplasia, has been noted in high-altitude dwellers.[86–88] Carotid body enlargement is also seen in some lowland dwellers with chronic hypoxemia secondary to emphysema.[88] Carotid chemodectomas, which are usually benign neoplasms, have a tenfold higher incidence in Peruvian high-altitude dwellers than in lowland inhabitants, and chronic hypoxia is believed to play a major role in their development.[89] These pathologic findings, however, cannot assign the primary role in chronic acclimatization to the carotid body alone. The role of central nervous system receptors in chronic acclimatization is also unclear, although a suprapontine location for a regulator involved in the "blunting" of the hypoxic response in chronically acclimatized cats has been documented by Tenney and Ou.[90]

An interesting finding is the relatively rapid return of the normal hypoxic ventilatory response in pregnant high-altitude natives. Moore and co-workers determined that these women had an increase in resting ventilation and an increase in arterial oxygen saturation (Sa_{O_2}) in comparison with values determined in a postpartum study.[91] The precise mechanism for this "normalized" hypoxic ventilatory response and its rapid reversal in the postpartum period is unknown. However, the results of studies of ventilatory acclimatization from one population cannot be applied to another. The hypoxic ventilatory response in Sherpas, for example, is subject to considerable scatter and is not significantly different from that of low-altitude sojourners. It is clear that the precise mechanism of ventilatory acclimatization by the adult human is not fully delineated. In addition, it must be stressed that most studies on this intriguing aspect of humans' adaptation to altitude have involved healthy adults rather than children. Although the mechanisms for acclimatization may be similar, both the ability to adapt and the speed of adaptation may be different in children.

CARDIAC AND PULMONARY VASCULAR RESPONSE AT ALTITUDE

Cardiovascular Adaptation

On acute exposure to the hypoxia of altitude, cardiac output increases. This increase is caused mostly by an increase in heart rate, whereas stroke volume is usually unchanged or mildly decreased.[92, 93]

Although there exists some evidence of increases in catecholamine levels in persons at altitude,[94] plasma catecholamine levels do not appear to increase under hypoxic conditions in the resting subject.[95] The combination of acute hypoxic exposure with exercise results in a marked increase in plasma catecholamine levels.[96] Parasympathetic tone may also be altered under hypoxic conditions.[97–99] Although the cardiac output increases on initial exposure to high altitude, continued upward sojourn results in a fall in cardiac output values over several days, and the cardiac output may fall below preascent levels with longer stays at high altitude. This is the result of a fall in stroke volume, and it is accentuated with exercise. The heart rate declines with longer sojourns at high altitude but does not return to the preascent value.[93]

There are two major postulates explaining the decrease in stroke volume seen during high-altitude acclimatization: (1) decreased venous return secondary to contracted total body water and plasma volume[100] and (2) left ventricular dysfunction resulting from persistent hypoxemia.[101] Alexander and Grover[102] could find no evidence of left ventricular dysfunction by M-mode echocardiography and concluded that a fall in plasma volume was primarily responsible for the decrease in left ventricular stroke volume at altitude. Furthermore, evidence from studies in animals suggests that chronic hypoxia does not lead to a decrease in myocardial force development.[103]

Both systemic blood pressure and peripheral vascular resistance increase during acute acclimatization.[93] With long-term (at least 1-year) residence at high altitude, however, there is a fall in systemic blood pressure, the systolic pressure being most affected.[104, 105]

There have been few studies of the systemic and pulmonary circulations in infants and children at high altitude. In a review of this topic, Penaloza and co-workers[106] pointed out several differences between children born and raised at sea level and those born and raised at high altitudes. Children native to high altitude had (1) long-term persistence of right ventricular preponderance on electrocardiograms; (2) increased right ventricular weight in relation to the left ventricle; (3) increased pulmonary artery pressure, pulmonary vascular resistance, and right ventricular work; (4) increases in pulmonary arterial muscle secondary to the presence of a muscular media in more peripheral pulmonary arterial branches; and (5) increased incidence of patent ductus arteriosus in infants.

Pulmonary Vascular Adaptation

Distinct hemodynamic and anatomic changes are seen in the pulmonary vasculature in highland natives as well as lowland sojourners at high altitude. Hypoxia leads to pulmonary vasoconstriction, with increases in pulmonary arterial pressure and pulmonary vascular resistance. The precise mechanism for this vasoconstriction is not known, although numerous mechanisms including a direct effect of oxygen on pulmonary vascular smooth muscle, neurohumoral effects, or the activities of intrinsic chemical mediators such as catecholamines, prostaglandins, angiotensin II, or serotonin have been suggested.[107] This increase in pulmonary vascular resistance raises pulmonary arterial pressure and leads to an improvement in the ventilation/perfusion ratio ($\dot{V}/\dot{Q}$).

In intact animals, the response of the pulmonary vasculature to acute hypoxia is characterized by a short latent period followed by a slow pressure rise over 5 to 10 min before stabilizing.[108, 109] Although von Euler and Liljestrand[109] believed that the pulmonary vascular effects of hypoxia were the result of its direct effect on the pulmonary vessels, the actions of various mediators, including histamine, serotonin, bradykinin, angiotensin II, and prostaglandins have been implicated in this process. None of these have specifically proved to be the mediator of hypoxic pulmonary vasoconstriction.[107] An increase in transmembrane calcium influx, resulting either from a change in membrane charge or from a decrease in intracellular high-energy phosphate stores caused by hypoxia, has also been suggested as the mechanism of hypoxic pulmonary vasoconstriction.[36, 108]

Continued residence at high altitude leads to pulmonary hypertension in man.[110] Rotta and associates[104] demonstrated that healthy high-altitude natives have higher pulmonary artery and right ventricular pressures and increased pulmonary vascular resistance and right ventricular work than are found in control subjects (sea-level dwellers). Temporary (1-year) residents of high-altitude areas have increases in these values also but to a lesser extent than do healthy high-altitude natives.

Hematologic Adaptation at Altitude

The two major hematologic alterations seen in response to chronic exposure to high altitude are polycy-

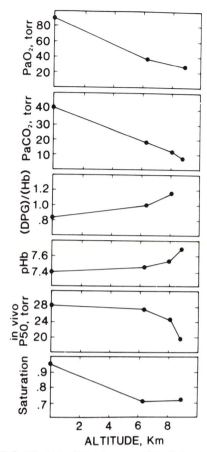

Figure 47–3. Effectors of blood oxygen (O_2) affinity at sea level and at high altitude. The net result, shown in the bottom panel, is a protected arterial O_2 saturation at extreme altitude. (From Winslow RM: Red cell function at extreme altitude. *In* West JB, Lahiri S [eds]: High Altitude and Man, pp. 59–72. Bethesda, MD: American Physiological Society, 1984.)

themia and altered hemoglobin oxygen affinity (Fig. 47–3). These aspects of adaptation have been reviewed.[111–113]

The rise in hematocrit after ascent to high altitude takes place within a few days. Erythropoietin levels, as might be expected, also rise quickly. Faura and co-workers[114] and Abbrecht and Littell[115] demonstrated a rapid (<24-h) rise in plasma and urine erythropoietin of subjects moved from sea level to high altitude. High-altitude natives have an increase in red cell mass, hematocrit, and total blood volume, whereas their plasma volume is decreased.

The polycythemia seen with exposure to altitude, although providing an increase in oxygen-carrying capacity, has disadvantages.[112] Blood viscosity is an exponential function of hematocrit, increasing dramatically above hematocrit values of 50% to 58%.[116] There is evidence of increased resistance to flow in pulmonary and systemic circulation, as well as a decrease in cardiac output as a result of polycythemia.[117–119] In the systemic microcirculation, blood flow is decreased to a point at which viscous properties of the blood may affect oxygen delivery to tissues.[120] For example, polycythemic subjects at high altitude who breathed 100% oxygen during exercise continued to have a reduction in maximal oxygen consumption, which is suggestive of a peripheral limitation of oxygen extraction. This limitation was believed to represent decreased muscle perfusion secondary to increased viscosity.[121] The optimal hematocrit at altitude probably varies with circumstances, exercise demands, and physical characteristics of each individual.[112]

Some investigators suggested that phlebotomy be considered to treat excessive polycythemia at altitude. They pointed out that decreased perfusion of the microcirculation may affect neurologic, cardiac, and peripheral muscular function. For example, coronary oxygen transport is stable over a wide hematocrit (20% to 60%); total body oxygen transport is stable within a hematocrit range of 40% to 60%.[119] Excessive polycythemia, however, interferes with coronary and peripheral oxygen transport and may therefore be deleterious.

Studies of the effectiveness of phlebotomy on polycythemic sojourners are few. Hemodilution has been advocated as an alternative to phlebotomy.[122] Sarnquist and co-workers[123] showed mild improvement in psychometric testing in three of four mountaineering subjects undergoing hemodilution. However, only a small hematocrit change was achieved (58% to 50.75%), and there was no significant change in work capacity, oxygen uptake, minute ventilation, or blood oxygen saturation. One subject experienced a hypersensitivity reaction during hemodilution. Transporting a suitable diluent to high altitude is logistically difficult, and the advantages may not be clinically warranted. Obviously, more study is necessary before routine hemodilution or phlebotomy can be recommended.

The potential advantage of a rightward-shifted oxyhemoglobin dissociation (OHD) curve at altitude is improved unloading of oxygen in the systemic capillary bed, where P_{O_2} is low. This shift, however, decreases the ability of blood to take up oxygen in the lungs, especially if the alveolar CO_2 is very low, which is the case at extremely high altitude. In fact, a leftward shift of the OHD curve (lower P_{50}) and higher affinity for oxygen is seen in some birds that can withstand extremes of altitude during migration, and there is evidence of decreased interaction of the hemoglobin from such species with organic phosphates such as 2,3-diphosphoglycerate (2,3-DPG).[124]

There is other evidence that a leftward shift of the OHD curve may improve survival at moderate altitude. Bartels and colleagues[125] exposed newborn rats and guinea pigs to lowered atmospheric pressures, simulating altitudes of 3000 or 5000 m. The rats showed a marked increase in red blood cell 2,3-DPG levels, a rightward shift in OHD curve (increased P_{50}), and an increased hemoglobin concentration at both altitudes. Guinea pigs, on the other hand, had less change in 2,3-DPG levels and P_{50} and more erythrocytosis at 5000 m. The guinea pigs fared better than the rats in terms of growth, and rats at high altitude showed more evidence of right ventricular hypertrophy. The investigators speculated that immaturity of the newborn rat, in comparsion with the newbron guinea pig, and the increased oxygen affinity of guinea pig hemoglobin levels resulted in improved survival of guinea pig newborns at high altitude. Eaton and collaborators[126] experimentally shifted the OHD curve of rats to the left and acutely exposed them to conditions of simulated high altitude (9180 m). Animals with the leftward-shifted OHD curve survived; 80% of control animals died within 90 min of exposure to the decreased barometric pressure.

There are therefore clinical and experimental data as well as physiologic argument in favor of either a rightward (decreased affinity) shift or a leftward (increased affinity) shift of the OHD curve in residents or sojourners at high altitude. Winslow pointed out that hemoglobin as a carrier of oxygen probably evolved before human evolutionary adaptations to high altitude and that the behavior of the OHD curve at high altitude is not fully understood, and there is no reason to believe that this behavior is "good or bad or a uniquely human property."[111]

AIR TRAVEL AND HIGH-ALTITUDE EXPOSURE IN PATIENTS WITH PULMONARY DISEASE

There are sparse data on the influence of high-altitude exposure on pre-existing cardiopulmonary disease. Hultgren,[127] as well as Hackett and Hornbein,[3] addressed this topic. The medical problems most likely to be exacerbated at high altitude are those in which either arterial desaturation or changes in the pulmonary vascular pressure and resistance are prominent. Examples of patients at risk include those with primary pulmonary hypertension, cyanotic congenital heart disease, and chronic pulmonary diseases such as cystic fibrosis. As previously discussed in this chapter, a variety of physiologic changes occur at high altitude, including decreases in Pa_{O_2} and Sa_{O_2}, changes in $\dot{V}/\dot{Q}$ characteristics, pulmonary hypertension, and changes in cardiac output. Of these, the decreases in Pa_{O_2} and Sa_{O_2} and pulmonary hypertension are probably most important in leading to exacerbations of sea-level illness in children.

Because of hypoxic pulmonary vasoconstriction, primary pulmonary hypertension may be acutely exacerbated at high altitude. As previously discussed, an increased pulmonary artery pressure may be instrumental in the development of HAPE. Cyanotic congenital heart disease may be accompanied by pulmonary hypertension, and hypoxic exposure places these patients at risk for worsening pulmonary hypertension and a decrease in an already low Pa_{O_2}.[128] In addition, polycythemia in these patients could adversely affect the pulmonary vascular endothelium in the presence of hypoxic vasoconstriction.

Patients with cystic fibrosis who have low oxyhemoglobin saturation at sea level exhibit further decreases in Pa_{O_2} and Sa_{O_2} at altitude. Because patients with advanced disease may experience loss of pulmonary vascular cross-sectional area, they may be at risk for complications of pulmonary hypertension, including acute right ventricular failure, on exposure to high altitude. Desmond and colleagues[129] suggested that patients with cystic fibrosis with forced expiratory flow between 25% and 75% of vital capacity (FEF_{25-75}) of more than 20% of the predicted normal value are most likely to have a $Pa_{O_2} > 50$ mm Hg at sea level and can consider air travel without supplemental oxygen. This Pa_{O_2} at sea level, however, may be too low to risk flying without oxygen; this recommendation is discussed later. Patients with bronchopulmonary dysplasia (BPD), particularly those who require oxygen at low altitude or who have evidence of pulmonary hypertension, are also at increased risk during high-altitude exposure. In addition, patients with unusual pulmonary malformations, such as unilateral pulmonary agenesis or unilateral agenesis of a pulmonary artery, are at increased risk for severe hypoxic pulmonary vasoconstriction and increased risk of HAPE.[130-131]

Exercise at high altitude in any of these patients is accompanied by a pronounced decrease in Sa_{O_2} and a decrease in work capacity, as is seen in healthy sea-level natives.[93] This combination of pre-existing pulmonary or pulmonary-vascular disease and a lowered Pa_{O_2} with its consequent changes in pulmonary vascular resistance may be dangerous.

AIR TRAVEL BY INDIVIDUALS WITH CARDIOPULMONARY DISEASE

Patients with pre-existent sea level illness may be faced with the possibility of air travel between sea level destinations. Although such patients might not necessarily choose to travel to an area of high altitude, they ascend to high altitudes while flying in modern pressurized aircraft. These patients are the same population discussed previously and include persons with cardiopulmonary disease such as cystic fibrosis or BPD. The relatively rapid fall in cabin pressure after airplane takeoff can lead to an increased risk of pneumothorax in some patients with chronic lung disease (e.g., patients with cystic fibrosis who have subpleural bullae); this risk may be increased when these patients cough.[132]

It is important for the physician to understand principles of modern aircraft pressurization, as well as availability of onboard oxygen, in order to advise patients of measures to prevent altitude-related illness. This subject has been reviewed by Liebman and co-authors[133] and is briefly summarized as follows.

Modern aircraft are pressurized by the creation of a pressure differential between the ambient barometric pressure, which varies with altitude, and the internal cabin environment. For example, a Boeing B-747 is capable of a differential pressure of 8.9 pounds per square inch (psi). (Although millimeters of mercury is a term more common to the physician, psi is the standard measurement used by the airline industry.) At a maximal flight altitude of 12,195 m (40,000 feet), the ambient barometric pressure is 2.72 psi (140 mm Hg). Thus the expected cabin altitude is 2.72 + 8.9 = 11.62 psi, equivalent to 1860 m (6100 feet), with an atmospheric P_{O_2} of 125, PA_{O_2} of 71, and Pa_{O_2} of 64 mm Hg in normal subjects. Other aircraft generally are not as successful at pressurizing their cabins, so the expected P_{O_2} in normal subjects could potentially be lower. In patients who have a widened alveolar-arterial oxygen gradient, the Pa_{O_2} may be even lower.

The actual altitude attained varies with each aircraft and is often lower than its rated maximum. The choice of altitude is based on wind speed when the aircraft is aloft, duration of flight, and other factors. However, the amount of pressure differential generated varies with the age of the aircraft and other factors, including consideration of passengers' comfort (a higher pressure differential results in increased cabin noise).

The U.S. Federal Aviation Administration requires only that operating aircraft be capable of maintaining a cabin altitude of no more than 2440 m (8000 feet) (Federal Aviation Administration, Department of Transportation, Regulation 25,841). At this altitude, the partial pressure of oxygen is 116 mm Hg. The PA_{O_2} and Pa_{O_2} are 59 and 55 mm Hg, respectively, assuming mild hyperventilation and a narrow alveolar-arterial oxygen gradient.[133] Studies by Cottrell[134] and Aldrette and Aldrette[135] suggested that cabin altitude during some commercial flights may actually exceed this 2440 m (8000-foot) mandated maximal altitude. Persons who have a widened alveolar-arterial oxygen gradient may indeed experience desaturation under these circumstances. Liebman and co-authors[133] suggested that a patient should have a Pa_{O_2} of 50 mm Hg or more before approval for air travel is given. This Pa_{O_2} at sea level, if accompanied by a normal or only mildly elevated Pa_{CO_2}, implies a widened alveolar-arterial oxygen gradient. Such a patient may have a very low Pa_{O_2} if the cabin altitude is 2440 m. Gong and associates[136] determined that Pa_{O_2} in adults with chronic obstructive airway disease subjected to lowered fraction of inspired oxygen simulates 1500-m (5000 foot) and 2440-m (8000-foot) altitudes. They noted that more than 90% of patients with sea-level Pa_{O_2} values of at least 68 mm Hg and 72 mm Hg had Pa_{O_2} levels of 55 mm Hg or higher at each simulated altitude. Recommendations about air travel for this group of patients are that oxygen should be administered to prevent hypoxemia in those at risk of having a resultant Pa_{O_2} of less than 55 mm Hg during a flight (i.e., those patients with a sea-level Pa_{O_2} of <72 mm Hg).[137]

Although most of the studies determining minimal Pa_{O_2} for safe air travel have involved adults, the author suggests that children with cystic fibrosis and other chronic obstructive lung diseases are physiologically similar and thus recommends that oxygen be administered to patients with mild to moderate disease rather than only to those with more severe disease. It may be necessary to determine a pediatric patient's Pa_{O_2} before deciding on the use of oxygen during a flight. An alternative method, at least for patients with cystic fibrosis, is to determine the patient's degree of airflow obstruction. Desmond and colleagues[129] reported that the Pa_{O_2} of such patients is correlated with the logarithm of the percentage predicted FEF_{25-75}. Although they based a suggestion for flying without supplemental oxygen on an adequate Pa_{O_2} (FEF_{25-75} of at least 20% predicted), their estimate allows for extrapolation to a Pa_{O_2} of approximately 70 mm Hg. Using this method, this author suggests that a patient with cystic fibrosis in whom the FEF_{25-75} is less than 50% predicted will have a Pa_{O_2} low enough to require the use of supplemental oxygen during commercial air travel.

Many (but not all) airlines can provide oxygen to passengers. The mode of oxygen supply varies, although nasal cannula at a preset rate (usually 2 or 4 l/min) is the most common available form. For reasons of airline safety and liability, patients are rarely permitted to provide their own oxygen. Oxygen supply en route must be arranged in advance of the flight and adds a moderate increase in cost. The patient's physician can expedite the arrangement of oxygen by speaking with the medical officer of the airline and prescribing the necessary amount of oxygen. The airline medical officer is often able to help determine the appropriate oxygen need for the patient after discussion with the physician. By arranging for supplemental oxygen during commercial air travel, the physician can lower the potential discomfort of a flight, thereby increasing its enjoyment as well as expanding the travel opportunities of pediatric patients with cardiopulmonary disease.

REFERENCES

1. Macfarlane A: Altitude and birth weight: Commentary. J Pediatr 111:842–844, 1987.
2. Hackett PH, Rennie D: The incidence, importance, and prophylaxis of acute mountain sickness. Lancet 2:1149–1155, 1976.
3. Hackett PH, Hornbein TF: Disorders of high altitude. In Murray JF, Nadel JA (eds): Textbook of Respiratory Medicine, pp. 1646–1663. Philadelphia: WB Saunders, 1988.
4. Singh I, Khanna PK, Srivastava ML, et al: Acute mountain sickness. N Engl J Med 280:175–184, 1969.
5. Johnson TS, Rock PB: Acute mountain sickness. N Engl J Med 319:841–845, 1988.
6. Hackett PH, Rennie D, Grover RF, Reeves JT: Acute mountain sickness and the edemas of high altitude: A common pathogenesis? Respir Physiol 46: 383–390, 1981.
7. Grubb RL, Raichle ME, Eichling JO, Ter-Pogossian MM: The effects of changes in Pa_{CO_2} on cerebral blood volume, blood flow, and vascular mean transit time. Stroke 5:630–639, 1974.
8. Hansen JE, Evans WO: A hypothesis regarding the pathophysiology of acute mountain sickness. Arch Environ Health 21:666–669, 1970.
9. King AB, Robinson SM: Ventilation response to hypoxia and acute mountain sickness. Aerosp Med 43:419–421, 1972.
10. Moore LG, Harrison GL, McCullough RE, et al: Low acute hypoxic ventilatory response and hypoxic depression in acute altitude sickness. J Appl Physiol 60:1407–1412, 1986.
11. Harvey TC, Raichle ME, Winterborn MH, et al.: Effect of carbon dioxide in acute mountain sickness: A rediscovery. Lancet 2:639–641, 1988.
12. Hackett PH, Rennie D: Acute mountain sickness. Semin Respir Med 5:132–139, 1983.
13. Severinghaus JW, Chiodi H, Eger E, et al: Cerebral blood flow in man at high altitude. Role of cerebrospinal fluid pH in normalization of flow in chronic hypocapnia. Circ Res 19:274–282, 1966.
14. Kety SS, Schmidt CF: The effects of altered arterial tensions of carbon dioxide and oxygen on cerebral blood flow and cerebral oxygen consumption of normal young men. J Clin Invest 27:484–492, 1948.
15. Robin ED: Permeability pulmonary edema. In Fishman AP, Renkin EM (ed): Pulmonary Edema, pp. 217–228. Bethesda, MD: American Physiological Society, 1979.
16. Maher JT, Cymerman A, Reeves JT, et al: Acute mountain sickness: Increased severity in eucapnic hypoxia. Aviat Space Environ Med 46:826–829, 1975.
17. Hultgren H, Marticorena E: Epidemiological observations in high altitude pulmonary edema [Abstract] Clin Res 16:142, 1968.
18. Hultgren HN, Marticorena E: High altitude pulmonary edema. Chest 74:372–376, 1978.
19. Wagner PD: Hypobaric effects on the pulmonary circulation and high altitude pulmonary edema. In Weir EK, Reeves JT (eds): Pulmonary Vascular Physiology and Pathophysiology, pp. 173–198. New York: Marcel Dekker, 1989.
20. Hultgren HN: High altitude pulmonary edema. In Staub NC (ed): Lung Water and Solute Exchange, pp. 437–469. New York: Marcel Dekker, 1978.
21. Scoggin CH, Hyers TM, Reeves JT, Grover RF: High-altitude pulmonary edema in children and young adults of Leadville, Colorado. N Engl J Med 297:1269–1272, 1977.
22. Gray GW: High altitude pulmonary edema. Semin Resp Med 5:141–150, 1983.

23. Grover RF, Hyers TM, McMurtry IF, Reeves JT: High-altitude pulmonary edema. In Fishman AP, Renkin EM (eds): Pulmonary Edema, pp. 229–240. Bethesda, MD: American Physiological Society, 1979.
24. Hultgren H, Spickard W, Lopez C: Further studies of high altitude pulmonary edema. Br Heart J 24:95–102, 1962.
25. Hultgren H, Spickard W, Hellriegel K, Houston CS: High altitude pulmonary edema. Medicine 40:289–313, 1961.
26. Schoene RB, Hackett PH, Henderson WR, et al: High-altitude pulmonary edema. Characteristics of lung lavage fluid. JAMA 256:63–69, 1986.
27. Hackett PH, Bertman J, Rodriguez G, Tenney J: Pulmonary edema fluid protein in high-altitude pulmonary edema. JAMA 256:36, 1986.
28. Dickinson JG: High altitude cerebral edema: Cerebral acute mountain sickness. Semin Respir Med 5:151–158, 1983.
29. Sutton JR, Lassen N: Pathophysiology of acute mountain sickness and high altitude pulmonary oedema. Bull Physiopathol Respir 15:1045–1052, 1979.
30. Callen WL, Perna JL, Field CJ: Acute mountain sickness [Letter]. N Engl J Med 320:1492, 1989.
31. Hackett PH: Mountain Sickness: Prevention, Recognition, and Treatment. New York: American Alpine Club, 1980.
32. Gray GW, Bryan AC, Frayser R, et al: Control of acute mountain sickness. Aerosp Med 42:81–84, 1971.
33. Swenson ER, Maren TH: Acute mountain sickness. N Engl J Med 320:1492–1493, 1989.
34. Cain SM, Dunn JE: Low doses of acetazolamide to aid accommodation of men to altitude. J Appl Physiol 21:1195–1200, 1966.
35. Levine BD, Yoshimuri K, Kobayashi T, et al: Dexamethasone in the treatment of acute mountain sickness. N Engl J Med 321:1707–1713, 1989.
36. McMurtry IF, Davidson AB, Reeves JT, Grover RF: Inhibition of hypoxic pulmonary vasoconstriction by calcium antagonists in isolated rat lungs. Circ Res 38:99–104, 1976.
37. Stanbrook HS, Morris KG, McMurtry IF: Prevention and reversal of hypoxic pulmonary hypertension by calcium antagonists. Am Rev Respir Dis 130:81–85, 1984.
38. Oelz, O, Maggiorini M, Ritter M, et al: Nifedipine for high altitude pulmonary oedema. Lancet 2:1241–1244, 1989.
39. Forwand SA, Landowne M, Follansbee JN, Hansen JE: Effect of acetazolamide on acute mountain sickness. N Engl J Med 279:839–845, 1968.
40. Larson EB, Roach RC, Schoene RB, Hornbein TF: Acute mountain sickness and acetazolamide. JAMA 248:328–332, 1982.
41. Johnson TS, Rock PB, Fulco CS, et al: Prevention of acute mountain sickness by dexamethasone. N Engl J Med 310:683–686, 1984.
42. Rock PB, Johnson TS, Larsen RF, et al: Dexamethasone as prophylaxis for acute mountain sickness. Effect of dose level. Chest 95:568–573, 1989.
43. Kruger H, Arias-Stella J: The placenta and the newborn infant at high altitudes. Am J Obstet Gynecol 106:586–591, 1970.
44. Unger C, Weiser JK, McCullough RE, et al: Altitude, low birth weight, and infant mortality in Colorado. JAMA 259:3427–3432, 1988.
45. Yip R: Altitude and birth weight. J Pediatr 111:869–876, 1987.
46. Jackson MR, Mayhew TM, Haas JD: The volumetric composition of human term placentae: Altitudinal, ethnic and sex differences in Bolivia. J Anat 152:173–187, 1987.
47. Jackson MR, Mayhew TM, Haas JD: On the factors which contribute to thinning of villous membrane in human placentae at high altitude I. Thinning and regional variation in thickness of trophoblast. Placenta 9:1–8, 1988.
48. Jackson MR, Mayhew TM, Haas JD: On the factors which contribute to thinning of the villous membrane in human placentae at high altitude. II. An increase in the degree of peripheralization of fetal capillaries. Placenta 9:9–18, 1988.
49. Moore LG, Rounds SS, Jahnigen D, et al: Infant birth weight is related to maternal arterial oxygenation at high altitude. J Appl Physiol 52:695–699, 1982.
50. Moore LG: Maternal O_2 transport responses to high altitude pregnancy. In Sutton JR, Houston CS, Coates G (eds): Hypoxia: The Tolerable Limits, pp. 207–219. Indianapolis, IN: Benchmark Press, 1988.

51. Haas JD, Moreno-Black G, Frongillo EA, et al: Altitude and infant growth in Bolivia: A longitudinal study. Am J Physiol Anthropol 59:251–262, 1982.
52. Frisancho AR, Borkan GA, Klayman JE: Pattern of growth of lowland and highland Peruvian Quechua of similar genetic composition. Hum Biol 47:233–243, 1975.
53. Frisancho AR, Baker PT: Altitude and growth: A study of the patterns of physical growth of a high altitude Peruvian Quechua population. Am J Phys Anthropol 32:279–292, 1970.
54. Yip R, Binkin NJ, Trowbridge FL: Altitude and childhood growth. J Pediatr 113:486–489, 1988.
55. Brody JS, Lahiri S, Simpser M, et al: Lung elasticity and airway dynamics in Peruvian natives to high altitude. J Appl Physiol 42:245–251, 1977.
56. Green M, Mead J, Turner JM: Variability of maximum expiratory flow-volume curves. J Appl Physiol 37:67–74, 1974.
57. Martin TR, Feldman HA, Fredberg JJ, et al: Relationship between maximal expiratory flows and lung volumes in growing humans. J Appl Physiol 65:822–828, 1988.
58. Cruz JC: Mechanics of breathing in high altitude and sea level subjects. Respir Physiol 17:146–161, 1973.
59. Mansell A, Powles A, Sutton J: Changes in pulmonary PV characteristics of human subjects at an altitude of 5,366 m. J Appl Physiol 49:79–83, 1980.
60. Jaeger JJ, Sylvester JT, Cymerman A, et al: Evidence for increased intrathoracic fluid volume in man at high altitude. J Appl Physiol 47:670–676, 1979.
61. Hoon RS, Balasubramanian V, Tiwari SC, et al: Changes in transthoracic electrical impedance at high altitude. Br Heart J 39:61–66, 1977.
62. Rahn H, Otis AB: Man's respiratory response during and after acclimatization to high altitude. Am J Physiol 157:445–462, 1949.
63. Rahn H, Otis AB: Alveolar air during simulated flights to high altitudes. Am J Physiol 150:202–221, 1947.
64. Gautier H, Milic-Emili J, Miserocchi G, Siafakas NM: Pattern of breathing and mouth occlusion pressure during acclimatization to high altitude. Respir Physiol 40:365–377, 1980.
65. Tenney SM, Remmers JE, Mithoefer JC: Interaction of CO_2 and hypoxic stimuli on ventilation. Q J Exp Physiol Cognate Med Sci 48:192–201, 1963.
66. Weil JV, Byrne-Quinn E, Sodal IE, et al: Hypoxic ventilatory drive in normal man. J Clin Invest 49:1061–1072, 1970.
67. Moore LG, Huang SY, McCullough RE, et al: Variable inhibition by falling CO_2 of hypoxic ventilatory response in humans. J Appl Physiol 56:207–210, 1984.
68. Loeschcke H: Central chemoreceptors. In Pallot DJ (ed): Control of Respiration, pp. 41–77. New York: Oxford University Press, 1983.
69. Morrill CG, Meyer JR, Weil JV: Hypoxic ventilatory depression in dogs. J Appl Physiol 38:143–146, 1975.
70. Heymans C, Bouckaert JT, Dautrebande L: Sinus carotidien et relexes respiratoire, II. Influences respiratoires relexes de l'acidose, de l'alcalose, de l'anhydride carbonique, de l'ion hydrogene et de l'anoxemie. Sinus carotidiens et echanges respiratoires dans less poumons et au dela des poumons. Arch Int Pharmacodyn Ther 39:400–448, 1930.
71. McDonald DM: Peripheral chemoreceptors. Structure-function relationships of the carotid body. In Hornbein TF (ed): Regulation of Breathing, Part I, pp. 105–319. New York: Marcel Dekker, 1981.
72. Lahiri S, DeLaney RG: Relationship between carotid chemoreceptor activity and ventilation in the cat. Respir Physiol 24:267–286, 1975.
73. Chiodi H: Respiratory adaptations to chronic high altitude hypoxia. J Appl Physiol 10:81–87, 1957.
74. Severinghaus JW, Bainton CR, Carcelen A: Respiratory insensitivity to hypoxia in chronically hypoxic man. Respir Physiol 1:308–334, 1966.
75. Lahiri S, Kao FF, Velasquez T, et al: Irreversible blunted respiratory sensitivity to hypoxia in high altitude natives. Respir Physiol 6:360–374, 1969.
76. Sorensen SC, Severinghaus JW: Irreversible respiratory insensitivity to acute hypoxia in man born at high altitude. J Appl Physiol 25:217–220, 1968.
77. Sorensen SC, Severinghaus JW: Respiratory sensitivity to acute hypoxia in man born at sea level living at high altitude. J Appl Physiol 25:211–216, 1968.
78. Lahiri S, Edelman NH: Peripheral chemoreflexes in the regulation of breathing of high altitude natives. Respir Physiol 6:375–385, 1969.
79. Lahiri S, DeLaney RG, Brody JS, et al: Relative role of environmental and genetic factors in respiratory adaptation to high altitude. Nature 261:133–135, 1976.
80. Lahiri S, Milledge JS, Chattopadhyay HP, et al: Respiration and heart rate of Sherpa highlanders during exercise. J Appl Physiol 23:545–554, 1967.
81. Lahiri S: Respiratory control in Andean and Himalayan high-altitude natives. In West JB, Lahiri S (eds): High Altitude and Man, pp. 147–162. Bethesda, MD: American Physiological Society, 1984.
82. Lahiri S: Alveolar gas pressures in man with life-long hypoxia. Respir Physiol 4:373–386, 1968.
83. Milledge JS, Lahiri S: Respiratory control in lowlanders and Sherpa highlanders at altitude. Respir Physiol 2:310–322, 1967.
84. Lahiri S: Respiratory control in Andean and Himalayan high-altitude natives. In West JB, Lahiri S (eds): High Altitude and Man, pp. 147–162. Bethesda, MD: American Physiological Society, 1984.
85. Huang SY, Ning XH, Zhou ZN, et al: Ventilatory function in adaptation to high altitude: Studies in Tibet. In West JB, Lahiri S (eds): High Altitude and Man, pp. 173–177. Bethesda, MD: American Physiological Society, 1984.
86. Arias-Stella J: Human carotid body at high altitude. Am J Pathol 55:82a, 1969.
87. Arias-Stella J, Valcarcel J: Chief cell hyperplasia in the human carotid body at high altitudes. Hum Pathol 7:361–373, 1976.
88. Heath D, Edwards C, Harris P: Postmortem size and structure of the human carotid body. Thorax 25:129–140, 1970.
89. Saldana MJ, Salem LE, Travezan R: High altitude hypoxia and chemodectomas. Hum Pathol 4:251–263, 1973.
90. Tenney SM, Ou LL: Hypoxic ventilatory response of cats at high altitude: An interpretation of "blunting." Respir Physiol 30:185–199, 1977.
91. Moore LG, Brodeur P, Chumbe O, et al: Maternal hypoxic ventilatory response, ventilation, and infant birth weight at 4,300 m. J Appl Physiol 60:1401–1406, 1986.
92. Vogel JA, Hansen JE, Harris CW: Cardiovascular responses in man during exhaustive work at sea level and high altitude. J Appl Physiol 23:531–539, 1967.
93. Vogel JA, Harley LH, Cruz JC, Hogan RP: Cardiac output during exercise in sea-level residents at sea level and high altitude. J Appl Physiol 36:169–172, 1974.
94. Cunningham WL, Becker EJ, Kreuzer F: Catecholamines in plasma and urine at high altitude. J Appl Physiol 20:607–610, 1965.
95. Manchanda SC, Maher JT, Cymerman A: Cardiac performance during graded exercise in acute hypoxia. J Appl Physiol 38:858–862, 1975.
96. Escourrou P, Johnson DG, Rowell LB: Hypoxemia increases plasma catecholamine concentrations in exercising humans. J Appl Physiol 57:1507–1511, 1984.
97. Hartley LH, Vogel JA, Cruz JC: Reduction of maximal exercise heart rate at altitude and its reversal with atropine. J Appl Physiol 36:362–365, 1974.
98. Hammill SC, Wagner WW, Latham LP, et al: Autonomic cardiovascular control during hypoxia in the dog. Circ Res 44:569–575, 1979.
99. Richalet JP, Vignon P, Rathat C, et al: Catecholamines and histamine at exercise in acute hypoxia (3823 and 4350 m): Effects of atropine. In Sutton JR, Houston CS, Coates G (eds): Hypoxia and Cold, p. 539. New York: Praeger, 1987.
100. Krzywicki HJ, Consolazio CF, Johnson HL, et al: Water metabolism in humans during acute high-altitude exposure (4300 m). J Appl Physiol 30:806–809, 1971.
101. Balasubramanian V, Mathew OP, Tiwari SC, et al: Alterations in left ventricular function in normal man on exposure to high altitude (3658 m). Br Heart J 40:276–285, 1978.
102. Alexander JK, Grover RF: Mechanism of reduced cardiac stroke volume at high altitude. Clin Cardiol 6:301–303, 1983
103. Maher JT, Goodman AL, Bowers WD, et al: Myocardial function

and ultrastructure in chronically hypoxic rats. Am J Physiol 223:1029–1033, 1972.

104. Rotta A, Canepa A, Hurtado A, et al: Pulmonary circulation at sea level and at high altitudes. J Appl Physiol 9:328–336, 1956.

105. Marticorena E, Ruiz L, Severino J, et al: Systemic blood pressure in white men born at sea level: Changes after long residence at high altitudes. Am J Cardiol 23:364–368, 1969.

106. Penaloza D, Arias-Stella J, Sime F, et al: The heart and pulmonary circulation in children at high altitudes. Pediatrics 34:568–582, 1964.

107. Fishman AP: Hypoxia on the pulmonary circulation: How and where it acts. Circ Res 38:221–231, 1976.

108. Reeves JT, Wagner WW, McMurtry IF, Grover RF: Physiological effects of high altitude on the pulmonary circulation. In Robertshaw D (ed): Environmental Physiology III, pp. 289–310. Baltimore, MD: University Park Press, 1979.

109. von Euler VS, Liljestrand G: Observations on the pulmonary arterial blood pressure in the cat. Acta Physiol Scand 12:301–320, 1947.

110. Lockhart A, Saiag B: Altitude and the human pulmonary circulation. Clin Sci 60:599–605, 1981.

111. Winslow RM: Red cell function at extreme altitude. In West JB, Lahiri S (eds): High Altitude and Man, pp. 59–72. Bethesda, MD: American Physiological Society, 1984.

112. Winslow RM: High-Altitude polycythemia. In West JB, Lahiri S (eds): High Altitude and Man, pp. 163–172. Bethesda, MD: American Physiological Society, 1984.

113. Hlastala MP: Interactions between O_2 and CO_2: The blood. In Sutton JR, Jones NL, Houston CS (eds): Hypoxia: Man at Altitude, pp. 17–23. New York: Thieme-Stratton, 1982.

114. Faura J, Ramos J, Reynafarje C, et al: Effect of altitude on erythropoiesis. Blood 33:668–676, 1969.

115. Abbrecht PH, Littell JK: Plasma erythropoietin in men and mice during acclimatization to different altitudes. J Appl Physiol 32:54–58, 1972.

116. Castle WB, Jandl JH: Blood viscosity and blood volume: Opposing influences upon oxygen transport in polycythemia. Semin Hematol 3:193–198, 1966.

117. Buick JC, Gledhill N, Froese AB, Spriet LC: Red cell mass and aerobic performance at sea level. In Sutton JR, Jones NC, Houston CS (eds): Hypoxia: Man at Altitude, pp. 43–50. New York: Thieme-Stratton, 1982.

118. Fan FC, Chen RY, Schuessler GB, Chien S: Effects of hematocrit variations on regional hemodynamics and oxygen transport in the dog. Am J Physiol 238:H545–552, 1980.

119. Jan KM, Chien S: Effect of hematocrit variations on coronary hemodynamics and oxygen utilization. Am J Physiol 233:H106–H113, 1977.

120. Whitmore RL: Rheology of the Circulation. Oxford, England: Pergamon, 1968.

121. Cerretelli P: Oxygen transport on Mount Everest: The effects of increased hematocrit on maximal O_2 transport. Adv Exp Med Biol 75:113–119, 1976.

122. Messmer K: Hemodilution Surg Clin North Am 55:659–678, 1975.

123. Sarnquist FH, Schoene RB, Hackett PH, Townes BD: Hemodilution of polycythemic mountaineers: Effects on exercise and mental function. Aviat Space Environ Med 57:313–317, 1986.

124. Petschow D, Wurdinger I, Baumann R, et al: Causes of high blood O_2 affinity of animals living at high altitude. J Appl Physiol 42:139–143, 1977.

125. Bartels H, Bartels R, Rathschlag-Schaefer AM, et al: Acclimatization of newborn rats and guinea pigs to 3000 to 5000 m simulated altitudes. Respir Physiol 36:375–389, 1979.

126. Eaton JW, Skelton TD, Berger E: Survival at extreme altitude: Protective effect of increased hemoglobin-oxygen affinity. Science 183:743–744, 1974.

127. Hultgren HN: High altitude medical problems. West J Med 131:8–23, 1979.

128. Waldman JD, Lamberti JJ, Mathewson JW, et al: Congenital heart disease and pulmonary artery hypertension. I. Pulmonary vasoreactivity to 15% oxygen before and after surgery. J Am Coll Cardiol 2:1158–1164, 1983.

129. Desmond KJ, Coates AL, Beaudry PH: Relationship between the partial pressure of arterial oxygen and airflow limitation in children with cystic fibrosis. Can Med Assoc J 131:325–326, 1984.

130. Hackett PH, Creagh CE, Grover RF, et al: High-altitude pulmonary edema in persons without the right pulmonary artery. N Engl J Med 302:1070–1073, 1980.

131. Levine SJ, White DA, Fels AO: An abnormal chest radiograph in a patient with recurring high altitude pulmonary edema. Chest 94:627–628, 1988.

132. Gong H Jr: Air travel and patients with chronic obstructive pulmonary disease. Ann Intern Med 100:595–597, 1984.

133. Liebman J, Lucas R, Moss A, et al: Airline travel for children with chronic pulmonary disease. Pediatrics 57:408–410, 1976.

134. Cottrell JJ: Altitude exposures during aircraft flight. Chest 93:81–84, 1988.

135. Aldrette SA, Aldrette LE: Oxygen concentrations in commercial aircraft flights. South Med J 76:12–14, 1983.

136. Gong H Jr, Tashkin DP, Lee EY, Simmons MS: Hypoxia-altitude simulation test. Evaluation of patients with chronic airflow obstruction. Am Rev Respir Dis 130:980–986, 1984.

137. AMA Commission on Emergency Medical Services. Medical aspects of transportation aboard commercial aircraft. JAMA 247:1007–1011, 1982.

48 ADULT RESPIRATORY DISTRESS SYNDROME

SANTIAGO-R. REYES DE LA ROCHA, M.D./ROBERT W. PRYOR, M.D.

Adult respiratory distress syndrome (ARDS) is the clinical expression of diffuse alveolar damage. It results in increased permeability of the alveolar-capillary membrane and seepage of protein-rich fluid into the interstitium or alveolar spaces. This pulmonary edema causes acute respiratory failure. First described by Ashbaugh and colleagues,[1] this syndrome has been described by numerous synonyms, which reflect the diversity of etiologic factors (Table 48–1).

The incidence of ARDS in the adult population is about 150,000 per year;[2] the number of cases affecting children is not known.[2,3] A mortality rate of 59% was esti-

Table 48–1. SYNONYMS FOR ADULT RESPIRATORY DISTRESS SYNDROME

Wet lung
Shock lung
Respirator lung
White lung syndrome
Stiff lung syndrome
Posttraumatic atelectasis
Capillary leak syndrome
Da Nang lung
Noncardiogenic pulmonary edema
Postperfusion lung
Posttransfusion lung

mated from five retrospective studies of ARDS in children;[3-8] the mortality rate is higher than 50% in adults.[9] A poorer outcome is reported in patients with gram-negative bacteremia,[10, 11] a poor response to positive end-expiratory pressure (PEEP),[12] or multiple-organ system failure.[10, 13] Among adults surviving ARDS, the prognosis for recovery of pulmonary function is good, although abnormalities in diffusing capacity and decrease in arterial oxygen concentration with exercise may persist.[14] Fanconi and colleagues[15] reported sequelae in nine children 0.9 to 4.2 years after ARDS. Three children had exertional dyspnea and cough; in two, chest radiographs were suggestive of fibrotic changes; and all nine had abnormalities in pulmonary function.[15]

Although a variety of insults may initiate the alveolar-capillary membrane injury (Table 48–2), the clinical features are similar, and there typically are four stages: initial (acute injury), latent period, acute respiratory failure, and complications from severe physiologic abnormalities.[10, 16] ARDS is characterized by (1) respiratory distress and hypoxemia in patients with previously normal lungs, (2) delay between precipitating event and onset of respiratory distress (6 to 72 h), (3) decreased lung compliance, (4) decreased lung volumes, (5) hypoxemia refractory to supplemental oxygen but improved by restoring lung volume (i.e., increase in functional residual capacity [FRC] with elevation of FRC above closing volume), and (6) delayed resolution or progression to chronic phase with alveolar/interstitial fibrosis and intractable respiratory failure.

Table 48–2. COMMON CONDITIONS ASSOCIATED WITH ADULT RESPIRATORY DISTRESS SYNDROME IN CHILDREN

Sepsis
Shock (e.g., septic, hypovolemic)
Asphyxia (immersion or strangulation)
Meningitis
Drug intoxication
Smoke inhalation
Fat embolism
Liver failure
Aspiration (gastric content)
Trauma
Burns
Chemical pneumonitis (e.g., hydrocarbon, talc)
Acidosis
Hemolytic uremic syndrome
Guillain-Barré syndrome

During the initial phase, some patients may hyperventilate, and hypocapnia may develop with respiratory alkalosis despite adequate arterial oxygen pressure/tension (Pa_{O_2}) values.[10] Initially, breath sounds and chest radiographs may be normal. In the latent phase, dyspnea with hyperventilation is usually seen, and the chest radiograph may show fine reticular infiltrates.[10] During the stage of acute respiratory failure, common findings include tachypnea, retractions, crackles, grunting respirations, hypoxemia secondary to ventilation/perfusion mismatch and intrapulmonary shunting, and diffuse bilateral infiltrates or haziness on chest radiographs. Also, decreased FRC, decreased pulmonary compliance, increased dead space, and variable levels of arterial carbon dioxide are observed. The stage of complications resulting from severe physiologic abnormalities has been referred to as the terminal stage when associated with intractable respiratory failure.[10] This stage is characterized by hypoxemia unresponsive to oxygen therapy and hypercapnia unresponsive to mechanical ventilation. In the more advanced stages of ARDS, fibrosis can produce a decrease in alveolar surface area and an increase in the thickness of the alveolar-capillary barrier, limiting the diffusion of oxygen across the alveolar-capillary membrane. Hypercapnia may also occur with advanced disease and fibrosis.[17]

PATHOLOGIC FINDINGS

The pathologic changes in the lungs in ARDS vary with the extent of the injury and the duration of the disease and can be divided into two stages:[17] (1) acute exudative stage and (2) chronic proliferative stage.

The *acute exudative stage* results from epithelial or endothelial damage and from interstitial and alveolar edema. During this stage, proteinosis or hemorrhagic fluid containing leukocytes, macrophages, cell debris, and remnants of surfactant fill the alveoli. Hyaline membranes are found in the alveoli and alveolar ducts. Pulmonary capillaries may be obstructed with plugs of leukocytes, fibrin deposits, or microthrombi.[17]

The *chronic proliferative stage* is characterized by epithelial lining cell changes, alveolar wall thickening, infiltration of cells (lymphocytes, plasma cells, and histiocytes) into the interstitium.[17] There is cellular proliferative phase with proliferation of the type II alveolar epithelial lining cells. Later, the cellularity decreases with subsequent fibrotic proliferative changes, disruption of the pulmonary parenchymal (alveolar) architecture, replacement of the hyaline membranes by proliferating fibroblasts, and the organization of alveolar fluid to form intra-alveolar fibrosis.[17]

PATHOLOGIC CORRELATION WITH RADIOGRAPHIC FINDINGS

Radiographic findings in ARDS are similar in children and adults.[3, 18] These changes are not specific and may vary depending on the time of the study. During the initial episode of respiratory distress, chest radiographs are often normal, or a fine reticular pattern can be observed.[18] Def-

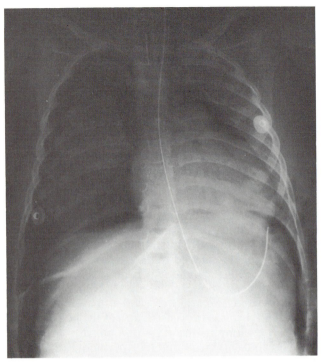

Figure 48–1. Early exudative phase of adult respiratory distress syndrome (ARDS) in an 18-month-old child. ARDS was induced by aspiration of baby powder.

inite radiographic abnormalities usually appear during the first 24 to 48 h after the clinical onset. These abnormalities consist of patchy, poorly defined pulmonary densities corresponding to pulmonary edema, which occurs during the acute exudative phase of ARDS[18] (Fig. 48–1).

In the event of death at this particular stage, the lungs have a liverlike appearance. Capillary congestion, interstitial edema, intra-alveolar edema, and hemorrhage can be observed microscopically.[19]

In the week after the initial (24 to 48 h) changes, the pulmonary densities may coalesce (Fig 48–2). At this stage, the lungs are heavy with gray discoloration. There is microscopic evidence of hyaline membranes, intra-alveolar fibrous exudate, and alveolar cell hyperplasia.[19] If the patient survives beyond the first week, the radiographic findings reflect the complications of the syndrome or its management, such as infection, oxygen toxicity, or barotrauma.[19]

Positive end-expiratory pressure (PEEP) has become the cornerstone modality of supportive therapy in ARDS. The earliest and most common radiographic sign of complications in patients on PEEP is pulmonary interstitial emphysema[20] (Fig. 48–3). Radiographic findings may consist of vesicular rarefactions, radiolucent halos around vessels and airways, lucent lines toward the hilum, pneumatoceles, and subpleural emphysematous changes.[20, 21] A worsening of the pulmonary status that requires higher levels of PEEP may cause development of pneumothorax, penumomediastinum, pneumoperitoneum, and subcutaneous emphysema[20, 21] (Fig. 48–4).

PATHOPHYSIOLOGY AND POSSIBLE PATHOGENIC MECHANISMS

The primary pathophysiologic feature of this syndrome is a noncardiogenic or permeability pulmonary edema. Under normal circumstances, hydrostatic pressure in the microvascular space is higher than in the interstitial space,

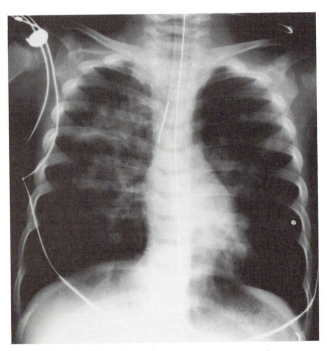

Figure 48–2. Whiteout of the chest radiograph in a 5-year-old child with a seizure disorder on day 1 of mechanical ventilation. ARDS was induced by aspiration pneumonia. Fraction of inspired oxygen (F_{IO_2}), 1.0; mean airway pressure (MAP), 16.5 cm H_2O; peak inspiratory pressure (PIP), 48 cm H_2O; positive end-expiratory pressure (PEEP), 12 cm H_2O.

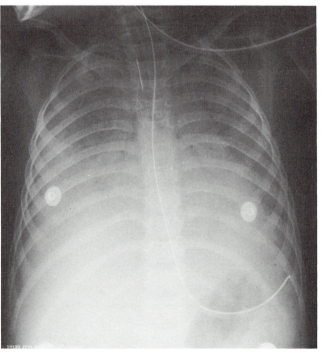

Figure 48–3. Pulmonary interstitial emphysema in a 5-year-old child with a seizure disorder on day 7 of mechanical ventilation. ARDS was induced by aspiration pneumonia. F_{IO_2}, 1.0; PIP, 55 cm H_2O; MAP, 20 cm H_2O; PEEP, 16 cm H_2O.

3. Alveolar collapse from surfactant depletion.

4. Iatrogenic pathogenic processes such as toxic effects of supplemental oxygen.

Leukocytes accumulate in the microvasculature with the release of toxic products such as oxygen radicals, lysosomal enzymes, and arachidonic acid metabolites. Fibrin microthrombi or hyperoxia may also cause alveolar-capillary injury with leukocyte accumulation, which may result in amplification of the initial injury.

Platelet aggregation may result in thromboxane release; subsequent pulmonary vasoconstriction leads to increased leukocyte adherence to endothelial cells. Proteolytic enzyme actions can result in destruction of pulmonary architecture and pulmonary fibrosis. These mechanisms do not initiate the alveolar-capillary injury; however, they may amplify it.

Surfactant depletion can result in alveolar collapse and worsening of the hypoxemia.

Processes that result from therapeutic interventions may affect the progression of the syndrome (e.g., exposure to high concentrations of oxygen).

Some of the various factors that can mediate injury to the alveolar-capillary membrane are discussed in detail next.

INFLAMMATION AND COAGULATION

It is important to understand the interaction of inflammation and coagulation in the pathogenesis of ARDS. These two complex processes tend to occur on surfaces; in coagulation, at the surface site, platelets interact with injured endothelium or underlying subendothelial tissues. In inflammation, macrophages and neutrophils interact with injured parenchymal cells or bacteria.

NEUTROPHIL-MEDIATED LUNG INJURY

There is considerable evidence of the importance of the neutrophil in the pathogenesis of ARDS.[22-25] For example, an increased number of neutrophils is observed in bronchoalveolar lavage fluid from patients with ARDS.[24, 26] Myeloperoxidase and elastase activities of neutrophils are also increased in patients with ARDS. The increase in neutrophils correlates with the degree of hypoxemia and protein permeability.[24]

In ARDS, granulocytes appear to marginate to the endothelium and localize adjacent to damaged endothelial cells.[17] This step coincides with the disappearance of neutrophils from the peripheral circulation apparently sequestered to the pulmonary microvasculature.[23, 24] Speculations on mechanisms of endothelial damage produced by neutrophils suggest lactoferrin as a potential agent for promoting adhesion of granulocytes to target cells.[27] Patients with ARDS have higher concentrations of lactoferrin and eosinophil cationic protein. Circulating levels of these specific granules are increased despite neutropenia and eosinopenia; this phenomenon is suggestive of increased leukocyte activity in ARDS.[28]

The recruitment of neutrophils to the lower respiratory tract seems to be partially mediated by complement acti-

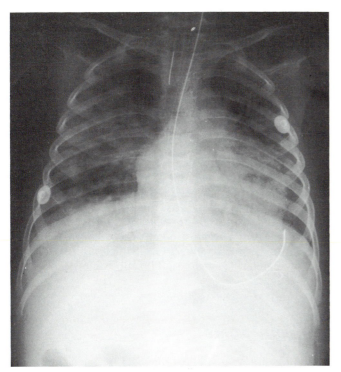

Figure 48–4. Pneumothorax, pneumomediastinum, pneumoperitoneum, subcutaneous emphysema in a 5-year-old child with a seizure disorder on day 7 of mechanical ventilation. ARDS was induced by aspiration pneumonia. FI_{O_2}, 1.0; PIP, 64 cm H_2O; MAP, 23.6 cm H_2O; PEEP, 18 cm H_2O.

causing the movement of fluid into the interstitial space. The alveolar-capillary membrane is normally relatively impermeable to protein, and so protein concentration is less in the interstitial space than in the microvascular space. The colloid osmotic pressure difference tends to move fluid from the interstitial space to the microvascular space. Because the hydrostatic forces are normally greater than the colloid osmotic forces, there is a net movement of fluid into the interstitial space, where the fluid is taken up by the pulmonary lymphatic vessels and returned to the circulation.[9] The lymphatic vessels can increase the normal clearance of interstitial fluid up to 10 times normal; however, when this capacity is exceeded, fluid accumulates in the lung, first around vessels and airways and then in the alveoli.[9]

The increased pulmonary vascular resistance in ARDS is attributed to alveolar hypoxia caused by occlusion of microvasculature with plugs of leukocytes, platelets, or fibrin and probably also caused by the effect of vasoconstrictor substances.[10] Right ventricular function can be altered by the increased vascular resistance and by PEEP.

The underlying pathogenic mechanisms leading to ARDS are not completely understood; however, more than one pathogenic process can occur simultaneously. According to Royall and Levin,[10] there are four categories of pathogenic processes:

1. Processes that may initiate the injury, such as leukocyte accumulation in the microvasculature, fibrin microthrombi, or hypoxia.

2. Processes that usually amplify the initial injury, seen as platelet aggregation and lysosomal enzyme release.

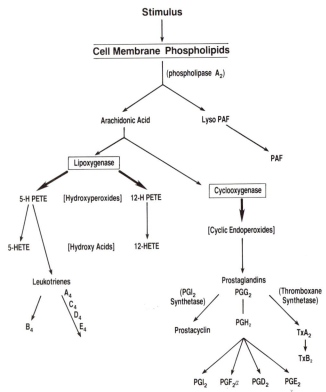

Figure 48-5. Scheme of the arachidonic acid metabolism. The cyclo-oxygenase pathway renders prostaglandins and thromboxanes, whereas the lipoxygenase pathway yields the leukotrienes.

Arachidonic acid is the substrate for the production of prostaglandins and thromboxanes (through the cyclooxygenase enzyme pathway) and for several hydroxy fatty acids and biologically active leukotrienes (through the action of the lipo-oxygenase pathway)[37] (Fig. 48-5). One lipo-oxygenase product, leukotriene B4, is a strong chemotactic agent capable of activating neutrophils to produce free oxygen radicals, which may result in pulmonary injury. Cyclooxygenase metabolites of arachidonic acid may also mediate pulmonary vasoconstriction and airway constriction in a process similar to ARDS.[37]

Thomboxanes, which are potent smooth muscle constrictors, have been associated with pulmonary vasoconstriction and marked increase in airway resistance. Other cyclooxygenase metabolites of arachidonic acid appear to be vasodilators. The most potent vasodilator in the lung circulation is prostacyclin (PGI_2), which is also an inhibitor of platelet aggregation. Thromboxane A_2 is also a platelet aggregator.

OXYGEN RADICALS

Neutrophils can injure lung cells by releasing highly reactive oxygen molecules known as free oxygen radicals. These free radicals are molecules of oxygen that have an odd number of electrons or an unpaired electron in the outer orbit[38-40] (see Chapter 94).

LYSOSOMAL ENZYMES

Within neutrophil granules, there are lysosomal enzymes capable of causing lung injury. These proteolytic enzymes include elastase, collagenase, cathepsins, lysozyme, cationic proteins, lactoferrin, and myeloperoxidase. Elastase and collagenase can digest vascular basement membrane, endothelial cartilage, and proteins such as elastin, collagen, and fibronectin.[25, 41] In addition, neutrophil-derived proteolytic enzymes can amplify the inflammatory process by activating complement and the Hageman factor,[42, 43] which can increase bradykinin production. These proteolytic enzymes may act synergistically with oxygen radicals in producing lung injury.[44]

SURFACTANT DEPLETION

Surfactant, a phospholipid produced by type II pneumocytes, reduces surface tension in the lungs and prevents alveolar collapse at low lung volumes. Although surfactant deficiency is not considered a primary etiologic factor in ARDS, the mechanisms that result in secondary surfactant depletion in ARDS may cause alveolar collapse and worsening of the hypoxemia. Some of the causes of secondary loss of surfactant include washout of phospholipids into the blood stream, inactivation of surfactant by plasma components, depletion by foaming and ventilation with large tidal volumes, and damage of type II pneumocytes.[10, 17, 26]

vation.[29-32] Activation of complement generates the peptide fragment C5a. C5a attracts neutrophils to the pulmonary circulation, thus inducing leukocyte aggregation. The aggregates of neutrophils are trapped or sequestered in the pulmonary microvasculature. Whether complement activation alone is sufficient to cause neutrophil activation and alveolar-capillary damage is an unresolved issue; other factors such as hypoxia or prostaglandin activity may contribute. Studies in animals have shown that complement activation combined with an additional stress factor was necessary to produce neutrophil migration to the alveoli and to increase permeability.[33] A second possible mechanism in pulmonary neutrophil migration is the elaboration of chemotactic factors by alveolar macrophages. These chemotaxins stimulate neutrophil locomotion.[34, 35] In addition, alveolar macrophages stimulated by hyperoxia produce factors that can promote neutrophil adhesiveness and neutrophil superoxide generation.[35, 36] There are three mechanisms by which neutrophils may mediate lung injury: (1) arachidonic acid metabolites, (2) oxygen radicals, and (3) lysosmal enzymes.

ARACHIDONIC ACID METABOLITES

Arachidonic acid is bound to the phospholipids of cell membranes. Phospholipases (especially phospholipase A_2) may promote the liberation of arachidonic acid and its metabolites at the time of injury to cell membranes.

PLATELET-ASSOCIATED LUNG INJURY

Pulmonary microembolization produced by aggregation of proteins and platelets has also been implicated in the pathogenesis of ARDS. The presence of these microaggregates in the circulation may explain the consumption of other plasma proteins such as antithrombin III and fibronectin.[45] The involvement of platelets in the development of ARDS is suggested by a progressive thrombocytopenia observed in as many as 50% of the patients with nontraumatic ARDS. A rising deficit of platelets parallels worsening of the hypoxemia.[46] The findings of several studies in which platelets labeled with chromium were used[47] indicate sequestration of platelets in the lungs. Platelets may be sequestered in the pulmonary microvasculature during the course of acute edematous lung injury and may interact in the pathogenic mechanisms. During aggregation, there is a release of vasoconstrictors such as thromboxane that also contribute to pulmonary hypertension and bronchoconstriction. This worsens the ventilation/perfusion mismatch. In addition, platelets may activate complement. This may further release metabolites of arachidonic acid and specific proteins that may, in turn, recruit neutrophils and stimulate them to generate toxic substances.

Endothelial cell injury may release thromboxane and platelets. If injury progresses, factors released by platelets (in a wound-healing effort) stimulate excessive fibroblast deposition and collagen, with subsequent pulmonary fibrosis.[46] Other agents such as fibrin may have an important role in producing altered capillary membrane permeability.[48] The interaction of platelets and leukocytes is suggested by studies demonstrating neutrophil phagocytic aggregation induced by platelets,[49] stimulation of neutrophil activity, and perhaps release of toxic neutrophil metabolites.[50] There is also an increase in neutrophil chemotaxis promoted by platelet products.[51] Platelet activating factor may be the link among leukocyte stimulation, platelet aggregation, and some of the pathogenic mechanisms in ARDS.[46]

MANAGEMENT

Although several innovative therapeutic interventions are currently in the experimental phase, treatment remains predominantly supportive. In addition to the treatment of underlying or precipitating conditions, the primary therapeutic goals are, when possible: (1) to maintain adequate tissue oxygenation, (2) to support the breathing workload, (3) to establish and maintain electrolyte balance, (4) to maintain adequate nutrition, and (5) to reduce or prevent secondary lung and airway injury from oxygen toxicity, barotrauma, infection, and other complications.[11]

MAINTENANCE OF ADEQUATE TISSUE OXYGENATION

The adequacy of oxygen delivery to the tissues is determined by tissue oxygen needs and by the availability of oxygen. In ARDS, metabolic demand and requirement for oxygen delivery are increased; there is also a change in the relationship of oxygen consumption to oxygen delivery. Because oxygen delivery is the product of cardiac index and oxygen content, tissue oxygenation depends not only on the arterial oxygen tension but also on cardiac output, hemoglobin concentration, and the ability of hemoglobin to release oxygen. Cardiac output can be improved by increasing the preload, decreasing the afterload, or enhancing cardiac contractility.[11] One of the therapeutic aims in ARDS is to maintain adequate cardiac function with the lowest effective intravascular volume (about 70% of maintenance requirements initially) and adequate amounts of glucose and electrolytes.[11]

Arterial blood oxygen content depends on both hemoglobin concentration and the percentage of oxygen saturation. It is important to optimize hemoglobin concentration and its dissociation characteristics. Hemoglobin performance is enhanced by reversing alkalemia to facilitate oxygen unloading. Hemoglobin and hematocrit should be restored to the normal range to ensure an oxygen content of 10 vol% to 13 vol%.[52] If hematocrit is boosted too high, the increase in blood viscosity could retard red blood cell passage through the capillaries and impair oxygen delivery.

Oxygen saturation should be kept above 90% (corresponding to Pa_{O_2} of approximately 60 mm Hg) without risking oxygen toxicity. The occurrence of oxygen toxicity depends on both the time of administration and the concentration of oxygen used. Excessive oxygen can also be detrimental because it can wash out alveolar nitrogen, producing absorption atelectasis with worsening of the intrapulmonary shunt.[53]

PEEP improves oxygenation by reducing ventilation/perfusion mismatching and by decreasing intrapulmonary shunting.[54] The use of PEEP increases the FRC, reversing the alterations in lung mechanics caused by the pulmonary edema.[52, 55] There is a linear relationship between PEEP and FRC over the range of 0 to 15 cm H_2O.[55] The increase in FRC reflects both an increase in volume of patent alveoli and reinflation of previously collapsed alveoli.[56] PEEP causes a redistribution of pulmonary blood flow toward better ventilated lung units and improves the ventilation/perfusion ratios. PEEP can increase Pa_{O_2} by elevation of the mean alveolar pressure and a reduction in the barrier to gas diffusion. It accomplishes this by thinning the edema fluid layer within the alveolus and redistributing lung water from the alveolar spaces to the interstitium. Another possible benefit of PEEP is the elevation of FRC above closing volume. When FRC falls below closing volume, air trapping occurs during normal tidal breathing. In ARDS, there is decreased lung compliance with reduction of FRC below closing volume.[54, 55]

PEEP can have adverse effects on lung and cardiac function. There is a level of PEEP above which no additional benefit is gained; beyond this level, gas exchange may be impaired as a result of alveolar overdistension, increased alveolar dead space, and detrimental effects on cardiac function.[54, 56] High levels of PEEP can reduce the cardiac output by decreasing venous return and lowering left ventricular end-diastolic volume or by displacing the intraventricular septum. Other possible mechanisms for reducing cardiac output are a decrease in myocardial perfusion by a theoretical myocardial depressor substance.[57]

Although not all patients respond to PEEP, PEEP is the only known standard therapy in ARDS that may improve the chance of survival.[53] The patients who do not respond to PEEP tend to have a poor prognosis.[12] There is no absolute upper level of PEEP. Most patients can be treated with levels below 20 cm H_2O, but PEEP should be carefully titrated, and the effect on both arterial oxygenation and cardiac function must be carefully evaluated. Royall and Levin[11] suggested several endpoints of PEEP therapy: (1) 90% arterial oxygen saturation with a hematocrit of 40% to 49% on a fraction of inspired oxygen (F_{IO_2}) of <0.5, a cardiac index of ≥4.5 l/min/sq m, and oxygen delivery of more than 600 ml/min/sq m, (2) a decrease in arterial oxygen with increased PEEP that cannot be explained by changes in cardiac function, and (3) inhibition of cardiac function that is not reversible with fluids and inotropy.

MECHANICAL VENTILATION (VENTILATORY ASSISTANCE)

The most common indication for mechanical ventilation is hypoxemia (Pa_{O_2}) < 60 mm Hg with F_{IO_2} > .50). Other indications for ventilatory assistance are evidence of intrapulmonary shunting (a poor response of arterial oxygen concentration to increases in F_{IO_2}), increased work of breathing,[53] and hypercapnia. There is some evidence that early intervention with PEEP in patients at risk for ARDS is helpful, although the mechanism of benefit is unclear.[53] Mechanical ventilation can be accomplished in children with ARDS with either volume-limited ventilators or time-cycled ventilators. If possible, intermittent mandatory ventilation (IMV) rather than controlled ventilation is preferable because the cardiovascular effects of PEEP are fewer with the former mode.[58] Synchronized IMV has not proved more effective than IMV.[59] Extracorporeal membrane oxygenation (ECMO) and high-frequency ventilation[60, 61] have been used to treat the hypoxemia and support adequate ventilation in patients with ARDS.

ECMO is a technique in which gas exchange is effected by an extracorporeal circuit. This is another attempt at decreasing the barotrauma and increasing inspired oxygen concentration in the lungs. It is a highly specialized procedure, and this technique should be performed only by clinicians with extensive experience with this modality.[60] The indications for ECMO in ARDS have not been clearly established.

Sedation and neuromuscular paralysis may be necessary in patients receiving assisted mechanical ventilation. Supportive care includes suctioning of secretions (time should be kept to less than 15 sec) with hyperventilation with 100% oxygen before and immediately after suctioning. Endotracheal tube adapters or swivel adaptors that seal around the suction catheter enable suctioning without the need to discontinue ventilatory support. Patients with large volumes of secretions and lobar atelectasis may benefit from chest physical therapy and bronchial drainage.[62] Oxygen saturation during these procedures should be monitored.

Hypoxemia should be avoided when patients are weaned from PEEP. Some guidelines for weaning based on criteria used in adults include (1) stable, nonseptic condition of the patient, (2) F_{IO_2} ≤ .40, (3) arterial blood oxygen tension ≥ 80 mm Hg, stable or increasing over 12 h, and (4) effective compliance (tidal volume/inspiratory hold pressures) ≥ 25 ml/cm H_2O, stable or improving for 12 h.[63]

NUTRITIONAL SUPPORT

Outcome is improved by nutritional support of the patient with ARDS. In contrast, overfeeding does have some adverse effects such as hepatic dysfunction, fatty liver degeneration, increased carbon dioxide (CO_2) production, and increased oxygen demands.[11] Intake of large carbohydrate loads and intravenous lipid infusion may worsen the respiratory status. The patient with ARDS does not have sufficient reserve to eliminate the increased load of CO_2 that may result from a large carbohydrate intake. Although the mechanism is not known, the use of intravenous lipids alters pulmonary gas exchange, can worsen hypoxemia, and is associated with elevated serum triglyceride levels.[64, 65] The use of intravenous lipid in excess of 3 g/kg/day can be associated with fat toxicity during parenteral nutrition. Serum triglyceride levels > 150 mg/dl are associated with decreased clearance because of saturation of enzyme systems.[66]

Initially, caloric requirements must be met to minimize the depletion of endogenous stores during the period of hypercatabolism from physiologic stress. Recommendations for nutritional support during this initial period are approximately 50 to 60 kCal/kg/day for infants and 35 to 40 kCal/kg/day for older children, with 1 to 3 g/kg/day or more from protein and the remaining calories from a mixture of glucose and fat.[11] A minimum of 4% and a maximum of 20% to 30% of fat are recommended.[11] Later in the course of ARDS, more calories are needed for repletion of losses, for growth, and for tissue repair. These caloric needs may be as high as 25% to 50% above the resting energy requirements.[11]

In patients with significant respiratory compromise, the use of hypertonic carbohydrate solutions such as dextrose may lead to increased CO_2 production, because excessive glucose is metabolized to fat in the liver.[67] A relatively new technique, bedside indirect calorimetry, determines the respiratory quotient and enables estimation of resting energy requirements for individualizing nutritional support.[68]

OTHER SUPPORTIVE MEASURES

Antacids

Common complications in patients with ARDS, as well as in other patients on mechanical ventilation, are gastritis and stress ulcers. These problems could be prevented by alkalinization of gastric secretions or the use of H1 blockers if the gastric pH is less than 4.5.

Vitamin E

Vitamin E has been advocated as a potential agent for modifying lung injury.[69] Although it is supposed to neutralize oxygen radicals, prevent aggregation of neutrophils and platelets, and protect the alveolar epithelial and endothelial membranes, there is not much evidence of actual benefit in ARDS.

Antibiotics

It is difficult to make the diagnosis of bronchopneumonia in patients with ARDS.[11, 70] Antibiotic coverage should be provided in the case of suspected or proven infection. Secondary infections could be treated with broad-spectrum agents to cover infectious agents such as *Staphylococcus* and *Pseudomonas* organisms.[11] A combination of nafcillin and an aminoglycoside can provide coverage for both these pathogens. If beta-lactamase–positive *Haemophilus influenzae* is present, the antibiotic choices include a third-generation cephalosporin.

Intravenous Fluids

Fluid therapy should sustain adequate tissue perfusion. Excessive administration of fluids should be avoided in order to prevent worsening of pulmonary edema or intrapulmonary shunt caused by overhydration. There is no agreement as to whether crystalloids or colloids should be used in patients with ARDS. Because colloids expand the intravascular volume with a smaller amount of fluid, many physicians prefer colloids such as albumin or packed red blood cells[53] in the treatment of ARDS.

Diuretics

A trial with diuretics may be desirable for the control of pulmonary edema if a deterioration in oxygenation, possibly caused by excessive fluid, occurs. Furosemide dosage of 1 mg/kg every 6 to 12 h is recommended.

Corticosteroids

Although the use of corticosteroids has been advocated by some authors, there are no specific recommendations for their use in ARDS. One review of the literature concluded that the current clinical data do not support the routine use of corticosteroids in ARDS,[11] despite some studies that suggest that they modify the pulmonary injury if administered within 4 h of the initial insult.

MONITORING IN ARDS

Monitoring in ARDS has the dual purpose of evaluating the course of the disease and the effects of therapy. Careful hemodynamic and respiratory monitoring also increases the chances of detecting and preventing complications. Improvement of tissue oxygenation is the primary aim of therapy. Cardiac output is an important variable in oxygen delivery. Frequent determinations of cardiac output, oxygen consumption, arterial blood gases, intrapulmonary shunt ($\dot{Q}_S/\dot{Q}_T$), and studies of lung compliance are important in the management of ARDS.[71, 72]

MONITORING ARTERIAL BLOOD GASES, CARDIAC OUTPUT, AND TISSUE OXYGENATION

The insertion of an indwelling arterial cannula is recommended to facilitate arterial blood gas sampling and to minimize chances of complications produced by trauma to the arteries from repetitive sampling. An arterial catheter also offers the advantage of monitoring arterial pressure and peripheral vascular resistance. Changes in arterial blood gases usually guide alterations in oxygen therapy and ventilator parameters. The data needed for calculation of the alveolar-arterial oxygen gradient ([A-a] D_{O_2}) are obtained from an arterial blood gas sample. The gradient is calculated using the alveolar gas equation:[71, 72]

$$(A - a)D_{O_2} = PA_{O_2} - Pa_{O_2},$$

$$PA_{O_2} = (PB - P_{H_2O}) (FI_{O_2}) - \frac{Pa_{CO_2}}{RQ}$$

where PB is barometric pressure, P_{H_2O} is water vapor pressure (47 mm Hg assuming saturation at 37°C), RQ is respiratory quotient (assumed to equal 0.8), and PA_{CO_2} = alveolar carbon dioxide pressure/tension (assumed to equal arterial carbon dioxide pressure/tension).

However, this determination is affected by the FI_{O_2}, PA_{O_2}, changes in cardiac output, and oxygen consumption. Similar information can be obtained from the arterial to alveolar oxygen ratio: Pa_{O_2}/PA_{O_2} (normal is >0.7). Because it is a ratio, it affords the advantage of no variational changes in the FI_{O_2} in contrast to $(A - a)D_{O_2}$.[72]

Central venous catheters are used to monitor right atrial venous pressure and to administer vasoactive medications. Central venous pressure reflects the pressure in the right atrium which indicates preload of the right ventricle. The information is useful in the calculation of pulmonary vascular resistance, which is increased in ARDS.[72]

A flow-directed pulmonary artery (Swan-Ganz) catheter allows vascular pressures distal to the balloon to be measured and provides information on (1) cardiac output, (2) wedge pressure, and (3) mixed venous oxygen saturation. All three determinations are essential for monitoring therapeutic interventions such as administration of intravenous fluids, PEEP, and vasopressor agents. The pulmonary capillary wedge pressure (PCWP) closely approximates the left ventricular end-diastolic pressure (LVEDP) and is a reasonable estimate of the pulmonary capillary hydrostatic pressure. The pulmonary catheter has a distal thermistor that enables determination of cardiac output by thermodilution, the measurement of right atrial pressure, and the collection of mixed venous blood samples, which are essential for calculation of the arteriovenous oxygen content difference, shunt fraction, and cardiac output by means of the Fick equation.[72, 73]

Right atrial pressure and PCWP are considered equivalent to the preload of the right and left ventricles respectively. A potential source of error is using LVEDP to approximate left ventricle end-diastolic volume, which represents the preload of the left ventricle and assumes that left ventricular compliance is normal. However, the latter is not usually the case in ARDS, especially if high PEEP is being used.

Direct measurement of cardiac output combined with filling pressure enables assessment of the effects of ventilator changes on cardiac function. Knowledge of the cardiac output is also necessary for calculating stroke volume, systemic vascular resistance, pulmonary vascular resistance, oxygen delivery, and oxygen consumption. Systemic and pulmonary vascular resistances indicate afterloads or the resistance that ventricles need to overcome to eject blood.[72, 74]

Myocardial function can be estimated as it relates to oxygen demand by calculation of the ventricular stroke work index.[74] These indexes are used for optimization of myocardial function to avoid myocardial work overload:

$$LVSWI = SVI \times (MAP - PAOP) \times 0.0136,$$
$$RVSWI = SVI \times (PAP - RAP) \times 0.0136,$$

where LVSWI is the left ventricular work index, SVI is the stroke volume index, RVSWI is the right ventricular work index, PAP is the pulmonary artery pressure, MAP is the mean arterial pressure, RAP is the mean right atrial pressure, and PAOP is the pulmonary artery opening (wedge) pressure.

Oxygen delivery indicates the amount of oxygen supplied to the body. Low values (<500 ml/min) are warning signals that either cardiac output or arterial oxygen content needs to be improved:[72]

$$\dot{Q}_{O_2} = \text{Cardiac Output} \times Ca_{O_2} \times 10,$$

where Ca_{O_2} is the arterial oxygen content (ml/dl). Determination of oxygen consumption ($\dot{V}_{O_2}$), the amount of oxygen used per minute, implies measures of inspired and expired O_2, CO_2, and minute ventilation. $\dot{V}_{O_2}$ can also be calculated with the Fick equation. In a stable patient at rest, it is a fixed value; a reduction indicates a decrease in work or in oxygen delivery, whereas an increase indicates expanding work:[72, 75]

$$\dot{V}_{O_2} = AVD_{O_2} \times \text{Cardiac Output} \times 10 \text{ (ml/dl/min)},$$

where AVD_{O_2} is the arteriovenous oxygen content difference.

AVD_{O_2} expresses the relationship between the supply of and the demand for oxygen. It is the difference in oxygen content in arterial and venous blood. Increases in cardiac output produce a decrease in AVD_{O_2}, indicating an inverse relationship between cardiac output and AVD_{O_2} in the presence of a constant $\dot{V}_{O_2}$:[72, 75]

$$AVD_{O_2} = Ca_{O_2} - Cv_{O_2} \text{ (ml/dl)},$$

where Ca_{O_2} is the arterial oxygen content and Cv_{O_2} is the mixed venous oxygen content.

Samples for calculating mixed venous oxygen content are obtained distal to the level of the pulmonary artery. Cv_{O_2} is determined by the amount of oxygen supplied to the tissues and the amount in the vena cava and coronary sinus:[72, 75]

$$Cv_{O_2} = (1.34 \times Hgb \times Sv_{O_2}) + (0.003 \times Pv_{O_2}) \text{ (ml/dl)},$$

where Sv_{O_2} is the oxygen saturation of mixed venous blood (%) and Pv_{O_2} is the partial pressure of mixed venous oxygen.

Sv_{O_2} is nonspecific but has a strong correlation with oxygen use. A normal value suggests that oxygen supply is adequate for the demand. Low values are suggestive of increased consumption or decreased supply. Sv_{O_2} reflects tissue oxygenation more accurately than assessment for lactic acidosis or metabolic acidosis.[72, 75]

The shunt fraction ($\dot{Q}_S/\dot{Q}_T$) is the best indicator of pulmonary dysfunction. The calculation is based on samples of arterial blood gases and pulmonary artery blood. Shunt fraction requires determination of Ca_{O_2}, Cv_{O_2}, capillary O_2 content (Cc_{O_2}), and PA_{O_2}. Because of continuous changes in physiologic parameters, the calculated shunt values are often inaccurate. However, the shunt fraction represents the most accurate and easily available technique for separating cardiovascular from pulmonary dysfunction:[72]

$$\frac{\dot{Q}_S}{\dot{Q}_T} = \frac{Cc'_{O_2} - Ca_{O_2}}{Cc'_{O_2} - C\bar{v}_{O_2}}.$$

MONITORING OF RESPIRATORY FUNCTION

Airway pressure is an important parameter in monitoring the mechanically ventilated patient because an excessive increase in airway pressure is a crucial factor in the production of air leakages. Increased peak airway pressure can be caused by greater flow resistance in the airways or resistance produced by increased elastic recoil of the lung and chest wall. Airway pressure is measured during the inspiratory phase for calculating pulmonary compliance and during the expiratory phase for calculating expiratory distending pressure. Decreased compliance in ARDS indicates deterioration, and higher airway pressure is needed to accomplish an effective ventilation. Increased compliance indicates an improved pulmonary condition.[72, 76]

Dynamic compliance is calculated by dividing the delivered tidal volume by the peak inspiratory pressure (PIP). However, because PIP is partially determined by airway resistance, dynamic compliance is not the best indicator of pulmonary compliance.[76] When PIP increases as a result of an elevation in airway resistance, dynamic compliance will decrease.

Static compliance (C_{ST}) is calculated by dividing the delivered tidal volume by the pressure when no gas flow is present. This is achieved by using the plateau pressure produced by occluding the expiratory limb of the ventilator circuit at the end of inspiration. This maneuver eliminates the airway resistance factor. When PEEP is being used, the pressure needs to be subtracted from the PIP in the denominator of the equation.[76] Frequent determinations of static compliance assist in the selection of the proper tidal volume and PEEP for optimizing ventilation and decreasing the possibility of barotrauma:[72, 76]

$$C_{ST} = \frac{TV}{PIP - PEEP},$$

where C_{ST} is static compliance, TV is tidal volume, and PIP is peak inspiratory pressure.

End-tidal CO_2 ($P_{ET_{CO_2}}$) approximates Ca_{O_2}. A rise in the gradient between Pa_{CO_2} and $P_{ET_{CO_2}}$ reflects an increase in alveolar dead space. $P_{ET_{CO_2}}$ is used to calculate minute volume, oxygen consumption, CO_2 production, and the respiratory quotient. Two available techniques for measuring $P_{ET_{CO_2}}$ are mass spectrometry and infrared analysis.[72]

GENERAL MONITORING

Monitoring of the heart rhythm and rate is an essential part of management of patients with ARDS. Bradycardia may impede adequate tissue perfusion, and tachycardia may lead to inadequate ventricular filling and coronary perfusion.[77]

Pulse Doppler oximetry for evaluating arterial oxygen saturation is a useful tool in the management of ARDS. Accurate pulse oximetry requires an effective pulse, hemoglobin of 7 g or more, and a nonpulsatile venous pressure. The venous pressure could lead to pitfalls in accuracy, because high levels of PEEP or an obstructed venous return may produce a pulsatile venous pressure. Chest radiographs are valuable for checking the position of catheters and tubes as well as to confirm clinical suspicions of new problems.[77]

COMPLICATIONS OF ARDS

INFECTION AND SEPSIS

Infection and sepsis are important precipitating conditions in ARDS as well as complications that frequently affect outcome. Bronchopneumonia, the most common cause of secondary infection in ARDS, can be caused by gram-negative and gram-positive bacteria, viruses, *Legionella* organisms, and fungi.[53, 70, 78] Establishing the diagnosis of bronchopneumonia in patients with ARDS is difficult because usual clinical radiographic findings may not be characteristic.[53, 70] The mortality rate associated with gram-negative bacterial pneumonia is high, even with antimicrobial therapy. On the basis of clinical studies of ARDS in adults, four categories of infection have been described:[70] (1) positive blood culture with known site of infection, (2) positive blood culture with unknown site of infection, (3) negative blood culture with known site of infection, and (4) "clinical sepsis" or sepsis syndrome with leukocytosis, fever, negative blood culture and no known site of infection. Patients with a positive blood culture and an unknown site of infection have the worst outcome. Those with positive blood culture and known site of infection have the best survival rates.

MULTIPLE-ORGAN FAILURE

Multiorgan system failure represents a primary life-threatening situation in ARDS. Although there are no specific figures for this condition in pediatric ARDS, an increased number of failing organs and longer duration of failure are directly related to morbidity and mortality.

Dysfunction of almost every organ system can be associated with ARDS.[78] Disseminated intravascular coagulation (DIC) has been reported in about 25% of patients with ARDS, and thrombocytopenia has been reported in 50% of the remaining patients without DIC.[79] Thrombocytopenia in ARDS results from consumption and sequestration of platelets; pulmonary artery catheter placement can be associated with increased platelet consumption.[79]

Renal impairment may also be associated with ARDS either from the initial insult or from the secondary pathophysiologic abnormalities. Possible mechanisms causing decreased urinary output and fluid retention include a decrease in renal blood flow (related to cardiac dysfunction and increased airway pressure), elevated levels of antidiuretic hormones, and the effects of nephrotoxic drugs.[80] Some reports have suggested that the use of IMV rather than controlled ventilation may minimize the effect of airway pressure on renal blood flow.[80] Careful assessment for signs of renal insufficiency is needed for early detection and intervention.[80]

Gastrointestinal complications such as gastritis and stress-induced ulcers with gastrointestinal bleeding are common in patients with ARDS.

PULMONARY BAROTRAUMA

Pulmonary barotrauma is partially dependent on increased airway pressure and can result from overdistension of alveoli with rupture at alveolar bases adjacent to a pulmonary vessel.[81] In a noncompliant lung, the gas can dissect through the perivascular sheath and cause interstitial and subcutaneous emphysema, pneumomediastinum, pneumothorax, pneumoperitoneum, and pneumopericardium.[4, 5, 82] Many factors contribute to pulmonary barotrauma, including increased mean airway pressure, high PIP, and PEEP.[11, 56, 78] The longer duration of mechanical support and the use of high mean airway pressure exacerbate the complications of pulmonary barotrauma. Measures to keep the airway pressure at a minimum may be of benefit in decreasing the incidence of pulmonary air leakage. Some of these measures include use of higher rates and lower tidal volumes to obtain adequate minute ventilation, use of intermittent mandatory ventilation rather than controlled ventilation (when possible), use of PEEP within the optimal range when lung compliance is best, and the prevention of coughing against the ventilator. Lyrene and Truog[4] reported air leakage in 66% of the children with ARDS in their series; there was no statistic difference in PIP or in levels of PEEP between the patients with and the patients without air leakages. Pollack and co-workers described barotrauma in 42% of their patients,[83] and Pfenninger and colleagues[5] in 40%, which occurred most commonly during days 6 and 7 after onset of ARDS; the children in this series received a level of PEEP between 8 and 15.[5] A sudden deterioration in clinical, hemodynamic, or ventilatory parameters should alert the clinician to the possibility that barotrauma may have occurred.

REFERENCES

1. Ashbaugh DG, Bigelow DB, Petty TL, Levine BE: Acute respiratory distress in adults. Lancet 2:319–323, 1967.
2. National Heart and Lung Institute (DHEW): Respiratory diseases. Task force report on problems, research approaches, needs. NIH Publication No. 73-432, pp. 167–180. Washington, DC: U.S. Government Printing Office, 1972.
3. Holbrook PR, Taylor G, Pollack MM, Fields HJ: Adult respiratory distress syndrome in children. Pediatr Clin North Am 27:677–685, 1980.
4. Lyrene R, Truog W: Adult respiratory distress syndrome in a pediatric intensive care unit: Predisposing conditions, clinical course and outcome. Pediatrics 67:790–795, 1981.
5. Pfenninger J, Gerber A, Tschappeler H, Zimmermann A: Adult respiratory distress syndrome in children. J Pediatr 101:352–357, 1982.
6. Nussbaum E: Adult-type respiratory distress syndrome in children: Experience in seven cases. Clin Pediatr 22:401–406, 1983.
7. Truog WE: ARDS in children: A critical care challenge. J Respir Dis 7:104–119, 1986.
8. Effmann EL, Merten DF, Kirks DR, et al: Adult respiratory distress syndrome in children. Radiology 157:69–74, 1985.
9. Murray JF: Division of Lung Diseases, National Heart, Lung, and Blood Institute, Conference Report: Mechanisms of acute respiratory failure. Am Rev Respir Dis 115:1071–1078, 1977.
10. Royall JA, Levin DL: Adult respiratory distress syndrome in pediatric patients: I. Clinical aspects; pathophysiology, pathology and mechanisms of lung injury. J Pediatr 112:169–180, 1988.
11. Royall JA, Levin DL: Adult respiratory distress syndrome in pediatric patients: II. Management. J Pediatr 112:335–347, 1988.
12. Lamy M, Fallat RJ, Koeniger E, et al: Pathologic features and mechanisms of hypoxemia in adult respiratory distress syndrome. Am Rev Respir Dis 114:267–284, 1976.
13. Fowler AA, Hamman RF, Good JT, et al: Adult respiratory distress syndrome: Risk with common predispositions. Ann Intern Med 98:593–597, 1983.
14. Alberts WM, Priest GR, Moser KM: The outlook for survivors of ARDS. Chest 84:272–274, 1983.
15. Fanconi S, Kraemer R, Weber J, et al: Long term sequelae in children surviving adult respiratory distress syndrome. J Pediatr 106:218–222, 1985.
16. Connors AF, McCaffree DR, Rogers RM: The adult respiratory distress syndrome. Dis Mon 27(4):1–75, 1981.
17. Bachofen M, Weibel ER: Structural alterations of lung parenchyma in the adult respiratory distress syndrome. Clin Chest Med 3:35–56, 1982.
18. Ovenfors CO, Hedgcock MW: Intensive care unit radiology: Problems of interpretation. Radiol Clin North Am 16:407–439, 1978.
19. Johnson TH, Altman AR, McCaffree RD: Radiologic considerations in the adult respiratory distress syndrome treated with positive end-expiratory pressure (PEEP). Clin Chest Med 3:89–100, 1982.
20. Johnson TH, Altman AR: Pulmonary interstitial gas: First sign of barotrauma due to PEEP therapy. Crit Care Med 7:532–535, 1979.
21. Altman AR, Johnson TH: Roentgenographic findings in PEEP therapy: Indications of pulmonary complication. JAMA 242:727–730, 1979.
22. Repine JE: Two blood cells and the adult respiratory distress syndrome. Sem Respir Med 8:6–11, 1986.
23. Zimmerman GA, Renzetti AD, Hill HR: Functional and metabolic activity of granulocytes from patients with adult respiratory distress syndrome—Evidence for activated neutrophils in the pulmonary circulation. Am Rev Respir Dis 127:290–300, 1983.
24. Weiland JE, Davis WB, Holter JF, et al: Lung neutrophils in the adult respiratory distress syndrome—Clinical and pathophysiologic significance. Am Rev Respir Dis 133:218–225, 1986.
25. Tate RM, Repine JE: Neutrophils and the adult respiratory distress syndrome. Am Rev Respir Dis 128:552–559, 1983.
26. Lee CT, Fein AM, Lippman M, et al: Elastolytic activity in pulmonary lavage fluid from patients with adult respiratory distress syndrome. N Engl J Med 304:192–196, 1981.
27. Vercellotti GM, Van Asbeck BS, Jacob HS: Oxygen radical-induced erythrocyte hemolysis by neutrophils: Critical role of iron and lactoferrin. J Clin Invest 76:956–962, 1985.
28. Hallgren R, Borg T, Venge P, Modig J: Signs of neutrophils and eosinophil activation in adult respiratory distress syndrome. Crit Care Med 12:14–18, 1984.
29. Parrish DA, Mitchell BC, Henson PM, Larsen GL: Pulmonary responses of fifth component of complement-sufficient and deficient mice to hyperoxia. J Clin Invest 74:956–965, 1984.
30. Larsen GL, McCarthy K, Webster RO, et al: A differential effect of C5a and C5a des Arg in the induction of pulmonary inflammation. Am J Pathol 100:179–192, 1980.
31. Hammerschmidt DE, Weaver LJ, Hudson LD, et al: Association of complement activation and elevated plasma-C5a with adult respiratory distress syndrome. Lancet 1:947–949, 1980.
32. Till GO, Johnson KJ, Kunkel R, Ward PA: Intravascular activation of complement and acute lung injury: Dependency on neutrophils and toxic oxygen metabolites. J Clin Invest 69:1126–1135, 1982.
33. Henson PM, Larsen GL, Webster RO, et al: Pulmonary microvascular alterations and injury induced by complement fragments: Synergistic effect of complement activation, neutrophil sequestration and prostaglandins. Ann N Y Acad Sci 384:287–300, 1982.
34. Fox RB, Hoidal JR, Brown DM, Repine JE: Pulmonary inflammation due to oxygen toxicity: Involvement of chemotactic factors and polymorphonuclear leukocytes. Am Rev Respir Dis 123:521–523, 1981.
35. Harada RN, Bowman CM, Fox RB, Repine JE; Alveolar macrophage secretions: Initiators of inflammation in pulmonary oxygen toxicity? Chest 81:52S–53S, 1982.
36. Bowman CM, Harada RN, Repine JE: Hyperoxia stimulates alveolar macrophages to produce and release a factor which increases neutrophil adherence. Inflammation 7:331–338, 1983.
37. Brigham KL: Mechanisms of lung injury. Clin Chest Med 3:9–24, 1982.
38. Saugstad OD: Oxygen radicals and pulmonary damage. Pediatr Pulmonol 1:167–175, 1985.
39. Johnson KJ, Ward PA: Role of oxygen metabolites in immune complex injury of lung. J Immunol 126:2365–2369, 1981.
40. Weiss SJ, Ward PA: Immune complex induced generation of oxygen metabolites by human neutrophils. J Immunol 129:309–313, 1982.
41. Rinaldo JE, Rogers RM: Adult respiratory distress syndrome: Changing concepts of lung injury and repair. N Engl J Med 306:900–909, 1982.
42. Plow EF, Edgington TS: Comparative immunochemical characterizations of products of plasmin and leukocyte protease cleavage of human fibrinogen. Thromb Res 12:653–665, 1978.
43. Snyderman R, Shin HS, Dannenberg AM: Macrophage proteinase and inflammation: The production of chemotactic activity from the fifth component of complement by macrophage proteinase. J Immunol 109:896–898, 1972.
44. Baird BR, Cheronis JC, Sandhaus RA, et al: O_2 metabolites and neutrophil elastase synergistically cause edematous injury in isolated rat lungs. J Appl Physiol 61:2224–2229, 1986.
45. Wilson RF, Mammen EF, Robson MC, et al: Antithrombin, prekallikrein and fibronectin levels in surgical patients. Arch Surg 121:635–640, 1986.
46. Heffner JE, Sahn JA, Repine JE: Role of platelets in the adult respiratory distress syndrome. Am Rev Respir Dis 135:482–492, 1987.

47. Carvalho ACA: Blood alterations in ARDs. *In* Zapol William, Falke KJ (eds): Acute Respiratory Failure, pp. 303–306. New York: Marcel Dekker, 1985.

48. Malik AB, Johnson A, Tahamont MV: Mechanisms of lung vascular injury after intravascular coagulation. Ann N Y Acad Sci 384:213–234, 1982.

49. Redl H. Hammerschmidt DE, Schlag G: Augmentation by platelets of granulocyte aggregation in response to chemotaxins: Studies utilizing an improved cell preparation technique. Blood 61:125–131, 1983.

50. Sakamoto H, Firkin FC, Chesteman CN: Stimulation of leukocyte phagocytic activity by the platelet release reaction. Pathology 16:126–130, 1984.

51. Deuel TF, Senior RM, Chang D, et al: Platelet factor 4 is chemotactic for neutrophils and monocytes. Proc Natl Acad Sci USA 78:4584–4587, 1981.

52. Kahlstron EJ: Adult respiratory distress syndrome in children. *In* Nussbaum E (ed): Pediatric Intensive Care, pp. 309–324. New York: Futura, 1984.

53. Nichols DG, Rogers MC: Adult respiratory distress syndrome. *In* Rogers MC (ed): Pediatric Intern Care, pp. 237–271. Baltimore, MD: Williams & Wilkins, 1987.

54. Dantzker DR: Gas exchange in the adult respiratory distress syndrome. Clin Chest Med 3:57–67, 1982.

55. Falke KJ, Pontoppidan H, Kumar A, et al: Ventilation with end-expiratory pressure in acute lung disease. J Clin Invest 51:2315–2323, 1972.

56. Shapiro BA, Cane RD, Harrison, RA: Positive end-expiratory pressure therapy in adults with special reference to acute lung injury: A review of the literature and suggested clinical complications. Crit Care Med 12:127–141, 1984.

57. Venus B, Jacobs HK: Alterations in regional myocardial blood flows during different levels of positive end-expiratory pressure. Crit Care Med 12:96–101, 1984.

58. Kirby RR, Perry JC, Calderwood KW, et al: Cardiorespiratory effects of high pressure end-expiratory pressure. Anesthesiology 43:533–539, 1975.

59. Hasten RW, Downs JB, Heenan TJ: A comparison of synchronized and non-synchronized intermittent mandatory ventilation. Respir Care 25:554–557, 1980.

60. Gattinoni L, Pesenti A, Mascheroni D, et al: Low frequency positive-pressure ventilation with extra corporeal CO_2 removal in severe acute respiratory failure. JAMA 256:881–886, 1986.

61. Froese AB: High-frequency ventilation: A critical assessment. *In* Shoemaker WC (ed): Critical Care: State of the Art, vol. 5, pp. A1–55. Fullerton, CA: Society of Critical Care Medicine, 1984.

62. Kirilloff LH, Owens GR, Rogers RM, Mazzocco MC: Does chest physical therapy work? Chest 88:436–444, 1985.

63. Weaver LJ, Haisch CE, Hudson LD, Carrico CJ: Prospective analysis of PEEP reduction. Am Rev Respir Dis 119(Suppl):182, 1979.

64. Periera GR, Fox WW, Stanley CA, et al: Decreased oxygenation and hyperlipemia during intravenous fat infusions in premature infants. Pediatrics 66:26–30, 1980.

65. Greene HL, Hazlett D, Demaree R: Relationship between intralipid-induced hyperlipemia and pulmonary function. Am J Clin Nutr 29:127–135, 1976.

66. American Academy of Pediatrics Committee on Nutrition: Use of intravenous fat emulsions in pediatric patients. Pediatrics 68:738–743, 1981.

67. Askanazi J, Rosenbaum SH, Hyman AL, et al: Respiratory changes induced by the large glucose loads of total parenteral nutrition. JAMA 243:1444–1447, 1980.

68. Pingleton SK, Harmon GS: Nutritional management in acute respiratory failure. JAMA 257:3094–3099, 1987.

69. Wolf HR, Seeger HW: Experimental and clinical results in shock lung treatment with vitamin E. Ann N Y Acad Sci 393:392–410, 1982.

70. Johanson WG: Bacterial infection in ARDS: Pathogenic mechanisms and consequences. *In* Shoemaker WC (ed): Critical Care: State of the Art, vol. 5, pp. H1–43, Fullerton, CA: Society of Critical Care Medicine, 1984.

71. Neff TA: Monitoring alveolar ventilation and respiratory gas exchange. Respir Care 30:413–421, 1985.

72. Oliver DL: Monitoring the patient with adult respiratory distress syndrome. Crit Care 1:505–521, 1987.

73. Matthay RA, Wiedemann HP, Matthay MA: Cardiovascular function in the intensive care unit: Invasive and noninvasive monitoring. Respir Care 30:432–455, 1985.

74. Stevens JH, Raffin TA, Mihm FG, et al: Thermodilution cardiac output measurement: Effects of the respiratory cycle on its reproducibility. JAMA 253:2240–2242, 1985.

75. Dantzker DR, Gutierrez G: Assessment of tissue oxygenation. Respir Care 30:456–462, 1985.

76. Bone RC: Monitoring respiratory mechanics in acute respiratory failure. Respir Care 28:597–604, 1983.

77. Goldenheim PD, Kazemi H: Cardiopulmonary monitoring of critically ill patients. N Engl J Med 311:717–720, 776–780, 1984.

78. Pingleton SK: Complications associated with the adult respiratory distress syndrome. Crit Care Med 13:786–791, 1985.

79. Bone RC, Francis PB, Pierce AK: Intravascular coagulation associated with the adult respiratory distress syndrome. Am J Med 61:585–589, 1976.

80. Steinhoff H, Falke K, Schwarzhoff W: Enhanced renal function associated with intermittent mandatory ventilation in acute respiratory failure. Intensive Care Med 8:69–74, 1982.

81. Macklin MT, Macklin CC: Malignant interstitial emphysema of the lungs and mediastinum as an important occult complication in many respiratory diseases and other conditions. Medicine 23:281–358, 1944.

82. Culpepper JA, Langler R, Parvner OJ: Complicatons of adult respiratory distress syndrome. Probl Crit Care 1:488–496, 1987.

83. Pollack MM, Fields AI, Holbrook PR: Cardiopulmonary parameters during high PEEP in children. Crit Care Med 8:372–376, 1980.

49 PULMONARY ASPIRATION

JOHN L. COLOMBO, M.D.

Aspiration of foreign materials into the lower respiratory tract is an event that occurs in normal people without apparent clinical significance. Alternatively, aspiration can be life-threatening, as in foreign body aspiration, large-volume hydrocarbon ingestion, and drowning.

Between these extremes is the relatively common occurrence of aspirating food, gastric contents, and oral secretions. If these substances have significant intrinsic toxicity or are aspirated in large enough quantities or with sufficient frequency, disease may result.

The major classifications of types of foreign materials aspirated and resultant pathologic process include (1) airway foreign body with acute obstruction of a large airway, (2) particulate materials that produce foreign body pneumonia and small airway obstruction, (3) toxic substances that produce chemical pneumonia, and (4) oropharyngeal flora that cause bacterial pneumonia and abscess. The focus of this chapter is on the pathogenesis, recognition, and management of disease caused by recurrent aspiration of foods, oral secretions, and gastric contents. Aspiration of gastric contents overlaps greatly with the important issue of gastroesophageal reflux and its relationship to the respiratory tract. This topic is discussed only briefly here because it is covered in detail in Chapter 57.

UNDERLYING DISORDERS PREDISPOSING TO ASPIRATION INJURY

Determinants of whether symptoms or illness develops from aspiration depend on the quantity and type of material aspirated, the frequency of aspiration, and host defense variables. The interaction of these factors and the possible relationship to future lung disease are still poorly understood. It appears that aspiration into the lungs is probably a common event that is usually well tolerated. It has been shown that normal adults aspirate oropharyngeal secretions during sleep.[1] A high incidence of aspiration has been shown among patients with tracheostomies[2] and endotracheal tubes.[3, 4] Several underlying factors are recognized to predispose persons to pulmonary aspiration injury. These factors are listed in Table 49–1 and include anatomic factors, esophageal dysfunction, and neuromuscular problems.

ANATOMIC FACTORS

Congenital abnormalities of the airway and the esophagus are a relatively infrequent cause of aspiration. Tracheoesophageal fistulas with esophageal atresia are usually diagnosed shortly after birth. The H-type tracheoesophageal fistula accounts for fewer than 5% of all such fistulas[5] but must be considered in infants or children with significant recurrent lung disease. The classic findings of choking or coughing with feedings, abdominal distention, and hypersalivation may be present in fewer than 50% of affected patients.[6, 7] In patients who have undergone repair of a tracheoesophageal fistula, development of a secondary fistula as well as esophageal motility abnormalities should also be considered. Laryngeal clefts can sometimes escape detection for weeks or even months after birth. Although rare, these should be looked for in any child with coughing during feedings because of the high morbidity and mortality rates associated with them.[8]

Among patients with tracheostomies, there appears to be an increased incidence of recurrent aspiration, possibly because of the tracheal attachment to the anterior

Table 49–1. DISORDERS LEADING TO PULMONARY ASPIRATION INJURY

Neuromuscular
Immaturity of swallowing reflex
Pharyngeal, laryngeal paralysis
Cerebral palsy
Dysautonomia
Muscular dystrophy
Myasthenia gravis
Altered consciousness
  (e.g., drug intoxication, general anesthesia, head trauma)
Seizures
Intracranial neoplasm
Hydrocephalus
Anatomic
Tracheoesophageal fistula
Laryngeal cleft
Tracheostomy
Endotracheal tube
Indwelling nasogastric tube
Oral or esophageal masses/stricture
  (e.g., foreign body, tumor)
Vascular ring
Micrognathia
Functional
Gastroesophageal reflux
Achalasia (cricopharyngeal)
Posttracheoesophageal fistula repair
Protracted vomiting
Collagen vascular diseases (scleroderma, dermatomyositis)
Miscellaneous
Gingivitis
Poor oral hygiene
Trauma to pharynx

neck, which prevents normal laryngeal closure with swallowing.[2]

Esophageal strictures, tumors, foreign bodies, and vascular rings can all predispose affected patients to aspiration. Congenital or acquired mass lesions of the oropharynx also increase the risk of aspiration by interfering with swallowing and airway protection.

ESOPHAGEAL DYSFUNCTION

This group of disorders is likely the most common cause of aspiration in children. Included in this category are gastroesophageal reflux, achalasia, hiatal hernia, and poor motility secondary to prior (repaired) tracheoesophageal fistula. Acquired lesions such as candidiasis and scleroderma are less common disorders included in this group.

NEUROMUSCULAR PROBLEMS

Any disorder that suppresses the level of consciousness, interferes with the swallowing or gag mechanism, or decreases the effectiveness of cough predisposes the affected person to injury from both acute and chronic aspiration. Many of these disorders are listed in Table 49–1.

The sucking and gagging reflexes are not mature until approximately 34 weeks' gestation and are abnormal in some term infants, particularly if there is any birth insult. Several investigators found aspiration occurring with swallowing by infants without anatomic abnormalities. This has been attributed to fatigue[9] or to transient pharyngeal incoordination.[10, 11] Any infant (premature or term) should be considered at higher risk for aspiration.

PATHOPHYSIOLOGY

Aspiration of foreign materials into the lungs appears to be a common event, and aspiration of saliva and solid food particles during sleep has been demonstrated in normal adults.[1, 12] All people have experienced symptomatic aspiration, which fortunately is self-limited after, perhaps, an embarrassing paroxysm of coughing. Pulmonary injury from aspiration as classically described by Mendelson[13] produces serious and potentially fatal consequences, depending on the amount and type of material aspirated.

Since the time of Mendelson's original description, many studies have helped define the determinants of pulmonary injury after aspiration. For obvious reasons, much of this knowledge comes from animal experiments. Extrapolation to humans and particularly to very young children is limited; however, results of animal studies and limited reports in humans have shown that the pH of the aspirate is one of the major elements. Lung injury increases significantly as the pH falls below 2.5. The volume of aspirate is also a major factor. In dogs, 1 ml/kg of acid aspiration produces only mild effects, whereas 2 ml/kg or more of acid aspiration causes serious effects and usually death.[14] Histologic findings include degeneration of bronchiolar epithelium, pulmonary edema and hemorrhage, focal atelectasis, exudation of fibrin, and acute inflammatory cellular infiltrate. Later findings include regeneration of bronchiolar epithelium, proliferation of fibroblasts, and fibrosis.

Aspiration of nonacidic gastric contents is also damaging, particularly when they contain milk or food particles.[15, 16] Distribution and injury occur rapidly. When gastric contents are instilled into the trachea of excised ventilated canine lungs, they may be seen on the lung surface within 12 to 18 sec, and extensive atelectasis develops within 3 min. Changes of acute pneumonia occur within hours, and chronic granulomatous changes develop within 48 h.[15, 17]

Nonacidic fluid aspiration (pH > 2.5) may have immediate effects on reflex airway closure, decreased oxygen tension/pressure, and decreased lung compliance. Atelectasis may occur secondary to surfactant washout or fluid filling of alveoli. The risk of atelectasis increases significantly if the solution is hypertonic or contains particulate matter.

Although both acute aspiration and chronic aspiration probably cause the lungs to be more susceptible to bacterial infection, it does not appear that infection plays a role in the initial lung injury. Animal and clinical studies have generally shown no benefit from routine usage of antibiotics with aspiration of foods or gastric contents.[17, 18] When oropharyngeal secretions are the major material aspirated, infection may be the primary pathologic process. Usually the actual episode of aspiration is not observed, and the disease process is insidious. Necrotizing pneumonia and possibly lung abscess or empyema develop over 7 to 14 days. The patient often presents only after these complications have already occurred. The predominant organisms involved in this process are usually combinations of aerobes and anaerobes.[19, 20]

CLINICAL FEATURES

Finding lower respiratory tract symptoms in any patient with a predisposing condition should arouse suspicion of aspiration-induced disease. A history of coughing or choking in relationship to feedings is useful but often is not present, particularly if very small amounts of material are aspirated, if aspiration occurs primarily during sleep, or if the cough reflex is depressed.

Signs and symptoms of aspiration include unexplainable chronic cough, wheezing or rattling breathing, tachypnea, and apnea. The clinical picture depends mainly on the frequency of aspiration, the quantity of aspirate, and the characteristics of the foreign material. In milder cases with infrequent or small amounts of aspirate, there may be no significant parenchymal lung disease but only findings of large airway hypersecretion, including particularly coarse expiratory crackles and wheezing or rattling. With chronic recurrent aspiration of even small quantities, children and particularly infants may have evidence of hyperinflation with subcostal retractions and increased chest anteroposterior diameter. Many of these patients are considered to have difficult-to-control "asthma." Chronic aspiration may eventually lead to chronic interstitial pneumonia and fibrosis. This group of patients are expected to have increased problems with infection, including exacerbation of symptoms with acute viral infections as well as occasional secondary bacterial infection with bronchiectasis and possibly abscess formation. Lung abscess, however, occurs infrequently in young children and is more common in older children and adults.

Although infectious pneumonia is probably less common than chemical or mechanical lung problems from aspiration, it still is a relatively frequent occurrence, particularly in high-risk patients. Aspiration of oral secretions containing a high bacterial concentration is most likely to produce this type of pneumonia. The typical patient has a combination of periodontal disease and either altered consciousness or dysphagia. The organisms responsible for this are, logically, those of the oral flora, and transtracheal aspiration or lung puncture typically reveals mixed cultures of both anaerobic and aerobic bacteria. The aerobic pathogens are more often found when aspiration occurs in a child residing in a medical institution.[20]

For conceptual purposes, it can be useful to classify pulmonary aspiration sequelae into syndromes. One such classification is listed in Table 49–2. There is certainly

Table 49–2. ASPIRATION SYNDROMES

Type	Material	Clinical and Radiographic Findings
Chemical pneumonitis Acute	Acid, hydrocarbons, toxic gases	Acute, massive: Dyspnea, hypoxemia, hypotension, bilateral patchy infiltrates often with development of adult respiratory distress syndrome picture
Chronic	Gastric contents, foods	Chronic: Cough, wheeze, failure to thrive, recurrent pneumonia (especially dependent areas), bronchial wall thickening and hyperinflation, interstitial pneumonia, fibrosis
Infection	Oropharyngeal secretions	Fever, cough, sputum, foul breath, dependent area consolidation, occasionally pleural effusion (empyema), abscess
Mechanical obstruction/ foreign body pneumonia	Foods, antacid suspension, inert fluids, foreign bodies	Dyspnea, wheeze, cough, apnea, hyperinflation, focal atelectasis/infiltrates

overlap between these syndromes, and any individual patient may suffer from acute or chronic consequences of more than one process.

DIAGNOSIS

To establish the diagnosis of aspiration-induced lung disease, two criteria should be met. First, it should be determined that aspiration is occurring in a patient. Second, because aspiration can occur without causing disease, it should be established that the patient's problems are a result of aspiration. The ideal test would not only quantify the amount of aspiration and give a marker of aspirated materials in the lungs but would also indicate that lung disease has been induced by these materials. Because there is no test or even a combination of tests that are specific and sensitive enough to accomplish these objectives, a great deal of clinical judgment is necessary on the basis of clues that can be revealed from the history and physical examination combined with appropriate tests. Frequently, the best the clinician can do is show that aspiration is at least occasionally occurring and then decide (often by exclusion) that aspiration is the most likely cause of a child's illness.

The caretakers of any child with recurrent respiratory symptoms should be asked about the relationship of symptoms to feedings. They may notice that the child becomes fatigued, has difficulty breathing, or simply loses interest after the first few ounces. The coughing or gagging may be minimal or even nonexistent in a child with neurologic impairment or tolerance as a result of frequent aspiration.

There is no substitute for observation of the child during feeding when the diagnosis of aspiration is being considered. A child should be observed closely for difficulty with sucking or swallowing and any associated coughing or choking. Nasopharyngeal reflex, indicating poor swallowing coordination, may also be observed. Inspection of the palate, tongue, and oropharynx for gross abnormality should be performed. In a toothless infant, simply inserting a finger into the mouth to test for strength and coordination of sucking as well as appropriate resistance to deep finger insertion is a valuable and important part of the physical examination. Finding either a hypoactive or hyperactive gag reflex on oropharyngeal examination is significant. Patients with swallowing abnormalities, upper esophageal motility problems, or tracheoesophageal fistula may have excess secretion accumulation in the mouth. Gaseous abdominal distension may also be noted with tracheoesophageal fistulas.

Although physical findings in the pulmonary examination are nonspecific for aspiration, it is important to examine the child before and after feedings for crackles and wheezing. These adventitious sounds may be more prominent in dependent areas of the lung in a child with recurrent aspiration. They may disappear rapidly after feeding if materials are effectively cleared from the airway.

The initial study for a patient with chronic or recurrent respiratory symptoms is the chest radiograph. Findings vary from normal to diffuse, severe involvement. The most typical findings involve infiltrates of dependent areas, particularly in the upper lobes and posterior areas of the lower lobe. There is often hyperinflation. In other children, there may be only bronchial wall thickening, and one hypothesis is that these children have a more effective clearance mechanism, aspirate smaller amounts of material, or both, with primary involvement of the larger airways only. Figures 49–1 to 49–3 show radiographs of patients with known aspiration.

In a group of 22 children with recurrent aspiration, the author and associates found that chest radiographs showed localized infiltrates involving two lobes or fewer in 41%, diffuse infiltrates in 27%, and bronchial wall thickening or only hyperinflation in 18%. Chest radiographs were normal in 14% of this group (Table 49–3).

The usual next step in evaluation is the barium esophagogram. When properly performed, this allows evaluation of the swallowing mechanism and direct aspiration into the trachea through the larynx, or regurgitation into the nasopharynx can be seen. Aspiration through a laryngoesophageal cleft can also be visualized, although this can appear quite similar to aspiration through the vocal cords with swallowing, and careful endoscopic examination is sometimes necessary for differentiating the two conditions. Tracheoesophageal fistula without esophageal atresia (H type) can be difficult to

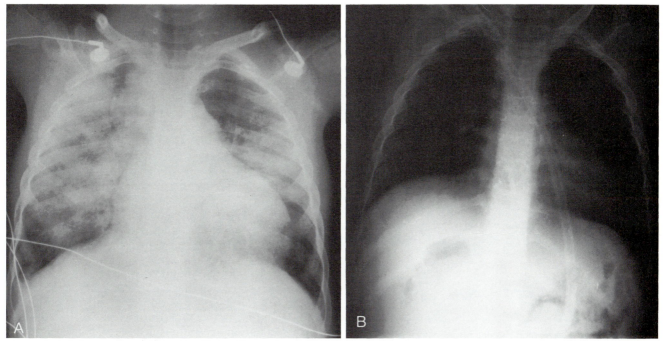

Figure 49–1. *A,* Chest radiograph showing diffuse infiltrates, hyperinflation, and mild cardiomegaly in a 5-year-old boy with dysautonomia and known chronic aspiration. *B,* Chest radiograph of same patient taken 18 months later after fundoplication and gastrostomy feeding tube placement.

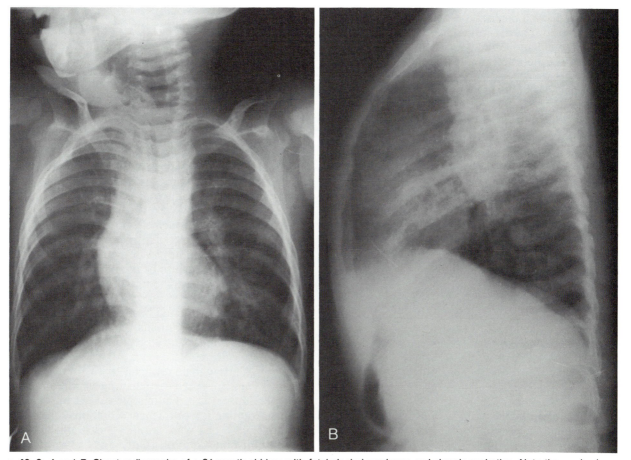

Figure 49–2. *A* and *B,* Chest radiographs of a 21-month-old boy with fetal alcohol syndrome and chronic aspiration. Note the predominance of posterior infiltrates.

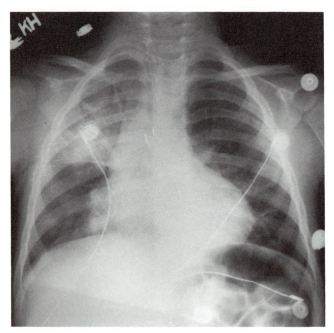

Figure 49–3. Chest radiograph showing predominance of right-sided and particularly right upper lobe infiltrates in a 5-year-old girl 24 h after aspiration secondary to codeine overdose and vomiting.

demonstrate. It is recommended that contrast material be injected through a catheter at various levels of the esophagus. The bolus injection should distend the esophagus and, it is hoped, open the fistula, which usually is directed cephalad from esophagus to trachea. Even with careful inspection and cineradiography, these fistulas can escape detection and sometimes are found only after repeated studies or at bronchoscopy with or without contrast instillation into the trachea.[5, 21]

Gastroesophageal reflux or hiatal hernia may also be detected with the barium esophagogram, but this test is relatively insensitive for detecting gastroesophageal reflux.[22, 23] Prolonged pH measurements of the lower esophagus, esophagoscopy with biopsy, and scintigraphy are more sensitive indicators of gastroesophageal reflux.[24, 25] However, documenting reflux alone does not establish this as a cause of aspiration or respiratory disease.

Radionuclide scintigraphy (milk scan) offers advantages over a barium esophagogram in detecting gastro-esophageal reflux and aspiration. Mixing a radioisotope with milk feedings offers a more physiologic approach and allows longer monitoring time. Using scintigraphy, some investigators have found aspiration in approximately 25% of children with respiratory tract symptoms that appeared suspicious for pulmonary aspiration.[25, 26] In 44 children studied by the same group with "near-miss" sudden infant death syndrome, 9 (20%) had positive scans for aspiration. Other investigators have found much lower incidence rates of positive aspiration scans.[27, 28] Variation in technical aspects of test performance and differences in populations studied probably account for much of the difference in reported frequencies of aspiration detection. Also, the lack of a gold standard for comparison makes it difficult to assess sensitivity and specificity. One technical consideration is the timing of a follow-up scan. In one study, investigators found that of 23 children with positive scans, 21 were positive at 2 h, whereas only six were found positive at 24 h.[25] Although the authors stated that they had ceased performing the 24-h scan, the finding of two additional patients positive at 24 h would make this procedure worthwhile because no further radiation exposure is necessary. However, it suggests that relying on only a late scan is extremely insensitive, probably relating to the half-life of the isotope and, to a lesser extent, mucociliary clearance from the larger airways.[27]

The finding of lipid-laden macrophages in respiratory secretions has been suggested as being indicative and even diagnostic of lipid aspiration.[29, 30] Quantification of these macrophages was reported to be a sensitive but relatively nonspecific test for aspiration-induced lung disease in adults.[31] Children with gastroesophageal reflux and chronic respiratory disease were more likely to have lipid-laden macrophages found in bronchial lavage fluid than were children with chronic respiratory disorders but without gastroesophageal reflux.[32] Although lipid-laden alveolar macrophages are found in many patients without suspected aspiration, quantification of lipid-laden macrophages in bronchial washings is reported to be useful in determining whether significant aspiration is occurring in children with lung disease.[33] When this test is considered, it should be remembered that endogenous lipoid pneumonia with high levels of lipid-laden macrophages can be found with bronchial obstruction.[34] Also children receiving large amounts of intravenous lipid infusion may exhibit high levels of lipid-laden macrophages.[35]

Bronchoscopy can also be used for diagnosis with gross detection of food, gastric contents, or other foreign materials. It has also been reported that the finding of erythema localized to subsegmental bronchi is highly suggestive of aspiration of gastric contents.[36] In samples of bronchoalveolar lavage, meat and vegetable fibers have also been microscopically detected.[12, 37]

For patients with an artificial airway in place, a variety of tests have been used for detecting aspiration. The most frequently used test requires placement of oral dye and visual examination of tracheal secretions for presence of staining.[2, 4, 38] The volume of dye used appears to be an important consideration. Only 16% of endotracheally intubated children were shown to aspirate when two to

Table 49–3. RADIOGRAPHIC FINDINGS IN CHRONIC ASPIRATION (N = 22 CHILDREN)

Variable	Number of Patients	%
Diffuse infiltrates	6	27
Normal inflation	4	18
Hyperinflation	2	9
Localized infiltrates (≤ lobes)	9	41
Normal inflation	6	27
Hyperinflation	3	14
Bronchial wall thickening only	2	9
Hyperinflation only	2	9
Normal	3	14

four drops of dye were instilled.[38] With larger aliquots (0.5 to 3.0 ml) of dye solution, approximately 80% of infants and children were found to aspirate with uncuffed endotracheal tubes.[3, 4] Assay for lactose concentration in tracheal aspirates has also been proposed to detect aspiration in lactose-fed, ventilator-dependent infants.[39] Microscopic examination for lipid can also be used in this group of patients.

The detection of high levels of immunoglobulin A and immunoglobulin G antibodies against bovine milk has been suggested to be helpful in diagnosing recurrent aspiration in young children fed cows' milk.[40]

MANAGEMENT

Whenever possible, an anatomic abnormality causing significant morbidity from aspiration should be corrected. Such a procedure includes the removal of the tracheostomy and endotracheal tubes when clinically feasible. Patients with neuromuscular impairment should be monitored closely for problems that may be caused by aspiration. When such patients are fed orally, parents should be warned to avoid feeding them any food particles of sufficient size to obstruct a large airway. In patients with significantly depressed cough and gag reflexes, insertion of a nasogastric feeding tube into the airway may occur without any immediate symptoms. Parents should be advised to consider this if they are changing such tubes at home. Attention to good oral hygiene and dental repair may help reduce the incidence of infectious aspiration pneumonia. In young children with immaturity of the swallowing reflex or with fatigue, feeding with nasogastric or gastrostomy tubes may protect the lungs until the problem improves. In some children, it may be advisable to give a few spoonfuls of soft food two to three times daily if tolerated so that the child can continue to develop the swallowing mechanism. Multiple medical and ethical issues must be considered in decisions of whether to use gastrostomy or jejunostomy feeding tubes or anti–gastroesophageal reflux procedure in patients with severe mental retardation or other poor prognoses.

When clinical or radiographic evidence is suggestive of a bacterial aspiration pneumonia, antibiotic selection depends on the specific circumstances. Of particular importance is whether the patient is institutionalized or has other underlying disorders. Usually broad anaerobic coverage is recommended; this topic is discussed in Chapter 32.

Although it is generally accepted that aspiration into the lower respiratory tract is relatively common, there remain many uncertainties regarding which determinants cause this to progress from inconsequential to minor, serious, and even fatal conditions. The relationship among types and quantities of materials aspirated, frequency of aspiration, and host defense mechanisms remains poorly understood. The questions of whether children aspirate more than adults do and how, if at all, such aspiration can influence lung development and respiratory function later in life remain largely unanswered. A review of available information and deficiencies in knowledge of this

subject has been published.[41] Increasing the knowledge in these areas is important in helping to differentiate aspiration that is potentially serious from aspiration that is truly benign.

REFERENCES

1. Huxley E, Viroslav J, Gray W, Pierce A: Pharyngeal aspiration in normal adults and patients with depressed consciousness. Am J Med 64:564–568, 1978.
2. Cameron J, Reynolds J, Zuidema G: Aspiration in patients with tracheostomies. Surg Gynecol Obstet 136:68–70, 1973.
3. Goodwin S, Graves S, Haberkern C: Aspiration in intubated premature infants. Pediatrics 75:85–88, 1985.
4. Browning D, Graves S: Incidence of aspiration with endotracheal tubes in children. J Pediatr 102:582–584, 1983.
5. LaSalle A, Andrassy R, Ver-Steeg K, Ratner I: Congenital tracheoesophageal fistula without esophageal atresia. J Thorac Cardiovasc Surg 78:583–588, 1979.
6. Andrassy R, Ko P, Hanson B, et al: Congenital tracheoesophageal fistula without esophageal atresia. A 22 year experience. Am J Surg 140:731–733, 1980.
7. Yazbeck S, Dubuc M: Congenital tracheoesophageal fistula without esophageal atresia. Can J Surg 26:239–241, 1983.
8. Evans J: Management of the cleft larynx and tracheoesophageal clefts. Ann Otol Rhinol Laryngol 94:627–630, 1985.
9. Cumming W, Reilly B: Fatigue aspiration. A cause of recurrent pneumonia in infants. Radiology 105:387–390, 1972.
10. Frank M, Gatewood O: Transient pharyngeal incoordination in the newborn. Am J Dis Child 111:178–181, 1966.
11. Matsaniotis N, Karpouzas J, Tzortzatou-Vallianou M, Tsagournis E: Aspiration due to difficulty in swallowing. Arch Dis Child 46:788–790, 1971.
12. Crausaz F, Favez G: Aspiration of solid food particles into lungs of patients with gastroesophageal reflux and chronic bronchial disease. Chest 93:376–378, 1988.
13. Mendelson C: The aspiration of stomach contents into the lungs during obstetric anesthesia. Am J Obstet Gynecol 52:191–205, 1946.
14. Greenfield L, Singleton R, McCaffree D, Coalson J: Pulmonary effects of experimental graded aspiration of hydrochloric acid. Ann Surg 170:74–86, 1969.
15. Moran T: Experimental food-aspiration pneumonia. Arch Pathol 52:350–354, 1951.
16. Moran T: Milk-aspiration pneumonia in human and animal subjects. Arch Pathol 55:286–301, 1953.
17. Hamelberg W, Bosomworth P: Aspiration pneumonitis: Experimental studies and clinical observations. Anesth Analg 43:669–676, 1964.
18. Bynum L, Pierce A: Pulmonary aspiration of gastric contents. Am Rev Respir Dis 114:1129–1136, 1976.
19. Bartlett J, Finegold S: Anaerobic infections of the lung and pleural space. Am Rev Respir Dis 110:56–77, 1974.
20. Brook I, Finegold S: Bacteriology of aspiration pneumonia in children. Pediatrics 65:1115–1120, 1980.
21. Kuhn J: The thorax. In Silverman F (ed): Caffey's Pediatric X-Ray Diagnosis: An Integrated Imaging Approach, p. 1186. Chicago: Year Book Medical Publishers, 1985.
22. Macfadyen U, Hendry G, Simpson H: Gastro-oesophageal reflux in near-miss sudden infant death syndrome or suspected recurrent aspiration. Arch Dis Child 58:87–91, 1983.
23. Leonidas J: Gastroesophageal reflux in infants: Role of the upper gastrointestinal series. AJR 143:1350–1351, 1984.
24. Orenstein S, Orenstein D: Gastroesophageal reflux and respiratory disease in children. J Pediatr 112:847–858, 1988.
25. McVeagh P, Howman-Giles R, Kemp A: Pulmonary aspiration studied by radionuclide milk scanning and barium swallow roentgenography. Am J Dis Child 141:917–921, 1987.
26. Boonyaprapa S, Alderson P, Garfinkel D, et al: Detection of pulmonary aspiration in infants and children with respiratory disease: Concise communication. J Nucl Med 21:314–318, 1980.

27. Heyman S, Kirkpatrick J, Winter H, Treves S: An improved radio-nuclide method for the diagnosis of gastroesophageal reflux and aspiration in children (milk scan). Radiology 131:479–482, 1979.
28. Fawcett H, Hayden C, Adams J, Swischuk L: How useful is gastro-esophageal reflux scintigraphy in suspected childhood aspiration? Pediatr Radiol 18:311–313, 1988.
29. Williams H, Freeman M: Milk inhalation pneumonia: The signifi-cance of fat filled macrophages in tracheal secretions. Aust Paediatr J 9:286–288, 1973.
30. Epstein R: Constituents of sputum: A simple method. Ann Intern Med 77:259–265, 1972.
31. Corwin R, Irwin R: The lipid-laden alveolar macrophage as a marker of aspiration in parenchymal lung disease. Am Rev Respir Dis 132:576–581, 1985.
32. Nussbaum E, Maggi J, Mathis R, Galant S: Association of lipid-laden alveolar macrophages and gastroesophageal reflux in chil-dren. J Pediatr 110:190–194, 1987.
33. Colombo J, Hallberg T: Recurrent aspiration in children: Lipid-laden alveolar macrophage quantitation. Pediatr Pulmonol 3:86–89, 1987.
34. Cohen A, Cline M: In vitro studies of the foamy macrophage of

35. Recalde A, Nickerson B, Vegas M, et al: Lipid-laden macrophages in tracheal aspirates of newborn infants receiving intravenous lipid infusions: A cytologic study. Pediatr Pathol 2:25–34, 1984.
36. Wolfe J, Bone R, Ruth W: Diagnosis of gastric aspiration by fiber-optic bronchoscopy. Chest 70:458–459, 1976.
37. Ristagno R, Kornstein M, Hansen-Flaschen J: Diagnosis of occult meat aspiration by fiberoptic bronchoscopy. Am J Med 80:154–156, 1986.
38. Goitein K, Rein A, Gornstein A: Incidence of aspiration in endo-tracheally intubated infants and children. Crit Care Med 12:19–21, 1984.
39. Hopper A, Kwong L, Stevenson D, et al: Detection of gastric con-tents in tracheal fluid of infants by lactose assay. J Pediatr 102:415–418, 1983.
40. Muller W, Rieger C, von der Hardt H: Increased concentrations of milk antibodies in recurrent pulmonary aspiration in infants and young children. Acta Paediatr Scand 74:660–663, 1985.
41. Platzker A (ed): Supplement: Aspiration hazards to the developing lung. Am Rev Respir Dis 131(5):S1–S66, 1985.

postobstructive endogenous lipoid pneumonia in man. Am Rev Respir Dis 106:69–78, 1972.

50 ATELECTASIS

KARL H. KARLSON, JR., M.D

Atelectasis is a term used to indicate a loss of volume in the lung. This volume loss may be subsegmental (includ-ing round or plate atelectasis), segmental, or lobar or may involve the whole lung. Because atelectasis is a phenom-enon secondary to changes in lung mechanics or airway obstruction, the diagnosis and treatment of atelectasis must be aimed at the primary cause. Certain conditions are more prone to complications by atelectasis than are others. In one study, Lecks and colleagues found segmen-tal atelectasis in 7% of hospitalized asthmatics.[1] Brooks and co-workers[2] found segmental or subsegmental atel-ectasis in 24% of hospitalized asthmatics, whereas mucus plugging or subsegmental atelectasis was found in 60% of asthmatics studied by Maxwell.[3] Muller and associates reported that asthma was the most common cause of mas-sive total lung atelectasis in their series of five patients.[4] Aspiration of a foreign body is also frequently associated with atelectasis. Foreign body aspiration, presenting as atelectasis on chest radiographs, was found in 27% and 15% of patients reported by Schloss[5] and Aytac[6] and their colleagues, respectively. Atelectasis or mucoid impaction that can lead to atelectasis was reported in 33% of cases of cystic fibrosis.[7]

Infections that are often complicated by atelectasis include pertussis, tuberculosis, and measles.[8] Quinn and co-authors found that 26% of children with respiratory syncytial virus infection acquired upper lobe atelectasis.[9] Atelectasis was also reported by Reines and colleagues in patients who suffered acute spinal cord injury.[10] Patients who have neuromuscular disease are also prone to acquire atelectasis; in one series, atelectasis developed in 85% of

patients despite mechanical ventilation.[11] Moylan and Shannon found that 46% of patients with bronchopul-monary dysplasia had atelectasis of the right upper lobe and hyperinflation of the right lower lobe.[12] Hyaline membrane disease in premature infants was found to be a significant risk factor for the development of atelecta-sis.[13] Compression of the airways in patients who have congenital cardiovascular, pulmonary, or extrapulmon-ary anomalies is associated with obstructive atelectasis in childhood, as are rare bronchial tumors.[14-19]

PATHOPHYSIOLOGY

The pathophysiologic processes of atelectasis can be the result of either airway obstruction or altered pulmonary mechanics. Conditions that cause airway obstruction lead to resorption of the gas distal to the obstruction and loss of lung volume in the affected area. Using a canine model of obstructive atelectasis, Dale and Rahn showed that the rate of absorption of the gas distal to an obstructed airway was dependent on the initial composition of the gas within the airways as well as the partial pressure of the gases within the blood.[20] Ford and colleagues analyzed the differences in translobar pressures during left lower-lobe atelectasis and whole-lung collapse at different lung vol-umes. They found that these deforming forces were sig-nificant and localized.[21]

Atelectasis can also be the result of altered pulmonary mechanics. Fung showed that volume loss leads to alve-olar collapse, except in plate atelectasis, in which external compression of portions of the lung parenchyma can occur while the rest of the lung maintains its resting volume.[22] Computed tomographic (CT) scans of adult volunteers undergoing general anesthesia showed that atelectasis did occur after volume loss.[23] Body position also affects airway closure and may contribute to the development of atelectasis.[24] Constant volume ventilation in dogs was associated with decreased lung compliance and atelectasis and was reversible with forced inhalations.[25] These findings correlate with the report of hypoxia and atelectasis in patients ventilated at a constant volume without sighs.[26] Exposure to 100% oxygen causes atelectasis by the rapid absorption of the pure gas.[27] Ford and colleagues showed that diaphragmatic dysfunction after abdominal surgery was associated with the development of postoperative atelectasis.[28] Surfactant plays an important role in alveolar stability, and its depletion was shown to be related to the presence of atelectasis in hyaline membrane disease.[29] Decreased surfactant has been proposed also as the mechanism by which atelectasis occurs in meconium aspiration syndrome.[30]

Blood flow to the atelectatic portion of the lung is decreased, according to Pirlo and colleagues.[31] They studied this phenomenon in a canine model of atelectasis in both open-chest and closed-chest preparations and found that the decreases in blood flow in both were similar.[31] From this, they concluded that changes in mechanical forces did not explain the decrease in blood flow and that hypoxic vasoconstriction was the cause. Thomas and Garrett showed that the strength of the hypoxic vasoconstrictive response determines the degree of shunting in canine atelectasis.[32] McFarlane and associates further demonstrated that although the primary cause of decrease in blood flow to an atelectatic lobe was hypoxic vasoconstriction, this response was significantly augmented by both increased partial pressure of carbon dioxide and mechanical factors.[33] Studying both open-chest and closed-chest canine models of atelectasis, Chen and co-workers also suggested that mechanical factors play a significant role in the shunt fraction occurring with atelectasis.[34]

The right middle-lobe syndrome was initially described by Brock and co-authors as an obstructive phenomenon; they found parabronchial lymph nodes compressing the right middle-lobe bronchus in patients with tuberculosis.[35] In contrast, using bronchograms to study right middle-lobe atelectasis, Culiner documented right middle-lobe atelectasis with no obstruction present.[36] The bronchoscopic wedge technique was used by Inners and co-workers to study the collateral ventilation of the right middle lobe.[37] They found higher resistance and longer time constants in the collateral ventilation in the right middle lobe and concluded that the right middle-lobe syndrome is the result of inefficient collateral ventilation.

CLINICAL MANIFESTATIONS

The clinical manifestations of atelectasis depend on the underlying cause as well as the degree of volume loss within the lung. When the atelectasis is relatively small and associated with little physiologic impairment, there may be no signs or symptoms. Cough may be the only symptom associated with mild cases. However, in atelectasis involving a significant portion of the lung, patients experience dyspnea. On physical examination, no signs may be elicited in cases involving small areas of the lung. Tachypnea occurs when substantial volume is lost, resulting in impaired gas exchange. Retractions accompany the tachypnea in patients in whom the atelectasis has caused a significant increase in the work of breathing, and use of accessory muscles of breathing may also be evident. Over the affected area, there may be dullness to percussion. Auscultation of the atelectatic area often reveals decreased breath sounds. A localized wheeze may be present in the area of partial obstruction, although this is not found in total obstruction. Crackles may also be present, particularly if the atelectatic area is infected. When there is significant volume loss in one hemithorax, shift of both the trachea and the mediastinum is evident. Cyanosis may occur in patients who have marked impairment of oxygenation as a result of the atelectasis.

DIAGNOSTIC APPROACHES

The chest radiograph remains the most important diagnostic tool in the evaluation of a patient with suspected atelectasis. Radiographic findings consistent with significant volume loss include shift of the interlobar fissures and may include elevation of the diaphragm or shift of the mediastinum accompanied by an increase in focal density.[38] Lobar atelectasis is apparent on radiographs. In segmental and subsegmental atelectasis or in cases in which the volume loss is relatively small, establishing the diagnosis is more difficult. The vertical fissure line has been described as a sign of partial volume loss in the right lower lobe and is a helpful clue to minor changes in volume.[39] Lacombe and colleagues reported that three or more left upper-lobe vessels seen on end along the left heart border on a plain chest film indicated loss of volume in the left lower lobe.[40]

CT has been found to be useful in the evaluation of atelectasis.[41–46] CT has also been useful in the evaluation of round atelectasis in which a characteristic pattern has evolved.[47–49] A "comet tail," a confluence of bronchi and blood vessels that converge toward the atelectasis, is found; there is pleural thickening over the atelectasis, and an air bronchogram in the center of the mass.

Ultrasonography of the chest has been limited by the air content of the lung parenchyma but occasionally may be a helpful adjunct to other diagnostic techniques. Erasmie and Lundell reported the use of ultrasonography to aid in the diagnosis of pneumonia and atelectasis in two children who appeared to have pericardial effusions.[50] Ultrasonography was also used in the evaluation of a child who had pulmonary sequestration that mimicked left lower-lobe atelectasis.[51]

DIFFERENTIAL DIAGNOSIS

Lobar atelectasis involving one or more lobes should be differentiated from lobar consolidation associated with pneumonia and from pleural fluid. The normal thymus can also mimic atelectasis in both upper lobes.[52] Lobar atelectasis should also be differentiated from a number of congenital anomalies that cause a focal opacification on the chest radiograph, such as pulmonary sequestration. When it involves an entire hemithorax, atelectasis must be differentiated from a mass lesion and from pleural fluid with or without an underlying pneumonia. When the entire hemithorax is atelectatic, a foreign body should be considered as a possible cause.[53] The differential diagnosis of obstructive atelectasis includes not only foreign body aspiration but also tumors, granulation tissue, mucus plugging, and external compression of the airway. Round atelectasis may suggest a congenital anomaly or a malignancy.

MANAGEMENT

Management of atelectasis is directed toward the underlying cause. This includes treatment of an underlying infection (e.g., tuberculosis) bronchoscopic removal of an aspirated foreign body, or correction of a congenital heart defect in order to relieve the obstruction to the airway. Several different respiratory therapy techniques have also been used for adjunctive treatment of atelectasis. Chest physiotherapy is often used to facilitate the removal of secretions from the respiratory tract and to aid in the resolution of atelectasis. Using radioisotope studies, Bateman and associates showed that there was more rapid elimination of the tracer in patients who received chest physiotherapy than in those who did not.[54] Finer and co-workers showed in a controlled study that chest physiotherapy effectively prevented postextubation atelectasis in neonates.[55] In a randomized, prospective study, however, Morran and associates found that postoperative atelectasis was not decreased in the group that received chest physiotherapy.[56] Reines and colleagues, in a prospective, randomized study of chest physical therapy in children after cardiac surgery, found that chest physiotherapy was actually associated with an increased incidence of atelectasis.[10] Chest physiotherapy is often augmented by the use of aerosolized bronchodilators to improve airway patency.[57] The combination of chest physical therapy and bronchodilator aerosols significantly reduced airway resistance in young cystic fibrosis patients who had no symptoms of lung disease.[58]

Incentive spirometry has been used increasingly as the method of choice for both treatment and prevention of atelectasis, particularly in postoperative patients.[59] In a controlled study of incentive spirometry in children after cardiac surgery, Krastins and colleagues showed that atelectasis was significantly reduced in patients who received incentive spirometry.[60] In a study of adults after cardiac surgery, Paul and Downs suggested that intermittent positive-pressure breathing may actually be associated with a decrease in functional residual capacity.[61] However, it remains a method that may prove effective for the treatment of children with chronic or recurrent atelectasis, particularly that associated with neurologic disease. Continuous positive airway pressure (CPAP) is another method of applying a distending pressure to the airway

and has been used extensively in obstructive sleep apnea. Duncan and colleagues reported the success with nasal CPAP in treatment of atelectasis refractory to standard therapy in adults.[62]

Despite the differences in the outcomes that have been reported, there appears to be a general uniformity in the management of postoperative atelectasis in the United States.[63] Intermittent positive-pressure ventilation is used less frequently than in the past, whereas CPAP is used by about 25% of hospitals surveyed. Incentive spirometry was used most often for both prevention and treatment of atelectasis and was often used in conjunction with chest physiotherapy.

In addition to respiratory therapy techniques, other methods have been developed for the management of atelectasis. Galvis and colleagues used an angiographic catheter passed into the trachea and guided to the affected area by position of the head[64] in infants who had atelectasis and found improvement after one or more of these procedures. A similar technique involving fluoroscopic guidance of a suction catheter was reported by Rode and colleagues in the successful treatment of atelectasis in infants.[65]

Bronchoscopy has been increasingly used to treat atelectasis since the advent of the pediatric flexible fiberoptic bronchoscope. Nussbaum used pediatric flexible bronchoscopy in 46 children under 2 years of age. He successfully treated the atelectasis in 29 children who were under 1 year of age and cleared the atelectasis in 59% of children between 1 and 2 years of age.[66] Fitzpatrick and others found that bronchoscopy was effective in treating atelectasis caused by mucus plugging.[67] However, Levy and associates reported their experience with rigid bronchoscopy in children and found that in patients who had atelectasis, there was no improvement after the procedure.[68] In adults, flexible fiberoptic bronchoscopy was not superior to conventional respiratory therapy in the treatment of acute atelectasis or in the prevention of postoperative atelectasis.[57, 69]

Bronchoscopy in patients with cystic fibrosis and lobar atelectasis did not significantly ameliorate the atelectasis.[70] Successful insufflation of an area of atelectasis in adults by means of a Swan-Ganz catheter passed through a flexible fiberoptic bronchoscope has been reported.[71] Instillation of acetylcysteine through a bronchoscope was reported by Perruchoud and colleagues[72] in 51 adult patients who had mucoid impaction; the atelectasis improved in 94% of the patients, although it recurred in 16%.

When surgery is used in the treatment of atelectasis, it is directed toward removal of the underlying cause, such as tumors or granulation tissue. Wood and co-workers reported the resection of acquired bronchial stenosis by an argon laser in four infants. This method may prove to be a useful adjunct or an alternative to surgery in children who have atelectasis that is caused by certain obstructive lesions.[73] Surgical removal of the affected lobe is a method that has been used in selected patients. Billig and Darling reported that bronchograms were important in selecting patients for surgery. They suggested that resection may benefit patients with right middle-lobe atelectasis who had abnormal bronchograms.[74]

Antibiotics currently are reserved for those patients who have demonstrated infections of the atelectatic area. Drinkwater and associates showed that in a pig model of atelectasis, there is decreased bacterial clearance.[75] Frederick and Pesanti showed in a rat model that the decreased clearance of bacteria may be related to the alterations in alveolar stability.[76] Although these studies suggested an increased likelihood of infection, there is no clinical evidence that this infection represents a significant problem in children who have atelectasis.

REFERENCES

1. Lecks HI, Whitney T, Wood D, Kravis LP: Newer concepts in occurrence of segmental atelectasis in acute bronchial asthma and status asthmaticus in children. J Asthma Res 4:65–74, 1966.
2. Brooks LJ, Cloutier MM, Afshani E: Significance of roentgenographic abnormalities in children hospitalized for asthma. Chest 82:315–318, 1982.
3. Maxwell GM: The problem of mucus plugging in children with asthma. J Asthma 22:131–137, 1985.
4. Muller W, Von der Hardt H, Rieger CH: Diagnostic implications and treatment of massive spontaneous atelectasis in childhood. Pediatr Pulmonol 2:65–69, 1986.
5. Schloss MD, Pham-Dang H, Rosales JK: Foreign bodies in the tracheobronchial tree—A retrospective study of 217 cases. J Otolaryngol 12:212–216, 1983.
6. Aytac A, Yurdakul Y, Ikizler C, et al: Inhalation of foreign bodies in children. J Thorac Cardiovasc Surg 74:145–151, 1977.
7. Waring WW, Brunt CH, Hilman BC: Mucoid impaction of the bronchi in cystic fibrosis. Pediatrics 39:166–175, 1967.
8. James U, Brimblecombe FSW, Wells JW: The natural history of pulmonary collapse in childhood. Q J Med 25:121–136, 1956.
9. Quinn SF, Erickson S, Oshman D, Hayden F: Lobar collapse with respiratory syncytial virus pneumonitis. Pediatr Radiol 15:229–230, 1985.
10. Reines HD, Sade RM, Bradford BF, Marshall J: Chest physiotherapy fails to prevent postoperative atelectasis in children after cardiac surgery. Ann Surg 195:451–455, 1982.
11. Schmidt-Nowara WW, Altman AR: Atelectasis and neuromuscular respiratory failure. Chest 85:792–795, 1984.
12. Moylan FM, Shannon DC: Preferential distribution of lobar emphysema and atelectasis in bronchopulmonary dysplasia. Pediatrics 63:130–134, 1979.
13. Whitfield JM, Jones MD Jr: Atelectasis associated with mechanical ventilation for hyaline membrane disease. Crit Care Med 8:729–731, 1980.
14. Stanger P, Lucas RV, Edwards JE: Anatomic factors causing respiratory distress in acyanotic congenital cardiac disease. Pediatrics 43:760–769, 1969.
15. Montgomery DP, Partridge JB: Vascular rings causing pulmonary collapse. Clin Radiol 32:277–280, 1981.
16. Danis RK: Tracheal diverticulum with recurrent apnea and segmental pulmonary atelectasis. J Pediatr Surg 17:182–183, 1982.
17. Iannaccone G, Capocaccia P, Colloridi V, Roggini M: Double right tracheal bronchus: A case report in an infant. Pediatr Radiol 13:156–158, 1983.
18. Wellons HA, Eggleston P, Golden GT, Allen MS: Bronchial adenoma in childhood. Am J Dis Child 130:301–304, 1976.
19. Mak H, Metz SJ, Stokes DC, et al: Recurrent wheezing and massive atelectasis in an adolescent. J Pediatr 102:955–962, 1983.
20. Dale WA, Rahn H: Rate of gas absorption during atelectasis. Am J Physiol 170:606–615, 1952.
21. Ford GT, Bradley CA, Anthonisen NR: Forces involved in lobar atelectasis in intact dogs. J Appl Physiol 48:29–33, 1980.
22. Fung YC: Stress, deformation, and atelectasis of the lung. Circ Res 37:481–496, 1975.
23. Hedenstierna G, Brismar B, Strandberg A, et al: New aspects on atelectasis during anaesthesia. Clin Physiol 3:127–131, 1985.
24. Leblanc P, Ruff F, Milic-Emili J: Effects of age and body position on "airway closure" in man. J Appl Physiol 28:448–451, 1970.
25. Mead J, Collier C: Relation of volume history of lungs to respiratory mechanics in anesthetized dogs. J Appl Physiol 14:669–678, 1959.
26. Bendixen HH, Hedley-Whyte J, Laver MB, Chir B: Impaired oxygenation in surgical patients during general anesthesia with controlled ventilation. N Engl J Med 269:991–996, 1963.
27. DuBois A, Turaids T, Mammen RE, Nobrega FT: Pulmonary atelectasis in subjects breathing oxygen at sea level or at simulated altitude. J Appl Physiol 21:828–836, 1966.
28. Ford GT, Whitelaw WA, Rosenal TW, et al: Diaphragm function after upper abdominal surgery in humans. Am Rev Respir Dis 127:431–436, 1983.
29. Avery ME, Mead J: Surface properties in relation to atelectasis and hyaline membrane disease. Am J Dis Child 97:517–523, 1959.
30. Clark DA, Nieman GF, Thompson JE, et al: Surfactant displacement by meconium free fatty acids: An alternative explanation for atelectasis in meconium aspiration syndrome. J Pediatr 110:765–770, 1987.
31. Pirlo AF, Benumof JL, Trousdale FR: Atelectatic lobe blood flow: Open vs. closed chest, positive pressure vs. spontaneous ventilation. J Appl Physiol 50:1022–1026, 1981.
32. Thomas HM, Garrett RC: Strength of hypoxic vasoconstriction determines shunt fraction in dogs with atelectasis. J Appl Physiol: Respir Environ Exercise Physiol 53:44–51, 1982.
33. McFarlane PA, Gardaz JP, Sykes MK: CO_2 and mechanical factors reduce blood flow in a collapsed lung lobe. J Appl Physiol 57:739–743, 1984.
34. Chen L, Williams JJ, Alexander CM, et al: The effect of pleural pressure on the hypoxic pulmonary vasoconstrictor response in closed chest dogs. Anesth Analg 67:763–769, 1988.
35. Brock RC, Cann RJ, Dickinson JR: Tuberculous mediastinal lymphadenitis in childhood: Secondary effects on the lungs. Guy's Hospital Report 87:295–317, 1937.
36. Culiner MM: The right middle lobe syndrome, a non-obstructive complex. Dis Chest 50:57–66, 1966.
37. Inners CR, Terry PB, Traystman RJ, Menkes HA: Collateral ventilation and the middle lobe syndrome. Am Rev Respir Dis 118:305–310, 1978.
38. Proto AV, Tocino I: Radiographic manifestations of lobar collapse. Semin Roentgenol 15:117–173, 1980.
39. Davis LA: The vertical fissure line. Pediatr Radiol 84:451–453, 1959.
40. Lacombe P, Lallemand D, Garel L, Sauvegrain J: Pulmonary vascular nodules: New sign of left lower lobe collapse in children. AJR 139:873–878, 1982.
41. Woodring JH: Determining the cause of pulmonary atelectasis: A comparison of plain radiography and CT. AJR 150:757–763, 1988.
42. Malmgren N, Laurin S, Ivancev K, Bekassy A: Mediastinal pseudomass: Pneumonia and atelectasis behind the left pulmonary ligament. Pediatr Radiol 17:451–453, 1987.
43. Adler J, Camerson DC: CT correlation in peripheral right upper lobe collapse. J Comput Assist Tomogr 12:510–511, 1988.
44. Flanagan JJ, Flower CD, Dixon AK: Compensatory emphysema shown by computed tomography. Clin Radiol 33:553–554, 1982.
45. Naidich DP, McCauley DI, Khouri NF, et al: Computed tomography of lobar collapse: 1. Endobronchial obstruction. J Comput Assist Tomogr 7:745–757, 1983.
46. Schlesinger AE, Smith MB, Genez BM, et al: Chest wall mesenchymoma (hamartoma) in infancy. CT and MR findings. Pediatr Radiol 19:212–213, 1989.
47. Tallroth K, Kiviranta K: Round atelectasis. Respiration 45:71–77, 1984.
48. Doyle TC, Lawler GA: CT features of rounded atelectasis of the lung. AJR 143:225–228, 1984.
49. Leone A, Danza FM, Vincenzoni M, et al: Rounded atelectasis: Consideration on its radiological diagnosis. Diagn Imaging Clin Med 55:293–300, 1986.
50. Erasmie U, Lundell B: Pulmonary lesions mimicking pericardial effusion on ultrasonography. Pediatr Radiol 17:447–450, 1987.
51. Morin C, Filiatrault D, Russo P: Pulmonary sequestration with histologic changes of cystic adenomatoid malformation. Pediatr Radiol 19:130–132, 1989.
52. Lanning P, Heikkinen E: Thymus simulating left upper lobe atelectasis. Pediatr Radiol 9:177–178, 1980.
53. Seibert RW, Seibert JJ, Williamson SL: The opaque chest: When to suspect a bronchial foreign body. Pediatr Radiol 16:193–196, 1986.
54. Bateman JR, Newman SP, Daunt KM, et al: Regional lung clear-

ance of excessive bronchial secretions during chest physiotherapy in patients with stable chronic airways obstruction. Lancet 1:294–297, 1979.

55. Finer NN, Moriartey RR, Boyd J, et al: Postextubation atelectasis: A retrospective review and a prospective controlled study. J Pediatr 94:110–113, 1979.

56. Morran CG, Finlay IG, Mathieson M, et al: Randomized controlled trial of physiotherapy for postoperative pulmonary complications. Br J Anaesth 55(11):1113–1117, 1983.

57. Marini JJ, Pierson DJ, Hudson LD: Acute lobar atelectasis: A prospective comparison of fiberoptic bronchoscopy and respiratory therapy. Am Rev Respir Dis 119:971–978, 1979.

58. Hardy KA, Wolfson MR, Schidlow DV, Shaffer TH: Mechanics and energetics of breathing in newly diagnosed infants with cystic fibrosis: Effect of combined bronchodilator and chest physical therapy. Pediatr Pulmonol 6:103–108, 1989.

59. Iverson LI, Ecker RR, Fox HE, May IA: A comparative study of IPPB, the incentive spirometer, and blow bottles: The prevention of atelectasis following cardiac surgery. Ann Thorac Surg 25:197–200, 1978.

60. Krastins I, Corey ML, McLeod A, et al: An evaluation of incentive spirometry in the management of pulmonary complications after cardiac surgery in a pediatric population. Crit Care Med 10:525–528, 1982.

61. Paul WL, Downs JB: Postoperative atelectasis: Intermittent positive pressure breathing, incentive spirometry, and face-mask positive end-expiratory pressure. Arch Surg 116:861–863, 1981.

62. Duncan SR, Negrin RS, Mihm FG, et al: Nasal continuous positive airway pressure in atelectasis. Chest 92:621–624, 1987.

63. O'Donohue WJ Jr: National survey of the usage of lung expansion modalities for the prevention and treatment of postoperative atelectasis following abdominal and thoracic surgery. Chest 87:76–80, 1985.

64. Galvis AG, White JJ, Oh KS: A bedside washout technique for atelectasis in infants. Am J Dis Child 127:824–827, 1974.

65. Rode H, Millar AJ, Stunden RJ, Cywes S: Selective bronchial intubation for acute post-operative atelectasis in neonates and infants. Pediatr Radiol 18:494–496, 1988.

66. Nussbaum E: Pediatric flexible bronchoscopy and its application in infantile atelectasis. Clin Pediatr 24:379–382, 1985.

67. Fitzpatrick SB, Marsh B, Stokes D, Wang KP: Indications for flexible fiberoptic bronchoscopy in pediatric patients. Am J Dis Child 137:595–597, 1983.

68. Levy M, Glick B, Springer C, et al: Bronchoscopy and bronchography in children. Experience with 110 investigations. Am J Dis Child 137:14–16, 1983.

69. Jaworski A, Goldberg SK, Walkenstein MD, et al: Utility of immediate postlobectomy fiberoptic bronchoscopy in preventing atelectasis. Chest 94:38–43, 1988.

70. Stern RC, Boat TF, Orenstein DM, et al: Treatment of prognosis of lobar and segmental atelectasis in cystic fibrosis. Am Rev Respir Dis 118:821–826, 1978.

71. Lee TS, Wright BD: Selective insufflation of collapsed lung with fiberoptic bronchoscopy and Swan-Ganz catheter. Intensive Care Med 7(5):241–243, 1981.

72. Perruchoud A, Ehrsam R, Heitz M, et al: Atelectasis of the lung: Bronchoscopic lavage with acetylcysteine. Experience in 51 patients. Eur J Respir Dis Suppl 111:163–168, 1980.

73. Wood RE, Azizkhan RG, Powers SK: Use of an argon laser to resect acquired bronchial stenosis in infants. Am Rev Respir Dis 37(Suppl):15, 1988.

74. Billig DM, Darling DB: Middle lobe atelectasis in children. Clinical and bronchographic criteria in the selection of patients for surgery. Am J Dis Child 123:96–98, 1972.

75. Drinkwater DC Jr, Wittnich C, Mulder DS, et al: Mechanical and cellular bacterial clearance in lung atelectasis. Ann Thorac Surg 32:235–243, 1981.

76. Frederick D, Pesanti EL: Intrapulmonary growth of *staphylococcus aureus* in rats during induced atelectasis. Infect Immun 55:2747–2753, 1987.

51 BRONCHOPULMONARY DYSPLASIA

BRAD E. ALPERT, M.D. / JULIAN L. ALLEN, M.D. / DANIEL V. SCHIDLOW, M.D.

Bronchopulmonary dysplasia (BPD) is a chronic lung disease that develops in some neonates who are exposed to positive airway pressure and high oxygen tension during the first week of life. This disease was originally recognized in 1967 by Northway and co-workers,[1] who described a group of premature infants with hyaline membrane disease (HMD) that followed an atypical course. Instead of the normal improvement at 2 to 4 days and complete resolution by 1 week of life, physical and radiographic evidence of pulmonary abnormalities persisted. Since then, BPD has been reported in full-term newborns and after other neonatal diseases, such as apnea, meconium aspiration, pneumonia, and congenital heart disease.[2]

Unfortunately, there is still no universally accepted definition of BPD.[3] The confusion results from the lack of a well-defined cause or specific diagnostic tests for this disease. Bancalari and associates recommend making the diagnosis of BPD when an infant requires positive-pressure ventilation for at least 3 days in the first week of life, has clinical signs of respiratory distress, requires supplemental oxygen to maintain an arterial oxygen tension (Pa_{O_2}) of 50 mm Hg for more than 28 days, and has radiographic evidence of BPD.[4] Tooley's criteria for the diagnosis of BPD include radiographic abnormalities at 30 days of age and at least one of the following: (1) a Pa_{O_2} of 60 mm Hg or less in room air; (2) an arterial carbon dioxide tension (Pa_{CO_2}) higher than 45 mm Hg; or (3) oxygen dependency.[5] Other authors have defined BPD as chronic lung disease in low-birth-weight infants who are respirator-dependent or oxygen-dependent at 1 month of age or older, regardless of radiographic changes.[6, 7]

The reported incidence of BPD ranges from 2.4% to 68%, with the overall approximation of 20% among premature infants with HMD.[2, 8] (Because HMD occurs at a rate of approximately 10 per 1000 live births, the overall incidence of BPD is approximately 2 per 1000 live births.) This range is broad as a result of several factors. First, the diagnostic criteria for BPD are not uniform and are often subjective. For example, oxygen dependency may not be defined objectively by a minimally acceptable Pa_{O_2}. Second, most studies are flawed by a selection bias, because patients at one institution may not be representative of the entire population at risk. Third, infants in whom BPD is developing and who die before the age of 1 month are often excluded from studies. Fourth, stratification for birth weight, sex, race, and site of the delivery (inside or outside the reporting institution) is often omitted. Fifth, treatment regimens, which vary widely among institutions, might affect the incidence.

In 1986, Farrell and Palta surveyed 16 neonatal intensive care units (NICUs) and found that the incidence of BPD varied from 3% to 33% (mean, 7%) of all premature infants and from 6% to 50% (mean, 20%) of those with HMD.[2] Transportation from another hospital had no effect on the incidence. Avery and colleagues retrospectively studied 1625 infants with birth weights between 700 and 1500 g who required supplemental oxygen at 28 days of age at eight major NICUs to determine whether the incidence of BPD differs among centers when birth weight, race, and sex are taken into consideration.[6] The percentage of survivors requiring oxygen at 28 days ranged from 21% to 42% and was highly dependent on birth weight. The group from Columbia Presbyterian Medical Center, which had the lowest incidence, instituted continuous positive airway pressure (CPAP) at 5 cm of water (H_2O) with nasal prongs soon after birth in all infants with respiratory distress. Hyperventilation was avoided, and endotracheal intubation was not performed until the Pa_{CO_2} rose to 60 mm Hg. This was the only center in which muscle relaxants were never used. In two other institutions in which the outcomes were worse, intubation and positive end-expiratory pressure were used from birth. Avery and colleagues[6] speculated that the decreased dependence on intubation at Columbia facilitated normal mucociliary clearance and lessened the possibility of airway injury, secondary infection, and aspiration. They concluded that the incidence of BPD does vary among centers and that differences in treatment regimens may account for some of the variation.

Kraybill and co-workers surveyed the outcome of 1095 (95.5%) of the 1147 infants (1.3 per 1000 live births) born in North Carolina in 1984 with birth weights of 501 to 1500 g.[7] Because this study was based on a well-defined population, selection bias was minimized. The incidence of BPD varied inversely with birth weight and widely among the 10 NICUs in the study. Because 22% of all infants weighing less than 1500 g acquired BPD, the overall incidence was 2.8 per 1000 live births. Only two thirds of the variation in outcome at 30 days could be explained by an unequal distribution of birth weights among the NICUs; therefore, Kraybill and co-workers also concluded that differences in treatment are important factors contributing to the development of this disease.

BPD is the most common chronic lung disease of childhood with the exception of asthma. The incidence is about 2 to 3 per 1000 live births and is highly dependent on birth weight. Among newborns who were intubated and who survived for 30 days, BPD developed in about 25% of those with birth weights between 1000 and 1500 g, 70% with birth weights between 700 and 1000 g, and almost 100% with birth weights of less than 700 g.[6, 7] The wide variation in its incidence among centers can be accounted for, at least in part, by differences in treatment regimens.[6]

PATHOGENESIS

The pathogenesis of BPD has been primarily attributed to oxygen toxicity and barotrauma. Oxygen toxicity is mediated through the production of hydrogen peroxide and oxygen free radicals, including singlet oxygen, superoxide, and the hydroxyl radical. (A free radical is an atom or molecule that has an unpaired electron in its outer orbit, which makes it highly reactive.) Oxygen radicals normally originate from several sources including the cytosol, mitochondria, endoplasmic reticulum, plasma and nuclear membranes, and peroxisomes,[9] and hyperoxia results in increased production. Fox and collaborators[10] postulated that alveolar macrophages are stimulated by hyperoxia to release chemotaxins for neutrophils that accumulate in the lung and release oxygen radicals.

Oxygen radicals can injure and kill cells by reacting with several cellular constituents. DNA and proteins with sulfhydryl-containing amino acids exposed in their tertiary structure are susceptible to damage. Probably the most important injury is lipid peroxidation of membrane polyunsaturated fatty acids, which results in the loss of membrane function and, eventually, of cellular integrity. The pathologic changes of oxygen toxicity in animal models are very similar to those of BPD.[11]

Cells have mechanisms to defend themselves against free radical damage. Cytochrome oxidase reduces oxygen without releasing large numbers of radicals. Superoxide can be eliminated by superoxide dismutases; glutathione peroxidase and catalase eliminate hydrogen peroxide and lipid peroxides. Vitamin E and ceruloplasmin also function as antioxidants. Injury occurs when these mechanisms are overwhelmed by excessive production of oxygen radicals. Oxygen toxicity has been the subject of several reviews.[9, 11-13]

Positive airway pressure has also been implicated in the pathogenesis of BPD; however, it is difficult to isolate its effects from oxygen toxicity. Both of these modalities were used together in most infants in whom BDP developed. Findings in several retrospective studies have implicated high airway pressure;[14-16] however, positive airway pressure has not been shown to contribute to the development of BPD in prospective studies in which investigators have controlled for other variables that might influence the outcome.[17-19]

Although the role of airway pressure in the pathogenesis of parenchymal damage in BPD remains controversial, substantial data support its role in the development

Table 51-1. THE POTENTIAL EFFECTS OF UNDERNUTRITION IN PREMATURE NEWBORNS OF VERY LOW BIRTH WEIGHT

Condition	Result
Poor caloric/energy reserves	Early onset of catabolic state
Respiratory distress syndrome	Inhibited/delayed surfactant production; decrease in respiratory muscle function
Effects on protection from hyperoxia/barotrauma	Decreases in epithelial integrity (vitamin A), defense against oxygen free radicals and lipid peroxidation (decreases in quantity of antioxidant enzymes, vitamin E stores, and PUFA in comparison with term infants), and lung biosynthesis/cell replication for repair of injury
Effects on lung repair and development of BPD	Decreases in lung biosynthesis, replacement of damaged cells, and replacement of damaged extracellular components (collagen, elastin)
Effects on lung growth	Decreases in lung biosynthesis/cell replication and lung structural maturation (alveolarization)
Effects on susceptibility to infection	Decreases in cellular, humoral defenses against pathogens, epithelial cell integrity, and clearance mechanisms

Adapted from Frank L, Sosenko IRS: Undernutrition as a major contributing factor in the pathogenesis of bronchopulmonary dysplasia. Am Rev Respir Dis 138:725–729, 1988.
PUFA, polyunsaturated fatty acid; BPD, bronchopulmonary dysplasia.

of airway damage. Nilsson demonstrated necrosis of the bronchial epithelium in premature rabbits after positive-pressure ventilation without supplemental oxygen.[19] Ackerman and associates observed pulmonary interstitial emphysema in premature baboons with HMD that received positive-pressure ventilation.[20] This occurred because these airways were more compliant than those containing the surfactant-deficient alveoli.

Bhutani and colleagues demonstrated that neonatal airways may be more susceptible to barotrauma because they are more compliant than adult airways.[21, 22] Panitch and co-authors compared the mechanics of airway smooth muscle from premature and adult sheep; they showed that immature smooth muscle was more compliant, generated less force when maximally stimulated, and had decreased acetylcholine-receptor sensitivity.[23] These properties may explain the propensity of premature infants who receive positive-pressure ventilation to acquire airway lesions, such as tracheomegaly and tracheomalacia.

Other factors have also been implicated in the pathogenesis of BPD. *Ureaplasma urealyticum,* which is commonly found in vaginal flora during pregnancy, can be transmitted to premature infants. Studies have demonstrated that this organism may cause a chronic subclinical pneumonia resulting in increased ventilation and oxygen requirements;[24, 25] however, its role in the development of BPD remains unclear. Persistence of a patent ductus arteriosus has been suspected to increase the risk of developing BPD. In a randomized, controlled trial in infants who weighed 1000 g or less, Cassady and associates did not find a decrease in the incidence when ductal ligation was performed during the first 24 h of life.[26] Pulmonary edema secondary to capillary leakage or to excessive fluid administration, pulmonary interstitial emphysema, and a family history of asthma have also been associated with the development of BPD.[27-29]

Cytomegalovirus is another infectious agent that has been implicated in the pathogenesis of BPD in some infants. Sawyer and colleagues studied 32 infants with acquired cytomegalovirus infection; twenty-four (75%) of these infants showed radiographic evidence of BPD in comparison with 12 (38%) of 32 control infants.[30]

Compromised nutritional status in the premature infant may contribute to the development of BPD.[31] Infants of very low birth weight have meager nonprotein energy reserves in comparison with normal-term newborns. Adequate protein and calories are required for cell growth, division, and repair. In addition, many other nutrients (including vitamins A and E) and trace minerals (such as iron, copper, zinc, selenium, and others) accumulate to a large extent during the third trimester of gestation. Copper, zinc, iron, and selenium are required cofactors for antioxidant enzymes, such as superoxide dismutase and glutathione peroxidase; however, the effect of deficiencies of these metals or antioxidants in the pathogenesis of BPD has not been studied extensively.[32, 33]

Vitamin E may provide additional antioxidant protection. In studies of animals, vitamin E deficiency increased the risk of oxygen toxicity, but pharmacologic doses provided no more protection than normal nutritional sources. In a controlled study of infants, vitamin E supplementation was not shown to be protective; however, the control group was not evaluated for vitamin E deficiency. Therefore, vitamin E supplementation may decrease the risk of oxygen toxicity only in vitamin E–deficient infants.[34] Table 51-1 summarizes the potential effect of undernutrition in infants of very low birth weight.

Premature infants have been shown to be deficient in retinol, the major circulating form of vitamin A, and its transport protein, retinol-binding protein. Vitamin A is essential for differentiation, integrity, and repair of respiratory epithelial cells, and a deficiency is characterized by loss of cilia and squamous metaplasia.[35] Hustead and associates found that the concentration of retinol at birth was lower in infants in whom BPD developed than in those in whom it did not.[36] Shenai and colleagues demonstrated that intramuscular supplementation of vitamin A to mechanically ventilated infants with HMD reduced the incidence of BPD.[37] These preliminary data indicate that vitamin A deficiency may play a substantial role in the pathogenesis of BPD.

Stocker speculated that the focal nature of the septal fibrosis in BPD might be accounted for by varying degrees of occlusion of small airways by necrotizing bronchiolitis.[38] The parenchyma distal to an unobstructed airway

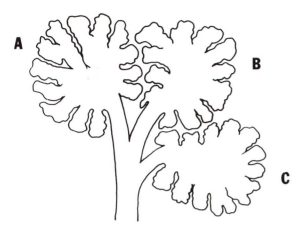

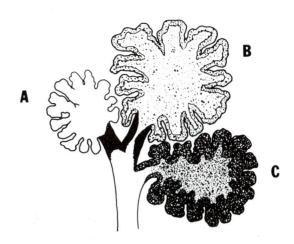

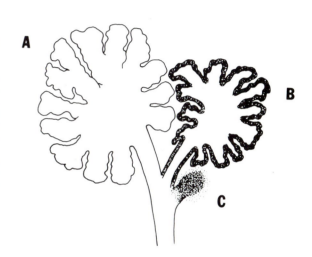

Figure 51–1. *Top left,* schematic drawing of normally expanded and aerated pulmonary lobules. *Top right,* acute bronchopulmonary dysplasia. *A,* Necrotizing bronchiolitis occludes the bronchiolar lumen, "protecting" the parenchyma distal to it from the high oxygen tension and pressure used in maintaining adequate oxygenation. *B,* The bronchiole is narrowed by mucosal hyperplasia and muscular hypertrophy, thereby reducing the amount of pressure and oxygen tension in the lobule distal to it. Alveolar cell hyperplasia, septal fibroplasia, and alveolar macrophage dysplasia, however, occur to a mild to moderate degree. *C,* The bronchiole is widely patent, exposing the distal sublobule to the full ventilatory pressure and oxygen tension. The alveolar lumina are largely obliterated by alveolar macrophages, alveolar cell hyperplasia, and marked septal fibroplasia. *Bottom right,* long-standing "healed" bronchopulmonary dysplasia (LSHBPD). *A,* With resolution of the necrotizing bronchiolitis that occluded the lumen of the bronchiole, the uninjured sublobule overexpands to compensate for the less expansile injured portions of lung (*B* and *C*). *B,* With resolution of the mild to moderate injury incurred by the parenchyma during the acute stages of bronchopulmonary dysplasia, the sublobule displays the hallmark of LSHBPD: septal fibrosis. *C,* The sublobule is virtually obliterated by organization of the severe acute bronchopulmonary dysplasia. (From Stocker JT: Pathologic features of long-standing "healed" bronchopulmonary dysplasia: A study of 28 3- to 40-month old infants. Hum Pathol 17:943–961, 1986.)

becomes most severely damaged because it is not protected from barotrauma and oxygen toxicity. A partially occluded bronchus affords some protection, resulting in less damage. When the airway is completely occluded, the parenchyma remains normal, and the airway eventually recanalizes[38] (Fig. 51–1).

PATHOLOGY

The pathologic features of BPD were first reported by Northway and co-workers[1] and have been further elucidated by several investigators.[8, 39–41] The morphologic findings can be separated into four overlapping stages.

Stage I (2 to 3 days) is the period of acute respiratory distress syndrome (RDS). HMD and RDS are synonymous. Hyaline membranes, hyperemia, atelectasis, and dilatation of lymphatic vessels are seen. There is metaplasia and necrosis of the bronchiolar mucosa and some patchy loss of ciliated epithelial cells.

Stage II (4 to 10 days) is the period of regeneration. There are persistent hyaline membranes, with necrosis and regeneration of the alveolar epithelium by type II pneumocytes. Early epithelialization of hyaline membranes by these cells is also seen. Septal walls are thick-

ened by edema and early fibroblastic proliferation. Nodular fibrotic foci, suggesting organization of alveolar exudation, and emphysematous coalescence of alveoli are frequently present. Bronchiolar mucosal necrosis and metaplasia become more pronounced, and eosinophilic deposits are seen in some airways. Obliterative bronchiolitis may occur and has been associated with cystic bronchiectasis. There is focal thickening of the capillary basement membrane, with replication of the pericapillary reticulum.

Stage III (10 to 20 days) is the period of transition to chronic disease. Fewer hyaline membranes are seen, and there is continued injury of alveolar epithelial cells with regeneration by type II pneumocytes. The septal walls are thickened by residual edema, fibrosis, and proliferation of myofibroblasts. Alveolar coalescence progresses to spheric groups of emphysematous alveoli, with surrounding atelectatic alveoli. There are widespread bronchial and bronchiolar mucosal metaplasia and hyperplasia. Bronchiolitis obliterans and cystic bronchiectasis may develop. Moderate amounts of alveolar macrophages and histiocytes are noted in the airways, along with large amounts of mucous secretions.

Stage IV (after 1 month) is the period of chronic disease. Capillaries are markedly separated from the alveolar epithelia by deposition of collagen and elastin fibers in the alveolar septa. Emphysematous alveoli are noted in association with marked smooth muscle hypertrophy in the bronchioles, whereas more normal airways are seen with areas of atelectasis. Alveolar epithelial cells are markedly heterotypic, and macrophages, histiocytes, and foam cells are increased. There are some perimucosal fibrosis and many areas of mucosal sloughing and metaplasia. Tortuous lymphatic vessels and early vascular changes of pulmonary hypertension are seen.

Stocker reported the pathologic features of BPD in infants 3 to 40 months old.[38] He found alveolar septal fibrosis to be the main residual feature. It involved less than 10% to as much as 75% of the parenchyma and was highly focal in nature; some areas were completely spared. Bronchial and bronchiolar muscular hyperplasia, glandular hyperplasia, and mild to moderate pulmonary hypertensive vascular disease were also present.

RADIOGRAPHIC MANIFESTATIONS

The radiographic manifestations of BPD, as first described by Northway and colleagues,[1] were divided into the same four stages as for the pathologic features; however, the stages are now rarely seen as such distinct entities. In stage I, the chest radiograph showed the typical pattern of HMD, with a generalized granular pattern and air bronchograms. Both lung fields were nearly completely opacified in stage II. In stage III, there were small, round, lucent areas that alternated with areas of irregular density, and the air bronchograms disappeared. In stage IV, there was enlargement of the radiolucent areas with thinner strands of radiodensity, hyperinflation, and frequently cardiomegaly.

The orderly progression of BPD through these stages is now uncommonly seen.[42] Because stage II rarely occurs, this radiographic appearance should suggest another process, such as pulmonary edema or hemorrhage. Stage III is infrequently seen as well and may develop without a period of parenchymal opacity. Stage IV is now often manifested by less marked hyperinflation and multiple fine, lacy densities rather than dense streaks and large lucencies. Cardiomegaly is generally less prominent.

Mortensson and Lindroth described the radiographic course of BPD for the first 4 to 6 years of life.[43] Of the 38 patients observed, 11 (29%) exhibited complete resolution of the initial pulmonary lesions. There was improvement in 26 (68%), and the condition worsened in 1 patient. The majority of the resolution occurred during the first year after termination of mechanical ventilation. Two of the 10 patients with early radiographic evidence of mild disease and 11 of the 14 with moderate to severe initial radiographic changes had abnormal chest radiographs (interstitial fibrosis or hyperinflation) at the end of the study. Other authors found similar progressive improvement in chest radiographs[44] (Fig. 51–2).

When the chest radiograph does not show a course that is generally improving over time, complications such as chronic aspiration, unrecognized or inadequately treated heart failure, airway lesions, and poorly controlled reactive airway disease should be considered.

LUNG MECHANICS AND PULMONARY FUNCTION TESTS

The pathologic changes in the parenchyma and airways of infants with BPD lead to functional abnormalities that have been quantitated by pulmonary function tests. With increased availability of infant pulmonary function testing, a number of studies of lung mechanics in BPD have appeared in the medical literature. However, comparisons are often difficult because the methodologies vary from study to study. Therefore, it is worthwhile to organize the data by the various techniques that have been used.

LUNG VOLUMES

Comparisons of lung volumes in BPD infants younger than 6 months relative to those of normal full-term and preterm controls yielded conflicting results. For example, Morray and associates[45] and Tepper and associates[46] found the mean functional residual capacity (FRC) (corrected for body weight) in 2- to 4-month-old infants with BPD to be 70% of that of control infants. Similarly, Bryan found FRC (corrected for body length) in BPD infants to be 60% of that of normal controls and 80% of that of infants with HMD who required ventilation but in whom BPD did not develop.[47] On the other hand, Kao and associates found that thoracic gas volume (TGV) was 20% to 50% higher in 2- to 3-month-old infants with BPD than in normal controls.[48–50] This discrepancy may have resulted from the use of different methods to measure lung volumes. Kao and co-workers used body plethysmography, whereas investigators reporting low values used helium dilution, which can produce underestimates of lung volumes in the presence of airway obstruction.

Some investigators found FRC in BPD infants older than 6 months to be normal,[45, 51] whereas others showed it to be increased by up to 60%.[47] A similar shift from low to relatively high FRC with growth was reported by Gerhardt and colleagues, who demonstrated that FRC increased rapidly after the age of 6 months in a longitudinal study of 39 infants.[52]

In summary, most studies show that lung volumes are low early in infancy and become normal or elevated later in infancy. It is possible that the helium dilution measurement artifact mentioned previously may be present to a greater extent in younger infants, inasmuch as the severity of airway obstruction in these infants seems to diminish with growth. Therefore, lung volumes may be underestimated to a greater extent in early infancy. Alternatively, some authors have speculated that with time, pulmonary fibrosis may become less important relative to airway disease; therefore, lung volumes increase disproportionately with growth.[53]

PULMONARY AND RESPIRATORY SYSTEM COMPLIANCE

Dynamic pulmonary compliance, measured by the esophageal balloon technique,[54] has been shown to be

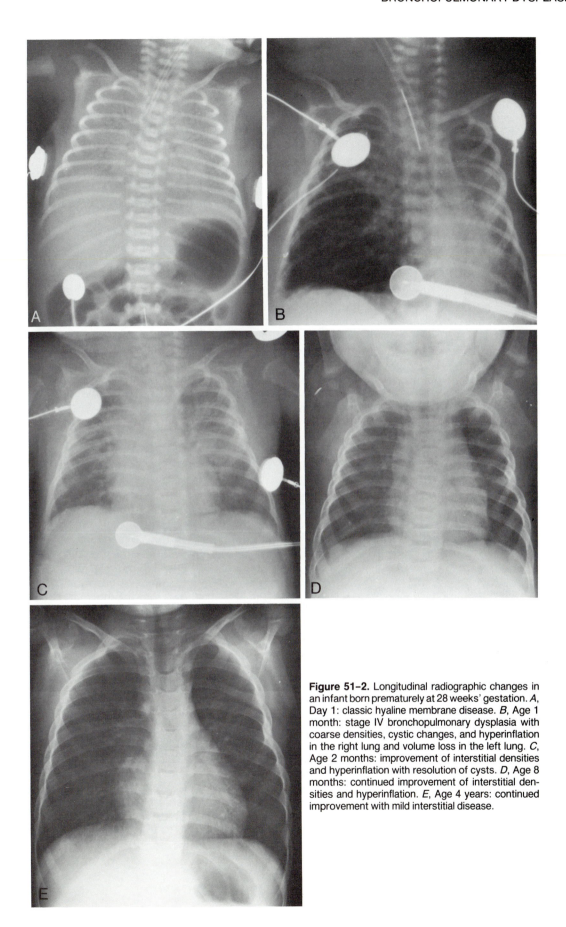

Figure 51–2. Longitudinal radiographic changes in an infant born prematurely at 28 weeks' gestation. *A*, Day 1: classic hyaline membrane disease. *B*, Age 1 month: stage IV bronchopulmonary dysplasia with coarse densities, cystic changes, and hyperinflation in the right lung and volume loss in the left lung. *C*, Age 2 months: improvement of interstitial densities and hyperinflation with resolution of cysts. *D*, Age 8 months: continued improvement of interstitial densities and hyperinflation. *E*, Age 4 years: continued improvement with mild interstitial disease.

decreased in young infants with BPD and to approach normal values with increasing age. Because pulmonary compliance is dependent on lung volume, the results of most studies are expressed as "specific" compliance (corrected for body weight, lung volume at FRC, or body length). Normal lung compliance is 1.2 to 2.0 ml/cm of H_2O/kg of body weight.[45, 52, 55] In studies of infants with BPD, authors have consistently reported dynamic specific compliance to be 30% to 50% of control values in infants 2 to 4 months of age.[45, 47, 52, 55] Because dynamic compliance measurements reflect not only lung tissue properties but also uneven distribution of ventilation to regions with differing time constants (frequency dependence of compliance), it is impossible to determine from these studies whether the diminished compliance is caused entirely by altered elastic properties of the lung parenchyma or by abnormal airway resistance.

Tepper and associates measured static compliance of the respiratory system by using the weighted spirometer technique in young (10 months postconceptional age) infants with BPD.[56] They, too, found compliance to be about 60% of control values. This suggests that changes in elastic properties alone can explain the low compliance seen in these infants, which is consistent with the pathologic hallmark of this disease, pulmonary fibrosis, as discussed previously.[38]

Results of one study suggested that the measurement of respiratory system compliance after the acute phase of HMD may have predictive value for the development of BPD.[57] In this study, the compliance of infants in whom BPD developed later was half that of those who did not develop BPD. As infants with BPD grow, a consistent pattern of improving specific compliance has been observed. Between the ages of 2 and 3 years, values of 80% to 90% of those of controls are seen.[45, 52]

AIRWAY FUNCTION

A hallmark of the injury to airways in patients with BPD is elevated airway resistance. Investigators have used the esophageal balloon technique[54] to measure pulmonary resistance and have reported values of more than twice those of controls in infants with BPD under 3 months of age.[45, 52, 55] Similarly, respiratory system resistance measured by the technique of passive expiratory flow-volume curves is elevated.[58] With growth, airflow resistance decreases. Gerhardt and associates found mean pulmonary resistance decreased from 160 to 33 cm H_2O/liter/sec between the ages of 1 and 36 months.[52] However, these data cannot distinguish the effects of lung and airway growth from resolution of airway obstruction per se. For this reason, a size-corrected evaluation of airway function, such as specific conductance (defined as the reciprocal of resistance divided by lung volume at FRC), is probably more useful. This is particularly important in the evaluation of a population of infants, such as those with BPD, in whom TGV may be low in early infancy and relatively high in later infancy (see previous discussion). Arad and co-workers measured specific conductance by plethysmography in 10-month-old infants with BPD and reported values of about 60% predicted.[51] In Gerhardt and co-authors' study, although resistance fell dramatically in the first 3 years of life, specific conductance rose only from 60% of predicted value to 70% predicted over the same time period.[52]

Tepper and associates[46] demonstrated a similar phenomenon by performing partial expiratory flow-volume curves and measuring size-corrected maximal flow rates at FRC (reported in units of FRCs/sec). Infants with BPD had flows that were 50% of control values at a mean postnatal age of 2 months. This value had not increased by the age of 10 months.

The anatomic sites of airflow obstruction in infants with BPD can be the central airways, the peripheral airways, or both. The previously mentioned studies concentrated on small-airway function. It is known that central airway function in infants with BPD can also be affected as a result of subglottic narrowing or acquired tracheobronchomalacia.[59-61] At present, there are no lung function tests that reliably distinguish central from peripheral airflow obstruction in these infants. McCubbin and colleagues[62] demonstrated large-airway collapse in BPD infants using computed tomographic scans of the chest; they found that the percentage of change in the tracheal cross-sectional area during tidal breathing was 63%, as opposed to 9% in control infants. There is some preliminary evidence that partial forced expiratory flow-volume curves contain information about central as well as peripheral airway function, and these curves may become useful in assessments of the central airways.[63, 64]

WORK OF BREATHING

In view of the foregoing abnormalities in mechanical properties of the respiratory system, it is not surprising that the work of breathing has been shown to be elevated in infants with BPD. Wolfson and associates[65] measured tidal breathing–pulmonary pressure-volume loops in infants with BPD and found work of breathing per minute to average 5.4 ± 0.65 kg cm/min/kg of body weight, roughly 10 times that of normal newborn infants.[54] Assuming a 4% mechanical efficiency of breathing,[66] this would require 5 kCal/kg of body weight per day to perform. Infants with BPD display inefficient ventilatory patterns, with markedly asynchronous chest wall motion.[67] Weinstein and Oh measured oxygen uptake and calculated that approximately an additional 10 kCal/kg/day were spent on work of breathing by infants with BPD in comparison with controls.[68] Thus in view of the fact that 25 kCal/kg/day of total caloric intake is allotted for growth,[69] it appears that the work of breathing in an infant with BPD may "steal" 20% to 40% of that amount. However, in two studies in which work of breathing and oxygen uptake were simultaneously measured in infants with BPD, a relationship between these two parameters was not shown.[70, 71] Thus the increased metabolic expenditure of infants with BPD may not be attributable to increased work of breathing alone.

AIRWAY REACTIVITY

The extent to which airflow obstruction in BPD is reversible by bronchodilators has been studied extensively and by a variety of methods. Infants without BPD who are younger than 18 months and who acquire viral infections and wheezing have in the past been regarded as having poor bronchodilator responsiveness. However, many studies have since called these conclusions into question. Infants with BPD have airway smooth muscle hypertrophy[72] and therefore might be expected to be more responsive to bronchodilator therapy. Results of many studies support this conjecture. Twenty percent to 30% decreases in airway, lung, and total respiratory system resistance have been reported in response to a variety of agents, including subcutaneous terbutaline,[73] nebulized metaproterenol,[74] salbutamol and ipratropium bromide,[58] and isoproterenol.[48] The early age (both postconceptional and postnatal) at which infants with BPD demonstrate bronchodilator responsiveness is remarkable. Gomez del Rio and associates demonstrated marked improvement in pulmonary resistance after isoetharine inhalation in infants as young as 3 days and whose gestational age was as low as 27 weeks.[72] Motoyama and colleagues measured maximal expiratory flow-volume curves in intubated infants and found significant improvement in maximal flows at low lung volumes after isoetharine inhalation in infants as young as 12 days and whose gestational age was as low as 26 weeks.[75]

Other agents have been shown to improve lung mechanics in infants with BPD; these include theophylline,[76] dexamethasone,[77] and both intravenous and oral diuretics.[49, 55, 78, 79] There is also evidence that diuretics and bronchodilators may have a synergistic effect in improving lung mechanics.[50]

The effect of hypoxia itself on airway function is often overlooked. Two studies demonstrated hypoxic airway constriction in infants with BPD.[80, 81]

LONG-TERM STUDIES

Long-term follow-up studies for children up to 6 to 10 years of age have been reported for children who had BPD as infants. The pulmonary function abnormalities of airway obstruction and airway hyperreactivity persist in these older children. Smythe and colleagues[82] reported the average vital capacity and forced expiratory volume in 1 sec (FEV_1) to be 70% and 67%, respectively, of the predicted values; the ratio of residual volume to total lung capacity (RV/TLC) averaged 41%, and two thirds of the children demonstrated abnormal bronchial reactivity in response to methacholine challenge. Wheeler and associates[83] reported that FVC and FEV_1 were low and that RV/TLC was high in children with a history of BPD in comparison with three height-matched control groups: (1) children with a history of prematurity and HMD, (2) children born prematurely without lung disease, and (3) normal term infants. These investigators found no significant differences in the lung function among the three control groups.[83] In contrast, Mansell and associates[84] found that children who had BPD did not have low FVC or FEV_1 or an elevated RV/TLC ratio in relation to controls who had had RDS or who were born prematurely without lung disease; however, they did find that the latter group of children had low FEV_1 in comparison with children born at term. Therefore, they speculated that the low

flow rates seen in older children with a history of BPD were related more to their prematurity per se than to either RDS or its treatment. It has been suggested that if prematurity is related to airflow obstruction, this obstruction may be modulated through increased airway reactivity. Bertrand and colleagues[29] found a markedly increased incidence of methacholine responsiveness among not only children who had a history of BPD but also children born prematurely without a history of lung disease. They demonstrated airway hyperreactivity in the full-term siblings and mothers of these infants, which suggests that familial airway hyperreactivity is very common in infants with BPD and may be a predisposing factor in the development of BPD.[29]

In summary, there are multiple abnormalities of lung function in infants with BPD. Lung volumes are low in early infancy but high in later infancy, and air trapping can persist into childhood. Compliance is low in infancy but normalizes with growth. Airway resistance is abnormal in infancy, and the work of breathing is elevated. Although airway function generally improves with growth, abnormalities persist into childhood. Abnormal airway reactivity is present from the onset of the development of BPD and persists into childhood in a large proportion of patients. Studies indicate that airway obstruction and airway hyperreactivity can persist into early adult life.[85]

LONG-TERM COMPLICATIONS OF BPD

Multiple disabilities can affect the child with BPD and have an impact on the family for years. Bonding is impaired because of prolonged hospitalization and frequent readmissions. Yu and associates found that 69% of these infants are readmitted during the first 2 years of life.[86] Many require complicated medical regimens, including bronchodilators and diuretics, aerosols, chest physiotherapy, apnea monitors, special diets, developmental programs, oxygen, and even mechanical ventilation at home. Noncompliance with therapy is a common problem because the parents become largely responsible for the complex medical and nursing needs of the child when discharged. The medical management of BPD is comprehensive, since it affects many organ systems (Table 51–2).

ASTHMA/REACTIVE AIRWAY DISEASE

Asthma/reactive airway disease is a frequent complication of BPD. This problem can develop very early in the neonatal period and continue for years. Once the infant leaves the nursery, the condition often causes exacerbations of respiratory symptoms and frequently leads to rehospitalization. Yu and associates found that wheezing developed in 13 (81%) of 16 hospital survivors with BPD during the first 2 years of life.[86] Smyth and collaborators evaluated nine children at a mean age of 8.4 years (range, 7.2 to 9.6 years). Six still had positive metacholine bronchoprovocation tests. Although asthma remained a common problem, symptoms had ameliorated with time.[82] Northway and colleagues studied 22 survivors with BPD

Table 51–2. LONG-TERM COMPLICATIONS ASSOCIATED WITH BRONCHOPULMONARY DYSPLASIA

Respiratory
Chronic respiratory distress
Respiratory acidosis
Bronchospasm
Recurrent pneumonia
Ventilator dependency
Tracheostomy
Subglottic stenosis
Tracheomegaly
Tracheomalacia
Bronchomalacia
Airway granulation tissue and pseudopolyps
Acquired lobar emphysema
Laryngospasm
Apnea
Atelectasis
Chronic hypoxemia
Sleep hypoxemia
Sudden death

Gastrointestinal
Gastroesophageal reflux
Aspiration
Behavioral feeding disorders
Oral movement disorder

Cardiovascular
Pulmonary hypertension
Right ventricular hypertrophy
Systemic hypertension
Left ventricular hypertrophy
Heart failure
Patent foramen ovale
Occult congenital heart disease
Systemic-to-pulmonary arterial shunts

Renal
Nephrocalcinosis

Neurologic
Developmental delay
Static encephalopathy
Progressive encephalopathy
Movement disorders
Seizures
Visual impairment
Hearing impairment
Oromotor feeding disorders

Metabolic
Metabolic alkalosis
Hypokalemia
Hypochloremia
Elevated metabolic rate
Failure to thrive
Rickets of prematurity

Table 51–3. CAUSES OF ACUTE DETERIORATION OR EXACERBATION OF RESPIRATORY SYMPTOMS IN INFANTS WITH BRONCHOPULMONARY DYSPLASIA

Aspiration
Atelectasis
Pneumonia
Respiratory syncytial virus infection
Bronchospasm
Tracheobronchomalacia
Laryngospasm
Endotracheal or tracheostomy tube complications
Subglottic stenosis
Seizure
Heart failure
Patent foramen ovale
Systemic-to-pulmonary artery shunts
Occult congenital heart disease

gastroesophageal reflux, and so it should be reserved for patients who have not responded adequately to other medications. Adequate oxygenation, with supplemental oxygen if required, should be ensured because hypoxia may exacerbate bronchoconstriction, as discussed previously.

Respiratory syncytial virus infection is a common exacerbating factor and may result in considerable morbidity, and even mortality, in infants with BPD. Groothuis and co-authors found that 11 (69%) of 16 infants with BPD who acquired this virus required hospitalization. All either were receiving home oxygen therapy or had received it within the past 3 months.[87] Infants with BPD have a more prolonged and severe course when infected with this virus, and ribavirin therapy is probably indicated for many of these infants.[88, 89]

Because the natural history of asthma and pulmonary functions in children with BPD is one of improvement over time, worsening of symptoms or pulmonary functions behooves the physician to search for additional causes for the deterioration (Table 51–3).

AIRWAY COMPLICATIONS

Endotracheal intubation and positive airway pressure can cause injury to the neonatal airway. After successful weaning from mechanical ventilation, extubation may fail because of upper airway obstruction resulting from subglottic edema, pseudomembranes, and stenosis.[90, 91] Excessive endotracheal tube size and prolonged or recurrent intubation increase the risk for these injuries. The necessity for reintubation because of subglottic edema may sometimes be avoided by treatment with racemic epinephrine and corticosteroids, although the latter medications are controversial.[92] Replacing the tube with a smaller one, which allows an air leakage, may permit the injury to resolve and subsequent extubation to be successful. If these maneuvers fail, surgical intervention with an anterior cricoidotomy, laryngotracheoplasty, or tracheostomy may be required.[93, 94]

The airway smooth muscle of premature infants is more compliant than that of term infants or adults.[23, 95, 96] Positive airway pressure can lead to dilatation of the tra-

at a mean age of 17.9 years (range, 13.9 to 23.1 years). Eleven still had pulmonary function tests indicative of asthma.[85]

Asthma and its management are discussed in Chapters 66 to 68. Many children with BPD have symptoms of severity sufficient to require chronic medications. The first-line drug is usually cromolyn sodium by inhalation. Beta-agonists may be added if needed. Theophylline has neurologic and cardiac side effects and can exacerbate

chea and bronchi, resulting in acquired tracheomegaly, tracheomalacia, bronchomalacia, and tracheal and bronchial stenosis.[59, 60, 97] Tracheomegaly results in an increase in the anatomic dead space and may be a factor in extubation failures because the minute ventilation required to maintain an adequate carbon dioxide tension and the work of breathing are increased. Tracheomegaly can be diagnosed from radiographic measurements of the trachea.[59] Tracheomalacia and bronchomalacia can cause wheezing, hyperinflation, atelectasis, and possibly cyanotic (BPD) spells.[60, 97]

It is important to auscultate over the trachea and larynx in order to differentiate large-airway sounds from bronchospasm. In the latter, heterophonous wheezes are heard over the peripheral lung fields. Extrathoracic tracheomalacia and subglottic narrowing produce inspiratory stridor, whereas intrathoracic tracheomalacia produces expiratory wheezes, which are often audible, relatively low-pitched, and usually less prominent when the infant is resting or sleeping. Auscultation reveals that the wheezing is loudest over the trachea, radiates to the periphery, and is homophonous. Tracheomalacia has been successfully treated with CPAP.[64, 98]

When an infant has both tracheomalacia and asthma, bronchodilators have the potential to either improve or worsen symptoms, and therapy should be individualized. Bronchodilators may lessen the degree of forced expiration resulting from asthma. Therefore, the collapsing pressure on the trachea is decreased, leading to an improvement in the symptoms of tracheomalacia. However, these drugs may increase the compliance of tracheal smooth muscle, which may worsen airway collapsibility and symptoms. Bronchoconstrictors, such as methacholine, may decrease compliance and collapsibility of the trachea and result in a clinical improvement; however, they may also induce asthma[63, 99] and must be used with caution. Other airway problems include granulation tissue, pseudopolyps, and inspissated secretions.[38, 60] Granulation tissue can completely occlude an airway and lead to atelectasis or cause a partial occlusion, which may result in an acquired lobar emphysema.[95]

Because airway complications are common in infants with BPD, a high index of suspicion is warranted. Difficulty with extubation, homophonous stridor or wheezing heard loudest over the central airway, worsening symptoms or lack of improvement with bronchodilators, persistent lobar or segmental atelectasis or hyperinflation, and unexplained episodes of respiratory distress are indications for airway endoscopy (laryngoscopy and bronchoscopy) in these patients.

GASTROESOPHAGEAL REFLUX

Gastroesophageal reflux occurs commonly in infants with BPD and may cause gastrointestinal sequelae, such as hematemesis, anemia, esophageal stricture, and perforation. In addition, it can lead to multiple respiratory complications, including diffuse interstitial disease caused by chronic aspiration, asthma, pneumonia, laryngospasm, chronic stridor, and apnea.[100, 101] Goodwin and co-workers demonstrated that 16 (80%) of 20 intubated premature infants aspirated orally placed Evan's blue dye,[102] demonstrating that an uncuffed endotracheal tube offers little protection and may even increase the risk of aspiration. Herbst and co-workers reported 14 infants (5 term and 9 premature) with apnea and gastroesophageal reflux who had radiographic changes in the chest similar to those of BPD that probably resulted from chronic aspiration.[103] Eight responded to medical management, and six required antireflux surgery. The apnea resolved, no new infiltrates were noted, and old infiltrates began to clear in all infants. These studies indicate that chronic lung disease that can mimic or exacerbate BPD may develop in intubated newborns with gastroesophageal reflux.

Hrabovsky and Mullett[104] reported 22 premature infants with documented gastroesophageal reflux who exhibited some or all of the following: vomiting, refusal of feedings, poor weight gain, irritability, increasing tracheal secretions, sudden episodic deterioration of pulmonary status, and radiographic evidence of worsening BPD. These problems usually began by 4 to 6 weeks of age. BPD was a major factor in the development of symptomatic gastroesophageal reflux, occurring in 14 (64%) of the 22 infants. This represents 18.4% of the population in the study with BPD; however, only 1.2% of premature infants without BPD had symptomatic gastroesophageal reflux. All of the infants with BPD required Nissen fundoplications because of failure of medical management, and all but one improved postoperatively. All 10 infants who could not be extubated preoperatively were successfully extubated within 1 week postoperatively. Giuffre and co-workers[105] similarly reported an improvement in growth and a decreasing oxygen requirement in infants with BPD who had surgery for symptomatic gastroesophageal reflux.

Gastroesophageal reflux has also been shown to be an etiologic factor in some cases of asthma.[106] The mechanism is thought to be a vagal reflex resulting from irritation of the esophagus by gastric acid. Although there are no studies specifically on infants with BPD, gastroesophageal reflux is probably an important factor in the exacerbation of reactive airways in these infants.

Recurrent pneumonia is a frequent complication of gastroesophageal reflux. It occurred in 5 (36%) of the 14 infants studied by Hrabovsky and Mullett.[104] Edwards[42] also noted that radiographically demonstrable pneumonia was frequently related to a clinically apparent episode of aspiration.

Obstructive apnea as a result of laryngospasm can occur as a result of gastroesophageal reflux.[103, 107] The proposed mechanism of this association is either irritation of the esophagus by acid, resulting in a vagal reflex, or direct stimulation of the vocal cords by vomitus.[103, 107] Central apnea can also occur when laryngeal chemoreceptors are stimulated by gastric contents that have undergone reflux.[108]

A high index of suspicion must be kept for gastroesophageal reflux because it is a frequent exacerbating factor in infants with BPD. In addition, Malfroot and co-workers[109] showed that chronic respiratory disease caused by gastroesophageal reflux frequently develops in the absence of gastrointestinal symptoms. When an infant with BPD has recurrent pneumonias, highly variable or persistently worsening appearance on chest radiographs, severe asthma, or failure to thrive, gastroesophageal reflux should be considered as a possible cause. A barium swallow, a radionuclide scan, and 24-h esophageal pH monitoring are the most useful studies for documenting this condition. However, there is no test for aspiration that is both sensitive and specific. Some investigators documented gastroesophageal reflux by scanning the lungs after a radionuclide study[110] or by examining bronchoalveolar lavage fluid for lipid-laden macrophages.[111] The diagnosis usually must be made clinically when gastroesophageal reflux is present in an appropriate setting. A modification of Bernstein's test has been suggested as a diagnostic study for eliciting laryngospasm.[102, 103]

Medical management consists of thickened feedings and positioning. When appropriate, nasojejunal feedings or hyperalimentation can be used. Because theophylline and caffeine decrease lower esophageal sphincter tone, they should be avoided, if possible. Nasogastric tubes and gastrostomies without a fundoplication increase the risk of gastroesophageal reflux. Antacids or H_2 blockers may improve lower gastroesophageal junction function by decreasing esophagitis. Bethanechol is usually contraindicated because it can cause bronchospasm, but metoclopramide may be of some value. Antireflux surgery is frequently necessary.

CARDIOVASCULAR COMPLICATIONS

Pulmonary hypertension, an important complication of BPD, can result in diminished right ventricular performance, cor pulmonale, and heart failure. It may contribute substantially to respiratory failure, growth retardation, and mortality.[112, 113] The evaluation of pulmonary hypertension is problematic. Noninvasive methods may not be sufficiently sensitive and specific, and, because of its attendant risks, cardiac catheterization is infrequently performed unless significant abnormalities are likely to be found.

The right ventricular systolic time interval (RVSTI), which is the ratio of the right ventricular pre-ejection period to the right ventricular ejection time, can be measured by M-mode echocardiography and has been used to evaluate pulmonary hypertension noninvasively. A ratio of more than 0.35 has been reported to be correlated with a pulmonary artery diastolic pressure of more than 20 mm Hg; a ratio of less than 0.30 suggests normality.[114] Ratios between these values are less informative. Much of the early enthusiasm for this method of evaluating pulmonary hypertension has waned because in more recent studies investigators have not found a close correlation with pressures measured during cardiac catheterization.[115, 116]

Halliday and colleagues studied 10 infants with BPD who required supplemental oxygen.[117] The mean Pa_{O_2} was 62 mm Hg, measured in arterialized capillary blood or transcutaneously, and the mean RVSTI was 0.32. The patients were then given 90% and 110% of their baseline fraction of inspired oxygen, which resulted in a mean Pa_{O_2} and RVSTI of 52 and 0.36 and of 72 and 0.30,

respectively. The RVSTI was correlated negatively with the Pa_{O_2}. Halliday and colleagues speculated that it was optimal to maintain a Pa_{O_2} of more than 55 mm Hg, because this level correlated with an RVSTI of less than 0.35.[117] This became the standard practice for many;[113, 118] however, an RVSTI of less than 0.30 was not attained until the Pa_{O_2} was approximately 90 mm Hg. Using echocardiography and cardiac catheterization, Berman and associates studied nine subjects with BPD.[115] The RVSTIs measured by these two methods were in close agreement but correlated poorly with pulmonary vascular resistance. Newth and associates confirmed these findings by demonstrating a poor correlation between echocardiographic RVSTI and pulmonary artery mean and diastolic pressures in six infants with BPD.[116] These data indicate that M-mode echocardiography has a limited role in the diagnosis of pulmonary hypertension in patients with BPD.

Right ventricular performance can be evaluated quantitatively and noninvasively by measuring the right ventricular ejection fraction (RVEF) with radionuclide angiography. Findings from the use of the RVEF have been shown to correlate well with pulmonary hypertension. Alpert and associates reported its use in a 3-year-old with BPD who was not clinically in heart failure but who had an RVEF of 26% (normal > 45%) in room air with an arterial oxygen saturation (Sa_{O_2}) of 86%. With supplemental oxygen, the Sa_{O_2} was 96% and the RVEF was 41%.[119] The child was given sufficient oxygen to maintain an Sa_{O_2} of at least 92% for 1 year, at which time her Sa_{O_2} in room air was 96% and the RVEF was 47%. This study showed that acute and long-term improvement in right ventricular performance could be demonstrated noninvasively. Although radionuclide angiography may be useful in older children, it is technically difficult to obtain reliable information in infants.

Cardiac catheterization has been used to diagnose pulmonary hypertension and its response to supplemental oxygen in patients with BPD. Berman and associates evaluated nine infants who were receiving oxygen and diuretics.[115] The pulmonary vascular resistance (PRV) was elevated in eight while in room air. When oxygen was given, the PVR decreased slightly in four and substantially in three. These nine infants and one additional child were observed for an average of 4.4 years.[120] Four were recatheterized because of a persistent oxygen requirement and were still found to have elevated PVR, although it had decreased in three patients. Abman and colleagues studied six oxygen-dependent patients with pulmonary hypertension in room air and then with supplemental oxygen, which increased the Sa_{O_2} to at least 96%. The mean pulmonary artery pressure decreased by a minimum of 10 mm Hg in all six and normalized in four. One patient in whom the pressure decreased from 30 to 20 mm Hg had an Sa_{O_2} of 92% in room air.[121] Goodman and co-workers found that all 15 of their patients with pulmonary hypertension responded to oxygen; the pressure normalized in 5 (33%).[112] Maximal vasodilation occurred when the Sa_{O_2} exceeded 95%. Of the 10 who remained hypertensive, 5 (50%) died. These data indicate that an Sa_{O_2} of at least 92% to 95% should be maintained for maximal vasodilation.

Systemic-to-pulmonary artery collateral vessels forming left-to-right shunts have been reported in infants with

BPD.[112, 122] Ascher and associates demonstrated such vessels arising from the descending aorta, the right subclavian artery, and the right internal mammary arteries in two ventilated patients. The vessels were ligated in one patient, who was then successfully extubated 3 days later.[122] Goodman and co-workers evaluated 15 patients with pulmonary hypertension by cardiac catheterization. Six (40%), including the only two patients who remained mechanically ventilated, had collateral vessels.[112] Tomashefski and others found dilated, tortuous bronchial arteries communicating through precapillary collateral channels with the pulmonary arterial circulation at autopsy in five of six infants with BPD over 30 postconceptional weeks of age.[123] The hemodynamic significance and management of these vessels have not been well defined, but such malformations have the potential to physiologically mimic a patent ductus arteriosus.

Abman and co-workers[124] found systemic hypertension, defined as a systolic pressure exceeding 113 mm Hg, in 13 (43%) of 30 infants with BPD on supplemental oxygen. However, they could not determine the cause of this disorder. Left ventricular hypertrophy (LVH) was present in three (23%) by electrocardiographic criteria. Antihypertensive therapy was necessary in six (46%) and resulted in normalization of the systolic pressure. The mean duration of treatment was 3.7 months, after which all infants remained normotensive.

LVH occurs in many children with BPD. Melnick and co-workers demonstrated it echocardiographically in six (67%) of nine patients.[125] The electrocardiograms were normal with the exception of two that showed evidence of septal hypertrophy. Melnick and co-workers also examined the hearts in seven consecutive autopsy specimens and found LVH in six; the right ventricles were normal.[125] Stocker found LVH in 6 (21%) and biventricular hypertrophy in an additional 8 (29%) of 28 autopsies performed on infants with BPD who died at 3 to 40 months of age.[38] The cause of the LVH has not been defined; however, it might result from systemic hypertension[124] or the increased left ventricular afterload caused by the exaggerated inspiratory decrease in pleural pressure that occurs in the presence of decreased lung compliance, increased airway resistance, or both.[126]

Berman and associates[120] and Abman and co-workers[127] diagnosed unsuspected congenital heart disease by cardiac catheterization in children with BPD. In addition, because the foramen ovale is anatomically patent in about 35% of normal children,[128] right-to-left shunting can occur if right atrial pressure rises as a result of pulmonary hypertension. An incompetent foramen found at autopsy or intracardiac shunting, demonstrated by contrast echocardiography or cardiac catheterization, has been documented in several children with BPD at the authors' institution (unpublished data). This lesion should be suspected in the presence of refractory hypoxemia or sudden fluctuations in Pa_{O_2}.

Hazinski and colleagues studied infants with BPD and found elevated levels of vasopressin, which can lead to hyponatremia and inappropriately concentrated urine osmolality.[129]

Nephrocalcinosis may develop in infants with BPD who have received furosemide for diuresis.[130] Furosemide increases urinary excretion of calcium. In contrast, thiazide diuretics decrease calcium excretion and may help prevent this complication.

The diagnosis of heart failure in BPD may be difficult and is often overlooked. The noninvasive studies discussed previously are frequently not diagnostic. Cardiomegaly is often not evident on chest radiograph because of hyperinflation, although a tilting up of the cardiac apex and enlargement of the main pulmonary artery may occur in the presence of right ventricular hypertrophy and pulmonary hypertension.[42] Therefore, the physician must have a high index of suspicion, because the signs and symptoms are similar to those of a pulmonary exacerbation. Two very important signs are hepatomegaly and inappropriate weight gain. Measurement of the edge of the liver below the costal margin to determine liver size is inaccurate even in normal children and more so when hyperinflation is present.[131] The liver span must be measured by percussion, palpation, or the scratch test.[132, 133] Radiographs[134] and ultrasonograms[133] can also be used. In infants, a span of more than 7 cm on physical examination is abnormal[131, 132, 135] and is probably indicative of volume overload.

The most important aspect of treatment is the administration of supplemental oxygen. An Sa_{O_2} of at least 95% should be maintained for maximal pulmonary vasodilation[112] except when retinopathy of prematurity is still a consideration. Diuresis and fluid restriction should be instituted. In general, a decrease in total body weight of 5% for mild heart failure and 10% for severe heart failure is necessary. Return of the liver to a normal size is an important sign of adequate volume depletion. Because digoxin increases hypoxic pulmonary vasoconstriction, its effect on cardiac contractility is offset. Therefore, it is not indicated for heart failure secondary to pulmonary hypertension unless left ventricular dysfunction is also present.

There is little information on the role of vasodilators, such as hydralazine[112] and nifedipine, in patients with BPD. Brownlee and co-workers studied the acute hemodynamic effects of either nifedipine administered by nasogastric tube or 95% oxygen in comparison with room air in six infants with BPD aged 7 to 26 months. Nifedipine resulted in a lower pulmonary vascular resistance and a higher cardiac output than did 95% oxygen.[136] Because these drugs are also systemic vasodilators and can potentially worsen the hemodynamic status, their use should be individualized. Their effects should be documented, optimally by cardiac catheterization. Patients who are not adequately responding to therapy should have a more extensive cardiac evaluation to document pulmonary hypertension and its responsiveness to oxygen and to look for systemic-to-pulmonary artery shunts, occult heart disease, right-to-left shunting through a foramen ovale, or left ventricular dysfunction.

GROWTH AND NUTRITION

Many infants with BPD fail to attain normal growth parameters even when these parameters are corrected for gestational age (Table 51–4). Markestad and Fitzhardinge

Table 51–4. POTENTIAL CAUSES OF GROWTH FAILURE IN INFANTS WITH BRONCHOPULMONARY DYSPLASIA

Elevated metabolic rate
Hypoxemia
Heart failure
Gastroesophageal reflux
Rickets of prematurity
Feeding disorders
Socioeconomic factors
Inadequate parenting skills and knowledge
Emotional deprivation as a result of prolonged hospitalization

observed the growth of 20 consecutive survivors with BPD for 2 years in an uncontrolled study.[44] Although the average weight and height were appropriate for gestational age at birth, they were at or below the third percentile at 40 weeks after conception. When the pulmonary status improved, an acceleration in growth rate occurred. By 2 years after term, the weight for both sexes was between the third and 10th percentiles, and the height was at the 10th to 25th percentiles for boys and at the 25th percentile for girls. The head circumference was at the 50th percentile. In a similar uncontrolled study, Yu and associates observed 16 patients with BPD.[86] At 2 years, the mean height was between the 10th and 25th percentiles, the weight was at the 10th percentile, and the head circumference was at the 50th percentile. Because these studies were not controlled, the effect of BPD as a factor causing growth retardation independently of prematurity cannot be determined.

In three controlled studies, researchers evaluated the effect of BPD on growth. Vohr and associates observed 26 infants with BPD (group A), 8 with similar neonatal courses but without BPD (group B), and 25 premature infants with benign courses (group C).[137] All three groups had similar mean weights and lengths for the first 3 years of life (at approximately the third to 25th percentiles, corrected for gestational age). At 4 and 12 months, significantly more infants were at less than the third percentile for weight in group A than in group C; however, this finding did not persist at 24 and 36 months.

Sauve and Singhal studied 179 patients with BPD and 112 controls who had been intubated during the first week of life, received supplemental oxygen for 15 days or less, and did not develop BPD.[138] Of those with BPD, 46%, 35%, and 25% were at or below the fifth percentile for weight, height, and head circumference, respectively, in comparison with 35%, 20%, and 20% of controls. The statistical significance of these differences was not tested.

Meisels and colleagues studied 37 premature infants, 20 with HMD and 17 with BPD. Subjects with conditions known to have exhibited developmental consequences were excluded from the study.[139] The patients with BPD had a significantly slower rate of growth in the second year, and 67% and 53% were at less than the 10th percentile for weight and length, respectively, in comparison with 35% and 25% of those with HMD. However, neither of these findings reached statistical significance. There was no difference in head circumference between the groups.[139]

Infants with BPD do not grow normally with regard to weight and length in comparison with term infants. The effect on growth is probably independent of prematurity, but this is still controversial. However, several complications associated with BPD have been shown to affect growth.

Gastroesophageal reflux can lead to growth retardation.[104, 105] Giuffre and colleagues showed that surgical correction of the reflux improves feeding and growth in infants with BPD.[105]

Poor weight gain can be the result of hypoxemia. Abman and co-workers observed 23 infants with BPD on supplemental oxygen with the transcutaneous Pa_{O_2} maintained above 55 mm Hg.[118] Their weight gain was poor. Girls grew at the 10th percentile, and the boys grew below the fifth percentile at a growth rate slower than normal. However, Groothuis and Rosenberg observed 22 patients with BPD who required oxygen at home to maintain an oxygen saturation higher than 92%.[140] In seven infants, the oxygen was abruptly and prematurely discontinued by the parents. Although rate of weight gain in these infants was equivalent to the remaining 15 before removal of the supplemental oxygen, it significantly decreased to a mean of 1.4 g/day as opposed to 16.0 g/day for those who continued to receive supplemental oxygen. Length and head circumference were not affected. Accelerated growth occurred when oxygen was restarted, but the infants failed to catch up with their peers.[140] These data indicate that a saturation of at least 92% or a Pa_{O_2} of about 70 mm Hg should be maintained.

Heart failure is a common complication of BPD that can result in growth retardation. Poor feeding, caused by hypoxemia and respiratory distress, and an increase in oxygen and caloric requirements might occur. Also, peripheral hypoxia may lead to inefficient use of nutrients.[141]

The oxygen consumption of infants with BPD may be increased, resulting in excessive caloric requirements.[68, 70, 142] Weinstein and Oh found that the mean resting caloric expenditure was 25% higher in infants with BPD (28 kCal/kg/day) than in controls (47 kCal/kg/day).[68] Similar results were found by Yeh and associates, who showed a 30% increase in infants with BPD in comparison with controls (70 vs. 58.5 kCal/kg/day).[143] Kurzner and co-workers studied 13 infants with BPD, 7 of whom were at less than the 10th percentile for length and weight, and 12 full-term healthy controls.[70, 142] They found an increase of approximately 50% in resting caloric consumption in the growth-failure group in comparison with both the normal infants with BPD and the controls.[70, 142] This 10- to 20-kCal/kg/day excess expenditure at rest, in addition to the augmented requirement that occurs with activity, would leave very little energy for growth in an infant with a normal caloric intake because only 20 to 30 kCal/kg/day are usually available for this purpose. The increased work of breathing resulting from their decreased dynamic compliance, increased airway resistance, and tachypnea probably accounts for these findings. Increasing the caloric intake of these infants by raising the caloric density of the formula may improve growth.

Infants with BPD are at high risk for rickets of prematurity, which is associated with growth delays in weight, length, and head circumference.[144, 145] However, Greer and McCormick reported that BPD is not an independent factor responsible for this entity, inasmuch as there was no difference in bone mineral content among 16 patients with BPD and 16 premature controls without BPD.[145] Neither group attained mineralization levels equivalent to those of term infants until 6 months of chronological age. Inadequate intake of calcium, phosphorus, and possibly vitamin D is thought to be the primary cause of this disease.

Other factors that can affect growth include lower socioeconomic status, suboptimal parenting skills and knowledge, and emotional deprivation as a result of prolonged and repeated hospitalization. Some infants with BPD seem to acquire an aversion to oral intake on a behavioral basis, possibly because of a delayed opportunity to suck and many negative oral stimuli, such as suctioning and intubation (unpublished data). A similar problem has been reported in children with congenital anomalies.[146] Severely neurologically impaired infants may also feed poorly. Perlman and Volpe described a movement disorder in infants with BPD that includes darting or thrusting tongue movements that may interfere with feeding.[147]

NEURODEVELOPMENTAL COMPLICATIONS

Neurodevelopmental disabilities have been reported in 0%[148] to 63%[149] of children with BPD; however, the effect of BPD, independent of prematurity and its consequences, remains controversial. Markestad and Fitzhardinge[44] found that 75% of infants with BPD were free of major developmental defects at 18 months after term. They proposed that the outcome was more closely associated with neonatal and perinatal events than with the presence of BPD. In the study by Vohr and associates,[137] the incidence of disability, including cerebral palsy, hydrocephalus, blindness, and developmental delay, was significantly higher in infants with BPD (52%) than in those without BPD (8%). Meisels and colleagues[139] reported that the developmental outcome of infants with BPD was significantly less optimal than that of infants with HMD in the second year of life; however, only 12% of the former could be considered developmentally retarded. Sauve and Singhal[138] evaluated 179 infants with BPD and 112 controls matched for birth weight and year of birth; 28.4% with BPD had abnormal scores on the Bayley Scales of Infant Development (<74), in comparison with 17.9% of controls. However, the difference was not significant. Although neurodevelopmental and hearing abnormalities occurred more frequently in those with BPD, none of the differences were found to be statistically significant.

In addition to static encephalopathies, Campbell and colleagues described a progressive encephalopathy in infants with BPD characterized by seizures, neurologic deterioration, and death.[150] Perlman and Volpe reported 10 infants with BPD who had movement disorders. The limb movements were rapid, random, and jerky and were more prominent distally. The infants also exhibited orobucco-lingual movements consisting of tongue thrusting, opening the mouth widely, lip puckering, and chewing.[147]

Sauve and Singhal reported a death rate after the initial hospital discharge of 11.2% in infants with BPD.[138] Some of these infants had sudden unexplained deaths.[38, 151] Garg and co-authors studied the hypoxic arousal response in 12 infants with BPD. Although the arousal response to an inspired oxygen tension of 80 mm Hg was normal in 11 (92%), 8 (67%) experienced prolonged apnea and bradycardia after the initial arousal. They speculated that some of these infants may die unexpectedly because of an inability to recover from a hypoxic event.[152]

The neurodevelopmental outcome of infants with BPD is encouraging, because only approximately one quarter are likely to have major deficits. In a study of 82 five-year-old survivors who weighed 500 to 999 g at birth, 59 (72%) had no functional handicap and 27 (33%) exhibited functional improvement since 2 years of age.[153] Because the disabilities of these premature infants improved over time, more long-term studies of children with BPD are needed to determine their ultimate outcome.

DIFFERENTIAL DIAGNOSIS

Although the diagnosis is usually not in question, several disorders should be considered in the differential diagnosis of BPD during the neonatal period.

The Wilson-Mikity syndrome occurs in premature infants.[154] Transient respiratory distress develops in approximately one third of these infants with normal chest radiographs in the first 48 h of life. Subsequently, 2 to 6 weeks of increasing respiratory distress is followed by a period of a few days to several weeks of more severe pulmonary symptoms, which then resolve over the ensuing weeks to months. During this period, the chest radiographs initially show diffuse interstitial infiltrates with small cystic areas. Later, cysts at the bases enlarge and coalesce. These changes resolve in 3 months to 2 years. This syndrome is pathologically distinct from BPD.

Pulmonary interstitial emphysema frequently complicates mechanical ventilation of premature infants. The radiographic appearance may be similar to that in stage III BPD, and some authors believe that it may be a factor in the pathogenesis of BPD.

Congenital heart disease with left-to-right shunting and anomalous pulmonary venous drainage with obstruction can result in respiratory failure. Pulmonary edema can lead to bilateral opacification of the lungs similar to that in stage II BPD. These conditions can be differentiated by clinical findings and echocardiography or cardiac catheterization.

Pulmonary hemorrhage may result in complete opacification of the lungs, resulting in a radiographic appearance similar to that of stage II BPD.

Viral pneumonia, especially when the cause is cytomegalovirus, can be radiographically similar to BPD. Antibody titers and viral cultures can help to differentiate the two.

Recurrent aspiration can cause diffuse interstitial infiltrates and can simulate or worsen BPD.[103] This is discussed in more detail in the section on gastroesophageal reflux.

Cystic fibrosis can manifest in the neonatal period with

respiratory distress, and a chest radiograph may show increased interstitial markings, hyperinflation, or atelectasis. Affected infants occasionally require mechanical ventilation as neonates. The diagnosis is made by elevated chloride and sodium levels, as determined by quantitative analysis of sweat electrolytes (see Chapter 70 for further details).

Pulmonary lymphangiectasia is a congenital diffuse overgrowth of the lung lymphatic vessels, which may occur in association with other anomalies, especially obstruction of pulmonary venous drainage. Chest radiographs reveal diffuse mottling and hyperinflation at birth, thus distinguishing it from BPD.

PREVENTION

Most aspects of prevention have already been addressed in the discussion of pathogenesis. Two other aspects of prevention—surfactant therapy and high-frequency ventilation—are mentioned only briefly because they are beyond the scope of this chapter.

Studies reporting the use of exogenous surfactant for the treatment of HMD date back to 1980. Since that time, several studies found that it improves the course of HMD; however, it has not resulted in a decreased incidence of BPD.[155] High-frequency oscillatory ventilation has also been found to be ineffective in preventing BPD.[156]

REFERENCES

1. Northway WH, Rosan RC, Porter DY: Pulmonary disease following respirator therapy of hyaline membrane disease: Bronchopulmonary dysplasia. N Engl J Med 276:357–368, 1967.
2. Farrell PM, Palta M: Bronchopulmonary dysplasia. In Farrell PM, Taussig LM (ed): Bronchopulmonary Dysplasia and Related Chronic Respiratory Disorders: Report of the Nineteenth Ross Conference on Pediatric Research, pp. 1–7. Columbus, OH: Ross Laboratories, 1986.
3. Recommendations of the workshop on bronchopulmonary dysplasia. J Pediatr 95:815–920, 1979.
4. Bancalari E, Abdenour GE, Feller R, et al: Bronchopulmonary dysplasia: Clinical presentation. J Pediatr 95:819–823, 1979.
5. Tooley WH: Epidemiology of bronchopulmonary dysplasia. J Pediatr 95:851–858, 1979.
6. Avery ME, Tooley WH, Keller JB, et al: Is chronic lung disease in low birth weight infants preventable? A survey of eight centers. Pediatrics 79:26–30, 1987.
7. Kraybill EN, Bose CL, D'Ercole AJ: Chronic lung disease in infants with very low birth weight: A population-based study. Am J Dis Child 141:784–788, 1987.
8. Anderson WR, Strictland MB: Pulmonary complications of oxygen therapy in the neonate: Postmortem study of bronchopulmonary dysplasia with emphasis on fibroproliferative obliterative bronchitis and bronchiolitis. Arch Pathol Lab Med 91:506–514, 1971.
9. Wispe JR, Roberts RJ: Molecular basis of pulmonary oxygen toxicity. Clin Perinatol 14:651–666, 1987.
10. Fox RB, Hoidal JR, Brown DM, et al: Pulmonary inflammation due to oxygen toxicity: Involvement of chemotactic factors and polymorphonuclear leukocytes. Am Rev Respir Dis 123:521–523, 1981.
11. Jenkinson SG: Oxygen toxicity. J Intensive Care Med 3:137–152, 1988.
12. Saugstad OD: Oxygen radicals and pulmonary damage. Pediatr Pulmonol 1:167–175, 1985.
13. Jackson RM: Pulmonary oxygen toxicity. Chest 88:900–905, 1985.
14. Taghizadeh A, Reynolds EO: Pathogenesis of bronchopulmonary dysplasia following hyaline membrane disease. Am J Pathol 82:241–264, 1976.
15. Berg TJ, Pagtakhan RD, Reed MH, et al: Bronchopulmonary dysplasia and lung rupture in hyaline membrane disease: Influence of continuous distending pressure. Pediatrics 55:51–54, 1975.
16. Heicher DA, Kasting DS, Harrod JR: Prospective clinical comparison of two methods for mechanical ventilation of neonates: Rapid rate and short inspiratory time versus slow rate and long inspiratory time. J Pediatr 98:957–961, 1981.
17. Bancalari E, Feller R, Gerhardt T, et al: Prospective evaluation of different IPPV settings in infants with RDS [Abstract]. Clin Res 28:870A, 1980.
18. Nilsson R, Grossman G, Robertson B: Lung surfactant and the pathogenesis of neonatal bronchiolar lesions induced by artificial ventilation. Pediatr Res 12:249–255, 1978.
19. Nilsson R: Lung compliance and lung morphology following artificial ventilation in the premature and full-term rabbit neonate. Scand J Respir Dis 60:206–214, 1979.
20. Ackerman NB, Coalson JJ, Kuehl TJ, et al: Pulmonary interstitial emphysema in the premature baboon with hyaline membrane disease. Crit Care Med 12:512–516, 1984.
21. Bhutani VK, Koslo RJ, Shaffer TH: The effect of tracheal smooth muscle tone on neonatal airway collapsibility. Pediatr Res 20:492–495, 1986.
22. Bhutani VK, Rubenstein SD, Shaffer TH: Pressure-volume relationships of tracheae in fetal newborn and adult rabbits. Respir Physiol 43:221–231, 1981.
23. Panitch HB, Allen JL, Ryan JP, et al: A comparison of preterm and adult airway smooth muscle mechanics. J Appl Physiol 66:1760–1765, 1989.
24. Holtzman RB, Hageman JR, Yogev R: Role of Ureaplasma urealyticum in bronchopulmonary dysplasia. J Pediatr 114:1061–1063, 1989.
25. Cassell GH, Crouse DT, Waites KB, et al: Does Ureaplasma urealyticum cause respiratory disease in newborns? Pediatr Infect Dis J 7:535–541, 1988.
26. Cassady G, Crouse DT, Kirklin JW et al: A randomized, controlled trial of very early prophylactic ligation of the ductus arteriosus in babies who weigh 1000g or less at birth. N Engl J Med 320:1511–1516, 1989.
27. Brown ER, Stark A, Sosenko I, et al: Bronchopulmonary dysplasia: Possible relationship to pulmonary edema. J Pediatr 92:982–984, 1978.
28. Nickerson BG, Taussig LM: Family history of asthma in infants with bronchopulmonary dysplasia. Pediatrics 65:1140–1144, 1980.
29. Bertrand J, Riley SP, Popkin J, et al: The long-term pulmonary sequelae of prematurity: The role of familial airway hyperreactivity and the respiratory distress syndrome. N Engl J Med 312:742–745, 1985.
30. Sawyer MH, Edwards DK, Spector SA: Cytomegalovirus infection and bronchopulmonary dysplasia in premature infants. Am J Dis Child 141:303–305, 1987.
31. Frank L, Sosenko IR: Undernutrition as a major contributing factor in the pathogenesis of bronchopulmonary dysplasia. Am Rev Respir Dis 138:725–729, 1988.
32. Lockitch G, Jacobson B, Quigley G, et al: Selenium deficiency in low birth weight neonates: An unrecognized problem. J Pediatr 114:865–870, 1989.
33. Bonta VW, Gawron ER, Warshaw JB: Neonatal red cell superoxide dismutase enzyme levels: Possible role as a cellular defense mechanism against pulmonary oxygen toxicity. Pediatr Res 11:754–757, 1977.
34. Bell EF: Prevention of bronchopulmonary dysplasia: Vitamin E and other antioxidants. In Farrell PM, Taussig LM (eds): Bronchopulmonary Dysplasia and Related Chronic Respiratory Disorders: Report of the Nineteenth Ross Conference on Pediatric Research, pp. 77–81. Columbus, OH: Ross Laboratories, 1986.
35. Lawson EE, Stiles AD: Vitamin A therapy for prevention of chronic lung disease in infants. J Pediatr 111:247–248, 1987.
36. Hustead VA, Gutcher GR, Anderson SA, Zachman RD: Relation-

ship of vitamin A (retinol) status to the lung disease in preterm infant. J Pediatr 105:610–615, 1984.

37. Shenai JP, Kennedy KA, Chytil F, Stahlman MT: Clinical trial of vitamin A supplementation in infants susceptible to bronchopulmonary dysplasia. J Pediatr 111:269–277, 1987.

38. Stocker JT: Pathologic features of long-standing "healed" bronchopulmonary dysplasia: A study of 28 3- to 40-month old infants. Hum Pathol 17:943–961, 1986.

39. Anderson WR, Engel RR: Cardiopulmonary sequelae of reparative stages of bronchopulmonary dysplasia. Arch Pathol Lab Med 107:603–608, 1983.

40. Thurlbeck WM: Morphologic aspects of bronchopulmonary dysplasia. J Pediatr 95:842–843, 1979.

41. Reid L: Bronchopulmonary dysplasia—Pathology. J Pediatr 95:836–841, 1979.

42. Edwards DK: Radiographic aspects of bronchopulmonary dysplasia. J Pediatr 95:823–829, 1979.

43. Mortensson W, Lindroth M: The course of bronchopulmonary dysplasia: A radiographic follow-up. Acta Radiol Diagn 27:19–22, 1986.

44. Markestad T, Fitzhardinge PM: Growth and development in children recovering from bronchopulmonary dysplasia. J Pediatr 98:597–602, 1981.

45. Morray JP, Fox WW, Kettrick RG, Downes JJ: Improvement in lung mechanics as a function of age in the infant with severe bronchopulmonary dysplasia. Pediatr Res 16:290–294, 1982.

46. Tepper RS, Morgan WJ, Cota K, Taussig LM: Expiratory flow limitation in infants with bronchopulmonary dysplasia. J Pediatr 109:1040–1046, 1986.

47. Bryan MH, Hardie MJ, Reilly BJ, Swyer PR: Pulmonary function studies during the first year of life in infants recovering from the respiratory distress syndrome. Pediatrics 52:169–178, 1973.

48. Kao LC, Warburton D, Platzker AC, Keens TG: Effect of isoproterenol inhalation on airway resistance in chronic bronchopulmonary dysplasia. Pediatrics 73:509–514, 1984.

49. Kao LC, Warburton D, Cheng MH, et al: Effect of oral diuretics on pulmonary mechanics in infants with chronic bronchopulmonary dysplasia: Results of a double-blind crossover sequential trial. Pediatrics 74:37–44, 1984.

50. Kao LC, Durand DJ, Phillips BL, Nickerson BG: Oral theophylline and diuretics improve pulmonary mechanics in infants with bronchopulmonary dysplasia. J Pediatr 111:439–444, 1987.

51. Arad I, Bar-Yishay E, Eyal F, et al: Lung function in infancy and childhood following neonatal intensive care. Pediatr Pulmonol 3:29–33, 1987.

52. Gerhardt T, Hehre D, Feller R, et al: Serial determination of pulmonary function in infants with chronic lung disease. J Pediatr 110:448–456, 1987.

53. O'Brodovich HM, Mellins RB: Bronchopulmonary dysplasia: Unresolved neonatal acute lung injury. Am Rev Respir Dis 132:694–709, 1985.

54. Cook CD, Sutherland JM, Segal S, et al: Studies of respiratory physiology in the newborn infant: III. Measurements of mechanics of respiration. J Clin Invest 36:440–448, 1957.

55. Kao LC, Warburton D, Sargent CW, et al: Furosemide acutely decreases airways resistance in chronic bronchopulmonary dysplasia. J Pediatr 103:624–629, 1983.

56. Tepper RS, Pagtakhan RD, Taussig LM: Noninvasive determination of total respiratory system compliance in infants by the weighted-spirometer method. Am Rev Respir Dis 130:461–466, 1984.

57. Dreizzen E, Migdal M, Praud JP, et al: Passive compliance of total respiratory system in preterm newborn infants with respiratory distress syndrome. J Pediatr 112:778–781, 1988.

58. Wilkie RA, Bryan MH: Effect of bronchodilators on airway resistance in ventilator-dependent neonates with chronic lung disease. J Pediatr 111:278–282, 1987.

59. Bhutani VK, Ritchie WG, Shaffer TH: Acquired tracheomegaly in very preterm neonates. Am J Dis Child 140:449–452, 1986.

60. Miller RW, Woo P, Kellman RK, Slagle TS: Tracheobronchial abnormalities in infants with bronchopulmonary dysplasia. J Pediatr 111:779–782, 1987.

61. Bhutani VK: Tracheobronchial abnormalities complicating bronchopulmonary dysplasia. J Pediatr 112:843–844, 1988.

62. McCubbin M, Frey EE, Wagener JS, et al: Large airway collapse in bronchopulmonary dysplasia. J Pediatr 114:304–307, 1989.

63. Panitch HB, Keklikian EN, Motley RA: Effect of altering smooth muscle tone on maximal expiratory flows in patients with tracheomalacia. Pediatr Pulmonol 9:170–176, 1990.

64. Panitch HB, Allen JL, Motley RA, et al: The effect of airway distending pressure on airway mechanics in infants with tracheobronchomalacia [Abstract]. Pediatr Res 27:361A, 1990.

65. Wolfson MR, Bhutani VK, Shaffer TH, Bowen FW: Mechanics and energetics of breathing helium in infants with bronchopulmonary dysplasia. J Pediatr 104:752–757, 1984.

66. Thibeault DW, Clutario B, Auld PAM: The oxygen cost of breathing in the premature infant. Pediatrics 37:954–959, 1966.

67. Allen JL, Wolfson MR, McDowell K, et al: Thoracoabdominal asynchrony in infants with airflow obstructions. Am Rev Respir Dis 141:337–342, 1990.

68. Weinstein MR, Oh W: Oxygen consumption in infants with bronchopulmonary dysplasia. J Pediatr 99:958–961, 1981.

69. Sinclair JC, Driscoll JM, Heird WC, Winters RW: Supportive management of the sick neonate: Parenteral calories, water and electrolytes. Pediatr Clin North Am 17:863–893, 1970.

70. Kurzner SI, Garg M, Bautista DB et al: Growth failure in bronchopulmonary dysplasia: Elevated metabolic rates and pulmonary mechanics. J Pediatr 112:73–80, 1988.

71. Kao LC, Durand DJ, Nickerson BG: Improving pulmonary function does not decrease oxygen consumption in infants with bronchopulmonary dysplasia. J Pediatr 112:616–621, 1988.

72. Gomez-Del Rio M, Gerhardt T, Hehre D, et al.: Effect of a beta-agonist nebulization on lung function in neonates with increased pulmonary resistance. Pediatr Pulmonol 2:287–291, 1986.

73. Sosulski R, Abbasi S, Bhutani VK, Fox WW: Physiologic effects of terbutaline on pulmonary function of infants with bronchopulmonary dysplasia. Pediatr Pulmonol 2:269–273, 1986.

74. Cabal LA, Larrazabal C, Ramanathan R, et al: Effects of metaproterenol on pulmonary mechanics, oxygenation, and ventilation in infants with chronic lung disease. J Pediatr 110:116–119, 1987.

75. Motoyama EK, Fort MD, Klesh K, et al: Early onset of airway reactivity in premature infants with bronchopulmonary dysplasia. Am Rev Respir Dis 136:50–57, 1987.

76. Rooklin AR, Moomjian AS, Shutack JG, et al: Theophylline therapy in bronchopulmonary dysplasia. J Pediatr 95:882–888, 1979.

77. Avery GB, Fletcher AB, Kaplan M, Brudno DS: Controlled trial of dexamethasone in respirator-dependent infants with bronchopulmonary dysplasia. Pediatrics 75:106–111, 1985.

78. Logvinoff MM, Lemen RJ, Taussig LM, Lamont BA: Bronchodilators and diuretics in children with bronchopulmonary dysplasia. Pediatr Pulmonol 1:198–203, 1985.

79. Engelhardt B, Elliott S, Hazinski TA: Short- and long-term effects of furosemide on lung function in infants with bronchopulmonary dysplasia. J Pediatr 109:1034–1039, 1986.

80. Teague WG, Pian MS, Heldt GP, Tooley WH: An acute reduction in the fraction of inspired oxygen increases airway constriction in infants with chronic lung disease. Am Rev Respir Dis 137:861–865, 1988.

81. Tay-Uyboco JS, Kwiatkowski K, Cates DB, et at: Hypoxic airway constriction in infants of very low birthweight recovering from moderate to severe bronchopulmonary dysplasia. J Pediatr 115:456–459, 1989.

82. Smyth JA, Tabachnik E, Duncan WJ, et al: Pulmonary function and bronchial hyperreactivity in long-term survivors of bronchopulmonary dysplasia. Pediatrics 68:336–340, 1981.

83. Wheeler WB, Castile RG, Brown ER, Wohl MEB: Pulmonary function in survivors of prematurity [Abstract]. Am Rev Respir Dis 129:A218, 1984.

84. Mansell AL, Driscoll JM, James LS: Pulmonary follow-up of moderately low birth weight infants with and without respiratory distress syndrome. J Pediatr 110:111–115, 1987.

85. Northway WH, Moss RB, Carlisle KB, et al: Late pulmonary sequelae of bronchopulmonary dysplasia. N Engl J Med 323:1793–1799, 1990.

86. Yu VY, Orgill AA, Lim SB, et al: Growth and development of very low birthweight infants recovering from bronchopulmonary dysplasia. Arch Dis Child 58:791–794, 1983.

87. Groothuis JR, Butierrez KM, Lauer BA: Respiratory syncytial virus infection in children with bronchopulmonary dysplasia. Pediatrics 82:199–203, 1988.

88. McMillan JA, Tristram DA, Weiner LB, et al: Prediction of the duration of hospitalization in patients with respiratory syncytial

virus infection: Use of clinical parameters. Pediatrics 81:22–26, 1988.

89. Hall CB, McBride JT, Gala CL, et al: Ribavirin treatment of respiratory syncytial virus infection in infants with underlying cardiopulmonary disease. JAMA 254:3047–3051, 1985.

90. Fan LL, Flynn JW, Pathak DR: Risk factors predicting laryngeal injury in intubated neonates. Crit Care Med 11:431–433, 1983.

91. Fan LL, Flynn JW: Laryngoscopy in neonates and infants: Experience with the flexible fiberoptic bronchoscope. Laryngoscope 91:451–456, 1981.

92. Supance JS: Antibiotics and steroids in the treatment of acquired subglottic stenosis: A canine model study. Ann Otol Rhinol Laryngol 92:377–382, 1983.

93. Pashley NRT: Anterior cricoidotomy for congenital and acquired subglottic stenosis in infants and children. J Otolaryngol 13:187–190, 1984.

94. Pashley NRT, Jaskunas JM, Waldstein G: Laryngotracheoplasty with costochondral grafts: A clinical correlate to graft survival. Laryngoscope 94:1493–1496, 1984.

95. Bhutani VK, Rubenstein D, Shaffer TH: Pressure-induced deformation in immature airways. Pediatr Res 15:829–832, 1981.

96. Greenholz SK, Hall RJ, Lilly JR, et al: Surgical implications of bronchopulmonary dysplasia. J Pediatr Surg 22:1132–1136, 1987.

97. Sotomayor JL, Godinez RI, Borden S, Wilmott RW: Large-airway collapse due to acquired tracheobronchomalacia in infancy. Am J Dis Child 140:367–371, 1986.

98. Wiseman NE, Duncan PG, Cameron CB: Management of tracheobronchomalacia with continuous positive airway pressure. J Pediatr Surg 20:489–493, 1985.

99. Panitch HB, Keklikian EN, Motley RA, et al: The effect of altering smooth muscle tone on maximal expiratory flows in patients with tracheomalacia. Pediatr Pulmonol 10:314–315, 1991.

100. Orenstein SR, Orenstein DM: Gastroesophageal reflux and respiratory disease in children. J Pediatr 112:847–858, 1988.

101. Neilson DW, Heldt GP, Tooley WH: Stridor and gastroesophageal reflux in infants. Pediatrics 85:1034–1039, 1990.

102. Goodwin SR, Graves SA, Haberkern CM: Aspiration in intubated premature infants. Pediatrics 75:85–88, 1985.

103. Herbst JJ, Minton SD, Book LS: Gastroesophageal reflux causing respiratory distress and apnea in newborn infants. J Pediatr 95:763–768, 1979.

104. Hrabovsky EE, Mullett MD: Gastroesophageal reflux and the premature infant. J Pediatr Surg 21:583–587, 1986.

105. Giuffre RM, Rubin S, Mitchell I: Antireflux surgery in infants with bronchopulmonary dysplasia. Am J Dis Child 141:648–651, 1987.

106. Berquist WE, Rachelefsky GS, Kadden M, et al: Gastroesophageal reflux-associated recurrent pneumonia and chronic asthma in children. Pediatrics 68:29–35, 1981.

107. Orenstein SR, Kocoshis SA, Orenstein DM, Proujansky R: Stridor and gastroesophageal reflux: Diagnostic use of intraluminal esophageal acid perfusion (Bernstein test). Pediatr Pulmonol 3:420–424, 1987.

108. Downing SE, Lee JC: Laryngeal chemosensitivity: A possible mechanism of sudden infant death. Pediatrics 55:640–649, 1975.

109. Malfroot A, Vandenplas Y, Verlinden M et al: Gastroesophageal reflux and unexplained chronic respiratory disease in infants and children. Pediatr Pulmonol 3:208–213, 1987.

110. McVeagh P, Howman-Giles R, Kemp A: Pulmonary aspiration studied by radionuclide milk scanning and barium swallow roentgenography. Am J Dis Child 141:917–921, 1987.

111. Nickerson BG: A test for recurrent aspiration in children. Pediatr Pulmonol 3:65–66, 1987.

112. Goodman G, Perkins RM, Anas NG, et al: Pulmonary hypertension in infants with bronchopulmonary dysplasia. J Pediatr 112:67–72, 1988.

113. Fouron JC, Le Guennec JC, Villemant D, et al: Value of echocardiography in assessing the outcome of bronchopulmonary dysplasia of the newborn. Pediatrics 65:529–535, 1980.

114. Hirschfeld SS: Cor pulmonale: Diagnosis and significance. *In* Farrell PM, Taussig LM (eds): Bronchopulmonary Dysplasia and Related Chronic Respiratory Disorders: Report of the Nineteenth Ross Conference on Pediatric Research, pp. 59–68. Columbus, OH: Ross Laboratories, 1986.

115. Berman W, Yabek SM, Dillon T, et al: Evaluation of infants with bronchopulmonary dysplasia using cardiac catheterization. Pediatrics 70:708–712, 1982.

116. Newth CJ, Gow RM, Rowe RD: The assessment of pulmonary arterial pressures in bronchopulmonary dysplasia by cardiac catheterization and M-mode echocardiography. Pediatr Pulmonol 1:58–62, 1985.

117. Halliday HL, Dumpit FM, Brady JP: Effects of inspired oxygen on echocardiographic assessment of pulmonary vascular resistance and myocardial contractility in bronchopulmonary dysplasia. Pediatrics 65:536–540, 1980.

118. Abman SH, Accurso FJ, Koops BL: Experience with home oxygen in the management of infants with bronchopulmonary dysplasia. Clin Pediatr 23:471–476, 1984.

119. Alpert BE, Gainey MA, Schidlow DV, Capitanio MA: Effect of oxygen on right ventricular performance evaluated by radionuclide angiography in two young patients with chronic lung disease. Pediatr Pulmonol 3:149–152, 1987.

120. Berman W, Katz R, Yabek SM, et al: Long-term follow-up of bronchopulmonary dysplasia. J Pediatr 109:45–50, 1986.

121. Abman SH, Wolfe RR, Accurso FJ, et al: Pulmonary vascular response to oxygen with severe bronchopulmonary dysplasia. Pediatrics 75:80–84, 1985.

122. Ascher DP, Rosen P, Null DM, et al: Systemic to pulmonary collaterals mimicking patent ductus arteriosus in neonates with prolonged ventilatory courses. J Pediatr 107:282–284, 1985.

123. Tomashefski JF, Oppermann HC, Vawter GF: Bronchopulmonary dysplasia: A morphometric study with emphasis on the pulmonary vasculature. Pediatr Pathol 2:469–487, 1984.

124. Abman SH, Warady BA, Lum GM, Koops BL: Systemic hypertension in infants with bronchopulmonary dysplasia. J Pediatr 104:929–931, 1984.

125. Melnick G, Pickoff AS, Ferrer PL, et al: Normal pulmonary vascular resistance and left ventricular hypertrophy in young infants with bronchopulmonary dysplasia: An echocardiographic and pathologic study. Pediatrics 66:589–596, 1980.

126. Bromberger-Barnea B: Mechanical effects of inspiration on heart functions: A review. Fed Proc 40:2172–2177, 1981.

127. Abman SH, Accurso FJ, Bowman CM: Unsuspected cardiopulmonary abnormalities complicating bronchopulmonary dysplasia. Arch Dis Child 59:966–970, 1984.

128. Hagen PT, Scholz DG, Edwards WD: Incidence and size of patent foramen ovale during the first 10 decades of life: An autopsy study of 965 normal hearts. Mayo Clin Proc 59:17–20, 1984.

129. Hazinski TA, Blalock WA, Engelhart B: Control of water balance in infants with bronchopulmonary dysplasia: Role of endogenous vasopressin. Pediatr Res 23:86–88, 1988.

130. Hufnagle KG, Khan SN, Penn D, et al: Renal calcifications: A complication of long-term furosemide therapy in preterm infants. Pediatrics 70:360–363, 1982.

131. Lawson EE, Grand RJ, Neff RK, Cohen LF: Clinical estimation of liver span in infants and children. Am J Dis Child 132:474–476, 1978.

132. Naveh Y, Berant M: Assessment of liver size in normal infants and children. J Pediatr Gastroenterol Nutr 3:346–348, 1984.

133. Fuller GN, Hargreaves MR, King DM: Scratch test in clinical examination of liver. Lancet 1 (8578):181, 1988.

134. Deligeorgis D, Yannakos D, Doxiadis S: Normal size of liver in infancy and childhood: X-ray study. Arch Dis Child 48:790–793, 1973.

135. Reiff MI, Osborn LM: Clinical estimation of liver size in newborn infants. Pediatrics 71:46–48, 1983.

136. Brownlee JR, Beekman RH, Rosenthal A: Acute hemodynamic effects of nifedipine in infants with bronchopulmonary dysplasia and pulmonary hypertension. Pediatr Res 24:186–190, 1988.

137. Vohr BR, Bell EF, Oh W: Infants with bronchopulmonary dysplasia: Growth patterns and neurologic and developmental outcome. Am J Dis Child 136:443–447, 1982.

138. Sauve RS, Singhal N: Long-term morbidity of infants with bronchopulmonary dysplasia. Pediatrics 76:725–733, 1985.

139. Meisels SJ, Plunkett JW, Roloff DW, et al: Growth and development of preterm infants with respiratory distress syndrome and bronchopulmonary dysplasia. Pediatrics 77:345–352, 1986.

140. Groothuis JR, Rosenberg AA: Home oxygen promotes weight gain in infants with bronchopulmonary dysplasia. Am J Dis Child 141:992–995, 1987.

141. Menon G, Poskitt EM: Why does congenital heart disease cause failure to thrive? Arch Dis Child 60:1134–1139, 1985.

142. Kurzner SI, Garg M, Bautista DB, et al: Growth failure in infants

with bronchopulmonary dysplasia: Nutrition and elevated resting metabolic expenditure. Pediatrics 81:379–384, 1988.

143. Yeh TF, McClenan DA, Ajayi OA, Pildes RS: Metabolic rate and energy balance in infants with bronchopulmonary dysplasia. J Pediatr 114:448–451, 1989.

144. Ryan S, Congdon PJ, Horsman A, et al: Bone mineral content in bronchopulmonary dysplasia. Arch Dis Child 62:889–894, 1987.

145. Greer FR, McCormick A: Bone mineral content and growth in very low birth-weight premature infants: Does bronchopulmonary dysplasia make a difference? Am J Dis Child 141:179–183, 1987.

146. Handen BL, Mandell F, Russo DC: Feeding induction in children who refuse to eat. Am J Dis Child 140:52–54, 1986.

147. Perlman JM, Volpe JJ: Movement disorder of premature infants with severe bronchopulmonary dysplasia: A new syndrome. Pediatrics 84:215–218, 1989.

148. Harrod JR, L'Heureux P, Wangensteen OD, Hunt CE: Long-term follow-up of severe respiratory distress syndrome treated with IPPB. J Pediatrics 84:277–285, 1974.

149. Northway WH: Observations on bronchopulmonary dysplasia. J Pediatr 95:815–818, 1979.

150. Campbell LR, McAlister W, Volpe JJ: Neurologic aspects of bronchopulmonary dysplasia. Clin Pediatr 27:7–13, 1988.

151. Werthammer J, Brown ER, Neff RK, et al: Sudden infant death syndrome in infants with bronchopulmonary dysplasia. Pediatrics 69:301–304, 1982.

152. Garg M, Kurzner SI, Bautista D, Keens TG: Hypoxic arousal responses in infants with bronchopulmonary dysplasia. Pediatrics 82:59–63, 1988.

153. Kitchen W, Ford G, Orgill A, et al: Outcome in infants of birth weight 500 to 999 g: A continuing regional study of 5-year-old survivors. J Pediatr 111:761–766, 1987.

154. Wilson MG, Mikity VG: A new form of respiratory disease in premature infants. Am J Dis Child 99:489–499, 1960.

155. Horbar JD, Soll RF, Sutherland JM, et al: A multicenter randomized, placebo-controlled trial of surfactant therapy for respiratory distress syndrome. N Engl J Med 320:959–965, 1989.

156. The HIFI Study Group: High-frequency oscillatory ventilation compared with conventional mechanical ventilation in the treatment of respiratory failure in preterm infants. N Engl J Med 320:88–93, 1989.

52 CONGENITAL ABNORMALITIES

MICHELLE LIERL, M.D.

BRONCHOGENIC CYST

Bronchogenic cysts are remnants of the primitive foregut, derived from abnormal budding of the embryonic tracheobronchial tree. The anomaly was first described by Blackader in 1911;[1] successful surgical resection was reported by Maier in 1948.[2] Bronchogenic cysts account for 14% to 22% of congenital cystic diseases of the lung[3-5] and represent approximately 10% of mediastinal masses in children.[2] There is no apparent racial or sex predilection for development of bronchogenic cyst, and no cases of familial recurrence have been reported.

PATHOPHYSIOLOGY

During the embryonic stage of development, the primitive foregut gives rise through a ventral outpouching to the tracheobronchial tree. The bronchi develop by a process of budding and branching between the 5th and 16th weeks of gestation. Anomalous buds can form at any stage of development and at any site along the tracheobronchial tree. Ectopic buds that develop normally and establish functional communication with the pulmonary parenchyma become accessory bronchi. Some ectopic buds, however, are arrested in an embryonic state of development and become bronchogenic cysts.

These cysts contain tissue normally found in the trachea and bronchi: mucous glands, smooth muscle, elastic tissue, and usually cartilage. Subcutaneous bronchogenic cysts, whose histologic features are otherwise typical of bronchogenic cysts, often do not contain cartilage.[6] The cyst wall, when uninfected, is thin and lined with secretory ciliated columnar or cuboidal epithelium (Fig. 52–1A). The cyst fluid is mucoid and clear or white unless hemorrhage into the cyst has occurred, in which case the contents are thick and brown. Calcium crystals may be seen,[7] and a high calcium oxalate content has been noted.[8, 9] On gross inspection, the bronchogenic cyst is bluish gray, white, or tan. The cyst may be single, multilocular, or multiple; up to 10 cysts may be present in one lung.[10] In a few cases, a systemic arterial supply has been noted,[11] but most reports contain no mention of anomalous blood supply.

Maier[2] classified bronchogenic cysts in five groups by location: (1) paratracheal cysts, which arise most often from the right lateral tracheal wall just above the carina; (2) carinal cysts, which are located at or just below the carina; (3) paraesophageal cysts, which are adjacent to or embedded in the wall of the esophagus, often anteriorly or anterolaterally (some authors refer to paratracheal, carinal, and paraesophageal cysts collectively as mediastinal cysts, which can compress the trachea or either of the main bronchi and frequently result in respiratory distress and hyperinflation); (4) hilar cysts, which arise from the main or lobar bronchi, can remain attached or in proximity to the bronchi, or can migrate into the lung parenchyma (the majority of intrathoracic bronchogenic cysts

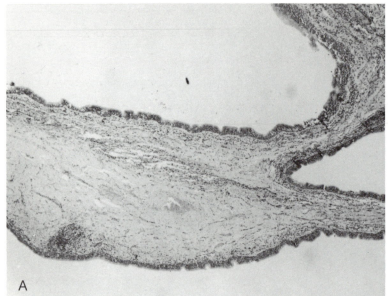
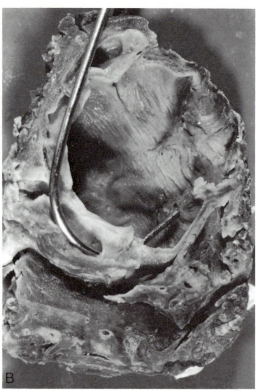

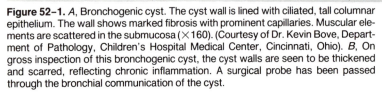

Figure 52–1. *A*, Bronchogenic cyst. The cyst wall is lined with ciliated, tall columnar epithelium. The wall shows marked fibrosis with prominent capillaries. Muscular elements are scattered in the submucosa (×160). (Courtesy of Dr. Kevin Bove, Department of Pathology, Children's Hospital Medical Center, Cincinnati, Ohio). *B*, On gross inspection of this bronchogenic cyst, the cyst walls are seen to be thickened and scarred, reflecting chronic inflammation. A surgical probe has been passed through the bronchial communication of the cyst.

belong to this group[12]); and (5) "miscellaneous" cysts, which include bronchogenic cysts that detach from the tracheobronchial tree during the course of embryonic development and migrate to various unusual sites. Pericardial, cervical, subcutaneous, and abdominal sites are the most common extrapulmonary locations of bronchogenic cysts. One sublingual bronchogenic cyst has been reported.[13]

About two thirds of bronchogenic cysts are attached to the tracheobronchial tree by a stalk of fibrous tissue or are embedded in the wall of the trachea or the bronchus.[14] Some of these cysts have a patent communication with the tracheobronchial tree (Fig. 52–1*B*). Progressive dilatation of the cyst with air can result in airway compression, or the cyst contents can become infected. Noncommunicating cysts can also progressively enlarge as they become distended with mucous secretions.[14] Even small (1.5- to 3.0-cm) bronchogenic cysts can cause significant airway compression.[14, 15] Large cysts can compress the normal pulmonary parenchyma, resulting in atelectasis, recurrent infection, and mediastinal shift.

In a few cases, malignancies, including embryonal rhabdomyosarcoma,[16] leiomyosarcoma,[17] and anaplastic carcinoma[18] have developed within bronchogenic cysts. In one unusual case, autoantibodies directed against an intrathoracic bronchogenic cyst apparently caused autoimmune hemolytic anemia.[19]

CLINICAL MANIFESTATIONS

The clinical manifestation of a bronchogenic cyst varies with its location and size. About 5% to 19% of bronchogenic cysts are asymptomatic.[10, 20, 21] Most symptomatic cases manifest in infancy or early childhood,[10, 14] although symptoms can develop at any age. Intrathoracic bronchogenic cysts present with respiratory distress, typically in infants, or with infectious complications, which occur more often in older children and adults.

Respiratory distress secondary to a bronchogenic cyst is usually caused by airway compression. Compression of the trachea results in episodes of cough, stridor, and wheezing; suprasternal and intercostal retractions; and diffuse air trapping. Symptoms are exacerbated by feeding and crying. Affected infants tend to hyperextend the neck in an attempt to alleviate the tracheal obstruction. Diffuse rales (crackles) can result from impairment of clearance of secretions.[15, 22, 23]

If one of the main or lobar bronchi is compressed, obstructive emphysema can develop in the lung or the lobe supplied by the bronchus. The clinical picture in affected infants is similar to that of congenital lobar emphysema.[24, 25] Progressive overinflation of the obstructed lung or lobe with compression of the normal lung, the heart, and the great vessels can result in rapidly progressive cardiorespiratory distress. Physical examination reveals patients to be tachypneic and, sometimes, cyanotic. Once hemithorax is hyperexpanded with decreased breath sounds, a localized wheeze may be heard over the obstructed bronchus. The trachea and the heart are shifted away from the hyperinflated hemithorax. In many of these cases, the bronchogenic cyst is not visible on chest radiograph[15, 24] and should be actively sought before infants are subjected to lobectomy for presumed congenital lobar emphysema. A less common manifestation of airway compression by a bronchogenic cyst is recurrent atelectasis of a lobe or a lung.[26]

Bronchogenic cysts whose size or location results in respiratory distress usually become symptomatic in infancy. In some cases, however, respiratory distress develops later in childhood or in adulthood, presumably because of increase in the size of the cyst.[21, 27] Persistent or recurrent pneumonia distal to a bronchogenic cyst can occur at any age and is usually caused by impairment of clearance of secretions past the cyst.[10] In some cases, the cyst itself becomes infected, and the clinical manifestations are similar to that of a pulmonary abscess. Rupture of an infected cyst results in pneumonia or empyema.[28]

Chest pain is a common symptom of bronchogenic cyst, especially in adult patients.[21] Hemoptysis also can occur and in some cases is the only symptom.[20] Pulmonary arterial compression by a bronchogenic cyst has been noted in several patients, who had chronic cough,[29] had dyspnea and pleuritic chest pain,[30] or were asymptomatic.[31, 32] Paraesophageal cysts also can be asymptomatic,[33] or they can manifest with symptoms of epigastric discomfort, dysphagia, and shoulder or back pain;[34–36] with wheezing, as a result of compression of the posterior trachea;[35] or with symptoms of infection, fever, chest pain, and dysphagia.[2, 20]

A cervical bronchogenic cyst can cause stridor, respiratory distress, tracheal displacement,[36] and recurrent infection[37] or can present as an asymptomatic mass, which may drain mucus through a cutaneous opening.[38, 39] Most recorded cases of pericardial bronchogenic cysts have been discovered in adult patients. Chest pain is the most common symptom.[40–42] Dysphagia, cough, dyspnea, cardiac arrhythmias, recurrent pericarditis, and right heart failure have also occurred in these patients.[40, 42, 43] Superior vena caval syndrome can result from compression of the superior vena cava by a large pericardial bronchogenic cyst.[41, 42, 44]

Abdominal bronchogenic cysts are reported rarely. Symptoms of nausea, vomiting, and epigastric pain have been reported in patients with intra-abdominal bronchogenic cysts,[45] whereas those with a transdiaphragmatic dumbbell configuration have exhibited respiratory symptoms.[46, 47]

Subcutaneous bronchogenic cysts are typically located in the suprasternal area, the lower neck, or the anterior chest wall.[6] A few have been reported over the shoulder, on the scapula[48] or on the chin.[49] A fistula to the skin often develops with these cysts, and mucoid material is periodically drained.

Associated anomalies—most often cardiac, respiratory, or skeletal—are occasionally noted in patients with bronchogenic cyst.[10, 14, 50]

DIAGNOSTIC PROCEDURES

Chest radiographs usually demonstrate an abnormality in patients with bronchogenic cysts, although the nature of the anomaly may not be evident. Many bronchogenic cysts are not visible on the chest radiographs, being obscured by mediastinal structures or by surrounding inflammation. Hyperinflation, pneumonitis, atelectasis, mediastinal deviation, or abnormal separation of the trachea and esophagus can be seen on chest radiographs. In newborns, bronchogenic cysts may manifest with opacification of the lung, secondary to retained amniotic fluid

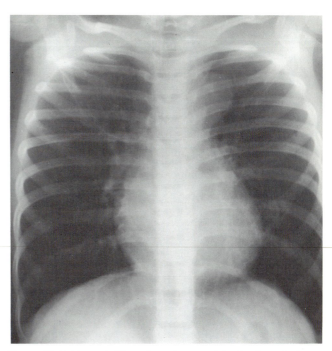

Figure 52–2. Unaerated bronchogenic cyst originating from the lateral wall of the lower trachea appears as a radiodense, smoothly rounded mass.

in the obstructed lung.[15] When the cyst is seen, its radiographic appearance is variable. Mediastinal cysts are usually opaque, smoothly contoured single masses. (Figs. 52–2, 52–3) On occasion, a mediastinal cyst, especially in the subcarinal location, communicates with the airway and thus is filled with air or has an air-fluid level.

Hilar cysts can be single, multiple, or multilocular and vary greatly in size. Many of these cysts communicate with the tracheobronchial tree. When seen in association with acute pneumonia, a bronchogenic cyst with an air-fluid level is difficult to distinguish from a lung abscess (Fig. 52–4), and an air-filled cyst has the appearance of a pneumatocele. Persistence of the lesion on follow-up radiographs is suggestive of a bronchogenic cyst. In some cases, a characteristic semilunar layer of calcium is seen in the dependent wall of the cyst.

The barium esophagogram is useful in the diagnosis of paraesophageal or cervical bronchogenic cysts (Fig. 52–3B).[10, 15] An anterior or anterolateral indentation in the esophagus, which moves upward on deglutition, is the characteristic finding.[51]

The computed tomographic (CT) scan can demonstrate mediastinal bronchogenic cysts that are not visible on plain chest radiographs.[52] Abdominal bronchogenic cysts can also be detected on CT scans.[45] High-density measurements are sometimes found on CT scans of fluid-filled bronchogenic cysts because of their high calcium content.[7-9] These "dense" cysts are sometimes misinterpreted as solid masses.

Bronchoscopy can be helpful in demonstrating extrinsic compression of the airway but sometimes causes a clinical deterioration of the patient's condition.[50] A communicating cyst or an obstructed, hyperinflated lung can expand further during instrumentation with the ventilating bronchoscope; fiberoptic bronchoscopy is preferable

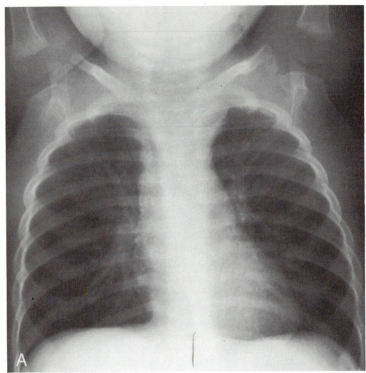

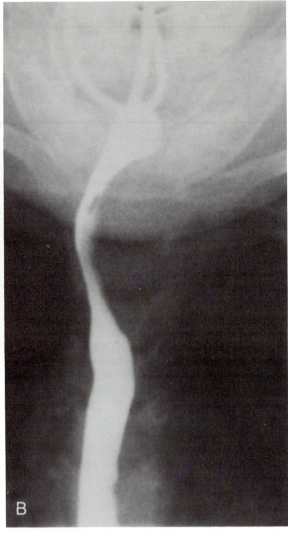

Figure 52–3. Bronchogenic cyst of the superior mediastinum. A rounded mass displaces the trachea to the right (*A*). Barium swallow examination (*B*) reveals similar displacement of the esophagus. Ultrasonography (not shown) demonstrated the cystic nature of the lesion, which at excision was found to be a typical bronchogenic cyst.

in these patients. Bronchography can sometimes demonstrate the bronchial communication of the cyst[10] or show poor filling of the obstructed bronchi.

Arterial angiography is generally not helpful in the diagnosis of bronchogenic cyst,[10] although it would detect the rare case with an anomalous systemic arterial supply. Digital subtraction angiography is a less invasive technique for ruling out anomalous vascularization. Magnetic resonance imaging (MRI) has been used to demonstrate a bronchogenic cyst;[53] anomalous systemic arteries can also be demonstrated by this method.

Subcutaneous bronchogenic cysts are usually diagnosed on histologic examination after excision.

DIFFERENTIAL DIAGNOSIS

The differential diagnosis of bronchogenic cyst includes other mass lesions of the middle mediastinum, such as enlargement of lymph nodes secondary to infection or neoplasm, primary malignancy, pericardial cyst, hemangioma, lipoma, esophageal duplication, varix, or leiomyoma. Anterior mediastinal masses such as cystic hygroma, thymoma, thyroid tumor, dermoid cyst, or teratoma can also resemble bronchogenic cysts, although the pattern of calcification in dermoids and teratomas can distinguish them from bronchogenic cysts in some cases. Posterior mediastinal masses, including neurenteric cyst and neurogenic tumors, are often associated with vertebral anomalies.[54] In many cases, however, only pathologic studies after excision of a mediastinal mass can distinguish among these anomalies.

Hyperinflation caused by a mediastinal bronchogenic cyst usually involves an entire lung; this feature helps distinguish it from congenital lobar emphysema, which usually involves only one lobe. An aerated parenchymal bronchogenic cyst must be differentiated from a pneumatocele, residual abscess cavity, or cavitary tuberculosis. In asymptomatic patients whose skin tests and sputum studies are negative for tuberculosis, a period of observation is indicated in order to determine whether the cystic lesion will resolve spontaneously.

An extralobar sequestration of the lung or an intralobar sequestration with a large cystic component can resemble a bronchogenic cyst radiographically. Unless the chest radiographic and CT appearances of the lesion are typical of a bronchogenic cyst, arterial angiography, digital subtraction angiography, or MRI should be performed in

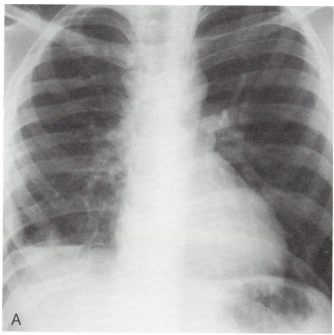

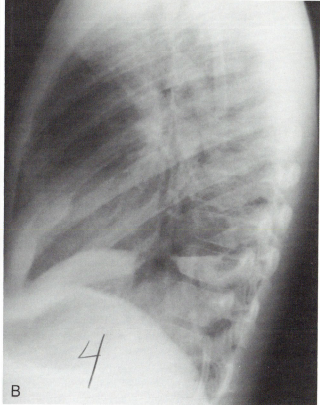

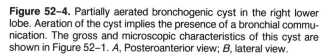

Figure 52–4. Partially aerated bronchogenic cyst in the right lower lobe. Aeration of the cyst implies the presence of a bronchial communication. The gross and microscopic characteristics of this cyst are shown in Figure 52–1. *A*, Posteroanterior view; *B*, lateral view.

order to rule out an anomalous systemic arterial supply. Although surgical resection is the treatment for both sequestration and bronchogenic cyst, the preoperative identification of an anomalous vessel decreases the risk of serious intraoperative hemorrhage.

TREATMENT

The treatment of choice for bronchogenic cysts is surgical excision. Even in asymptomatic patients, elective excision of the cyst should be performed in order to prevent later complications of airway obstruction, infection, or malignancy.[16, 28, 55]

At surgery for congenital lobar emphysema, a mediastinal bronchogenic cyst should be sought. Paratracheal cysts are often not seen until the mediastinal pleura is opened and the pulmonary root is retracted anteriorly.[15, 56] If a bronchogenic cyst is excised, lobectomy is often not necessary, although in some cases irreversible deformity of the bronchial cartilage, secondary to compression by the cyst, necessitates lobectomy.

Many parenchymal bronchogenic cysts are infected at the time of diagnosis. Resection in these cases should be preceded by appropriate antibiotic therapy. Lobectomy may be necessary in some cases if prolonged obstruction and infection have resulted in severe bronchiectasis.

Some authors have reported short-term success in treating bronchogenic cysts in adults with transbronchial[57] or mediastinoscopic[58] aspiration; the patients were observed postoperatively for only a few months. Other authors[38, 48, 59, 60] noted recurrence of bronchogenic cysts after aspira-

tion or partial excision, and they recommended complete resection.

Air transportation at high altitudes should be avoided by patients with known bronchogenic cysts because these cysts can expand by as much as 30% at the cabin pressure usually maintained in commercial jets. Similarly, the use of nitrous oxide for inhalation anesthesia should be avoided in patients with bronchogenic cysts; nitrous oxide is more soluble than nitrogen and can diffuse into the cyst, causing it to expand.[61] Positive pressure ventilation should also be minimized in patients with communicating bronchogenic cysts because of the potential for rapid expansion of the cyst.

PROGNOSIS

Without surgery, the mortality rate among symptomatic infants is 100%,[22, 50] whereas with surgical excision, the mortality rate is 0% to 14%.[10, 22, 50] Infants with marked emphysema of a lung secondary to a bronchogenic cyst exhibit a gradual resolution of the emphysema postoperatively.[12, 25] A residual area of bronchomalacia can contribute to continued symptoms, which often resolve spontaneously over several months. Bronchial stenting is occasionally necessary.

PULMONARY SEQUESTRATION

A pulmonary sequestration is a mass of nonfunctioning, embryonic lung tissue that has no communication with the normal bronchial system and is usually supplied by an aberrant systemic artery. Intralobar sequestrations are located within the visceral pleura and are partly or totally surrounded by normal lung. Extralobar sequestrations are located outside the pleura of the normal lung and have a separate pleural covering. The overall incidence of pulmonary sequestration is not well defined, but sequestrations have been found in 1.1% to 1.8% of all resected pulmonary specimens.[62] In most published series and reviews of sequestration, authors have noted a slightly higher incidence among males, especially in extralobar sequestrations; however, in an analysis of 546 cases of sequestration published between 1862 and 1975, Savic and associates[63] found no significant difference in incidence between the genders. In their review, 400 (73%) of the sequestrations were intralobar and 133 (24%) were extralobar; 6 cases (1%) involved both intralobar and extralobar sequestrations, and 2 (0.3%) involved bilateral intralobar sequestrations. In the remaining five cases (0.9%), an entire lung was sequestered.

PATHOPHYSIOLOGY

Several theories have been advanced in attempts to explain the developmental events resulting in sequestration. The reader is referred to excellent articles by Carter[62] and Iwai and colleagues[64] for succinct reviews of these theories, most of which seem less plausible in light of more current data. The theory most consistent with the available data was initially proposed by Eppinger and Schaunstein[65] and more recently supported by Halasz and co-authors.[66] These authors[65, 66] postulated that the sequestered lung tissue is derived from an accessory lung bud, which originates from the primitive foregut caudal to the primary lung bud. Both the primary and the accessory lung buds carry blood vessels of the splanchnic plexus, the network of vessels that arise from the dorsal and ventral aortas and surround the embryonic foregut. The network of vessels carried with the developing lung bud is called the postbranchial pulmonary plexus. Its connections with the aorta normally degenerate at the 8-mm stage of embryonic development, and its arterial supply is then derived solely from the sixth aortic arch, which becomes the pulmonary artery.

Branches of the pulmonary artery develop in tandem with the branches of the bronchopulmonary tree, to form the normal pulmonary vascular system. Meanwhile, the anomalous lung bud, in an arrested state of development, maintains its primitive systemic arterial supply. It is overtaken by the rapidly growing normal lung and either becomes surrounded by it, which results in an intralobar sequestration, or remains separate from but adjacent to the normal lung, which results in an extralobar sequestration. Rare cases in which otherwise typical extralobar sequestrations have been supplied by a branch of the pulmonary artery are easily accommodated by this theory, simply by the postulate that an anastomosis with the pulmonary arterial system occurred and the systemic vessel then degenerated. Theories based on a causative role of the systemic vessel in the development of the sequestration[67–69] cannot account for these cases. Halasz

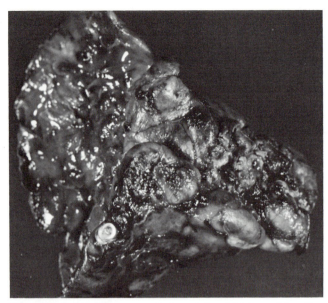

Figure 52–5. Intralobar sequestration of the right lower lobe. Two anomalous vessels are seen entering the sequestered lung along its posteroinferior margin. The medial half of the lobe consists of sequestered tissue; the lateral half is normal lung parenchyma. Bronchi extend around, but do not enter, the sequestered segment.

and co-authors' theory also accounts for the findings of patent or atretic connections between the esophagus and the sequestration, reported in 3.7% of intralobar and 10% of extralobar sequestrations.[63, 66, 70]

Intralobar sequestrations are most commonly located in the posterior basal segment of the lower lobe; in Savic and associates' review,[63] 98% of all intralobar sequestrations occurred in the lower lobes; 58% of these were on the left side. Two percent of cases occurred in the upper lobes, and one case was reported in the middle lobe. Extralobar sequestrations are most often (77%) located between the diaphragm and the lower lobe; 83% of these have been on the left side. Extralobar sequestrations have also been found between the upper and lower lobes and in paracardiac, mediastinal, infrapericardial, infradiaphragmatic, and abdominal locations. Intra-abdominal sequestrations are more common on the left side and have been described in perigastric, pararenal,[71] and supra-adrenal[72] locations.

Intralobar sequestrations appear macroscopically as pale, grayish-red areas, easily distinguished from the surrounding normal parenchyma (Fig. 52–5). The pleura adjacent to the sequestration is often adherent to the mediastinum, the diaphragm, or the thoracic wall. In some cases, there is a small patent connection with the normal tracheobronchial tree, so that some air enters the sequestration. The texture is variable, ranging from elastic to firm, depending on the amount of air and fluid contained within the cysts. Extralobar sequestrations vary in color from gray to dark red and are uniformly firm in texture with a smooth, shiny surface. Communication with the tracheobronchial tree is not present; hence there is no aeration.

Intralobar sequestrations are characterized histologically by bronchiectasis and varying degrees of cystic

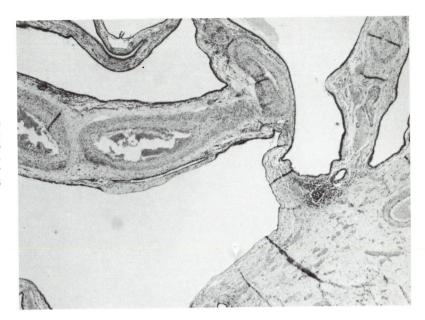

Figure 52-6. Intralobar sequestration. On histologic examination, the sequestration shown in Figure 52-5 is composed of markedly ectatic bronchial cysts with no normal alveolar structures. One of the anomalous systemic arteries is shown (center left) ($\times$ 160). (Courtesy of Dr. Kevin Bove, Department of Pathology, Children's Hospital Medical Center, Cincinnati, Ohio.)

changes. The cysts contain mucus or mucopurulent material and are lined by ciliated columnar or cuboidal epithelium (Fig. 52-6). The cyst walls may contain bits of cartilage, muscle, or bronchial glands. Some alveolar structures are usually present with varying degrees of atelectasis or emphysema.[64] Multifocal proliferative epithelial changes and dysplastic changes[73] and frank carcinoma[74] have been reported within intralobar sequestrations in adult patients. Inflammatory changes are frequently present; cultures may reveal bacterial, fungal, or tuberculous infection. Histologic examination of extralobar sequestrations reveals atelectatic embryonal lung tissue with dysplastic and hyperplastic elements.[75] Single or multiple cysts are often present.

The arterial supply of intralobar sequestrations has been of systemic origin in all reported cases, whereas 4% of extralobar sequestrations are supplied by a branch of the pulmonary artery.[63] The most common site of origin of the anomalous artery is the thoracic aorta, followed by the abdominal aorta and the intercostal arteries.[76] The supplying artery occasionally arises from the subclavian, innominate, internal thoracic, pericardiophrenic, celiac, gastric, or suprarenal arteries or from the ascending aorta. About 15% of reported patients have had more than one anomalous artery.[62, 63] The diameters of the anomalous arteries have ranged from 1 to 15 mm; the arteries supplying intralobar sequestrations tend to be larger than those associated with extralobar sequestrations. Histologic examination reveals that the arteries usually have predominantly elastic fibers characteristic of pulmonary arteries, despite their systemic origins. Arteriosclerosis is often noted in these vessels, even in children.

The venous drainage of intralobar sequestrations is generally via the pulmonary veins, although a few cases with systemic venous drainage have been described.[62] Conversely, extralobar sequestrations most often have systemic venous drainage, but on occasion there is drainage into the pulmonary venous system.

Other congenital anomalies have been noted in association with 14% of intralobar sequestrations and with 59%

of extralobar sequestrations.[63] The most frequent serious associated anomalies are diaphragmatic hernias, which are present in about 40% of all reported cases of extralobar sequestration and 3% of intralobar sequestrations.[63] Other anomalies that occur with some frequency include pulmonary and foregut malformations, eventration or paralysis of the diaphragm, hydrothorax, anasarca, and anomalies of the heart, the pericardium, and the great vessels.[62, 63, 77, 78] Bronchiectasis of the adjacent normal lung is a frequently reported finding in intralobar sequestration; however, it is not certain whether this is a congenital anomaly or a secondary change resulting from chronic infection of the sequestered tissue. Pectus excavatum and other thoracic skeletal anomalies have been associated with several cases of intralobar sequestration.

CLINICAL MANIFESTATIONS

Intralobar sequestrations are rarely detected during infancy; however, about one third of reported cases have manifested before the age of 10 years, usually with symptoms of chronic or recurrent pulmonary infection.[79] Productive cough, fever, hemoptysis, recurrent pneumonia, and chest pain are typical presenting complaints. A few patients with large supplying arteries have decreased exercise tolerance or frank congestive heart failure, caused by a large systemic arterial-to-pulmonary venous shunt through the sequestration.[80] Physical examination may reveal dullness to percussion and decreased breath sounds in the area of sequestration. Digital clubbing and cyanosis are occasionally present. Skeletal abnormalities such as pectus excavatum, thoracic asymmetry, and rib anomalies are noted in some patients. In one patient, an intrathoracic bruit was heard in the region of the sequestration.[70]

Less commonly, patients have emphysema, hemothorax, or pneumothorax, usually in association with a history of recurrent pulmonary infections.[81] One patient with a communicating stalk between the sequestration

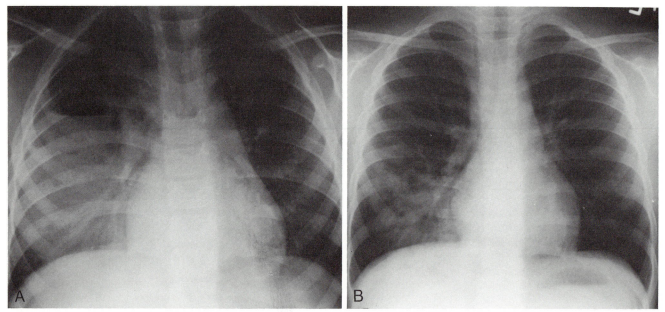

Figure 52–7. Intralobar pulmonary sequestration. The patient, a 6-year-old girl, had a 3-month history of recurrent pneumonia. *A,* The initial chest radiograph shows extensive consolidation in the right lower lobe, with an air-fluid level suggestive of abscess formation. *B,* After appropriate antibiotic therapy, the patient is clinically well, but the chest radiograph reveals persistent right lower lobe infiltrates.

and esophagus had massive esophageal bleeding after a long history of persistent localized pneumonia.[82] About 15% of intralobar sequestrations remain asymptomatic and are detected on routine chest radiographs.

Extralobar sequestrations are often discovered during the neonatal period in infants with other congenital anomalies. Many of these infants are premature, and there may be a history of polyhydramnios.[75] There is no known association with any specific teratogen. The associated anomalies dominate the clinical picture, and the sequestration is discovered incidentally at thoracotomy or autopsy. A few cases of a large extralobar sequestration presented with respiratory distress in an otherwise normal infant.[83] Extralobar sequestrations that are not diagnosed in newborns are often asymptomatic and detected on routine radiographs. Infection of the sequestration can occur, especially if there is a communication with the esophagus or the stomach. Intra-abdominal sequestrations, when infected, are accompanied by fever and abdominal pain. One such sequestration was initially thought to be a pancreatic pseudocyst because of the high amylase content in aspirated fluid.[71] Mahadevia[84] reported the case of a boy who complained of chest and shoulder pain and was found to have a necrotizing arteritis throughout an extralobar sequestration, with no associated pulmonary or systemic vasculitis.

DIAGNOSIS

Plain radiographs of the chest reveal an intralobar sequestration as a solid, multicystic, or simple cystic mass, most often located posteromedially in a lower lobe. Air-fluid levels are present in many cysts (Fig. 52–7). The long axis of the mass often points posteromedially toward the

aorta. Extralobar sequestrations appear as uniform densities that are oval, triangular, or fusiform and are most often located in the posteromedial lower lobe, just above the diaphragm. Calcifications are occasionally present in both intralobar and extralobar sequestrations. Bronchoscopy usually reveals no abnormalities, although in cases with chronic infection there may be bronchitis or bronchiectasis in the lung adjacent to the sequestration. Bronchography demonstrates the normal bronchi curving around the sequestration, and no contrast material enters the sequestration itself. In rare cases, a small amount of contrast material does enter and outlines a cyst within the sequestration.

The definitive step in the diagnosis of sequestration is the demonstration of the systemic arterial supply. This can sometimes be achieved by radioisotope study of the lung; after an intravenous injection of radioisotope, an area with systemic blood supply shows peak activity several seconds later than does the lung tissue with normal pulmonary blood supply.[85] Once the systemic blood supply has been demonstrated, however, it is essential that the number and location of the anomalous vessels be defined because the accidental severance of an unsuspected anomalous artery is a potential cause of intraoperative mortality.[86, 87] Angiography of the thoracic and abdominal aorta, either by direct aortic catheterization (Fig. 52–8) or by digital subtraction angiography, is the most straightforward and accurate approach. Even with aortography, there have been a few cases in which an anomalous artery, usually small and originating from an intercostal artery, was missed and identified only during surgery.[63] If aortic angiography fails to demonstrate a systemic arterial supply to an area of suspected sequestration, a lung scan can be performed after injection of a radioisotope into the thoracic aorta at the conclusion of

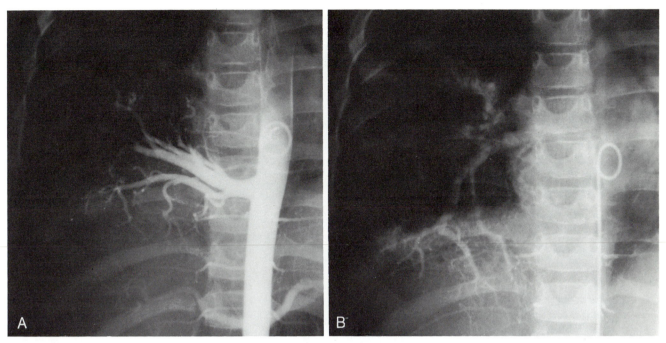

Figure 52–8. *A,* Aortic angiography of the patient described in Figure 52–7 demonstrates an anomalous artery arising from the descending aorta and supplying the right lower lobe of the lung. *B,* The venous return from the sequestration is seen entering the left antrium, as is typical of intralobar sequestration.

the angiogram. Early uptake seen in the area of the sequestration indicates the presence of a systemic blood supply that has not appeared on the angiogram.[88]

CT scan[89, 90] and MRI[91] have been advocated as less invasive means of identifying the anomalous artery. These procedures are useful in cases of a relatively large anomalous artery, especially if it originates directly from the aorta. Additional smaller vessels, present in 15% of sequestrations, may be missed by CT scan or MRI.

DIFFERENTIAL DIAGNOSIS

An unaerated sequestration may have a radiologic appearance similar to those of pulmonary and mediastinal neoplasms, aortic aneurysms, and bronchogenic, enterogenic, and pericardial cysts. Sequestrations containing air-filled cysts may resemble pneumatoceles, emphysematous blebs and bullae, infantile lobar emphysema, congenital cystic adenomatoid malformation, or Bochdalek's hernia; those with air-fluid levels in cysts may be mistaken for pneumonia with abscess formation or for partially aerated bronchogenic cysts.[92, 93] Sequestrations can be distinguished from most of these entities by the demonstration of a systemic blood supply. CT scan may be helpful in distinguishing bronchogenic cysts from sequestrations by showing a stalk connecting the bronchogenic cyst to the trancheobronchial tree. Chronic pulmonary infection distal to an aspirated foreign body or an area of bronchiectasis may result in neovascularization of the infected tissue by ingrowth of systemic arteries. In general, this acquired systemic vascularization consists of several small vessels rather than the one or two large ves-

sels that typically supply a sequestration; however, it may be impossible to make the distinction between true sequestration and so-called pseudosequestration secondary to chronic infection preoperatively.[94] Resection is the treatment of choice in either case.

Systemic arterialization of the lung is also seen in arteriovenous malformations, pulmonary artery aplasia, and systemic arterial supply to normal lung;[95] these entities can usually be distinguished from sequestration by clinical manifestation and radiologic characteristics.

TREATMENT

Resection is the treatment of choice for intralobar and extralobar sequestrations, including those that are asymptomatic and discovered by chance, because of the risk of subsequent serious infection.[62] In cases of acute infection, a preoperative course of antibiotics should be given. The resected tissue should be sent for mycobacterial and fungal cultures, in addition to aerobic and anaerobic bacterial cultures; postoperative antibiotic therapy can be guided by the results of these studies.

Resection of the involved lobe is necessary for intralobar sequestration; extralobar sequestrations can often be removed without disrupting the normal lung. Intraoperative and postoperative mortality rates are low, except in the subset of patients who present in infancy with extralobar sequestration associated with other congenital anomalies, many of which prove to be lethal. The chief cause of intraoperative mortality has been hemorrhage secondary to accidental severance of a systemic artery. Postoperative complications include emphysema, hemo-

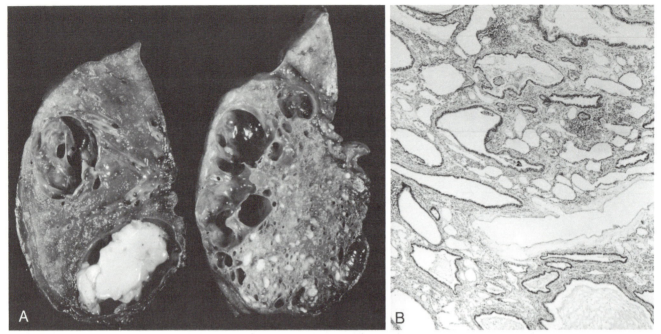

Figure 52–9. Congenital cystic adenomatoid malformation of the left lower lobe. *A*, Most of the pulmonary parenchyma is replaced by thin-walled cysts, varying from 0.1 to 4.0 cm in diameter. Many of the cysts are filled with a pale yellow gelatinous material. No communication with the bronchial tree is demonstrated. *B*, The cysts are lined with respiratory epithelium. Inflammatory changes and bronchial cartilage are not prominent in the cyst walls; this finding helps distinguish this lesion from cystic bronchiectasis. Numerous irregularly shaped tubular structures, lined with cuboidal epithelium, are present in the stroma (× 160). (Courtesy of Dr. Kevin Bove, Department of Pathology, Children's Hospital Medical Center, Cincinnati, Ohio.)

thorax, bronchopleurocutaneous fistula, and bronchopleural fistulae; the incidence of each of these complications has been 1% or less among reported cases.[63]

The long-term prognosis, in the absence of other debilitating congenital anomalies, is excellent.

CONGENITAL CYSTIC ADENOMATOID MALFORMATION OF THE LUNG

Since congenital cystic adenomatoid malformation of the lung (CCAML) was first described in 1949, approximately 200 cases have been described in the English-language literature. In surgical series, CCAML has accounted for 22% to 40% of all resected congenital lung anomalies.[96–99] The occurrence of CCAML is sporadic; there is no association with race, sex, or maternal age and no familial predisposition.

PATHOPHYSIOLOGY

The gross pathologic appearance of CCAML is of an enlarged, firm mass without normal lobar configuration. Sectioning reveals solid material interspersed with cysts of variable number and size (Fig. 52–9*A*). In some cases, no cysts are present. The blood supply to a CCAML is usually of pulmonary arterial origin.

The histologic characteristics of CCAML as described by Kwittken and Reiner[100] are widely used as diagnostic criteria. Solid "adenomatous" areas consist of closely packed tubular structures, which resemble terminal bronchioles; there are no mature alveoli. Electron microscopy

shows that the cuboidal epithelium lining the tubules consists predominantly of type 2 pneumocytes.[101] Thus the adenomatous areas of CCAML bear a close resemblance to the histologic appearance of the normal fetal lung at about 20 weeks' gestation. A generally accepted theory postulates that a developmental arrest, at about 20 weeks' gestation, results in failure of the fetal mesenchyme to develop into the respiratory bronchioles and alveoli.[102]

Interspersed with the adenomatous areas are cysts, of which two distinct types have been described. One type, resembling a dilated version of the tubular structures, is lined by a single layer of cuboidal epithelium, and its walls contain no elastic tissue or smooth muscle. The other type of cyst has a characteristic appearance that is included in Kwittken and Reiner's[100] criteria for CCAML. These cysts are lined with a pseudostratified columnar epithelium with papillary projections into the lumen (Fig. 52–9*B*). Large amounts of elastic tissue, and often smooth muscle, are present in the walls of the cysts. Clumps of tall, columnar, mucin-secreting cells resembling intestinal mucosa cells occur in the epithelium lining the lumen of some cysts.

The number and size of the cysts found in CCAML vary from none (solid CCAML) to mostly cystic.[103, 104] Stocker and associates[105] describe three types of CCAML. The type I lesion is composed of large cysts interspersed with enlarged alveolar structures with little or no adenomatous component; type II is mixed cystic and adenomatous; and type III is entirely adenomatous.

Cartilage and mucous glands are not found in CCAML. This characteristic helps distinguish cases of chronically infected multicystic CCAML from areas of cystic bronchiectasis. Inflammation is not present in CCAML resected from infants, but it is invariably found in older patients.[106, 107] Malignancies, such as rhabdomyosarcoma, rarely develop within CCAML.[108]

The normal lung tissue surrounding a CCAML is compressed, atelectatic, and often hypoplastic. The mediastinum is frequently shifted away from the mass lesion. Compression of the heart and the great vessels can result in hydrops fetalis. Compression of the esophagus, with impairment in swallowing, may contribute to the polyhydramnios often seen in infants with CCAML.[109] Other mechanisms that may account for the development of polyhydramnios include excessive secretion of fluid from the CCAML and impaired absorption of fluid from the compressed normal lung.[101, 110]

CLINICAL PRESENTATION

Patients with CCAML present either as neonates with severe, progressive respiratory distress or as older children or adults with recurrent pulmonary infections. The neonatal presentation is more easily recognized. The pregnancy is often complicated by hydramnios, severe preeclampsia, or hydrops fetalis.[103, 104] Prematurity and stillbirth are common, particularly among infants who are hydropic[103, 104] and those with solid CCAML.[111] Neonates with mixed solid and cystic CCAML have respiratory distress, which is usually evident at birth or soon after and is rapidly progressive. These infants have a strong potential for survival if surgical resection is performed promptly.

Most infants with CCAML are otherwise normal, but other pulmonary defects and cardiac, gastrointestinal, and genitourinary anomalies have been described in about 20% of patients.[105, 106, 110, 112, 113]

Between 50% and 65% of patients with CCAML present after the neonatal period.[114, 115] The cystic lesions in these patients probably have less communication with the tracheobronchial tree and therefore do not progressively expand and cause respiratory distress.[98] These patients develop recurrent pulmonary infection resulting from impairment in the clearance of secretions from the abnormal tissue. On occasion, CCAML remains asymptomatic and is discovered incidentally on a chest radiograph.[107] A few patients have presented with spontaneous pneumothorax.[115, 116]

DIAGNOSTIC APPROACH

The chest radiograph is usually diagnostic, especially in association with the typical neonatal manifestation of progressive respiratory distress. Immediately after birth, the lesion may appear solid on the chest radiograph because of delayed clearing of fetal lung fluid from the cysts. As the lung fluid is cleared, the cysts become aerated and progressively expand.[117, 118] The surrounding normal lung becomes increasingly atelectatic, and mediastinal shift occurs. In the most characteristic radiographic appearance, CCAML is multicystic, interspersed with solid areas (Fig. 52–10). A single large cyst or an entirely solid lesion can also be seen. The lesion is usually unilateral and affects only one lobe, although an entire lung is occasionally involved. When a multicystic lesion is seen in the left thorax, a barium swallow or barium enema can be helpful in distinguishing CCAML from a diaphragmatic hernia.

Thoracic CT scan with contrast material can be useful in differentiating fluid-filled cysts from solid lesions. Ultrasonography can also be used to distinguish between cystic and solid lesions, when they are adjacent to the chest wall, and can reveal CCAML in the fetus. Adzik and colleagues[111] described two categories of CCAML that are identifiable prenatally by ultrasonography. The microcys-

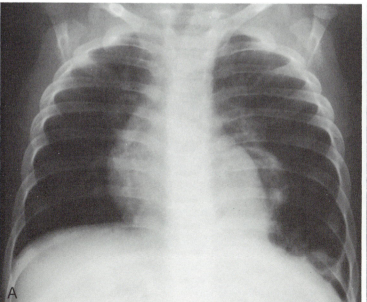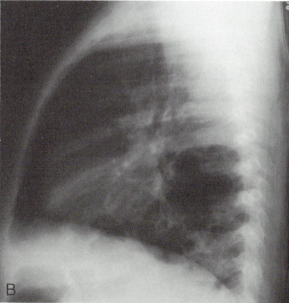

Figure 52–10. Congenital cystic adenomatoid malformation. The patient, a 16-month-old boy, had fever, tachypnea, and a history of chronic cough. Chest radiographs reveal an irregular multicystic lesion in the left lower lobe. The pathologic features of the malformation are seen in Figure 52–9. *A*, Posteroanterior view; *B*, lateral view.

tic lesions have a poor prognosis; many affected infants are hydropic and may be stillborn. However, if the diagnosis is made prenatally and the lesion is resected immediately after birth, some infants can survive. Macrocystic CCAML is usually not associated with hydrops, and the condition of the infants at delivery tends to be more stable. These patients have a relatively good prognosis with early resection of the lesion. In older patients with recurrent pulmonary infection and cystic lesions shown on chest radiographs, bronchography is useful in distinguishing CCAML from localized bronchiectasis. MRI can also be helpful in these cases.[119]

In some cases, angiography may be necessary for distinguishing CCAML from a pulmonary sequestration. The blood supply to CCAML is almost always of pulmonary origin; the vessels within the lesion show a characteristic irregular spacing.[106]

DIFFERENTIAL DIAGNOSIS

As mentioned earlier, diaphragmatic hernia, bronchiectasis, and pulmonary sequestration are the most frequent considerations in the differential diagnosis of CCAML. When CCAML involves a single cyst and is paramediastinal in location, it can be difficult or impossible to distinguish from a bronchogenic cyst. Also, a single large cyst in CCAML sometimes mimics congenital lobar emphysema on chest radiographs. Surgical resection is the treatment of choice for each of these lesions.

Cystic lesions seen on chest radiographs in the area of resolving pneumonia may represent postpneumonic pneumatoceles or abscesses. Review of previous chest radiographs, when available, can resolve the question of whether these cystic lesions are congenital or acquired. If previous radiographs are not available and if the patient is clinically well, the lesions can be observed with serial chest radiographs for several months after the completion of antibiotic therapy; pneumatoceles and abscess cavities spontaneously resolve.

Mesenchymal cystic hamartoma of the lung[120] is characterized by multiple, sometimes bilateral, slowly progressive lesions composed of nodules and cysts. The nodules are composed of primitive mesenchymal cells; they contain hypertrophic systemic arteries and plexi of anastomosing airways. The cysts are lined by respiratory epithelium with an underlying layer of mesenchymal cells. Mark[120] suggested that some cases diagnosed as CCAML or other pulmonary cystic lesions, including cases in which malignancies have subsequently developed,[108, 121–123] may actually have been cases of mesenchymal cystic hamartoma.

Mesothelial cysts and cystic lymphangiectasis are rare congenital pulmonary lesions that may have radiographic appearances similar to that of CCAML.

TREATMENT

Surgical resection of the abnormal tissue is the treatment of choice. Symptomatic infants should undergo immediate resection. Because of the progressive expansion of the lesion, efforts to stabilize an infant and delay surgery are usually unsuccessful. An advantage of early resection is the decompression of normal lung tissue, which provides maximal potential for growth of new lung parenchyma. When CCAML has been diagnosed prenatally, delivery in a tertiary care center with surgical resection immediately after delivery maximizes the infant's chance of survival.[111]

Some controversy exists over the advisability of segmental resection versus lobectomy. Lilly and co-authors[97] contended that segmental resection can be performed safely by skilled surgeons and anesthesiologists and spares normal lung tissue. Other authors, however, believe that the complication rate after segmental resection is unacceptably high.[96, 106, 107, 124]

It is essential that all abnormal tissue be resected because residual CCAML may enlarge and require reoperation.[115, 121]

PROGNOSIS

The long-term prognosis after surgical resection of CCAML is relatively good. Merenstein,[125] in a review of 48 cases of CCAML, found that 14 of 16 surgically treated patients survived, whereas 16 of 32 medically treated patients died. Wolf and collaborators[115] reported a 94% survival rate among 32 surgically treated patients. In the immediate postoperative period, respiratory distress often persists because of hypoplasia of the normal lung. As atelectatic areas re-expand and new lung tissue is formed, the respiratory distress gradually resolves. Frenckner and Freyschuss[126] studied pulmonary function in five patients 2 to 11 years after lobectomy for CCAML. The patients were 1 day old to 11 years old at the time of the resection. The average quantity of lung tissue resected was 24%; however, the decreases from predicted lung volumes and in carbon monoxide diffusing capacity were only 10% and 8%, respectively, which implies that compensatory growth of new lung tissue had occurred.

CONGENITAL LOBAR EMPHYSEMA

Congenital lobar emphysema (CLE) is a condition characterized by progressive overinflation, usually of one lobe, with compression of the remainder of the lung and the mediastinal structures. By definition, in CLE there is no acquired intraluminal obstructive lesion such as aspirated foreign body or inspissated mucus. The pathologic features were first described by Overstreet.[127] In 1943, the first successful surgical resection of CLE was performed by Gross and Lewis.[128] In more recent surgical series, CLE has been listed as the diagnosis in 14% to 31% of infants requiring pulmonary resections.[129–131] The occurrence of CLE is usually sporadic, although occasional familial recurrence has been noted.[132, 133] Murray,[134] in a collective view of 166 cases of CLE, reported a male-to-female ratio of 2:1.

PATHOPHYSIOLOGY

On gross inspection of the lung in CLE, the involved lobe or segment is massively overdistended, smooth, and pale pink. The hyperinflated lobe does not deflate, even

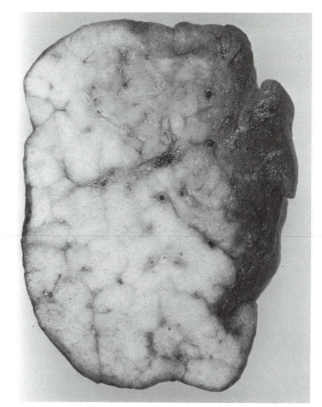

Figure 52–11. Congenital lobar emphysema. On sectioning, the massively enlarged right upper lobe was found to have a homogeneous, finely spongy surface. Prominent white interlobular septae are seen. Normal bronchial and bronchiolar structures are present throughout the lobe.

when the lobar bronchus is transected and manual compression is applied. The cut surface of the emphysematous lobe has a uniform, spongy appearance (Fig. 52–11). The upper and middle lobes are involved more often than the lower lobes. In most cases, only a single lobe is involved, but two or more emphysematous lobes have been reported in a few patients.[135-137]

The histologic appearance of CLE is variable, indicating that the clinical entity of CLE may encompass an assortment of anatomic aberrations. Most authors have described alveoli as anatomically normal but overdistended. Others have noted disruption of alveolar septa, forming cystlike spaces (Fig. 52–12).[138, 139] Boren[140] discussed the possible significance of alveolar fenestrations, thought to be either tears in the alveolar wall or enlarged pores of Kohn, in the pathogenesis of emphysema. In some cases, abnormal collagen deposition has been noted in the alveolar walls and the supporting stroma.[138, 141, 142] The increased rigidity of the alveolar walls may interfere with normal deflation and thus result in emphysema in affected patients.

In most reported cases the number of alveoli in the affected lobe is thought to be normal. A variant, first described by Hislop and Reid[143] and Munnell and associates[144] as "polyalveolar lobe," is characterized by a striking increase in the number of alveoli and the alveolar-to-arterial ratio. The alveoli are not emphysematous; thus this condition would be more accurately classified as lobar giantism rather than CLE. The polyalveolar lobe may represent a significant subset of cases classified as CLE; Tapper and colleagues,[145] in a retrospective pathologic review of sixteen cases of CLE, found six of these specimens to have a fivefold increase in the number of alveoli.

The elastic tissue in the emphysematous lobe is normal.[134] The pulmonary vessels are anatomically normal, although widely spaced and often compressed.[132, 145, 146] In one case, markedly dilated septal lymphatic vessels traversed the emphysematous lobe.[147]

An obstructive abnormality of the bronchus seems to be the most obvious explanation for the development of CLE, especially in cases in which alveolar architecture appears normal. However, in 50% of cases of CLE, no bronchial abnormality can be demonstrated.[134] Extrinsic bronchial compression, as in vascular ring, hilar adenopathy, or bronchogenic cyst, accounts for 2% of cases of CLE; 48% of cases are associated with intraluminal bronchial obstruction.

Figure 52–12. Congenital lobar emphysema. Histologic examination of the specimen shown in Figure 52–11 revealed striking emphysematous changes. The alveoli were hyperinflated, and destruction of alveolar septal walls, alveolar fenestrations, and coalescence of adjacent alveoli are seen (× 160). (Courtesy of Dr. Kevin Bove, Department of Pathology, Children's Hospital Medical Center, Cincinnati, Ohio.)

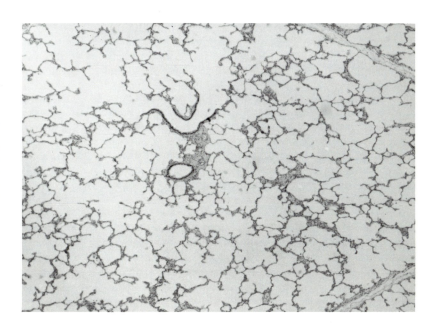

Various intrinsic bronchial abnormalities, including abnormal mucosal folds, bronchial stenosis, and bronchial kinking or rotation, have been found in patients with CLE. Bronchomalacia, however, is the most common abnormality. The bronchomalacia may be focal, involving the lobar bronchus, or diffuse, involving peripheral airways throughout the affected lobe. The abnormal cartilage has been variously described as absent, hypoplastic, flaccid, or immature. Diffuse bronchomalacia of the entire bronchial tree has been found in a few cases; this condition may account for the tendency of some patients to have persistent wheezing or diffuse generalized emphysema, after lobectomy for CLE.[132, 148–150]

CLINICAL MANIFESTATIONS

Congenital lobar emphysema manifests in the form of progressive, severe respiratory distress in infants and in the form of wheezing, cough, or recurrent chest infection in older children.

In the majority of patients with CLE, symptoms develop in infancy. Half the patients are symptomatic within the first few days of life, and most of the remaining patients exhibit symptoms by the age of 4 months.[136] Intermittent bouts of dyspnea, tachypnea, wheezing, cough, and cyanosis are precipitated by feeding, crying, or excitement. The respiratory symptoms progressively worsen, eventually becoming persistent and severe. Acute development of severe respiratory distress, necessitating emergency surgical intervention, occurs in about 12% of patients, often in association with an acute upper respiratory infection.[132]

Physical examination reveals tachypnea, nasal flaring, intercostal retractions, and sometimes cyanosis. The hemithorax of the affected side is hyperinflated and hyperresonant to percussion, with decreased breath sounds and vocal fremitus. The apical cardiac pulse and the trachea may be shifted away from the hyperinflated side. Abnormal prominence of the liver or the spleen can result from flattening of the diaphragm on the affected side. On chest radiographs, a progressively expanding area of hyperlucency is seen. The mediastinum is shifted away from the abnormal side, and the surrounding normal lung becomes increasingly compressed.

Older children with CLE tend to have milder symptoms. Some children manifest diffuse wheezing, which may reflect an anatomic abnormality of the airways such as bronchomalacia rather than true asthma. Other patients acquire recurrent pulmonary infection secondary to impairment in the clearance of secretions. In occasional patients, CLE is asymptomatic and is discovered incidentally in late childhood.[141] Rare cases of CLE manifesting in adulthood have been reported.[148, 151] However, it can be difficult to distinguish CLE from acquired emphysema in adult patients.

DIAGNOSTIC PROCEDURES

The chest radiograph in CLE shows findings typical of lobar hyperinflation. The affected lobe is enlarged and markedly hyperlucent, but lung markings are visible throughout the lobe; this characteristic distinguishes CLE from a cystic lesion, diaphragmatic hernia, or pneumothorax. Serial chest radiographs show increasing hyperinflation of the emphysematous lobe, with progressive atelectasis of the ipsilateral normal lung, mediastinal shift away from the emphysematous side, and compression of the contralateral lung (Fig. 52–13). In neonates, chest radiographs often initially reveal an opaque, fluid-filled lobe that gradually becomes radiolucent as the fluid is absorbed.[139, 152]

Fluoroscopy is useful for distinguishing obstructive hyperinflation or CLE from compensatory hyperinflation secondary to atelectasis. In primary emphysema, the hyperinflation persists during exhalation, and the diaphragm on the affected side moves poorly. The mediastinum shifts toward the emphysematous side during inspiration and away from it during exhalation.[153]

After the diagnosis of primary lobar emphysema is made, the remaining question is whether the emphysema represents CLE (which necessitates lobectomy) or is secondary to a potentially remediable bronchial obstruction such as inspissated mucus or foreign body. Bronchoscopy should be performed in older children with lobar emphysema because an acquired obstruction such as an aspirated foreign body is a more likely cause than CLE for emphysema in these patients. In infants with suspected CLE, however, rigid bronchoscopy with the ventilating bronchoscope can lead to rapid deterioration because the positive-pressure ventilation causes increasing hyperinflation of the affected lobe. Fiberoptic bronchoscopy may be a safer alternative but should be attempted only in patients who are clinically stable. Bronchography also can result in rapid deterioration of the patient and is not often helpful; the bronchial tree of the affected lobe tends not to fill, even if no bronchial obstruction is found at resection.[146] When the bronchi do fill, they show widely separated segments.

Less invasive techniques can be helpful in screening for causes of extrinsic bronchial compression. The barium swallow is useful for ruling out vascular ring or mediastinal mass. Thoracic CT scan with contrast can show a small subcarinal or perihilar bronchogenic cyst that may not be visible on the chest radiograph.[154] The CT scan also demonstrates the typical widely separated vascular pattern of CLE and sometimes identifies an area of localized bronchial narrowing.[155] MRI can be used to detect abnormal mediastinal structures or anomalous blood vessels.[156]

Ventilation/perfusion scanning of the lung is usually not necessary in the diagnosis of CLE; however, it can be helpful in distinguishing CLE from compensatory emphysema. In CLE, matched defects in ventilation and perfusion are found, whereas in compensatory emphysema, ventilation and perfusion of the emphysematous lobe are normal.[153, 157]

DIFFERENTIAL DIAGNOSIS

CLE must be differentiated from compensatory emphysema, reversible obstructive emphysema, large cystic lesions, diaphragmatic hernia, and pneumothorax.

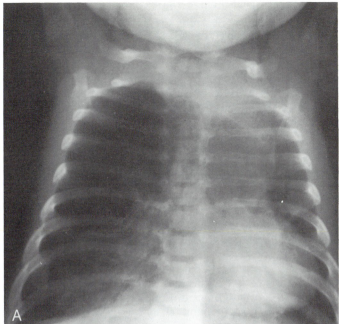
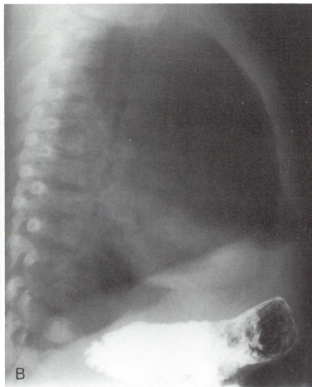

Figure 52–13. Congenital lobar emphysema. The patient, a newborn, had progressive respiratory distress. Chest radiographs show a hyperlucent right upper lobe that herniates across the midline into the left hemithorax. The right middle and lower lobes and the left lung are compressed. The heart is shifted to the left. The pathologic appearance of the right upper lobe is shown in Figure 52–11 and 52–12. *A,* Posteroanterior view; *B,* lateral view.

The unilateral hyperlucent lung (Swyer-James) syndrome, in which obliterative bronchiolitis and markedly decreased pulmonary blood flow to one lung follow a severe episode of pneumonia, shares some radiographic characteristics with CLE. The affected lung appears hyperlucent on chest radiographs, and the mediastinum shifts toward the normal side on exhalation. However, the volume of the hyperlucent lung is slightly decreased, and there is no compression of normal lung tissue. The hyperlucency of the lung appears to be secondary to the decrease in perfusion rather than to emphysema.[158] Congenital absence of the pulmonary artery also results in hyperlucency of a lung secondary to decreased vascular markings.

A syndrome of acquired lobar emphysema in infants with bronchopulmonary dysplasia was described by Cooney and co-authors.[159] Two subsets of patients were identified; those with normal lung perfusion scans, who were successfully weaned from the ventilator and eventually showed complete resolution of the emphysema, and those with markedly decreased perfusion of the emphysematous lobe, who required lobectomy.

TREATMENT

For infants with typical CLE and progressive respiratory distress, immediate surgical intervention is indicated. Without surgery, the mortality rate among these patients is 50%, and 75% of the survivors have persistent respiratory distress.[135] However, older children with mild

or no symptoms have been managed conservatively without serious sequelae.[153, 160, 161] Patients who have both congenital heart disease and CLE usually require surgical correction of both conditions. In cases in which only the cardiovascular defect has been corrected, in hopes that the CLE would then resolve, lobectomy has been necessary in the early postoperative period.[162] Pierce and co-workers,[163] however, defined a subgroup of infants with congenital heart disease and mild lobar emphysema, with no mediastinal shift or significant compression of normal lung, who responded well to treatment of the heart disease alone.

The surgical treatment of choice is lobectomy. When two lobes are involved, staged lobectomies, with removal of the more hyperinflated lobe first, have been successful.[135, 136] The administration of inhalation anesthesia for the patient with CLE can be complicated by rapid expansion of the emphysematous lobe and sudden deterioration of the patient's condition. Thus positive pressure ventilation should not be initiated until just before thoracotomy. When the chest wall is opened, the emphysematous lobe often herniates through the wound, thus ameliorating the compression of other intrathoracic structures.

PROGNOSIS

The mortality rate among surgically treated patients is about 7%.[134] Most of these deaths have been related to concomitant heart disease or hypoxic brain damage. In some patients, diffuse, often fatal emphysema develops postoperatively,[148, 150] and some patients have recurrent wheezing.[132, 150]

In long-term follow-up of pulmonary function after lobectomy for CLE, some investigators have found evidence of compensatory lung growth.[145, 164, 165] Other studies of pulmonary functions, however, reveal persistent defects, including increased functional residual volume, increased total lung capacity, and decreased midexpiratory flow rates.[160, 166] Despite the abnormaliteis on pulmonary function testing, most surgically treated patients are asymptomatic.

TRACHEOESOPHAGEAL FISTULA

Tracheoesophageal fistula (TEF) is a relatively common congenital pulmonary anomaly, occurring in 1 in 4000 to 5000 live births.[167] There is no difference in incidence between the sexes and no apparent genetic predisposition in most cases, although a few kindreds with two or more affected infants have been reported.

PATHOPHYSIOLOGY

The embryologic basis for the development of TEF is not fully understood. The septum between the embryonic trachea and esophagus normally begins to form at the level of the future carina and progresses cephalad. Most authors have postulated that the typical carinal TEF results from primary failure of septal development at the carinal level. An alternative theory holds that normal septation occurs and is followed by necrosis and fistula formation secondary to localized vascular insufficiency.[168] Holder and Ashcraft[169] offered an in-depth discussion of the embryologic development of TEF. Several anatomic variants of TEF occur, most of which are associated with esophageal atresia. The most common form of TEF, accounting for approximately 85% of cases, is proximal esophageal atresia and distal TEF (Fig. 52–14A). In these cases, the proximal esophageal pouch usually extends 1.0 to 3.5 cm below the superior constrictor muscle. The pouch is often dilated, with a luminal diameter of 10 mm or more. It has the normal two layers of striated muscle. In many cases, there is a fibrous attachment of the proximal esophageal pouch to either the distal esophageal pouch or the posterior tracheal wall.[169] The gap between the proximal and distal esophageal pouches is variable, averaging about 2 cm in length[167] but ranging from a few millimeters to several centimeters. When there is no fibrous attachment between the proximal and distal pouches, the gap tends to be longer.

The wall of the distal esophageal pouch is thin with a thickness of about 1 mm, although both the normal layers of smooth muscle are present. The proximal end of the distal pouch tends to be of much smaller diameter than the distal end of the proximal pouch, and this feature poses technical problems with anastomosis. The distal pouch also tends to have a relatively poor blood supply, of which a significant portion is derived from lateral vessels that can be disrupted during surgery.

The fistula originates from the apex of the distal esophageal segment and enters the posterior trachea at or just above the carina in most cases.[167] The tracheal end of the fistula can be located anywhere from 2 cm above the carina to the proximal 2 cm of either main bronchus. The tracheal orifice of the fistula is usually crescent shaped and easier to see endoscopically than the esophageal orifice, which is a longitudinal slit.[168] The mucosa of the fistula is typically esophageal along its entire length. Esophageal muscular elements are also present. In some cases, esophageal mucosa and muscular elements are present in the membranous wall of the trachea around the fistula opening. Enoksen and associates[170] described a 51-year-old patient in whom these muscular elements appeared to have exerted a protective effect by functioning as a sphincter around the tracheal orifice of the TEF. In other cases, tracheal mucosa, mucous glands, and rudimentary cartilage rings extend through part of the fistula.[168] In about 1.2% of cases, the fistula is not patent.[171]

A much rarer anatomic variant is esophageal atresia with TEF originating from the proximal pouch (Fig. 52–14B). The fistula extends from the apex of the proximal esophageal pouch to the carina or the midportion of the trachea; in some cases the fistula consists of a side-to-side communication. An even rarer variant is esophageal atresia with both a proximal and a distal TEF.[172] The proximal fistula enters the trachea near or below the midpoint; the distal fistula enters near the carina (Fig. 52–14C).

About 10% of cases of esophageal atresia are not associated with a TEF.[167] Conversely, about 3% of cases of TEF exist without esophageal atresia (Fig. 52–14D). In this form, often referred to as H-type fistula, the trachea and the esophagus are anatomically normal except for the fistula, which usually runs upward from the esophagus to the middle or upper trachea. Because of the upward course of the fistula, aspiration does not occur with every swallow. Fluids tend to cross the fistula more readily than solids. A rare and rapidly fatal variant of TEF consists of tracheal atresia, esophageal atresia, and distal TEF (Fig. 52–14E). Affected infants are in severe neonatal respiratory distress and have no audible cry. Immediate tracheostomy can be life-saving in these infants.[173] With proximal tracheal atresia or aplasia and TEF (Fig. 52–14F), patients are able to ventilate the lungs via the proximal esophagus. However, massive aspiration of feedings occurs.[174]

The pulmonary problems associated with TEF and/or esophageal atresia result from aspiration by several mechanisms: (1) esophageal atresia precludes swallowing of oral secretions and feedings, which spill over from the proximal esophageal pouch and are aspirated; (2) in the case of H-type fistula or esophageal atresia with proximal TEF, feedings enter the trachea via the fistula; (3) in esophageal atresia with a distal TEF and, to a lesser extent, in some cases of H-type fistula, there is reflux of the acidic gastric contents through the fistula into the trachea; and (4) even after operative repair of the esophageal atresia and TEF, many patients are prone to recurrent aspiration because of esophageal abnormalities such as anastomotic stricture, esophageal dysmotility, and gastroesophageal reflux.

Aspiration pneumonia occurs more often in patients

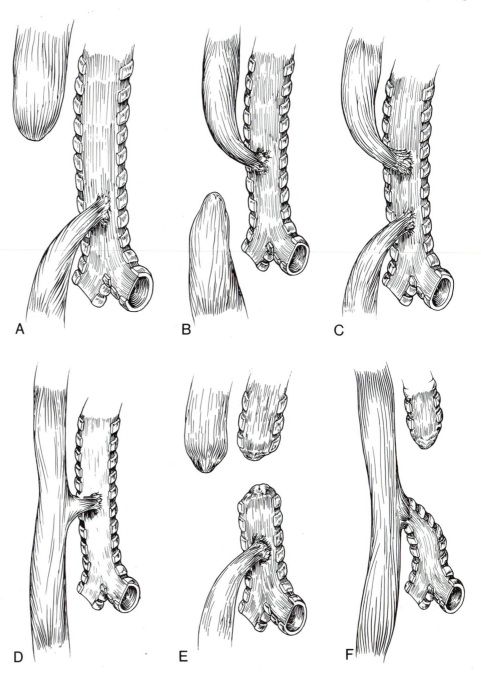

Figure 52–14. Diagrams of anatomic variants of tracheoesophageal fistula (TEF). *A*, Esophageal atresia with distal TEF. *B*, Esophageal atresia with proximal TEF. *C*, Esophageal atresia with both proximal and distal TEF. *D*, H-type TEF. *E*, Esophageal atresia, tracheal atresia, and distal TEF. *F*, Tracheal atresia and distal TEF.

with TEF associated with esophageal atresia and may be massive. In patients with H-type fistula and in postoperative patients with recurrent aspiration, the volumes of aspirated material may be smaller. Chronic airway inflammation with bouts of infection can eventually result in bronchiectasis (Fig. 52–15) or obliterative bronchiolitis.[175] Another cause of respiratory distress in patients with a distal TEF is massive dilatation of the stomach by air with consequent elevation of the diaphragm and pulmonary compression. Examination of the tracheal mucosa reveals extensive areas of squamous metaplasia in about 80% of children who die of TEF.[176] The absence of ciliated epithelium over large areas of the trachea may impair the clearance of secretions, contributing significantly to the development of recurrent pneumonia in these patients.

CLINICAL MANIFESTATIONS

Infants with TEF and esophageal atresia are symptomatic from birth. Presenting symptoms include excessive oral secretions, inability to accept passage of a nasogastric tube, respiratory distress, and immediate regurgitation of feedings.

The diagnosis of TEF usually becomes obvious within the first day or two after birth, although in some cases the concurrent presence of other major congenital anomalies or prematurity clouds the clinical picture. About one third of infants with TEF and esophageal atresia are premature.[167] It has been theorized that premature delivery is precipitated by hydramnios,[177] which complicates the pregnancy in about one third of the cases of TEF with esophageal atresia.[178] About half of patients with TEF and

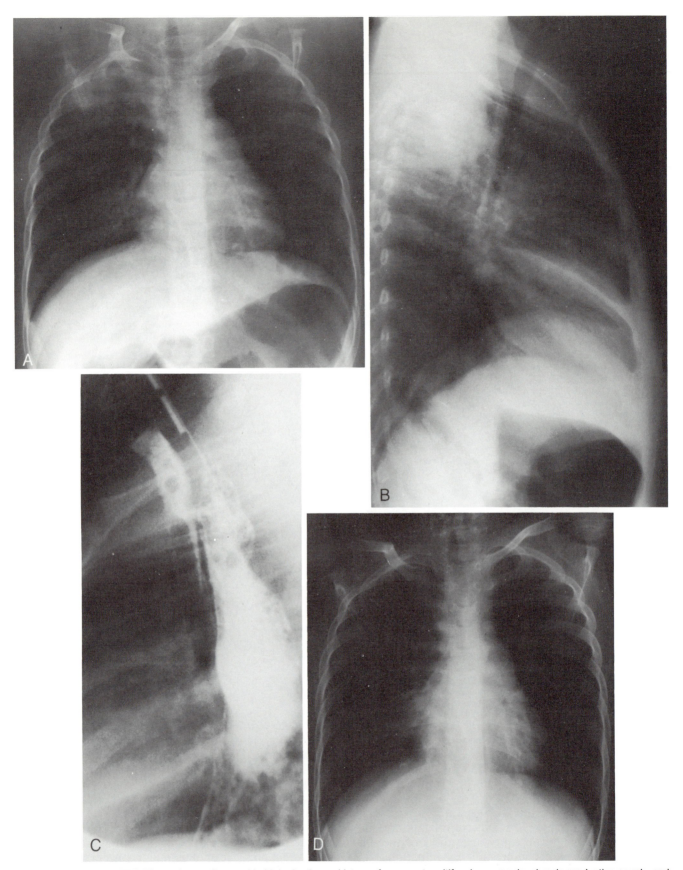

Figure 52–15. H-type TEF. The patient, a 6-year-old girl, had a 1-year history of recurrent multifocal pneumonia, chronic productive cough, and intermittent wheezing. The initial chest radiographs (*A*, posteroanterior view; *B*, lateral view) show right upper lobe and right middle lobe infiltrates and atelectasis and increased peribronchial markings in the left lower lobe. *C*, Cine-esophagography demonstrates an H-type TEF. At operation, the diameter of the fistula was found to be 1.2 cm. *D*, Postoperatively, the patient continued to have occasional lower respiratory infections which responded well to chest physiotherapy and oral antibiotics. Chest radiograph at 8 years of age shows persistent right middle lobe atelectasis and saccular bronchiectasis of the left lower lobe (confirmed by computed tomographic scan).

esophageal atresia have associated anomalies, most often involving the cardiovascular, renal, gastrointestinal, or central nervous systems.[167]

The manifestation of H-type fistula tends to be more subtle. Affected infants are usually full-term and may have no associated anomalies, although congenital heart defects, imperforate anus, arm and hand anomalies, and cleft lip and palate are sometimes found. These infants have intermittent dysphagia and choking, especially during liquid feedings, and recurrent bouts of bronchitis and pneumonia. The abdomen tends to be distended and hypertympanic because of passage of air across the fistula into the gastrointestinal tract. The diagnosis of H-type fistula can be delayed for months to years. In occasional patients, the anomaly is not detected until adulthood,[170] although most affected adult patients have been symptomatic since infancy.

DIAGNOSTIC PROCEDURES

Esophageal atresia with or without TEF is readily detected through the passage of a radiopaque nasogastric tube, which typically stops 10 to 13 cm from the tip of the nose.[179] The tube often coils in the proximal pouch and can be seen on the routine chest radiograph (Fig. 52–16). If any question about the condition remains, a small amount (about 0.25 or 0.5 ml) of contrast material can be instilled through the tube to demonstrate the atresia. It is important that water-soluble contrast material be used and that the contrast material be removed back out of the esophagus immediately after the radiographic studies in order to prevent aspiration.

The chest radiograph often shows associated aspiration pneumonia. If air is seen in the stomach or bowel in the presence of esophageal atresia, a distal TEF is present. If the abdomen is airless, the patient has either isolated esophageal atresia or esophageal atresia with a proximal TEF (see Fig. 52–16). Severe aspiration pneumonia on the chest radiograph is suggestive of the possibility of a proximal TEF; the fistula can be demonstrated by the instillation of a small amount of contrast material into the proximal esophageal pouch. In the rare patient with esophageal atresia and both proximal and distal TEFs, gaseous distention of the gastrointestinal tract and aspiration pneumonia are seen on the chest radiograph; the diagnosis can be confirmed by careful contrast studies.

With H-type fistula, the diagnosis is best made by contrast esophagogram and fluorography, with the use of soluble contrast material (see Fig. 52–15C). Several repetitions may be needed to demonstrate the fistula, even with the best technique.[167] Dysmotility of the distal esophagus is often evident even when the fistula is not visualized. When an H-type TEF is suspected but cannot be demonstrated radiographically, endoscopic examination can be helpful. The tracheal end of the fistula is usually located in the upper third of the posterior tracheal wall, appearing as a pit or crescent-shaped aperture. Colored or radiopaque dye or a flexible catheter can be introduced into the tracheal aperture and then observed, endoscopi-

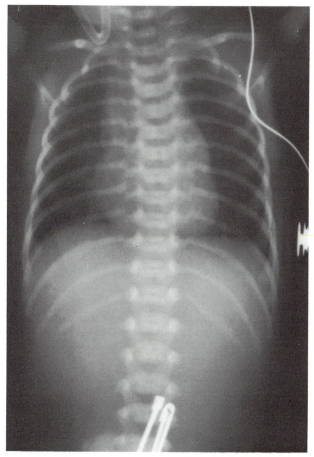

Figure 52–16. Esophageal atresia. The patient, a newborn, had a history of polyhydramnios. A nasogastric tube could not be passed to the stomach; the proximal esophagus is dilated. The abdomen is airless, indicating that there is no distal TEF.

cally or radiographically, passing into the esophagus or the stomach.

MANAGEMENT

TEF with esophageal atresia was among the earliest pulmonary anomalies to be described, and hundreds of cases have been reported in the world literature; however, the condition was almost uniformly fatal until 1943, when the first complete repair of esophageal atresia and TEF was performed by Haight and Towsley.[180] Since that time, improvements in surgical and anesthetic techniques, as well as in pre- and postoperative supportive care, have improved survival.

Preoperative stabilization is essential, especially in sick premature infants, in infants with significant pneumonia, and in infants with severe associated anomalies. Patients with esophageal atresia should have a nasogastric tube placed in the proximal esophageal pouch; the nasogastric tube as well as the oropharynx should be suctioned every 15 min to prevent aspiration of oral secretions.[167] Assisted ventilation, administration of intravenous fluids, hyperalimentation, and administration of antibiotics should be performed as needed; several days of supportive care are often necessary for stabilizing the infant for corrective surgery.

The infant with a distal TEF should be kept in an upright position in order to decrease the gastric acid reflux through the fistula. Some surgeons routinely perform a gastrostomy immediately after diagnosis to decompress the stomach and thus diminish the gastroesophageal reflux.[169] Other surgeons perform a preliminary gastrostomy only when massive gastric dilatation is compromising the infant's respiratory status or threatening gastric perforation.[167]

When severe associated anomalies, prematurity, or respiratory distress renders an infant too ill to survive complete repair of TEF and esophageal atresia, a staged operative approach is beneficial.[171] In the first stage, the TEF is ligated and divided, and a gastrostomy is placed. The infant can then be fed via the gastrostomy without reflux of feedings into the lungs. Careful and frequent suctioning of the oropharynx and the proximal esophageal pouch must be continued until the esophageal atresia can be repaired.[167, 179] The staged approach is also useful when a long gap exists between the esophageal segments. After placement of the gastrostomy and ligation of the TEF, daily dilatations of the proximal esophageal pouch are performed in an attempt to stretch it. Some surgeons have had success with this approach,[181, 182] whereas others have not found it to be effective.[167] Other methods for stretching the proximal and distal pouches have been tried with some success and are summarized by Holder.[183] In the event that these maneuvers fail to achieve adequate length of the esophageal segments, a technique of circular myotomies developed by Livaditis and collaborators[184] and successfully applied by de Lorimier and Harrison[185] can add length to the proximal pouch.

In some patients, it is impossible to bring the two esophageal segments close enough together for anastomosis. In these patients, the fistula is divided and the proximal esophageal pouch is brought out on the neck in a cervical esophagostomy so that secretions can drain. The patients are fed via the gastrostomy until about the age of 2 years, when a conduit from the proximal esophagus to the stomach can be fashioned from a segment of colon or stomach. These esophageal replacements do not function as well as a true esophagus.

When primary repair of esophageal atresia and TEF is possible, the procedure consists of two major parts: (1) the fistula is ligated and divided, usually just caudal to the tracheal entry, and a small diverticulum often remains on the posterior trachea; then (2) the esophageal pouches are opened and anastomosed. It is important that the anastomosis be performed under minimal tension to decrease the likelihood of anastomotic breakdown or leakage. In-depth discussions of the details and controversial points of operative technique are found in the writings of Holder and Ashcraft,[169] Touloukian and colleagues,[186] de Lorimier and Harrison,[185] Hicks and Mansfield,[179] and Ein and Friedberg.[167]

Meticulous postoperative nursing care is essential after repair of esophageal atresia, TEF, or both. Upright positioning should be maintained to decrease gastroesophageal reflux. Usually the esophagus is too edematous to allow swallowing in the immediate postoperative period; thus frequent oropharyngeal suctioning must be continued. A nasogastric tube should not be passed during the immediate postoperative period because of the risk of disrupting the anastomosis. Some surgeons place a transanastomotic nasogastric catheter during the esophageal anastomosis,[167] whereas others prefer to use a gastrostomy tube. When saliva begins to appear in gastric aspirates, small feedings can be started, usually by a slow constant infusion via gastrostomy or nasogastric catheter.

Postoperative complications are frequent. Anastomotic leakage occurs to some extent in 7% to 50% of patients after esophageal anastomosis.[167, 187] The presence of leakage is indicated by saliva in the chest tube drainage. Major leakages manifest with sepsis, shock, and acute respiratory distress. The chest radiograph often reveals a right pneumothorax. Small leakages can be more subtle, manifesting with mediastinitis or pneumonia. When an anastomotic leakage is diagnosed, tube feedings should be discontinued, chest tube drainage instituted, and the infant positioned upright. With good supportive care, most leakages heal, sometimes leaving a stricture. In severe cases it is sometimes necessary to reoperate, closing the distal esophageal segment and creating a cervical esophagostomy.[187]

Anastomotic strictures, another frequent complication of esophageal atresia repair, can develop at any time. Because the distal esophageal pouch is of smaller diameter than the proximal pouch, there is always some narrowing of the esophagus at the anastomotic site. Contraction and scarring of the healing anastomosis can result in the formation of a stricture sufficiently tight to impair swallowing. Dysphagia, frequent regurgitation of feedings, failure to thrive, and aspiration pneumonia can result. Treatment is dilatation of the stricture; often, repeated dilatations must be performed for several days to months at gradually lengthening intervals. It is unusual for strictures to continue to recur after the ages of 1 to 2 years. Unusual persistence or severity of stricture formation is suggestive of the possibility of gastroesophageal reflux.[167, 187]

Recurrence of the tracheoesophageal fistula occurs in 4% to 10% of cases,[167, 179, 187] usually in association with an anastomotic leakage. Holder[183, 188] speculated that in many children, small, recurrent TEFs may go undiagnosed because of subtle findings. The manifestation of a recurrent TEF is similar to that of an H-type TEF. Patients choke with feedings, especially with liquids, and have recurrent bouts of bronchitis and pneumonia. Respiratory distress can develop during crying because of gastroesophageal reflux through the fistula. Abdominal distention is common. Recurrent TEFs do not close spontaneously; surgical repair is necessary.

Tracheomalacia at the fistula site is common, resulting in a brassy cough and impaired clearance of secretions.[188] The area of malacic tracheal cartilage is often positioned between the aortic arch and the innominate artery anteriorly and the proximal esophageal pouch posteriorly. During feedings, when the esophageal pouch dilates, the malacic trachea can be compressed, resulting in sudden apnea. Ein and Friedberg[167] recommended aortopexy and innominate artery suspension from the sternum for relief of this syndrome. An alternative treatment is stenting of the trachea. Tracheomalacia usually resolves by the age of 2 years.

Even after full recovery from surgical correction of TEF and esophageal atresia, esophageal dysfunction is usually present and persistent. Kirkpatrick and co-authors[189] and Desjardins and co-authors[190] documented the absence of normal peristalsis in the distal esophageal segment. Esophageal dysmotility results in dysphagia and regurgitation of feedings, sometimes with recurrent aspiration pneumonia. Recurrent bouts of bronchitis or pneumonia occur in about half of postoperative TEF patients.[188] Most children learn to compensate for their esophageal dysfunction as they grow older by swallowing small amounts of well-chewed food and washing it down with liquids. Gastroesophageal reflux is also a frequent problem in these patients. Up to 60% of patients continue to have significant gastroesophageal reflux even into adulthood.[191]

Foreign bodies, usually food, are frequently impacted in the esophagus. Because of the disparity in sizes between the proximal and distal esophageal segments, folds of redundant proximal pouch tissue are often present. Swallowed chunks of food can be trapped in these folds, resulting in dysphagia and coughing. The treatment is endoscopic removal. As the child grows older and learns to chew food thoroughly, food impactions become less frequent.

The rate of postoperative complications is lower among patients with H-type TEF than among patients with associated esophageal atresia. Postoperative strictures, anastomotic leakages, and recurrence of the TEF are uncommon. Patients with H-type TEF do tend to have incoordination of the pharyngeal muscles, resulting in aspiration of feedings. This problem usually improves with age.

PROGNOSIS

Without surgery, TEF with esophageal atresia is uniformly fatal. Patients with H-type TEF can survive for many years without surgery, especially if the fistula is small. However, significant chronic pulmonary disease usually develops when the diagnosis and treatment of H-type fistula are delayed.

In infants in whom TEF is promptly diagnosed and who receive appropriate surgical intervention, the prognosis is variable. Term infants with no other major anomalies generally do well; about 95% survive.[179, 188, 191, 192] Among slightly premature infants and infants with moderate pneumonia or congenital anomalies in addition to the TEF, the survival rate is about 70%. Among extremely premature infants and infants with severe pneumonia or congenital anomalies, the survival rate is less than 10%.[192] Many of these infants do not survive to have corrective surgery or die in the immediate postoperative period. Early postoperative deaths are usually related to sepsis, whereas preoperative and late postoperative deaths are more often related to associated anomalies and prematurity.[188, 193] Overall, in a series of 82 patients with TEF and esophageal atresia, Holder and Ashcraft[188] found that 79% of the patients were alive and taking food by mouth 3½ to 15 years postoperatively.

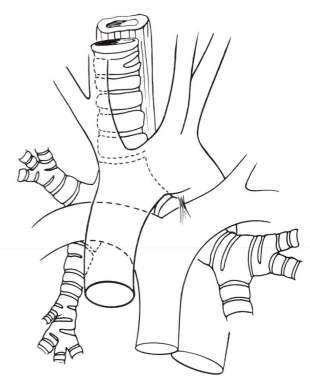

Figure 52–17. Normal mediastinal anatomy (diagram). Note the intimate relationship of the trachea and main bronchi to the aorta and its branches, the pulmonary arteries, and the esophagus.

VASCULAR COMPRESSION OF THE AIRWAY

In the normal mediastinum, the heart and the great vessels are positioned close to the trachea, the main stem bronchi, and the esophagus (Fig. 52–17). Abnormal location or dilatation of the vascular structures can result in compression of the airway, the esophagus, or both, with corresponding symptoms of respiratory distress and dysphagia. Several variations of the normal vascular anatomy have been described; the overall incidence is about 3% of the general population.[194] Some of these variations are of no functional consequence; some are usually asymptomatic but cause significant obstructive symptoms in occasional affected persons; and some cause significant symptoms in the majority of affected persons (Table 52–1). Abnormal dilatation of the pulmonary arteries, as in congenital heart disease with left-to-right shunt or absent pulmonary valve syndrome, can also encroach upon the airway. The term *vascular ring* is commonly used in referring to syndromes of vascular compression of the airways, although not all of these anomalies are characterized by a complete ring of vascular structures encircling the trachea and esophagus.

PATHOGENESIS AND PATHOPHYSIOLOGY

The embryologic basis for the development of the various aortic arch anomalies can best be conceptualized by recalling the normal sequence of aortic arch development

Table 52–1. VARIANTS OF MEDIASTINAL VASCULAR ANATOMY THAT CAUSE TRACHEOBRONCHIAL AND ESOPHAGEAL COMPRESSION

Usually Symptomatic
Double aortic arch
Pulmonary artery sling (aberrant left pulmonary artery)
Right aortic arch with left ductus arteriosus originating from descending aorta
Left aortic arch with right ductus arteriosus originating from descending aorta

Sometimes Symptomatic
Right aortic arch with aberrant left subclavian artery and left ductus arteriosus
Left aortic arch with aberrant right subclavian artery and right ductus arteriosus

Occasionally Symptomatic
Anomalous innominate artery
Aberrant subclavian artery
Dilated pulmonary arteries

(Fig. 52–18). The ventral aortic root becomes the ascending aorta; the left fourth branchial arch persists as the aortic arch, and the left dorsal aortic root becomes the descending aorta. The proximal part of the right fourth branchial arch forms the base of the right subclavian artery; the remainder of the right fourth arch and the aortic root regress. The third arches develop into the proximal portions of the carotid arteries. The proximal parts of the sixth arches become the pulmonary arteries; the distal part of the left sixth arch persists as the ductus arteriosus. (Throughout this section, the term *ductus arteriosus* refers to both the ductus arteriosus and the ligamentum arteriosum.) All the other branchial arches normally regress completely. Persistence of vessels that normally regress and regression of vessels that normally persist may occur in various combinations, accounting for the known variations in anatomy.

The most common form of symptomatic vascular ring is the double aortic arch (Fig. 52–19). This aortic anomaly occurs when the fourth branchial arches and the dorsal aortic roots persist on both sides. Usually, both aortic arches are patent; they may be equal in size, but more often the right arch is larger than the left. On occasion, the left arch or, very rarely, the right arch has an atretic segment, located either between the origins of the carotid and subclavian arteries or distal to the origin of the subclavian artery.

The right-sided aortic arch is present in approximately 1 in 2500 people.[195] There are two major subgroups in the right aortic arch with differing embryologic origins and clinical significance. The more common of the two is the right aortic arch with aberrant left subclavian artery and left ductus arteriosus.[195] The developmental basis for the variant is probably similar to that of the double aortic arch with an atretic segment of the left arch between the left carotid and subclavian arteries, except that in this case the atretic segment regresses completely. The vascular ring formed by this anomaly is looser than that formed by the double aortic arch and is more likely to be asymptomatic.

In right aortic arch with mirror-image branching, the anatomy of the arch and of the innominate, carotid, and subclavian arteries is the mirror image of the anatomy of the normal left-sided arch, except that the ductus arteriosus is usually on the left. This pattern is almost always associated with congenital heart disease, most commonly tetralogy of Fallot, truncus arteriosus, and ventricular septal defect. It is thought that during embryonic development, the cardiac abnormality results in direction of

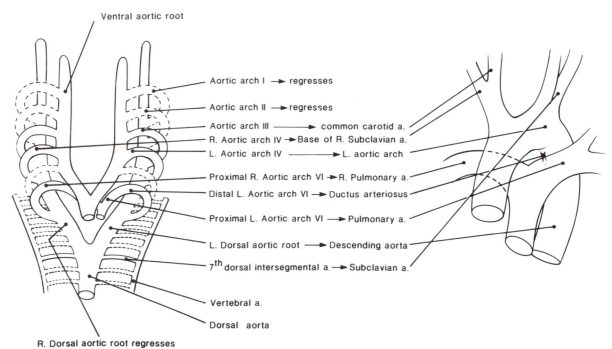

Figure 52–18. Embryologic development of the mediastinal vessels (diagram). The embryonic vascular system is symmetric, with paired ventral and dorsal aortic roots connected by the branchial arches. Some elements of this primitive system regress; others persist and develop into the normal mediastinal vascular structures. a, artery; R, right; L, left.

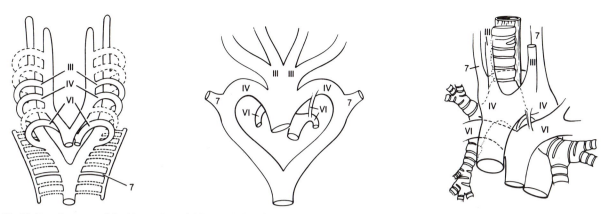

Figure 52-19. Development of double aortic arch (diagram). The fourth branchial arches and dorsal aortic roots persist on both sides. The result is a ring (often tight) of aortic structures encircling the tracheal and esophagus.

aortic blood flow to the right (rather than to the left); this stimulates the right arch to remain patent, while the left arch regresses.[195] The ductus arteriosus usually connects the left subclavian artery to the left pulmonary artery; a vascular ring is not formed. On occasion, however, the ductus connects the upper descending aorta to the left pulmonary artery; a vascular ring is therefore present. Usually in these cases, the upper descending aorta crosses over behind the esophagus to descend on the left side, thus further compressing the esophagus.[196] This situation accounts for more cases of symptomatic vascular ring than does the right aortic arch with aberrant left subclavian artery and left ductus arteriosus.[197] The associated congenital heart disease often contributes to the respiratory distress of affected infants. The left-to-right shunting may result in dilatation of the pulmonary arteries and left atrium, adding to the tracheobronchial compression caused by the vascular ring.[197, 198]

The left aortic arch with right ductus arteriosus connecting the upper descending aorta to the right pulmonary artery occurs less frequently than the corresponding right arch anomaly; in most cases, the aorta crosses behind the esophagus to descend on the right.[196, 199–201] During embryologic development, the left ductus arteriosus regresses while the right one persists; blood flows from the pulmonary artery through the right ductus arteriosus and the right dorsal aortic root, stimulating the right dorsal aortic root to remain patent. The remnant of dorsal aortic root distal to the ductus arteriosus is called the diverticulum of Kommerell (Fig. 52–20). The left aortic arch with aberrant right subclavian artery and right ductus arteriosus originating from the right subclavian artery is also a relatively rare form of vascular ring.[196, 202, 203] The developmental origin is presumably identical to that of the corresponding right arch anomaly; that is, the portion of the primitive right aortic arch between the right common carotid and subclavian arteries regresses while the right ductus arteriosus and dorsal aortic root persist (Fig. 52–21). In two reported cases, hypoplasia or complete absence of the left pulmonary artery was associated with this anomaly; whether this was the cause or the effect of the absent left ductus arteriosus is open to conjecture.

Pulmonary artery sling is a relatively rare anomaly but usually produces severe symptoms. In this condition, the left pulmonary artery is absent; the left lung is supplied by a large collateral artery that arises from the right pulmonary artery, passing between the esophagus and trachea to reach the left lung (Fig. 52–22). This anomaly is thought to arise embryologically in response to regression or primary agenesis of the left pulmonary artery during the primitive lung-bud stage when the two lungs are still confluent. A collateral vessel then grows into the left lung

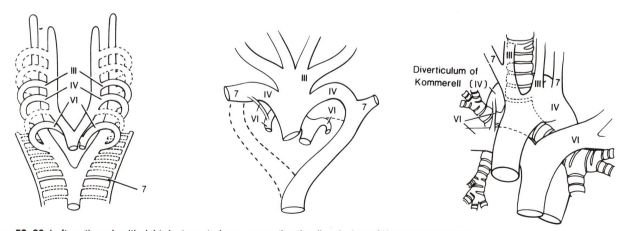

Figure 52-20. Left aortic arch with right ductus arteriosus connecting the diverticulum of Kommerell to the right pulmonary artery. A complete vascular ring is formed.

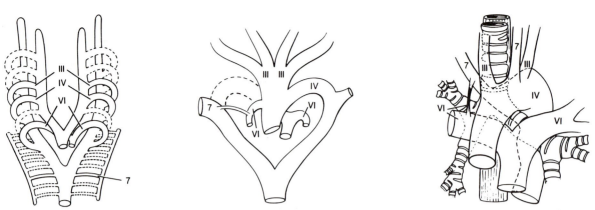

Figure 52–21. Aberrant right subclavian artery with right ductus arteriosus connecting the aberrant subclavian artery to the right pulmonary artery. A loose vascular ring is formed.

from the circulation of the right lung; as the lungs separate and grow, the collateral vessel is carried cephalad with the left hilum until it courses between the trachea and the esophagus.[195]

About half the cases of pulmonary artery sling are associated with severe tracheal stenosis caused by complete cartilage rings, with absence of the pars membranacea.[204] The cause of the tracheal stenosis is not known; in general, long segments of the trachea are involved. In an often-associated bronchial configuration, the right upper lobe bronchus branches more distally than normal, so that the right main stem bronchus is the same length as the left; both main stem bronchi have horizontal courses (Fig. 52–23).[204] Other cardiovascular anomalies are associated with pulmonary artery sling in about 50% of cases.

An aberrant right subclavian artery, without an associated right ductus arteriosus, forms an incomplete vascular ring. This is a common anatomic variant, occurring in about 1 of every 200 persons, and is asymptomatic in most cases. During embryologic development, the ventral segment of the right aortic arch degenerates, but the dorsal segment, distal to the right subclavian artery, persists. The right dorsal aortic root is then gradually absorbed into the left aortic arch until the right subclavian artery

originates just caudal to the left subclavian artery[195] and passes behind the esophagus to reach the right arm. The corresponding anomaly with a right-sided aortic arch and aberrant left subclavian artery, without an associated left ductus arteriosus, is very rare.

Anterior compression of the trachea is occasionally caused by the innominate artery, originating to the left of the trachea and crossing diagonally to the right (Fig. 52–24). This condition accounted for 8% of surgically treated vascular compression syndromes in two series.[194, 196] There has been considerable controversy over the significance of the "anomalous" innominate artery in the pathogenesis of tracheal obstruction. Without question, the majority of affected persons are not clinically ill; indeed, in one study it was found that the innominate artery originated totally or partially to the left of the trachea in 96% of children undergoing angiography for congenital heart disease, none of whom had symptoms of airway compression.[205] In the same study, 30% of asymptomatic children under 2 years of age exhibited indentation of the tracheal air column on lateral chest radiographs at the level of the innominate artery. These findings suggest that the term *anomalous innominate artery* is a misnomer because the anatomic location of the

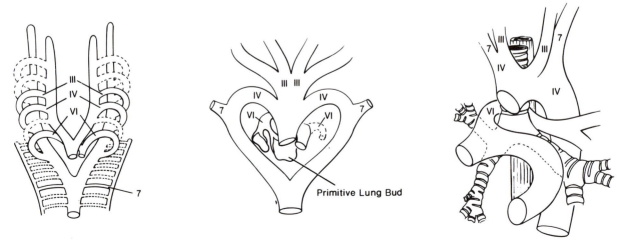

Figure 52–22. Aberrant left pulmonary artery (pulmonary artery sling). An anomalous vessel arising from the right pulmonary artery courses between the trachea and esophagus to supply the left lung. The anomalous vessel probably develops as a collateral, in response to degeneration of the left pulmonary artery during the lung-bud stage of embryonic development.

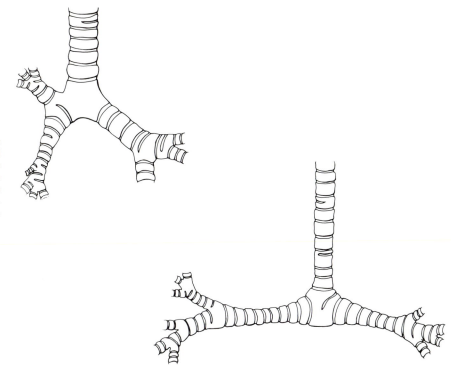

Figure 52–23. The normal configuration of the trachea and main bronchi (*left*) is contrasted with the distal takeoff of the right upper lobe bronchus and horizontal ("inverted T") course of the bronchi, often associated with complete cartilage-ring tracheal stenosis (*right*). This condition is found in approximately half of patients with pulmonary artery sling.

artery in affected children is actually normal. Some children, however, have significant tracheal compression at the site of the innominate artery crossing and are severely symptomatic. In these children, symptoms are often relieved by aortopexy, in which the aorta is sutured to the sternum, pulling the innominate artery away from the trachea.[206-210] It has been postulated that these patients have significant tracheal compression because the innominate artery is more taut than normal; it could also be theorized that the tracheal cartilages of affected children are unusually compliant, so that they are easily compressed. There is an increased incidence of innominate artery compression of the trachea in children with dilatation of other mediastinal structures, such as the esophagus or the heart; this is probably caused by crowding.[211]

Vascular compression of the airways may also occur as

a result of pulmonary arterial dilatation. Congenital heart disease with left-to-right shunting and poststenotic dilatation of the pulmonary arteries secondary to pulmonic valvular stenosis[197,198] frequently cause some degree of tracheobronchial compression, which in severe cases may be clinically significant. The "absent pulmonary valve syndrome" is a rare syndrome associated, as the name implies, with absence of the pulmonary valve, right ventricular outflow tract obstruction, and massive dilatation of the pulmonary arteries.[212,213] Usually a malalignment type of ventral septal defect is also present. Airway compression by the dilated proximal pulmonary arteries is a prominent feature of the syndrome; one study[213] also demonstrated abnormal branching of the entire pulmonary arterial system, with compression of the intrapulmonary bronchi.

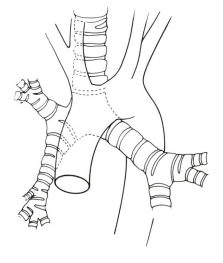

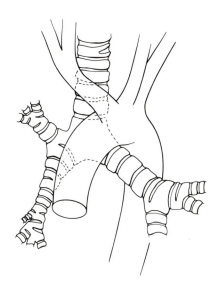

Figure 52–24. The normal (*left*) and anomalous (*right*) positions of the innominate artery.

All the anomalies discussed result in some combination of tracheal and esophageal compression. Complete vascular rings generally compress both the trachea and the esophagus to a significant degree. The aberrant subclavian artery compresses only the esophagus. The "anomalous" innominate artery compresses only the trachea. Pulmonary artery sling indents the right main stem bronchus or the bronchus intermedius anterosuperiorly, the trachea posteriorly, and the esophagus anteriorly; airway symptoms usually predominate inasmuch as the esophagus is free to expand posteriorly.

The consequences of tracheal compression are obstruction of airflow and of mucus clearance. The compression is usually intrathoracic, so that airflow obstruction is predominantly expiratory, resulting in air trapping, pulmonary hyperinflation, and expiratory wheezing. With increasingly severe compression, inspiratory obstruction becomes evident, with stridor and retractions. Bronchial compression, secondary to pulmonary artery sling or dilated pulmonary arteries, results in distal hyperinflation, with or without a localized wheeze; on occasion, distal atelectasis occurs. Impaired clearance of mucus is evidenced by coarse crackles (rales) or diffuse wheezing; recurrent bronchopulmonary infections are common.

With severe esophageal compression, dysphagia and regurgitation occur. The compressed segment of the esophagus is unable to expand posteriorly to accommodate a bolus of food; hence the anterior wall of the esophagus must bulge forward, indenting the membranous portion of the trachea. Thus cough and respiratory distress are often exacerbated during feeding in patients with complete vascular rings. Aspiration pneumonia frequently adds to the patient's respiratory compromise.

Infants with tracheal compression caused by a vascular ring or an anomalous innominate artery sometimes have apneic episodes that seem to be associated with coughing or swallowing. It has been postulated that a reflex mechanism is involved in these apneic episodes.[214] There seems to be little correlation between the severity of tracheal compression seen at tracheoscopy and the occurrence of apnea. However, the apnea usually resolves after aortopexy, even in infants with mild tracheal compression, which implies a causative role of tracheal compression in the pathogenesis of this so-called reflex apnea.[209, 210]

CLINICAL MANIFESTATIONS

The age at presentation of patients with vascular rings or other airway compression syndromes varies inversely with the severity of the compression. Patients with double aortic arch often are symptomatic at birth, and nearly all have exhibited significant symptoms by the age of 3 months. Occasional patients with double aortic arch present later in childhood, with recurrent pneumonia or atelectasis as the only manifestation. Pulmonary artery sling also causes symptoms within the first 3 months of life in most patients. The looser forms of complete vascular rings tend to manifest later in infancy or childhood, as does innominate artery compression. Aberrant subclavian artery, if symptomatic at all, usually begins to cause

significant dysphagia after an affected patient begins to eat solid foods. Loose vascular rings sometimes are clinically silent until adulthood, when they present with dysphagia. Possibly the late development of symptoms relates to the development of atherosclerosis in the ring vessels, making them less compliant.[215]

Except in the case of aberrant subclavian artery, respiratory symptoms usually dominate the clinical picture. Stridor or wheezing is the most frequent presenting complaint, occurring in 50% to 65% of affected patients. Recurrent respiratory infections, cyanosis, and dysphagia each occur in 20% to 30% of patients.[194, 196] Affected infants often assume a characteristic posture, with the neck hyperextended; this seems to partially alleviate the tracheal obstruction. On physical examination, both inspiratory stridor and expiratory wheezing may be evident; a prolonged expiratory phase and hyperexpansion of the chest are often seen. Suprasternal retractions are frequently present. With aspiration pneumonia or inspissated mucus, intercostal and subcostal retractions, diffuse wheezing, or rales may also develop. Cyanosis, cough, and tachypnea may be present at rest or may develop only during feeding or crying. The respiratory distress is usually exacerbated by feedings. Dysphagia is often present from infancy but becomes more evident when a patient begins to eat solid foods.

The syndrome of reflex apnea has occurred in association with both double aortic arch and anomalous innominate artery. It may occur as the sole presenting complaint, but more often it is associated with some degree of respiratory distress or cough.[209, 210] Affected infants typically become apneic during feeding, coughing, or crying. They are described as limp and "lifeless" in many cases, but they may hyperextend the neck. The apneic episode may or may not resolve spontaneously.[207] Sudden death from reflex apnea might be difficult to distinguish from the idiopathic sudden infant death syndrome if tracheal compression was not severe enough to cause significant obstructive symptoms.

DIAGNOSIS

The diagnosis of vascular ring must begin with a high index of suspicion because there are no pathognomonic findings on history, physical examination, or routine chest radiographs (Table 52–2). The diagnosis should be considered in patients with chronic respiratory distress, especially if it is exacerbated by feeding or associated with dysphagia; in patients with impaired mucus clearance and recurrent bronchopulmonary infections; and in infants with reflex apnea. Careful scrutiny of the routine chest radiograph may provide clues to the diagnosis of vascular ring. Hyperinflation of the lungs is often evident. In the case of pulmonary sling, the right lung may be selectively hyperinflated, and the lower trachea is often pulled to the right. With double aortic arch or right aortic arch anomalies, the right-sided aortic arch can often be detected on routine chest radiographs (Fig. 52–25A). High-kilovoltage filtered magnification films or tomograms may be helpful in discerning the location of the aortic arch or

Table 52–2. DIFFERENTIAL DIAGNOSIS OF VASCULAR COMPRESSION OF THE AIRWAY

Structural Defects of Airways
Primary tracheomalacia or bronchomalacia
Tracheal or bronchial stenosis
Laryngomalacia
Vocal cord paralysis or spasm
Intratracheal or Bronchial Obstruction
Foreign body
Polyp
Hemangioma
Cyst
Broncholith
Extrinsic Airway Compression
Paratracheal or parabronchial lymphadenopathy
Mediastinal lymphadenopathy or tumor
Bronchogenic or enterogenic cyst
Esophageal foreign body
Congenital lobar emphysema
Congenital goiter
Predisposition to Bronchopulmonary Infection
Immunodeficiency syndrome
Cystic fibrosis
Immotile cilia syndrome
Asthma
Recurrent Aspiration
Esophageal dysfunction: gastroesophageal reflux, achalasia, esophageal stricture, esophageal duplication, hiatus hernia
Tracheoesophageal fistula, H type
Neuromuscular disorders
Seizure disorder
Congestive Heart Failure With Pulmonary Edema
Infectious Process
Bronchiolitis; prolonged course
Visceral larva migrans

arches and in identifying areas of tracheal compression. These techniques also demonstrate the stenotic trachea and the horizontal course of the main stem bronchi in pulmonary artery sling associated with complete cartilage rings. Lateral airway films may demonstrate the anterior indentation of the trachea associated with vascular ring and innominate artery compression (Fig. 52–26A); this is not a reliable finding, however, inasmuch as both false-positive and false-negative observations are common.

Barium esophagogram is most helpful for diagnosing vascular ring; it demonstrates characteristic esophageal filling defects in each of the vascular compression syndromes except for the anomalous innominate artery, in which the esophagogram is normal (Fig. 52–26B). Pulmonary artery sling is the only vascular compression syndrome in which an anterior esophageal filling defect is seen. This defect is not present in every case of pulmonary artery sling, however. Double aortic arch causes a characteristic double concavity indenting both sides of the esophagus; usually the right concavity is a little higher than the left (Fig. 52–25B). On the lateral esophagogram, a large posterior compression, caused by the upper descending aorta, is always present (Fig. 52–25C); a smaller anterior defect, caused by the compression of the trachea, is sometimes noted.

With aberrant right subclavian artery, a posterior filling defect is seen slanting upward at about a 70-degree angle,

from the level of T-4 on the left to T-2 on the right. The anteroposterior esophagogram may resemble that seen with double aortic arch; however, with double aortic arch the concavities are more rounded, and the right-sided concavity is only slightly higher than the left. On the lateral view, a shallow and relatively long filling defect is seen, in contrast to the deeper and more sharply circumscribed posterior defect seen with double aortic arch. When a right ductus arteriosus originates from the aberrant right subclavian artery, the junction of the left aortic arch and the prominent right dorsal aortic root produces a large posterior esophageal impression, which slants downward slightly from left to right.

In a patient with a left aortic arch and right-sided descending aorta, the anteroposterior esophagogram demonstrates the normal left-sided indentation caused by the aortic arch and a shallower, slightly lower right-sided indentation caused by the upper descending aorta; the lateral view demonstrates a sharply circumscribed posterior indentation. With right aortic arch and left descending aorta, the findings are opposite those just described. In these cases, the presence or absence of a ductus arteriosus does not affect the findings on esophagogram.

Tracheoscopy and bronchoscopy demonstrate extrinsic pulsatile compression of the airways. The tracheal compression is anterior or anterolateral in all the vascular compression syndromes except for pulmonary artery sling. Pulmonary artery sling results in pulsatile indentation of the posterior membranous portion of the trachea and also of the anterosuperior wall of the right main stem bronchus. The dilated pulmonary arteries associated with congenital heart disease or absent pulmonary valve syndrome compress the left main stem bronchus and the right bronchus intermedius.

Tracheoscopy is also useful in identifying associated anomalies, such as tracheomalacia or bronchomalacia at the site of compression, which may account for delay in resolution of symptoms after surgery. Complete cartilage-ring stenosis of the trachea, frequently associated with pulmonary artery sling, is readily identified at tracheoscopy; in fact the trachea is often too stenotic to permit advancement of the bronchoscope below the cords. Correction of the vascular anomaly in these cases, without correction of the tracheal stenosis, does not relieve the airway compromise.[204]

Another important role of tracheobronchoscopy is to rule out the presence of a foreign body, hemangioma, polyp, or nonpulsatile extrinsic compression caused by a bronchogenic cyst, lymphadenopathy, large thymus, or mediastinal tumor. In patients with significant respiratory distress whose only apparent vascular anomaly is aberrant subclavian artery or anomalous innominate artery, it is imperative that other causes of airway obstruction be ruled out before the symptoms are attributed to these usually benign variants.

Angiography or other vascular imaging studies should always be performed in cases of suspected vascular ring.[216-218] The course of the aorta and of its patent branches is clearly demonstrated by aortography (Fig. 52–27), but small vessels (i.e., small patent ductus arteriosus or atretic aortic arch) often are not visible on aortograms.

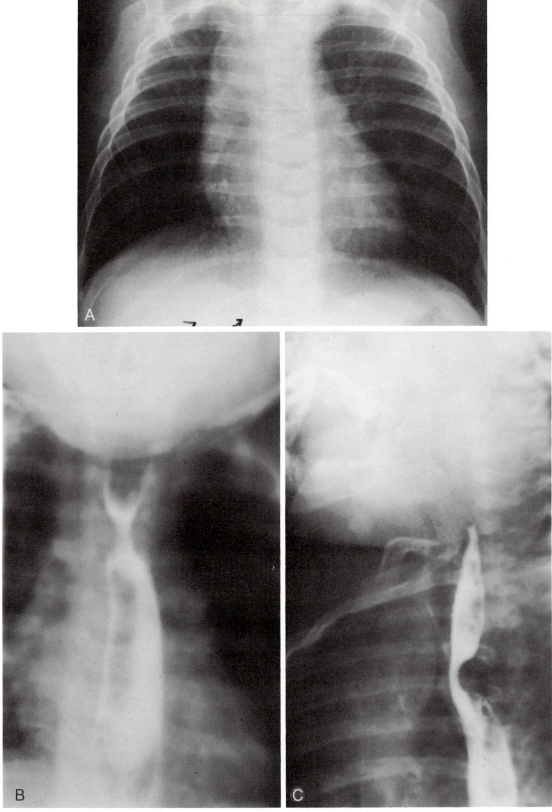

Figure 52–25. Double aortic arch. The patient, a 7-month-old child, had inspiratory stridor. *A*, Posteroanterior chest radiograph demonstrates widening of the mediastinum on the right, suggestive of a right-sided or double aortic arch. Note the loss of the lower tracheal shadow (the "missing segment sign"). *B*, Cine-esophagography (posteroanterior view) reveals bilateral fixed indentations of the esophagus. *C*, On the lateral view a deep, sharply circumscribed posterior indentation of the esophagus is seen; tracheal compression is evident at the same level.

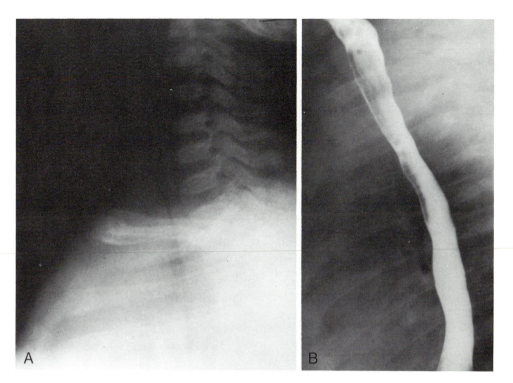

Figure 52–26. Anomalous innominate artery. The patient, a 3-month-old infant, was evaluated because of stridor and intermittent cyanosis. *A*, Lateral view of the trachea reveals marked anterior tracheal compression at the level of the clavicular head. *B*, Cine esophagogram demonstrates no compression of the esophagus.

In some types of vascular ring, the correct diagnosis (and hence optimal planning of the operative approach) can be made only by putting together the information gleaned from the esophagogram, the angiogram, and the endoscopy (Table 52–3). Cardiac catheterization can be performed along with the aortic angiograms to rule out associated cardiac malformations.

Certain clues can help in interpretation of the angiogram. If a right aortic arch is present, left anterior oblique

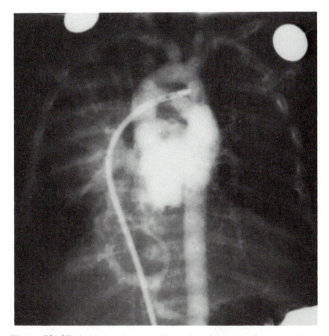

Figure 52–27. Angiography reveals cardiac dextroversion and a double aortic arch in a 4-week-old infant with congestive heart failure. In addition, an anomalous artery can be seen arising from the descending aorta and supplying a pulmonary sequestration in the right lower lobe.

views should be carefully examined for evidence of a small left aortic arch[218] (Fig. 52–28). If an aberrant subclavian artery is demonstrated and the patient has symptoms of tracheal compression, a ductus arteriosus connecting the aberrant subclavian artery to the ipsilateral pulmonary artery should be suspected. In these cases, a bulbous dorsal aortic root is usually seen extending medially. The aberrant subclavian artery originates from this aortic root, rather than from the dorsalateral part of the aortic arch as it does in cases without an associated ductus arteriosus. Lateral or oblique views are best for demonstrating the ductus arteriosus in these cases;[218] if a ductus arteriosus cannot be seen, a ligamentum arteriosum is probably present. A prominent right diverticulum of Kommerell, associated with a left aortic arch, represents a remnant of the right dorsal aortic root. It may be associated with a right ductus arteriosus[198, 201] or an atretic right aortic arch; the opposite holds true for a left diverticulum of Kommerell associated with right aortic arch.[219]

In digital subtraction angiography, contrast material is injected intravenously; the heart and great vessels are then visualized with the aid of an image intensifier. When performed by a skilled clinician, this relatively noninvasive technique can be as accurate as aortography in delineating the anatomy of vascular rings (Fig. 52–29).[217, 220]

Thoracic CT scans demonstrate pulmonary artery sling[221, 222] and can be used as a noninvasive alternative to angiography in order to confirm this diagnosis. Many patients with pulmonary artery sling eventually require cardiac catheterization and angiography, however, inasmuch as approximately 50% of these patients have other cardiovascular anomalies. Other vascular ring anomalies can sometimes be identified by CT scanning, although the definition of the vascular anatomy is not as consistently accurate as that achieved with angiography.

MRI is a noninvasive technique that can accurately

Table 52–3. SITES OF TRACHEAL AND ESOPHAGEAL COMPRESSION BY VASCULAR RINGS

Vascular Anomaly	Tracheal Compression	Esophageal Compression
Double aortic arch	Anterior and lateral	Posterior and lateral
Pulmonary artery sling	Posterior	Anterior
Right aortic arch with left ductus originating from descending aorta	Right anterolateral	Right lateral and posterior
Left aortic arch with right ductus originating from descending aorta	Left anterolateral	Left lateral and posterior
Right aortic arch, aberrant left subclavian artery and left ductus	Right anterolateral	Right lateral and posterior
Left aortic arch, aberrant right subclavian artery and right ductus	Left anterolateral	Left lateral and posterior
Anomalous innominate artery	Anterior	None
Aberrant subclavian artery	None	Posterior

demonstrate the anatomic relationships of the mediastinal vessels. Like angiography, MRI is incapable of showing the ligamentum arteriosum.[223, 224]

TREATMENT AND PROGNOSIS

Conservative medical management may suffice for relatively loose vascular rings that are mildly or moderately symptomatic. Medical management consists of bronchial drainage to facilitate mucus clearance, antibiotics as needed for infection, humidified air and supplemental oxygen as needed for exacerbations of respiratory distress resulting from intercurrent infection, and soft or liquid diet if dysphagia is a significant problem.

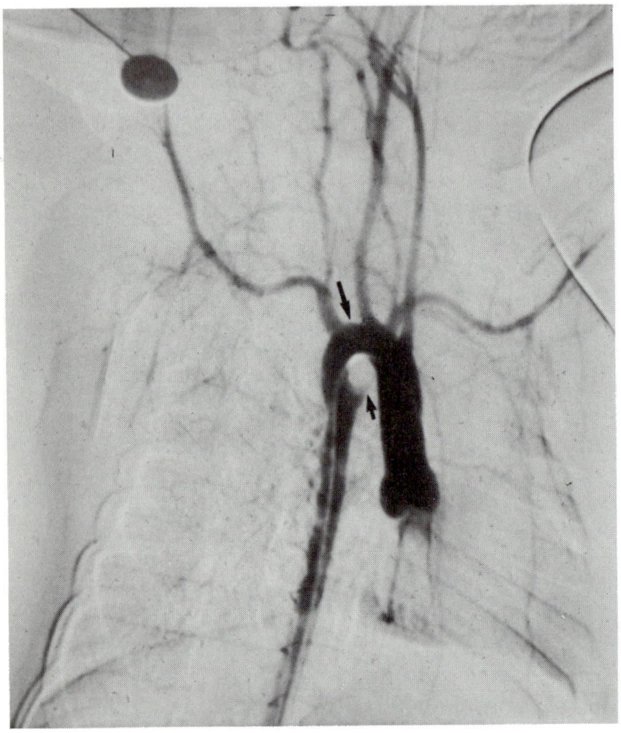

Indications for surgical intervention include reflex apnea, severe respiratory distress, recurrent bronchopulmonary infections, and significant dysphagia with secondary failure to thrive or recurrent aspiration pneumonia. The surgical techniques involved in correction of the vascular compression syndromes are described briefly. In double aortic arch, the smaller of the two arches is divided; if the arches are equal in size, the anterior arch is divided. In right aortic arch with left ductus arteriosus, the ductus arteriosus is divided. In the case of aberrant subclavian artery with or without an associated ductus arteriosus or ligamentum arteriosus, the aberrant subclavian artery is divided along with the ductus or ligamentum

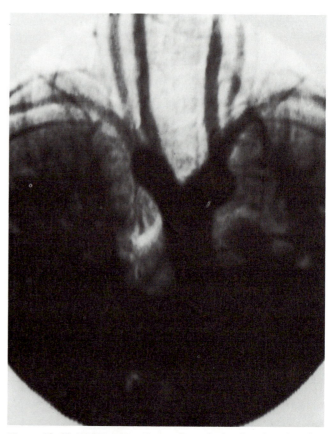

Figure 52–28. Double aortic arch with atretic segment of left arch. The long arrow points to the right aortic arch; the short arrow shows the patent dorsal segment of the left arch. The presence of an atretic left arch can easily be missed by angiography unless appropriate oblique views are obtained.

Figure 52–29. Digital subtraction angiography is a less invasive alternative to arterial angiography for demonstrations of double aortic arch (shown here) or other aortic arch anomalies.

arteriosus. Before dividing any large vessel, the surgeon should routinely perform a trial occlusion of the vessel while the anesthesiologist monitors the patient's carotid pulses and general cardiovascular status.[196] There have been cases in which the aorta was mistaken for the anomalous vessel and divided, resulting in the rapid demise of the patient.[225] Innominate artery compression is usually relieved by aortopexy, in which the ascending aorta is sutured to the sternum. On occasion, these sutures later become detached, and the procedure must be repeated.[226]

In the case of cyanotic congenital heart disease with secondarily dilated pulmonary arteries and left atrium, treatment should be directed primarily at the underlying cardiac defect. If correction of the underlying defect is not possible, relief of the airway obstruction can sometimes be achieved by pulmonary arteriopexy, in which the pulmonary artery is sutured to the anterior chest wall.[197, 198] In the absent pulmonary valve syndrome, the prognosis has generally been very poor with a high operative mortality rate; a surgical technique[212] in which hypothermic circulatory arrest is used to allow extensive resection and plication of the aneurysmal pulmonary arteries shows some promise.

In each of the conditions just mentioned, the airway should be examined via bronchoscope during the operative procedure in order to determine whether the compression is adequately relieved and to assess the degree of residual tracheomalacia. The postoperative course is often difficult; respiratory distress, usually secondary to tracheobronchomalacia at the site of compression, may persist for weeks or months. In severe cases, a tracheostomy tube may be necessary for creating an internal stent for the trachea. In most cases, the malacic cartilages gradually stiffen and the respiratory distress resolves,[194, 196] but occasionally the tracheomalacia or bronchomalacia persists indefinitely. External stenting of the malacic segment with a rib graft[227-229] or Marlex mesh[226] or an internal stent with an extended tracheostomy tube[230, 231] is often quite effective in these cases. Long-term follow-up of pulmonary function after surgical correction of vascular ring reveals residual upper airway or peripheral airway obstruction in about half the patients[232, 233] and bronchial hyperreactivity in the majority of patients.[233]

Pulmonary artery sling is corrected by dividing the aberrant left pulmonary artery at its origin and reattaching it to the left side of the main pulmonary artery trunk. Complete cartilage ring tracheal stenosis, if present, must also be corrected. Often the stenotic segment is too long for simple resection. Tracheoplasty techniques with the use of cartilaginous or membranous grafts are being developed with some success.[234, 235] In patients with pulmonary artery sling, tracheomalacia is usually not a problem postoperatively. Long-term results of surgical repair of pulmonary artery sling can be excellent,[236, 237] although in some cases the reimplanted left pulmonary artery does not remain patent.[229]

ARTERIOVENOUS FISTULA

Arteriovenous fistulas (AVFs) of the lung are rare malformations characterized by abnormal communications between pulmonary arterial and venous vessels. The true incidence of pulmonary AVF is unknown. In a series of 15,000 consecutive autopsies, only three cases of pulmonary AVFs were found.[238]

Most pulmonary AVFs are congenital, but they may become clinically evident at any age. Stringer and associates[239] in a collective review of 140 cases of AVF, found that approximately 23% of the patients were symptomatic in infancy; 48% presented during childhood (up to 18 years of age), and an additional 23% became symptomatic by the age of 40. Forty percent to 65% of patients with congenital pulmonary AVF have Rendu-Osler-Weber syndrome (hereditary hemorrhagic telangiectasia);[240] conversely, about 15% of all patients with Rendu-Osler-Weber syndrome have pulmonary AVF.

Occasionally, AVF is an acquired anomaly, secondary to trauma, hepatic cirrhosis, metastatic carcinoma, actinomycosis, or schistosomiasis.

PATHOGENESIS AND PATHOLOGY

The pathogenesis of AVF is uncertain. Anabtawi and colleagues[241] postulated a developmental defect in the septa separating the fetal arterial and venous plexi, so that a normal capillary bed does not develop. Stork[242] and Hodgson and co-workers[243] theorized that the capillary walls are structurally defective. Exposure of the abnormal vessels to pulmonary arterial pressures results in gradually increasing dilatation of a segment or segments of the capillary bed until a typical fistula sac has formed. This process may occur over the course of years, accounting for the development of clinically apparent AVF in previously asymptomatic adults.

An AVF appears macroscopically as a pulsating sac, usually in a subpleural location, with arterial and venous vessels opening into the center. The size is variable, up to several centimeters in diameter. Utzon and Brandrup[244] described three types of AVFs: (1) solitary or a few isolated fistulas; (2) multiple discrete fistulas; and (3) widespread telangiectatic anastomoses throughout both lungs. In a review of 350 cases of AVF, Bosher and collaborators[245] found that single AVFs were present in 65% of the patients. Although AVFs can be located in any part of the lung, the lower lobes are involved more often than the upper lobes. The blood supply to a pulmonary AVF is occasionally systemic, originating from the aorta, a bronchial artery, or a chest wall artery.

Histologic studies show dilated arterial and venous vessels, which may be connected by a single fistula sac or by a tangle of abnormal, distended vessels. The walls of the fistula sac are usually thin, although variable degrees of intimal fibrosis may be seen.[244] Thrombi or endarteritis occasionally develop within an AVF.

PATHOPHYSIOLOGY AND CLINICAL PRESENTATION

Because the blood traversing an AVF does not encounter an alveolar-capillary interface, no gas exchange occurs, and the unoxygenated blood is returned to the systemic circulation. The clinical significance of this phenomenon depends on the volume of blood shunted through the lesion. Small AVFs have no clinical effect and may be discovered in asymptomatic persons on routine chest radiographs. Fistulas 2 cm in diameter or multiple smaller fistulas can cause a clinically significant decrease in systemic oxygenation. The earliest symptom associated with an AVF is dyspnea on exertion. With shunts of 20% of the total blood flow, increasing dyspnea, cyanosis, polycythemia, and clubbing of the fingers and toes develop. Shunts of up to 79% through an AVF have been documented.[246]

In the rare cases of pulmonary AVF with a systemic arterial supply, congestive heart failure can occur if the systemic-to-pulmonary shunt is large. In cases involving a pulmonary arterial supply, however, cardiovascular parameters such as heart rate, cardiac index, blood pressure, intracardiac pressures, pulmonary vascular resistance, and electrocardiographic findings have been found to be normal.[247–250] Chest pain on the side of the lesion is occasionally described by patients with pulmonary AVF.[256]

Central nervous system symptoms are common in patients with pulmonary AVFs.[251] Tinnitus, headache, and dizziness can occur secondary to hypoxemia and polycythemia. Parodoxical embolization of infectious or thrombotic material to the central nervous system results in serious complications, such as brain abscess or stroke, in about 5% of patients.[252] Brain abscess or meningitis occurs most often in the third to fifth decades of life[253] and can be the presenting symptom of AVF.[254, 255]

Patients with Rendu-Osler-Weber syndrome have multiple capillary telangiectasias, which tend to bleed. Symptoms of hemoptysis, epistaxis, and gastrointestinal or genitourinary bleeding are common. Central nervous system symptoms such as headache, vertigo, numbness, paresis,

syncope, and confusion can also occur.[257] Patients with pulmonary AVF associated with Rendu-Osler-Weber syndrome are more likely to have multiple fistulas, rapid fistula growth, and complications than are patients with simple pulmonary AVF.[250] Multiple pulmonary AVFs, even in the absence of Rendu-Osler-Weber syndrome, are associated with a higher rate of serious complications such as polycythemia,[250] central nervous system complications,[258] hemoptysis, and hemothorax.[259] Pregnancy also seems to be associated with an increased rate of AVF growth and complications.[260]

The physical examination may reveal cyanosis, clubbing of the nails, or both. Auscultation of the chest often reveals a continuous extracardiac murmur, with or without a thrill. The intensity of the murmur increases during inspiration and is maximized by Müller's maneuver (forced inspiration against a closed glottis). These maneuvers create a negative intrathoracic pressure that distends the extra-alveolar blood vessels, thus increasing the blood flow through the fistula. Similarly, during exhalation and with the Valsalva maneuver, intrathoracic pressure is increased, the fistula is relatively compressed, and the murmur becomes less audible. The phenomenon of orthocyanosis (cyanosis in the upright position, which resolves in the supine position) has been described in patients with AVF.[261] The decreased intrathoracic pressure in the upright position results in increased shunting of blood through the AVF.

DIAGNOSTIC APPROACHES

On the routine chest radiograph, an AVF appears as a circumscribed nodule, round or serpiginous in shape (Fig. 52–30A). Fewer than 5% of the lesions are calcified. Selective tomograms often demonstrate the feeding and drain-

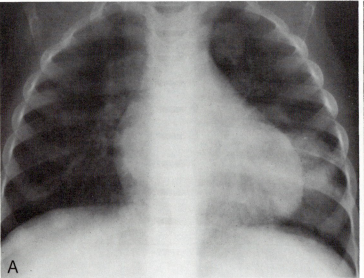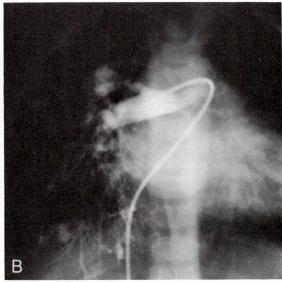

Figure 52–30. Multiple pulmonary arteriovenous malformations. The patient, a child with Rendu-Osler-Weber syndrome, had mucosal telangiectasia and cyanosis. The plain chest radiograph (A) reveals several pulmonary densities of varying size. Pulmonary angiography (B) demonstrates multiple arteriovenous malformations throughout both lungs. Balloon embolizations of several of these malformations were performed; however, the remaining malformations continued to grow, and the patient became profoundly cyanotic. She died of a massive gastrointestinal hemorrhage.

ing vessels. CT with contrast is useful in demonstrating the vascularity of the lesion as well as delineating the course of the blood vessels.[240] Examination under fluoroscopy may reveal pulsation of the nodule. An increase in size of the lesion with Müller's maneuver and a decrease in size with the Valsalva maneuver can also be documented fluoroscopically.

Lung perfusion scanning, a relatively noninvasive screening test, is sometimes helpful. After the intravenous injection of technetium-labeled albumin microaggregates, the pulmonary capillary bed filters out the microaggregates and appears as a "hot" area on the lung scan. The AVF, if large enough, may appear as a "cold spot" on the scan, or uptake may be seen in the brain and kidneys, indicating the presence of a right-to-left shunt.[262, 263] Perfusion scans are not sensitive, however, for the detection of small AVFs.[264]

Contrast echocardiography is another method for demonstrating the presence of a right-to-left shunt in patients with suspected pulmonary AVF.[265] Bubbles of contrast material (saline or indocyanine green dye) after intravenous injection are seen in the right atrium and then disappear into the pulmonary circulation. Normally, the pulmonary capillary bed filters out the contrast material, but in the presence of a pulmonary AVF, the contrast material reappears in the left atrium after a lag period of a few heart beats. This lag period distinguishes a pulmonary AVF from an intracardiac lesion such as atrial or ventricular septal defect, in which the contrast material appears immediately in the left cardiac chambers.

Angiography, although more invasive, is still the most accurate method for diagnosing AVFs and locating the feeding and draining vessels. Angiography of both lungs should always be performed preoperatively in patients with pulmonary AVF so as to ensure that all the lesions have been identified (Fig. 52–30B).[240] Digital subtraction angiography, where available, is a less invasive angiographic method.[266]

DIFFERENTIAL DIAGNOSIS

In asymptomatic patients who present only with an abnormal chest radiograph, the differential diagnosis includes a long list of disease entities that can cause discrete nodular pulmonary lesions. Tuberculosis, primary or metastatic neoplasm, bronchial adenoma, hamartoma, coccidioidomycosis, histoplasmosis, bronchogenic cyst, and pulmonary venous varix all can have similar radiographic appearances. Fluoroscopy and tomography usually demonstrate the vascular nature of the lesion; angiography confirms the diagnosis of AVF.

In patients with polycythemia, the differential diagnosis includes polycythemia vera. However, with polycythemia vera, there is no cyanosis or digital clubbing. The spleen may be enlarged, and there is an increased number of white blood cells and immature cells in the peripheral blood.

Patients with cyanosis, digital clubbing, and a continuous murmur are usually first suspected to have cyanotic congenital heart disease. The normal results of electrocardiography and cardiac catheterization, however, rule out

this diagnosis. Pulmonary angiography can be performed at the time of the cardiac catheterization to establish the diagnosis of AVF.

TREATMENT

There is some controversy concerning which patients with pulmonary AVF should be treated with surgical resection of the lesion. Some authors[256, 257] advocate excision even of small asymptomatic pulmonary AVFs because of the potential for serious complications. Others[247, 258] recommend excision of only AVFs that are symptomatic, are enlarging, or have a systemic blood supply. The goal of surgical therapy is to completely excise the AVF while preserving as much pulmonary tissue as possible, because repeated resections may be necessary if other AVFs develop. Segmental wedge resections are often effective, but lobectomy is occasionally required for removing the entire lesion.

The preoperative evaluation should include the measurement of cardiac ejection fraction and shunt fraction. A Swan-Ganz balloon can be wedged in the feeding artery of the AVF to determine the degree of improvement in shunt fraction and arterial oxygen pressure/tension that will be attained by surgical excision.[267] If only partial improvement is obtained despite adequate wedging of the balloon, other unidentified AVFs may be present. The shunt fraction can also be rechecked intraoperatively to ensure that all fistulous tissue has been removed.[268, 269]

In patients who have multiple AVFs throughout both lungs, complete surgical removal of the AVFs is impossible. Dines and associates[250] recommended conservative surgical excision of the largest lesions in these patients, if the fistulas are localized enough to be resected. An alternative treatment for multiple pulmonary AVFs or for the patient who is a poor surgical candidate is therapeutic embolization of the lesions.[248] This technique, pioneered by Taylor and colleagues,[270] involves selective catheterization of the feeding artery of the AVF, followed by release of a steel coil or balloon.[271, 272] The foreign object ablates the blood flow through the artery, and the fistula undergoes infarction. Particulate agents used in treatment of systemic AVFs should not be used for embolization of pulmonary AVFs because there is no capillary bed to filter out the particles; systemic embolization could occur.[273]

CONGENITAL DIAPHRAGMATIC HERNIA

Defects in diaphragmatic development vary in size and position; their clinical manifestations range from asymptomatic to life-threatening. The major types of diaphragmatic hernia include (1) Bochdalek's hernia (posterolateral defect), (2) Morgagni's hernia (retrosternal defect), (3) eventration of the diaphragm, and (4) hiatus hernia.

PATHOPHYSIOLOGY

The diaphragm develops between the 8th and 10th weeks of fetal life, separating the coelomic cavity into abdominal and thoracic compartments. The septum transversum develops beneath the heart and extends from the sternum to the dorsal foregut mesentery, forming the central portion of the diaphragm. A defect in the septum transversum can result in Morgagni's hernia. Factors that increase intra-abdominal pressure, such as obesity, excessive coughing, and abdominal trauma, are thought to increase the likelihood that abdominal contents will herniate through such a defect.[274-276] Most hernias of Morgagni occur on the right side, probably because left-sided defects are often occluded by the heart and pericardium. The hernia contains portions of liver, omentum, or bowel.

The lateral and posterior portions of the diaphragm are formed by the pleuroperitoneal folds. The fusion of the diaphragm to the lateral and posterior chest wall usually occurs later on the left side than on the right, the posterior segment being the last to close; hence most hernias of Bochdalek are located posteriorly and on the left side. Normally, the posterolateral portion of the diaphragm closes just before the midgut rotates back into the abdominal cavity. If the midgut returns to the abdomen early or if the diaphragmatic development is delayed, the bowel protrudes through the pleuroperitoneal sinus into the thorax. The diaphragm is then unable to close. The space-occupying effect of the bowel in the thorax results in hypoplasia of the ipsilateral lung and often the contralateral lung. The pulmonary hypoplasia is characterized primarily by a striking decrease in the number of alveoli,[277, 278] although the pulmonary arterial tree is also proportionately decreased (Fig. 52–31).

The primative diaphragm is initially composed only of folds of pleura and peritoneum. Muscular fibers subsequently migrate between the two membranous layers of the septum transversum. Failure of the muscular layer to develop results in eventration of the diaphragm. The entire hemidiaphragm or a portion of the diaphragm can be involved. Eventration can also result from denervation of the diaphragm, secondary to birth-related or surgical phrenic nerve injuries, with subsequent muscular atrophy.

Hiatal hernias occur when an abnormally large crural defect allows the stomach to slide up into the chest. Free gastroesophageal reflux then occurs, resulting in esophagitis, frequent vomiting, and often recurrent aspiration.

CLINICAL PRESENTATION AND DIAGNOSIS

Herniation through the foramen of Bochdalek is the most common form of diaphragmatic hernia, occurring in 1 of every 3000 births. About 80% of Bochdalek's hernias occur on the left side; rare cases of bilateral Bochdalek's hernias have been reported.[279-282] Wolff[282] noted several cases of familial occurrence.

Infants with Bochdalek's hernia usually present at or soon after birth with severe cardiorespiratory distress. The physical examination reveals a scaphoid abdomen and thoracic asymmetry. The side of the thorax that contains the hernia is often enlarged and hyperresonant, moves poorly with respirations, and has decreased or no breath

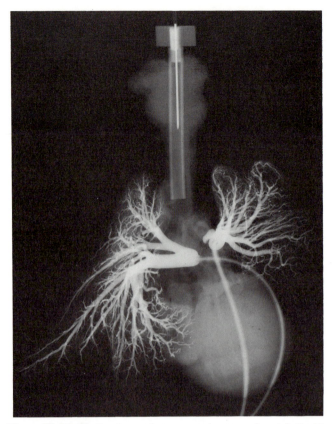

Figure 52–31. Postmortem pulmonary angiograms of an infant with Bochdalek's hernia reveal the marked hypoplasia of the arterial system of the left lung. The right lung is also hypoplastic.

sounds. The cardiac impulse is displaced away from the involved side. Bowel sounds are occasionally heard in the thorax. The infant is tachypneic, tachycardic, and cyanotic; blood gases reveal hypercapnia, hypoxia, and acidosis.

Smaller Bochdalek's hernias result in mild symptoms and are sometimes present for several months before diagnosis.[283]

The radiographic findings are virtually always diagnostic in cases of Bochdalek's hernia (Fig. 52–32). Typically, one hemithorax is filled with ringlike lucencies; the ipsilateral lung is severely compressed. The mediastinum is displaced away from the side of the hernia, and the contralateral lung is partially atelectatic. The diaphragmatic shadow is not seen on the affected side, and little or no intestinal gas is present. These two features are important in distinguishing diaphragmatic hernia from congenital cystic adenomatoid malformation, in which the diaphragm and abdominal gas pattern appear normal.

Morgagni's hernias are much less common than Bochdalek's hernias and generally manifest at a later age.[283] Many Morgagni's hernias are discovered incidentally on chest radiographs in asymptomatic persons. Some patients have intermittent nonspecific abdominal symptoms or acute intestinal obstruction. Less often, cough, dyspnea, and chest pain are the presenting symptoms.

Morgagni's hernias containing liver or omentum appear as a solid mass on the chest radiograph whereas those containing bowel are often partially lucent (Fig. 52–

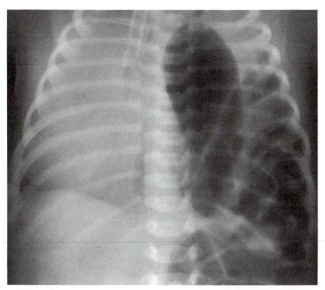

Figure 52-32. Bochdalek's hernia. The patient, a newborn, had severe respiratory distress and a scaphoid abdomen. The chest radiograph reveals loops of bowel in the left hemithorax. The left lung is atelectatic; the heart and mediastinum are shifted to the right, and the right lung is severely compressed. The infant died during attempted surgical repair.

33). The presence of a mixed solid and lucent mass in the typical retrosternal location is practically diagnostic of Morgagni's hernia. A barium enema or upper gastrointestinal contrast study can confirm the presence of intestine in the lesion. Hernias containing liver or omentum must be differentiated from tumors of the anterior mediastinum. A liver scan can demonstrate the presence of liver in the liver sac.[284] A barium enema sometimes reveals abnormal elevation or angulation of the transverse colon when omentum is trapped in the hernial sac.

The manifestation of diaphragmatic eventration varies with the extent of involvement. Small localized areas of eventration are often asymptomatic, whereas total eventration can produce a clinical picture identical to that of Bochdalek's hernia. Patients with intermediate degrees of eventration have repeated bronchopulmonary infections or mild respiratory insufficiency.[285] The chest radiograph reveals diaphragmatic elevation; fluoroscopy demonstrates paradoxical respiratory movements of the eventrated segment of the diaphragm.

TREATMENT AND PROGNOSIS

Most authors recommend surgical repair of Morgagni's hernias, even in asymptomatic patients, because of the risk of acute strangulation, which occurs in about 10% of untreated cases.[274-276] Indications for repair of diaphragmatic eventration include recurrent pulmonary infection, significant respiratory insufficiency, and suspicion of associated congenital thoracic anomalies.[285] Intraoperative or postoperative complications are rare in patients with Morgagni's hernia or diaphragmatic eventration. The long-term prognosis for these patients is good.

The mortality rate among patients with large Bochdalek's hernias is 100% without surgical correction. Even with immediate surgical intervention, the mortality rate is high (35% to 66%)[286, 287] because of the severe lung hypoplasia that is invariably associated with the anomaly.[277, 278] Pulmonary insufficiency and persistent fetal circulation are the most frequent causes of postoperative deaths; severe associated congenital anomalies contribute to mortality in some cases.[285] Some authors advocate a preoperative stabilization period to improve acid-base balance and cardiovascular function.[277, 287] Extracorporeal membrane oxygenation (ECMO) has been used to treat patients with Bochdalek's hernia and severe ventilatory failure, improving the survival rate to about 50% among these otherwise moribund patients.[288, 289] Stolar and coauthors[290] recommended that the use of ECMO be reserved for those infants who achieve satisfactory blood gas values during the immediate postoperative "honeymoon" period but then develop refractory persistent fetal circulation and respiratory failure. Infants who are never able to achieve satisfactory blood gases are excluded from the use of ECMO, on the assumption that the pulmonary

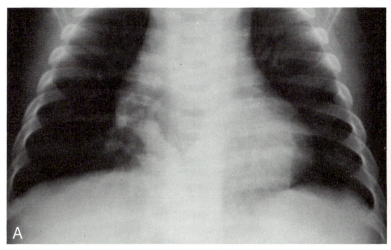
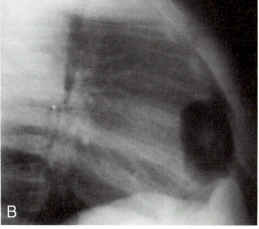

Figure 52-33. Foramen of Morgagni hernia. The patient, a 6-month-old infant, had symptoms of intermittent intestinal obstruction. *A,* Posteroanterior chest radiograph shows a cystic, solid lesion at the right cardiophrenic angle. *B,* The lateral view readily demonstrates the anteromedial diaphragmatic defect, through which an intestinal segment has herniated.

tissue is inadequate for survival. When these criteria are applied, 86% of the infants selected for ECMO survive.

The long-term prognosis for patients surviving surgical correction of diaphragmatic hernias is good. Wohl and co-workers[291] studied 19 patients whose diaphragmatic hernias had been repaired during infancy 6 to 18 years earlier. All the patients showed normal somatic growth; pulmonary function values were normal in most subjects. Three patients had moderately increased residual volumes, and five had moderately decreased forced expiratory volume in 1 sec. A moderate decrease in perfusion to the lung on the side of the hernia was found in all patients.

CONGENITAL PULMONARY LYMPHANGIECTASIS

Congenital pulmonary lymphangiectasis is a rare, usually lethal anomaly characterized by markedly dilated, hypertrophic lymphatic vessels throughout both lungs. Fewer than 100 cases have been reported in the world literature. No racial predisposition has been evident, but males are affected almost twice as often as females.[292, 293] Two cases of familial occurrence have been reported.[292, 294]

PATHOPHYSIOLOGY

In the normal fetal lung between 12 and 16 weeks' gestation, the subpleural and interlobular connective tissue is prominent and contains large lymphatic channels. Ordinarily, the connective tissue diminishes, and the lymphatic channels become smaller between 16 and 20 weeks' gestation. In congenital pulmonary lymphangiectasis, it appears that the connective tissue and lymphatic channels retain their fetal proportions, whereas the rest of the lung develops normally.[295] In cases of pulmonary lymphangiectasis associated with obstruction of the pulmonary veins, venous congestion probably results in increased lymphatic flow, stimulating the lymphatic vessels to remain dilated. In the majority of patients with congenital pulmonary lymphangiectasis, however, no cause for the persistent lymphatic dilation is apparent.

Noonan and associates[296] described three forms of congenital pulmonary lymphangiectasis. In the first and rarest form, dilation of the pulmonary lymphatic vessels occurs as part of a generalized lymphangiectasis. Hemihypertrophy and intestinal lymphangiectasis are prominent features of this syndrome. Pulmonary lymphangiectasis can also be seen in a syndrome of diffuse angiomatosis, involving predominantly the bones.[297, 298] In the second form, pulmonary lymphatic dilation occurs as a consequence of pulmonary venous obstruction. The primary anomaly in these cases is total anomalous pulmonary venous return or another congenital cardiovascular defect.[292, 293] The third and most common form of congenital pulmonary lymphangiectasis is thought to represent a primary developmental defect of the pulmonary lymphatic vessels. The cardiovascular system is normal in these cases, and the lymphangiectasis is limited to the lungs.

The lungs in cases of congenital pulmonary lymphangiectasis are bulky, stiff, and prominently lobulated. A dense network of subpleural lymphatic vessels is sometimes visible to the naked eye. The subpleural surface is often studded with cystlike dilated lymphatic segments up to 3 mm in diameter and filled with clear fluid.[295, 296] On sectioning, the lung parenchyma is found to be riddled with dilated lymphatic vessels. The amount of connective tissue in the interlobular septa is increased, which accounts for the accentuated lobulation of the lungs.[295] Microscopic examination reveals the dilated lymphatic vessels and increased amounts of connective tissue in perivascular, interlobular, and subpleural areas.[292, 295] The lymphatic vessels are thin-walled, lined with a single layer of endothelial cells. Scattered areas of patchy atelectasis and pneumonia are found in some cases.[293]

The mechanisms accounting for the severe respiratory distress in patients with congenital pulmonary lymphangiectasis are not entirely understood. A major factor appears to be a decrease in pulmonary compliance resulting from dilation of the lymphatic vessels and thickened bands of connective tissue. Results of blood gas analyses on affected infants are consistent with hypoventilation secondary to restriction of ventilatory movement.[296] The cause of intermittent bouts of increased respiratory distress, often associated with wheezing, is unclear. Pulmonary edema resulting from altered lymphatic function has been proposed as an explanation for these episodes.[296]

CLINICAL PRESENTATION

Neonates with congenital pulmonary lymphangiectasis frequently have meconium-stained amniotic fluid or other signs of fetal distress.[295] About one third of these infants are premature.[293] Cardiovascular anomalies, asplenia, urinary tract anomalies, cutaneous defects, and other congenital abnormalities are sometimes associated with congenital pulmonary lymphangiectasis. The most frequently associated cardiovascular anomaly is total anomalous pulmonary venous return. Hypoplastic left heart, obstructed left ventricle, antrioventricular canal, and septal defects have also been found.

Most infants are symptomatic from birth, although an occasional patient appears normal for the first few days to weeks of life. The onset of respiratory distress tends to occur earliest in infants whose pulmonary lymphangiectasis is secondary to cardiovascular anomalies. Most of these infants are severely symptomatic within a few hours of birth, and few survive beyond 1 or 2 weeks of age.[293, 296] Many infants with primary pulmonary lymphangiectasis are stillborn or are in severe neonatal respiratory distress. A subset of these infants, however, appears well initially and develops progressive respiratory distress at 1 to 4 weeks of age.[293] In some patients, chest radiographs taken before onset of pulmonary symptoms are normal, raising the possibility that the pulmonary lymphangiectasis is an acquired anomaly in these patients. Even in the late-onset groups of patients, survival beyond a few months of age is rare. The pulmonary involvement tends to be less severe in patients with systemic lymphangiectasis or angiomatosis. Long-term survival has been reported in these patients.[297-299]

Patients with congenital pulmonary lymphangiectasis have tachypnea, intercostal retractions, and marked cyanosis. Hyperexpansion of the lungs, wheezing, and decreased breath sounds are present either continuously or intermittently. There is no response to bronchodilator medications.[296] The course can be complicated by the development of pneumothorax[294] or chylothorax.[300] In most cases, however, the course is one of progressive respiratory failure. Congestive heart failure is a frequent occurrence in patients with congenital heart disease.

DIAGNOSTIC APPROACHES

The chest radiograph in congenital pulmonary lymphangiectasis has the appearance of pulmonary venous congestion. In some cases, a reticular pattern interspersed with small cystic areas is seen. Nonspecific findings, including diffuse hyperinflation of the lungs, areas of atelectasis, and patchy infiltrates are often seen. Electrocardiograms show right axis deviation, right ventricular hypertrophy, and sometimes right atrial hypertrophy.[292,296] Blood gas analyses demonstrate elevated arterial carbon dioxide tension and low oxygen saturation, which are consistent with hypoventilation. Cardiac catheterization frequently reveals pulmonary arterial hypertension.

The differential diagnosis includes congenital heart disease with congestive heart failure, hyaline membrane disease, meconium aspiration syndrome, and pneumonia. The diagnosis of pulmonary lymphangiectasis can be made with certainty only by means of lung biopsy or autopsy.

TREATMENT

No specific treatment is available for congenital pulmonary lymphangiectasis. France and Brown[292] suggested that atrial septostomy might benefit some patients with pulmonary venous obstruction by partially relieving the obstruction. However, successful treatment of pulmonary lymphangiectasis by this method has not been reported. The disease is universally fatal in infancy except in occasional cases associated with systemic lymphangiectasis or angiomatosis.

REFERENCES

Bronchogenic Cyst

1. Blackader AD, Evans DJ: A case of mediastinal cyst producing compression of the trachea, ending fatally in an infant of nine months. Arch Pediatr 28:194–200, 1911.
2. Maier HC: Bronchiogenic cysts of the mediastinum. Ann Surg 127:476–502, 1948.
3. Buntain WL, Isaacs H, Payne VC, et al: Lobar emphysema, cystic adenomatoid malformation, pulmonary sequestration, and bronchogenic cyst in infancy and childhood: A clinical group. J Pediatr Surg 9:85–93, 1974.
4. Haller JA, Golladay ES, Pickard LR, et al: Surgical management of lung bud anomalies: Lobar emphysema, bronchogenic cyst, cystic adenomatoid malformation, and intralobar pulmonary sequestation. Ann Thorac Surg 28:33–43, 1979.
5. Wesley JR, Heidelberger KP, DiPietro MA, et al: Diagnosis and management of congenital cystic disease of the lung in children. J Pediatr Surg 21:202–207, 1986.
6. Fraga S, Helwig EB, Rosen SH: Bronchogenic cysts in the skin and subcutaneous tissue. Am J Clin Pathol 56:230–238, 1971.
7. Yernault JC, Kuhn G, Dumortier P, et al: "Solid" mediastinal bronchogenic cyst: Mineralogic analysis. AJR 146:73–74, 1986.
8. Mendelson DS, Rose JS, Efremidis SC, et al: Bronchogenic cysts with high CT numbers. AJR 140:463–465, 1983.
9. Nakata H, Sato Y, Nakayama T, et al: Bronchogenic cyst with high CT number: Analysis of contents. J Computer Assist Tomog 10:360–362, 1986.
10. Ramenofsky ML, Leape LL, McCauley RGK: Bronchogenic cyst. J Pediatr Surg 14:219–224, 1979.
11. Bressler S, Wiener D: Bronchiogenic cyst associated with an anomalous pulmonary artery arising from the thoracic aorta. Surgery 35:815–819, 1954.
12. Weichert RF, Lindsey ES, Pearce CW, Waring WW: Bronchogenic cyst with unilateral obstructive emphysema. J Thorac Cardiovasc Surg 59:287–291, 1970.
13. Bailey BM: A detached bronchogenic cyst occurring in the tongue of a neonate. Br J Oral Surg 20:288–293, 1982.
14. DuMontier C, Graviss ER, Silberstein MJ, McAlister WH: Bronchogenic cyst in children. Clin Radiol 36:431–436, 1985.
15. Eraklis AJ, Griscom NT, McGovern JB: Bronchogenic cysts of the mediastinum in infancy. New Engl J Med 281:1150–1155, 1969.
16. Krous HF, Sexauer CL: Embryonal rhabdomyosarcoma arising within a congenital bronchogenic cyst in a child. J Pediatric Surg 16:506–508, 1981.
17. Bernheim J, Griffel B, Versano S, Bruderman I: Mediastinal leiomyosarcoma in the wall of a bronchial cyst [Letter]. Arch Pathol Lab Med 104:221, 1980.
18. Lozano FM, Martinez BG, More SL, Rodriguez AV: Carcinoma arising in a calcified bronchogenic cyst. Respiration 42:135–137, 1981.
19. Burmester HB, Douglas WK, Lodge KV, et al: Case report: Auto-immune haemolytic anaemia caused by a bronchial cyst. Clin Lab Haematol 2:145–151, 1980.
20. Rogers LF, Osmer JC: Bronchogenic cyst. A review of 46 cases. AJR 91:273–283, 1964.
21. Gourin A, Garzon AA, Rosen Y, Lyons HA: Bronchogenic cysts: Broad spectrum of presentation. NY State J Med 76:714–719, 1976.
22. Opsahl T, Berman EJ: Bronchogenic mediastinal cysts in infants: Case report and review of literature. Pediatrics 30:372–377, 1962.
23. Isdale JM, Levin SE, Chappell J, et al: Bronchogenic cysts of the infantile mediastinum. S Afr Med J 47:1871–1874, 1973.
24. Gerami S, Richardson R, Harrington B, Pate JW: Obstructive emphysema due to mediastinal bronchogenic cysts in infancy. J Thorac Cardiovasc Surg 58:432–434, 1969.
25. Crawford DB, Oh KS, Shermeta DW: Case reports: Neonatal respiratory distress due to a bronchogenic cyst. Br J Radiol 48:494–496, 1975.
26. Ikard RW: Bronchogenic cyst causing repeated left lung atelectasis in an adult. Ann Thorac Surg 14:434–439, 1972.
27. Ofoegbu RO: Intraparenchymal bronchogenic cyst in adults. Thorac Cardiovasc Surg 30:298–301, 1982.
28. Schmidt CA, Gordon R, Ahn C: Bronchogenic cysts presenting subsequent to intrapleural rupture. West J Med 134:212–214, 1981.
29. Selke AC, Belin RP, Durnin R: Bronchogenic cyst in association with hypoplasia of the left pulmonary artery. J Pediatr Surg 10:541–543, 1975.
30. Watts WJ, Rotman HH, Patten GA: Pulmonary artery compression by a bronchogenic cyst simulating congenital pulmonary artery stenosis. Am J Cardiol 53:347–348, 1984.
31. Burke DW, Folger GM, Magilligan DJ: Pulmonary arterial compression caused by bronchogenic cyst. Angiology 30:780–783, 1979.
32. Folger GM, Lewis JW: Cardiovascular findings with bronchogenic cyst. Angiology 32:29–33, 1981.
33. Van Suu D, Carpathios J, Bogedain W: Paraesophageal bronchogenic cysts: Case reports. Am Surg 32:65–68, 1966.

34. Lilly JO, Bruni H, McHardy G: Bronchogenic cyst of the esophagus: Report of a case and review of the literature. Gastrointest Endosc 18:31–32, 1971.

35. Farman J, Laster W, Rose JS, Faegenburg D: Bronchogenic cysts involving esophagus. NY State J Med 76:1507–1511, 1976.

36. Harmand D, Grosdidier J, Hoeffel JC: Multiple bronchogenic cysts of the esophagus. Am J Gastroenterol 75:321–323, 1981.

37. Touloukian RJ: Air filled bronchogenic cyst presenting as a cervical mass in the newborn. J Pediatr Surg 17:311–312, 1982.

38. McManus K, Holt GR, Aufdemorte TM, Trinkle JK: Bronchogenic cyst presenting as deep neck abscess. Otolaryngol Head Neck Surg 92:109–114, 1984.

39. Dubois P, Belanger R, Wellington JL: Bronchogenic cyst presenting as a supraclavicular mass. Can J Surg 24:530–531, 1981.

40. Leagus CJ, Gregorski RF, Crittenden JJ, et al: Giant intrapericardial bronchogenic cyst: A case report. J Thorac Cardiovasc Surg 52:581–587, 1966.

41. Gomes MN, Hufnagel CA: Intrapericardial bronchogenic cysts. Am J Cardiol 36:817–822, 1975.

42. Gayet C, Villard J, Andre-Fouet X, et al: Case report: Superior vena caval thrombosis and recurrent pericarditis caused by a bronchogenic cyst. J Cardiovasc Surg 25:86–89, 1984.

43. Watson AJ, Chaudhary BA: Cardiac arrhythmias and abnormal chest roentgenogram. Chest 92:335–336, 1987.

44. Rammohan G, Berger HW, Lajam F, et al: Superior vena cava syndrome caused by bronchogenic cyst. Chest 68:599–601, 1975.

45. Sumiyoshi K, Shimuzu S, Enjoji M, et al: Bronchogenic cyst in the abdomen. Virchows Archiv [A] 408:93–98, 1985.

46. McGlynn TJ, Burnside JW, Gatenby RA: Symptomatic abdominal bronchogenic cyst mimicking acute ischemic heart disease. Heart Lung 10:109–111, 1981.

47. Amendola MA, Shirazi KK, Brooks J, et al: Transdiaphragmatic bronchopulmonary foregut anomaly: "Dumbbell" bronchogenic cyst. AJR 138:1165–1167, 1982.

48. Van der Putte SCJ, Toonstra J: Cutaneous "bronchogenic" cyst. J Cutan Pathol 12:404–409, 1985.

49. Ambiavagar PC, Rosen Y: Cutaneous ciliated cyst of the chin. Arch Dermatol 115:895–896, 1979.

50. Grafe WR, Goldsmith EI, Redo SF: Bronchogenic cyst of the mediastinum in children. J Pediatr Surg 1:384–393, 1966.

51. Agha FP, Master K, Kaplan S, et al: Multiple bronchogenic cysts in the mediastinum. Br J Radiol 48:54–57, 1975.

52. Caudill JL, Lloyd TV: Use of computed tomography in evaluation of acute respiratory distress in a 4.5-month-old with bronchogenic cyst. Clin Pediatr 26:601–604, 1987.

53. Brasch RC, Gooding CA, Lallemand DP, et al: Magnetic resonance imaging of the thorax in childhood. Radiology 150:463–467, 1984.

54. Marks C, Marks P: The embryologic basis of tracheobronchopulmonary maldevelopment. Int Surg 72:109–114, 1987.

55. Estrera AS, Landay MJ, Pass LJ: Mediastinal carinal bronchogenic cyst: Is its mere presence an indication for surgical excision? South Med J 80:1523–1526, 1987.

56. Ryckman FC, Rosenkrantz JG: Thoracic surgical problems in infancy and childhood. Surg Clin North Am 65:1423–1454, 1985.

57. Schwartz DB, Beals TF, Wimbish KJ, et al: Transbronchial fine needle aspiration of bronchogenic cysts. Chest 88:573–575, 1985.

58. Ginsberg RJ, Atkins RW, Paulson DL: A bronchogenic cyst successfully treated by mediastinoscopy. Ann Thorac Surg 13:266–268, 1972.

59. Constant E, Davis DG, Edminster R: Bronchogenic cyst of the suprasternal area: Case report. Plast Reconstr Surg 52:88–90, 1973.

60. Miller DC, Walter JP, Guthaner DF, et al: Recurrent mediastinal bronchogenic cyst: Cause of bronchial obstruction and compression of superior vena cava and pulmonary artery. Chest 74:218–220, 1978.

61. Murray JF: Anaesthesia for congenital bronchogenic lung cyst resection. Anaesth Intensive Care 11:172–173, 1983.

Pulmonary Sequestration

62. Carter R: Pulmonary sequestration. Ann Thorac Surg 7:68–88, 1969.

63. Savic B, Birtel FJ, Tholen W, et al: Lung sequestration: Report of seven cases and review of 540 published cases. Thorax 34:96–101, 1979.

64. Iwai K, Shindo G, Hajikano H, et al: Intralobar pulmonary sequestration, with special reference to developmental pathology. Am Rev Respir Dis 107:911–920, 1973.

65. Eppinger H, Schaunstein W: Krankheiten der Lungen. Ergeb d Allg Path u Path Anat 8:267–365, 1902.

66. Halasz NA, Lindskog GE, Liebow AA: Esophagobronchial fistula and bronchopulmonary sequestration: Report of a case and review of the literature. Ann Surg 155:215–220, 1962.

67. Pryce DM: Lower accessory pulmonary artery with intralobar sequestration of lung: A report of seven cases. J Pathol Bacteriol 58:457–467, 1946.

68. Bruwer A, Clagett OT, McDonald JR: Anomalous arteries to the lung associated with congenital pulmonary abnormality. J Thorac Surg 19:957–972, 1950.

69. Smith RA: A theory of the origin of intralobar sequestration of the lung. Thorax 11:10–24, 1956.

70. Kilman JW, Battersby JS, Taybi H, Vellios F: Pulmonary sequestration. Arch Surg 90:648–657, 1965.

71. Morris SJ: An amylase-containing subdiaphragmatic bronchopulmonary sequestration. Aust N Z J Surg 53:487–490, 1983.

72. Baker EL, Gore RM, Moss AA: Retroperitoneal pulmonary sequestration: Computed tomographic findings. AJR 138:956–957, 1982.

73. Gottrup S, Lund C: Intralobar pulmonary sequestration: A report of 12 cases. Scand J Respir Dis 59:21–29, 1978.

74. Bell-Thompson J, Missier P, Sommers SC: Lung carcinoma arising in bronchopulmonary sequestration. Cancer 44:334–339, 1979.

75. Stocker JT, Kagan-Hallet K: Extralobar pulmonary sequestration. Analysis of 15 cases. Am J Clin Pathol 72:917–925, 1979.

76. Delarue NC, Pearson FG, Cooper JD, et al: Developmental bronchopulmonary disease in adults: Practical clinical considerations. Can J Surg 24:23–29, 1981.

77. Valle AR, White ML: Subdiaphragmatic aberrant pulmonary tissue. Dis Chest 13:63–68, 1947.

78. Rodgers BM, Harman PK, Johnson AM: Bronchopulmonary foregut malformations: The spectrum of anomalies. Ann Surg 203:517–524, 1986.

79. Buntain WL, Wooley MM, Mahour GH, et al: Pulmonary sequestration in children: A twenty-five year experience. Surgery 81:413–420, 1977.

80. Ransom JM, Norton JB, Williams GD: Pulmonary sequestration presenting as congestive heart failure. J Thorac Cardiovasc Surg 26:378–380, 1978.

81. Mannix EP, Haight C: Anomalous pulmonary arteries and cystic disease of the lung. Medicine 34:193–231, 1955.

82. Arroyo JG, James G: Bronchopulmonary sequestration as a rare cause of acute, massive intraesophageal bleeding. South Med J 76:241–242, 1983.

83. Werthammer JW, Hatten HP, Blake WB: Upper thoracic extralobar pulmonary sequestration presenting with respiratory distress in a newborn. Pediatr Radiol 9:116–117, 1980.

84. Mahadevia PS: Necrotizing vasculitis in an extralobar sequestrated lung [Letter]. Arch Pathol Lab Med 104:114, 1980.

85. Kawakami K, Tada S, Katsuyama N, Mochizuki S: Radionuclide study in pulmonary sequestration. J Nucl Med 19:287–289, 1978.

86. Harris HA, Lewis I: Anomalies of the lungs with special reference to the danger of abnormal vessels in lobectomy. J Thorac Surg 9:666–671, 1940.

87. Douglass R: Anomalous pulmonary vessels. J Thorac Surg 17:712–716, 1948.

88. Johnson F, Laird T: Radionuclide evaluation of a communicating bronchopulmonary foregut malformation. Pediatr Radiol 7:175–177, 1978.

89. Miller PA, Williamson BR, Minor GR, Buschi AJ: Pulmonary sequestration: Visualization of the feeding artery by CT. J Comput Assist Tomogr 6:828–830, 1982.

90. Paul DJ, Mueller CF: Pulmonary sequestration. J Comput Assist Tomogr 6:163–165, 1982.

91. Naidich DP, Rumancik WM, Lefleur RS, et al: Intralobar pulmonary sequestration: MR evaluation. J Comput Assist Tomogr 11:531–533, 1987.

92. Guest JL, Yeh TJ, Ellison LT, Ellison RG: Pulmonary parenchymal air space abnormalities. Ann Thorac Surg 1:102–104, 1965.

93. Hutchin P: Congenital cystic disease of the lung. Rev Surg 28:79–87, 1971.

94. Scully RE, Mark EJ, McNeely BU: Case records of the Massachusetts General Hospital: Weekly clinicopathological exercises, Case 48-1983. New Engl J Med 309:1374–1381, 1983.
95. Flisak ME, Chandrasekar AJ, Marsan RE, Ali MM: Systemic arterialization of lung without sequestration. AJR 138:751–753, 1982.

Congenital Cystic Adenomatoid Malformation of the Lung

96. Buntain WL, Isaacs H, Payne VC, et al: Lobar emphysema, cystic adenomatoid malformation, pulmonary sequestration, and bronchogenic cyst in infancy and childhood: A clinical group. J Pediatr Surg 9:85–93, 1974.
97. Lilly JR, Wesenberg RL, Shikes RH: Segmental lung resection in the first year of life. Ann Thorac Surg 22:16–22, 1976.
98. Haller JA, Golladay ES, Pickard LR, et al: Surgical management of lung bud anomalies: Lobar emphysema, bronchogenic cyst, cystic adenomatoid malformation and intralobar pulmonary sequestration. Ann Thorac Surg 28:33–43, 1979.
99. Wesley JR, Heidelberger KP, DiPietro MA, et al: Diagnosis and management of congenital cystic disease of the lung in children. J Pediatr Surg 21:202–207, 1986.
100. Kwittken J, Reiner L: Congenital cystic adenomatoid malformation of the lung. Pediatrics 30:759–768, 1962.
101. Olson JL, Mendelsohn G: Congenital cystic adenomatoid malformation of the lung. Arch Pathol Lab Med 102:248–251, 1978.
102. Alt B, Shikes RH, Stanford RE, Silverberg SG: Ultrastructure of congenital cystic adenomatoid malformation of the lung. Ultrastruct Pathol 3:217–228, 1982.
103. Van Dijk C, Wagenvoort CA: The various types of congenital adenomatoid malformation of the lung. J Pathol 110:131–134, 1973.
104. Ostor AG, Fortune DW: Congenital cystic adenomatoid malformation of the lung. Am J Clin Pathol 70:595–604, 1978.
105. Stocker JT, Madewell JE, Drake RM: Congenital cystic adenomatoid malformation of the lung: Classification and morphologic spectrum. Hum Pathol 8:155–171, 1977.
106. Miller RK, Sieber WK, Yunis EJ: Congenital adenomatoid malformation of the lung. Pathol Annu 15:387–402, 1980.
107. Avitabile AM, Greco MA, Hulnick DH, Feiner HD: Congenital cystic adenomatoid malformation of the lung in adults. Am J Surg Pathol 8:193–202,1984.
108. Ueda K, Gruppo R, Unger F, et al: Rhabdomyosarcoma of lung arising in congenital cystic adenomatoid malformation. Cancer 40:383–388, 1977.
109. Kohler HG, Rymer BA: Congenital cystic malformation of the lung and its relation to hydramnios. J Obstet Gynaecol Br Commonw 80:130–134, 1973.
110. Krous HF, Harper PE, Perlman M: Congenital cystic adenomatoid malformation in bilateral renal agenesis. Arch Pathol Lab Med 104:368–370, 1980.
111. Adzick NS, Harrison MR, Glick PL, et al: Fetal cystic adenomatoid malformation: Prenatal diagnosis and natural history. J Pediatr Surg 20:483–488, 1985.
112. Roloff DW, Baillie EE, Weaver DK: Macrobullous medullary polycystic kidney and cystic lung disease. Am J Dis Child 121:318–324, 1971.
113. Weber ML, Rivard G, Perreault G: Prune belly syndrome associated with congenital cystic adenomatoid malformation of the lung [Letter]. Am J Dis Child 132:316–317, 1978.
114. Bale PM: Congenital cystic malformation of the lung: A form of congenital bronchiolar ("adenomatoid") malformation. Am J Clin Pathol 71:411–420, 1979.
115. Wolf SA, Hertzler JH, Philippart AL: Cystic adenomatoid dysplasia of the lung. J Pediatr Surg 15:925–930, 1980.
116. Gaisie G, Oh KS: Spontaneous pneumothorax in cystic adenomatoid malformation. Pediatr Radiol 13:281–283, 1983.
117. Tucker TT, Smith WL, Smith JA: Fluid-filled cystic adenomatoid malformation. AJR 129:323–325, 1977.
118. Rychman FC, Rosenkrantz JG: Thoracic surgical problems in infancy and childhood. Surg Clin North Am 65:1423–1454, 1985.
119. Cohen MD, Scales RL, Eigen H, et al: Evaluation of pulmonary parenchymal disease by magnetic resonance imaging. Br J Radiol 60:223–230, 1987.
120. Mark EJ: Mesenchymal cystic hamartoma of the lung. New Engl J Med 315:1255–1259, 1986.
121. Stephanopoulos C, Catsaras H: Myxosarcoma complicating a cystic hamartoma of the lung. Thorax 18:144–145, 1963.
122. Svennevig JL, Bugge-Asperheim B, Boye NP: Carcinoma arising in a lung cyst. Scand J Thorac Cardiovasc Surg 13:153–155, 1979.
123. Weinberg AG, Currarino G, Moore GC, Votteler TP: Mesenchymal neoplasia and congenital pulmonary cysts. Pediatr Radiol 9:179–182, 1980.
124. Nishibayashi SW, Andrassy RJ, Woolley MM: Congenital cystic adenomatoid malformation: A 30-year experience. J Pediatr Surg 16:704–706, 1981.
125. Merenstein GB: Congenital cystic adenomatoid malformation of the lung: Report of a case and a review of the literature. Am J Dis Child 118:772–776, 1969.
126. Frenckner B, Freyschuss U: Pulmonary function after lobectomy for congenital loba emphysema and congenital cystic adenomatoid malformation. Scand J Thorac Cardiovasc Surg 16:293–298, 1982.

Congenital Lobar Emphysema

127. Overstreet RM: Emphysema of a portion of the lung in the early months of life. Am J Dis Child 57:861–870, 1939.
128. Gross RE, Lewis JE: Defect of the anterior mediastinum: Successful surgical repair. Surg Gynecol Obstet 80:549–554, 1945.
129. Buntain WL, Isaacs H, Payne VC, et al: Lobar emphysema, cystic adenomatoid malformation, pulmonary sequestration, and bronchogenic cyst in infancy and childhood: A clinical group. J Pediatr Surg 9:85–92, 1974.
130. Haller JA, Golladay ES, Pickard LR, et al: Surgical management of lung bud anomalies: Lobar emphysema, bronchogenic cyst, cystic adenomatoid malformation, and intralobar pulmonary sequestration. Ann Thorac Surg 28:33–43, 1979.
131. Wesley JR, Heidelberger KP, DiPietro MA, et al: Diagnosis and management of congenital cystic disease of the lung in children. J Pediatr Surg 21:202–207, 1986.
132. Hendren WH, McKee DM: Lobar emphysema of infancy. J Pediatr Surg 1:24–39, 1966.
133. Wall MA, Eisenberg JD, Campbell JR: Congenital lobar emphysema in a mother and daughter. Pediatrics 70:131–133, 1982.
134. Murray GF: Congenital lobar emphysema. Surg Gynecol Obstet 124:611–625, 1967.
135. Floyd FW, Repici AJ, Gibson ET, McGeorge CK: Bilateral congenital lobar emphysema surgically corrected. Pediatrics 31:87–96, 1963.
136. May RL, Meese EH, Timmes JJ: Congenital lobar emphysema: Case report of bilateral involvement. J Thorac Cardiovasc Surg 48:850–854, 1964.
137. Lincoln JC, Stark J, Subramanian S, et al: Congenital lobar emphysema. Ann Surg 173:55–62, 1971.
138. Bolande RB, Schneider AF, Boggs JD: Infantile lobar emphysema. AMA Arch Pathol 289–294, 1956.
139. Franken EA Jr, Buehl I: Infantile lobar emphysema: Report of two cases with unusual roentgenographic manifestation. AJR 98:354–357, 1966.
140. Boren HG: Alveolar fenestrae: Relationship to the pathology and pathogenesis of pulmonary emphysema. Am Rev Respir Dis 85:328–344, 1962.
141. Leape LL, Longino LA: Infantile lobar emphysema. Pediatrics 34:246–255, 1964.
142. Janovski NA, Balacki JA, Keenan FD: Congenital segmental lobar emphysema. Med Ann DC 38:249–254, 1969.
143. Hislop A, Reid L: New pathological findings in emphysema of childhood. 1. Polyalveolar lobe with emphysema. Thorax 25:682–690, 1970.
144. Munnell ER, Lambird PA, Austin RL: Polyalveolar lobe causing lobar emphysema of infancy. Ann Thorac Surg 16:624–628, 1973.
145. Tapper D, Schuster S, McBride J, et al: Polyalveolar lobe: Anatomic and physiologic parameters and their relationship to congenital lobar emphysema. J Pediatr Surg 15:931–937, 1980.
146. Kennedy JH, Rothman BF: The surgical treatment of congenital lobar emphysema. Surg Gynecol Obstet 121:253–260, 1965.
147. Allen RP, Taylor RL, Reiquam CW: Congenital lobar emphysema with dilated septal lymphatics. Radiology 86:929–931, 1966.
148. Campbell D, Bauer AJ, Hewlett TH: Congenital localized emphysema. J Thorac Cardiovasc Surg 41:575–586, 1961.
149. Ehrenhaft JL, Taber RE: Progressive infantile emphysema. Surgery 34:412–425, 1953.
150. Sloan H: Lobar obstructive emphysema in infancy treated by lobectomy. J Thorac Surg 26:1–20, 1953.

151. Mallory TB, Castleman B, Towne VW (eds): Weekly clinicopath-ological exercises: Case records of the Massachusetts General Hospital, Case #36041. New Engl J Med 242:149–154, 1950.

152. DeLuca FG, Wesselhoeft CW Jr, Frates R: Congenital lobar emphysema documented by serial roentgenograms. J Pediatr 82:859–862, 1973.

153. Man DW, Hamdy MH, Hendry GM, et al: Congenital lobar emphysema: Problems in diagnosis and management. Arch Dis Child 58:709–712, 1983.

154. Engle WA, Lemons JA, Weber TR, Cohen MD: Congenital lobar emphysema due to a bronchogenic cyst. Am J Perinatol 1:196–198, 1984.

155. Pardes JG, Auh YH, Blomquist K, et al: Case report: CT diagnosis of congenital lobar emphysema. J Comput Assist Tomogr 7:1095–1097, 1983.

156. Fletcher BD, Dearborn DG, Mulopulos GP: MR imaging in infants with airway obstruction: Preliminary observations. Radiology 160:245–249, 1986.

157. Padilla L, Orzel JA, Kreins CM, Weiland FL: Congenital lobar emphysema: Segmental lobar involvement demonstrated on ventilation and perfusion imaging. J Nucl Med 26:1343–1344, 1985.

158. Cumming GR, Macpherson RI, Chernick V: Unilateral hyperlucent lung syndrome in children. J Pediatr 78:250–260, 1971.

159. Cooney DR, Menke JA, Allen JE: Acquired lobar emphysema: A complication of respiratory distress in premature infants. J Pediatr Surg 12:897–904, 1977.

160. Eigen H, Lemen RJ, Waring WW: Congenital lobar emphysema: Long-term evaluation of surgically and conservatively treated children. Am Rev Respir Dis 113:823–831, 1976.

161. Morgan WJ, Lemen RJ, Rojas R: Acute worsening of congenital lobar emphysema with subsequent spontaneous improvement. Pediatrics 71:844–848, 1983.

162. Cottom DG, Myers NA: Congenital lobar emphysema. Br Med J 1:1394–1396, 1957.

163. Pierce WS, DeParedes CG, Friedman S, Waldhausen JA: Concomitant congenital heart disease and lobar emphysema in infants: Incidence, diagnosis, and operative management. Ann Surg 172:951–956, 1970.

164. McBride JT, Wohl ME, Strieder DJ, et al: Lung growth and airway function after lobectomy in infancy for congenital lobar emphysema. J Clin Invest 66:962–970, 1980.

165. Frenckner B, Freyschuss U: Pulmonary function after lobectomy for congenital lobar emphysema and congenital cystic adenomatoid malformation. Scand J Thorac Cardiovasc Surg 16:293–298, 1982.

166. DeMuth GR, Sloan H: Congenital lobar emphysema: Long-term effects and sequelae in treated cases. Surgery 59:601–607, 1966.

Tracheoesophageal Fistula

167. Ein SH, Friedberg J: Esophageal atresia and tracheoesophageal fistula. Review and update. Otolaryngol Clin North Am 14:219–249, 1981.

168. Lister J: The blood supply of the oesophagus in relation to oesophageal atresia. Arch Dis Child 39:131–137, 1964.

169. Holder TM, Ashcraft KW: Esophageal atresia and tracheo-esophageal fistula. Curr Probl Surg (August):1–68, 1966.

170. Enoksen A, Lovaas J, Haavik PE: Congenital tracheo-oesophageal fistula in the adult. Scand J Thorac Cardiovasc Surg 13:173–176, 1979.

171. Koop CE, Hamilton JP: Atresia of the esophagus: Increased survival with staged procedures in the poor-risk infant. Ann Surg 162:389–401, 1965.

172. Goodwin CD, Ashcraft KW, Holder TM, et al: Esophageal atresia with double tracheoesophageal fistula. J Pediatr Surg 13:269–273, 1978.

173. Sankaran K, Bhagirath CP, Bingham WT, et al: Tracheal atresia, proximal esophageal atresia, and distal tracheoesophageal fistula: Report of two cases and review of literature. Pediatrics 71:821–823, 1983.

174. Altman RP, Randolph JG, Shearin RB: Tracheal agenesis: Recognition and management. J Pediatr Surg 7:112–118, 1972.

175. Hardy KA, Schidlow DV, Zaeri N: Obliterative bronchiolitis in children. Chest 93:460–466, 1988.

176. Emery JL, Haddadin AJ: Squamous epithelium in respiratory tract of children with tracheo-oesophageal fistula. Arch Dis Child 46:236–242, 1971.

177. Scott JB, Wilson JK: Hydramnios as an early sign of oesophageal atresia. Lancet 2:569–572, 1957.

178. Waterston DJ, Bonham-Carter RE, Aberdeen E: Congenital tracheo-oesophageal fistula in association with oesophageal atresia. Lancet 2:55–57, 1963.

179. Hicks LM, Mansfield PB: Esophageal atresia and tracheoesophageal fistula: Review of thirteen years' experience. J Thorac Cardiovasc Surg 81:358–363, 1981.

180. Haight C, Towsley HA: Congenital atresia of the esophagus with tracheoesophageal fistula: Extrapleural ligation of fistula and end-to-end anastomosis of esophageal segments. Surg Gynecol Obstet 76:672–688, 1943.

181. Howard R, Myers NA: Esophageal atresia: A technique for elongating the upper pouch. Surgery 58:725–727, 1965.

182. Johnston PW: Elongation of the upper segment in esophageal atreas: Report of a case. Surgery 58:741–744, 1965.

183. Holder TM: Current trends in the management of esophageal atresia and tracheoesophageal fistula. Am Surg 44:31–36, 1978.

184. Livaditis A, Radberg L, Odensjo G: Esophageal end-to-end anastomosis: Reduction of anastomotic tension by circular myotomy. Scand J Thorac Cardiovasc Surg 6:206–214, 1972.

185. de Lorimier AA, Harrison MR: Long gas esophageal atresia: Primary anastomosis after esophageal elongation by bougienage and esophagomyotomy. J Thorac Cardiovasc Surg 79:138–141, 1980.

186. Touloukian RJ, Pickett LK, Spackman T, Biancani P: Repair of esophageal atresia by end-to-side anastomosis and ligation of the tracheoesophageal fistula: A critical review of 18 cases. J Pediatr Surg 9:305–310, 1974.

187. Daum R: Postoperative complications following operation for oesophageal atresia and tracheo-oesophageal fistula. Prog Pediatr Surg 1:209–237, 1970.

188. Holder TM, Ashcraft KW: Developments in the care of patients with esophageal atresia and tracheoesophageal fistula. Surg Clin North Am 61:1051–1061, 1981.

189. Kirkpatrick JA, Cresson SL, Pilling GP: The motor activity of the esophagus in association with esophageal atresia and tracheoesophageal fistula. AJR 86:884–887, 1961.

190. Desjardins JG, Stephens CA, Moes CAF: Results of surgical treatment of congenital tracheo-esophageal fistula with a note on cine-fluorographic findings. Ann Surg 160:141–145, 1964.

191. Orringer MB: Esophageal atresia: Discussion. J Thorac Cardiovasc Surg 74:341, 1977.

192. Waterston DJ, Bonham-Carter RE, Aberdeen E: Oesophageal atresia: Tracheo-oesophageal fistula. A study of survival in 218 infants. Lancet 1:819–823, 1962.

193. Blyth B, Davidson JR: Tracheo-oesophageal fistula in Christchurch: A review. N Z Med J 97:42–44, 1984.

Vascular Compression of the Airway

194. Smith RJ, Smith MC, Glossop LP, et al: Congenital vascular anomalies causing tracheoesophageal compression. Arch Otolaryngol 110:82–87, 1984.

195. Stewart JR, Kincaid OW, Edwards JE: An Atlas of Vascular Rings and Related Malformations of the Aortic Arch System. Springfield, IL: Charles C Thomas, 1964.

196. Roesler M, de Leval M, Chrispin A, Stark J: Surgical management of vascular ring. Ann Surg 197:139–146, 1983.

197. Berlinger NT, Long C, Foker J, Lucas RV: Tracheobronchial compression in acyanotic congenital heart disease. Ann Otol Rhinol Laryngol 92:387–390, 1983.

198. Berlinger NT, Lucas RV, Foker J: Pulmonary arteriopexy to relieve tracheobronchial compression by dilated pulmonary arteries. Ann Otol Rhinol Laryngol 93:473–476, 1984.

199. Ergin MA, Jayaram N, LaCorte M: Left aortic arch and right descending aorta: Diagnostic and therapeutic implications of a rare type of vascular ring. Ann Thorac Surg 31:82–85, 1981.

200. Whitman G, Stephenson LW, Weinberg P: Vascular ring: Left cervical aortic arch, right descending aorta, and right ligamentum arteriosum. J Thorac Cardiovasc Surg 83:311–315, 1982.

201. Minami K, Sagoo KS, Matties W, et al: Left aortic arch, retroesophageal aortic segment, right descending aorta and right patent ductus arteriosus—A very rare "vascular ring" malformation. Thorac Cardiovasc Surg 34:395–397, 1986.

202. Berman W, Yabek SM, Dillon T, et al: Vascular ring due to left aortic arch and right descending aorta. Circulation 63:458–460, 1981.

203. McKay R, Stark J, de Leval M: Unusual vascular ring in infant with pulmonary atresia and ventricular septal defect. Br Heart J 48:180–183, 1982.
204. Berdon WE, Baker DH, Wung JT, et al: Complete cartilage-ring tracheal stenosis associated with anomalous left pulmonary artery: The ring-sling complex. Radiology 152:57–64, 1984.
205. Strife JL, Baumel AS, Dunbar JS: Tracheal compression of the innominate artery in infancy and childhood. Radiology 139:73–75, 1981.
206. Gross RE, Neuhauser EBD: Compression of the trachea by an anomalous innominate artery: An operation for its relief. Am J Dis Child 75:570–574, 1948.
207. Mustard WT, Bayliss CE, Fearon B, et al: Tracheal compression by the innominate artery in children. Ann Thorac Surg 8:312–319, 1969.
208. Moes CA, Izukawa T, Trusler GA: Innominate artery compression of the trachea. Arch Otolaryngol 101:733–738, 1975.
209. Ardito JM, Tucker GF, Ossoff RH, DeLeon SY: Innominate artery compression of the trachea in infants with reflex apnea. Ann Otol Rhinol Laryngol 89:401–405, 1980.
210. Wenig BL, Abramson AL: Innominate artery compression of the trachea. Bull N Y Acad Med 60:525–531, 1984.
211. Berdon WE, Baker DH, Bordiuk J: Innominate artery compression of the trachea in infants with stridor and apnea. Radiology 92:272–278, 1969.
212. Stellin G, Jonas RA, Goh TH, et al: Surgical treatment of absent pulmonary valve syndrome in infants: Relief of bronchial obstruction. Ann Thorac Surg 36:468–475, 1983.
213. Rabinovitch M, Grady, S, David I, et al: Compression of intrapulmonary bronchi by abnormally branching pulmonary arteries associated with absent pulmonary valves. Am J Cardiol 50:804–813, 1982.
214. Fearon B, Shortreed R: Tracheobronchial compression by congenital cardiovascular anomalies in children: Syndrome of apnea. Ann Otol Rhinol Laryngol 72:949–969, 1963.
215. Adkins RB, Maples MD, Graham BS, et al: Dysphagia associated with an aortic arch anomaly in adults. Am Surg 52:238–245, 1986.
216. Keith HH: Vascular rings and tracheobronchial compression in infants. Pediatr Ann 6:540–591, 1977.
217. Tonkin IL, Gold RE, Moser D, Laster RE: Evaluation of vascular rings with digital subtraction angiography. AJR 142:1287–1291, 1984.
218. Bertolini A, Pelizza A, Panizzon G, et al: Vascular rings and slings: Diagnosis and surgical treatment of 49 patients. J Cardiovasc Surg 28:301–312, 1987.
219. Pirtle T, Clarke E: Vascular ring: Unusual cause of unilateral obstructive pulmonary hyperinflation. AJR 140:1111–1112, 1963.
220. Otero-Cagide M, Moodie DS, Sterba R, Gill CC: Digital substraction angiography in the diagnosis of vascular rings. Am Heart J 112:1304–1308, 1986.
221. Rheuban KS, Ayres N, Still G, Alford B: Pulmonary artery sling: A new diagnostic tool and clinical review. Pediatrics 69:472–475, 1982.
222. Moncada R, Demos TC, Churchill R, Reynes C: Chronic stridor in a child: CT diagnosis of pulmonary vascular sling. J Comput Assist Tomogr 7:713–715, 1983.
223. Bisset GS, Strife JL, Kirks DR, Bailey WW: Vascular rings: MR imaging. AJR 149:251–256, 1987.
224. Kersting-Sommerhoff BA, Sechtem UP, Fisher MR, Higgins CB: MR imaging of congenital anomalies of the aortic arch. AJR 149:9–13, 1987.
225. Beavan TED, Fatti L: Ligature of aortic arch in the neck. Br J Surg 34:414–416, 1947.
226. Filler RM, Buck JR, Bahoric A, Steward DJ: Treatment of segmental tracheomalacia and bronchomalacia by implantation of an airway splint. J Pediatr Surg 17:597–603, 1982.
227. Vasko JS, Ahn C: Surgical management of secondary tracheomalacia. Ann Thorac Surg 6:269–272, 1968.
228. Johnston MR, Loeber N, Hillyer P, et al: External stent for repair of secondary tracheomalacia. Ann Thorac Surg 30:291–296, 1980.
229. Nakayama DK, Harrison MR, de Lorimier AA, et al: Reconstructive surgery for obstructing lesions of the intrathoracic trachea in infants and small children. J Pediatr Surg 17:854–868, 1982.
230. Page BA, Klein EF: Tracheal stent as an aid in weaning from mechanical ventilation in tracheomalacia. Anesthesiology 47:300–301, 1977.
231. Martin WM, Shapiro RS: Long custom-made tracheostomy tube in severe tracheomalacia. Laryngoscope 91:355–362, 1981.
232. Marmon LM, Bye MR, Haas JM, et al: Vascular rings and slings: Long-term follow-up of pulmonary function. J Pediatr Surg 19:683–690, 1984.
233. Bertrand JM, Chartrand C, Lamarre A, Lapierre JG: Vascular ring: Clinical and physiological assessment of pulmonary function following surgical correction. Pediatr Pulmonol 2:378–383, 1986.
234. Lobe TE, Hayden CK, Nicolas D, Richardson CJ: Successful management of congenital tracheal stenosis in infancy. J Pediatr Surg 22:1137–1142, 1987.
235. Hauft SM, Perlman JM, Siegel MJ, Muntz HR: Tracheal stenosis in the sick premature infant. Am J Dis Child 142:206–209, 1988.
236. Campbell CD, Wernly JA, Koltip PC, et al: Aberrant left pulmonary artery (pulmonary artery sling): Successful repair and 24 year followup report. Am J Cardiol 45:316–320, 1980.
237. Stark J, Roesler M, Chrispin A, de Leval M: The diagnosis of airway obstruction in children. J Pediatr Surg 20:113–117, 1985.

Arteriovenous Fistula
238. Sloan RD, Cooley RN: Congenital pulmonary arteriovenous aneurysm. AJR 70:183–210, 1953.
239. Stringer CJ, Stanley AL, Bates RC, Summers JE: Pulmonary arteriovenous fistula. Am J Surg 89:1054–1080, 1955.
240. Moser RJ, Tenholder MF: Diagnostic imaging of pulmonary arteriovenous malformations. Chest 89:586–589, 1986.
241. Anabtawi IN, Ellison RG, Ellison LT: Pulmonary arteriovenous aneurysms and fistulas: Anatomical variations, embryology, and classification. Ann Thorac Surg 1:277–285, 1965.
242. Stork WJ: Pulmonary arteriovenous fistulas. AJR 74:441–454, 1955.
243. Hodgson CH, Burchell HB, Good CA, Clagett OT: Hereditary hemorrhagic telangiectasia and pulmonary arteriovenous fistula. N Engl J Med 261:625–636, 1959.
244. Utzon F, Brandrup F: Pulmonary arteriovenous fistulas in children. Acta Paediatr Scand 62:422–432, 1973.
245. Bosher LH, Blake DA, Byrd BR: An analysis of the pathologic anatomy of pulmonary arteriovenous aneurysms with particular reference to the applicability of local excision. Surgery 45:91–104, 1959.
246. Friedlich A, Bing RJ, Blount SG Jr: Physiological studies in congenital heart disease: Circulatory dynamics in the anomalies of venous return to the heart including pulmonary arteriovenous fistula. Bull Johns Hopkins Hosp 86:20–57, 1950.
247. Moyer JH, Glantz G, Brest AN: Pulmonary arteriovenous fistulas: Physiologic and clinical considerations. Am J Med 32:417–435, 1962.
248. Gomes MR, Bernatz PE, Dines DE: Pulmonary arteriovenous fistulas. Ann Thorac Surg 7:582–593, 1969.
249. Mansour KA, Hatcher CR, Logan WD, Abbott OA: Pulmonary arteriovenous fistula. Am Surg 37:203–208, 1971.
250. Dines DE, Arms RA, Bernatz PE, Gomes MR: Pulmonary arteriovenous fistulas. Mayo Clin Proc 49:460–465, 1974.
251. Sisel RJ, Parker BM, Bahl OP: Cerebral symptoms in pulmonary arteriovenous fistula. Circulation 41:123–128, 1970.
252. Meacham WF, Scott HW: Congenital pulmonary arteriovenous aneurysm complicated by *Bacteroides* abscess of brain: Successful surgical management. Ann Surg 147:404–408, 1958.
253. Tyler HR: Brain abscess and pulmonary arteriovenous fistulae. Trans Am Neurol Assoc 98:314–317, 1973.
254. Thompson RL, Cattaneo SM, Barnes J: Recurrent brain abscess: Manifestation of pulmonary arteriovenous fistula and hereditary hemorrhagic telangiectasia. Chest 72:654–655, 1977.
255. Feneley MP, Burns MW: Cerebral abscess: Manifestation of pulmonary arteriovenous malformations. Aust N Z J Med 13:280–282, 1983.
256. Mattila S, Meurala H, Jarvinen A, Ketonen P: Pulmonary arteriovenous fistulas. Scand J Thorac Cardiovasc Surg 16:165–168, 1982.
257. Prager RL, Laws KH, Bender HW: Arteriovenous fistula of the lung. Ann Thorac Surg 36:231–239, 1983.
258. Sluiter-Eringa H, Orie NG, Sluiter HJ: Pulmonary arteriovenous fistula: Diagnosis and prognosis in noncompliant patients. Am Rev Respir Dis 100:177–188, 1969.

259. Shumacker HB, Waldhausen JA: Pulmonary arteriovenous fistulas in children. Ann Surg 158:713–720, 1963.
260. Hoffman R, Rabens R: Evolving pulmonary nodules: Multiple pulmonary arteriovenous fistulas. AJR 120:861–864, 1974.
261. Hoeppner VH: Orthocyanosis: A sign of pulmonary arteriovenous malformation. Thorax 37:952–953, 1982.
262. Lewis AB, Gates GF, Stanley P: Echocardiography and perfusion scintigraphy in the diagnosis of pulmonary arteriovenous fistula. Chest 73:675–677, 1978.
263. Spies WG, Spies SM, Mintzer RA: Radionuclide imaging in diseases of the chest (Part 2). Chest 83:250–255, 1983.
264. Harding JA, Velchik MG: Pulmonary scintigraphy in a patient with multiple pulmonary arteriovenous malformations and pulmonary embolism. J Nucl Med 26:151–154, 1985.
265. Hernandez A, Strauss AW, McKnight R, Hartmann AF: Diagnosis of pulmonary arteriovenous fistula by contrast echocardiography. J Pediatr 93:258–261, 1978.
266. Reekers JA, Smeets RW: Digital subtraction angiography and pulmonary vascular anomaly: Two case reports. Eur J Radiol 5:199–201, 1985.
267. Harrow EM, Beach PM, Wise JR, et al: Pulmonary arteriovenous fistula: Preoperative evaluation with a Swan-Ganz catheter. Chest 73:92–94, 1978.
268. Purcell GR, Manners JM, Cockburn JS: Pulmonary arteriovenous fistula: A shunt equation exercise during thoracotomy. Anaesthesia 32:777–783, 1977.
269. Bruya TE, Keppel JF, D'Silva R, Barker AF: Longitudinal evaluation of a patient with arteriovenous fistulas: Use of FRC-TLC shunt technique. Chest 76:603–605, 1979.
270. Taylor BG, Cockerill EM, Manfredi F, Klatte EC: Therapeutic embolization of the pulmonary artery in pulmonary arteriovenous fistula. Am J Med 64:360–365, 1978.
271. Terry PB, Barth KH, Kaufman SL, White RI: Balloon embolization for treatment of pulmonary arteriovenous fistulas. N Engl J Med 302:1189–1190, 1980.
272. Hatfield DR, Fried, AM: Therapeutic embolization of diffuse pulmonary arteriovenous malformations. AJR 137:861–863, 1981.
273. Kaufman SL, Kumar AA, Roland JM, et al: Transcatheter embolization in the management of congenital arteriovenous malformations. Radiology 137:21–29, 1980.

Congenital Diaphragmatic Hernia
274. Boyd DP: Diaphragmatic hernia through the foramen of Morgagni. Surg Clin North Am 41:839–846, 1961.
275. Bentley G, Lister J: Retrosternal hernia. Surgery 57:567–575, 1965.
276. Baran EM, Houston HE, Lynn HB, O'Connell EJ: Foramen of Morgagni hernias in children. Surgery 62:1076–1081, 1967.
277. Bohn D, Tamura M, Perrin D, et al: Ventilatory predictors of pulmonary hypoplasia in congenital diaphragmatic hernia, confirmed by morphologic assessment. J Pediatr 111:423–431, 1987.
278. George DK, Cooney TP, Chiu BK, Thurlbeck WM: Hypoplasia and immaturity of the terminal lung unit (acinus) in congenital diaphragmatic hernia. Am Rev Respir Dis 136:947–950, 1987.
279. Levy JL, Guynes WA, Louis JE, Linder LH: Bilateral congenital diaphragmatic hernias through the foramina of Bochdalek. J Pediatr Surg 4:557–559, 1969.
280. Conde J, Mendoza E, Rafel E, Parra DM: Congenital bilateral posterolateral and anterior diaphragmatic defects. J Pediatr Surg 14:185–186, 1979.
281. Furuta Y, Nakamura Y, Miyamoto K: Bilateral congenital posterolateral diaphragmatic hernia. J Pediatr Surg 22:182–183, 1987.
282. Wolff G: Familial congenital diaphragmatic defect. Review and conclusions. Hum Genet 54:1–5, 1980.
283. Allen MS, Thomson SA: Congenital diaphragmatic hernia in children under one year of age: A 24 year review. J Pediatr Surg 1:157–161, 1966.
284. Comer TP, Schmalhorst WR, Arbegast NR: Foramen of Morgagni hernia diagnosed by liver scan. Chest 63:1036–1038, 1973.
285. Groff DB, Caprio A, Behrle F: Early repair of diaphragmatic hernia to correct associated anomalies. Am Surg 43:610–612, 1977.
286. Nguyen L, Guttman FM, de Chadarevian JP, et al: The mortality of congenital diaphragmatic hernia: Is total pulmonary mass inadequate, no matter what? Ann Surg 198:766–770, 1983.
287. Cartlidge PH, Mann NP, Kapila L: Preoperative stabilization in congenital diaphragmatic hernia. Arch Dis Child 61:1226–1228, 1986.
288. Redmond C, Heaton J, Calix J, et al: A correlation of pulmonary hypoplasia, mean airway pressure, and survival in congenital diaphragmatic hernia treated with extracorporeal membrane oxygenation. J Pediatr Surg 22:1143–1149, 1987.
289. Langham MR, Krummel TM, Bartlett RH, et al: Mortality with extracorporeal membrane oxygenation following repair of congenital diaphragmatic hernia in 93 infants. J Pediatr Surg 22:1150–1154, 1987.
290. Stolar C, Dillon P, Reyes C: Selective use of extracorporeal membrane oxygenation in the management of congenital diaphragmatic hernia. J Pediatr Surg 12:207–211, 1988.
291. Wohl ME, Griscom NT, Strieder DJ, et al: The lung following repair of congenital diaphragmatic hernia. J Pediatr 90:405–414, 1977.

Congenital Pulmonary Lymphangiectasis
292. France NE, Brown RJ: Congenital pulmonary lymphangiectasis: Report of 11 examples with special reference to cardiovascular findings. Arch Dis Child 46:528–532, 1971.
293. Felman AH, Rhatigan RM, Pierson KK: Pulmonary lymphangiectasia: Observation in 17 patients and proposed classification. AJR 116:548–558, 1972.
294. Scott-Emuakpor AB, Warren ST, Kapur S, et al: Familial occurrence of congenital pulmonary lymphangiectasis. Am J Dis Child 135:532–534, 1981.
295. Laurence KM: Congenital pulmonary lymphangiectasis. J Clin Pathol 12:62–69, 1959.
296. Noonan JA, Walters LR, Reeves JT: Congenital pulmonary lymphangiectasis. Am J Dis Child 120:314–319, 1970.
297. Koblenzer PJ, Bukowski MJ: Angiomatosis (hamartomatous hem-lymphangiomatosis): Report of a case with diffuse involvement. Pediatrics 28:65–76, 1961.
298. Scully RE, Galdabini JJ, McNeely BU: Case records of the Massachusetts General Hospital: Weekly clinicopathological exercises, Case #30-1980. New Engl J Med 303:270–276, 1980.
299. Mann TP: Hemihypertrophy left side of body: Congenital lymphatic oedema of left arm. Radiological enlargement of heart shadow. Proc R Soc Med, 48:330–331, 1955.
300. Gardner TW, Domm AC, Brock CE, Pruitt AW: Congenital pulmonary lymphangiectasis. Clin Pediatr 22:75–78, 1983.

53 CHILDHOOD NEAR-DROWNING

DAVID F. WESTENKIRCHNER, M.D. / HOWARD EIGEN, M.D.

Drowning is the cause of 140,000 deaths annually; nearly 10,000 of them are in the United States. Of drowning victims in the United States, approximately 50% are under the age of 15 years, and 40% are 4 years old or younger. Drowning is the third most common cause of death in infants and children, after motor vehicle accidents and perinatal mortality. The incidence of near-drowning is unknown, but it is estimated to be two to three times that of drowning.

The most common site for childhood near-drowning is the backyard swimming pool. Pearn and Nixon found that 74% of swimming pool accidents occur in private, in-ground backyard pools.[1] Other common sites include bathtubs, canals, lakes, ponds, the ocean, and bays. Also reported are immersions in buckets of cleaning solution, which adds the toxicity of the cleaning agent to that of the water aspiration. In near-drowning incidents outside the home, there is a male predominance of three to one; in bathtub incidents, female infants predominate. Incidents occurring in private swimming pools usually involve white male infants and toddlers; those occurring in lakes, ponds, canals and ocean involve mostly black male school-age children. An important factor in near-drowning incidents involving children is lack of proper adult supervision, which may be complicated by improper access barriers.

PATHOPHYSIOLOGY

Drowning is immersion that results in asphyxia and death, either during immersion or within 1 day of the episode. Near-drowning is immersion of such severity that the victim requires medical attention at a hospital but not severe enough to result in death within the first day.

A well-defined sequence of stages in response to immersion has been described by various investigators.[2, 3] Initially there is a period of panic and violent struggling with breath-holding for 1 to 2 min. This is followed both by a suspension of movement and by exhalation. Third, reflex swallowing of large amounts of water occurs. This is followed by relaxation of the larynx with flooding of the lungs and, lastly, asphyxia and death. In most cases water is aspirated into the lungs, but in approximately 10% of victims, laryngospasm and "dry" drowning occurs.

Theoretically, there should be differences between salt- and fresh-water drowning on the basis of the tonicity of the fluid entering the alveolar spaces. Swann and co-workers pioneered experimental investigation of drowning and focused on profound electrolyte changes seen in drowned dogs.[4] They demonstrated marked shifts of water from the lung into the circulation in fresh-water drowning. This resulted in volume expansion, hemodilution, hemolysis, and hyperkalemia with ventricular fibrillation. In contrast, salt-water drowning caused a shift of water from the circulation into the lung. This resulted in volume depletion, hemoconcentration, hyperelectrolytemia, and hypotension with shock. Further experiments by Modell and associates demonstrated a relationship between the volume of fluid aspirated and the severity of blood volume changes.[5, 6] When large volumes of fluid were aspirated, hemoconcentration or hemodilution as well as electrolyte abnormalities did take place. However, at low volumes of fluid aspiration such as those encountered clinically, the changes were not severe and were transient in animals that survived the initial insult. At this low level of aspirant, the animals did not exhibit clinically significant electrolyte abnormalities, nor did ventricular fibrillation develop. Subsequently, studies in human near-drowning victims indicate that electrolyte disturbances are mild, if present at all.[7] Similarly, there are few abnormalities in serum hemoglobin values or blood volume. The importance of immediate therapy for electrolyte disturbances has been overestimated.

The most striking and clinically significant changes are in blood gas and acid-base status because of respiratory insufficiency. Hypoxemia, hypercapnia, and combined metabolic and respiratory acidosis are common clinical manifestations. In experimental animals, a decrease in the partial pressure of arterial oxygen and pH and an increase in the partial pressure of arterial carbon dioxide was observed 3 min after aspiration, regardless of the quantity of fluid aspirated.[8]

Hypoxemia is the most damaging result of near-drowning. The immediate effect of immersion is hypoventilation and lack of oxygen breathing. When laryngospasm is simulated in dogs by endotracheal tube occlusion, the arterial oxygen tension (Pa_{O_2}) drops precipitously to 40 mm Hg after 1 min to 10 mm Hg after 3 min, and to 4 mm Hg after 5 min.[9] After retrieval from the water, this immediate cause of hypoxemia is reversed to varying degrees, but effects related to the aspiration of fluid into the lungs result in further hypoxemia. Most drowning victims aspirate only relatively small volumes, but the water aspirated may contain mud, sand, algae, chemicals, or vomitus or a combination of these materials. Such intraluminal obstruction by aspirated particles, as well as by the water itself, results in areas of nonventilated alveoli, contributing to intrapulmonary shunting and hypoxemia. Intrapulmonary shunting or perfusion of nonventilated alveoli can also occur because of atelectasis or because of fluid filling the alveolar spaces. Destruction of normal surfactant by the aspirated water results in higher surface tension of the alveoli at small volumes and contributes to atelectasis. Organic and inorganic contents of the aspirated fluid, irrespective of the type of water aspirated, produce local inflammatory lesions in the alveolar capillary membrane, leading to outpouring of plasma-rich exudate into the alveolus and deposition of proteinaceous material within the alveolar space. This alveolar pulmonary edema further complicates intrapulmonary shunting and hypoxemia. Ventilation/perfusion mismatching also contributes to the development of arterial hypoxemia. This mismatching can be based on intraluminal airways obstruction from aspirated particles, as noted earlier, or on interstitial pulmonary edema. In addition, active bronchospasm may contribute to narrowing of the small airways secondary to irritation from the aspirated water or aspirated particles.

In summary, moderate to severe degrees of arterial hypoxemia are the most damaging of respiratory abnormalities that develop after pulmonary edema. Modell and associates evaluated near-drowing victims on their arrival in the emergency room and found moderate arterial hypoxemia ($Pa_{O_2} < 80$ mm Hg) in 50 of 81 patients, irrespective of the fraction of inspired oxygen (FI_{O_2}), which ranged from that of room air to 100% inspired oxygen.[10] This hypoxemia results whether the incident occurs in salt or fresh water. The major mechanisms of hypoxemia in near-drowning, as indicated earlier, are intrapulmonary shunting from atelectasis or fluid-filled alveoli and ventilation/perfusion mismatch from airway narrowing that results from interstitial pulmonary edema and bronchospasm.

The other major organ system damaged by the asphyxial episode is the central nervous system.[3] Central nervous system dysfunction, most likely caused by hypoxemia, is present in a significant percentage of near-drowning patients. Unfortunately, there is a misconception that children who have experienced near-drowning are less likely to suffer irreversible cerebral damage than are near-drowning adult victims. Central nervous system damage results primarily from the onset-related hypoxemia and ischemia, but secondary insult may occur after near-drowning because of abnormalities of cerebral blood flow, perfusion pressure changes, and metabolic consequences.

MANAGEMENT

Therapy of near-drowning victims is directed at restoration of oxygenation, ventilation, circulation, and acid-base balance, as well as at protection of the central nervous system from further insult. When the victim is rescued after immersion, immediate and effective cardiopulmonary resuscitation must be begun. Mouth-to-mouth resuscitation should begin in the water, if possible. If an effective pulse is not present, closed chest cardiac massage must be instituted and continued until an adequate blood pressure is documented. Oxygen must be administered as soon as possible and continued during transport to the hospital emergency department. All near-drowning victims should be admitted to the hospital regardless of their apparent condition. Delayed deaths caused by the accumulation of atelectatic areas, sudden pulmonary edema, and hypoxemia have been noted in near-drowning victims who left the scene of immersion or were discharged from the emergency room. Even asymptomatic patients should be observed for at least 24 h in the hospital. The majority of patients show clinical evidence of a significant episode of tachypnea, tachycardia, bibasilar crackles, wheezing, and depressed level of consciousness; fewer patients exhibit severe aspiration with seizures, coma, or circulatory collapse.[11] Initial chest radiographs usually demonstrate varying degrees of interstitial and alveolar pulmonary edema, and most show some nodular confluent infiltrates in the medial third of the lung fields bilaterally.

Evaluation normally takes place as therapy is initiated. If the patient is breathing spontaneously, 100% oxygen should be administered by humidified face mask, regardless of the patient's clinical appearance. Arterial blood should be analyzed, and changes in oxygen therapy should be based on these results. According to Modell and associates, 70% of near-drowning victims have metabolic acidosis.[10] If the patient is hypotensive or unresponsive, sodium bicarbonate should be administered intravenously in a dose of 1 mEq/kg body weight.

The airway should be cleared of debris and patency maintained. As mentioned earlier, near-drowning victims swallow large amounts of fluids and are at extremely high risk for aspiration of vomitus. The stomach should be emptied immediately by placement of a nasogastric tube. If immediate intubation is required, the airway should be protected during the procedure by the use of manual cricoid pressure. The course of further treatment depends on the evaluation of Pa_{O_2}, arterial carbon dioxide tension (Pa_{CO_2}), and pH. The correction of these abnormalities is often all that is necessary to reestablish an effective cardiac output and enable return of consciousness. Indications for endotracheal intubation and institution of mechanical ventilation include ventilatory failure and oxygenation failure. A Pa_{CO_2} higher than 60 mm Hg is a reasonable criterion for institution of ventilatory assistance. Failure of oxygenation despite supplemental oxygen delivery is another indication for endotracheal intubation. One method of assessing lung function is to calculate the alveolar-arterial oxygen difference. This establishes the effective intrapulmonary shunt; patients with an alveolar-arterial gradient of more than 350 should benefit from intubation and ventilation. Another practical method is to determine the Pa_{O_2}/FI_{O_2} ratio. In normal persons, this ratio is higher than 400. Patients who are unable to maintain a Pa_{O_2}/FI_{O_2} ratio higher than 200 to 250 are candidates for intubation and mechanical ventilation.

In selected patients, continuous positive airway pressure (CPAP) may be maintained by face mask while the patient breathes spontaneously. Glasser and co-workers[11] quoted success with this technique. The principal risk associated with mask CPAP is abdominal distension with subsequent vomiting or aspiration. Mask CPAP should be considered only in alert or mildly sedated patients.

The goals of mechanical ventilation include improvement of intrapulmonary shunting and ventilation/perfusion mismatching to reverse arterial hypoxemia. Mechanical ventilation alone may be effective in reversing hypercapnia and in reducing oxygen requirements. However, the application of positive end-expiratory pressure (PEEP) is often needed because of the loss of alveolar volume secondary to atelectasis and fluid filling of alveolar spaces. PEEP is useful in stabilizing airways and alveoli by restoring functional residual capacity and by recruiting functional gas exchange interface. This can result in a reduction in intrapulmonary shunt, improvement in ventilation/perfusion matching, and increased lung compliance, which in turn lead to improved oxygenation. The level of PEEP applied should be no higher than that necessary to permit reduction in supplemental oxygen fraction to a nontoxic level, usually thought to be 50% or less inspired oxygen.

Application of high levels of PEEP ($>$ 14 cm) may reduce cardiac output because of a reduction of systemic venous return. Placement of a Swan-Ganz catheter in the pulmonary artery enables constant monitoring of cardiac output by thermodilution, measurement of pulmonary capillary wedge pressure, and determination of oxygen delivery to assess the optimal PEEP level for each patient. In all cases, placement of an intra-arterial catheter for blood sampling and monitoring of systemic blood pressure is necessary. Withdrawal of positive pressure ventilation should proceed cautiously. Patients with neurologic sequelae or persistent pulmonary problems may require prolonged mechanical ventilation.

Other considerations in the regimen of respiratory care include bronchodilators, antibiotics, and steroids. If bronchospasm is present on clinical examination, bronchodilators such as intravenous aminophylline or nebulized albuterol may produce dramatic results. Although the water aspirated by near-drowning victims is frequently contaminated, early use of antibiotics is not advisable. The best course is to monitor near-drowning patients carefully with blood cultures, white blood cell counts, sputum cultures, and analysis of vital signs. The choice of antibiotics should be based on sputum and blood cultures and on any special circumstances of the drowning incident or the hospital course. The use of steroids has been advocated for their anti-inflammatory effect, but there is no clinical or experimental evidence that their use is beneficial in the near-drowning victims, and they are not recommended.

Management of cardiac and circulatory abnormalities should proceed according to standarized protocols. Particular attention should be paid to reversal of primary hypoxemia, acidosis, and electrolyte abnormalities because of their contribution to dysrhythmias. Fluid resuscitation from circulatory shock should involve administration of colloid solution to maintain an adequate circulating blood volume. Although it seems desirable to keep the patient "dry" in order to reduce pulmonary edema, care must be taken not to compromise other organ systems. The use of vasoactive agents in the treatment of shock is often necessary in the severely affected victims.

Central nervous system dysfunction resulting from cerebral hypoxemia is present in a significant percentage of near-drowning victims. As mentioned earlier, this dysfunction is related both to initial hypoxemia and acidosis and to continuing neuronal injury related to local metabolic derangements within the brain, cerebral blood flow abnormalities, and perhaps further insults from ongoing hypoxemia and acidosis. Numerous therapeutic interventions have been carried out in an attempt to improve neurologic outcome. The first therapeutic approach to limiting damage resulting from cerebral hypoxemia must be aimed at increasing oxygen supply. If this is not possible, therapy must be directed toward reducing the level of oxygen supply demanded by the brain. Therapies include abolishing activation metabolism or synaptic transmission within the brain and reducing residual basal metabolism of processes that maintain structural neuronal integrity. Therapies also have been directed at inhibition of ongoing damage by the use of calcium channel blockers, prostaglandin inhibitors, and free radical scavengers. The area of cerebral resuscitation for ischemic hypoxic damage to the central nervous system is an exciting one and beyond the scope of this chapter.

PROGNOSIS

There has been a misconception that pediatric near-drowning patients do well from the standpoint of neurological recovery. Fandel and Bancalari, in a review of near-drowning victims in Florida, stated that 12% of all patients suffered neurologic damage, but two thirds of those who survived mechanical ventilation were affected.[12] Patients arriving at the hospital who are fully conscious with reactive pupils at the time of rescue are in little danger of poor neurologic outcome if their course is not complicated. However, patients who arrive in the emergency room still requiring cardiopulmonary resuscitation (CPR) with an initial pH of less than 7 uniformly have a very poor neurologic outcome. Nonetheless, even in patients with apparently poor prognosis, vigorous attempts should be made for cerebral salvage. Cold water may mitigate cerebral anoxia, and the initial history is often in error as to the duration of the immersion, circumstances of rescue, and circumstances of transportation. Improved care at all levels as well as use of specialized centers for the intensive care of children will certainly increase the number of neurologically intact survivors.[13]

As always, prevention results in the best outcome. Prevention of immersion incidents is central to decreasing mortality and morbidity from drowning and near-drowning. It is estimated that only 12% of Americans who swim for pleasure are competent swimmers and that 65% of drowning victims were unable to swim. The number of backyard swimming pools in the United States is estimated to be increasing at a rate of 50,000 each year. There is also a dramatic increase in the number of public aquatic recreation facilities, including community pools, water slide facilities, and wave pools. Although not yet reflected in injury statistics, the availability of such facilities, and their promotion to children and their families may increase the already unacceptable number of near-drowning episodes and drowning victims. Important factors for prevention of immersion incidents are (1) community education program to alert adults to the magnitude of the problem; (2) proper supervision of infants and children in pools and bathtubs; (3) effective barriers limiting access to swimming pools; (4) mandatory CPR certification for all pool owners; (5) mandatory swimming lessons for all children; and (6) proper use of life preservers and aquatic recreation vehicles. It is important that all children be taught to swim correctly and to know the limits of their abilities; young children must be made aware of the potential dangers of the water or else they are likely to put themselves at risk by attempting to swim beyond their capabilities. Community education on all aspects of water safety is an essential part of parents' and physicians' duties.

REFERENCES

1. Pearn JH, Nixon J: Swimming pool immersion accidents: An analysis from the Brisbane drowning study. Med J Aust 1:432–437, 1977.
2. Levin DL: Near-drowning. Crit Care Med 8:590–595, 1980.
3. Orlowski JP: Drowning, near-drowning, and ice-water submersions. Pediatr Clin North Am 34:75–92, 1987.
4. Swann HG, Brucer M, Moore C, et al: Fresh water and sea water drowning: A study of the terminal cardiac and biochemical events. Tex Rep Biol Med 5:423–437, 1947.
5. Modell JH, Moya F: Effects of volume of aspirated fluid during chlorinated fresh water drowning. Anesthesiology 27:662–672, 1966.
6. Modell JH, Moya F, Newby EJ, et al: The effects of fluid volume in sea water drowning. Ann Intern Med 67:68–80, 1967.
7. Gilfoil MP, Carvajal HF: Near-drowning in children. Tex Med 73:39–44, 1977.
8. Ruiz BC, Calderwood HW, Modell JH, et al: Effect of ventilatory patterns on arterial oxygenation after near-drowning with fresh water. Anesth Analg 52:570–576, 1973.
9. Modell JH, Kuck EJ, Ruiz BC, et al: Effect of intravenous vs. aspirated distilled water on serum electrolytes and blood gas tensions. J Appl Physiol 32:579–584, 1972.
10. Modell JH, Davis JH, Giammona ST, et al: Blood gas and electrolyte changes in human near-drowning victims. JAMA 203:337–343, 1968.
11. Glasser KL, Civetta JM, Flor RJ: The use of spontaneous ventilation with constant-positive airway pressure in the treatment of salt water near drowning. Chest 67:355–357, 1975.
12. Fandel I, Bancalari E: Near-drowning in children: Clinical aspects. Pediatr 58:573–579, 1976.
13. Quan L, Wentz KR, Gore EJ, et al: Outcome and predictors of outcome in pediatric submersion victims receiving prehospital care in King County, Washington. Pediatrics 86:586–593, 1990.

54 PULMONARY EDEMA
JOHN STEVENS, M.D. / HOWARD EIGEN, M.D.

Pulmonary edema is a condition in which there is an abnormal accumulation of fluid in the interstitium and, perhaps, the airspaces of the lungs. Numerous clinical conditions can cause pulmonary edema. An understanding of the basic physiologic principles of liquid and solute transport in the lungs enables physicians to predict which conditions lead to edema formation.

PHYSIOLOGIC ASPECTS

In 1896, Ernest Starling first proposed the physiologic basis for filtration of liquid and protein across a semipermeable barrier.[1] Subsequently, Starling's equation was formulated as a method of predicting net flow of liquid across a semipermeable membrane in terms of hydrostatic and osmotic pressures and the permeability of the barrier. The equation is written as

$$Qf = K[(P_{mv} - P_{pmv}) - \sigma(\pi_{mv} - \pi_{pmv})],$$

where Qf is the net transvascular flow of liquid; K is the conductance coefficient of water across the barrier; P_{mv}

and P_{pmv} are the microvascular hydrostatic and perimicrovascular hydrostatic pressures, respectively; σ is the reflection coefficient of protein that describes the relative permeability of the membrane to protein (a value of 1 = totally impermeable); and π_{mv} and π_{pmv} represent the microvascular and perimicrovascular protein colloid osmotic pressures, respectively.

To facilitate the rapid exchange of oxygen and carbon dioxide, the alveolar walls of the lung are very thin, consisting of capillary endothelium, interstitial space, and alveolar epithelium. Pulmonary edema is most likely to form in the alveolar interstitium, where most of the pulmonary capillary bed is located. The Qf in the normal lung is positive. Staub estimated that 10 to 20 ml of fluid is filtered and removed by lymphatic vessels every hour in normal adults.[2] The area of microcirculation of the lung, which consists of arterioles ($< 75\ \mu m$ in diameter), alveolar capillaries (10 to 12 μm in diameter), and venules ($\leq 200\ \mu m$ in diameter) is the major site of this transvascular flow.[3] The σ for the pulmonary microcirculation is approximately 0.9, indicating that protein, as well as liquid, crosses into the interstitial space. This normal transendothelial liquid and protein movement has been shown to occur through leaky endothelial intercellular junctions.[4]

Once liquid and protein enter the interstitial space, a negative pressure gradient from the alveolar interstitial space to the extra-alveolar space draws the filtered liquid proximally from the lung periphery toward the hilum via the lymphatic vessels so as to return it to the systemic circulation.[5, 6, 7]

Under normal circumstances, the liquid and protein that reach the interstitial space do not enter the alveolar airspace. Ultrastructural studies have shown that epithelial cells are interconnected with tight junctions, in contrast to the endothelial junctions.[4, 8] Taylor and Gaar,[6] using measurements of transfer of solutes from air to blood, demonstrated that the epithelial cells have highly impermeable membranes. Estimates are that the alveolar airway protein coefficient is nearly 1.[9]

The lung has a number of mechanisms to counter the development of pulmonary edema: (1) as Qf rises, P_{pmv} also rises to oppose further fluid movement; (2) any increase in interstitial fluid effectively decreases the π_{pmv} by simple dilution, thereby increasing the colloid osmotic gradient opposing flow from the intravascular to the perivascular compartments; and (3) the lung can counter increased Qf by increasing the rate of lymphatic flow. Studies in animals have shown that when edema begins to develop, lymphatic flow increases several times over base line.[10]

PATHOPHYSIOLOGY

Pulmonary edema occurs when transvascular filtration exceeds lymphatic drainage. From Starling's equation, it is evident that excess Qf can occur with (1) an increase in microvascular pressure ($\uparrow P_{mv}$); (2) a decrease in perimicrovascular pressure ($\downarrow P_{pmv}$); (3) an increase in capillary membrane permeability ($\uparrow K$ or $\downarrow \sigma$); or (4) a decrease in colloid osmotic pressure ($\downarrow \pi_{mv}$). Starling's equation does not predict two other causes of pulmonary edema: (1) blockage of the lymphatic drainage and (2) a change in the vascular surface area available for fluid and protein exchange.

An increase in the microvascular pressure (P_{mv}) can result in high-pressure pulmonary edema, also referred to as hydrostatic or cardiogenic edema. Any congenital or acquired heart disease causing an increase in left atrial pressure may result in this type of edema when the increased left atrial pressure is transmitted back to the microcirculation of the lung, increasing P_{mv} and Qf. This type of edema is characterized microscopically by vascular congestion, extravasation of red blood cells, and fluid that is low in protein. Congenital causes are most prevalent in pediatric patients and include left heart outflow obstructive entities such as hypoplastic left heart syndrome and congenital mitral valve stenosis. By increasing blood flow to the lungs, left-to-right shunts, such as that seen with a ventricular septal defect or an arterioventricular canal, also increase P_{mv} and subsequently Qf, causing edema formation. Acquired cardiac problems causing pulmonary edema in children include cardiomyopathies of numerous origins and rheumatic heart disease.

Fluid overload from excess fluid administration in any patient can lead to an increased P_{mv} and Qf, causing pulmonary edema. High-pressure pulmonary edema can also result from a decrease in P_{pmv}, which results in a larger pressure gradient from the microvascular space to the perimicrovascular space. This mechanism may, in part, account for the pulmonary edema associated with prematurity and upper airway obstruction. Premature birth is often associated with a deficiency of pulmonary surfactant. Clements[11] and Pattle[12] initally proposed that lack of adequate surfactant could result in interstitial pressures sufficiently negative to cause pulmonary edema. This large negative interstitial pressure is most likely secondary to the generation of large transpulmonary pressure, inasmuch as the airspaces are unstable without adequate surfactant. Preterm lamb lung has reduced interstitial pressure around extra-alveolar vessels, which is most likely secondary to insufficient surfactant.[13] In attempts to overcome an upper airway obstruction, significant transpulmonary pressure gradients can develop, leading to pulmonary edema.

As predicted by Starling's equation, an increase in the permeability of the microvascular endothelium ($\uparrow K$, $\downarrow \sigma$) results in an increase in the transvascular filtration of fluid and protein into the interstitium of the lung, which is often referred to as increased-permeability pulmonary edema. This type of edema fluid, in contrast to that of high-pressure pulmonary edema, is rich in protein.[14, 15] Numerous experimental models have been devised to investigate increased-permeability pulmonary edema. The infusion of *Escherichia coli* endotoxin is one of the most thoroughly investigated methods of inducing reversible lung changes. The changes induced by *E. coli* endotoxin are believed to be representative of the classic pathophysiologic alteration seen with this type of edema. Studies in sheep by Bernard and associates[16] and Heflin and Brigham[17] showed that initially there is a rise in pulmonary artery pressure, followed by a rise in lymphatic flow that is accompanied by a decrease in the relative protein concentration of the lymph fluid. These changes are similar to those seen in high-pressure pulmonary edema. After a couple of hours of endotoxin infusion, pulmonary artery pressure decreases, and lung lymphatic flow increases to very high levels. This occurrence is associated with a rise in the relative protein concentration of lymphatic fluid to normal levels, indicating an increase in the permeability of the transvascular membrane to protein ($\downarrow \sigma$) as well as to fluid ($\uparrow K$). It appears that the effect of endotoxin is mediated in part by the release of toxic oxygen radicals from degranulated neutrophils.[16, 17]

The most common clinical example of increased-permeability pulmonary edema is adult respiratory distress syndrome (ARDS). Bachofen and Weibel[18, 19] investigated the pathologic structural alterations of the patients with ARDS who had died. The changes were classified as acute or chronic in nature. The acute stage, which comprises the first 20 h of symptoms, is characterized pathologically by focal damage and destruction of the microvascular and alveolar barriers in conjunction with significant interstitial and alveolar edema. The edema fluid is hemorrhagic in appearance and contains erthrocytes, leukocytes, cellular debris, fibrin strands, and globules of surfactant. The chronic stage is characterized by proliferation of type 2 cells, alveolar septal thickening, alveolitis, and progressive fibrosis.

As predicted by Starling's equation, Qf increases if there is a decrease in π_{mv}. This phenomenon has been documented in numerous experimental studies such as that by Guyton and Lindsey,[20] who found an increase in lung lymphatic flow with plasma protein depletion. This has also been found to be the case in clinical studies. However, the effect of plasma protein depletion on lymphatic flow is much more clinically evident in the presence of coexistent high-pressure or increased-permeability pulmonary edema.[21]

Starling's equation does not predict the effect of inadequate lymphatic drainage on the formation of pulmonary edema. It has been shown both experimentally[22] and clinically[23] that if lymphatic drainage is obstructed, as with malignant lymphatic infiltration or surgical ligation, pulmonary edema develops.

The effect on Qf of changes in the surface area over which filtration occurs is independent of Starling's equation. Such an increase in filtration surface area should increase the total Qf, whereas the protein concentration remains unchanged. This has been shown to be the case in experimental studies, such as that of Coates and associates.[24] They investigated the effects of exercise on lung lymphatic flow in sheep and found lymphatic flow increased to three times that of base line in response to the recruitment of more capillaries with exercise.

For practical purposes, the clinical causes of pulmonary edema are often divided pathophysiologically into those related to either high-pressure or increased-permeability pulmonary edema. In reality, many clinical causes of edema cannot be labeled as only one or the other but are a mixture of the two with, at times, the added influence of other factors such as a low plasma osmotic pressure or an increase in the filtration surface area.

SPECIFIC CLINICAL CAUSES OF PULMONARY EDEMA

ADULT RESPIRATORY DISTRESS SYNDROME

ARDS was first described by Ashbaugh and colleagues[25] in 1967, when they reported on 12 cases of acute pulmonary edema in adults, without apparent cardiac dysfunction, that was precipitated by catastrophic events such as trauma, lung contusion, fat embolism, and acute pancreatitis. Although all these original patients were adults, retrospective studies of pediatric patients indicate a rate of 8.5 to 10.4 cases per 1000 intensive care admissions.[26-30] Of the numerous causes of ARDS (Table 54–1), the most common is sepsis.[31] Conners and co-workers[32] delineated the progression of ARDS in four stages: acute injury, a latent period, acute respiratory failure, and severe physiologic abnormalities. Whatever the acute injury, some alteration of the transvascular pulmonary microcirculation membrane is effected. However, during the initial phase, few clinical abnormalities may be apparent. Some patients hyperventilate; however, oxygen saturation,

Table 54–1. CAUSES OF ADULT RESPIRATORY DISTRESS SYNDROME

Direct Lung Injury
Pneumonia: viral, bacterial, and so forth
Inhalation of noxious gases
Pulmonary aspiration
Pulmonary contusion
Radiation pneumonitis

Secondary Lung Injury
Shock: any cause
Sepsis
Trauma, burns
Disseminated intravascular coagulation
Massive blood transfusion
Drug overdose
Diabetic ketoacidosis
Uremia
Pancreatitis
Increased intracranial pressure
Post–cardiopulmonary bypass
Posthemodialysis
Postcardioversion
Paraquat ingestion

Adapted from Royall JA, Levin DC: Adult respiratory distress syndrome in pediatric patients: Clinical aspects, pathophysiology, pathology, and mechanisms of lung injury. J Pediatr 112:169, 1988. Reproduced with permission from Mosby–Year Book, Inc.

chest radiographs, and other physical findings can be normal. A latent period lasting 6 to 48 h then follows, during which patients appear to be recovering from the acute insult but after which acute respiratory failure ensues. Patients appear tachypneic and cyanotic, and rales are heard on auscultation. Chest radiographs show bilateral diffuse hazy infiltrates. Arterial blood gas analysis reveals gradually increasing hypercapnia and progressive hypoxemia that responds poorly to supplemental oxygen. In most cases, this progression of events results in the need for mechanical ventilation, which heralds the onset of the final stage of severe physiologic abnormalities. In the pediatric cases reported, mortality rates from 28.5% to 94.4% have been noted.[26-30] In patients who survive, the need for mechanical ventilation may be quite prolonged. However, follow-up studies of adult patients with ARDS indicate a good long-term pulmonary prognosis.[33, 34] The long-term pulmonary outlook for pediatric patients, although not as clearly delineated, appears to be good.[26, 28]

NEONATAL LUNG DISEASE

Pulmonary edema is often found to complicate a number of the different types of lung disease of neonates. This scenario has been most intensively studied in infants with hyaline membrane disease (HMD) and bronchopulmonary dysplasia (BPD).[35] Bland delineated the conditions that may contribute to the development of pulmonary edema after premature birth:[36] excess fetal lung liquid at birth; elevated lung vascular pressures, especially in the presence of a patent ductus arteriosus; increased surface tension secondary to surfactant deficiency, causing low perimicrovascular pressures; low plasma protein osmotic pressure; abnormal leakage of the alveolar epithelium and capillary endothelium; and, possibly, inadequate lymphatic drainage from increased intrathoracic pressures. With the continued need for high supplemental oxygen concentrations and mechanical ventilation, some infants with HMD go on to develop BPD. Infants with BPD have a persistence of the abnormally increased pulmonary permeability[37] noted in HMD, which can cause an ongoing complication with pulmonary edema. In view of these conditions in infants with HMD and BPD, it is evident why diuretics often prove useful in their management.[38]

NEUROGENIC CAUSES

Although seizures are the events that most frequently incite neurogenic pulmonary edema, a number of different diseases and injuries to the central nervous system (CNS) such as head trauma, intracerebral hemorrhage, pituitary or intracerebral tumors, subdural hematomas, and hydrocephalus secondary to bacterial meningitis can cause this disorder.[39] In most cases, the pulmonary edema develops within a few hours after the CNS insult. Patients typically appear dyspneic, with tachypnea, tachycardia, and inspiratory crackles noted on examination. Chest radiographs show a characteristic bilateral alveolar filling process. Initially, this may be attributed to aspiration, but when the appearance on chest radiographs improves rapidly over 1 to 2 days, neurogenic pulmonary edema becomes the most likely diagnosis.

A delayed onset form of neurogenic pulmonary edema has been noted.[40] The signs and symptoms of pulmonary edema typically develop slowly over 12 h to several days after the CNS insult.

The pathogenesis of neurogenic pulmonary edema is not well understood but is thought to be most likely secondary to both high-pressure[41] and increased-permeability pulmonary edema.[42]

UPPER AIRWAY OBSTRUCTION

Since the first case report by Oswalt and co-authors[43] in 1977, pulmonary edema complicating acute upper airway obstruction has been reported in a variety of clinical situations, including upper airway obstruction secondary to endotracheal tube obstruction,[44] postoperative subglottic edema,[45] croup and epiglottitis,[46, 47] laryngospasm,[48, 49] hanging,[48] choking,[50] and anatomic anomalies.[51, 52] Although pulmonary edema complicating acute upper airway obstruction is thought to be rare, Soliman and Richer[53] noted that 7% of their pediatric patients had associated pulmonary edema. Pulmonary edema developed in 12% of patients with epiglottitis reported by Kanter and Watchko.[47] In all these patients, however, the edema developed after intubation; hence this situation complicated the relief of an upper airway obstruction.[54–56]

The mechanism of these two causes of pulmonary edema is not clear. In upper airway obstruction alone, the large negative intrathoracic pressure generated in an attempt to overcome the obstruction may significantly decrease the perimicrovascular pressure, thereby drawing fluid across the capillary and alveolar membranes. It is postulated that when the upper airway obstruction is acutely relieved, as with intubation, any positive end-expiratory pressure provided by the obstruction during exhalation is removed; this causes a sudden increase in systemic venous return, which in turn produces a sudden increase in pulmonary microvascular pressure and results in edema.[57]

The onset of pulmonary edema with upper airway obstruction or with the relief of the obstruction is quite variable and, as yet, not predictable. If the edema is detected early, most patients can be treated effectively with the usual measures (to be discussed).

EXPOSURE TO HIGH ALTITUDE

High-altitude pulmonary edema (HAPE) occurs in 1% to 2% of climbers who attempt to climb Mt. McKinley, which has a height of 6192 m.[58] Typical affected climbers are young and in good health. Within the first 4 days of a rapid ascent to 3000 to 4000 m, fatigue, dyspnea at rest, dry cough, a marked decrease in exercise tolerance, and insomnia develop. If a climber does not rest at this point but ascends further, the symptoms may progress to full-blown pulmonary edema, coma, and death. The best way to avoid HAPE is to allow for proper acclimatization to the high altitudes. When a climber is above 3000 m, the rate of ascent should be no more than 300 m per day. The best treatment is descent.[58] The pathophysiologic changes leading to HAPE have not been clearly delineated, but current evidence seems to indicate that some mechanism, perhaps hypoxemia, leads to increased permeability of the capillary and alveolar membranes.[58]

CLINICAL MANIFESTATION

The clinical manifestations of both high-pressure and increased-permeability pulmonary edema are often quite similar. The clinical course can be divided into two phases: interstitial edema and alveolar edema.

Under close observation, patients are noted to be symptomatic even in the early stages of interstitial edema. As the interstitial spaces begin to fill with edema fluid, the peripheral airways become compressed, stimulating stretch receptors. This compression causes the initial signs of tachypnea and wheezing. The wheezing has been shown to be secondary to airway compression and not to reactive airway disease.[59] The increase in interstitial fluid has been shown to cause an alteration in the elastic recoil properties of the lung, which is associated with a reduction in the static and dynamic lung compliance.[60] These changes decrease tidal volume and increase the tachypnea. As the volume of interstitial fluid increases, patients become progressively more dyspneic, diaphoretic, and anxious. Hypoxemia may or may not be present at this point.

The phase of alveolar edema begins as the excess interstitial fluid penetrates the alveoli. At this point, the patient may begin producing pink, frothy sputum, after which atelectasis may be apparent on chest radiograph. With significant ventilation/perfusion mismatching, hypoxemia is always present in this phase, but patients are often hypocapnic. If the edema is the result of high microvascular pressure secondary to an underlying cardiac dysfunction, further physical signs may include an S_3 gallop, jugular venous distention, and peripheral edema.

In increased-permeability edema, such as that seen with ARDS, the cause may not always be apparent at the onset of the patient's symptoms. As the disease progresses, however, the cause usually becomes apparent. The alterations in pulmonary mechanics with increased-permeability pulmonary edema, especially in ARDS, are often more severe than the corresponding alterations with high-pressure pulmonary edema. Thus many patients with increased-permeability pulmonary edema show signs of greater respiratory distress and hypoxemia than do those with high-pressure pulmonary edema.

If the underlying cause and the pulmonary edema itself, either high-pressure or increased-permeability edema, are not treated, many patients go on to experience increasing hypoxemia, respiratory failure, and death.

RADIOLOGIC DETECTION OF PULMONARY EDEMA

Many techniques have been devised to quantify pulmonary edema. Those with the most clinical applicability include the chest radiograph, soluble gas technique, computed tomography, and double-indicator dilution. In reviews of these and other methods of pulmonary edema detection, the chest radiograph has continued to be the standard against which all other methods are assessed.[61-64] Being inexpensive, noninvasive, and readily reproducible, although somewhat lacking in sensitivity, it is the technique most commonly employed for quantifying pulmonary edema. The characteristics and distribution of the changes noted on chest radiographs often enable differentiation between high-pressure and increased-permeability pulmonary edema. In a study by Milne and collaborators,[65] this distinction was made on chest radiographs with 80% to 90% accuracy in cases of pulmonary edema resulting from heart disease, chronic renal failure, or iatrogenic overhydration and acute lung injury, which caused increased-permeability pulmonary edema.

In high-pressure pulmonary edema, blood vessels not normally perfused at rest are recruited. This is first evident as increased upper zone perfusion. As the edema progresses, the presence of fluid around the bronchioles, vessels, and interlobar septa becomes evident in the form of perivascular and peribronchial cuffing. With the onset of septal edema, Kerley A and B lines appear. Harley showed that the Kerley B lines appear at a mean left atrial pressure of 17 to 20 mm Hg.[66] In more advanced edema, significant alveolar flooding occurs and is evident as a perihilar haze that may progress to diffuse confluent, patchy infiltrates.

In increased-permeability pulmonary edema, as with ARDS, initial changes on chest radiographs may be secondary to an underlying pulmonary disorder such as pulmonary contusion, pneumonia, or aspiration. If the inciting cause is not pulmonary in origin, however, the initial changes are usually not seen until 6 to 48 h after the acute injury. At this time, fine reticular infiltrates consistent with the presence of interstitial pulmonary fluid may be noted. With the onset of obvious respiratory distress, bilateral hazy infiltrates become evident. Finally, with further progression and the oxygen toxicity and barotrauma that result from the required respiratory support, chronic lung changes with fibrosis develop.

Cardiomegaly is often seen in conjunction with high-pressure pulmonary edema, especially in the presence of an underlying cardiac abnormality. In increased-permeability pulmonary edema, the heart size is usually normal, and the signs of pulmonary venous congestion seen with high-pressure edema are absent.

TREATMENT

The foremost objective in the treatment of pulmonary edema is to correct the hypoxemia. Supplemental oxygen is indicated when a patient is unable to maintain an adequate hemoglobin oxygen saturation of more than 94% or an arterial oxygen tension of 70 to 75 mm Hg when breathing room air. If this level of oxygenation cannot be maintained while the patient breathes a fractional inspired oxygen (FI_{O_2}) concentration of 0.6 to 0.7 or if excessive work of breathing is noted, intubation and mechanical ventilation are indicated. Mechanical ventilation decreases the work of breathing and allows for adequate oxygenation at lower, less toxic FI_{O_2} concentrations. It also allows for the application of positive end-expiratory pressure (PEEP).

PEEP improves oxygenation in either form of pulmonary edema by improving ventilation/perfusion mismatching and decreasing intrapulmonary shunting.[67,68] In pulmonary edema, there is collapse of alveoli and reduction of the functional residual capacity (FRC). PEEP is believed to recruit alveoli and increase FRC, thereby decreasing intrapulmonary shunting.[69,70] The level of PEEP needed depends on the severity of the pulmonary edema and any underlying pulmonary abnormality. In general the best level of PEEP to use is one that allows for maximal oxygenation at the lowest level of FI_{O_2} concentration without significantly compromising cardiac output. If high levels of PEEP are required, placement of a pulmonary artery catheter is useful for monitoring cardiac output. With cardiac support, high levels of PEEP (> 20 cm H_2O) can be used in pediatric patients.[71]

To facilitate the treatment of pulmonary edema and its resultant hypoxemia, differentiation between high-pressure and increased-permeability pulmonary edema and identification of the underlying cause are needed. Usually with an adequate history, a thorough physical examination and a chest radiograph, the differentiation can be achieved. Once the underlying cause of either type of pulmonary edema is identified, aggressive, specific treatment is needed.

In the nonspecific treatment of high-pressure pulmonary edema, such as that resulting from cardiac failure, an effort is made to decrease the elevated microvascular hydrostatic pressure by decreasing cardiac preload or afterload or both and by increasing cardiac output. Mechanical modalities used to reduce cardiac preload include (1) placing the patient in the upright position, thereby shifting 25% of the pulmonary blood volume to more dependent body parts;[72] (2) placing rotating tourniquets on the upper arms and thighs; (3) phlebotomy; (4) plasmapheresis; and (5) fluid restriction.

Medical therapy is often indicated in the treatment of high-pressure pulmonary edema. Morphine, by relieving anxiety, effecting arteriolar dilation, and increasing venous capacitance, reduces both preload and afterload.[73] Diuretics are useful in reducing fluid overload. Furosemide has been shown to reduce capillary wedge pressure and improve lung function before its diuretic effect takes place.[74] It is often useful to augment cardiac output with digoxin, dobutamine, or dopamine. In an effort to reduce afterload, vasodilators such as nitroprusside can be administered.

In the treatment of increased-permeability pulmonary edema, such as ARDS secondary to sepsis or other causes, it is very important to identify the underlying causes, and treat it appropriately. The use of corticosteroids in the treatment of ARDS remains controversial. In studies of animals, corticosteroids have been shown to protect against lung injury if given before the inciting insult.[75] Schumer[76] reported a decrease in mortality rate with the use of steroids and antibiotics in a prospective study of 172 patients in septic shock. In subsequent studies, investigators found not only a lack of benefit but also an increase in the fatality rate when the corticosteroids were used in cases of acute lung injury.[77,78] Other investigations have indicated that corticosteroids may be useful in patients with prolonged ARDS[79] or when ARDS is complicated by ideopathic pulmonary fibrosis.[80] Further studies are needed in order to delineate the role, if any, of corticosteroids in the treatment of this disease.

Hemorrhagic shock often complicates ARDS that is caused by sepsis. The indicated volume replacement with either colloid or crystalloid may further complicate the pulmonary edema. A definite advantage of one agent over the other has not been established.[81,82] With either agent, close monitoring of cardiac output and pulmonary artery wedge pressure is needed.

REFERENCES

1. Starling EH: On the absorption of fluids from the connective tissue spaces. J Physiol 19:312–326, 1896.
2. Staub NC: Pulmonary edema: Physiologic approaches to management. Chest 74:559–564, 1978.
3. Staub NC: Pathophysiology of pulmonary edema. In Staub NC, Taylor AE (eds): Edema, p. 719. New York: Raven Press, 1984.
4. Schneeberger EE, Karnovsky MJ: Substructure of intercellular functions in freeze-fractured alveolar-capillary membranes of mouse lung. Circ Res 38:404–411, 1976.
5. Schneeberger EE: Segmental differentiation of endothelial intercellular junctions in intra-acinar arteries and veins of the rat lung. Circ Res 49:1102–1111, 1981.
6. Taylor AE, Gaar KA: Estimation of equivalent pore radii of pulmonary capillary and alveolar membranes. Am J Physiol 218:1133–1140, 1970.
7. Gee MH, Williams DO: Effect of lung inflation in perivascular cuff fluid volume in isolated dog lung lobes. Microvasc Res 19:209, 1980.
8. Bhattacharya J, Gropper MA, Staub NC: Interstitial fluid pressure gradient measured by micropuncture in excised dog lung. J Appl Physiol 56:271–277, 1984.
9. Staub NC: Pulmonary edema. Physiol Rev 54:678–811, 1974.
10. Drake RE, Scott RL, Gabel JC: Relationship between weight gain and lymph flow in dog lungs. Am J Physiol 14:H125–H130, 1983.
11. Clements JA: Pulmonary edema and permeability of alveolar membranes. Arch Environ Health 2:280–283, 1961.
12. Pattle RE: Properties, function and origin of the alveolar lining layer. Nature 175:1125–1126, 1955.
13. Raj JU: Alveolar liquid pressure measured by micropuncture in isolated lungs of mature and immature fetal rabbits. J Clin Invest 79:1579–1588, 1987.
14. Fein A, Grossman RF, Jones JG, et al: The value of edema fluid protein measurements in patients with pulmonary edema. Am J Med 67:32–38, 1979.
15. Vreim CR, Snashall PD, Demling RH, et al: Lung lymph and free interstitial fluid protein composition in sheep with edema. Am J Physiol 230:1650–1653, 1976.
16. Bernard GR, Lucht WD, Niedermeyer ME, et al: Effect of N-acetylcysteine on the pulmonary response to endotoxin in the awake sheep and upon in vitro granulocyte function. J Clin Invest 73:1772–1784, 1984.
17. Heflin AC, Brigham KL: Prevention by granulocyte depletion of increased vascular permeability of sheep lung following endotoxemia. J Clin Invest 68:1253–1260, 1981.
18. Bachofen M, Weibel ER: Alterations of the gas exchange apparatus in adult respiratory insufficiency associated with septicemia. Am Rev Respir Dis 116:589–615, 1977.
19. Bachofen M, Weibel ER: Structural alterations of lung parenchyma in the adult respiratory distress syndrome. Clin Chest Med 3:35–56, 1982.
20. Guyton AC, Lindsey AW: Effect of elevated left atrial pressure and decreased plasma protein concentration on the development of pulmonary edema. Circ Res 7:649–657, 1959.
21. da Luz PL, Shubin H, Weil MH, et al: Pulmonary edema related to changes in colloid osmotic and pulmonary artery wedge pressure in patients after acute myocardial infarction. Circulation 51:350–357, 1975.
22. Magno M, Szidon JP: Hemodynamic pulmonary edema in dogs with acute and chronic lymphatic ligation. Am J Physiol 231:1777–1782, 1976.
23. Hurley JV: Current views on mechanisms of pulmonary oedema. J Pathol 125:59–79, 1978.
24. Coates G, O'Brodovich H, Jefferies AL, Gray GW: Effects of exercise on lung lymph flow in sheep and goats during normoxia and hypoxia. J Clin Inves 74:133–141, 1984.
25. Ashbaugh DG, Bigelow DB, Petty TL, et al: Acute respiratory distress in adults. Lancet 2:319–323, 1967.
26. Effmann EL, Merten DF, Kirks DR, et al: Adult respiratory distress syndrome in children. Radiology 157:69–74, 1985.
27. Holbrook PR, Taylor G, Pollack MM, Fields A: Adult respiratory distress syndrome in children. Pediatr Clin North Am 27:677–685, 1980.
28. Lyrene RK, Truog WE: Adult respiratory distress syndrome in a pediatric intensive care unit: Predisposing conditions, clinical course, and outcome. Pediatrics 67:790–795, 1981.
29. Nussbaum E: Adult-type respiratory distress syndrome in children. Clin Pediatr (Phila) 22:401–406, 1983.
30. Pfenninger J, Gerber A, Tschäppelor H, Zimmermann A: Adult respiratory distress syndrome in children. J Pediatr 101:352–357, 1982.
31. Royall JA, Levin DC: Adult respiratory distress syndrome in pediatric patients: Clinical aspects, pathophysiology, pathology and mechanisms of lung injury. J Pediatri 112:169–180, 1988.
32. Conners AF Jr, McCaffree DR, Rogers RM: The adult respiratory distress syndrome. Dis Mon 27:1–75, 1981.
33. Lakshminarayan S, Hudson LD: Pulmonary function following the adult respiratory distress syndrome. Chest 74:489–490, 1978.
34. Alberts WM, Priest GR, Moser KM: The outlook for survivors of ARDS. Chest 84:272–274, 1983.
35. O'Brodovich HM, Mellins RB: Bronchopulmonary dysplasia. Am Rev Respir Dis 132:694–709, 1985.
36. Bland RD: Pathogenesis of pulmonary edema after premature birth. Adv Pediatr 34:175–221, 1987.
37. Jefferies AL, Coates G, O'Brodovich H: Pulmonary epithelial permeability in hyaline membrane disease. N Engl J Med 311:1075–1080, 1984.
38. Kao LC, Warburton D, Cheng MH, et al: Effect of oral diuretics on pulmonary mechanics in infants with chronic bronchopulmonary

dysplasia: Results of a double-blind crossover sequential trial. Pediatrics 74:37–44, 1984.

39. Colice GL: Neurogenic pulmonary edema. Clin Chest Med 6:473–489, 1985.

40. Fisher A, Aboul-Nasr HT: Delayed nonfatal pulmonary edema following sub-arachnoid hemorrhage. J Neurosurg 51:856–859, 1979.

41. Ducker TB: Increased intracranial pressure and pulmonary edema: I. Clinical study of 11 patients. J Neurosurg 28:112, 1968.

42. Hucker H, Schafer U, Meinen K: Early morphological alterations of the rat lung with increased intracranial pressure: I. A light and electron microscopic study. Virchows Arch [A] 362:331–342, 1974.

43. Oswalt CE, Gated GA, Holmstrom FMG: Pulmonary edema as a complication of acute airway obstruction. JAMA 238:1833, 1977.

44. Warner LO, Beach TP, Martino JD: Negative pressure pulmonary oedema secondary to airway obstruction in an intubated infant. Can J Anaesth 35:507–510, 1988.

45. Scherer R, Dreyer P, Jorch G: Pulmonary edema due to partial upper airway obstruction in a child. Intensive Care Med 14:661–662, 1988.

46. Travis KW, Todres ID, Shannon DC: Pulmonary edema associated with croup and epiglottitis. Pediatrics 59:695–698, 1977.

47. Kanter RK, Watchko JF: Pulmonary edema associated with upper airway obstruction. Am J Dis Child 138:356–358, 1984.

48. Barin ES, Stevenson IF, Donnelly GL: Pulmonary oedema following acute upper airway obstruction. Anaesth Intensive Care 14:54–57, 1986.

49. Lee KW, Downes JJ: Pulmonary edema secondary to laryngospasm in children. Anesthesiolgy 59:347–349, 1983.

50. Sofer S, Bar-Ziv J, Mogle P: Pulmonary oedema following choking: Report of two cases. Eur J Pediatr 143:295–296, 1985.

51. Roa NL, Moss KS: Treacher-Collins syndrome with sleep apnea: Anesthetic considerations. Anesthesiology 60:71–73, 1984.

52. Brown RE Jr: Negative pressure pulmonary oedema. *In* Berry FA (ed): Anesthetic Management of Difficult and Routine Pediatric Patients, pp. 169–178. New York: Churchill-Livingstone, 1986.

53. Soliman MG, Richer P: Epiglottitis and pulmonary oedema in children. Can Anaesth Soc J 25:270–275, 1978.

54. Galvis AG: Pulmonary edema complicating relief of upper airway obstruction. Am J Emerg Med 5:294–297, 1987.

55. Sofer S, Bar-Ziv J, Scharf SM: Pulmonary edema following relief of upper airway obstruction. Chest 86:401–403, 1984.

56. Rao CC, McNiece WL, Krishna G: Acute pulmonary edema after removal of an esophageal foreign body in an infant. Crit Care Med 14:988–989, 1986.

57. Galvis AG, Stool SE, Bluestone CD: Pulmonary edema following relief of acute upper airway obstruction. Ann Otol Rhinol Laryngol 89:124–128, 1980.

58. Schoene RB: High-altitude pulmonary edema: Pathophysiology and clinical review. Ann Emerg Med 16:987–992, 1987.

59. Snapper JR, Shellen JR: Effects of pulmonary edema on lung mechanics. Semin Respir Med 4:289, 1983.

60. Staub NC, Nagano H, Pearce ML: Pulmonary edema in dogs, especially the sequence of fluid accumulation in lungs. J Appl Physiol 22:227–240, 1967.

61. Staub NC, Hogg JC: Conference report of a workshop on the measurement of lung water. Crit Care Med 8:752–759, 1980.

62. Staub NC: Clinical use of lung water measurements: Report of a workshop. Chest 90:588–594, 1986.

63. Miniati M, Pistolesi M, Milne NC, et al: Detection of lung edema. Crit Care Med 15:1146, 1987.

64. Massimo P, Massimo M, Pistolesi M, et al: The chest roentgenogram in pulmonary edema. Clin Chest Med 6:315–344, 1985.

65. Milne ENC, Pistolesi M, Miniati M, Giuntini C: The radiologic distinction of cardiogenic and noncardiogenic edema. AJR 144:879–894, 1985.

66. Harley HRS: The radiological changes in pulmonary venous hypertension, with special reference to the root shadows and lobular pattern. Br Heart J 23:75–87, 1961.

67. Prewitt RM, McCarthy J, Wood LD: Treatment of acute low pressure pulmonary edema in dogs: Relative effects of hydrostatic and oncotic pressure, nitroprusside and positive end-expiratory pressure. J Clin Invest 67:409–418, 1981.

68. Wood LD, Prewitt RM: Cardiovascular management in acute hypoxemic respiratory failure. Am J Cardiol 47:963–972, 1981.

69. Andersen JB, Qvist J, Kann T: Recruiting collapsed lung through collateral channels with positive end-expiratory pressure. Scand J Respir Dis 60:260–266, 1979.

70. Shapiro BA, Cane RD, Harrison RA: Positive end-expiratory pressure therapy in adults with special reference to acute lung injury: A review of the literature and suggested clinical correlations. Crit Care Med 12:127–141, 1984.

71. Pollack MM, Fields AI, Holbrook RP: Cardiopulmonary parameters during high PEEP in children. Crit Care Med 8:372–376, 1980.

72. Gauer OH, Thron HL: Postural changes in the circulation. *In* Hamilton WF (ed): American Physiological Society Handbook of Physiology, Section 2: Circulation, vol. III, p. 2409. Baltimore: Williams & Williams, 1965.

73. Zelis R, Mansour EJ, Capone RJ, et al: The cardiovascular effects of morphine: The peripheral capacitance and resistance vessels in human subjects. J Clin Invest 54:1247–1258, 1974.

74. Biddle TL, Yu PN: Effect of furosemide on hemodynamics and lung water in acute pulmonary edema secondary to myocardial infarction. Am J Cardiol 43:86–90, 1979.

75. Sheagren JN: Septic shock and corticosteroids. N Engl J Med 305:456–458, 1981.

76. Schumer W: Steroids in the treatment of clinical septic shock. Ann Surg 184:333–341, 1976.

77. Kreger BE, Craven DE, McCabe WR: Gram-negative bacteremia IV: Re-evaluaton of clinical features and treatment of 612 patients. Am J Med 68:344–355, 1980.

78. Luce JM, Marks JD, Montgomery AB, et al: Methylprednisone does not prevent the adult respiratory distress syndrome or improve mortality in patients with septic shock [Abstract]. Am Rev Respir Dis 135(Suppl):A5, 1987.

79. Hooper RG, Kearl RA: Established ARDS treated with a sustained course of adrenocortical steroids. Chest 97:138–143, 1990.

80. Ashbaugh DG, Maier RV: Idiopathic pulmonary fibrosis in adult respiratory distress syndrome. Arch Surg 120:530–535, 1985.

81. Sturm J, Carpenter M, Lewis FR, et al: Water and protein movement in the sheep lung after septic shock: Effect of colloid versus crystalloid resuscitation. J Surg Res 26:233, 1979.

82. Nylander WA Jr, Hammon JW Jr, Roselli RJ, et al: Comparison of the effects of saline and homologous plasma infusion on lung fluid balance during endotoxemia in the unanesthetized sheep. Surgery 90:221–228, 1981.

55 VENOUS THROMBOSIS AND PULMONARY EMBOLUS IN CHILDHOOD

KAREN S. McCOY, M.D. / NEIL J. GROSSMAN, M.D.

BACKGROUND AND INCIDENCE

It is generally believed that venous thrombosis and pulmonary embolus (PE) rarely occur in childhood; however, a growing literature and clinical experience indicate that these conditions are strikingly underdiagnosed in pediatrics.

PE in adults continues to be a significant and well-recognized cause of morbidity and mortality, particularly in hospitalized patients.[1] Among children, the incidence is lower, but consideration of the diagnosis by pediatricians is uncommon. The true incidence of the problem among adults is unknown, and incidence figures available undoubtedly reflect a severity selection bias. The best available information indicates that at least 5 million episodes of deep vein thrombosis (DVT) occur each year in the United States. Approximately 500,000 to 700,000 episodes of PE are diagnosed each year in the United States (in approximately 10% of cases of DVT). Of the total episodes of PE, approximately 10% (or 50,000) are fatal. For each PE episode diagnosed, there are probably several that remain subclinical and are unsuspected. Because of the strong association of certain risk factors with the development of PE in adults and the consequent heightened awareness, the likelihood of diagnosing an actual episode is much higher than in pediatric medicine. The reasons for this difference lie in the general lack of awareness by pediatricians of these conditions among children. The incidence of PE in unselected autopsies of children has been estimated at 8%.[2] In cases in which PE was found, the diagnosis had rarely been suspected, and if considered, therapy had been initiated even less frequently. With the advent of ever-increasing acuity in pediatric hospital-based and outpatient care as a result in part of newer technology, a new set of pediatric risk factors is being recognized. The relationship of these newly recognized problems to pediatrics and the place of this diagnosis in this ever more technologically based field are reviewed in this chapter.

The classic adultlike manifestation of an episode of DVT in pediatric patients does occur,[3] but it is more rare than among older patients.[4] Some of the useful findings and diagnostic entities available to internists, how these relate to the pediatric patient, and how they can be modified to be useful in practice are reviewed. Optimal use of the diagnostic options available in internal medicine requires an understanding of the nature of the problem in adult medicine, which provides a framework for relating to pediatric practice.

DEEP VENOUS THROMBOSIS

The natural history of DVT and relationship between DVT and the development of PE are well recognized. The progression in adults usually involves a minor platelet-based thrombus that becomes adherent to a venous structure in a lower extremity, usually at a valve, with subsequent propagation of the thrombus into the iliofemoral venous system. In adults, 95% of clinically significant thromboses arise in the lower extremities, whereas propagation and embolization of thrombi from a superior venous system are rare.[5] In the absence of indwelling catheters, thrombi formed in an upper extremity, in hepatic and renal veins, and in the right atrium are unlikely to embolize.[5] In contrast, when an indwelling venous catheter initiates thrombus formation, embolization is more likely.[6] Thrombi derived from the calf veins alone and not propagating into the area above the knee are also relatively unlikely to embolize. Fortunately, only 15% to 20% of thrombi below the knee extend; this is more likely to occur early (within 48 h) after thrombus formation.[7] Central catheter-associated thrombus formation resulting from the marked increase in the use of central long-term catheters in the pediatric population is responsible for a huge increase in the incidence of potential embolism in pediatric patients.[8-10]

The presence of coagulation abnormalities that result in increased tendency to form clots is as infrequent in adult practice as it is in pediatrics. Alpha$_1$-antitrypsin deficiency, alpha$_2$-macroglobulinemia, homocysteinuria, and deficiencies of antithrombin III, protein C, and protein S are identified as potential causes of a hypercoagulable state, and recurrent unexplained episodes of thrombus formation should be investigated as possible signs of such a defect.[11, 12] Nonetheless, identified coagulation abnormalities probably account for 10% or fewer of the DVTs seen in clinical practice. Therefore, identifying at-risk patients is dependent on recognizing certain clinical risk factors and anticipating the event.[13] Some of the clin-

Table 55–1. FACTORS PREDISPOSING PATIENTS TO DEEP VENOUS THROMBOSIS AND PULMONARY EMBOLISM

Previous history
Postoperative/postpartum states
Immobilization
Obesity
Malignancy
Infection
Cardiac failure
Dehydration
Polycythemia
Trauma
Steroids or corticotropins
Estrogens
Nephrotic syndrome
Femoral venipuncture
Ventriculovenous shunts
Deep venous catheters
Chemotherapy: L-asparaginase, vincristine

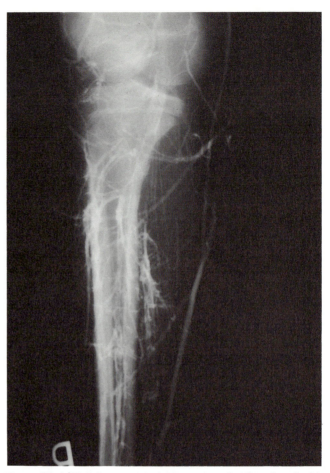

Figure 55–1. Right lower extremity venogram of patient described in Figures 55–2 and 55–3. A filling defect of the popliteal vein is shown. There is a failure to visualize the continuation of the popliteal veins despite numerous collaterals.

ical entities recognized as high risk in adult medicine are similarly important in pediatrics. These include surgery or fracture involving a lower extremity,[14] prolonged administration of anesthesia, burn injury, pregnancy or the postpartum period, prior thrombosis with residual venous obstruction, right ventricular failure, prolonged bed rest for any reason, obesity, malignancy, ingestion of estrogen-containing compounds, ingestion of exogenous corticosteroids,[15, 16] nephrotic syndrome,[12, 17] and treatment with chemotherapeutic agents, such as L-asparaginase and vincristine (Table 55–1). Particular mention should be made of surgery for scoliosis, severe dehydration, serious nutritional deficiency, the presence of ventriculoatrial shunts,[18] cyanotic congenital heart disease, and polycythemia. The highest increase in pediatric thrombosis has occurred among the numerous children with indwelling catheters, particularly if they have had previous episodes of thrombosis and have altered vascular anatomy.[19] With the advent of tunnel catheters and completely implanted catheters to allow frequent and humane intravenous treatment of children with cancer, hemophilia, cystic fibrosis, immunodeficiency, and profound nutritional disorders and prolonged postneonatal treatment for medical and surgical problems, there has been a sharp rise in awareness of the potential for thrombus formation to interfere with these devices and enhance the possibility of embolization.[10] According to figures from the pediatric oncology experience, approximately 85% to 90% of these patients now undergo placement of long-term central catheters. Of these patients, 25% to 50% suffer infection or thrombus formation; the majority of these complications are thought to be isolated infection in immunocompromised patients. In a substantial minority of patients, however, thrombus is either an isolated finding or generated by a septic focus.[20] These problems may be heralded by mechanical difficulty with infusion through the catheter, by fever, or by both or by signs of embolization.

When DVT is suspected on clinical grounds (local heat, tenderness, and swelling in a lower extremity), it is present only 50% of the time. Furthermore, of high-risk patients who are observed closely, only 50% acquire DVT.

Because clinical findings as predictors are essentially as reliable as chance when DVT is suspected, it is of paramount importance to have readily available accurate diagnostic tests to confirm or refute the diagnosis. The performance of lower extremity contrast venography is still the gold standard in evaluating for the presence of DVT even in an adult population. In many facilities it may be the only available test, and certainly it is the test with which newer ones must be compared in order to define their accuracy and practical usefulness. Notable characteristics and limitations of each technique are stated.

When lower extremity contrast venography is used, the major limitation is the ability of the operator to fill and visualize the vessel system adequately. Note the findings on venography in Figure 55–1. Radiofibrinogen leg scanning can be used at the bedside but is practical only up to the midthigh. A period of 24 h is required in order to allow deposition of the labeled material, which must still be occurring, to detect the clot. The results are obscured by the presence of local cellulitis.

Impedance plethysmography involves the use of impedance change as a result of insufflation of a lower extremity with a sphygmomanometer. The success of the technique is extremely dependent on the operator. Doppler ultrasonography, radiovenography, phleborrheography, indium-labeled platelet infusion, and angioscopy are additional techniques currently used in adults; they are not yet validated in relation to contrast venography but may offer convenient alternatives in the future. Only radiofibrinogen leg scanning and impedance plethysmography are validated in relation to contrast venography.

In pediatric medicine, none of these techniques, except contrast venography, is readily available, nor have they been validated in relation to contrast venography. Unfortunately, clinical diagnosis (notably unreliable) continues to be the method most frequently used in pediatrics.

The availability of high-quality technical and interpretive evaluation by echocardiography is essential for the appropriate diagnosis and management of catheter-associated thrombus formation. When this technique is performed by experienced clinicians, the identification of thrombi as small as 4 mm is possible. When concerns persist and echocardiogram is nondiagnostic, "catheterograms" may be necessary and beneficial.

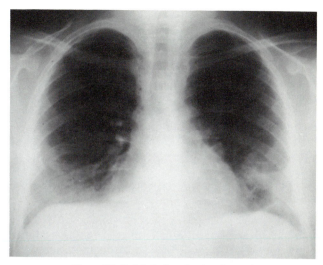

Figure 55–2. Admission chest radiograph.

EVALUATION FOR PULMONARY EMBOLUS

Demonstration of DVT or catheter-associated thrombus along with clinical suspicion leads to the need to evaluate the patient for possible PE. Clinical evidence or lack of it is unreliable in establishing the presence or absence of PE. Some patients with definite PE have no clinical manifestations or complaints.[14] Among adults with PE, the predominating symptoms are the sudden onset of dyspnea, tachypnea, an overwhelming sense of impending doom, heart palpitations, and, in those with infarction, pleuritic chest pain and hemoptysis delayed until 12 to 36 h after embolization. Signs manifested by patients with PE are as variable as those seen with DVT. In pediatric practice, the onset of symptoms related to pulmonary embolus is commonly confused with a worsening of the underlying (usually pulmonary) problem or the development of infection.[21] At least 50% of adult patients with PE exhibit no evidence of venous thrombosis. Among the common signs are unexplained tachycardia and tachypnea, low-grade fever (usually no higher than 38.3°C) unless infected thrombus and, less frequently, hemoptysis are involved. The diagnosis is therefore highly dependent on the ability to demonstrate the PE with supportive laboratory tests.

Abnormal findings may be few and nonspecific. The ordinary chest radiograph may be normal or abnormal; effusion is present in varying degrees, and infiltrates, if present, may take any shape (Fig. 55–2). The electrocardiogram may be normal, show tachycardia alone or rightward changes in axis and right ventricular strain pattern. Arterial gases likewise may be normal or may show hypoxia or even hypocapnia, especially if the patient has baseline lung dysfunction or a massive embolus. Sputum should be obtained in order to evaluate for the presence of bleeding or infection, but it is frequently difficult to obtain in small children.

Ventilation/perfusion scans are indicated in most patients. If they are negative and normal, PE is ruled out.

If a patient has obstructive lung disease, the ventilation component is abnormal and therefore nondiagnostic, but the perfusion component may be helpful. A normal perfusion scan in a patient with known lung disease effectively rules out PE; an abnormal perfusion scan with a localized defect along with a normal ventilation scan is suggestive, but not diagnostic, of PE with a confidence of about 90% (Fig. 55–3). In the patient described in Figures 55–1 to 55–3, ventilation was normal, the arteriogram was confirmatory, and the patient did well on anticoagulant therapy despite a single recurrence when sodium warfarin (Coumadin) was discontinued. Scans showing both ventilation and perfusion comoponents to be abnormal are nondiagnostic and require definitive confirmation

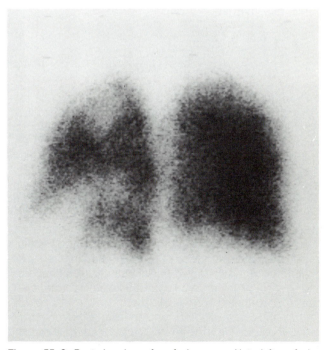

Figure 55–3. Posterior view of perfusion scan. Note left perfusion defects (absence of perfusion in left apex and left base). Ventilation scan (not shown) was normal.

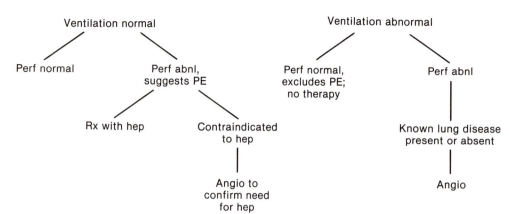

Figure 55–4. Diagnosis sequence in evaluating for pulmonary embolus. Perf, perfusion; abnl, abnormal; PE, pulmonary embolism; hep, heparin; Angio, angiography.

with angiography. Of the patients undergoing evalution for PE, approximately 20% of adults require pulmonary angiography, and the percentage of pediatric patients is even higher. If the ventilation/perfusion scan is suggestive in an appropriate clinical settting, no further diagnostic tests need be undertaken. If, however, a contraindication to anticoagulation exists, angiography is appropriate before initiating such therapy.

Other diagnostic alternatives in evaluating for PE are even less likely to be useful than for DVT, particularly in pediatrics. The ventilation/perfusion scan and, when necessary, the pulmonary angiogram, although not foolproof, remain the diagnostic tests of choice and are the only tests available in many pediatric settings. The diagram in Figure 55–4 represents an appropriate sequence for pediatric evaulations. The evaluation of adults is being attempted with Indium-labeled platelets, which have the same shortcomings as for the evaluation of lower extremity venous obstruction. Angioscopy, digital subtraction angiography, and magnetic resonance imaging are not recognized as useful, nor are they likely to be widely applicable, in pediatrics.

TREATMENT

From the experience gained in the 1980s, it is clear that PE occurs in a variety of clinical situations in pediatric practice and that this occurrence appears to parallel the situations in adult medicine. Investigators have also recognized the emergence of a group of patients who in early childhood and even infancy manifest emboli, either massive or multiple, secondary to the presence of long-term central venous indwelling catheters. Children with cancer, hemophilia, cystic fibrosis, immunodeficiency, and other primary diagnoses who frequently require intravenous treatment are among the newly recognized groups with these problems. Also of note are the large numbers of children with prolonged postneonatal chronic medical and surgical problems who continue to have central catheters for prolonged periods of time.

Once the diagnosis of PE or significant DVT or central catheter-associated thrombus is established, a specific plan of therapy must be devised. The approach to classical DVT or established PE is fairly standard. In addition to appropriate general measures to limit dislodgement, aug-

ment oxygenation, and control pain, initial therapy is anticoagulation with heparin. Heparin therapy works by altering the structure of antithrombin III, potentiating the thrombosis-inhibiting acition of antithrombin III. Intravenous heparin is administered as a bolus (50 to 100 $\mu g/$ kg), then by continuous infusion (20 to 20 $\mu g/kg/h$) to keep the partial thromboplastin time 55 to 60 sec. The desired result is the prevention of propagation of already established clots. Organization and adherence of a clot to the vessel wall require an average of 7 to 10 days. Vitamin K antagonists, such as sodium warfarin (Coumadin), may be started anytime after heparin is begun but ordinarily are not relied on as the sole anticoagulant therapy until the clot is expected to be stabilized. Vitamin K antagonists interfere with synthesis of factors II, VII, IX, and X and therefore require several days before maximal effect is achieved. Oral doses of sodium warfarin (2.5 to 10 mg/ day) are adjusted to keep prothrombin time twice normal.

Management of pediatric patients with catheter-associated thrombus formation is dependent on the size of the thrombus and the overall clinical status of the child. Thrombolytic agents, such as urokinase, work by generating active plasmin, leading to lysis of fibrin in clots. The best results are achieved when therapy is instituted early, and the overall efficacy is irrefutable. Intravenous infusion of urokinase, 600-unit/kg bolus, followed by a continuous infusion of urokinase, 500 to 2000 units/kg/h, is recommended.[22] In the rare patient with a very large, mobile thrombus attached to the tip of the catheter, immediate cardiovascular surgery to remove the thrombus may be the only prudent approach.[23, 24]

All of the aforementioned therapies are directed at the prevention of further propagation and embolization of thrombi. In established pulmonary emboli, treatment beyond anticoagulant and supportive therapy has not been definitively shown to be beneficial.[25] The usefulness of thrombolytic or other medical therapy in this situation is not yet clearly established. The patient with severe pulmonary embarrassment caused by PE may well be considered for thrombolytic therapy to speed resolution of pulmonary vascular obstruction.[25, 26] Surgical therapy is reserved for massive embolization unresponsive to cardiopulmonary resuscitation, pressors, and initiation of anticoagulant therapy in which hemodynamic or oxygenation status are unacceptable. Timely surgical intervention, when available, may be life-saving.[23, 26]

Fat embolus and embolization of sheared catheters

may result in pulmonary arterial occlusion and symptoms consistent with pulmonary embolus. In the former situation, the occurrence is rare, and the clinical manifestation is often clear-cut because of the patient's history.[27] Sheared catheter emboli occur frequently and clearly require surgical resolution.[28] One of the authors cared for a premature infant with a history of cavoatrial catheter embolus who later developed progressive occlusion of the superior and inferior vena cavae.

Overall, the increase in the incidence of pediatric PE is clear, as is the need to consider this diagnosis in hospitalized and chronically ill children. The need for awareness of the clinical predisposing factors, the need for rapid diagnostic assessment, the limitations of testing modalities, and the therapies available must be constantly reviewed.

REFERENCES

 1. Colman RW, Rubin RN: Update on pulmonary embolism—Modern management. Dis Mon 29(2):1–41, 1982.
 2. Emery JL: Pulmonary embolism in children. Arch Dis Child 37:385, 1962.
 3. Carson C, Johnson RL, Stanford P, et al: Deep vein thrombosis and pulmonary embolism of unknown etiology in a 16-year-old male. J Adolesc Health Care 3:51–52, 1982.
 4. Wise RC, Todd JK: Spontaneous, lower-extremity venous thrombosis in children. Am J Dis Child 126:766–769, 1973.
 5. Havig O: Source of pulmonary emboli. Acta Chir Scand 478(Suppl):42–47, 1977.
 6. Goldstein MF, Nestico P, Olshan AR: Superior vena cava thrombosis and pulmonary embolus. Arch Intern Med 142:1726–1728, 1982.
 7. Moser KM, LeMoine JR: Is embolic risk conditioned by location of deep venous thrombosis? Arch Intern Med 94:439–444, 1981.
 8. Matthew DJ, Levin M: Pulmonary thromboembolism in children. Intensive Care Med 12:404–406, 1986.
 9. Wesley JR, Keens TG, Miller SW, Platzker AC: Pulmonary embolism in the neonate: Occurrence during the course of total parenteral nutrition. J Pediatr 93:113–115, 1978.
10. Ducatman BS, McMichan JC, Edwards WD: Catheter-induced lesions of the right side of the heart. JAMA 253:791–795, 1985.
11. Winter JH, Fenech A, Ridley W, et al: Familial antithrombin III deficiency. Q J Med 51:373–395, 1982.
12. Mehls O, Andrassy K, Koderisch J, et al: Hemostasis and thromboembolism in children with nephrotic syndrome: Differences from adults. J Pediatr 110:862–867, 1987.
13. Jones DR, MacIntyre IM: Venous thromboembolism in infancy and childhood. Arch Dis Child 50:153–155, 1975.
14. Joffe S: Postoperative deep vein thrombosis in children. J Pediatr Surg 10:539–540, 1975.
15. Cosgriff SW: Thromboembolic complications associated with ACTH and cortisone therapy. JAMA 147:924–926, 1951.
16. Cosgriff SW, Diefenbach AF, Vogt W: Hypercoagulability of the blood associated with ACTH and cortisone therapy. Am J Med 9:752–756, 1950.
17. Sullivan MJ, Hough DR, Agodoa LC: Peripheral arterial thrombosis due to the nephrotic syndrome: The clinical spectrum. South Med J 76:1011–1016, 1983.
18. Hougen TJ, Emmanoulides GC, Moss AJ: Pulmonary valvular dysfunction in children with ventriculovenous shunts for hydrocephalus: A previously unreported complication. Pediatrics 55:836–841, 1975.
19. Chakravarthy A, Edwards WD, Fleming CR: Fatal tricuspid valve obstuction due to a large infected thrombus attached to a Hickman catheter. JAMA 257:801–803, 1987.
20. Dorfman GS, Cronan JJ, Tupper TB, et al: Occult pulmonary embolism: A common occurrence in deep venous thrombosis. AJR 148:263–266, 1987.
21. Bernstein D, Coupey S, Schonberg SK: Pulmonary embolism in adolescents. Am J Dis Child 140:667–671, 1986.
22. Fraschini G, Jadeja J, Lawson M, et al: Local infusion of urokinase for the lysis of thrombosis associated with permanent central venous catheters in cancer patients. J Clin Oncol 5:672–678, 1987.
23. Clarke DB, Abrams LD: Pulmonary embolectomy: A 25 year experience. J Thorac Cardiovasc Surg 92:442–445, 1986.
24. Moreno-Cabral RJ, Breitweser JA: Pulmonary embolectomy in the neonate. Chest 84:502–504, 1983.
25. Marder VJ: The use of thrombolytic agents: Choice of patient, drug administration, laboratory monitoring. Ann Intern Med 90:802–808, 1979.
26. Delaplane D, Scott JP, Riggs, TW, et al: Urokinase therapy for a catheter-related right atrial thrombus. J Pediatr 100:149–152, 1982.
27. ten Duis HJ, Nijsten MW, Klasen HJ, Binnendijk B: Fat embolism in patients with an isolated fracture of the femoral shaft. J Trauma 28:383–390, 1988.
28. Drizin GS, Fein AM, Lippmann ML: Clinical pulmonary embolism from migration of a retained transvenous permanent pacemaker electrode. Crit Care Med 10:788–789, 1982.

56 RESPIRATORY FOREIGN BODY

ANN M. KOSLOSKE, M.D., M.P.H.

Aspiration of a foreign object is a common hazard of infancy and childhood. Although this injury is rarely fatal, 271 deaths were reported in 1984 in the United States in children under 5 years of age who choked on food or a foreign object.[1] In the first 12 months of life, most such deaths result from an object wedged at the vocal cords or in the trachea.[2] In children aged 1 to 4 years, impaction of a solid piece of food (e.g., hot dog) in the upper esophagus, with closure of the upper airway by compression, is the most frequent mechanism of food-related asphyxiation.[3, 4] Fortunately, most respiratory foreign bodies are small enough to pass through the vocal

Table 56–1. TYPES OF FOREIGN BODIES ASPIRATED BY 145 CHILDREN

Foreign Body	No. (and %) of Children	
Peanut or other nut	69	(48%)
Seed, husk, bean	29	(20%)
Plastic toy/fragment	8	(6%)
Raw carrot, apple, potato	7	(5%)
Popcorn	5	(3%)
Stone	3	(2%)
Chicken bone	3	(2%)
Amorphous debris	3	(2%)
Pen/pencil cap	2	(1.3%)
Pin	2	(1.3%)
Earring	2	(1.3%)
Miscellaneous*	12	(8%)
Total	145	(99.9%)

From New Mexico series, 1976–1988.
*One each: aluminum foil, cinder, crayon, juniper twig, magnet, orange peel, screw, styrofoam, thistle, timothy grass, trail mix, tumbleweed tuft.

cords and the subglottic trachea, and they lodge in a main stem or lobar bronchus. Of the children who aspirate foreign bodies, two thirds are boys, and 80% are under 3 years of age.[5, 6] Children at this age lack molar teeth to chew nuts and other small particulate foods finely enough to swallow them. At the moment of choking, many children are laughing or running with an object in the mouth.[2] Peanuts and other nuts account for about half of all the foreign bodies aspirated by children throughout the world.[5-10] Other common foreign objects include small vegetable fragments, pins, toys and plastic fragments, seeds, and popcorn. Table 56–1 lists the respiratory foreign bodies removed in the author's series at the University of New Mexico.

DIAGNOSIS

HISTORY

Inhalation of a foreign body triggers a violent cough reflex initially, but the child may have ceased coughing by the time he or she reaches the emergency room. Pyman[8] described a latent period that follows inhalation of a foreign body. After the initial irritation, surface sensory receptors of the respiratory tract undergo normal physiologic adaptation, and coughing may cease temporarily. Coughing may recur later with movement of the foreign body or because of secretions that accumulate in the airways. The latent period may vary from hours to years. Pyman documented such a latent period, which often caused a delay in diagnosis, in 10% of 230 children.[8] The observations of Manning and associates at the University of Michigan[11] supported the concept of the latent period. Of 51 children with a respiratory foreign body,[12] 34 (66.7%) had a history of coughing, but only 3 (6%) were described as still coughing during physical examination. In contrast, a history of wheezing was documented in 26 infants (51%), and the wheezing persisted in 23 (45%) during the physical examination.

In 80% to 90% of cases, a choking episode is witnessed,[13, 14] leading to a trip to the physician's office or the emergency room. Should the choking go unwitnessed, however, the child may exhibit unexplained wheezing or an episode of pneumonia that fails to clear with appropriate treatment. The physician who treats young children must maintain a high index of suspicion for the presence of a respiratory foreign body and must consider bronchoscopy in such instances. The adage "All that that wheezes is not asthma" is most applicable to infants and young children.

PHYSICAL EXAMINATION

The classical physical findings are unilateral decreased breath sounds as a result of decreased aeration of the lung, and unilateral wheezes resulting from partial occlusion of a bronchus. During examination, however, most children are breathing rapidly and may be crying; wheezes are often transmitted over both sides of the chest. In a detailed study of 157 Canadian children with foreign body aspiration, the diagnositc clinical triad of cough, wheezing, and diminished or absent breath sounds was evaluated.[14] Of these children 75% exhibited one or more of the diagnostic triad, but the triad was complete in only 39% of the children. Patients in whom the diagnosis was made after 1 day of aspiration were more likely to have the complete triad than were those diagnosed earlier (47% versus 31%).[14] Because most children presented with a history of choking, the importance of the history and of early diagnosis by bronchoscopy was emphasized.

CHEST RADIOGRAPH

Because only 10% of aspirated objects are radiopaque,[15] the radiographic diagnosis depends on unilateral changes in aeration caused by partial or complete obstruction of a bronchus. Inspiratory chest radiographs are insufficient for establishing the diagnosis because they are normal in 20% of patients with bronchial foreign bodies.[15, 16] Children suspected of retaining a respiratory foreign body should receive at least one supplementary diagnostic maneuver: expiratory views, decubitus views, or fluroscopy. These studies enable observation of aeration throughout the respiratory cycle. Kirks estimated that 80% of infants with a bronchial foreign body have obstructive emphysema, 20% have obstructive atelectasis, and fewer than 1% have normal aeration.[15] The cross-sectional area of a bronchus normally increases with inspiration and decreases with expiration. The most common radiographic abnormality, obstructive emphysema, occurs because air can pass around the object within the bronchus on inspiration but is trapped during expiration (Fig. 56–1). Obstructive emphysema is sometimes a subtle finding; the side of the pathologic process may be difficult to identify. Swischuk outlined two rules for radiologists to follow in such cases: (1) the lung with diminished blood flow is the abnormal lung, whether it is large and hyperlucent or small and hyperlucent, and (2) the lung that changes shape the least, or does not change at all,

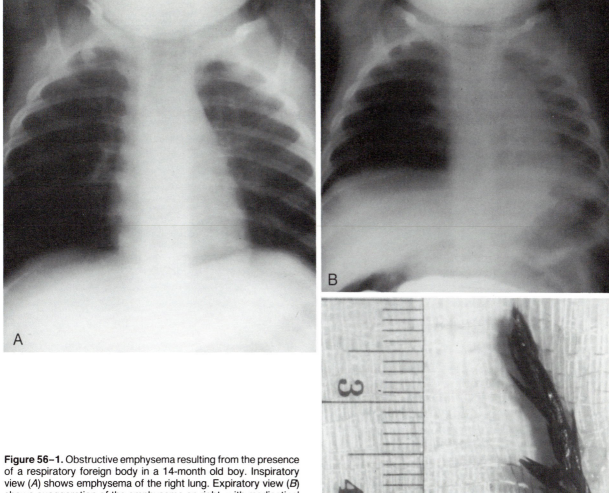

Figure 56–1. Obstructive emphysema resulting from the presence of a respiratory foreign body in a 14-month old boy. Inspiratory view (*A*) shows emphysema of the right lung. Expiratory view (*B*) shows exaggeration of the emphysema on right, with mediastinal shift to the left. The foreign body (*C*), a juniper twig, was removed from right main stem bronchus.

between inspiration and expiration is the abnormal lung.[17]

Obstructive atelectasis either results from an object wedged within a bronchus, causing collapse distally, or occurs as a later finding, after the aspirated object elicits enough mucosal reaction to occlude the bronchus (Fig. 56–2). On occasion, massive, total atelectasis of a lung ("white-out") occurs with aspiration of an object into a main stem bronchus.[12] Many infants with such gross disturbances of aeration are cyanotic, breathing with marked retractions and effort. Pneumomediastinum or pneumothorax can result and may distract attention from the underlying problem.[17]

Completely normal radiographic findings may be observed after aspiration. Reed documented normal radiographic findings in 14 (17%) of 81 children after aspi-

ration of nonradiopaque foreign objects.[16] Typical instances, illustrated in Figure 56–3, include (1) tracheal foreign bodies, (2) bilateral foreign bodies, and (3) seeds and other flat foreign bodies, which may cause minimal obstruction to airflow during inspiration or expiration. Such seeds may migrate and float within the airways, causing changing clinical findings and leading to a delay in diagnosis. Esclamado and Richardson reported a missed diagnosis in almost half of children with laryngotracheal foreign bodies,[18] 58% of whom had normal chest radiographs. Two thirds of the children with delayed diagnosis had subsequent complications (usually subglottic edema) and required intubation or tracheostomy.[18] Radiographic views of the neck, when obtained, were usually suggestive of the diagnosis of laryngotracheal foreign body. The inevitable conclusion of specialists who care

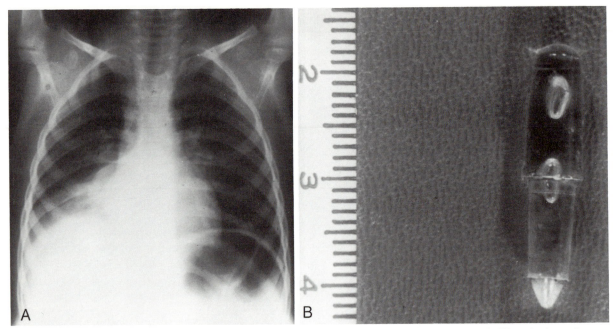

Figure 56–2. *A*, Obstructive atelectasis of right lower lobe and right middle lobe in a 35-month-girl. The foreign body (*B*), a plastic peg from a game, was removed at bronchoscopy. The tip had occluded the bronchus intermedius.

for young children was stated by Kirks: "Bronchoscopy is mandatory if there is a convincing history of foreign body aspiration, regardless of radiologic findings.[15]

PATHOPHYSIOLOGY OF THE RESPIRATORY FOREIGN BODY

In addition to changes in airflow, the foreign body incites local injury and inflammation. The degree of focal bronchitis and distal pneumonia may be a function of the type of foreign body aspirated. Inert objects of plastic or metal may remain in the airways for days, weeks, or even months without producing an infection, in contrast to peanuts and other nuts, which contain oils that may cause severe irritation. In a series from the Children's Hospital of Denver, 35 nut aspirations were compared with 38 non–nut aspirations. The incidence of pneumonia was significantly higher among nut aspirations (20% versus 8%; $p < .01$).[19]

It is generally thought that aspirations into the right main stem bronchus are more common than the left, on an anatomical basis, i.e., smaller angle from the midline leading to a "straighter shot" into the right main bronchus, assuming an upright child. In our own series (Fig. 56–4) there was a slight predominance of right-sided foreign bodies. Rothmann and Boeckman reported equal frequencies: 102 objects in the right bronchial tree, 100 in the left.[6] Other reports,[20, 21] however, have shown a left-sided predominance. Saijo and collaborators demonstrated a right-sided predominance in adults and a left-sided predominance in children under 6 years of age, especially in aspirations involving peanuts.[9] The reasons for these differences are not clear. The pediatric airway is dynamic, and factors in addition to the bronchial angle from the axis probably determine the final site of lodgement of the aspirated foreign body.

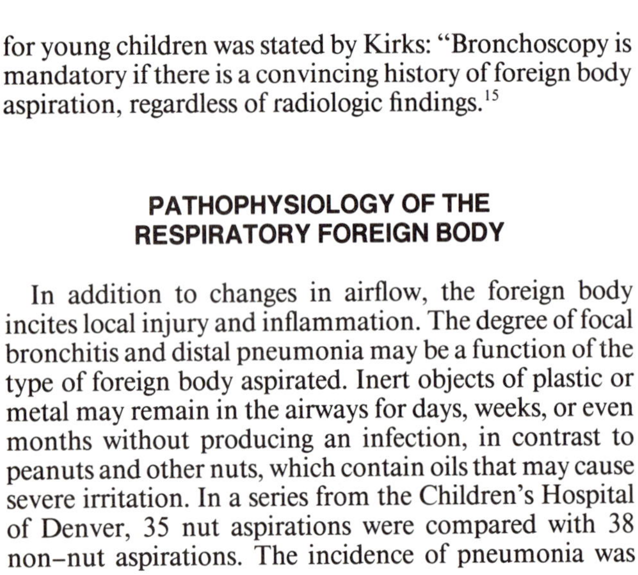

REMOVAL OF THE FOREIGN BODY

Respiratory foreign bodies should be removed while the patient is under general anesthesia, by means of the rigid pediatric ventilating bronchoscope. The introduction in the 1970s of pediatric instruments that contain the Hopkins rod-lens system has facilitated extraction of aspirated objects. Controlled ventilation and a superb view (Fig. 56–5) are maintained throughout the extraction procedure. The flexible fiberscope, a useful diagnostic instrument, has no use in the extraction of aspirated foreign objects from young children because it has no channel for ventilation.[22, 23]

The bronchoscopic extraction of a foreign body is a delicate procedure that should be carried out by an endos-

Figure 56–3. Normal radiographic findings in the author's series of infants, after aspiration of (1) a tracheal foreign body (a cinder), (2) bilateral foreign bodies (crayon fragments), and (3) a migrating watermelon seed. (From Musemeche CA, Kosloske AM: Normal radiographic findings after foreign body aspiration: When the history counts. Clin Pediatr (Phila) 25:624–625, 1986.)

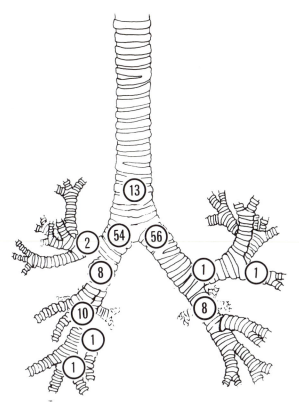

Figure 56-4. Anatomic site of 155 respiratory foreign bodies in 145 children. (New Mexico series, 1976–1988).

copist and an anesthesiologist experienced in the management of the pediatric airways. Mistakes based on inexperience may lead to traumatic extractions or even major complications, such as cardiopulmonary arrest during the procedure. The first chance to remove a foreign body is the best chance.[24] Thus if expert pediatric endos-

copy is not available in a community, a child with a respiratory foreign body should be transferred to a center where such expertise is available.

Although bronchoscopy is an urgent procedure, most children with a respiratory foreign body are stable enough to be prepared for general anesthesia. Only 3% to 6% of children require immediate bronchoscopy because of acute respiratory distress, usually from laryngeal or tracheal obstruction.[6, 21]. If a child has a full stomach, it is much safer to defer bronchoscopy for a few hours than to risk aspiration of gastric contents while the child is under general anesthesia.

An intravenous infusion is begun, and an appropriate antibiotic is given if the child has signs and symptoms of pneumonia. Even without pneumonia, an intravenous dose of antibiotic just before bronchoscopy is advisable if the foreign body has been in the airways for more than 24 h. Atropine should always be given before bronchoscopy for foreign body extraction. During the procedure, the patient should be monitored by pulse oximetry, in addition to electrocardiography and blood pressure monitoring. General anesthesia is usually induced by a combination of inhalation agents and oxygen, administered by face mask, along with intravenous muscle relaxants. A pediatric laryngoscope is inserted, and the vocal cords and upper airway may be sprayed with topical lidocaine (Xylocaine). The bronchoscope is slipped atraumatically into the airway.

As the bronchoscope is advanced into the trachea, the telescope provides a magnified view of the airway. The aspirated foreign object is usually sighted in the right or the left main stem bronchus. A variety of instruments are available for extraction. The techniques preferred by this author depend on the shape and type of foreign body: the Fogarty catheter technique[25] (Fig. 56–5B) is used for removal of peanuts and other spherical foreign bodies,

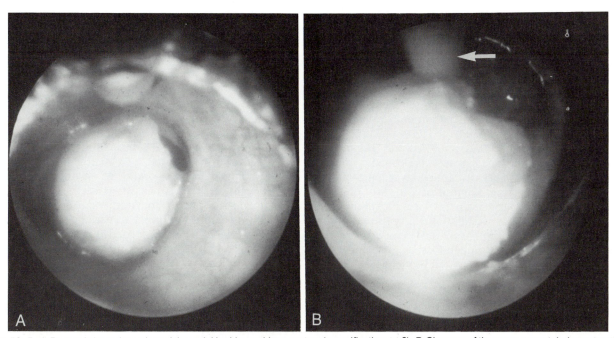

Figure 56-5. *A,* Peanut in bronchus, viewed through Hopkins rod-lens system (magnification, × 6). *B,* Close-up of the same peanut during extraction. A Fogarty catheter (*arrow*) has been passed beyond the peanut at start of extraction process. Details of the technique are described elsewhere.[25]

and a forceps is used for removal of seeds, husks, and other flat foreign bodies. Occasionally the Dormia basket is successful for removal of larger foreign bodies (e.g., sharp stones, screws) that may defy extraction by standard methods. An optical forceps with the grasper built into the outer sheath of the bronchoscope is the instrument preferred by many endoscopists.[5, 22] Removal of foreign bodies requires ingenuity, facility with the pediatric endoscopes, and, most crucial, familiarity with the pediatric airway. The skill and experience of the endoscopist are more important than the instrument chosen for the extraction.

After the respiratory foreign body has been extracted, the endoscopist should take a second look into the airways because multiple foreign bodies are present in 5% of patients.[26] Pooled secretions distal to the site of foreign body impaction may be suctioned away and submitted for cultures.

Most foreign bodies lodge in one or the other main stem bronchus (Fig. 56–5) and are readily extracted by the techniques just described. For a few very large or very small objects, special techniques may be required for extraction. Tracheal foreign bodies that appear to be too large to remove without risk of injury to the vocal cords may be retrieved through a technique described by Swensson and associates,[27] who performed a tracheostomy with the ventilating bronchoscope in place. The foreign body was grasped with a forceps, brought from the carina to the level of the tracheostomy, and extracted with a forceps via the tracheostoma. Small peripheral foreign bodies that are visible in segmental bronchi, which are out of reach of the ventilating bronchoscope, may be disimpacted by a Fogarty catheter balloon[22] and then grasped by a forceps or another instrument. Even smaller foreign bodies in subsegmental bronchi, too distant to be visible, may be retrieved endoscopically by the combination of techniques described by Hight and colleagues,[28] which included fluoroscopy, use of endobronchial contrast material, use of topical vasoactive medications, and a variety of retrieval instruments. Thoracotomy and bronchotomy are almost never necessary for extraction of a respiratory foreign body.

In the 1970s, a group from Denver used a nonendoscopic method for removal of foreign bodies; this method was a series of treatments consisting of inhalation of a bronchodilator followed by postural drainage and percussion.[29] Bronchoscopy was performed if the postural drainage method was unsuccessful after 4 days.[29] Because of reports of cardiopulmonary arrest associated with this technique,[19, 29, 30] however, it cannot be recommended. The original investigators abandoned it in favor of bronchoscopy as the primary treatment for removal of respiratory foreign bodies.[31, 32] Inhalation with postural drainage may be used safely in instances when endoscopy has failed to retrieve a small peripheral foreign body lodged in a lobar, segmental, or subsegmental bronchus.[33]

PERIOPERATIVE MANAGEMENT

After bronchoscopy, children often have some degree of croup from glottic or subglottic edema, particularly if the extraction procedure was lengthy. Such patients may benefit from humidification (e.g., a croup tent) and bronchodilators. Antibiotics should be used when there is evidence of pneumonia or bronchitis. In the 1960s and 1970s, tracheostomy was performed on 2% to 3% of children with aspirated foreign bodies[6] because of severe associated edema of the upper airway. Management today consists of endotracheal intubation until the edema subsides; tracheostomy is almost never necessary.

PERSISTENCE OF FOREIGN BODIES

On occasion inhaled foreign objects may escape diagnosis and remain within the airways for weeks or months. The result is an intense focal bronchitis with distal bronchiectasis and abscess formation. The clinical manifestation is recurrent pneumonia with hemoptysis. The most notorious of such persistent foreign bodies is the grass head (inflorescence). Jewett and Butsch described "the treacherous timothy grass"[34] as leading to chronic bronchiectasis. Hilman and co-workers classifed the mechanical configuration of two types of grasses: the lodging type, in which the grass head remained in the air passages, and the extrusive type, in which the grass head migrated distally by a ratchet effect, penetrating lung parenchyma, pleura, and intercostal muscles and even extruding through the skin of the chest wall.[35] The bronchiectasis from a persistent foreign body may require pulmonary resection for cure. A bronchogram or a computed tomographic scan[36] may confirm the diagnosis and delineate the extent of disease. Lobectomy is not always necessary; segmental resection or wedge resection may be possible for preservation of normal pulmonary parenchyma. An example from one of the children at the author's institution with bronchiectasis from such a chronic foreign body, cured by wedge resection, is shown in Figure 56–6.

EMERGENCY MANAGEMENT OF A CHOKING CHILD

Most children who have choked on a foreign body are able to breathe and speak. They should be taken immediately to the hospital for removal of the object. All first aid maneuvers are unnecessary and potentially dangerous. There has been controversy regarding optimal first aid maneuvers in the rare instance in which a choking child is cyanotic and unable to breathe or speak.[37] After review of the data, the Committee on Accident and Poison Prevention of the American Academy of Pediatrics in 1988 made the following recommendations:[38] if the choking victim is an infant under 1 year of age, the Heimlich maneuver should not be carried out because of risk of injury to intra-abdominal organs. The treatment of choice is by back blows and chest thrusts. The infant is placed face down on the rescuer's forearm or lap, with the infant's head firmly supported and held lower than the trunk. Four back blows are rapidly administered with the heel of the rescuer's hand between the infant's shoulder blades. If the obstruction is not relieved, the infant is turned to a supine position, and the rescuer, using two fin-

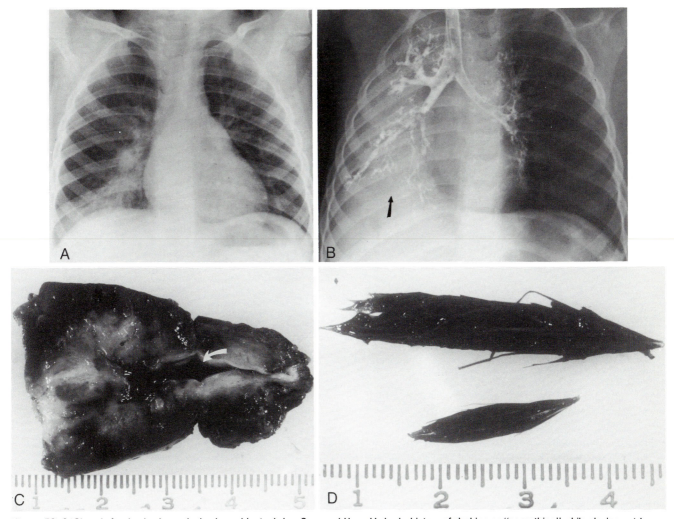

Figure 56–6. Chronic foreign body producing bronchiectasis in a 2-year-old boy. He had a history of choking on "something" while playing outdoors. A productive cough, recurrent pneumonia, and finger clubbing developed over the next 9 months. Chest film (*A*) shows right lower lobe infiltrate. Bronchogram (*B*) shows nonfilling of anterior basilar segment (*arrow*) of right lung. The resected segment (*C*) contained a bronchiectatic cavity (*arrow*) with an aspirated grasshead (*D*). Recovery was complete after operation and included resolution of severe clubbing.

gers, applies four rapid chest thrusts (similar to external cardiac compressions) over the infant's sternum. If breathing is not resumed, the victim's mouth is opened, and the tongue is grasped and drawn forward. A visible foreign body is manually extracted by a finger sweep. Blind finger sweeps, however, may cause further obstruction and should be avoided. If no spontaenous breathing occurs, mouth-to-mouth resuscitation should be initiated. The back blows and chest thrusts should be repeated while emergency medical services are en route to the scene. Henry Heimlich does not agree with this and recommends that his manuever be used even for infants. He believes that abdominal thrusts and back slaps can injure viscera and drive foreign bodies deeper into the bronchus (personal communication.) The current Pediatric Advanced Life Support course endorses the Academy's position.

If the choking victim is a child over 1 year of age, the Heimlich maneuver is the initial treatment of choice. Six to 10 abdominal thrusts are applied until the foreign body is expelled. The child may be placed supine with the rescuer kneeling beside the child, or, alternatively, the child may be in a standing or sitting position, with the rescuer behind and arms wrapped around the child.[37] A sharp upward and inward thrust is applied, 6 to 10 times, just above the umbilicus. If the Heimlich maneuver does not relieve the obstruction, the child's mouth is opened and the tongue drawn forward, in an attempt to visualize the foreign body. No blind finger sweeps should be used. If these maneuvers are unsuccessful, mouth-to-mouth ventilation should be attempted and the Heimlich maneuver repeated while emergency medical services are en route.

PREVENTION

Many accidents involving aspiration of foreign bodies are preventable. Most laypersons are unaware of the danger of feeding peanuts and small particulate foods to young children. The morbidity and mortality rates and the cost of these accidents might be reduced to half if parents would simply slice hotdogs into small pieces for young children and avoid giving them nuts altogether. Governmental regulations properly enforced could prevent tragedies associated with aspirations of foreign bodies.[3] The United States Consumer Product Safety Commission is empowered to recall and to prevent importation of hazardous toys and other products. Criminal penalties exist for willful violation of the Consumer Product Safety Act. In the United States, most manufacturers are keenly aware of product liability. Products such as the Christmas bow have been modified for safety reasons.[39] Warning labels on foods that are dangerous to young children (e.g., hotdogs, peanuts, popcorn), similar to warning labels on drugs, cigarettes, or hazardous household products, have been proposed.[4] Physicians who treat children must become activists in the arena of public education for prevention of accidents involving aspiration of foreign bodies.

REFERENCES

1. Accident Facts, 1987 ed, p. 8. Chicago: National Safety Council, 1987.
2. Weston JT: Airway foreign body fatalities in children. Ann Otol Rhinol Laryngol 74:1144–1148, 1965.
3. Baker SP, Fisher RS: Childhood asphyxiation by choking or suffocation. JAMA 244:1343–1346, 1980.
4. Harris CS, Baker SP, Smith GA, et al: Childhood asphyxiation by food: A national analysis and overview. JAMA 251:2231–2235, 1984.
5. Black RE, Choi KJ, Syme WC, et al: Bronchoscopic removal of aspirated foreign bodies in children. Am J Surg 148:778–781, 1984.
6. Rothmann BF, Boeckman CR: Foreign bodies in the larynx and tracheobronchial tree in children: A review of 225 cases. Ann Otol Rhinol Laryngol 89:434–436, 1980.
7. Kosloske AM: Bronchoscopic extraction of aspirated foreign bodies in children. Am J Dis Child 136:924–927, 1982.
8. Pyman C: Inhaled foreign bodies in childhood: A review of 230 cases. Med J Aust 1:62–68, 1971.
9. Saijo S, Tomioka S, Takasaka T, et al: Foreign bodies in the tracheobronchial tree: A review of 110 cases. Arch Otorhinolaryngol 225:1–7, 1979.
10. Schloss MD, Pham-Dang H, Rosales JK: Foreign bodies in the tracheobronchial tree—A retrospective study of 217 cases. J Otolaryngol 12:212–216, 1983.
11. Manning PB, Wesley JR, Polley TZ Jr, et al: Esophageal and tracheobronchial foreign bodies in infants and children. Pediatr Surg Int 2:346–351, 1987.
12. Seibert RW, Siebert JJ, Williamson SL: The opaque chest: When to suspect a bronchial foreign body. Pediatr Radiol 16:193–196, 1986.
13. Blazer S, Naveh Y, Friedman A: Foreign body in the airway: A review of 200 cases. Am J Dis Child 134:68–71, 1980.
14. Wiseman NE: The diagnosis of foreign body aspiration in childhood. J Pediatr Surg 19:531–535, 1984.
15. Kirks DA: Practical Pediatric Imaging: Diagnostic Radiology in Infants and Children, pp. 518–521. Boston: Little, Brown, 1984.
16. Reed MH: Radiology of airway foreign bodies in children. J Can Assoc Radiol 28:111–118, 1977.
17. Swischuk LE: Emergency Radiology of the Acutely Ill or Injured Child, 2nd ed, pp. 96–105. Baltimore: Williams & Wilkins, 1986.
18. Esclamado RM, Richardson MA: Laryngotracheal foreign bodies in children: A comparison with bronchial foreign bodies. Am J Dis Child 141:259–262, 1987.
19. Law D, Kosloske AM: Management of tracheobronchial foreign bodies in children: A reevaluation of postural drainage and bronchoscopy. Pediatrics 58:362–367, 1976.
20. Cohen SR, Herbert WI, Lewis GB Jr, et al: Foreign bodies in the airway: Five-year retrospective study with special reference to management. Ann Otol Rhinol Laryngol 89:437–442, 1980.
21. Vane DW, Pritchard J, Colville CW, et al: Bronchoscopy for aspirated foreign bodies in children: Experience in 131 cases. Arch Surg 123:885–888, 1988.
22. Johnson DG: Esophagoscopy. In Welch KJ, Randolph JG, Ravitch MM, et al (eds): Pediatric Surgery, 4th ed, pp. 677–681, Chicago: Year Book Medical, 1986.
23. Wood RE, Gauderer MW: Flexible fiberoptic bronchoscopy in the management of tracheobronchial foreign bodies in children: The value of a combined approach with open tube bronchoscopy. J Pediatr Surg 19:693–698, 1984.
24. Gans SL: Discussion of Wood RE, Gauderer MWL: Flexible fiberoptic bronchoscopy in the management of tracheobronchial foreign bodies in children. The value of a combined approach with open tube bronchoscopy. J Pediatr Surg 19:697, 1984.
25. Kosloske AM: The Fogarty balloon technique for removal of foreign bodies from the tracheobronchial tree. Surg Gynecol Obstet 155:72–73, 1982.
26. McGuirt WF, Holmes KD, Feehs R, et al: Tracheobronchial foreign bodies. Laryngoscope 98:615–618, 1988.
27. Swensson EE, Rah KH, Kim MC, et al: Extraction of large tracheal foreign bodies through a tracheostoma under bronchoscopic control. Ann Thorac Surg 39:251–253, 1985.
28. Hight DW, Philippart AI, Hertzler JH: The treatment of retained peripheral foreign bodies in the pediatric airway. J Pediatr Surg 16:694–699, 1981.
29. Cotton EK, Abrams G, Vanhoutte J, et al: Removal of aspirated foreign bodies by inhalation and postural drainage. Clin Pediatr (Phila) 12:270–276, 1973.
30. Kosloske AM: Tracheobronchial foreign bodies in children: Back to the bronchoscope, and a balloon. Pediatrics 66:321–323, 1980.
31. Cotton E, Yasuda K: Foreign body aspiration. Pediatr Clin North Am 31:937–941, 1984.
32. Janik JS, Burrington JD, Wayne ER, et al: Foreign body aspiration in children. Colo Med 83:10–11, 1986.
33. Campbell DN, Cotton EK, Lilly JR: A dual approach to tracheobronchial foreign bodies in children. Surgery 91:178–182, 1982.
34. Jewett TC Jr, Butsch WL: Trials with treacherous timothy grass. J Thorac Cardiovasc Surg 50:124–126, 1965.
35. Hilman BC, Kurzweg FT, McCook WW Jr, et al: Foreign body aspiration of grass inflorescences as a cause of hemoptysis. Chest 78:306–309, 1980.
36. Berger PE, Kuhn JP, Kuhns LR: Computed tomography and the occult tracheobronchial foreign body. Radiology 134:133–135, 1980.
37. Standards and guidelines for cardiopulmonary resuscitation (CPR) and emergency cardiac care (ECC). Part IV: Pediatric basic life support. JAMA 255:2954–2960, 1986.
38. American Academy of Pediatrics Committee on Accident and Poison Prevention: First aid for the choking child. Pediatrics 81:740–742, 1988.
39. Buntain WL, Benton JW, Gutierrez JF: Christmas bow tragedies. South Med J 72:1471–1472, 1979.
40. Musemeche CA, Kosloske AM: Normal radiographic findings after foreign body aspiration: When the history counts. Clin Pediatr (Phila) 25:624–625, 1986.

57 GASTROESOPHAGEAL REFLUX AND RESPIRATORY SEQUELAE

JOHN J. HERBST, M.D. / BETTINA C. HILMAN, M.D.

There is a general agreement that there are important interactions between gastroesophageal reflux (GER) and a variety of disorders of the respiratory system, but there is frequent disagreement as to whether these interactions reflect a cause-and-effect relationship or merely simultaneous events. GER is common in childhood, and some reflux is physiologic.[1-4] Respiratory symptoms associated with GER in children are also common, and GER and respiratory symptoms may occur independently in the same patient. In this chapter, the pathophysiologic features of such relationships are described, and situations in which respiratory problems affect GER and in which GER causes respiratory problems are delineated. The usefulness of various tests in evaluating patients with respiratory problems possibly caused by GER and the use of various methods of treatment are also discussed.

PATHOPHYSIOLOGY

PHYSIOLOGY OF REFLUX

Basic information about normal esophageal physiology is helpful in the understanding of the pathophysiologic processes of GER and the rationale for the use of the various studies of esophageal function. Sometimes GER is a physiologic event in normal children, occurring rarely during sleep but commonly after meals.[2] Episodes of reflux may occur up to 5.8 times per hour and for up to 33% of the time in the first 2 h after a meal; however, more than 0.3% of episodes of reflux per hour or reflux for more than 0.5% of the time during sleep more than 2 h after a meal is abnormal. In contrast to adults, in whom heartburn is one of the most common symptoms, vomiting occurs in more than 90% of children with GER.[3,4] Spitting of small amounts of formula after feedings is so common in infants that parents often dismiss it as normal "wet burps" unless they are specifically questioned. The frequency of vomiting in children is related to the fact that the reservoir capacity of the esophagus in infants is only about 5 to 6 ml, and intake per kilogram of body weight may be three times higher in an infant than in an adult,[4] in whom the reservoir capacity of the esophagus is about 180 ml.

Several mechanisms normally inhibit reflux (Fig. 57–1, Table 57–1). The lower esophageal sphincter is an approximately 2.5-cm region of increased tone at the distal end of the esophagus that is partially within the abdomen and partially in the thorax.[5] The intra-abdominal position of the lower esophageal sphincter is important because abdominal pressure can also compress the sphincter, which counteracts the tendency of the transmitted intra-abdominal pressure to force gastric contents into the esophagus. In patients who respond to medical therapy of GER, the intra-abdominal portion of the sphincter tends to be longer than in patients requiring surgery.[6] If the sphincter is in the thorax, as with a hiatal hernia, the negative intrathoracic pressure surrounding the sphincter tends to reduce sphincter competence.[7]

The normal position of the esophagus produces an acute angle between the distal esophagus and the fundus, creating a flap valve mechanism that enhances sphincter competence.[7, 8] The distal esophagus usually has a collapsed H-shaped potential opening, which is similar to a choke valve.[8] Small variations in length of the circumferential smooth muscle produce large variations in cross-sectional area. In chronic inflammation or fibrosis (e.g., esophagitis), this mechanism may malfunction. The esophageal sphincter is not in a state of constant contraction. With deglutition, there is relaxation that is mediated by the vagus nerve, whereby relaxation occurs before the peristaltic wave reaches the sphincter. The lower esophageal sphincter (LES) is a zone of increased intraluminal pressure in the distal 1 to 3 cm of esophagus that is not an identifiable anatomic structure, as is the pyloric sphincter. Many of the problems of GER are related to abnormalities in function of the LES. Reflux may occur across a chronically lax sphincter; this is an uncommon condition usually associated with severe esophagitis.[9] Reflux frequently occurs with a spontaneous brief relaxation of LES pressure that is not related to swallowing. Reflux may also occur with increased LES pressure if there is increased abdominal pressure (e.g., during cough).[9]

Material from reflux may be returned to the stomach by primary peristaltic waves, which are initiated by swallowing, or by secondary waves, which are stimulated by esophageal distention. Normal esophageal motility is assumed for these mechanisms to operate. Patients with abnormal esophageal motility may have poor esophageal clearance that prolongs the effects of acid gastric material

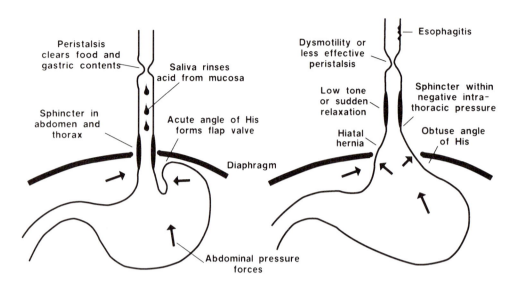

Figure 57–1. Esophageal function. GER, gastroesophageal reflux.

in the esophagus and increases the risk that esophagitis will develop. Also, esophagitis is associated with altered motility and persistently low sphincter pressure.[6, 10-12] Tertiary esophageal waves are ineffectual, uncoordinated, or simultaneous contractions that are commonly seen in patients with esophagitis. Final traces of acid are washed from the esophagus by swallowed saliva, which has little capacity to neutralize gastric acidity.[7, 13] This last mechanism is especially important during reflux that occurs during sleep because less saliva is made and swallowing occurs less frequently during sleep.[14]

Esophageal clearance mechanisms and the reaction of the esophagus to material from reflux have major influences on the type and severity of symptoms caused by GER. With normal or minimally abnormal esophageal mucosa and clearance, few or no symptoms may result when gastric contents that flow into the esophagus are quickly removed. When esophageal clearance is compromised, a spectrum of symptoms of varying severity may result. Ineffectiveness in removal of acid gastric contents prolongs their contact with the esophageal mucosa and increases both esophageal inflammation and the likelihood of aspiration during vomiting. The resulting severe esophagitis may further contribute to severe heartburn and pain associated with high-pressure tertiary waves. Jolley and associates[15] reported an association between duration of reflux episode during sleep and the presence of respiratory symptoms. There are certainly some relation-ships among subtle malfunctions of the superior esophagus sphincter, pharyngeal clearance mechanisms, and the frequency of aspiration of gastric contents after reflux to the upper esophagus.

MECHANISMS OF GER-RELATED RESPIRATORY DISEASE

The pharynx is a passage for movement of air into the lungs and food into the esophagus; incoordination enables spillage of saliva, food, and gastric material from reflux into the trachea. Coordinated movement of air across the nasopharynx into the trachea occurs approximately 30 times per minute in infants during feeding. Sucking occurs every 1.25 sec in prolonged bursts; swallowing occurs every 4 to 5 sucks. The integration of swallowing and sucking is an exceedingly complex and sophisticated control process.[16] Aspiration of refluxed material with failure of nasopharyngeal clearance mechanisms is thought to be the major mechanism for pulmonary symptoms related to GER. Coughing, choking, and dyspnea are obvious sequelae to aspiration. Aspiration can cause pneumonia, but it may also lead to irritation of airways and reactive airway disease.[17] The occurrence of aspiration implies that there is some defect, deficiency, or overwhelming of the pharyngeal clearing mechanisms[18, 19] (Table 57–2). An association between GER and reactive

Table 57–1. FACTORS ENCOURAGING GASTROESOPHAGEAL REFLUX

Intrathoracic LES
Obtuse gastroesophageal angle
Scarred or inflamed choke valve mechanism
Inappropriate relaxation of LES
LES hypotension
Increased abdominal pressure

LES, lower esophageal sphincter.

Table 57–2. MECHANISMS FOR RESPIRATORY PROBLEMS CAUSED BY GASTROESOPHAGEAL REFLUX

Aspiration (mechanical)
Bronchospasm and laryngospasm
Involved structures
 Chemoreceptors
 Vagus nerve
 Brainstem
 Higher central nervous system centers

airway disease caused by a vagally mediated mechanism was postulated in the 1930s.[19] There are chemoreceptors in the esophagus and the larynx; stimulation of these receptors with infused acid can produce reactive airway disease which implies a neural reflex mechanism.[20, 21] Many patients with no pulmonary symptoms may exhibit reflux, vomiting, and failure to thrive as the major symptoms. In other patients, vomiting may be absent or minimal, and aspiration is the predominant problem. A causal relationship between GER and pulmonary symptoms is often difficult to document because symptomatic events may be episodic and must be differentiated from aspiration of food and saliva.

Laryngospasm that causes partial or complete obstruction of the airway may be mediated by neural reflexes, as may central apnea and bradycardia.[22, 23] This phenomenon is most commonly seen in premature infants, in whom the stimulation of receptors in the pharynx and esophagus by a nasogastric tube or a suction catheter also frequently slows respirations and heartbeat.[24]

Pulmonary disease, especially during acute exacerbation, or severe disease is usually associated with increased respiratory efforts. The subsequent wide changes in intrathoracic pressure during respiration and the increased abdominal pressure during expiration tend to compromise LES competence. Overexpansion of the lungs, which occurs in asthma, lowers the diaphragm and may interfere with the flap valve mechanism produced by the angulated entrance of the esophagus into the stomach.[7] These mechanisms are especially important during coughing, wheezing, or choking, during which there are marked changes in abdominal and thoracic pressure.

INTERACTION OF RESPIRATORY AND ESOPHAGEAL DYSFUNCTION

It is obvious from the preceding description that several types of interactions between esophageal and respiratory dysfunction may occur. GER may produce respiratory symptoms, respiratory problems may cause or aggravate GER, and there may be a vicious cycle in which the two problems reinforce each other. In addition, subtle problems of pharyngeal incoordination that normally would be clinically unimportant can cause major problems if the poorly coordinated pharyngeal clearance mechanisms are suddenly overwhelmed by gastric material from reflux. The reflux-induced inflammation of the upper esophagus and pharynx sensitizes chemoreceptors, leading to bronchospasm and other respiratory symptoms.

RESPIRATORY PROBLEMS CAUSED BY GER

ASPIRATION PNEUMONIA AND LUNG ABSCESS

Aspiration pneumonia is the most obvious pulmonary sequela of GER (Table 57–3). Coughing and choking are characteristically associated with vomiting near the end of or soon after meals and are followed by the development

Table 57–3. RESPIRATORY PROBLEMS CAUSED BY GASTROESOPHAGEAL REFLUX

Aspiration pneumonia
Lung abscess
Wheezing/reactive airway disease
Laryngospasm
Stridor
Chronic cough
Choking spells
Apnea
  Obstructive
  Central
Hiccups

of pulmonary infiltrates. Coughing is a protective mechanism, and Carré reported that patients with GER and nighttime cough are less likely to develop pulmonary infiltrates.[25] It is difficult to document individual episodes of aspiration because their occurrence is usually infrequent. (Many studies are flawed because it is assumed that all pulmonary problems in patients with GER are caused by aspiration.) GER has been convincingly implicated in some cases of pneumonia and lung abscess, recurrent granulomatous pneumonia, bronchiectasis, chronic bronchitis, and pulmonary fibrosis.[18, 26, 27] In infants and older patients who are usually recumbent, the right upper lobe is commonly the predominant site of aspiration, whereas in ambulatory patients, the lower lobes are usually the involved areas.

There is no strong correlation between the severity of vomiting or heartburn and the severity of respiratory problems. A cause-and-effect relationship between GER and respiratory sequelae is more common among children with problems of delayed development.[10, 22, 28, 29] Among patients with trisomy 21, there is a high incidence of pneumonia and GER.[29-31] It is proposed that problems of incoordination in pharyngeal clearance mechanisms may predispose children with impaired neuromuscular development to aspiration.

Patients who have undergone repair of esophageal atresia are at special risk for GER and recurrent pneumonia secondary to GER.[32, 33] The motility in the distal esophagus of these patients is abnormal, and approximately two thirds of the patients have pathologic GER. Control of GER usually improves or eliminates the respiratory problems; this observation provides support for the notion of causal relationship.[34]

Patients with GER-related pulmonary disease often have prolonged reflux while asleep, which may cause more esophagitis, increase the sensitivity of chemoreceptors, and a decrease in esophageal sphincter pressure.[15]

REACTIVE AIRWAY DISEASE

Evidence for a causal relationship between GER and reactive airway disease comes from individual case reports and studies of the frequency of reflux and asthma as well as likelihood of both occurring in the same patient. Studies have shown that abnormal GER occurs in 20% to 80% of children with asthma; this incidence is dramatically higher than that among normal children.[35-40] Although asthma might induce GER rather than be caused by it, patients with documentation of more severe reflux are more likely to have severe reactive airway disease.[36, 39] In some patients, onset of wheezing has been correlated with individual GER episodes.[36] Several investigators have reported improvement of pulmonary problems after effective treatment of GER with medical or surgical methods.[15, 31, 35, 36] Children with steroid-dependent and nocturnal asthma are especially likely to have GER.[39, 40]

Several studies involving adults and children have demonstrated bronchospasm after infusion of acid into the esophagus, in contrast to lack of bronchospasm after infusion of water.[20, 21, 41] One study in adults showed that acidification of the esophagus potentiated the bronchospasm caused by agents such as methacholine, a known bronchoconstricting agent.[42] During these studies, there was no assurance that microaspiration did not occur as the esophagus was perfused with acid. Evidence that neural reflexes are important in bronchospasm caused by GER is derived from animal studies in which vagal blockade prevented bronchospasm after esophageal acidification.[43, 44]

There is compelling evidence that GER can cause bronchospasm that may not be associated with aspiration, often in patients whose asthma is uncontrolled, nonatopic, or primarily nocturnal.[18, 39, 40] The relationship of reflux esophagitis to GER-induced asthma is unclear. Esophagitis is a reflection of prolonged acidic stimulation of the esophagus. The chemoreceptors in the inflamed esophagus may be more sensitive than normal to various stimuli. The pain of esophagitis may augment the bronchospasm through reflexes in the central nervous system. It is unknown whether acid is the major stimulus or whether flow of food or spices from reflux also stimulates the receptors.

UPPER AIRWAY PROBLEMS; APNEA, AIRWAY OBSTRUCTION, SUDDEN INFANT DEATH SYNDROME

Sudden episodes of partial or complete upper airway obstruction as a result of laryngospasm have been found to be associated with GER.[24] Episodes of upper airway obstruction have been associated with apnea, bradycardia, and episodes of apparently life-threatening events.[24, 45] GER has also been proposed as a possible mechanism in some cases of sudden infant death syndrome.[23] Incomplete airway obstruction has been associated with stridor, cough, and choking episodes. Findings from animal studies suggest that laryngospasm is mediated via neural reflexes and that mechanical blockage of the airway by gastric contents from reflux is of minor importance.[46, 47] Symptoms of obstruction tend to be most severe in infants, in whom airways are narrow and muscular support of airway patency is limited.

The cause-and-effect relationship between GER and obstructive apnea or partial airway obstruction in some patients with stridor is postulated on the basis of several studies with small groups of patients who were carefully observed in order to demonstrate such an association.[22, 24, 45, 48, 49] Unfortunately, apnea and partial upper airway obstruction are common, and an association with GER cannot be demonstrated in all patients.

Improvement or cessation of episodes of respiratory arrest after medical or surgical correction of GER has been noted in several studies.[23, 24, 44, 45, 48-50] Improvement was noted in some patients who also had other congenital abnormalities of the upper airway. Careful monitoring revealed a temporal relationship in some patients between onset of symptoms and presence of acid gastric contents in the esophagus.[24] The spilling of reflux material into airways has also been documented scintigraphically in some children.[51, 52]

Nasal airflow thermistors were used to show that infusion of acid, but not formula or water, into the esophagus could cause obstructive apnea in some patients.[24] This finding implies that a neural reflex involving pH-sensitive receptors, rather than factors related to mechanical obstruction, was operative.

Some authors have challenged the association between GER and apnea because they noted poor correlation of apnea with episodes of reflux.[54, 54] In these studies, many episodes of GER detected by pH monitoring might have been masked because of neutralization of gastric contents by food. The authors contended that the data suggested that some episodes of stridor and obstructive apnea are caused by GER, and they acknowledged that in many cases there is no causal relationship. GER can also cause some episodes of central apnea, via neural reflexes, especially in very young or premature infants. The mechanism is presumed to be the same as in the central apnea that often occurs with placement of nasogastric feeding tubes.[46, 47]

Hiccups (singultus) is a sudden involuntary spasm of the diaphragm. This symptom may be caused by esophageal distention with reflux material and esophagitis; other problems not related to GER such as acute gastric distention or pericardial irritation are also known causes.[55, 56] Thus GER can be associated with problems caused by decreased muscular tone (apnea) or increased muscular tone (asthma, cough, laryngospasm, hiccups).

INDUCTION OF GER BY RESPIRATORY DISORDERS AND THEIR MANAGEMENT

Just as GER can cause respiratory problems, respiratory disease and its management can cause reflux through numerous mechanisms. Respiratory problems can cause or augment GER in a variety of clinical situations through changes in thoracic and abdominal pressure, the effects of positioning for respiratory therapy, and alterations of acid production and sphincter pressures. Coughing, wheezing, and forced expiratory maneuvers in such disorders as pneumonia, bronchopulmonary dysplasia, asthma, or bronchiectasis increase abdominal pressure and promote reflux. Especially in patients with hyperreactive airway disease, the associated therapy often encourages GER, which then increases respiratory problems, initiating a vicious cycle of events. Overexpansion of the lungs with flattening of the diaphragm may also compromise antireflux mechanisms. Among patients with cystic fibrosis, a high incidence of GER and esophagitis has been noted.[57, 58] In patients with chronic pulmonary diseases such as cystic fibrosis, the marked increases in intrathoracic negative pressure on inhalation can promote the development of GER, especially if there is a hiatal hernia that places the sphincter within the thorax. Although obstructive apnea, stridor, and hiccups can be caused by GER, the sudden negative intrathoracic pressures produced by these problems can trigger GER regardless of the original etiologic process.

Therapy in patients with respiratory problems may also have effects leading to incompetency of the lower esophageal sphincter. Theophylline, a drug used to treat asthma, has several effects, including a decrease in pressure on the LES.[59–62] In toxic doses, theophylline causes gastric irritation and vomiting, which is difficult to distinguish from GER in young children. Beta-adrenergic drugs such as isoproterenol, metaproterenol, and albuterol that are also used to treat reactive airway disease can cause a decrease in the LES pressure.[63–66] Theophylline and other xanthines such as caffeine can make gastric contents from reflux more toxic by stimulating acid secretion.[67]

Smoking is conducive to reflux by decreasing the LES pressure. This effect appears to be related to the actions of nicotine on adrenergic stimulation.[68–69] In adolescents who actively smoke, LES pressure may be decreased as a result of the action of nicotine on adrenergic stimulation.

Other therapeutic measures can also trigger GER. Bronchial drainage and chest physiotherapy induce reflux as a result of positioning patients with the esophagus in a dependent position (the opposite of positions recommended for control of GER).[70, 71] The forced expiration and coughing during chest physical therapy also induce reflux by dramatically increasing abdominal pressures.

As the importance of nutrition in chronic lung disease receives increasing recognition, different forms of enteral supplemental nutrition are being successfully used, especially in patients with cystic fibrosis. The presence of a nasogastric tube interferes with esophageal sphincter competence; esophagitis and, in rare instances, stricture formation may result from the provision of enteral supplemental nutrition in patients with chronic lung disease.[72] The use of nocturnal enteral feedings in patients with cystic fibrosis was successful in one study even though significant GER occurred.[73] In another study, a short period of aggressive gavage improved nutrition and GER in infants with failure to thrive who had failed conventional antireflux therapy.[74] It is reasonable to elevate the head of the bed for patients with GER symptoms who are receiving gavage, and if heartburn or other symptoms continue, initiation of more aggressive medical therapy is indicated.

Placement of a gastrostomy tube can obviate the discomfort of a nasogastric tube while providing an access for enteral feeding. The development of procedures for percutaneous endoscopic placement of gastrostomy tubes in children is useful in gastrostomy feedings, not only for patients with severe dysphagia, but also as a means for providing adequate enteral nutrition for patients with consistent poor appetite or prolonged inadequate intake.

This type of gastrostomy placement avoids the need for abdominal surgery and the discomfort of a nasogastric tube.[75] It has been demonstrated in animals and in humans that the placement of a gastrostomy tube is conducive to reflux, probably by altering the angle of the esophagus as it enters the stomach.[75-77] The clinician should be alert to symptoms in patients with respiratory disease that may be caused by GER. Also, treatment of respiratory disorders may induce reflux and cause disease in the upper gastrointestinal tract that may exaggerate the respiratory problems.

DIAGNOSIS

Numerous pulmonary tests have been developed for evaluating lung function, and numerous gastroenterologic tests have been developed for documenting GER and evaluating esophageal function. Demonstration of initial disease in one system that is caused by dysfunction of the other system is difficult in the research setting and is impossible in many individual patients. Detailed and repeated history taking is of primary importance, especially in evaluating symptoms that occur only occasionally and are often absent during short periods of intense, sophisticated monitoring. Once alerted as to which factors are important, parents or other caretakers can often provide valuable insights into sequence and timing of symptoms. Tests used for diagnosing GER are outlined in Table 57–4.

DIAGNOSTIC TESTS

The first step in the diagnosis of GER is to document the presence of pathologic reflux; the *history* or simple observation may make the possibility obvious.[4] The most common symptom, vomiting, may not be present, or it may be accepted as normal and thus overlooked by the parents. Symptoms suggestive of reflux may not always be caused by GER. In infants, vomiting may be caused by food intolerance, pyloric stenosis, intestinal obstruction, compression of esophagus (e.g., vascular ring), or other causes. Coughing and choking may be caused by aspiration of gastric contents, deglutition problems, or both.

Some reflux is physiologic, and so the challenge is to distinguish between physiologic and pathologic reflux. The child should be observed for reflux during and after feeding. Several tests can document the presence of

Table 57–4. TESTS FOR DIAGNOSING GASTROESOPHAGEAL REFLUX

History and physical examination
Upper gastrointestinal series
Monitoring esophageal pH
Short-term Tuttle test
Prolonged monitoring
Gastric scintiscan
Esophageal endoscopy
Esophageal biopsy
Esophageal motility studies
Ultrasonography

abnormal or excessive GER. An *upper gastrointestinal series* or an *esophagogram* can help identify GER, detect other problems that can cause similar problems (such as a vascular ring or distal intestinal obstruction), and identify complications of GER (e.g., esophageal stricture). The observation time is short; in different studies, GER was detected in 50% to 85% of patients with GER, and false-positive results were noted in 25% to 30% of patients.[78–80] The experience of the radiologist performing the study is important. Perhaps the greatest value of the test is in ruling out many problems that cause similar symptoms.

Monitoring of esophageal pH after a meal of apple juice or sugar water *(Tuttle test)* identifies more than 90% of patients with reflux, but approximately 25% of patients identified by the Tuttle test have false-positive results.[79, 81, 82] The Tuttle test is a direct test for the presence of acid gastric contents (pH < 4) in the esophagus, in which the pH is normally neutral. In the diagnostic study, a pH probe is placed approximately 3 cm above the LES, and 300 ml of unsweetened apple juice or dilute hydrochloric acid are swallowed or placed in the stomach through a nasogastric tube. The esophageal pH is monitored for a minimum of 30 to 60 min. Two or more episodes of reflux are considered abnormal. An unbuffered or acid feeding is necessary. In the original test in adults, 0.1 N of hydrochloric acid was used because regular feeding can buffer gastric pH and make reflux undetectable for up to an hour after feedings.

Prolonged monitoring of esophageal pH for 18 to 24 h is considered the most sensitive test by many investigators and distinguishes normal and abnormal reflux correctly in more than 95% of cases.[79, 83, 84] Unfortunately, it is time consuming and costly and often requires hospitalization. Besides demonstrating abnormal GER, this test also has the advantage of documenting the frequency and duration of reflux episodes in the different positions while awake and asleep and enables therapy to be more individualized. The results can be quantified, and responses to therapy can be objectively measured.

A *gastric scintiscan,* or scanning over the esophagus after feeding of radioactive technetium, is a widely available test[85–88] that is extremely sensitive for detecting GER, but the specificity of the test is not very high.[45, 52, 87] The appearance of gastric material in the lungs on scintiscan is strong evidence of reflux and aspiration, but this finding is rare.

Esophagoscopy and *esophageal biopsy* can confirm the presence of significant reflux by demonstrating esophagitis.[79, 89–93] Many patients, especially infants, do not exhibit visible esophagitis, presumably because of decreased acid production in infancy and the fact that formula buffers gastric acidity for almost an hour after feedings.[90] Esophagoscopy is a direct method for visualization of complications of GER, such as esophageal strictures, or for the documentation of gross esophagitis. Visualization of the esophageal epithelium by endoscopy is more sensitive in the detection of esophagitis than is barium swallow. The absence of visual changes in esophageal epithelium on esophagoscopy does not rule out GER; histologic examination of esophageal biopsy specimens may be the only

way to detect esophageal inflammation in most patients. Fiberoptic endoscopy can easily be accomplished in outpatients with sedation and local anesthesia applied to the pharyngeal mucosa.

In a properly oriented, adequate biopsy specimen, changes in esophageal epithelium may indicate the presence of significant GER, even though no inflammatory cells are present. These histologic findings include an increase in the proliferating basal cells in the stratified squamous epithelium to more than 15% of the thickness of the esophageal mucosa and an increase in the length of the dermal peg to more than 65% of the thickness of esophageal mucosa. Esophageal biopsies directed by endoscopy yield specific results. Hypertrophy of the basal layer and extension of the dermal papilla in the stratified squamous epithelium of the esophagus are indicative of reflux with approximately 90% specificity.[79, 91–93] These findings are more readily visible in biopsy specimens that are obtained with a properly oriented Rubin suction biopsy tube or a similar instrument than in much smaller grasp biopsy specimens obtained through an endoscope, which are difficult to orient properly for sectioning.[93] The presence of polymorphonuclear neutrophils or eosinophils is evidence of more severe esophagitis, as is actual esophageal ulceration.[89–93]

Esophageal motility studies can provide information regarding sphincter tone and peristalsis but does not detect reflux. There is no strong correlation between reflux and LES pressure, although in patients with severe esophagitis, the pressure is low.[7, 11, 93, 94]

Ultrasonography can detect reflux of fluid into the esophagus, but experience with this modality in documenting reflux in children is extremely limited.[95]

Documenting a temporal relationship between GER and respiratory symptoms represents a second and more difficult level of evaluation (Table 57–5). A history of coughing and choking just after feeding and preceded by

Table 57–5. DEMONSTRATION OF TEMPORAL OR CAUSAL RELATIONSHIP BETWEEN RESPIRATORY SYMPTOMS AND GASTROESOPHAGEAL REFLUX

History
Demonstration of aspiration
  Upper gastrointestinal series
  Scintiscan
  Tracheal aspirate
    Gross inspection
    Lipid-laden macrophages
    Lactose assay
Reflux (pH) and acute symptom observed/recorded
  Monitoring esophageal pH
  Recording symptoms
    Cough, choking
    Stridor
    Wheeze
    Apnea
    Central obstruction
Induction of gastroesophageal reflux and symptoms
  Perfusion of esophagus with acid
  Observation: Subjective
  Polysonography
Improvement with treatment of gastroesophageal reflux

spitting of formula is extremely suggestive. If monitoring of esophageal pH is combined with observation, the physician can easily determine whether cough, apnea, stridor, or wheezing episodes occur after episodes of reflux or whether the coughing or wheezing precedes reflux.[24, 35, 52] A regular diet neutralizes gastric acidity for a period of time, and so the best evaluation of the immediate postprandial period requires use of acidified food such as apple juice or unbuffered liquids such as sugar water.[2] Respiratory symptoms may not occur instantaneously after reflux or with each bout of reflux. The temporal relationship of GER and respiratory symptoms may be further documented by combining the pH monitoring with several pulmonary function tests or monitoring of nasal airflow, pulse oximetry, or end–tidal carbon dioxide concentrations.[21]

CAUSAL OR TEMPORAL RELATIONSHIP WITH GER

Demonstrating a causal relationship between GER and respiratory symptoms represents a higher level of diagnostic specificity. A thorough history can be helpful. Demonstration of aspiration of gastric contents into the lungs is strong evidence of a causal relationship between the pulmonary problems and reflux. On occasion, this demonstration can be accomplished by noting aspiration of barium into the trachea during fluoroscopy after reflux or by noting the presence of a nucleotide in the lungs on a scintiscan. Direct aspiration of milk from the trachea or from an endotracheal or tracheostomy tube is strong evidence of a direct association, if aspiration and dysphagia during ingestion of the material can be ruled out. Assay of endotracheal suction fluid for the presence of lactose can reveal small amounts of milk that are not grossly visible.[96] Staining of tracheal aspiration samples for lipid-laden macrophages can reveal evidence of chronic, intermittent aspiration of gastric contents from reflux.[97]

Exacerbation of respiratory symptoms after induced or simulated reflux can provide strong evidence of a causal relationship. Thus demonstration of apnea and increasing respiratory effort after the infusion of a dilute acid into the esophagus but continuation of normal respiration after infusion of water or milk is strong evidence that the apnea is related to the presence of acid in gastric contents from reflux.[24, 52] Also, apnea during wakefulness is much more likely to be caused by GER than is apnea during sleep.[50]

In Bernstein's test, 0.1 N of hydrochloric acid or saline is infused into the proximal esophagus via a nasoesophageal tube.[98] It is not a test of reflux per se, but it was originally devised to simulate reflux and demonstrate that chest pain or other symptoms in adults were caused by GER. The test has been adapted for use in children to demonstrate that stridor or chest pain may occur after acidification of the esophagus.[52, 98] Such findings strongly suggest that the symptom was caused by GER. The finding of prolonged mean duration of reflux during sleep in the late postprandial period is strong evidence that GER and respiratory symptoms are causally related.[15] Prompt

Table 57–6. THERAPY OF GASTROESOPHAGEAL REFLUX

Treat respiratory symptoms
  Postural drainage before meals
  Induced cough before meals
Drugs that encourage gastroesophageal reflux
  Theophylline
  Beta-adrenergic agents
Positional therapy
Frequent small feedings
Enteral feeding
Thickened feedings
Prokinetic drugs
  Metoclopramide
  Bethanechol
  Cisapride*
  Domperidone*
Drugs that decrease gastric acid
  Cimetidine
  Ranitidine
  Famotidine
  Omeprazole
Drugs that neutralize gastric acid
  Antacids with alginic acid (Gaviscon)
Therapy to minimize aspiration
  Enteric feedings
  Fundoplication gastrostomy
Surgery of GER
  Nissen fundoplication

*Not available in the United States.

improvement of chronic respiratory symptoms after effective control of GER can provide strong circumstantial evidence of causality.[18, 24] Improvement may be immediate after surgical procedures for reflux, whereas improvement is more likely to be slower and less dramatic with medical therapy.

THERAPY

GER may be the primary problem or may be secondary to respiratory disease. Therapeutic strategies include treatment of the underlying respiratory disease, the respiratory sequelae of GER, GER itself, and its intestinal complications. Treatment of respiratory diseases is discussed only in the context of their effects on GER (Table 57–6).

RESPIRATORY THERAPY

Aggressive treatment of respiratory diseases to reduce forceful breathing efforts is important in the treatment of GER. Effective treatment of reactive airway disease and improved control of infection in patients with chronic diseases such as asthma, bronchopulmonary dysplasia, bronchiectasis, and cystic fibrosis will reduce major swings in intrathoracic and intra-abdominal pressure that are conducive to reflux, while simultaneously improving the primary pulmonary disease. Scheduling postural therapy and forced coughing sessions for before rather than after meals can markedly ameliorate reflux and vomiting in these patients.

Theophylline and beta-adrenergic drugs decrease the LES pressure and promote reflux; the clinical problem is more pronounced with theophylline.[59, 61, 63–65] When GER symptoms are made worse with theophylline therapy, it is reasonable to be more aggressive with the use of inhaled beta-adrenergic agents that cause fewer problems with GER and to discontinue theophylline. Avoidance of alcohol, tobacco, and caffeine, all of which increase gastric acidity or impede sphincter competence, is advisable in adolescents but is usually not a concern in younger patients.[67–69]

POSITIONING

Positioning is one of the oldest therapies in the management of GER and is based on the intuitive concept of keeping the gastroesophageal junction elevated to prevent reflux.[99] This type of treatment helps relieve symptoms of heartburns in adults and older children and is based on the assumption that the horizontal position may precipitate heartburn. Traditionally, positioning often was done only for a short period after meals. Prolonged pH monitoring studies have shown that reflux episodes usually occur without vomiting in children. Among patients with GER, reflux is especially frequent during sleep. In normal patients, reflux is very infrequent during sleep and most frequent after meals.[2] Thus patients with significant reflux should undergo positioning for as much of the day as possible.

The most effective position is prone with the head elevated 30 degrees.[100, 101] This position can easily be maintained by having a patient straddle a padded peg on an inclined plane or by the use of a harness to keep the patient from sliding. Positioning the patient supine with head elevated is not effective. Beyond 8 to 10 months of age, positional therapy is usually limited to keeping the patient upright during the day and raising the head of the bed 8 to 10 inches during sleep, because older patients do not readily tolerate being confined in the 30-degree head-elevated position for long periods of time.

Sitting upright is a minor improvement over the horizontal supine position. Orenstein and co-workers demonstrated that placing children under 6 weeks of age in an infant seat, a traditional form of therapy, caused more reflux on pH monitoring than did the horizontal and prone position.[102] It is assumed that the poor truncal tone in very young infants leads to slumping, causing increased abdominal pressure and GER. In older children, the authors and other investigators have noted improvement during pH monitoring in the upright position.[100]

FEEDING STRATEGIES

Changing the feeding schedule to smaller, more frequent feedings is a simple measure that is often overlooked. One extreme approach to small, frequent feedings is to use constant nasogastric feedings. Ferry and associates showed this approach can be effective in approximately half of patients who do not respond to conventional treatment.[74]

Use of thickened feedings has been encouraged since the early 1960s with empirical success in controlling symptoms.[1] Results of studies of esophageal pH monitoring with the use of thickened feedings are not in agreement.[103, 104] Some authors noted decreased acid exposure to the distal esophagus but did not always take into account the buffering capacity of thickened feedings. Using gastric scintiscan to document the number of reflux episodes and the number of vomiting episodes, Orenstein and co-workers found that the number of reflux episodes were unchanged with thickened feedings, which gives credence to negative findings.[105] However, the children receiving thickened feedings had fewer episodes of visible emesis, the total volume of emesis was lower, and the children were less irritable and slept more in the 2-h postprandial period. The addition of 15 ml of dried cereal powder per ounce of formula provides a 30 calorie/ounce formula that requires larger nipple holes but can be swallowed easily.[105]

PROKINETIC DRUGS

Drugs such as metoclopramide, bethanechol, domperidone, and cisapride are frequently used to treat GER.[106–122] Only the first two drugs are available in the United States at present. Justification for their use is based on several types of data. Improvement in various parameters of reflux noted on prolonged pH monitoring after a single dose of medication is one type of study.[111, 112, 114] This type of study may or may not be associated with clinical improvement. Improvement in esophageal pH monitoring studies after a course of drug therapy provides more convincing data, but usually the infants receive nondrug therapy as well, and the effect of the other therapy and the expected improvement with increasing age are confounding variables. Improvement in clinical scores obtained by independent observers and a double-blind placebo control protocol has been used only occasionally.[115]

Metoclopramide (Reglan), one of the most frequently used drugs in North America, is available in a liquid form for convenient oral administration. Infrequent side effects of this drug include methemoglobinemia (cited in rare reports) and occasional extrapyramidal signs, such as tremors that disappear when the dose is reduced.[119] If continued use of metoclopramide is critical, the tremors can be controlled with the use of antihistamines. Results of a pharmacokinetic study suggest that a dose of 0.15 mg/kg/dose every 6 h provides adequate drug levels.[118] Administration of the drug just before eating appears not to be warranted. These dosages should not be increased in newborns and occasionally need to be decreased in very small premature infants.

Domperidone, which has been available in Europe since the early 1980s can increase gastric motility at least acutely.[112, 113] Cisapride appears to be very promising, and several European controlled studies in children have shown a beneficial effect, including improvement of nighttime cough in patients with GER.[114, 116]

Use of antacids or H2-blockers can raise intragastric pH and significantly relieve heartburn.[120] It is also assumed that effective treatment of heartburn helps heal esophagitis, raises the esophageal sphincter pressure, and improves esophageal clearance of acid gastric contents. Several studies of the use of H2-blockers in adults provided inconsistent results concerning improvement of the esophagitis.[120] A multicenter study in Italian children showed that a 12-week course of cimetidine was associated with histologic improvement of esophagitis in children.[121] The improvement was more marked in patients with more severe esophagitis. Symptom scores also improved more in the children who received therapy than in the children who received placebo. It was unclear to what extent the clinical score reflected improvement in heartburn and pain as opposed to symptoms such as spitting and vomiting.

The greatest experience in children is with cimetidine, but ranitidine and famotidine are available in liquid oral preparations and are often used in older patients, even though they have not been approved for use in children. Omeprazole has been shown to be effective in treatment of esophagitis in adults.[122] It is a very potent inhibitor of gastric acid secretion, inhibiting H^+/K^+ adenosine triphosphatase at the secretory surface of the gastric parietal cell. The effectiveness and safety of this drug in children has not been demonstrated, and it should not be used routinely in children.

It is reasonable to use antacids in place of H2-blockers, but effective therapeutic doses are often associated with diarrhea, and frequent administration of the antacid is required. The diarrhea can be minimized by substituting the use of aluminum- for magnesium-containing antacids. Gaviscon, a combination of an antacid and an alginic acid that expands and tends to float at the top of the stomach and form a plug, has been shown to be effective.[123, 124] Severe esophagitis is much more common after the age of 6 months; this phenomenon is possibly related to the facts that formula feedings keep gastric contents above a pH of 4 for nearly an hour after feeding and that infants younger than 6 months are traditionally fed very frequently. In addition, gastric acid secretion appears to be lower in infants than in older children.[125] Patients with esophagitis have abnormal motility that may compromise sphincter competence and acid clearance; effective therapy should result in improvement of esophageal function.[6, 11, 126] The authors usually administer H2-blockers in cases of known or suspected esophagitis, but they administer it in conjunction with other therapy.

An aggressive approach to medical therapy usually results in improvement in symptoms, and if pulmonary problems such as cough, choking, apnea, or reactive airway disease are present and are related even partially to GER, they also improve. Improvement or control of GER often brings about only partial improvement in respiratory symptoms, especially asthma; positive results can be measured by documenting a decrease in need for asthma medications.[18] In reactive airway disease, GER may be only one of several stimuli causing bronchoconstriction. In other cases, long-lasting disease, such as bronchiectasis, may have developed, and resolution of pulmonary problems may be slow or incomplete. Patients with severe or chronic central nervous system disorders such as cerebral palsy often have problems with deglutition, GER, and respiratory symptoms. Problems in one of these three areas can aggravate problems in the other two, and treatment should be directed toward all problems.

SURGICAL MANAGEMENT

Use of a nasogastric or gastrostomy tube is often considered in children with chronic gagging, repeated aspiration, or poor feeding habits. Because placement of a gastrostomy tube has been shown to aggravate or cause GER, the physician must choose between creating a Stamm gastrostomy and antireflux procedure or merely creating a gastrostomy, possibly a percutaneous endoscopic gastrostomy.[76, 127-129] In the presence of esophagitis or if severe reflux is noted on prolonged esophageal monitoring, both a surgically placed gastrostomy and a reflux procedure are recommended. If GER is mild or within normal limits, a percutaneous endoscopic gastrostomy tube is placed. If placement of the gastrostomy tube aggravates or causes reflux, the patient is treated aggressively with medical therapy for GER, and an antireflux procedure is considered only if the patient does not respond. Some authors recommend the routine use of percutaneous endoscopic gastrostomy and reserve a surgical antireflux procedure for patients whose GER symptoms are not controlled with aggressive medical therapy.[127, 128] Those authors view the percutaneous endoscopic gastrostomy procedure as one with few risks that has a minimal recovery time and accept the fact that some patients would subsequently require an abdominal antireflux procedure.

When symptoms of GER persist despite a prolonged effort of at least 6 weeks with aggressive medical management or if there are recurrent and ongoing life-threatening complications of GER, a surgical antireflux procedure should be considered. Several surgical series of more than 150 patients without operative mortality have been reported.[70, 129-135] According to the experience of the authors, reflux can be controlled in 90% of the cases without surgery. Some investigators reported that repeat surgical procedures were needed in as many as 24% of the cases, although a failure rate of about 10% is more common.[132-135] Nissen fundoplication or a variation is presently the procedure most frequently performed. Control of GER does not guarantee cure of respiratory symptoms. In a series of 91 patients undergoing surgery for GER and respiratory problems, respiratory symptoms were well controlled in patients without other concomitant problems. In the presence of other problems, mainly neurologic, complete resolution of respiratory problems occurred in only 54% of the patients. This experience further illustrates the difficulty in demonstrating causality between GER and respiratory problems.

The late follow-up of children who have undergone antireflux procedures is very satisfying. Although 50% of adults experience return of heartburn within 60 months of surgery, normal pH levels were demonstrated in more than 90% of a group of children after prolonged follow-up.[136, 137] There were, however, minor problems (such as mild bloating from gas, slower eating, and mild swallowing disorders) that were not disabling and support the contention that the procedure should not be routinely recommended for control of minor symptoms. Carré noted that more than 60% of all patients with GER are well by the age of 18 months even without specific therapy.[3] The remainder improve more slowly, although in 5% a stricture develops, and about 5% die of inanition and chronic pneumonia in the absence of therapy. Developments in medical therapy such as prokinetic agents and antacid therapy have resulted in further improvement in the outcome of medical therapy. A review of in the authors' experience indicated that all children who failed medical therapy and were referred for reflux surgery had significant associated problems, whereas in a previous series, it was noted that only 35% of patients had associated problems.[31] The implication is that surgical therapy is increasingly being reported only in the most refractory cases.

REFERENCES

1. Carré IJ: Pediatric Gastroenterology. Oxford, England: Blackwell Scientific, 1975.
2. Jolley SG, Herbst JJ, Johnson DG, et al: Patterns of postcibal gastroesophageal reflux in symptomatic infants. Am J Surg 138:946–950, 1979.
3. Carré IJ: Natural history of partial thoracic stomach ("hiatus hernia") in children. Arch Dis Child 34:344–353, 1959.
4. Herbst JJ: Development of gastroesophageal reflux. In Lebenthal E (ed): Textbook of Gastroenterology and Nutrition in Infancy, 2nd ed, pp. 803–813. New York: Raven Press, 1989.
5. Boix-Ochoa J, Canals J: Maturation of the lower esophagus. J Pediatr Surg 11:749–756, 1976.
6. Herbst JJ, Book LS, Johnson DG, et al: The lower esophageal sphincter in gastroesophageal reflux in children. J Clin Gastroenterol 1:119–123, 1979.
7. Boix-Ochoa J: Address of honored guest: The physiologic approach to the management of gastric esophageal reflux. J Pediatr Surg 21:1032–1039, 1986.
8. Chrispin AR, Friedland GW, Wright DE: Some functional characteristics of the oesophageal vestibule in infants and children. Thorax 22:188–192, 1967.
9. Dodds WJ, Dent J, Hogan WJ, et al: Mechanisms of gastroesophageal reflux in patients with reflux esophagitis. N Engl J Med 307:1547–1552, 1982.
10. Byrne WJ, Campbell M, Ashcraft E, et al: A diagnostic approach to vomiting in severely retarded patients. Am J Dis Child 137:259–262, 1983.
11. Welch RW, Luckmann K, Ricks P, et al: Lower esophageal sphincter pressure in histologic esophagitis. Dig Dis Sci 25:420–426, 1980.
12. Arana J, Tovar JA: Motor efficiency of the refluxing esophagus in basal conditions and after acid challenge. J Pediatr Surg 24:1049–1054, 1989.
13. Helm JF, Dodds WJ, Pelc LR, et al: Effect of esophageal emptying and saliva on clearance of acid from the esophagus. N Engl J Med 310:284–288, 1984.
14. Orr WC, Johnson LF, Robinson MG: Effects of sleep on swallowing, esophageal peristalsis, and acid clearance. Gastroenterology 86:814–819, 1984.
15. Jolley SG, Herbst JJ, Johnson DG, et al: Esophageal pH monitoring during sleep identifies children with respiratory symptoms from gastroesophageal reflux. Gastroenterology 80:1501–1506, 1981.
16. Herbst JJ: Development of suck and swallow. In Lebenthal E (ed): Textbook of Human Gastrointestinal Development, 2nd ed, pp. 229–239. New York: Raven Press, 1989.
17. Christie DL, O'Grady LR, Mack DV: Incompetent lower esophageal sphincter and gastroesophageal reflux in recurrent acute pulmonary disease of infancy and childhood. J Pediatr 93:23–27, 1978.
18. Euler AR, Byrne WJ, Ament ME, et al: Recurrent pulmonary disease in children: A complication of gastroesophageal reflux. Pediatrics 63:47–51, 1979.
19. Bray GW: Recent advances in the treatment of asthma and hay fever. Practitioner 133:368–379, 1934.
20. Herve P, Denjean A, Jian R, et al: Intraesophageal perfusion of acid increases the bronchomotor response to methacholine and to isocapnic hyperventilation in asthmatic subjects. Am Rev Respir Dis 134:986–989, 1986.
21. Davis RS, Larsen GL, Grunstein MM: Respiratory response to intraesophageal acid infusion in asthmatic children during sleep. J Allergy Clin Immunol 72:393–398, 1983.
22. Ramenofsky ML, Leape LL: Continuous upper esophageal pH monitoring in infants and children with gastroesophageal reflux, pneumonia, and apneic spells. J Pediatr Surg 16:374–378, 1981.
23. Leape LL, Holder TM, Franklin JD, et al: Respiratory arrest in infants secondary to gastroesophageal reflux. Pediatrics 60:924–928, 1977.
24. Herbst JJ, Minton SD, Book LS: Gastroesophageal reflux causing respiratory distress and apnea in newborn infants. J Pediatr 95:763–768, 1979.
25. Carré IJ: Pulmonary infections in children with a partial thoracic stomach ('hiatus hernia'). Arch Dis Child 35:481–483, 1960.
26. McVeagh P, Howman-Giles R, Kemp A: Pulmonary aspiration studied by radionuclide milk scanning and barium swallow roentgenography. Am J Dis Child 141:917–921, 1987.
27. Knoblich R: Pulmonary granulomatosis caused by vegetable particles. Am Rev Respir Dis 99:380–389, 1969.
28. Sondheimer JM, Morris BA: Gastroesophageal reflux among severely retarded children. J Pediatr 94:710–714, 1979.
29. Cadman D, Richards J, Feldman W: Gastroesophageal reflux in severely retarded children. Dev Med Child Neurol 20:95–98, 1978.
30. Hillemeier C, Buchin PJ, Gryboski J: Esophageal dysfunction in Down's syndrome. J Pediatr Gastroenterol Nutr 1:101–104, 1982.
31. Jolley SG, Herbst JJ, Johnson DG, et al: Surgery in children with gastroesophageal reflux and respiratory symptoms. J Pediatr 96:194–198, 1980.
32. Fonkalsrud EW: Gastroesophageal fundoplication for reflux following repair of esophageal atresia: Experience with nine patients. Arch Surg 114:48–51, 1979.
33. Werlin SL, Dodds WJ, Hogan WJ, et al: Esophageal function in esophageal atresia. Dig Dis Sci 26:796–800, 1981.
34. Jolley SG, Johnson DG, Roberts CC, et al: Patterns of gastroesophageal reflux in children following repair of esophageal atresia and distal tracheoesophageal fistula. Pediatr Surg 15:857–862, 1980.
35. Berquist WE, Rachelefsky GS, Kadden M, et al: Gastroesophageal reflux–associated recurrent pneumonia and chronic asthma in children. Pediatrics 68:29–35, 1981.
36. Hoyoux C, Forget P, Lambrechts L, et al: Chronic bronchopulmonary disease and gastroesophageal reflux in children. Pediatr Pulmonol 1:149–153, 1985.
37. Gustafsson PM, Kjellman NI, Tibbling L: Oesophageal function and symptoms in moderate and severe asthma. Acta Paediatr Scand 75:729–736, 1986.
38. Baer M, Maki M, Nurminen J, et al: Esophagitis and findings of long-term esophageal pH recording in children with repeated lower respiratory tract symptoms. J Pediatr Gastroenterol Nutr 5:187–190, 1986.
39. Martin ME, Grunstein MM, Larsen GL: The relationship of gastroesophageal reflux to nocturnal wheezing in children with asthma. Ann Allergy 49:318–322, 1982.
40. Shapiro GG, Christie DL: Gastroesophageal reflux in steroid-dependent asthmatic youths. Pediatrics 63:207–212, 1979.
41. Andersen LI, Schmidt A, Bundgaard A: Pulmonary function and acid application in the esophagus. Chest 90:358–363, 1986.
42. Denjean A, Herve P, Simonneau G, et al: Effects of acid infusion into the esophagus on airflow obstruction and bronchial hyperreactivity in adult asthmatic patients. Chest 87(Suppl):201S–202S, 1985.
43. Rudolph CD, Heyman MB, Rose DB, et al: Lack of association between gastroesophageal reflux and delayed gastric emptying in young infants. Gastroenterology 88:1562, 1985.
44. Mansfield LE, Hameister HH, Spaulding HS, et al: The role of the vagus nerve in airway narrowing caused by intraesophageal hydrochloric acid provocation and esophageal distention. Ann Allergy 47:431–434, 1981.
45. Sacre L, Vandenplas Y: Gastroesophageal reflux associated with

respiratory abnormalities during sleep. J Pediatr Gastroenterol Nutr 9:28–33, 1989.

46. Downing SE, Lee JC: Laryngeal chemosensitivity: A possible mechanism for sudden infant death. Pediatrics 55:640–649, 1975.

47. Harned HS, Myracle J, Ferreiro J: Respiratory suppression and swallowing from introduction of fluids into the laryngeal region of the lamb. Pediatr Res 12:1003–1009, 1978.

48. Orenstein SR, Kocoshis SA, Orenstein DM, et al: Stridor and gastroesophageal reflux: Diagnostic use of intraluminal esophageal acid perfusion (Bernstein test). Pediatr Pulmonol 3:420–424, 1987.

49. Nielson DW, Heldt GP, Tooley WH: Stridor and gastroesophageal reflux in infants. Pediatrics 85:1034–1039, 1990.

50. Spitzer AR, Boyle JT, Tuchman DN, et al: Awake apnea associated with gastroesophageal reflux: A specific clinical syndrome. J Pediatr 104:200–205, 1984.

51. Heyman S, Kirkpatrick JA, Winter HS, et al: An improved radionuclide method for the diagnosis of gastroesophageal reflux and aspiration in children (milk scan). Radiology 131:479–482, 1979.

52. McVeagh P, Howman-Giles R, Kemp A: Pulmonary aspiration studied by radionuclide milk scanning and barium swallow roentgenography. Am J Dis Child 141:917–921, 1987.

53. Walsh JK, Farrell MK, Keenan WJ, et al: Gastroesophageal reflux in infants: Relation to apnea. J Pediatr 99:197–201, 1981.

54. Ariagno RL, Guilleminault C, Baldwin R, et al: Movement and gastroesophageal reflux in awake term infants with "near miss" SIDS, unrelated to apnea. J Pediatr 100:894–897, 1982.

55. Shay SS, Myers RL, Johnson LF: Hiccups associated with reflux esophagitis. Gastroenterology 87:204–207, 1984.

56. Gluck M, Pope CE: Chronic hiccups and gastroesophageal reflux disease: The acid perfusion test as a provocative maneuver. Ann Intern Med 105:219–220, 1986.

57. Scott RB, O'Loughlin EV, Gall DG: Gastroesophageal reflux in patients with cystic fibrosis. J Pediatr 106:223–227, 1985.

58. Bendig DW, Seilheimer DK, Wagner ML, et al: Complications of gastroesophageal reflux in patients with cystic fibrosis. J Pediatr 100:536–540, 1982.

59. Goyal RK, Rattan S: Mechanism of the lower esophageal sphincter relaxation: Action of prostaglandin E_1 and theophylline. J Clin Invest 52:337–341, 1973.

60. Berquist WE, Rachelefsky GS, Kadden M, et al: Effect of theophylline on gastroesophageal reflux in normal adults. J Allergy Clin Immunol 67:407–411, 1981.

61. Stein MR, Towner TG, Weber RW, et al: The effect of theophylline on the lower esophageal sphincter pressure. Ann Allergy 45:238–241, 1980.

62. Vandenplas Y, de Wolf D, Sacre L: Influence of xanthines on gastroesophageal reflux in infants at risk for sudden infant death syndrome. Pediatrics 77:807–810, 1986.

63. Zfass AM, Prince R, Allen FN, et al: Inhibitory beta adrenergic receptors in the human distal esophagus. Am J Dig Dis 15:303–310, 1970.

64. Christensen J: Effects of drugs on esophageal motility. Arch Intern Med 136:532–537, 1976.

65. DiMarino AJ, Cohen S: Effect of an oral beta$_2$-adrenergic agonist on lower esophageal sphincter pressure in normals and in patients with achalasia. Dig Dis Sci 27:1063–1066, 1982.

66. Berquist WE, Rachelefsky GS, Rowshan N, et al: Quantitative gastroesophageal reflux and pulmonary function in asthmatic children and normal adults receiving placebo, theophylline, and metaproterenol sulfate therapy. J Allergy Clin Immunol 73:253–258, 1984.

67. Foster LJ, Trudeau WL, Goldman AL: Bronchodilator effects on gastric acid secretion. JAMA 241:2613–2615, 1979.

68. Dennish GW, Castell DO: Inhibitory effect of smoking on the lower esophageal sphincter. N Engl J Med 284:1136–1137, 1971.

69. Rattan S, Goyal RK: Effect of nicotine on the lower esophageal sphincter: Studies on the mechanism of action. Gastroenterology 69:154–159, 1975.

70. Lilly JR, Randolph JG: Hiatal hernia and gastroesophageal reflux in infants and children. J Thorac Cardiovasc Surg 55:42–54, 1968.

71. Foster AC, Voyles JB, Murphy SA: Twenty-four-hour pH monitoring in children with cystic fibrosis: Association of chest physical therapy to gastroesophageal reflux [Abstract]. Pediatr Res 17:188A, 1983.

72. Spiliopoulos A, Megevand R: Oesophagite peptique stenosante apres sondage oeso-gastrique. Helv Chir Acta 47:527–532, 1980.

73. Scott RB, O'Loughlin EV, Gall DG: Gastroesophageal reflux in patients with cystic fibrosis. J Pediatr 106:223–227, 1985.

74. Ferry GD, Selby M, Pietro TJ: Clinical response to short-term nasogastric feeding in infants with gastroesophageal reflux and growth failure. J Pediatr Gastroenterol Nutr 2:57–61, 1983.

75. Grunow JE, al-Hafidh A, Tunell WP: Gastroesophageal reflux following percutaneous endoscopic gastrostomy in children. J Pediatr Surg 24:42–44, 1989.

76. Jolley SG, Tunell WP, Hoelzer DJ, et al: Lower esophageal pressure changes with tube gastrostomy: A causative factor of gastroesophageal reflux in children? J Pediatr Surg 21:624–627, 1986.

77. Canal DF, Vane DW, Goto S, et al: Reduction of lower esophageal sphincter pressure with Stamm gastrostomy. J Pediatr Surg 22:54–57, 1987.

78. Arasu TS, Wyllie R, Fitzgerald JF, et al: Gastroesophageal reflux in infants and children—comparative accuracy of diagnostic methods. J Pediatr 96:798–803, 1980.

79. Meyers WF, Roberts CC, Johnson DG, et al: Value of tests for evaluation of gastroesophageal reflux in children. J Pediatr Surg 20:515–520, 1985.

80. McCauley RG, Darling DB, Leonidas JC, et al: Gastroesophageal reflux in infants and children: A useful classification and reliable physiologic technique for its demonstration. AJR 130:47–50, 1978.

81. Euler AR, Ament ME: Detection of gastroesophageal reflux in the pediatric-age patient by esophageal intraluminal pH probe measurement (Tuttle test). Pediatrics 60:65–68, 1977.

82. Tuttle SG, Grossman MI: Detection of gastro-esophageal reflux by simultaneous measurement of intraluminal pressure and pH. Proc Soc Exp Biol 98:225–227, 1958.

83. Euler AR, Byrne WJ: Twenty-four-hour esophageal intraluminal pH probe testing: A comparative analysis. Gastroenterology 80:957–961, 1981.

84. Vandenplas Y, Sacre-Smits L: Continuous 24-hour esophageal pH monitoring in 285 asymptomatic infants 0–15 months old. J Pediatr Gastroenterol Nutr 6:220–224, 1978.

85. Blumhagen JD, Rudd TG, Christie DL: Gastroesophageal reflux in children: Radionuclide gastroesophagography. AJR 135:1001–1004, 1980.

86. Fisher RS, Malmud LS, Roberts GS, et al: Gastroesophageal (GE) scintiscanning to detect and quantitate GE reflux. Gastroenterology 70:301–308, 1976.

87. Heyman S, Kirkpatrick JA, Winter HS, et al: An improved radionuclide method for the diagnosis of gastroesophageal reflux and aspiration in children (Milk scan). Radiology 131:479–482, 1979.

88. Gonzalez-Fernandez F, Arguelles-Martin F, Rodriguez de Quesada B, et al: Gastroesophageal scintigraphy: A useful screening test for GE reflux. J Pediatr Gastroenterol Nutr 6:217–219, 1987.

89. Biller JA, Winter HS, Grand RJ, et al: Are endoscopic changes predictive of histologic esophagitis in children? J Pediatr 103:215–218, 1983.

90. Leape LL, Bhan I, Ramenofsky ML: Esophageal biopsy in the diagnosis of reflux esophagitis. J Pediatr Surg 16:379–384, 1981.

91. Ismail-Beigi F, Horton PF, Pope CE: Histological consequences of gastroesophageal reflux in man. Gastroenterology 58:163–174, 1970.

92. Shub MD, Ulshen MH, Hargrove CB, et al: Esophagitis: A frequent consequence of gastroesophageal reflux in infancy. J Pediatr 107:881–884, 1985.

93. Black DD, Haggitt RC, Orenstein SR, et al: Esophagitis in infants. Gastroenterology 98:1408–1414, 1990.

94. Dodds WJ, Dent J, Jogan WJ, et al: Mechanisms of gastroesophageal reflux in patients with reflux esophagitis. N Engl J Med 307:1547–1552, 1982.

95. Naik DR, Moore DJ: Ultrasound diagnosis of gastroesophageal reflux. Arch Dis Child 59:366–367, 1984.

96. Hopper AO, Kwong LK, Stevenson DK, et al: Detection of gastric contents in tracheal fluid of infants by lactose assay. J Pediatr 102:415–418, 1983.

97. Williams HE, Freeman M: Milk inhalation pneumonia: The significance of fat filled macrophages in tracheal secretions. Aust Paediatr J 9:286–288, 1973.

98. Berezin S, Medow MS, Glassman M, et al: Use of intraesophageal

acid perfusion test in provoking nonspecific chest pain in children. J Pediatrics 115:709–712, 1989.

99. Carré IJ: Postural treatment of children with a partial thoracic stomach (hiatus hernia). Arch Dis Child 35:569–580, 1960.

100. Meyers WF, Herbst JJ: Effectiveness of positioning therapy for gastroesophageal reflux. Pediatrics 69:768–772, 1982.

101. Orenstein SR, Whitington PF: Positioning for prevention of infant gastroesophageal reflux. J Pediatr 103:534–537, 1983.

102. Orenstein SR, Whitington PF, Orenstein DM: The infant seat as treatment for gastroesophageal reflux. N Engl J Med 309:760–763, 1983.

103. Bailey DJ, Andres JM, Danek GD, et al: Lack of efficacy of thickened feeding as treatment for gastroesophageal reflux. J Pediatr 110:187–189, 1987.

104. Ramenofsky ML, Leape LL: Continuous upper esophageal pH monitoring in infants and children with gastroesophageal reflux, pneumonia, and apneic spells. J Pediatr Surg 16:374–378, 1981.

105. Orenstein SR, Magill HL, Brooks P: Thickening of infant feedings for therapy of gastroesophageal reflux. J Pediatr 110:181–186, 1987.

106. Euler AR: Use of bethanechol for the treatment of gastroesophageal reflux. J Pediatr 96:321–324, 1980.

107. Thanik KD, Chey WY, Shah AN, et al: Reflux esophagitis: Effect of oral bethanechol on symptoms and endoscopic findings. Ann Intern Med 93:805–808, 1980.

108. Sondheimer JM, Mintz HL, Michaels M: Bethanechol treatment of gastroesophageal reflux in infants. J Pediatr 104:128–131, 1984.

109. Strickland AD, Chang JH: Results of treatment of gastroesophageal reflux with bethanechol. J Pediatr 103:311–315, 1983.

110. Saco LS, Orlando RC, Levinson SL, et al: Double-blind controlled trial of bethanechol and antacid versus placebo and antacid in the treatment of erosive esophagitis. Gastroenterology 82:1369–1373, 1982.

111. Orenstein SR, Lofton SW, Orenstein DM: Bethanechol for pediatric gastroesophageal reflux: A prospective, blind, controlled study. J Pediatr Gastroenterol Nutr 5:549–555, 1986.

112. Grill BB, Hillemeier AC, Semeraro LA, et al: Effects of domperidone therapy on symptoms and upper gastrointestinal motility in infants with gastroesophageal reflux. J Pediatr 106:311–316, 1985.

113. De Loore I, Van Ravensteyn H, Ameryckx L: Domperidone drops in the symptomatic treatment of chronic paediatric vomiting and regurgitation: A comparison with metoclopramide. Postgrad Med J 55:40–42, 1979.

114. Rode H, Stunden RJ, Millar AJ, Cywes S: Esophageal pH assessment of gastroesophageal reflux in 18 patients and the effect of two prokinetic agents: Cisapride and metoclopramide. J Pediatr Surg 22:931–934, 1987.

115. Vandenplas Y, Deneyer M, Verlinden M, et al: Gastroesophageal reflux incidence and respiratory dysfunction during sleep in infants: Treatment with cisapride. J Pediatr Gastroenterol Nutr 8:31–36, 1989.

116. Saye Z, Forget PP: Effect of cisapride on esophageal pH monitoring in children with reflux-associated bronchopulmonary disease. J Pediatr Gastroenterol Nutr 8:327–332, 1989.

117. Machida HM, Forbes DA, Gall DG, et al: Metoclopramide in gastroesophageal reflux of infancy. J Pediatr 112:483–487, 1988.

118. Kearns GL, Butler HL, Lane JK, et al: Metoclopramide pharmacokinetics and pharmacodynamics in infants with gastroesophageal reflux. J Pediatr Gastroenterol Nutr 7:823–829, 1988.

119. Terrin BN, McWilliams NB, Maurer HM: Side effects of metoclopramide as an antiemetic in childhood cancer chemotherapy. J Pediatr 104:138–140, 1984.

120. Richter JE: Gastro-Esophageal Reflux Disease. Mount Kisco, NY: Futura, 1985.

121. Cucchiara S, Gobio-Casali L, Balli F, et al: Cimetidine treatment of reflux esophagitis in children: An Italian multicentric study. J Pediatr Gastroenterol Nutr 8:150–156, 1989.

122. Hetzel DJ, Dent J, Reed WD, et al: Healing and relapse of severe peptic esophagitis after treatment with omeprazole. Gastroenterology 95:903–912, 1988.

123. Weldon AP, Robinson MJ: Trial of Gaviscon in the treatment of gastro-oesophageal reflux of infancy. Aust Paediatr J 8:279–281, 1972.

124. Forbes D, Hodgson M, Hill R: The effect of Gaviscon and metoclopramide in gastroesophageal reflux in children. J Pediatr Gastroenterol Nutr 5:556–559, 1986.

125. Johnson RJ: Functional development of the stomach. Annu Rev Physiol 47:199–215, 1985.

126. Kahrilas PJ, Dodds WJ, Hogan WJ, et al: Esophageal peristaltic dysfunction in peptic esophagitis. Gastroenterology 91:897–904, 1986.

127. Langer JC, Wesson DE, Ein SH, et al: Feeding gastrostomy in neurologically impaired children: Is an antireflux procedure necessary? J Pediatr Gastroenterol Nutr 7:837–841, 1988.

128. Gauderer MW: Feeding gastrostomy or feeding gastrostomy plus antireflux procedure? J Pediatr Gastroenterol Nutr 7:795–796, 1988.

129. Fonkalsrud EW, Foglia RP, Ament ME, et al: Operative treatment for the gastroesophageal reflux syndrome in children. J Pediatr Surg 24:525–529, 1989.

130. Johnson DG, Jolley SG, Herbst JJ, et al: Surgical selection of infants with gastroesophageal reflux. J Pediatr Surg 16:587–594, 1981.

131. Ashcraft KW, Holder TM: Pediatric Esophageal Surgery. Orlando, FL: Grune & Stratton, 1986.

132. Ashcraft KW, Goodwin CD, Amoury RW, et al: Thal fundoplication: A simple and safe operative treatment for gastroesophageal reflux. J Pediatr Surg 13:643–647, 1978.

133. Leape L: Gastroesophageal reflux. In Gellis SS (eds): Proceedings of the 76th Ross Conference on Pediatric Research, pp. 30–35. Columbus, OH: Ross Laboratories, 1979.

134. Tunell WP, Smith EI, Carson JA: Gastroesophageal reflux in childhood: The dilemma of surgical success. Ann Surg 197:560–565, 1983.

135. Opie JC, Chaye H, Fraser GC: Fundoplication and pediatric esophageal manometry: Actuarial analysis over 7 years. J Pediatr Surg 22:935–938, 1987.

136. Woodward ER, Thomas HF, McAlhany JC: Comparison of crural repair and Nissen fundoplication in the treatment of esophageal hiatus hernia with peptic esophagitis. Ann Surg 173:782–792, 1971.

137. Harnsberger JK, Corey JJ, Johnson DG, et al: Long-term follow-up surgery for gastroesophageal reflux in infants and children. J Pediatr 102:505–508, 1983.

58 HEMOPTYSIS

BERYL J. ROSENSTEIN, M.D.

Hemoptysis, defined as the expectoration of blood or blood-tinged sputum, is potentially life-threatening but, fortunately, an unusual occurrence in the pediatric age group. Over a 10-year period at a large pediatric referral center, hemoptysis was diagnosed in only 40 children.[1] In seven of these children, hemoptysis was the sole presenting manifestation; in the remaining patients, hemoptysis was associated with other symptoms, often fever and cough. The amount of bleeding was usually small; only two children experienced a blood loss in excess of 200 ml. Because hemoptysis often is a sign of significant underlying disease and may be life-threatening, patients with bleeding should undergo a rapid and complete evaluation. If the blood loss is more extensive than blood-tinged sputum or mild bleeding, the evaluation is best performed in a hospital setting in collaboration with consultants who have expertise in pediatric pulmonology and pediatric endoscopy.

The majority of children who are brought to medical attention because of "spitting up blood" have an identifiable source of bleeding outside the lower respiratory tract, usually epistaxis, gingivitis, pharyngeal ulceration, or trauma to the oropharynx.[2, 3] At times, it may be difficult to differentiate hemoptysis from hematemesis (Table 58–1).[4] In hematemesis, the blood is dark red or brownish in color, may contain food particles, and has an acid pH; bleeding is usually preceded by nausea or accompanied by retching. In hemoptysis, the blood is usually bright red and frothy, may be mixed with sputum, and has an alkaline pH; such bleeding may be preceded by a gurgling noise in the large airways and is usually accompanied by coughing. Older patients with bleeding in the lung may describe a vague sensation that enables them to localize the site of the bleeding. It is sometimes difficult to determine the origin of bleeding when both coughing and vomiting are present. In infants, swallowed blood originating

in the lungs may be vomited in the absence of coughing. Therefore, the possibility that the source of bleeding is in the respiratory tract should be considered in children with unexplained hematemesis, particularly if there are chest radiograph abnormalities. Children under the age of 6 years rarely expectorate sputum, and, in this age group, the presence of hemoptysis may not be apparent unless the amount of bleeding is large.

The lung receives its blood supply from two major sources: the larger, lower pressure pulmonary arterial circulation and the smaller, higher pressure systemic bronchial arterial circulation. These two circulations are often linked by arterial and venous collateral vessels. Bleeding from either source can cause moderate to massive hemoptysis, but because of the pressure gradient from the systemic to the pulmonary circulation, bronchial arterial bleeding is often massive. Children who have a hard, forceful cough may produce sputum that has small streaks of blood on the surface but that is not mixed with blood. This finding may be seen in association with respiratory tract infections and is usually of little clinical significance.

The treatment of hemoptysis is the management of the underlying disorder, making a correct etiologic diagnosis mandatory. In adults, hemoptysis is a relatively common occurrence. The leading causes are chronic bronchitis and bronchiectasis, lung cancer, and tuberculosis.[4] However, almost any disease that affects the respiratory tract can result in hemoptysis. The number of disorders associated with hemoptysis is not as large in children as in adults but is nevertheless extensive (Table 58–2). The most common cause is infection, followed by aspiration of a foreign body.[1] Many of the underlying conditions occur infrequently and may be difficult to diagnose.

EVALUATION

Evaluation of the patient with hemoptysis should begin with a detailed history and physical examination. History should be elicited as to underlying illnesses, fever, cough, sputum production, stridor, wheezing, dyspnea, joint pain, weight loss, menstrual history, family illnesses, recent trauma, prior episodes of bleeding, choking episodes, medication use, substance abuse, exposure to toxins, and travel to areas endemic for parasitic infestations and mycobacterial disease. History of travel is especially pertinent because of the large-scale immigration from Southeast Asia to the United States. Some patients with

Table 58–1. DIFFERENTIATION OF HEMOPTYSIS FROM HEMATEMESIS

Variable	Hemoptysis	Hematemesis
Color	Bright red and frothy	Dark red or brown
pH	Alkaline	Acid
Consistency	May be mixed with sputum	May contain food particles
Symptoms	Preceded by gurgling noise; accompanied by coughing	Preceded by nausea Accompanied by retching

Table 58–2. CAUSES OF HEMOPTYSIS IN CHILDREN

Infection	**Autoimmune Disorders**
Bacterial	Wegener's granulomatosis
Lung abscess	Pulmonary hemosiderosis
Necrotizing pneumonia	Milk allergy
Tuberculosis	Goodpasture's syndrome
Bronchiectasis (cystic fibrosis,	Collagen vascular disease
immune deficiency, immotile	**Trauma**
cilia)	*Compression or Crush Injury*
Fungal	* Iatrogenic*
Actinomycosis	Postsurgical
Aspergillosis	Diagnostic lung puncture
Coccidioidomycosis	Transbronchial biopsy
Histoplasmosis	*Inhalation of Toxins*
Parasitic	**Neoplastic Conditions**
Echinococcosis (hydatid disease)	*Endobronchial Metastases*
Paragonimiasis	*Primary Lung Tumors*
Strongyloidiasis	Benign (hamartoma, neurogenic
Foreign Bodies	tumors)
Congenital Defects	Malignant (bronchial adenoma,
Cardiovascular	bronchogenic carcinoma,
Congenital heart defects	pulmonary blastoma)
Absent pulmonary artery	*Endometriosis*
Arteriovenous malformation	**Drug Induced**
Hemangiomatous malformation	Propylthiouracil
Telangiectasia (Osler-Weber-	**Pulmonary Embolism**
Rendu syndrome)	**Hemoglobinopathy With**
Other	**Pulmonary Infarct**
Pulmonary sequestration	**Factitious**
Bronchogenic cyst	
Intrathoracic enteric cyst	
Vasculitis	
Periarteritis nodosa	

hemoptysis, however, are otherwise asymptomatic and give an entirely negative history.

In a child with presumed hemoptysis, it must first be determined whether the blood originated from the lungs or lower airways or from the mouth, upper airway, or gastrointestinal tract. Careful examination of the nasopharynx and oral cavity for bleeding sites is essential. Nasopharyngoscopy and laryngoscopy may be helpful. Pertinent physical findings include saddle-nose deformity, bruits, thrills, unequal chest wall movement and air entry, abnormal breath sounds (especially localized wheezing heard with bronchial lesions and foreign bodies), pleural rub, heart murmur, hypertension, digital clubbing, lymphadenopathy, hepatosplenomegaly, hemangiomas, telangiectases, neuropathies, deep venous thrombosis, and evidence of trauma to the head, neck, or chest.

RADIOGRAPHIC EVALUATION

If the source of bleeding is not apparent on the basis of the history and physical examination, a chest radiograph is the next step in the evaluation.[5] The most common abnormalities found on check radiographs are atelectasis and parenchymal and interstitial infiltrates. Other helpful findings include localized air trapping, pulmonary nodules, hilar adenopathy, pleural effusion, pneumothorax, cardiomegaly, and foreign bodies. Ring shadows and parallel lines represent thick-walled bronchi and suggest bronchiectasis. Preferential blood flow to the upper lobes

is an early radiographic feature of pulmonary venous obstruction. In one third of children with hemoptysis, the initial radiograph is normal; however, a pulmonary source for the bleeding is eventually identified in half of patients with negative chest radiographs.[1]

Inspiratory and expiratory films are helpful in evaluating for the presence of a partially obstructing endobronchial foreign body. The lung on the side of the foreign body exhibits air trapping on expiration in relation to the normal side. On a decubitus view, the side that does not deflate normally in the dependent position is the side with air trapping. With complete obstruction secondary to a foreign body, there is obstructive atelectasis or pneumonia. High-kilovoltage films can be helpful for better visualization of the upper airway and in defining mass lesions. Fluoroscopy can be used to (1) confirm questionable parenchymal lesions on plain film; (2) localize an identified lesion or mass on a chest radiograph to lung parenchyma, pleura, chest wall, mediastinum, or vascular structures; or (3) identify and localize a suspected bronchial foreign body causing air trapping when findings are equivocal or not apparent on chest radiographs. An esophagogram may be helpful in localizing a mass to the middle mediastinum. On the basis of the results of the radiographic evaluation, the diagnostic workup may require a number of laboratory and imaging procedures.

LABORATORY EVALUATION

A variety of laboratory tests (Table 58–3) may be helpful. These include a complete blood count and indices; eosinophil count; erythrocyte sedimentation rate; urinal-

Table 58–3. LABORATORY TESTS FOR EVALUATING HEMOPTYSIS IN CHILDREN

Cytology
Bronchial secretions: for malignant cells, hemosiderin-laden macrophages
Pleural fluid
Hematology
Complete blood count
Eosinophil count
Erythrocyte sedimentation rate
Prothrombin/partial thromboplastin time
Microbiologic Studies
Gastric aspirate: for ova, parasites, hemosiderin-laden macrophages, mycobacteria
Sputum stain: for bacteria (Gram's stain), fungi (potassium hydroxide), mycobacteria (fluorochrome)
Sputum culture: for bacteria, fungi, mycobacteria
Stool sample: for ova and parasites
Renal Function Studies
Creatinine clearance
Renal biopsy: for histologic study and immunofluorescence stains
Urinalysis
Serologic Studies
Antiglomerular basement membrane antibody
Antinuclear antibody test
Lupus erythematosus cell preparation
Tests for bacteria, fungi, parasites
Serum Immunoglobulins
Skin Test Reactions
Cow's milk constituents
Aspergillus, Echinococcus, mycobacteria
Sweat Test

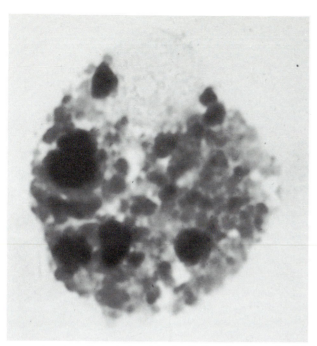

Figure 58–1. Gastric aspirate, stained with Prussian blue, showing a hemosiderin-laden macrophage in an infant with idiopathic pulmonary hemosiderosis.

Table 58–4. DIAGNOSTIC IMAGING AND NUCLEAR MEDICINE STUDIES USEFUL IN THE EVALUATION OF HEMOPTYSIS

Angiography
Digital subtraction
Pulmonary
Thoracic
Bronchography (in Conjunction With Bronchoscopy)
Computed Tomography
Chest and Upper Airway Radiography
Fluoroscopy
High-kilovoltage films
Inspiration-expiration films
Plain films
Magnetic Resonance Imaging
Ventilation/Perfusion Scanning
Radionuclide scan with radiolabeled red blood cells

ysis; arterial blood gas measurements; skin test for *Mycobacterium, Aspergillus,* and *Echinococcus;* clotting studies; sputum cytologic studies; and cultures for bacteria, fungi, and mycobacteria. Gastric aspirates can be examined for ova, parasites, and hemosiderin-laden macrophages (hemosiderosis) (Fig. 58–1) and cultured for mycobacteria. Other helpful procedures include measurement of sweat electrolyte concentration (cystic fibrosis); milk precipitins in serum (milk allergy, hemosiderosis); and antinuclear antibody, lupus erythematosus cell preparation, and rheumatoid factor (collagen vascular disease). In patients with hemoptysis and renal involvement (Goodpasture's syndrome, collagen vascular disease, Wegener's granulomatosis), renal function studies, measurement of antiglomerular basement membrane antibody, and renal biopsy may be needed for a definitive diagnosis.

DIAGNOSTIC IMAGING

Computed tomography (CT) may reveal radiographically unrecognized parenchymal infiltrates or foreign bodies and is usually the procedure of choice for further defining the anatomy of an abnormality found on chest radiograph (Table 58–4).[5] It can outline the extent of a mass and properly localize it to the anterior, middle, or posterior mediastinum, lung parenchyma, pleura, chest wall, or spine. The trachea and major proximal bronchi are well defined. CT is good for the detection of cystic bronchiectasis, broncholithiasis, and endobronchial obstruction secondary to adenoma or blood clot. The use of intravenous contrast identifies vascular structures and can show whether a suspected mass is vascular in nature. The internal characteristics of a mass can be identified;

calcification, hemorrhage, and fat can be differentiated by their relative densities. It may also be useful in guiding diagnostic procedures.

Magnetic resonance imaging (MRI) gives superior soft tissue contrast resolution and is useful in the evaluation of the mediastinum and hila.[5] Because vessels can be distinguished from other mediastinal structures, this technique can be used to demonstrate arteriovenous malformations and congenital anomalies of the pulmonary arteries. Thoracic vessels and spinal cord contents can be imaged directly without the need for intravenous or intrathecal contrast. Disadvantages include the need for sedation in young children, loss of spatial resolution, long acquisition time, impact of respiratory motion, and inability to detect calcification.

Conventional angiography is useful for the evaluation of congenital malformations of the lungs and abnormalities of pulmonary vessels (i.e., pulmonary sequestration, arteriovenous malformations, pulmonary embolus, and congenital anomalies of the pulmonary vessels). A small percentage of pulmonary arteriovenous malformations are systemically supplied by intercostal and bronchial arteries and are detected only by thoracic angiography. Digital subtraction angiography can be used to define the blood supply to a pulmonary sequestration or arteriovenous malformation (Fig. 58–2).

Ultrasonography is of limited value in the evaluation of the chest; however, it may be helpful in distinguishing between a cystic mass and a solid intrathoracic mass.

Ventilation/perfusion scanning is helpful in evaluating regional lung perfusion and ventilation. This procedure can reveal a decrease in pulmonary blood flow (i.e., pulmonary artery agenesis or hypoplasia, and pulmonary embolus). The hallmark of a pulmonary embolus is ventilation without perfusion (ventilation/perfusion mismatch).

A technetium radionuclide scan with radiolabeled red blood cells can be used to identify active bleeding sites (even with bleeding rates as low as 0.1 ml/min)[6] or ectopic gastric mucosa.

ENDOSCOPY

If, after laboratory and radiographic evaluation, the source of hemoptysis is still not apparent or if bleeding is

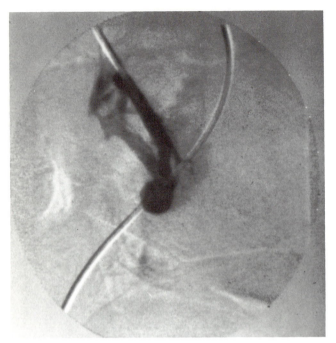

Figure 58–2. Digital angiogram outlining the arterial supply and venous drainage of a pulmonary arteriovenous malformation. (Courtesy of Dr. Floyd Osterman.)

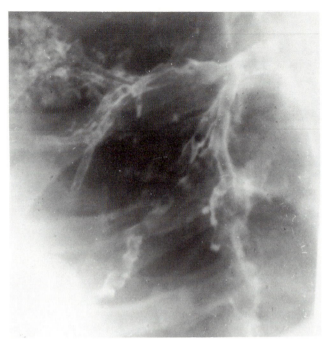

Figure 58–3. Bronchogram in a 17-year-old girl with a 1-year history of intermittent hemoptysis. There is irregular cystic dilatation of the right upper lobe bronchi consistent with bronchiectasis.

recurrent or substantial, endoscopy is indicated.[7-9] Localization of a bleeding site is best accomplished when bronchoscopy is performed during active bleeding. The availability of the flexible fiberoptic bronchoscope has been a major advance. In comparison with the rigid bronchoscope, this instrument has increased maneuverability and is tolerated more readily and for longer periods. The fiberoptic bronchoscope can usually be passed transnasally with the use of sedation instead of general anesthesia. It can be used to visualize subsegmental airways that are beyond the reach of the rigid bronchoscope. There is still a role, however, for the rigid bronchoscope; it is better for removing foreign bodies and for maintaining a secure airway while providing adequate suctioning in patients who have massive bleeding.

Bronchoscopy is particularly useful for the detection of foreign bodies and the diagnosis of infection and endobronchial lesions. Material can be obtained for cultures, stains, and cytologic studies. Old blood can be removed by saline lavage of segmental bronchi, and the airway can then be re-examined. The need for bronchography has been virtually eliminated by the availability of CT and high-kilovoltage radiography. In rare cases it may be indicated as an adjunct to fiberoptic bronchoscopy to define type, site, and extent of bronchiectasis[10, 11] (Fig. 58–3) or to identify a congenital abnormality of the bronchus. It may also be used to differentiate an extrinsic from an intrinsic defect in the airway.

SPECIFIC CONDITIONS

PULMONARY EMBOLUS

Pulmonary embolism is rare but probably underreported in the pediatric age group.[12] The most common presenting complaint is pleuritic pain (84%), followed by dyspnea (58%), cough (47%), and hemoptysis (32%).[12] Tachypnea and fever are common. The most common laboratory abnormality is arterial hypoxemia. Half of affected patients have an abnormal chest radiograph, and half have signs of a deep venous thrombosis of a lower extremity. Antecedent events include oral contraceptive use, trauma to a lower extremity, and recent abortion. Other risk factors include surgery, prolonged immobilization, systemic infection, intravenous drug abuse, and collagen vascular disease.[12] Abortion and oral contraceptive use are major risk factors in adolescent girls, whereas trauma to the lower extremities is the major risk factor in adolescent boys.[12] Ventilation/perfusion scan (decreased perfusion) (Fig. 58–4) and MRI can be helpful in suggesting the diagnosis, but pulmonary arteriography is the definitive diagnostic procedure.[5]

NEOPLASMS

Primary tumors of the lung are not common in children but may manifest with hemoptysis.[13] The most common benign lesions are inflammatory pseudotumors, hamartomas, and neurogenic tumors. With benign lesions, the most common presenting symptoms are fever and cough. Hemoptysis is present in 5% of affected patients.[13] One third of all patients with benign tumors are asymptomatic.

The most common malignant lesions are bronchial adenoma, bronchogenic carcinoma, and pulmonary blastoma. The most common clinical manifestations are cough and recurrent pneumonitis. Hemoptysis is present in 10% to 15% of patients with malignant lesions, including one third of those with bronchial adenomas.[13] Only 10% of patients with malignant lesions are asymptomatic.

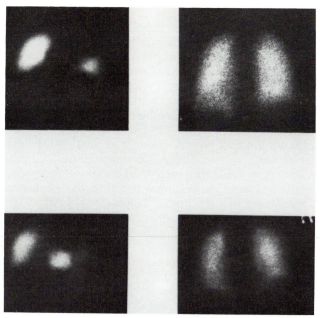

Figure 58–4. Ventilation/perfusion scans showing symmetric ventilation (right panels) and decreased perfusion to the right lung (left panels) in a patient with a pulmonary embolus. (Courtesy of Dr. Elias Zerhouni.)

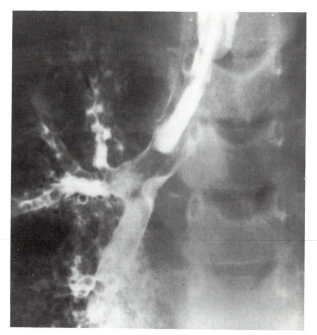

Figure 58–5. Filling defect at the level of the origin of the right upper lobe bronchus in an 8-year-old patient with a bronchial adenoma. (Courtesy of Dr. John Dorst.)

Radiographs may show a solitary mass lesion or evidence of airway obstruction with atelectasis and pneumonitis (Fig. 58–5). Calcification may be seen in a small percentage of lesions. Most malignant lesions can be visualized at bronchoscopy (Fig. 58–6), especially those producing airway obstruction. Pleural fluid is unusual but, if present, may provide cytologic confirmation of the diagnosis.

CARDIOVASCULAR LESIONS

Hemoptysis is not uncommon as a complication of congenital heart disease, although the incidence has decreased since the advent of early corrective surgery. It has been most frequently described in cyanotic patients with pulmonary vascular obstruction, including Eisenmenger's complex, enlarged bronchial arterial circulation, and pulmonary venous congestion. In a review of 42 patients seen at the Johns Hopkins Hospital with hemoptysis complicating congenital heart disease, the most frequent diagnosis was extreme pulmonic stenosis (mostly tetralogy with outflow atresia).[14] In some patients, atresia of the right ventricular outflow tract was associated with absence or extreme hypoplasia of the main pulmonary artery. The age at onset of hemoptysis varied from 4 to 47 years and in most cases originated from the lung with decreased flow, namely the side supplied by bronchial vessels. There are three major pathologic changes: thrombosis in small pulmonary vessels, increased size and tortuosity of the bronchial arteries, and relative hypoplasia of the pulmonary arterial walls. All three may contribute to hemoptysis, but the enlargement of bronchial artery collateral vessels is thought to be the major cause of hemoptysis in patients with decreased pulmonary arterial flow. Treatment depends on the underlying pathologic process but may include angiographic embolotherapy, surgical resection of the involved lung, or ligation of

bleeding vessels. Hemoptysis is also seen in patients with pulmonary vascular obstructive disease. In the past, this was most commonly seen as a late complication after a systemic-pulmonary artery anastomotic procedure for cyanotic malformations associated with pulmonic stenosis. In these cases, episodes of hemoptysis are rare in children under 10 years of age, but the incidence rises sharply in the second decade of life. Clinically, the episodes are usually low or moderate in degree and recur at unpredictable intervals. In patients with Eisenmenger's complex, hemoptysis, secondary to thromboembolism, may occur in association with pregnancy or the use of oral contraceptives.

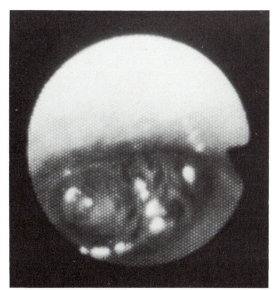

Figure 58–6. A bronchial adenoma seen at bronchoscopy in a 13-year-old boy with a 2-year history of recurrent left lower lobe pneumonia and a 7-month history of hemoptysis.

FOREIGN BODIES

In children with hemoptysis, it is always important to be aware of the possibility of foreign body aspiration, even in the absence of a suggestive history.[15] Although most aspirations of foreign bodies occur in children younger than 4 years, teenagers with retained aspirated foreign bodies may exhibit hemoptysis.[16–18] The major complication of foreign body aspiration is bronchial obstruction, which may result in atelectasis, abscess formation, pneumonia, and bronchiectasis. Hemoptysis is secondary to the extensive neovascularization that may occur in the bronchiectatic portion of the lung.[18]

In many patients, the initial choking episode is either not observed or not remembered, and there may be a long latent period between the episode of aspiration and the appearance of symptoms.[15] The likelihood that an aspirated foreign body is the cause of hemoptysis is increased if the episode of hemoptysis is accompanied by pronounced coughing, localized wheezing, and locally diminished or absent breath sounds. On examination, there may be localized rales or wheezes, but some patients have a normal examination. Patients commonly have recurrent or incomplete clearing of a focal infiltrate. Chest radiographs may be normal (20% of cases) or may show localized air trapping, atelectasis, or signs of unresolved pneumonia. A radiopaque object is seen in approximately 15% of cases. Fluoroscopy may reveal unequal aeration, asymmetric diaphragmatic movement, or mediastinal shift. Inspiratory and expiratory films may be useful in demonstrating localized air trapping. Foreign bodies may also be identified by CT. However, normal radiographic findings do not eliminate the need for bronchoscopy, at which time the diagnosis is usually confirmed. A flexible fiberoptic bronchoscope may be used for diagnosis, but for removal of foreign bodies, a rigid bronchoscope is more useful. Because there may be more than one foreign body, it is important to examine both sides during bronchoscopy.

HEMOSIDEROSIS

Idiopathic pulmonary hemosiderosis (IPH) is an unusual and often baffling cause of hemoptysis in children.[19] It is a disorder of unknown cause characterized by recurrent episodes of diffuse intra-alveolar hemorrhage. Although familial cases have been reported,[20] the inheritance pattern is not clear. Affected patients usually present during infancy and early childhood with hemoptysis, respiratory distress (cough, dyspnea, wheezing), diffuse parenchymal infiltrates (Fig. 58–7), and iron-deficiency anemia.[19, 20] Eventually patients may show evidence of digital clubbing and pulmonary hypertension. In some infants, cor pulmonale secondary to upper airway obstruction related to hypertrophy of the tonsils and adenoids develops.[21] It is one of the few conditions in which refractory iron-deficiency anemia occurs without an obvious bleeding site.

Hemosiderosis may occur as a primary condition or in association with glomerulonephritis (Goodpasture's syndrome), collagen vascular disease, immunoglobulin An

(IgA) deficiency and, in rare cases, cow's milk protein allergy.[22] The diagnosis of pulmonary hemosiderosis is suggested by the clinical picture along with finding iron-laden macrophages in bronchial or gastric washings (see Fig. 58–1) and is confirmed by demonstrating iron-laden macrophages in lung biopsy material. Nuclear scanning of the lungs after injection of radiolabeled red blood cells can be used to confirm that lung infiltrates are secondary to intrapulmonary hemorrhage. Patients with hemosiderosis should have an immunologic evaluation for collagen vascular disease. Renal function studies, including renal biopsy and measurement of antiglomerular basement membrane antibody are useful in the evaluation of Goodpasture's syndrome. The measurement of circulating precipitins to constituents of cow's milk are used to evaluate patients with hemosiderosis for milk allergy.

Treatment depends on associated disorders. In patients with cow's milk allergy, all dairy products should be eliminated from the diet. Patients with Goodpasture's syndrome and collagen vascular disease are treated with immunosuppressive agents.

In patients with IPH, the course is variable but the prognosis is poor.[23] Average survival is about 2.5 years after the onset of symptoms. Survival is not correlated with disease severity at onset but may be better in girls and patients who present after 5 years of age.[23] Steroids are often used in IPH along with other immunosuppressive agents (azathioprine, cyclophosphamide, and chlorambucil), although their efficacy has not been firmly established.[23] Patients with persistent pulmonary infiltrates may benefit from an iron-chelating agent such as deferoxamine.

INFECTIONS

Hemoptysis can occur with a variety of pulmonary infections including necrotizing pneumonia,[1] tuberculosis,[1] aspergillosis,[24] coccidioidomycosis, actinomycosis,[25] histoplasmosis,[26] and parasitic infestations.[27, 28] On a worldwide basis, echinococcosis[27] and paragonimiasis[28] are probably the most common causes of hemoptysis in children. Bronchiectasis may be seen after infections of the lower respiratory tract (measles, adenovirus, tuberculosis) (see Fig. 58–3), after aspiration of a foreign body, with allergic bronchopulmonary aspergillosis, and with genetic disorders such as cystic fibrosis, immotile cilia syndrome, immunodeficiencies, and alpha$_1$-antitrypsin deficiency.[29] About 5% of patients with bronchiectasis have significant hemoptysis.[29] This diagnosis should be considered when hemoptysis occurs in conjunction with pulmonary infiltrates, cough, purulent sputum, and localized abnormal breath sounds. Plain radiography, CT, and ventilation/perfusion scans may aid in the diagnosis. Bronchoscopy may be helpful in confirming the diagnosis and in obtaining material for stains and culture. Bronchography is not usually performed but may be helpful in conjunction with bronchoscopy[10, 11] (see Fig. 58–3). In children with suspected infection, serologic studies, cultures, and skin testing all may aid in determining a specific cause. In some cases, needle aspiration of a lesion or open-lung biopsy is necessary.

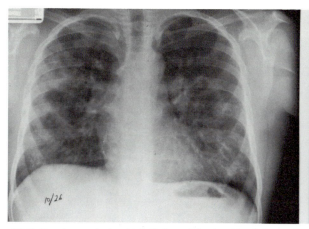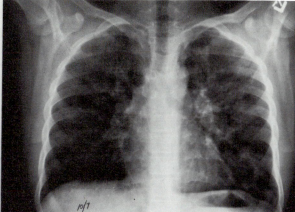

Figure 58–7. Development of multiple fluffy nodular densities (left panel) secondary to intra-alveolar bleeding in a 12-year-old patient with pulmonary hemosiderosis. (Courtesy of Dr. John Dorst.)

CONGENITAL DEFECTS

A variety of congenital defects other than congenital heart disease may be associated with mild to moderate hemoptysis in children. These include arteriovenous malformations[30] (see Fig. 58–2), extralobar bronchopulmonary sequestration[31] (Fig. 58–8), hemangiomatous malformation[32] (Fig. 58–9), intrathoracic gastrogenic cysts,[33] and hereditary hemorrhagic telangiectasia (Osler-Weber-Rendu disease).[34] Massive bleeding in an infant or a young child is suggestive of arteriovenous malformation or intrathoracic cystic malformation.

Conventional angiography and digital subtraction angiography can be used to define the blood supply to these lesions[5] (see Figs. 58–2, 58–8). A small percentage of pulmonary arteriovenous malformations are systemically supplied by intercostal and bronchial arteries. In such cases, a thoracic angiogram is needed in order to outline the vascular pattern. Treatment of these lesions consists of localized resection of involved tissue, ligation of vessels, or embolization therapy.

RENAL DISEASE

There are a number of disorders involving vasculitis or autoimmune mechanisms in which hemoptysis is seen in association with combined renal and pulmonary dis-

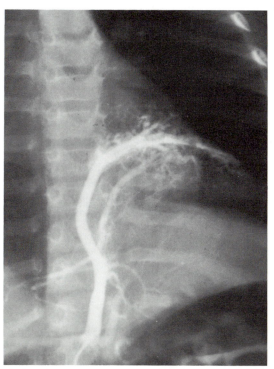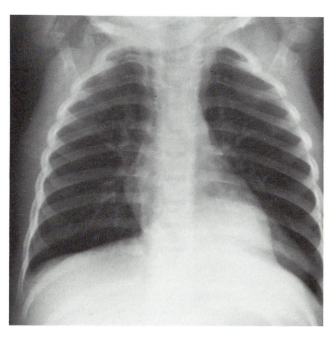

Figure 58–8. A 17-month-old child with a rounded density in the left lower lobe posterior to the heart (right panel). A selective thoracic aortogram (left panel) demonstrates systemic vascular supply from the thoracic aorta to a sequestration. (Courtesy of Dr. John Dorst.)

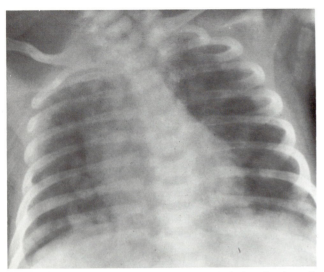

Figure 58–9. Multiple pulmonary hemangiomas in the lung in a 1-month-old infant with cutaneous, central nervous system, and bladder hemangiomas. (Courtesy of Dr. John Dorst.)

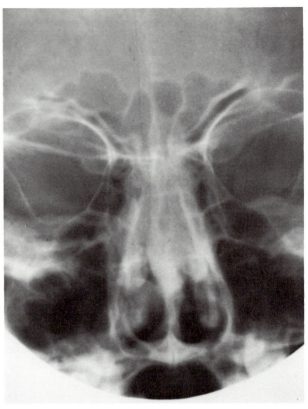

Figure 58–10. Thickening of the mucosa of the ethmoid sinuses and erosion of the nasal septum in the patient with Wegener's granulomatosis. (Courtesy of Dr. John Dorst.)

ease.[35–37] Goodpasture's syndrome is an autoimmune disorder in which patients have glomerulonephritis, anemia, and pulmonary hemorrhage.[37] There may be pulmonary infiltrates. It usually occurs in males 15 to 30 years of age and may occasionally show a familial pattern. The pulmonary and renal involvement are not always concurrent; either can appear first, weeks to months before the clinical recognition of the other.[35] There may be hemosiderin-laden macrophages in the sputum. Circulating antiglomerular basement membrane antibody can be demonstrated by radioimmunoassay in about 90% of patients.[35] The diagnosis is confirmed by demonstrating IgG and C3 deposition in lung or renal tissue. Treatment consists of immunosuppression.

Systemic vasculitis, of which periarteritis is the most commonly recognized type, may manifest with wheezing, dyspnea, and hemoptysis.[35] Other clinical features include polyarthralgia, weight loss, hypertension, fever, abdominal pain, and peripheral neuropathy. Renal involvement occurs in 80% to 90% of patients at some point in the illness and is usually heralded by hematuria.[35]

Wegener's granulomatosis consists of necrotizing lesions of the upper and lower respiratory tracts and focal glomerulonephropathy.[35] It is one of the most prevalent forms of pulmonary vasculitis. Manifestations in the upper respiratory tract include epistaxis, intractable rhinitis, sinusitis (Fig. 58–10), and a saddle-nose deformity. Involvement in the lower tract is a necrotizing pneumonitis. Nodular lung densities may eventually cavitate (Fig. 58–11) and produce massive pulmonary bleeding. The radiographic appearance of the pulmonary lesions tends to change rapidly, a feature useful in differentiating Wegener's granulomatosis from tumors or infectious granulomas.[35] Mucocutaneous involvement can be prominent. The renal lesion is a form of necrotizing glomerulitis manifested by hematuria, proteinuria, and, eventually, renal insufficiency. Biopsy of the ethmoid sinus or kidney (necrotizing granulomas) can be diagnostic, and in the kidney, there is focal deposition of IgG, IgM, and C3 in the glomeruli and small vessels.[35]

Allergic granulomatosis (Churg-Strauss syndrome) is probably a variant of Wegener's granulomatosis characterized by necrotizing angiitis of small arteries and veins, extravascular granulomas, and eosinophilic infiltration of the lungs.[35]

Collagen vascular disorders, of which systemic lupus erythematosus is the model, may be complicated by diffuse alveolar hemorrhage.[36] Affected patients usually have hemoptysis, diffuse pulmonary infiltrates (Fig. 58–12), fever, and dyspnea in the context of clinically active lupus.[36] The bleeding may be massive. Because most of these patients are immunosuppressed, lung biopsy should be performed to rule out opportunistic infections.[36] Histologic examination reveals intra-alveolar hemorrhage with or without interstitial pneumonitis. Vasculitis is rarely seen; it probably occurs on an immunologic basis. Management includes evaluation for infection and initiation of antibiotics and corticosteroids pending the results of lung biopsy.

CYSTIC FIBROSIS

In patients with cystic fibrosis and bronchiectasis or chronic suppurative *Pseudomonas* bronchitis, there is dilatation, increased tortuosity, and hyperplasia of the bronchial arteries[38] (Fig. 58–13). Anastomoses develop

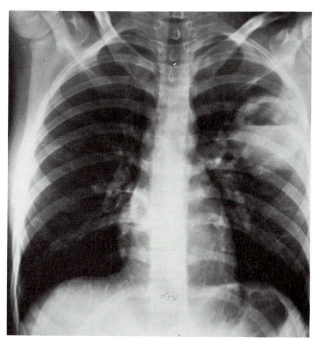

Figure 58–11. A thick-walled cavity with an air-fluid level in the left upper lobe in a 15-year-old patient with Wegener's granulomatosis. (Courtesy of Dr. John Dorst.)

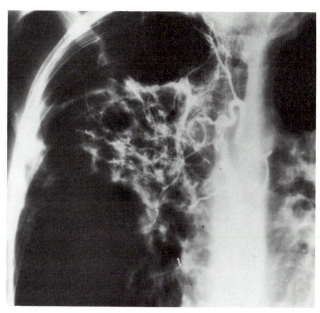

Figure 58–13. This patient with cystic fibrosis had recurrent episodes of hemoptysis for 18 months. A selective right bronchial arteriogram shows hypervascularity and marked enlargement of the bronchial arteries supplying the right upper lobe. Bleeding was controlled by gelatin-sponge embolization of the involved arteries.

between the bronchial and pulmonary circulations in the walls of larger bronchi in chronically infected segments of lung. The right upper lobe is the most common site of bleeding. Secondary to exacerbations of pulmonary infection, there may be erosion of bronchial arteries and episodes of moderate to massive hemoptysis. Although episodes may subside spontaneously, recurrences are common. Bronchoscopy during active bleeding remains

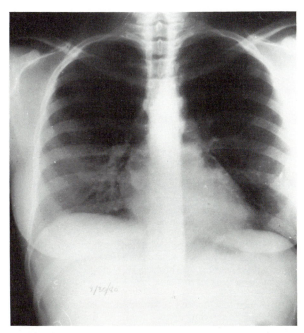

Figure 58–12. In this 16-year-old girl with lupus erythematosus, hemoptysis and respiratory failure developed. Chest radiograph shows an interstitial infiltrate in the right middle and lower lobes.

the most reliable means of identifying the area of bleeding[38, 39] but may not always be possible. Identification of a hypervascular area of lung by arteriography may also help localize the bleeding site.

Conservative treatment consists of bed rest, sedation, temporary withholding of chest physiotherapy, and intravenous antibiotics. Blood losses should be replaced and vitamin K administered if there is prolongation of the prothrombin time.

Percutaneous bronchial artery embolization is now accepted as the standard procedure for treating episodes of hemoptysis in patients with cystic fibrosis.[39] Indications for embolotherapy include either massive acute bleeding (300 ml over 24 h) or chronic bleeding (75–100 ml/day) recurring over weeks or months. Selective bronchial arteriography is performed before embolization to assess the size and distribution of the bronchial arteries and the possibility of a common origin of radiculomedullary branches to the spinal cord. Visualization of spinal cord arteries arising from any underlying bronchial vessel is an absolute contraindication to embolization. The injection of embolizing material (Gelfoam, Ivalon, bucrylate) and subsequent flow within the artery being occluded are monitored fluoroscopically through the use of injections of contrast material. Embolization is terminated when, on repeated arteriography, 90% or more of the peripheral branches have been occluded and marked stasis of flow in the main segment is achieved.

The usual approach is to embolize the bronchial arteries in the area identified as the site of bleeding as well as to attempt to occlude any other abnormal, obviously enlarged bronchial arteries that can be found. With this technique, immediate cessation of bleeding can be achieved in more than 90% of patients.[39] On long-term follow-up, recurrent episodes of minor bleeding can be expected in 70% of patients and major rebleeding in 20%.[38, 39] This is probably related to ongoing vascularization of infected areas as well as revascularization of previously occluded areas through collateral channels from adjacent patent bronchial arteries.[40]

Complications of the procedure include transient fever, chest pain, back pain, and dysphagia.[38, 39] Bowel necrosis secondary to inadvertent embolization of the superior mesenteric area has been reported. Chest physiotherapy can usually be resumed within 24 to 48 h. In rare instances in unstable patients with cystic fibrosis and massive hemoptysis, pulmonary resection may be indicated.[41]

MISCELLANEOUS

A number of unusual causes of hemoptysis must be considered in pediatric patients. Hemoptysis may occur secondary to inhalations of resins during occupational exposure[42] and has also been reported in thyrotoxic adolescents in whom a clinical picture of purpura, nephritis, severe anemia, and hemoptysis develops (secondary to pulmonary cavitation) during treatment with propylthiouracil.[43]

In rare cases, recurrent episodes of hemoptysis may coincide with the onset of menses in patients with bronchopulmonary endometriosis.[44] Chest radiographs are usually normal. The clinical diagnosis is based on the association of unexplained hemoptysis coincident with menses, but the bleeding site can be localized by CT at the time of bleeding.[44]

Factitious bleeding is one of the most baffling of all causes of hemoptysis in children.[45] This represents a form of Münchausen's syndrome by proxy in which blood other than the patient's own is presented as evidence of hemoptysis. Innovative detective work may be needed in such cases including video monitoring and the typing of blood from the patient and caretakers.

MANAGEMENT

Management of patients with hemoptysis depends almost entirely on the underlying cause and extent of bleeding. Once the underlying cause is found, treatment is directed at the source. In children with massive bleeding (more than 8 ml/kg/24 h), an aggressive approach is mandatory. Arterial blood gases should be monitored. Once the airway is established, vigorous suctioning may be necessary. Supplemental oxygen, transfusions, and mechanical ventilation may be required. Bronchoscopy is useful, both diagnostically and therapeutically.[7-9] It can be used to localize the bleeding site, protect and maintain the airway, and prevent asphyxiation. In patients with active bleeding, the open, ventilating bronchoscope is preferable. It allows for simultaneous ventilation and inspection of the airway and is better than the flexible bronchoscope for suctioning and clearing the airway. Lavage with iced saline solution or topical application of a vasoconstrictor may be helpful. Control of massive bleeding may require endoscopic tamponade with a balloon catheter, emboli-

zation of involved arteries, or thoracotomy with a direct surgical approach to the source of bleeding.

REFERENCES

1. Tom LW, Weisman RA, Handler SD: Hemoptysis in children. Ann Otol Rhinol Laryngol 89:419–424, 1980.
2. Metz SJ, Rosenstein BJ: Uncovering the cause of hemoptysis in children. J Respir Dis 5(6):43–51, 1984.
3. Turcios NL, Vega M: The child with hemoptysis. Hosp Pract (Off Ed) 22:214, 217–218, 1987.
4. Putnam JS, Tellis CJ: Hemoptysis. Prim Care 5:67–80, 1978.
5. Ablin DS, Newell JD: Diagnostic imaging for evaluation of the pediatric chest. Clin Chest Med 8:641–660, 1987.
6. Coel MN, Druger G: Radionuclide detection of the site of hemoptysis. Chest 81:242–243, 1982.
7. Selecky PA: Evaluation of hemoptysis through the bronchoscope. Chest 73:741–745, 1978.
8. Smiddy JF, Elliott RC: The evaluation of hemoptysis with fiberoptic bronchoscopy. Chest 64:158–162, 1973.
9. Fitzpatrick SB, Marsh B, Stokes D, et al: Indications for flexible fiberoptic bronchoscopy in pediatric patients. Am J Dis Child 137:595–597, 1983.
10. Jones DK, Cavanagh P, Shneerson JM, et al: Does bronchography have a role in the assessment of patients with haemoptysis? Thorax 40:668–670, 1985.
11. Lundgren R, Hietala S, Adelroth E: Diagnosis of bronchial lesions by fiber-optic bronchoscopy combined with bronchography. Acta Radiol 23:231–234, 1982.
12. Bernstein D, Coupey S, Schonberg SK: Pulmonary embolism in adolescents. Am J Dis Child 140:667–671, 1986.
13. Hartman GE, Shochat SJ: Primary pulmonary neoplasms of childhood: A review. Ann Thor Surg 36:108–119, 1983.
14. Haroutunian LM, Neill CA: Pulmonary complications of congenital heart disease: Hemoptysis. Am Heart J 84:540–559, 1972.
15. Pyman C: Inhaled foreign bodies in childhood. Med J Aust 1:62–68, 1971.
16. Hilman BC, Kurzweg FT, McCook WW, et al: Foreign body aspiration of grass inflorescences as a cause of hemoptysis. Chest 78:306–309, 1980.
17. Pattison CW, Leaming AJ, Townsend ER: Hidden foreign body as a cause of recurrent hemoptysis in a teenage girl. Ann Thorac Surg 45:330–331, 1988.
18. Scully RE, Mark EJ, McNeely BU: Case records of the Massachusetts General Hospital. N Engl J Med 309:1374–1381, 1983.
19. Levy J, Kolski GB, Scanlin TF: Hemoptysis and anemia in a 3-year-old boy. Ann Allergy 55:439–440, 486–489, 1985.
20. Beckerman RC, Taussig LM, Pinnas JL: Familial idiopathic pulmonary hemosiderosis. Am J Dis Child 133:609–611, 1979.
21. Boat TF, Polmar SH, Whitman V, et al: Hyperreactivity to cow milk in young children with pulmonary hemosiderosis and cor pulmonale secondary to nasopharyngeal obstruction. J Pediatr 87:23–29, 1975.
22. Heiner DC: Respiratory diseases and food allergy. Ann Allergy 53:657–664, 1984.
23. Chryssanthopoulos C, Cassimos C, Panagiotidou C: Prognostic criteria in idiopathic pulmonary hemosiderosis in children. Eur J Pediatr 140:123–125, 1983.
24. Borkin MH, Arena FP, Brown AE, et al: Invasive aspergillosis with massive fatal hemoptysis in patients with neoplastic disease. Chest 78:835–839, 1980.
25. Old L Jr, Stokes TL: Shock from massive hemoptysis due to pulmonary actinomycosis in a child. Va Med Mon 99:142–147, 1972.
26. Zeiss J, Woldenberg LS, Morgan R, et al: Pulmonary histoplasmoma presenting as massive hemoptysis. Pediatr Infect Dis J 6:689–691, 1987.
27. Carcassonne M, Aubrespy P, Dor V, et al: Hydatid cysts in childhood. Prog Pediatr Surg 5:1–35, 1973.
28. Fischer GW, McGrew GL, Bass JW: Pulmonary paragonimiasis in childhood. JAMA 243:1360–1362, 1980.
29. Lewiston NJ: Bronchiectasis in childhood. Pediatr Clin North Am 31:865–878, 1984.
30. Hoffman WS, Weinberg PM, Ring E, et al: Massive hemoptysis sec-

ondary to pulmonary arteriovenous fistula. Chest 77:697–700, 1980.

31. Telander RL, Lennox C, Sieber W: Sequestration of the lung in children. Mayo Clin Proc 51:578–584, 1976.

32. Kings GL: Multifocal haemangiomatous malformation: A case report. Thorax 30:485–488, 1975.

33. Chang SH, Morrison L, Shaffner L, et al: Intrathoracic gastrogenic cysts and hemoptysis. J Pediatr 88:594–596, 1976.

34. Reyes-Mujica M, Lopez-Corella E, Perez-Fernandez L, et al: Osler-Weber-Rendu disease in an infant. Hum Pathol 19:1243–1246, 1988.

35. Scully RE, Mark EJ, McNeely BU: Case records of the Massachusetts General Hospital. N Engl J Med 314:834–844, 1986.

36. Carette S, Macher AM, Nussbaum A, et al: Severe, acute pulmonary disease in patients with systemic lupus erythematosus: Ten years of experience at the National Institutes of Health. Semin Arthritis Rheum 14:52–59, 1984.

37. Ekholdt PF, Gulsvik A, Digranes S, et al: Recurrent diffuse pulmonary hemorrhage with minor kidney lesions. Eur J Respir Dis 66:353–359, 1985.

38. Church NR: Bronchial Artery Embolization for the Treatment of

39. Fellows KE, Khaw KT, Schuster S, et al: Bronchial artery embolization in cystic fibrosis: Technique and long-term results. J Pediatr 95:959–963, 1979.

40. Tomashefski JF, Cohen AM, Doershuk CF: Long-term histopathologic follow-up of bronchial arteries after therapeutic embolization with polyvinyl alcohol (Ivalon) in patients with cystic fibrosis. Hum Pathol 19:555–561, 1988.

41. Marmon L, Schidlow D, Palmer J, et al: Pulmonary resection for complications of cystic fibrosis. J Pediatr Surg 18:811–815, 1983.

42. Herbert FA, Orford R: Pulmonary hemorrhage and edema due to inhalation of resins containing tri-mellitic anhydride. Chest 76:546–551, 1979.

43. Cassorla FG, Finegold DN, Parks JS, et al: Vasculitis, pulmonary cavitation, and anemia during antithyroid drug therapy. Am J Dis Child 137:118–122, 1983.

44. Elliot DL, Barker AF, Dixon L: Catamenial hemoptysis: New methods of diagnosis and therapy. Chest 87:687–688, 1985.

45. Shafer N, Shafer R: Factitious diseases including Munchausen's syndrome. NY State J Med 80:594–604, 1980.

Massive Hemoptysis in Cystic Fibrosis. Rockville, MD: Cystic Fibrosis Foundation, 1983.

59 PULMONARY HEMOSIDEROSIS

JACOV LEVY, M.D. / ROBERT WILMOTT, M.D.

Pulmonary hemosiderosis is a disease characterized by alveolar hemorrhage and accumulation of iron within the alveolar macrophages as hemosiderin. Pulmonary hemosiderosis may occur either as a primary disease of the lungs or as a secondary complication of cardiac disease or systemic vasculitis. Idiopathic pulmonary hemosiderosis is the most prevalent form. It is an uncommon childhood disease consisting of spontaneous pulmonary hemorrhage associated with iron-deficiency anemia, which is more common in childhood than are the secondary forms of pulmonary hemosiderosis.[1] It is generally accepted that there are four variants of primary (idiopathic) pulmonary hemosiderosis: (1) an isolated form; (2) a form associated with allergy to cow's milk; (3) a form associated with either myocarditis or pancreatitis; and (4) a form associated with progressive (proliferative) glomerulonephritis (Goodpasture's syndrome).[2] Two forms of secondary pulmonary hemosiderosis have been described: one form results from increased left atrial pressure and the other is associated with collagen vascular diseases.[2] The association of pulmonary hemorrhage with glomerulonephritis and the presence of antiglomerular basement membrane antibodies is termed Goodpasture's syndrome. This disease is more prevalent in men, with a male-to-female ratio of approximately 3:1,[3] and it usually occurs in young adults. Cases have been reported in childhood[4,5] but never in infancy. In addition, pulmonary hemosiderosis can also be caused by ingestion of certain medications or

chemicals, and it has been described in association with systemic disorders such as diabetes mellitus and celiac disease.[6–9]

Idiopathic pulmonary hemosiderosis usually manifests in infancy or childhood, and the incidences in the sexes are equal.[1,6] Its rarity is illustrated by the fact that only five cases were described in Scandinavia during a period of 23 years.[10] A more recent report suggests a yearly incidence of 9.24 cases per million children in Sweden.[11] A group of 30 children was reported from Greece over a period of 20 years, but these patients may represent a cluster of cases related to an environmental factor.[12] Several familial cases have been reported[13,14] and may represent a manifestation of an inherited immunopathologic abnormality.

PATHOPHYSIOLOGY

GENERAL PATHOLOGY

The characteristic pathologic manifestation of pulmonary hemosiderosis is that of hemosiderin-laden macrophages in both the interstitium and the alveolar spaces of the lung.[1] Macroscopic examination usually reveals frank intra-alveolar hemorrhage (Fig. 59–1A). Microscopic findings (Fig. 59–1B) include alveolar epithelial cell hyperplasia and degeneration with epithelial sloughing.[15] A large number of iron-laden macrophages (sideroblasts)

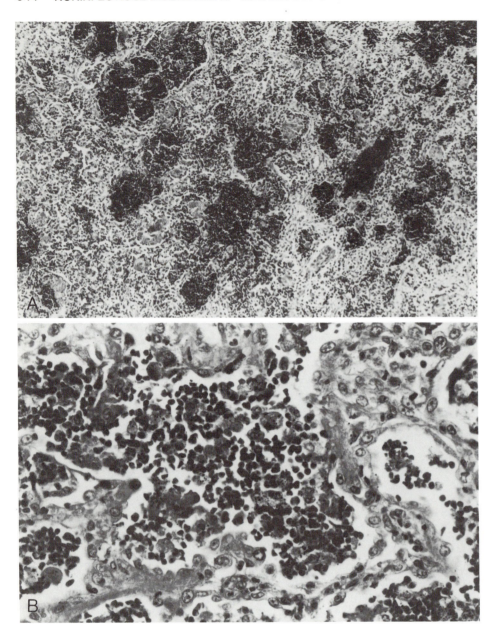

Figure 59–1. *A*, Low-power view of a lung biopsy that shows extensive intra-alveolar hemorrhage. *B*, Higher magnification shows intra-alveolar hemorrhage associated with hemosiderin-laden macrophages.

can usually be identified with various degrees of interstitial fibrosis and mast cell accumulation.[16] Elastin fiber degeneration and sclerotic vascular changes have also been described,[17] as have chronic perilymphangitis and mild hypertrophy of bronchial artery muscle.[15] If vasculitis is found, hemosiderosis may be the result of a systemic vascular disease. The general morphologic characteristics of the lung parenchyma usually remain intact in hemosiderosis. Detailed ultrastructural studies have shown focal interruptions of the pulmonary capillary basement membrane,[9, 18] a defect that may predispose to bleeding into the alveolar spaces.[9] Extensive damage to the capillary endothelium and its basement membrane have been observed. Capillary endothelial cells are swollen to the extent of obliterating the intercellular gaps in the most extreme cases.[19] Capillary endothelial basement membrane may show focal thickening without evidence of electron-dense deposits on the membrane.[19] Collagen may accumulate within the basement membrane, although fibroblasts are seldom seen.[20] Immunofluorescence studies of the lungs reveal deposits of fibrinogen and fibrin with, in most cases, no evidence of immunoglobulin or complement.[21] In Goodpasture's syndrome, which is mediated by a cytotoxic antibody, immunofluorescent staining has shown linear deposition of immunoglobulin and complement on the basement membrane. In one case, antibasement membrane antibodies were found in the serum, but the disease was limited to the lung, and there was no renal involvement.[22]

In a lung biopsy specimen of a patient with pulmonary hemosiderosis and antibasement membrane antibodies in the serum, the alveolar basement membrane and the elastic laminae of the pulmonary vessels showed fine deposits of iron with small quantities of calcium.[23] It has been speculated that the hemosiderin-containing macrophages may undergo necrosis with release of iron-containing substances that damage the basement membrane, causing further hemorrhage.[24] This theory may explain why symptoms may persist even when antibodies have disappeared from the serum and why the pathologic picture can occur without evidence of any immunologic (or other) mechanism.

PATHOLOGIC CLASSIFICATION

Pulmonary hemosiderosis can be classified into three groups according to the suspected pathogenesis.[25] In the first group, there are antibodies against anatomic constituents of the lung, such as the alveolar basement membrane in Goodpasture's syndrome. Goodpasture's syndrome is characterized by linear deposition of immunoglobulin G (IgG) and complement on the capillary basement membrane of both the lung and the kidney by immunofluorescence, indicating a type II hypersensitivity reaction. There is no evidence of immune complexes in the serum of these patients. Antibasement membrane antibodies that bind to renal and lung tissue can be demonstrated in the serum in 90% of cases.[22]

In a second group of diseases, there may be involvement of soluble immune complexes. There are several reports of diffuse pulmonary hemorrhage in immune complex nephritis and systemic lupus erythematosus.[25] An electron-microscopic study of the lung in such patients revealed proteinaceous deposits on the capillary basement membrane that were consistent with immune complex deposition.[26]

A third group consists of cases of pulmonary hemosiderosis without evidence of any immune mechanism in the pathogenesis.[18, 25, 27]

PATHOGENESIS

The pathogenesis of pulmonary hemosiderosis is unclear. Early theories included anatomic defects of elastin fibers, abnormal acid mucopolysaccharides, hyperplastic alveolar capillaries, and impaired vasomotor control; however, none of these theories have been confirmed.[1, 6] The disease is sometimes associated with cow's milk allergy.[28] However, most patients do not manifest clinical symptoms of allergy to cow's milk, nor are there antibodies to cow's milk proteins in the sera. Autoimmunity is accepted as the etiologic factor in Goodpasture's syndrome[22] and may be involved in the formation of soluble immune complexes in other forms. Most children with idiopathic pulmonary hemosiderosis have no evidence of an immune process.

There are many clinical reports of patients with pulmonary hemosiderosis and abnormal immunologic findings. Three patients have been described with idiopathic pulmonary hemosiderosis associated with decreased (or absent) levels of IgA in serum and secretions.[2] In contrast, an adult patient was reported with pulmonary hemosiderosis, IgA monoclonal gammopathy, and IgA deposits

along the alveolar basement membrane.[29] Increased serum IgG_4 was found in one patient with hemosiderosis,[30] but this IgG subclass is known to be elevated in allergic patients. Viral infection was suspected in several patients in whom increased titers of cold agglutinating antibodies were found, but cultures from these patients failed to grow pathogenic viruses.[1] Studies of hemostasis and coagulation have been normal in patients with pulmonary hemosiderosis, and impaired coagulation does not appear to be a common cause. The familial occurrence of pulmonary hemosiderosis in two sibling pairs suggested a genetic factor in the pathogenesis. The grandmother of one of these pairs also had hemoptysis and iron-deficiency anemia.[13, 14] Thirteen of 26 children with pulmonary hemosiderosis from central Greece, where intermarriage is common, showed a familial tendency without a clear pattern of inheritance.[31] These reports indicate that a genetic factor may play a role in the occurrence of the disease, but the precise mode of inheritance is unclear.

Environmental factors also may account in part for the cause of pulmonary hemosiderosis. Cow's milk protein is believed to have a major role in causing pulmonary hemosiderosis in those children with cow's milk allergy, although the mechanism has not been fully elucidated. Heiner and associates reported the presence of precipitins to cow's milk in the sera of children with pulmonary hemosiderosis[28] and noted that the disease became milder when cow's milk was excluded from the diet. Some milk-sensitive patients with pulmonary hemosiderosis also have nasopharyngeal obstruction from lymphoid hyperplasia that may lead to cor pulmonale.[32] A child with Down's syndrome and cor pulmonale was observed to have specific IgD antibody responses to cow's milk proteins that increased with dietary challenges and correlated with clinical symptoms.[33]

A toxic cause is suggested by an epidemiologic study from Greece,[12] where an unidentified environmental agent, possibly an insecticide, appeared to cause pulmonary bleeding in 30 children. Other toxic causes include penicillamine, reported to cause Goodpasture's syndrome in patients treated for Wilson's disease,[34] toxic hydrocarbons,[35] and resin powder containing trimellitic anhydride.[36] In experimental studies of rats injected with a number of imidazole compounds, reversible pulmonary bleeding develops and leads to extensive pulmonary hemosiderosis.[36]

CLINICAL MANIFESTATIONS

The clinical picture of pulmonary hemosiderosis is characterized by either an insidious onset with anemia, pallor, weakness, and lethargy or a fulminant onset with recurrent acute hemoptysis. There are usually transient infiltrates on the chest radiograph when bleeding is heavy. In children with an insidious onset, weight gain is usually poor, or there may be weight loss. Patients may present with any one of these symptoms, and the diagnosis may not become evident for some time. On physical examination, there is striking variation in signs according to the severity of the disease.[2] Pallor, shortness of breath, coughing, rales, wheezing, altered breath sounds, and rhonchi are common abnormalities. The liver and spleen are enlarged in 20% of patients. Fever occurs in many patients with iron-deficiency anemia.[1]

Recurrent episodes of pulmonary bleeding over several years may cause signs of chronic respiratory disease that include dyspnea, finger clubbing, and pulmonary hypertension. Pulmonary hypertension may lead eventually to death from right-sided heart failure,[6] although it is more common for patients to die from uncontrolled hemorrhage.[37] The various secondary forms of pulmonary hemosiderosis differ from the idiopathic form in the accompanying physical signs. Children with the form associated with cow's milk allergy may have chronic rhinitis, recurrent otitis media, chronic cough, wheezing, croup, vomiting, diarrhea, occult blood in the stool, and growth retardation.[28] These symptoms, including hemosiderosis, usually disappear when cow's milk products are excluded from the diet. Some patients with cow's milk allergy present later with adenoidal and tonsillar hypertrophy, which may lead to chronic upper airway obstruction and cor pulmonale from chronic hypoxia and hypercapnia.[32]

Pulmonary hemosiderosis has other less common clinical associations. Myocarditis, with cardiomegaly and inflammatory infiltrates of the myocardium, has been reported in a small number of patients with pulmonary hemosiderosis, corneal ulceration, and diabetes mellitus.[38] It is difficult to establish whether the myocardial disease was primary, secondary, or unrelated to pulmonary hemosiderosis. Hemosiderosis sometimes complicates chronic left-sided heart failure because of increased pulmonary venous pressure,[2] and a similar mechanism may operate in myocarditis.

Some patients have pancreatic exocrine deficiency associated with pulmonary hemorrhage;[2, 7] the reason for this association is unknown. In Goodpasture's syndrome, hemoptysis may precede the symptoms of glomerulonephritis by weeks, or even months, and the pulmonary hemorrhage may be acute or chronic. Children with antiglomerular basement membrane antibodies usually have the characteristic renal disease without pulmonary involvement. The mortality rate in Goodpasture's syndrome is higher than that in idiopathic pulmonary hemosiderosis, and death may be caused by either renal disease or massive pulmonary hemorrhage.[39]

Pulmonary hemosiderosis sometimes occurs with collagen vascular diseases or as an early manifestation of a systemic vasculitis.[40, 41] The vascular changes of polyarteritis may be limited to the lungs.[2] Pulmonary hemorrhage has been reported in children with systemic lupus erythematosus,[42-44] rheumatoid arthritis,[2, 45, 46] and Wegener's granulomatosis,[47] and in a syndrome of chronic meningitis, polyarthritis, and lymphadenitis.[48] Several patients with anaphylactoid purpura,[2] thrombocytopenic purpura,[44] microangiopathic hemolytic anemia,[6] and pulmonary lymphangioleiomyomas[49] have also been described. Adult patients with pulmonary hemosiderosis associated with celiac syndrome were shown to have total villous atrophy of the small bowel mucosa, which responded to a gluten-free diet.[50, 51] It is interesting to note that over a long period of follow-up, one of these patients had antibasement membrane antibodies in the serum and recurrent hemoptysis without any evidence of renal disease. This case may represent a disease with antibodies directed against the basement membrane of the lung and small intestine. A 4-year-old boy was described with idiopathic pulmonary hemosiderosis and circulating antibodies against gliadin, reticulin, and various avian antigens. Jejunal biopsy revealed a subtotal villous atrophy, and the symptoms resolved on a 15-month gluten-free diet.[8]

DIAGNOSTIC APPROACHES

Patients with pulmonary hemosiderosis typically have a microcytic hypochromic anemia with a low serum iron. It is thought that the iron is sequestered by the alveolar macrophages and that it is unavailable for hemoglobin synthesis.[52] Increased indirect bilirubin concentrations, urobilinogen, and reticulocyte count are sometimes caused by mild hemolysis. Some patients have a positive direct Coombs' test, and others have positive serum cold agglutinins; in such cases the disease appears to have an immunologic mechanism. Eosinophilia occurs in about 20% of patients.[2]

The stool usually contains occult blood derived from material swallowed after clearance from the lungs by the mucociliary system. Hemosiderin-laden macrophages can be identified in the gastric fluid by staining gastric aspirates with Prussian blue. Similar cells can be identified in the sputum and in bronchoalveolar lavage fluid.

Immunologic studies may reveal anti–cow's milk antibodies of the IgG, IgE, or IgD isotypes,[32] circulating antiglomerular basement membrane antibodies,[22] and antinuclear antibodies.[2] Reduced levels of complement components C3 and CH_{50} are commonly observed in patients with immune complex disease. Immunoglobulins should be measured routinely to investigate for the association with IgA deficiency.[2]

Chest radiographs show abnormalities ranging widely from fine reticulonodular shadowing to large confluent shadows and atelectasis (Fig. 59–2). Other findings include emphysema, hilar adenopathy, and radiographic findings resembling pulmonary edema (Fig. 59–3). Longitudinal studies of a patient with acute bleeding revealed soft shadows with the appearance of acinar consolidation initially and a reticular pattern developing after 2 to 3 days.[53, 54] The latter changes correspond to the period when alveolar macrophages are clearing the alveoli of red blood cells. If there is no more bleeding, the radiographic appearance returns to normal within 2 weeks. However, interstitial fibrosis develops if the process is repeated. A mixed reticular and alveolar pattern indicates that new bleeding has occurred in the presence of a chronic organizing process. Pleural effusions are very rare,[55] and spontaneous pneumothorax has been reported only once.[56]

Pulmonary function tests show impaired diffusion, decreased compliance, and severe airflow obstruction.[57] Total lung capacity is normal or increased. During an acute episode of hemorrhage, the arterial oxygen tension and oxygen saturation may decrease substantially because of intrapulmonary shunting, usually without any

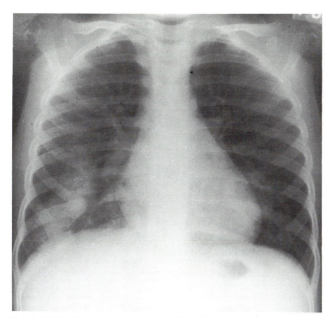

Figure 59–2. The chest radiograph of a 4-year-old boy with idiopathic pulmonary hemosiderosis showing a mild increase in interstitial markings and a large confluent shadow in the right lower zone, together with infiltrates in the right middle lobe and the lingula.

change in the arterial carbon dioxide tension. Ewan and associates[58] found an increase in the single-breath carbon monoxide uptake (DL_{CO}) during acute pulmonary bleeding. The increased uptake was attributed to the affinity of carbon monoxide for sequestered hemoglobin. Patients with acute pulmonary hemorrhage were found to have an increased DL_{CO} as well as changes on the chest radiograph.[59]

The hemorrhagic process in pulmonary hemosiderosis can be demonstrated by radioisotope scanning with autologous red blood cells labeled with chromium 51, iron 59, or technetium 99m.[60, 61] Carbon 15–labeled carbon monoxide clearance has also been used to detect the presence of increased quantities of hemoglobin in the lungs, but this method requires the use of a cyclotron to produce the isotope.[58] Bronchoalveolar lavage has been used to diagnose diffuse alveolar hemorrhage[62, 63] and can be performed in all patients. The lavage effluent in patients with diffuse bleeding is usually bloody and contains hemosiderin-laden macrophages. It is usually necessary for 48 h to pass from time of bleeding until hemosiderin-laden macrophages are evident.[64]

The diagnostic approach to a patient suspected of having pulmonary hemosiderosis should include examination of the gastric fluid for the presence of hemosiderin-laden macrophages. Only in cases with negative results and strong clinical evidence is an open-lung biopsy indicated. Transbronchial biopsy (which is difficult to perform in children) or bronchoalveolar lavage are alternative approaches that may lead to confirmation of the diagnosis with less risk and discomfort.

DIFFERENTIAL DIAGNOSIS

The differential diagnosis of patients with hemoptysis, fever, respiratory distress, and anemia should include bacterial pneumonia, septicemia, tuberculosis, bronchiectasis, pulmonary malignancy, Gaucher's disease, and Wegener's granulomatosis. If hematuria is present, collagen vascular disease, blood dyscrasia, or massive hemoglobinuria secondary to hemolysis should also be considered.

MANAGEMENT

The management of patients with pulmonary hemosiderosis is directed first at finding underlying causes such as cow's milk allergy, heart disease, collagen vascular disease, blood dyscrasia, or exposure to known toxins. If an underlying cause can be identified, it should be treated promptly. Exclusion of milk from the diet and adenotonsillectomy should be considered in patients with cow's milk allergy and adenotonsillar hypertrophy. A small number of patients show a direct relationship between the amount of milk consumed and the severity of their pulmonary symptoms,[2] and such children should not consume any dairy products.

If respiratory distress is evident, arterial blood gases should be determined because oxygen administration may be indicated. Mechanical ventilation with positive end-expiratory pressure is used when severe pulmonary involvement leads to respiratory failure. The patient

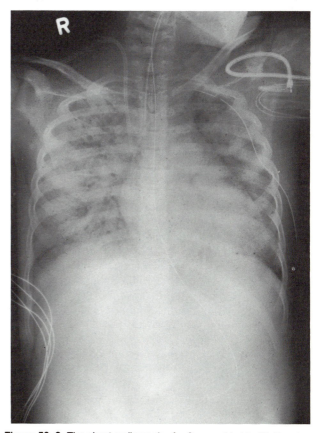

Figure 59–3. The chest radiograph of a 9-year-old girl with Goodpasture's syndrome. There was extensive bilateral alveolar hemorrhage with diffuse opacification of both lung fields. The patient required intubation, mechanical ventilation, and a left thoracostomy for a pneumothorax.

should also undergo transfusion if the anemia is severe. Most authors agree that the use of corticosteroids or other immunosuppressants leads to improvement in some patients,[65-67] although they are not effective for acute bleeding. Intravenous adrenocorticotrophic hormone (10 to 25 units daily), methylprednisolone (2 mg/kg/day), or hydrocortisone (8 mg/kg/day) are recommended initially, followed by maintenance oral prednisone at a dose of 1 to 2 mg/kg/day. Maintenance treatment with corticosteroids is often prolonged because of recurrent disease, and the regimen should be individualized according to the symptoms, hemoglobin concentrations, and findings on chest radiographs. Goran[68] reported a favorable response to prolonged inhalation treatment with the nonabsorbable glucocorticoid budesonide. Immunosuppressants that are used to treat pulmonary hemosiderosis include azathioprine, cyclophosphamide, and chlorambucil. Azathioprine can be given at a dose of 2 to 5 mg/kg/day, usually in combination with prednisone.

Heiner and colleagues successfully treated patients who have hemosiderosis associated with IgA deficiency by repeated transfusions with plasma or blood.[2] The patients manifested a rapid improvement of the clinical symptoms, which suggests that the immunodeficiency plays an important role in this form of disease. Iron-chelating agents, such as desferrioxamine, have been used in an attempt to control iron deposition in the lung tissue.[69] This treatment is given as intramuscular injections every 8 h at a dose of 25 mg/kg/day. Continuous subcutaneous infusion by pump is a better alternative that is less painful. However, the authors believe that iron-chelation therapy is of limited value.

Plasmapheresis and plasma exchange are used in patients with Goodpasture's syndrome as well as those with idiopathic pulmonary hemosiderosis, usually during the acute phase of the disease. These treatments may be combined with immunosuppressants, anticoagulants, or steroids.[5, 47, 70] Plasmapheresis may occasionally be indicated in patients without antibasement membrane antibodies, because some such patients respond empirically to this therapy.[71] Bilateral nephrectomy may lead to resolution of the pulmonary hemorrhage in patients with Goodpasture's syndrome and severe symptoms.[39]

One patient with pulmonary hemosiderosis and abundant mast cells demonstrated by open-lung biopsy responded to treatment with disodium cromoglycate.[16] The clinical value of cromoglycate in pulmonary hemosiderosis is unproven, but it should be considered if excessive numbers of mast cells are present in the biopsy specimen. Patients with pulmonary hemosiderosis may die of pulmonary hypertension in an advanced stage of the disease, but one patient was reported to have a temporary improvement in pulmonary hypertension after treatment with nitroglycerin.[72] The use of other pulmonary vasodilators such as nifedipine and tolazoline should be evaluated in such patients.

PROGNOSIS

The prognosis of patients with idiopathic pulmonary hemosiderosis is difficult to establish because of the rarity and the variability of this disease. One early series reported an average period of 2½ years between diagnosis and death, although many patients with longer survival were reported.[1] The prognosis has probably improved with the use of modern therapy, and some patients have a spontaneous recovery. Those with antibasement membrane antibodies have a less favorable prognosis; an average survival time of 6 months was reported in older series.[73-75] A more recent publication describes a much better prognosis in patients treated early with immunosuppressive therapy.[39]

REFERENCES

1. Soergel KH, Sommers SC: Idiopathic pulmonary hemosiderosis and related syndromes. Am J Med 32:499–511, 1962.
2. Heiner DC: Pulmonary hemosiderosis. *In* Kendig EL, Chernick V (eds): Disorders of the Respiratory Tract in Children, pp. 430–442. Philadelphia: WB Saunders, 1983.
3. Proskey AJ, Weatherbee L, Easterling R, et al: Goodpasture's syndrome: A report of five cases and a review of the literature. Am J Med 48:162–173, 1970.
4. Ozsoylu S, Hisconmex G, Berkel I, et al: Goodpasture's syndrome: Pulmonary hemosiderosis with nephritis. Clin Pediatr (Phila) 15:358–360, 1976.
5. Levin M, Rigden SP, Pincott JR, et al: Goodpasture's syndrome: Treatment with plasmapheresis, immunosupression, and anticoagulation. Arch Dis Child 58:697–702, 1983.
6. Morgan PG, Turner-Warwick M: Pulmonary hemosiderosis and pulmonary hemorrhage. Br J Dis Chest 75:225–242, 1981.
7. Yodaiken RE, Pardo V: Diabetic capillaropathy. Hum Pathol 6:455–465, 1975.
8. Reading R, Watson JG, Platt JW, Bird AG: Pulmonary hemosiderosis and gluten. Arch Dis Child 62:513–515, 1987.
9. Joshi VV, Costello D, Dadzie CKA, Simpser M: Reader's forum. Ultrastruct Pathol 6:271–272, 1984.
10. Gutteberg TJ, Moe PJ, Noren CE: Diagnosis and therapeutic studies in idiopathic pulmonary hemosiderosis. Acta Paediatr Scand 68:913–914, 1979.
11. Kjellman B, Elinder G, Garwicz S, Svan H: Idiopathic pulmonary hemosiderosis in Swedish children. Acta Pediatr Scandia 73:584–588, 1984.
12. Cassimos CD, Chryssanthopoulos C, Panagiotidou C: Epidemiologic observations in idiopathic pulmonary hemosiderosis. J Pediatr 102:698–702, 1983.
13. Breckenridge RL Jr, Ross JS: Idiopathic pulmonary hemosiderosis: A report of familial occurrence. Chest 75:636–639, 1979.
14. Beckerman RC, Taussig LM, Pinnas JL: Familial idiopathic pulmonary hemosiderosis. A J Dis Child 133:609–611, 1979.
15. Soergel KH, Sommers SC: The alveolar epithelial lesion of idiopathic pulmonary hemosiderosis. Am Rev Respir Dis 85:540–552, 1962.
16. Dolan J, McGuire S, Sweeney E, et al: Mast cells in pulmonary hemosiderosis. Arch Dis Child 59:276–278, 1984.
17. Mohri N, Noda M: Idiopathic pulmonary hemosiderosis: An autopsy case. Acta Pathol Jpn 15:75, 1965.
18. Hyatt RW, Adelstein ER, Halazun JF, Lukens JN: Ultrastructure of the lung in idiopathic pulmonary hemosiderosis. Am J Med 52:822–829, 1972.
19. Corrin B, Jagusch M, Dewar A, et al: Five structural changes in idiopathic pulmonary hemosiderosis. J Pathol 153:249–256, 1987.
20. Gonzalez-Crussi F, Hull MT, Grosfeld JL: Idiopathic pulmonary hemosiderosis: Evidence of capillary basement membrane abnormality. Am Rev Respir Dis 114:689–698, 1976.
21. Dolan CJ, Srodes CH, Duffy FD: Idiopathic pulmonary hemosiderosis. Electron microscopic, immunofluorescent and iron kinetic studies. Chest 68:577–580, 1975.
22. Wilson CB, Dixon FJ: Antiglomerular basement membrane antibody-induced glomerulonephritis. Kidney Int 3:74–89, 1973.
23. Brambilla CG, Brambilla EM, Stoebner P, Dechelette E: Idiopathic pulmonary hemorrhage. Ultrastructural and mineralogic study. Chest 81:120–123, 1982.

24. Teplitz C, Farrugia R, Irwin RS: Idiopathic pulmonary hemosiderosis (IPH): Ultrastructural observations on the role of interstitial ferritin diffusion and hemosiderin localization in the pathogenetic progression of IPH. Am Rev Respir Dis 119(Suppl. 2):176, 1979.

25. Thomas HM III, Irwin RS: Classification of diffuse intrapulmonary hemorrhage. Chest 68:483–484, 1975.

26. Kuhn C: Systemic lupus erythematosus in a patient with ultrastructural lesions of the pulmonary capillaries previously reported in the review as due to idiopathic pulmonary hemosiderosis. Am Rev Respir Dis 106:931–932, 1972.

27. Irwin RS, Cottrell TS, Hsu KC, et al: Idiopathic pulmonary hemosiderosis: An electron microscopic and immunofluorescent study. Chest 65:41–45, 1974.

28. Heiner DC, Sears JW, Kniker WT: Multiple precipitins to cow's milk in chronic respiratory disease. Am J Dis Child 103:634–654, 1962.

29. Nomura S, Kanoh T: Association of idiopathic pulmonary hemosiderosis with IgA monoclonal gammopathy. Thorax 42:696–697, 1987.

30. Oxelius VA: Immunoglobulin G (IgG) subclasses and human disease. Am J Med 76:7–18, 1984.

31. Matsaniotis N, Karpouzas J, Apostolopoulou E, et al: Idiopathic pulmonary haemosiderosis in children. Arch Dis Child 43:307–309, 1968.

32. Boat TF, Polmar SH, Whitman V, et al: Hyperreactivity to cow's milk in young children with pulmonary hemosiderosis and cor pulmonale secondary to nasopharyngeal obstruction. J Pediatr 87:23–29, 1975.

33. Galant S, Nussbaum E, Wittner R, et al: Increased IgD milk antibody responses in a patient with Down's syndrome, pulmonary hemosiderosis and cor pulmonale. Ann Allergy 51:446–449, 1983.

34. Sternlieb I, Bennett B, Scheinberg IH: D-Penicillamine induced Goodpasture's syndrome in Wilson's disease. Ann Intern Med 82:673–676, 1975.

35. Beirne GJ, Brennan JT: Glomerulonephritis associated with hydrocarbon solvents. Arch Environ Health 25:365–369, 1972.

36. Ahmad D, Morgan WK, Patterson R, et al: Pulmonary hemorrhage and haemolytic anemia due to trimellitic anhydride. Lancet 2:328–330, 1979.

37. Grill C, Szogi S, Bogren H: Fulminant idiopathic pulmonary hemosiderosis. Acta Med Scand 171:329–334, 1962.

38. Murphy KJ: Pulmonary hemosiderosis associated with myocarditis with bilateral penetrating corneal ulceration and with diabetes mellitus. Thorax 20:341–347, 1965.

39. Briggs WA, Johnson JP, Teichman S, et al: Antiglomerular basement membrane antibody mediated glomerulonephritis and Goodpasture's syndrome. Medicine 58:348–361, 1979.

40. Eagen JW, Memoli VA, Roberts JL, et al: Pulmonary hemorrhage and systemic lupus erythematosus. Medicine 57:545–560, 1978.

41. Byrd RB, Trunk G: Systemic lupus erythematosus presenting as pulmonary hemosiderosis. Chest 64:128–129, 1973.

42. Nadorra RL, Landing BH: Pulmonary lesions in childhood onset systemic lupus erythematosus: Analysis of 26 cases and summary of the literature. Pediatr Pathol 7:1–18, 1987.

43. Ramirez RE, Glasier C, Kirks D, et al: Pulmonary hemorrhage associated with systemic lupus erythematosus in children. Radiology 152:409–412, 1984.

44. Buchanan GR, Moore GC: Pulmonary hemosiderosis and immune thrombocytopenia. Initial manifestations of collagen-vascular disease. JAMA 246:861–864, 1981.

45. Smith BS: Idiopathic pulmonary haemosiderosis and rheumatoid arthritis. Br Med J 1:1403–1404, 1966.

46. Lemley DE, Katz P: Rheumatoid-like arthritis presenting as idiopathic pulmonary hemosiderosis. J Rheumatol 13:954–957, 1986.

47. Kincaid-Smith P, d'Apice AJF: Plasmapheresis in rapidly progressive glomerulonephritis. Am J Med 65:564–566, 1978.

48. Fajardo JE, Geller TJ, Koenig HM, Kleine ML: Chronic meningitis polyarthritis, lymphadenitis and pulmonary hemosiderosis. J Pediatr 101:738–740, 1982.

49. Corrin B, Liebow AA, Friedman PJ: Lymphangiomyomatosis: A review. Am J Pathol 79:348–382, 1975.

50. Wright PH, Menzies IS, Pounder RE, Keeling PW: Adult idiopathic pulmonary haemosiderosis and coeliac disease. Q J Med 50:95–102, 1981.

51. Wright PH, Buxton-Thomas M, Keeling PWN, Kreel L: Adult idiopathic pulmonary haemosiderosis: A comparison of lung function changes and the distribution of pulmonary disease in patients with and without coeliac disease. Br J Dis Chest 77:282–292, 1983.

52. DeGowin RL, Sorensen LB, Charleston DB, et al: Retention of radioiron in the lungs of a woman with idiopathic pulmonary hemosiderosis. Ann Intern Med 69:1213–1220, 1968.

53. Theros EG, Reeder MM, Eckert JF: An exercise in radiologic-pathologic correlation. Radiology 90:784–791, 1968.

54. Albelda SM, Gefter WB, Epstein DM, Miller WT: Diffuse pulmonary hemorrhage: A review and classification. Radiology 154:289–297, 1985.

55. Slonim L: Goodpasture's syndrome and its radiological features. Australas Radiol 13:164–172, 1969.

56. Nickol KH: Idiopathic pulmonary haemosiderosis presenting with spontaneous pneumothorax. Tubercle 41:216–218, 1960.

57. Turner-Warwick M, Dewar A: Pulmonary hemorrhage and pulmonary hemosiderosis. Clin Radiol 33:361–370, 1982.

58. Ewan PW, Jones HA, Rhodes CG, Hughes JM: Detection of intrapulmonary hemorrhage with carbon monoxide uptake. Application in Goodpasture's syndrome. N Engl J Med 295:1391–1396, 1976.

59. Bowley NB, Hughes JM, Steiner RE: The chest x-ray in pulmonary capillary hemorrhage: Correlation with carbon monoxide uptake. Clin Radiol 30:413–417, 1979.

60. Miller T, Tanaka T: Nuclear scan of pulmonary hemorrhage in idiopathic pulmonary hemosiderosis. AJR 132:120–121, 1979.

61. Kurzweil PR, Miller DR, Freeman JE, et al: Use of sodium chromate Cr[51] in diagnosing childhood idiopathic pulmonary hemosiderosis. Am J Dis Child 138:746–748, 1984.

62. Drew WL, Finley TN, Golde DW: Diagnostic lavage and occult pulmonary hemorrhage in thrombocytopenic immunocompromised patients. Am Rev Respir Dis 116:215–221, 1977.

63. Stover DE, Zaman MB, Hajdu SI, et al: Bronchoalveolar lavage in the diagnosis of diffuse pulmonary infiltrates in the immunosuppressed host. Ann Intern Med 101:1–7, 1984.

64. Sherman JM, Winnie G, Thomassen MJ, et al: Time course of hemosiderin production and clearance by human pulmonary macrophages. Chest 86:409–411, 1984.

65. Browning JR, Houghton JD: Idiopathic pulmonary hemosiderosis. Am J Med 20:374–382, 1956.

66. Steiner B: Immunoallergic lung purpura treated with azathioprine and with splenectomy and azathioprine. Helv Paediatr Acta 24:413–419, 1969.

67. Yeager H, Powell D, Weinberg RM, et al: Idiopathic pulmonary hemosiderosis. Ultrastructural studies and response to azathioprine. Arch Intern Med 136:1145–1149, 1976.

68. Goran E: Budesonide inhalation to treat idiopathic pulmonary hemosiderosis. Lancet 1:981–982, 1985.

69. Cavalieri S: Desferrioxamine with corticosteroids in case of idiopathic pulmonary hemosiderosis. Francastoro 56:389, 1963.

70. Lockwood CM, Pussell B, Wilson CB, Peters DK: Plasma exchange in nephritis. Adv Nephrol Necker Hosp 8:383–418, 1979.

71. Pozo-Rodriguez F, Freire-Campo JM, Gutierrez-Millet V, et al: idiopathic pulmonary haemosiderosis treated by plasmapheresis. Thorax 35:399–400, 1980.

72. Frankel LR, Smith DW, Pearl RG, Lewiston NJ: Nitroglycerin-responsive pulmonary hypertension in idiopathic pulmonary hemosiderosis. Am Rev Respir Dis 133:170–172, 1986.

73. Bacani RA, Velasquez F, Kanter A, et al: Rapidly progressive glomerulonephritis. Ann Intern Med 69:463–485, 1968.

74. Benoit FL, Rulon DB, Theil GB, et al: Goodpasture's syndrome: A clinicopathologic entity. Am J Med 37:424–444, 1964.

75. Leonard CD, Nagle RB, Striker GE, et al: Acute glomerulo-nephritis with prolonged oliguria. An analysis of 29 cases. Ann Intern Med 73:703–711, 1970.

60 THE IMMOTILE CILIA SYNDROME

DANIEL V. SCHIDLOW, M.D. / HOWARD PANITCH, M.D. /
SHEILA M. KATZ, M.D., M.B.A.

The immotile cilia syndrome (ICS) is a genetic disease characterized by chronic disease of the upper and lower respiratory tract, male infertility, and situs inversus of the viscera in 50% of affected patients (constituting the so-called Kartagener's syndrome).

The pathophysiologic basis of this condition resides in a lack of effective ciliary motility as a result of ultrastructural and functional defects of cilia.

HISTORIC PERSPECTIVE

ICS has been known since the beginning of the 20th century. Siewert,[1] in 1904, described the case of a young man with situs inversus, bronchiectasis, chronic cough, and purulent bronchorrhea whose symptoms had started in early infancy. Oeri,[2] in 1909, reported a 46-year-old woman with chronic lung disease and situs inversus, and in 1923 Gunther[3] reported a 19-year-old woman with situs inversus and bronchiectasis; one sister also had chronic bronchitis and situs inversus, and two others were healthy. In 1933, Kartagener[4] first recognized the clinical triad of situs inversus, chronic sinusitis, and bronchiectasis as a distinct clinicopathologic entity and postulated that a congenital deficiency or weakness of the bronchial wall was the cause of the bronchiectasis. Many authors, including Kartagener himself, later recognized that affected patients within a sibship could have sinobronchial disease and normal visceral situs, whereas others could manifest the complete expression of the syndrome.[5-10] In 1960 Arge[11] reported the association of male infertility with immobility of spermatozoa and chronic respiratory symptoms. It was, however, approximately 15 years later that the most significant contributions to the understanding of the disease were made, when Pedersen and Rebbe,[12] as well as Afzelius and colleagues,[13] demonstrated ultrastructural abnormalities of the sperm tails of infertile men, which rendered the flagella immobile. Camner and associates[14] reported the concomitant presence of sperm abnormalities, congenitally nonfunctioning cilia, and Kartagener's syndrome. The term *immotile cilia* was subsequently coined by Afzelius,[15] and various ultrastructural abnormalities were described by Eliasson and co-workers,[16] Sturgess and co-authors,[17, 18] and other investigators.[19-21] The terms *primary cilia dyskinesia* and *dyskinetic cilia syndrome* were later proposed by Rossman and co-authors[22-26] to indicate that cilia usually show not lack of movement but rather disorganized motion.

GENETICS

This syndrome follows an autosomal recessive pattern of inheritance without sex predilection.[27] Exact calculations of the incidence and prevalence of the disease are difficult not only because of misdiagnosis of mild cases but also because situs inversus, which occurs randomly in 50% of patients with ICS, can occur as an isolated entity without ciliary abnormalities. The incidence of ICS is approximately 1 in 16,000 live births, and that of Kartagener's syndrome is 1 in 32,000[28] (because only 50% of all patients have the visceral abnormality). On the basis of autosomal recessive inheritance alone, the carrier rate in the general population would be approximately 1 in 60 persons.[28] These incidence rates, however, may vary greatly, depending on the geographic area, the closeness of the community, and the degree of intermarriage. The incidence of situs inversus alone in the general population is approximately 1 in 8000.[28]

As with other autosomal recessive diseases, known heterozygote carriers have a risk of one in four of producing an affected child in each subsequent pregnancy resulting from the union of two known carriers.

There is no prenatal diagnostic test, and no specific gene or mutations have been identified. It is possible that the diagnosis of situs inversus could be made in utero by means of fetal ultrasonography.

NORMAL CILIARY ANATOMY

Cilia are found in various parts of the body: as organelles in the tail of sperm, in the ciliated epithelium lining fallopian tubes and vasa efferentia, in the ependymal lining of the central nervous system, and in the respiratory tract from the posterior third of the nose to the bronchioles, including the middle ear and paranasal sinuses. Cilia involved in the transport of mucus are short (5–7 μm) and are present in groups. In the mammalian respiratory tract, there may be 200 cilia per cell,[29] with a density of approximately eight cilia per square micron at the apex of the cell.[30] In general, ciliary activity is generated by many

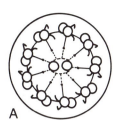
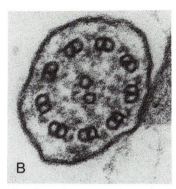

Figure 60–1. Transverse section of a cilium shows normal axonemal ultrastructure. Nine pairs of microtubules encircle a central pair. The outer and inner dynein arms are attached to the A subunit. Nexin links extend from the A subunit to the B subunit. Radial spokes originate in the A subunit and end in thicker spoke heads. *A*, Diagram. *B*, Actual photomicrograph.

small patches of regularly beating cilia ranging in size from one or two cells to four cells.[31] There is a steady increase in the dens████ █f ██ █.om the alveolar margins toward the trachea. The rate of ciliary beating increases from 7 Hz in the peripheral airways to 18 Hz in the main lobar bronchus.[30] The mean ciliary beat frequency in the human trachea is approximately 22 Hz at 37°C but is affected by temperature and relative humidity.[30–32] This beat frequency results in a mucus transport rate of 20 to 30 μm/sec. In healthy adult humans, 10 ml of mucus is expelled from the trachea per day.[32]

Ciliary ultrastructure is remarkably constant throughout different species. The cilium shares a unit membrane with the cell. The cell membrane is responsible for controlling the ionic environment of the cilium and regulating the concentrations of adenosine triphosphate (ATP) and divalent cations.

The cytoplasmic contents of the cilium are collectively referred to as the axoneme. Cross-sectional study of the ciliary shaft yields the characteristic 9 + 2 formation of microtubular doublets (Fig. 60–1). The two central doublets are separate, complete microtubules. The outer nine doublets, however, are composed of one complete microtubule (designated the A subunit) and one incomplete, laterally attached microtubule (the B subunit).[33] The main structural protein of these doublets is tubulin.

Attached to each A subunit and recurring periodically along its length are paired sets of curved arms that extend toward the adjacent B subunit in a clockwise manner.[34] The outer arms are longer than the inner arms. These structures, called dynein arms, are composed of approximately nine polypeptides, including two ATPase heavy chains per arm.[33] The ATPase is highly specific for ATP, and it must couple with Mg^{++} in order for ciliary motion to occur. Dynein is permanently associated with its A microtubule and, as is discussed, forms temporary bridges with the adjacent B microtubule.

A second type of link between the peripheral doublets exists as straplike bands between A microtubules of adjacent doublets or between adjacent A and B microtubules.[30] These are called nexin links. Their role in ciliary motility appears to be to limit the sliding of the peripheral

doublets and to help maintain the normal 9 + 2 arrangement of the axoneme.[34, 35]

Extending from the A microtubule centrally, and connecting the peripheral doublets to the central microtubules, are projections called radial links or spokes.[30, 34, 35] The heads of these radial links appear to make connections with short, curved rods that extend laterally from the central microtubules and that recur at constant intervals along the length of each microtubule, forming an incomplete central sheath.[30] These structures appear to be important in controlling the sliding of the cilium.[33, 35]

The cilium undergoes structural changes along its length. At its tip, the peripheral doublets become singlets by losing the B subunit, and radial links are no longer present. At the base, the central microtubules end at the level of the cell surface, and each doublet becomes a triplet by gaining a third (C) incomplete microtubule attached to the B subunit. Specialized roots anchor the cilium to the cell surface (Fig. 60–2).

NORMAL CILIARY FUNCTION AND MUCUS CLEARANCE

The hypothesis of how cilia bend favored by most investigators is one of sliding filaments, akin to the actin-myosin system of skeletal muscle contraction. There are

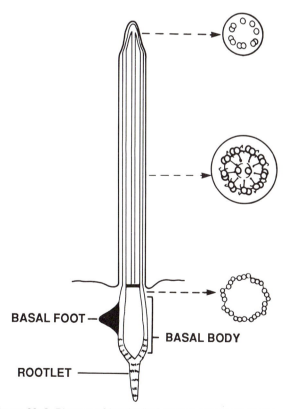

Figure 60–2. Diagram of longitudinal section across cilium shows the basal foot pointed in the direction of effective beat, the ciliary root anchoring the cilium to the cytoplasm, and the tubular structures running in parallel. Transverse views: At the tip of the cilium, the diameter is reduced and the microtubular composition is variable. No arms are noted. At the base, there are no central tubules, and the peripheral units are triplets rather than doublets.

BASAL FOOT

BASAL BODY

ROOTLET

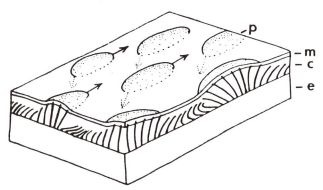

Figure 60–3. Diagram of an area of ciliated epithelium (e) propelling a thin sheet of mucus (m). Cilia (c) perform curved recovery strokes in periciliary fluid beneath mucus but penetrate the lower side of mucus during their erect effective strokes. Effective cilia lift up mucus a little in these areas of application of propulsive force (p). Mucus is propelled in the direction of the solid arrows, but metachronal waves that propel it move in the direction of the dotted arrows. (From Sleigh MA: Ciliary function in mucus transport. Chest 80(6 Suppl):791–795, 1981, by permission of Chest, Park Ridge, Illinois.)

two systems that operate within the axoneme: The first is the force-generating system, consisting of the dynein arms and peripheral doublets; the second is a control system consisting of the radial spokes, nexin links, and central complex, all of which convert the sliding filaments into ciliary bending.[33]

Sliding occurs when the dynein arm from one A subunit (doublet n) attaches to the B subunit of the adjacent microtubule (doublet n + 1) and undergoes a configurational change so that the n + 1 doublet slides tipward. Hydrolysis of ATP is necessary for the dynein arm to detach and therefore start the cycle over.[33, 36] In the absence of radial spokes and nexin links, ciliary elongation rather than bending occurs[34, 37] as the peripheral doublets slide without the restrictions imposed by these structures. When intact, the radial spoke heads appear to detach and to reattach to sites on the central complex,[30] thereby limiting sliding and perhaps propagating bending. This control system is thought to turn off and on active sliding of peripheral doublets on opposite halves of the axoneme at different times throughout the ciliary beat cycle.[33, 36]

The beat cycle is divided into two parts: the effective stroke and the recovery or preparatory stroke. Mucus-propelling cilia normally rest between beats,[29, 31, 32] at the end of the effective stroke, so that the tip is in the direction of mucus flow. The cilium moves in a whiplike manner, bent close to the cell surface in the recovery phase and fully extended in the effective stroke phase. The net effect of these movements is to propel fluid in the direction of the effective stroke (Fig. 60–3).

Lucas and Douglas[38] suggested a two-layer system in which the cilia of the respiratory tract work: an underlying sol layer in which the cilia move and an upper gel layer consisting of mucus. This basic hypothesis has been upheld with few revisions. Fluid dynamics result in a much greater propulsive force exerted on the mucus layer during the effective stroke than on the periciliary layer during the recovery stroke.[30, 32, 39]

The cilia of respiratory epithelium display coordination in their transport of mucus. In normal persons, cilia from one cell are arranged with their foot processes in approximately the same direction,[30, 40] which is also the direction of the effective stroke. When the epithelium over which a coordinated wave of fluid passes is examined, all cilia lying in parallel with the wave crests are in the same stage of their ciliary beat or are synchronous. Cilia lying at an angle to the wave crests are in different phases of their beat and so are metachronous.[30] Adjacent cilia influence each other[30, 32] so that the closely packed cilia of mucus-transporting epithelium become coordinated in a metachronal wave (see Fig. 60–3).

Effective mucociliary clearance depends on properly functioning cilia that beat in a coordinated manner, a periciliary fluid layer whose height should be almost that of a fully extended cilium, and mucus whose viscoelastic properties are fairly narrowly constrained. Alterations in any of these components can result in impaired mucociliary clearance.

ABNORMALITIES OF CILIARY STRUCTURE IN IMMOTILE CILIA SYNDROME

Patients with ICS may display a variety of genetically determined abnormalities, summarized in Figure 60–4. Specific ciliary defects are genetically determined and present in all members of a sibship regardless of severity of clinical picture or visceral situs.

The initial abnormality described was the total absence of dynein arms (Fig. 60–5). Other defects include partial or complete absence of outer and inner dynein arms, absence of radial spokes and nexin links, and absence of

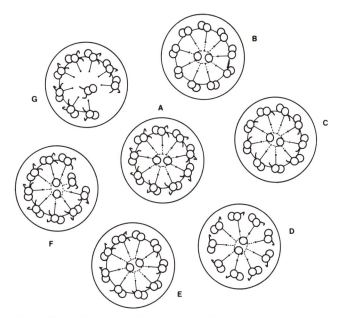

Figure 60–4. Diagrams of transverse sections of cilia showing ultrastructural abnormalities seen in the ICS: A, Normal structure; B, Complete absence of dynein arms; C, Absence of outer dynein arms; D, Absence of inner dynein arms–nexin links; E, Partial absence of inner and outer dynein arms; F, Radial spoke defect; G, Tubular transposition.

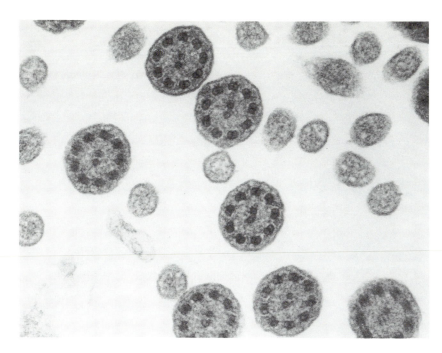

Figure 60–5. Cilia from a patient with Kartagener's syndrome showing lack of dynein arms (uranyl acetate, lead citrate).

the central microtubular pair with transposition of a peripheral microtubule into the center of the axoneme[13, 41–47] (Fig. 60–6). Case reports documented total absence of microtubules within cilia, absence of the entire axoneme, replacement of ciliated epithelium with brush-border cells containing microvilli, abnormal ciliary length, and abnormal ciliary function with normal ciliary ultrastructure.[19, 20, 40, 48]

Random ciliary orientation, which fails to generate metachronal waves and unidirectional movement of mucus, can be detected on ultrastructural examination. The transverse axonemal axis of two or more adjacent cilia is determined by drawing a straight line through the two central doublets, and the relative angle is calculated. Angles of more than 25 degrees are considered abnormal (Fig. 60–7A). Sections along the base of several cilia show disorientation of the basal feet, also indicative of asynchrony (Fig. 60–7B).

Ciliary biopsy specimens from normal subjects contain approximately 4% ultrastructurally abnormal cilia.[26] Some of these defects include extra doublets (2.6%), missing central microtubules with translocation of a peripheral doublet (0.6%), and compound or multiple cilia (0.8%). In contrast, biopsy specimens of patients with the ICS show a much higher proportion of abnormal cilia: In the same study,[26] 95.5% of the cilia in patients with deficiency of dynein arms were abnormal; in patients with radial spoke defects, 72.5% of the cilia were abnormal; and in those with no central microtubules and peripheral microtubular translocation, 31.5% of the cilia were abnormal.

Ciliary abnormalities and altered mucus transport can occur as a result of infection or chronic inflammation.[49–52] The alterations usually comprise fewer than 10% of the cilia sampled, are frequently heterogeneous, and are reversible. They include deformity of ciliary membranes, formation of compound cilia, as well as abnormal

number and arrangement of microtubules (Figs. 60–8, 60–9, 60–10). Axonemal lesions involving dynein arms, nexin links, and radial spokes are very rarely seen. Table 60–1 summarizes the lesions thought to be hereditary and those regarded as nonspecific.

Artifactual distortion of cilia, resulting from problems of fixation and staining, may render ultrastructural interpretation of cilia difficult and lead to erroneous diagnosis of abnormalities. The normal axonemal architecture may lack clarity and, as a consequence, be misinterpreted as absent. In addition, cytoplasmic ciliary membranes may be distorted because of fixation. As a result of chronic inflammation, cilia are often totally denuded, and pseudostratified ciliated columnar epithelium is completely replaced by cuboidal or squamous metaplasia, rendering evaluation of cilia impossible. To avoid such problems, whenever possible, the biopsy should be obtained from a minimally inflamed region. If this cannot be ascertained on gross examination, a frozen section (one portion placed in glutaraldehyde for electron microscopy) can swiftly reveal the presence of cilia and the degree of chronic inflammation. Within seconds after the biopsy is performed, the specimen must be placed into fresh glutaraldehyde. The specimen is then processed carefully by standard dehydration and embedding techniques and sectioned by an ultramicrotome. A calibrated, high-resolution electron microscope is optimal for examination of cilia. The conventional range of magnification is from 5000 to 70,000 times.

ABNORMALITIES IN MUCOCILIARY CLEARANCE IN IMMOTILE CILIA SYNDROME

On the average, one third of cells studied from patients with Kartagener's syndrome may display motile cilia,[24, 25,]

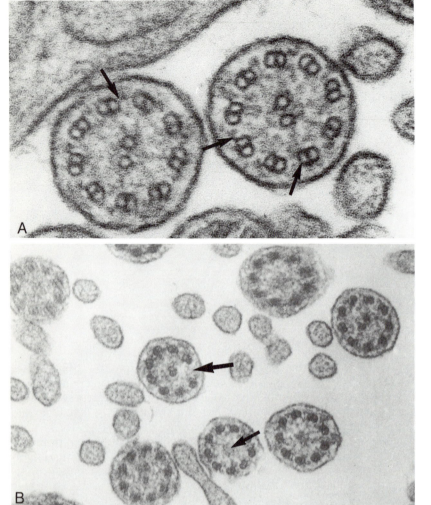

Figure 60–6. *A*, Electron micrograph of cross sections of nasal cilia demonstrate heterogeneity of alterations of dynein arms, including intact dynein arms, stubs of dynein arms, and absent dynein arms. *B*, Ciliary transposition. Absent central microtubular pair and central displacement of a peripheral doublet.

[53, 54] although the pattern of movement is abnormal and ineffective in producing movement of the mucus layer.[12] Indeed, complete ciliary immotility is the exception rather than the rule.[52, 55] Motion analysis of the ciliary beat cycle from patients with Kartagener's syndrome or clinical evidence of ciliary dyskinesia has enabled the recognition of the association of abnormal beat patterns with certain ultrastructural defects.[24, 25]

Cilia that lack dynein arms display two types of multiplanar asynchronous movements: an egg beater–like rotation of the midsection of the axoneme or a vibrational pattern in which only the distal half of the axoneme bends in several planes. In addition, the beat frequency of these cilia is approximately half that of normal. Immotile cilia with no dynein arms from patients with ICS may be activated *in vitro* by the addition of exogenous ATPase,[22] resulting in both movement and an increase in beat frequency.

Cilia with no radial spokes display a floppy appearance, rotating about two points of the axoneme at different rates in a corkscrew manner. The beat frequency of these cilia is approximately two-thirds normal.[24]

Cilia with a translocation defect display a third pattern of dyskinesia. They move with a grabbing-type motion

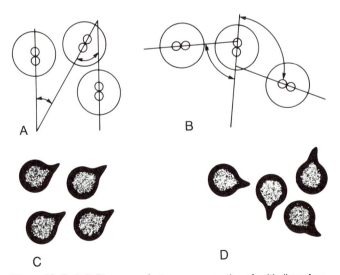

Figure 60–7. *A, B,* Diagrams of a transverse section of epithelium. Axonemal axis is represented by a straight line drawn across the two central doublets. Normal angles (*A*) between neighboring cilia range from 0 degrees to 25 degrees. Angles larger than 25 degrees reflect axonemal disorientation (*B*). *C, D,* Diagram of transverse section across the basal bodies shows normal orientation (*C*) and random orientation (*D*) characteristic of the disordered motility seen in ICS.

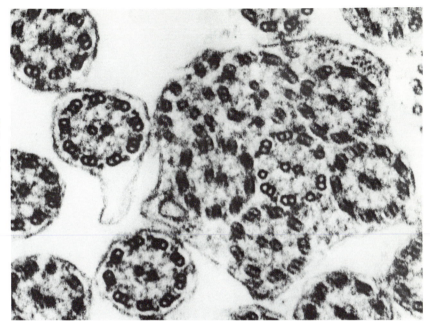

Figure 60-8. A compound cilium consists of six total central axonemes and one partial axoneme. This is from a patient who suffers from chronic bronchitis. Notice that the central axonemal structure has three peripheral microtubules that lack the doublet pair (uranyl acetate, lead citrate).

toward the apex of the axoneme, whereas the base remains rigid. They move with a normal beat frequency, although movement is in several planes and no metachronicity is present.[24]

In addition, a quivering, ineffective hypermotility has been described in some cilia with normal ultrastructure of patients with ICS.[54, 55] All these abnormalities are summarized in Figures 60–11 and 60–12.

The lack of effective ciliary movement demonstrated in these patients results in defective mucociliary clearance. Several studies in which aerosolized radioisotopes were deposited in the central airways have demonstrated a marked reduction of clearance of the particles in patients with ICS.[23, 56] In one study, at the end of 2 h, normal subjects retained 38% ± 22% of the initial dose of particles, whereas those with ICS retained 92% ± 8%.[56] All studies demonstrated the effectiveness of coughing, which can remove 30% ± 15% of particles from the airways of patients with ICS.

CLINICAL MANIFESTATIONS

NOSE AND SINUSES

The severity of clinical manifestations varies from patient to patient, ranging from very mild rhinorrhea and sinus disease to frequent exacerbations of sinobronchial

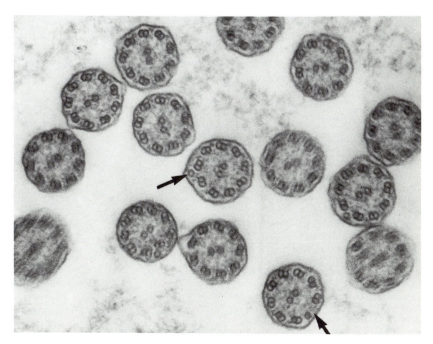

Figure 60-9. Cilia from a patient suffering from chronic bronchitis without Kartagener's syndrome shows secondary abnormalities of abnormal number and positioning of microtubules. Notice the ectopic microtubules and absent microtubules (uranyl acetate, lead citrate).

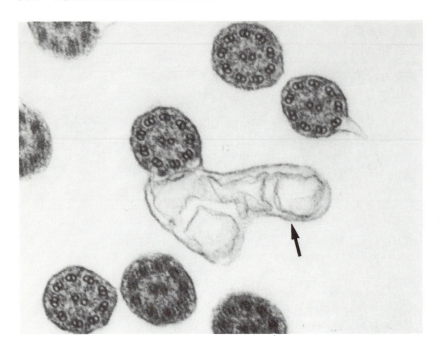

Figure 60–10. The central cilium from a patient who suffers from chronic bronchitis without immotile cilia syndrome demonstrates a cytoplasmic bleb. This finding is seen in secondary ciliary abnormalities and is not artifactual, providing the specimen is properly fixed and processed. Notice the intact dynein arms, nexin links, and radial spokes (uranyl acetate, lead citrate).

inflammation and pneumonia that require aggressive therapy. Even within a sibship in which two or more persons are affected and share similar ciliary defects, the seriousness of the clinical picture is not uniform. Chronic inflammation of the nasal and paranasal mucosa is the most common and constant manifestation of this condition. In older children and adolescents, mucopurulent rhinorrhea, sensation of fullness, and pain over paranasal sinuses (usually ethmoid and maxillary) are common. These symptoms characteristically tend to respond to the administration of antimicrobial agents and recur quickly after discontinuation of these drugs. For some patients, paranasal sinus involvement causes the most disabling symptoms that necessitate repeated therapeutic interventions.

Opacification of all sinus cavities is a common radiographic feature. Thickening of the mucosa and the presence of fluid levels can be detected by computed tomography (CT). As in other diseases with chronic sinus disease, such as cystic fibrosis, the frontal sinuses are frequently hypoplastic.

Table 60–1. GENETIC AND ACQUIRED CILIARY DEFECTS

Major Ciliary Abnormalities Associated With Immotile Cilia Syndrome
Total absence of dynein arms
Partial absence or fragmentation of inner or outer dynein arms, or both
Absence of radial spokes
Combined absence of inner dynein arm and spoke head
Absence of nexin links
Microtubular transposition
Agenesis of axonemes
Acquired (Secondary, Nonspecific) Abnormalities
Compound cilia
Cytoplasmic blebs and outer membrane disruption
Axonemal disorganization
Shed or internalized cilia

As a result of these inflammatory changes, it is common for these patients to have nasal obstruction, postnasal drip, snoring during sleep, anosmia, halitosis, and hyponasal speech.

NASAL POLYPS

The pathogenesis of polyps formation is unclear. It is probably related to chronic mucosal irritation. The incidence of nasal polyps is approximately 20% in large series.[58]

EAR DISEASE

Chronic otitis media with periodic acute exacerbations is present in most if not all patients. Conductive hearing loss is very common. Almost all of the authors' patients have eventually undergone insertion of tympanostomy tubes to relieve middle-ear pressure, provide adequate drainage, and restore hearing.

LOWER RESPIRATORY TRACT

The original description of the syndrome included bronchiectasis as one of the main clinical features. Initially, it was believed that there was a congenital weakness of the bronchial wall.[1] It is clear now that bronchiectasis develops slowly over time as a result of chronic mucus impaction, infection, and inflammation. Hence it is uncommon to find this abnormality in young children. It is possible that bronchiolectasis is present very early, but it is difficult to detect abnormality by noninvasive means. Eventually, however, most older patients with ICS have bronchiectasis as part of the clinical picture. Turner and

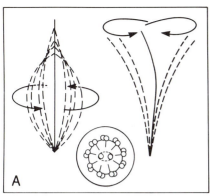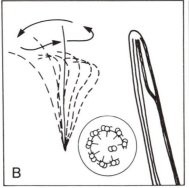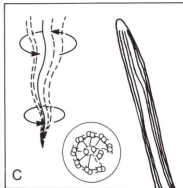

Figure 60–11. Diagrams of patterns of ciliary beating and corresponding ultrastructural abnormalities. *A,* Absence of dynein arms—rotational (left) and vibrational (right) waveform. *B,* Radial spoke defect. Transposition of peripheral doublet toward the center of the axoneme seen in (*A*) transverse section and (*B*) longitudinal section. Biphasic rotational waveform. *C,* Translocation defect. Absent central pair of microtubules and translocation of a peripheral pair to the center of the axoneme seen in (*A*) transverse section and (*B*) longitudinal section. There is a "grabbing" motion toward the apex of the axoneme while the base remains rigid. (Adapted from Rossman C, Forrest J, Lee R, et al: The dyskinetic cilia syndrome: Abnormal ciliary motility in association with abnormal ciliary ultrastructure. Chest 80(Suppl):860–865, 1981, by permission of the publisher.)

colleagues[57] studied 21 patients aged 1 to 21 years and found bronchiectasis in 30% of them. The clinical experience of the authors has been similar, and as medical intervention takes place in a more opportune manner because of earlier diagnosis, it is possible that this incidence may decrease further.

PRIMARY CILIARY DYSKINESIA

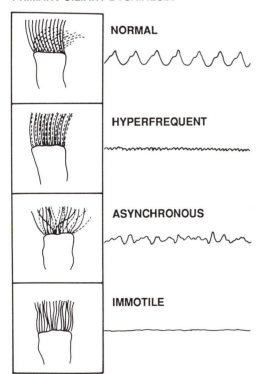

NORMAL

HYPERFREQUENT

ASYNCHRONOUS

IMMOTILE

Figure 60–12. Schematic drawing of patterns of ciliary beating and corresponding microphoto-oscillographic curves. Normal beating, hypermotile (hyperfrequent) cilia characterized by very frequent beat with small amplitude, asynchronous beating, and immotile cilia. (From Pedersen M, Nielsen MH, Mygind N: Primary ciliary dyskinesia: A preliminary comparison between ciliary motility and ultrastructure. Mod Probl Paediatr 21:68–78, 1982, by permission of the publisher, S. Karger, AG, Basel, Switzerland.)

Lower respiratory tract symptoms may be present early in the neonatal period as respiratory distress, atelectasis, or pneumonia.[59] Later in life, productive cough, expectoration of thick, purulent yellowish-green sputum, recurrent bouts of bronchitis and pneumonia, or atelectasis can occur with some frequency, particularly in untreated patients.

In the authors' experience, most of these patients exhibit signs of airway reactivity that is totally or partially responsive to the administration of bronchodilator drugs. Scattered wheezes and rhonchi are frequently heard on auscultation. Rales can be heard over areas of bronchiectasis. These are more common in the lower than in the upper lobes probably because of the effect of gravity.

Pulmonary function ranges from mild obstructive disease of the small airways to moderately severe, irreversible obstructive disease and air trapping in patients with more extensive changes. Obstructive disease is manifested by decreased forced vital capacity, forced expiratory volume in 1 sec, and maximal mid-expiratory flow rates as well as flows at low lung volumes (forced expiratory flows at 75% and 50% of vital capacity). Pulmonary function remains remarkably stable, usually with only very slow deterioration.

The radiographic appearance of the chest ranges from mild inflammatory interstitial disease to areas of bronchiectasis, peribronchial thickening, subsegmental or lobar atelectasis, and overaeration.[59] CT and bronchography may identify specific areas where the bronchi are dilated (Fig. 60–13). The presence of dextrocardia and abdominal situs inversus is indicative of the diagnosis of ICS (discussed later). Otherwise, the chest radiograph presents no distinct characteristics specific of ICS.

DIGITAL CLUBBING

This finding is a nonspecific manifestation of chronic lung disease and bronchiectasis. It is seen in approximately 20% of all patients with ICS,[60] particularly older patients with more advanced disease. In the authors'

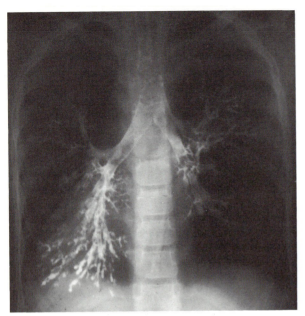

Figure 60–13. Bronchogram in a patient with Kartagener's syndrome. There is total reversal (mirror image) of the thoracic anatomy and bronchiectasis in the right lower lobe.

experience, severe digital clubbing is rare; most affected patients have relatively mild changes.

MALE REPRODUCTIVE SYSTEM

The ultrastructural abnormalities typical of this disease render the spermatozoa unable to migrate or fertilize the ovum. Fertility has been reported in several male patients with Kartagener's syndrome, but the issue of paternity was not explored in any of the cases (i.e., semen samples were not examined). In one report,[61] investigators described a patient with abnormal respiratory cilia and normal, motile spermatozoa who fathered a child. This phenomenon is the exception rather than the rule. The overwhelming majority of male patients are infertile on the basis of sperm immotility. Although the number of spermatoza is normal, their forward propulsion is impaired.

FEMALE REPRODUCTIVE SYSTEM

The fallopian tubes are lined with ciliated epithelium. Ultrastructural abnormalities of the reproductive system have been described in the syndrome.[62] There is no conclusive evidence that fertility is diminished, even though some reports suggest that.[63] The incidence of ectopic pregnancy is not increased.[63] One of the explanations that have been offered for this apparent lack of functional abnormality is that tubal muscular movement may play an important role in the propulsion of the ovum, which overcomes the obstacle posed by ciliary dysfunction.

VISCERAL SITUS

Fifty percent of patients with ICS have mirror-image configuration of their viscera (total situs inversus). The pathophysiologic origin of this abnormality remains unclear. The current hypothesis offered by Afzelius is that ciliary beating would cause the embryonic organs to rotate in a right helix, leading to a normal visceral position. In the absence of normal ciliary activity, visceral orientation would take place at random. Therefore, in 50% of patients, total transposition of the viscera would result. This theory, although attractive, does not explain other conditions or syndromes of abnormal organ position such as isolated situs inversus and polysplenia syndrome. Furthermore, in a series of Polynesian patients reported by Wakefield and Waite,[64] dynein arms were absent in all patients who had normal visceral situs. One other possibility is the existence of a gene that determines reversal of visceral situs and is close to the gene that determines ciliary abnormality. There is experimental evidence of such a recessive gene in an inbred strain of mice, in which 50% of homozygotic animals have situs inversus.[65,66] It is likely that other genetic determinants play a role in the pathogenesis of visceral malrotation in patients with ICS.

MANIFESTATIONS IN OTHER ORGAN SYSTEMS

The presence of cilia in microtubular structures in organ systems other than the respiratory and reproductive systems raises the question of potential manifestations in other organs.

CENTRAL NERVOUS SYSTEM

The ependyma of the brain and spinal cord have a ciliated epithelium. Hence in theory at least, patients with ICS could have disorders of circulation of cerebral spinal fluid. A slight enlargement of the ventricular size and possibly of the sulci has been described by Afzelius.[41] Greenstone and colleagues[67] reported a 12-year-old boy with ICS in whom hydrocephalus developed in the neonatal period, and they speculated about the possible relationship between ciliary abnormality and these findings. The evidence for abnormalities in the central nervous system, however, remains scant and inconclusive.

OCULAR FINDINGS

Cilia can be found in the corneal endothelium, the trabecular meshwork, the choroid, and the retina. Corneal abnormalities were reported in 9 of a series of 10 patients.[68] The findings, however, seem to be without significance and point to some abnormality in the development of the cornea.[68] No abnormalities in the circulation of aqueous humor, light and color sensitivity (rods and cones are modified ciliated cells), or other parts of the eye have been reported. Other familial ocular changes have been described, but the association with ICS in these cases seems accidental.[69]

LEUKOCYTE FUNCTION

Because neutrophils have a cytoplasmic microtubular system, the possibility of a defect in neutrophil migration has been explored in patients with ICS and microtubular abnormalities in cilia. The concern is that abnormal leukocyte function could contribute to the severity of respiratory infection in these patients.

Caleb and associates[70] first reported abnormal leukocyte migration in a patient with ICS. Corkey and colleagues[71] reported neutrophil function in 14 patients with ICS with a variety of ultrastructural ciliary defects. No significant abnormality was detected in migration or other phagocytic functions. Corkey and colleagues concluded that abnormalities in neutrophil function play no role in the severity of respiratory infection. In a series of patients with ICS, Valerius and colleagues found only slightly reduced neutrophil chemotaxis in one patient; bactericidal activity was normal, and ingestion of bacteria was decreased. Valerius and colleagues suggested that the abnormalities in ICS are related primarily to motility, possibly secondary to a microtubular defect.[72] Wolberg and associates[73] found normal granulocytic function with reduced chemotaxis and intramembranous particles. Although evidence is inconclusive, there seems to be reduced leukocyte migration in patients with ICS. The clinical relevance of this finding is unclear at this time.

DIAGNOSIS

ICS should be suspected in children who have recurrent sinobronchial disease, particularly those with severe mucopurulent rhinitis, otitis media, sinusitis, and chronic cough.

The diagnostic workup should include a complete personal and family history as well as a pedigree in order to trace the disease to other family members. An important element of the history is the time of onset of symptoms because ICS is one of very few diseases that can cause symptoms early in the neonatal period. The presence of situs inversus, particularly when associated with respiratory disease in a child, should alert the clinician to the possibility of ICS.

The diagnosis can be confirmed by the finding of abnormal electron-microscopic appearance of cilia on a biopsy of respiratory epithelium. Caution must be exercised to obtain appropriate samples and to have them examined by an electron microscopist familiar with this condition and the proper processing of specimens. To ensure availability of a proper sample, it is preferable that two biopsy specimens be obtained from different areas of the respiratory tree (e.g., nose and trachea).

Studies of mucociliary clearance in patients with ICS show diminished velocity of mucus removal, evidenced by decreased elimination of radioactively tagged particles. The saccharin test can also be used to measure muco-

ciliary transport. After a saccharin particle is placed on the anterior portion of the inferior turbinate, a sweet flavor is perceived in approximately 20 min in normal individuals. In persons with abnormal mucociliary transport, this time is greatly prolonged. In the authors' experience, this test is not very reliable and is subject to a variety of technical problems such as interference from sneezing, forceful inhalation and mucosal swelling.

Ciliary motion can also be studied by analyzing ciliary beat frequency and waveform by direct videocinematography or oscillographic techniques.[24, 54, 55] These methods can be useful but are available in only a few institutions. Ciliary motion analysis is particularly useful in patients in whom the biopsy results are inconclusive or technically unsatisfactory. This kind of analysis was used in an elegant study by Rossman and Newhouse, and in their laboratory it is used as a first approach in the diagnosis of a patient with ICS.[40]

In mature adolescent and adult males, analysis of the ejaculate discloses immotile sperm. Structural abnormalities in sperm tail are usually identical to those in respiratory mucosa; hence electron-microscopic examination of the sperm may yield a definitive diagnosis. Exceedingly rare exceptions are the cases of patients in whom sperm motility is normal, whereas the respiratory epithelium shows the characteristic changes of ICS.[61]

The radiographic changes of the chest in patients with ICS without situs inversus are not specific and only suggestive of the diagnosis. Opacification of all paranasal sinuses is a common feature, which, although characteristic, is not pathognomonic of this condition and is seen in other diseases such as cystic fibrosis and immunoglobulin deficiency.

Bronchoscopic examination usually discloses the presence of chronically inflamed mucosa, which may bleed easily on contact, and mucopurulent secretions, particularly abundant in areas of bronchiectasis or atelectasis. This technique may confirm the reversal of the bronchial anatomy in patients with situs inversus. Bronchograms are useful in the delineation of anatomic changes of the respiratory tree, particularly in the diagnosis of saccular bronchiectasis. The latter is particularly important if surgical resection is being considered.

DIFFERENTIAL DIAGNOSIS

The differential diagnosis is summarized in Table 60–2.

The signs and symptoms of cystic fibrosis may be very similar to those of ICS. History of meconium ileus and signs of pancreatic insufficiency suggest the diagnosis of cystic fibrosis. It is common clinical knowledge that the bronchiectatic changes in the lung are worse in the upper lobes in cystic fibrosis and in the middle lobes in ICS. Measurement of sweat electrolytes (quantitative analysis of sweat chloride) and genetic studies (i.e., detection of known mutations) would help in the differential diagnosis (see Chapters 69 and 70).

Patients with immunoglobulin deficiency (Bruton's agammaglobulinemia, hypogammaglobulinemia G or A)

Table 60–2. DIFFERENTIAL DIAGNOSIS OF THE IMMOTILE CILIA SYNDROME

Variable	Immotile Cilia Syndrome	Cystic Fibrosis	Allergy	Immune Deficiency	Young's Syndrome	Asplenia/Polysplenia
Onset of symptoms	Birth	Birth	Infancy	Infancy	Adult life	Birth/infancy
Genetics	Autosomal recessive	Autosomal recessive	?	Depends on condition	?	Autosomal recessive (?)
Situs abnormality	Yes (50%)	No	No	No	No	Yes
Rhinorrhea	+++	+	++/+++	++/+++	+	—
Sinusitis	+++	++	++	+++	+++	—
Otitis media	+++		++	+++	+ (?)	—
Bronchiectasis	Lower lobes > upper lobes	Upper lobes > lower lobes	Rare in lower lobes, right middle lobes (asthma)	Lower lobes > upper lobes	Lower lobes > upper lobes	—
Nasal polyps	++	+++	+	—	—	
Spermatozoa	Immotile	Absent	N	N	Absent	N
Other clinical findings	Males with situs inversus: lower right testicle	Malabsorption, abnormal food sweat test	Skin atopy, allergy	Opportunistic infections, autoimmune phenomenon ↑ lymph nodes (HIV) ↓ lymphoid tissue (B cell deficiency)	Dilated epididymis	Cardiovascular abnormalities, intestinal malrotation, other anomalies
Digital clubbing	+/++	+++	—	−/+ (if bronchiectasis)	+	—

HIV, human immunodeficiency virus; N, normal; +, mild; ++, moderate; +++, severe

usually have recurrent sinusitis, otitis, bronchitis, and pneumonia. Bronchiectasis may occur, particularly in the lower lobes. Like patients with ICS, patients with immunoglobulin deficiency require almost ongoing antibiotic therapy to control their symptoms. The symptoms tend to appear after the age of 3 or 4 months and vary in severity. Unlike patients with ICS, these patients may acquire infections in other organ systems, particularly with opportunistic microorganisms as well as autoimmune phenomena. Combined immunodeficiencies and disorders of cellular immunity, such as the bare lymphocyte syndrome,[74] can potentially cause bronchiectasis and severe respiratory disease (see Chapter 75).

Children with severe respiratory allergies may have symptoms suggestive of ICS in the absence of situs inversus. In these patients, careful history, biopsy of cilia, and other studies help rule out the diagnosis of ICS.

Young's syndrome is characterized by chronic sinusitis, bronchitis, bronchiectasis, and male sterility. Affected patients have progressive obstructive azoospermia. Mucociliary clearance is delayed, but ciliary ultrastructure is normal. The pattern of inheritance is unclear, as is the pathogenesis of this disease.[75-78]

Other syndromes of abnormal visceral position can be confused with Kartagener's syndrome. These include the syndrome of asplenia and polysplenia.[79] In asplenia, the liver lies symmetrically in the middle of the abdomen, and there are other abnormalities such as a right- or left-sided stomach, systemic venous anomalies, cardiac malformations, bilateral trilobed lungs, and eparterial bronchi. In polysplenia, the most common malformations include a symmetrically placed midline liver and systemic venous anomalies, most commonly an interrupted inferior vena cava with azygous (bilateral left-sidedness) continuation, bilobed lungs, and bilateral hyperaterial bronchi. Usually the cardiac malformations in asplenia are severe and life-threatening. Ciliary abnormalities have been reported in patients with polysplenia.[80-82]

Situs inversus, asplenia, and polysplenia have been reported to occur within families.[84] The presence of discordant visceral situs (i.e., lack of perfect mirror image), liver in the midline, venous malformations, and cardiac defects in the absence of severe respiratory symptoms help differentiate these syndromes from ICS.

The Williams-Campbell syndrome, or congenital deficiency of bronchial cartilage, can lead to the development of bronchiectasis.[84] Onset of symptoms in the neonatal period and familial occurrence have been reported. Affected children, however, do not have other characteristics of ICS.

MEDICAL TREATMENT

The aim of treatment is the prevention of progression of lung disease and its complications. Chest physical therapy, postural drainage, and aerosol therapy with bronchodilator agents are useful in relieving airway obstruction.

Antimicrobial therapy is the hallmark of the treatment. Most patients require ongoing or intermittent administration of antibiotics to keep infection under control. Upon discontinuation of this kind of therapy, many patients

characteristically experience recrudescence of the sinobronchial symptoms. Intravenous antibiotic therapy may be necessary for controlling exacerbations of bronchitis, sinusitis, and pneumonia.

The choice of drugs depends on the infecting microorganisms and their sensitivities. The most frequent oral antibiotics used are ampicillin, cephalosporin, and sulfa drugs. Antistaphylococcal drugs (cloxacillin, dicloxacillin) and oral quinolones can be useful, depending on the presence of staphylococcal or pseudomonal infection.

Intravenous cephalosporins, semisynthetic penicillins, or aminoglycosides can be used when indicated. No experience with the use of aerosolized antimicrobial drugs in this disease has been reported.

Paranasal sinus disease is one of the most difficult problems to treat, particularly in younger children. Antimicrobial agents, local and systemic decongestants, intranasal corticosteriods, antihistamines, and antiflammatory analgesic drugs are all used in the treatment of sinusitis.

SURGICAL TREATMENT

Pulmonary resections should be considered if there is abscess formation or if a specific area of the lung is causing recurrent exacerbations and cannot be controlled by medical treatment. Tympanostomy and insertion of ventilating tubes may be necessary in many patients with ICS and otitis media. Paranasal sinus surgery is necessary in some patients to improve drainage from the sinuses.

PROGNOSIS

Although ICS is a chronic and potentially progressive disease, the clinical picture tends to be rather stable. Patients as old as 88 years who have Kartagener's syndrome have been recorded in the literature.[85] The quality of life depends on the severity of symptoms, the onset of complications, and the ability of medical treatment to control the symptoms. Early diagnosis allows for treatment or prevention of complications and improved quality of life.

REFERENCES

1. Siewert AK: Uber einen fall von bronchiectasie bei einem Patienten mit situs inversus viscerum. Berl Klin Wochenschr 41:139–141, 1904.
2. Oeri R: Zur Kasuistik des situs viscerum inversus totalis. Frankfurter Z Pathol 3:393–397, 1909.
3. Gunther H: Die biologische bedeutung der inversionen. Biol Zentralbl 43:175–213, 1923.
4. Kartagener M: Zur pathogenese der bronchiektasien. I Mitteilung: Bronchiectasien bei situs viscerum inversus. Betr Klin Tuberk 83:498–501, 1933.
5. Bergstrom WH, Cook CD, Scannell J, Berenberg W: Situs inversus, bronchiectasis and sinusitis. Pediatrics 6:573–580, 1950.
6. Kartagener M, Mully K: Bronchiectasien bei situs inversus. Schweiz Z Tuberk, 13:166–191, 1956.
7. Kartagener M, Stucki P: Bronchiectasis with situs inversus. Arch Pediatr 79:193–207, 1962.
8. Hartline JV, Zelkowitz PS: Kartagener's syndrome in childhood. Am J Dis Child 121:349–352, 1971.

9. Karman S, Lewitt Y, Terracina S: Kartagener's syndrome in two siblings. Harefuah 91:338–339, 1976.
10. Rott HD, Warnatz H, Pasch-Hilgers R, Weikl A: Kartagener's syndrome in sibs: Clinical and immunologic investigations. Hum Genet 43:1–11, 1978.
11. Arge E: Transposition of the viscera and sterility in men. Lancet 278:412–414, 1960.
12. Pedersen H, Rebbe H: Absence of arms of the axoneme of immotile human spermatozoa. Biol Reprod 12:541–544, 1975.
13. Afzelius BA, Eliasson R, Johnsen O, Lindholmer C: Lack of dynein arms in immotile human spermatozoa. J Cell Biol 66:225–232, 1975.
14. Camner P, Mossberg B, Afzelius BA: Evidence for congenitally nonfunctioning cilia in the tracheobronchial tract in two subjects. Am Rev Respir Dis 112:807–809, 1975.
15. Afzelius BA: A human syndrome caused by immotile cilia. Science 193:317–319, 1976.
16. Eliasson R, Mossberg B, Camner P, Afzelius BA: The immotile-cilia syndrome: A congenital ciliary abnormality as an etiologic factor in chronic airway infections and male sterility. N Engl J Med 296:1–6, 1977.
17. Sturgess J, Chao J, Wong J, et al: Cilia with defective radial spokes. A cause of human respiratory disease. N Engl J Med 300:53–56, 1979.
18. Sturgess JM, Chao J, Turner JA: Transposition of ciliary microtubules: Another cause of impaired ciliary motility. N Engl J Med 303(6):318–322, 1980.
19. Herzon FS, Murphy S: Normal ciliary ultrastructure in children with Kartagener's syndrome. Ann Otol Rhinol Laryngol 89:81–83, 1980.
20. Schidlow DV, Katz SM: Immotile cilia syndrome. N Engl J Med 308(10):595, 1983.
21. Rooklin AR, McGeady SJ, Mikaelian DO, et al: The immotile cilia syndrome: A cause of recurrent pulmonary disease in children. Pediatrics 66:526–531, 1980.
22. Forrest JB, Rossman CM, Newhouse MT, Ruffin R: Activation of nasal cilia in immotile cilia syndrome. Am Rev Respir Dis 120:514–515, 1979.
23. Rossman CM, Forrest JB, Ruffin RE, Newhouse MT: Immotile cilia syndrome in persons with and without Kartagener's syndrome. Am Rev Respir Dis 121:1011–1016, 1980.
24. Rossman CM, Forrest JB, Lee RM, Newhouse MT: The dyskinetic cilia syndrome: Ciliary motility in immotile cilia syndrome. Chest 78:580–582, 1980.
25. Rossman CM, Forrest JB, Lee RM: et al: The dyskinetic cilia syndrome: Abnormal ciliary motility in association with abnormal ciliary ultrastructure. Chest 80(Suppl.):860–865, 1981.
26. Rossman CM, Lee RM, Forrest JB, Newhouse MT: Nasal ciliary ultrastructure and function in patients with primary ciliary dyskinesia compared with that in normal subjects and in subjects with various respiratory diseases. Am Rev Respir Dis 129:161–167, 1984.
27. Sturgess JM, Thompson MW, Czegledy-Nagy E, et al: Genetic aspects of immotile cilia syndrome. Am J Med Genet 25(1):149–160, 1986.
28. Rott HD: Kartagener's syndrome and the syndrome of immotile cilia. Hum Genet 46:249–261, 1979.
29. Sleigh MC: Ciliary function in mucus transport. Chest 80(6 Suppl):791–795, 1981.
30. Sleigh MC: The nature and action of respiratory tract cilia in respiratory defense mechanisms. In Brain JD, Proctor DF, Reid LM (eds): Book Title, pp. 247–288. New York: Marcel Dekker, 1977.
31. Sanderson MJ, Sleigh MA: Ciliary activity of cultured rabbit tracheal epithelium: Beat pattern and metachrony. J Cell Sci 47:331–347, 1981.
32. Sleigh MA, Blake JR, Liron N: The propulsion of mucus by cilia. Am Rev Respir Dis 137:726–741, 1988.
33. Satir P: The generation of ciliary motion. J Protozool 31(1):8–12, 1984.
34. Afzelius BA: Disorders of ciliary motility. Hosp Pract (Off Ed) 21:73–80, 1986.
35. Yarnal JR, Golsish JA, Ahmad M, Tomashefski JF: The immotile cilia syndrome: Explanation for many a clinical mystery. Postgrad Med 71(2):195–217, 1982.
36. Satir P: Structural basis of ciliary movement. Environ Health Perspect 35:77–82, 1980.
37. Satir P, Sale WS: Tails of tetrahymena. J Protozool 24:498–501, 1977.
38. Lucas AM, Douglas LC: Principles underlying ciliary activity in the respiratory tract: II. A comparison of nasal clearance in man, monkey and other mammals. Arch Otolaryngol 20:518–541, 1934.
39. Sleigh MA: The integrated activity of cilia: Function and coordination. J Protozool 31(1):16–21, 1984.
40. Rossman CM, Newhouse MT: Primary ciliary dyskinesia: Evaluation and management. Pediatr Pulmonol 5:36–50, 1988.
41. Afzelius BA: The immotile-cilia syndrome and other ciliary diseases. Int Rev Exp Pathol 19:1–43, 1979.
42. Chao J, Turner JA, Sturgess JM: Genetic heterogeneity of dynein-deficiency in cilia from patients with respiratory disease. Am Rev Respir Dis 126:302–305, 1982.
43. Lungarella G, Fonzi L, Burrini AG: Ultrastructural abnormalities in respiratory cilia and sperm tails in a patient with Kartagener's syndrome. Ultrastruct Pathol 3:319–323, 1982.
44. Afzelius BA: Genetical and ultrastructural aspects of the immotile-cilia syndrome. Am J Hum Genet 33:852–864, 1981.
45. Schneeberger EE, McCormac J, Issenberg HJ, et al: Heterogeneity of ciliary morphology in the immotile-cilia syndrome in man. J Ultrastruct Res 73:34–43, 1980.
46. Neustein HB, Nickerson B, O'Neal M: Kartagener's syndrome with absence of inner dynein arms of respiratory cilia. Am Rev Respir Dis 122:979–981, 1980.
47. Afzelius BA, Eliasson R: Flagellar mutants in man: On the heterogeneity of the immotile cilia syndrome. J Ultrastruct Res 69:43–52, 1979.
48. Gordon RE, Kattan M: Absence of cilia and basal bodies with predominance of brush cells in the respiratory mucosa from a patient with immotile cilia syndrome. Ultrastruct Pathol 6:45–49, 1984.
49. Howell JT, Schochet S, Goldman AS: Ultrastructural defects of respiratory tract cilia associated with chronic infections. Arch Pathol Lab Med 104:52–55, 1980.
50. Lungarella G, Fonzi L, Pacini E: Atypical cilia in rabbit bronchial epithelial cells induced by elastase: An ultrastructural study. J Pathol 131:379–383, 1980.
51. Carson JL, Collier AM, Hu SS: Acquired ciliary defects in nasal epithelium of children with acute viral upper respiratory infections. N Engl J Med 312:463–468, 1985.
52. Corbeel L, Cornillie F, Lauweryns J, et al: Ultrastructural abnormalities of bronchial cilia in children with recurrent airway infections and bronchiectasis. Arch Dis Child 56:929–933, 1981.
53. Petersen M, Morkassel E, Nielsen MH, Mygind N: Kartagener's syndrome: Preliminary report on cilia structure, function, and upper airway symptoms. Chest 80:858–860, 1981.
54. Pedersen M, Mygind N: Ciliary motility in the "immotile cilia syndrome." First results of microphoto-oscillographic studies. Br J Dis Chest 74:239–244, 1980.
55. Pedersen M, Nielsen MH, Mygind N: Primary ciliary dykinesia: A preliminary comparison between ciliary motility and ultrastructure. Mod Probl Paediatr 21:68–78, 1982.
56. Mossberg B, Afzelius BA, Eliasson R, Camner P: On the pathogenesis of obstructive lung disease: A study on the immotile cilia syndrome. Scand J Respir Dis 59:55–65, 1978.
57. Turner JA, Corkey CW, Lee JY, et al: Clinical expressions of immotile cilia syndrome. Pediatrics 67(6):805–810, 1981.
58. Corkey CWB, Levison H, Turner JA: The immotile cilia syndrome. Am Rev Respir Dis 124:544–548, 1981.
59. Nadel HR, Stringer DA, Levison H, et al: The immotile cilia syndrome: Radiological manifestations. Radiology 154(3):651–655, 1985.
60. Whitelaw A, Evans A, Corrin B: Immotile cilia syndrome: A new cause of neonatal respiratory distress. Arch Dis Child 56:432–435, 1981.
61. Moryan A, Guay AT, Kurtz S, Nowak PJ: Familial ciliary dyskinesis: A cause of infertility without respiratory disease. Fertil Steril 44(4):539–542, 1985.
62. Marchini M, Losa GA, Nara S, et al: Ultrastructural aspects of endometrial surface in Kartagener's syndrome. Fertil Steril 57:461–463, 1992.
63. Afzelius BA, Eliasson R: Male and female infertility problems in the immotile-cilia syndrome. Eur J Respir Dis 127:144–147, 1983.
64. Wakefield SJ, Waite D: Abnormal cilia in Polynesians with bronchiectasis. Am Rev Respir Dis 121:1003–1010, 1980.

65. Layton WM Jr: Random determination of a developmental process. J Hered 67:336–338, 1976.
66. Layton WM Jr: Heart malformations in mice homozygous for a gene causing situs inversus. Birth Defects 14(7):277–293, 1978.
67. Greenstone MA, Jones RW, Dewar A, et al: Hydrocephalus and primary ciliary dyskinesia. Arch Dis Child 59(5):481–482, 1984.
68. Svedbergh B, Jonsson V, Afzelius B: Immotile-cilia syndrome and the cilia of the eye. Graefes Arch Klin Exp Ophthalmol 215:265–272, 1981.
69. Segal PL, Kikiela M, Mrzygold S, Zeromska-Zbierska I: Kartagener's syndrome with familial eye changes. Am J Opthalmol 55:1043–1049, 1963.
70. Caleb M, Lecks H, South MA, Norman ME: Kartagener's syndrome and abnormal cilia [letter]. N Engl J Med 297:1012–1013, 1977.
71. Corkey CW, Minta JO, Turner JA, Biggar WD: Neutrophil function in the immotile cilia syndrome. J Lab Clin Med 99:838–844, 1982.
72. Valerius NH, Knudsen BB, Pedersen M: Defective neutrophil motility in patients with primary ciliary dyskinesia. Eur J Clin Invest 13:489–494, 1983.
73. Wolburg H, Dopfer R, Schieferstein G, Theil D: Immotile cilia syndrome: Reduced chemotaxis and reduced number of intramembranous particles in granulocytes. Klin Wochenschr 62:1044–1046, 1984.
74. Sugiyama Y, Maeda H, Okumura K, Takaku F: Progressive sinobronchiectasis associated with the "bare lymphocyte syndrome" in an adult. Chest 89(3):398–401, 1986.
75. Handelsman DJ, Conway AJ, Boylan LM, Turtle JR: Obstructive azoospermia and chronic sinopulmonary infections. N Engl J Med 310:3–9, 1984.
76. Lau KY, Lieberman J: Young's syndrome. An association between male sterility and bronchiectasis. West J Med 144:744–746, 1986.
77. Neville E, Brewis R, Yeates WK, Burridge A: Respiratory tract disease and obstructive azoospermia. Thorax 38:929–933, 1983.
78. Pavia D, Agnew JE, Bateman JR, et al: Lung mucociliary clearance in patients with Young's syndrome. Chest 80:892–895, 1981.
79. Van Mierop LH, Gessner IH, Schiebler GL: Asplenia and polysplenia syndrome. Birth Defects 8:74–82, 1972.
80. Schidlow DV, Katz SM, Turtz MG, et al: Polysplenia and Kartagener syndrome in a sibship: Association with abnormal respiratory cilia. J Pediatr 100:401–403, 1982.
81. Teichberg S, Markowitz J, Silverberg M, et al: Abnormal cilia in a child with the polysplenia syndrome and extrahepatic biliary atresia. J Pediatr 100:399–401, 1982.
82. Gershoni-Baruch R, Gottfried E, Pery M, et al: Immotile cilia syndrome including polysplenia, situs inversus, and extrahepatic biliary atresia. Am J Med Genet 33:390–393, 1989.
83. Niikawa N, Kohsaka S, Mizumoto M, et al: Familial clustering of situs inversus totalis, and asplenia and polysplenia syndromes. Am J Med Genet 16:43–47, 1983.
84. Wayne KS, Taussig LM: Probable familial congenital bronchiectasis due to cartilage deficiency (Williams-Campbell syndrome). Am Rev Respir Dis 114:15–22, 1976.
85. Amjad H, Richburg FD, Adler E: Kartagener syndrome. JAMA 227:1420–1422, 1974.

61 OBSTRUCTIVE SLEEP APNEA SYNDROME

MAYNARD C. DYSON, M.D. / ROBERT C. BECKERMAN, M.D.

Charles Dickens offered the now classic description of Joe, the "fat and redfaced boy, in a state of somnolency," in *The Posthumous Papers of the Pickwick Club*[1] more than 150 years ago. This condition has found its way into the medical literature as the Pickwickian syndrome.

Case reports of the association between obesity and hypersomnolence have appeared in the literature since 1816,[2, 3] but not until the 1960s did the development of polysomnographic recording with the ability to monitor electroencephalography (EEG), electrocardiography (EKG), airflow, and chest wall movements permit an understanding of the basic and clinical aspects of sleep. With this understanding came the recognition of the interaction of sleep stages and apnea. Further advances in instrumentation, such as continuous monitoring of oxygen saturation and end-tidal carbon dioxide (CO_2) levels during sleep, led to the finding that sleep apnea was associated with significant hypoxemia and hypoventilation. These advances in turn led to recognition that daytime drowsiness correlated not with daytime blood gas values but with the frequency and severity of sleep arousals.[4] In addition, a wide spectrum of patients, which included more than the classic hypersomnolent, obese patients,

came to be recognized as suffering from obstructive sleep apnea syndrome (OSAS), or sleep-disordered breathing.

As polysomnography was applied to the study of children, both similarities and differences were noted between the ways in which the condition affects children and adults. In children, congenital malformations, continuing growth, and physiologic immaturity contribute to the unique aspects of OSAS. The pathophysiology, diagnosis, and treatment of OSAS are discussed, with emphasis on the aspects unique to children.

PATHOPHYSIOLOGY

The definition of sleep apnea offered by Guilleminault and associates in 1975[5] has been widely but not universally accepted.[6, 7] They defined the condition as 30 or more apneic episodes of at least 10 sec duration within 8 h, occurring during both rapid-eye-movement (REM) and non-REM sleep phases. However, patients with clinically significant OSAS generally have apneic episodes longer than 15 sec, significant arterial oxygen desaturation, and up to several hundred episodes per night.[8] Sleep

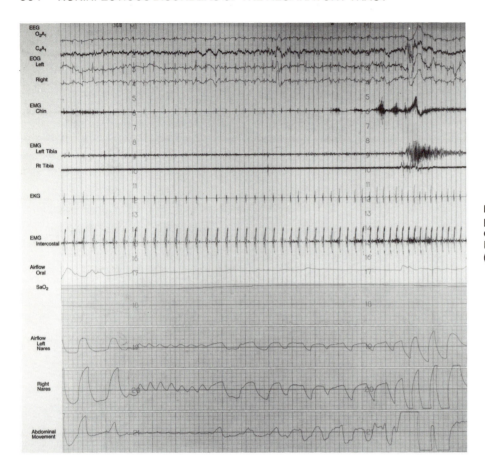

Figure 61–1. Central apnea. A 12-sec period of apnea/hypopnea occurred at the onset of rapid eye movement (REM) sleep. Note the lack of both electromyographic (EMG) activity and abdominal movement.

apneas are further classified as central, obstructive, and mixed. Central apnea occurs when there is no apparent respiratory effort (Fig. 61–1), in contrast to obstructive apnea, which is associated with apparent, often vigorous inspiratory efforts (Figs. 61–2A, 62–2B). These efforts are ineffective, however, because of the lack of airway patency. Obstructive apnea is thus caused by the lack of a patent airway and the consequent lack of effective airflow.

Central and obstructive apnea differ significantly from each other. In children, the obstructive episodes usually cause more of a change in oxygenation and heart rate[9] than do central episodes. In addition, obstructive sleep apnea generally begins at a later age than does central apnea, except in children with congenital abnormalities. Because of the different causes, therapeutic approaches for these two classes of apnea have little in common. Mixed apnea is, as the name implies, a combination of central and obstructive apnea in the same episode. In this chapter, the discussion is limited to obstructive sleep apnea.

OSAS is a syndrome of complete or partial obstruction causing significant physiologic derangement that may have a wide variety of clinically adverse effects. Children who have clinical features of OSAS may not have frequent periods of total airflow cessation, but they may have partial airway obstruction in association with significant symptoms.[10] Although OSAS is characterized by periods of prolonged obstruction, many patients have additional associated episodes of central and mixed apnea. Mixed apnea typically has a central apnea com-

ponent followed by an obstructive component, which is terminated when the airway opens and effective respirations are restored.[5] Elimination of the obstructive component frequently eliminates all apneas, including the central component of the mixed apneas. Only after the obstructive component has been relieved can it be determined with certainty whether there is a primary central component.

Mixed apneas demonstrate the possible interactions among anatomic, peripheral, and central neurologic factors. The initial central apnea results from inadequacy of a ventilatory drive to initiate a respiratory effort. The obstructive component occurs as the ventilatory drive increases and the muscles of inspiration create an increasingly negative pressure. Obstruction occurs because the muscles maintaining upper airway patency are unable to prevent collapse of the airway tissues.

Several sets of paired muscles are involved in this process, and their interaction is only partially understood (Fig. 61–3). The genioglossus muscle attaches the tongue anteriorly to the mandible and acts to thrust the tongue forward, holding it out of the pharynx. The hyoid bone floats in the neck, anterior to the pharynx. The hyoglossus and geniohyoid muscles attach the hyoid bone to the anterior mandible and tongue, and the thyrohyoid membrane attaches the bone to the thyroid cartilage. The vector resulting from the tensing of these muscles is directed anteriorly, serving to stiffen and open the airway. Studies have shown that in inspiration, pharyngeal muscles act in a coordinated manner to maintain patency.[11] When these

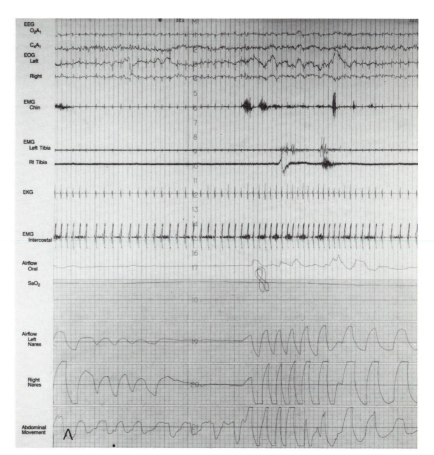

Figure 61-2. Obstructive apnea. *A*, Graph of a 10-sec period of obstructive sleep apnea that resulted in desaturation to 88%. Note continuing intercostal EMG activity and abdominal movement.

A

Illustration continued on following page

constrictions are either inadequate or uncoordinated, the upper airway may collapse and obstruction may result. Factors causing the cross-sectional area in the pharynx to be smaller than normal, such as congenital malformations and enlarged tonsils or adenoids, place increased demand on these mechanisms. The obstructive component is terminated when the dilator mechanisms break apart the pharyngeal tissues; arousal may be required in order to accomplish this process. This condition may manifest clinically as gasping and restless sleep.

Sleep is classified as either REM or non-REM (Table 61–1). Non-REM sleep is divided into four stages on the basis of EEG and clinical criteria. A person going to sleep usually first enters stages I and II, also referred to as unsteady non-REM sleep. During these stages, breathing typically exhibits a periodic nature. Ventilation decreases slightly with a small rise in carbon dioxide pressure (P_{CO_2}) and a decrease in oxygen pressure (P_{O_2}). As sleep progresses, a state of steady non-REM sleep is entered in stages III and IV. During stages III and IV, breathing is very regular, and ventilation decreases further. Studies in adults have shown increases in Pa_{CO_2} of 3 to 7 mm Hg and decreases in Pa_{O_2} of 3.5 to 9.4 mm Hg.[12]

One to two hours after the onset of sleep and after stages III and IV, an adult enters REM sleep. Children may enter REM sleep from stage II without going through stages III and IV. When REM sleep begins, there is initially a marked decrease in ventilation and then an increase, which may be accompanied by gross movements. During REM sleep, the degree of pharyngeal hypotonia is highest.

Although results of studies of airway mechanics are somewhat variable, it is generally agreed that the upper airway resistance is highest during the REM stage. Some patients experience apnea primarily during REM sleep, but significant obstructive episodes can occur in any stage and in fact may prevent a patient from reaching REM sleep. REM sleep, the sleep state in which dreaming occurs, can be reached only by passing through the earlier stages. It is essential for the sleeper to attain REM sleep in order to avoid the effects of sleep deprivation. Thus if the sleeper is aroused frequently, REM sleep may never be reached, and the effects of sleep deprivation may result.

Both adults and children exhibit decreased responses to both hypercapnic and hypoxic drives in all stages of sleep. With the exception of the late apneic response to hypoxia that is present in neonates, the responses to hypoxia and hypercapnia are qualitatively similar in children and adults. However, the anatomy of children differs significantly from that of adults. In infants and young children, the cross-sectional area of the pharynx is smaller. Because resistance varies with the fourth power of the radius, small changes in radius result in large changes in resistance.

In children suffering from OSAS who have no congenital abnormalities, the nasopharyngeal area may be smaller than in their age-controlled peers. As both the bony and soft tissues (including lymphoid tissue) develop, the area of the nasopharynx changes. Although the cross-sectional area of the bony nasopharynx increases in a manner approximately parallel to body height, the mean airway area size declines until the age of 5 or 6 years.[13]

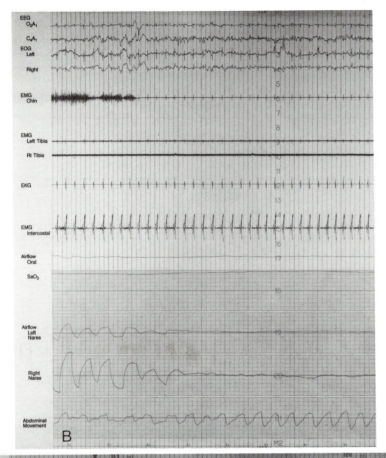

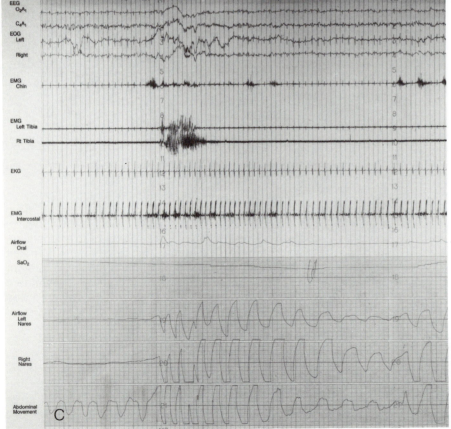

Figure 61–2 *Continued B, C*, Graphs of a 39-sec period of obstructive sleep apnea that resulted in desaturation to 66%. Note the increasing activity in the intercostal EMG and abdominal movement until airflow is established.

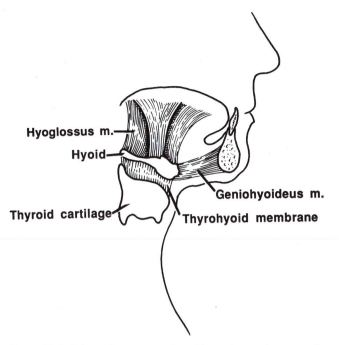

Figure 61–3. Schematic representation of the major attachments maintaining pharyngeal patency (m, muscle).

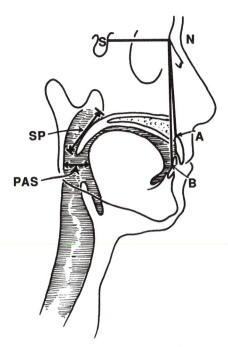

Figure 61–4. Representation of common cephalometric measurements. Shown are the posterior air space (PAS), soft palate (SP), and points of measurement for the sphenoid-nasal-maxillary angle (S-N-A) and sphenoid-nasal-mandibular angle. (S-N-B).

This decrease in area results from the relatively rapid growth of the pharyngeal soft tissues, primarily the adenoidal and tonsillar tissue, during early life.

Cephalometry is a radiographic technique that allows the study of these anatomic changes. In cephalometry, radiography is used in a more standardized manner than a routine lateral neck film. The technique involves obtaining a lateral film of the nasopharyngeal area under standard conditions with the head in a neutral position, the tongue relaxed, and the patient upright, 5 feet from the source of the x-ray and in a device to hold the head in a true lateral position. Many measurements can be obtained from these views (Fig. 61–4), but the length of the soft palate, the depth of the posterior airway space, and the sphenoid-nasal-maxillary and sphenoid-nasal-mandibular angles are commonly examined.[14, 15]

In adults, normal values for cephalometric parameters

are well established. Although these measurements do not enable a specific diagnosis of OSAS to be made, they may be used as supportive data and may aid in selection of surgical approaches. However, there have been no controlled prospective studies of the importance of cephalometry in predicting either prognosis or response to therapy in children. Nevertheless, because a large percentage of facial growth is completed early in life, further studies in the field may prove helpful.

Thus sleep apnea is the final result of many factors, including airway size, sleep stage, physiologic balance of muscle forces, and sensitivity of respiratory drives. Not only are the causal factors complex, but the effects of maturation in children make it difficult to predict the natural course of the disorder in an individual patient.

Table 61–1. STAGES AND CHARACTERISTICS OF SLEEP

Stage	Electroencephalographic Findings	Ocular Movement	Muscular Movement
Awake	Alpha activity, low amplitude	REMs may be present	Highest level of tone
Stage I	Low amplitude, mixed frequency	Slow or no eye movement	Decreased from awake level
Stage II	Sleep spindles and high-amplitude, low-frequency signals begin to appear	None	Further decrease
Stage III	Increasing % of high-amplitude, low-frequency cycles	None	Further decrease
Stage IV	High-amplitude, low-frequency cycles; >50% sleep spindles	None	Same as in stage III
REM	Low-amplitude, mixed-frequency cycles; alpha activity	Bursts of REM activity	Lowest with transient increases during REM activity

REM, rapid eye movement. Transition between sleep stages is gradual, and at a given time the stage may be classified by its dominant activity or as transitional.

The natural history of OSAS is important and may vary, depending on the age of the child and the mode of presentation. Infants with an apparently life-threatening event[16] (ALTE) may have obstructive sleep apnea.[16, 17] Some infants with an ALTE demonstrate obstructive or mixed apneas on polysomnography, but these episodes may disappear in 2 to 3 months. This outcome seems to be most likely if the episode is preceded by symptoms of infection of the upper respiratory tract and no underlying anatomic or neurologic abnormality is present. In some infants between 3 and 12 weeks of age with an ALTE, snoring[18] and obstructive sleep apnea develop. There have been no large prospective studies of the different manifestations and the development of OSAS. Experience suggests that in most infants who have one ALTE and are otherwise normal, clinically significant OSAS does not develop later in childhood. In most studies of adults in which the natural history of OSAS has been examined, investigators have found that snoring has been present since adolescence or early childhood;[19] this finding is suggestive of some compromise of the airways. Thus although only a minority of children who experience obstruction with an acute illness go on to develop OSAS, the majority of adult patients have experienced gradual development of symptoms, over years.

One of the reasons why acute obstruction in infants may not portend sleep apnea in adulthood may be that infants suffer from a unique difficulty: almost 50% are unable to establish mouth breathing within 25 sec of nasal obstruction.[20] This failure leaves such infants especially vulnerable to obstructive episodes. Blockage of the nasal passages that might result only in habitual mouth breathing in an older child may cause serious obstruction in an infant. In the presence of conditions such as choanal atresia, infections of the upper respiratory tract, and reflux into the nose, the obstruction may develop into an ALTE.

Beyond infancy, snoring is almost constantly associated with childhood sleep apnea.[21-23] Infants may not be able to generate enough airflow to produce the snoring sound, and so obstruction may occur without warning in neonates. However, snoring has been reported to develop as early as the age of 4 months. The incidence of snoring is dependent on age, being higher in older age groups. Studies in adults have produced estimates of a 30% to 60% incidence of snoring, whereas estimates of incidence in children are in the range of 3% to 5%. The presence of snoring in a child warrants consideration of OSAS.

Snoring itself is caused by vibrating palatal and pharyngeal tissue and does not always mean that there is clinically significant obstruction to airflow. Snoring can serve not only as an alerting signal but also as a crude measure of airflow and its interruption.[24] The history of snoring may be quite impressive; the noise may be described as disturbing the patient's entire family. The recording of the sound while the child sleeps can be helpful in evaluating sleep apnea. Evaluation involves an informal listening to an audio recording. Although no studies of the subjective ratings of tape recordings have been made, computer analysis of the recorded sounds has shown strong correlation of these ratings with polysomnographic findings.[25] The typical pattern of an obstructive episode is one of snoring interrupted by brief periods of silence and followed by louder, more rapid breathing. This pattern may be cyclic in nature and reminiscent of periodic apnea in preterm infants.

Current data from adults suggest that snoring is associated with morbidity in a high percentage of cases, even when frank apnea may not be present, and a similar situation may exist in children.[10] Some children do not meet the criteria of cessation of airflow or hypoxia and yet may suffer from typical symptoms of OSAS such as daytime somnolence, hyperactivity, and failure to thrive.[7, 26] In these cases, the increased respiratory effort apparently interferes with progression of sleep stages. Snoring secondary to obstruction may also increase the work of breathing, which in turn increases the metabolic rate. One manifestation of this increase may be profuse sweating at night.[27]

EVALUATION

HISTORY

A careful history of sleep-associated symptoms is the first step in detecting OSAS (Table 61–2). In taking such a history, it is important to ascertain the sleeping arrangements in a patient's home. Snoring is more likely to be reported for a child who sleeps in the same room as the parents than for a child who sleeps in another room. Likewise, an older child, who may not take naps or who may go to sleep at the same time as the parents, is less likely to be heard than is a younger child who falls asleep while adults are still awake.

Infections of the upper respiratory tract may increase the frequency and severity of snoring episodes, and allergic diathesis may add a seasonal component to the history. The age at onset and progression of fluctuations in severity of sleep disturbances should be noted. Also, snoring is not the only relevant observation during sleep. Sleeping in odd positions, such as with the knees drawn up under the body or with the head hanging off the side of the bed, suggests an effort to alleviate airway obstruction by hyperextending the neck or allowing gravity to pull the tongue and jaw forward. Sleep position is also important

Table 61–2. BEHAVIORS AND SYMPTOMS ASSOCIATED WITH OBSTRUCTIVE SLEEP APNEA SYNDROME

Difficulty breathing during sleep
Apnea during sleep
Snoring
Chronic rhinorrhea
Mouth breathing when awake
Frequent infections of the upper respiratory tract
Frequent nausea or vomiting
Difficulty swallowing
Sweating when asleep
Poor appetite
Recurrent middle ear disease
Pathological shyness, social withdrawal
Delayed development
Speech problems
Hyperactivity
Increased difficulty breathing during infections of the upper respiratory tract

because worsening of obstruction in certain positions may be a clue to the site of blockage. For example, the supine position may cause the tonsils and tongue to fall back and occlude the pharynx. It has been shown that a sleep history that includes snoring and sleep disturbances is correlated quite strongly with positive findings on polysomnography.[22]

Thus in children with a chief complaint of sleep disturbance, OSAS should be considered as a possible diagnosis. Because of the myriad of secondary effects, OSAS also needs to be considered in children with many other symptoms, including failure to thrive, developmental delays, hypotonia, and cor pulmonale.[26, 27]

The presence or absence of daytime symptoms depends on the frequency and severity of the nighttime apneas and arousals.[4] Behavioral changes are often quite troublesome. Such changes may take the form of hyperactivity rather than hypersomnolence, presumably because of an inability to concentrate. In school-age children, this problem may translate into school failure[28] or may result in a diagnosis of a learning disorder. Psychological testing (including tests directed at sleep, such as the Multiple Sleep Latency Test) may be useful in detecting the contribution of OSAS to behavioral problems. Nighttime events such as enuresis[29] and nightmares have been attributed to OSAS. All these symptoms are nonspecific, but when they are the chief complaints, the possibility of OSAS should be considered.

A complete review of systems and the medical history should be obtained. Many conditions are associated with OSAS (Table 61–3), and although some, such as congenital malformations, are obvious to the examiner, others can be detected only through careful history taking. Allergic rhinitis, sinusitis, and tonsillitis all cause swelling of

Table 61–3. CONDITIONS PREDISPOSING TO OBSTRUCTIVE SLEEP APNEA SYNDROME

Chromosomal Abnormalities
Trisomy 21
Any trisomy or deletion causing micrognathia or hypotonia
Congenital Malformations
Complex
Pierre Robin syndrome
Treacher Collins syndrome
Apert's syndrome
Beckwith's syndrome
Focal
Cleft palate
Choanal atresia or stenosis
Neurologic
Vocal cord paresis or paralysis
Dandy-Walker syndrome
Extrinsic Masses
Ectopic thyroid
Rhabdomyosarcoma
Enlarged tonsils or adenoids
Systemic Conditions
Allergic disease
Sickle cell disease
Gastroesophageal reflux
Metabolic disorders
  Hypocalcemia
  Gaucher's disease
  Hurler's disease
  Morbid obesity

the tissues in the nasopharyngeal area and may thus be associated with OSAS. Sickle cell disease may also be associated with lymphoid tissue enlargement and thereby play a role in the development of OSAS.[30]

The medical history should include a record of the use of medication. Medications with a sedative effect, most commonly antihistamines, are often used in childhood and may be used particularly in children with OSAS in an effort to relieve upper airway obstruction. Although the effects of common antihistamines on OSAS have not been evaluated, sedatives, narcotics, and ethanol have been associated with obstruction in adults, and such an association may be true in some children for antihistamines. It is prudent for children to avoid these medications and use instead nonsedating medications for allergic rhinitis, such as topical nasal cromolyn sodium or beclomethasone.

The very early onset of OSAS may be suggestive of a congenital abnormality such as a subglottic hemangioma, a laryngeal web, or choanal stenosis.[31, 32] If the symptoms continue when the child is awake as well as asleep, a fixed or variable extrathoracic airway narrowing should be suspected. Fixed obstructions include ectopic thyroid,[33] tracheal ring, and tracheal stenosis. Laryngomalacia is the most common variable obstruction in childhood. In contrast to the situation of uncomplicated OSAS, in which symptoms worsen when the patient is asleep, activity may make laryngomalacia worse, particularly at high airflows.[34] If the child is able to perform the test, a maximal flow-volume curve during inspiration and expiration may help in the evaluation of type and severity of obstruction. A forced partial expiratory curve may demonstrate fixed obstruction to the expiratory flow in infants, but there is no way to obtain an equivalent to the inspiratory limb of a full flow-volume curve. OSAS not associated with an anatomic obstruction, either fixed or variable, should demonstrate no abnormality in these pulmonary function tests in fully awake children.

PHYSICAL EXAMINATION

Physical examination of children with OSAS in the awake state is quite variable. Results of the examination are usually entirely normal, but this outcome should not be interpreted as ruling out the possibility of OSAS. First, the facies and habitus should be observed. A retrognathic or hypognathic profile should arouse the suspicion that the tongue is being pushed back because of a lack of space in the oropharynx and is thus compromising the airway.[31] Long, narrow facies may be associated with OSAS because of a narrowing of the pharynx. Many malformation syndromes have been associated with sleep apnea. Some of these are associated with a small pharynx,[35] as in Treacher Collins syndrome, or a small oral cavity,[31] as in Pierre Robin syndrome. Isolated cleft palate may be associated with sleep apnea, probably because of abnormal insertion of pharyngeal muscles. Some syndromes such as Down's syndrome may be accompanied by obstruction caused both by physical factors such as a relatively large tongue, and by functional factors, such as hypotonia.

The growth pattern may take any of several forms.

Morbid obesity (more than 150% of predicted weight) is an increased risk factor for OSAS. However, OSAS can also be a cause of delayed skeletal development and poor weight gain.[36] The mechanism of this delay is not understood. However, the delay may result from an interruption of the release of growth hormone that occurs predominantly in REM sleep.[27] Another possible explanation for the poor weight gain is the increased work of breathing and subsequent increased caloric expenditure.

Affected children should be observed while breathing quietly. Airflow from the nostrils may be qualitatively evaluted either by having the child breathe on a mirror or by holding a wisp of cotton in front of each nostril. The nasal passages should be closely examined and signs of infection or allergic rhinitis noted. Nasal septal deviations and polyps should be ruled in or out only after an adequate examination with a nasal speculum. Infants should be examined for the possibility of choanal atresia, which may be either unilateral or bilateral and complete or partial in nature.[31] The diagnosis can be made by passing a No. 8 French catheter through the nose into the nasopharynx. If it cannot be passed, rhinoscopy or instillation of barium in the nose with the patient supine further defines the anatomy. At present, computed tomography (CT) of the area provides the least invasive way of accurately investigating the nasopharyngeal area and is the procedure of choice.

Next, the presence of respiratory stridor, a hoarse voice, or an abnormal cry should be noted. These symptoms may indicate lesions of the vocal cords, such as polyps, paresis, or paralysis. The mouth should be examined, particularly with regard to malocclusion and the size of the tongue in relation to the oral cavity. The palate should be palpated in order to rule out a submucous cleft. Tonsillar size is pertinent, but relying on it alone leads to both false-positive and false-negative diagnoses.[34, 37] This uncertainty may exist because obstruction can occur at other sites or because the physical examination may not reveal the full size of the tonsils. Even in cooperative children only the upper poles may be visible, and the greater mass of the tonsils may extend down into the pharyngeal space ("iceberg tonsils"). At this level, large tonsils interfere with pharyngeal patency and cause intermittent, position-dependent obstruction. Abnormally copious secretions may play a role in OSAS by irritating the larynx or being aspirated, causing laryngospasm or repeated pneumonia.

Because assessing the nasopharyngeal space and the adenoids is difficult by direct visualization, nasolaryngoscopy with a fiberoptic laryngoscope is a reasonable extension of the physical examination for the physician who is familiar with this technique. However, endoscopy is not the only way of obtaining information about the nasopharynx. Moreover, what is seen during the awake state does not necessarily reflect the sleeping condition. For example, estimations of pharyngeal size on physical examination are difficult in awake children because the walls are mobile structures that are quite plastic. Also, the size and shape of the pharynx may be quite different in the sleep state than in the awake state. In one study, the pharynxes of children with OSAS who were examined under anesthesia were narrower than those of controls.

However, in the children with OSAS, the pharynxes were not shallower, and the soft palates were not longer.[37] However, other authors using different techniques have reached different conclusions.[24, 35] These contradictory conclusions probably indicate that anatomic variation is but one factor in OSAS.

Severe and long-standing OSAS may be associated with pulmonary hypertension.[38, 39] This may be suspected if signs of right-sided heart failure, such as peripheral edema and a loud, fixed, split S2 signal, are found. Evaluation for evidence of pulmonary hypertension should be approached in a stepwise manner. EKG is seldom helpful; it is the least sensitive form of evaluation, positive only after secondary right ventricular hypertrophy has developed. Similarly, chest radiographs show changes in the cardiac silhouette only after significant right ventricular hypertrophy has occurred. Echocardiography, including flow-directed Doppler recording, usually provides the evidence needed for evaluating the possibility of pulmonary hypertension. Cardiac catheterization is the gold standard of testing and has added greatly to the understanding of cor pulmonale; however, it is far too invasive as a first step. Cardiac catheterization has provided evidence that pulmonary hypertension may change dramatically between the obstructed sleep and awake states and with the addition of supplemental oxygen.[39, 40] Patients who have congenital heart disease with a left-to-right shunt may be at risk of an adverse interaction with OSAS, which heightens the possibility of pulmonary hypertension. This possibility may affect the timing of corrective surgery to prevent irreversible pulmonary hypertension. In patients with Down's syndrome, OSAS and congenital heart disease are frequently present in the same patient.[41, 42] Systemic hypertension,[40] pectus excavatum, and digital clubbing have been associated with OSAS but are uncommon. A large pulsus paradoxus may be present during episodes of obstruction.[39]

LABORATORY EVALUATION

Routine laboratory tests are not sensitive and thus are helpful in assessing only severe cases of OSAS. In such severe cases, hypoventilation or hypoxemia may affect a variety of laboratory values. Pa_{CO_2} from either a capillary or an arterial blood gas specimen is usually normal but may be at the upper limits of normal or elevated even when a patient is awake. The presence of hypercapnia or hypoxia when the patient is awake is unusual enough that it should prompt consideration of entities other than uncomplicated OSAS. These include congenital hypoventilation syndrome (Ondine's curse), Pickwickian syndrome, chest wall deformity, neurologic disease, and any airway or lung diseases resulting in ventilation/perfusion mismatching.

RADIOGRAPHIC EXAMINATION

Radiographic examination of the sinuses and nasopharynx may be helpful in assessing patients with OSAS. Clinical studies have reached conflicting conclusions about whether plain lateral neck films are useful. In two studies, investigators found no significant correlation between sleep apnea and the estimation of pharyngeal, adenoidal, or tonsillar size.[43, 44] Neither of these studies, however, involved the use of polysomnography in assessing sleep apnea, and so the final classification of the presence or absence of OSAS may be questioned. Cephalometry, as described previously, provides more standardization of airway measurements than do routine lateral radiographs of the head and neck. Studies with cephalometry have shown correlations in various parameters for groups of patients,[45, 46] but no single technique enables a definitive diagnosis in an individual patient.

Other ways of assessing the upper airway include fluoroscopy, CT (both static and cine-CT), magnetic resonance imaging (MRI), and acoustic impedance. Fluoroscopy can reveal the site of obstruction but may be difficult to perform when a child is asleep, the state that would ideally be studied.[46] CT of the nasopharynx has shown differences in the cross-sectional area of the hypopharynx in adults[46] as a group. Whether children exhibit these differences is unknown. The new technique of cine-CT has the advantage of evaluating the dynamics of the upper airway, although, like fluoroscopy, it may be difficult to perform under natural sleep conditions. MRI is a static technique but has the advantage of enabling views to be examined in different projections. Acoustic impedance technology provides a measure of the cross-sectional area over the length of the pharynx, but at present it is not generally available for clinical use.

Although all these techniques are useful for ruling out congenital abnormalities or masses or in performing studies on groups of patients to improve the understanding of OSAS, they cannot be used to diagnose OSAS in individual patients. This is because the pharyngeal structures are dynamic and deformable and may change in relation to each other as a result of many factors, including muscle tone and body position.

PHYSIOLOGIC LABORATORY MONITORING

If the history, physical examination, and other studies are suggestive of sleep apnea, a physician may select from several studies to confirm the diagnosis. The cornerstone of diagnosis is documentation of clinically significant obstruction to airflow during sleep. The simplest step is to have the parents record the night's events on a tape recorder. Particular attention needs to be paid to snoring and the interruption of airflow. Parents should note variation in the child's position because this may suggest posterior displacement of the tongue, nasal septal deviation, or lymphoid tissue or redundant pharyngeal tissue, each of which can cause positional occlusion of the airway.

During naps in the office, pulse oximetry can be used to screen for oxygen desaturation. If hypoxemia is documented it is significant, but a negative study cannot be used to rule out OSAS. Also, pulse oximetry alone does not document the cause of the hypoxemia, nor does it reflect airflow. Moreover, some symptomatic children do not become hypoxemic even if they exhibit hypercapnia.

A pneumogram, which records heart rate and chest wall movement, is of limited usefulness in evaluating OSAS. During an obstructive apneic episode, chest wall excursions continue and often increase as the drive to overcome the obstruction increases. It is difficult to judge from a pneumogram whether the chest wall movement is abnormal, and often movement artifact further complicates interpretation. Thus only episodes severe enough to cause bradycardia or tachycardia may be detected, but these are difficult to differentiate from changes that occur during sleep without obstruction.

The most accurate way of diagnosing obstructive sleep apnea is by noctural polysomnography. This technique involves the simultaneous measurement of multiple physiologic parameters. At the minimum, EKG pulse oximetry, chest wall movement, and airflow are measured. Airflow is sensed by a thermistor or thermocouple, but if an end-tidal CO_2 level is being measured, fluctuations in that parameter may also reflect alterations in airflow. Airflow must be sensed at both nares and at the mouth if an accurate measurement is to be made. Measurement of extraocular movement and EEG recording is necessary if the sleep stage is to be ascertained. Unless a complete EEG is needed for investigating the possibility of seizures, two channels of EEG recordings are adequate for evaluation of sleep phase and stage.

Additional electrodes may be placed in order to record other parameters if clinically indicated. If gastroesophageal reflux is considered a possible cause of apnea or oxygen desaturation, an esophageal pH probe can be placed. All of the channels are then recorded simultaneously on a multichannel recorder, enabling correlation of clinical and physiologic events (Fig. 61–5). Audiovisual recording should be available in order to assess sleep behavior and should be conducted in a manner that allows synchronization with the other parameters. A wide range of information is supplied by a properly performed sleep study. The frequency of obstructive episodes and information about whether they are associated with desaturation, arousal, or cardiovascular instability are primary in the assessment of OSAS. Primary causes such as esophageal reflux and seizures may be diagnosed. In addition, observation of body position in sleep, such as hyperextension of the neck or a preference for lying on one side, may provide insight into the nature of the obstruction. An accurate study is important not only in making the diagnosis of OSAS but also in planning appropriate therapy and determining its efficacy.

A sleep study with full polysomnography is technically demanding and requires familiarity with the equipment and ability to work with patients in a calm and reassuring manner. The environment itself must be free of distracting sounds and sights and regulated to a comfortable temperature. If young children have been deprived of several hours of sleep, a daytime nap study 2 to 4 h after sleep often provides the needed information. Sedation is sometimes administered in an effort to induce sleep during the day. Although chloral hydrate is not generally considered a respiratory depressant, children with OSAS may be more susceptible to any blunting of respiratory reflexes, and every effort should be made to avoid using sedatives to accomplish a sleep study. Studies obtained under these

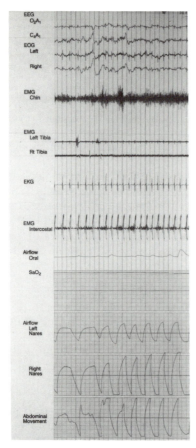

Figure 61–5. Normal polysomnogram. Tracing of a period of normal sleep. Note the continuing EMG activity and airflow synchronous with abdominal movement.

conditions should clearly indicate the presence of medication and be interpreted with caution, because of the possibility of interaction with respiratory drive. If the history is suggestive of sleep apnea, a full sleep study should be performed when the shorter nap study is unrevealing. However, even a full overnight sleep study may not duplicate the environmental conditions at home. Studies have shown that more than one night is needed to establish a base line for adults, whereas children usually can establish a stable base line on the first night.

DIFFERENTIAL DIAGNOSIS

A variety of other conditions may mimic OSAS. As mentioned earlier, any condition narrowing the airway such as vascular rings, ectopic thyroid,[33] tracheal stenosis, laryngeal stenosis, or laryngomalacia may secondarily cause stridor or obstruction at night. Unusual conditions such as seizures[47] or the tetany of hypocalcemia[48] may cause episodes of disorganized breathing and stridor. These can be distinguished from OSAS by polysomnography. Children with cerebral palsy may have disorganized breathing, depending on the extent of pharyngeal involvement and its effects on pharyngeal musculature. Asthmatic children may experience acute onset of short-

ness of breath, especially in the early morning. Usually the history can reveal the difference between the inspiratory stridor and snoring of OSAS and the primarily expiratory wheezing of asthma. In addition, asthma persists after patients have awakened, whereas the airway obstruction of OSAS is relieved on awakening.

Gastroesophageal reflux, which may be produced by one of several mechanisms, occasionally leads to night-time coughing or stridor that may be confused with OSAS. Gastric secretions reaching the pharynx may cause protective coughing or laryngospasm.[49] Chronic irritation of pharyngeal and nasal tissues may also cause swelling, further aggravating the tendency of these tissues to cause obstruction. Irritation of the esophagus can cause a reflex irritation with a cough. A history of excessive spitting or vomiting or, in older children, pain consistent with esophagitis should prompt consideration of reflux.

TREATMENT

Although many diagnostic techniques used to study adults have been applied to children, not all are applicable. Moreover, the therapeutic modalities commonly used are markedly different in children and adults. Adult subjects have been treated with centrally acting drugs, nocturnal oxygen, nasal continuous positive airway pressure (CPAP), and nasopharyngeal surgery. Most affected children can be successfully treated with simple tonsillectomy, adenoidectomy, or both.[50]

Therapy is directed at the abnormality noted. If a specific area of airway narrowing such as tracheal or choanal stenosis can be identified, it may be surgically corrected. Uvulopalatopharyngoplasty has been used primarily in adults and consists of excision of part of the soft palate and lateral pharyngeal walls. The experience in children has been quite limited, but the procedure may yield good results. Unfortunately, at present there are no criteria for deciding who may respond to this therapy. It should therefore probably be reserved for patients who have failed to respond to other interventions.

Similarly, specific craniofacial abnormalities such as Arnold-Chiari malformation, Treacher Collins syndrome, Crouzon's disease, or Apert's syndrome may require major surgical intervention to the skull or the midfacial area.[32] The postoperative period for this type of major surgery is critical because of the vulnerability of the airway during this time. Such surgery should be performed only at centers with personnel experienced in the critical care of children and by a team of surgeons who have had extensive experience in craniofacial surgery. Patients with severe cases of obstructive sleep apnea may need to be stabilized before definitive surgery is attempted. Likewise, children with severe failure to thrive or cor pulmonale may also need temporary measures such as tracheostomy, or maximal medical therapy in the form of digitalis and diuretics. With the exception of cases in which a permanent tracheostomy is indicated for improving pulmonary toilet, tracheostomies are seldom the definitive treatment of choice in children with OSAS.

In an effort to find alternatives to surgery, a number of

medical therapies have been attempted. Therapy with drugs that stimulate the central nervous system (CNS), such as methylxanthines, has been less effective in OSAS than in central apnea syndromes.[51] Protriptyline, a tricyclic antidepressant, has been shown to ameliorate OSAS in adults,[52] but whether this treatment is applicable to children is unknown. Long-term nocturnal administration of oxygen may decrease nighttime desaturation and the absolute number of apneic episodes.[53] Unfortunately, the daytime symptoms are not improved by nocturnal oxygen. The administration of CPAP through a fitted nasal mask at night has also been attempted in order to "prop" open the nasopharynx area.[54,55] Initial administration of CPAP during a sleep study enables the physician to titrate the minimal pressure needed for achieving the desired result. Complications of CPAP are minimal, such as irritation of the eyes or skin. The major reason for the failure of CPAP is behavioral: preschool and mentally delayed children may not tolerate wearing the mask and may require other intervention. However, when major surgery is being considered for relieving symptoms, CPAP should be given every opportunity to succeed, because often over time the airway enlarges and symptoms become milder.

The efficacy of CPAP is illustrated by the case of a 4½-year-old, mildly obese male, J.B., who had snored since the age of 1½ years and suffered from daytime drowsiness. Sleep studies conducted at age 4½ years had revealed 134 obstructive episodes during 8 hours of sleep, with hypercapnia (alveolar carbon dioxide pressure in the 60s) and oxygen saturations as low as 50%. The patient underwent a tonsilloadenoidectomy and, 6 months later, a repeated adenoidectomy and uvulectomy. These procedures resulted in temporary, partial improvement of symptoms. A repeat sleep study (see Fig. 61-5) showed continuous and periodic obstructive apnea episodes. CPAP by mask was applied during a sleep study, and at a critical pressure of 14 to 15 cm H_2O, the obstructive breathing pattern and oxygen desaturation (<90%) were eliminated. The child rapidly adjusted to the mask at home and requested it regularly before going to sleep. With the use of nasal CPAP, the parents reported that the child exhibited almost no snoring, less enuresis, and more daytime alertness. This case illustrates that CPAP can be practical, especially if the child is not mentally retarded, can cooperate, and appreciates the effectiveness of the intervention.

Fortunately, in most cases, removing the tonsils and adenoids provides relief.[8, 27, 56, 57] Uniformly good results have been reported in series of patients without specific craniofacial anomalies.[27, 50, 57] However, it may be impossible to know beforehand whether this surgery is sufficient therapy in a particular patient. No one measurement or set of measurements uniformly predicts the response to this procedure for the child with midface hypoplasia or retrognathia. Nevertheless, most children who have OSAS should undergo a simple adenotonsillectomy before other, more complicated surgical procedures because the response is often good. When surgery of any kind is indicated, preoperative sedation should be avoided because it may precipitate sudden, unexpected obstruction.[58] Adenotonsillectomy cases must be closely

monitored because edema and sedation may also act to precipitate obstruction in the first 24 h after surgery. Effectiveness cannot be judged for several weeks after surgery[59] in some cases because of residual swelling and in others because long-standing changes of pulmonary hypertension may be slow to resolve. If after 6 weeks there is significant residual OSAS, additional therapy such as uvulopalatopharyngoplasty or nighttime CPAP may be tried.

Children who have been treated for OSAS should continue to be observed in adulthood because some will have symptoms of OSAS years later.[60] Whether this is a continuing condition or a recurrence in adult life is unknown. Thus periodically taking a history for such signs as snoring may alert the physician to the need for further study.

REFERENCES

1. Dickens C: The Posthumus Papers of the Pickwick Club, p. 44. New York: Dodd, Mead 1944.
2. Kryger MH: Fat, sleep and Charles Dickens: Literary and medical contributions to the understanding of sleep apnea. Clin Chest Med 6:555–562, 1985.
3. Hill W: On some causes of backwardness and stupidity in children. Br Med J 2:711–712, 1889.
4. Gastaut H, Tassinari CA, Duron B: Polygraphic study of the episodic diurnal and nocturnal (hypnic and respiratory) manifestations of the Pickwick syndrome. Brain Res 2:167–186, 1966.
5. Guilleminault C, Tilkian A, Dement W: The sleep apnea syndromes. Annu Rev Med 27:465–484, 1976.
6. Berry DT, Webb WB, Block AJ: Sleep apnea syndrome: A critical review of the apnea index as a diagnostic criterion. Chest 86:529–531, 1984.
7. Swift AC: Upper airway obstruction, sleep disturbance and adenotonsillectomy in children. J Laryngol Otol 102:419–422, 1988.
8. Strohl KP, Cherniack NS, Gothe B: Physiologic basis of therapy for sleep apnea. Am Rev Respir Dis 134:791–802, 1986.
9. Kahn A, Blum D, Waterschoot P, et al: Effects of obstructive sleep apneas on transcutaneous oxygen pressure in control infants, siblings of sudden infant death syndrome victims, and near miss infants: Comparison with the effects of central sleep apneas. Pediatrics 70:852–857, 1982.
10. Guilleminault C, Winkle R, Korobkin R, Simmons B: Children and nocturnal snoring: Evaluation of the effects of sleep related respiratory resistive load and daytime functioning. Eur J Pediatr 139:165–171, 1982.
11. Remmers JE, deGroot WJ, Sauerland EK, Anch AM: Pathogenesis of upper airway occlusion during sleep. J Appl Physiol 44:931–938, 1978.
12. Krieger J: Breathing during sleep in normal subjects. Clin Chest Med 6:577–594, 1985.
13. Jeans WD, Fernando DCJ, Maw AR, Leighton BC: A longitudinal study of the growth of the nasopharynx and its contents in normal children. Br J Radiol 54:117–121, 1981.
14. Guilleminault C, Riley R, Powell N: Obstructive sleep apnea and abnormal cephalometric measurements. Chest 86:793–794, 1984.
15. Fletcher EC: Abnormalities of Respiration During Sleep: Diagnosis, Pathophysiology, and Treatment, p. 128. Orlando, FL: Grune & Stratten, 1986.
16. Guilleminault C, Ariagno R, Coons S, et al: Near-miss sudden infant death syndrome in eight infants with sleep apnea–related cardiac arrhythmias. Pediatrics 76:236–242, 1985.
17. Guilleminault C, Ariagno RL, Forno LS, et al: Obstructive sleep apnea and near miss SIDS: 1. Report of an infant with sudden death. Pediatrics 63:837–843, 1979.
18. Guilleminault C, Souquet M, Ariagno R, et al: Five cases of near-miss sudden infant death syndrome and development of obstructive sleep apnea syndrome. Pediatrics 73:71–78, 1984.

19. Whitcomb M, Clark R, Altman M, Ralstin JH: Central and obstructive sleep apnea. Chest 73:857–860, 1978.
20. Swift PF, Emery J: Clinical observations on response to nasal occlusion in infancy. Arch Dis Child 48:947–951, 1973.
21. Guilleminault C, Eldridge F, Simmons F, Dement W: Sleep apnea in eight children. Pediatrics 58:23–30, 1976.
22. Brouillette R, Hanson D, David R, et al: A diagnostic approach to suspected obstructive sleep apnea in children. J Pediatr 105:10–14, 1984.
23. Orr W, Moran W: Diagnosis and management of obstructive sleep apnea. Arch Otolaryngol 111:583–588, 1985.
24. Wong H: The problem of the snoring child and obstructive apnea syndrome. J Singapore Paediatr Soc 30:1–6, 1988.
25. Potsic WP: Comparison of polysomnography and sonography for assessing regularity of respiration during sleep in adenotonsillar hypertrophy. Laryngoscope 97:1430–1437, 1987.
26. Brouillette R, Fernbach S, Hunt C: Obstructive sleep apnea in infants and children. J Pediatr 100:31–40, 1982.
27. Lind M, Lundell B: Tonsillar hyperplasia in children. Arch Otolaryngol Head Neck Surg 108:650–654, 1982.
28. Mandel EM, Reynolds CF: Sleep disorders associated with upper airway obstruction in children. Pediatr Clin North Am 28:897–903, 1981.
29. Maddern BR, Reed HT, Ohene-Frempong K, Beckerman RC: Obstructive sleep apnea syndrome in sickle cell disease. Ann Otol Rhinol Laryngol 98:174–178, 1989.
30. Weider DJ, Hauri PJ: Nocturnal enuresis in children with upper airway obstruction. Int J Pediatr Otorhinolaryngol 9:173–182, 1985.
31. Cozzi F, Pierro A: Glossoptosis-apnea syndrome in infancy. Pediatrics 75:836–843, 1985.
32. Holinger LD, Weiss KS: Diagnosis and management of airway obstruction in craniofacial anomalies. Otolaryngol Clin North Am 14:1005–1017, 1981.
33. Chanin L, Greenberg L: Pediatric upper airway obstruction due to ectopic thyroid: Classification and case reports. Laryngoscope 98:422–427, 1988.
34. Apley J: The infant with stridor. Arch Dis Child 28:423–435, 1953.
35. Shprintzen RJ, Croft C, Berkman MD, Rakoff SJ: Pharyngeal hypoplasia in Treacher Collins syndrome. Arch Otolaryngol 105:127–131, 1979.
36. Everett A, Koch W, Saulsbury F: Failure to thrive due to obstructive sleep apnea. Clin Pediatr (Phila) 26:90–92, 1987.
37. Bodsky L, Moore L, Stanievich JF: A comparison of tonsillar size and oropharyngeal dimensions in children with obstructive adenotonsillar hypertrophy. Int J Pediatr Otorhinolaryngol 13:149–156, 1987.
38. Levy AM, Tabakin BS, Hanson JS, Narkewicz RM: Hypertrophied adenoids causing pulmonary hypertension and severe congestive heart failure. N Engl J Med 277:506–511, 1967.
39. Tilkian A, Guilleminault C, Schroeder J, et al: Hemodynamics in sleep-induced apnea. Ann Intern Med 85:714–719, 1976.
40. Ross RD, Daniels SR, Loggie JM, et al: Sleep apnea–associated hypertension and reversible left ventricular hypertrophy. J Pediatr 111:253–255, 1987.
41. Rowland T, Nordstrom L, Bean M, Burkhardt H: Chronic upper airway obstruction and pulmonary hypertension in Down's syndrome. Am J Dis Child 135:1050–1052, 1981.
42. Loughlin G, Wynne J, Victorica B: Sleep apnea as a possible cause of pulmonary hypertension in Down syndrome. J Pediatr 98:435–437, 1981.
43. Laurikainen E, Erkinjuntti M, Alihanka J, et al: Radiological parameters of the bony nasopharynx and the adenotonsillar size compared with sleep apnea episodes in children. Int J Pediatr Otorhinolaryngol 12:303–310, 1987.
44. Mahboubi S, Marsh RR, Potsic WP, Pasquariello PS: The lateral neck radiograph in adenotonsillar hyperplasia. Int J Pediatr Otorhinolaryngol 10:67–73, 1985.
45. Guilleminault C, Heldt G, Powell N, Riley R: Small upper airway in near-miss sudden infant death syndrome infants and their families. Lancet 2:402–407, 1986.
46. Suratt PM, Dee P, Atkinson RL, et al: Fluoroscopic and computed tomographic features of the pharyngeal airway in obstructive sleep apnea. Am Rev Respir Dis 127:487–492, 1983.
47. Navelet Y, Wood C, Robieux I, Tardieu M: Seizures presenting as apnoea. Arch Dis Child 64:357–359, 1989.
48. Hidalgo HA, Davis SH: Intermittent stridor and hypocalcemia in childhood. Pediatr Pulmonol 7:110–111, 1989.
49. Newman LJ, Russe J, Glassman MS, et al: Patterns of gastroesophageal reflux (GER) in patients with apparent life-threatening events. J Pediatr Gastroenterol Nutr 8:157–160, 1989.
50. Ahlqvist-Rastad J, Hultcrantz E, Svanholm H: Children with tonsillar obstruction: Indications for and efficacy of tonsillectomy. Acta Paediatr Scand 77:831–835, 1988.
51. Espinoza H, Antic R, Thornton AT, McEvoy RD: The effects of aminophylline on sleep and sleep-disordered breathing in patients with obstructive sleep apnea syndrome. Am Rev Respir Dis 136:80–84, 1987.
52. Brownell LG, West P, Sweatman P, et al: Protriptyline in obstructive sleep apnea. N Engl J Med 307:1037–1042, 1982.
53. Gold AR, Schwartz AR, Bleecker ER, Smith PL: The effect of chronic nocturnal oxygen administration upon sleep apnea. Am Rev Respir Dis 134:925–929, 1986.
54. Guilleminault C, Nino-Murcia G, Heldt G, et al: Alternative treatment to tracheostomy in obstructive sleep apnea syndrome: Nasal continuous positive airway pressure in young children. Pediatrics 78:797–802, 1986.
55. Guilleminault C: Obstructive sleep apnea syndrome and its treatment in children: Areas of agreement and controversy. Pediatr Pulmonol 3:429–436, 1987.
56. Eliaschar I, Lavie P, Halperin E, et al: Sleep apneic episodes as indications for adenotonsillectomy. Arch Otolaryngol 106:492–496, 1980.
57. Frank Y, Kravath RE, Pollak CP, Weitzman ED: Obstructive sleep apnea and its therapy: Clinical and polysomnographic manifestation. Pediatrics 71:737–742, 1983.
58. Weinberg S, Kravath R, Phillips L, et al: Episodic complete airway obstruction in children with undiagnosed obstructive sleep apnea. Anesthesiology 60:356–358, 1984.
59. Levin DL, Muster AJ, Pachman LM, et al: Cor pulmonale secondary to upper airway obstruction. Chest 68:166–171, 1975.
60. Guilleminault C, Partinen M, Praud JP, et al: Morphometric facial changes and obstructive sleep apnea in adolescents. J Pediatr 44:997–999, 1989.

62 PNEUMOTHORAX
WARREN J. WARWICK, M.D.

The presence of air in the thoracic cavity outside the lung parenchyma is always abnormal. Pneumothorax, as this condition is called, may be defined as spontaneous (occurring without obvious cause) or traumatic (caused by a direct or an indirect injury to the lung parenchyma). It can be further divided into two functional types: static and tension pneumothorax. In the static type, air enters the thoracic space but does not continue to accumulate and eventually is absorbed by the pleural circulation. In the tension type, air continues to accumulate, increases in volume and pressure, compresses the lung, and interferes with respiration.

PATHOPHYSIOLOGY

SPONTANEOUS PNEUMOTHORAX

Pneumothorax rarely occurs in the absence of pathologic processes in the lung. Regardless of the underlying disease, all cases of spontaneous pneumothorax have a single cause: partial obstruction of one of the peripheral airways. The accumulated air causes partial collapse and may again block the leaking airway. Large amounts of subpleural air cause such symptoms as shortness of breath and chest pain.

If the ball-valve partial obstruction is in one of the larger peripheral airways, the leakage may not seal as the lung collapses. In this case, the increased amount of subpleural air bypasses the obstruction during inspiration and is again trapped during expiration. Each deeper inspiratory effort accentuates the process. Eventually the air pressure in the pleural space compresses the opposite lung. The tension pneumothorax process leads to hypoxia and, if not arrested, to asphyxia and death. In the midsized airways, this tension pneumothorax can progress rapidly, and death can occur within minutes.

TRAUMATIC PNEUMOTHORAX

Any form of trauma to the lungs can tear the airways or parenchyma and cause air to leak into the thorax. If the tear is small, the subsequent pneumothorax is usually stable, and the air is reabsorbed by the pleural vessels. If the tear is large, a tension pneumothorax is likely to develop, and surgical treatment is required.

CLINICAL MANIFESTATIONS

SPONTANEOUS PNEUMOTHORAX

The clinical manifestations of pneumothorax vary, depending on the age and the state of consciousness of the patient, whether the pneumothorax is spontaneous or traumatic, and whether it is a static or a tension pneumothorax.

Pneumothorax in infancy and early childhood is almost always associated with a clinically active pulmonary disease or with specific trauma. In infants on ventilators who show unexpected clinical deterioration, pneumothorax should be suspected.[1] The presence of hypoxia with tachycardia and tachypnea in an infant or a young child with active pulmonary disease or with the potential for the development of a traumatic pneumothorax should raise suspicion of pneumothorax in the differential diagnosis. Lack of response to symptomatic treatment of hypoxemia, tachycardia, and tachypnea increases the suspicion of a pneumothorax.

In a child or an adolescent, pleuritic pain in the upper chest, with or without shortness of breath, may be associated with the rupture of a bleb in the apices of the lung with the release of a small quantity of air into the pleural space. A pattern of sudden onset and short duration of chest pain is common before the development of pneumothorax in patients who are at risk for pneumothorax. Some patients exhibit the same pain pattern and have little, if any, shortness of breath and only a slight increase in pulse or respiratory rate; chest radiographs of such patients may show a 20% to 30% incidence of pneumothorax. Often the diagnosis of pneumothorax may be missed if chest radiographs are not taken. Adolescents and older children who experience sudden onset of persistent chest pain, especially if high in the chest, in association with shortness of breath may have pneumothorax, even if there is no known underlying disease process. Patients who experience sudden onset of chest pain with progressive shortness of breath, especially in association with hypoxia and tachypnea, should be suspected of having a tension pneumothorax.

TRAUMATIC PNEUMOTHORAX

Trauma capable of rupturing, tearing, or puncturing an airway can be quite diverse. Obvious examples include penetration of the thorax by any object and any form of direct blunt trauma to the chest or upper abdomen. Common medical therapies are occasionally the cause of traumatic pneumothorax, such as bronchoscopy, airway suctioning, ventilatory therapy, positive airway pressure, aspiration of the pleural space of the lung, insertion of jugular or supraclavicular intravenous lines, and any thoracic surgical procedure.

PHYSICAL FINDINGS

Breathlessness, tachypnea, and tachycardia accompanied by hypoxia are suggestive of pneumothorax, regardless of the patient's age. When these symptoms are associated with acute onset of chest pain, whether the pain is pleuritic or not, suspicion of pneumothorax should be high. Physical examination is usually but not always helpful. The chest wall on the side of the pneumothorax typically appears fuller, is less mobile, and may be hyperresonant. The trachea may be shifted away from the pneumothorax. Tactile fremitus is absent, and breath sounds are reduced or absent in comparison with the nonaffected side. Subcutaneous emphysema over the neck or upper chest is highly suggestive of pneumothorax; exceptions are seen on rare occasions, and symmetric physical findings may be indicative of bilateral pneumothorax.

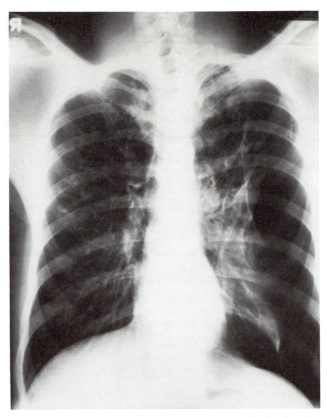

Figure 62–1. Pneumothorax: bilateral parietal pleural adhesions in a patient with advanced cystic fibrosis. (Courtesy of Dr. Martha N. Frantz.)

RADIOGRAPHIC EVALUATION

Every patient, regardless of age, in whom pneumothorax is considered should undergo diagnostic imaging to confirm the diagnosis. The initial order should be inspiratory and expiratory anteroposterior or posteroanterior chest films plus a lateral view. Although an inspiratory film is sufficient for making the diagnosis in cases of moderate and severe pneumothorax, an expiratory film is essential when there is a minimal air leakage. This is true especially in the presence of factors predisposing a patient to bleb formation with lucent areas in the apices of the lungs. In such a patient, it can be difficult to identify the thin lines that separate the hyperinflated lung tissue from the air external to the lung. Occasional useful signs include the anterior junction line, a highly specific sign of bilateral pneumothorax in neonates;[2] the medial stripe; and a large hyperlucent hemithorax.[3] The latter may be a helpful sign on a posteroanterior chest radiograph when the air is between lobes or on a lateral chest radiograph when the air is between the anterior or posterior chest wall and the lungs (Fig. 62–1).

When pneumothorax is suspected but not clearly identified, air is occasionally loculated between lobes or between the lung tissue and the mediastinum. Computed tomography of the chest may be necessary for proving the presence of pneumothorax in such atypical manifestations. The precise location of air leakages can also be identified from the presence of bubbles in water-soluble contrast material in the pleural space.[4]

LABORATORY FINDINGS

Laboratory tests can aid in the diagnosis of pneumothorax: arterial blood gas analysis can confirm hypoxemia, often with an increase in the alveolar-arterial oxygen difference. In left-sided pneumothorax, an electrocardiogram may show precordial T wave inversion and a shift of the QRS axis.

Rapidly progressive hypoxemia in a patient in whom pneumothorax is suspected may be caused by tension pneumothorax. In these circumstances, emergency diagnosis and therapy can be accomplished simultaneously with the insertion of a large-bore trochar or needle through the superior chest wall. Immediate elimination of air under pressure confirms the diagnosis and provides temporary but life-saving therapy.

DIFFERENTIAL DIAGNOSIS

Pneumothorax is rarely confused with other diseases or disorders except during infancy, when congenital abnormalities can mimic a pneumothorax. The most common congenital abnormalities confused with pneumothorax are those involving a large cyst,[5] a diaphragmatic hernia, and gas-distended structures extending into the thorax.[6, 7] Auscultation of the chest may locate bowel sounds in the thorax. Lateral views of the chest and abdominal radiographs or auscultation of bowel sounds in the thorax may help identify abnormal location of abdominal viscera. Differential diagnosis of underlying disease is important in both the management and the prediction of recurrence of pneumothorax. The instillation of radiopaque material into the gastrointestinal tract may also confirm the diagnosis of diaphragmatic hernia.

Aspiration of both small and large foreign bodies[8] as well as liquid material may lead to a pneumothorax. Hydrocarbon ingestion in children may also be associated with a pneumothorax.[9] Pneumothorax occurs in about 5% of children hospitalized for asthma and is clinically suspected in only about half of occurrences.[10] Spontaneous pneumothorax is a rare complication of bronchiolitis.[11]

Bronchiectasis, regardless of underlying disease or predisposing factors, has a strong association with pneumothorax. Pneumothorax is a common complication of bronchiectasis in patients with cystic fibrosis. The risk of recurrence is about 50% per year and is independent of the site of the first occurrence.[12]

In one fourth of children in whom pulmonary edema complicates the course of croup or epiglottitis, pneumothorax is likely to develop.[13] Near-drowning with aspiration pneumonia may be also associated with pneumothorax.[14]

Tension pneumothorax is a rare complication of the rapid growth of a pulmonary hydatid cyst.[15] Spontaneous pneumothorax may also occur in some patients with histiocytosis X.[16] Rapidly progressive acute respiratory insufficiency in children with acute lymphoblastic leukemia may be associated with a syndrome of pulmonary alveolar septal calcinosis, pneumomediastinum, and pneumothorax.[17] Both Hodgkin's disease and non-Hodgkin's lymphoma have also been associated with the development of a pneumothorax; the risk is higher in patients treated with radiotherapy.[18] On rare occasions, intrapulmonary metastases can cause a pneumothorax.[19]

Pneumothorax occurs in 30% of children with measles and mediastinal or subcutaneous emphysema, with an increased mortality rate.[20] Catamenic pneumothorax is a very rare complication of endometriosis. Pneumothorax can occur as a complication of any pyogenic or suppurative pulmonary infection, including infections by such diverse agents as *Staphylococcus aureus, Streptococcus pneumoniae, Bordetella pertussis,* and *Mycobacterium tuberculosis. Chlamydia trachomatis* is a rare etiologic agent.[21]

Infarction of the main pulmonary artery in infancy can lead to subpleural cyst formation with pneumothorax in late infancy.[22] Blunt trauma to the thorax can injure any of the airways at any age.[23] In infancy and early childhood, when the thorax is very flexible, such injury can occur without other obvious injury. In older children, physical signs of thoracic trauma, such as rib fractures, are usually present.[24, 25] Internal trauma (such as barotrauma from conventional pressure-cycle or volume-cycle ventilators or jet ventilators) and penetrating injury (from bronchoscopy, airway suctioning, insertion of a feeding tube, or cardiac catheterization) may cause a pneumothorax.[26–28] Penetrating external injury (gunshot, knife wound, thoracentesis, percutaneous lung biopsy, or pleural biopsy)

may also cause a pneumothorax but is associated with an obvious wound.[29]

The difference between the partial pressure of air in the alveolar space and the mixed venous blood normally keeps the pleural space free of air so that any air leakage is eventually absorbed. Breathing 100% oxygen rapidly washes nitrogen from the lungs and blood and decreases the total venous gas pressure to about 145 mm Hg, increasing the gradient for uptake of nitrogen from the pleural space. This gradient enables the blood traversing the pleura to absorb the pleural air.

Immediate surgical exploration is indicated when pneumothorax develops because of trauma to a large airway. Intermediate treatment is to block the bronchus proximal to the leak or to insert an endotracheal tube into the main stem bronchus opposite the pneumothorax.[29, 30]

Mildly symptomatic pneumothorax usually requires no intervention other than close observation. Attention must be directed toward identifying the underlying pathophysiologic process and directing treatment to prevent a recurrence.

Any pneumothorax involving more than 25% of the lung usually occupies enough space to be symptomatic, and insertion of a chest tube is required in order to evacuate the intrapulmonary air. After the air is evacuated and the lung has re-expanded, the chest tube should be clamped and the patient observed. In most patients, the pneumothorax does not recur. In cases of continued air leakages, the chest tube should be maintained on closed suction until the leakage has stopped. Then the tube may be clamped again and the patient observed.

Tension pneumothorax requires immediate insertion of the chest tube and suction. Suction must be maintained until the air leakage stops. If the air leakage remains large, immediate surgery is indicated. If the air leakage diminishes, surgical intervention may be deferred. All patients with persistent tension pneumothorax should be considered for thoracotomy with oversewing or stapling of the area of the leakage and localized pleurectomy or pleural abrasion.

COMPLICATIONS

Because infectious diseases are among the common causes of pneumothorax, infection of the pleural space and even empyema may occur. In this event, diagnosis of the infective organism and specific intravenous antibiotic therapy are indicated. The same chest tube used to remove air from the thoracic space may be used to drain the purulent material from the pleural space. Bleeding into the pleural space, especially in traumatic pneumothorax, usually stops after chest tube insertion. Continuing loss of blood may require surgical exploration.

Pleural adhesions are another common complication of pneumothorax. These adhesions may cause thoracic pain. Adhesions may provide some benefit for the patient during subsequent pneumothorax because the adhesions may prevent the complete collapse of the lung. Patients with cystic fibrosis or pulmonary cystic lymphangiectasia who are potential candidates for lung or heart-lung transplantation may not be considered candidates for future lung transplantation, if surgery is performed for the treatment of pneumothorax. Any patient considering the possibility of a lung or heart-lung transplantation in the future should consult with a transplant surgeon before any thoracic surgery for the treatment of the pneumothorax.

PROGNOSIS

The immediate prognosis for pneumothorax, when death is prevented, is usually good; however, the long-term prognosis for the patient is dependent on the underlying disorder. Because patients with cystic fibrosis usually experience recurrences, prophylactic treatment is necessary for preventing subsequent pneumothoraces and their complications. It is likely that subsequent pneumothorax will be tension pneumothorax and life-threatening.

When future pneumothorax is expected because of the chronic and uncontrollable nature of the underlying disorder, binding the diseased lung to the thoracic cage by the formation of scar tissue should prevent or reduce such recurrences. The formation of scar tissue can be stimulated by either surgical or chemical methods.

Two surgical techniques, pleural abrasion and pleurectomy, have been successful in preventing recurrences of pneumothorax; each has strong advocates. Either of these techniques is the surgical treatment of choice when pneumothorax must be prevented. Both pleural abrasion and pleurectomy are safe, and both may be compatible, if performed to a limited degree, with later double-lung or heart-lung transplantation in most patients.

Scar tissue can also be produced by chemical agents such as tetracycline, quinacrine, talc, nitrogen mustard, and bleomycin, but these techniques have not been as reliable as surgical procedures discussed earlier. The chemical agents also produce severe pain, which can exceed the pain from a surgical procedure. The chemical treatment of the pleura cannot be used in a limited area and thus is contraindicated when there is a potential for future lung or heart-lung transplantation. Chemical treatment of the pleura also is associated with scarring of the lung and the diaphragm and reducing the mobility of the diaphragm, whereas diaphragmatic function remains normal in patients who undergo pleural abrasion or pleurectomy.[13] Chemical agents are not recommended in the treatment of pneumothorax because of the uncontrolled injury to the pleura, especially in patients with cystic fibrosis.

REFERENCES

1. Greenough A, Milner AD: High frequency ventilation in the neonatal period. Eur J Pediatr 146:446–449, 1987.
2. Markowitz RI: The anterior junction line: A radiographic sign of bilateral pneumothorax in neonates. Radiology 167:717–719, 1988.
3. Grim P 3rd, Keenan WJ: Two uncommon radiographic signs of an anterior neonatal pneumothorax: Correlated with clinical finding. Clin Pediatr (Phila) 25:440–444, 1986.
4. Babbitt DP, Sty JR, Glicklich M, et al: A precise technique to localize pulmonary-pleural air leaks. Radiology 144:412–413, 1982.
5. Fan LL, Strain JD, Foley C, et al: Radiological case of the month: Giant pulmonary cyst simulating pneumothorax. Am J Dis Child 142:189–190, 1988.
6. Langer JC, Filler RM, Bohn DJ, et al: Timing of surgery for congenital diaphragmatic hernia: Is emergency operation necessary? J Pediatr Surg 23:731–734, 1988.
7. Berman L, Stringer D, Ein SH, et al: The late-presenting pediatric Bochdalek hernia: A 20-year review. J Pediatr Surg 23:735–739, 1988.
8. Stanisavljevic B, Stefanovic P: Incidence of pneumothorax caused by foreign bodies inhaled in the lower respiratory tract in children. J Fr Otorhinolaryngol 30:75–78, 1981.
9. Marandian MH, Sabouri M, Youssefian H, et al. Pneumatoceles and pneumothorax following accidental hydrocarbon ingestion in children. Ann Pediatr (Paris) 28:687–691, 1981.
10. Brooks LJ, Cloutier MM, Afshani E: Significance of roentgenographic abnormalities in children hospitalized for asthma. Chest 82:315–318, 1982.
11. Pollack J: Spontaneous bilateral pneumothorax in an infant with bronchiolitis. Pediatr Emerg Care 3:33–35, 1987.
12. Rich RH, Warwick WJ, Leonard AS: Open thoracotomy and pleural abrasion in the treatment of spontaneous pneumothorax in cystic fibrosis. J Pediatr Surg 13:237–242, 1978.
13. Kanter RK, Watchko JF: Pulmonary edema associated with upper airway obstruction. Am J Dis Child 138:356–358, 1984.
14. Wunderlich P, Rupprecht E, Trefftz F, et al: Chest radiographs of near-drowned children. Pediatr Radiol 15:297–299, 1985.
15. Stewart MP, Cunningham MS: Tension pneumothorax complicating pulmonary hydatid disease in childhood. Clin Pediatr (Phila) 26:422–424, 1987.
16. Benoit Y: Bilateral pneumothorax as an early sign in a child with histiocytosis X. Acta Paediatr Belg 34:43–45, 1981.
17. Sinniah D, Landing BH, Siegel SE, et al: Pulmonary alveolar septal calcinosis causing progressive respiratory failure in acute lymphoblastic leukemia in childhood. Pediatr Pathol 6:439–448, 1986.
18. Yellin A, Benfield JR: Pneumothorax associated with lymphoma. Am Rev Respir Dis 134:590–592, 1986.
19. Siegel MJ, McAlister WH: Unusual intrathoracic complications in Wilms tumor. AJR 134:1231–1234, 1980.
20. Odita JC, Akamaguna AI: Mediastinal and subcutaneous emphysema associated with childhood measles. Eur J Pediatr 142:33–36, 1984.
21. Lebel MH, Lamarre A, Rousseau E: Pneumothorax: New manifestation of Chlamydia trachomatis infection in infancy. Pediatr Pulmonol 3:362–363, 1987.
22. Stocker JT, McGill LC, Orsini EN: Post-infarction peripheral cysts of the lung in pediatric patients: A possible cause of idiopathic spontaneous pneumothorax. Pediatr Pulmonol 1:7–18, 1985.
23. King DR: Trauma in infancy and childhood: Initial evaluation and management. Pediatr Clin North Am 32:1299–1310, 1985.
24. Bender TM, Oh KS, Medina JL, Girdany BR: Pediatric chest trauma. J Thorac Imaging 2:60–67, 1987.
25. Viano DC, Lau IV: A viscous tolerance criterion for soft tissue injury assessment. J Biomech 21:387–399, 1988.
26. Wetmore SJ, Key JM, Suen JY: Complications of laser surgery for laryngeal papillomatosis. Laryngoscope 95:798–801, 1985.
27. Ostfeld E, Ovadia L: Bilateral tension pneumothorax during pediatric bronchoscopy. Int J Pediatr Otorhinolaryngol 7:301–304, 1984.
28. Hickey PR, Hansen DD, Norwood WI, et al: Anesthetic complications in surgery for congenital heart disease. Anesth Analg 63:657–664, 1984.
29. Zalesnyĭ SA, Nemets VD: Vremennaia okkliuziia bronkha pri lechenii piopnevmotoraksa u detei [Temporary occlusion of the bronchus in the treatment of pyopneumothorax in children]. Vestn Khir 135:113–115, 1985.
30. Baraka A, Dajani A, Maktabi M, et al: Selective contralateral bronchial intubation in children with pneumothorax or bronchopleural fistula. Br J Anaesth 55:901–904, 1983.

63 SUDDEN INFANT DEATH SYNDROME

ROBERT C. BECKERMAN, M.D. / PETE GOYCO, M.D.

The term *sudden infant death syndrome* (SIDS) refers to the sudden death of any infant or young child that is unexpected according to the medical history and in which a thorough postmortem examination and death scene investigation fail to demonstrate an adequate cause of death.[1]

Although many hypotheses have been postulated as explanations for SIDS, attention has been focused on abnormalities of cardiovascular and respiratory regulation as important components in the pathophysiologic origins of SIDS. Consequently, any discussion on SIDS requires that terms used to define pathologic processes be used consistently. Thus a glossary of terms commonly used in discussions of disorders of breathing is included at the end of this chapter. These definitions were adopted at the 1986 National Institutes of Health Consensus Development Conference on Infantile Apnea and Home Monitoring.[2]

EPIDEMIOLOGY

Information from epidemiologic investigations in SIDS may elucidate risk factors for sudden death in a defined population and, subsequently, as a basis for prevention. Retrospective studies may help focus prospective studies in order to better characterize the infants at risk and possibly allow for early intervention and prevention. However, certain limitations of epidemiologic research must be recognized. Epidemiologic methods and their application to clinical practice are reviewed in Chapter 4.

Findings of epidemiologic studies are suggestive of various associations between SIDS and perinatal events, both prenatal and postnatal, some of which are discussed in this chapter. In addition, Shannon and Kelly[3] reviewed and analyzed the published epidemiologic studies with regard to whether the risk factors existed during pregnancy, labor, or delivery; during the neonatal period; or at the time of death. Shannon and Kelly recognized the limitations of most of the epidemiologic studies and suggested that SIDS is probably one final outcome of several disease processes.

Although SIDS may occur during the first month of life, the peak incidence is between 2 and 4 months of age; 80% of cases occur before the age of 5 months.[4] The estimated incidence of SIDS in the United States is approximately 1.5 to 2.0 per 1000 live births and has remained unchanged despite reductions in the rates of infant mortality.[5] Rates of death from SIDS are higher for blacks and Alaskan natives than for whites and children of Asian descent.

In the evaluation of presumed risk factors for SIDS, it is difficult to establish an association between a particular factor and the sudden, unexpected death of an infant. Because infants who eventually die of SIDS cannot be prospectively identified, it is not possible to establish an adequate control group from the general population. In addition, with regard to a retrospective review of records, most epidemiologic studies do not mention whether the interviewer had previous knowledge of which group the study subjects belonged to.[6-8]

Lewak[9] reported risk factors associated with an increased incidence of SIDS: (1) maternal age of less than 25 years; (2) inadequate prenatal care; (3) an interval of <12 months since the preceding pregnancy; (4) maternal smoking during pregnancy; (5) gestation of <40 weeks; and (6) lower socioeconomic status. However, no single factor was sensitive or specific enough to predict SIDS. In fact, the presence of all these risk factors carried only a 10% probability that an infant would die, and all risk factors were present in only one of five SIDS victims. In a study by Naeye and associates,[6] when only the most discriminative variables were evaluated, SIDS occurred in only 1% of infants at highest risk.

The National Institute of Child Health and Human Development Cooperative Epidemiological Study of SIDS Risk Factors revealed an incidence of 1.7 cases per 1000 live births; 88% of the victims were under 5.5 months of age.[10] In this study, SIDS was established as the cause of death only after a detailed review of the gross autopsy, microscopic slides, and death investigation reports by a panel of expert pathologists. The study identified 757 cases of SIDS, accounting for 37.9% of all postneonatal infant deaths. Of the potential maternal risk factors studied, the strongest links were made with age of less than 20 years at first pregnancy, cigarette smoking, and use of illegal drugs during pregnancy. Among infant factors, there appeared to be indirect associations with prematurity, low birth weight, and a recent illness, notably one affecting the gastrointestinal tract.

Most SIDS deaths occur during the winter, which coincidentally represents the predominant season for infections of the respiratory tract.[11] However, a well-defined association between SIDS and an infective organism, either bacterial or viral, has not yet been proved. Most SIDS deaths occur while the children are not being observed: usually at night or during periods associated with sleep.[12]

In a 1988 review, Bentele and Albani[13] identified four major groups of infants considered to be at high risk for SIDS: (1) survivors of apparent life-threatening events (ALTE); (2) subsequent siblings of SIDS victims; (3) premature infants; and (4) infants of drug-dependent mothers.

Among infants with a history of ALTE, the rates of morbidity and risk for SIDS appear to be increased, although these infants account for only a small number of the total SIDS cases.

Although most data suggest that the risk for SIDS among subsequent siblings of SIDS victims is four times higher than that for the general population,[14] Peterson and colleagues[15] found no statistically sufficient difference when siblings from families of SIDS victims were matched against siblings from families in which maternal age and birth rank were comparable. In addition, risk for SIDS was not affected by birth order in subsequent siblings.

Among premature infants, those with prenatal and perinatal complications appear to be at increased risk. Werthammer and co-authors[16] reported that the risk for infants with bronchopulmonary dysplasia was increased sevenfold in comparison with a control population of infants without bronchopulmonary dysplasia. However, another study attributed the deaths of all but one infant with bronchopulmonary dysplasia to conditions other than SIDS, such as chronic lung disease or congenital heart defects.[17]

Maternal use of illegal drugs, such as heroin and methadone, during pregnancy has been associated with increased risk for SIDS.[18] This association suggests a mechanism for SIDS that is based on the effect of narcotics on the brainstem regulation of breathing. Cocaine use by the mother during pregnancy has also been associated with an increased risk for SIDS,[19] but this increased risk may also reflect maternal socioeconomic factors.[20]

Results of some studies have suggested that infants of multiple-birth pregnancies may be at increased risk for SIDS. However, a study by Peterson and colleagues[21] failed to show any significant difference in risk between siblings of multiple births and subsequent siblings of singleton SIDS victims, although the risk was approximately twice that of infants in the general population. Any increased risk for SIDS in infants of multiple-birth pregnancies may be related to a lower birth weight, not to the multiple pregnancy itself.[22] Although SIDS can occur in families, there is no evidence to support a genetic influence in SIDS.

PATHOLOGY

A diagnosis of SIDS cannot be made until a thorough postmortem examination fails to demonstrate an adequate cause of death; however, there are different beliefs as to what constitutes a thorough postmortem examination. Some authors advocate a detailed death-scene investigation as part of the complete postmortem evaluation of a SIDS death, believing that it may reveal or rule out potentially preventable causes of death.[23, 24]

Wigglesworth and collaborators[25] suggested that the two basic prerequisites for an adequate postmortem examination in a suspected SIDS case are a detailed clinical history and prompt access to the deceased infant. Information from persons close to the infant should include a description of the circumstances of the fatal event and a medical history of the infant that includes data about gestation, birth, immunizations, and recent health problems. In addition, information about recent illnesses in immediate relatives and about previous infant deaths in the family must be gathered.

The postmortem examination should include a general description of the infant (including body position at the time of death) and of the internal organs, as well as histopathologic examination of specimens of the heart, lungs, liver, kidneys, adrenal glands, thymus, thyroid gland, brain, and skeletal muscle. Blood and cerebrospinal fluids should be obtained for cultures, as should appropriate tissues for metabolic studies when inborn errors of metabolism are suspected. The history and physical features of the infant may indicate the need for additional studies.

In the past, SIDS investigators considered apnea to be the terminal event in SIDS. This belief gave rise to the apnea hypothesis of SIDS and encouraged investigators to search for morphologic markers of chronic hypoxia, which could be a result of repeated apneic episodes. First described by Naeye and associates,[26-30] these markers of chronic hypoxia include (1) an increase in the medial mass of the small pulmonary arteries; (2) retention of periadrenal brown fat; (3) persistence of hepatic extramedullary hematopoiesis; (4) hyperplasia of chromaffin tissue in the adrenal medulla; (5) proliferation of astroglial cells in the brainstem; (6) abnormalities in the development of the carotid body; and (7) right ventricular hypertrophy.

The finding of brainstem gliosis on microscopic sections of the brains of SIDS victims has been the only marker consistently found in a large percentage of SIDS infants. However, the proliferation of astroglial cells is a nonspecific response to injury and may be merely coincidental, unrelated to the SIDS death and not a result of recurrent apnea and chronic hypoxia.

Nonetheless, not being able to establish a causal relationship between SIDS and pathologic changes in the brainstem does not rule out a defect in the neural control of respiration and cardiovascular function during sleep at a critical stage in the development of an infant. The mechanism of death could be an apneic episode with hypoxia and a secondary cardiac arrhythmia, a fulminant cardiac arrhythmia, or an impaired arousal response to an apneic episode.[31]

Another pathologic marker of SIDS reported by many investigators is the presence of intrathoracic petechiae, believed to be a result of an increased negative pressure within the thorax.[32] These petechiae have been observed on the surfaces of the heart, the lungs, and the thymus gland in approximately 80% of SIDS victims.[33] Beckwith indicated that thymic petechiae tend to spare the cervical lobe of the thymus gland, which is not subject to changes in intrathoracic pressures.[34] This finding supported the idea that increased negative intrathoracic pressures produced by respiratory efforts in the presence of an upper airway obstruction represent the final event in most SIDS victims.

Investigators have described a variety of pathologic findings in SIDS infants, among them a lower number of myelinated vagal fibers. This finding suggests abnormal development of the vagus nerve secondary to chronic hypoxia or an abnormal role of the vagus nerve in the control of respiration.[35] Other investigators have found elevated levels of hypoxanthine in the vitreous humor of SIDS victims, also a consequence of chronic hypoxia.[36] To date, however, no specific pathologic marker for SIDS has been described.

PATHOPHYSIOLOGY

Although the causative factors in SIDS remain unknown, current investigators attempt to link the sudden deaths to abnormalities in cardiorespiratory control at a time of important maturational changes in these infants. Thus it is hoped that by identifying such abnormalities in an infant population at risk, the incidence of SIDS can be altered.

For many years, it was thought that an apneic event during sleep was the triggering factor in SIDS; however, researchers in prospective studies who have attempted to correlate the occurrence of apneic events in future SIDS victims have failed to establish any such association.[37] Southall and colleagues[38] demonstrated that two-channel cardiorespiratory recordings of infants during the first 6 weeks of life are not useful predictors of infants at risk for SIDS. In addition, epidemiologic data from a National Institute of Child Health and Human Development study indicate that only a few parents of infants who died of SIDS are able to report a history of apnea or ALTE at any time before the SIDS event.[39]

These findings, however, do not imply that apnea may not be part of the sequence of events leading to SIDS. In fact, according to one current theory, SIDS occurs when a susceptible infant cannot arouse himself or herself adequately from a prolonged apneic event, cardiac arrhythmia, or shock. Thus SIDS would be the result not of the apneic event itself but of an abnormal arousal response caused by defective regulation of some aspect of cardiorespiratory control.[40]

Although ALTE survivors account for only a small fraction of SIDS victims, they have been the subjects of cardiorespiratory control studies because of the belief that they are at a higher risk for SIDS. Some investigators have found that these infants have more episodes of short obstructive apneas, mixed apneas, and periodic breathing during sleep than do control infants.[41–43] However, values of the two groups tend to overlap, which indicates that information obtained from tracings of cardiorespiratory patterns of infants, even those who are thought to be at higher risk, should not be used to predict SIDS.

Investigators have studied another aspect of cardiorespiratory regulation, the ventilatory response to hypoxia and hypercapnia, by assessing the adequacy of ventilatory chemoreceptor function. Whereas peripheral control of breathing is exerted mainly through hypoxia and its effect on aortic and carotid body chemoreceptors, central respiratory control is primarily exerted through hypercapnia and changes in hydrogen ion concentration in the fluid that surrounds the central chemoreceptor zones in the brainstem. Carotid bodies respond first to alterations in blood pH, arterial oxygen tension, and arterial carbon dioxide tension (Pa_{CO_2}) because they are bathed by the high systemic blood flow. Hypercapnia and acidosis stimulate the carotid body receptors and lead to hyperventilation. In contrast, when the Pa_{CO_2} is less than 30 mm Hg, a decrease in the stimulus to breathe leads to an apneic pause. Physiologically, there is a lag time of approximately 60 sec before the excitatory receptors in the brainstem respond to the alterations in blood pH, an important fact during periods of metabolic acidosis.[44]

These studies have produced conflicting results; investigators have been unable to discriminate between controls and infants thought to be at risk.[45,46] The expense and technical difficulties of these tests, as well as their poor predictive value for SIDS, rule out their use in clinical practice.

The most likely hypothesis for explaining SIDS remains a deficient arousal or gasping response in a child who is susceptible to a sleep-related asphyxia related to factors such as an upper respiratory infection[47] or pharyngeal hypotonia during sleep.[48] The infant's inability to arouse himself or herself appropriately leads to prolonged central apnea and, subsequently, to respiratory arrest, cardiac arrhythmia, shock, and eventually sudden death. Some evidence from studies of heart rate and heart rate variability in ALTE survivors suggests that some SIDS cases could be the result of abnormal autonomic activity of the heart that predisposes infants to a fatal cardiac arrhythmia.[49] However, this hypothesis also remains speculative.

Moreover, not all instances of sudden death in infancy can be considered SIDS. For example, fulminant sepsis, aspiration,[50] botulism,[51] and child abuse[52] can result in ALTE episodes and sudden infant death. In those cases, finding the cause of death changes the presumptive diagnosis of SIDS. In addition, Emery and co-authors[53] postulated that of children who die suddenly and unexpectedly, approximately 10% have a previously undetected inborn error of metabolism. Of these, disorders of fatty acid oxidation, such as long- and medium-chain acylcoenzyme A dehydrogenase deficiency, carnitine deficiency, and ethylmalonic-adipic aciduria are commonly implicated.[54,55]

MANAGEMENT

The characteristics of SIDS infants and their mothers described in epidemiologic studies lack the specificity to serve as predictors of higher risk for SIDS. Therefore, it has been difficult to develop adequate strategies for prevention.

In addition, tests for studying abnormalities of breathing in infants are useful only as records of the cardiac and respiratory pattern, not of other aspects of cardiorespiratory regulation. Moreover, it is difficult to distinguish abnormalities in the respiratory pattern of infants from maturational changes of cardiorespiratory control. Thus pneumocardiographic recordings should not be used as screening tests for SIDS. However, they can be useful in confirming the diagnoses of apnea of prematurity and apnea of infancy, conditions that can be corrected pharmacologically with respiratory stimulants, specifically the xanthines theophylline and caffeine.

Although it is clear that their role in predicting SIDS is limited, it is likely that most pediatricians and family physicians encounter infants who survive an ALTE. The management of ALTE survivors should begin with a complete history (emphasizing the circumstances surrounding the event, medical history, and family history) and a complete physical examination, which includes a detailed neurodevelopment assessment. This initial information helps determine the severity of the event and indicates a more specific management course. A capillary or arterial blood sample and a pulse oximetry reading may also provide useful information of the infant's acid-base status and oxygenation status, respectively.

After assessing the severity of the event, the physician must decide on further management. If the episode is not considered severe and the infant appears well, it is appropriate to admit the child to the hospital for a few days of observation and monitoring. If the hospital course is uneventful, the parents can be reassured of the unlikelihood of subsequent episodes. However, if the information obtained is indicative of a more severe episode, the child may require an extensive hospital workup that includes a chest radiograph, an electrocardiogram, an electroencephalogram, a pneumocardiogram or a polysomnogram, blood gas measurements, a complete blood count, and a measurement of serum electrolytes, including calcium and phosphorus.[56]

Nevertheless, physicians must realize that the information obtained from this evaluation may not establish a diagnosis or alter the course of therapy. Studies of ALTE survivors indicate that a definable cause is found in fewer than half of all cases that come to medical attention. The most commonly found causes include gastroesophageal reflux, seizures, infection, upper airway obstruction, structural abnormalities of the central nervous system, congenital airway anomalies, and congenital heart disease.[57]

If the cause of an ALTE is found, appropriate management can be instituted. However, if a cause cannot be found, management is more complex because decisions must be based on observations made by biased subjects, most likely parents.

Parents of ALTE survivors depend on physicians for emotional support. In addition, parental counseling by other health providers, such as social workers, psychologists, or psychiatrists, may be necessary. Physicians must also establish an adequate follow-up program with frequent visits and serial measurements of weight, height, and head circumference to assess growth and maturation of the infant.

Sometimes, as a result of an ALTE, a decision is made to monitor a child. However, several factors have contributed to the fact that the use of home monitors has not decreased the incidence of SIDS: investigators' inability to select the proper candidates for monitoring, the technical limitations of the monitors themselves, parental noncompliance with a monitoring regime, or a combination of these factors.[58, 59]

Although there are no specific guidelines for patient selection in apnea monitoring, likely candidates for monitoring include survivors of a severe ALTE, infants with very low birth weights, infants with bronchopulmonary dysplasia (especially if oxygen dependent), infants with artificial airways, and infants with central hypoventilation who require oxygen or ventilatory support.[57] There are additional instances when monitoring is not as clearly indicated but parental anxiety becomes an important factor in the decision. One such case is the monitoring of a subsequent sibling of a SIDS victim. Although data are conflicting as to whether these infants are a particularly high risk for SIDS, parental concern may be a deciding factor in instituting monitoring.

If a decision is made to monitor a child, parents must understand that the available monitors are designed only to detect episodes of central apnea and not to detect purely obstructive apneas or defects of cardiorespiratory regulation. They should not believe that monitoring an infant will make their lives easier; instead, they should recognize that it is a full-time job that requires constant dedication by the caretakers. It does not prevent all infant deaths, and it may become a source of family stress and anxiety caused by the financial burden and by the changes in family dynamics as the continuously monitored child becomes the central focus of the family. Supervision is constantly needed because monitors can pose accidental risks to the infants from electrical shock or from becoming entangled with the wires that keep them attached to the monitors.

Physicians and caretakers alike must realize that the currently available monitors have technologic limitations that restrict their use. The commonly used monitors measure signals produced by the movement of the chest with respiratory excursions and are unable to detect obstructive apnea or shallow breathing. Also, on occasion they falsely interpret as respiratory movements the transthoracic impedance changes produced by a compensatory increase in cardiac stroke during bradycardia associated with a central apneic event.[11]

False alarms by monitors, most commonly caused by loosening of a monitor lead as a result of the child's movements, can be a source of additional anxiety to the family.[60] Frequent or nightly alarms, even if not caused by apneic episodes, can make the decision to terminate monitoring a difficult one. In some cases, a monitor with event recording and data storage may be helpful in "diagnosing" false alarms and in determining the significance of perceived events.

Most infants over 8 months of age need not be monitored because the risk for SIDS after this age is low; however, infants with predisposing conditions, such as bronchopulmonary dysplasia, may benefit from prolonged monitoring. Absence of monitor alarms in a child who shows adequate catch-up growth and development while properly monitored should be an indicator for discontin-

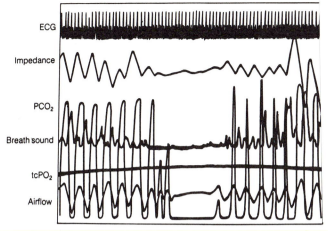

Figure 63–1. Central apnea: cessation of airflow and respiratory efforts. ECG, electrocardiogram, PCO$_2$, carbon dioxide pressure; tcPO$_2$, total capacity oxygen pressure.

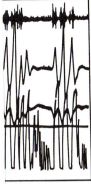

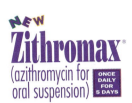

Please see full prescribing information attached.

ratory pauses of 3-
n between pauses.

uation of monitoring. This step requires education and preparation of the caretakers, and the decision must be made jointly by them and the physician. A program of close follow-up can facilitate the transition.

Infants who are being treated for apnea with xanthines may be monitored until the dose of medication is outgrown and subtherapeutic serum levels are reached. Alternatively, the medication may be stopped while the infants continue to be monitored, usually for 2 to 4 weeks. Uneventful monitoring at subtherapeutic xanthine serum levels or while the infant is no longer receiving medication should indicate that monitoring could be discontinued. At this point, these infants should be considered at low risk for sudden death.

GLOSSARY

Apnea: Cessation of airflow; the respiratory pause may be central, obstructive, or mixed.
Central Apnea: Cessation of airflow and respiratory efforts (Fig. 63–1).

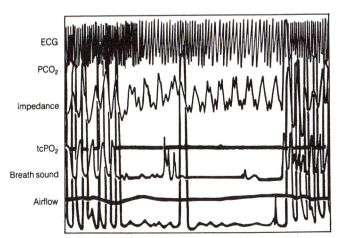

Figure 63–2. Obstructive apnea: cessation of airflow with continued respiratory efforts. Abbreviations as in Figure 63–1.

Obstructive Apnea: Cessation of airflow with continued respiratory efforts; usually caused by upper respiratory obstruction (Fig. 63–2).
Mixed Apnea: Central apnea followed by respiratory movements without airflow.
Pathologic Apnea: A respiratory pause that lasts longer than 20 sec or is associated with cyanosis, bradycardia, marked pallor, or hypotonia.
Apnea of Infancy: Pathologic apnea in infants who are older than 37 weeks' gestation at the onset of the condition.
Periodic Breathing: A respiratory pattern in which there are at least three respiratory pauses of 3- to 10-sec duration with less than 20 sec of respiration between pauses; it is seen commonly in premature infants and may be occasionally a forerunner of prolonged apnea (Fig. 63–3).
Apnea of Prematurity: Periodic breathing with pathologic apnea in a premature infant younger than 37 weeks' gestation.
Apparent Life-Threatening Event (ALTE): An episode that an observer believes is life-threatening and that is characterized by some combination of apnea, change in skin color, marked change in muscle tone, choking, or gagging.

REFERENCES

1. Bergman AB, Beckwith JB, Ray CG (eds): Sudden Infant Death Syndrome: Proceedings of the Second International Conference on Causes of Sudden Death in Infants. Seattle: University of Washington Press, 1970.
2. National Institutes of Health Consensus Development Conference on Infantile Apnea and Home Monitoring, Sept. 29 to Oct. 1, 1986: Consensus Statement. Pediatrics 79:292–299, 1987.
3. Shannon DC, Kelly DH: SIDS and apnea of infancy. In Chernick V, Kendig EL (eds): Disorders of the Respiratory Tract in Children, pp. 939–956. Philadelphia: WB Saunders, 1990.
4. Peterson DR: The epidemiology of sudden infant death syndrome. In Culbertson JL, Krous HF, Bendell RD (eds): Sudden Infant Death Syndrome: Medical Aspects and Psychological Management, pp. 3–17. Baltimore: Johns Hopkins University Press, 1988.
5. Infant Apnea and Home Monitoring. National Institutes of Health Publication No. 87-2905, pp. 3–11, 1986,
6. Naeye RL, Ladis B, Drage JS: Sudden infant death syndrome: A prospective study. Am J Dis Child 130:1207–1210, 1976.
7. Arsenault PS: Maternal and antenatal factors in the risk of sudden infant death syndrome. Am J Epidemiol 111:279–284, 1980.

8. Biering-Sorensen F, Jorgensen T, Hilden J: Sudden infant death in Copenhagen 1956–1971 [Parts I and II]. Acta Paediatr Scand 67:129–137, 1978; 68:1–9, 1979.

9. Lewak N: Sudden infant death syndrome risk factors. Clin Pediatr (Phila) 18:404–411, 1979.

10. Hoffman HJ, Damus K, Hillman L, Krongrad E: Risk factors for SIDS: Results of the National Institute of Child Health and Human Development SIDS Cooperative Epidemiological Study. Ann N Y Acad Sci 533:13–30, 1988.

11. Shannon DC, Kelly DH: SIDS and near-SIDS [Parts I and II]. N Engl J Med 306:959–965, 1022–1028, 1982.

12. Harper RM: State-related physiological changes and risk for the sudden infant death syndrome. Aust Paediatr J 22(Suppl 1):55–58, 1986.

13. Bentele KHP, Albani M: Are there tests predictive for prolonged apnoea and SIDS? A review of epidemiological and functional studies. Acta Paediatr Scand Suppl 342:1–21, 1988.

14. Irgens LM, Skjaerven R, Peterson DR: Prospective assessment of recurrence risk in sudden infant death syndrome siblings. J Pediatr 104:349–351, 1984.

15. Peterson DR, Sabotta EE, Daling JR: Infant mortality among subsequent siblings of infants who died of sudden infant death syndrome. J Pediatr 108:911–914, 1986.

16. Werthammer J, Brown E, Neff RK, Taeusch HW: Sudden infant death syndrome in infants with bronchopulmonary dysplasia. Pediatrics 69:301–304, 1982.

17. Sauve RS, Singhal N: Long-term morbidity of infants with bronchopulmonary dysplasia. Pediatrics 76:725–733, 1985.

18. Chavez CJ, Ostrea EM, Styker JC, Smialek Z: Sudden infant death syndrome among infants of drug-dependent mothers. J Pediatr 95:407–409, 1979.

19. Chasnoff I, Hunt C, Kletter R, Kaplan D: Increased risk of SIDS and respiratory pattern abnormalities in cocaine-exposed infants. Pediatr Res 20:425A, 1986.

20. Bauchner H, Zuckerman B, McClain M, et al: Risk of sudden infant death syndrome among infants with *in utero* exposure to cocaine. J Pediatr 113:831–834, 1988.

21. Peterson DR, Chinn NM, Fisher LD; The sudden infant death syndrome: Repetitions in families. J Pediatr 97:265–267, 1980.

22. Valdes-Dapena M: Sudden Unexplained Infant Death, 1969 through 1975: An Evolution in Understanding. U.S. Department of Health, Education, and Welfare Publication 80-5255, pp. 1–25. Washington, DC: U.S. Government Printing Office, 1980.

23. Taylor EM, Emery JL: Two-year study of the causes of postperinatal deaths classified in terms of preventability. Arch Dis Child 57:668–673, 1982.

24. Bass M, Kravath RE, Glass L: Death-scene investigation in sudden infant death. N Engl J Med 315:100–105, 1986.

25. Wigglesworth JS, Keeling JW, Rushton DI, et al: Pathological investigations in cases of sudden death. J Clin Pathol 40:1481–1483, 1987.

26. Naeye RL: Pulmonary arterial abnormalities in the sudden-infant-death-syndrome. N Engl J Med 289:1167–1170, 1973.

27. Naeye RL: Hypoxemia and the sudden infant death syndrome. Science 186:837–838, 1974.

28. Naeye RL, Whalen P, Ryser M, Fisher R: Cardiac and other abnormalities in the sudden infant death syndrome. Am J Pathol 82:1–8, 1976.

29. Naeye RL, Fisher R, Ryser M, Whalen P: Carotid body in the sudden infant death syndrome. Science 191:567–569, 1976.

30. Naeye RL: Brain-stem and adrenal abnormalities in the sudden infant death syndrome. Am J Clin Pathol 66:526–530, 1976.

31. Kinney HC, Filiano JJ: Brainstem research in sudden infant death syndrome. Pediatrician 15:240–250, 1988.

32. Werne J, Garrow I: Sudden apparently unexplained death during infancy: I. Pathologic findings in infants found dead. Am J Pathol 29:633–675, 1953.

33. Krous HF: Pathological considerations of sudden infant death syndrome. Pediatrician 15:231–239, 1988.

34. Beckwith JB: Observations on the pathological anatomy of the sudden infant death syndrome. *In* Bergman AB, Beckwith JB, Ray CG (eds): Sudden Infant Death Syndrome: Proceedings of the Second International Conference on Causes of Sudden Death in Infants, pp. 83–107. Seattle: University of Washington Press, 1970.

35. Sachis PN, Armstrong DL, Becker LE, et al: The vagus nerve and sudden infant death syndrome: A morphometric study. J Pediatr 98:278–280, 1981.

36. Rognum TO, Saugstad OD, Oyasaeter S, Olaisen B: Elevated levels of hypoxanthine in vitreous humor indicate prolonged cerebral hypoxia in victims of sudden infant death syndrome. Pediatrics 82:615–618, 1988.

37. Southall DP, Richards JM, Rhoden KJ, et al: Prolonged apnea and cardiac arrhythmias in infants discharged from neonatal intensive care units: Failure to predict an increased risk for sudden infant death syndrome. Pediatrics 70:844–851, 1982.

38. Southall DP, Richards JM, de Swiet M, et al: Identification of infants destined to die unexpectedly during infancy: Evaluation of predictive importance of prolonged apnoea and disorders of cardiac rhythm or conduction. Br Med J 286:1092–1096, 1983.

39. Krongrad E: Post neonatal risk factors: The NIH Cooperative Epidemiological Study of Sudden Infant Death Syndrome (SIDS) Risk Factors. Proceedings of the American Pediatric Society—Society for Pediatric Research, Washington DC, May 1982.

40. Hunt CE, Brouillette RT: Sudden infant death syndrome: 1987 perspective. J Pediatr 110:669–678, 1987.

41. Guilleminault C, Ariagno RL, Forno LS, et al: Obstructive sleep apnea and near miss for SIDS: I. Report of an infant with sudden death. Pediatrics 63:837–843, 1979.

42. Kahn A, Blum D, Rebuffat E, et al: Polysomnographic studies of infants who subsequently died of sudden infant death syndrome. Pediatrics 82:721–727, 1988.

43. Kelly DH, Shannon DC: Periodic breathing in infants with near-miss sudden infant death syndrome. Pediatrics 63:355–360, 1979.

44. Levitzky MG: The control of breathing. In Pulmonary Physiology (2nd ed), pp. 176–194. New York: McGraw-Hill, 1986.

45. Hunt CE: Abnormal hypercarbic and hypoxic sleep arousal responses in near-miss SIDS infants. Pediatr Res 15:1462–1464, 1981.

46. Coleman JM, Mammel MC, Reardon C, Boros SJ: Hypercarbic ventilatory responses of infants at risk for SIDS. Pediatr Pulmonol 3:226–230, 1987.

47. Steinschneider A: Prolonged apnea and the sudden infant death syndrome: Clinical and laboratory observations. Pediatrics 50:646–654, 1972.

48. Tonkin S: Sudden infant death syndrome: Hypothesis of causation. Pediatrics 55:650–661, 1975.

49. Leistner HL, Haddad GG, Epstein RA, et al: Heart rate and heart rate variability during sleep in aborted sudden infant death syndrome. J Pediatr 97:51–55, 1980.

50. Herbst JL, Book LS, Bray PF: Gastroesophageal reflux in the "near-miss" sudden infant death syndrome. J Pediatr 92:73–75, 1978.

51. Arnon SS, Midura TF, Damus K, et al: Intestinal infection and toxic production by *Clostridium botulinum* as one cause of sudden infant death syndrome. Lancet 1:1273–1277, 1978.

52. Berger D: Child abuse simulating "near-miss" sudden infant death syndrome. J Pediatr 95:554–556, 1979.

53. Emery, JL, Howat AJ, Variend S, Vawter GF: Investigation of inborn errors of metabolism in unexpected infant deaths. Lancet 2:29–31, 1988.

54. Howat AJ, Bennett MJ, Variend S, et al: Defects of metabolism of fatty acids in the sudden infant death syndrome. Br Med J 290:1771–1773, 1985.

55. Harpey JP, Charpentier C, Coude M, et al: Sudden infant death syndrome and multiple acyl-coenzyme A dehydrogenase deficiency, ethylmalonic-adipic aciduria, or systemic carnitine deficiency. J Pediatr 110:881–884, 1987.

56. Lewis JM, Ganick DJ: Initial laboratory evaluation of infants with "presumed near-miss" sudden infant death syndrome. Am J Dis Child 140:484–486, 1986.

57. Bokulic RE, Beckerman RC: Apnea and SIDS: The home monitoring controversy. J Respir Dis 10(8):73–89, 1989.

58. Apnoea monitors and sudden infant death: Report from the Foundation for the Study of Infant Death and the British Paediatric Respiratory Group. Arch Dis Child 60:76–80, 1985.

59. Meny RG, Blackmon L, Fleischmann D, et al: Sudden infant death and home monitors. Am J Dis Child 142:1037–1040, 1988.

60. Cain LP, Kelly DH, Shannon DC: Parents' perceptions of the psychological and social impact of home monitoring. Pediatrics 66:37–41, 1980.

64 THORACIC TRAUMA

ROBERT HOPKINS, M.D.

Thoracic trauma is classified as either blunt or penetrating. The blunt type is more common in younger children and in rural settings. Penetrating trauma, however, is more common in adolescents and in urban surroundings. The majority of thoracic trauma victims are males.

A 20-year experience with thoracic trauma in children was reported by Meller and colleagues.[1] In their report, blunt thoracic trauma was most commonly caused when motor vehicles struck pedestrians and was more common in younger children. Penetrating trauma, caused more often by gunshot wounds than by stabbings, was seen more often in older children and adolescents, especially after 9 years of age.

Mayer and associates reported a 2-year detailed study of pediatric trauma from the Primary Children's Medical Center, Salt Lake City.[2] Thoracic injuries were present in 40% of pediatric patients with multiple trauma (injury to at least two body areas). Thoracic trauma accounted for 40% of all injuries and only 9% of deaths; head trauma played a role in all deaths or disabilities.

Rates of mortality from thoracic trauma vary greatly from one series to another. In younger children, it is reported to be as high as 25%,[3] and in older children it ranges from 7% to 14%.[1,2,4–6] Injury to other organ systems drastically increases these figures. Injuries to two other major subsystems increase mortality rates to 58%[4] and injury to three other subsystems increases mortality rates to almost 100%.[4,7]

DEVELOPMENTAL ASPECTS

The respiratory system in children is different from that in adults in many important ways. First, ossification of the thoracic cage continues from prenatal life through the third decade of life. This prolonged cartilaginous state has important implications for the frequency of rib fractures and flail chest. Second, the chest wall in infants and children is highly compliant. The age at which thoracic compliance reaches adult levels has not been clearly established. Sharp and associates studied changes in chest wall compliance over a wide age range[8] and found that compliance of the chest in children was 50% of adult values at 8 years of age, reaching 78% of adult values at 12 years of age and 92% of adult values at 16 years of age. This is of some importance because the absence of rib fractures in a pediatric thoracic trauma victim does not preclude the possibility of severe intrathoracic injury.

TRAUMATIC ASPHYXIA

Blunt thoracic trauma involving chest compression is termed *traumatic asphyxia.* The most common cause is a vehicle's wheels rolling over the chest. The common scenario is of a child playing in the driveway and unaware of the moving vehicle until the injury occurs.[9,10] Child abuse may also produce traumatic asphyxia.[11] The victims of this kind of injury die within minutes unless associated injuries can be successfully managed. Treatment of traumatic asphyxia requires attention to maintenance of airway, adequate ventilation, circulatory support, and frequent reassessment. Adjacent organ systems must be assessed for damage. Pulmonary contusion, tension pneumothorax, hemothorax, and airway disruption are associated thoracic injuries that must be detected quickly.

Many children require only observation in an intensive care unit. However, the potential for serious intra-abdominal or intrathoracic injury mandates intense observation, frequent reassessment, and careful monitoring.

Injuries are caused by both the blunt thoracic trauma and its transmitted forces. These forces cause injury when a person inspires deeply and closes the glottis at the time of the injury. The closed glottis increases the transmission of the crushing forces through the valveless vena cava. In one study, pneumatic compression of thoraces in dogs with the glottis open (control group) resulted in very little increase in superior vena cava pressures; however, the same compression to thoraces with glottic closure resulted in vena cava pressure 10 times higher than that of controls.[12]

RIB FRACTURES

Despite the elasticity of the developing thoracic cage, rib fractures from blunt trauma do occur. Meller and colleagues,[1] Smyth,[4] and Levy[11] described incidences of 28%, 58%, and 86%, respectively. The series by Meller and associates is remarkable in that 90% of the patients with rib fractures had associated injuries, although some of these injuries were from penetrating trauma.

Crushing injuries, including roll-over injuries, are common causes of rib fractures, as is child abuse in young infants. Fractures of the first rib should alert the clinician to the presence of considerable blunt force.[13] Injuries associated with first-rib fracture include tracheobronchial rupture, brachial plexus trauma, disruption of major vessels, and maxillofacial trauma.

Treatment of rib fractures includes rest, analgesics, and chest physiotherapy to prevent atelectasis.

FLAIL CHEST

Flail chest is the result of the isolation of a segment of chest wall as a result of multiple rib fractures, sternal fracture, or costochondral separations. Because of the compliance of the chest in children, a tremendous force must be applied to the chest wall to produce a flail segment.[14] Such a large force often produces contusion of the underlying lung and results in paradoxical movement of the flail segment (moving inward during inspiration and bulging outward with expiration). Pathophysiologic derangements include decreased ventilation secondary to (1) increased work of breathing as a result of inefficient movement of the discontinuous chest wall, (2) hypoventilation as a result of splinting from pain, (3) hypoxemia from ventilation/perfusion mismatch as a result of pulmonary contusion, (4) decreased compliance of the contused lung, (5) altered pleural pressures from damage to respiratory muscles, and (6) decreased clearance of bronchial secretions.[15] Efforts to breathe are mechanically inefficient and result in increased oxygen demand. Respiratory muscle fatigue may lead to acute respiratory failure.

Treatment must be directed at several areas, including (1) pain control, (2) management of the flail segment, and (3) care of the pulmonary contusion. Pain control is achieved by analgesics and possibly by epidural analgesics. Management of the flail segment is a minor component of the overall care. Towel rolls or sandbags decrease paradoxical movement of the flail segment and improve cough effectiveness. In most cases, surgical fixation of a child's ribs is not necessary; pain control and meticulous tracheobronchial toilet are usually adequate. Close monitoring of fluid therapy, attention to pulmonary secretions, and humidified oxygen may be sufficient for managing the pulmonary contusion. Mechanical ventilation, if needed at all, is usually not required for more than 2 to 3 days. Indications for mechanical ventilation include (1) need for general anesthesia, (2) shock, and (3) respiratory failure. Controlled ventilation is preferred because intermittent mandatory ventilation does not stabilize the chest wall. Several reported series of adult trauma victims have shown that mechanical ventilation may not be necessary in most cases.[16, 17]

PNEUMOTHORAX

Pneumothorax is one of the most common sequelae of either blunt or penetrating thoracic trauma. According to published series, pneumothoraces occur in 15% to 40% of patients with pediatric chest trauma.[1, 4, 6] Traumatized children with a pneumothorax may be asymptomatic or in severe distress. Physical findings include ipsilateral prominence of the hemithorax and decreased breath sounds. Additional physical findings include subcutaneous emphysema and ipsilateral hyperresonance.

Diagnosis is confirmed by chest radiograph. Treatment is by evacuation of air from the pleural space. Indications for chest tube insertion include (1) pneumothorax of more than 15%, (2) clinical signs of respiratory distress in any size of pneumothorax, and (3) the need for general anesthesia with positive-pressure ventilation in the presence of pneumothorax.[18] Tension pneumothorax is a special case that results from a disruption of the pleural space and progressive accumulation of air. This air cannot escape, and the pleural pressure increases. This accumulation of pleural air results in compression of the ipsilateral lung, shift of the mediastinal structures, decrease in venous return to the thorax, and compression of the contralateral lung. Tension pneumothorax is a potentially life-threatening emergency and must be recognized and treated promptly. For a more detailed discussion, the reader is referred to Chapter 62.

HEMOTHORAX

Hemothorax is the result of accumulation of blood in the intrapleural space. The source of this blood is major vessel injury, usually a result of penetrating trauma. However, hemothorax may occur in younger children because of intercostal artery injury from blunt trauma. Hemothorax may also occur in association with pneumothorax. Isolated hemothorax is seen in about 10% of thoracic trauma patients in published series.[1, 4, 6] Hemopneumothorax is much more common, occurring in about 10% to 20% of reported patients.[1, 4, 6]

Physical examination usually reveals a patient in moderate to severe respiratory distress, dullness to percussion over the ipsilateral hemithorax, decreased breath sounds, and a tracheal shift away from the affected side. There may be signs of shock if a sufficient quantity of blood has been lost in the pleural space. Diagnosis is further confirmed by chest radiograph. A film of the patient upright must be obtained to demonstrate a fluid level. A film of the patient recumbent may show only a diffuse haziness over the affected lung.

Treatment is chest tube drainage of the hemothorax. Needle drainage can help establish the diagnosis but is not adequate for complete evacuation of the pleural space. The re-expanded lung often compresses an injured intercostal vessel, and bleeding ceases. Bleeding from a larger vessel, however, continues. Thoracotomy may be required to achieve hemostasis. Chest tube drainage of 1 to 2 ml/kg/h requires thoracotomy. Before insertion of a chest tube, adequate venous access should be established because continued loss of blood creates the need for volume replacement.

CHYLOTHORAX

The thoracic duct enters the thorax to the right of the aorta, crosses the midline at midesophagus, and joins the venous system at the confluence of the left internal jugular vein and the left subclavian vein. Disruption of the thoracic duct results in accumulation of chyle in the mediastinum with subsequent rupture into the pleural space.[18] Injury to the thoracic duct can occur during thoracic procedures that require esophageal mobilization or during ligation of a patent ductus arteriosus. Blunt trauma involving hyperextension of the spine places the thoracic duct at risk of injury. Diagnosis of chylothorax should be suspected in a trauma patient with a pleural effusion. Pleural fluid is usually cloudy and contains fat.

Initial treatment consists of chest tube drainage and either oral feedings of medium-chain triglycerides or total parenteral nutrition. These nutritional regimens decrease thoracic duct flow. Continuing loss of chyle results in depletion of lymphocytes and an increased risk of opportunistic infections. To avoid this situation, surgical ligation of the thoracic duct should be performed if nonoperative therapy is unsuccessful after 4 to 6 weeks.

DISRUPTION OF TRACHEOBRONCHIAL TREE

Injuries to the tracheobronchial tree are more common in the adolescent because of the increased incidence of penetrating chest trauma among older pediatric patients.[1] However, crushing chest injuries in younger children can also result in ruptures of major airways.[3]

Several clinical signs and situations should raise the suspicion of major airway injury: (1) hemoptysis, (2) massive subcutaneous or mediastinal emphysema, (3) tension pneumothorax, (4) widespread atelectasis, and (5) persistent air leakage through a chest tube placed for pneumothorax.

Bronchoscopy to locate the tracheobronchial tree injury should be performed if a patient is clinically stable. For unstable patients, urgent thoracotomy and repair of the laceration are indicated. Massive injury may necessitate resection of the involved lung. Complications of repair include disruption of suture lines and late tracheal or bronchial stenosis.

PULMONARY CONTUSION

Pulmonary contusion, like many thoracic injuries, is more thoroughly described in the adult literature.[19] It does, however, occur in children. Pulmonary contusion is the result of a blunt, compression-decompression injury to the chest wall. The underlying pulmonary parenchyma undergoes alveolar-capillary disruption, which results in hemorrhage and edema. Movement of fluid from injured capillaries into the alveolar space and interstitium results in decreased pulmonary compliance and hypoxemia.

The frequency of pulmonary contusion in children with thoracic trauma varies greatly. In a study of children in Belfast, Smyth reported a 62% occurrence.[4] In studies from Columbus, Ohio,[3] and Detroit,[1] investigators reported occurrences of 18% and 4%, respectively. Despite this wide range, it is apparent that pulmonary contusion must be considered in blunt thoracic trauma in children.

Manifestations vary, depending on the extent of thoracic injuries as well as of other injuries in multisystem trauma. A child may be asymptomatic or have only chest pain. Tachypnea and increased effort in breathing develop with a clinically significant contusion. Initial auscultation reveals inspiratory crackles; however, as consolidation progresses, the breath sounds become more bronchial in quality. Initial chest radiographs may be normal; however, over a period of 6 to 12 h, patchy infiltrates develop and are followed by lobar consolidation. If the plain chest radiograph is not definitive, CT scans of the chest clearly define a pulmonary contusion.[20] Arterial blood gases reveal hypoxemia and a widened alveolar-arterial oxygen gradient.

Treatment is supportive. There is no benefit demonstrated by prophylactic mechanical ventilation.[17] Standard criteria for beginning mechanical ventilation should be used. Meticulous attention to fluid balance and pulmonary toilet, coupled with careful monitoring of cardiopulmonary status, may obviate the need for mechanical ventilation. There is no clear indication for steroid therapy. Antibiotics should be used only if clinically indicated, although studies in adults indicate a high occurrence of pneumonia in patients with pulmonary contusion.

TRAUMATIC PSEUDOCYSTS

Pulmonary contusion is the usual lung injury in blunt chest trauma. A less common entity is the pulmonary pseudocyst.[21] The exact cause of this lesion is uncertain. Shearing stresses or an acute increase in bronchial pressures may result in these cystic-appearing, air-filled cavities.

Most examples in the literature have occurred in young children. Symptoms are nonspecific and include cough, hemoptysis, and chest pain. Differential diagnosis includes lung abscess; however, the presence of hemoptysis in a trauma victim with a cystic pulmonary lesion should raise the suspicion of a traumatic pulmonary pseudocyst.

No treatment is necessary. Rupture is rare. Radiographic evidence of the pseudocyst usually disappears over 4 to 6 weeks.

DIAPHRAGM INJURIES

Diaphragm injuries result from either blunt or penetrating thoracic trauma. These injuries can present in either a devastating or a subtle manner and may include diaphragmatic disruption, herniation, and paralysis.

Falls, compression injuries, and gunshot wounds to the lower chest can lead to traumatic rupture of the diaphragm.[1, 11] Many of the signs and symptoms are caused by herniation of abdominal contents into the thorax.[18] Dyspnea, chest pain, diminished breath sounds, and tracheal shift may be present. However, patients may be relatively asymptomatic if no abdominal viscera have entered the chest. Herniation of abdominal contents is more common on the left, perhaps because of the blocking effect of the liver on the right; however, herniation of the liver, stomach, and spleen have been described. Herniation of abdominal viscera may not occur immediately after injury, and diaphragmatic rupture may not be detected for years. Chest pain secondary to incarcerated bowel or other ischemic viscera can lead to the diagnosis.

Traumatic diaphragmatic injuries occur in fewer than 5% of thoracic injuries, but clinical suspicion should be high in cases of compression injuries, falls, and penetrating injuries in the lower thorax. Tracheal shift, diminished chest movement, decreased breath sounds, and bowel sounds in the chest are all suggestive physical findings.

Plain chest radiograph may demonstrate the stomach or bowel loops in the left hemithorax. Radiographic visibility of a nasogastric tube in the left hemithorax confirms the diagnosis.[14] Administration of oral contrast agents, if the likelihood of visceral disruption is small, may also help to demonstrate stomach or bowel loops in the chest. CT scanning after the administration of oral-contrast agents can help to differentiate thoracic viscera, pleural effusion, and diaphragmatic disruption. The stomach may be mistaken for a normal left hemidiaphragm, and abdominal contents may mimic a pleural effusion if the costophrenic angle is obscured, which is important because pleural effusions may be associated with esophageal disruption. Decubitus views of the chest with injured side up or examination of draining pleural fluid can help to differentiate abdominal contents from pleural effusions. A partially or completely herniated liver may be confused with an elevated hemidiaphragm. A liver-spleen radionuclide scan helps confirm a thoracic herniation of the liver.

Damage to the phrenic nerve from blunt or penetrating thoracic trauma can lead to hemidiaphragmatic paralysis. Diminished chest movement, paradoxical thoracoabdominal respiratory motion, and decreased breath sounds are all signs of diaphragm paralysis. Radiographic evidence includes an elevated hemidiaphragm and paradoxical diaphragmatic movement on fluoroscopy.

Treatment of traumatic rupture of the diaphragm is surgical, requiring either an abdominal or a thoracic approach. The transabdominal approach is usually recommended because there is a high incidence of associated abdominal visceral injuries. A thoracic approach yields better exposure and is recommended for right-sided injuries. Abdominal injuries may be repaired through the diaphragm defect.

Diaphragmatic paralysis resulting from blunt trauma may resolve spontaneously, or plication of the affected hemidiaphragm may ultimately be required. Plication may be required earlier if the phrenic nerve is destroyed by penetrating trauma.

ESOPHAGEAL INJURIES

Esophageal injury from blunt thoracic trauma is unusual in children. A high index of suspicion is essential because of the potential morbidity and mortality.

Clinical signs that should raise suspicion of esophageal injury include (1) cardiovascular collapse that is not suspected from the extent of apparent injuries, (2) mediastinal or subcutaneous emphysema, (3) hydropneumothorax, and (4) mediastinal crunch. Radiographic findings from a portable chest film are mediastinal widening, pleural effusion, and pleural air.[14] A pneumothorax caused by esophageal tear usually implies a large esophageal perforation.

Esophageal disruption is confirmed by radiographic contrast study. Esophagoscopy may be necessary if radiographic studies are negative and a high degree of suspicion still exists. The most common cause of iatrogenic esophageal injury in children is instrumentation.[18] Insertion of nasogastric tubes may cause perforation at the normal sites of esophageal narrowing: (1) the pharyngoesophageal junction, (2) the aortic arch, or (3) the diaphragm. Attempts at tracheal intubation may also lead to perforation of the cervical esophagus. Sudden increases in esophageal pressure, such as thoracic compression, may also cause esophageal rupture.

Rapid diagnosis and treatment are essential because mediastinitis, empyema, and sepsis are potential complications. Treatment depends on the anatomic site of injury. High esophageal injury, almost always a result of nasogastric tube insertion, may be treated with observation and broad-spectrum antibiotics. Primary repair, drainage, and intravenous antibiotics are needed for repair of a cervical esophageal injury. Perforation of the thoracic esophagus requires thoracotomy, chest tube drainage, and intravenous antibiotics.

CARDIAC INJURIES

Blunt chest trauma may injure the heart. Consequences range from anatomic disruption to mild tissue injury. Major injuries may include chamber rupture, papillary muscle injury, ventricular septum rupture, and valvar injury. Mild tissue injury produces characteristic biochemical, histopathologic, and electrophysiologic changes.

The major injuries noted previously are associated with high rates of mortality. Symptoms and signs of major blunt cardiac trauma include chest pain, dyspnea, tachycardia, hypotension, distended neck veins, cardiac murmurs, and acute congestive heart failure. Pericardial tamponade or hemorrhage may complicate these injuries. The most common major injury is atrial disruption. High-speed vehicular accidents are the most common cause of these blunt cardiac injuries. The association of multisystem trauma makes diagnosis more difficult, and a high index of suspicion aids in the detection of these injuries. This high index of suspicion is augmented by the chest radiograph, echocardiography, and even cardiac catheterization.

Treatment consists of immediate thoracotomy or sternotomy. Initial pericardial decompression by a pericardial window, performed under local anesthesia, was recommended by Calhoun and co-authors.[22] The potentially catastrophic consequences of a pericardial tamponade and the vasodilation of general anesthesia can thus be avoided.

Cardiac contusion is focal blunt injury to the myocardium, resulting in cellular injury or death. Lethal arrhythmias may be associated with cardiac contusion. Tellez and associates[23] reported the largest series of children (*N*

Table 64–1. BLUNT CARDIAC TRAUMA IN 39 CHILDREN WITH MULTIPLE-SYSTEM INJURY

Electrocardiogram (22/30, or 56%)
Persistent sinus tachycardia
ST-T wave abnormalities
Low-voltage QRS
Conduction abnormalities
Premature ventricular contractions
Junctioned rhythm
Ventricular tachycardia

Echocardiographic (9/39, or 23%)
Hypodynamic left ventricle
Hyperdynamic left ventricle
Hyperdynamic septal wall motion
Mild mitral regurgitation
Mild tricuspid regurgitation
Pericardial effusion

Radionuclide Angiographies (12/35 or 34%)

Enzymes (3/39 or 7.7%)

*Right ventricular ejection fraction (11/12). †Left ventricular ejection fraction (1/12). ‡Muscle-brain creatine phosphokinase fraction.

= 39) with cardiac contusion. All were victims of falls or motor vehicle accidents, and multiple-system injury occurred in one third of the children. Elevated cardiac enzymes (muscle-brain creatine phosphokinase), electrocardiograms, echocardiogram, and radionuclide angiography were used to detect cardiac contusion. These studies revealed a number of abnormalities but no injuries of clinical significance (Table 64–1).

A prudent approach to children with blunt chest wall trauma is immediate and continuous cardiac rhythm monitoring and careful assessment of cardiac status for structural injury.

REFERENCES

1. Meller JL, Little AG, Shermeta DW: Thoracic trauma in children. Pediatrics 74:813–819, 1984.
2. Mayer T, Walker ML, Johnson DG, Matlak ME: Causes of morbidity and mortality in severe pediatric trauma. JAMA 245:719–721, 1981.
3. Kilman JW, Charnock E: Thoracic trauma in infancy and childhood. J Trauma 9:863–873, 1969.
4. Smyth BT: Chest trauma in children. J Pediatr Surg 14:41–47, 1979.
5. Bickford BJ: Chest injuries in childhood and adolescence. Thorax 17:240–243, 1962.
6. Sinclair MC, Moore TC: Major surgery for abdominal and thoracic trauma in childhood and adolescence. J Pediatr Surg 9:155–162, 1974.
7. Mayer T, Matlak ME, Johnson DG, et al: The modified injury severity scale in pediatric multiple trauma patients. J Pediatr Surg 15:719–726, 1980.
8. Sharp JT, Druz WS, Balagot RC, et al: Total respiratory compliance in infants and children. J Appl Physiol 29:775–779, 1970.
9. Bell MJ, Ternberg JL, Bower RJ: Low velocity vehicular injuries in children—"run-over" accidents. Pediatrics 66:628–631, 1980.
10. Haller JA, Donahoo JS: Traumatic asphysxia in children: Pathophysiology and management. J Trauma 11:453–457, 1971.
11. Levy JL Jr: Management of crushing chest injuries in children. South Med J 65:1040–1044, 1972.
12. Williams JS, Minken SL, Adams JT: Traumatic asphyxia—reappraised. Ann Surg 167:384–392, 1968.
13. Harris GJ, Soper RT: Pediatric first rib fractures. J Trauma 30:343–345, 1990.
14. Jones KW: Thoracic trauma. In Mayer TA (ed): Emergency Management of Pediatric Trauma, pp. 254–271. Philadelphia: WB Saunders, 1985.
15. Todd TR, Shamji F: Pathophysiology of chest wall trauma. In Roussos C, Macklem PT (ed): The Thorax (Part B), Lung Biology in Health and Disease, Vol. 29, pp. 979–997. New York: Marcel Dekker, 1985.
16. Trinkle JK, Richardson JD, Franz JL, et al: Management of flail chest without mechanical ventilation. Ann Thorac Surg 19:355–363, 1975.
17. Richardson JD, Adams L, Flint LM: Selective management of flail chest and pulmonary contusion. Ann Surg 196:481–487, 1982.
18. Eichelberger MR, Anderson KD: Sequelae of thoracic injury in children. In Eichelberger MR, Pratsch GL (eds): Pediatric Trauma Care, pp. 59–68. Rockville, MD: Aspen, 1988.
19. Trinkle JK, Furman FW, Hinshaw MA, et al: Pulmonary contusion: Pathogenesis and effect of various resuscitative measures. Ann Thorac Surg 16:568–573, 1973.
20. Sivit CJ, Taylor GA, Eichelberger MR: Chest injury in children with blunt abdominal trauma: Evaluation with CT. Radiology 171:815–818, 1989.
21. Santon GH, Mahendra T: Traumatic pulmonary pseudocysts. Ann Thorac Surg 27:359–362, 1979.
22. Calhoon JH, Hoffman TH, Trinkle JK, et al: Management of blunt rupture of the heart. J Trauma 26:495–502, 1986.
23. Tellez DW, Hardin WD, Takahashi M, et al: Blunt cardiac injury in children. J Pediatr Surg 22:1123–1128, 1987.

65 THORACOPULMONARY NEOPLASIA AND LUNG COMPLICATIONS OF CHILDHOOD CANCER

JAN WATTERSON, B.A. / PAUL KUBIC, M.D. / LOUIS P. DEHNER, M.D. / JOHN R. PRIEST, M.D.

Malignant neoplasms of childhood, especially rhabdomyosarcoma, Wilms' tumor, Ewing's sarcoma, and osteosarcoma, metastasize to the lungs with some degree of frequency. However, primary pulmonary tumors of benign and malignant types are very rare, as shown by Hartman and Shochat in their comprehensive review of 230 pediatric cases.[1] Fewer than 2% of all primary malignant neoplasms in childhood originate in the lung or the thoracic cavity.[2] The purpose of this chapter is to present a broad differential diagnosis of intrathoracic masses, neoplastic lesions, and pulmonary consequences of systemic neoplasia. Tumors and tumorlike lesions involving the pulmonary parenchyma (Table 65–1)[3–14] and the tracheobronchial tree (Table 65–2),[15–35] are considered as well as the principal lesions of the mediastinum (anterior, middle, and posterior) (Table 65–3)[36–53] and of the chest wall, diaphragm, and pleura (Table 65–4).[54–62] We review in some detail primary pulmonary conditions and disorders with substantial lung involvement, but we mention only as part of the differential diagnosis the vertebral, chest wall, esophageal, or cardiac lesions that encroach on the respiratory tract. In addition, the pulmonary consequences of systemic neoplasia and its treatment are discussed. A glossary of terms used in this chapter is included.

Unlike neoplastic disease of the chest in adults, in which the epidemiologic factors are well understood in some instances by the strong association with certain environmental exposures (e.g., tobacco smoke, asbestos fibers), relatively little is known about the epidemiologic factors of thoracopulmonary neoplasia in children. Children with primary immunodeficiency syndromes develop lymphoreticular neoplasms that often involve the mediastinum or lung. Neurofibromatosis underlies occasional tumors in the chest. Several cases of rhabdomyosarcoma and other sarcomas arising in presumed congenital lung cysts or cystic adenomatoid malformations have been reported,[63–68] including two cases in the authors' experiences in which these diseases occurred in the setting of a familial predisposition to cancer.

PATHOPHYSIOLOGY

Disordered pulmonary physiologic processes caused by neoplastic and related disease in the chest result from the direct mass effects of the lesion in most cases, such as tracheal compression or lung parenchymal volume replacement by tumor or pleural effusion. Some lymphoreticular proliferations such as leukemia or Löffler's syndrome produce diffuse interstitial infiltration of lung parenchyma. "Remote" effects of systemic or distant neoplasia occasionally involve the lungs, as in pulmonary hemorrhage secondary to disseminated intravascular coagulation, which may accompany acute monocytic, monoblastic, or promyelocytic leukemias and their treatment. Catecholamine secretion from neurogenic tumors (neuroblastoma or pheochromocytoma) may produce a cardiomyopathy with secondary cor pulmonale as the presenting manifestation. In addition, pulmonary function can be compromised by the direct toxic effects of chemotherapy and radiotherapy.[37] In the case of bleomycin, the pathophysiologic process of the toxicity is probably an excessive accumulation of the drug in pulmonary epithelial cells, resulting in damage from an excess of free oxygen radicals, and an inflammatory or fibrotic reaction to this damage.[69]

CLINICAL MANIFESTATIONS

The clinical manifestations of thoracopulmonary neoplasia are usually caused by direct compressive, obstructive, or space-occupying effects. Easily understood symptoms are cough, dyspnea, and venous obstruction (superior vena cava syndrome). Pain may accompany the pleuritis secondary to tumor invasion of the chest wall, parietal pleura, or peripheral pulmonary parenchyma and visceral pleura, but pain is rare in exclusively bronchopulmonary disease. Systemic symptoms such as fever, anorexia, weight loss, malaise, or pruritis are associated with thoracic neoplasia. Pulmonary osteodystrophy or

Table 65–1. PROLIFERATIVE AND NEOPLASTIC DISEASES OF THE PEDIATRIC CHEST: LUNG PARENCHYMA*

Benign Lesions	Malignant Lesions
Malformations/Hamartomas	***Primary Neoplasms in Lung Parenchyma***
Cystic adenomatoid malformation (cystic hamartoma)	Pleuropulmonary blastoma
Bronchogenic cyst	Rhabdomyosarcoma
Sequestration cyst[3, 4]	Myxosarcoma
Arteriovenous malformation	Leiomyosarcoma
Hemangioma/lymphangioma	Fibrosarcoma
Lymphangiomyomatosis	Extraskeletal Ewing's sarcoma
Fibroleiomyomatous hamartoma	Plasmacytoma
Chondromatous hamartoma	Intravascular bronchioloalveolar tumor
Lymphoreticular Proliferations and Infectious/Reactive Lesions	Primary pulmonary lymphoma
Langerhans cell histiocytosis (histiocytosis X)	Pseudolymphoma
Eosinophilic pneumonia	Teratoma
Round pneumonia[5]	Neurogenic tumor[11]
Pyogenic abscess	Hemangiopericytoma[12, 13]
Mycotic abscess	Endodermal tumor resembling fetal lung[14]
Hydatid cyst (echinococcal cyst)[3]	***Metastases to Lung Parenchyma***
Plasma-cell granuloma (inflammatory pseudotumor)	Wilms' tumor
Pseudolymphoma[6]	Osteogenic sarcoma
Tumors	Ewing's sarcoma
Chondroma	Rhabdomyosarcoma
Leiomyoma	Hepatoblastoma
Neurofibromas/neurilemomas[7]	Hepatocellular carcinoma
Conditions Associated With Systemic Malignancy	Malignant germ cell tumor
Opportunistic infections	Lymphoreticular malignancy
Hypereosinophilia syndrome	Central nervous system tumor
Disseminated intravascular coagulation/pulmonary hemorrhage	Renal clear-cell sarcoma
Excess catecholamine secretion	Neuroblastoma
Pseudometastases	Other rare tumors
Therapy-related toxicities	
Chemotherapy	
Radiation therapy	
Bone marrow transplantation	
Granulocyte transfusions	
Second malignant neoplasm[8]	
Pulmonary embolism[9, 10]	

*Pleural effusions are listed separately in Table 65–5.

digital clubbing has been associated with intrathoracic Hodgkin's disease in young patients.[70]

Thoracic neoplasms occasionally produce remote symptoms that do not immediately suggest the site of primary disease. For example, thoracic spinal cord compression from a neurogenic or vertebral neoplasm may manifest as weakness in a lower extremity that progresses to bowel or bladder dysfunction.[71] Autoimmune phenomena may be indicative of lymphoreticular malignancies of the mediastinum. Memory loss that was reversible (Ophelia syndrome) is one of the most peculiar of the reported remote effects of otherwise silent thoracic Hodgkin's disease.[72] Similarly, unexplained cholestatic jaundice has been reported in otherwise occult mediastinal non-Hodgkin's lymphoma.[73]

In rare circumstances, pulmonary symptoms can be caused by a lung neoplasm, even if no typical radiographic evidence suggests the diagnosis. Particularly with endobronchial lesions (see Table 65–2), there may be few, if any, radiographic findings, and the diagnosis must be made by bronchoscopy. Benign-appearing lung cysts may represent primary or metastatic malignant parenchymal disease.[74–76] The association of sarcomas with congenital lung cysts has been mentioned earlier.[63–68]

Pulmonary embolism is rare in children but has occasionally been associated with osteogenic sarcoma with or without endocardial metastases.[9]

DIAGNOSTIC APPROACHES

Because neoplastic intrathoracic disease most often produces mass lesions or significant replacement of lung parenchyma, the process is usually apparent on plain chest radiographs. Computed tomographic (CT) scanning provides better anatomic localization of masses than does conventional radiography and has replaced plane tomography. In addition, the CT scan is more sensitive than conventional radiography for metastatic disease to the lung and mediastinum,[77] which is often clinically silent. Magnetic resonance imaging provides the benefits of (1) axial, sagittal, and coronal views; (2) differentiation of tissue densities; and (3) exquisite detail of the vertebral column and neural foramina (of importance in neurogenic tumors of the posterior mediastinum).

Table 65–2. PROLIFERATIVE AND NEOPLASTIC DISEASE OF THE PEDIATRIC CHEST: AIRWAYS

Benign Lesions	Malignant Lesions
Hamartoma	***Primary Neoplasms***
Hemangioma/lymphangioma (cystic hygroma)	Bronchial adenoma group
Endobronchial chondromatous hamartoma[15]	Carcinoid
Infectious/Reactive Lesions	Bronchial tumors of salivary gland type (mucoepidermoid tumor, low-grade mucoepidermoid carcinoma)
Plasma-cell granuloma (inflammatory) pseudotumor)	Adenoid cystic carcinoma (cylindroma)
Papillomatosis[16]	Bronchogenic carcinoma (squamous cell carcinoma, adenocarcinoma, small-cell/oat-cell undifferentiated carcinoma, large-cell undifferentiated carcinoma)
Bronchiolitis obliterans after bone marrow transplantation[17]	
Tumors	
Mucous gland adenoma	Sarcoma
Chondroma[18]	Papillomatosis with malignant transformation[26, 27]
Myoblastoma (granular cell tumor)[19–21]	Squamous cell carcinoma of larynx[28–30]
Leiomyoma[22, 23]	Non-Hodgkin's lymphoma[31–33]
Teratoma[24]	Intravascular bronchoalveolar tumor[34, 35]
Lipoblastoma[25]	

Ultrasonography helps define pleural effusions and cardiovascular complications of neoplasia such as the occlusion of the superior or inferior vena cava by a tumor thrombus. Fluoroscopy, often with barium swallow, occasionally provides information on dynamic relationships among mediastinal structures. Gallium radionuclide scanning may identify lymphoreticular proliferations.[78] Angiography is occasionally useful when major vessels are compromised or when vascular hamartomas or neoplasms are suspected. Bronchoscopy is useful when

Table 65–3. PROLIFERATIVE AND NEOPLASTIC DISEASES OF THE PEDIATRIC CHEST: MEDIASTINUM*

Benign Lesions	Malignant Lesions
Anterior Mediastinum	**_Anterior Mediastinum_**
Thymic lesions	
Large thymus (normal, poststress rebound, true massive hyperplasia, follicular or lymphoid hyperplasia)	Thymic malignancies
	Lymphoreticular malignancies
	Hodgkin's lymphoma
Ectopic thymus	Non-Hodgkin's lymphoma
Thymic cysts	Lymphoid leukemia
Thymolipoma	Myeloid leukemia
Thymoma	Malignant thymoma
Langerhans cell histiocytosis (histiocytosis X)	Malignant germ-cell tumor (malignant teratoma)
Extramedullary hematopoiesis[36]	Soft tissue sarcoma
Histoplasmosis	Carcinoid
Teratoma	
Lipoma/lipoblastoma	
Hemangioma/lymphangioma/cystic hygroma	
Myofibromatosis (fibromatosis, desmoid tumors)	
Ectopic thyroid	
Neurofibromatosis	
Middle Mediastinum	**_Middle Mediastinum_**
Lymphoreticular proliferations and infectious/reactive lesions of hilar lymph nodes	Mediastinal nodal structures
	Lymphoreticular malignancies
Histoplasmosis	Hodgkin's lymphoma
Fibrosing mediastinitis (collagenosis)	Non-Hodgkin's lymphoma
	Lymphoid leukemia
Plasma-cell granuloma	Myeloid leukemia
Giant lymph node hyperplasia (Castleman's disease)	Metastases of systemic malignancies (see Table 65–1)
Sarcoidosis	Tumors of the heart, pericardium, and great vessels
Chemotherapy extravasation[37]	
Tumors of the heart, pericardium, and great vessels[38–40]	Soft tissue sarcoma[46]
Neurofibromatosis	
Posterior Mediastinum	**_Posterior Mediastinum_**
Neurogenic tumors (ganglioneuroma, schwannoma, pheochromocytoma, neurofibroma)[7, 41]	Neurogenic malignancies
	Neuroblastoma
	Ganglioneuroblastoma
Malformations	Neurofibrosarcoma (malignant schwannoma)[7, 47]
Bronchogenic cysts[3, 42]	
Neurenteric cysts (split notochord syndrome)[3, 43]	Pheochromocytoma (paraganglioma), malignant[48, 49]
Esophageal duplications[3, 42]	Pigmented neuroectodermal tumor of infancy[50]
Intrathoracic meningocele[44]	
Hemangioma/lymphangioma	Lymphoreticular malignancies (paraspinal nodes)
Ectopic thymus	Sarcomas[46, 51, 52]
Extramedullary hematopoiesis	Chordoma[53]
Plasma-cell granuloma	
Lipoma[45]	

*Pleural effusions are listed separately in Table 65–5.

Table 65–4. PROLIFERATIVE AND NEOPLASTIC DISEASES OF THE PEDIATRIC CHEST: CHEST WALL, DIAPHRAGM, AND PLEURA*

Benign Lesions	Malignant Lesions
Malformations/Hamartomas	**_Primary Neoplasms_**
Diaphragmatic herniations[54]	Mesothelioma
Mesenchymal hamartoma	Chest wall sarcomas (Ewing's sarcoma, Askin tumor, peripheral neuroepithelial tumor, osteosarcoma, chondrosarcoma, and fibrosarcoma, rhabdomyosarcoma, extrarenal Wilms' sarcoma)
Hemangioma/lymphangioma	
Vascular/cartilaginous hamartoma of ribs[55]	
Lymphoreticular Proliferations and Infectious/Reactive Lesions	Rhabdomyosarcoma (diaphragm)
Langerhans cell histiocytosis (histiocytosis X)	Hemangiopericytoma[59]
Osteomyelitis[56]	Primary lymphoma of bone (reticulum cell sarcoma)[60]
Extramedullary hematopoiesis (pleural)	Malignant mesenchymoma[61, 62]
Tumors	**_Metastases to Chest Wall, Diaphragm, and Pleura_**
Cartilaginous/bony tumors of the thoracic cage and vertebral column (chondroma, enchondroma, osteoid osteoma, osteoblastoma, osteochondroma, aneurysmal bone cyst, fibrous dysplasia)[3, 57, 58]	
Pleural fibroma (solitary fibrous tumors of pleura)	
Myofibromatosis (generalized fibromatosis, musculoaponeurotic fibromatosis)	
Lipoblastoma[25]	

*Pleural effusions are listed separately in Table 65–5.

the tracheobronchial tree is the suspected site of involvement; this method occasionally identifies endobronchial lesions or extrinsic bronchial compression not suggested by imaging studies. Bronchoscopy should be strongly considered when obstructive airway disease is not readily reversible with traditional asthma pharmacotherapy. Bronchoalveolar lavage is being used increasingly, especially for identifying opportunistic infections in patients with cancer[79–81] and has demonstrated eosinophils in acute eosinophilic pneumonia[82, 83] and Reed Sternberg cells in advanced Hodgkin's disease.[84]

Laboratory investigations may provide pertinent diagnostic findings such as the confirmation of acute leukemia. Elevated levels of alpha-fetoprotein and human chorionic gonadotropin are virtually diagnostic of a malignant germ-cell tumor, even if the predominant histologic finding is a mature teratoma. Serologic studies may differentiate mediastinal histoplasmosis from a lymphoreticular neoplasm.[85]

Laboratory studies provide adjunctive, but not diagnostic, data for several different types of diseases. For example, elevated urinary or serum catecholamines indicate the presence of a secreting neurogenic tumor, but histologic confirmation is still required. Serum ferritin and neuron-specific enolase are important prognostic markers for neuroblastoma. Peripheral blood hematologic studies are essential for lymphoreticular proliferations, such as leukemia, lymphoma, hypereosinophilia, and Langerhans cell histiocytosis (histiocytosis X). Severe chronic hemolysis is occasionally associated with paraspinal mediastinal nodules of extramedullary hematopoiesis;[86] the peripheral blood studies may obviate the need for a surgical diagnosis.[87] Lactate dehydrogenase activity has prognostic significance in non-Hodgkin's lymphomas[88] and malignant germ-cell tumors.[89]

A tissue diagnosis is ultimately necessary for virtually all thoracic neoplasms. Except for lymphoreticular disease diagnosed in peripheral blood, bone marrow, or extrathoracic lymph nodes, the tissue is obtained from the chest. The diagnostic approach should be planned jointly by the pulmonologist, the surgeon, the hematologist or oncologist, and the pathologist to ensure adequate sampling and proper handling and study of the specimens. Lymphoreticular neoplasms are not managed primarily by surgery, and so a limited surgical approach is appropriate. Thoracentesis alone may be sufficient for diagnosing a lymphoreticular neoplasm with pleural effusion, but extreme caution must be used because infectious processes have been reported to produce pleural effusions containing T lymphoblasts that are indistinguishable from lymphoblastic leukemia or lymphoma.[90] Alternatively, a formal thoracotomy is the principal approach for most benign tumors and nonlymphoid malignant solid tumors. However, if major resection of a malignant tumor is potentially dangerous, is disfiguring, or may cause functional impairment, a limited surgical approach followed by aggressive chemoradiotherapeutic treatment may be more desirable. This initial approach can be followed by more limited, delayed surgery to achieve a potential cure with preservation of anatomy and function.[91]

Major advances in classification and treatment of childhood leukemias and lymphomas have resulted from detailed clinicopathologic studies.[92-94] In addition to routine histologic and cytochemical studies, the neoplasm should be evaluated by cytogenetic studies, immunohistochemistry studies, and immunoglobulin gene and T receptor gene rearrangements of lymphoreticular neoplasms. Many of these studies require special processing of fresh tissues, hence the need for preoperative coordination. Electron microscopy is especially helpful in the differential diagnosis of small round-cell tumors when it is performed in conjunction with immunohistochemistry. Oncogene studies, cytogenetic studies, and ploidy analysis by flow cytometry on appropriately prepared fresh tissue provide important prognostic data in the case of neuroblastoma.

DIFFERENTIAL DIAGNOSIS OF THORACOPULMONARY PROLIFERATIVE AND NEOPLASTIC DISEASE

The proliferative and neoplastic diseases of the chest are discussed on the basis of the following anatomic divisions: lung parenchyma (see Table 65-1), respiratory airways (see Table 65-2), mediastinum (see Table 65-3), and chest wall, diaphragm, and pleura (see Table 65-4). Diseases associated with or causing pleural effusions are

Table 65-5. THORACOPULMONARY NEOPLASTIC PROCESSES ASSOCIATED WITH PLEURAL EFFUSIONS IN CHILDREN

Benign	Malignant
Lymphangiomatosis[95-97]	Acute lymphoblastic leukemia with hypereosinophilia[103]
Langerhans cell histiocytosis (histiocytosis X)[98, 99]	Acute lymphoblastic leukemia/lymphoma syndrome[99, 104]
Histoplasmosis[90]	Hodgkin's disease[12, 105]
Hemangiomatosis[100]	Non-Hodgkin's lymphoma[32, 99, 106-108]
Churg-Strauss syndrome[101]	Endodermal sinus tumor[109, 110]
Complications of radiotherapy[102]	Cervical teratoma[111]
Complications of chemotherapy (Table 65-6)	Pleural mesothelioma[112]
Pulmonary embolism[9]	Pheochromocytoma[48]
	Wilms' tumor[113]
	Ewing's sarcoma[114, 115]
	Rhabdomyosarcoma[46]
	Clear-cell sarcoma*
	Malignant mesenchymoma[62, 99]
	Malignant histiocytosis[99]
	Squamous cell carcinoma[99]

*J. R. Priest: Personal experience, 1985.

listed in Table 65-5.[9, 12, 32, 46, 48, 62, 90, 95-115] Benign lesions, although distorted occasionally by large size, typically remain confined to the regional anatomic boundaries, whereas malignancies often transgress defined borders so that assignment to a specific organ or topographic site becomes arbitrary and is based on probable tissue and site of origin. Similarly, the distinction between the anterior, middle, and posterior portions of the mediastinum (see Table 65-3) is difficult when a mass is very large (Fig. 65-1).

Many conditions listed in Tables 65-1 through 65-4 represent those neoplasms and other pathologic processes that are discussed in the text. The other conditions are presented for the sake of the differential diagnosis and are not discussed but are referenced within the tables.

LUNG PARENCHYMA

Benign Lesions

MALFORMATIONS/HAMARTOMAS

Various congenital malformations of thoracic structures should be considered in the differential diagnosis of chest masses in children (see Chapter 52). Adenomatoid malformation of the cystic and solid types and bronchogenic cyst are discussed later in terms of the putative association with pulmonary rhabdomyosarcoma, pleuropulmonary blastoma, and other sarcomas.[63-68]

Developmental abnormalities of large and small vessels are a diverse and complex group of disorders that range from arteriovenous malformations and fistulae (large vessels) to hemangiomas and lymphangiomas (small vessels); all are rare in lung parenchyma.[95-97, 116] Arteriovenous fistulae of the lung may occur in children with Osler-Weber-Rendu syndrome (hereditary hemorrhagic telangiectasia). Cyanosis, digital clubbing, and polycythemia may occur in these patients.[117, 118] Diffuse pulmonary heman-

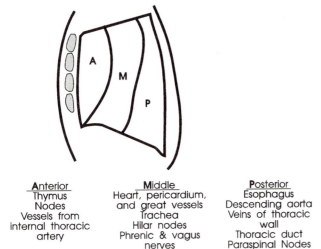

Anterior	Middle	Posterior
Thymus	Heart, pericardium,	Esophagus
Nodes	and great vessels	Descending aorta
Vessels from	Trachea	Veins of thoracic
internal thoracic	Hilar nodes	wall
artery	Phrenic & vagus	Thoracic duct
	nerves	Paraspinal Nodes
		Sympathetic nerve
		trunks

Figure 65–1. Mediastinal compartments and their contents.

giomatosis in an infant can be associated with hemoptysis and platelet trapping.[119] The involved lobe has a pathologic appearance similar to that of infantile hemangioendothelioma of the liver. Extensive hemangiomas may be life-threatening through bleeding, mass effect, or diffuse coagulopathy. The successful use of interferon-α in several cases may represent an important therapeutic advance.[120–122]

Sclerosing hemangioma of the lung is a somewhat disputed entity because it may represent, not a vascular neoplasm, but rather a lesion of type II pneumocytes.[123] Regardless of whether the lesion is endothelial or epithelial in origin, it has been rarely observed, even in young children, as a solitary lung nodule. The complex papillary lesion is one of several histologic appearances (Fig. 65–2).

Pulmonary lymphangiomyomatosis (lymphangioleiomyomatosis) is a rare disorder affecting young women. Radiographically identical lesions are found in patients with tuberous sclerosis. Dyspnea on exertion is the presenting sign; chest radiographs are often normal at diagnosis.[124, 125] A lung biopsy demonstrates the proliferation of spindle cells through the interstitium and along and within intraparenchymal lymphatic channels.

Fibroleiomyomatous hamartoma is also a disorder affecting females, usually of middle age, but a 9-year-old girl was reported with this lesion; she was being treated for rhabdomyosarcoma, and metastatic tumor was suspected. The nodules are multiple and are composed of smooth muscle and fibrous and glandular tissue.[126]

Hamartomas (chondromatous hamartomas) are the most common benign parenchymal tumor of the lung and are diagnosed in adults with an asymptomatic coin lesion. A few cases have been reported in children.[15, 127–130]

LYMPHORETICULAR PROLIFERATIONS AND INFECTIOUS/REACTIVE LESIONS

Langerhans cell histiocytosis (histiocytosis X) is an idiopathic disorder that expresses itself variously from silent, isolated organ involvement (e.g., solitary eosino-

philic granuloma of bone or lung or isolated cutaneous histiocytosis X) to severe, extensive multisystem disease and organ failure (Letterer-Siwe syndrome). Pulmonary histiocytosis X occurs most often in young adult and teenage males.[98, 131] The course is usually indolent, and the disease may remain stable, regress, or progress to honeycomb lung. Diabetes insipidus may be the only extrapulmonary manifestation. Pleural effusion is a rare finding, and spontaneous pneumothorax may be the presenting manifestation even with a normal chest radiograph. Diffuse interstitial or reticulonodular infiltrates are the classic radiographic finding; hilar adenopathy may also occur. Several cases of isolated pulmonary histiocytosis X in infants and young children have been reported with various clinical courses. The disease is usually more aggressive in infants than in older children.[132–134]

Pulmonary histiocytosis is typical in children younger than 5 years of age as part of systemic disease, and pulmonary symptoms are generally mild in comparison with the systemic manifestations.[98] In a review of 127 patients in a single institution, Greenberger and colleagues reported pulmonary disease in 53% of young patients with multisystem disease.[135] The course of the disease depends almost entirely on the systemic involvement; pulmonary infiltrates contribute little to the overall clinical condition. The diagnosis of Langerhans cell histiocytosis is predicated in all the various clinical circumstances on the demonstration of Birbeck granules in the cytoplasm of histiocytes by electron microscopy or the expression of CD1 on cell membranes.

Eosinophilic pneumonias are a somewhat diverse group of conditions that may occur with benign or malignant systemic illnesses.[136–138] Eosinophilic pulmonary infiltrations may occur with or without peripheral blood eosinophilia. Bronchoalveolar lavage may identify eosinophilic pneumonia in the absence of other signs of eosinophilia.[82, 83] The pulmonary involvement may be transient and "wandering" (Löffler's syndrome) or may be severe and acute or chronic.[82] Conditions associated with pulmonary infiltration include many intestinal parasitoses ("tropical eosinophilia," filariasis, visceral and cutaneous larva migrans), fungal infections (aspergillosis),[139] toxic exposure (nickel), periarteritis nodosa, Churg-Strauss syndrome (systemic vasculitis, asthma, and eosinophilia),[101] and exposure to certain drugs.[136, 137] The implicated drugs that children may be given include aspirin, beclomethasone, carbamazepine, cephalosporins, cromolyn sodium, imipramine, methotrexate, nitrofurantoin, penicillin, sulfonamides, and tetracycline.[137] In children in the United States, atopic disease is the most common cause of moderate eosinophilia (absolute eosinophil count, 500 to 1500 cells/μl), and pulmonary infiltration would not be expected. Parasitic infection is the most common cause of exaggerated eosinophilia (eosinophil count 1500 to 75,000/μl).[140] Pulmonary infiltrates are reported in approximately 50% of children with eosinophilia associated with visceral larva migrans.[141] Eosinophilic pneumonia associated with systemic malignancies is discussed later. In chronic reactive airway disease, eosinophils are characteristically found in the airway mucosa and lumen[142] but not in the lung parenchyma.

Plasma-cell granuloma (inflammatory pseudotumor,

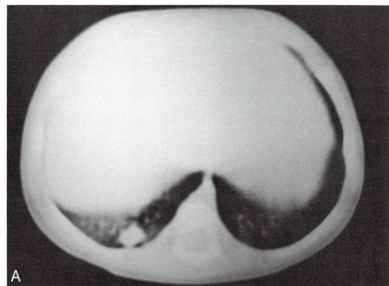

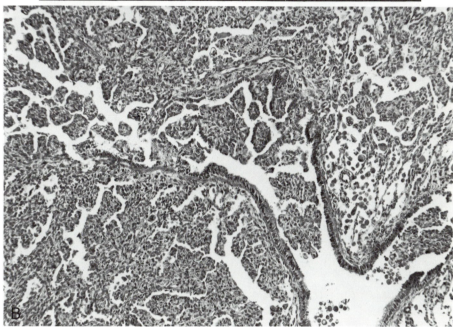

Figure 65–2. Sclerosing hemangioma. *A,* Chest computed tomogram (CT) of a 1-year-old girl, showing right lower lobe nodule discovered incidentally on chest radiograph for upper respiratory congestion. *B,* Complex papillary projections involve a bronchiole and surrounding parenchyma. The lining cells are epithelial rather than endothelial in type. Hematoxylin and eosin, ×150. (Washington University Illustration #89-8692)

inflammatory myofibroblastic tumor) is an idiopathic tumefaction of the lung that occurs predominantly in children.[1, 143–145] In fact, it was described as the most common "benign" tumor of the lung in children in the review by Hartman and Shochat.[1] A solitary density of variable size and with calcification in 25% to 30% of cases is the radiographic appearance. The lesion may be an incidental finding on radiographs, or a patient may have cough, chest pain, fever, weight loss, or hemoptysis. Esophageal obstruction has also been reported.[146] A circumscribed firm mass measuring 3 to 4 cm in diameter and consisting of a mixture of spindle cells (myofibroblasts), plasma cells, and lymphocytes is the characteristic pathologic finding (Fig. 65–3). The locally invasive nature and the occasional recurrences[147] suggest that the plasma-cell granuloma may be neoplastic rather than a postinflammatory process.

BENIGN TUMORS

Even in adults, benign neoplasms of the lung are uncommon, and in children they are extremely rare. The combination of pulmonary chondroma, gastric leiomyosarcoma, and extra-adrenal (often thoracic) paraganglioma (chemodectoma) is known as Carney's triad and has been reported in a child.[148] If the plasma-cell granuloma is excluded, the leiomyoma, neurofibroma, and neurilemoma (schwannoma) are the remaining entities.[11, 149] Fibromatosis of the lung occurs only in infants with congenital generalized fibromatosis.

CONDITIONS ASSOCIATED WITH SYSTEMIC MALIGNANCY

A number of pulmonary conditions have been associated with systemic malignancy in children. The most

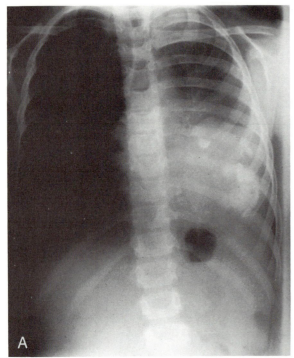

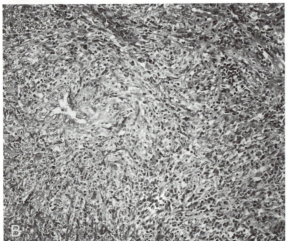

Figure 65–3. Plasma cell granuloma (inflammatory pseudotumor). A, Chest radiograph of a 6-year-old girl with fever and cough. B, Spindle-cell proliferation and a mixed inflammatory infiltrate. An entrapped bronchiole is surrounded by the process. Hematoxylin and eosin, ×160.

common are opportunistic infections in the immuno-compromised child (see Chapters 36 and 75).

Hypereosinophilic syndrome (exaggerated peripheral eosinophilia) with pulmonary symptoms and radiographic findings may be the presenting manifestation of acute lymphoblastic leukemia; at least 15 such cases have been reported in children.[103,150,151] White blood cell counts have ranged from 14,000 to 200,000 cu mm with 25% to 75% mature eosinophils without circulating lymphoblasts. In one patient, the initial bone marrow test revealed only 6% lymphoblasts, but a second bone marrow test 2 weeks later revealed 50% lymphoblasts.[103] Corticosteroid is a common therapy for eosinophilic pneumonia but should be avoided until acute lymphoblastic leukemia is excluded from the differential diagnosis.

Acute eosinophilic leukemia is exceedingly rare and is not a recognized subtype of the acute myeloid leukemias. The authors saw a 12-year-old boy with acute eosinophilic leukemia who had asthmatic symptoms (cough, wheezing) that resolved as the leukemia was lysed.

Disseminated intravascular coagulation is a frequent concomitant of the promyelocytic, monocytic, and monoblastic subtypes of acute myelogenous leukemia. Indeed, this profound bleeding disorder is often the presenting manifestation of acute promyelocytic leukemia and nearly always occurs with treatment. Both pulmonary hemorrhage and adult respiratory distress syndrome may be associated with the disseminated intravascular coagulation that occurs in acute promyelocytic leukemia.[152]

Excess catecholamine secretion leading to a cardiomyopathy with symptoms of respiratory distress has been associated with pheochromocytoma[41] and neuroblastoma[153] in children.

Pseudometastasis is a designation for a discrete lung lesion appearing in children being treated for a systemic malignancy when the suspected pulmonary lesions are nonneoplastic.[154–156] Among 39 children with lung nodules and malignant disease, Cohen found that 26 had metastatic disease and 13 had benign lesions (7 with histoplasmosis, 2 with "round" pneumonia, and 1 each with inflammatory pseudotumor, "round" atelectasis, radiation pneumonitis, and fibroleiomyomatous hamartoma.[127,154] Septic emboli have also been mistaken initially as metastases.[157–159] Bleomycin-induced pulmonary fibrosis may also manifest as isolated pulmonary nodules.[160–162]

The spectrum of pulmonary toxicity of chemotherapy in children is the same as in adults. Most of the agents used to treat pediatric malignancies are relatively nontoxic to the lungs; however, bleomycin and the nitrosoureas are predictably damaging at high cumulative doses. It is disturbing to note that progressive pulmonary fibrosis may continue up to 17 years after chemotherapy in children given carmustine.[163,164] High-dose cytosine arabinoside therapy is used increasingly and has been associated with acute lung injury syndrome in 13 of 103 adults; 9 of these patients died.[165] The literature on drug-induced pulmonary disease is extensive and beyond the scope of this discussion but is summarized in several thorough reviews.[166–169] Cooper and associates and other authors emphasized that interstitial lung disease (pneumonitis and fibrosis), hypersensitivity lung disease, and acute lung injury syndrome (noncardiogenic pulmonary edema, adult respiratory distress syndrome) are the three major clinical manifestations of drug-induced toxicity (Table 65–6).[168–172] The diagnosis of these syndromes is made only after other causes with similar clinical features are carefully ruled out. There are no specific histologic or biochemical markers for these toxicities, and affected patients are typically undergoing complex therapies that predispose them especially to infectious complications (see Chapter 36). A lung biopsy may be required in order to rule out an infectious cause. Acute alveolar injury with or without organization is the common histologic finding. Cooper and Matthay identified possible predisposing factors to chemotherapy-induced lung disease: the drug, its

Table 65-6. CLINICAL MANIFESTATIONS OF CHEMOTHERAPY-INDUCED PULMONARY DISEASE

	Interstitial Lung Disease	Hypersensitivity Pneumonitis	Acute Lung Injury
Drugs	Bleomycin* Busulfan* Carmustine (BCNU) Chlorambucil Cyclophosphamide* Lomustine (CCNU) Melphalan Methotrexate* Mitomycin* Semustine (methyl CCNU) Vinblastine with mitomycin Vincristine with mitomycin	Azothioprine Bleomycin* Methotrexate* Procarbazine* 6-Mercaptopurine	Bleomycin* Cyclophosphamide* Cytosine arabinoside Methotrexate* Mitomycin* Teniposide (VM-26)
Symptoms	Dyspnea, nonproductive cough, fatigue, malaise	Fever, chills, headaches, myalgias, dyspnea, nonproductive cough	Tachypnea, hypoxemia, respiratory failure
Time Course	Weeks to months	Hours to days	Immediate to hours

Adapted from (1) Cooper JAD, White DA, Matthay RA: Drug-induced pulmonary disease. Part 1: Cytotoxic drugs. Am Rev Respir Dis 133:321–340, 1986; (2) Cooper JAD Jr, Matthay RA: Drug-induced pulmonary disease. Dis Mon 33(2):66–120, 1987; (3) Cooper JAD Jr, Zitnik RJ, Matthay RA: Mechanisms of drug-induced pulmonary disease. Am Rev Med 39:395–404, 1988; (4) Ganick DJ, Peters ME, Hafez G-R: Acute bleomycin toxicity. Am J Pediatr Hematol Oncol 2(3):249–252, 1980; and (5) Jones SE, Moore M, Blank N, Castellino RA: Hypersensitivity to procarbazine (Matulane) manifested by fever and pleuropulmonary reaction. Cancer 29(2):498–500, 1972.

*Associated with pleural effusions.

cumulative dose and route of administration, concurrent oxygen therapy, pulmonary radiation therapy, antecedent lung disease, age of the patient, coincident use of transfusions or other drugs, and renal impairment.[169]

Bleomycin is probably the most toxic of the commonly used antineoplastic agents.[167, 173] It is a component of curative regimens for young patients with malignant germ-cell tumors (vinblastine or VP-16, bleomycin, and cisplatin) or Hodgkin's disease (doxorubicin [Adriamycin], bleomycin, vinblastine, dacarbazine); both regimens are widely applied. Bleomycin toxicity is probably associated with excessive production of reactive oxygen radicals as a result of drug-induced imbalance in pulmonary oxidant-antioxidant systems.[169] The toxicity is dose related. Pulmonary damage is usually heralded by a decrease in the diffusing capacity of carbon monoxide during a course of chemotherapy.[69, 174, 175] This complication can usually be avoided if the total cumulative dose is less than 150 to 200 U/sq m. The drug is excreted in urine, and fatal pulmonary toxicity was reported in a patient with renal insufficiency who received only 60 U.[176] Bleomycin toxicity is usually chronic, but acute toxicity and death were reported in a child.[171]

Bleomycin toxicity is potentiated by pulmonary radiation and oxygen therapy. With patients who have received bleomycin and who are under anesthesia, extreme care should be taken to limit their inspired oxygen concentration to 22% to 25%.[177] In one center, in the first five young adult men to receive standard cumulative doses of bleomycin for testicular cancer, acute lung injury developed within 3 to 5 days of surgery for dissection of retroperitoneal nodes; all died. In these cases, the mean intraoperative inspired oxygen concentration was 39% and did not exceed 45%. Subsequent patients were managed with less than 25% oxygen and did well.[178] Intraoperative fluid restriction also appears to be important in preventing oxygen-related damage.[177, 178]

Radiation therapy is potentially very toxic to the lung.[179] The total radiation dose, the number of fractions into which this dose is divided, total elapsed time (days) of therapy course, and the volume of lung tissue irradiated are the most important factors determining toxicity. A total dose of 1800 to 2000 cGy whole-lung irradiation in 10 to 12 fractions over 12 to 16 days is probably safe in patients not receiving chemotherapy. Clinical radiation pneumonitis is estimated to occur in 5% of patients receiving 2650 cGy to the whole lung (20 fractions in 4 weeks) and in 50% of patients receiving 3050 cGy (20 fractions in 4 weeks).[102] Tolerable radiation doses are approximately 20% less when chemotherapy is given.[102, 180] However, of 153 children with Wilms' tumor who received 1200-cGy whole-lung irradiation (150 cGy/day; eight doses over a 10-day period) and chemotherapy, 19 developed interstitial pneumonitis.[181] Clinical radiation toxicity is biphasic: acute radiation pneumonitis is manifested by unproductive cough and dyspnea on exertion (and in rare instances by pain, fever, or hemoptysis) beginning 2 to 6 months after the irradiation; these symptoms usually abate, and some degree of permanent radiation fibrosis ensues in the next 6 to 12 months and is usually asymptomatic.[102] In severe cases, serious permanent respiratory compromise occurs: dyspnea, orthopnea, cyanosis, cor pulmonale, and digital clubbing.[102] Radiographic changes follow essentially the same time course and progress from an acute alveolar or interstitial alteration to a chronic stage of fibrosis, pleural thickening, and volume reduction in severe cases.[102] Pleural effusions occur in about 10% of patients with severe, acute radiation pneumonitis. Spontaneous pneumothorax is a rare but recognized complication.[102, 182, 183]

Because many children (60%) now survive childhood malignancy, increasing attention is paid to the late effects of curative therapy. The pulmonary toxicity of individual chemotherapeutic agents (see Table 65-6) and of radiation has been discussed previously, but there have been few comprehensive studies of pulmonary function in long-term survivors. In three studies, investigators assessed pulmonary function in 101 long-term survivors of Wilms' tumor.[184-186] The pulmonary function of the patients who received actinomycin D alone could not be differentiated from normal. Those who also received chest radiation (1100 to 1300 cGy) had, in general, reduced lung volumes, reduced dynamic compliance, and variable decreases in diffusing capacity of carbon monoxide. Most of those who received 2000 cGy had marked thoracic hypoplasia.[185] Despite these changes detected by formal pulmonary function tests, no patients in these studies were disabled or had dyspnea.

Two studies addressed pulmonary function in survivors of disease other than Wilms' tumor.[187, 188] Miller and co-workers suggested that in a wide variety of diagnoses, an age of less than 3 years at diagnosis predisposed patients to pulmonary abnormalities even in the absence of thoracic irradiation.[187] Shaw and co-workers studied 38 acute lymphoblastic leukemia survivors. All had received methotrexate, and 10 had received cyclophosphamide; 33 had received chemotherapy alone. Two had received total body irradiation, and 3 had received spinal irradiation. By a questionnaire survey, 17 of the 38 reported mild to moderate intolerance of exercise, in contrast to no such reports in a control group of 150 normal children. There were reductions in vital capacity, total lung capacity, and residual lung volume in 65% of the patients. Again there was a suggestion that occurrence of disease at younger ages (less than 8 years at diagnosis) led to a higher incidence of late pulmonary effects.[188]

Interstitial pneumonitis is a serious complication occurring in about 25% to 35% of patients undergoing bone marrow transplantation and is often fatal.[189-191] In addition to chemotherapy, transplantation often involves whole-body irradiation (approximately 750 to 1200 cGy over 1 to 5 days) as part of the immediate pretransplantation preparative regimen. Other important factors in the development of interstitial pneumonitis are cytomegalovirus and herpes virus, older age, severe graft-versus-host disease, specific graft-versus-host prophylactic regimen, and pretransplantation performance status.[189]

Acute lung injury after granulocyte transfusions was reported when such transfusions first came into wide use.[192, 193] There may have been a temporal association with the use of amphotericin in the affected patients, but this association has been questioned.[194-196] Pulmonary reactions to granulocyte transfusions appear to be more likely when one or more of the following factors is present: gram-negative bacteremia and a severely ill host,[192, 197] concomitant use of amphotericin,[192] allosensitization to leukocyte antigens,[193, 196] or granulocytes collected by nylon-wool fiber technique (in contrast to the currently used continuous-flow centrifugation technique).[198]

Malignant Lesions

Primary Lesions of Lung Parenchyma

Primary malignant tumors of pneumogenic mesenchyma are rare in childhood in contrast to the pediatric cancers of hematopoietic, neuroectodermal, renal, adre-

nal, soft tissue, or osseous origin, which are far more common. Hartman and Shochat reviewed 230 primary pulmonary neoplasms in children; only 39 of the 151 malignant tumors were parenchymal in origin.[1] Manivel and co-authors suggested pleuropulmonary blastoma or childhood pulmonary blastoma as the unifying nosologic entity for a group of malignant pleuropulmonary mesenchymal neoplasms of children.[199] Eleven children (five boys and six girls), aged 2½ to 12 years, were described. Most had fever, cough, dyspnea, and chest or abdominal pain. Massive unilateral multilobulated tumors arising from the periphery of the affected lobe, mediastinum, or pleura were discovered at surgery. On gross examination, the mass had a uniform, gray-white appearance with a glistening myxoid surface in the unfixed state (Fig. 65–4). Cysts were identified in some cases. The histologic pattern was variable with blastomatous islands surrounded by a loose mesenchyma, scattered large anaplastic cells, spindle-cell sarcoma, and heterologous foci of rhabdomyosarcoma, chondrosarcoma, or liposarcoma (Fig. 65–5). Neoplastic glandular and tubular elements were not identified, which differentiated this neoplasm from the pulmonary blastoma of adults. The pleuropulmonary blastoma is a highly malignant neoplasm; 7 of 11 children died less than 2 years after diagnosis. No consistently useful therapeutic regimen could be described from this series of cases. Early metastases to the brain were a distinct feature of this disease in comparison to other childhood cancers.

Rhabdomyosarcoma of the lung parenchyma is a very rare entity,[200] whereas metastatic rhabdomyosarcoma of the lungs is relatively common. Crist and associates reviewed the intrathoracic soft tissue sarcomas in the Intergroup Rhabdomyosarcoma Study (I and II pilot); only 3 of 646 neoplasms arose in lung parenchyma (two alveolar rhabdomyosarcomas and one undifferentiated sarcoma).[46] Of particular interest are several individual reports of rhabdomyosarcoma in association with congenital abnormalities of the lung.[63-67] The authors are aware of two unpublished cases of rhabdomyosarcoma in lung cysts in cousins (M. C. O'Leary, W. G. Woods, personal communication, 1987). In addition to the peculiar association with lung cysts, a familial predisposition to cancer existed in three patients known to the authors: the two cousins just mentioned and one subject in the study by Allen and colleagues.[65] A brother of one of these patients later developed a pleuropulmonary blastoma.[199] In the family whose children are reported by Allen and Manivel and their colleagues, there were numerous other cancers, including a rhabdomyosarcoma of the bladder in a young person of this family. The implication of these rare reports of rhabdomyosarcomas in congenital lung malformations for the average child with such a malformation is unclear; an index of suspicion regarding potential malignant change may be warranted if there is a familial predisposition to cancer. Pathologic examination reveals that the cysts are lined by respiratory epithelium, a cambium layer of primitive cells, and an outer layer of differentiating rhabdomyoblasts (Fig. 65–6). Myxosarcoma,[201] mesenchymal hamartoma,[202] and other sarcomas[68] have also been reported in the wall of presumed congenital lung cysts.

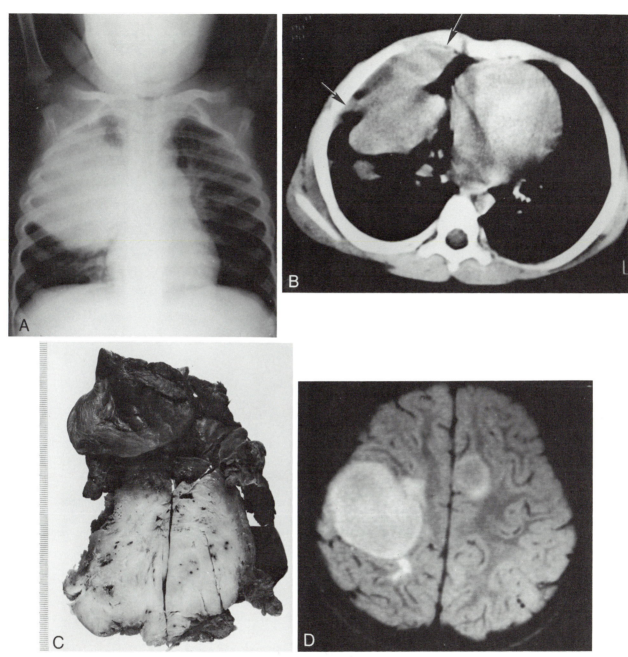

Figure 65–4. Pleuropulmonary blastoma. *A*, Chest radiograph of a 3-year-old boy being evaluated for fever and "pneumonia." Strong family history for sarcomas, including a sister with rhabdomyosarcoma in lung cyst (see Fig. 65–6). *B*, Chest CT scan showing large mass. Configuration at pleural interface *(arrows)* suggests pleural origin or infiltration. *C*, Pleuropulmonary blastoma, replacing a portion of the lung. Focal areas of hemorrhage and necrosis are present in an otherwise homogenous, gray-white solid mass. *D*, Magnetic resonance imaging (MRI) head scan, which had been normal at diagnosis, showing brain metastases 6 months after diagnosis; chest disease was still under control. (See also Fig. 65–5.)

Primary leiomyosarcoma of the lung has been described in 10 children.[203] The age range was newborn to 11 years; presenting symptoms were dyspnea, cough, anorexia, hemoptysis, fever, and pneumonia. The tumor was predominantly a monotonous spindle-cell pattern replacing the affected parenchyma. Complete resection is the recommended treatment, but the success of additional therapies and the ultimate prognosis cannot be determined from the few case reports. Intrapulmonary fibrosarcomas are rare low-grade malignancies and occur primarily in adults.[204] Eleven cases in children have been reported and were reviewed by Pettinato and co-work-

ers.[205] Both leiomyosarcomas and fibrosarcomas are compact spindle-cell neoplasms with scattered mitotic figures. Electronic microscopy and immunohistochemistry may be necessary for differentiating these neoplasms from each other.

Extraskeletal Ewing's sarcoma is a neoplasm of uncertain histogenesis that most often occurs in the second decade of life. It is believed by some authors to arise from primitive neuroectodermal cells. The extraskeletal sites are protean,[206] and one case with a malignant course was reported to arise in lung parenchyma in a 23-year-old.[207]

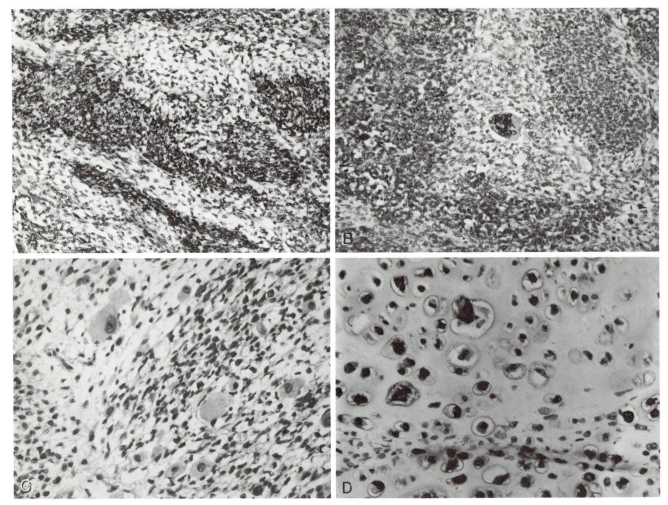

Figure 65–5. Pleuropulmonary blastoma. Several histologic findings are typical in a single tumor. *A*, Blastematous foci resembling Wilms' tumor (×150). *B*, An isolated anaplastic cell in a blastematous background (×150). *C*, Large eosinophilic cells representing rhabdomyoblasts (×250). *D*, Malignant-appearing islands of cartilage are the usual microscopic findings. Hematoxylin and eosin, ×250. (See also Fig. 65–4.)

Plasmacytoma, the isolated, monoclonal immunoglobulin-secreting tumor related to systemic multiple myeloma, is rare in children, but a 14-year-old with a solitary plasmacytoma in lung parenchyma was described.[208]

The intravascular, bronchiolar, and alveolar tumor of the lung (IVBAT) is an unusual tumor of possible vascular endothelial origin.[34] The tumor usually manifests as multiple, slowly growing pulmonary nodules. Cases in young patients (ages 12, 13, 17, and 19 years) have been reported.[34, 35]

Primary pulmonary lymphoma (non-Hodgkin's) is rare regardless of age. In a review of 36 patients at Memorial Sloan Kettering Cancer Center, one case was diagnosed in a 12-year-old child.[209] Other cases in children, ages 5, 14, and 15 years, have been reported.[210,211] Primary Hodgkin's disease of the lung is even more rare but has been reported in children and young adults.[74, 212] Pseudolymphoma of the lung is an incompletely understood, probably reactive process that can occur in young adults. It may be difficult to distinguish from lymphoma and may recur locally.[6]

Malignant teratoma arising in lung parenchyma (as opposed to mediastinum) is only rarely reported.[213–215] In fact, the lung is one of the least common sites for a primary teratoma.

Metastases to Lung Parenchyma

Childhood malignancies with metastases to the lungs are far more common than primary parenchymal neoplasms. The authors' experience indicates that more than 95% of all lung malignancies in children are metastatic in nature. In most patients, the primary site is known; however, the authors have seen embryonal rhabdomyosarcoma of the common bile duct first manifesting with pulmonary metastases. With few exceptions, the metastatic disease is asymptomatic and is discovered during diagnostic or follow-up studies related to the primary disease. The childhood cancers with a predilection for lung metastasis are Wilms' tumor, osteogenic sarcoma, skeletal or extraskeletal Ewing's sarcoma, rhabdomyosarcoma, other soft tissue sarcomas, hepatoma (hepatoblastoma and hepatocellular carcinoma), and malignant gonadal and extragonadal germ-cell tumors. Much less common is metastatic pulmonary parenchymal involvement with Hodgkin's and non-Hodgkin's lymphomas, acute

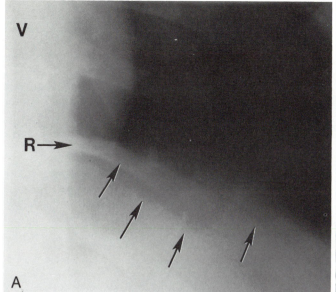

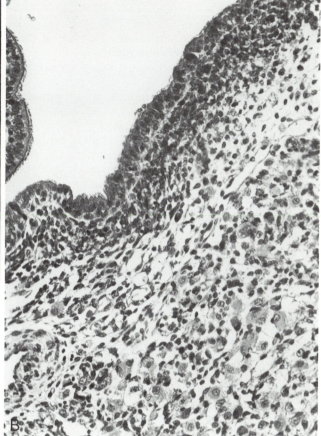

Figure 65–6. Rhabdomyosarcoma in a cystic adenomatoid malformation. *A,* Fluoroscopic spot film of medial left lower lung (V, vertebral column; R, 11th left rib) showing inferior margins of irregular air-filled cyst *(arrows).* The patient was a 2-year-old girl with repeated spontaneous pneumothoraces; she is the sister of the patient described in Fig. 65–4. *B,* Pulmonary cyst with a lining of respiratory epithelium, showing a condensed zone of small neoplastic cells beneath the surface (cambium layer) and larger rhabdomyoblasts beneath the cambium layer. Hematoxylin and eosin, ×300. (Washington University Illustration #89-8698)

myelogenous and lymphoblastic leukemias, the various central nervous system tumors of childhood, clear-cell sarcoma (bone-metastasizing renal tumor of childhood), and neuroblastoma. Peripheral T cell lymphomas (helper or suppressor cell lymphomas) occur but are rare in children; however, they have a particular predilection for involvement of the lung parenchyma.[216] Extraneural metastases of primary central nervous system tumors in children are rare, but, with increasingly effective approaches to diagnosis and treatment of the primary central nervous system lesions, extraneural metastases are being reported. Medulloblastoma, ependymoma, primitive neuroectodermal tumor, glioblastoma, meningioma, and intracranial germinoma and nongerminoma have been reported to metastasize to the lung.[217–221] Nasopharyngeal carcinoma (lymphoepithelioma),[222, 223] chondroblastoma,[224] and ameloblastoma[225] have been reported to metastasize to lung parenchyma. Parenchymal metastases may be manifest as cavitary lesions, which are suggestive of nonmalignant processes.[75, 76]

There are several circumstances in which metastases of systemic cancer to the lung may be of particular interest to the pulmonologist. Respiratory failure secondary to pulmonary vascular leukostasis and subsequent parenchymal infiltration is a serious problem in acute myelogenous leukemia, especially when there is hyperleukocytosis (white blood cell count >100,000/μl).[226] Dyspnea with tachypnea, rales, nonhypercapneic respiratory fail-

ure, and diffuse interstitial infiltrates are the features of pulmonary leukostasis.[226] Respiratory symptoms may develop or worsen as treatment proceeds.[227, 228] Pulmonary radiation and leukapheresis may ameliorate this life-threatening complication.[226, 228]

Isolated pulmonary relapse in the presence of bone marrow and central nervous system remission has occurred in children with acute lymphoblastic leukemia.[229, 230] Both interstitial and nodular infiltrates are present on chest radiographs, and lung biopsy is required in order to differentiate recurrent leukemia from an infectious cause or from occult pulmonary hemorrhage.[231]

Spontaneous pneumothoraces have been reported in 5% to 15% of patients with lung metastases of osteogenic sarcoma.[232, 233] In one study, there was a suggestion that chemotherapy increases the likelihood of pneumothorax.[232] In contrast, pneumothorax occurred in none of 64 patients in the same institution with testicular cancer metastatic to the lung. Spontaneous pneumothorax is a recognized complication after mantle-field irradiation for Hodgkin's disease.[182]

Surgery is potentially curative for persistent or recurrent pulmonary metastases of osteogenic sarcoma, Wilms' tumor, and malignant germ-cell tumors if the disease has not extended into the peribronchial tissues or mediastinum. Substantially improved control of disease results from single or multiple thoracotomies for osteogenic sarcoma.[234–237] In metastatic malignant germ-cell tumors (malignant teratomas), chemotherapy may eradicate disseminated malignant tissue, but mature teratomatous elements with only limited proliferative potential may remain at the sites of metastases. Excision of these residual masses (the "growing teratoma syndrome")[238] has become an essential part of a curative approach to affected patients.[238–241]

There are several pulmonary thoracic complications of Wilms' tumor. Tumor thrombus in the vena cava extending to the right atrium is well described,[242, 243] and combined thoracoabdominal resection, including cardiopulmonary bypass, is indicated in some instances.[242, 244] Pre-resection chemotherapy is advocated by other authors for shrinking the tumor, which in turn enables a more limited resection.[245, 246] Fatal preoperative and intraoperative tumor embolization to the pulmonary arteries has been reported.[10, 247] Metastases to the lung from Wilms' tumor are potentially curable both at diagnosis[248] or as recurrent disease.[249] Surgical resection of recurrent pulmonary nodules is generally recommended if those are the only sites of disease.[250] In two reported cases of Wilms' tumor, nonmalignant pulmonary nodules appeared 5 months and 2 years, respectively, after diagnosis and initiation of therapy.[155, 156] These nodules were composed of benign-appearing mesenchymal tissue and fibrosis, which conceivably represented the residual stroma of the Wilms' tumor. These cases emphasize the importance of aggressive diagnosis and treatment of apparent metastatic disease to the lung in children with systemic malignancy. Not all lung nodules in such children represent recurrent malignancy; rather, some represent the aforementioned pseudometastases.

Neuroblastoma does not typically metastasize to lung parenchyma,[251, 252] but a syndrome of recurrent extensive pulmonary metastases, ranging from multiple large nodules to miliary neuroblastoma and metastatic interstitial pneumonitis, has been reported after bone marrow transplantation for neuroblastoma.[253, 254]

THE AIRWAYS

Benign Processes

HAMARTOMAS

Hemangiomas and lymphangiomas (cystic hygromas) with exclusive or prominent involvement of the larynx are hamartomatous vascular malformations. They often manifest in the neonatal period, and most are diagnosed by 1 year of age. Recurrent croup, hoarseness, cough, hemoptysis, wheezing, and dysphagia may be presenting symptoms. Cutaneous hemangiomas occur in 50% of patients with subglottic hemangiomas.[255] Although hemangiomas usually spontaneously regress by 12 to 18 months of age, treatment is often necessary for laryngeal and subglottic involvement. Hemangiomas may respond to steroids[255] or interferon-α[120, 121] if needed for widespread disease, but laser surgery has proved very useful for the airway portions of both hemangiomas[256] and lymphangiomas.[257] Because of late effects, radiation therapy is no longer acceptable except in extremely extensive, progressive cases.

INFECTIOUS/REACTIVE LESIONS

Plasma-cell granuloma (inflammatory pseudotumor, inflammatory myofibroblastic tumor) of the trachea or bronchus accounted for 6 of the 230 primary pulmonary mass lesions in the review of pulmonary tumors by Hartman and Shochat.[1] The plasma-cell granuloma in this site has the pathologic features of its parenchymal counterpart.[1, 143, 144, 146]

TUMORS

Endobronchial and endotracheal tumors are very rare; mucous gland adenoma[1, 258] is mentioned here to emphasize that it is the only truly benign type of bronchial "adenoma," which should in general be considered malignant and is discussed next.

Malignant Lesions: Primary Neoplasms

Malignant neoplasms of the airway in children are as rare as the benign tumors. The most common neoplasms among these rare tumors are the so-called bronchial adenomas, which include bronchial carcinoids; there are about 20 pediatric cases in the English-language literature (Fig. 65–7). Less commonly reported are the low-grade mucoepidermoid carcinoma or bronchial tumor of salivary gland type (Fig. 65–8), and the very rare adenoid cystic carcinoma. These tumors manifest with fever, cough, wheezing, hemoptysis, or unremitting or recurrent pneumonias. Most often, they are discovered on bronchoscopy or CT scanning. Several reviewers collected the world's literature on carcinoid,[21, 259] mucoepidermoid carcinoma,[260, 261] and adenoid cystic carcinoma.[1] Bronchial carcinoid in children may behave in the same indolent manner as its counterpart in adults or may be aggressive and fatal. There is one example in the pediatric literature of a bronchial mucoepidermoid carcinoma with regional lymph node metastases.[260]

Bronchogenic carcinoma of the various adult types (squamous cell, small cell, large cell, and adenocarcinoma) is exceedingly rare in children. Several reviews indicated that there have been perhaps 20 to 30 cases.[1, 21, 262, 263]

Sarcomas of the respiratory tree are the subject of several reports. Leiomyosarcoma occurs in the airway as well as the lung parenchyma.[203] Fibrosarcomas of the bronchus are low-grade malignancies with a favorable outcome; 10 cases in children have been identified.[205] Rhabdomyosarcomas of the larynx[264–266] and bronchus[267] and unclassified spindle-cell sarcoma of the bronchus[3] have also been reported.

MEDIASTINUM

Benign Lesions

ANTERIOR MEDIASTINUM

The thymus is prominent from birth through the first 5 years of life; despite its size, it rarely causes pulmonary symptoms. In an otherwise normal young child, a thymus that appears large on radiographs should be regarded as

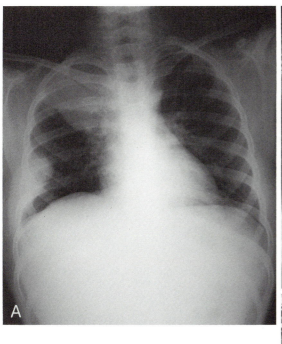

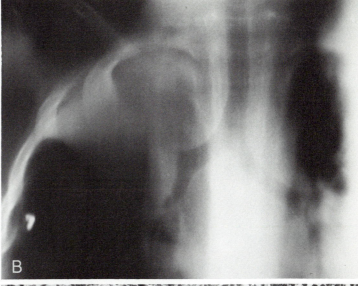

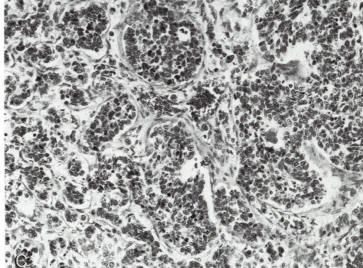

Figure 65–7. Bronchial adenoma: carcinoid. *A*, Chest radiograph of a 9-year-old girl evaluated for Cushing's syndrome with obesity, buffalo hump, and striae; the film reveals right upper lobe collapse and destructive lesion of the right sixth rib with associated soft tissue mass. *B*, Right upper chest tomogram showing complete obstruction at takeoff of right upper lobe bronchus. *C*, Circumscribed nests of small uniform cells with delicate nuclear chromatin. Hematoxylin and eosin, ×300. (Washington University Illustration #89-8696)

normal if it conforms to one of several well-recognized pediatric thymic silhouettes (Fig. 65–9).[77] The thymus involutes rapidly in young children who are physiologically or pharmacologically stressed, and poststress thymic rebound or hyperplasia is recognized after cessation of the stress.[77, 268–270] Radiographically worrisome thymomegaly is recognized even in older children and young adults after chemotherapy for malignancy; it may occur during[271] or a few months after chemotherapy or radiotherapy.[271–282] Chest CT scans reveal this phenomenon more often than do plain chest radiographs.[274] Thymic biopsies reveal normal corticomedullary architectural features with the expected immunophenotypic distribution of lymphocytes.[271, 278–280] A particular dilemma is presented in the childhood neoplasms with a predilection for mediastinal relapse or metastasis (of which Hodgkin's disease, lymphoblastic lymphoma, and malignant germ cell tumors are three examples). Caution is advised in the presumption that a tumor has recurred in the thymus of patients who have recently completed chemotherapy and are otherwise doing well.

Large thymuses in children are occasionally resected in order to rule out a neoplasm; among 19 such cases reviewed by Lack, 17 were histologically normal and were within normal weight limits for age on the basis of standard morphometric data.[283] Two cases represented true thymic hyperplasia (large size with normal microscopic appearance).[283] True hyperplasia is amenable to successful surgical extirpation,[283, 284] but the need for doing so has been questioned.[3]

Follicular or lymphoid hyperplasia of the thymus is a separate condition in which lymphoid follicles with germinal centers are present and is the abnormality typically seen in myasthenia gravis[285] with or without associated thymoma.

Ectopic or aberrant thymus is a rare form of mediastinal mass in children and an even rarer cause of respiratory distress. Abnormal embryologic development allows thymic tissue to appear ectopically in the nasopharynx, neck, chest, or abdomen.[286] In rare instances, paratracheal posterior mediastinal aberrant thymus causes respiratory distress.[287–289] (Fig. 65–10).

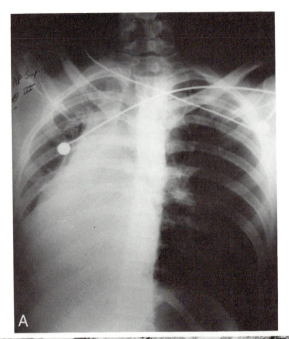

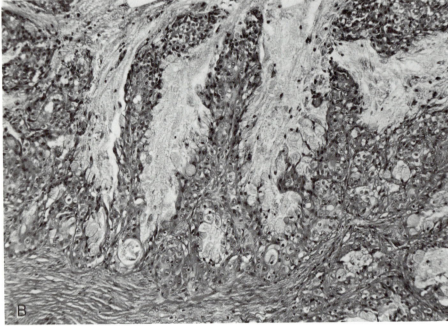

Figure 65–8. Mucoepidermoid carcinoma of the bronchus. *A*, Chest radiograph of a 14-year-old male with bouts of pneumonia. *B*, Copious mucus production is accompanied by the proliferation of bland-appearing mucinous and intermediate cells, which are the findings in a low-grade mucoepidermoid carcinoma. Hematoxylin and eosin, ×150. (Washington University Illustration #89-7751)

Thymic cysts are a rare cause of anterior mediastinal mass (and may occur at other sites of aberrant thymic tissue). The diagnosis requires thoracotomy especially to distinguish simple cysts from a cystic thymoma, Hodgkin's disease, or teratoma.[290–293]

Thymolipoma is a rare, benign, encapsulated anterior mediastinal tumor in which large islands of fat are interspersed with normal thymic tissue.[42, 294, 295] Although rare, most cases occur in children or young adults.[295] Respiratory distress may occur, or the lesion may be found incidentally on chest radiographs.

Thymoma is rare in children, most often has an aggressive course, and is therefore discussed with the malignant neoplasms.

Langerhans cell histiocytosis (histiocytosis X) was dis-

cussed earlier in reference to parenchymal lung involvement, but this proliferative disorder may manifest as an isolated anterior mediastinal mass.[296] In other cases, it is the initial manifestation of multisystem involvement, as in one 15-month-old patient.[297]

Histoplasmosis is an important cause of benign anterior and middle mediastinal masses in children because its clinical manifestation simulates lymphoma. Most masses resulting from *Histoplasma capsulatum* infection are in the middle mediastinum and are discussed in the following section; conversely, most lymphomas are in the anterior mediastinum and are discussed with the malignant processes.

Anterior mediastinal teratoma may be classified as either mature ("benign"), frankly malignant, or imma-

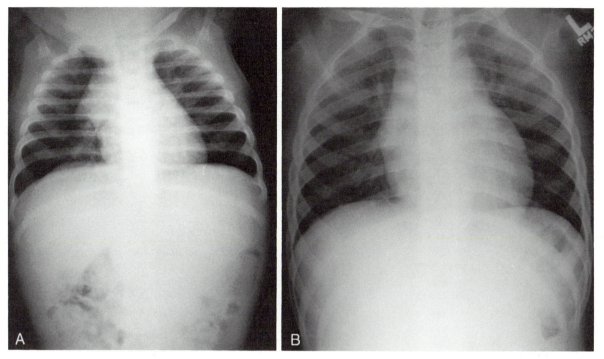

Figure 65–9. Unusual thymic silhouettes. *A*, Right sail sign in a 7-month-old. *B*, Prominent thymus in a 4-year-old. This configuration is probably acceptable to age 5 years in an otherwise normal child.

ture with an indeterminate prognosis. Carter and associates reviewed the literature and suggested that patients under 15 years of age with immature teratomas do well, whereas this same neoplasm in older patients behaves in a malignant manner.[298] Cervical teratomas may extend into the anterior mediastinum in newborns; these lesions may be associated with fetal hydrops, profound respiratory distress, polyhydramnios, and pleural effusions.[111]

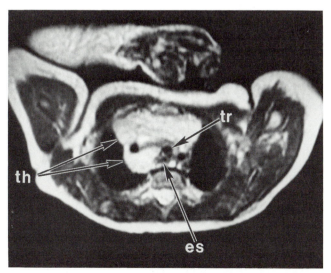

Figure 65–10. Ectopic thymus in a 4-month-old child with cough and stridor. Bronchoscopy revealed extrinsic compression of the distal trachea from the right. MRI scan reveals posterior extension of thymus (th) adjacent to trachea (tr). Stridor was relieved after surgical removal of this paratracheal tissue, which was histologically normal thymus. (es, esophagus).

Anterior mediastinal lipomas (composed of adult fat cells) and lipoblastomas (composed of fetal fat cells resembling hibernomas) are rare benign tumors amenable to surgical cure. The lipoblastomas occur usually in children under 3 years of age,[299] whereas lipomas have occurred only in children over three years of age.[300]

Hemangiomas (hemangioendotheliomas) and lymphangiomas are hamartomatous vascular proliferations that can occur in the anterior, middle, or posterior mediastinum. The terms *hemangiomatosis* and *lymphangiomatosis* refer to the anatomic extent of the disease and imply no differences in the microscopic appearance. Hemangiomas are found in very young children, and rarely is the mediastinum the only site of disease.[301–305] Lymphangiomas (cystic hygromas) occur more often in older children in the neck with some mediastinal extension, but rare isolated mediastinal tumors occur even in older patients.[306] Chylothorax can occur with lymphangiomas.[95, 96, 306] Patients may present with respiratory distress or the lymphangioma may be discovered incidentally. The radiographic features are nonspecific, and the nature of the lesion is determined at surgery. Necrotic, hemorrhagic neuroblastoma in the mediastinum and the supraclavicular area has been reported to simulate cystic hygroma.[307]

Myofibromatoses (desmoid tumors) are benign proliferations of myofibroblasts and occur in a number of distinct clinical syndromes.[308–310] The musculoaponeurotic fibromatosis of the shoulder girdle is considered in the section on chest wall, diaphragm, and pleura. Fibromatosis of the mediastinum is rare in children. Although histologically benign, fibromatoses often have exceedingly ill-defined borders thus defying complete surgical resection and leading to a locally aggressive course.

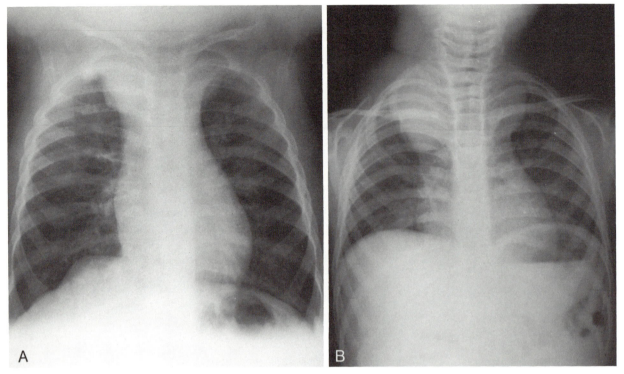

Figure 65–11. Neurofibromatosis of anterior mediastinum. *A,* Chest radiograph of boy with known neurofibromatosis at age 1 year. Neck masses and intrathoracic disease were present. *B,* Radiograph of same patient at age 3 years. Partial resection of neurofibromas was undertaken at ages 3 and 3½ years. Disease progressed, and the patient died of unresectable and extensive neck and superior thoracic involvement at age 8 years.

Ectopic thyroid tissue is rare in the chest[311] but has been reported as a substernal mass causing severe respiratory distress.[312]

Neurofibromatosis (von Recklinghausen's disease) usually spares the anterior mediastinum except in rare and devastating cases of extensive plexiform neurofibromas engulfing mediastinal structures and causing respiratory compromise (Fig. 65–11). The potential for this process should be anticipated in patients with neurofibromatosis and segmental cervical or mediastinal hypertrophy in whom highly vascular plexiform neurofibromas may be present; such lesions often lie deep to regions of hyperpigmented skin (darker than café au lait spots).[313, 314] Vagus nerve neurofibromas are discussed with the middle mediastinum.

MIDDLE MEDIASTINUM

The middle mediastinum contains the trachea and bronchi, paratracheal and parabronchial lymphoid tissue, and the heart and great vessels. Neoplasia of the airways is summarized in Table 65–2 and has been discussed in the section on airways.

Benign lymphoreticular proliferations and inflammatory or reactive lesions of the lymph nodes surrounding the airways constitute a complex and important group of pediatric conditions to be contrasted with the many malignant lesions in the same sites (see Table 65–3). Of particular importance is histoplasmosis, which affects the hilar nodes and the thymus. This condition simulates lymphoma, indistinguishable from the presenting clinical syndrome of fever, anorexia, weight loss, anemia, night sweats, and elevated sedimentation rate; lung infiltrates and nodal calcifications are seen in both conditions.[85, 90, 315] Respiratory compromise (tracheal compression) and pleural effusion may also be seen in both conditions and raises the disturbing possibility of emergency radiotherapy (for lymphoma) without biopsy.[90, 315] In the case reported by Brodeur and colleagues, the pleural fluid contained T lymphoblasts indistinguishable from the malignant T lymphoblasts of typical childhood T lymphoblastic lymphoma.[90] In a series of 37 cases, Gaebler and associates emphasized that histoplasmosis involved the middle mediastinum (21 of 21 cases) more often than did malignant lymphoma (8 of 16 cases). Malignant lymphoma more often affected the anterior mediastinum (11 of 16 cases) than did histoplasmosis (1 of 21 cases). In addition, high titers ($\geq 1:32$) to *Histoplasma* yeast or mycelial antigens or both differentiated patients with histoplasmosis from those with lymphoma.[85] Isolated anterior mediastinal histoplasmosis has been recognized.[315] A biopsy is strongly recommended when the diagnosis is unclear and when biopsy can be performed safely. Difficulties with anesthesia and the impact of empiric radiation on ultimate diagnosis in critically ill patients with mediastinal masses are discussed with the malignant mediastinal masses.[312]

Fibrosing mediastinitis is a serious late complication of histoplasmosis and similar infectious processes (see Table 65–3) in the middle mediastinum. Extensive and progressive fibrotic and granulomatous reactions beginning in paratracheal lymph nodes may lead to widespread, life-threatening mediastinal fibrosis and are thought to represent a hypersensitivity response in the particular host, perhaps in conjunction with especially heavy inhalation exposures.[316] Pulmonary infarction was the presenting manifestation of mediastinal fibrosis in two children.[317] Malignant neoplasms causing extensive mediastinal fibrosis (nodular sclerosing Hodgkin's disease and certain non-Hodgkin's lymphomas) may pose a diagnostic problem even when biopsy specimens are examined.[318, 319]

Plasma-cell granuloma (inflammatory pseudotumor) has been discussed as an entity in lung parenchyma (Table 65–1). It occasionally involves the middle[144, 290] and posterior[146] divisions of the mediastinum and may be difficult to differentiate from fibrosing mediastinitis in the absence of granulomas.[3]

Giant lymph node hyperplasia (Castleman's disease) is a rare, benign proliferation of lymph nodes, usually in the paratracheal region. It is often associated with systemic symptoms and hyperimmunoglobulinemia, which usually disappears with surgical removal. The cause is unknown.[320–322]

Neurofibromatosis associated with unilateral or rare bilateral vagus nerve neurofibromas has been reported.[323]

POSTERIOR MEDIASTINUM

The posterior mediastinum is the site of the most common benign chest masses of childhood. Most of these lesions are paravertebral and are neurogenic or malformative in origin (Table 65–3). With CT scans, magnetic resonance imaging, and urine screening for catecholamine secretion, these benign lesions are often presumptively diagnosed in advance and must be treated surgically.

Hemangiomas and lymphangiomas (cystic hygromas) occur rarely as isolated posterior thoracic masses and have been discussed with anterior mediastinal masses.[302–304]

Posterior mediastinal ectopic thymus tissue may cause respiratory distress in infants and is discussed with the thymus (anterior mediastinum).[287, 324, 325]

Extramedullary hematopoiesis in chronic hemolytic anemias can cause extensive parpasinal widening progressing to spinal cord compression.[36, 86, 326–328] It occurs more often in adults, but it has been reported in young adults.[329]

Plasma-cell granuloma (inflammatory pseudotumor) has been discussed with lung parenchymal lesions[144] (Table 65–1) and can occur in the posterior mediastinum, causing esophageal obstruction.[146]

Malignant Processes

Primary intrathoracic malignancies in children most often involve the anterior mediastinum (thymic involvement with leukemia or lymphoma) and posterior mediastinum (neuroblastoma).[290]

ANTERIOR MEDIASTINUM

Many of the lymphoreticular malignancies of childhood can be expressed prominently or exclusively in the thymus. The morphologic, cytochemical, immunophenotypic, genotypic, and molecular genetic diversities and specificities for many of these processes are known but are beyond the scope of this discussion. Such precise classifications are essential for accurate diagnosis, prognosis, and therapy. These neoplasms may also manifest with pleural effusions (see Table 65–5).

Thymic involvement in children most often occurs in Hodgkin's disease, non-Hodgkin's lymphoblastic lymphoma (early T cell disease), and the leukemia/lymphoma syndrome (T cell or non–T cells acute lymphoblastic leukemia with prominent organomegaly). Mature T lymphomas (helper or suppressor cell lymphomas; peripheral T cell lymphomas) occur in the thymus on rare occasions in teenagers and have a tendency for parenchymal lung involvement.[216] Undifferentiated or small, noncleaved B cell lymphomas (classic monomorphic Burkitt type or pleomorphic type) rarely involve the mediastinum and have a predilection for Waldeyer's ring, the ileocecal region, and the bone marrow.[107, 108, 330] Somewhat more differentiated B cell non-Hodgkin's lymphomas (e.g., diffuse histiocytic lymphoma) frequently involve the thymus.[318, 319, 331]

The acute and chronic myelogenous leukemias seldom involve the thymus.[332, 333] The rare exceptions are monocytic leukemias, which have protean manifestations and may include anterior mediastinal masses.[334, 335] Chronic lymphocytic proliferations virtually never occur in childhood.

Respiratory distress and the superior vena cava syndrome are often the presenting signs of lymphoreticular thymic malignancies (Fig. 65–12). Histoplasmosis may also manifest with tracheal compression, although it involves the paratracheal nodes more often than the thymus.[85] Patients with severe respiratory compromise from thymic enlargement may require emergency radiation therapy or corticosteroids before undergoing biopsy. Although oncologists and radiotherapists always prefer a biopsy-proven diagnosis, such biopsies may pose an additional risk to these patients, and general anesthesia must be given with extreme care.[336–342] The alert and distressed but compensated patient may protect airway patency through physiologic, negative-pressure pulmonary mechanics only to have the airway collapse and be unsupportable after anesthesia commences.[339, 340] Fine-needle aspiration or biopsy of accessible lymph nodes with local anesthesia are alternatives to general anesthesia in high-risk patients.

Löffler and colleagues analyzed the impact of emergency prebiopsy radiation for respiratory distress on subsequent pathologic diagnosis in 19 patients.[312] In 8 of 19 patients, a pathologic diagnosis could not be made after emergency radiation. Five of these eight patients were under 20 years of age. A full course of empiric chemoradiotherapy for a presumed malignant diagnosis was given to all eight. In four patients a diagnosis was never established, and these patients were well 4½ to 8 years after treatment. In the four other patients, a diagnosis was made only after relapse of the malignancy (Hodgkin's lymphoma, lymphoblastic lymphoma, diffuse histiocytic lymphoma, seminoma). The three patients with lymphoma died despite having received definitive therapy for their presumed (later determined correct) diagnoses. The patient with seminoma was cured by appropriate germ-cell therapy administered after relapse.[312] Brodeur and

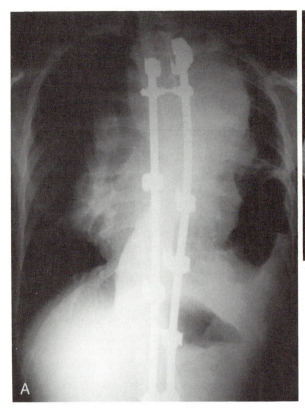

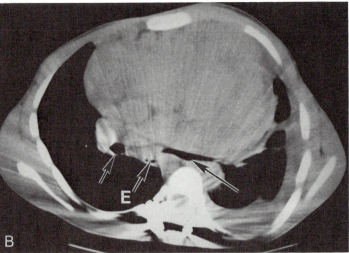

Figure 65–12. Hodgkin's disease with subcarinal bilateral bronchial compression. *A,* Fifteen-year-old male with familial scoliosis had experienced recent onset of cough and dyspnea when reclining. Chest radiograph shows large mediastinal mass, tracheal deviation, and left pleural effusion. *B,* Chest CT scan 3 cm below the carina shows anterior mediastinal mass with extreme compression of right bronchus intermedius and bifurcation of left main stem bronchus *(arrows).* Esophagus (E) is also displaced to right. The patient underwent biopsy of the supraclavicular node under local anesthesia.

associates reported a patient with histoplasmosis that caused a pleural effusion containing T lymphoblasts; this case emphasizes the difficulty of achieving diagnostic precision.[90]

The problem of residual or recurring masses after therapy for malignant anterior mediastinal masses has been discussed previously with benign thymomegaly. Such masses are not rare, are usually benign, and can be observed in otherwise well patients.[271, 272]

Thymoma is a rare but serious cause of anterior mediastinal enlargement in children and may cause cough, dyspnea, or superior vena cava syndrome.[343-345] Most thymomas in adults are benign, but in children they are often aggressive. Myasthenia gravis, aplastic anemia, and immunodeficiency are occasionally found in children with thymoma. Although the prognosis is usually guarded,[293, 346] some patients do well.[293, 347]

Malignant germ-cell tumors (malignant teratomas) constitute a heterogeneous but important group of anterior mediastinal tumors.[348, 349] The mature (benign) and immature teratomas have been discussed previously. Immature teratomas tend to respond to treatment in patients under 15 years of age but are more aggressive in older patients.[298] Markedly elevated levels of serum alpha-fetoprotein and human chorionic gonadotropin are indicative of a malignant teratoma (except for slightly increased alpha-fetoprotein with some mature teratomas or physiologic markedly increased alpha-fetoprotein in newborns). Lactate dehydrogenase is a nonspecific marker as well. Malignant teratomas contain one or more malignant histologic subtypes: embryonal carcinoma,[348]

endodermal sinus tumor (yolk sac tumor),[109, 350, 351] choriocarcinoma,[348] and germinoma (seminoma);[352] malignant tumors may also include mature or immature elements, but the presence of any malignant element dictates the expected behavior of the entire neoplasm.

The anterior mediastinum is a rare site for malignant soft tissue sarcomas in children (rhabdomyosarcoma, extraosseous Ewing's sarcoma, liposarcoma).[46, 353] The Intergroup Rhabdomyosarcoma Study identified only 10 mediastinal tumors among 646 total cases;[46] the specific mediastinal sites were not reported.

Carcinoid occurs very rarely within the thymus in children.[354] More likely, carcinoids are endobronchial (see Table 65–2).

MIDDLE MEDIASTINUM

Primary middle mediastinal malignancies in children most often involve the lymphoreticular diseases discussed previously (anterior mediastinum) and tumors of the heart, pericardium, and great vessels.[38-40] Sarcomas may arise from the aorta. These tumors represent a diverse histogenetic group, yet most neoplasms have a spindle-cell pattern. The authors have seen two examples of hemangiopericytoma of the great vessels in young children[355] (Fig. 65–13).

Metastatic disease to the middle mediastinum is not often considered pulmonary disease even though airway compression or superior vena cava syndrome occasionally occurs. Diseases metastasizing to hilar nodes are

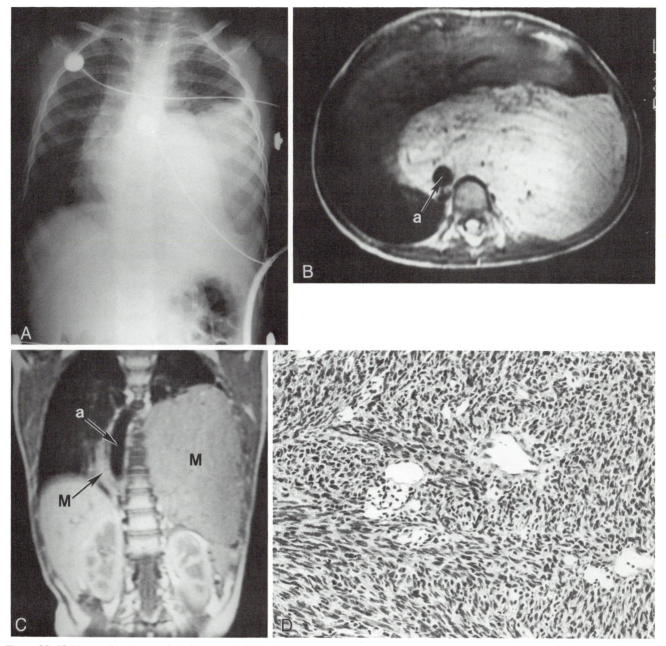

Figure 65–13. Hemangiopericytoma. *A*, Chest radiograph of a 4-year-old boy with a 1-day history of respiratory distress, showing large left lower thoracic density with some tracheal displacement. *B*, Axial MRI scan showing mass crossing midline and partially surrounding the descending aorta, causing it to deviate to right (a). *C*, Coronal MRI scan showing mass (M) in relation to descending aorta (a). *D*, Hemangiopericytoma of the aorta, showing a dense, spindle-cell proliferation with interspersed small vascular channels surrounded by neoplastic cells. The mass measured 12 × 12 × 8 cm. Hematoxylin and eosin, ×300. (Washington University Illustration #89-8697)

essentially those metastasizing to lung parenchyma, which were discussed earlier (see Table 65–1).

POSTERIOR MEDIASTINUM

The posterior mediastinum is the site of the most common childhood thoracic tumors, most of which are neurogenic in origin. Although not easily confused with pulmonary disease of the thorax, some of their unique features merit discussion.

Neuroblastoma and ganglioneuroblastoma constitute 75% to 90% of primary malignant posterior mediastinal tumors.[290, 356] Most occur in children under 4 years of age[356] (Fig. 65–14). They are often asymptomatic[357] but may cause spinal cord compression,[357–359] Horner's syndrome,[357] chronic diarrhea,[357] pain,[357] and the opsomyoclonus syndrome.[360] The outlook for children with thoracic neuroblastoma and ganglioneuroblastoma (50% to 88% survival rate) is better than that for children with tumors at other sites,[357–359, 361–363] but some authors believe that this phenomenon is attributable to the favorable prognostic influence of the low stage and young age at

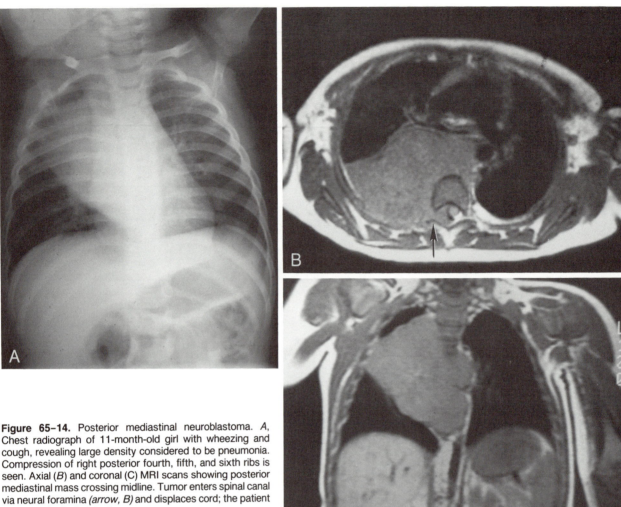

Figure 65–14. Posterior mediastinal neuroblastoma. *A,* Chest radiograph of 11-month-old girl with wheezing and cough, revealing large density considered to be pneumonia. Compression of right posterior fourth, fifth, and sixth ribs is seen. Axial (*B*) and coronal (C) MRI scans showing posterior mediastinal mass crossing midline. Tumor enters spinal canal via neural foramina *(arrow, B)* and displaces cord; the patient was neurologically intact.

which most of these children present.[364] The unusual association of cystic fibrosis and thoracic neuroblastoma has been reported in two infants.[365]

Paraspinal nodal involvement with spinal cord compression is an unfortunate consequence of many lymphoreticular malignancies. Nodular, central densities on chest radiographs should not be assumed to be hilar adenopathy; magnetic resonance imaging readily identifies paraspinal tumor with extension through neural foramina.[366] Early treatment with chemotherapy, radiation, or laminectomy may prevent spinal cord injury.[358, 359, 367–369]

CHEST WALL, DIAPHRAGM, AND PLEURA

Benign Lesions

Neoplastic disease of the chest wall, diaphragm, and pleura (see Table 65–4) can usually be identified by modern imaging techniques as arising from these anatomic structures. Such lesions can compromise pulmonary function through bulk mass effect and by causing pleural effusions (see Table 65–5).

MALFORMATIONS AND HAMARTOMAS

Mesenchymal hamartoma (mesenchymoma) is a benign overgrowth of skeletal elements of the chest wall occurring in neonates and infants under 1 year of age.[370–372] Respiratory compromise may be fatal. Wide surgical excision is generally recommended, but a more conservative approach has been suggested because the lesion may remain stable as the infant grows.[370]

Hemangioma and lymphangioma of the lung (see Table 65–1) and mediastinum (see Table 65–3) have been discussed earlier. Isolated hemangiomatosis of the pleura with recurrent life-threatening bloody pleural effusions and Kasabach-Merritt syndrome was reported in an infant who ultimately improved after cyclophosphamide therapy.[100]

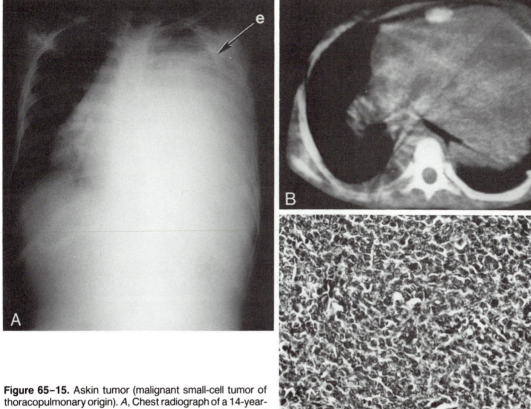

Figure 65–15. Askin tumor (malignant small-cell tumor of thoracopulmonary origin). *A,* Chest radiograph of a 14-year-old boy with dyspnea and asymmetry of the left external chest wall (e, effusion). *B,* Chest CT scan showing massive tumor with intra- and extrathoracic extensions (ex). *C,* Uniformly cellular neoplasm consisting of small cells. The tumor was immunoreactive for neuron-specific enolase and synaptophysin. Hematoxylin and eosin, ×120.

LYMPHORETICULAR, REACTIVE, AND INFECTIOUS PROLIFERATIONS

Langerhans cell histiocytosis has been discussed with diseases of the lung parenchyma (see Table 65–1) and the mediastinum (see Table 65–3). Bone lesions (eosinophilic granuloma of bone) can involve the ribs and be associated with pleural effusions.[98]

Extramedullary hematopoiesis causing isolated pleural masses without adjacent gross bony changes occurs occasionally in severe beta-thalassemia (intermedia and homozygous) and hemoglobin E thalassemia.[86]

TUMORS

Pleural fibromas (solitary fibrous tumors of the pleura) are very rare in children, but many cases in adults have been reviewed.[3, 373] These lesions are considered by some authors as benign mesotheliomas,[373] but they may be locally aggressive.[374]

Myofibromatosis (generalized fibromatosis, musculoaponeurotic fibromatosis) is a group of uncommon benign fibroblastic or myofibroblastic proliferations that can occur in the chest wall.[308–310] Congenital lesions of the chest wall occur,[373] and shoulder girdle lesions may appear in the second decade of life.[375] These lesions may be locally invasive, unresectable, and fatal if they entangle the airways. When surgical treatment is not possible, radiation and chemotherapy have been suggested.[376–378]

Malignant Lesions

PRIMARY NEOPLASMS

Primary malignant mesothelioma of the pleura in children is extraordinarily rare.[112, 379–381] Four cases have been reported as second tumors after Wilms' tumor with or without chest radiation.[382]

Sarcomas of the chest wall are a diverse pathologic group. The osseous (rib) and extraosseous Ewing's sarcoma, small-cell tumors of the thoracopulmonary region in childhood (Askin's tumor), and peripheral neuroepithelial tumors of the chest wall are similar-appearing and possibly related neoplasms[52, 114, 115, 383–387] (Fig. 65–15).

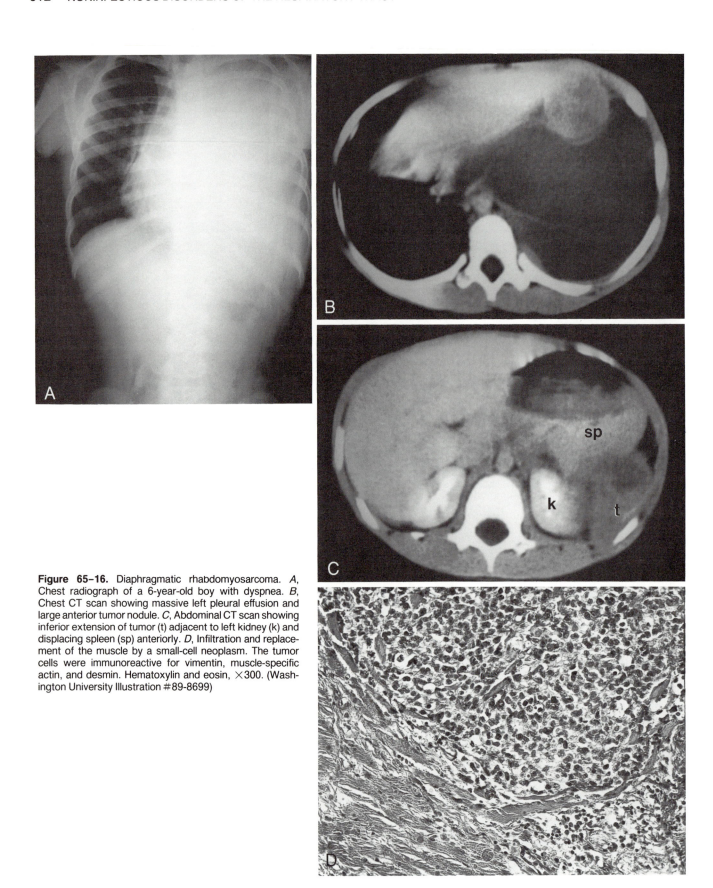

Figure 65–16. Diaphragmatic rhabdomyosarcoma. *A,* Chest radiograph of a 6-year-old boy with dyspnea. *B,* Chest CT scan showing massive left pleural effusion and large anterior tumor nodule. *C,* Abdominal CT scan showing inferior extension of tumor (t) adjacent to left kidney (k) and displacing spleen (sp) anteriorly. *D,* Infiltration and replacement of the muscle by a small-cell neoplasm. The tumor cells were immunoreactive for vimentin, muscle-specific actin, and desmin. Hematoxylin and eosin, ×300. (Washington University Illustration #89-8699)

Rhabdomyosarcoma, undifferentiated sarcomas, fibrosarcoma, synovial sarcoma, chondrosarcoma, osteogenic sarcoma, and extrarenal Wilms' tumor are less often encountered in this site.[384, 386, 388-391] These lesions may occur from infancy to adolescence and require aggressive multimodal therapy. Repetitive, iatrogenic pneumothorax with lung collapse has been used by one group as a means of preventing radiation pneumonitis during thoracic cage irradiation in such patients.[392]

Rhabdomyosarcoma of the diaphragm is a rare but distinct neoplasm that may manifest with respiratory distress, including pleural effusion[46, 393] (Fig. 65-16).

METASTASES TO CHEST WALL, DIAPHRAGM, AND PLEURA

Metastases of systemic malignancies to soft tissues of the chest wall are rare. Metastases to the ribs or vertebrae may occur with the many diseases that metastasize to bone. Metastatic malignancies to the pleura are more common in adults with carcinomas, which often metastasize to the pleura. However, among the common pediatric malignancies, Hodgkin's disease, non-Hodgkin's lymphoma, central nervous system tumors, rhabdomyosarcoma, Ewing's sarcoma, neuroblastoma (including stage IVS), and Wilms' tumor are known to metastasize to the pleura.[46, 115, 218, 357, 359, 370, 383, 394-397] Metastatic diseases causing pleural effusions are listed in Table 65-5. There is increasing understanding of the use of intracavitary chemotherapy to control pleural disease, and several safe agents are available.[398-400]

GLOSSARY

Tumor: A lump or mass without the implication of a proliferative or neoplastic process.

Neoplasia: An autonomous proliferation of tissue; the histologic examination may reveal either benign or malignant features. The clinical course invariably reflects the pathologic nature of the neoplasm.

Malignant: Histologic malignancy diagnosed on the basis of the presence of cytologic abnormalities, mitotic activity, degree of cellularity, invasiveness, and the potential to metastasize. It is also recognized that some neoplasms are not clearly benign or malignant and that their potential to behave aggressively is, therefore, borderline.

Benign: Histologic benignancy, so designated on the basis of pathologic critiera such as slight deviation in cytologic features and degree of cellularity. Benign tumors usually have circumscribed and often encapsulated borders. By definition, benign tumors lack the ability to metastasize, but they may locally infiltrate and expand into adjacent structures so as to compromise function and even, by local effects, threaten life.

Hamartoma: Tumefactions of developmental origin that represent an excessive proliferation of a particular cell type native to the structure of origin. The proliferation is histologically normal or nearly normal. Hamartomas are clinically benign in a pathologic sense and yet rarely have an aggressive or life-threatening clinical course through local damage. The growth of hamartomas eventually stabilizes or they even regress, but benign neoplasms have the capacity to continue to proliferate.

REFERENCES

1. Hartman GE, Shochat SJ: Primary pulmonary neoplasms of childhood: A review. Ann Thorac Surg 36:108–119, 1983.
2. Sutow WW: Malignant Solid Tumors in Children: A Review. New York: Raven Press, 1981.
3. Dehner LP: Pediatric Surgical Pathology. Baltimore, MD: Williams & Wilkins, 1987.
4. Sieber WK: Lung cysts, sequestration and bronchopulmonary dysplasia. In Welch KJ, Randolph JG, Ravitch MM, et al (eds): Pediatric Surgery, pp. 649–650. Chicago: Year Book Medical Publishers, 1986.
5. Rose RW, Ward BH: Spherical pneumonias in children simulating pulmonary and mediastinal masses. Radiology 106:179–182, 1973.
6. Koss MN, Hochholzer L, Nichols PW, et al: Primary non-Hodgkin's lymphoma and pseudolymphoma of lung: A study of 161 patients. Hum Pathol 14:1024–1038, 1983.
7. Ackerman LV, Taylor FH: Neurogenous tumors within the thorax. A clinicopathological evaluation of forty-eight cases. Cancer 4:669–691, 1951.
8. Kowalski P, Rodziewicz B, Pejcz J: Bilateral bronchioloalveolar carcinoma of the lungs in a 7 year old girl treated for Hodgkin's disease. Tumori 75:449–451, 1989.
9. Booth AJ, Tweed CS: Case report: Fatal pulmonary embolism due to osteogenic sarcoma in a child. Clin Radiol 40:533–535, 1989.
10. Zakowski MF, Edwards RH, McDonough ET: Wilms' tumor presenting as sudden death due to tumor embolism. Arch Pathol Lab Med 114:605–608, 1990.
11. Bartley TD, Arean VM: Intrapulmonary neurogenic tumors. J Thorac Cardiovasc Surg 50:114–123, 1965.
12. Yousem SA, Hochholzer L: Primary pulmonary hemangiopericytoma. Cancer 59:549–555, 1987.
13. Meade JB, Whitwell F, Bickford BJ, Waddington JK: Primary haemangiopericytoma of lung. Thorax 29:1–15, 1974.
14. Manning JT Jr, Ordoñez NG, Rosenberg HS, Walker WE: Pulmonary endodermal tumor resembling fetal lung. Arch Pathol Lab Med 109:48–50, 1985.
15. Fudge TL, Ochsner JL, Mills NL: Clinical spectrum of pulmonary hamartomas. Ann Thorac Surg 30:36–39, 1980.
16. Cohen SR, Geller KA, Seltzer S, Thompson JW: Papilloma of the larynx and tracheobronchial tree in children. A retrospective study. Ann Otol Rhinol Laryngol 89:497–503, 1980.
17. Ralph DD, Springmeyer SC, Sullivan KM, et al: Rapidly progressive air-flow obstruction in marrow transplant recipients. Possible association between obliterative bronchiolitis and chronic graft-versus-host disease. Am Rev Respir Dis 129:641–644, 1984.
18. Shermeta DW, Carter D, Haller JA Jr: Chondroma of the bronchus in childhood: A case report illustrating problems in diagnosis and management. J Pediatr Surg 10:545–548, 1975.
19. Oparah SS, Subramanian VA: Granular cell myoblastoma of the bronchus: Report of 2 cases and review of the literature. Ann Thorac Surg 22:199–202, 1976.
20. Sawada K, Fukuma S, Karasawa K, Suchi T: Granular cell myoblastoma of the bronchus in a child: A case report. Jpn J Surg 11:111–114, 1981.
21. Lack EE, Harris GB, Eraklis AJ, Vawter GF: Primary bronchial tumors in childhood. A clinicopathologic study of six cases. Cancer 51:492–497, 1983.
22. Taylor TL, Miller DR: Leiomyoma of the bronchus. J Thorac Cardiovasc Surg 57:284–288, 1969.
23. Yellin A, Rosenman Y, Lieberman Y: Review of smooth muscle tumours of the lower respiratory tract. Br J Dis Chest 78:337–351, 1984.
24. Jamieson MP, McGowan AR: Endobronchial teratoma. Thorax 37:157–159, 1982.
25. Stringel G, Shandling B, Mancer K, Ei SH: Lipoblastoma in infants and children. J Pediatr Surg 17:277–280, 1982.

26. Chaput M, Ninane J, Gosseye S, et al: Juvenile laryngeal papillomatosis and epidermoid carcinoma. J Pediatr 114:269–272, 1989.

27. Kawanami T, Bowen A: Juvenile laryngeal papillomatosis with pulmonary parenchymal spread. Case report and review of the literature. Pediatr Radiol 15:102–104, 1985.

28. Gindhart TD, Johnston WH, Chism SE, Dedo HH: Carcinoma of the larynx in childhood. Cancer 46:1683–1687, 1980.

29. Laurian N, Sadov R, Strauss M, Kessler E: Laryngeal carcinoma in childhood. Report of a case and review of the literature. Laryngoscope 94:684–687, 1984.

30. Shvero J, Hadar T, Segal K, et al: Laryngeal carcinoma in patients 40 years of age and younger. Cancer 60:3092–3095, 1987.

31. Cohen SR, Thompson JW, Siegel SE: Non-Hodgkin's lymphoma of the larynx in children. Ann Otol Rhinol Laryngol 96:357–361, 1987.

32. Carr T, Stevens RF, Marsden HB, et al: An unusual presentation of non-Hodgkin's lymphoma (NHL) in a child. Eur J Surg Oncol 12:193–195, 1986.

33. Morgan K, MacLennan KA, Narula A, et al: Non-Hodgkin's lymphoma of the larynx (Stage IE). Cancer 64:1123–1127, 1989.

34. Dail DH, Liebow AA, Gmelich JT, et al: Intravascular, bronchiolar, and alveolar tumor of the lung (IVBAT). An analysis of twenty cases of a peculiar sclerosing endothelial tumor. Cancer 51:452–464, 1983.

35. Miettinen M, Collan Y, Halttunen P, et al: Intravascular bronchioloalveolar tumor. Cancer 60:2471–2475, 1987.

36. Tokumitsu S, Tokumitsu K, Kohnoe K, et al: Extramedullary hematopoiesis presenting as mediastinal tumor. Acta Pathol Jpn 30:315–322, 1980.

37. Watterson J, Heisel M, Cich JA, Priest JR: Intrathoracic extravasation of sclerosing agents associated with central venous catheters. Am J Pediatr Hematol Oncol 10:249–251, 1988.

38. Chan HSL, Sonley MJ, Möes CA, et al: Primary and secondary tumors of childhood involving the heart, pericardium, and great vessels. A report of 75 cases and review of the literature. Cancer 56:825–836, 1985.

39. Schmaltz AA, Apitz J: Primary heart tumors in infancy and childhood. Report of four cases and review of literature. Cardiology 67:12–22, 1981.

40. Barnes WSF, Craft AW, Hunter AS, Stiller CA: Primary malignant cardiac tumors in children. Pediatr Hematol Oncol 3:347–351, 1986.

41. Schaffer MS, Zuberbuhler P, Wilson G, et al: Catecholamine cardiomyopathy: An unusual presentation of pheochromocytoma in children. J Pediatr 99:276–279, 1981.

42. Ravitch MM: Mediastinal cysts and tumors. In Welch KJ, Randolph JG, Ravitch MM, et al: (eds): Pediatric Surgery, pp. 602–618. Chicago: Year Book Medical Publishers, 1986.

43. Bentley JFR, Smith JR: Developmental posterior enteric remnants and spinal malformations. Arch Dis Child 35:76–86, 1960.

44. Weimann RB, Hallman GL, Bahar D, Greenberg SD: Intrathoracic meningocele. Case report and review of the literature. J Thorac Cardiovasc Surg 46:40–49, 1963.

45. Grosfeld JL, Weinberger M, Kilman JW, Clatworthy HW Jr: Primary mediastinal neoplasms in infants and children. Ann Thorac Surg 12:179–190, 1971.

46. Crist WM, Raney RB, Newton W, et al: Intrathoracic soft tissue sarcomas in children. Cancer 50:598–604, 1982.

47. Kent EM, Blades B, Valle AR, Graham EA: Intrathoracic neurogenic tumors. J Thorac Surg 13:116–161, 1944.

48. Hodgkinson DJ, Telander RL, Sheps SG, et al: Extra-adrenal intrathoracic functioning paraganglioma (pheochromocytoma) in childhood. Mayo Clin Proc 55:271–276, 1980.

49. Odze R, Bégin LR: Malignant paraganglioma of the posterior mediastinum. A case report and review of the literature. Cancer 65:564–569, 1990.

50. Misugi K, Okajima H, Newton WA Jr, et al: Mediastinal origin of a melanotic progonoma or retinal anlage tumor. Ultrastructural evidence for neural crest origin. Cancer 18:477–484, 1965.

51. Pokorny WJ, Sherman JO: Mediastinal masses in infants and children. J Thorac Cardiovasc Surg 68:869–875, 1974.

52. Kozlowski K, Beluffi G, Cohen DH, et al: Primary bone tumours in infants. Short literature review and report of 10 cases. Pediatr Radiol 15:359–367, 1985.

53. Clemons RL, Blank RH, Hutcheson JB, Ruffolo EH: Chordoma presenting as a posterior mediastinal mass. A choristoma. J Thorac Cardiovasc Surg 63:922–924, 1972.

54. Anderson KD: Congenital diaphragmatic hernia. In Welch KJ, Randolph JG, Ravitch MM, et al (eds): Pediatric Surgery, pp. 589–593. Chicago: Year Book Medical Publishers, 1986.

55. McCarthy EF, Dorfman HD: Vascular and cartilaginous hamartoma of the ribs in infancy with secondary aneurysmal bone cyst formation. Am J Surg Pathol 4:247–253, 1980.

56. Waldvogel FA, Papageorgiou PS: Osteomyelitis: The past decade. N Engl J Med 303:360–370, 1980.

57. Joseph WL, Fonkalsrud EW: Primary rib tumors in children. Am Surg 38:338–342, 1972.

58. Marcove RC, Huvos AG: Cartilaginous tumors of the ribs. Cancer 27:794–801, 1971.

59. Wiener MF, Chou WH: Primary tumors of the diaphragm. Arch Surg 90:143–152, 1965.

60. Howat AJ, Thomas H, Waters KD, Campbell PE: Malignant lymphoma of bone in children. Cancer 59:335–339, 1987.

61. Mayer CMH, Favara BE, Holton CP, Rainer WG: Malignant mesenchymoma in infants. Am J Dis Child 128:847–850, 1974.

62. Darling DB, Segi K, MacMahon HE: Malignant mesenchymoma of pleura in infancy. Report of a case. JAMA 199:848–849, 1967.

63. Ueda K, Gruppo R, Unger F, et al: Rhabdomyosarcoma of lung arising in congenital cystic adenomatoid malformation. Cancer 40:383–388, 1977.

64. Krous HF, Sexauer CL: Embryonal rhabdomyosarcoma arising within a congenital bronchogenic cyst in a child. J Pediatr Surg 16:506–508, 1981.

65. Allan BT, Day DL, Dehner LP: Primary pulmonary rhabdomyosarcoma of the lung in children. Report of two cases presenting with spontaneous pneumothorax. Cancer 59:1005–1011, 1987.

66. Williams RA: Embryonal rhabdomyosarcoma occurring in cystic adenomatoid malformation. Pediatr Pathol 5:118–119, 1986.

67. Shariff S, Thomas JA, Shetty N, D'Cunha S: Primary pulmonary rhabdomyosarcoma in a child, with a review of the literature. J Surg Oncol 38:261–264, 1988.

68. Hedlund GL, Bisset GS III, Bove KE: Malignant neoplasms arising in cystic hamartomas of the lung in childhood. Radiology 173:77–79, 1989.

69. Eigen H, Wyszomierski D: Bleomycin lung injury in children. Pathophysiology and guidelines for management. Am J Pediatr Hematol Oncol 7:71–78, 1985.

70. Kuritzky P, Conti DR, Vance JW: Cavitary pulmonary Hodgkin disease. Association with digital clubbing. JAMA 234:1166–1167, 1975.

71. Baten M, Vannucci RC: Intraspinal metastatic disease in childhood cancer. J Pediatr 90:207–212, 1977.

72. Carr I: The Ophelia syndrome: Memory loss in Hodgkin's disease. Lancet 1:844–845, 1982.

73. Watterson J, Priest JR: Jaundice as a paraneoplastic phenomenon in a T-cell lymphoma. Gastroenterology 97:1319–1322, 1989.

74. Bergeron C, Dauriac C, Desrues B, et al: Image pulmonaire excavée revelatrice d'une maladie de Hodgkin. Ann Med Interne (Paris) 140:53–55, 1989.

75. Leone G, Castellana M, Rabitti C, et al: Escavative pulmonary Hodgkin's lymphoma: Diagnosis by cutting needle biopsy. Eur J Haematol 44:139–141, 1990.

76. Traweek ST, Rotter AJ, Swartz W, Azumi N: Cystic pulmonary metastatic sarcoma. Cancer 65:1805–1811, 1990.

77. Silverman FN (ed): Caffey's Pediatric X-Ray Diagnosis: An Integrated Imaging Approach. Chicago: Year Book Medical Publishers, 1985.

78. Sty JR, Starshak RJ, Miller JH: Pediatric nuclear medicine. Norwalk, CT: Appleton-Century-Crofts, 1987.

79. Stokes DC, Shenep JL, Parham D, et al: Role of flexible bronchoscopy in the diagnosis of pulmonary infiltrates in pediatric patients with cancer. J Pediatr 115:561–567, 1989.

80. Heurlin N, Lönnqvist B, Tollemar J, Ehrnst A: Fiberoptic bronchoscopy for diagnosis of opportunistic pulmonary infections after bone marrow transplantation. Scand J Infect Dis 21:359–366, 1989.

81. Leskinen R, Taskinen E, Volin L, et al: Use of bronchoalveolar lavage cytology and determination of protein contents in pulmonary complications of bone marrow transplant recipients. Bone Marrow Transplant 5:241–245, 1990.

82. Allen JN, Pacht ER, Gadek JE, Davis WB: Acute eosinophilic pneumonia as a reversible cause of noninfectious respiratory failure. N Engl J Med 321:569–574, 1989.

83. Greenburg M, Schiffman RL, Geha DG: Acute eosinophilic pneumonia. N Engl J Med 322:635, 1990.

84. Wisecarver J, Ness MJ, Rennard SI, et al: Bronchoalveolar lavage in the assessment of pulmonary Hodgkin's disease. Acta Cytol 33:527–532, 1989.

85. Gaebler JW, Kleiman MB, Cohen M, et al: Differentiation of lymphoma from histoplasmosis in children with mediastinal masses. J Pediatr 104:706–709, 1984.

86. Weatherall DJ, Clegg JB: The Thalassaemia Syndromes. Oxford, England: Blackwell Scientific Publications, 1981.

87. Da Costa JL, Loh YS, Hanam E: Extramedullary hemopoiesis with multiple tumor-simulating mediastinal masses in hemoglobin E-thalassemia disease. Chest 65:210–212, 1974.

88. Magrath I, Lee YJ, Anderson T, et al: Prognostic factors in Burkitt's lymphoma. Importance of total tumor burden. Cancer 45:1507–1515, 1980.

89. Bosl GJ, Geller NL, Cirrincione C, et al: Multivariate analysis of prognostic variables in patients with metastatic testicular cancer. Cancer Res 43:3403–3407, 1983.

90. Brodeur GM, Wilber RB, Melvin SL, Murphy SB: Histoplasmosis mimicking childhood non-Hodgkin lymphoma. Med Pediatr Oncol 7:77–81, 1979.

91. Rao BN, Hayes FA, Thompson EI, et al: Chest wall resection for Ewing's sarcoma of the rib: An unnecessary procedure. Ann Thorac Surg 46:40–44, 1988.

92. Drexler HG, Gignac SM, Minowada J: Routine immunophenotyping of acute leukaemias. Blut 57:327–339, 1988.

93. Foon KA, Gale RP, Todd RF III: Recent advances in the immunologic classification of leukemia. Semin Hematol 23:257–283, 1986.

94. Griesser H, Tkachuk D, Reis MD, Mak TW: Gene rearrangements and translocations in lymphoproliferative diseases. Blood 73:1402–1415, 1989.

95. Berberich FR, Bernstein ID, Ochs HD, Schaller RT: Lymphangiomatosis with chylothorax. J Pediatr 87:941–942, 1975.

96. Morphis LG, Arcinue EL, Krause JR: Generalized lymphangioma in infancy with chylothorax. Pediatrics 46:566–575, 1970.

97. Ducharme JC, Belanger R, Simard P, Bazinet HP: Chylothorax, chylopericardium with multiple lymphangioma of bone. J Pediatr Surg 17:365–367, 1982.

98. Carlson RA, Hattery RR, O'Connell EJ, Fontana RS: Pulmonary involvement by histiocytosis X in the pediatric age group. Mayo Clin Proc 51:542–547, 1976.

99. Ishii E, Yamada S, Kano S, et al: Pulmonary and pleural involvements at initial diagnosis in children with malignant neoplasm. Am J Pediatr Hematol Oncol 11:281–285, 1989.

100. Hurvitz CH, Greenberg SH, Song CH, Gans SL: Hemangiomatosis of the pleura with hemorrhage and disseminated intravascular coagulation. J Pediatr Surg 17:73–75, 1982.

101. Lanham JG, Elkon KB, Pusey CD, Hughes GR: Systemic vasculitis with asthma and eosinophilia: A clinical approach to the Churg-Strauss syndrome. Medicine 63:65–81, 1984.

102. Gross NJ: Pulmonary effects of radiation therapy. Ann Intern Med 86:81–92, 1977.

103. Nelken RP, Stockman JA III: The hypereosinophilic syndrome in association with acute lymphoblastic leukemia. J Pediatr 89:771–773, 1976.

104. Chilcote RR, Coccia P, Sather HN, et al: Mediastinal mass in acute lymphoblastic leukemia. Med Pediatr Oncol 12:9–16, 1984.

105. Johnson DW, Hoppe RT, Cox RS, et al: Hodgkin's disease limited to intrathoracic sites. Cancer 52:8–13, 1983.

106. Alford BA, Coccia PF, L'Heureux PR: Roentgenographic features of American Burkitt's lymphoma. Radiology 124:763–770, 1977.

107. Ziegler JL, Magrath IT, Deisseroth AB, et al: Combined modality treatment of Burkitt's lymphoma. Cancer Treat Rep 62:2031–2034, 1978.

108. Brecher ML, Gardner RV, Ettinger LJ, et al: High-dose cyclophosphamide and intermediate-dose methotrexate for the treatment of far-advanced Burkitt's lymphoma. Am J Pediatr Hematol Oncol 7:117–124, 1985.

109. Kuzur ME, Cobleigh MA, Greco FA, et al: Endodermal sinus tumor of the mediastinum. Cancer 50:766–774, 1982.

110. Hijiya N, Horikawa R, Matsushita T, et al: Malignant mediastinal germ-cell tumors in childhood: A report of two cases achieving long-term disease-free survival. Am J Pediatr Hematol Oncol 11:437–440, 1989.

111. Jordan RB, Gauderer MW: Cervical teratomas: An analysis. Literature review and proposed classification. J Pediatr Surg 23:583–591, 1988.

112. Brenner J, Sordillo PP, Magill GB: Malignant mesothelioma in children: Report of seven cases and review of the literature. Med Pediatr Oncol 9:367–373, 1981.

113. Patel CC, Rees A, Bertolone SJ: Intracardiac extension of Wilms' tumor. Am J Pediatr Hematol Oncol 11:46–50, 1989.

114. Staalman CR: Ewing's sarcoma in rib. A report on 7 cases with special emphasis to the early roentgen findings. J Belge Radiol 65:329–337, 1982.

115. Thomas PR, Foulkes MA, Gilula LA, et al: Primary Ewing's sarcoma of the ribs. A report from the Intergroup Ewing's Sarcoma Study. Cancer 51:1021–1027, 1983.

116. Swank DW, Hepper NG, Folkert KE, Colby TV: Intrathoracic lymphangiomatosis mimicking lymphangioleiomyomatosis in a young woman. Mayo Clin Proc 64:1264–1268, 1989.

117. Mulliken JB, Young AE: Vascular Birthmarks. Hemangiomas and Malformations. Philadelphia: WB Saunders, 1988.

118. Dines DE, Arms RA, Bernatz PE, Gomes MR: Pulmonary arteriovenous fistulas. Mayo Clin Proc 49:460–465, 1974.

119. Koerper MA, Addiego JE Jr, deLorimier AA, et al: Use of aspirin and dipyridamole in children with platelet trapping syndromes. J Pediatr 102:311–314, 1983.

120. White CW, Sondheimer HM, Crouch EC, et al: Treatment of pulmonary hemangiomatosis with recombinant interferon alpha-2a. N Engl J Med 320:1197–1200, 1989.

121. Orchard PJ, Smith CM III, Woods WG, et al: Treatment of haemangioendotheliomas with alpha interferon. Lancet 2:565–567, 1989.

122. White CW: Treatment of hemangiomatosis with recombinant interferon alfa. Semin Hematol 27 (Suppl. 4):15–22, 1990.

123. Satoh Y, Tsuchiya E, Weng S, et al: Pulmonary sclerosing hemangioma of the lung. A type II pneumocytoma by immunohistochemical and immunoelectron microscopic studies. Cancer 64:1310–1317, 1989.

124. Bradley SL, Dines, DE, Soule EH, Muhm JR: Pulmonary lymphangiomyomatosis. Lung 158:69–80, 1980.

125. Taylor JR, Ryu J, Colby TV, Raffin TA: Lymphangioleiomyomatosis. Clinical course in 32 patients. N Engl J Med 323:1254–1260, 1990.

126. Hull MT, Gonzalez-Crussi F, Grosfeld JL: Multiple pulmonary fibroleiomyomatous hamartomata in childhood. J Pediatr Surg 14:428–431, 1979.

127. Poirier TJ, Van Ordstrand HS: Pulmonary chondromatous hamartomas. Report of seventeen cases and review of the literature. Chest 59:50–55, 1971.

128. Oldham HN, Young WG Jr, Sealy WC: Hamartoma of the lung. J Thorac Cardiovasc Surg 53:735–742, 1967.

129. Jones CJ: Unusual hamartoma of the lung in a newborn infant. Arch Pathol 48:150–154, 1949.

130. Gudbjerg CE: Pulmonary hamartoma. AJR 86:842–849, 1961.

131. Corrin B, Basset F: A review of histiocytosis X with particular reference to eosinophilic granuloma of the lung. Invest Cell Pathol 2:137–146, 1979.

132. Aftimos S, Nassar V, Najjar S: Primary pulmonary histiocytosis in an infant. Am J Dis Child 128:851–852, 1974.

133. Berlow ME, Markarian M, Heitzman ER, Raasch BN: Diffuse pulmonary disease in a 2½-year-old child. JAMA 248:875–876, 1982.

134. McDowell HP, MacFarlane PI, Martin J: Isolated pulmonary histiocytosis. Arch Dis Child 63:423–426, 1988.

135. Greenberger JS, Crocker AC, Vawter G, et al: Results of treatment of 127 patients with systemic histiocytosis (Letterer-Siwe syndrome, Schuller-Christian syndrome and multifocal eosinophilic granuloma). Medicine 60:311–338, 1981.

136. Liebow AA, Carrington CB: The eosinophilic pneumonias. Medicine 48:251–285, 1969.

137. Schatz M, Wasserman S, Patterson R: Eosinophils and immunologic lung disease. Med Clin North Am 65:1055–1071, 1981.

138. Meeker DP: Pulmonary infiltrates and eosinophilia revisited. Cleve Clin J Med 56:199–211, 1989.

139. Pulmonary eosinophilia [Editorial]. Lancet 335 (8688):512, 1990.
140. Lukens JN: Eosinophilia in children. Pediatr Clin North Am 19:969–981, 1972.
141. Mok CH: Visceral larva migrans. A discussion based on review of the literature. Clin Pediatr 7:565–573, 1968.
142. Bousquet J, Chanez P, LaCoste JY, et al: Eosinophilic inflammation in asthma. N Engl J Med 323:1033–1039, 1990.
143. Monzon CM, Gilchrist GS, Burgert EO, et al: Plasma cell granuloma of the lung in children. Pediatrics 70:268–274, 1982.
144. Berardi RS, Lee SS, Chen HP, Stines GJ: Inflammatory pseudotumors of the lung. Surg Gynecol Obstet 156:89–96, 1983.
145. Bahadori M, Liebow AA: Plasma cell granulomas of the lung. Cancer 31:191–208, 1973.
146. Hutchins GM, Eggleston JC: Unusual presentation of pulmonary inflammatory pseudotumor (plasma cell granuloma) as esophageal obstruction. Am J Gastroenterol 71:501–504, 1979.
147. Maier HC, Sommers SC: Recurrent and metastatic pulmonary fibrous histiocytoma/plasma cell granuloma in a child. Cancer 60:1073–1076, 1987.
148. Dajee A, Dajee H, Hinrichs S, Lillington G: Pulmonary chondroma, extra-adrenal paraganglioma, and gastric leiomyosarcoma. Carney's triad. J Thorac Cardiovasc Surg 84:377–381, 1982.
149. Yannopoulos K, Stout AP: Smooth muscle tumors in children. Cancer 15:958–971, 1962.
150. Tan AM, Downie PJ, Ekert H: Hypereosinophilia syndrome with pneumonia in acute lymphoblastic leukaemia. Aust Paediatr J 23:359–361, 1987.
151. Gaynon PS, Gonzalez-Crussi F: Exaggerated eosinophilia and acute lymphoid leukemia. Am J Pediatr Hematol Oncol 6:334–337, 1984.
152. Cordonnier C, Vernant JP, Brun B, et al: Acute promyelocytic leukemia in 57 previously untreated patients. Cancer 55:18–25, 1985.
153. Halperin DS, Oberhansli I, Siegrist CA, et al: Intrathoracic neuroblastoma presenting with neonatal cardiorespiratory distress. Chest 85:822–823, 1984.
154. Cohen M, Smith WL, Weetman R, Provisor A: Pulmonary pseudometastases in children with malignant tumors. Radiology 141:371–374, 1981.
155. Omar R, Davidian MM, Marcus JR, Rose J: Significance of the "maturation" of metastases from Wilms' tumor after therapy. J Surg Oncol 33:239–242, 1986.
156. Alvarez Silvan AM, Gonzalez del Castillo J, Martinez Caro A, et al: Maturation of Wilms' tumor pulmonary metastases to benign fibromas after therapy. Med Pediatr Oncol 12:218–220, 1984.
157. Stine KC, Friedman HS, Kurtzberg J, et al: Pulmonary septic emboli mimicking metastatic rhabdomyosarcoma. J Pediatr Surg 24:491–493, 1989.
158. Shaw PJ, Eden OB: Pulmonary infection mimicking metastases in Ewing's sarcoma. Pediatr Hematol Oncol 7:213–215, 1990.
159. Yang YM, Wheeler VR, Mankad VN: Pulmonary lipid nodules after intralipid infusion in a child with rhabdomyosarcoma and Staphylococcus epidermidis sepsis. Am J Pediatr Hematol Oncol 12:231–236, 1990.
160. Nachman JB, Baum ES, White H, Crussi FG: Bleomycin-induced pulmonary fibrosis mimicking recurrent metastatic disease in a patient with testicular carcinoma: Case report of the CT scan appearance. Cancer 47:236–239, 1981.
161. Scharstein R, Johnson JF, Cook BA, Stephenson SR: Bleomycin nodules mimicking metastatic osteogenic sarcoma. Am J Pediatr Hematol Oncol 9:219–221, 1987.
162. McCrea ES, Diaconis JN, Wade JC, Johnston C: Bleomycin toxicity simulating metastatic nodules to the lung. Cancer 48:1096–1100, 1981.
163. O'Driscoll BR, Hasleton PS, Taylor PM, et al: Active lung fibrosis up to 17 years after chemotherapy with carmustine (BCNU) in childhood. N Engl J Med 323:378–382, 1990.
164. Limper AH, McDonald JA: Delayed pulmonary fibrosis after nitrosourea therapy. N Engl J Med 323:407–409, 1990.
165. Andersson BS, Luna MA, Yee C, et al: Fatal pulmonary failure complicating high-dose cytosine arabinoside therapy in acute leukemia. Cancer 65:1079–1084, 1990.
166. Gockerman JP: Drug-induced interstitial lung diseases. Clin Chest Med 3:521–536, 1982.
167. Ginsberg SJ, Comis RL: The pulmonary toxicity of antineoplastic agents. Semin Oncol 9:34–51, 1982.
168. Cooper JA, White DA, Matthay RA: Drug-induced pulmonary disease. Part 1: Cytotoxic drugs. Am Rev Respir Dis 133:321–340, 1986.
169. Cooper JA Jr, Matthay RA: Drug-induced pulmonary disease. Dis Mon 33:61–120, 1987.
170. Cooper JA Jr, Zitnik RJ, Matthay RA: Mechanisms of drug-induced pulmonary disease. Annu Rev Med 39:395–404, 1988.
171. Ganick DJ, Peters ME, Hafez GR: Acute bleomycin toxicity. Am J Pediatr Hematol Oncol 2:249–252, 1980.
172. Jones SE, Moore M, Blank N, Castellino RA: Hypersensitivity to procarbazine (Matulane®) manifested by fever and pleuropulmonary reaction. Cancer 29:498–500, 1972.
173. Rubin P: The Franz Buschke Lecture: Late effects of chemotherapy and radiation therapy: A new hypothesis. Int J Radiat Oncol Biol Phys 10:5–34, 1984.
174. McKeage MJ, Evans BD, Atkinson C, et al: Carbon monoxide diffusing capacity is a poor predictor of clinically significant bleomycin lung. J Clin Oncol 8:779–783, 1990.
175. Comis RL: Detecting bleomycin pulmonary toxicity: A continued conundrum. J Clin Oncol 8:765–767, 1990.
176. McLeod BF, Lawrence HJ, Smith DW, et al: Fatal bleomycin toxicity from a low cumulative dose in a patient with renal insufficiency. Cancer 60:2617–2620, 1987.
177. Goldiner PL, Schweizer O: The hazards of anesthesia and surgery in bleomycin-treated patients. Semin Oncol 6:121–124, 1979.
178. Goldiner PL, Carlon GC, Cvitkovic E, et al: Factors influencing postoperative morbidity and mortality in patients treated with bleomycin. Br Med J 1:1664–1667, 1978.
179. Gross NJ: The pathogenesis of radiation-induced lung damage. Lung 159:115–125, 1981.
180. Kun LE, Moulder JE: General principles of radiation therapy. In Pizzo PA, Poplack DG (eds): Principles and Practice of Pediatric Oncology, pp. 233–254. Philadelphia: JB Lippincott, 1989.
181. Green DM, Finklestein JZ, Tefft ME, Norkool P: Diffuse interstitial pneumonitis after pulmonary irradiation for metastatic Wilms' tumor. A report from the National Wilms' Tumor Study. Cancer 63:450–453, 1989.
182. Desablens B, Venet P, Muir JF: Pneumothorax apres radiotherapie pour maladie de Hodgkin. Ann Med Interne (Paris) 140:52–53, 1989.
183. Pezner RD, Horak DA, Sayegh HO, Lipsett JA: Spontaneous pneumothorax in patients irradiated for Hodgkin's disease and other malignant lymphomas. Int J Radiat Oncol Biol Phys 18:193–198, 1990.
184. Littman P, Meadows AT, Polgar G, et al: Pulmonary function in survivors of Wilms' tumor. Patterns of impairment. Cancer 37:2773–2776, 1976.
185. Benoist MR, Lemerle J, Jean R, et al: Effects on pulmonary function of whole lung irradiation for Wilms' tumour In children. Thorax 37:175–180, 1982.
186. Wohl ME, Griscom NT, Traggis DG, Jaffe N: Effects of therapeutic irradiation delivered in early childhood upon subsequent lung function. Pediatrics 55:507–516, 1975.
187. Miller RW, Fusner JE, Fink RJ, et al: Pulmonary function abnormalities in long-term survivors of childhood cancer. Med Pediatr Oncol 14:202–207, 1986.
188. Shaw NJ, Tweeddale PM, Eden OB: Pulmonary function in childhood leukaemia survivors. Med Pediatr Oncol 17:149–154, 1989.
189. Weiner RS, Bortin MM, Gale RP, et al: Interstitial pneumonitis after bone marrow transplantation. Assessment of risk factors. Ann Intern Med 104:168–175, 1986.
190. Vega RA, Franco CM, Abdel-Mageed AM, Ragab AH: Bone marrow transplantation in the treatment of children with cancer. Current Status. Hematol Oncol Clin North Am 1:777–800, 1987.
191. Clark JG, Crawford SW, Madtes DK, Sullivan KM: Obstructive lung disease after allogeneic marrow transplantation. Clinical presentation and course. Ann Intern Med 111:368–376, 1989.
192. Wright DG, Robichaud KJ, Pizzo PA, Deisseroth AB: Lethal pulmonary reactions associated with the combined use of amphotericin B and leukocyte transfusions. N Engl J Med 304:1185–1189, 1981.
193. Strauss RG, Connett JE, Gale RP, et al: Controlled trial of prophylactic granulocyte transfusions during initial induction chemotherapy for acute myelogenous leukemia. N Engl J Med 305:597–603, 1981.

194. Dana BW, Durie BG, White RF, Huestis DW: Concomitant administration of granulocyte transfusions and amphotericin B in neutropenic patients: Absence of significant pulmonary toxicity. Blood 57:90–94, 1981.
195. Forman SJ, Robinson GV, Wolf JL, et al: Pulmonary reactions associated with amphotericin B and leukocyte transfusions. N Engl J Med 305:584–585, 1981.
196. Dutcher JP, Kendall J, Norris D, et al: Granulocyte transfusion therapy and amphotericin B: Adverse reactions? Am J Hematol 31:102–108, 1989.
197. DeGregorio MW, Lee WMF, Ries CA: Pulmonary reactions associated with amphotericin B and leukocyte transfusions. N Engl J Med 305:585, 1981.
198. Boxer LA, Ingraham LM, Allen J, et al: Amphotericin-B promotes leukocyte aggregation of nylon-wool-fiber-treated polymorphonuclear leukocytes. Blood 58:518–523, 1981.
199. Manivel JC, Priest JR, Watterson J, et al: Pleuropulmonary blastoma. The so-called pulmonary blastoma of childhood. Cancer 62:1516–1526, 1988.
200. Thomas WJ, Koenig HM, Ellwanger FR, Lightsey AL: Primary pulmonary rhabdomyosarcoma in childhood. Am J Dis Child 135:469–471, 1981.
201. Stephanopoulos C, Catsaras H: Myxosarcoma complicating a cystic hamartoma of the lung. Thorax 18:144–145, 1963.
202. Weinberg AG, Currarino G, Moore GC, Votteler TP: Mesenchymal neoplasia and congenital pulmonary cysts. Pediatr Radiol 9:179–182, 1980.
203. Jimenez JF, Uthman EO, Townsend JW, et al: Primary bronchopulmonary leiomyosarcoma in childhood. Arch Pathol Lab Med 110:348–351, 1986.
204. Guccion JG, Rosen SH: Bronchopulmonary leiomyosarcoma and fibrosarcoma. A study of 32 cases and review of the literature. Cancer 30:836–847, 1972.
205. Pettinato G, Manivel JC, Saldana MJ, et al: Primary bronchopulmonary fibrosarcoma of childhood and adolescence: Reassessment of a low-grade malignancy. Clinicopathologic study of five cases and review of the literature. Hum Pathol 20:463–471, 1989.
206. Stuart-Harris R, Wills EJ, Philips J, et al: Extraskeletal Ewing's sarcoma: A clinical, morphological and ultrastructural analysis of five cases with a review of the literature. Eur J Cancer Clin Oncol 22:393–400, 1986.
207. Palmer RN, Saini N, Guccion J: Ewing's-like sarcoma appearing as a primary pulmonary neoplasm. Arch Pathol Lab Med 105:277–278, 1981.
208. Baroni CD, Mineo TC, Ricci C, et al: Solitary secretory plasmacytoma of the lung in a 14-year-old boy. Cancer 40:2329–2332, 1977.
209. L'Hoste RJ Jr, Filippa DA, Lieberman PH, Bretsky S: Primary pulmonary lymphomas. A clinicopathologic analysis of 36 cases. Cancer 54:1397–1406, 1984.
210. Sery Z: Pulmonary resection in children. Surgery 54:810–814, 1963.
211. Veliath AJ, Khanna KK, Subhas BS, et al: Primary lymphosarcoma of the lung with unusual features. Thorax 32:632–636, 1977.
212. Radin AI: Primary pulmonary Hodgkin's disease. Cancer 65:550–563, 1990.
213. Pound AW, Willis RA: A malignant teratoma of the lung in an infant. J Pathol 98:111–114, 1969.
214. Gautam HP: Intrapulmonary malignant teratoma. Am Rev Respir Dis 100:863–865, 1969.
215. Prauer HW, Mack D, Babic R: Intrapulmonary teratoma 10 years after removal of a mediastinal teratoma in a young man. Thorax 38:632–634, 1983.
216. Greer JP, York JC, Cousar JB, et al: Peripheral T-cell lymphoma: A clinicopathologic study of 42 cases. J Clin Oncol 2:788–798, 1984.
217. Hoffman HJ, Duffner PK: Extraneural metastases of central nervous system tumors. Cancer 56:1778–1782, 1985.
218. Duffner PK, Cohen ME: Extraneural metastases in childhood brain tumors. Ann Neurol 10:261–265, 1981.
219. Liote HA, Vedrenne C, Schlienger M, et al: Late pleuropulmonary metastases of a cerebral ependymoma. Chest 94:1097–1098, 1988.
220. Campbell AN, Chan HS, Becker LE, et al: Extracranial metastases in childhood primary intracranial tumors. Cancer 53:974–981, 1984.
221. Watterson J, Priest JR: Control of extraneural metastasis of a primary intracranial non-germinomatous germ cell tumor. J Neurosurg 71:601–604, 1989.
222. Pick T, Maurer HM, McWilliams NB: Lymphoepithelioma in childhood. J Pediatr 84:96–100, 1974.
223. Ahmad A, Stefani S: Distant metastases of nasopharyngeal carcinoma: A study of 256 male patients. J Surg Oncol 33:194–197, 1986.
224. Kyriakos M, Land VJ, Penning HL, Parker SG: Metastatic chondroblastoma. Report of a fatal case with a review of the literature on atypical, aggressive, and malignant chondroblastoma. Cancer 55:1770–1789, 1985.
225. Ramadas K, Jose CC, Subhashini J, et al: Pulmonary metastases from ameloblastoma of the mandible treated with cisplatin, Adriamycin and cyclophosphamide. Cancer 66:1475–1479, 1990.
226. Lester TJ, Johnson JW, Cuttner J: Pulmonary leukostasis as the single worst prognostic factor in patients with acute myelocytic leukemia and hyperleukocytosis. Am J Med 79:43–48, 1985.
227. Myers TJ, Cole SR, Klatsky AU, Hild DH: Respiratory failure due to pulmonary leukostasis following chemotherapy of acute non-lymphocytic leukemia. Cancer 51:1808–1813, 1983.
228. Mangal AK, Growe GH: Extensive pulmonary infiltration by leukemic blast cells treated with irradiation. Can Med Assoc J 128:424–426, 1983.
229. Corbaton J, Muñoz A, Madero L, Camerero C: Pulmonary leukemia in a child presenting with infiltrative and nodular lesions. Pediatr Radiol 14:431–432, 1984.
230. Wells RJ, Weetman RM, Ballantine TV, et al: Pulmonary leukemia in children presenting as diffuse interstitial pneumonia. J Pediatr 96:262–264, 1980.
231. Golde DW, Drew WL, Klein HZ, et al: Occult pulmonary haemorrhage in leukaemia. Br Med J 2:166–168, 1975.
232. Smevik B, Klepp O: The risk of spontaneous pneumothorax in patients with osteogenic sarcoma and testicular cancer. Cancer 49:1734–1737, 1982.
233. McKenna RJ, Schwinn CP, Soong KY, Higinbotham NL: Sarcomata of the osteogenic series (osteosarcoma, fibrosarcoma, chondrosarcoma, parosteal osteogenic sarcoma, and sarcomata arising in abnormal bone). An analysis of 552 cases. J Bone Joint Surg 48-A:1–26, 1966.
234. Beron G, Euler A, Winkler K: Pulmonary metastases from osteogenic sarcoma: Complete resection and effective chemotherapy contributing to improved prognosis. Eur Paediatr Haematol Oncol 2:77–85, 1985.
235. Meyer WH, Schell MJ, Kumar AP, et al: Thoracotomy for pulmonary metastatic osteosarcoma. An analysis of prognostic indicators of survival. Cancer 59:374–379, 1987.
236. Goorin AM, Delorey MJ, Lack EE, et al: Prognostic significance of complete surgical resection of pulmonary metastases in patients with osteogenic sarcoma: Analysis of 32 patients. J Clin Oncol 2:425–431, 1984.
237. Putnam JB Jr, Roth JA, Wesley MN, et al: Survival following aggressive resection of pulmonary metastases from osteogenic sarcoma: Analysis of prognostic factors. Ann Thorac Surg 36:516–523, 1983.
238. Logothetis CJ, Samuels ML, Trindade A, Johnson DE: The growing teratoma syndrome. Cancer 50:1629–1635, 1982.
239. Vugrin D, Whitmore WF Jr, Bains M, Golbey RB: Role of chemotherapy and surgery in the treatment of thoracic metastases from nonseminomatous germ cell testis tumor. Cancer 50:1057–1060, 1982.
240. Tiffany P, Morse MJ, Bosl G, et al: Sequential excision of residual thoracic and retroperitoneal masses after chemotherapy for stage III germ cell tumors. Cancer 57:978–983, 1986.
241. Donohue JP, Rowland RG: The role of surgery in advanced testicular cancer. Cancer 54:2716–2721, 1984.
242. Nakayama DK, Norkool P, deLorimier AA, et al: Intracardiac extension of Wilms' tumor. Ann Surg 204:693–697, 1986.
243. Ritchey ML, Kelalis PP, Breslow N, et al: Intracaval and atrial involvement with nephroblastoma: Review of National Wilms' Tumor Study-3. J Urol 140 (Pt. 2):1113–1118, 1988.
244. Hunt TM, Firmin RK, Johnstone MJ: Management of a patient with Wilms's tumour extending into the right heart chambers: A case report and a review of other published reports. Br Heart J 60:165–168, 1988.

245. Bracken RB, Sutow WW, Jaffe N, et al: Preoperative chemotherapy for Wilms tumor. Urology 19:55–60, 1982.
246. Bürger D, Moorman-Voestermans CG, Mildenberger H, et al: The advantages of preoperative therapy in Wilms' tumor. A summarized report on clinical trials conducted by the International Society of Paediatric Oncology (SIOP). Z Kinderchir 40:170–175, 1985.
247. Shurin SB, Gauderer MW, Dahms BB, Conrad WG: Fatal intraoperative pulmonary embolization of Wilms' tumor. J Pediatr 101:559–562, 1982.
248. D'Angio GJ, Evans A, Breslow N, et al: The treatment of Wilms' tumor: Results of the Second National Wilms' Tumor Study. Cancer 47:2302–2311, 1981.
249. Grundy P, Breslow N, Green DM, et al: Prognostic factors for children with recurrent Wilms' tumor: Results from the Second and Third National Wilms' Tumor Study. J Clin Oncol 7:638–647, 1989.
250. Sutow WW, Breslow NE, Palmer NF, et al: Prognosis in children with Wilms' tumor metastases prior to or following primary treatment. Results from the first National Wilms' Tumor Study. Am J Clin Oncol 5:339–347, 1982.
251. Towbin R, Gruppo RA: Pulmonary metastases in neuroblastoma. AJR 138:75–78, 1982.
252. Stigall R, Smith WL, Franken EA, et al: Intrapulmonic metastatic neuroblastoma. Ann Radiol (Paris) 22:223–227, 1979.
253. Glorieux P, Bouffet E, Philip I, et al: Metastatic interstitial pneumonitis after autologous bone marrow transplantation. A consequence of reinjection of malignant cells? Cancer 58:2136–2139, 1986.
254. Graeve JL, de Alarcon PA, Sato Y, et al: Miliary pulmonary neuroblastoma. A risk of autologous bone marrow transplantation? Cancer 62:2125–2127, 1988.
255. Hawkins DB, Crockett DM, Kahlstrom EJ, MacLaughlin EF: Corticosteroid management of airway hemangiomas: Long-term follow-up. Laryngoscope 94:633–637, 1984.
256. Mizono G, Dedo HH: Subglottic hemangiomas in infants: Treatment with CO$_2$ laser. Laryngoscope 94:638–641, 1984.
257. Cohen SR, Thompson JW: Lymphangiomas of the larynx in infants and children. A survey of pediatric lymphangioma. Ann Otol Rhinol Laryngol 95(Pt. 2):1–20, 1986.
258. Emory WB, Mitchell WT Jr, Hatch HB Jr: Mucous gland adenoma of the bronchus. Am Rev Respir Dis 108:1407–1410, 1973.
259. Andrassy RJ, Feldtman RW, Stanford W: Bronchial carcinoid tumors in children and adolescents. J Pediatr Surg 12:513–517, 1977.
260. Seo IS, Warren J, Mirkin LD, et al: Mucoepidermoid carcinoma of the bronchus in a 4-year-old child. A high-grade variant with lymph node metastasis. Cancer 53:1600–1604, 1984.
261. Helin I, Tedgard U, Dejmek A, Lindgren S: Muco-epidermoid tumour of the bronchus. Int J Pediatr Otorhinolaryngol 7:289–295, 1984.
262. Niitu Y, Kubota H, Hasegawa S, et al: Lung cancer (squamous cell carcinoma) in adolescence. Am J Dis Child 127:108–111, 1974.
263. McWhirter WR, Stiller CA, Lennox EL: Carcinomas in childhood. A registry-based study of incidence and survival. Cancer 63:2242–2246, 1989.
264. Abramowsky CR, Witt WJ: Sarcoma of the larynx in a newborn. Cancer 51:1726–1730, 1983.
265. Diehn KW, Hyams VJ, Harris AE: Rhabdomyosarcoma of the larynx: A case report and review of the literature. Laryngoscope 94:201–205, 1984.
266. Dodd-O JM, Wieneke KF, Rosman PM: Laryngeal rhabdomyosarcoma. Case report and literature review. Cancer 59:1012–1018, 1987.
267. Fallon G, Schiller M, Kilman JW: Primary rhabdomyosarcoma of the bronchus. Ann Thorac Surg 12:650–654, 1971.
268. Rizk G, Cueto L, Amplatz K: Rebound enlargement of the thymus after successful corrective surgery for transposition of the great vessels. AJR 116:528–530, 1972.
269. Caffey J, Silbey R: Regrowth and overgrowth of the thymus after atrophy induced by the oral administration of adrenocorticosteroids to human infants. Benjamin Knox Rachford Lecture. Pediatrics 26:762–770, 1960.
270. Gelfand DW, Goldman AS, Law EJ, et al: Thymic hyperplasia in

children recovering from thermal burns. J Trauma 12:813–817, 1972.
271. Cohen M, Hill CA, Cangir A, Sullivan MP: Thymic rebound after treatment of childhood tumors. AJR 135:151–156, 1980.
272. Bell BA, Esseltine DW, Azouz EM: Rebound thymic hyperplasia in a child with cancer. Med Pediatr Oncol 12:144–147, 1984.
273. Ford EG, Lockhart SK, Sullivan MP, Andrassy RJ: Mediastinal mass following chemotherapeutic treatment of Hodgkin's disease: Recurrent tumor or thymic hyperplasia? J Pediatr Surg 22:1155–1159, 1987.
274. Woodhead PJ: Thymic enlargement following chemotherapy. Br J Radiol 57:932–934, 1984.
275. Tartas NE, Korin J, Dengra CS, et al: Diffuse thymic enlargement in Hodgkin's disease. JAMA 254:406, 1985.
276. Radford JA, Cowan RA, Flanagan M, et al: The significance of residual mediastinal abnormality on the chest radiograph following treatment for Hodgkin's disease. J Clin Oncol 6:940–946, 1988.
277. Jochelson M, Mauch P, Balikian J, et al: The significance of the residual mediastinal mass in treated Hodgkin's disease. J Clin Oncol 3:637–640, 1985.
278. Shin MS, Ho KJ, Diffuse thymic hyperplasia following chemotherapy for nodular sclerosing Hodgkin's disease. An immunologic rebound phenomenon? Cancer 51:30–33, 1983.
279. Düe W, Dieckmann KP, Stein H: Thymic hyperplasia following chemotherapy of a testicular germ cell tumor. Immunohistological evidence for a simple rebound phenomenon. Cancer 63:446–449, 1989.
280. Stolar CJ, Garvin JH Jr, Rustad DG, et al: Residual or recurrent chest mass in pediatric Hodgkin's disease. A surgical problem? Am J Pediatr Hematol Oncol 9:289–294, 1987.
281. Choyke PL, Zeman RK, Gootenberg JE, et al: Thymic atrophy and regrowth in response to chemotherapy: CT evaluation. AJR 149:269–272, 1987.
282. Uematsu M, Kondo M, Tsutsui T, et al: Residual masses on follow-up computed tomography in patients with mediastinal non-Hodgkin's lymphoma. Clin Radiol 40:244–247, 1989.
283. Lack EE: Thymic hyperplasia with massive enlargement. Report of two cases with review of diagnostic criteria. J Thorac Cardiovasc Surg 81:741–746, 1981.
284. Katz SM, Chatten J, Bishop HC, Rosenblum H: Massive thymic enlargement. Report of a case of gross thymic hyperplasia in a child. Am J Clin Pathol 68:786–790, 1977.
285. Levine GD, Rosai J: Thymic hyperplasia and neoplasia: A review of current concepts. Hum Pathol 9:495–515, 1978.
286. Martin KW, McAlister WH: Intratracheal thymus: A rare cause of airway obstruction. AJR 149:1217–1218, 1987.
287. Bar-Ziv J, Barki Y, Itzchak Y, Mares AJ: Posterior mediastinal accessory thymus. Pediatr Radiol 14:165–167, 1984.
288. Malone PS, Fitzgerald RJ: Aberrant thymus: A misleading mediastinal mass. J Pediatr Surg 22:130–131, 1987.
289. Shackelford GD, McAlister WH: The aberrantly positioned thymus. A cause of mediastinal or neck masses in children. AJR 120(2):291–296, 1974.
290. King RM, Telander RL, Smithson WA, et al: Primary mediastinal tumors in children. J Pediatr Surg 17:512–520, 1982.
291. Raila FA, McKerchar B: Thymic cysts simulating loculated pneumomediastinum in the newborn. Br J Radiol 50:286–287, 1977.
292. Nogues A, Tovar JA, Suñol M, et al: Hodgkin's disease of the thymus: A rare mediastinal cystic mass. J Pediatr Surg 22:996–997, 1987.
293. Welch KJ, Tapper D, Vawter GP: Surgical treatment of thymic cysts and neoplasms in children. J Pediatr Surg 14:691–698, 1979.
294. Almog CH, Weissberg D, Herczeg E, Pajewski M: Thymolipoma simulating cardiomegaly: A clinicopathological rarity. Thorax 32:116–120, 1977.
295. Boetsch CH, Swoyer GB, Adams A, Walker JH: Lipothymoma. Report of two cases. Dis Chest 50:539–543, 1966.
296. Siegal GP, Dehner LP, Rosai J: Histiocytosis X (Langerhans' cell granulomatosis) of the thymus. A clinicopathologic study of four childhood cases. Am J Surg Pathol 9:117–124, 1985.
297. Nakata H, Suzuki H, Sato Y, et al: Histiocytosis X with anterior mediastinal mass as its initial manifestation. Pediatr Radiol 12:84–85, 1982.

298. Carter D, Bibro MC, Touloukian RJ: Benign clinical behavior of immature mediastinal teratoma in infancy and childhood: Report of two cases and review of the literature. Cancer 49:398–402, 1982.

299. Dudgeon DL, Haller JA Jr: Pediatric lipoblastomatosis: Two unusual cases. Surgery 95:371–372, 1984.

300. Kleinhaus S, Ducharme JC: Mediastinal lipoma in children. Surgery 66:790–793, 1969.

301. Seybold WD, McDonald JR, Clagett OT, Harrington SW: Mediastinal tumors of blood vascular origin. J Thorac Surg 18:503–517, 1949.

302. Awotwi JD, Zusman J, Waring WW, Beckerman RC: Benign hemangioendothelioma—A rare type of posterior mediastinal mass in children. J Pediatr Surg 18:581–584, 1983.

303. Tarr RW, Page DL, Glick AG, Shaff MI: Benign hemangioendothelioma involving posterior mediastinum: CT findings. J Comput Assist Tomogr 10:865–867, 1986.

304. Bedros AA, Munson J, Toomey FE: Hemangioendothelioma presenting as posterior mediastinal mass in a child. Cancer 46:801–803, 1980.

305. Niedzwiecki G, Wood BP: Thymic hemangioma. Am J Dis Child 144:1149–1150, 1990.

306. Brown LR, Reiman HM, Rosenow EC III, et al: Intrathoracic lymphangioma. Mayo Clin Proc 61:882–892, 1986.

307. Ganick DJ, Kodroff MB, Marrow HG, et al: Thoracic neuroblastoma presenting as a cystic hygroma. Arch Dis Child 63:1270–1271, 1988.

308. MacKenzie DH: The fibromatoses: A clinicopathological concept. Br Med J 4:277–281, 1972.

309. Allen PW: The fibromatoses: A clinicopathological classification based on 140 cases. Am J Surg Pathol 1:255–270, 1977.

310. Dehner LP, Askin FB: Tumors of fibrous tissue origin in childhood. A clinicopathologic study of cutaneous and soft tissue neoplasms in 66 children. Cancer 38:888–900, 1976.

311. Kaplan M, Kauli R, Lubin E, et al: Ectopic thyroid gland. A clinical study of 30 children and review. J Pediatr 92:205–209, 1978.

312. Loeffler JS, Leopold KA, Recht A, et al: Emergency prebiopsy radiation for mediastinal masses: Impact on subsequent pathologic diagnosis and outcome. J Clin Oncol 4:716–721, 1986.

313. Riccardi VM: Von Recklinghausen neurofibromatosis. N Engl J Med 305:1617–1627, 1981.

314. Raffensperger J, Cohen R: Plexiform neurofibromas in childhood. J Pediatr Surg 7:144–151, 1972.

315. Woods WG, Singher LJ, Krivit W, Nesbit ME Jr: Histoplasmosis simulating lymphoma in children. J Pediatr Surg 14:423–425, 1979.

316. Scully RE, Mark EJ, McNeely WF, McNeely BU: Case Records of the Massachusetts General Hospital (Case 6-1989). N Engl J Med 320:380–389, 1989.

317. Katzenstein AL, Mazur MT: Pulmonary infarct: An unusual manifestation of fibrosing mediastinitis. Chest 77:521–524, 1980.

318. Trump DL, Mann RB: Diffuse large cell and undifferentiated lymphomas with prominent mediastinal involvement. A poor prognostic subset of patients with non-Hodgkin's lymphoma. Cancer 50:277–282, 1982.

319. Miller JB, Variakojis D, Bitran JD, et al: Diffuse histiocytic lymphoma with sclerosis: A clinicopathologic entity frequently causing superior venacaval obstruction. Cancer 47:748–756, 1981.

320. Yabuhara A, Yanagisawa M, Murata T, et al: Giant lymph node hyperplasia (Castleman's disease) with spontaneous production of high levels of B-cell differentiation factor activity. Cancer 63:260–265, 1989.

321. Keller AR, Hochholzer L, Castleman B: Hyaline-vascular and plasma-cell types of giant lymph node hyperplasia of the mediastinum and other locations. Cancer 29:670–683, 1972.

322. Ballow M, Park BH, Dupont B, et al: Benign giant lymphoid hyperplasia of the mediastinum with associated abnormalities of the immune system. J Pediatr 84:418–420, 1974.

323. Newman A, So SK: Bilateral neurofibroma of the intrathoracic vagus associated with von Recklinghausen's disease. AJR 112:389–392, 1971.

324. Saade M, Whitten DM, Necheles TF, et al: Posterior mediastinal accessory thymus. J Pediatr 88:71–72, 1976.

325. Cohen MD, Weber TR, Sequeira FW, et al: The diagnostic dilemma of the posterior mediastinal thymus: CT manifestations. Radiology 146:691–692, 1983.

326. Cross JN, Morgan OS, Gibbs WN, Cheruvanky I: Spinal cord compression in thalassaemia. J Neurol Neurosurg Psychiatry 40:1120–1122, 1977.

327. Sorsdahl OS, Taylor PE, Noyes WD: Extramedullary hematopoiesis, mediastinal masses, and spinal cord compression. JAMA 189:343–347, 1964.

328. Bate CM, Humphries G: Alpha-beta thalassaemia. Lancet 1:1031–1034, 1977.

329. Luyendijk W, Went L, Schaad HD: Spinal cord compression due to extramedullary hematopoiesis in homozygous thalassemia. Case report. J Neurosurg 42:212–216, 1975.

330. Levine PH, Kamaraju LS, Connelly RR, et al: The American Burkitt's lymphoma registry: Eight years' experience. Cancer 49:1016–1022, 1982.

331. Bunin NJ, Hvizdala E, Link M, et al: Mediastinal nonlymphoblastic lymphomas in children: A clinicopathologic study. J Clin Oncol 4:154–159, 1986.

332. Liu HW, Wong KL, Chan TY, et al: Superior vena cava syndrome: A rare presenting feature of acute myeloid leukemia. Acta Haematol 79:213–216, 1988.

333. Gardella S, Cervantes F, Blade J, et al: Acute myeloblastic leukaemia presenting with superior vena cava syndrome due to mediastinal mass. Acta Haematol 71:174–177, 1984.

334. Peterson L, Dehner LP, Brunning RD: Extramedullary masses as presenting features of acute monoblastic leukemia. Am J Clin Pathol 75:140–148, 1981.

335. Schwarzmeier JD, Bettelheim P, Radaszkiewicz T, et al: Acute leukemia with mediastinal mass, lymphadenopathy, and monocytic precursor cells. Am J Hematol 22:313–321, 1986.

336. Azizkhan RG, Dudgeon DL, Buck JR, et al: Life-threatening airway obstruction as a complication to the management of mediastinal masses in children. J Pediatr Surg 20:816–822, 1985.

337. Mandell GA, Lantieri R, Goodman LR: Tracheobronchial compression in Hodgkin lymphoma in children. AJR 139:1167–1170, 1982.

338. Kirks DR, Fram EK, Vock P, Effmann EL: Tracheal compression by mediastinal masses in children: CT evaluation. AJR 141:647–651, 1983.

339. Prakash UB, Abel MD, Hubmayr RD: Mediastinal mass and tracheal obstruction during general anesthesia. Mayo Clin Proc 63:1004–1011, 1988.

340. Halpern S, Chatten J, Meadows AT, et al: Anterior mediastinal masses: Anesthesia hazards and other problems. J Pediatr 102:407–410, 1983.

341. Merrick HW, Martin JT, Woldenberg LS, Driscoll PL: Massive intraoperative atelectasis secondary to untreated mediastinal Hodgkin's disease: Report of the hazard and review of the literature. J Surg Oncol 41:60–64, 1989.

342. Ferrari LR, Bedford RF: General anesthesia prior to treatment of anterior mediastinal masses in pediatric cancer patients. Anesthesiology 72:991–995, 1990.

343. Montaldo P, Massimo L, Cornaglia-Ferraris P: Thymoma in children: Clinical and immunological features in three cases. Eur Paediatr Haematol Oncol 2:203–208, 1985.

344. Furman WL, Buckley PJ, Green AA, et al: Thymoma and myasthenia gravis in a 4-year-old child. Case report and review of the literature. Cancer 56:2703–2706, 1985.

345. Maggi G, Giaccone G, Donadio M, et al: Thymomas. A review of 169 cases, with particular reference to results of surgical treatment. Cancer 58:765–776, 1986.

346. Dehner LP, Martin SA, Sumner HW: Thymus related tumors and tumor-like lesions in childhood with rapid clinical progression and death. Hum Pathol 8:53–66, 1977.

347. Chatten J, Katz SM: Thymoma in a 12-year-old boy. Cancer 37:953–957, 1976.

348. Brodeur GM, Howarth CB, Pratt CB, et al: Malignant germ cell tumors in 57 children and adolescents. Cancer 48:1890–1898, 1981.

349. Hawkins EP, Finegold MJ, Hawkins HK, et al: Nongerminomatous malignant germ cell tumors in children. A review of 89 cases from the Pediatric Oncology Group, 1971–1984. Cancer 58:2579–2584, 1986.

350. Truong LD, Harris L, Mattioli C, et al: Endodermal sinus tumor of the mediastinum. A report of seven cases and review of the literature. Cancer 58:730–739, 1986.

351. Gooneratne S, Keh P, Sreekanth S, et al: Anterior mediastinal endodermal sinus tumor in a female infant. Cancer 56:1430–1433, 1985.

352. Raghavan D, Barrett A: Mediastinal seminomas. Cancer 46:1187–1191, 1980.

353. Castleberry RP, Kelly DR, Wilson ER, et al: Childhood liposarcoma. Report of a case and review of the literature. Cancer 54:579–584, 1984.

354. Wick MR, Scott RE, Li CY, Carney JA: Carcinoid tumor of the thymus. A clinicopathologic report of seven cases with a review of the literature. Mayo Clin Proc 55:246–254, 1980.

355. Simonton SC, Watterson J, Swanson P, et al: Hemangiopericytoma of the mediastinum in children. Manuscript in preparation, 1992.

356. Bower RJ, Kiesewetter WB: Mediastinal masses in infants and children. Arch Surg 112:1003–1009, 1977.

357. Adam A, Hochholzer L: Ganglioneuroblastoma of the posterior mediastinum: A clinicopathologic review of 80 cases. Cancer 47:373–381, 1981.

358. Traggis DG, Filler RM, Druckman H, et al: Prognosis for children with neuroblastoma presenting with paralysis. J Pediatr Surg 12:419–425, 1977.

359. Punt J, Pritchard J, Pincott JR, Till K: Neuroblastoma: A review of 21 cases presenting with spinal cord compression. Cancer 45:3095–3101, 1980.

360. Farrelly C, Daneman A, Chan HS, Martin DJ: Occult neuroblastoma presenting with opsomyoclonus: Utility of computed tomography. AJR 142:807–810, 1984.

361. Carachi R, Campbell PE, Kent M: Thoracic neural crest tumors. A clinical review. Cancer 51:949–954, 1983.

362. Goon HK, Cohen DH, Harvey JG: Review of thoracic neuroblastoma. Aust Paediatr J 20:17–21, 1984.

363. Young DG: Thoracic neuroblastoma/ganglioneuroma. J Pediatr Surg 18:37–41, 1983.

364. Moskal MJ, Green AA, Hayes A, George S: Why children with thoracic neuroblastoma have a favorable prognosis [Abstract C-288]. Proc Am Assoc Cancer Res, Am Soc Clin Oncol 21:391, 1980.

365. Moss RB, Blessing-Moore J, Bender SW, Weibel A: Cystic fibrosis and neuroblastoma. Pediatrics 76:814–817, 1985.

366. Brown LM, Daeschner C III, Timms J, Crow W: Granulocytic sarcoma in childhood acute myelogenous leukemia. Pediatr Neurol 5:173–178, 1989.

367. Hayes FA, Thompson EI, Hvizdala E, et al: Chemotherapy as an alternative to laminectomy and radiation in the management of epidural tumor. J Pediatr 104:221–224, 1984.

368. Allen JC: Management of metastatic epidural disease in children. J Pediatr 104:241–242, 1984.

369. Young RF, Post EM, King GA: Treatment of spinal epidural metastases. Randomized prospective comparison of laminectomy and radiotherapy. J Neurosurg 53:741–748, 1980.

370. Campbell AN, Wagget J, Mott MG: Benign mesenchymoma of the chest wall in infancy. J Surg Oncol 21:267–270, 1982.

371. McLeod RA, Dahlin DC: Hamartoma (mesenchymoma) of the chest wall in infancy. Radiology 131:657–661, 1979.

372. Brand T, Hatch EI, Schaller RT, et al: Surgical management of the infant with mesenchymal hamartoma of the chest wall. J Pediatr Surg 21:556–558, 1986.

373. Briselli MF, Soule EH, Gilchrist GS: Congenital fibromatosis. Report of 18 cases of solitary and 4 cases of multiple tumors. Mayo Clin Proc 55:554–562, 1980.

374. Stout AP, Himadi GM: Solitary (localized) mesothelioma of the pleura. Ann Surg 133:50–64, 1951.

375. Enzinger FM, Shiraki M: Musculo-aponeurotic fibromatosis of the shoulder girdle (extra-abdominal desmoid). Analysis of thirty cases followed up for ten or more years. Cancer 20:1131–1140, 1967.

376. Hill DR, Newman H, Phillips TL: Radiation therapy of desmoid tumors. AJR 117:84–89, 1973.

377. Rock MG, Pritchard DJ, Reiman HM, et al: Extra-abdominal desmoid tumors. J Bone Joint Surg 66:1369–1374, 1984.

378. Kiel KD, Suit HD: Radiation therapy in the treatment of aggressive fibromatoses (desmoid tumors). Cancer 54:2051–2055, 1984.

379. Grundy GW, Miller RW: Malignant mesothelioma in childhood. Report of 13 cases. Cancer 30:1216–1218, 1972.

380. Kauffman SL, Stout AP: Mesothelioma in children. Cancer 17:539–544, 1964.

381. Brenner J, Sordillo PP, Magill GB, Golbey RB: Malignant mesothelioma of the pleura. Review of 123 patients. Cancer 49:2431–2435, 1982.

382. Austin MB, Fechner RE, Roggli VL: Pleural malignant mesothelioma following Wilms' tumor. Am J Clin Pathol 86:227–230, 1986.

383. Askin FB, Rosai J, Sibley RK, et al: Malignant small cell tumor of the thoracopulmonary region in childhood. A distinctive clinicopathologic entity of uncertain histogenesis. Cancer 43:2438–2451, 1979.

384. Shamberger RC, Grier HE, Weinstein HJ, et al: Chest wall tumors in infancy and childhood. Cancer 63:774–785, 1989.

385. Schmidt D, Harms D, Burdach S: Malignant peripheral neuroectodermal tumours of childhood and adolescence. Virchows Arch [PA] 406:351–365, 1985.

386. Raney RB Jr, Ragab AH, Ruymann FB, et al: Soft-tissue sarcoma of the trunk in childhood. Results of the Intergroup Rhabdomyosarcoma Study. Cancer 49:2612–2616, 1982.

387. Marina NM, Etcubanas E, Parham DM, et al: Peripheral primitive neuroectodermal tumor (peripheral neuroepithelioma) in children. A review of the St. Jude experience and controversies in diagnosis and management. Cancer 64:1952–1960, 1989.

388. Hachitanda Y, Tsuneyoshi M, Daimaru Y, et al: Extraskeletal myxoid chondrosarcoma in young children. Cancer 61:2521–2526, 1988.

389. Grosfeld JL, Weber TR, Weetman RM, Baehner RL: Rhabdomyosarcoma in childhood: Analysis of survival in 98 cases. J Pediatr Surg 18:141–146, 1983.

390. Greager JA, Patel MK, Briele HA, et al: Soft tissue sarcomas of the adult thoracic wall. Cancer 59:370–373, 1987.

391. Madanat F, Osborne B, Cangir A, Sutow WW: Extrarenal Wilms' tumor. J Pediatr 93:439–443, 1978.

392. Ortega JA, Stowe SM, Shore NA, et al: Prevention of radiation pneumonitis by controlled pneumothorax in childhood rhabdomyosarcoma of the chest wall. Int J Radiat Oncol Biol Phys 11:2033–2034, 1985.

393. Federici S, Casolari E, Rossi F, et al: Rhabdomyosarcoma of the diaphragm in a 4-year-old girl. Z Kinderchir 41:303–305, 1986.

394. Glasauer FE, Yuan RHP: Intracranial tumors with extracranial metastases. Case report and review of the literature. J Neurosurg 20:474–493, 1963.

395. Magill HL, Sackler JP, Parvey LS: Wilms' tumor metastatic to the mediastinum. Pediatr Radiol 12:62–64, 1982.

396. Robinson B, Kingston J, Nogueira Costa R, et al: Chemotherapy and irradiation in childhood Hodgkin's disease. Arch Dis Child 59:1162–1167, 1984.

397. Evans AE, Baum E, Chard R: Do infants with stage IV-S neuroblastoma need treatment? Arch Dis Child 56:271–274, 1981.

398. Markman M: Intracavitary chemotherapy. CRC Crit Rev Oncol Hematol 3:205–233, 1985.

399. Brenner DE: Intraperitoneal chemotherapy: A review. J Clin Oncol 4:1135–1147, 1986.

400. Hausheer FH, Yarbro JW: Diagnosis and treatment of malignant pleural effusion. Semin Oncol 12:54–75, 1985.

V Asthma

66 ASTHMA: AN INFLAMMATORY DISEASE

SHIRLEY MURPHY, M.D.

One of the traditional hallmarks of asthma has been eosinophilia in sputum.[1] Immunofluorescence studies have localized these increased numbers of eosinophils to the respiratory epithelium of patients dying of asthma.[2] Until the 1980s, knowledge about histologic changes in asthma was limited to information about patients dying of status asthmaticus. The pathologic processes in fatal asthma include mucosal and submucosal edema of the bronchi and bronchioles, thickening of the basement membrane, a profuse leukocyte infiltration (predominantly eosinophils), intraluminal mucus plugs, and smooth muscle hyperplasia.[3] Current scientific information supports the concept that asthma, even in mild cases, is an inflammatory disease of airway hyperresponsiveness and airflow limitation resulting from this inflammatory response.

EVIDENCE THAT ASTHMA IS AN INFLAMMATORY DISEASE

The ultrastructural characteristics of the airways in nonfatal asthma were first described by Cutz and colleagues[4] in two asthmatic children undergoing open lung biopsy during clinical remission. The investigators compared these findings with lung tissue from two children who had died in status asthmaticus. Bronchial changes were comparable in the two groups of patients, and the specimens showed goblet-cell hyperplasia, mucus plugging, and increased collagen deposition beneath the epithelial basement membrane. The only differences that the investigators found were a higher number of submucosal eosinophils and more extensive denudation of the epithelium in the children with fatal asthma.

Laitinen and colleagues[5] studied bronchial epithelial changes associated with mild to moderate asthma in bronchial biopsy specimens and found epithelial cell disruption even in patients with mild asthma. Their findings were expanded and supported by Lundgren,[6] who, using bronchoscopy and scanning electron microscopy, demonstrated large areas of ciliary loss and cells with abnormal cilia in patients with mild to moderate asthma.

An alternative approach to biopsy has been to use bronchoalveolar lavage (BAL) fluid to analyze cell types and numbers and to quantify cell-derived products. In many studies, interpretation of the results and the extrapolation to actual changes occurring in the airway wall have been difficult.[7, 8]

To understand the role of the inflammatory response in asthma, Beasley and associates[9] completed a detailed cellular and ultrastructural examination of bronchial biopsies and bronchial lavage fluid from allergic subjects with mild asthma. To explore the relationship between allergen-induced changes in bronchial reactivity and cellular events in the bronchial wall during the late phase of the asthmatic reaction, they repeated the sampling procedures 18 h after provocation with inhaled allergen.

In their study, eight atopic asthmatic patients (mean provocation dose of histamine that caused a 20% drop [PD_{20}] in forced expiratory volume in 1 sec [FEV_1] was 0.90 mg/ml) and four nonasthmatic control subjects underwent fiberoptic bronchoscopy. A single 50-ml bronchial wash was obtained, followed by endobronchial biopsy at the subcarinae. These procedures were repeated in the asthmatic subjects 18 h after provocation with inhaled allergen or methacholine. Subsequently, all subjects underwent bronchial reactivity testing with inhaled histamine. The number of epithelial cells in lavage fluids was higher in the asthmatic subjects (7.23×10^4/ml) than in the nonasthmatic subjects (1.48×10^4/ml, $p = .048$); there was a significant inverse correlation between lavage epithelial cell count and bronchial reactivity. In asthmatic subjects, there was an extensive deposition of collagen beneath the epithelial basement membrane. Eosinophils, monocytes, and platelets were observed in contact with the vascular endothelium. Mast cell degranulation and mucosal infiltration by eosinophils, which showed morphologic evidence of activation, were also found in these asthmatic subjects.

The high degree of correlation between the epithelial cell count in the lavage fluids and the degree of airway responsiveness to inhaled histamine observed in this study provides significant support for the hypothesis that epithelial cell loss may be fundamental to the pathogenesis of bronchial asthma.[9] It is also likely that the damage to and the loss of ciliated respiratory epithelium lead to the defect in mucociliary clearance that has been documented in asthma, which may contribute to the accumulation of mucus and to airflow obstruction. Loss of epithelial cells may expose submucosal cells to increased allergen penetration and other inflammatory stimuli. In addition, the influx of inflammatory cells may result in the release of products, such as oxygen radicals, major basic protein, and lysosomal enzymes, that are toxic to epithelial cells.

The appearance of dense subepithelial collagen also supports the severity of the tissue disruption in apparently mild asthma and the persistence of such changes in the absence of clinical disease. This abnormal collagen deposition may result in a diffusion barrier and nutrient deprivation of the epithelium, which are similar to the effects of diabetic microangiopathy and may further aggravate the disease process.

Varying degrees of inflammatory cell infiltration were observed in the mucosa of the asthmatic subjects. The active recruitment of inflammatory cells into the bronchial wall was evidenced by the finding of numerous leukocytes in the vascular lumina, adherent to or emigrating from the vessel walls of the bronchial microvasculature. It is interesting that the eosinophils in the lamina propria were exclusive to the asthmatic group. These eosinophils, irrespective of bronchial challenge with allergen, showed morphologic features of activation, as indicated by a marked heterogeneity in granular contents.

The mast cells in the bronchial lamina propria exhibited various stages of degranulation in the asthmatic subjects but not in the control subjects. This finding in subjects with mild asthma supports the concept that mast cell degranulation and mediator release occur continuously within the bronchial mucosa of atopic asthmatic subjects. Mast cells obtained from BAL fluid of such subjects also exhibited increased spontaneous release of histamine.

Beasley and associates concluded from their study that "allergic asthma is accompanied by extensive inflammatory changes in the airways, even in mild clinical and subclinical disease."[9]

THE LINK BETWEEN THE LATE-PHASE ASTHMATIC REACTIONS AND INFLAMMATION

Inhalation challenge with antigen in patients with asthma results in immediate bronchoconstriction. Many asthmatic patients undergo a second bronchoconstrictive response 4 to 12 h after the first; the second is known as the late-phase or delayed asthmatic response. The early response can be rapidly reversed by beta$_2$-agonists; the late reaction responds poorly to these agents, and bronchospasm is prolonged and more severe. Symptoms in patients with asthma more closely resemble the late rather than the immediate response to antigen, which emphasizes the importance of the late asthmatic response. After a late-phase reaction, the airways become hyperreactive to multiple stimuli, including histamine, exercise, cold air, and methacholine. Immediate asthmatic responses

occurring without a late asthmatic response do not produce this increase in nonspecific hyperreactivity.

The exact pathogenesis of the late-phase response is still under investigation. However, mast cell degranulation and release of bronchospastic mediators are thought to play a role in the immediate response. The participation of the mast cell in the late-phase response is less clearly defined. It appears that mediators released from mast cells attract other inflammatory cells into the airways. Of particular importance is the finding that there are increased numbers of eosinophils in the airways during the late-phase response (including neutrophils, macrophages, and lymphocytes). These inflammatory cells may also play an important role in sustaining the reaction.

Several animal models have been used to study the late-phase asthmatic response. Abraham and co-workers[10] induced early and late asthmatic responses in sheep sensitive to *Ascaris suum*. In this model, inhalation of cromolyn sodium by nebulization before antigen challenge blocked both the early and the late responses. The intravenous injection of methylprednisolone 3 h after antigen challenge blocked the late response to the same degree as inhaled cromolyn given before challenge.[10] Larson,[11] in an IgE-mediated *Alternaria*-induced late asthmatic reaction in rabbits, also showed that prechallenge inhalation of cromolyn blocks the immediate and late asthmatic reactions. Corticosteroids block only the development of the late response. This consistent ability of cromolyn sodium to block both the early and late asthmatic responses and to prevent the increase in bronchial hyperreactivity suggests a role for the mast cell in initiating the response.

PATHOPHYSIOLOGY OF AIRWAY RESPONSIVENESS

Airway hyperresponsiveness is defined as an exaggerated bronchoconstrictive reaction of the airways on exposure to a small quantity of a nonspecific stimulus that does not evoke bronchoconstriction in a normal subject.[12] It is a key feature of asthma and relates closely to the severity of disease, the frequency of symptoms, and the amount of medications required to achieve adequate control.[13] Increased airway responsiveness may follow exposure to allergens, viral infections of the upper respiratory tract, and exposure to some industrial chemicals. Increased airway responsiveness is clinically manifested by increases in cough and asthma symptoms and an increased diurnal variation in peak expiratory flow rate.

Nonspecific airway responsiveness is measured in the laboratory by stimulation with pharmacologic agents or physical stimuli, such as exercise or cold air. Methacholine and histamine are the pharmacologic agents used most often to assess the degree of nonspecific airway responsiveness. The stimuli used to provoke a response are administered by inhalation in increasing concentrations, and with each dose, spirometry is performed. The administration of the stimulus is stopped when the FEV_1 drops 20% from base line. The concentration or dose that causes a 20% drop in FEV_1 is the PD_{20}.

The precise relationship among inflammation, bronchial responsiveness, and the symptoms of asthma is still uncertain. As association between the presence of inflammatory cells in the airways and hyperresponsiveness of the airways has been demonstrated in humans after inhaling ozone,[14] toluene diisocyanate,[15] and allergens.[16] Although the inflammatory cell type has varied with different stimuli, the result of increased airways responsiveness has been the same, which indicates that the consequence of the inflammatory response is the development of airway hyperresponsiveness. Such inflammation may increase bronchial responsiveness and may lower the threshold at which other triggering stimuli (e.g., exercise, smoke) precipitate bronchonconstriction. Also, the inflammation may contribute directly to the asthma by sensitizing sensory nerve endings.

Currently, only the anti-inflammatory agents cromolyn, nedocromil, and inhaled corticosteroids have been shown to decrease airway hyperresponsiveness when taken over a period of several months. Theophylline and the beta$_2$-agonists have not been shown to decrease hyperresponsiveness.

THE CELLS OF INFLAMMATION IN ASTHMA

MAST CELLS

For many years, mast cells have been thought to play a pivotal role in asthma. Mast cells are located both superficially between epithelial cells and in the bronchial mucosa. Activation of the mast cell through immunoglobulin E (IgE) receptors or other nonspecific mechanisms causes the release of mediators, including histamine, leukotrienes, prostaglandins, and platelet activating factor (PAF). These mediators cause smooth muscle contraction, vasodilation, and recruitment of other inflammatory cells.

The mast cell may have a role in the persistence of the asthmatic response. Mast cells obtained by BAL from atopic asthmatic patients have a greater response *in vivo* to inhaled allergens than do mast cells from normal persons, as measured by the histamine and tryptase levels in the lavage fluids.[17] In addition, spontaneous mast cell activation is greater in atopic asthmatic patients than in normal persons, even though the number of mast cell numbers recovered in the lavage fluid is not higher.[18]

It appears that mast cells have an important role in the early asthmatic response, possibly through the release of histamine. However, their role in the late response and the development of bronchial hyperreactivity is questioned. Cromolyn has been shown, through studies in animals and humans, to be a mast cell stabilizer. However, mast cell stabilizers more potent than cromolyn have been developed, and they do not block the late response. Beta$_2$-agonists have been shown to be more potent than cromolyn in stabilizing mast cells, and they have no effect in suppressing the late asthmatic response or the bronchial reactivity that follows. Corticosteroids, cromolyn, and nedocromil given to asthmatic patients are also able to decrease bronchial hyperreactivity.

Although mast cells are involved in immediate asthmatic responses to both allergens and exercise and may recruit other inflammatory cells, they themselves are unlikely to play a critical role in the development of bronchial reactivity.

ALVEOLAR MACROPHAGES

Alveolar macrophages may be activated by IgE-dependent mechanisms. This possibility has given rise to the hypothesis that these potent cells may be involved in the asthmatic response. In asthmatic subjects, an increased amount of IgE is bound to many of these cells, and the number of the IgE-bearing cells is higher in asthmatic patients than in normal persons.[19] Macrophages from patients with asthma release increased amounts of mediators, including prostaglandins, PAF, and leukotriene B$_4$.[20] Studies have been conducted with immunohistochemical techniques and monoclonal antibodies to monocytes and macrophages in tissues from asthmatic patients. Through the use of a panmacrophage marker, it was found that asthmatic patients have an higher number of macrophages than do normal controls. In addition, some of these cells were in an activated state and could release enzymes such as metalloproteinases; these enzymes have the capacity to degrade extracellular matrix macromolecules. Although the macrophage has IgE receptors and certainly the ability to cause destruction, its role in asthma needs further clarification.

NEUTROPHILS

Neutrophils can be recruited into the lung and airways by a variety of chemoattractants. They have the capacity to release mediators, proteases, and oxygen radicals, which could induce airway responsiveness. However, in asthmatic humans the neutrophil appears to play a less important role.

Most studies conducted to establish the role of the neutrophil in asthma have been performed in animals. Fabbri and co-workers[21] demonstrated a temporal association in dogs between the development of airway hyperresponsiveness and the presence of neutrophils in biopsies of airways and in BAL fluid after inhalation of ozone. In rabbits sensitized to *Alternaria tenius,* the development of the late asthmatic response and of airway hyperresponsiveness was associated with the influx of neutrophils into the airways.[22] Neutrophils are important in the development of airway hyperresponsiveness in rabbits and dogs, but their role in human asthma is less clear.

EOSINOPHILS

One of the hallmarks of asthma has long been eosinophilia in sputum. It was initially postulated that eosinophils limit the inflammation after immediate hypersensitivity reactions by neutralizing some mediators of anaphylaxis. However, more recent research has implicated eosinophils as contributors to the pathogenesis of asthma.[23]

Eosinophils contain several potentially toxic compounds, the importance of which lies in the ability to kill parasites. Four cationic proteins compose the bulk of the eosinophil granule: eosinophil peroxides, eosinophil-derived neurotoxin, eosinophil cationic protein, and major basic protein (MBP). MBP is localized to the core of the granule and has been shown to be toxic to the respiratory epithelium. When applied to guinea pig tracheal rings, MBP induced dose-dependent epithelial damage, desquamation of epithelial cells, and impairment of ciliary activity. These changes were also produced in human bronchial epithelium. The histopathologic changes induced by MBP include shedding of the bronchial epithelium down to the lamina propria, which is also reported as a frequent finding in pathologic studies of asthma.[2] In addition, elevated levels of MBP have been found in the sputum of asthmatic patients.[24]

Davis and co-workers[25] examined eosinophil-mediated injury to lung parenchymal cells and interstitial matrix. Guinea pig peritoneal eosinophils and human eosinophils obtained from a patient with chronic eosinophilic pneumonia caused spontaneous cytolysis of lung fibroblasts, epithelial cells, and mesothelial cells. In addition, the investigators demonstrated that eosinophil granules contain a collagenase capable of cleaving human collagen types I and III, providing further evidence for potential of eosinophils to injure lung framework tissues.[25]

In addition to MBP, the other cationic proteins have also been shown to be toxic to guinea pig tracheal epithelium in vitro.[26] In another group of human experiments, antigen was instilled locally into a subsegmental portion of the airway of an asthmatic patient and was followed by lavage after 48 h and 96 h. The total number of cells increased about 1.5-fold after 48 h, but there was no further increase at 96 h. The number of eosinophils increased markedly after 48 h from 9.6×10^5 to 35×10^5 cells and remained elevated at 96 h.[27]

Metzger and co-workers preformed BAL after bronchoprovocation challenges in 12 asthmatic patients. The total number of cells obtained from a single lavage site increased 46% after bronchoprovocation; the percentage of macrophages was reduced, but those of eosinophils and neutrophils increased.[28] Electron microscopy performed on the lavage fluids revealed mast cell degranulation after bronchoprovocation. Eosinophils also exhibited degranulation with loss of central cores and small granules. The lavage macrophages appeared activated and were noted to contain eosinophil granules.[29]

Release of eosinophils from the bone marrow is controlled by several factors, including those released by epithelial cells, granulocyte-macrophage colony–stimulating factor, interleukin-3, and interleukin-5. These factors can support colony growth and maturation of eosinophils as well as recruit eosinophils from bone marrow and activate them.[30]

Study findings suggest that eosinophils pass through at least one stage before they can release a maximal number of mediators. Agents capable of eosinophil priming include leukotriene B$_4$, PAF, and interleukin-5. Circulating eosinophils from subjects with blood eosinophilia display a range of densities upon separation; hypodense cells predominate.[31] It is thought that in asthma, hypodense

eosinophils are in an activated state because of their increased oxygen consumption and increased spontaneous release of their granule content. Once activated, the eosinophil can release a number of potent mediators of lipid metabolism, including PAF, leukotriene B$_4$, and especially leukotriene C$_4$.[32]

LYMPHOCYTES

Lymphocytes are known for their role in asthma: as B cells, they produce IgE. However, T cells may also have a role. An increased proportion of peripheral blood T lymphocytes from patients with acute, severe asthma have been shown to be activated, as measured by increased expression of human lymphocyte antigen DR (HLA-DR) and interleukin-2R.[33] T lymphocytes from patients with allergic asthma produce higher amounts of interleukin-2 in response to mite antigen than those of nonallergic persons. This effect is decreased after the patient has undergone immunotherapy.[34]

In addition, T lymphocytes may have a regulatory role in the production of IgE. T cell factors such as interleukin-4 alone or in combination with interleukin-5 enhance antigen-driven B lymphocyte synthesis of IgE. This effect of T cells can be blocked by interferon-γ.[35] An additional regulatory effect of T cells is shown by the inhibition of in vitro IgE synthesis by lymphocytes in atopic patients after cocultivation with T lymphocytes from normal subjects.[36]

PLATELETS

Several abnormalities of platelet function have been demonstrated in asthmatic patients.[37] Platelets can release a number of mediators, including serotonin, thromboxane, and lipo-oxygenase products. Their possible role in asthma received attention through the discovery of a mediator, PAF, which is a potent bronchoconstrictor in animal species, including primates. A hypothesis proposed by Morley and collaborators[37] was that platelet activation and the release of PAF may be important in the pathogenesis of asthma.

Indeed, the inhalation of PAF by humans produces prolonged increases in airway responsiveness to methacholine. PAF is generated from membrane phospholipase A$_2$ and is produced by several inflammatory cells, including macrophages, neutrophils, eosinophils, and mast cells.[38]

THE EPITHELIUM

Epithelial damage is a prominent postmortem finding in asthma, and bronchial biopsy specimens have shown that epithelial disruption may occur even in patients with mild asthma (Fig. 66–1). Two separate functions of the epithelium may be important in the pathogenesis of asthma: as a barrier in which changes in permeability occur after injury and as a mediator-generating cell with the capabilities to induce inflammation.

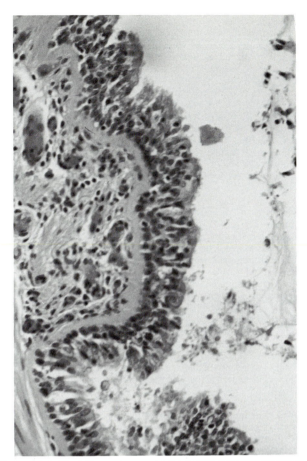

Figure 66-1. The inflammatory response in asthma is illustrated in this airway section from a patient with mild asthma who died in an accident. There is a submucosal infiltration of eosinophils and a marked deposition of collagen below the basement membrane.

CHANGES IN EPITHELIAL PERMEABILITY

The effects of epithelial loss and its relationship to the development of airway hyperreactivity in asthma have been studied by several investigators. Laitinen and colleagues, using electron microscopy studies of bronchial biopsies from patients with mild asthma, could find no definite correlation between the extent of the epithelial damage and the clinical severity of asthma or the degree of airway hyperresponsiveness.[5] In at least two studies, investigators have reported the presence of increased numbers of bronchial epithelial cells recovered through BAL from asthmatic subjects in comparison with normal subjects and have established a positive correlation between the epithelial cell numbers and the degree of airway responsiveness.[9, 39]

Increased permeability of the bronchial mucosa has been proposed as a factor contributing to the pathogenesis of asthma. This hypothesis has been difficult to document. Investigators who measured mucosal permeability by measuring the total clearance of technetium 99m–diethylenetriamine penta-acetic acid (DTPA) showed that there was decreased mucociliary clearance in asthmatic patients; this finding implied that DTPA passed through the mucosa, indicating greater than normal mucosal permeability in asthma.[33]

Most hypotheses that relate epithelial damage and airway hyperresponsiveness are based on the belief that epithelial damage results in exposure of afferent nerve receptors and in increased reflex bronchonconstriction through vagal or local reflexes involving sensory afferent nerve fibers.[40]

MICROVASCULAR LEAKAGE

Increased amounts of plasma proteins are found in the airways of asthmatic patients and are indicative of increased microvascular leakage.[41] Albumin can alter the rheologic properties of airway mucus by increasing its viscosity through formation of viscous protein-glycoprotein complexes, decreasing mucociliary clearance.

Edema of the airway wall is regarded as an important feature of asthma. The mechanisms responsible for microvascular leakage involve autocoid- and neuropeptide-induced contraction of postcapillary venule endothelial cells. In bronchial biopsy specimens obtained from asthmatic subjects, the presence of large gaps between the endothelial cells of the submucosal venules provides direct evidence of this contraction. Plasma leakage occurs between the cell gaps.[42]

Microvascular leakage is a characteristic of many types of inflammation; it is important in the pathogenesis of asthma and might be caused by the same mediators of inflammation that induce bronchospasm. Many of the inflammatory mediators in asthma, including histamine, bradykinin, leukotrienes, and PAF, can cause microvascular leakage in airways. In addition, stimulation of the vagus nerve and capsaicin through release of sensory neuropeptides, as with substance P, can cause microvascular leakage.[43] Edema may contribute to the epithelial shedding by lifting of epithelial cells. Edema of the airways may also lead to increased responsiveness because submucosal thickening enhances the increased airway resistance that occurs with constriction of airway smooth muscle.

EPITHELIAL BASEMENT MEMBRANE

Thickening and hyalinization of the epithelial basement membrane is consistently referred to in studies of the histopathologic processes in asthmatic airways. This appears to occur regardless of age and has been found in patients with mild asthma.[9] Careful studies of bronchial tissue have shown that the basement membrane itself is not thickened, but collagen is deposited beneath it. This has been mistakenly referred to as basement membrane thickening. Increased subepithelial collagen deposition occurs in young asthmatic patients and even those with very mild asthma.[45]

The subepithelial collagen consists of collagen types III and V together with fibrin. This suggests a fibroblast source for the excess collagen.[44] The effect of inflammatory processes on collagen deposition is unclear. There are many sources of mitogenic stimuli for fibroblasts. Also, nothing is known at present about the effects of anti-inflammatory treatment on collagen thickness and the relevance of the collagen thickness to the degree of airway responsiveness.[44]

EPITHELIAL MEDIATOR RELEASE

Human tracheal and bronchial epithelia release a number of mediators when stimulated, including prostaglandin E_2, 15-hydroxyeicosatetraenoic acid (HETE), and 8,15 di-HETE.[45] In addition, epithelial cells have been shown to produce leukotriene B_4 and may release a relaxing factor (epithelium-derived relaxing factor [EDRF]) that causes smooth muscle relaxation. Experiments have shown that when epithelium is removed from canine bronchi, the *in vitro* sensitivity of the bronchial smooth muscle to histamine is enhanced because of loss of EDRF.[46]

Thus several mechanisms cause epithelial damage and may contribute to bronchial hyperresponsiveness: (1) easier access of irritant factor to nerve endings, (2) enhanced penetration of allergen particles to mediator-secreting cells in the submucosa, and (3) decreased production of epithelium-derived bronchodilator substances.

REFERENCES

1. Naylor B: The shedding of the mucosa of the bronchial tree in asthma. Thorax 17:69–72, 1962.
2. Filley WV, Holley KE, Kephart GM, Gleich GJ: Identification by immunofluorescence of the eosinophil granule major basic protein in lung tissue of patients with bronchial asthma. Lancet 2:11–16, 1982.
3. Takizawa, T, Thurlbeck WM: Muscle and mucus glands size in the major bronchi of patients with chronic bronchitis, asthma and asthmatic bronchitis. Am Rev Respir Dis 104:331–336, 1971.
4. Cutz E, Levison H, Cooper DM: Ultrastructure of airways in children with asthma. Histopathology 2:407–421, 1978.
5. Laitinen LA, Heino M, Laitinen A, et al: Damage of the airway epithelium and bronchial reactivity in patients with asthma. Am Rev Respir Dis 131:599–606, 1985.
6. Lundgren R: Scanning electron microscopic studies of bronchial mucosa before and during treatment with beclomethasone dipropionate inhalations. Scand J Respir Dis [Suppl] 101:179–187, 1977.
7. Godard P, Bousquet J, Lebel B, Michel FB: Bronchoalveolar lavage in the asthmatic. Bull Eur Physiopathol Respir 23:73–83, 1987.
8. Flint KC, Leung KB, Hudspith BN, et al: Bronchoalveolar mast cells in extrinsic asthma: A mechanism for the initiation of antigen specific bronchoconstriction. Br Med J 291:923–926, 1985.
9. Beasley R, Roche W, Roberts J, Holgate S: Cellular events in the bronchi in mild asthma and after bronchial provocation. Am Rev Respir Dis 139:806–817, 1989.
10. Abraham WM, Delehunt JC, Yerger L, Marchette B: Characterization of a late phase pulmonary response after antigen challenge in allergic sheep. Am Rev Respir Dis 128:839–844, 1983.
11. Larson GL: Late-phase reactions: Observations on pathogenesis and prevention. J Allergy Clin Immunol 76:665–669, 1985.
12. Barnes PJ: New concepts in the pathogenesis of bronchial hyperresponsiveness and asthma. J Allergy Clin Immunol 83:1013–1026, 1989.
13. Juniper EF, Frith PA, Hargreave FE: Airway responsiveness to histamine and methacholine: Relationship to minimum treatment to control symptoms of asthma. Thorax 36:575–579, 1981.
14. Stelzer J, Bigby BG, Stulbarg M, et al: O_3-induced changes in bronchial reactivity to methacholine and airway inflammation in humans. J Appl Physiol 60:1321–1326, 1986.
15. Boschetto P, Zocca E, Milani GF, et al: Bronchoalveolar neutrophilia during the late, but not early, asthmatic reactions induced by toluene diisocyanate (TDI). J Allergy Clin Immunol 77:244, 1986.
16. De Monchy JG, Kaufman HF, Venge P, et al: Bronchoalveolar eosinophilia during allergen-induced late asthmatic reaction. Am Rev Respir Dis 131:373–376, 1985.
17. Wenzel SE, Fowler AA, Schwartz LB: Activation of pulmonary mast cells by bronchoalveolar allergen challenge. Am Rev Respir Dis 137:1002–1008, 1988.
18. Rankin JA, Kaliner M, Reynolds HY: Histamine levels in bronchoalveolar lavage from patients with asthma, sarcoidosis and idiopathic pulmonary fibrosis. J Allergy Clin Immunol 79:371–377, 1987.
19. Capron M, Jouault T, Prin L: Functional study of a monoclonal antibody to IgE-Fc receptor of eosinophils, platelets, and macrophages. J Exp Med 164:72–89, 1986.
20. Godard P, Chainteuil J, Damon M, et al: Functional assessment of alveolar macrophages: Comparison of cells from asthmatics and normal subjects. J Allergy Clin Immunol 70:88–93, 1982.
21. Fabbri LM, Aizawa H, Alpert SE, et al: Airway hyperresponsiveness and changes in cell counts in bronchoalveolar lavage after ozone exposure in dogs. Am Rev Respir Dis 129:288–291, 1984.
22. Murphy KR, Wilson MC, Irvin CG, et al: The requirement for polymorphonuclear leukocytes in the late asthmatic response and heightened airways reactivity in an animal model. Am Rev Respir Dis 134:62–68, 1986.
23. Gleich GJ, Flavahan NA, Fujisawa T, Vanhoutte PM: The eosinophil as a mediator of damage to respiratory epithelium: A model for bronchial hyperreactivity. J Allergy Clin Immunology 81:776–781, 1988.
24. Dor PJ, Ackerman SJ, Gleich GJ: Charcot-Leyden crystal protein and eosinophil granule major basic protein in sputum of patients with respiratory diseases. Am Rev Respir Dis 130:1072–1077, 1984.
25. Davis WB, Fells GA, Sun XH, et al: Eosinophil-mediated injury to lung parenchymal cells and interstitial matrix. J Clin Invest 74:269–278, 1984.
26. Motojima S, Frigas E, Loegering DA, Gleich GJ: Toxicity of eosinophil cationic proteins for guinea pig tracheal epithelium *in vitro*. Am Rev Respir Dis 139:801–805, 1989.
27. Metzger WJ, Hunninghake GW, Richerson HB: Late asthmatic responses: Inquiry into mechanisms and significance. Clin Rev Allergy 3:145–165, 1985.
28. Metzger WJ, Nugent K, Richerson HB, et al: Methods for bronchoalveolar lavage in asthmatic patients following bronchoprovocation and local antigen challenge. Chest 87:16s–19s, 1985.
29. Worden K, Metzger WJ, Knopp W, et al: Dissolution of eosinophil granules in bronchial lavage obtained from allergic asthmatics during bronchoprovocation and seasonal exposure. Proc Ann EMSA 41:798–799, 1983.
30. Lopez AF, Williamson DJ, Gamble JR, et al: Recombinant human granulocyte-macrophage colony–stimulating factor stimulates *in vitro* mature human neutrophil and eosinophil function, surface receptor expression and survival. J Clin Invest 78:1220–1228, 1986.
31. Fukuda T, Dunnette SL, Reed CE, et al: Increased numbers of hypodense eosinophils in the blood of patients with bronchial asthma. Am Rev Respir Dis 132:981–985, 1985.
32. Shaw RJ, Walsh GM, Cromwell O, et al: Activated human eosinophils generate SRS-A leukotrienes following IgG-dependent stimulation. Nature 316:150–152, 1985.
33. Djukanovic R, Roche WR, Wilson JW, et al: Mucosal inflammation in asthma. Am Rev Respir Dis 142:434–457, 1990.
34. Hsieh KH: Altered interleukin-2 (IL-2) production and responsiveness after hyposensitization to house dust. J Allergy Clin Immunol 76:188–194, 1985.
35. Romagnani S, Del Prete G, Maggi E, et al: Role of interleukins in induction and regulation of human IgE synthesis. Clin Immunol Immunopathol 50:S13–S23, 1989.
36. Saxon A, Morrow C, Stevens RH: Subpopulations of circulating B cells and regulatory T cells involved in *in vitro* immunoglobulin E production in atopic patients with elevated serum immunoglobulin E. J Clin Invest 65:1457–1468, 1980.
37. Morley J, Sanjar S, Page CP: The platelet in asthma. Lancet 2:1142–1144, 1984.

38. Barns PJ, Chung KF, Page CP: Platelet-activating factor as a mediator of allergic disease. J Allergy Clin Immunol 81:919–934, 1988.
39. Wardlaw AJ, Dunnette S, Gleich GJ, et al: Eosinophils and mast cells in bronchoalveolar lavage in subjects with mild asthma: Relationship to bronchial hyperreactivity. Am Rev Respir Dis 137:62–69, 1988.
40. Barnes PJ: Neural control of human airway in health and disease. Am Rev Respir Dis 134:1289–1314, 1986.
41. Brogan TD, Ryley HC, Neale L, Yassa J: Soluble proteins of bronchopulmonary secretions from patients with cystic fibrosis, asthma and bronchitis. Thorax 30:72–79, 1975.
42. Laitinen LA, Laitinen A: Mucosal inflammation and bronchial hyperreactivity. Eur Respir J 1:488–489, 1988.
43. Persson CGA: Leakage of macromolecules from the tracheobronchial microcirculation. Am Rev Respir Dis 135:S71–S75, 1987.
44. Roche WR, Beasley R, Williams JH, Holgate ST: Subepithelial fibrosis in the bronchi of asthmatics. Lancet 1:520–524, 1989.
45. Henderson WR: Lipid-derived and other chemical mediators of inflammation in the lung. J Allergy Clin Immun 79:543–553, 1987.
46. Flavahan NA, Aarhus LL, Rimele TJ, Vanhoutte PM: Respiratory epithelium inhibits bronchial smooth muscle tone. J Appl Physiol 58:834–838, 1985.

67 THE MANAGEMENT OF ACUTE EXACERBATION OF CHILDHOOD ASTHMA

SHIRLEY MURPHY, M.D. / H. WILLIAM KELLY, PHARM.D.

In the United States, acute exacerbations of asthma are responsible for more hospital visits and missed school days than is any other chronic disease of childhood. Both the prevalence and the severity of this disease are increasing around the world.[1]

Retrospective studies of asthma deaths have identified risk factors that may be predictive of which patients are at risk.[2] These include absence of readily available treatment during a severe attack, underestimation of the severity of the attack, underuse of steroids with overreliance on bronchodilators, and chronic poor control of the asthma.

Results of studies in adult asthmatic patients have shown repeatedly that 80% of deaths occurred as a result of poor education, supervision, and management of patients.[3, 4] Results of a further study of childhood asthma deaths in New Zealand suggested that deaths in children were largely preventable.[5, 6] Fletcher and associates analyzed 35 childhood asthmatic deaths in England and found that although 18 patients (51%) had been chronically undertreated, the major factor in 57% was suboptimal management of the final attack as a result of delay in seeking medical attention, inadequate medical response and treatment, or both.[7]

If mortality rates are to be reduced, physicians must teach families to recognize acute, severe asthma, must develop crisis plans for home management and transport, and must have a protocol for managing asthmatic children in the emergency room and the hospital. In this chapter, the focus is on assessing children with asthma; suggested protocols for management in the home, emergency department, and the hospital; and the rationale for the therapies chosen and the dosages suggested.

Exacerbations of asthma are acute episodes of airflow obstruction manifested by shortness of breath, increased coughing, wheezing, increased respiratory rate, a feeling of tightness in the chest, or any combination of these symptoms. Respiratory distress is common and, if untreated, may lead to respiratory failure and death.

The best strategy for the management of acute exacerbations of asthma is prevention or early intervention. In the early treatment of asthma exacerbations, three procedures are important: (1) early recognition of worsening lung function (monitored by peak expiratory flow rate [PEFR]), (2) prompt communication between the patient and the physician with regard to steps for preventing further deterioration; and (3) intensification of prescribed asthma medications. In many episodes of acute asthma, a short course of systemic corticosteroids can reverse an otherwise refractory asthmatic exacerbation and can prevent a visit to the emergency room or hospitalization.[8, 9]

Some patients are at risk for the development of life-threatening asthma. Such patients should be identified and should have extensive education, crisis plans, close monitoring, and adequate access to emergency care. These patients include those who have undergone previous intubation for asthma, have been hospitalized for asthma two or more times in the past year, have made three or more emergency care visits for asthma within the past year, have been hospitalized or received emergency care within the past month; are currently using systemic steroids, or have been previously admitted to an intensive care unit.

Initial treatment of an exacerbation of asthma can begin at home. If symptoms and objective measures do not improve rapidly, treatment should be continued in a setting in which close observation, frequent treatments, and repeated measurements of lung function (e.g., PEFR), oxygen saturations, and blood gas measurements

Table 67-1. ESTIMATION OF SEVERITY OF ACUTE EXACERBATION OF ASTHMA IN CHILDREN

Characteristic	Respiratory Rate		
	Normal to <1 SD for Age	*Normal to <2 SD for Age*	*Normal to >2 SD for Age*
Alertness	Normal	Normal	May be decreased
Dyspnea	Absent or mild; speaks in complete sentences	Moderate; speaks in phrases or partial sentences	Severe; speaks only in single words or short phrases
Pulsus paradoxus	<10 mm Hg	10–20 mm Hg	20–40 mm Hg
Accessory muscle use	No intercostal to mild indrawing	Moderate intercostal indrawing with tracheosternal retractions; use of sternocleidomastoid muscles	Severe intercostal retractions; tracheosternal retractions with nasal flaring
Color	Good	Pale	Possibly cyanotic
Auscultation	End expiratory wheeze only	Wheeze during entire expiration and inspiration	Decreased air movement
Sa_{O_2}	>95%	90%–95%	<90%
Pa_{CO_2}	<35 mm Hg	<40 mm Hg	>40 mm Hg
PEFR	70%–90% predicted	30%–70% predicted	<30% predicted

SD, Standard deviation; Sa_{O_2}, oxygen saturation; Pa_{CO_2}, arterial carbon dioxide tension; PEFR, peak expiratory flow rate.

can be made if necessary. In addition, care should be given by clinicians who are qualified to manage patients with respiratory distress and who can recognize impending respiratory failure.

The principal goal in treatment of the acute exacerbation of asthma is the rapid reversal of airflow obstruction, which can best be achieved by the frequent administration of inhaled beta$_2$-agonist. In addition, the early addition of systemic corticosteroids improves the response in patients who incompletely respond to beta$_2$-agonist. Hypoxemia, if present, must be corrected with administration of supplemental oxygen. Close monitoring of the patient's condition and response to treatment is an essential part of care and, if the patient is over 4 years of age and can cooperate, should include PEFR measurement.

ASSESSMENT

A brief history pertinent to an exacerbation should be obtained. It should include the time of onset and possible causes of the exacerbation. The severity of symptoms before this episode should be ascertained, along with all current medications, time of last administered dose, and any recent use of systemic corticosteroids. The history should identify any previous hospitalizations and visits to the emergency room and documentation of loss of consciousness, intubation, and mechanical ventilation. Documentation of any other medical conditions or underlying lung disease is also important.

In the assessment of infants and children with an acute asthmatic exacerbation, several objective and subjective parameters may be used in combination to most accurately characterize the severity of the airway obstruction. These parameters are listed in Table 67-1. It is often difficult for physicians and parents to determine the severity of the airway obstruction in the infants and small children with asthma. However, by using a combination of the parameters, a fairly accurate assessment can be made and treatment instituted promptly. In order to understand the physiologic basis of these signs and symptoms, a brief discussion of the overall pathophysiologic processes of the acute exacerbation of asthma is necessary.

PATHOPHYSIOLOGY

A definition of asthma is important because an exacerbation of asthma is a worsening of the underlying disease: "Asthma is a pulmonary disease with the following characteristics: 1) airway obstruction that is reversible either spontaneously or with treatment; 2) airway inflammation, and 3) increased airway responsiveness to a variety of stimuli."[10]

The physiologic changes in asthma are the result of inflammatory events in the airways, which include cellular infiltration and the release of inflammatory mediators. Although airflow obstruction is the major underlying pathophysiologic process in asthma, other physiologic changes contribute to the clinical events during acute exacerbations. During acute asthma, airways narrow because of bronchospasm, mucosal edema, and mucus plugging. Air is trapped behind occluded or narrowed small airways. Functional residual capacity rises, and the asthmatic patient breathes at close to total lung capacity. The work of breathing increases, and accessory muscles of respiration (e.g., sternocleidomastoid muscles) must be used. The use of the accessory muscles of respiration is more strongly correlated with the severity of acute asthma exacerbation than is wheezing. Hypoxemia is always present during severe asthma exacerbations because of mismatching of ventilation and perfusion (V/Q); this V/Q mismatching can persist for many days.[11]

During the initial stages of an exacerbation of asthma, alveolar ventilation is maintained, and carbon dioxide (CO_2) levels are decreased. As increasing airflow obstruction occurs and the forced expiratory volume in 1 sec (FEV_1) or PEFR decreases to less than 25% of the values predicted, there is alveolar hypoventilation and an increase in arterial CO_2. During a severe asthma exacerbation, hypoxemia and pulmonary hyperinflation may lead to an increase in pulmonary vascular resistance. Negative pleural pressures become more negative with hyperinflation, and pulmonary hyperinflation can produce an increased afterload on the left ventricle. These changes in pleural pressure and lung volumes are clinically apparent in a pulsus paradoxus. It is important to remember that the basis of these changes is airway inflammation with resultant edema, brochospasm, and increased production of mucus.

ESTIMATION OF SEVERITY OF ACUTE EXACERBATION OF ASTHMA IN CHILDREN

Overall alertness or response to environment and to parents may help determine the level of fatigue of a patient. Respiratory rate is variable in children and should be assessed when a patient is at rest or sleeping because activity can markedly increase the respiratory rate.[12]

Dyspnea, measured according to the parents' or physicians' impression of the degree of a child's breathlessness, can help determine the degree of airway obstruction. This can be semiquantified by having the child say a sentence with one breath or count to 10 with one breath. As the child improves, he or she will be able to count higher or say more words without needing to take another breath.

Pulsus paradoxus is the difference in fluctuation of systolic blood pressure between inspiration and expiration; systolic blood pressure falls with inspiration and rises with expiration. It can best be measured in children by a sphygmomanometer and stethoscope as the difference between the systolic blood pressure at which sporadic, faint pulse sounds are first heard and the pressure at which all sounds are heard.[12] No attempt should be made to correlate pulsus paradoxus with phase of respiration. One limitation in children is that the heart rate is often so fast in small children that systolic blood pressure is difficult to measure without an arterial catheter. However, if the pulsus paradoxus is higher than 20 mm Hg, moderate to severe obstruction is present.[13]

Accessory muscle use is strongly correlated with airway obstruction in children. It has been shown that the use of the sternocleidomastoid muscles is correlated with a PEFR or FEV_1 of less than 50% of that predicted.[14] In addition, parents and health professionals, such as school nurses, can be taught to watch for intercostal retractions and use of other accessory muscles. The alae nasi flare when both nares are enlarged during inspiration. Such flaring indicates that accessory muscles are being recruited for inspiration. It is an excellent sign of dyspnea.

Wheezing indicates partial obstruction and may be caused by single or multiple points of a narrowing within the airways. Wheezing is probably the least sensitive indicator of airflow obstruction. A louder wheeze is usually thought to be a sign of more airway obstruction; however, the obstruction may be so extensive that not enough airflow for wheezing is being generated. Therefore, quietness in the chest may indicate severe obstruction.

V/Q inequalities in the lung lead to hypoxemia in acute asthma. One of the measurements that is predictive of the need for hospitalization in asthma is an oxygen saturation (Sa_{O_2}) of less than 91% of breathing room air. This is easily measured with a pulse oximeter and can be used in small infants.

The best objective measurement of airflow obstruction in an acute asthmatic episode is PEFR. This rate quantifies the degree of obstruction and is a measure of the response of a patient to bronchodilator medication. It can be used with any child aged 4 years or older. Because only a short blast of air is required, PEFR can be used in children with acute obstruction.

Only patients with a PEFR of less than 25% of that predicted are at risk for significant hypercapnia.[15] It is often difficult for physicians and parents to determine the severity of the airway obstruction in infants and small children with asthma. However, by using a combination of the parameters in Table 67–1, a fairly accurate assessment can be made and treatment instituted promptly.

HOME MANAGEMENT

Many patients who have moderate to severe asthma have at-home equipment and medications necessary for treating and monitoring an acute asthmatic exacerbation. In addition, patients who live in rural settings may have to manage an acute asthmatic exacerbation at home.

Figure 67–1 provides a protocol for home management of an acute exacerbation. The severity of the asthmatic episode should be assessed on the basis of the child's general activity level, response to the environment, pulse rate, respiratory rate, degree of airflow obstruction, and use of accessory muscles. In addition, PEFR measurements should be obtained in children older than 5 years. Patients may be treated with inhalation of a selective beta$_2$-agonist delivered by a metered-dose inhaler (MDI) with or without a spacer device.

After the first nebulizer treatment, a patient should be assessed for improvement in airflow movement, heart rate, respiratory rate, and PEFR. If there is no improvement in symptoms and PEFR remains extremely low (less than 30% of base line), the patient should seek immediate medical care. If PEFR has improved to more than 70% to 90% of base line, the beta$_2$-agonist should be continued every 2 h for three doses. Additional medications, such as oral theophylline, may also be administered at this time. It is important that the patient be assessed continually and that the physician be kept informed of the patient's status. The degree of care provided in the home depends on both the physician's and the patient's experience and the availability of emergency care.

OFFICE OR EMERGENCY ROOM MANAGEMENT

Many pediatricians and family practitioners prefer to treat an acute exacerbation of asthma in their offices. An air compressor for nebulizing medications, a Mini-Wright Peak Flow Meter or spirometer for objectively monitoring airflow obstruction, and supplemental oxy-

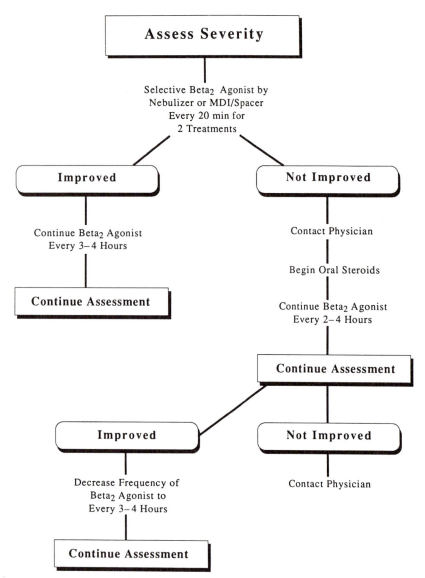

Figure 67–1. Acute asthma in childhood: home management.

gen should be available. If the patient fails to improve with nebulized beta$_2$-agonists given every 20 min for 1 h in the office setting (PEFR < 70% of that predicted), the patient should be transferred to an emergency room for further treatment and monitoring. Figure 67–2 provides a flow diagram for acute management in the physician's office and the emergency room.

A child in the physician's office or the emergency room with an acute asthmatic attack should be assessed clinically as to the severity of the asthma; the assessment should be based on the child's general activity level, response to the environment, color, pulse rate, degree of pulsus paradoxus, use of accessory muscles, and airflow obstruction (measured by auscultation). In addition, PEFR measurement should be determined in children over 5 years of age, and continuous measurement of oxygenation with a pulse oximeter is also helpful.

Initial treatment should be with a selective beta$_2$-agonist, such as albuterol,[16-23] delivered by nebulizer, preferably with oxygen. Nebulized treatments should be given

every 20 min for 1 h, and then the patient should be reassessed. There is no evidence that theophylline adds to the bronchodilation achieved with beta$_2$-agonist in the first 4 h in the emergency room.[16, 17] If the patient is significantly improved (PEFR > 70% of that predicted), the beta$_2$-agonist treatment may be decreased to every 1 to 2 h, and the patient should be observed at least for 2 h. If after that time the patient is stable, he or she may be discharged to home, and education, medication, and a follow-up plan should be instituted.

If the patient is not significantly improved after the initial hour of beta$_2$-agonist treatment (PEFR < 70% of that predicted), nebulized treatments are continued every 20 min for 2 h. Oral or intravenous steroids should be added to the regimen.[24-27] The severity of the patient's condition should be continually assessed, and a decision should be made in 2 h as to whether the patient's treatment can be continued in the emergency room, whether hospitalization is necessary, or whether discharge to home is possible. If improved, a patient should be observed in the emer-

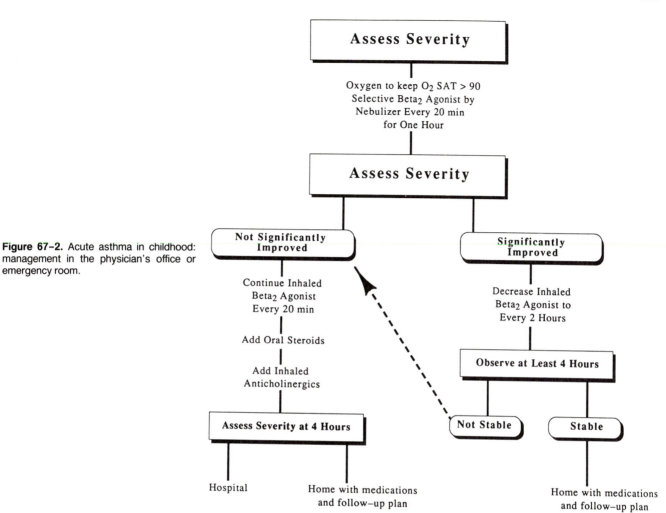

Figure 67–2. Acute asthma in childhood: management in the physician's office or emergency room.

gency room for at least 2 h more to ensure maintenance of improvement.

HOSPITAL MANAGEMENT

Upon admission to the hospital from the hospital emergency room or an outlying emergency room, the severity of the illness should be assessed (Fig. 67–3). In addition to clinical parameters and PEFR, this assessment may include an arterial blood gas measurement. The physician must decide whether the patient requires intensive therapy and close monitoring in an intensive care unit or intermediate care unit or whether the patient is stable enough to be managed on a general hospital floor. If stable enough for a general room (PEFR > 30% of that predicted, arterial carbon dioxide tension $[Pa_{CO_2}] < 40$ mm Hg, and $Sa_{O_2} \geq 90\%$), the patient should be treated initially with nebulized beta$_2$-agonists every 1 to 2 h and with oral or intravenous steroids every 6 h, oral sustained-release theophylline every 12 h, or intravenous aminophylline.[28-31] In addition, the patient should be monitored closely for signs of either increasing severity or improvement; in children over 5 years of age, monitoring should include PEFR measurement. If the patient is improved in the next 24 to 48 h, the patient may be discharged, and education and a continued management plan should be instituted. If the patient's condition deteriorates (PEFR < 40% of that predicted, $Pa_{CO_2} > 40$ mm Hg), he or she should be transferred to an intensive care unit.

Intensive care unit management requires the help of a specialist and includes blood gas assessment, continuous pulse oximetry, and frequent monitoring of PEFR. The patient admitted to the intensive care unit should be given oxygen and be treated with continuous nebulized albuterol,[28, 32, 33] intravenous steroids[24-27] every 6 h, and intravenous aminophylline given by continuous infusion.[29-31] The addition of anticholinergic medications may be considered at this time by the specialist.[34-40] Nebulized ipratropium bromide (not currently available in the United States) has been shown to be the most effective.

The patient in the intensive care unit must be continuously assessed. If the patient is not improving (PEFR < 25% of that expected, $Pa_{CO_2} > 45$ mm Hg), an arterial catheter should be inserted for continous monitoring of blood pressure, heart rate, and blood gas levels. If the patient does not improve, a trail of intravenous terbutaline may be given. If a trial of intravenous terbutaline does not result in an improvement and the patient is having progressive increase in fatigue, the patient should be

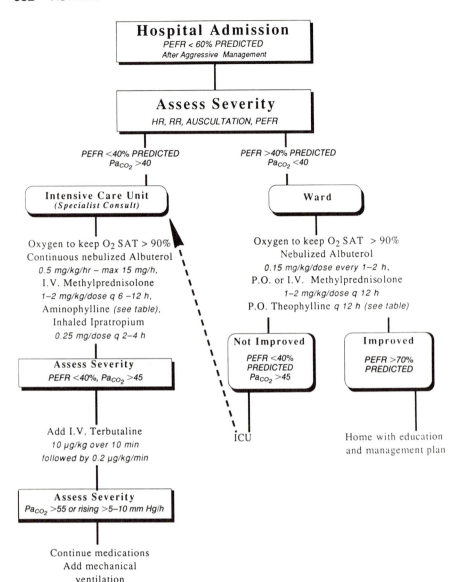

Figure 67-3. Acute asthma in childhood: hospital management. PEFR, peak expiratory flow rate; HR, heart rate; RR, respiratory rate; Pa_{CO_2}, carbon dioxide tension; SAT, saturation; I.V., intravenous; P.O., per orum; q, every; ICU, intensive care unit.

mechanically ventilated. Ventilation of an asthmatic patient is difficult and always requires the assistance of a qualified specialist.

MEDICATIONS

The therapy for acute exacerbations of asthma in children has undergone a number of changes. Although the same classes of drugs (sympathomimetic agents, anticholinergic agents, methylxanthines, and corticosteroids) have been available since the early 1960s, results of investigations since the early 1980s have defined the relative importance of each drug class. Dosage schedules and routes of administration have also been more firmly established so that current recommendations are based on extensive scientific evidence. Some issues are still unresolved, and they are also discussed in this section.

The cornerstone of therapy of acute asthmatic exacerbations is early aggressive intervention aimed at treating both the bronchospasm and the underlying inflamma-

tion. Therefore, as indicated in Figure 67-1, therapy should begin in the home. Most deaths from acute, severe asthma occur before patients reach a clinic or a hospital, usually as a result of inadequate assessment of the severity by the patients, which results in undertreatment.[7] A review of 3358 pediatric emergency room visits over a 16-month period underscores the problem of inadequate assessment and underuse of appropriate therapies.[41] The investigators found that objective measurements of severity were performed erratically, bronchodilators were often administered in inadequate doses, and corticosteroids were unused; all these factors led to a high hospital admission rate. Therefore, it is essential to remember that patients die as a result of underuse of medications and only extremely rarely of toxicity.

In one investigation, institution of an organized treatment protocol in an adult emergency department increased the efficiency of care of acute asthma, as shown by a decrease in the hospital admission rate and a decrease in average length of stay.[42] Open communication between patients and clinicians, education, and readily available access to the health care system are also essential components of therapy. May and co-workers[43] demonstrated that an intensive outpatient treatment program that emphasized teaching patients aggressive self-management with objective measurement (PEFR monitoring) and easier access to the health care team resulted in a reduction in the number of days in the hospital and a reduction in readmission rates. These studies should remind clinicians that an organized approach to the delivery of care and to education of and understanding by patients are as important to improving outcome in acute asthma as knowing how to administer the appropriate drug therapy.

OXYGEN

All patients arriving at the emergency room with acute severe asthma should be administered oxygen.[44] Hypoxemia is a universal finding in acute severe asthma (see Pathophysiology section) and occurs with and without hypercapnia.[45] Besides producing air hunger and anxiety, hypoxia has been associated with bronchoconstriction[46] and increased bronchial reactivity,[47] which may be deleterious in acute asthma. In addition, bronchodilator therapy can initially worsen the V/Q mismatch from pulmonary vascular dilation, producing an increase in hypoxemia. This phenomenon can occur with both aerosol and systemic administration of sympathomimetic agents, although it is not universally found with aerosol administration.[18, 48] Pulse oximetry may be used to monitor oxygen therapy.[49] There is evidence that patients with Sa_{O_2} of less than 91% have a poor outcome despite responding well to initial therapy.[49] Most of these patients have recurrences of wheezing and require hospitalization, whereas those with an initial Sa_{O_2} of at least 95% rarely experience relapse after discharge.

Enough oxygen should be administered to maintain Sa_{O_2} of more than 93%. There has been some concern that the administration of oxygen could result in an increase in arterial carbon dioxide tension (Pa_{CO_2}) in some patients. This appears to be a problem only in adults with chronic obstructive pulmonary disease and not in acute severe asthma.[50] Low oxygen flow rates typically produced by nasal cannulae are often inadequate when a patient is hyperventilating and thereby entraining large amounts of room air. During the initial stages of therapy, air entrainment may increase as the severe obstruction is reversed and the tidal volume increases. Thirty-five percent oxygen delivered by mask has been demonstrated to be both safe and effective in the initial therapy of acute, severe asthma.[50]

BETA-AGONISTS

The beta-adrenergic agonists are the most potent bronchodilators and the drugs of first choice in the setting of acute asthmatic exacerbations.[26, 44] The literature clearly indicates that a greater improvement in pulmonary functions can be produced with significantly fewer adverse effects when beta-agonists are given by the aerosol route

than when they are administered by the systemic route.[22] No advantage to systemic administration has been found in acute, severe asthma even in hospitalized patients with the most severe obstruction.[22, 26] Fanta and collaborators[17] observed that aerosolized administration of isoproterenol produced a significantly greater improvement in FEV_1 than did subcutaneous epinephrine in patients with severe obstruction (i.e., baseline $FEV_1 \leq 35\%$ of that predicted). The two treatments produced a similar improvement in patients with baseline FEV_1 values 35% higher than those predicted.

The results of a double-blind crossover trial by Appel and associates[51] suggested that subcutaneous epinephrine would improve PEFR in patients not initially responsive to aerosolized metaproterenol, but aerosolized metaproterenol would not improve PEFR in patients unresponsive to subcutaneous epinephrine. Each patient received the initial treatment every 30 min for three doses, and then, after 1 hour, the other treatment was administered. The duration of action of metaproterenol would be expected to provide some carryover beta$_2$-agonist activity into the epinephrine treatment period, but not vice versa,[52] and the relative beta$_2$-agonist dose achieved by a 15-mg dose of metaproterenol is considerably less than that achieved by the 2.5-mg dose of isoproterenol used by Fanta and collaborators[17] or the 5-mg dose of albuterol that is currently recommended;[52] these facts call the relevance of Appel and associates' findings[51] into question.

The airway obstruction and hypoxemia are potent cardiac stimulants resulting in tachycardia and premature atrial and ventricular contractions.[22, 26] Because the relief of the pathophysiologic processes in acute severe asthma results in a decreased heart rate and an improvement in abnormal rhythms, some authors have questioned the need to use selective beta$_2$-agonists, particularly when the aerosol route of administration is used.[26] A critical review of the available literature revealed that selective beta$_2$-agonists produce significantly less cardiac stimulation than do the nonselective agents even when both are administered as an aerosol.[53]

Two studies of aerosolized beta-agonists in children with acute, severe asthma aptly illustrate the difference between selective and nonselective agents. Garra and co-workers[54] compared aerosolized isoproterenol and metaproterenol administered every 30 min for 2 h and followed by hourly administration over 6 h. These authors reported significant increases in heart rate; in many cases, the rate approached 200 beats per minute after administration of both drugs. In addition, the heart rates of patients treated with metaproterenol were persistently elevated between treatments, which is consistent with the longer elimination half-life for metaproterenol.[52] However, both of the beta-agonists (isoproterenol and metaproterenol) act as nonselective beta-agonists,[22] although some authors mistakenly list metaproterenol as a beta$_2$-selective agent.[44] Schuh and co-workers[21] investigated two dosages of the beta$_2$-selective agent albuterol (0.05 and 0.15 mg/kg/dose, each given every 20 min for 3 h and found only 20% and 16% increases in heart rates for the low-dose and high-dose groups, respectively (i.e., mean maximal heart rates of 133 and 134 beats per minute); no heart rate exceeded 160 beats per minute. The patients in the high-dose group achieved a 130% mean improvement in FEV_1 over base line after 1 h, in contrast to the 70% improvement seen in the patients receiving metaproterenol in the study by Garra and co-workers.[54]

Some authors suggested that an MDI attached to a spacer device is an acceptable alternative to wet nebulization for delivering beta$_2$-agonists in acute, severe asthma.[26, 55] This raises an interesting question because use of an MDI with a spacer device has the advantage of being less expensive and, in many hospitals, not requiring the assistance of a respiratory therapist. However, the currently available data suggest that the nebulizer is the delivery method of choice. This conclusion is based on a review of studies of aerosol delivery as well as on comparisons of response in acute, severe asthma. Essentially, if two different delivery systems can deliver the same dose to the lungs, they will produce the same effects. Lung deposition studies indicate that approximately 10% of the starting dose from either form of delivery reaches the lung.[104] According to this estimate, calculation of the dose equivalence of the two delivery techniques is straightforward for albuterol:

By MDI, 0.1 mg/puff $\times$ 0.1
$$= 0.01 \text{ mg/puff that reaches airways;}$$

By nebulizer, 2.5 mg $\times$ 0.1
$$= 0.25 \text{ mg/treatment that reaches airways.}$$

Therefore, 25 puffs from MDI yields the same amount as 2.5 mg by nebulizer. For terbutaline,

By MDI, 0.25 mg/puff $\times$ 0.1
$$= 0.25 \text{ mg/puff that reaches airways;}$$

By nebulizer, 5 mg $\times$ 0.1
$$= 0.5 \text{ mg/treatment that reaches airways.}$$

Therefore, 20 puffs from MDI yield the same amount as 5 mg by nebulizer.

In an excellent review, Newman explained that the problem with this type of comparison is that the delivery by both methods can be altered by inhalation technique.[56] Slow, deep inhalation and breath holding improve deposition by either technique. With MDIs, deposition may be further improved by using a large volume spacer device. Greater delivery of a given dose in a jet nebulizer can be achieved by diluting the dose in a larger volume or by using closed systems and intermittent systems with a valve that allows nebulization only during inhalation. Tapping the sides of the nebulizer decreases the amount of drug trapped on the walls and baffles of the nebulizer. Most important, flow rates of the compressed gas into the nebulizer can significantly alter the percentage of respirable (5-μm–diameter) droplets produced. With these caveats in mind, Newman reviewed seven studies of deposition from MDIs and showed a range of 5% to 18% mean airway deposition between studies; ranges often exceed 10% within the individual studies.[56] The same was true for the eight nebulizer studies.[56]

Results of physiologic studies (i.e., tests after pulmo-nary function response) have been inconsistent. In studies of stable asthmatic patients and normal controls, investigators have reported dose-response curves that are consistent with greater lung deposition produced by MDI or by MDI with a spacer than by nebulizer.[23, 57, 58] However, studies in patients with acute, severe asthma have not shown that an MDI with a spacer provides a greater deposition, as measured by degree of bronchodilation. In the only study in which equivalent dosages by each method were used, Morgan and co-authors[59] reported identical responses to terbutaline in a crossover trial of 18 asthmatic adults. In two other well-controlled studies, larger doses of terbutaline administered by nebulizer showed more improvement than smaller doses given by MDI,[60, 61] as would be expected. In other trials, investigators have evaluated different delivery techniques with albuterol, but they did not use equivalent doses by each technique and were not as rigorous in their design, and so it is hard to draw any firm conclusion.[55, 62–64] However, it is unlikely that albuterol would provide results significantly different from those produced by terbutaline. In conclusion, if these drugs are given in equivalent dosages, it appears that the physiologic responses are identical, regardless of aerosol delivery technique.

In clinical practice, however, many patients with acute obstruction of the airways are unable to use MDIs efficiently, and children under 6 years of age are unlikely to use MDIs efficiently even when stable. Patients with acute obstruction are generally unable to control inspiratory flow rates and coordinate inspiration with activation of the canister. In all studies showing good results from use of an MDI with a spacer, trained personnel also assisted the patients with administration.[30, 31, 34–36] Thus use of an MDI does not obviate the requirement of assistance from respiratory therapists or trained nurses. In addition, the oxygen mixture can be used as the driving gas in the nebulizer, which also simplifies administration. Therefore, wet nebulization is the preferred route of administration of aerosol beta$_2$-agonists in children with acute, severe asthma because of the ease of administering the high dosages required to treat this condition.

The optimal dosage of aerosolized beta$_2$-agonists in acute, severe asthma of childhood is unknown. Both *in vitro* and *in vivo* studies suggest that the dose-response curve of bronchial smooth muscle is shifted to the right as the contractile stimulus is increased, so that higher dosages of beta$_2$-agonists are required in order to produce the same degree of bronchodilation in acute, severe asthma, in contrast to stable asthma.[22] The duration of action of aerosolized beta$_2$-agonists is also considerably shorter in acute, severe asthma than in stable, chronic asthma and this can also affect the dose-response characteristics.[22, 52] Robertson and colleagues[20] first demonstrated the importance of duration of action in determining the optimal dosing frequency of aerosolized beta$_2$-agonists in acute, severe asthma. They found that 0.05 mg/kg of aerosolized albuterol given every 20 min produced a significantly greater improvement in FEV_1 than did 0.15 mg/kg given hourly (i.e., the same total dose administered per hour). As illustrated in Figure 67–4, the difference was attributable to the decline in FEV_1 that began within 20 min of administering the hourly dose.

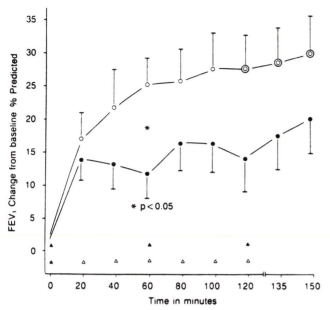

Figure 67–4. Forced expiratory flow in 1 second (FEV$_1$), percentage predicted plus standard error of the mean before and at 20-min intervals after 0.15 mg/kg (filled triangles) and 0.05 mg/kg (open triangles) of albuterol in group 1 (filled circles) and group 2 (open circles). Wheezing scores (dotted circles) were significantly lower ($p < .01$) in group 2 than in group 1. (From Robertson CF, Smith F, Beck R, et al: Response to frequent low doses of nebulized salbutamol in acute asthma. J Pediatr 106:672–674, 1985.)

It makes little sense to arbitrarily wait 1 h between treatments as the obstruction worsens. Since Robertson and colleagues' study,[20] the relatively short duration of action has been confirmed through the use of bronchoprovoca-tion studies in patients with stable asthma.[52] Portnoy and Aggarwal[33] and Kelly and collaborators[28] also showed that many hospitalized patients with severe obstruction respond to continuously nebulized beta$_2$-agonists after failing treatment of standard intermittent dosing.[28, 32, 33] The delivery device that the authors use for administering continuously nebulized albuterol is shown in Figure 67–5.

Two follow-up studies by Schuh and co-workers[21] also illustrated important concepts. They compared the low-dose (0.05 mg/kg up to 1.7 mg/dose every 20 min) regimen with a higher dosage (0.15 mg/kg up to 5 mg/dose every 20 min). The high-dose group exhibited significantly more improvement in FEV$_1$ (132%) than did the low-dose group (58% improvement); there was no difference in adverse effects. In another study, Robertson and colleagues[20] compared the standard hourly albuterol dose (0.15 mg/kg up to 5 mg/dose) to a higher hourly dose (0.3 mg/kg up to 10 mg/dose). They found that the higher dose produced more improvement in FEV$_1$ than did the lower dose. Like the every–20-min dosing regimen described previously, the high-dose hourly regimen produced steady, continuous improvement with less of the fluctuation produced by the low-dose hourly regime. This result is consistent with the finding that both peak effect and duration of action of aerosolized beta$_2$-agonists are dose dependent.[22, 52] Thus a number of alternative treatments are possible if the patient is not optimally responding to standard doses of the aerosolized beta$_2$-agonist; either increase the hourly dose or increase the frequency of administration, or both. For optimal delivery of the aerosol beta$_2$-agonist, dilution to a final volume of 3.5 to 4.5 ml in the nebulizer with an oxygen flow rate of 6 to 7

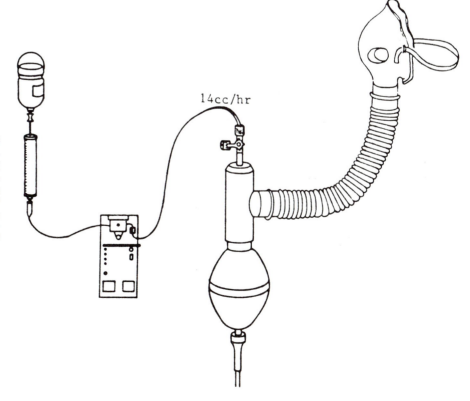

Figure 67–5. Setup for administration of continuous inhalation of albuterol, developed by Richard Levin, RRT. Ideal I-med flow into nebulizer, 14 ml/h. Example: Albuterol dose is 0.5 mg/kg/h (5 mg/ml); dose for a child weighing 20 kg is 10 mg/h (2 ml/h); total dose for 8 h at 14 ml/h is 112 ml; dose of albuterol at 2 ml/h is 16 ml; therefore, total dose (112 ml) − 2 ml/h dose (16 ml) = 96 ml normal saline.

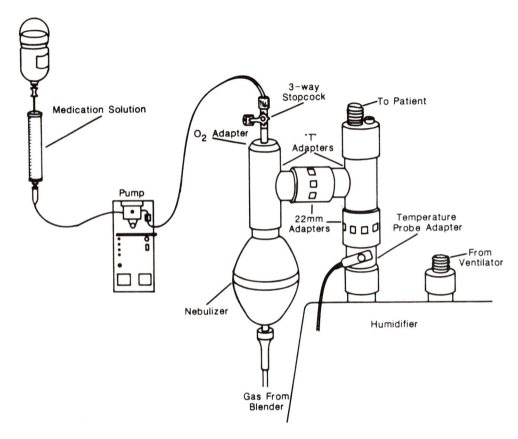

Figure 67–6. Setup for administration of continuous inhalation of albuterol through a ventilator circuit. Developed by Richard Levin, RRT.

l/min is recommended.[21,65] Figure 67–6 illustrates the setups that the authors have used for administering continuous nebulized albuterol through a ventilator circuit.

Despite their relatively long elimination half-lives, the selective beta$_2$-agonists (albuterol and terbutaline) produce few significant side effects even when administered continuously for prolonged periods.[8, 21, 32, 33] Significant hypokalemia does not occur as long as the patients receive standard maintenance dosages of potassium intravenously.[28] Because of the beta$_2$ selectivity, tachycardia is generally mild and is easily monitored in hospitalized patients. The greatest degree of tachycardia generally occurs in the first 60 to 80 min after administration of beta-agonists and then gradually improves despite continued administration.[21, 65] This probably reflects cardiac beta$_2$-receptor down-regulation,[53] as well as improvement in airway obstruction, but improvement in airway obstruction is the most significant factor. Beta$_2$-agonists can also elevate serum lactate levels,[66] and this can potentially worsen the lactic acidosis produced by the hypoxemia and the increased work of breathing in patients with severe obstruction. In the authors' experience, this has not been a significant problem. The serum lactate levels generally decrease over time, despite ongoing administration of high-dose aerosolized beta$_2$-agonist, when the obstruction and hypoxemia are corrected.

METHYLXANTHINES

The controversy surrounding the use of theophylline for acute, severe asthma has been reviewed.[29, 31] Rossing and associates[16] first demonstrated that intravenous ami-

nophylline was a significantly less potent bronchodilator than either parenteral or aerosolized sympathomimetics given as a single agent in the management of acute asthma in the emergency room. The same investigators then demonstrated that aminophylline added to optimal doses of aerosolized beta-agonists did not cause any perceptible increase in bronchodilation.[17] In a meta-analysis of 13 studies in which the efficacy of aminophylline for acute, severe asthma was evaluated, only one trial demonstrated an unequivocal beneficial response.[67] However, this was the only double-blind, placebo-controlled trial of aminophylline in hospitalized patients in which the patients were evaluated over a 24-h period.[30] Results of other studies have also indicated a delayed response in which maximal benefit from theophylline occurred 18 to 24 h after initiation of aminophylline.[31] This is most likely caused by the decrease in concentration of inflammatory and bronchoconstrictive mediators, shifting the theophylline concentration response curve back to the left so that the usual therapeutic concentrations can exert an effect.

Most of the aminophylline (or theophylline) studies have been conducted in the emergency room and/or the first 4 hours in the hospitalized patients.[21, 67] These studies unequivocally show that theophylline provides no added benefit and possibly increases adverse effects with optimal doses of aerosolized beta$_2$-agonists in the initial management of acute, severe asthma. The role of theophylline in the management of hospitalized patients is less clear. The double-blind, placebo-controlled study in children by Pierson and co-workers[30] demonstrated a positive significant benefit for aminophylline. However, a double-blind, placebo-controlled trial of aminophylline in hospitalized adults showed no beneficial effect.[68] In that study, the patients were evaluated over 32 h. The only differences between trials were the ages of the populations and the drugs used (the longer acting, selective beta₂-agonist albuterol in the latter trial[68] and isoproterenol and isoetharine in the study by Pierson and co-workers[30]). Thus until further studies are completed, aminophylline is still recommended for the therapy of hospitalized children with acute, severe asthma.

Because of its propensity for producing significant serious side effects (i.e., seizures, encephalopathy, gastrointestinal bleeding, and cardiac arrhythmias), theophylline should not be used unless serum theophylline concentrations can be monitored in an expeditious manner. Either intravenous aminophylline or oral sustained-release theophylline may be used. There is no advantage to the intra-

venous route of administration unless the patient is vomiting and unable to take oral medication. The authors recommend adjusting the dosages to maintain a steady-state theophylline concentration between 10 and 15 mg/l. See Table 67-2 for dosage and monitoring recommendations.

ANTICHOLINERGIC AGENTS

There has been a resurgence of interest in anticholinergic agents with the introduction of the more broncho-selective quaternary derivatives such as ipratropium bromide.[38, 39] Unlike sympathomimetic agents and methylxanthines, anticholinergic agents are not physiologic

Table 67-2. DOSAGES OF DRUGS IN ACUTE CHILDHOOD ASTHMA

Drug	Form	Available Dosage	Comment
Inhaled Beta₂-Agonist			
Albuterol (Ventolin, Proventil)			If no improvement, switch to nebulizer.
Metered dose inhaler	90 μg/puff, 200 puffs	2 inhalations every 5 min for total of 12 puffs	If improvement, decrease frequency to 4 puffs every hour
Nebulizer solution	0.5% (5 mg/ml)	0.15 mg/kg/dose up to 5 mg every 20 min for 1–2 h (minimum dose, 1.25 mg/dose)[21]	If improvement, decrease frequency to 1 to 2 h
		0.5 mg/kg/h by continuous nebulization (maximum, 15 mg/h)[28, 32, 33]	If no improvement, use by continuous inhalation
Systemic Beta₂-Agonist			
Epinephrine hydrochloride	1:1000 (1 mg/ml)	0.01 mg/kg up to 0.5 mg subcutaneously every 20 min for 3 doses	Inhaled beta₂-agonist preferred
Terbutaline (Bricanyl, Brethine)	1 mg/ml solution for injection	Subcutaneous 0.01 mg/kg up to 0.5 mg every 2–6 h as needed; intravenous 10 μg/kg over 10 min as loading dose, followed by 0.2 μg/kg/min, increasing as necessary[102]	Inhaled beta₂-agonist preferred
Methylxanthines			
Theophylline*	Aminophylline (80% anhydrous theophylline)	*Loading Dose* If theophylline concentration known: every 1 mg/kg dose produces 2 μg/ml increase in concentration If theophylline concentration is unknown: if no previous theophylline, administer 9 mg/kg aminophylline; if previous theophylline administered >6 h ago, administer 6 mg/kg aminophylline; if <6 hours ago, administer 3 mg/kg aminophylline If previous sustained-release theophylline administered >12 h ago, administer 6 mg/kg aminophylline; if <12 h ago, administer 3 mg/kg aminophylline *Infusion rates to obtain a mean steady-state concentration of 15 μg/ml* At ages 1–6 months, 0.5 mg/kg/h aminophylline; 6 months–1 year, 1.0 mg/kg/h aminophylline; 1–9 years, 1.5 mg/kg/h aminophylline; 10–16 years, 1.2 mg/kg/h aminophylline	

Table continued on following page

Table 67–2. DOSAGES OF DRUGS IN ACUTE CHILDHOOD ASTHMA *Continued*

Drug	Form	Available Dosage	Comment
Corticosteroids			
Hydrocortisone (various manufacturers)	Intravenously	4–6 mg/kg/dose every 6 h for 24–48 h, then 4 mg/kg/day	
Methylprednisolone (various manufacturers)	Intravenously	1–2 mg/kg/dose every 6 h for 24–48 h, then 1–2 mg/kg/day	
Prednisone tablets	Oral (5, 10, 20 mg)	1 mg/kg/dose every 6 h for 24–48 h, then 1–2 mg/kg/day every 12 h	Duration dependent on clinical course (see text)
Prednisolone (Pediapred Liquid)	Oral (1 mg/ml)	1 mg/kg/dose every 6 h for 24 h, then 1–2 mg/kg/day every 12 h	Duration dependent on clinical course (see text)
Prednisone (Prelone Liquid)	Oral (15 mg/5 ml)	1 mg/kg/dose every 6 h for 24 h, then 1–2 mg/kg/day every 12 h	Duration dependent on clinical course (see text)
Anticholinergics			
Ipratropium bromide (Atrovent)	18 μg/puff 0.025% solution	5–10 inhalations with a spacer device every 4–6 h; 250 mg every 4–6 h	Not approved by FDA for use in children; not available in United States
Atropine SO$_4$ (various manufacturers)	0.5% (5 mg/ml) 1.0% (10 mg/ml) ophthalmic solution	0.025–0.05 mg/kg max 5 mg in nebulized doses every 6 h	Not recommended because of absorption and side effects
Glycopyrrolate (Robinul)	0.2 mg/ml injectable solution	0.025–0.05 mg/kg in nebulized doses every 6 h	Not approved for this use

FDA, Food and Drug Administration (United States).
*Monitor theophylline blood levels 1 h after loading dose and then 6, 12, and 24 h. Monitor at 6 and 12 h after any dosage adjustment or every 24 h during continuous intravenous infusion. If oral sustained-release theophylline is used, monitor levels at 4–8 h after a dose. Monitor every 24 h while patient is in hospital.

antagonists of smooth muscle contraction. They competitively inhibit acetylcholine activity at the muscarinic receptor at the neuromuscular junction.[38] Therefore, they produce bronchodilation only if the bronchoconstriction is mediated by cholinergic input. Because the bronchospasm in asthma is produced by mediators with a direct effect on smooth muscle as well as indirect effects (i.e., irritant receptor stimulation producing cholinergic reflex–mediated constriction), anticholinergic agents would never be considered as primary therapy of acute, severe asthma. A recent review of 18 trials of anticholinergics in acute severe asthma revealed mixed results.[69]

Despite proven efficacy as a bronchodilator,[37] nebulized atropine sulfate has not added significant bronchodilation to aerosolized beta-agonists in acute, severe asthma, even when administered in doses that produced significant systemic effects.[69] Atropine sulfate is completely absorbed when administered orally or by inhalation, and so it cannot be recommended for use in acute, severe asthma.[70]

Studies of nebulized ipratropium bromide added to aerosolized beta-agonists generally show that the combination produces more bronchodilation than do beta-agonists alone.[69] The mean maximal improvement in pulmonary functions has been 40% greater with the combination than with beta-agonist therapy, but this has been found only in studies of adult patients.[35, 71] The mean improvement reported in two pediatric studies was only 20% greater than with beta-agonist therapy alone.[34, 36] In these two studies, frequent administration of high-dose albuterol (0.15 mg/kg every 20 min) produced a 70% or greater further improvement over the low-dose regimen.[21, 65] It remains to be seen whether ipratropium bromide will produce further bronchodilation when added to high-dose inhaled albuterol. In addition, despite the further improvement in bronchodilation, the administration

of ipratropium bromide did not result in any significant difference in overall outcome (i.e., number of patients admitted to a hospital or length of hospital stay) in any of the pediatric studies.

The authors recommend anticholinergic agents in patients who apparently do not respond optimally to aerosolized beta$_2$-agonist. Unfortunately, ipratropium bromide in a 0.25-mg dose is not available as a nebulizer solution in the United States, and so multiple puffs from an MDI with a spacer would be needed. An equivalent dose would be approximately 10 inhalations from the MDI. An alternative would be 0.025- to 0.05-mg/kg doses of glycopyrrolate injectable solution by nebulization every 6 h.[69] Glycopyrrolate is also a quaternary ammonium derivative of atropine that produces long-lasting bronchodilation when administered in nebulized doses.[40, 69]

CORTICOSTEROIDS

The use of corticosteroids in acute severe asthma has been surrounded by controversy over the years.[72, 73] However, every double-blinded, placebo-controlled trial of corticosteroids in acute severe asthma, shows that systemic corticosteroids are essential in the treatment of acute, severe exacerbation requiring hospitalization. For more detail on the mechanisms of action and dose response characteristics of corticosteroids for acute severe asthma, the reader should refer to Chapter 81 or the review by Kelly and Murphy.[74]

Short bursts of systemic corticosteroids (i.e., 1 to 2 mg/kg of oral prednisone daily for 3 to 5 days) have been shown to result in a decrease in hospitalization rates and emergency room visits for children with moderate to severe asthma who do not achieve normalization of pulmonary functions after intensive nebulized beta$_2$-agonists.[24, 75, 76] Prescriptions for oral prednisone started during viral infections of the upper respiratory tract or for acute exacerbations not responding to nebulized albuterol should be considered for all patients with chronic moderate to severe asthma who have a history of frequent emergency room visits and hospitalizations.

The utility of initiating corticosteroids upon presentation to the emergency room or clinic remains controversial. Littenberg and Gluck[25] reported significantly fewer admissions among adult patients who were given a single dose of intravenous methylprenisolone before bronchodilator therapy was instituted than among those who received placebo. However, some of the patients had prolonged stays (up to 12 h) in the emergency room before the acute episode of asthma was controlled, and the investigators did not control any of the other therapies. Investigators in previous studies had failed to detect any effect on airway obstruction in acute asthma in the first 6 h after administration of methylprednisolone.[75, 76] However, a single-dose study in hospitalized asthmatic children showed that a peak improvement in PEFR occurred 4 to 6 h after an oral prednisone dose.[79]

Stein and Cole[80] performed a double-blind, placebo-controlled trial similar to that of Littenberg and Gluck,[25] except that they also controlled the bronchodilator therapy so that it was the same in all patients. They did not find any difference in either rate of improvement or number of admissions between the two groups of patients. However, a double-blind, placebo-controlled trial by Tal and colleagues[81] demonstrated a significant reduction of admissions to the hospital among infants and toddlers presenting to the emergency room with acute asthma. The decision to admit or discharge the patients was made after only 3 h of therapy in the emergency room.

Although the studies just described and the results of delays in administering corticosteroids in acute asthma support the position for early insititution, it appears that little would be lost by waiting until the response to 1 h of intensive aerosolized beta$_2$-agonists is determined. Therefore, routine administration of a single dose of systemic corticosteroids to every asthmatic patient in the emergency room would be unwarranted. However, every patient who does not achieve a full response to nebulized beta$_2$-agonists, whether eventually admitted to the hospital or discharged to home, probably should receive a course of systemic corticosteroids. The corticosteroids should be initially given in divided doses (at a minimum of every 12 h). Parenteral therapy is unnecessary even if patients are hospitalized unless they are unable to take oral medications. The duration of therapy is determined by the course of the exacerbation, and full dosage (1 to 2 mg/kg/day) should be administered until pulmonary functions approach normal and then either be stopped or be quickly tapered off over 2 to 4 days.

MISCELLANEOUS THERAPIES

The therapies mentioned here should be considered rather heroic measures and be used only in children who fail the standard therapy of high-dose, inhaled, selective beta$_2$-agonists and systemic corticosteroids. It is recommended that both aerosolized anticholinergic agents and theophylline be started before any of these therapies is instituted. It is assumed that for patients receiving these therapies, either respiratory failure is impending—arterial carbon dioxide tension (Pa$_{CO_2}$) > 45 mm Hg or is increasing despite optimal therapy—or the patients are being mechanically ventilated. None of these therapies should be attempted without the consultation of a pediatric pulmonologist, an intensivist, or an allergist familiar with treating severe asthma.

Intravenous beta-agonists, particularly isoproterenol, have been recommended since the early 1970s for the treatment of severe status asthmaticus in children.[82, 83] It has been contended that intravenous isoproterenol prevents intubation and mechanical ventilation in asthmatic children with impending respiratory failure who failed to respond to standard therapy.[82, 83] These studies were uncontrolled and consisted of reports of a series of treated cases. Standard therapy at the time consisted of two injections of epinephrine, intravenous aminophylline, and intravenous hydrocortisone without inhaled beta-agonist. The patients demonstrated an initial rapid drop in Pa$_{CO_2}$ over the first 2 h, but Pa$_{CO_2}$ only gradually improved to normal over 24 to 48 h. A follow-up trial again demonstrated an improvement in Pa$_{CO_2}$, but isoproterenol was not found to decrease the incidence of mechanical ventilation among children with impending respiratory failure.[84]

None of the published reports of intravenous isoproterenol were controlled clinical trials,[82–87] and inhaled beta-agonists in relatively low doses were used in only two.[84, 86] In addition, there have been reports of myocardial ischemia and fatal myocardial necrosis in children receiving intravenous isoproterenol for asthma.[88, 89] Bohn and associates,[90] in another uncontrolled study, indicated that the selective beta$_2$-agonist albuterol given intravenously produced a smoother response with less cardiac toxicity than did intravenous isoproterenol in children. A number of controlled clinical trials with both intravenous terbutaline and albuterol have variously shown those drugs to be no better than intravenous aminophylline[91–94] or aerosolized beta$_2$-agonists[95–100] in hospitalized patients with severe obstruction. Thus there have been no controlled studies providing unequivocal evidence that intravenous beta$_2$-agonists are superior or would provide further benefit when added to optimal aerosolized therapy. The older reports on isoproterenol are no longer relevant in view of the current understanding of the treatment of acute, severe asthma.

Patients requiring mechanical ventilation may be at risk for barotrauma from high-peak airway pressures. Bronchodilator therapy must be continued in these patients. Aerosolized beta$_2$-agonists may also be administered into the ventilator circuits either intermittently or continously. Figure 67–6 illustrates the method that the authors use for delivering continuous beta$_2$-agonists in a ventilator circuit. The dose of aerosol through a nebulizer may need to be increased. One study demonstrated that only 1% of a nebulized dose of beta$_2$-agonist reaches the patient's lungs via a ventilator circuit.[101] Both halothane and isoflurane inhalational anesthetics have been shown to produce bronchodilation in ventilated asthmatic children.[102, 103] Continuous intravenous infusion of 1 to 2.5 mg/kg of ketamine per hour has also been reported to be useful.[104, 105]

REFERENCES

1. Halfon N, Newacheck PW: Trends in the hospitalization for acute asthma, 1970–1984. Am J Public Health 76:1308–1311, 1986.
2. Bateman JR, Clarke SW: Sudden death in asthma. Thorax 34:40–44, 1979.
3. Ellis ME, Friend JA: How well do asthma clinic patients understand their asthma? Br J Dis Chest 17:43–48, 1985.
4. British Thoracic Association: Death from asthma in two regions of England. Br Med J 285:1251–1255, 1982.
5. Sears MR, Rea HH, Beaglehole R: Asthma mortality in New Zealand: A two-year national study. N Z Med J 98:271–275, 1985.
6. Carswell F: Thirty deaths from asthma. Arch Dis Child 60:25–28, 1985.
7. Fletcher HJ, Ibrahim SA, Speight N: Survey of asthma deaths in the Northern region, 1970–85. Arch Dis Child 65:163–167, 1990.
8. Deshpande A, McKenzie SA: Short course of steroids in home treatment of children with acute asthma. Br Med J 293:169–171, 1986.
9. Storr J, Barry W, Barrell E, et al: Effect of a single oral dose of prednisolone in acute childhood asthma. Lancet 1:879–882, 1987.
10. National Asthma Education Project Guidelines for the Treatment of Asthma. Bethesda, MD: National Institutes of Health, National Heart, Lung, Blood Institute, Division of Lung Diseases, August 1991.
11. Roca J, Ramis LI, Rodriguez-Roisin R, et al: Serial relationships between ventilation-perfusion inequality and spirometry in acute severe asthma requiring hospitalizations. Am Rev Respir Dis 137:1055–1061, 1988.
12. Waring WW: The history and physical examination. In Kendig EL, Chernick V (eds): Disorders of the Respiratory Tract in Children, p. 63. Philadelphia: WB Saunders, 1983.
13. Galant SP, Groncy CE, Shaw KC: The value of pulsus paradoxus in assessing the child with status asthmaticus. Pediatrics 61:46–51, 1978.
14. Commey JO, Levison H: Physical signs in childhood asthma. Pediatrics 58:537–541, 1976.
15. Martin TG, Elenbaas RM, Pingleton SH: Use of peak expiratory flow rates to eliminate unnecessary arterial blood gases in asthma. Ann Emerg Med 11:70–73, 1982.
16. Rossing TH, Fanta CH, McFadden ER: A controlled trial of the use of single versus combined drug therapy in the treatment of acute episodes of asthma. Am Rev Respir Dis 123:190–194, 1981.
17. Fanta CH, Rossing TH, McFadden ER: Treatment of acute asthma: Is combination therapy with sympathomimetics and methylxanthines indicated? Am J Med 80:5–10, 1986.
18. Becker AB, Nelson NA, Simons FE: Inhaled salbutamol (albuterol) vs. injected epinephrine in the treatment of acute asthma in children. J Pediatr 102:465–469, 1983.
19. Tinkelman DG, Vanderpool GE, Carroll MS, et al: Comparison of nebulized terbutaline and subcutaneus epinephrine in the treatment of acute asthma. Ann Allergy 50:398–401, 1983.
20. Robertson CF, Smith F, Beck R, et al: Response to frequent low doses of nebulized salbutamol in acute asthma. J Pediatr 106:672–674, 1985.
21. Schuh S, Parkin P, Rajan A, et al: High versus low dose, frequently administered nebulized albuterol in children with severe, acute asthma. Pediatrics 83:513–518, 1989.
22. Kelly HW: New beta₂-adrenergic agonist aerosols. Clin Pharm 4:393–403, 1985.
23. Nelson HS, Spector SL, Whitsett TL, et al: The bronchodilator response to inhalation of increasing doses of aerosolized albuterol. J Allergy Clin Immunol 72:371–375, 1983.
24. Harris J, Weinberger MM, Nassif E, et al: Early intervention with short courses of prednisolone to prevent progression of asthma in ambulatory patients incompletely responsive to bronchodilators. J Pediatr 110:627–633, 1987.
25. Littenberg B, Gluck EH: A controlled trial of methylprednisolone in the emergency treatment of acute asthma. N Engl J Med 314:150–152, 1986.
26. McFadden ER: Therapy of acute asthma. J Allergy Clin Immunol 84:151–158, 1989.
27. Harrison BD, Stokes TC, Hart GJ, et al: Need for intravenous hydrocortisone in addition to oral prednisolone in patients admitted to hospital with severe asthma without ventilatory failure. Lancet 1:181–184, 1986.
28. Kelly HW, McWilliams BC, Katz R, Murphy S: Safety of frequent high-dose nebulized terbutaline in children with acute, severe asthma. Ann Allergy 64:229–233, 1990.
29. Self TH, Ellis RF, Abou-Shala N, Amarshi N: Is theophylline use justified in acute exacerbations of asthma? Pharmacotherapy 9:260–266, 1989.
30. Pierson WE, Bierman CW, Stamm SJ, et al: Double-blind trial of aminophylline in status asthmaticus. Pediatrics 48:642–646, 1971.
31. Kelly WH, Murphy S: Should we stop using theophylline for the treatment of the hospitalized patient with status asthmaticus? DICP, Ann Pharmacother 23:995–998, 1990.
32. Moler FW, Hurwitz ME, Custer JR: Improvement in clinical asthma score and PaCO₂ in children with severe asthma treated with continuously nebulized terbutaline. J Allergy Clin Immunol 81:1101–1109, 1988.
33. Portnoy J, Aggarwal J. Continuous terbutaline nebulization for the treatment of severe exacerbations of asthma in children. Ann Allergy 60:368–371, 1988.
34. Beck R, Robertson C, Galdes-Sebaldt, M, Levison H: Combined salbutamol and ipratropium bromide by inhalation in the treatment of severe acute asthma. J Pediatr 107:605–608, 1985.
35. O'Driscoll BR, Taylor RJ, Horsley MG, et al: Nebulized salbutamol with and without ipratropium bromide in acute air flow obstruction. Lancet 1:1418–1420, 1989.
36. Reisman J, Galdes-Sebalt M, Kazim F, et al: Frequent administration by inhalation of salbutamol and ipratropium bromide in the initial management of severe acute asthma in children. J Allergy Clin Immunol 81:16–20, 1988.
37. Cavanaugh MJ, Cooper DM: Inhaled atropine sulfate: Dose-response characteristics. Am Rev Respir Dis 114:517–524, 1976.
38. Gross NJ, Skorodin MS: State of the art: Anticholinergic antimuscarinic bronchodilators. Am Rev Respir Dis 129:856–870, 1984.
39. Davis A, Vickerson F, Worsley G, et al: Determination of dose-response relationship for nebulized ipratropium in asthmatic children. J Pediatr 105:1002–1005, 1984.
40. Walker FB, Kaiser DL, Kowal MB, Suratt PM: Prolonged effect of inhaled glycopyrrolate in asthma. Chest 91:49–51, 1987.
41. Canny GJ, Reisman J, Healy R, et al: Acute asthma: Observations regarding the management of a pediatric emergency room. Pediatrics 83:507–512, 1989.
42. Schneider SM: Effect of a treatment protocol on the efficiency of care of the adult acute asthmatic. Ann Emerg Med 15:703–706, 1986.
43. Mayo PH, Richman J, Harris HW: Results of a program to reduce admissions for adult asthma. Ann Intern Med 112:864–871, 1990.
44. Rubin BK, Marcushamer S, Priel I, App EM: Emergency management of the child with asthma. Pediatr Pulmonol 8:45–57, 1990.
45. Hori T: Pathophysiological analysis of hypoxaemia during acute severe asthma. Arch Dis Child 60:640–643, 1985.
46. Libby DM, Briscoe WA, King TK: Relief of hypoxia-related bronchoconstriction by breathing 30 percent oxygen. Am Rev Respir Dis 123:171–175, 1981.
47. Ahmed T, Marchette B: Hypoxia enhances nonspecific bronchial reactivity. Am Rev Respir Dis 132:839–844, 1985.
48. Douglas JG, Rafferty P, Fergusson RJ, et al: Nebulized salbutamol without oxygen in severe acute asthma: How effective and how safe? Thorax 40:180–183, 1985.
49. Geelhoed GC, Landau LI, LeSouef PN: Predictive valve of oxygen saturation in emergency evaluation of asthmatic children. Br Med J 297:395–396, 1988.
50. Ford DJ, Rothwell RP: "Safe oxygen" in acute asthma: Prospective trial using 35% Ventimask prior to admission. Respir Med 83:189–194, 1989.
51. Appel D, Karpel JP, Sherman M: Epinephrine improves expiratory flow rates in patients with asthma who do not respond to

inhaled metaproterenol sulfate. J Allergey Clin Immunol 84:90–98, 1989.

52. Jenne JW, Ahrens RC: Pharmacokinetics of beta-adrenergic compounds. In Jenne JW, Murphy S (eds): Drug Therapy for Asthma: Research and Clinical Practice, pp 213–258. New York: Marcel Dekker, 1987.

53. Reed MT, Kelly HW: Sympathomimetics for acute severe asthma: Should only beta-2-selective agonists be used? DICP: Ann Pharmacother 24:868–873, 1990.

54. Garra B, Shapiro GG, Dorsett CS, et al: A double-blind evaluation of the use of nebulized metaproterenol and isoproterenol in hospitalized asthmatic children and adolescents. J Allergy Clin Immunol 60:63–68, 1977.

55. Benton G, Thomas RC, Nickerson BG, et al: Experience with a metered-dose inhaler with a spacer in the pediatric emergency department. Am J Dis Child 143:678–681, 1989.

56. Newman SP: Aerosol deposition considerations in inhalation therapy. Chest 88(Suppl):152–160, 1985.

57. Madsen EB, Bundgaard A, Hidinger KG: Cumulative dose-response study comparing terbutaline pressurized aerosol administered via a pear-shaped spacer and terbutaline in a nebulized solution. Eur J Clin Pharmacol 23:27–30, 1982.

58. Cushley MJ, Lewis RA, Tattersfield AE: Comparison of three techniques of inhalation on the airway response to terbutaline. Thorax 38:908–913, 1983.

59. Morgan MD, Singh BV, Frame MH, Williams SJ: Terbutaline aerosol given through pear spacer in acute severe asthma. Br Med J 285:849–850, 1982.

60. Freelander M, Van Asperen PP: Nebuhaler versus nebulizer in children with acute asthma. Br Med J 288:1873–1874, 1984.

61. Beasley CR, O'Donnell TV: Pear-shaped spacer nebuhaler compared with nebulized solution for terbutaline administration in acute severe asthma. N Z Med J 98:854–855, 1985.

62. Tarala RA, Madsen BW, Paterson JW: Comparative efficacy of salbutamol by pressurized aerosol and wet nebulizer in acute asthma. Br J Clin Pharmacol 10:393–397, 1980.

63. Cayton RM, Webber B, Paterson JW, Clark TJ: A comparison of salbutamol given by pressure-packed aerosol or nebulization via IPPB in acute asthma. Br J Dis Chest 72:222–224, 1978.

64. Morley TF, Marozsan E, Zappasodi SJ, et al: Comparison of beta-adrenergic agents delivered by nebulizer vs. metered-dose inhaler with InspirEaze in hospitalized asthmatic patients. Chest 94:1205–1210, 1988.

65. Schuh S, Reider MJ, Canny G, et al: Nebulized albuterol in acute childhood asthma: Comparison of two doses. Pediatrics 86:509–513, 1990.

66. Nelson HS: Adrenergic therapy of bronchial asthma. J Allergy Clin Immunol 77:771–785, 1986.

67. Littenberg B: Aminophylline treatment in severe, acute asthma: A meta-analysis. JAMA 259:1678–1684, 1988.

68. Self T, Abou-Shala N, Burns R, et al: Inhaled albuterol and oral prednisone in hospitalized adult asthma: Does theophylline add any benefit? Am Rev Respir Dis 141(4):A21, 1990.

69. Kelly HW, Murphy S: Should anticholinergics be used in acute severe asthma? DICP 24:409–416, 1990.

70. Harrison LI, Smallridge RC, Lasseter KC, et al: Comparative absorption of inhaled and intramuscularly administered atropine. Am Rev Respir Dis 134:254–257, 1986.

71. Ward MJ, MacFarlane JT, Davies D: A place for ipratropium bromide in the treatment of severe acute asthma. Br J Dis Chest 79:374–378, 1985.

72. Fiel SB: Should corticosteroids be used in the treatment of acute, severe asthma? I. A case for the use of corticosteroids in acute, severe asthma. Pharmacotherapy 5:327–331, 1985.

73. Mok J, Kattan J, Levison H: Should corticosteroids be used in the treatment of acute, severe asthma? II. A case against the use of corticosteroids in acute, severe asthma. Pharmacotherapy 5:331–335, 1985.

74. Kelly HW, Murphy S: Corticosteroids for acute severe asthma. Ann Pharmacother 25:72–79, 1991.

75. Deshpande A, McKenzie SA: Short course of steroids in home treatment of children with acute asthma. Br Med J 293:169–171, 1986.

76. Loren ML, Chai H, Leung P, et al: Corticosteroids in the treatment of acute exacerbations of asthma. Ann Allergy 45:67–71, 1980.

77. McFadden ER, Kiser R, deGroot WJ, et al: A controlled study of the effects of single doses of hydrocortisone on the resolution of acute attacks of asthma. Am J Med 60:52–59, 1976.

78. Collins JV, Clark TJ, Brown D, Townsend J: The use of corticosteroids in the treatment of acute asthma. Q J Med 44:259–273, 1975.

79. Storr J, Barry W, Barrell E, et al: Effect of a single oral dose of prednisolone in acute childhood asthma. Lancet 1:879–882, 1987.

80. Stein LM, Cole RP: Early administration of corticosteroids in emergency room treatment of acute asthma. Ann Intern Med 112:822–827, 1990.

81. Tal A, Levy N, Bearman JE: Methylprednisolone therapy for acute asthma in infants and toddlers: A controlled clinical trial. Pediatrics 86:350–356, 1990.

82. Wood DW, Downes JJ, Scheinkepf H, Lecks HI: Intravenous isoproterenol in the management of respiratory failure in childhood status asthmaticus. J Allergy Clin Immunol 50:75–81, 1972.

83. Downes JJ, Wood DW, Harwood I, et al: Intravenous isoproterenol infusion in children with severe hypercapnia due to status asthmaticus: Effects on ventilation, circulation, and clinical score. Crit Care Med 1:63–68, 1973.

84. Parry WH, Martorano F, Cotton EK: Management of life threatening asthma with intravenous isoproterenol infusions. Am J Dis Child 130:39–42, 1976.

85. Wood DW, Downes JJ: Intravenous isoproterenol in the treatment of respiratory failure in childhood status asthmaticus. Ann Allergy 31:607–610, 1973.

86. Herman JJ, Noah ZL, Moody RR: Use of intravenous isoproterenol for status asthmaticus in children. Crit Care Med 11:716–720, 1983.

87. Klaustermeyer WB, DiBernardo RL, Hale FC: Intravenous isoproterenol: Rationale for bronchial asthma. J Allergy Clin Immunol 55:325–333, 1975.

88. Matson JR, Loughlin GM, Strunk RC: Myocardial ischemia complicating the use of isoproterenol in asthmatic children. J Pediatr 92:776–778, 1978.

89. Kurland G, Williams J, Lewiston NJ: Fatal myocardial toxicity during continuous infusion intravenous isoproterenol therapy of asthma. J Allergy Clin Immunol 63:407–411, 1979.

90. Bohn D, Kalloghlian A, Jenkins J, et al: Intravenous salbutamol in the treatment of status asthmaticus in children. Crit Care Med 12:892–896, 1984.

91. Johnson AJ, Spiro SG, Pidgeon J, et al: Intravenous infusion of salbutamol in severe acute asthma. Br Med J 1:1013–1015, 1978.

92. Williams SJ, Parrish RW, Seaton A: Comparison of intravenous aminophylline and salbutamol in severe asthma. Br Med J 4:685, 1975.

93. Evans WV, Monie RD, Crimmins J, Seaton A: Aminophylline, salbutamol and combined intravenous infusions in acute severe asthma. Br J Dis Chest 74:385–389, 1980.

94. Hambleton G, Stone MJ: Comparison of IV salbutamol with IV aminophylline in the treatment of severe, acute asthma in childhood. Arch Dis Child 54:391–392, 1979.

95. Lawford P, Jones BJM, Milledge JS: Comparison of intravenous and nebulized salbutamol in initial treatment of severe asthma. Br Med J 1:84, 1978.

96. Edmunds AT, Godfrey S: Cardiovascular response during severe acute asthma and its treatment in children. Thorax 36:534–540, 1981.

97. Williams SJ, Winner SJ, Clark TJ: Comparison of inhaled and intravenous terbutaline in acute severe asthma. Thorax 36:629–631, 1981.

98. Bloomfield P, Carmichael J, Petrie GR, et al: Comparison of salbutamol given intravenously and by intermittent positive-pressure breathing in life-threatening asthma. Br Med J 1:848–850, 1979.

99. Pierce RJ, Payne CR, Williams SJ: Comparison of intravenous and inhaled terbutaline in the treatment of asthma. Chest 79:506–511, 1981.

100. Van Renterghem D, Lamont H, Elinck W, et al: Intravenous versus nebulized terbutaline in patients with acute severe asthma: A double-blind randomized study. Ann Allergy 59:313–316, 1987.

101. Fuller HD, Dolovich MB, Posmituck G, et al: Pressurized aerosol versus jet aerosol delivery to mechanically ventilated patients: Comparison of dose to the lungs. Am Rev Respir Dis 141:440–444, 1990.

102. O'Rourke PP, Crone RK: Halothane in status asthmaticus. Crit Care Med 10:341–343, 1982.
103. Johnston RG, Noseworthy TW, Friesen EG: Isoflurane therapy for status asthmaticus in children and adults. Chest 97:698–701, 1990.
104. Strube PJ, Hallam PL: Ketamine by continuous infusion in status asthmaticus. Anaesthesia 41:1017–1019, 1986.
105. Rock MJ, Reyes de la Rocha S, L'Hammedieu CS, et al: Use of ketamine in asthmatic children to treat respiratory failure refractory to conventional therapy. Crit Care Med 14:514–516, 1986.

68 EXERCISE-INDUCED ASTHMA

R. MICHAEL SLY, M.D.

During the second century A.D., Aretaeus the Cappadocian wrote, "If from running, gymnastic exercises, or any other work, the breathing becomes difficult, it is called Asthma. . . ."[1] This adverse effect that exercise can have in asthmatic subjects was not reemphasized in the medical literature until the 17th century, when Sir John Floyer, an asthmatic physician, observed that the effect depended on how strenuous the exercise was.[2] In 1864, Salter recognized a relationship between exercise-induced asthma and the temperature of the inspired air and speculated that "rapid passage of fresh and cold air over the bronchial mucous membrane" might stimulate airways either directly or by causing irritability of the nervous system.[3] In 1946, Herxheimer reported the results of measurement of pulmonary function before and after exercise in six subjects with exercise-induced asthma.[4] Having found bronchoconstriction in these subjects after both exercise and voluntary hyperventilation, he concluded that hypocapnia and respiratory alkalosis resulting from inappropriate hyperventilation after exercise caused the exercise-induced asthma; this hypothesis was later disproved.

Jones found that exercise could have opposite effects on pulmonary function in asthmatics, depending on the duration of exercise.[5] Strenuous exercise such as running for 1 to 2 minutes often causes bronchodilation, but if exercise is continued for 6 to 12 min, it usually produces airway obstruction, often with coughing and wheezing. Bronchodilation after brief exercise is of short duration with return of forced expiratory volume in 1 sec (FEV_1) or peak expiratory flow rate (PEFR) to the pre-exercise baseline within 5 min.[5, 6] Such bronchodilation is more extreme when it follows pre-exercise airway obstruction, and it is enhanced further by pretreatment with a beta-adrenergic agonist.[5, 7–9] The combination of brief exercise and a bronchodilator causes more bronchodilation than does either alone.

The airway obstruction that follows strenuous exercise for 6 to 12 min may begin during exercise but often is manifested by decreases in FEV_1 or PEFR below the pre-exercise values only after completion of exercise and usually becomes most extreme 5 to 10 min after completion of exercise (Fig. 68–1). Mild exercise-induced asthma may resolve within a few minutes, but pulmonary function may not return to the pre-exercise base line for 1 h after more severe exercise-induced asthma. A late-phase asthmatic response may occur 3 to 6 h after exercise in asthmatic subjects who have recovered from the early response to exercise, and late-phase responses may be most likely in patients with the slowest rates of recovery from the early response (Fig. 68–2).[10, 11] Late-phase responses have been reported in as many as 40% of subjects with exercise-induced asthma.[10, 11] Apparent late-phase responses may also occur when the early response has been prevented by inhalation of hot, humid air during exercise.[12] This observation and similar recurrences of airway obstruction 2 to 4 h after methacholine-induced bronchoconstriction followed by recovery in the same subjects suggest that apparent late-phase responses to exercise may often be caused by spontaneous changes in airway obstruction that result from withholding of medications.[12, 13]

The reported frequency of exercise-induced asthma among asthmatic subjects has varied with conditions of exercise, parameters measured, and definition of exercise-induced asthma. Increased bronchial reactivity after challenge with allergen increases the likelihood of an episode of exercise-induced asthma.[14] Single tests have disclosed abnormal responses to exercise in 70% to 90% of asthmatic patients. Under appropriate conditions, abnormal responses are probably demonstrable in virtually all asthmatic patients.[15–19] Abnormal responses to exercise are more easily detectable when some airway obstruction is present even before exercise.[17] Severity of exercise-induced asthma is unrelated to pre-exercise pulmonary function, however.[9, 17]

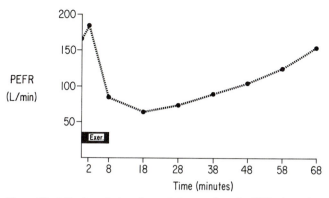

Figure 68–1. Peak expiratory flow rate in an asthmatic child before, during, and after running on a treadmill up a 15% grade at 3 miles per hour for 8 min, indicating the response typical in asthma. Bronchodilation often follows the first 1 to 2 min of exercise. Bronchoconstriction usually follows more prolonged exercise, becoming most extreme 5 to 10 min after the completion of exercise.

PHYSIOLOGIC FEATURES OF NORMAL EXERCISE

The conformational changes in actin and myosin manifested as muscular contraction involve the use of the free energy of hydrolysis of the terminal phosphate bond of adenosine triphosphate (ATP).[20] Adenosine diphosphate and creatine phosphate react to form ATP and creatine to prevent depletion of ATP by exercise. Mitochondrial production of ATP requires oxygen as the terminal oxidant. As workloads increase, oxygen consumption increases from resting levels of 3.5 ml/kg/min to a maximum of 50 ml/kg/min.[21] The maintenance of an adequate supply of oxygen during exercise depends on pulmonary adjustments to maintain arterial oxygen content, increased cardiac output, and redistribution of the cardiac output to the exercising muscles.

During exercise in which work rate increases in increments, minute ventilation and rates of oxygen uptake and carbon dioxide (CO_2) output increase linearly to approximately 60% of maximal work capacity.[22] Arterial pH and CO_2 and oxygen tensions remain unchanged during moderate exercise. Thereafter, minute ventilation increases more rapidly and is more closely related to CO_2 output than to oxygen uptake. This more rapid increase in ventilatory response as maximal work capacity is approached is caused by an increase in production of CO_2 by the buffering of lactic acid by bicarbonate and by the increase in hydrogen ion concentration that is caused by the reduction in concentration of bicarbonate. The effect of the increased hydrogen ion concentration on ventilation is mediated by chemoreceptors found in the carotid bodies and the medulla oblongata.[22] Further enhancement of minute ventilation by metabolic acidosis at highest work rates causes hypocapnia with respiratory compensation for the metabolic acidosis.

While arterial oxygen partial pressure remains constant during exercise with incremental increases in work rate, ideal alveolar oxygen partial pressure decreases during moderate exercise, causing a decrease in the alveolar-arterial difference in oxygen pressure, probably because of better matching of perfusion to ventilation with improved perfusion of the apices of the lungs.[20] During heavy work, the alveolar-arterial oxygen pressure difference increases, possibly because of incomplete equilibration between alveolar gas and end-capillary blood at high work rates and an increase in the shunt fraction of perfused blood.

Exercise at a constant work rate elicits an immediate increase in minute ventilation, which is followed by a more gradual increase to a steady-state level.[22] Ventilation usually reaches steady state within 3 min of light exercise but may continue to increase without reaching steady state at work rates heavy enough to cause metabolic acidosis with respiratory compensation.

Minute ventilation is the sum of alveolar ventilation and dead space ventilation, but physiologic dead space as a fraction of tidal volume decreases during exercise.

Cardiac input increases linearly with oxygen uptake during exercise because of increases in both cardiac rate and stroke volume. The increase in stroke volume is caused by increased diastolic filling of the ventricles and increased force of contraction, resulting in decreased ventricular volume at the end of systole.[20] Increases in heart rate during exercise are linear with increasing work rate

Figure 68–2. Reported duration of inhibition of exercise-induced asthma after inhalation or oral adminstration of various drugs at usual doses. Studies have failed to show a longer inhibitory effect for some drugs, such as inhaled isoproterenol or metaproterenol. The duration of action of other drugs may appear limited because effects have not been studied over longer periods. The effect of inhaled terbutaline has not been studied beyond 1 h, for example. (Modified from Sly RM: Exercise-induced asthma. *In* Current Views in Allergy and Immunology [audiovisual program]. Atlanta: School of Medicine, Medical College of Georgia, in cooperation with the American Academy of Allergy and Immunology, 1981.)

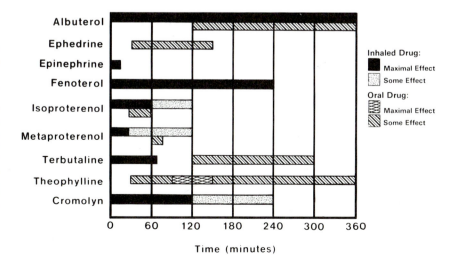

Table 68-1. AVERAGE HEART RATES BY AGE

Age (Years)	Maximal Heart Rate (Beats/Minute)					
	100%	*95%*	*90%*	*85%*	*80%*	*75%*
5	206	196	185	175	165	155
10	202	192	182	172	162	152
15	198	188	178	168	158	149
20	194	184	175	165	155	146
25	191	181	172	162	153	143
30	187	178	168	159	150	140
35	183	174	165	156	146	137
40	180	171	162	153	144	135

From Johnson WR, Buskirk ER: Science and Medicine of Exercise and Sports, 2nd ed, p. 125. New York: Harper & Row, 1974.

up to an age-dependent maximum at exhaustion[23] (Table 68-1).

Redistribution of peripheral blood flow largely because of local reduction of vascular resistance can shunt as much as 80% of the cardiac output to exercising muscle, in comparison with the 15% typically distributed to skeletal muscle at rest.[20]

Thus although pulmonary and cardiovascular adjustments can satisfy the increased demand for oxygen during moderate exercise, they may be inadequate for the oxygen requirements of heavy exercise.[20] Anaerobic glycolysis with production of lactic acid consequently becomes necessary for supplementing aerobic energy transfer.

Strenuous exercise for 5 min at a constant workload sufficient to increase heart rate to 90% of maximum for age during the last 2 min of exercise causes decreases in FEV_1 of less than 15% and decreases in maximal midexpiratory flow rate of less than 25% in most normal subjects.[16] Mean decreases in PEFR after treadmill or free-range running for 6 min are less than 4%; a decrease of 15% is more than two standard deviations above the mean.[15, 17, 24, 25] A study of the effect of free-range running for 6 min in 548 twelve-year-old children with no histories of wheezing, eczema, or allergic rhinitis and no family histories of asthma disclosed a mean decrease in PEFR of 2.5% and a mean decrease plus two standard deviations of 14.7%.[24] Walking on a treadmill at 3 miles per hour up a 10-degree grade elicits a mean increase in PEFR of 5% ($\pm$ 4.7) after 2 min and a decrease of 2.1% ($\pm$ 3.0) after 9 min in normal children.[26] Thus decreases in PEFR of as little as 10% after treadmill walking and 15% after running are abnormal responses to exercise.

PATHOPHYSIOLOGY

The mechanism or mechanisms through which exercise causes airway obstruction in asthmatic subjects remains unknown, but extensive study has eliminated some possibilities and has provided support for others. The observation that airway obstruction could follow hyperventilation as well as exercise in asthmatic subjects suggested mediation by a mechanical effect of hyperpnea or by hypocapnia.[4] Although there was a suggestion that exercise was more likely to cause airway obstruction when

associated with relatively high rates of ventilation, there was no correlation between patients most susceptible to exercise-induced asthma and those most susceptible to hyperventilation-induced airway obstruction.[27] It was demonstrated that isocapnic hyperpnea had no effect on pulmonary function despite matching of minute ventilation to that achieved during sufficient treadmill running to cause a decrease of 34% in FEV_1 in eight asthmatic subjects;[28] this finding ruled out mediation by mechanical effects of hyperpnea. Permitting end-tidal CO_2 to fall to 20 mm Hg during hyperventilation with rebreathing elicited a decrease of only 6% in FEV_1. End-tidal CO_2 5 min after completion of exercise, when pulmonary function was measured, was reduced to a mean of only 28.9 mm Hg, and hyperventilation with an end-tidal CO_2 tension of 30 mm Hg caused no significant change in pulmonary function.[28] Mechanical effects of neither hyperpnea nor hypocapnia could account for the abnormal response to exercise.

Futher investigation indicated lactic acidosis could not be the cause of exercise-induced asthma. Infusion of sodium bicarbonate during cycloergometer exercise to prevent any change in arterial pH did not change the bronchoconstrictive response in asthmatic subjects.[29] Furthermore, infusion of at least as much lactate as that produced during exercise did not cause airway obstruction.

Several investigators reported that inhalation during exercise of air that was warmed to body temperature and fully humidified prevented exercise-induced asthma.[30-32] Inhalation of air at subfreezing temperatures enhanced the bronchoconstrictive effect of exercise.[33] Respiratory heat exchange calculated from minute ventilation, the difference in temperature of inspired and expired air, and the difference in water content of inspired and expired air was strongly correlated with the decreases in FEV_1 that followed cycloergometer exercise in asthmatic adults.[34] Reasoning that the effect of hyperventilation on pulmonary mechanics should also depend on the condition of the inspired air, the investigators demonstrated isocapnic hyperventilation with air at -12°C that contained no water vapor caused a mean decrease of 37% in FEV_1 in asthmatic subjects, but hyperventilation with air at 37°C that contained 44 mg H_2O per liter of air caused no change in pulmonary function.[35] Failure of hyperpnea to elicit airway obstruction in the earlier study of asthmatic subjects apparently had been a result of the rebreathing technique used, which had entailed inhalation of warm, humid air.[28]

Nasal breathing, which warms and humidifies inspired air, or wearing a cold weather mask, which forms a reservoir in which the previous exhalation warms and humidifies air immediately before inhalation, minimizes exercise-induced asthma.[36, 37]

Cooling of airways by inhalation of subfreezing dry air during exercise was indicated by decreases in retrotracheal temperature of 2.5°C to 3°C in both asthmatic and normal subjects.[38] Inhalation of air at 25°C to 27°C that contained 6 mg of water vapor per liter of air caused decreases of 1.5°C during exercise. Measurement of changes in temperature with thermocouples in the airways of normal subjects has confirmed significant decreases in temperature during hyperventilation with subfreezing dry air even in segmental bronchi.[39] The site at which inspired air reaches body temperature and full saturation with water depends on rate and depth of inspiration as well as on temperature and water content of the inspired air. During quiet breathing, most heat transfer and water transfer occur in the upper airways. Airways are cooled during an increase in ventilation associated with exercise as they warm and humidify relatively cool, dry air, supplying latent heat of vaporization. Asthmatic subjects differ from normal subjects in their responses to these effects.

These data suggested cooling might trigger release of chemical mediators of bronchoconstriction from mast cells. Exercise-induced asthma, however, can occur without respiratory heat loss, and inhalation of ultrasonically nebulized distilled water can also cause airway obstruction in asthmatic subjects.[40, 41]

Inhalation of ultrasonically nebulized hypertonic saline or hypertonic dextrose can cause bronchoconstriction in asthmatic subjects, but isotonic saline and isotonic dextrose do not.[42] Hyperosmolar solutions can cause release of histamine and can augment anti-immunoglobulin E– (IgE–) mediated release of histamine from human lung mast cells in vitro.[43] In patients in whom cold, dry air has caused rhinorrhea, nasal congestion, or sneezing, examination of nasal washings has disclosed associated increases in concentrations of histamine and other mediators with increased nasal fluid osmolality.[44, 45] Accordingly, local changes in osmolarity associated with increased ventilation with relatively dry air during exercise likely cause release of histamine and other mediators from mast cells in the airways, which causes exercise-induced asthma.[46]

Previous indirect evidence implicated mediator release as a cause of exercise-induced asthma. Response to exercise depends on how recently the subject has exercised. Repeating identical exercises at intervals of 1 h or less causes progressively smaller decrements in PEFR even without significant changes in the pre-exercise base line.[47] Increasing the interval between periods of exercise to 2 h restores the usual abnormal responsiveness. Occurrence of this refractory period after exercise is consistent with exhaustion of a supply of mediators that requires regeneration for restoration of the abnormal responsiveness, although nasal challenge with allergen repeated at intervals of 30 min does not deplete mast cell–derived mediators in some patients with allergic rhinitis.[48] During the refractory period that follows exercise, some but not all patients with allergic asthma also exhibit the bronchoconstrictive effect of inhalation of nebulized extracts of allergens.[49] Asthmatic subjects whose airways exhibit a refractory period 1 hour after exercise-induced asthma also exhibit a refractory period to the bronchoconstrictive effects of inhalation of aerosolized hypertonic saline.[50] Bronchoconstriction induced by hypertonic saline is also followed by a period during which the subjects exhibit a refractory period to effects of both hypertonic saline and exercise, implying similar mechanisms for the refractory states.

Furthermore, repeated inhalation challenge with adenosine monophosphate attenuates subsequent responsiveness to exercise.[51] If bronchoconstriction provoked by inhalation of adenosine monophosphate is caused by mediator release, as some evidence suggests, progressive loss of responsiveness both to successive challenges with adenosine monophosphate and to exercise may be caused at least in part by mediator depletion.

However, exercise-induced airway obstruction has not been associated with significant changes in recovery of histamine, tryptase, prostaglandin D_2, and leukotriene C_4 in bronchoalveolar lavage fluid.[52] Mast cells recovered by bronchoalveolar lavage after exercise have contained no less histamine than those recovered before exercise, which is suggestive of no mediator depletion by exercise.[52]

Bronchoconstrictor prostaglandins such as prostaglandins D_2 and $F_{2\alpha}$ and thromboxane A_2 are apparently not primarily responsible for exercise-induced asthma, inasmuch as pretreatment with the cyclooxygenase inhibitor indomethacin does not modify exercise-induced asthma.[53, 54] Release of inhibitory prostaglandins such as prostaglandin E_2 or prostacycline during bronchoconstriction induced by exercise may afford protection against subsequent exercise challenge because pretreatment with indomethacin abolishes the refractory state. Pretreatment with indomethacin also abolishes the protective effect of inhaled furosemide against exercise-induced airway obstruction, which is suggestive of the role of prostaglandin E_2 in the mediation of this protective effect of furosemide.[55] The failure of indomethacin to prevent a refractory period after eucapnic hyperventilation with dry air indicates that exercise and eucapnic hyperventilation are not equivalent with regard to tolerance to repeated challenge.[54]

The rate and extent of rewarming of the airways after exercise can modify exercise-induced asthma, possibly through a direct effect on airway smooth muscle or by obstruction from reactive hyperemia.[56] In normal subjects, exercise while breathing dry, frigid air followed by inhalation of frigid air or air at ambient room temperature and humidity during recovery elicited no significant change in FEV_1. A significant decrease in FEV_1, however, followed inhalation of fully saturated air at body temperature for 5 min after exercise. In asthmatic subjects, breathing cold dry air during cycloergometer exercise elicited airway obstruction regardless of whether air breathed during the 5 min after exercise was cold dry air, room air, or fully saturated air at body temperature; however, significantly greater decreases in FEV_1 followed recovery from exercise while they breathed saturated air at body temperature.[56] Furthermore, a gradual return to normal rates of ventilation after isocapnic hyperventilation with cold dry air minimizes the resultant airway obstruction in asthmatic subjects, in comparison with a rapid reduction in the rate of ventilation.[56]

The refractory period that follows exercise may be at least partly caused by demonstrable decreased cooling of the airway with repeated exercise and slower rewarming in central airways, possibly because of some continued dilatation of the bronchial vasculature after reactive hyperemia that follows exercise.[57]

DIAGNOSIS

A history of coughing, dyspnea, or wheezing after exercise is suggestive of exercise-induced asthma, but absence of such a history does not exclude this possbility. Documentation requires measurement of pulmonary function before and after strenuous exercise.

A medical history and a physical examination before exercise should be conducted to identify anyone at increased risk from strenuous exercise, including patients with evidence of ischemic heart disease, cardiac arrhythmia, congenital heart disease, hypertension, or pulmonary disease that may impair oxygen saturation. It is prudent to defer strenuous exercise when pulmonary function is not at least 80% of the usual values and when FEV_1 is not at least 65% of the predicted normal amount.[58]

Medications that may affect the response to exercise should be withheld for as long as necessary to minimize or to eliminate that effect unless the purpose is to evaluate response to exercise during treatment. Medications to be withheld include most inhaled beta-agonists for at least 8 h before exercise and slow-release, oral beta-agonists for at least 12 h. Inhaled antimuscarinic agents should be withheld for at least 8 h. Theophylline should be withheld long enough to decrease serum concentrations to less than 5 μg/ml. For most children, this duration would be 8 hr for plain theophylline tablets or liquid preparations, but it could be 12 to 24 h or even longer for a slow-release preparation of theophylline, depending on the product and conditions of its administration.[59] Cromolyn should be withheld at least 6 h; some authors have recommended 24 h.[58] Adrenal corticosteroids may modify response to exercise, but it may be acceptable to continue them at a stable dosage.

Either a motor-driven treadmill or a cycloergometer is satisfactory for the exercise challenge. Precautions must be taken to prevent children from falling from a treadmill. It is sometimes more difficult to induce children to maintain a constant rate of exercise on the cycloergometer than on the treadmill. Either of these methods is preferable to running back and forth in a hallway or running up and down a hill or a stairway, during which less energy is expended during descent.

Exercise is generally safe for children without complicating cardiovascular or pulmonary disease, but some authors have recommended continual electrocardiographic monitoring during exercise, and monitoring of pulse rate is necessary to ensure that exercise is sufficiently strenuous for adequate challenge.[58] Monitoring of both room temperature and relative humidity is also necessary.

Pulmonary function should be measured before and after exercise with a Wright Peak Flow Meter or a spirometer that meets the minimal standards of the American Thoracic Society.[60] Changes in peak expiratory flow rate or FEV_1 are most relevant, but changes in forced expiratory flow between 25% and 75% of vital capacity may be important when there has been little change in FEV_1.

The exercise should be sufficiently strenuous to increase heart rate to 90% of the predicted maximum (Table 68–1) or to increase oxygen consumption to 30 ml/kg/min.[58] For most asthmatic children under 14 years of age, running for 6 min on a motor-driven treadmill at 3 to 4 miles per hour up a 15% upgrade while breathing through the mouth at room temperature of 23°C to 25°C and relative humidity of less than 40% is sufficient to elicit significant airway obstruction. Some authors have recommended a stepped stress protocol, starting with 2 min of exercise at 2.5 miles per hour with the treadmill flat, followed by 2 min at a rate and an incline expected to increase heart rate to 70% of the predicted maximum and then 5 to 8 min at a faster rate and a steeper incline expected to increase heart rate to 90% of the predicted maximum.[58] It is best to complete the evaluation as quickly as possible in some children who soon tire of this procedure.

Pulmonary function should be measured immediately before exercise, within 1 min after the completion of exercise, and at intervals of 5 to 10 min thereafter until the nadir of PEFR or FEV_1 or a completion of recovery is observed, depending on the purpose of the evaluation. After the nadir is reached or significant airway obstruction is established, inhalation of a beta-agonist can reverse the airway obstruction rapidly.

Results are usually expressed as a percentage decrease:

$$100 \times \frac{\text{Pre-Exercise Value} - \text{Postexercise Value}}{\text{Pre-Exercise Value}}.$$

The greatest decrease in PEFR or FEV_1 usually occurs 5 to 10 min after the completion of exercise. A decrease of at least 15% confirms exercise-induced asthma.[24]

Failure to elicit significant bronchoconstriction in the laboratory does not exclude the possibility of exercise-induced asthma, proof of which may require challenge on more than one occasion. Exercise during inhalation of air that is colder and drier than that of the laboratory is more likely to cause bronchoconstriction.

In an early investigation, treadmill exercise that caused significant airway obstruction in children with asthma caused none in children with cystic fibrosis or primary pulmonary tuberculosis; this finding suggests that the phenomenon might be unique to asthma.[26] Subsequent investigation has disclosed abnormal responses to exercise in a few children with cystic fibrosis, but changes in pulmonary function have been much less frequent and less extreme than in children with asthma.[61, 62] In a few children with atopic dermatitis, PEFR has decreased by more than 20% after running, but some of these children have subsequently had recurrent asthma unrelated to exercise.[63] As many as 40% of children with allergic rhinitis and no history of asthma may have abnormal responses to exercise; it is not known how many of them later experience asthma unrelated to exercise.[64] A few healthy siblings and parents of children with asthma also have slightly abnormal responses to exercise.[65, 66] Significant obstructive changes in pulmonary function after exercise are most frequent and most extreme in patients with asthma, but abnormal responses are sometimes demonstrable years after remission of overt asthma.[9, 67, 68]

Isocapnic hyperventilation during breathing of subfreezing, dry air can cause small but significant decreases in FEV_1 in healthy adults at levels of ventilation that exceed those associated with strenuous exercise.[69] Small decreases in rates of flow at 30% of vital capacity occur at rates of ventilation similar to those associated with strenuous exercise.

MANAGEMENT

Acupuncture can inhibit exercise-induced asthma in some subjects, and posthypnotic suggestion that exercise will be effortless or will cause no breathing difficulty is somtimes effective.[26, 70, 71] The mechanism of protection is unknown, but hypnosis may minimize the increase in ventilation associated with exercise. Pharmacologic therapy and the warming and humidification of inspired air are more dependable in modifying exercise-induced asthma.

DRUG THERAPY

Bronchodilators. Bronchodilators may be helpful in the management of exercise-induced asthma in at least four ways. First, bronchodilators may cause sufficient improvement in pulmonary function to compensate for any obstruction induced by subsequent exercise. Second, bronchodilators may enhance the bronchodilating effect of the first 1 to 2 min of exercise.[5, 7-9] Third, bronchodilators may inhibit exercise-induced asthma, whatever its mechanism, causing a parallel shift of the stimulus-response curve to the right, so that an increase in the exercise challenge with an increase in rate of ventilation may overcome the protective effect of the inhaled beta-agonist.[72] Finally, bronchodilators have been used most frequently to relieve exercise-induced asthma after it has occurred. It is usually impossible to be certain of the mechanism of protection afforded by a bronchodilator. After pre-exercise treatment with a bronchodilator and before achievement of peak bronchodilation, the increasing bronchodilating effect of the drug appears to minimize exercise-induced asthma because of the changing baseline pulmonary function. Waning bronchodilation after achievement of peak bronchodilation tends to minimize the apparent protective effect from later challenge.

Inhaled albuterol is the treatment of choice for prevention of exercise-induced asthma because of convenience, rapid bronchodilation, and prolonged protection. The usual dose of 180 μg delivered from a metered-dose inhaler affords protection for 4 h in most patients and 6 h in many.[73-78] Protection is evident within a few minutes after inhalation.

Oral albuterol can also inhibit exercise-induced asthma for 2 to 6 h after administration.[76] Oral metaproterenol inhibits exercise-induced asthma for 1 h after administration but not for 2 h.[79, 80]

There is also remarkable discordance between bronchodilation and inhibition of exercise-induced asthma after inhalation of metaproterenol.[80-82] Although inhaled metaproterenol inhibits exercise-induced asthma in most patients within 15 min after treatment and in many for 1 h, it does not usually afford protection for 2 h despite continued bronchodilation.

Inhaled terbutaline inhibits exercise-induced asthma for at least 1 h but has not been studied for a longer duration of effect.[83, 84] Oral terbutaline is protective for 2 to 5 h.[85, 86]

Epinephrine and isoproterenol afford protection within a few minutes after inhalation, and one study disclosed protection for as long as 2 h after inhalation of isoproterenol.[8, 87]

Inhalation of fenoterol has usually been found to be protective for 4 h,[88] but one study disclosed protection for 2 h and none at 4 h,[89] whereas another study showed partial protection for as long as 7 h after treatment.[90]

Bitolterol mesylate inhibits exercise-induced asthma 45 min after inhalation but has not been evaluated at other intervals.[91]

Inhaled salmeterol, which is not yet available commercially, can inhibit exercise-induced airway obstruction for at least 12 h.[92]

Oral ephedrine affords modest protection 1.5 to 2.5 h after administration but is far less effective than beta-adrenergic agonists.[8, 93]

Theophylline can inhibit exercise-induced asthma 0.5 to 6 h after oral administration.[8, 85, 93-95] The degree of protection is usually correlated with the serum theophylline concentration and is maximal at peak concentrations. Slow-release preparations of theophylline are probably protective much longer than 6 h.

Although antimuscarinic agents can cause bronchodilation, evaluations of their effect on exercise-induced asthma have produced conflicting results.[8, 94-102] Atropine has been administered by intravenous, intramuscular, subcutaneous, and inhalational routes; ipratropium bromide and oxitropium bromide, by inhalation. Treatment has sometimes afforded protection, but more often it has not. The conflict has been resolved by the observation that inhalation of aerosolized atropine at doses that abolish response to inhaled methacholine shifts to the right the stimulus-response curve for eucapnic hyperventilation with subfreezing air in asthmatic patients.[103] Thus the effects of muscarinic blockade can be overcome by increasing the intensity of the stimulus. Pre-exercise treatment with atropine at doses that ranged from 0.25 to 6 mg did not abolish the obstructive response to hyperventilation. The lack of any difference in the protective effect across this wide range of doses indicates that cholinergic mechanisms do not play a major role in exercise-induced asthma.[103]

Cromolyn. Single doses of cromolyn sodium can inhibit exercise-induced asthma and bronchoconstriction induced by hyperventilation with cold, dry air.[95, 104-108] The effect is to shift the stimulus-response curve to the right.[106] Whereas the usual doses of 2 mg by metered-dose inhaler and 20 mg by Spinhaler are most effective during the first 2 h after inhalation, large doses afford better and larger protection.[107, 108]

Other Drugs. Inhalation of nedocromil sodium and minocromil can inhibit exercise-induced asthma 30 min later.[109-111] Controlled studies have disclosed no protective effect of ketotifen against exercise-induced asthma.[112, 113] Studies of calcium channel blockers have yielded somewhat conflicting findings of effects on exercise-induced asthma. Sublingual nifedipine and inhaled verapamil have provided protection, but inhaled diltiazem has had little effect.[114-117]

Antihistamines have generally failed to inhibit exercise-induced asthma, although thiazinaminium by intramuscular injection can be effective.[118] Terfenadine, however, affords protection 4 h after administration of large doses (120 or 180 mg).[119] Apparent ineffectiveness of other antihistamines may have been attributable to limitation of dosage because of side effects.

Adrenal Corticosteroids. Adrenal corticosteroids have had variable effects on exercise-induced asthma. Prednisone, 5 mg four times a day for 13 doses, has afforded partial protection in asthmatic children, but most investigators have found oral or inhaled steroids to be protective in only a few patients.[7, 26, 120, 121] Treatment with inhaled budesonide for 1 to 4 weeks, however, causes progressively increasing protection.[122, 123]

Pharmacologic Therapy. For protection conferred by usual dosages of drugs available for prevention of exercise-induced asthma, an inhaled beta-agonist is recommended because it provides rapid bronchodilation and protection (see Fig. 68–2). Inhaled albuterol may provide the longest lasting protection of the inhaled beta-agonists. Slow-release preparations of theophylline may provide even longer protection at an adequate dosage.

When a single drug does not provide sufficient protection, combinations of a beta-agonist with cromolyn or a beta-agonist with theophylline may afford better protection.[85, 106, 124]

CONDITIONING OF INSPIRED AIR

Nasal breathing to warm and humidify the inspired air can minimize the bronchoconstrictive effect of exercise, but strenuous exercise usually requires mouth breathing.[36] A cold-weather mask can form a reservoir in which the expired breath warms and humidifies the inspired air, also producing a protective effect.[37] A muffler wrapped around the nose and mouth can serve the same function in cold weather.

EXERCISE THERAPY

Warm Up. Warming up can improve tolerance to subsequent exercise. This phenomenon is not entirely accounted for by the refractory period of at least 1 h that follows exercise-induced asthma because 30-sec sprints repeated at intervals of 2.5 min without provoking bronchoconstriction can also enhance tolerance for a 6-min run 20 min later.[47, 125]

Physical Conditioning. Programs of general physical conditioning can improve cardiovascular fitness in asthmatic children and adults,[126-130] although some studies have failed to disclose such a beneficial effect, possibly because of the nature of the program or inadequate participation by some subjects.[131-133] One controlled study disclosed less exercise-induced bronchoconstriction in asthmatic children after a 6-week program of physical training, but the exercise challenge was not adjusted for the improvement in fitness observed.[128] Other investigators have not found any change in frequency or severity of exercise-induced asthma after such programs at least with adjustment for improvement in work capacity.[126, 129, 133, 134] Investigators have, however, often noted decreases in the frequency and severity of overt asthma with decreased requirements for medications in participants in such programs.[126, 130, 134-136] Increased self-confidence and improvement in psychological adjustment among patients have also been observed.[135-137]

Type of Exercise. Response to exercise depends on the type of exercise. Free-range running is most likely to cause airway obstruction in patients with asthma, swimming is least likely, and walking and cycling are intermediate.[47, 138] These differences may be attributable largely to different effects on ventilation. Leg and arm work elicit similar degrees of bronchoconstriction when workloads are adjusted to cause similar increases in heart rate and minute ventilation.[139] This does not entirely account for the more modest effect of swimming. Swimming causes less bronchoconstriction than does running when minute ventilation and oxygen consumption are matched during breathing of dry or humid air.[140]

SUMMARY

Strenuous exercise in cold, dry air can cause airway obstruction in virtually every asthmatic patient. Specific mechanisms remain unknown, but release of mediators from luminal mast cells is likely, and rapid rewarming of airways after completion of exercise may be important.

Whatever the mechanism, such obstruction can be minimized or prevented. Inhaled albuterol is the treatment of choice for prevention of exercise-induced asthma; cromolyn is helpful when protection is required for only 1 to 2 h. Increasing the dose of either of these drugs or use of both together can enhance protection. Theophylline can also afford protection and can be used with either a beta-agonist or cromolyn for better protection. Large doses of nonsedating antihistamines may also be helpful. Concurrent treatment with budesonide and other inhaled corticosteroids may also have some protective effect.

Nasal breathing or use of a scarf or a muffler over the nose and mouth to increase humidity and warmth of the inspired air can afford protection in cold weather.

Warm-up exercises before the main exercise can minimize subsequent exercise-induced asthma. Programs of physical conditioning are helpful to the extent that they improve cardiovascular fitness; the results are that asthmatic patients may tolerate somewhat more strenuous exercise without increase in ventilation sufficient to cause significant airway obstruction.

With appropriate management, most patients should be able to tolerate most forms of exercise, but when these precautions are impossible or insufficient, repeated brief exercise for 1 to 2 min at a time is more tolerable than prolonged, strenuous exercise.

REFERENCES

1. Adams F (Ed and Trans): The Extant Works of Aretaeus the Cappadocian, p. 316. London: Sydenham Society, 1856.
2. Floyer J: A Treatise of the Asthma. London: R Wilkin, 1698.
3. Salter HH: On Asthma: Its Pathology and Treatment. pp. 132–153. Philadelphia: Blanchard & Lea, 1864.
4. Herxheimer H: Hyperventilation asthma. Lancet 1:83–87, 1946.
5. Jones RS, Buston MH, Wharton MJ: The effect of exercise on ventilatory function in the child with asthma. Br J Dis Chest 56:78–86, 1962.
6. Sly RM: Exercise and the asthmatic child. Pediatr Digest 14:42–49, 1972.
7. Jones RS: Assessment of respiratory function in the asthmatic child. Br Med J 2:972–975, 1966.
8. Jones RS, Wharton MJ, Buston MH: The place of physical exercise and bronchodilator drugs in the assessment of the asthmatic child. Arch Dis Child 38:539–545, 1963.
9. Sly RM: Exercise-related changes in airway obstruction: Frequency and clinical correlates in asthmatic children. Ann Allergy 28:1–16, 1970.
10. Lee TH, Nagakura T, Papageorgiou N, et al: Exercise-induced late asthmatic reactions with neutrophil chemotactic activity. N Engl J Med 308:1502–1505, 1983.
11. Iikura Y, Inui H, Nagakura T, Lee, TH: Factors predisposing to exercise-induced late asthmatic responses. J Allergy Clin Immunol 75:285–289, 1985.
12. Zawadski DK, Lenner KA, McFadden ER, Jr: Reexamination of the late asthmatic response to exercise. Am Rev Respir Dis 137:837–841, 1988.
13. Mussaffi H, Springer C, Godfrey S: Increased bronchial responsiveness to exercise and histamine after allergen challenge in children with asthma. J Allergy Clin Immunol 77:48–52, 1986.
14. Karjalainen J: Exercise response in 404 young men with asthma: No evidence for a late asthmatic reaction. Thorax 46:100–104, 1991.
15. Silverman M, Anderson SD: Standardization of exercise tests in asthmatic children. Arch Dis Child 47:882–889, 1972.
16. Eggleston PA, Guerrant JL: A standardized method of evaluating exercise-induced asthma. J Allergy Clin Immunol 58:414–425, 1976.
17. Kattan M, Keens TG, Mellis CM, Levison H: The response to exercise in normal and asthmatic children. J Pediatr 92:718–721, 1978.
18. Haynes RL, Ingram RH Jr, McFadden ER Jr: An assessment of the pulmonary response to exercise in asthma and an analysis of the factors influencing it. Am Rev Respir Dis 114:739–752, 1976.
19. Godfrey S: Exercise-induced asthma: In Clark TJH, Godfrey S (eds): Asthma, pp. 57–78, London: Chapman & Hall, 1983.
20. Wasserman K, Whipp BJ: Exercise physiology in health and disease. Am Rev Respir Dis 112:219–249, 1975.
21. Eggleston PA: Exercise-induced asthma. In Bierman CW, Pearlman DS (eds): Allergic Diseases of Infancy, Childhood, and Adolescence, pp. 605–611. Philadelphia: WB Saunders, 1980.
22. Wasserman K: Breathing during exercise. N Engl J Med 298:780–785, 1978.
23. Johnson WR, Buskirk ER (eds): Science and Medicine of Exercise and Sports, 2nd ed, p. 125. New York: Harper & Row, 1974.
24. Burr ML, Eldridge BA, Borysiewicz LK: Peak expiratory flow rates before and after exercise in schoolchildren. Arch Dis Child 49:923–926, 1974.
25. Anderson SD, Silverman M, Konig P, Godfrey S: Exercise-induced asthma. Br J Dis Chest 69:1–39, 1975.
26. Heimlich EM, Strick L, Busser RJ: An exercise response test in childhood asthma. J Allergy 37:103, 1966.
27. Sly RM: Induction of increased airway obstruction by exercise or voluntary hyperventilation in asthmatic children. Ann Allergy 30:668–675, 1972.
28. McFadden ER Jr, Sterns DR, Ingram RH Jr, Leith DE: Relative contributions of hypocarbia and hyperpnea as mechanisms in postexercise asthma. J Appl Physiol 42:22–27, 1977.
29. Strauss RH, Ingram RH Jr, McFadden ER Jr: A critical assessment of the roles of circulating hydrogen ion and lactate in the production of exercise-induced asthma. J Clin Invest 60:658–664, 1977.
30. Weinstein RE, Anderson JA, Kvale P, Sweet LC: Effects of humidification on exercise-induced asthma. J Allergy Clin Immunol 57:250–251, 1976.
31. Chen WY, Horton DJ: Heat and water loss from the airways and exercise-induced asthma. Respiration 34:305–313, 1977.
32. Bar-Or O, Neuman I, Dotan R: Effects of dry and humid climates on exercise-induced asthma in children and preadolescents. J Allergy Clin Immunol 60:163–168, 1977.
33. Strauss RH, McFadden ER Jr, Ingram RH Jr, Jaeger JJ: Enhancement of exercise-induced asthma by cold air. N Engl J Med 297:743–747, 1977.
34. Deal EC Jr, McFadden ER Jr, Ingram RH Jr, et al: Role of respiratory heat exchange in production of exercise-induced asthma. J Appl Physiol 46:467–475, 1979.
35. Deal EC Jr, McFadden ER Jr, Ingram RH Jr, Jaeger JJ: Hyperpnea and heat flux: Initial reaction sequence in exercise-induced asthma. J Appl Physiol 46:476–483, 1979.
36. Shturman-Ellstein R, Zeballos RJ, Buckley JM, Souhrada JF: The beneficial effect of nasal breathing on exercise-induced bronchoconstriction. Am Rev Respir Dis 118:65–73, 1978.
37. Schachter EN, Lach E, Lee M: The protective effect of a cold weather mask on exercise-induced asthma. Ann Allergy 46:12–16, 1981.
38. Deal EC Jr, McFadden ER Jr, Ingram RH Jr, Jaeger JJ: Esophageal temperature during exercise in asthmatic and nonasthmatic subjects. J Appl Physiol 46:484–490, 1979.
39. McFadden ER Jr, Denison DM, Waller JF, et al: Direct recordings of the temperatures in the tracheobronchial tree in normal man. J Clin Invest 69:700–705, 1982.
40. Ben-Dov I, Bar-Yishay E, Godfrey S: Exercise-induced asthma without respiratory heat loss. Thorax 37:630–631, 1982.
41. Allegra L, Bianco S: Non-specific broncho-reactivity obtained with an ultrasonic aerosol of distilled water. Eur J Respir Dis (Suppl) 106:41–49, 1980.
42. Eschenbacher WL, Boushey HA, Sheppard D: Alteration in osmolarity of inhaled aerosols cause bronchoconstriction and cough, but absence of a permeant anion causes cough alone. Am Rev Respir Dis 129:211–215, 1984.
43. Eggleston PA, Kagey-Sobotka A, Schleimer RP, Lichtenstein LM: Interaction between hyperosmolar and IgE-mediated histamine release from basophils and mast cells. Am Rev Respir Dis 130:86–91, 1984.
44. Togias AG, Naclerio RM, Proud D, et al: Nasal challenge with cold, dry air results in release of inflammatory mediators. J Clin Invest 76:1375–1381, 1985.
45. Togias AG, Proud D, Lichtenstein LM, et al: The osmolality of nasal secretions increases when inflammatory mediators are released in response to inhalation of cold, dry air. Am Rev Respir Dis 137:625–629, 1988.
46. Anderson SD: Is there a unifying hypothesis for exercise-induced asthma? J Allergy Clin Immunol 73:660–665, 1984.
47. James L, Faciane J, Sly RM: Effect of treadmill exercise on asthmatic children. J Allergy Clin Immunol 57:408–416, 1976.
48. Naclerio RM, Meier HL, Kagey-Sobotka A, et al: In vivo model for the evaluation of topical antiallergic medications. Arch Otolaryngol 110:25–27, 1984.
49. Weiler-Ravell D, Godfrey S: Do exercise- and antigen-induced asthma utilize the same pathways? J Allergy Clin Immunol 67:391–397, 1981.
50. Belcher NG, Rees PJ, Clark TJ, Lee TH: A comparison of the refractory periods induced by hypertonic airway challenge and exercise in bronchial asthma. Am Rev Respir Dis 135:822–825, 1987.
51. Finnerty JP, Polosa R, Holgate ST: Repeated exposure of asthmatic airways to inhaled adenosine 5′-monophosphate attenuates bronchoconstriction provoked by exercise. J Allergy Clin Immunol 86:353–359, 1990.
52. Broide DH, Eisman S, Ramsdell JW, et al: Airway levels of mast cell–derived mediators in exercise-induced asthma. Am Rev Respir Dis 141:563–568, 1990.
53. O'Bryne PM, Jones GL: The effect of indomethacin on exercise-induced bronchoconstriction and refractoriness after exercise. Am Rev Respir Dis 134:69–72, 1986.
54. Margolskee DJ, Bigby BG, Boushey HA: Indomethacin blocks air-

way tolerance to repetitive exercise but not to eucapnic hyperpnea in asthmatic subjects. Am Rev Respir Dis 137:842–846, 1988.

55. Pavord ID, Wisniewski A, Tattersfield AE: Inhaled furosemide and exercise-induced asthma: Evidence of a role for inhibitory prostanoids [Abstract]. Am Rev Respir Dis 143:A210, 1991.

56. McFadden ER Jr, Lenner KA, Strohl KP: Postexertional airway rewarming and thermally induced asthma. J Clin Invest 78:18–25, 1986.

57. Gilbert IA, Fouke JM, McFadden ER Jr: The effect of repetitive exercise on airway temperatures. Am Rev Respir Dis 142:826–831, 1990.

58. Eggleston PA, Rosenthal RR, Anderson SA, et al: Guidelines for the methodology of exercise challenge testing of asthmatics. J Allergy Clin Immunol 64:642–645, 1979.

59. Hendeles L, Massanari M, Weinberger M: Update on the pharmacodynamics and pharmacokinetics of theophylline. Chest 88 (Suppl): 103S–111S, 1985.

60. American Thoracic Society: Standardization of spirometry—1987 update. Am Rev Respir Dis 136:1285–1298, 1987.

61. Day G, Mearns MB: Bronchial lability in cystic fibrosis. Arch Dis Child 48:355–359, 1973.

62. Skorecki K, Levison H, Crozier DN: Bronchial lability in cystic fibrosis. Acta Paediatr Scand 65:39–44, 1976.

63. Price JF, Cogswell JJ, Joseph MC, Cochrane GM: Exercise-induced bronchoconstriction, skin sensitivity, and serum IgE in children with eczema. Arch Dis Child 51:912–917, 1979.

64. Bierman EW, Kawabori I, Pierson WE: Incidence of exercise-induced asthma in children. Pediatrics 56:847–850, 1975.

65. Konig P, Godfrey S: Prevalence of exercise-induced bronchial lability in families of children with asthma. Arch Dis Child 48:513–518, 1973.

66. Verity CM, Vanheule B, Carswell F, Hughes AO: Bronchial lability and skin reactivity in siblings of asthmatic children. Arch Dis Child 59:871–876, 1984.

67. Jones RH, Jones RS: Ventilatory capacity in young adults with a history of asthma in childhood. Br Med J 2:976–978, 1966.

68. Konig P, Godfrey S, Abrahamov A: Exercise-induced bronchial lability in children with a history of wheezy bronchitis. Arch Dis Child 47:578–580, 1972.

69. O'Cain CF, Dowling NB, Slutsky AS, et al: Airway effects of respiratory heat loss in normal subjects. J Appl Physiol 49:875–880, 1980.

70. Fung KP, Chow OK, So SY: Attenuation of exercise-induced asthma by acupuncture. Lancet 2:1419–1422, 1986.

71. Ben-Zvi Z, Spohn WA, Young SH, Kattan M: Hypnosis for exercise-induced asthma. Am Rev Respir Dis 125:392–395, 1982.

72. Rossing TH, Weiss JW, Breslin FJ, et al: Effects of inhaled sympathomimetics on the obstructive response to respiratory heat loss. J Appl Physiol 52:1119–1123, 1982.

73. Silverman M, Konig P, Godfrey S: Use of serial exercise tests to assess the efficacy and duration of action of drugs for asthma. Thorax 28:574–578, 1973.

74. Sly RM, Puapan P, Ghazanshahi S, Midha R: Exercise-induced bronchospasm: Evaluation of albuterol aerosol. Ann Allergy 34:7–14, 1975.

75. Anderson SD, Seale JP, Rozea P, et al: Inhaled and oral salbutamol in exercise-induced asthma. Am Rev Respir Dis 114:493–500, 1976.

76. Francis PW, Krastins IR, Levison H: Oral and inhaled salbutamol in the prevention of exercise-induced bronchospasm. Pediatrics 66:103–108, 1980.

77. Higgs CM, Laszlo G: The duration of protection from exercise-induced asthma by inhaled salbutamol and a comparison with inhaled reproterol. Br J Dis Chest 77:262–269, 1983.

78. Berkowitz R, Schwartz E, Bukstein D, et al: Albuterol protects against exercise-induced asthma longer than metaproterenol sulfate. Pediatrics 77:173–178, 1986.

79. Sly RM, Mayer J: Exercise-induced bronchospasm: Evaluation of metaproterenol syrup. Ann Allergy 27:158–163, 1969.

80. Konig P, Eggleston PA, Serby CW: Comparison of oral and inhaled metaproterenol for prevention of exercise-induced asthma. Clin Allergy 11:597–604, 1981.

81. Sly RM, Heimlich EM, Ginsburg J, et al: Exercise-induced bronchospasm. Evaluation of metaproterenol. Ann Allergy 26:253–258, 1968.

82. Schoeffel RE, Anderson SD, Seale JP: The protective effect and duration of action of metaproterenol aerosol on exercise-induced asthma. Ann Allergy 46:273–275, 1981.

83. Rosenthal RR, Campbell J, Norman PS: The protective effects of inhaled terbutaline and isoproterenol on exercise induced bronchospasm [Abstract]. Am Rev Respir Dis 119(suppl):79, 1979.

84. Henriksen JM, Dahl R: Effects of inhaled budesonide alone and in combination with low-dose terbutaline in children with exercise-induced asthma. Am Rev Respir Dis 128:993–997, 1983.

85. Shapiro GG, McPhillips JJ, Smith K, et al: Effectiveness of terbutaline and theophylline alone and in combination in exercise-induced bronchospasm. Pediatrics 67:508–513, 1981.

86. Sly RM, O'Brien SR: Effect of oral terbutaline on exercise-induced asthma. Ann Allergy 48:151–155, 1982.

87. Sly RM, Heimlich EM, Busser RJ, Strick L: Exercise-induced bronchospasm: Evaluation of isoproterenol, phenylephrine and the combination. Ann Allergy 25:324–327, 1967.

88. Anderson SD, Rozea PJ, Dolton R, et al: Inhaled and oral bronchodilator therapy in exercise induced asthma. Aust N Z J Med 5:544–550, 1975.

89. Konig P, Hordvik NL, Serby CW: Fenoterol in exercise-induced asthma: Effect of dose on efficacy and duration of action. Chest 85:462–464, 1984.

90. Agostini M, Barlocco G, Mastella G: Protective effect of fenoterol spray, ipratropium bromide plus fenoterol spray, and oral clenbuterol, on exercise-induced asthma in children. Eur J Respir Dis (suppl) 128:529–532, 1983.

91. Walker SB, Bierman CW, Pierson WE, et al: Bitolterol mesylate in exercise-induced asthma. J Allergy Clin Immunol 77:32–36, 1986.

92. Newnham D, Ingram C, Earnshaw J, et al: Duration of action of inhaled salmeterol against exercise induced asthma [Abstract]. Am Rev Respir Dis 143:A29, 1991.

93. Badiei B, Faciane J, Sly RM: Effect of theophylline, ephedrine, and their combination upon exercise-induced airway obstruction. Ann Allergy 35:32–36, 1975.

94. Bierman CW, Shapiro GG, Pierson WE, Dorsett CS: Acute and chronic theophylline therapy in exercise-induced bronchospasm. Pediatrics 60:845–849, 1977.

95. Pollock J, Kiechel F, Cooper D, Weinberger M: Relationship of serum theophylline concentration to inhibition of exercise-induced bronchospasm and comparison with cromolyn. Pediatrics 60:840–844, 1977.

96. McNeill RS, Nairn JR, Millar JS, Ingram CG: Exercise-induced asthma. Q J Med 35:55–67, 1966.

97. Sly RM, Heimlich EM, Busser RJ, Strick L: Exercise-induced bronchospasm: Effect of adrenergic or cholinergic blockade. J Allergy 40:93–99, 1967.

98. Borut TC, Tashkin DP, Fischer TJ, et al: Comparison of aerosolized atropine sulfate and SCH 1000 on exercise-induced bronchospasm in children. J Allergy Clin Immunol 60:127–133, 1977.

99. Rachelefsky GS, Tashkin DP, Katz RM, et al: Comparison of aerosolized atropine, isoproterenol, atropine plus isoproterenol, disodium cromoglycate and placebo in the prevention of exercise-induced asthma. Chest 73:1017S–1019S, 1978.

100. Deal EC Jr, McFadden ER Jr, Ingram RH Jr, Jaeger JJ: Effects of atropine on potentiation of exercise-induced bronchospasm by cold air. J Apply Physiol 45:238–243, 1978.

101. Chen WY, Brenner AM, Weiser PC, Chai H: Atropine and exercise-induced bronchoconstriction. Chest 79:651–656, 1981.

102. Taytard A, Vergeret J, Guenard H, et al: Prevention of exercise-induced asthma by oxitropium bromide. Eur J Clin Pharmacol 33:455–458, 1987.

103. Griffin MP, Fung KF, Ingram RH Jr, McFadden ER Jr: Dose-response effects of atropine on thermal stimulus-response relationships in asthma. J Appl Physiol 53:1576–1582, 1982.

104. Sly RM: Effect of cromolyn sodium on exercise-induced airway obstruction in asthmatic children. Ann Allergy 29:362–366, 1971.

105. Breslin FJ, McFadden ER Jr, Ingram RH Jr: The effects of cromolyn sodium on the airway response to hyperpnea and cold air in asthma. Am Rev Respir Dis 122:11–16, 1980.

106. Latimer KM, O'Byrne PM, Morris MM, et al: Bronchoconstriction stimulated by airway cooling: Better protection with combined inhalation of terbutaline sulphate and cromolyn sodium than with either alone. Am Rev Respir Dis 128:440–443, 1983.

107. Bar-Yishay E, Gur I, Levy M, et al: Duration of action of sodium

cromoglycate on exercise induced asthma: Comparison of 2 formulations. Arch Dis Child 58:624–627, 1983.

108. Patel KR, Wall RT: Dose-duration effect of sodium cromoglycate aerosol in exercise-induced asthma. Eur J Respir Dis 69:256–260, 1986.

109. Debelic M: Nedocromil sodium and exercise-induced asthma in adolescents. Eur J Respir Dis 69(Suppl 147):266–267, 1986.

110. Thomson NC, Roberts JA: Nedocromil sodium attenuates exercise-induced asthma. Eur J Respir Dis 69(Suppl 147):297–298, 1986.

111. Roberts JA, Thomson NC: Attenuation of exercise-induced asthma by pretreatment with nedocromil sodium and minocromil. Clin Allergy 15:377–381, 1985.

112. Tanser AR, Elmes J: A controlled trial of ketotifen in exercise-induced asthma. Br J Dis Chest 74:398–402, 1980.

113. Petheram IS, Moxham J, Bierman CW, et al: Ketotifen in atopic asthma and exercise-induced asthma. Thorax 36:308–312, 1981.

114. Barnes PJ, Wilson NM, Brown MJ: A calcium antagonist, nifedipine, modifies exercise-induced asthma. Thorax 36:726–730, 1981.

115. Cerrina J, Denjean A, Alexandre G, et al: Inhibition of exercise-induced asthma by a calcium antagonist, nifedipine. Am Rev Respir Dis 123:156–160, 1981.

116. Patel KR: Calcium antagonists in exercise-induced asthma. Br Med J 282:932–933, 1981.

117. Foresi A, Corbo GM, Ciappi G, et al: Effect of two doses of inhaled diltiazem on exercise-induced asthma. Respiration 51:241–247, 1987.

118. Zielinski J, Chodosowska E: Exercise-induced bronchoconstriction in patients with bronchial asthma: Its prevention with an antihistaminic agent. Respiration 34:31–35, 1977.

119. Patel KR: Terfenadine in exercise induced asthma. Br Med J 288:1496–1497, 1984.

120. Konig P, Jaffe P, Godfrey S: Effect of corticosteroids on exercise-induced asthma. J Allergy Clin Immunol 54:14–19, 1974.

121. Yazigi R, Sly RM, Frazer M: Effect of triamcinolone acetonide aerosol upon exercise-induced asthma. Ann Allergy 40:322–325, 1978.

122. Henriksen JM, Dahl R: Effects of inhaled budesonide alone and in combination with low-dose terbutaline in children with exercise-induced asthma. Am Rev Respir Dis 128:993–997, 1983.

123. Venge P, Henriksen J, Dahl R, Hakansson L: Exercise-induced asthma and the generation of neutrophil chemotactic activity. J Allergy Clin Immunol 85:498–504, 1990.

124. Woolley MJ: Duration of action of terbutaline and sodium crom-

oglycate alone and in combination on exercise-induced asthma [Abstract]. Am Rev Respir Dis 137(Suppl):340, 1988.

125. Schnall RP, Landau LI: Protective effects of repeated short sprints in exercise-induced asthma. Thorax 35:828–832, 1980.

126. Fitch KD, Morton AR, Blanksby BA: Effects of swimming training on children with asthma. Arch Dis Child 51:190–194, 1976.

127. Leisti S, Finnila MJ, Kiuru E: Effects of physical training on hormonal responses to exercise in asthmatic children. Arch Dis Child 54:524–528, 1979.

128. Henriksen JM, Nielsen TT: Effect of physical training on exercise-induced bronchoconstriction. Acta Paediatr Scand 72:31–36, 1983.

129. Nickerson BG, Bautista DB, Namey MA, et al: Distance running improves fitness in asthmatic children without pulmonary complications or changes in exercise-induced bronchospasm. Pediatrics 71:147–152, 1983.

130. Bundgaard A, Ingemann-Hansen T, Halkjaer-Kristensen J, et al: Short-term physical training in bronchial asthma. Br J Dis Chest 77:147–152, 1983.

131. Vavra J, Macek M, Mrzena B, et al: Intensive physical training in children with bronchial asthma. Acta Paediatr Scand [Suppl]217:90–92, 1971.

132. Graff-Lonnevig V, Bevegard S, Eriksson BO, et al: Two years' follow-up of asthmatic boys participating in a physical activity programme. Acta Paediatr Scand 69:347–352, 1980.

133. Fitch KD, Blitvich JD, Morton AR: The effect of running training on exercise-induced asthma. Ann Allergy 57:90–94, 1986.

134. Sly RM, Harper RT, Rosselot I: The effect of physical conditioning upon asthmatic children. Ann Allergy 30:86–94, 1972.

135. McElhenney TR, Petersen KH: Physical fitness for asthmatic boys. JAMA 185(2):142–143, 1963.

136. Tuberculosis and Health Association of Hennepin County: Physical conditioning program for asthmatic children. J School Health 37:107–110, 1967.

137. Scherr MS, Frankel L: Physical conditioning program for asthmatic children. JAMA 168:1996–2000, 1958.

138. Fitch KD, Morton AR: Specificity of exercise in exercise-induced asthma. Br Med J 4:577–581, 1971.

139. Strauss RH, Haynes RL, Ingram RH Jr, McFadden ER Jr: Comparison of arm versus leg work in induction of acute episodes of asthma. J Appl Physiol 42:565–570, 1977.

140. Bar-Yishay E, Gur I, Inbar O, et al: Differences between swimming and running as stimuli for exercise-induced asthma. Eur J Appl Physiol 48:387–397, 1982.

VI Cystic Fibrosis

69 GENETIC ASPECTS OF CYSTIC FIBROSIS

KATHERINE W. KLINGER, PH.D.

The generally accepted incidence of cystic fibrosis (CF) in the United States is 1 in 2000–2500 in Caucasian populations. The CF gene is inherited in an autosomal recessive manner;[1] the carrier frequency is approximately 1 in 25. Several explanations have been proposed for the persistence of the CF gene at such relatively high levels, including heterozygote advantage[2] and random drift.[3]

In 1985 the cystic fibrosis gene was linked first to the paraoxonase polymorphism[4] and then to a DNA polymorphism.[5] As is common in linkage studies, additional markers more tightly linked to the CF locus were rapidly identified.[6, 7] The known chromosomal assignment of the linked markers then allowed the assignment of the CF gene to the long arm of chromosome 7. Advances in molecular biology and physiology have added to the understanding of CF pathophysiology and enabled the cloning and characterization of the CF gene.[8–10]

The gene associated with CF was cloned in 1989 and is called cystic fibrosis transmembrane conductance regulator (CFTR).[10] The DNA sequence predicts a protein product of approximately 170 kD composed of two homologous repeated units. Each unit is composed of six transmembrane domains and a nucleotide binding fold in which the two units are separated by a large polar R-domain. The predicted structure places CFTR in the class of related proteins that includes multidrug resistance,

bovine adenylcyclase, yeast STE6 protein, and several bacterial transport proteins.[10, 11]

As a result of intensive efforts to identify causative CF mutations,[12] it is now possible to determine carrier status and provide diagnosis in most at-risk families, to consider the implications of population screening, and to draw some inferences regarding specific mutations and different manifestations of the disease.

MOLECULAR GENETIC DIAGNOSIS

For many years, genetic counseling with regard to CF was largely limited to providing statistical estimates of risk based on gene frequency and mendelian odds (Table 69–1). Before the identification of polymorphic markers linked to the CF gene, there was no reliable test for heterozygote detection. Prenatal diagnosis was limited to the analysis of microvillar enzymes in amniotic fluid. This was very useful for predictive prenatal diagnosis in families with a risk of 1 in 4 but was not absolutely diagnostic.[13–16]

Discovery of polymorphic markers closely linked to the CF locus enabled accurate (>99%) prediction of CF gene inheritance in at-risk families.[17, 18] The segregation of these markers in families was initially followed by analyzing

Table 69–1. MENDELIAN RISK OF CYSTIC FIBROSIS (CF) CARRIER STATUS IN RELATIVES OF CF PROBANDS AND SUBSEQUENT RISK TO CF OFFSPRING

Relationship to Proband	Probability of Heterozygosity (Ff)	Probability of ff Child of Ff Parents	Mendelian Risk	Probability of Unrelated Heterozygous Spouse (Ff)	Chance of Affected Child
None*	1/25	1/4	1/100	1/25	1/2500
Parent	1	1/4	1/4	1	1/4
Sibling	2/3	1/4	1/6	1/25	1/150
Aunt or uncle	1/2	1/4	1/8	1/25	1/200
	2/3	1/4	1/6	1/25	1/150

*No family history of CF; risk based on the gene frequency in the population.

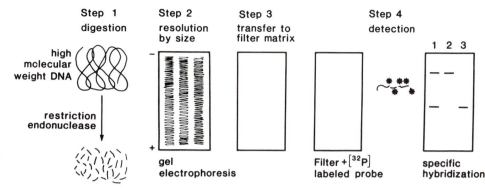

Figure 69–1. Restriction endonuclease analysis of DNA. The basic steps entail digestion and resolution of the resultant DNA fragments, followed by the identification of specific DNA fragments by means of a [P32]-labeled probe *(asterisks).* A characteristic digestion pattern is obtained for each individual in the example given; the DNA probe has detected a restriction fragment length polymorphism (RFLP) for the enzyme. Individual 1 is heterozygous for the RFLP, individual 2 is homozygous for the large fragment, and individual 3 is homozygous for the small fragment.

restriction fragment length polymorphisms (RFLPs) by means of the Southern blot assay (Fig. 69–1).

The general approach is based on restriction endonuclease analysis. Restriction endonucleases are enzymes that create double-stranded breaks in the DNA backbone when a specific nucleotide sequence, the recognition site, is present. It has been estimated that 1 nucleotide of every 200 nucleotide pairs in the human genome varies among individuals. Most of this variation is neither advantageous nor harmful but merely represents interindividual polymorphism. If the neutral polymorphism generates a change in a restriction enzyme recognition site, a different-sized DNA fragment is generated at that locus when the DNA is digested with the restriction enzyme. The result is referred to as an RFLP if it occurs at a frequency of 1% or higher.

Human DNA (usually prepared from a small sample of peripheral blood) is digested with a restriction endonuclease to generate small DNA fragments, which are separated according to size by agarose gel electrophoresis (see Fig. 69–1). The fragments are transferred to a nylon filter (or equivalent matrix) in a procedure known as the Southern blot.[19] Specific DNA fragments are detected by hybridization to a radioactive single-copy DNA probe, or specific hybridization can be detected through the use of nonisotopic systems. DNA sequences linked to the gene of interest are used as probes for genes of unknown function. The coding functions of many linked DNA sequences are not known, and they are referred to as anonymous.

An example of linkage analysis is shown in Figure 69–2. The segregation pattern of the linked alleles within the family must be established for linkage analysis. This usually requires documentation of the previous birth of an affected child for the analysis of a recessive disease, such as CF. In part A, the CF genotypes of the parents and the affected child are known a priori, and the large DNA fragment detected by the linked probe segregates with the disease gene. The DNA pattern illustrated predicts that the daughter is a normal homozygote and that the second son will be a carrier of the disease gene. In part B, the disease gene is segregating with the large DNA fragment in the mother, who is homozygous for the linked polymorphism. This limits the predictive information that can be generated. The daughter has inherited the disease-linked

allele from the father. The maternal alleles cannot be discriminated, and so the daughter is either a heterozygote or affected. This result does not allow prenatal diagnosis, but it would establish carrier status in a clinically unaffected sibling. Conversely, the second son is either a normal homozygote or a heterozygote. This information is useful for prenatal diagnosis but is not helpful for carrier detection. Although such partial information is useful to families, Figure 69–2B illustrates the need for highly polymorphic probes, so that a marker for which both parents

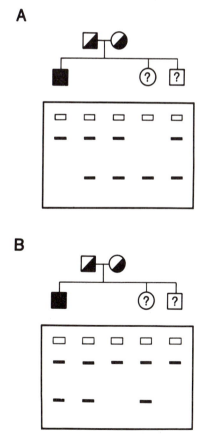

Figure 69–2. Assignment of genotype by RFLP analysis through the use of a linked DNA probe. Two different segregation patterns are shown (A and B). The diagnostic implications of each pattern are discussed in text.

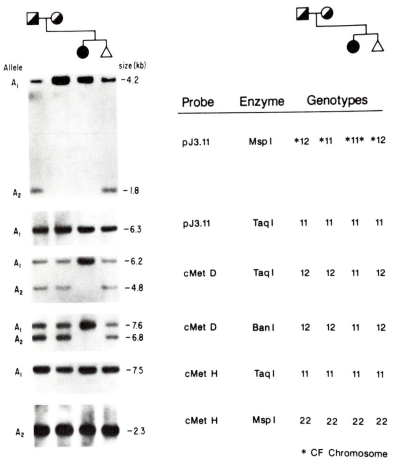

Probe	Enzyme	Genotypes			
pJ3.11	Msp I	*12	*11	*11*	*12
pJ3.11	Taq I	11	11	11	11
cMet D	Taq I	12	12	11	12
cMet D	Ban I	12	12	11	12
cMet H	Taq I	11	11	11	11
cMet H	Msp I	22	22	22	22

* CF Chromosome

Figure 69–3. Example of cystic fibrosis (CF) marker analysis. *Left,* Hybridization patterns obtained through DNA from CF family members, and the indicated probe-enzyme pairs. Only the relevant portion of the autoradiographs is shown. Allele sizes for each probe-enzyme polymorphism are shown to the right of the bands on the autoradiographs. *Right,* Assignment of marker alleles and determination of CF phase. On the basis of marker segregation, the test individual is predicted to be a CF gene carrier (CF maternal chromosome, normal paternal chromosome). Half-solid square, heterozygous male; half-solid circle, heterozygous female; solid circle, affected female; open triangle, test subject.

are informative can be used, as illustrated in Figure 69–3. With the identification of many linked polymorphisms flanking the CF locus (shown in Fig. 69–3), virtually every at-risk family is informative, and a fully accurate prediction of gene status can be given. The Southern blotting technique is very accurate but is relatively slow and labor intensive, requiring about 1 week to complete.

More recently, Southern blot analysis has largely been superseded by the polymerase chain reaction (PCR) technique for analysis of genetic polymorphisms linked to CF (Fig. 69–4). In PCR analysis DNA polymerase is used to synthesize many copies of DNA at a specific locus from a very small amount of starting DNA, a process known as amplification. The starting material can be very complex, as in total human DNA prepared for genetic disease diagnosis. Specificity of the amplification reaction is achieved by the choice of a pair of oligonucleotide primers, each complementary to sequences flanking the region to be amplified. The primers serve as starting points for the DNA polymerase enzyme, and they initiate DNA synthesis in opposing directions. Starting with 1 μg or less of total genomic DNA and 25 cycles of amplification, the target DNA can be amplified more than one millionfold in about 2 h. PCR analysis is much faster than the Southern blotting technique, and much less material is required. However, the technique does require detailed sequence information about the polymorphisms or mutations being studied, in order to design the PCR primers and allele specific oligonucleotides (to be described).

For PCR detection of a polymorphism or mutation, the sample DNA is first amplified *in vitro* by the PCR method[20] and then analyzed either directly or after restriction endonuclease digestion on agarose gels[21-24] by use of allele specific primers[25] or by hybridization with allele specific oligonucleotide (ASO) probes.[26] PCR assays to detect polymorphisms recognized by the linked markers *met d* and *met H*, XV2c, KM19, MP6d-9, J3.11, and CS.7 have been described[21, 22, 27-30] and are in common use. The limitations to linkage analysis are that (1) it is an indirect assay, (2) an affected family member must be present, (3) the family must be informative for the linked polymorphic markers, and (4) in general, the test is applicable only to people with a family history of the disease. Although direct detection of the most common causative CF mutations has largely replaced linkage analysis, linkage analysis remains a useful tool in at-risk families who have a history of CF but in whom a known CF mutation is not segregating. Finally, as a result of linkage disequilibrium,[31] chromosomes with certain combination of polymorphic alleles (haplotypes) are more likely to carry a CF mutation than others; therefore, RFLP information can be used to help determine risk in persons uninformative for known CF mutations.

The identification of the CF gene in 1989 enabled direct detection of CF mutations. The first CF mutation described was a three–base-pair deletion in exon 10. This deletion results in the removal of one phenylalanine and is known as ΔF508.[9] This is the most common mutation

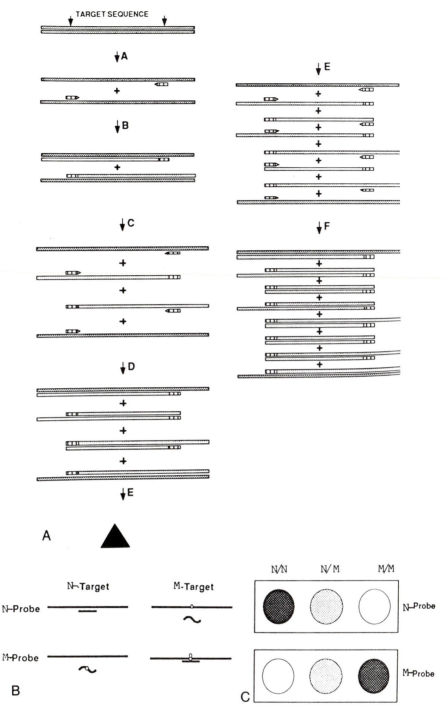

Figure 69-4. *A*, DNA amplification by the polymerase chain reaction. In step A, genomic DNA is heated to separate its strands. When cooled, synthetic oligonucleotide primers rapidly hybridize to their matched complementary sequences on the genomic DNA, binding to each of the separated strands in an orientation that directs the action of DNA polymerase toward the region to be amplified (target sequence). In step B, DNA polymerase uses the primers to begin the synthesis of DNA, and the genomic DNA serves as a template. The amount of DNA at the center of the figure is twice the amount present initially. This is the last step in the first cycle of amplification. In step C, DNA is heated and cooled, to allow the primers to bind to their target sequences. The newly synthesized DNA also serves as a target for the binding of primers. In step D, DNA polymerase extends each of the bound primers. When this occurs on the DNA products of the previous step, synthesis is terminated as the polymerase reaches the end of the template strand. This produces a DNA molecule of a defined size, bounded by the position of the two primers. This molecule rapidly becomes predominant. At the end of the second cycle, the DNA has quadrupled. The amplification process is continued by heating, cooling, and primer hybridization and by primer extension with DNA polymerase. In this third cycle, a DNA molecule in which the ends of both strands are defined by the locations of the primers appears. This molecule is the final product at the end of the amplification process. *B* and *C*, DNA analysis with allele-specific oligonucleotide (ASO) probes. In these examples, the DNA being analyzed either contains the normal human gene (N) or a mutant gene (M). Synthetic ASO probes are made with either the normal sequence or the mutant sequence. Part *B* shows how the probes are used to detect the presence of the normal or mutant DNAs. The ASO probe for the N allele *(upper left)* can hybridize to its exactly complementary sequence, whereas this probe fails to hybridize to the M target *(upper right)*. Similarly, the ASO probe designed to exactly match the M allele *(lower left)* fails to hybridize to the N target but is able to bind to the M allele *(lower right)*. Thus the pattern of binding of each probe reflects the composition of the DNA being tested. Part *C* depicts the visual pattern of binding of ASO probes to DNA samples. Three DNA samples, one with only the N allele (from a homozygous normal individual), one with both the N and M alleles, and one with only the M allele have been amplified and spotted in duplicate to two filters. These filters are then separately treated with either the ASO probe for the N allele or for the M allele. The binding of the probes is detected either through the use of radioactive isotopes or through nonradioactive methods. Comparison of the amount of hybridization for each probe then enables the investigator to infer the genotype of the original DNA sample.

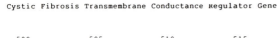

Cystic Fibrosis Transmembrane Conductance Regulator Gene

```
        500          505          510          515
    ProGlyThrIleLysGluAsnIleIlePheGlyValSerTyrAspGluTyrArgTyrArg
1621: CCTGGCACCATTAAAGAAAATATCATCTTTGGTGTTTCCTATGATGAATATAGATACAGA
      GGACCGTGGTAATTTCTTTTATAGTAGAAACCACAAAGGATACTACTTATATCTATGTCT
                               |/
                               |/
    GlyThrIleLysGluAsnIleIleGlyValSerTyrAspGluTyrArgTyrArg
      GGCACCATTAAAGAAAATATCATTGGTGTTTCCTATGATGAATATAGATACAGA
      CCGTGGTAATTTCTTTTATAGTAACCACAAAGGATACTACTTATATCTATGTCT
```

(CF Mutation ΔPhe-508)

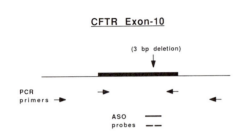

CFTR Exon-10

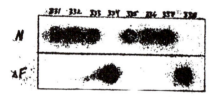

Figure 69–5. Polymerase chain reaction (PCR) assay for ΔF508 mutation. The sequence that contains the mutation is shown in the upper panel, a schematic of the PCR process is shown in the middle panel, and an ASO dot blot showing homozygous non-ΔF508 individuals (331,332,333,335,336,337) and homozygous ΔF508 individuals (334,338) is shown in the lower panel. ΔF, ASO probe specific for the phenylalanine deletion; N, ASO probe specific for the normal sequence at this locus.

in Northern European–derived populations (including the United States) and accounts for 70% to 75% of CF chromosomes.[9, 32] On the basis of a frequency of the ΔF508 mutation of 70%, approximately 49% of CF patients are homozygous for the deletion, 42% have one chromosome with the deletion and one chromosome with a different CF mutation, and about 9% have two non-ΔF508 CF mutations.

The three–base-pair ΔF508 deletion is easily detected in PCR-based assays, and these assays are routinely performed for diagnostic purposes. The deletion can be detected through the use of a number of different PCR-based formats. The first assays described were PCR-ASO assays, in which hybridization to alleles specific for the normal or mutant form of the gene are used to assign genotype (Fig. 69–5).[9, 33] Assays based on allele specific primers[34] and on direct detection by gel electrophoresis of the alternative-sized PCR products or the heteroduplex (i.e., a double-stranded molecule in which one strand lacks the three–base-pair deletion and the other pair has the deletion) have also been described.[35, 36]

The availability of direct detection of many carriers and cases of CF raises the issue of how to use this new diag-

nostic capability. The test is very specific: if the ΔF508 mutation is found in two copies, the individual has CF. If one copy of the deletion is found in an otherwise healthy adult or in a healthy relative of a CF patient, that person can be presumed to be a carrier of CF. The current assay has better specificity than sensitivity, and this raises issues with regard to carrier screening, as discussed later. Twenty-five percent of CF chromosomes do not carry the ΔF508 mutation but do carry another CF mutation instead. Thus unless it is known that the ΔF508 mutation (or another known CF mutation to be described) is segregating in the family being tested, a "negative result" (i.e., one in which the ΔF508 mutation is not detected) does not rule out the presence of the CF gene. In this case, rather than a precise diagnosis of normal genotype, it is necessary to calculate the residual risk of an undetected CF mutation.

The ΔF508 analysis is extremely useful and accurate for prenatal diagnosis and carrier detection in families with a history of CF. The majority of these families are either fully or partially informative, as described earlier, and linkage analysis can resolve matters for families that are uninformative. Many laboratories recommend CF mutation analysis for relatives of CF patients and for the spouses of those relatives. Although a small residual risk of CF carrier status remains in the non–blood relative spouse whose test for known CF mutations is negative, the relative risk has been significantly adjusted, in comparison with no testing at all. These concepts are described in Table 69–2.

CF mutation testing has also been helpful in resolving equivocal diagnoses of CF. The sweat electrolyte (chloride) test is one of the gold standards of CF diagnosis but does have limitations.[37, 38] Mutation analysis has been helpful in clarifying CF inheritance in individuals with borderline sweat chloride tests in families that already have an affected child. Similarly, if an individual has intermediate sweat chloride levels, some signs or symptoms of CF or congenital bilateral absence of the vas deferens (CBAVD) and no family history but has inherited one copy of a known CF mutation, the probability that this individual does have CF is very high, whereas if the individual has inherited no copies of a known CF muta-

Table 69–2. RISK IMPLICATIONS OF ΔF508
MUTATIONS TESTING

Parent 1*	Carrier Risk†	Parent 2*	Carrier Risk	Pregnancy Risk
NN	1:75	NN	1:75	1.22500
		Unknown	1:25	1:7500
		NF	1:1	1:300
Unknown	1:25	NN	1:75	1:7500
		Unknown	1:25	1:2500
		NF	1:1	1:90
NF‡	1:1	NN	1:75	1:300
		Unknown	1:25	1:100
		NF	1:1	1:4

*Assuming that neither parent has a family history of cystic fibrosis (CF).
†Assuming a 1:25 carrier frequency in the population.
‡This would also be the case if parent 1 has a CF-affected relative and has a positive test for ΔF508

tion, he or she is more likely to be normal. The relationship between the frequency of fetal ultrasound abnormalities consistent with meconium ileus, echogenic bowel, and obstructed bowel and subsequent detection of one or two copies of CF mutations is less clear.

CARRIER SCREENING

The cloning of the CF gene and the characterization of the ΔF508 mutation immediately raised the prospect of population screening to prospectively identify carriers. A direct DNA test could be applied to detect one or more CF mutations in the absence of any family history of CF. The pros and cons of population screening programs have been widely discussed,[39-41] and there is currently no consensus among geneticists as to whether population screening should be undertaken. Whenever a populationwide screening program is proposed, numerous health care, social, and economic issues must be addressed. Statements by advisory panels of the American Society of Human Genetics and the National Institutes of Health called for initial caution, with the development of pilot programs to study laboratory (quality assurance, sensitivity of the assay, and so forth), educational, and counseling aspects of screening. There is consensus that carrier testing should be offered to couples in which either partner has a close relative affected with CF, that carrier testing should be voluntary and confidential, that informed consent should be required, that education and counseling should be included, that there should be equal access to testing, and that laboratory quality control should be addressed. Concerns about possible discrimination in the workplace and in insurability have also been raised.[42, 43]

Many concerns also revolve around the *sensitivity* of a CF carrier test because a test that fails to detect 15% to 25% of CF chromosomes presents significant genetic counseling challenges when applied to a large population. A 75% detection rate means that on the basis of a carrier frequency of 1 in 25, the chance of having an affected child is approximately 1 in 39,000 if tests of both partners are negative, whereas the risk remains relatively high (1 in 396) if one partner's test is negative and the other's is positive. Because of the high carrier frequency, 1 in 15 to 1 in 20 couples (approximately 5.2%) would have a substantially high risk of having an affected child (1 in 396, in contrast to 1 in 2500 if no testing were done), and no definitive assay is available for clarifying the risk. It would be difficult for the current health care system in the United States to handle the counseling burden imposed by such a test. At the time of the initial policy statements on carrier screening,[42, 43] it was hoped that additional mutations that would raise the sensitivity to 90% to 95% would rapidly be found. At this detection level, the false-negative rate would be no worse than the population-based risk of an affected child (1 in 2500). As discussed later, this has unfortunately turned out not to be the case, and additional consideration must therefore be given to when carrier screening is appropriate. Information from pilot programs underway in Great Britain and Denmark (where ΔF508 accounts for more than 90% of CF chromosomes) may help guide programs in the United States,

although differences in health care delivery between countries may complicate direct extrapolation of the European experience. An excellent review of the issues surrounding carrier screening for CF can be found in the Office of Technology Assessment report.[44]

ADDITIONAL MUTATIONS

When the CF gene (CFTR) was originally identified and the ΔF508 mutation characterized, it was hoped that at most a few additional mutations would account for the remaining 25% of CF chromosomes. It is now clear that there exist many mutations in the CFTR gene, each of which gives rise to the clinical phenotype recognized as CF. By mid-1992, more than 200 mutations had been reported by the Cystic Fibrosis Gene Analysis Consortium. The various CF mutations identified are distributed throughout the gene, but they do cluster in several regions, especially the nucleotide-binding domains (Fig. 69–6). Most of the non-ΔF508 mutations discovered to date are rare, but several occur with sufficient frequency to be useful for diagnosis. Together, ΔF508, G551D, G542X, and R553X analyses detect 80% to 85% of CF chromosomes in non-Ashkenazic Caucasians in the United States (Table 69–3). A mutation called R117H, although less common, appears to be associated with milder forms of the disease. It is still possible that one or two mutations that account for the remaining 15% of CF chromosomes will be discovered. However, it would not be surprising if no additional high-frequency mutations are identified. Considerable variation in the frequency of the various mutations exists across population and ethnic groups; ΔF508 represents only about 46% of Southern European, 30% of black, and 30% of Ashkenazic CF chromosomes.[45-47] Analysis of six mutations, including ΔF508, W12824, N1303K, and 3849 + 10-kb C-T, detects approximately 96% of Ashkenazic CF chromosomes.[48] It is extremely important to have accurate information about the ethnic background of patients in order to obtain the most accurate risk predictions. The world frequency of CFTR mutations available from data from the CF Genetic Analysis Consortium in May 1992 is shown in Table 69–4.

CLINICAL CORRELATIONS

The clinical manifestation of CF varies both within and between families. Although most patients have progressive pulmonary disease and pancreatic insufficiency, about 15% of patients are pancreatic sufficient.[49] Pulmonary disease tends to be milder among pancreatic-sufficient patients.[50] There has been great interest in determining whether the various clinical phenotypes could be correlated with the presence of specific mutations. Pancreatic-sufficient patients are a more genetically heterogeneous group than are pancreatic-insufficient patients and have different haplotypes at the closely-linked markers.[9, 51, 52] This association of the pancreatic-sufficient phenotype with non-ΔF508 mutations continues to hold true: in general, ΔF508 is considered a severe mutation.

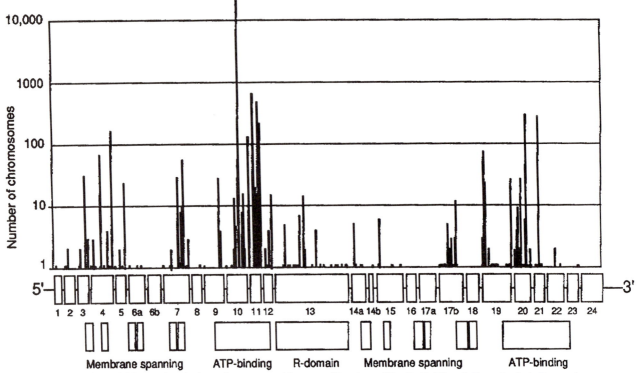

Figure 69-6. Distribution of CF mutations in the various exons of the gene. (Courtesy of the Cystic Fibrosis Gene Analysis Consortium, compiled by L. C. Tsui, Toronto.)

However, even within homozygous ΔF508 patients, there is considerable clinical variation, and two pancreatic-sufficient patients homozygous for ΔF508 have been reported.[53] No association has been observed between pulmonary function and specific mutations.[54, 55]

Both environment and genes outside the CF locus may influence the clinical severity of the disease. An increasing number of individuals with atypical CF (e.g., those with borderline sweat chloride levels or those whose symptoms are confined to a single component of CF such as CBAVD, as well as the rare asymptomatic adult) have been analyzed for mutations in the CFTR gene. The somewhat surprising results show that many of these individuals carry CF mutations identical to those of persons with more classical and severe CF. Perhaps equally surprising is the identification of some patients who are

Table 69-3. CYSTIC FIBROSIS MUTATION

Characteristic	n	%
Patients genotyped	3493	19
Of percentage genotyped		
Homozygous for ΔF508		48.1
Compound heterozygous for ΔF508		36.1
Mutations other than ΔF508		15.8
Most frequent mutations		
ΔF508	2940	84.2
G542X	111	3.2
G551D	101	2.9
W1282X	57	1.6
N1303K	48	1.3
R553X	46	1.4

Data from National Cystic Fibrosis Foundation Registry, 1991.

Table 69-4. WORLD FREQUENCY OF CFTR MUTATION

Mutation	Chromosomes	
	Found	*Screened (%)*
ΔF508	20,153	29,983 (67.2)
G542X	674	20,118 (3.4)
G551D	492	20,827 (2.4)
N1303K	306	16,739 (1.8)
W1282X	300	14,408 (2.1)
R553X	248	19,600 (1.3)
621+1G→T	186	14,056 (1.3)
1717−1G→A	151	13,715 (1.1)
R117H	82	10,460 (0.8)
R1162X	74	8699 (0.9)
ΔI507	58	12,465 (0.5)
R347P	54	10,307 (0.5)
R560T	47	11,527 (0.4)
1078delT	34	3192 (1.1)
G85E	32	4801 (0.7)
R334W	31	8733 (0.3)
A455E	31	7048 (0.4)
3659delC	29	3634 (0.8)
3849+10kbC→T	28	1955 (1.4)
3095insT	27	1313 (2.1)
711+1G→T	25	2860 (0.9)
S549N	21	12,516 (0.2)
Y122X	19	6535 (0.3)
2184delA	18	2598 (0.7)
Y1092X	15	3118 (0.5)
S549R(T→C)	15	5616 (0.3)
1898+1G→A	14	1589 (0.9)
V520F	14	6890 (0.2)
2789+5G→A	14	1305 (1.1)
Q493X	12	4317 (0.3)
3849+4A→G	11	1120 (1.0)
R347H	10	15,060 (0.1)

Data from Cystic Fibrosis Genetic Analysis Consortium, May 1992.

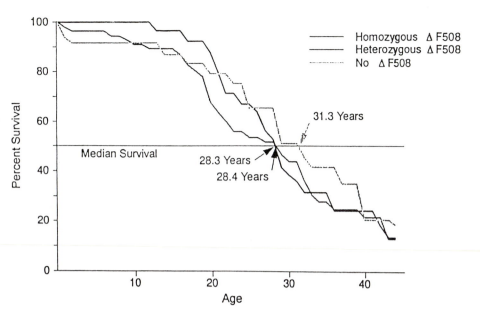

Figure 69-7. Survival curve for cystic fibrosis patients by genotype. Of the patients on the National CF Registry for 1991, 3493 (19%) were genotyped. Survival rates for patients homozygous for ΔF508 (48%), compound heterozygous for ΔF508 (36%), and with neither allele being ΔF508 (16%) are shown. (Data from the National CF Foundation, 1991.)

homozygous for nonsense mutations and who therefore produce either no protein or extremely truncated protein and yet have very mild phenotypes, whereas others have more typical disease.[47] The factors that modulate disease severity between individuals of identical genotype are as yet unknown. There is debate as to whether adults who are essentially diagnosed by molecular analysis rather than by classical clinical presentation should, in fact, be given the label "CF." However, these individuals and their carrier relatives are at risk for having more severely affected offspring should their partners carry a more severe CF mutation. Thus these individuals should receive counseling about CF. Much more data will be required in order to understand the full complexities of CF. Although the various mutations provide fascinating clues to the function of protein domains, it is too early to predict prognosis on the basis of the mutation inherited by a particular patient (Fig. 69–7).

FUTURE DIRECTIONS

The discovery of the CF gene has not only enabled improvements in diagnosis of the disease but has also opened the possibility of increased understanding of the pathophysiologic processes of the disease and improvements in therapy. Complementation of the CF chloride transport defect has been achieved in cultured cells through the use of full-length CFTR complementary DNA.[56,57] Thus it may be possible in the future to treat CF either with gene therapy or with protein replacement therapy.

Several naturally occurring CF mutations have been examined for their effect on protein biologic processes in transfection studies with *in vitro* cultured cells.[58] Surprisingly, ΔF508 results in a failure of the protein to mature. Glycosylation and subsequent movement to the cell membrane do not occur, and the protein remains trapped in the endoplasmic reticulum or the Golgi apparatus. Other mutations tested also prevent maturation (e.g.,

ΔI507), whereas R334W, a rare mutation in transmembrane 6 domain, allows protein maturation. The discovery that the majority of cases of CF appear to result from a lack of protein maturation raises the possibility of therapy with drugs that alter subcellular localization. In 1992, three groups independently succeeded in creating mouse models for CF by inactivating the mouse CFTR gene.[59–62] The disease pathology in these mice is strikingly similar to human CF. These mice should prove invaluable for further understanding of the molecular pathophysiology of the disease, advancement of pharmacologic protein replacement, gene therapy, and perhaps ultimately a cure for CF.

REFERENCES

 1. Boat T, Welsh MJ, Beaudet A: Cystic fibrosis. *In* Scriver S, Beaudet A, Sly W, Valle D (eds): The Metabolic Basis of Inherited Disease, pp. 2649–2660. New York: McGraw Hill, 1989.
 2. Anderson CM, Allan J, Johansen PG: Comments on the possible existence and nature of a heterozygote advantage in cystic fibrosis. Bibl Paediatr 86:381–387, 1967.
 3. Wright SW, Morton NE: Genetic studies on cystic fibrosis in Hawaii. Am J Hum Genet 20:157–169, 1968.
 4. Eiberg H, Mohr J, Schmiegelow K, et al: Linkage relationships of paraoxonase (PON) with other markers: Indication of PON-cystic fibrosis synteny. Clin Genet 28:265–271, 1985.
 5. Tsui LC, Buchwald M, Barker D, et al: Cystic fibrosis locus defined by a genetically linked polymorphic DNA marker. Science 230:1054–1057, 1985.
 6. White R, Woodward S, Leppert M, et al: A closely linked genetic marker for cystic fibrosis. Nature 318:382–384, 1985.
 7. Wainwright BJ, Scambler PJ, Schmidtke J, et al: Localization of cystic fibrosis locus to human chromosome 7cen-q22. Nature 318:384–385, 1985.
 8. Rommens JM, Iannuzzi MC, Kerem B, et al: Identification of the cystic fibrosis gene: Chromosome walking and jumping. Science 245:1059–1065, 1989.
 9. Kerem B, Rommens JM, Buchanan JA, et al: Identification of the cystic fibrosis gene: Genetic analysis. Science 245:1073–1080, 1989.
10. Riordan JR, Rommens JM, Kerem B, et al: Identification of the cystic fibrosis gene: Cloning and characterization of complementary DNA. Science 245:1066–1072, 1989.
11. Hyde SC, Emsley P, Hartshorn MJ, et al: Structural model of the

ATP-binding proteins associated with cystic fibrosis, multidrug resistance and bacterial transport. Nature 346:362–365, 1990.

12. Cystic Fibrosis Genetic Analysis Consortium: Worldwide survey of the ΔF508 mutation. Am J Hum Genet 47:354–359, 1990.

13. Brock DJH, Hayward C: Amniotic fluid arginine esterases as markers for cystic fibrosis. Lancet 1:619–620, 1982.

14. Carbarns N, Gosden C, Brock DJ: Microvillar peptidase activity in amniotic fluid: Possible use in the prenatal diagnosis of cystic fibrosis. Lancet 1:329–331, 1983.

15. Brock DJ, Bedgood D, Hayward C: Prenatal diagnosis of cystic fibrosis by assay of amniotic fluid microvillar enzyme. Hum Genet 65:248–251, 1984.

16. Brock DJ: Prenatal screening and heterozygote detection. In Lawson D (ed): Cystic Fibrosis: Horizons, pp. 1–12. Chichester, England: Wiley, 1984.

17. Beaudet A, Bowcock A, Buchwald M, et al: Linkage of cystic fibrosis of two tightly linked DNA markers: Joint report from a collaborative study. Am J Hum Genet 39:681–693, 1986.

18. Estivill X, Farrall M, Scambler PJ, et al: A candidate for the cystic fibrosis locus isolated by selection for methylation-free islands. Nature 326:840–845, 1987.

19. Southern E: Detection of specific sequences among DNA fragments separated by gel electrophoresis. J Mol Biol 98:503–517, 1975.

20. Saiki RK, Gelfand DH, Stoffel S, et al: Primer-directed enzymatic amplification of DNA with a thermostable DNA polymerase. Science 239:487–491, 1988.

21. Rosenbloom CL, Kerem BS, Romens JM et al: DNA amplification for detection of the XV-Zc polymorphism linked to cystic fibrosis. Nucleic Acids Res 17:7117, 1989.

22. Feldman GL, Williamson R, Beaudet AL, O'Brien WE: Prenatal diagnosis of cystic fibrosis by DNA amplification for detection of KM19 polymorphism. Lancet 2:102, 1988.

23. Northrup H, Rosenbloom C, O'Brien WE, Beaudet AL: Additional polymorphism for D7S8 linked to cystic fibrosis including detection by DNA amplification. Nuc Acids Res 17:1784, 1989.

24. Orita M, Suzuki Y, Sekiya T, Hayashi K: Rapid and sensitive detection of point mutations and DNA polymorphisms using the polymerase chain reaction. Genomics 5:874–879, 1989.

25. Wu DY, Ugozzoli L, Pal BK, Wallace RB: Allele-specific enzymatic amplification of β-globin genomic DNA for diagnosis of sickle cell anemia. Proc Natl Acad Sci USA 86:2757–2760, 1989.

26. Studencki AB, Conner BJ, Impraim CC, et al: Discrimination among human beta A, beta S, and beta C-globin genes using allele-specific oligonucleotide hybridization probes. Am J Hum Genet 37:42–51, 1985.

27. Horn GT, Richards B, Merrill JJ, Klinger KW: Characterization and rapid diagnostic analysis of DNA polymorphisms closely linked to the cystic fibrosis locus. Clin Chem 36:1614–1619, 1990.

28. Stanier P, Estivill X, Lench N, Williamson R: Detection of a rare-cutter RFLP in a CpG-rich island near the cystic fibrosis locus. Hum Genet 80:309–310, 1988.

29. Williams C, Williamson R, Coutelle C, et al: Same-day first-trimester antenatal diagnosis for cystic fibrosis by gene amplification. Lancet 2:102–103, 1988.

30. Huth A, Estivill X, Gradc K, et al: Polymerase chain reaction for detection of the pMP6d-9/MspI RFLP, a marker closely linked to the cystic fibrosis mutation. Nucleic Acids Res 17:7118, 1989.

31. Beaudet AL, Feldman GL, Fernbach SD, et al: Linkage disequilibrium, cystic fibrosis, and genetic counseling. Am J Hum Genet 44:319–326, 1989.

32. Lemna WK, Feldman GL, Kerem BS, et al: Mutation analysis for heterozygote detection and the prenatal diagnosis of cystic fibrosis. N Engl J Med 322:291–296, 1990.

33. Klinger K, Horn GT, Stanislovitis P: Cystic fibrosis mutations in the Hutterite brethren. Am J Hum Genet 46:983–987, 1990.

34. Wagner M, Schloesser M, Reiss J: Direct gene diagnosis of cystic fibrosis by allele-specific polymerase chain reactions. Mol Biol Med 7:359–364, 1990.

35. Tsui LC: Communication to the CF Gene Analysis Consortium, 1991.

36. Chong GL, Thibodeau SN: A simple assay for the screening of the cystic fibrosis allele in carriers of the Phe[508] deletion mutation. Mayo Clin Proc 65:1072–1076, 1990.

37. Diagnosis of cystic fibrosis in premature infants [Editorial]. Lancet 1:24–25, 1987.

38. Littlewood JM: The sweat test. Arch Dis Child 61:1041–1043, 1986.

39. ten Kate LP: Carrier screening in CF [Letter]. Nature 342:131, 1989.

40. Goodfellow P: Cystic fibrosis: Steady steps lead to the gene [Editorial]. Nature 341:102–103, 1989.

41. Gilbert F: Is population screening for cystic fibrosis appropriate now? Am J Hum Genet 46:394–395, 1990.

42. The American Society of Human Genetics statement on cystic fibrosis screening. Am J Hum Genet 46:393, 1990.

43. Workshop on Population Screening for the Cystic Fibrosis Gene: Statement from the National Institutes of Health workshop on population screening for the cystic fibrosis gene. N Engl J Med 323:70–71, 1990.

44. U.S. Congress, Office of Technology Assessment, Cystic Fibrosis and DNA tests: Implications of carrier screening, OTA-BA-532. Washington, DC: U.S. Government Printing Office, August 1992.

45. Estivill X, Chillon M, Casals T, et al: ΔF508 detection of major cystic fibrosis mutation. Lancet 2:972, 1989.

46. Novelli G, Sangiuolo F, Dallapiccola B, et al: ΔF508 gene deletion and prenatal diagnosis of cystic fibrosis in Italian and Spanish families. Prenat Diagn 10:413–414, 1990.

47. Cutting GR, Kasch LM, Rosenstein BJ, et al: Two cystic fibrosis patients with mild pulmonary disease and nonsense mutations in each CFTR gene. Am J Hum Genet 47(Suppl):A213, 1990.

48. Shoshani T, Augarten A, Gazit E, et al: Association of a nonsense mutation (W1282X), the most common mutation in the Ashkenazi Jewish cystic fibrosis patients in Israel, with presentation of severe disease. Am J Hum Genet 50:222–228, 1992.

49. Shwachman H: Gastrointestinal manifestations of cystic fibrosis. Pediatr Clin North Am 22:787–805, 1975.

50. Gaskin K, Gurwitz D, Durie P, et al: Improved respiratory prognosis in patients with cystic fibrosis with normal fat absorption. J Pediatr 100:857–862, 1982.

51. Gasparini P, Novelli G, Estivill X, et al: The genotype of a new linked DNA marker MP6d-9 is related to the clinical course of cystic fibrosis. J Med Genet 27:17–20, 1990.

52. Dean M, White MB, Amos J, et al: Multiple mutations in highly conserved residues are found in mildly affected cystic fibrosis patients. Cell 61:863–870, 1990.

53. Davies KE: Complementary endeavors [Editorial]. Nature 348:110–111, 1990.

54. Santis G, Osborne L, Knight RA, Hodson ME: Linked marker haplotypes and the ΔF508 mutation in adults with mild pulmonary disease and cystic fibrosis. Lancet 335:1426–1429, 1990.

55. Johansen HK, Nir M, Hoiby N, et al: Lack of correlation between clinical parameters and genotypes as defined by the ΔF508 in Danish cystic fibrosis patients. Pediatr Pulmonol S5:201, 1990.

56. Rich DP, Anderson MP, Gregory RJ, et al: Expression of cystic fibrosis transmembrane conductance regulator corrects defective chloride channel regulation in cystic fibrosis airway epithelial cells. Nature 347:358–363, 1990.

57. Drumm ML, Pope HA, Cliff WH, et al: Correction of the cystic fibrosis defect in vitro by retrovirus-mediated gene transfer. Cell 62:1227–1233, 1990.

58. Cheng SH, Gregory RJ, Marshall J, et al: Defective intracellular transport and processing of CFTR is the molecular basis of most cystic fibrosis. Cell 63:827–834, 1990.

59. Snouwaert JN, et al: An animal model for cystic fibrosis made by gene targeting. Science 257:1083–1088, 1992.

60. Clark LL, et al: Defective epithelial chloride transport in a gene-targeted mouse model of cystic fibrosis. Science 257:1125–1128, 1992.

61. Dorin JR, et al: Cystic fibrosis in the mouse by targeted insertional mutagenesis. Nature 359:211–215, 1992.

62. Colledge WH, et al: Cystic fibrosis mouse with intestinal obstruction. Lancet 340:680, 1992.

70 CLINICAL MANIFESTATIONS OF CYSTIC FIBROSIS

BETTINA C. HILMAN, M.D. / NORMAN J. LEWISTON, M.D.

Cystic fibrosis (CF) is a complex metabolic disorder characterized by dysfunction of the exocrine glands, including sweat glands, the pancreas, and mucous glands of the respiratory, gastrointestinal, and reproductive tracts. It is the most common lethal genetic disease in the United States among Caucasians of European ancestry. The gene for CF was first localized to the long arm (q) of chromosome 7 in 1985 by linkage analysis of DNA fragments with restriction fragment length polymorphisms.[1-4] In 1989 the CF gene was identified and cloned.[5-7] In Chapter 69, the genetic aspects of CF are discussed in detail.

The CF gene, a large gene composed of approximately 250,000 base pairs distributed among at least 24 exons, codes for a protein, cystic fibrosis transmembrane conductance regulator (CFTR), which contains 1480 amino acids.[5-7] From the analysis of the complementary DNA sequence, the CFTR is considered a membrane-bound protein; a schematic model of the CFTR protein is seen in Figure 70-1. The structure suggests a cell membrane transport function[6] consisting of a domain with membrane-spanning segments and a nucleotide-binding domain or fold (NBF). The CFTR protein is similar to the transport proteins of the P glycoprotein family. As shown in Figure 70-1, CFTR has six membrane-spanning helices in each half of the molecule connected to a cytosolic NBF. A large, highly charged domain (R domain) linking the two halves of the protein contains potential sites for phosphorylation by cyclic adenosine monophosphate (cAMP)-dependent protein kinase and protein kinase C.[6] How CFTR relates to the pathophysiologic features of CF is still unknown but is discussed further in the section on pathophysiology.

The major mutation among Caucasians from the United States and northern Europe is a three–base-pair deletion that corresponds to a single deletion of the amino acid, phenylalanine, at the ΔF508 position of the CFTR.[7-9] As of spring of 1992, approximately 200 mutations have been discovered, but most of the non-ΔF508 mutations are rare. Testing for 10 to 12 of these mutations, including the ΔF508, will detect approximately 85% to 90% of the CF mutations.[8] The ΔF508 mutation with three-point mutations (G551D, G542X, and R5553X) can be detected in 80% to 85% of CF chromosomes in non-Ashkenazic Caucasians in the United States. The ΔF508 mutation represents only 30% of the black population and of Ashkenazic Caucasians in the United States. There appears to be some correlation between particular mutations present in a given patient and the severity of the disease, although the spectrum of the severity associated with any given mutation makes it difficult to utilize this information clinically for prognostic purposes.[8]

Several investigators utilizing techniques of in situ hybridization and immunohistochemistry to detect the pattern of expression of the CFTR messenger RNA and protein in different organs have confirmed that for the most part, the tissues that express CFTR are also those in affected organ systems.[8] The CF gene is also expressed in the kidneys and uterus at fairly high levels.[8] CFTR protein has been found to be more abundant in the submucosal glands of the airways in patients with CF, in contrast to normal cells, in which the CFTR protein seems to be most abundant in the apical membrane surface of the epithelial cells of the respiratory, gastrointestinal, reproductive, and sweat glands.[8] Although there is controversy about the

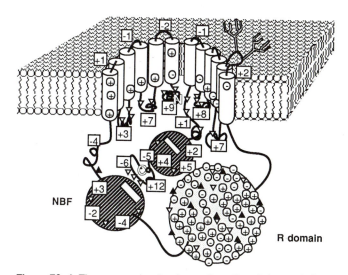

Figure 70-1. The proposed molecular configuration of the cystic fibrosis transmembrane conductance regulator. NBF, nucleotide binding fold. (From Riordan JR, Rommens JM, Kerem BS, et al: Identification of the cystic fibrosis gene: Chromosome walking and jumping. Science 245:1066-1073, 1989.)

location of the ΔF508 mutant protein, in some tissues and in many cutured cells, the ΔF508 CFTR seems to be improperly processed, remaining trapped within the cell cytoplasm and becoming degraded before reaching its destination.[8] It is hypothesized that the ΔF508 mutation results in a failure of the CFTR to mature; glycosylation and subsequent movement to the cell membrane do not occur, and the protein remains trapped in the endoplasmic reticulum or the Golgi apparatus.[10] The significance of these results suggests that even if a modest amount of the mutant protein is present in the proper location, drug therapies designed to stimulate it to function might be effective therapeutically.[8] In contrast, if only very small amounts of the mutant protein are present, other mechanisms of therapy would be needed to bypass this altered CFTR.[8]

Because of the multisystem involvement, CF can masquerade as other disorders. The spectrum of clinical manifestations in CF is broad because of the extent and severity of involvement of the various organ systems, the type of gene mutation, and the age at clinical manifestation. Since the early 1940s, when CF was recognized as a distinct clinical syndrome, therapeutic management, prognosis, and basic understanding of this challenging disorder have continued to change. As a result of improved diagnosis (including recognition of milder forms of CF) and improved treatment, the median life expectancy of patients with CF, according to data in the CF Foundation patient registry, is 29.4 years. In patients surviving the neonatal period, the predominant cause of morbidity and major cause of mortality is chronic progressive bronchopulmonary disease.

PATHOPHYSIOLOGY

Investigative efforts into the basic cellular pathophysiology in CF demonstrated altered ion transport in exocrine epithelial tissues with impairment of conductance of chloride ions and reduced permeability of apical epithelia to chloride.[11-14] The major defect in CF is thought to be in the intracellular pathways for the regulation of the chloride channel or in the structure of the channel itself.

Research studies have revealed that the CFTR is a chloride channel and that it is activated by a combination of phosphorylation by protein kinase A and binding of ATP, and under those conditions, CFTR can allow the passage of chloride through the membrane.[8] A number of other functions of CFTR have also been identified, including a role in intracellular acidification, the transport of intracellular vesicles, and possibly even transport of ATP itself.[8]

The genetic defect results in a disturbance in the movement of other ions and water across cellular membranes. The flow of water across epithelial membranes occurs in response to an osmotic gradient resulting from the active transport of sodium and chloride. CF tissues show alteration in the hydration of the periciliary fluid of respiratory mucus. In the sweat gland ducts, the epithelium is chloride impermeable, which causes the salt concentration of sweat to be increased. Like the sweat glands, the airway epithelia are relatively impermeable to chloride and dem-

onstrate an abnormally high sodium absorption. It is not certain whether the increased rate of Na^{++} absorption in airway epithelia is a direct result of altered regulation by CFTR or an indirect consequence of the reduced chloride permeability.

NEONATAL SCREENING

Until the recognition of immunoreactive trypsin (IRT), there was no valid test for screening newborns for CF that could easily be incorporated into existing metabolic screening programs for newborns. IRT has been found to be elevated in the blood of newborns with CF, presumably because of a secretory obstructive effect on the pancreas.[15] The IRT assay has 99% sensitivity and a false-positive rate of only 0.2% to 0.5% and appears to identify even CF patients whose pancreatic function is grossly intact.[16] Screening for CF through the use of IRT can be performed on dried blood spots and can be easily incorporated into current metabolic screening programs for newborns. There is still some reluctance to participate in widespread neonatal screening for CF in the general population because making the presumptive diagnosis in an asymptomatic infant would cause considerable anxiety for the family.

DIAGNOSIS

Clinical findings on presentation vary with age, the type of genetic mutations, the involvement of the various organ systems, and the presence and type of complications.

The more characteristic clinical findings include

1. Quantitative abnormalities of electrolytes in eccrine sweat glands with elevated sweat electrolytes (sodium, chloride, and potassium).

2. Pancreatic exocrine insufficiency.

3. Chronic and recurrent sinobronchial and bronchopulmonary infection, which result in chronic progressive bronchopulmonary disease and irreversible lung damage.

4. Focal biliary cirrhosis or multilobular biliary cirrhosis (Fig. 70–2).

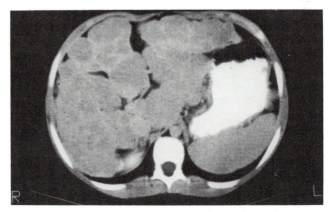

Figure 70–2. Computed tomographic scan of the abdomen demonstrating alternating areas of high and low attenuation of the liver suggestive of nodular biliary cirrhosis in a 9-year-old white girl with cystic fibrosis. The computed tomographic scan of the liver suggestive of nodular cirrhosis was later confirmed by liver biopsy.

5. Intestinal abnormalities, including intestinal obstruction of the newborn (meconium ileus), fecal impaction, and intussusception.

A high index of suspicion is the first requirement in the diagnosis of this complex and clinically variable syndrome. The age at manifestation varies from birth to adulthood. Approximately 10% to 15% of infants with CF have intestinal obstruction resulting from meconium ileus at birth, often complicated by intestinal atresia, volvulus, or perforation. If in utero perforation has occurred, meconium peritonitis may result, with intraperitoneal calcifications or pseudocyst formation. Septic peritonitis may be present at birth. Infants with meconium ileus exhibit abdominal distention, failure to pass meconium, and vomiting within the first 24 to 48 h of life. Abdominal radiographs show gastric distention with distended loops of small intestine, often with the characteristic "soap bubble" appearance as a result of air trapping in the meconium.[17] Air-fluid levels may not always be present on the abdominal films when the meconium is hyperviscid. Meglumine diatrizoate (Gastrografin) enema can demonstrate the microcolon and may help relieve the intestinal obstruction by drawing fluid into the lumen of the intestine.[18] Abnormalities in intestinal mucous gland secretions contribute to the underlying pathophysiologic processes of meconium ileus, and pancreatic insufficiency is not a prerequisite. A number of biochemical alterations of the small intestine have been described, including chloride impermeability of the epithelial membranes, alterations of the brush-border enzymes, transport defects,

increased permeability, and impaired secretions of some gut hormones.[19] In the intestine, in contrast to the sweat glands and airways, membrane chloride impermeability appears not to be increased by Ca^{++}-mediated pathways.[20]

Tables 70–1, 70–2, and 70–3 outline the respiratory, gastrointestinal, hepatobiliary, and urogenital manifestations in CF.

The most reliable diagnostic test for CF is the quantitative analysis of sweat electrolytes after collection of sweat by the pilocarpine iontophoresis method of Gibson and Cooke[21] (Table 70–4). When the sweat test is improperly performed, it may lead to false-positive and false-negative interpretations. A sufficient quantity of sweat (at least 50 mg and preferably 75 to 100 mg) is needed for the accurate quantitative analysis of sodium and chloride. No

Table 70–1. RESPIRATORY MANIFESTATIONS IN CYSTIC FIBROSIS

Upper Respiratory Tract
Recurrent otitis media
Pansinusitis
Nasal polyps

Lower Respiratory Tract
Chronic cough
(early: dry, hacking; later: productive)
  Mucoid → Purulent
  May be paroxysmal → Vomiting

Recurrent Respiratory Infections
Bronchiolitis (sequelae: bronchiolectasis, bronchiolitis obliterans)
Bronchitis (sequela: bronchiectasis)
Pneumonitis (alveolitis or interstitial) (sequelae: chronic interstitial lung disease, fibrosis, honeycomb lung disease on chest radiograph at end stage)

Complications of Chronic Lung Disease
Atelectasis
Mucoid impaction
Alteration of growth (poor weight gain or weight loss)
Increase in anteroposterior diameter of "barrel" chest
Scoliosis, kyphosis
Clubbing of digits
Hypertrophic pulmonary osteoarthropathy
Pneumothorax
Hemoptysis
Allergic bronchopulmonary aspergillosis
Dyspnea on exertion; decrease in exercise tolerance
Hypoxemia, pulmonary hypertension leading to cor pulmonale leading to cardiorespiratory failure
Respiratory failure
Death

Table 70–2. GASTROINTESTINAL AND HEPATOBILIARY MANIFESTATIONS OF CYSTIC FIBROSIS

Intestinal Involvement
Intestinal obstruction
Newborn: meconium ileus may be associated with meconium peritonitis, intestinal atresia, or volvulus
Older patients: fecal impaction
Intussusception: Ileocecal area is common site
Edema of duodenal mucosa with thickened mucosal folds on upper GI series

Pancreatic Involvement
Pancreatic Exocrine Insufficiency
Maldigestion of fats, proteins, carbohydrates, and fat soluble vitamins leading to steatorrhea, and increased fecal nitrogen loss
Abnormal stools (poorly formed, large, bulky, foul-smelling, greasy, floating stools)
Rectal prolapse
Failure to thrive with voracious appetite
Hypoproteinemia/edema
Abdominal distention
Flatulence or foul-smelling flatus
Recurrent abdominal pain
Recurrent pancreatitis
Vitamin A deficiency (dry skin)
Vitamin K deficiency (hypoprothrombinemia)
Vitamin B complex (e.g., cheilosis)
Pancreatic Islet Dysfunction
Glucose intolerance, chemical or clinical diabetes mellitus
Incidence increases with age
Decreased production of glucagon; lower glucagon fasting level
Ketosis less frequent
Usually low insulin requirements

Hepatobiliary Involvement
Cirrhosis (focal biliary cirrhosis, multilobular cirrhosis; complications: portal hypertension, splenomegaly, hypersplenism, esophageal varices leading to GI bleeding)
Fatty liver (steatosis)
  Ascites
  Hepatic failure
Gallbladder
  Cholecystitis
  Nonvisualizing or "microgallbladder"
  Cholelithiasis (usually associated with clinical pancreatic exocrine insufficiency; incidence increases with age)

Salivary Gland Involvement
Altered physiochemical secretions
Submandibular gland hypertrophy
Recurrent parotid swelling

GI, gastrointestinal.

Table 70-3. UROGENITAL MANIFESTATIONS IN CYSTIC FIBROSIS

Males	Females
Frequently sterile (defective development of Wolffian duct system)	Decrease in fertility (in some)
Vas deferens absent or abnormal (blind endings of vasa efferentia)	Increase in viscosity of cervical mucus
Epididymis atropic or absent	Increase in dry weight of cervical mucus
Abnormalities of seminal fluid	No midcycle increase in water or sodium (absence of "ferning")
Increase in citric acid	Increase in endocervical polyps
Increase in acid phosphatase (acid pH)	Secondary sexual development (breast development and onset of menarche may be delayed depending on severity of disease)
Decrease in fructose	
Decrease in volume	
Increase in turbidity	
Increase in concentration of potassium, zinc, magnesium, and calcium	Secondary amenorrhea, varies with severity of disease*
Testes normal	
Spermatogenesis normal	
Sexual development normal or delayed depending on severity	
Sexual behavior not altered	
Increased incidence of inguinal hernia	
Increased incidence of hydrocele	
Increased incidence of undescended testicles	

*May or may not be seen with severe disease.

single criterion is sufficient for confirming the diagnosis of CF; however, a sweat chloride of >60 mEq/l in children and adolescents is consistent with the diagnosis. The diagnosis of CF requires interpretation of information drawn from history, physical examination, and consistent laboratory results.

Stern and associates[22] proposed a new system of diagnostic criteria for CF; obstructive azoospermia (absence of sperm in semen with normal spermatogenesis on testicular biopsy) is included as a major criterion, and unexplained azoospermia on semen analysis is included only as a minor criterion. Other major criteria are positive quantitative sweat electrolytes and chronic obstructive pulmonary disease (COPD) with *Pseudomonas* infection of the airways. Minor criteria include positive family history for CF, unexplained COPD before the age of 20 years, and borderline-positive sweat electrolytes. The authors suggested that the presence of two major or one major and one minor criteria establishes the diagnosis of CF, if the two criteria involve different organ systems.[22]

Because chronic progressive bronchopulmonary disease is eventually seen in almost all CF patients and is the most common cause of recurrent illnesses, the major focus of management in CF is directed toward the treatment of the respiratory involvement and its complications. Table 70-5 outlines the nonpulmonary problems and plan for management.

Table 70-4. SWEAT ELECTROLYTE ANALYSIS IN CYSTIC FIBROSIS

Recommendations for Diagnostic Sweat Test
1. Stimulate sweating in local sweat glands in two or more different sites on the forearm: pilocarpine iontophoresis (Gibson and Cooke method[21]); Use cotton gauze free of sodium and chloride to absorb sweat
2. Analyze only adequate samples of sweat (above 50 mg and preferably 75–100 mg)
3. Minimum of two separate samples of sweat for analysis
4. Quantitative analysis of electrolytes
    Sodium and potassium by flame photometry
    Chloride titration techniques, electrometric method by Cotlove chloridometer or chemical (e.g., Schales and Schales method)
5. Electrolyte analysis in laboratory frequently performing these studies with regular quality control for accuracy of collection and analytic techniques

Causes of False-Positive Sweat Tests
1. Laboratory errors
    Contamination in collection
    Error in dilution or other technical errors
2. Conditions that may be associated with elevated electrolytes
    Untreated adrenal insufficiency
    Autonomic dysfunction
    Ectodermal dysplasia
    Glucose 6-phosphatase deficiency
    Hypothyroidism
    Malnutrition
    Mucopolysaccharidosis
    Glycogen storage disease (type I)
    Fucosidosis
    Hereditary nephrogenic diabetes insipidus
    Mauriac syndrome
    Pseudohypoaldosteronism
    Familial cholestasis

Factors Influencing Concentration of Electrolytes in Sweat
1. Sample size
2. Age
3. Clinical status (dehydration, edema, circulatory failure, respiratory distress, malnutrition)
4. Local conditions
    Exhaustion of glands by repeated stimulation of same area and humidity
    Drugs applied topically to induce sweating
    Area of body where sweat is collected
    Duration of sweat-collection period
5. Diet, especially salt intake
6. Time of day and season of year
7. Individual differences

RESPIRATORY DISEASE AND ITS COMPLICATIONS

The spectrum of respiratory manifestations and complications in CF is outlined in Table 70-1. There is wide intersubject variability in the age at onset, the extent of respiratory involvement, the severity of dysfunction, the type of complications, and the rate of progression of clinical and laboratory findings. With time, respiratory involvement occurs in all patients. The clinical course is characterized by progressive chronic pulmonary disease, with recurrent acute exacerbations and varying periods of stabilization.

Cough is one of the initial clinical findings in CF; the cough may initially be dry, hacking, and nonproductive and can be mistaken for a symptom of allergic respiratory

Table 70–5. NONPULMONARY PROBLEMS AND PLAN FOR TREATMENT IN CYSTIC FIBROSIS

Problem	Plan
Eccrine Sweat Gland Involvement	
Electrolytes (sodium, chloride, and potassium) elevated in 98%–99% of patients	Prompt recognition: replacement of electrolyte losses
Heat prostration or salt-depletion syndrome possible during febrile episodes or in elevated environmental temperatures	Prevention: supplemental salt and potassium during hot weather; avoid excessive temperatures
Pancreatic Involvement	
Exocrine insufficiency; variable symptoms of abnormal (frequent, poorly formed, bulky, or greasy) stools, flatulence/foul-smelling flatus, and abdominal distention	Supplemental pancreatic enzymes before meals and snacks to control stools, achieve satisfactory weight gain; supplemental vitamins (vitamins K and E, and multiple vitamins); high caloric diet with increased protein; hospitalization usually required for acute episodes
Weight usually below height percentile; degree of pulmonary disease primary determinant of weight	
May have recurrent pancreatitis	
Glucose intolerance and chemical/clinical diabetes mellitus	Dietary limitation of the free sugars; supplemental insulin in some cases
Intestinal Involvement	
Fecal impaction common	Regulation of stools by encouraging pancreatic enzyme compliance; n-acetylcysteine in cola by mouth may be of benefit; iso-osmotic solutions containing polyethylene glycol and electrolytes, similar to those used for bowel cleansing before colonoscopy
Intussusception	Reduction by meglumine diatrizoate (Gastrografin) enema
Gastroesophageal reflux with or without symptoms of esophagitis	Positioning at night; antacids, cimetidine, or ranitidine; metoclopramide hydrochloride
Hepatobiliary Involvement	
Focal biliary cirrhosis usually not associated with clinical findings	Intermittent sclerotherapy of varices; use of shunts if massive recurrent bleeding from varices; avoid salicylates; liver transplantation
Multilobular biliary cirrhosis complications of portal hypertension, esophageal varices, gastrointestinal bleeding and hypersplenism, ascites and hepatic failure	
Gallbladder Involvement	
Gallbladder abnormalities (small or hypoplastic)	Compliance with pancreatic enzymes; avoid excess fat in diet; may require surgical removal of calculi; may require cholescystectomy
Cholecystitis, cholelithiasis	
Urogenital Involvement	
Secondary sex characteristics possibly delayed	Improve nutritional status
Secondary amenorrhea possibly present in the more severely involved	
Increased viscosity and dry weight of cervical mucus in females	
Sterility in most males because of developmental failure of wolffian duct derivatives	

disease. With intercurrent or chronic infection and destructive changes in the airways, cough becomes productive of sputum. Clinical findings suggestive of acute respiratory infection or an exacerbation of chronic endobronchial infection are increased cough (with or without fever); increased production of sputum, change in color or the amount of sputum, or both; decreased appetite; decreased exercise tolerance; and weight loss or failure to gain expected weight. When the endobronchial infection is controlled and the secretions obstructing the airways are removed, the respiratory symptoms subside or improve. Persistence of respiratory symptoms is related to the residual airway obstruction and irreversible airway and lung damage.

Hyperinflation and patchy atelectasis on the chest radiograph are often the earliest manifestations of obstruction of the small airways from increased secretions and mucus plugging. Obstruction of the larger airways as a result of mucoid impaction of dilated bronchi is often seen on plain chest radiographs; however, the extensive dilatation of subsegmental bronchi (bronchiectasis) and

the mucoid impaction are best depicted on selected chest tomograms (Fig. 70–3) or computed tomography of the chest. Brasfield and colleagues proposed a scoring system for evaluating chest radiographs in CF based on five categories: air trapping, linear markings resulting from thickening of bronchial walls, nodular cystic lesions, large lesions (such as segmental or lobar atelectasis), and overall severity.[23]

Pulmonary function studies that reflect small-airway dysfunction are the first to show abnormalities in patients with CF. As pulmonary involvement progresses in CF, abnormalities in pulmonary function studies reflect the obstruction of larger airways with an increase in airway resistance and a decrease in forced expiratory volume in 1 sec (FEV_1) and peak expiratory flow rates. Loss of elastic recoil and air trapping in CF result in elevation of residual volume (RV), functional residual capacity (FRC), and RV/TLC ratio. Vital capacity (VC) is reduced in CF because of the restrictive component of the lung disease; however, the total lung capacity (TLC) may be normal because of the increase in RV. Pulmonary function stud-

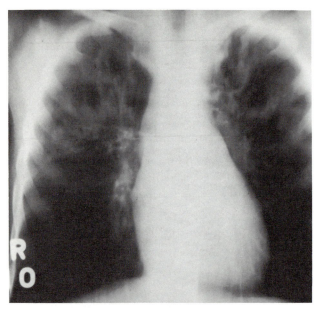

Figure 70-3. Tomogram of the chest of a 10-year-old white boy with cystic fibrosis with extensive dilation of subsegmental bronchi (bronchiectasis) and mucoid impaction.

ies also provide objective documentation of improvement in obstructive lung disease in patients with CF during and after hospitalization for acute exacerbations of the chronic pulmonary disease. The rate and magnitude of improvement in pulmonary function among patients with CF vary, depending on the severity of the exacerbation and the underlying pulmonary disease at the time of hospital admission. The pulmonary functions that most closely reflected clinical improvement in hospitalized patients with CF reported by Redding and co-workers were VC, RV/TLC, and FEV_1; these lung functions were the first to improve in relation to pulmonary functions.[24] Although volume-adjusted expiratory flow rates, such as maximal flow at 25% of VC ($\dot{V}_{max25\%VC}$) and forced expiratory flow between 25% and 75% of VC ($FEF_{25\%-75\%}$), are sensitive indicators of early pulmonary function abnormalities in CF, these studies were too variable to be used in serially monitoring lung function in CF patients with moderate or severe lung disease during hospitalization.

DIGITAL CLUBBING

Digital clubbing, an enlargement of the soft tissue at the distal end of the digit (Fig. 70–4), is often seen in patients with CF and is related to the chronic lung disease or to the liver disease. The exact cause of the clubbing is not known; however, the progression of clubbing in CF appears to parallel the progression of destructive lung disease. The documentation of the presence and quantification of severity of digital clubbing is facilitated by a method of measuring casts of the index finger proposed by Waring and co-authors.[25] Digital clubbing may be seen alone or in association with hypertrophic pulmonary osteoarthropathy syndrome (tenderness and pain over the distal long bones with periosteal elevation on radiograph with or without effusions in the adjacent joints).

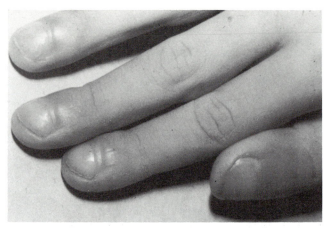

Figure 70-4. Digital clubbing in a 12-year-old patient with cystic fibrosis.

NASAL POLYPS, RHINOSINUSITIS

Nasal polyps occur in approximately 10% of younger CF patients and in up to 40% of the older CF patients. Nasal polyps tend to be multiple and may block nasal passages, requiring removal (Fig. 70–5); there is a tendency for the nasal polyps to recur after resection. Radiographic abnormalities of the sinuses have been found in CF patients of all ages, over 90% among adult patients; the most common abnormality is chronic pansinusitis.

SERIOUS RESPIRATORY COMPLICATIONS

The incidence and severity of respiratory complications in patients with CF vary among individuals and with age. Serious respiratory complications that have a significant impact on morbidity in CF are hemoptysis, pneumothorax, cor pulmonale, and respiratory failure. Hemoptysis results from the erosion of enlarged, tortuous, thin-walled bronchial vessels that develop in response to the increased vascularity of the peribronchial

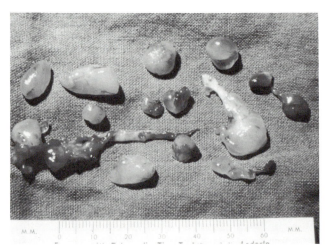

Figure 70-5. Multiple nasal polyps removed from a 13-year-old white boy with cystic fibrosis. Patient had had three previous nasal polypectomies.

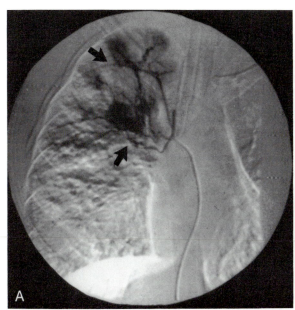
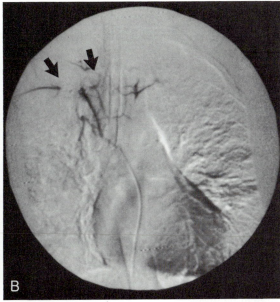

Figure 70–6. *A,* Bronchial arteriography via femoral artery by digital substractive angiography (DSA) technique demonstrating a bleeding site in the right upper lobe of a bronchial artery in a 9-year-old white girl with hemoptysis and bronchiectasis secondary to cystic fibrosis. *B,* Bronchial arteriography, DSA technique, postbronchial artery embolization with absorbable gelatin sponge (Gelfoam) in a 9-year-old white girl with CF and hemoptysis.

tissue from chronic inflammation of the airways. The bronchial arteries form bronchopulmonary arterial anastomoses. Bronchial arteriography can demonstrate the enlarged, tortuous bronchial vessels, which are direct shunts between the bronchial and pulmonary circulation. The extravasation of contrast during bronchial arteriography can help localize the bleeding site if performed during an episode of major bleeding (Fig. 70–6*A*).

For the majority of patients with CF, hemoptysis occurs as intermittent episodes of minor bleeding or only blood-streaked mucus. Continued hemoptysis of more significant amounts if often associated with an exacerbation of bronchopulmonary infection. These episodes usually subside after treatment with intensive, appropriate intravenous antibiotic therapy. In a small percentage of CF patients, massive or life-threatening bleeding from enlarged arteries can occur. Bronchial artery embolization with an absorbable gelatin sponge (Gelfoam) may be necessary for controlling the episodes of massive bleeding (Fig. 70–6*B*). Hemoptysis may resolve in the majority of cases after bronchial embolization.[26] When episodes of massive hemoptysis cannot be controlled or recur, lobar resection may be necessary in some patients with CF.

Spontaneous pneumothorax (Fig. 70–7) occurs most often with moderate or severe pulmonary involvement; recurrences are common on the same or opposite side and may be bilateral. Apical blebs and bullae are frequently seen on chest radiograph before a pneumothorax develops. A pneumothorax results from the rupture of subpleural blebs into the pleural space; the size of the pneumothorax depends on the amount of air escaping through the ruptured pleura. If a ball-valve mechanism occurs at the point of communication and the air entering the pleural space cannot escape, pressure within the pneumothorax may exceed the atmospheric pressure and cause a tension pneumothorax.

The most common presenting symptoms of a patient with a pneumothorax are chest pain and dyspnea; the pain is sharp and "pulling" and is aggravated by deep breathing. Severe dyspnea and cyanosis of abrupt onset suggest the presence of a tension pneumothorax. Decreased breath sounds and vocal fremitus, tachypnea,

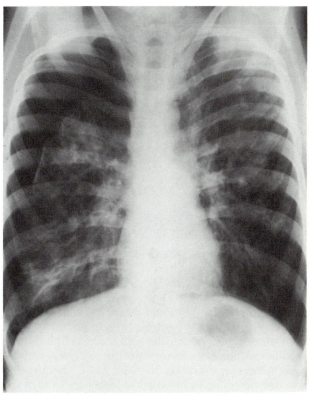

Figure 70–7. Radiograph of spontaneous pneumothorax in a 9-year-old white boy.

labored breathing, cyanosis, neck vein distention, and pleural friction rub are physical findings that may be associated with a pneumothorax. Mediastinal or tracheal shift away from the side of the pneumothorax is a sign of significant lung collapse. With a tension pneumothorax, signs of severe impairment of ventilatory capacity and circulatory collapse may be seen. The development of a tension pneumothorax requires immediate insertion of a chest tube to expand the collapsed lung and establish normal ventilation.

A small pneumothorax may be asymptomatic and discovered only on chest radiograph; however, the patient should be observed in the hospital until complete resolution. Larger pneumothoraces require closed-chest tube thoracostomy. To prevent recurrences, sclerosing agents can be instilled into the pleural space to produce chemical pleurodesis; open thoracotomy can be performed with surgical pleurodesis and oversewing of the visible blebs; or partial pleurectomy can be performed. Concerns about future candidacy for lung transplantation have favored limited surgical pleurodesis.

There are problems in the early detection and management of cor pulmonale (pulmonary hypertension with right ventricular hypertrophy [RVH]) in patients with CF. The clinical diagnosis of cor pulmonale is made on the basis of physical findings related to cardiac enlargement or cardiac failure that results from chronic pulmonary hypertension. Reliance on clinical criteria alone results in late diagnosis. The mechanism of pulmonary hypertension in cor pulmonale is related to hypoxemia and reactive pulmonary vasoconstriction as well as the anatomic alteration in pulmonary vascular architecture.[27] Cardiac functions detectable by various laboratory tests can be used to define cor pulmonale; however, there are limitations of functional criteria to establish the diagnosis because cardiac function varies with time. The standard scalar electrocardiogram may be normal in cor pulmonale. The following functional tests are used in the assessment of cor pulmonale:

1. Chest radiograph for cardiac enlargement.
2. Cardiac catheterization for pulmonary arterial, right ventricular, and right atrial pressures.
3. Angiography for chamber size, volume measurements, ejection calculations, and arterial oxygen saturation.
4. Echocardiography for systolic time interval measurements.
5. Radionuclide angiography for ejection fraction calculations to detect ventricular dysfunction.

The laboratory tests used for the demonstration of RVH are late manifestations of pulmonary hypertension and cor pulmonale. Because of the marked pulmonary hyperinflation in patients with CF, there is difficulty in visualization of the pulmonary valve on which some of the M-mode echocardiographic measurements of RVH rely. Pulmonary hypertension with increased pulmonary vascular resistance can result from contraction of vascular smooth muscle, decreases in pulmonary vessel caliber secondary to changing mechanical forces, and loss of vascular structures. With chronic pulmonary vasoconstriction, both reversible (early) muscular and irreversible

(late) intimal changes in pulmonary arteries and veins develop. Because hypoxemia plays a role in the development of pulmonary hypertension, supplemental oxygen (at the lowest flow rate to maintain an oxygen pressure/tension above 60 mm Hg) is used in the management of CF patients with advanced pulmonary disease. Nocturnal hypoxemia may be an early sign of advancing pulmonary disease, and supplemental low-flow oxygen at night is usually recommended for maintaining oxygen saturation above 90%.[28]

MANAGEMENT

Because of the complexity of the respiratory involvement and its complications, comprehensive management of CF patients requires the expertise of physicians and other health care professionals from a variety of disciplines. Table 70–6 lists the respiratory problems in CF and their management plans. Treatment should be individualized, and the severity and extent of respiratory involvement, the types of complications, and degree of expected compliance by the patient with therapeutic recommendations should be taken into consideration. Treatment can be divided into several categories:

1. Treatment of acute respiratory illnesses and acute exacerbations of chronic bronchopulmonary disease.
2. Treatment of complications of respiratory involvement.
3. Prophylactic/stabilization measures (e.g., segmental bronchial drainage [Figs. 70–8A, 70–8B] and chest physical therapy; influenza vaccine immunization annually).
4. Generalized supportive treatment (e.g., nutritional to provide adequate calories to support growth and increased work of breathing secondary to pulmonary disease and compensation for losses secondary to the maldigestion resulting from pancreatic exocrine insufficiency; education of patient and family about the disease and its treatment; genetic counseling; educational/vocational counseling; psychosocial counseling and supportive services to promote the development of competent coping skills).

Aggressive treatment of bronchopulmonary infections is an essential part of the comprehensive treatment of CF. Prompt recognition and treatment of acute respiratory infections with appropriate antibiotics are important in minimizing destructive changes in the airways, interstitium, and lung parenchyma. The treatment or control of respiratory staphylococcal infections is usually successful because of the availability of a wide spectrum of highly effective antibiotics, many of which can be taken orally for long periods of time. The treatment of respiratory infections resulting from *Pseudomonas* organisms such as *Pseudomonas aeruginosa* poses many difficulties: (1) the persistence of *Pseudomonas* organisms even after aggressive treatment with drugs with *in vitro* sensitivity, (2) the necessity for higher doses of aminoglycosides to maintain therapeutic blood levels in patients with CF, (3) the potential renal and otovestibular toxicity of aminoglycosides and the need for frequent monitoring of blood levels to

Table 70–6. RESPIRATORY PROBLEMS AND PLAN FOR MANAGEMENT IN PATIENTS WITH CYSTIC FIBROSIS

Problem	Plan
Pansinusitis (present radiographically in most patients); degree of symptoms varies	Antibiotics for acute episodes of sinusitis
Nasal polyps with varying degrees of obstruction	Removal with obstruction and recurrent infections
Chronic recurrent bronchopulmonary infections (cough, increased sputum, clubbing of fingers)	Segmented bronchial drainage; chest physical therapy; appropriate antibiotic therapy for microorganisms and severity of infection
Atelectasis	Intensive segmental bronchial drainage, chest physical therapy, and appropriate antibiotics; bronchoscopy role controversial
Hemoptysis	Treatment of associated infection; supplemental vitamin K; bronchial embolization for massive bleeding; resection may be necessary for massive continued bleeding; discontinuation of N-acetyl-cysteine aerosol and chest physical therapy over involved area until bleeding ceases; avoid aspirin
Hyperreactive airway disease	Aerosol bronchodilators (caution: bronchodilators may increase airway collapse and reduce efficacy of cough in some patients)
Pneumothorax (chest pain, aggravated by deep breathing, dyspnea, or cyanosis; may be asymptomatic, detected only on chest radiograph)	Recognition: careful observation if small (less than 10%–15%); chest tube for large pneumothorax; prevention of recurrence; avoid intermittent positive-pressure breathing
Pulmonary hypertension/cor pulmonale; may be associated with evidence of fluid retention, enlarged tender liver, dyspnea, and orthopnea	Prevention: supplement low-flow oxygen to correct nocturnal hypoxemia; continuous oxygen to alleviate chronic hypoxemia without suppressing ventilatory drive; diuretics as needed; benefit of digitalis controversial
Hypertrophic pulmonary osteoarthropathy; may be associated with pain, tenderness, swelling, and effusion of joints; pain worse with exercise and cold weather	No specific treatment; nonsteroidal anti-inflammatory agents may be beneficial
Respiratory failure	Hospitalization for acute episode, improvement in "pulmonary toilet," and intensive intravenous antibiotic therapy of bronchopulmonary infection; use of assisted ventilation should be individualized

adjust dosage, (4) the increased clearance of penicillins, especially those with antipseudomonal activity, (5) the development of resistant organisms, and (6) the necessity of parenteral administration of antipseudomonal antibiotics (with the exception of ciprofloxacin, a quinolone antibiotic).

For the treatment of acute respiratory infections, antibiotics should be appropriate for the suspected pathogens. The use of segmental bronchial drainage, chest physical therapy, and inhalation therapy at the time of acute exacerbations is an important aspect of treatment to decrease airway obstruction. The type of aerosol medications that should be used is controversial but usually includes a bronchodilator with or without the mucolytic agent N-acetyl-cysteine. Delivery of aerosolized aminoglycosides to lower respiratory tract infection by inhalation is a way to achieve high antibiotic concentration at the site of infection. Smith and colleagues demonstrated the safety and efficacy of tobramycin aerosol delivered by ultrasonic nebulizer (DeVilbiss Ultraneb 99/100) in minimizing the gradual decay in pulmonary function in patients with CF.[29, 30]

Several investigational studies and clinical experiences provide evidence that antimicrobial therapy for *P. aeruginosa* at the time of exacerbations of chronic endobronchial infection is beneficial in reducing the morbidity and improving pulmonary functions of patients with CF. The optimal antibiotic regimen for the treatment of the exacerbations of the endobronchial infections in CF remains controversial. Although results of some investigations

support the efficacy of intravenous single-drug therapy with an antipseudomonal penicillin or ceftazidime, a third-generation cephalosporin, results of other studies show the need for a combined drug regimen to cover the various strains of *P. aeruginosa* and to reduce the development of drug resistance. An antipseudomonal penicillin or ceftazidime in combination with an aminoglycoside is the most frequently used intravenous antibiotic treatment for the exacerbations of endobronchial infections in CF. The interpretation of clinical trials that address short-term efficacy may be misleading as supporting evidence of a particular antibiotic regimen for the treatment of the exacerbations of bronchopulmonary infections. Before choosing specific antibiotics for the treatment of endobronchial infections, the clinician should consider the duration and cost of therapy, the incidence of adverse reactions, and the likelihood of the development of resistant organisms. The duration of the intravenous antipseudomonal antibiotics varies because of the severity of the underlying lung disease, the individual differences in the time required for improvement in the clinical and laboratory parameters, the ability to maintain venous access, the degree of compliance with length of therapy by patient and parents, and the availability of cost reimbursement or coverage for drug treatment. Beta-lactam antibiotics vary in frequency of hypersensitivity and other adverse reactions.

With the rising costs of hospitalization for intravenous antibiotics, medical care providers have been forced to use alternative methods of delivering effective antipseu-

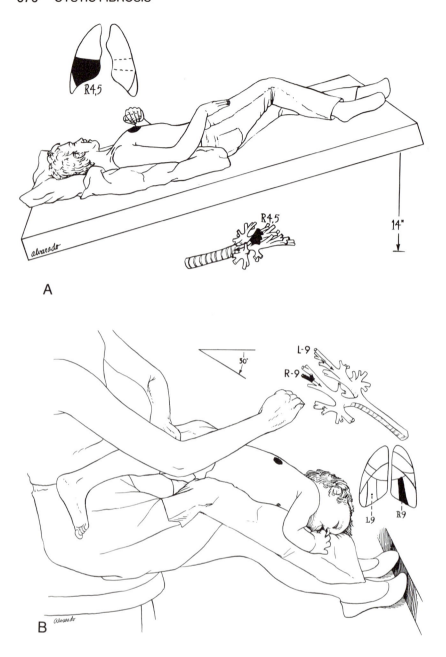

A

B

Figure 70–8. *A*, A position for segmental bronchial drainage of the right middle lobe. The patient lies head down on the left side and is rotated 45 degrees backwards. The therapist or the older patient claps over the right nipple. The area for clapping of the right middle lobe, R4-R5, is shown in the diagram. *B*, Positioning for drainage of the lateral basal segment of the right lower lobe in an infant. The infant is placed over the extended legs of the therapist in a head-down position toward the left side. A pillow may be used over the therapist's legs. The therapist claps over the uppermost portion of the lower ribs. The area for clapping of the right lateral basal segment, R9, is shown in the diagram. To drain the left lateral basal segment, L9, the infant should be rotated upward from a prone position toward the right side in the same head-down postion, and the therapist should clap over the left side of the chest.

domonal therapy. One alternative is home intravenous antibiotic therapy directed toward *Pseudomonas* organisms. Current pharmacokinetic data suggest that the antipseudomonal penicillins should optimally be given every 4 h. This dosing frequency is not practical for home intravenous antibiotic use. One advantage of ceftazidime over the antipseudomonal penicillins is the less frequent dosing interval (every 8 h, in comparison with every 4 h), which is an advantage for home intravenous antibiotic therapy.

With frequent exacerbations of endobronchial infection, patients with CF are at increased risk of the development of hypersensitivity or other adverse drug reactions and of drug resistance to β-lactam antibiotics and aminoglycosides. *P. aeruginosa* has at least three mechanisms for acquiring drug resistance: acquisition of plas-

mid DNA that encodes β-lactamase and the production of aminoglycoside-modifying enzymes, the production of a chromosomal β-lactamase that is inducible and can emerge rapidly after contact with certain β-lactam compounds, and regulation of genes to change its lipopolysaccharides and enzymes.

Until the availability of ciprofloxacin, there was no alternative to IV antipseudomonal antibiotics for the treatment of exacerbations of endobronchial infection resulting from *P. aeruginosa*. Ciprofloxacin also is effective against *Haemophilus influenzae* and *S. aureus*. Although ciprofloxacin is a highly effective drug and an alternative to parenteral antipseudomonal therapy in some older CF patients (over 18 years of age), its effectiveness often decreases with repeated use. At present, the duration of ciprofloxacin therapy should be limited to 4 weeks, although repeated courses may be appropriate in patients with advanced disease and strains of *P. aeruginosa* resistant to the β-lactams and aminoglycosides. There are no data from which to judge the usefulness of ciprofloxacin as a prophylactic agent (or as a continuous therapy) in CF patients with stable bronchopulmonary disease or mild exacerbations. Pharmacologic interactions of ciprofloxacin can occur with theophylline and other drugs. There have been few clinical trials with ciprofloxacin in younger patients because the fluoroquinolones are toxic to proliferating cartilage in experimental animals.

Colonization and infection with *Pseudomonas cepacia* are among the most challenging problems in the management of patients with CF.[31] *P. cepacia,* a plant pathogen that causes opportunistic infection in CF patients, is an aerobic, nonfermenting, nonglucose oxidizing, gram-negative bacteria. The association of *P. cepacia* with the pulmonary disease in CF was first noted during a study of aminoglycoside resistance in isolates of *Pseudomonas* organisms from sputum cultures. The epidemiologic features of *P. cepacia* in the CF population, including the initial means of colonization and the mode and extent of transmissibility of the organisms among patients, is still not well defined.

A wide spectrum of clinical patterns has been reported in CF patients colonized with *P. cepacia;* these patterns range in severity from a fulminant necrotizing pneumonia or septicemia with fever and a rapid clinical deterioration to a prolonged period of colonization before clinically significant infection develops. Other CF patients have a more intermediate course after *P. cepacia* colonization, with a progressive decline over months or years, weight loss, and repeated hospitalizations for bronchopulmonary disease.[32]

Treatment of *P. cepacia* endobronchial infection in CF is perplexing; most isolates are resistant to the aminoglycosides and a broad range of other antibiotics, including many of the antipseudomonal penicillins. Although many strains of *P. cepacia* show sensitivities to the ureidopenicillins and ceftazidime *in vitro,* the *in vivo* response to intravenous therapy with these β-lactam antibiotics is highly variable.

Advances in therapy are continually being reevaluated as better understanding of the pathophysiology has been gained since the cloning of the CF gene and the availability of an animal model for CF. New pharmacologic approaches include the use of amiloride and ATP/UTP, which work in different ways to bypass the chloride channel defect in the airway epithelial cells. Trials with DNase, an enzyme that digests the DNA in the airway mucus of affected patients, have resulted in improved mucus viscosity and mucociliary clearance of airway secretions. Investigation into drugs that would activate the mutant of CFTR is under way.

Gene therapy is being actively pursued for CF. Recombinant vectors utilizing the adenovirus system look promising. Studies have demonstrated a high efficiency of CFTR gene transfer to airway epithelial cells in a rat model, and the use of retroviruses to transfer CFTR in monkeys is under investigation.[8] Other approaches to gene therapy include the use of adeno-associated virus (AAV) and the use of DNA protein complexes to directly enter the CF cells.

The management of respiratory failure in patients with CF poses the most difficult dilemma in management. Assisted ventilation is usually considered an accepted mode of therapy for acute respiratory failure, even when superimposed on COPD. However, the results in CF patients are poorer than those reported for other forms of COPD because of differences in the natural history of the disease and response to current therapy. Some complications of assisted ventilation (e.g., pneumothorax and pneumomediastinum) occur more frequently in CF than in other forms of COPD. A patient with CF whose condition is progressively deteriorating despite optimal therapy with intravenous antibiotics and intensive bronchial drainage and chest physical therapy is usually not a good candidate for assisted ventilation.[33] Alternatively, the patient with adequate baseline pulmonary status and a sudden onset of acute respiratory failure is a good candidate for mechanical ventilation.

The use of mechanical ventilation in patients with CF should be individualized after consideration of several factors:

1. Severity and extent of the pulmonary disease.
2. Types and severity of complications.
3. Type of onset of respiratory failure.
4. Probability of return to baseline pulmonary status if current episode of respiratory failure resolves.
5. Natural history of disease.
6. Decision of patients or parents of patients who are minors.
7. Acceptability and availability of heart-lung or double-lung transplantation.

It is important for all patients in respiratory failure to receive appropriate antibiotic therapy directed toward the endobronchial infections, intensive segmental bronchial drainage and chest physical therapy, nutritional support, fluids for optimizing electrolyte status and hydration (while avoiding fluid overload), cautious supplemental oxygen (for providing optimal oxygenation without exacerbation of hypercapnia), and general medical and psychosocial supportive care.

PROGNOSIS

Survival of patients with CF has improved considerably since the 1960s. Females with CF have a slightly lower median survival than do males with CF. According to the CF Foundation's patient data registry, the mean survival for males in 1991 was 30.6 years, in contrast to 28.2 years for females.[34] Increasing numbers of women with CF have had successful pregnancies, although there is a potential risk of pulmonary deterioration with pregnancy. Prepregnancy nutritional, cardiac, and pulmonary statuses are most closely related to potential increased risks of pulmonary deterioration in females with CF. Although most infants born to CF mothers are healthy, the mean birth weight of the infants may be lower than for the normal population, and there is a chance of 1 in 40 to 50 that such infants will have CF.

In a study of prognostic factors for CF that reviewed data on 622 patients with CF born in Victoria, Australia, from 1955 to 1980, sex did not appear to have prognostic significance.[35] Analysis of the Australian CF data demonstrated that presentation with predominantly respiratory symptoms was associated with a worse prognosis and that failure to reverse extensive disease at diagnosis or deterioration of the lung disease in the first year after diagnosis was associated with a less favorable course in patients with CF.

Because of the heterogeneity among individuals affected by CF, prognosis is highly variable, depending on the extent and severity of involvement of the type and severity of complications. Major advances in the knowledge and understanding of the pathophysiologic processes and basic abnormalities in CF have contributed to the improvement in symptomatic treatment, increased survival age, and improved quality of life of affected patients. Successful heart-lung and double-lung transplantations have been reported in CF, which offers another source of hope for help in end-stage disease in patients with CF. The identification of the CF gene and the use of possible gene-transfer techniques to correct the apparent CF defect are also exciting possibilities for the future and should serve as an impetus to CF patients and caregivers to maximize control of pulmonary disease.

PSYCHOSOCIAL ASPECTS

The early 1980s marked an astonishing change in the psychological literature associated with CF.[36] Before this time, most of the studies dealt with the seriousness of CF and the effect of catastrophic illness on the functioning of a small number of patients. Subsequently, researchers compared cohorts of CF patients with normal controls and control groups of patients with other chronic illnesses, using standard psychological testing instruments. There was a virtual outpouring of findings that CF patients were emotionally like other people except that they worried more about their health. In spite of fairly good marks on psychological testing, CF continues to produce areas of psychological concern in patients and their families. Many of these concerns relate to the age of the patient. These are now reviewed by age grouping.

PRENATAL

The ability to provide genotype analysis to the parents and CF probands aids in predicting probabilities of outcome of pregnancies in those at high risk of CF. See Chapter 69 for additional information on the genetic aspects of CF.

INFANCY AND EARLY CHILDHOOD

Infants with meconium ileus and children who manifest severe respiratory or digestive symptoms usually pre-cipitate in their parents the clinical syndrome of FAGS (fear, anger, grief, and sadness as the implications of the disease become known). In spite of increased publicity, most of the parents of newly diagnosed CF patients have never heard of the disease. The initial approach to the family by an experienced care provider is extremely important because most of the literature on CF available in libraries and fund-raising offices is gloomy. Lines of communication and medical support systems should be established early in this process. It is especially important for the parents of newly diagnosed patients to be introduced to families of other CF patients in their vicinity and with children of comparable age (with some judicious pre-screening of the resource families, of course).

In spite of the anger and grief at the initial diagnosis, early childhood is almost a honeymoon period for CF patients. Careful attention to medical problems can make almost all of these patients feel much better. It is during this time that family health habits are established, and all concerned are encouraged not to "leave well enough alone" as the child develops. Children quickly learn to rebel at chest physiotherapy sessions or to refuse to eat the expensive nutritional supplements. In this regard, regular checkups at a CF center may be of considerable value in reducing stress on the parents.

LATE CHILDHOOD AND ADOLESCENCE

As CF patients mature and begin the period of withdrawal from parental control, compliance with the medical regimen may become an overwhelming issue. The child, of course, views the therapy as only another imposition by the parents and therefore fair game for limit testing. Unfortunately, in many patients the adolescent years and the consequent somatic growth acceleration mark the first real evidence of CF. Menarche may be delayed, and patients may fall behind their peers in stature. Adolescent girls seem to be at more risk than boys for real deterioration in health. The reasons for this are not known but may involve the effects of estrogen and progesterone on the viscosity of mucus. The majority of CF patients take the adolescent years in stride.[37] Those in poor health or in whom the withdrawal process precipitates major family stress may benefit from formal counseling.

EARLY ADULTHOOD

With current therapy, most CF patients are well enough for higher education or vocational training.[38] Problems develop when patients attempt to use this training for full-time employment. Although many persons with CF have exemplary attendance and performance records at work, it is likely for most that sick days and medical expenses are much higher than for their peers. Smoking in the work place, unsympathetic supervisors, or stringent attendance policies are particularly difficult for CF patients. Finding a marriage partner is much less a problem than might be imagined. Issues of sexual adequacy, financial burdens because of health, and fear of separation all may require counseling and supportive services from the CF caregiver.

THE ADULT CF PATIENT

As the number of CF patients in their 30s and 40s and beyond increases, new problems are brought to the attention of the health care system. Couples in which a partner has CF and is quite healthy often inquire about the advisability of having children. Although most men with CF are sterile, women with CF can and do bear children. This may prove a burden to their personal health. Increasing availability of *in vitro* fertilization and surrogate parenting has made parenting available to a larger number of couples. The effect of sick infants on parents' health and the long-term impact of rearing a child may tax the counseling skill of the primary caregiver.

REFERENCES

1. Knowlton RG, Cohen-Haguenauer O, Van Cong N, et al: A polymorphic DNA marker linked to cystic fibrosis is located on chromosome 7. Nature 318:380–382, 1985.
2. White R, Woodward S, Leppert M, et al: A closely linked marker for cystic fibrosis. Nature 318:382–384, 1985.
3. Wainwright BJ, Scambler PJ, Schmidtke J, et al: Localization of cystic fibrosis locus to human chromosome 7 cenq22. Nature 318:384–385, 1985.
4. Tsui LC, Buchwald M, Barker O, et al: Cystic fibrosis locus defined by a genetically linked polymorphic DNA marker. Science 230:1054–1057, 1985.
5. Rommens JM, Iannuzzi MC, Kerem BS, et al: Identification of the cystic fibrosis gene: Chromosome walking and jumping. Science 245:1059–1065, 1989.
6. Riordan JR, Rommens JM, Kerem B, et al: Identification of the cystic fibrosis gene: Cloning and characterization of complementary DNA. Science 245:1066–1073, 1989.
7. Kerem BS, Rommens JM, Buchanan JA, et al: Identification of the cystic fibrosis gene: Genetic analysis. Science 245:1073–1080, 1989.
8. Collins FS: The CF gene: Perceptions, puzzles, and promises. Pediatr Pulmonol Suppl 8:63–64, 1992.
9. Tsui L-C, Rommens JM, Kerem BS, et al: Molecular genetics of cystic fibrosis. Pediatr Pulmonol Suppl 5:58–59, 1990.
10. Cheng SH, Gregory RJ, Marshall J, et al: Defective intracellular transport and processing of CFTR is the molecular basis of most cystic fibrosis. Cell 63:827–834, 1990.
11. Quinton PM, Bijman J: Higher bioelectric potentials due to decreased chloride absorption in the sweat glands of patients with cystic fibrosis. N Engl J Med 308:1185–1189, 1983.
12. Knowles M, Gatzy J, Boucher R: Relative ion permeability of normal and CF nasal epithelium. J Clin Invest 71:1410–1417, 1983.
13. Wine J: Basic aspects of cystic fibrosis. *In* Moss R (ed): Cystic Fibrosis, pp. 1–25. Clifton, NJ: Humana Press, 1990.
14. Welsh M: Abnormal regulation of ion channels in cystic fibrosis epithelia. FASEB J 4:2718–2725, 1990.
15. Heeley A, Heeley M, King D, et al: Screening for cystic fibrosis by dried blood spot trypsin assay. Arch Dis Child 57:18–21, 1982.
16. Wilcken B, Brown A, Urwin R, Brown D: Cystic fibrosis screening by dried blood spot trypsin assay: Results in 75,000 newborn infants. J Pediatr 102:383–387, 1983.
17. Caniano D, Beaver B: Meconium ileus: A 15-year experience with 42 neonates. Surgery 102:669–703, 1987.
18. Noble HH: Treatment of uncomplicated meconium ileus by Gastrografin enema: A preliminary report. Pediatr Surg 4:190, 1969.
19. Dalzell A, Freestone N, Billington D, Heap D: Small intestinal permeability and orocoecal transit time in cystic fibrosis. Arch Dis Child 65:585–588, 1990.
20. DeJonge H: The molecular basis of chloride channel dysregulation in cystic fibrosis. Acta Paediatr Scand 363:14–19, 1989.
21. Gibson L, Cooke R: H test for concentration of electrolytes in sweat in CF utilizing pilocarpine by iontophoresis. Pediatrics 23:545–549, 1959.
22. Stern R, Boat T, Doershuk C: Obstructive azoospermia as a diagnostic criterion for the CF syndrome. Lancet 1:1401–1404, 1982.
23. Brasfield D, Hicks G, Joong S, et al: The chest roentgenogram in cystic fibrosis: A new scoring system. Pediatrics 63:24–29, 1979.
24. Redding G, Restuccia R, Cotton E, et al: Serial changes in pulmonary function in children hospitalized with cystic fibrosis. Am Rev Respir Dis 126:31–36, 1982.
25. Waring W, Wilkinson R, Wiebe R, et al: Quantitation of digital clubbing in children. Am Rev Respir Dis 117:639, 1978.
26. Cohan R, Doershuk C, Stern R: Bronchial artery embolization to control hemoptysis in cystic fibrosis. Radiology 175:401–405, 1990.
27. Moss A: The cardiovascular system in cystic fibrosis. Pediatrics 70:728–741, 1982.
28. Stern R, Borkat G, Hirschfeld S, et al: Heart failure in cystic fibrosis. Treatment and prognosis of cor pulmonale with failure of the right side of the heart. Am J Dis Child 134:267–272, 1980.
29. Smith AL, Ramsey BW, Hedges DL, et al: Safety of aerosol tobramycin administration for 3 months to patients with cystic fibrosis. Pediatr Pulmonol 7:265–271, 1989.
30. Smith AL: Aerosol aminoglycoside administration. Pediatr Pulmonol Suppl 6:79–80, 1991.
31. Goldmann D, Klinger J: *Pseudomonas cepacia:* Biology, mechanisms of virulences, epidemiology. J Pediatr 108:806–812, 1986.
32. Isles A, Maclusky I, Corey M, et al: *Pseudomonas cepacia* infection in cystic fibrosis: An emerging problem. J Pediatr 104:206–210, 1084.
33. Davis PB, di Sant'Agnese PA: Assisted ventilation for patients with cystic fibrosis. JAMA 239:1851–1854, 1978.
34. CF Patient Data Registry, 1991.
35. Hudson I, Phelan P: Are sex, age at diagnosis, or mode of presentation prognostic factors for cystic fibrosis? Pediatr Pulmonol 3:288–297, 1987.
36. Lewiston N: Psychosocial impact of cystic fibrosis: Semin Respir Med 6:321–332, 1985.
37. Kellerman J, Zeltza L, Ellenberg L, et al: Psychosocial effects of illness in adolescence. I: Anxiety, self-esteem, and perception of control. J Pediatr 97:126–131, 1980.
38. Shepard S, Hovell M, Harwood I, et al: A comparative study of the psychosocial assets of adults with cystic fibrosis and their healthy peers. Chest 97:1310–1316, 1990.

71 IMMUNOPATHOGENESIS OF CYSTIC FIBROSIS LUNG DISEASE

RICHARD B. MOSS, M.D.

Immunologic aspects of cystic fibrosis (CF) are diverse and complex. This chapter focuses on the pathogenesis of CF lung disease. It is useful to consider CF lung disease as a series of discrete stages, each of which involves its own aspects of microbial-host interactions. The intention of this schema is not to propose that these stages are distinct features of CF lung disease—it is clear that varying degrees of overlap and interaction occur among the processes described next—but to provide the reader with an evolutionary concept of CF lung disease that can help guide thoughts about stage-based interventions. For other reviews of immunologic aspects of CF, the reader is referred to several monographs[1-3] and reviews.[4-7]

STAGE I: ADHERENCE

The earliest events that occur in the process of mucosal infection involve adherence of pathogenic organisms to epithelial structures as a result of specific binding between adhesive structures on the surface of microorganisms (adhesins) and respective molecular ligands on the cell surface (adhesin receptors).[8, 9] The primary pathogen in CF, *Pseudomonas aeruginosa* (PA), probably adheres to respiratory epithelium or mucus of CF patients via adhesins on projecting polar pili (fimbriae) or within the alginate secreted and loosely associated with the cell lipopolysaccharide (LPS) capsule.[10-14] This earliest stage in the pathogenesis of CF lung infection represents a potential turning point: If adhesion could be prevented, the clinical course of the disease could likely be dramatically ameliorated.[15]

Little is known about the central questions regarding bacterial adherence to the respiratory epithelium of CF patients. How does the genetic defect in the CF transmembrane regulator protein (CFTR) lead to bacterial colonization? Does the connection lie in an alteration of periciliary fluid and mucociliary transport, changes in adhesin receptors, or alterations of other host defenses? Does it depend on prior injury to the epithelium (e.g., by viral infection), or is it related to malnutrition?[16-20] Does the emergence of PA reflect an adherence advantage relative to other bacteria or a subsequent adaptive advantage that eventually leads to overgrowth of other colonizing microbes?

Injury clearly increases adherence of PA to human respiratory epithelium.[16, 20] Loss of cell-associated fibronectin via excess protease activity may also increase adherence.[21] Fibronectin-cleaving proteolytic activity has been found in the saliva and bronchial secretions of CF patients,[22, 23] but this activity likely represents a secondary effect, inasmuch as similar changes are seen in postoperative patients and patients with tracheostomy before gram-negative bacillary colonization.[24, 25] Moreover, bronchial fibronectin-cleaving activity in CF patients is correlated with age, disease progression, and prior PA colonization.[23]

The role of secretory immunity in preventing adherence in CF has not been investigated. Alterations in the structure of secretory immunoglobulin A (IgA) and diminished secretory component in the respiratory fluids of CF patients may result in diminished antiadhesive properties,[26] but the observed changes are consistent with inflammatory effects of increased proteolytic activity and loss of epithelium.

Although PA adherence may be mediated by alginate as well as pili, it is uncertain whether alginate-mediated adherence is important in the pathogenesis of CF lung disease, because in initial PA colonization, smooth phenotypes express little alginate.[27] Such strains have been shown to typically adhere via pilin adhesins. Exposure of ciliary receptors to direct contact with pili adhesins via loss of periciliary fluid is perhaps the most parsimonious explanation of the adherence phase in CF lung infection.[28, 29] Such an effect could directly follow from reduced Cl^- secretion and excessive Na^+ reabsorption present in the respiratory epithelia of CF patients, which presumably causes dehydration of the periciliary fluid.[30, 31] If so, then rehydration (e.g., with amiloride aerosol) could prevent colonization, but as yet no data are available for answering this critical question.[32]

According to an alternative adhesion hypothesis, adhesin receptors are in mucus overlying the epithelium.[33, 34] Such mucus adhesin receptors may bind pili from nonmucoid PA or alginate from mucoid PA. Bacteria associated with colonization in CF (PA, *Staphylococcus aureus, Haemophilus influenzae,* and *Enterobacteriaceae*) bind to glycosphingolipids present at unknown sites in human lung tissue,[35] as seen in adhesion of other bacteria to other mucosae.[36] The primary defect in CF might offer an opportunity for bacterial adhesins to bind altered or exposed ligands in or overlying the respiratory mucosa in CF patients. Colonization would be afforded to a select spectrum of bacteria with a proper adhesin repertoire. Eventual dominance by PA could then be a secondary consequence of subsequent events such as early viral infection or antibiotic treatment as well as phenotypic adaptability of PA to the lung microenvironment of CF patients. This scenario is compatible with evidence from studies for the emergence of PA in early childhood after onset of clinical respiratory illness and treatment interventions, particularly antimicrobial treatment of *S. aureus*.[37, 38]

STAGE II: COLONIZATION

After adherence, local bacterial multiplication, aided by secretion of virulence factors, occurs if nonspecific host defenses such as local soluble antimicrobial factors and mucociliary clearance are insufficient. Colonization of airways might follow aspiration or descending colonization from the upper respiratory tract. PA grows in endobronchial interadherent clusters or microcolonies at the site of early lung lesions in CF.[28, 39, 40] Microcolony formation presents obstacles to early nonimmune phagocytosis by resident pulmonary macrophages and protects PA from soluble host defense factors.[39, 41] The transition to chronic PA colonization involves bacterial adaptations resulting in further modulation of host defense responses.[42–46] Table 71–1 summarizes effects of PA products on the colonized CF host that facilitate chronic colonization.

Perhaps the most remarkable adaptations of PA to the airways microenvironment in CF patients are the markedly increased production of alginate (which is responsible for conversion to the mucoid phenotype) and a downregulation of LPS serotype-specific O side chains. The lat-

Table 71–1. EFFECTS OF *PSEUDOMONAS AERUGINOSA* PRODUCTS ON HOST DEFENSES

PA Product	Effect	Reference
Pigments		
Pyocyanin, 1-OH-phenazine, 2-alkyl-4-OH-quinolines, rhamnolipid	↓Ciliary function	282–284
Pyocyanin, 1-OH-phenazine	↓Mucociliary clearance	285
Pyocyanin	↓Neutrophil O_2 production	179
Rhamnolipid	Altered Cl^- transport	286
Pyocyanin	↓Lymphocyte mitogen-induced proliferation;	287
	↓IL-2 production and IL-2 receptor expression	75
Rhamnolipid	↓Neutrophil chemotaxis	180
Proteases		
Elastase, alkaline protease	↓Neutrophil chemotaxis and O_2 consumption	181
	↓Neutrophil myeloperoxidase-dependent chemiluminescence	182
	↓Neutrophil phagocytosis of PA (no effect on *Staphylococcus aureus*)	183
	↑Mucus secretion	288
	↓Lymphocyte mitogen-induced proliferation; cleavage of IL-2	122
	↓Natural killer cell function	289
	Cleavage of CD4	290
	Cleavage of multiple lymphocyte CD antigens	291
	Cleavage of interferon-γ	121
Elastase	Cleavage of IgG, IgA, alpha$_1$-PI, complement proteins, lysozyme	184, 185, 292–295
Other Products		
Exotoxin A	↓Lymphocyte mitogen-induced proliferation	53, 296
	Cytotoxic for PMO	124
Leukocidin	Cytotoxic for neutrophils	297
Phospholipase C	Hydrolysis of surfactant	44
Alginate	Microcolony formation	39
	↑Required concentration of opsonic antibody	298
	↓Pulmonary clearance	164
	Adherence to mucin; ↓neutrophil phagocytosis	299
	↑Monocyte IL-1 secretion	118
Lipopolysaccharide	Opsonic immunodeterminant	300
	B cell mitogen	111

PA, *Pseudomonas aeruginosa;* O_2, oxygen; IL-2, interleukin-2; Ig, immunoglobulin; PMO, pulmonary macrophage; IL-1, interleukin-1.

ter change is responsible for an increased sensitivity to the action of serum complement and for a loss of serotype-specific agglutination *in vitro*.[27,47-49] Interruption of muco-ciliary clearance by PA phenazine pigments (see Table 71-1), enhanced use of iron for metabolism, and secretion of exoenzymes (elastase, alkaline protease, exotoxin A, phospholipase C, and exotoxin S) may also interfere with host defenses and cause direct tissue damage.[44,50-54] For example, PA strains expressing exotoxin A, exoenzyme S, or proteases have increased pathogenicity in the agar bead animal model of chronic PA endobronchitis in comparison with their nonsecretory isogeneic variants.[55-57] The long-term clinical impact of exoproducts in the lungs of CF patients is called into question, however, by results of studies that show their neutralization by antibodies produced in the months after onset of chronic colonization.[58] In addition, decreased virulence and decreased production of virulence factors by PA strains isolated from CF patients have been reported.[59,60] These data suggest that as PA establishes itself in the airways of CF patients, there is a gradual reduction in production of virulence factors. The reasons for all these remarkable phenotypic adaptations remain obscure but undoubtedly result from local microenvironmental factors.

Pier and colleagues reported that older CF patients without PA colonization had opsonic serum antibodies to PA alginate, whereas CF patients with PA colonization, as well as non-CF controls, did not.[61] Moreover, opsonic antialginate antibodies are protective in animal model PA endobronchial challenge studies.[62] Thus these antibodies might be anticolonization factors. Confirmation of this effect in humans is awaited; in one study, only a minority of CF patients without PA colonization had opsonic alginate-specific antibodies,[63] which implies that other factors are also responsible for escape from chronic PA colonization in these patients.

STAGE III: INFECTION

The transition from colonization to infection occurs along a temporal gradient controlled by two factors. The first is the growth of colonizing microbes beyond a threshold density, usually taken to be $>10^5$ colony-forming units per milliliter of biologic fluid on a mucosal surface. Presumably, microbial density is proportional to local tissue damage from virulence factors. The second factor is the host response, which initially involves nonspecific inflammatory components but soon includes elements of a specific immune response.[7,64] This host response is traditionally detected by rises in leukocyte counts, acute phase reactants, and systemic antibodies (sero-conversion), but it could also be detected by the occurrence of localized antibody responses, cell-mediated immunity, or other immune mechanisms such as cytokine production.

PRIMARY IMMUNITY

No convincing evidence for a primary defect in host immune or inflammatory systems has been found in CF.[65,66] Although many changes in immune functions have been observed, they are likely caused by secondary effects of disease or infection.[65-68] However, lack of gross malfunction does not rule out subtle abnormalities. The ion transport regulatory defects representing the fundamental effects of CFTR mutation in CF were described in exocrine tissues, including sweat ducts and acini, and in respiratory epithelial cells.[31,69] It has been shown that lymphocytes of CF patients express a hallmark biochemical defect: a lack of cyclic adenosine monophosphate–dependent protein kinase–induced transmembrane Cl⁻ conductance.[70,71] It is therefore possible that lymphocyte immune functions may also be directly affected. For example, reduced allogeneic cell–mediated cytotoxicity by blood mononuclear cells of CF patients might result in increased susceptibility to viral infection or in reduced early T cell response to PA.[72,73]

PRIMARY IMMUNE RESPONSES

Reduced antigen penetration or presentation by accessory cells responsible for induction of immune responses may occur in CF; this process could account for hypo-gammaglobulinemia observed in many young patients.[74] Alternatively, virulence factors released by PA, such as immunosuppressive phenazine pigments, could reduce immune responses.[75] Reduced mucosal antigen presentation in CF is further suggested by results of studies of antibody responses to mucosal microbial antigens. CF patients who do not have colonization with PA have reduced levels of naturally predominant serum IgG$_2$ antibodies to PA LPS.[76] CF patients also have low natural antibody levels to *H. influenzae* type b capsular polysaccharide.[77] Low levels of antibodies to *S. aureus* capsular polysaccharides and cell wall teichoic acid have been noted.[78,79] Deficient mucosal antigen penetration resulting in poor systemic responses is not inconsistent with normal antibody responses after parenteral immunization, which bypasses the mucosal barrier.[80-82] Interestingly, although secondary antibody responses to immunization with a polyvalent PA LPS vaccine in CF patients with PA colonization were brisk,[83] systemic antibody responses to a PA cell wall vaccine composed mostly of LPS in CF patients without PA colonization were described as poor to some serotypes and lower than those evoked by pulmonary infection. Unfortunately, this often-cited vaccine study contained no immunologic data.[84] More relevant to the mucosal barrier hypothesis were the poor antibody responses to intranasally administered PA LPS vaccine in CF patients with PA colonization. Although normal human responses to this route of vaccination are not known, intranasal PA LPS immunization induced brisk antibody responses in rabbits.[85] Collectively, these studies raise important questions about mucosal antigen presentation in CF that require further study.

RESPONSE TO PA COLONIZATION

There is usually a lapse of several months between when sputum cultures become positive for PA and when

Table 71–2. IMMUNOGENS OF *PSEUDOMONAS AERUGINOSA* IN COLONIZED CYSTIC FIBROSIS PATIENTS

Moiety	Reference
Lipopolysaccharide	
O side chains	87, 92, 93
Core	92, 301, 302
Alginate	61, 303–306
Proteases (elastase, alkaline protease)	86, 92, 102, 104, 105, 307, 308
Exoenzyme S	309
Outer membrane porin proteins	88, 91, 301
Cell envelope: flagellin	310
Cell envelope: "common antigen"	311
Phospholipase C (heat-labile hemolysin)	102, 104
Iron-regulated outer membrane proteins	52

a humoral immune response occurs.[86–88] This time lapse may represent a sluggish immune response to mucosally presented antigen. Rises in serum antibodies to PA LPS before detection of PA in sputum cultures have also been reported.[89, 90] This could represent sampling error (in which obtained cultures do not accurately reflect colonization of the lower respiratory tract), cross-reactivity between antigens of PA and other microbes, or assay differences.[91]

Despite reduced production of LPS side chains by mucoid PA in the lungs of CF patients, there is an increasing antibody response to these antigens throughout the illness.[87, 92, 93] This antibody response indicates continued immunogenicity of low levels of LPS O side-chain antigens in mucoid PA.[94–96] It is interesting in this regard that passive infusion of a hyperimmune globulin rich in opsonic PA LPS antibodies had beneficial effects in a pilot study of CF patients with pulmonary exacerbations.[97]

Antibody responses (mainly IgG and IgA) to a wide variety of conserved, expressed, and accessible PA components have been reported (Table 71–2).[98–101] No antibody responses to low–molecular-weight phenazine pigments and related compounds have been reported. Antibody responses to PA surface antigens may precede antibody responses to secretory products after colonization.[86, 91, 102, 103] An exception to this is the early response to the heat-labile PA hemolysin, phospholipase C.[104] Antibodies to PA antigens in CF patients with PA colonization usually reach a "hyperimmune" level, which may vary considerably between individuals, and then plateau. A correlation has been found between rising levels of antibodies to PA LPS and exotoxin A and worsening prognosis.[92, 101, 102, 105, 106]

In most patients with CF, hyperimmunoglobulinemia G and A develops.[107] Despite the vigor of the antibody response to PA in CF, only a minor portion of the hyperimmunoglobulinemia is caused by specific antibody formation.[108] Hypergammaglobulinemia may be caused mainly by PA-derived polyclonal B cell mitogens, including alginate and LPS.[109–111]

Antibodies to PA antigens rise during episodes of pulmonary exacerbation and fall in response to anti-PA therapy, which is indicative of a pathogenic role for PA.[90, 104, 112, 113]

PULMONARY MACROPHAGE

The resident phagocyte, the pulmonary macrophage (PMO), may not be appropriately activated and phagocytosing in the lungs of CF patients.[114–116] However, CF PMOs phagocytize normally *in vitro*.[114, 117] Also, indirect evidence of PMO activation in the lungs of CF patients comes from detection of elevated levels of free interleukin-1β in bronchial lavage fluid of CF patients (a finding not specific to CF) as well as increased plasma levels of tumor necrosis factor α, interleukin-1α, and interleukin-1β.[118, 119] Any paralysis of CF PMO could result from diminished activating lymphokine production (particularly interferon-γ) by T cells in the lungs of CF patients, possibly because of suppression of lymphokine secretion by PA exoproducts.[75] CF PMO can be activated by incubation with supernatants from stimulated normal lymphocytes *in vitro*.[120] Lymphokines may also be susceptible to local inactivation by PA exoproducts.[121, 122] Perhaps such suppression accounts for decreased helper function of freshly isolated peripheral blood T cells of CF patients *in vitro*.[72, 123] Yet other possible causes of PMO paralysis are suppression of PMO phagocytosis by exotoxin A,[124] insufficient opsonization of PA resulting from poor antigen penetration to accessory cells necessary for antibody induction, or suppression by nonopsonizing antibodies or immune complexes.

With regard to opsonization, nonspecific complement opsonins would be expected to play a major role, at least early in the course of the disease. There are no data on complement-mediated defenses in lung fluids of CF patients before onset of infection. After onset of PA infection, local complement function is greatly impaired by unbuffered proteolytic activity in lung fluids of CF patients, as discussed later.

MODULATION OF IMMUNE RESPONSES BY PA

Once PA infection is established and clearance by PMO fails, the stage is set for a vicious cycle of inflammatory cell recruitment, activation, degranulation, and bystander tissue damage.[6, 7, 125, 126] The ongoing modulation of host immune responses by PA is one of the most fascinating and clinically frustrating aspects of CF. Many independent and potentially interactive mechanisms for failure of immune clearance have been reported and are summarized in Table 71–3.

Proteolytic Degradation of Host Defense Molecules

Neutrophilic infiltration into and around airways is the single most impressive immunopathologic event in CF lung disease. Normally present in very low numbers, neutrophils quickly become the predominant inflammatory cell type in the lungs of CF patients, reaching enormous numbers and localized in a bronchocentric manner around PA microcolonies.[40, 46, 114, 117, 127, 128] After activation and discharge of neutrophil proteases in a frustrated attempt at phagocytosis, proteolytic activity in the air-

Table 71–3. EFFECTS OF THE HOST-MICROBIAL INTERACTION BETWEEN *PSEUDOMONAS AERUGINOSA* AND THE CYSTIC FIBROSIS PATIENT

Action	Reference
Proteolysis of Host Defense Molecules	145, 167, 176–179,
IgG, IgA, sIgA	188, 196, 197, 203
C1-9, C3bi	
C3b receptor, C3bi receptor	
Fcγ receptor I	
Alpha$_1$-PI	
Altered Immunoglobulin and Antibody	76, 77, 131–137
Isotype	
Relative decrease of IgG$_1$	
Relative/absolute increase of IgG$_2$, IgG$_3$,	
IgG$_4$	
Altered Glycosylation of IgG, Reduced	159, 160, 162
Intracellular Neutrophil Killing of PA	
Change in PA Phenotype	
Decreased LPS O side-chain production	27, 47–49
Increased serum sensitivity	
Poly- or nonagglutinability	
Increased alginate production (mucoid	
phenotype)	
Microcolony formation	39
Antiphagocytic	164
Decreased bacteremic virulence *in vivo*	59
Decreased production of virulence factors *in*	59, 60
vitro	
Proteases	
Flagellar motility	
Exotoxin A	
Exoenzyme S	
Phospholipase C (heat-labile hemolysin)	
Increased expression of iron-binding outer	50–52
membrane proteins	
Immune Complex Formation	
Type III hypersensitivity disease	92, 101, 112, 228–
	234, 238–243
Decreased opsonophagocytosis of PA	166
Regulation by neutrophil elastase	244
IgE Antibody Response	112, 271, 272

Ig, immunoglobulin; PI, protease inhibitor; PA, *Pseudomonas aeruginosa*; LPS, lipopolysaccharide.

ways rapidly exceeds the buffering capacity of host antiproteases, and a succession of disastrous consequences ensues. Among these are degradation of critical host defense molecules such as immunoglobulins, complement components, phagocyte receptors for opsonins, and antiproteases.[126] These consequences are discussed in detail later in the section on inflammation.

Altered Antibody Isotype

Chronic antigenic stimulation can lead to a switch in isotype predominance of responding antibody.[129] In general, this process is at least partly controlled by regulatory T cell–derived lymphokines.[130] In CF, it appears that chronic PA infection contributes to increased levels of minor immunoglobulin (IgG$_2$, IgG$_3$, and IgG$_4$) protein and production of nonopsonic IgG$_2$ and IgG$_4$ PA LPS-specific antibodies.[76, 77, 107, 131–141]

The induction of nonopsonizing IgG isotypes accounts for the presence of antigen-specific blocking antibodies for PMO opsonophagocytosis of PA present in unfragmented antibodies in peripheral blood of CF patients with

PA colonization[142–145] and explains the induction of similar activities in the agar bead animal model of chronic PA endobronchitis or parenteral hyperimmunization with PA LPS.[146, 147] It may also account for why IgG-blocking factors in the blood and sputum of PA-colonized CF patients inhibit serum bactericidal activity for autologous PA.[148–150] Serum and bronchial fluids of CF patients, and PA LPS IgG antibodies isolated from them, have a greater opsonophagocytic inhibitory effect on PMO than on neutrophils.[151, 152] Under certain conditions, however, inhibition of neutrophil phagocytosis by CF serum can be shown.[63, 153–155] Isotype switch appears to have a more profound inhibitory effect on PMOs than on neutrophils because of (1) the inability of the PMO to enhance opsonophagocytosis by complement-mediated mechanisms[156] and (2) a more restricted Fcγ receptor repertoire.[157, 158]

Altered Glycosylation of IgG

CF IgG is abnormally glycosylated.[159, 160] IgG has a conserved N-linked glycosylation site at aspargine 297 of the C$_H$2 domain.[161] There may also be idiotype-dependent N-linked oligosaccharides on Fab hypervariable region sites. It seems likely that altered IgG glycosylation is a secondary effect of disease.[159] Altered immunoglobulin glycosylation could affect antibody function because minor changes in carbohydrate structure, which serve to hold the C$_H$2 domains in proper spatial separation, can alter Fc-mediated immune functions.[161] Altered glycosylation of CF IgG may play a role in depressed neutrophil bactericidal activity for PA.[162]

Changes in PA Phenotype

PA undergoes a tremendous phenotypic evolution in the airways microenvironment of CF patients. Genotyping studies confirm the clonality of serially cultured PA from lungs of CF patients despite widely variant phenotypes.[163] The most consistent changes, discussed previously here, include increased alginate production and decreased LPS side-chain production. Whether these changes contribute directly to PA persistence is uncertain.[164, 165] The roles of other PA products in modifying host defenses have been discussed previously (see Table 71–1).

Immune Complex Formation

Most attention on immune complex (IC) in CF has focused on its proinflammatory effects (see later discussion), but the IC may also exert immunosuppressive effects on PMO and neutrophil phagocytosis and killing of PA.[153, 166] Suppression is probably caused by altered antibody isotype and consequent high content of nonopsonic antibody.[166]

STAGE IV: INFLAMMATION

If immune responses are ineffective in clearing infection, activation of amplifying inflammatory mechanisms results in bystander damage to host tissues.

NEUTROPHIL-MEDIATED INFLAMMATION

Studies on lung inflammation in CF have centered on the neutrophil, the major inflammatory cell type in the airways and peribronchial tissues of CF patients.[46, 114, 117, 127, 128, 167] The initial basis for neutrophil influx into the airways is uncertain. Candidate mechanisms include release of chemotactic bacterial formyl peptides or LPS,[168] complement activation with generation of C5a anaphylotoxin,[169] PMO release of leukotriene B$_4$,[170–172] and LPS-induced interleukin-1 production by PMO.[118, 173] The presence of extraordinary numbers of neutrophils in the airways is reflected in high levels of sputum DNA released from neutrophils as they die.[64, 174] The contribution of DNA to abnormal sputum viscosity in CF has led to the proposed use of recombinant human deoxyribonuclease (DNase) as a therapeutic mucolytic agent; in vitro, DNase is much more effective than any other mucolytic agent,[175] and aerosolized DNase clinical trials were initiated in 1992.

It is not certain why neutrophils fail in their task of clearing endobronchial PA in CF, but multiple mechanisms appear to be involved. First, it is likely that PA microcolonies are too large to be ingested and are further protected by antiphagocytic properties of alginate.[39, 41] This would result in ineffective phagocytosis with a high degree of extracellular release of neutrophil proteases and oxidants. Second, proteolytic inactivation of neutrophil opsonic receptors (FcγRI, C3bR) and complement opsonins bound to PA (C3bi) appear to play a major role in blocking efficient killing of PA in the airways.[126, 176–178] Third, neutrophil bactericidal activity is probably depressed by PA exoproducts.[179–183] Finally, reduction of neutrophil PA killing by nonopsonic antibodies also contributes to this devastating suppression of host defense.[63, 166]

Neutrophil neutral proteases and reactive intermediates of oxygen metabolism are strongly implicated in lung tissue damage in CF patients. A role for PA-derived elastase has been proposed by Fick and colleagues.[169, 184–186] However, other authors have not found free PA-derived elastase activity in lung fluids of CF patients, and antibodies to PA elastase arise in the first year after colonization and neutralize its bioactivity.[54, 58, 187–189] An important unsettled question is the relative contribution of specific neutrophil proteases and oxidants, because focused therapeutic interventions directed against inflammatory mediators are entering clinical trials.

Protease-Antiprotease Imbalance: Causes and Consequences

Increased proteolytic activity in CF lung fluids was first noted by Lieberman and Kurnich in 1963.[174] Interest reawakened in the 1980s with increasing recognition of elastase-antielastase imbalance as a major inflammatory mechanism for lung damage in emphysema.[190] Extremely high levels of free proteolytic activity are present in the airways of CF patients.[169, 186–188, 191–193] Most if not all of it is caused by neutrophil elastase, a major lysosomal granule exoproduct.[187–188, 194] Neutrophil elastase is normally buffered by alpha$_1$-protease inhibitor, or alpha$_1$-PI (alpha$_1$-antitrypsin).[195] In lung fluids of CF patients, antiprotease activity is low or nil, and alpha$_1$-PI and another major airway antiprotease, secretory leukocyte protease inhibitor (SLPI) are found in complexed, inactivated forms.[167, 188, 196, 197] Because the neutrophil burden in bronchiectatic lungs is huge, representing up to one half of the entire marginating pool,[198] it is not surprising that the antiprotease system is overwhelmed in CF. Degradation of IgG and IgA, as well as of opsonic receptors and bacterially bound complement, results from unbuffered elastase activity.[176–178, 186] Thus host defenses are foiled at the same time that lung tissue is attacked and degraded.[193]

Clinical trials of alpha$_1$-PI, recombinant human SLPI, and synthetic antielastases such as ICI 200,880 should define the extent to which buffering of free neutrophil elastase can impede or halt progressive lung injury in CF.[199, 200]

Oxidant Damage

A second mechanism of neutrophil-mediated lung inflammation in CF is extracellular release of toxic oxygen radicals.[201] Buffers include intracellular enzymes such as catalase, superoxide dismutase, and glutathione peroxidase as well as extracellular scavengers such as ceruloplasmin and vitamins C and E. There is excess neutrophil-derived oxidant activity in the airways of CF patients.[167, 188, 202–204] Neutrophils in CF patients with significant lung disease respond to nonspecific stimuli with enhanced oxidative responses.[205, 206] A correlation between CF opsonins that induce neutrophil oxidative responses and clinical severity has been reported.[207]

Anti-Inflammatory Therapy

The idea that host inflammatory mediators rather than bacterial virulence factors cause most lung damage in CF is supported by results of studies in animal models of chronic PA lung infections and underlies current therapeutic trials of nonspecific steroidal and nonsteroidal anti-inflammatory drugs.[208–210] Antibiotics, by reducing the burden of PA in the airways, may exert major effects indirectly by reducing the stimulus to neutrophil influx, as reflected in sputum DNA and elastase levels.[64, 197] Plasma elastase complexed to alpha$_1$-PI rises during pulmonary exacerbations and falls in response to antibiotic treatment in CF.[211]

IMMUNE COMPLEX DISEASE

Persistence of foreign antigens and ongoing antibody responses inevitably lead to IC formation. It is not surprising that local and circulating ICs are a consistent feature of CF lung disease.[92, 101, 112, 212–224] ICs are formed in the lungs and contain antigens from colonizing respiratory pathogens, including PA LPS and proteases, along with corresponding IgG and IgA antibodies.[101, 216, 219, 225–227] Deposition of IC in numerous tissues, including those of the respiratory tract, gastrointestinal tract, skin, joints, and kidneys, has been reported.[212, 213, 228–231] It is uncertain whether ICs play a significant immunopathologic role in progression of CF lung disease.[232-234] CF patients, unlike patients with some IC-mediated diseases, rapidly dispose of ICs via reticuloendothelial uptake.[235]

Circulating IC levels rise with pulmonary exacerbations,[112, 217] and these rises are correlated with progression of lung disease and poor prognosis.[92, 101, 106, 221-224] Pseudomonal antigen-antibody complexes trigger mediator release from human platelets *in vitro*.[236] In the agar bead model of chronic PA endobronchitis, alginate has been implicated in pulmonary IC deposition and tissue damage.[237] As CF patients age, there appears to be an increase in extrapulmonary manifestations of IC-mediated disease. These manifestations include episodic arthropathies, present in 5% to 10% of CF patients, and rarer instances of cutaneous leukoclastic vasculitis.[228, 231, 238-243]

In the lung, local IC could play a proinflammatory role in neutrophil recruitment and activation.[65, 214] As noted previously, however, IC might also exert an immunosuppressive effect and contribute to bacterial persistence.[166] Doring and associates suggested that IC-activated neutrophils, by secreting elastase, cleave IgG in IC and thereby down-regulate IC-induced inflammation by removing the effector IgG Fc region. Elastase-treated ICs lose their capacity to induce a neutrophil respiratory burst.[244]

Systemic glucocorticosteroid therapy may be clinically beneficial in CF and suppresses the rise in IgG and IC seen in untreated CF patients.[208, 245, 246] In contrast, in one study, inhaled steroids had no effect on IC levels or disease manifestations, possibly because of inadequate dosage or poor penetration to sites of inflammation.[220]

ALLERGIC BRONCHOPULMONARY INFLAMMATION

IgE antibody–mediated allergic inflammation is involved in a number of clinical manifestations of CF.[247] Typical allergic disease (e.g., allergic rhinitis and asthma) caused by common environmental allergens (e.g., pollen, dust mite) occurs with expected frequency in CF and is not independently associated with progression of lung disease.[248] Less well appreciated, with an uncertain role in CF, are IgE antibody responses to microbial antigens.[249-252]

In CF, the most significant allergic responses occur after endobronchial colonization with *Aspergillus fumigatus* (AF) mold.[253] A combined IgG/IgE systemic immune response is associated with manifestations of allergic bronchopulmonary aspergillosis (APBA) in 10% to 15% of CF patients.[254-259] In addition to overt ABPA, a variety of immune responses to AF are observed in most CF patients, which indicates that subclinical infection occurs frequently.[260-266] An immunohistopathologic study of CF with APBA showed a prominent eosinophilic infiltrate with exocytosis of eosinophil granular proteins, activated helper T cells, and AF hyphae in inflamed peribronchial tissues.[267] These changes are distinct from the immunohistopathologic processes of CF without ABPA, which is typified by a bronchocentric necrotizing neutrophilic and plasmacytic infiltrate.[268]

The immunoregulatory processes underlying the pathologic changes of ABPA in CF are complex. Activation of IgE-secreting B cells is accompanied by an increased T cell suppressor activity, which depresses lymphoproliferative responses to non-AF antigens.[269] Despite this increased suppressive activity, supernatants of AF-stimulated T cells from CF patients with ABPA enhance allogeneic B cell IgE synthesis.[270] This suggests an increased AF-driven, IgE-specific lymphokine dysregulation in CF with ABPA.

IgE antibody responses in CF patients to PA, *S. aureus*, and *H. influenzae* occur but have not been examined immunopathologically.[112, 271-273] Immediate skin test responses after intradermal injection of PA extract in CF patients was found to be caused by anaphylotoxin-dependent histamine release rather than by IgE.[274]

STAGE V: DESTRUCTION

Chronic inflammation impairs function and eventually destroys tissue structure. In addition to protease and oxidant attack on lung tissue, lung disease in CF also involves excessive laying down of excess fibrotic tissue. CF sputum contains an unidentified fibrogenic activity that meets the criteria of a competence factor, providing a signal early in G1 phase of the cell growth cycle. This activity was greater in sputum from CF patients than in that from patients with respiratory syncytial virus infection.[275]

Currently, lung transplantation offers realistic hope to CF patients with end-stage lung disease.[276, 277] As expected from current knowledge of CFTR function, non-CF donor lungs do not acquire CF ion transport defects postoperatively.[278, 279] CF patients do as well postoperatively as other lung transplant recipients.[277] However, it is hoped that "transplantation" in CF will eventually be understood to mean not the late replacement of a ruined organ but the early functional transfer of normal CFTR DNA or protein into the airway epithelium of CF patients, the ultimate therapy short of germ-line genetic manipulation.[280, 281]

REFERENCES

1. Shapira E, Wilson GB (eds): Immunological Aspects of Cystic Fibrosis. Boca Raton, FL: CRC Press, 1984.
2. Hoiby N (ed): *Pseudomonas aeruginosa* infection. Antibiot Chemother, vol. 42. Basel, Switzerland: S Karger, 1989.
3. Moss RB (ed): Cystic Fibrosis: Infection, Immunopathology, and Host Response. Clifton, NJ: Humana Press, 1990.
4. Fick RB: Pathogenesis of the *Pseudomonas* lung lesion in cystic fibrosis. Chest 96:158–164, 1989.
5. Doring G, Albus A, Hoiby N: Immunological aspects of cystic fibrosis. Chest 94:109S–115S, 1988.
6. Zach MS: Lung disease in cystic fibrosis—An updated concept. Pediatr Pulmonol 8:188–202, 1990.
7. Elborn JS, Shale DJ: Lung injury in cystic fibrosis. Thorax 45:970–973, 1990.
8. Beachley EH: Bacterial adherence: Adhesin-receptor interactions mediating the attachment of bacteria to mucosal surfaces. J Infect Dis 143:325–345, 1981.
9. Roberts DD: Interactions of respiratory pathogens with host cell surface and extracellular matrix components. Am J Respir Cell Mol Biol 3:181–186, 1990.

10. Woods DE, Strauss DC, Johanson WO Jr, et al: Role of pili in adherence of *Pseudomonas aeruginosa* to mammalian buccal epithelial cells. Infect Immun 29:1146–1151, 1980.

11. Ramphal R, Sadoff JC, Pyle M, Silipigni JD: Role of pili in the adherence of *Pseudomonas aeruginosa* to injured tracheal epithelium. Infect Immun 44:38–40, 1984.

12. Ramphal R, Pier GB: Role of *Pseudomonas aeruginosa* mucoid exopolysaccharide in adherence to tracheal cells. Infect Immun 47:1–4, 1985.

13. Paranchych W, Sastry PA, Volpel K, et al: Fimbriae (Pili): Molecular basis of *Pseudomonas aeruginosa* adherence. Clin Invest Med 9:113–118, 1986.

14. Irvin RT, Doig P, Lee KK, et al: Characterization of the *Pseudomonas aeruginosa* pilus adhesin. Infect Immun 57:3720–3726, 1989.

15. Hanson LA, Andersson B, Carlsson B, et al: Defense of mucous membranes by antibodies, receptor analogues and nonspecific host factors. Infection 13:S166–S170, 1985.

16. Johanson WG, Higuchi JH, Chaudhuri TR, Woods DE: Bacterial adherence to epithelial cells in bacillary colonization of the respiratory tract. Am Rev Respir Dis 121:55–63, 1980.

17. Ramphal R, Small PM, Shands JW, et al: Adherence of *Pseudomonas aeruginosa* to tracheal cells injured by influenza infection or by endotracheal intubation. Infect Immun 27:614–619, 1980.

18. Ramphal R, Pyle M: Adherence of mucoid and nonmucoid *Pseudomonas aeruginosa* to acid-injured tracheal epithelium. Infect Immun 41:345–351, 1983.

19. Boyd RL, Ramphal R, Rice R, Mangos JA: Chronic colonization of rat airways with *Pseudomonas aeruginosa*. Infect Immun 39:1403–1410, 1983.

20. Niederman MS, Merrill WW, Ferranti RD, et al: Nutritional status and bacterial binding in the lower respiratory tract in patients with chronic tracheostomy. Ann Intern Med 100:795–800, 1984.

21. Woods DE, Straus DC, Johanson WG, Bass JA: Role of fibronectin in the prevention of adherence of *Pseudomonas aeruginosa* to buccal cells. J Infect Dis 143:784–790, 1981.

22. Woods DE, Bass JA, Johanson WG, Straus DC: Role of adherence in the pathogenesis of *Pseudomonas aeruginosa* lung infection in cystic fibrosis patients. Infect Immun 30:694–699, 1980.

23. Suter S, Schaad UB, Morgenthaler JJ, et al: Fibronectin-cleaving activity in bronchial secretions of patients with cystic fibrosis. J Infect Dis 158:89–100, 1988.

24. Niederman MS, Merrill WW, Polomski LM, et al: Influence of sputum IgA and elastase on tracheal cell bacterial adherence. Am Rev Respir Dis 133:255–260, 1986.

25. Dal Nogare AR, Toews GB, Pierce AK: Increased salivary elastase precedes gram-negative bacillary colonization in postoperative patients. Am Rev Respir Dis 135:671–675, 1987.

26. Wallwork, JC, McFarlane H: The SIgA system and hypersensitivity in patients with cystic fibrosis. Clin Allergy 6:349–358, 1976.

27. Pier GB, Desjardins D, Aguilar R, et al: Polysaccharide surface antigens expressed by nonmucoid isolates of *Pseudomonas aeruginosa* from cystic fibrosis patients. J Clin Microbiol 24:189–196, 1986.

28. Marcus H, Baker NR: Quantitation of adherence of mucoid and nonmucoid *Pseudomonas aeruginosa* to hamster tracheal epithelium. Infect Immun 47:723–729, 1985.

29. Franklin AL, Todd T, Gurman G, et al: Adherence of *Pseudomonas aeruginosa* to cilia of human tracheal epithelial cells. Infect Immun 55:1523–1525, 1987.

30. Boucher RC, Knowles MR, Stutts MJ, Gatz JT: Epithelial dysfunction in cystic fibrosis lung disease. Lung 161:1–17, 1983.

31. Quinton PM: Cystic fibrosis: A disease in electrolyte transport. FASEB J 4:2709–2717, 1990.

32. Knowles MR, Church NL, Waltner WE, et al: A pilot study of aerosolized amiloride for the treatment of lung disease in cystic fibrosis. N Engl J Med 322:1189–1194, 1990.

33. Ramphal R, Pyle M: Evidence for mucins and sialic acid as receptors for *Pseudomonas aeruginosa* in the lower respiratory tract. Infect Immun 41:339–344, 1983.

34. Ramphal R, Guay C, Pier GB: *Pseudomonas aeruginosa* adhesins for tracheobronchial mucin. Infect Immun 55:600–603, 1987.

35. Krivan HC, Roberts DD, Ginsburg V: Many pulmonary pathogenic bacteria bind specifically to the carbohydrate sequence GalNAcβ1–4Gal found in some glycolipids. Proc Natl Acad Sci USA 85:6157–6161, 1988.

36. O'Hanley P, Low D, Romero I, et al: Gal-Gal binding and hemolysin phenotypes and genotypes associated with uropathogenic *Escherichia coli*. N Engl J Med 313:414–420, 1985.

37. Abman SH, Reardon MC, Harbeck RJ, et al: Early bacteriologic, immunologic and clinical courses of young infants with cystic fibrosis identified by newborn screening. Pediatr Pulmonol 1(Suppl):124, 1987.

38. Abman SH, Ogle JW, Butler-Simon N, et al: Role of respiratory syncytial virus in early hospitalizations for respiratory distress of young infants with cystic fibrosis. J Pediatr 113:826–830, 1988.

39. Costerton JW, Lam J, Lam K, Chan R: The role of microcolony mode of growth in the pathogenesis of *Pseudomonas aeruginosa* infections. Rev Infect Dis 5:S867–S873, 1983.

40. Baltimore RS, Christie CD, Smith GJ: Immunohistopathologic localization of *Pseudomonas aeruginosa* in lungs from patients with cystic fibrosis. Am Rev Respir Dis 140:1650–1661, 1989.

41. Pedersen SS, Kharazmi A, Esperen F, Hoiby N: *Pseudomonas aeruginosa* alginate in cystic fibrosis sputum and the inflammatory response. Infect Immun 58:3363–3368, 1990.

42. Speert DP: Host defenses in patients with cystic fibrosis: Modulation by *Pseudomonas aeruginosa*. Surv Synth Pathol Res 4:14–33, 1985.

43. Pier GB: Pulmonary disease associated with *Pseudomonas aeruginosa* in cystic fibrosis: Current status of the host-bacterium interaction. J Infect Dis 151:575–580, 1985.

44. Vasil ML: *Pseudomonas aeruginosa*: Biology, mechanisms of virulence, epidemiology. J Pediatr 108:800–805, 1986.

45. Cole P, Wilson R. Host-microbial interrelationships in respiratory infection. Chest 95:217S–221S, 1989.

46. Fick RB, Hata JS: Pathogenetic mechanisms in lung diseases caused by *Pseudomonas aeruginosa*. Chest 95:206S–213S, 1989.

47. Hancock RE, Mutharia LM, Chan L, et al: *Pseudomonas aeruginosa* isolates from patients with cystic fibrosis: A class of serum-sensitive, nontypable strains deficient in lipopolysaccharide o-side chains. Infect Immun 42:170–177, 1983.

48. Penketh A, Pitt T, Roberts D, et al: The relationship of phenotype changes in *Pseudomonas aeruginosa* to the clinical condition of patients with cystic fibrosis. Am Rev Respir Dis 127:605–608, 1983.

49. Ojeniyi B, Back L, Hoiby N: Polyagglutinability due to loss of O-antigenic determinants in *Pseudomonas aeruginosa* strains isolated from cystic fibrosis patients. Acta Pathol Microbiol Immunol Scand [B]93:7–13, 1985.

50. Sokol PA, Woods DE: Relationship of iron and extracellular virulence factors to *Pseudomonas aeruginosa* lung infections. J Med Microbiol 18:125–133, 1984.

51. Sriyosachati S, Cox CD: Siderophore-mediated iron acquisition from transferrin by *Pseudomonas aeruginosa*. Infect Immun 52:885–891, 1986.

52. Anwar H, Brown MRW, Day A, Weller PH: Outer membrane antigens of mucoid *Pseudomonas aeruginosa* isolated directly from the sputum of a cystic fibrosis patient. FEMS Microbiol Lett 24:235–239, 1984.

53. Pollack M: The role of exotoxin A in *Pseudomonas* disease and immunity. Rev Infect Dis 5:S979–S984, 1983.

54. Doring G, Obernesser HJ, Botzenhart K, et al: Proteases of *Pseudomonas aeruginosa* in patients with cystic fibrosis. J Infect Dis 147:744–750, 1983.

55. Woods DE, Cryz SJ, Friedman RL, Iglewski BH: Contribution of toxin A and elastase to virulence of *Pseudomonas aeruginosa* in chronic lung infections of rats. Infect Immun 36:1223–1228, 1982.

56. Woods DE, Sokol PA: Use of transposon mutants to assess the role of exoenzyme S in chronic pulmonary disease due to *Pseudomonas aeruginosa*. Eur J Clin Microbiol 4:163–169, 1985.

57. Nicas TI, Frank DW, Stenzel P, et al: Role of exoenzyme S in chronic *Pseudomonas aeruginosa* lung infections. Eur J Clin Microbiol 4:175–179, 1985.

58. Doring G, Goldstein W, Roll A, et al: Role of *Pseudomonas aeruginosa* exoenzymes in lung infections of patients with cystic fibrosis. Infect Immun 49:557–562, 1985.

59. Luzar MA, Montie TC: Avirulence and altered physiological prop-

erties of cystic fibrosis strains of *Pseudomonas aeruginosa.* Infect Immun 50:572–576, 1985.

60. Schaffer MS, Sokol PA, Rabin HR, et al: Phenotypic comparison of *Pseudomonas aeruginosa* clinical isolates [abstract]. Presented at the annual meeting of the American Society of Microbiology, 1986.

61. Pier GB, Saunders JM, Ames P, et al: Opsonophagocytic killing antibody to *Pseudomonas aeruginosa* mucoid exopolysaccharide in older noncolonized patients with cystic fibrosis. N Engl J Med 317:793–798, 1987.

62. Pier GB, Small GJ, Warren HB: Protection against mucoid *Pseudomonas aeruginosa* in rodent models of endobronchial infections. Science 249:537–540, 1990.

63. Eichler I, Joris L, Hsu YP, et al: Nonopsonic antibodies in cystic fibrosis: *Pseudomonas aeruginosa* lipopolysaccharide-specific immunoglobulin G antibodies from infected patients' sera inhibit neutrophil oxidative responses. J Clin Invest 84:1794–1804, 1989.

64. Smith AL, Redding G, Doershuk C, et al: Sputum changes associated with therapy for endobronchial exacerbation in cystic fibrosis. J Pediatr 112:547–554, 1988.

65. Moss RB: Immunology of cystic fibrosis: Immunity, immunodeficiency, and hypersensitivity. *In* Lloyd-Still JD (ed): Textbook of Cystic Fibrosis, pp. 109–151. Boston: Wright-PSG Publishing, 1983.

66. Moss RB, Lewiston NJ: Immunopathology of cystic fibrosis. *In* Shapira E, Wilson GB (eds): Immunological Aspects of Cystic Fibrosis, pp. 5–27. Boca Raton, FL: CRC Press, 1984.

67. Sorensen RU, Ruuskanen O, Miller K, Stern RC: B-lymphocyte function in cystic fibrosis. Eur J Respir Dis 64:524–533, 1983.

68. Smith MJ, Morris L, Stead RJ, et al: Lymphocyte subpopulations and function in cystic fibrosis. Eur J Respir Dis 70:300–308, 1987.

69. Welsh MJ: Abnormal regulation of ion channels in cystic fibrosis epithelia. FASEB J 4:2718–2725, 1990.

70. Chen JH, Schulman H, Gardner P: A cAMP-regulated chloride channel in lymphocytes that is affected in cystic fibrosis. Science 243:657–660, 1989.

71. Bubien JK, Kirk KL, Rado TA, Frizzell RA: Cell cycle dependence of chloride permeability in normal and cystic fibrosis lymphocytes. Science 248:1416–1419, 1990.

72. Knutsen AP, Slavin RG, Roodman ST, et al: Decreased T helper cell function in patients with cystic fibrosis. Int Arch Allergy Appl Immunol 85:208–212, 1988.

73. Powderly WG, Schreiber JR, Pier GB, Markham RB: T cells recognizing polysaccharide-specific B cells function as contrasuppressor cells in the generation of T cell immunity to *Pseudomonas aeruginosa.* J Immunol 140:2746–2752, 1988.

74. Wheeler WB, Williams M, Matthews WJ, Colten HR: Progression of cystic fibrosis lung disease as a function of serum immunoglobulin G levels: A 5 year longitudinal study. J Pediatr 104:695–699, 1984.

75. Nutman J, Berger M, Chase PA, et al: Studies on the mechanism of T cell inhibition by the *Pseudomonas aeruginosa* phenazine pigment pyocyanine. J Immunol 138:3481–3487, 1987.

76. Moss RB, Hsu YP, Sullivan MM, Lewiston NJ: Altered antibody isotype in cystic fibrosis: Possible role in opsonic deficiency. Pediatr Res 20:453–459, 1986.

77. Moss RB, Hsu YP, Van Eede PH, et al: Altered antibody isotype in cystic fibrosis: Impaired natural antibody response to polysaccharide antigens. Pediatr Res 22:708–713, 1987.

78. Hollsing AE, Granstrom M, Strandvik B: Prospective study of serum staphylococcal antibodies in cystic fibrosis. Arch Dis Child 62:905–911, 1987.

79. Albus A, Fournier JM, Wolz C, et al: *Staphylococcus aureus* capsular types and antibody response to lung infection in patients with cystic fibrosis. J Clin Microbiol 26:2505–2509, 1988.

80. Hilman BC, Jamison RM, Kirkpatrick CJ: Reactivity and antibody response to vaccination with bivalent influenza A/Victoria/ 75-A/New Jersey 76 vaccines in children with chronic pulmonary diseases. J Infect Dis 136:S638–S644, 1977.

81. Matthews WJ, Williams M, Oliphint B, et al: Hypogammaglobulinemia in patients with cystic fibrosis. N Engl J Med 302:245–249, 1980.

82. Adlard P, Bryett K: Influenza immunization in children with cystic fibrosis. J Int Med Res 15:344–351, 1987.

83. Pennington JE, Reynolds HY, Wood RE, et al: Use of a *Pseudomonas aeruginosa* vaccine in patients with acute leukemia and cystic fibrosis. Am J Med 58:629–636, 1975.

84. Langford DT, Hiller J: Prospective, controlled study of a polyvalent *pseudomonas* vaccine in cystic fibrosis—Three year results. Arch Dis Child 59:1131–1134, 1984.

85. Wood RE, Pennington JE, Reynolds HY: Intranasal administration of a *Pseudomonas* lipopolysaccharide vaccine in cystic fibrosis patients. Pediatr Infect Dis 2:367–369, 1983.

86. Doring G, Hoiby N: Longitudinal study of immune response to *Pseudomonas aeruginosa* antigens in cystic fibrosis. Infect Immun 42:197–201, 1983.

87. Fomsgaard A, Hoiby N, Shand GH, et al: Longitudinal study of antibody response to lipopolysaccharides during chronic *Pseudomonas aeruginosa* lung infection in cystic fibrosis. Infect Immun 56:2770–2778, 1988.

88. Kubesch P, Von Specht BU, Tummler B: Immune response in cystic fibrosis to outer membrane proteins of *Pseudomonas aeruginosa.* Zentralbl Bakteriol Mikrobiol Hyg [A] 269:395–410, 1988.

89. Brett MM, Ghoneim AT, Littlewood JM: Serum IgG antibodies in patients with cystic fibrosis with early *Pseudomonas aeruginosa* infection. Arch Dis Child 62:357–361, 1987.

90. Brett MM, Ghoneim AT, Littlewood JM: Prediction and diagnosis of early *Pseudomonas aeruginosa* infection in cystic fibrosis: A follow-up study. J Clin Microbiol 26:1565–1570, 1988.

91. Shand GH, Pedersen SS, Tilling R, et al: Use of immunoblot detection of serum antibodies in the diagnosis of chronic *Pseudomonas aeruginosa* lung infection in cystic fibrosis. J Med Microbiol 27:169–177, 1988.

92. Moss RB, Hsu YP, Lewiston NJ, et al: Association of systemic immune complexes, complement activation, and antibodies to *Pseudomonas aeruginosa* lipopolysaccharide and exotoxin A with mortality in cystic fibrosis. Am Rev Respir Dis 133:648–652, 1986.

93. Przyklenk B, Bauernfeind A: Significance of immunologic factors in cystic fibrosis. Scand J Gastroenterol 143:103–109, 1988.

94. Fomsgaard A, Conrad RS, Galanos C, et al: Comparative immunochemistry of lipopolysaccharides from typable and polyagglutinable *Pseudomonas aeruginosa* strains isolated from patients with cystic fibrosis. J Clin Microbiol 26:821–826, 1988.

95. Cochrane DM, Brown MR, Weller PH: Lipopolysaccharide antigens produced by *Pseudomonas aeruginosa* from cystic fibrosis lung infection. FEMS Microbiol Lett 50:241–245, 1988.

96. Fomsgaard A, Freudenberg MA, Galanos C: Modification of the silver staining technique to detect lipopolysaccharide in polyacrylamide gels. J Clin Microbiol 28:2627–2631, 1990.

97. Van Wye JE, Collins MS, Baylor M, et al: *Pseudomonas* hyperimmune globulin passive immunotherapy for pulmonary exacerbations in cystic fibrosis. Pediatr Pulmonol 9:7–18, 1990.

98. Pedersen SS, Hoiby N, Shand GH, Pressler T: Antibody response to *Pseudomonas aeruginosa* antigens in cystic fibrosis. Antibiot Chemother 42:130–153, 1989.

99. Schiotz PO, Hoiby N, Permin H, Wiik A: IgA and IgG antibodies against surface antigens of *Pseudomonas aeruginosa* in sputum and serum from patients with cystic fibrosis. Acta Pathol Microbiol Scand [C] 87:229–233, 1979.

100. Brett MM, Ghoneim AT, Littlewood JM: An ELISA to detect antipseudomonal IgA antibodies in sera of patients with cystic fibrosis. J Clin Pathol 41:1130–1134, 1988.

101. Van Bever HP, Gigase PL, De Clerck LS, et al: Immune complexes and *Pseudomonas aeruginosa* antibodies in cystic fibrosis. Arch Dis Child 63:1222–1228, 1988.

102. Hollsing A, Granstrom M, Vasil ML, et al: Prospective study of serum antibodies to *Pseudomonas aeruginosa* exoproteins in cystic fibrosis. J Clin Microbiol 25:1868–1874, 1987.

103. Kubesch P, Lingner M, Grothues D, et al: Strategies of *Pseudomonas aeruginosa* to colonize and persist in the cystic fibrosis lung. Scand J Gastroenterol 143:77–80, 1988.

104. Granstom M, Ericsson A, Strandvik B, et al: Relation between antibody responses to *Pseudomonas aeruginosa* exoproteins and colonization/infection in patients with cystic fibrosis. Acta Paediatr Scand 73:772–777, 1984.

105. Klinger JD, Straus DC, Hilton CB, Bass JA: Antibodies to proteases and exotoxin A of *Pseudomonas aeruginosa* in patients with

cystic fibrosis: Demonstration by radioimmunoassay. J Infect Dis 138:49–58, 1978.

106. Dasgupta MK, Lam J, Doring G, et al: Prognostic implications of circulating immune complexes and *Pseudomonas aeruginosa*-specific antibodies in cystic fibrosis. J Clin Lab Immunol 23:25–30, 1987.

107. Moss RB: Hypergammaglobulinemia in cystic fibrosis: The role of *Pseudomonas* endobronchial infection. Chest 91:522–526, 1987.

108. Hoiby N, Hertz JB: Quantitative studies on immunologically specific and nonspecific absorption of *Pseudomonas aeruginosa* antibodies in serum from cystic fibrosis patients. Acta Pathol Microbiol Immunol Scand [C] 89:185–192, 1981.

109. Garzelli C, Campa M, Colizzi V, et al: Evidence for autoantibody production associated with polyclonal B-cell activation by *Pseudomonas aeruginosa*. Infect Immun 35:13–19, 1982.

110. Daley L, Pier GB, Liporace JD, Eardley DD: Polyclonal B cell stimulation and interleukin 1 induction by the mucoid exopolysaccharide of *Pseudomonas aeruginosa* associated with cystic fibrosis. J Immunol 134:3089–3093, 1985.

111. Calame KL: Mechanisms that regulate immunoglobulin gene expression. Annu Rev Immunol 3:159–195, 1985.

112. Moss RB, Hsu YP, Lewiston NJ: ^{125}I-C1q binding and specific antibodies as indicators of pulmonary disease activity in cystic fibrosis. J Pediatr 99:215–222, 1981.

113. Petersen NT, Hoiby N, Mordhorst CH, et al: Respiratory infections in cystic fibrosis patients caused by virus, chlamydia and mycoplasma—Possible synergism with *Pseudomonas aeruginosa*. Acta Paediatr Scand 70:623–628, 1981.

114. Thomassen MJ, Demko CA, Wood RE, et al: Ultrastructure and function of alveolar macrophages from cystic fibrosis patients. Pediatr Res 14:715–721, 1980.

115. Sordelli DO, Cassino RJ, Macri CN, et al: Phagocytosis of *Candida albicans* by alveolar macrophages from patients with cystic fibrosis. Clin Immunol Immunopathol 22:153–158, 1982.

116. Cichocki T, Litwin JA, Szotowa W, et al: Histochemical observations on the pulmonary macrophages in cystic fibrosis. Z Kinderheildk 116:127–136, 1974.

117. Cassino RJ, Sordelli DO, Macri CN, et al: Pulmonary nonspecific defense mechanisms in cystic fibrosis. I. Phagocytic capacity of alveolar macrophages and neutrophils. Pediatr Res 14:1212–1215, 1980.

118. Wilmott RW, Kassab JT, Kilian PL, et al: Increased levels of interleukin-1 in bronchoalveolar washings from children with bacterial infections. Am Rev Respir Dis 142:365–368, 1990.

119. Suter S, Schaad UB, Roux-Lombard P, et al: Relation between tumor necrosis factor-alpha and granulocyte elastase-α1-proteinase immune complexes in the plasma of patients with cystic fibrosis. Am Rev Respir Dis 140:1640–1644, 1989.

120. Thomassen MJ, Demko CA, Sorensen RU, et al: *Pseudomonas aeruginosa* phagoyctosis by normal human alveolar macrophages: Influence of in vitro activation on inhibitory effect of cystic fibrosis serum. CF Club Abstr 22:163, 1981.

121. Horvat RT, Parmely MJ: *Pseudomonas aeruginosa* alkaline protease degrades human gamma interferon and inhibits its bioactivity. Infect Immun 56:2925–2932, 1988.

122. Theander TG, Kharazmi A, Pedersen BK, et al: Inhibition of human lymphocyte proliferation and cleavage of interleukin-2 by *Pseudomonas aeruginosa* proteases. Infect Immun 56:1673–1677, 1988.

123. Lahat N, Rivlin J, Iancu TC: Functional immunoregulatory T-cell abnormalities in cystic fibrosis patients. J Clin Immunol 9:287–295, 1989.

124. Pollack M, Anderson SE Jr: Toxicity of *Pseudomonas aeruginosa* exotoxin A for human macrophages. Infect Immun 19:1092–6, 1978.

125. Cole P, Wilson R: Host-microbial interrelationships in respiratory infection. Chest 95:217S–221S, 1989.

126. Berger M: Inflammation in the lung in cystic fibrosis. *In* Moss RB (ed): Cystic Fibrosis: Infection, Immunopathology, and Host Response, pp. 119–142. Clifton, NJ: Humana Press, 1990.

127. Barton AD, Ryder K, Lourenco RV, et al: Inflammatory reaction and airway damage in cystic fibrosis. J Lab Clin Med 88:423–426, 1976.

128. Spock A, Lanning CF, Klystra JA, Bell D: Composition of lavage fluid from patients with cystic fibrosis. CF Club Abstr 20:85, 1979.

129. Aalberse RC, Van der Gaag R, Van Leeuwen J: Serologic aspects of IgG4 antibodies. I. Prolonged immunization results in an IgG4-restricted response. J Immunol 130:722–726, 1983.

130. Finkelman FD, Holmes J, Katona IM, et al: Lymphokine control of in vivo immunoglobulin isotype selection. Annu Rev Immunol 8:303–333, 1990.

131. Shakib F, Stanworth DR, Smalley CA, Brown GA: Elevated serum IgG4 levels in cystic fibrosis patients. Clin Allergy 6:237–240, 1976.

132. Maguire O, Tempany E: Comparison of IgG subclass levels in pediatric and adolescent CF patients. *In* Sturgess J (ed): Perspectives in Cystic Fibrosis, p. 26a. Toronto: Imperial Press, 1980.

133. Moss RB, Hsu YP, Leahy M, Halpern G: IgG4 antibody to *Pseudomonas aeruginosa* in cystic fibrosis. *In* Kerr JW, Ganderton MA (eds): Proceedings of Invited Symposia, XI International Congress of Allergology and Clinical Immunology, pp. 351–355. London: Macmillan, 1983.

134. Fick RB, Olchowski J, Squier SU, et al: Immunoglobulin G subclasses in cystic fibrosis. IgG2 response to *Pseudomonas aeruginosa* lipopolysaccharide. Am Rev Respir Dis 133:418–422, 1986.

135. Shryock TR, Molle JS, Klinger JD, Thomassen MJ: Association with phagocytic inhibition of anti-*Pseudomonas aeruginosa* immunoglobulin G antibody subclass levels in serum from patients with cystic fibrosis. J Clin Microbiol 23:513–516, 1986.

136. Pressler T, Mansa B, Jensen T, et al: Increased IgG2 and IgG3 concentration is associated with advanced *Pseudomonas aeruginosa* infection and poor pulmonary function in cystic fibrosis. Acta Paediatr Scand 77:576–582, 1988.

137. Moss RB, Joris L, Eichler I, et al: *Pseudomonas aeruginosa* endobronchial infection in cystic fibrosis induces nonopsonic IgG2 and IgG4 lipopolysaccharide-specific antibodies. Pediatr Res 25:185A, 1989.

138. Moss RB: Antibody and immune complex production in cystic fibrosis. Pediatr Pulmonol S1:95–98, 1987.

139. Moss RB: IgG subclasses in respiratory disorders: Cystic fibrosis. Monogr Allergy 19:202–209, 1986.

140. Moss RB: The role of IgG subclass antibodies in chronic infection: The case of cystic fibrosis. N Engl Reg Allergy Proc 9:57–61, 1988.

141. Hodson ME, Morris L, Batten JC: Serum immunoglobulin G subclasses in cystic fibrosis related to the clinical state of the patient. Eur Respir J 1:701–705, 1988.

142. Biggar WD, Holmes B, Good RA: Opsonic defect in patients with cystic fibrosis of the pancreas. Proc Natl Acad Sci USA 68:1716–1719, 1971.

143. Boxerbaum B, Kagumba A, Matthews LW: Selective inhibition of phagocytic activity of rabbit alveolar macrophages by cystic fibrosis serum. Am Rev Respir Dis 108:777–783, 1973.

144. Thomassen MJ, Boxerbaum B, Demko CA, et al: Inhibitory effect of cystic fibrosis serum on *Pseudomonas* phagocytosis by rabbit and human alveolar macrophages. Pediatr Res 13:1085–1088, 1979.

145. Fick RB, Naegel GP, Matthay RA, Reynolds HY: Cystic fibrosis *Pseudomonas* opsonins. Inhibitory nature in an *in vitro* phagocytic assay. J Clin Invest 68:899–914, 1981.

146. Winnie GB, Klinger JD, Sherman JM, Thomassen MJ: Induction of phagocytic inhibitory activity in cats with chronic *Pseudomonas aeruginosa* pulmonary infection. Infect Immun 38:1088–1093, 1982.

147. Shryock TR, Sherman JM, Klinger JD, Thomassen MJ: Phagocytic inhibitory activity in serum of cats immunized with *Pseudomonas aeruginosa* lipopolysaccharide. Curr Microbiol 12:91–96, 1985.

148. Hoiby N, Olling S: *Pseudomonas aeruginosa* infection in cystic fibrosis. Bactericidal effect of serum from normal individuals and patients with cystic fibrosis on *P. aeruginosa* strains from patients with cystic fibrosis or other diseases. Acta Pathol Microbiol Scand [C] 85:107–114, 1977.

149. Thomassen MJ, Demko CA: Serum bactericidal effect on *Pseudomonas aeruginosa* isolates from cystic fibrosis patients. Infect Immun 33:512–518, 1981.

150. Schiller NL, Millard RL: *Pseudomonas*-infected cystic fibrosis

patient sputum inhibits the bactericidal activity of normal human serum. Pediatr Res 17:747–52, 1983.

151. Thomassen MJ, Demko CA, Wood RE, Sherman JM: Phagocytosis of *Pseudomonas aeruginosa* by polymorphonuclear leukocytes and monocytes: Effect of cystic fibrosis serum. Infect Immun 38:802–805, 1982.

152. LeBlanc CM, Bortolussi R, Issekutz AC, Gillespie T: Opsonization of mucoid and non-mucoid *Pseudomonas aeruginosa* by serum from patients with cystic fibrosis assessed by a chemiluminescence assay. Clin Invest Med 5:125–128, 1982.

153. Hornick DB: Pulmonary host defense: Defects that lead to chronic inflammation of the airway. Clin Chest Med 9:669–678, 1988.

154. Holland EJ, Loren AB, Scott PJ, et al: Demonstration of neutrophil dysfunction in the serum of patients with cystic fibrosis. J Clin Lab Immunol 6:137–139, 1981.

155. Moss R, Hsu YP, Larrick J: Opsonization of *Pseudomonas aeruginosa* by human polyclonal, murine monoclonal, and cystic fibrosis-derived human monoclonal antibodies. CF Club Abstr 26:23, 1985.

156. Berger M, Norvell T, Tosi M, et al: Lack of complement receptor expression by alveolar macrophages correlates with poor enhancement of phagocytosis of *P. aeruginosa* by complement. Pediatr Res 27:154A, 1990.

157. Naegel GP, Young KR, Reynolds HY: Receptors for human IgG subclasses on human alveolar macrophages. Am Rev Respir Dis 129:413–418, 1984.

158. Unkeless JC, Scigliano E, Freedman V: Structure and function of human and murine receptors for IgG. Annu Rev Immunol 6:251–281, 1988.

159. Margolies R, Boat TR: The carbohydrate content of IgG from patients with cystic fibrosis. Pediatr Res 17:931–935, 1983.

160. Hornick DB, Squier SU, Fick RB: Altered immunochemistry of cystic fibrosis IgG and proteolysis by *Pseudomonas* elastase. Clin Res 34:934A, 1986.

161. Rademacher TW, Homans SW, Parekh RB, Dwek RA: Immunoglobulin G as a glycoprotein. Biochem Soc Symp 51:131–148, 1986.

162. Schoderbek WE, Fick RB: Importance of IgG2 Cγ2 carbohydrate in cellular bactericidal processes. Clin Res 35:489A, 1987.

163. Ogle JW, Janda JM, Woods DE, Vasil ML: Characterization and use of a DNA probe as an epidemiological marker for *Pseudomonas aeruginosa*. J Infect Dis 155:119–126, 1987.

164. Govan JR, Fyfe JA, Baker NR: Heterogeneity and reduction in pulmonary clearance of mucoid *Pseudomonas aeruginosa*. Rev Infect Dis 5:S874–S879, 1983.

165. Blackwood LL, Pennington JE: Influence of mucoid coating on clearance of *Pseudomonas aeruginosa* from lungs. Infect Immun 32:443–448, 1981.

166. Hornick DB, Fick RB: The immunoglobulin G subclass composition of immune complexes in cystic fibrosis. J Clin Invest 86:1285–1292, 1990.

167. Davis WB, Fells GA, Chernick MS, et al: A role for neutrophils in the derangements of the bronchial wall characteristic of cystic fibrosis. Am Rev Respir Dis 127(Suppl):207, 1983.

168. Kharazmi A, Schiotz PO, Hoiby N, et al: Demonstration of neutrophil chemotactic activity in the sputum of cystic fibrosis patients with *Pseudomonas aeruginosa* infection. Eur J Clin Invest 16:143–148, 1986.

169. Fick RB, Robbins RA, Squier SU, et al: Complement activation in cystic fibrosis respiratory fluids: *In vivo* and *in vitro* generation of C5a and chemotactic activity. Pediatr Res 20:1258–1268, 1986.

170. Cromwell O, Walport MJ, Morris HR, et al: Identification of leukotrienes D and B in sputum from cystic fibrosis patients. Lancet 2:164–165, 1981.

171. Martin TR, Altman LC, Albert RK, Henderson WR: Leukotriene B4 production by the human alveolar macrophage: A potential mechanism for amplifying inflammation in the lung. Am Rev Respir Dis 129:106–111, 1984.

172. Zakrzewski JT, Barnes NC, Costello JF, Piper PJ: Lipid mediators in cystic fibrosis and chronic obstructive pulmonary disease. Am Rev Respir Dis 136:779–782, 1987.

173. Movat HZ, Cybulsky MI, Colditz IG, et al: Acute inflammation in gram-negative infection: Endotoxin, interleukin 1, tumor necrosis factor, and neutrophils. Fed Proc 46:97–104, 1987.

174. Lieberman J, Kurnick NB: Proteolytic enzyme activity and the role of DNA in cystic fibrosis sputum. Pediatrics 31:1028–1032, 1963.

175. Shak S, Capon DJ, Hellmiss R, et al: Recombinant human DNase I reduces the viscosity of cystic fibrosis sputum. Proc Natl Acad Sci USA 87:9188–9192, 1990.

176. Anderson DC, Dombrowski M, Parrish D, et al: Pulmonary proteases target complement and IgG Fc receptors of neutrophils in cystic fibrosis. Pediatr Res 23:561A, 1988.

177. Berger M, Sorensen RU, Tosi MF, et al: Complement receptor expression on neutrophils at an inflammatory site, the *Pseudomonas*-infected lung in cystic fibrosis. J Clin Invest 84:1302–1313, 1989.

178. Tosi MF, Zakem H, Berger M: Neutrophil elastase cleaves C3bi on opsonized *Pseudomonas* as well as CR1 on neutrophils to create a functionally important opsonin receptor mismatch. J Clin Invest 86:300–308, 1990.

179. Miller KM, Dearborn DG, Sorensen RU: In vitro effect of synthetic pyocyanine on neutrophil superoxide production. Infect Immun 55:559–563, 1987.

180. Shryock TR, Silver SA, Banschbach MW, Kramer JC: Effect of *Pseudomonas aeruginosa* heat-stable hemolysin on neutrophil chemotaxis. CF Club Abstr 24:143, 1983.

181. Kharazmi A, Doring G, Hoiby N, Valerius NH: Interaction of *Pseudomonas aeruginosa* alkaline protease and elastase with human polymorphonuclear leukocytes in vitro. Infect Immun 43:161–165, 1984.

182. Kharazmi A, Hoiby N, Doring G, Valerius NH: *Pseudomonas aeruginosa* exoproteases inhibit human neutrophil chemiluminescence. Infect Immun 44:587–591, 1984.

183. Kharazmi A, Eriksen HO, Doring G, et al: Effect of *Pseudomonas aeruginosa* proteases on human leukocyte phagocytosis and bactericidal activity. Acta Pathol Microbiol Immunol Scand [C] 94:175–179, 1986.

184. Fick RB, Baltimore RS, Squier SU, Reynolds HY: IgG proteolytic activity of *Pseudomonas aeruginosa* in cystic fibrosis. J Infect Dis 151:589–598, 1985.

185. Fick RB, Squier SU: Biochemical definition of the synergism between *Pseudomonas* elastase, α1-protease inhibitor and neutrophil elastase. Clin Res 34:577A, 1986.

186. Fick RB, Naegel GP, Squier SU, et al: Proteins of the cystic fibrosis respiratory tract. Fragmented immunoglobulin G opsonic antibody causing defective opsonophagocytosis. J Clin Invest 74:236–248, 1984.

187. Suter S, Schaad UB, Roux L, et al: Granulocyte neutral proteases and *Pseudomonas* elastase as possible causes of airway damage in patients with cystic fibrosis. J Infect Dis 149:523–531, 1984.

188. Goldstein W, Doring G: Lysosomal enzymes from polymorphonuclear leukocytes and proteinase inhibitors in patients with cystic fibrosis. Am Rev Respir Dis 134:49–56, 1986.

189. Tournier JM, Jacquot J, Puchelle E, Bieth JG: Evidence that *Pseudomonas aeruginosa* elastase does not inactivate the bronchial inhibitor in the presence of leukocyte elastase. Am Rev Respir Dis 132:524–528, 1985.

190. Janoff A: Elastases and emphysema. Current assessment of the protease-antiprotease hypothesis. Am Rev Respir Dis 132:417–433, 1985.

191. Schiotz PO, Clemmensen I, Hoiby N: Immunoglobulins and albumin in sputum from patients with cystic fibrosis. A study of protein stability and presence of proteases. Acta Pathol Microbiol Immunol Scand [C] 88:275–280, 1980.

192. Jackson AH, Hill SL, Afford SC, Stockley RA: Sputum sol-phase proteins and elastase activity in patients with cystic fibrosis. Eur J Respir Dis 65:114–124, 1984.

193. Bruce MC, Poncz L, Klinger JD, et al: Biochemical and pathologic evidence for proteolytic destruction of lung connective tissue in cystic fibrosis. Am Rev Respir Dis 132:529–535, 1985.

194. Falloon J, Gallin JI: Neutrophil granules in health and disease. J Allergy Clin Immunol 77:653–662, 1986.

195. Gadek JE, Fells GA, Zimmerman RL, et al: Antielastases of the human alveolar structures: Implications for the protease-antiprotease theory of emphysema. J Clin Invest 68:889–898, 1981.

196. Tournier JM, Jacquot J, Puchelle E, et al: Elastase and proteinase inhibitors in sputum from patients with cystic fibrosis. Am Rev Respir Dis 127:207, 1983.

197. Suter S, Schaad UB, Tegner H, et al: Levels of free granulocyte elas-

tase in bronchial secretions from patients with cystic fibrosis: Effect of antimicrobial treatment against *Pseudomonas aeruginosa*. J Infect Dis 153:902–909, 1986.

198. Currie DC, Saverymuttu SH, Peters AM, et al: [111]Indium-labelled granulocyte accumulation in respiratory tract of patients with bronchiectasis. Lancet 1:1335–1339, 1987.

199. Hubbard RC, Fells G, Chernick M, et al: Aerosolization of α1-antitrypsin to establish a functional antineutrophil elastase defense of the respiratory epithelium in cystic fibrosis. Clin Res 38:485A, 1990.

200. Sponer M, Nick HP, Schnebli HP: Sensitivity of human elastase inhibitors to bacterial proteinases. Pediatr Pulmonol 5(Suppl):249–250, 1990.

201. Ward PA: Host defense mechanisms responsible for lung injury. J Allergy Clin Immunol 78:373–378, 1986.

202. Schwartz BA, Smith C, Clawson CC, et al: Altered lower respiratory tract environment in cystic fibrosis increases the potential for oxidant mediated injury by alveolar macrophages. Am Rev Respir Dis 129:A318, 1984.

203. Cantin A, Begin R: Chloride mediated oxidant synthesis in cystic fibrosis bronchial secretions. Am Rev Respir Dis 137(Suppl):301, 1988.

204. Mohammed JR, Mohammed BS, Pawluk LJ, et al: Purification and cytotoxic potential of myeloperoxidase in cystic fibrosis sputum. J Lab Clin Med 112:711–720, 1988.

205. Graft DF, Mischler E, Farrell PM, Busse WW: Granulocyte chemiluminescence in adolescent patients with cystic fibrosis. Am Rev Respir Dis 125:540–543, 1982.

206. Roberts RL, Stiehm ER: Increased phagocytic cell chemiluminescence in patients with cystic fibrosis. Am J Dis Child 143:944–950, 1989.

207. Bender JG, Florman AL, Van Epps DE: Correlation of serum opsonic activity in cystic fibrosis with colonization and disease state: Measurement of opsonins to *Pseudomonas aeruginosa* by neutrophil superoxide anion generation. Pediatr Res 22:383–388, 1987.

208. Auerbach HS, Williams M, Kirkpatrick JA, Colten HR: Alternate-day prednisone reduces morbidity and improves pulmonary function in cystic fibrosis. Lancet 2:686–688, 1985.

209. Sordelli DO, Cerquetti MC, El-Tawil G, et al: Ibuprofen modifies the inflammatory response of the murine lung to *Pseudomonas aeruginosa*. Eur J Respir Dis 67:118–127, 1985.

210. Konstan MW, Vargo KM, Davis PB: Ibuprofen attenuates the inflammatory response to *Pseudomonas aeruginosa* in a rat model of chronic pulmonary infection. Am Rev Respir Dis 141:186–192, 1990.

211. Hollsing AE, Lantz B, Bergstrom K, et al: Granulocyte elastase-α1-antiproteinase complex in cystic fibrosis: Sensitive plasma assay for monitoring pulmonary infections. J Pediatr 111:206–211, 1987.

212. McFarlane H, Holzel A, Brenchley P, et al: Immune complexes in cystic fibrosis. Br Med J 1:423–428, 1975.

213. Schiotz PO, Hoiby N, Juhl F, et al: Immune complexes in cystic fibrosis. Acta Pathol Microbiol Immunol Scand [C] 85:57–64, 1977.

214. Schiotz PO, Nielson H, Hoiby N, et al: Immune complexes in the sputum of patients with cystic fibrosis suffering from chronic *Pseudomonas aeruginosa* lung infection. Acta Pathol Microbiol Immunol Scand [C] 86:37–40, 1978.

215. Moss RB, Lewiston NJ: Immune complexes and humoral response to *Pseudomonas aeruginosa* in cystic fibrosis. Am Rev Respir Dis 121:23–29, 1980.

216. Berdischewsky M, Pollack M, Young LS, et al: Circulating immune complexes in cystic fibrosis. Pediatr Res 14:830–833, 1980.

217. Church JA, Jordan SC, Keens TG, Wang CI: Circulating immune complexes in patients with cystic fibrosis. Chest 80:405–411, 1981.

218. Manthei U, Taussig LM, Beckerman RC, Strunk RC: Circulating immune complexes in cystic fibrosis. Am Rev Respir Dis 126:253–257, 1982.

219. Pitcher-Wilmott RW, Levinsky RJ, Matthew DJ: Circulating soluble immune complexes containing *Pseudomonas* antigens in cystic fibrosis. Arch Dis Child 57:577–581, 1982.

220. Schiotz PO, Jorgensen M, Flensborg EW, et al: Chronic *Pseudo-*

monas aeruginosa lung infection in cystic fibrosis. Acta Pediatr Scand 72:283–287, 1983.

221. Wisnieski JJ, Todd EW, Fuller RK, et al: Immune complexes and complement abnormalities in patients with cystic fibrosis. Increased mortality associated with circulating immune complexes and decreased function of the alternative complement pathway. Am Rev Respir Dis 132:770–776, 1985.

222. Hodson ME, Beldon I, Batten JC: Circulating immune complexes in patients with cystic fibrosis in relation to clinical features. Clin Allergy 15:363–370, 1985.

223. Disis ML, McDonald TL, Colombo JL, et al: Circulating immune complexes in cystic fibrosis and their correlation to clinical parameters. Pediatr Res 20:385–390, 1986.

224. Dasgupta MK, Zuberbuhler P, Abbi A, et al: Combined evaluation of circulating immune complexes and antibodies to *Pseudomonas aeruginosa* as an immunologic profile in relation to pulmonary function in cystic fibrosis. J Clin Immunol 7:51–58, 1987.

225. Moss RB, Hsu YP: Pulmonary origin of immune complexes in cystic fibrosis. Am Rev Respir Dis 125(Suppl):59, 1982.

226. Moss RB, Hsu YP: Isolation and characterization of circulating immune complexes in cystic fibrosis. Clin Exp Immunol 47:301–308, 1982.

227. Doring G, Buhl V, Hoiby N, et al: Detection of proteases of *Pseudomonas aeruginosa* in immune complexes isolated from sputum of cystic fibrosis patients. Acta Pathol Microbiol Immunol Scand [C] 92:307–312, 1984.

228. Soter NA, Mihm MC, Colten HR: Cutaneous necrotizing venulitis in patients with cystic fibrosis. J Pediatr 95:197–201, 1979.

229. Abramowsky CR, Swinehart GL: The nephropathy of cystic fibrosis: A human model of chronic nephrotoxicity. Hum Pathol 13:934–939, 1982.

230. Davis CA, Abramowsky CR, Swinehart G: Circulating immune complexes and the nephropathy of cystic fibrosis. Hum Pathol 15:244–247, 1984.

231. Fick RB, Hornick DB, Huston DP: Immunopathologic description of acute arthritis in cystic fibrosis. Clin Res 35:562A, 1987.

232. Hoiby N, Schiotz PO: Immune complex mediated tissue damage in the lungs of cystic fibrosis patients with chronic *Pseudomonas aeruginosa* infection. Acta Paediatr Scand [Suppl] 301:63–73, 1982.

233. Lewiston NJ, Moss RB: Immune complexes in cystic fibrosis: Keys to new clinical insight. J Respir Dis 7:60–66, 1986.

234. Hoiby N. Doring G, Schiotz PO: Pathogenic mechanisms of chronic *Pseudomonas aeruginosa* infections in cystic fibrosis patients. Antibiot Chemother 39:60–76, 1987.

235. Mantzouranis E, Rosen FS, Colten HR: Reticuloendothelial clearance in cystic fibrosis and other inflammatory lung diseases. N Engl J Med 319:338–343, 1988.

236. Permin H, Skov PS, Norn S, et al: Platelet ^{3}H-serotonin releasing immune complexes induced by *Pseudomonas aeruginosa* in cystic fibrosis. Allergy 37:93–100, 1982.

237. Woods DE, Bryan LE: Studies on the ability of alginate to act as a protective immunogen against infection with *Pseudomonas aeruginosa* in animals. J Infect Dis 151:581–588, 1985.

238. Newman AJ, Ansell BM: Episodic arthritis in children with cystic fibrosis. J Pediatr 94:594–596, 1979.

239. Schidlow DV, Goldsmith DP, Palmer J, Huang NN: Arthritis in cystic fibrosis. Arch Dis Child 59:377–379, 1984.

240. Rush PJ, Shore A, Coblentz C, et al: The musculoskeletal manifestations of cystic fibrosis. Semin Arthritis Rheum 15:213–225, 1986.

241. Fradin MS, Kalb RE, Grossman ME: Recurrent cutaneous vasculitis in cystic fibrosis. Pediatr Dermatol 4:108–111, 1987.

242. Bourke S, Rooney M, Fitzgerald M, Bresnihan B: Episodic arthropathy in adult cystic fibrosis. Q J Med 264:651–659, 1987.

243. Dixey J, Redington AN, Butler RC, et al: The arthropathy of cystic fibrosis. Ann Rheum Dis 47:218–223, 1988.

244. Doring G, Goldstein W, Botzenhart K, et al: Elastase from polymorphonuclear leucocytes: A regulatory enzyme in immune complex disease. Clin Exp Immunol 64:597–605, 1986.

245. Lewiston NJ, Moss RB: Prolonged corticosteroid therapy in cystic fibrosis. CF Club Abstr 22:131, 1981.

246. Lewiston NJ, Moss RB: Circulating immune complexes decrease during corticosteroid therapy in cystic fibrosis. Pediatr Res 16:354A, 1982.

247. Lewiston NJ, Moss RB: Allergic phenomena in cystic fibrosis. *In* Shapira E, Wilson GB (eds): Immunological Aspects of Cystic Fibrosis, pp. 125–147. Boca Raton, FL: CRC Press, 1984.

248. Wilmott RW: The relationship between atopy and cystic fibrosis. *In* Moss RB (ed): Cystic Fibrosis: Infection, Immunopathology, and Host Response, pp. 29–46. Clifton, NJ: Humana Press, 1990.

249. Welliver RC, Sun M, Rinaldo D, Ogra PL: Respiratory syncytial virus-specific IgE responses following infection: Evidence for a predominantly mucosal response. Pediatr Res 19:420–424, 1985.

250. Welliver RC, Wong DT, Sun M, McCarthy N: Parainfluenza virus bronchiolitis. Epidemiology and pathogenesis. Am J Dis Child 140:34–40, 1986.

251. Berger M, Kirkpatrick CH, Goldsmith PK, Gallin JI: IgE antibodies to *Staphylococcus aureus* and *Candida albicans* in patients with the syndrome of hyperimmunoglobulin E and recurrent infections. J Immunol 125:2437–2443, 1980.

252. Greenberger PA: Allergic bronchopulmonary aspergillosis. J Allergy Clin Immunol 74:645–653, 1984.

253. Knutsen AP, Slavin RG: Allergic bronchopulmonary aspergillosis in patients with cystic fibrosis. *In* Moss RB (ed): Cystic Fibrosis: Infection, Immunopathology, and Host Response, pp. 103–118. Clifton, NJ: Humana Press, 1990.

254. Nelson LA, Callerame ML, Schwartz RH: Aspergillosis and atopy in cystic fibrosis. Am Rev Respir Dis 120:863–873, 1979.

255. Brueton MJ, Ormerod LP, Shah KP, Anderson CM: Allergic bronchopulmonary aspergillosis complicating cystic fibrosis in childhood. Arch Dis Child 55:348–353, 1980.

256. Voss MJ, Bush RK, Mischler EH, Peters ME: Association of allergic bronchopulmonary aspergillosis and cystic fibrosis. J Allergy Clin Immunol 69:539–546, 1982.

257. Laufer P, Fink JN, Bruns WT, et al: Allergic bronchopulmonary aspergillosis in cystic fibrosis. J Allergy Clin Immunol 73:44–48, 1984.

258. Schonheyder H, Jensen T, Hoiby N, Koch C: Clinical and serological survey of pulmonary aspergillosis in patients with cystic fibrosis. Int Arch Allergy Appl Immunol 85:472–477, 1988.

259. Maguire S, Moriarty P, Tempany E, Fitzgerald M: Unusual clustering of allergic bronchopulmonary aspergillosis in children with cystic fibrosis. Pediatrics 82:835–839, 1988.

260. Galant SP, Rucker RW, Groncy CE, et al: Incidence of serum antibodies to several *Aspergillus* species and to *Candida albicans* in cystic fibrosis. Am Rev Respir Dis 114:325–331, 1976.

261. Schonheyder H, Jensen T, Hoiby N, et al: Frequency of *Aspergillus fumigatus* isolates and antibodies to *Aspergillus* antigens in cystic fibrosis. Acta Pathol Microbiol Immunol Scand [B] 93:105–112, 1985.

262. Forsyth KD, Hohmann AW, Martin AJ, Bradley J: IgG antibodies to *Aspergillus fumigatus* in cystic fibrosis: A laboratory correlate of disease activity. Arch Dis Child 63:953–957, 1988.

263. Zeaske R, Bruns WT, Fink JN, et al: Immune responses to *Aspergillus* in cystic fibrosis. J Allergy Clin Immunol 82:73–77, 1988.

264. El-Dahr J, Fink R, Arruda L, et al: IgE and IgG antibody responses to *Aspergillus* in patients with cystic fibrosis. J Allergy Clin Immunol 83:212, 1989.

265. Hutcheson PS, Slavin RG, Rejent AJ: Variability in parameters of allergic bronchopulmonary aspergillosis in cystic fibrosis patients. J Allergy Clin Immunol 83:177, 1989.

266. Hutcheson PS, Jarmoc LM, Kodesch LM, et al: A longitudinal study of aspergillus sensitivity in cystic fibrosis patients. J Allergy Clin Immunol 79:262, 1989.

267. Slavin RG, Bedrossian CW, Hutcheson PS, et al: A pathologic study of allergic bronchopulmonary aspergillosis. J Allergy Clin Immunol 81:718–725, 1988.

268. Jarmoc LM, Maton MC, Hutcheson PS, et al: The immunopathology of cystic fibrosis with and without allergic bronchopulmonary aspergillosis. J Allergy Clin Immunol 81:185, 1988.

269. Knutsen AP, Slavin RG: In vitro T cell responses in patients with cystic fibrosis and allergic bronchopulmonary aspergillosis. J Lab Clin Med 113:428–435, 1989.

270. Knutsen AP, Mueller KR, Hutcheson PS, Slavin RG: T- and B-cell dysregulation of IgE synthesis in cystic fibrosis patients with allergic bronchopulmonary aspergillosis. Clin Immunol Immunopathol 55:129–138, 1990.

271. Shen J, Brackett R, Fischer T, et al: Specific *Pseudomonas* immunoglobulin E antibodies in sera of patients with cystic fibrosis. Infect Immun 32:967–968, 1981.

272. Cohen BA, Cropp GJ, Welliver RC: Salivary *Pseudomonas*-specific IgE in cystic fibrosis. Am Rev Respir Dis 137(Suppl):302, 1988.

273. Tee RD, Pepys J: Specific serum IgE antibodies to bacterial antigens in allergic lung disease. Clin Allergy 12:439–450, 1982.

274. Skov PS, Norn S, Schiotz PO, et al: *Pseudomonas aeruginosa* allergy in cystic fibrosis. Allergy 35:23–29, 1980.

275. Ackerman UL, Hadley KJ, Eigen H, Antony VB: Cystic fibrosis tracheobronchial effluent stimulates proliferation of lung fibroblasts in vitro. Chest 95:234S–236S, 1989.

276. Scott J, Higenbottam T, Hutter J, et al: Heart-lung transplantation for cystic fibrosis. Lancet 2:192–194, 1988.

277. Lewiston NJ, Starnes V, Theodore J: Heart-lung and lung transplantation for cystic fibrosis. *In* Moss RB (ed): Cystic Fibrosis: Infection, Immunopathology, and Host Response, pp. 231–247. Clifton, NJ: Humana Press, 1990.

278. Alton EW, Batten J, Hodson M, et al: Absence of electrochemical defect of cystic fibrosis in transplanted lung. Lancet 1:1026, 1987.

279. Quittell LM, Fiel SB, Schidlow DV, Cavarrocchi N: Transplanted lungs retain normal potential difference in cystic fibrosis. Am Rev Respir Dis 137(Suppl):302, 1988.

280. Drumm ML, Pope HA, Cliff WH, et al: Correction of the cystic fibrosis defect *in vitro* by retrovirus-mediated gene transfer. Cell 62:1227–1233, 1990.

281. Rich DP, Anderson MP, Gregory RJ, et al: Expression of cystic fibrosis transmembrane conductance regulator corrects defective chloride channel regulation in cystic fibrosis airway epithelial cells. Nature 347:358–363, 1990.

282. Wilson R, Pitt T, Taylor G, et al: Pyocyanin and 1-hydroxyphenazine produced by *Pseudomonas aeruginosa* inhibit the beating of human respiratory cilia in vitro. J Clin Invest 79:221–229, 1987.

283. Wilson R, Munro N, Hastie A, et al: *Pseudomonas aeruginosa* produces low molecular weight molecules that damage human respiratory epithelium *in vitro* and slow mucociliary transport in the guinea pig trachea *in vivo*. Chest 95:214S, 1989.

284. Hingley ST, Hastie AT, Kueppers F, et al: Ciliostatic factors from *Pseudomonas aeruginosa*. Chest 95:214S–215S, 1989.

285. Wilson R, Sykes DA, Watson D, et al: Measurement of *Pseudomonas aeruginosa* phenazine pigments in sputum and assessment of their contribution to sputum sol toxicity for respiratory epithelium. Infect Immun 56:2515–2517, 1988.

286. Stutts MJ, Schwab JH, Chen MG, et al: Effects of *Pseudomonas aeruginosa* on bronchial epithelial ion transport. Am Rev Respir Dis 134:17–21, 1986.

287. Sorensen RU, Klinger JD, Cash HA, et al: In vitro inhibition of lymphocyte proliferation by *Pseudomonas aeruginosa* phenazine pigments. Infect Immun 41:321–330, 1984.

288. Klinger JD, Tandler B, Liedtke CM, Boat TF: Proteinases of *Pseudomonas aeruginosa* evoke mucin release by tracheal epithelium. J Clin Invest 74:1669–1678, 1984.

289. Pedersen BK, Kharazmi A: Inhibition of human natural killer cell activity by *Pseudomonas aeruginosa* alkaline protease and elastase. Infect Immun 55:986–989, 1987.

290. Pedersen BK, Kharazmi A, Theander TG, et al: Selective modulation of the CD4 molecular complex by *Pseudomonas aeruginosa* alkaline protease and elastase. Scand J Immunol 26:91–94, 1987.

291. Doring G, Hadam MR: Selective alterations of lymphocyte surfaces by proteinases. Pediatr Pulmonol 2(Suppl):123, 1988.

292. Schultz DR, Miller KD: Elastase of *Pseudomonas aeruginosa*: Inactivation of complement components and complement-derived chemotactic and phagocytic factors. Infect Immun 10:128–135, 1974.

293. Morihara K, Tsuzuki H, Oda K: Protease and elastase of *Pseudomonas aeruginosa*: Inactivation of human plasma α1-proteinase inhibitor. Infect Immun 24:188–193, 1979.

294. Doring G, Obernesser HJ, Botzenhart K: Extracellular toxins of *Pseudomonas aeruginosa*. II. Effect of two proteases on human immunoglobulins IgG, IgA, and secretory IgA. Zentralbl Bakteriol [A] 249:89–98, 1981.

295. Jacquot J, Tournier JM, Puchelle E: In vitro evidence that human airway lysozyme is cleaved and inactivated by *Pseudomonas aeruginosa* elastase and not by human leukocyte elastase. Infect Immun 47:555–560, 1985.

296. Holt PS, Misfeldt ML: Variables which affect suppresion of the immune response induced by *Pseudomonas aeruginosa* exotoxin A. Infect Immun 52:96–100, 1986.

297. Scharmann W, Jacob F, Porstendorfer J: Cytotoxic action of leukocidin from *Pseudomonas aeruginosa* on human polymorphonuclear leukocytes. J Gen Microbiol 93:303–308, 1976.

298. Baltimore RS, Mitchell M: Immunologic investigations of mucoid strains of *Pseudomonas aeruginosa:* Comparison of susceptibility to opsonic antibody in mucoid and nonmucoid strains. J Infect Dis 141:238–247, 1980.

299. Vishwanath S, Ramphal R, Guay C, et al: Respiratory mucin inhibition of the opsonophagocytic killing of *Pseudomonas aeruginosa.* Infect Immun 56:2218–2222, 1988.

300. Young LS: Human immunity to *Pseudomonas aeruginosa.* II. Relationship between heat-stable opsonins and type-specific lipopolysaccharides. J Infect Dis 126:277–287, 1972.

301. Hancock RE, Mouat EC, Speert DP: Quantitation and identification of antibodies to outer-membrane proteins of *Pseudomonas aeruginosa* in sera of patients with cystic fibrosis. J Infect Dis 149:220–226, 1984.

302. Jacobson MA, Radolf JD, Young LS: Human IgG antibodies to *Pseudomonas aeruginosa* core lipopolysaccharide determinants are detected in chronic but not acute *Pseudomonas* infection. Scand J Infect Dis 19:649–660, 1987.

303. Pier GB, Matthews WJ, Eardley DD: Immunochemical characterization of the mucoid exopolysaccharide of *Pseudomonas aeruginosa.* J Infect Dis 147:494–503, 1983.

304. Bryan LE, Kureishi A, Rabin HR: Detection of antibodies to *Pseudomonas aeruginosa* alginate extracellular polysaccharide in animals and cystic fibrosis patients by enzyme-linked immunosorbent assay. J Clin Microbiol 18:276–282, 1983.

305. Speert DP, Lawton D, Mutharia LM: Antibody to *Pseudomonas aeruginosa* mucoid exopolysaccharide and to sodium alginate in cystic fibrosis serum. Pediatr Res 18:431–433, 1984.

306. Baltimore RS, Fick RB, Fino L: Antibody to multiple mucoid strains of *Pseudomonas aeruginosa* in patients with cystic fibrosis, measured by an enzyme-linked immunosorbent assay. Pediatr Res 20:1085–1090, 1986.

307. Jagger KS, Robinson DL, Franz MN, Warren RL: Detection by enzyme-linked immunosorbent assays of antibody specific for *Pseudomonas* proteases and exotoxin A in sera from cystic fibrosis patients. J Clin Microbiol 15:1054–1058, 1982.

308. Cukor G, Blacklow NR, Nowak NA, et al: Comparative analysis of serum antibody responses to *Pseudomonas aeruginosa* exotoxin A by cystic fibrosis and intensive care unit patients. J Clin Microbiol 18:457–462, 1983.

309. Steinbach SF, Lile J, Loh B, et al: Antibody response in cystic fibrosis to *Pseudomonas* exoenzyme S. CF Club Abstr 27:73, 1986.

310. Hoiby N, Hertz JB, Sompolinsky D: Antibody response in patients with *Pseudomonas aeruginosa* infection to a 'common antigen' from *P. aeruginosa* analysed by means of quantitative immunoelectrophoretic methods. Acta Pathol Microbiol Immunol Scand [C] 88:149–154, 1980.

311. Fernandes PB, Kim C, Cundy KR, Haung NN: Antibodies to cell envelope proteins of *Pseudomonas aeruginosa* in cystic fibrosis patients. Infect Immun 33:527–532, 1981.

72 UPPER RESPIRATORY TRACT DISEASE IN CYSTIC FIBROSIS

LINDA GAGE-WHITE, M.D.

Disease of the nose and paranasal sinuses dominates the upper respiratory problems of patients with cystic fibrosis (CF). This includes a high incidence of nasal polyposis and, in most patients, opacification of the maxillary, ethmoid, and sphenoid sinuses. CF can also cause delayed development of the frontal sinuses.[1] The ears are usually spared, despite the histologic similarity of middle ear mucosa and nasal mucosa.[2]

It is important to treat the upper respiratory disease as well as the pulmonary disease of patients with CF. Chronic nasal obstruction increases airway resistance, leads to mouth breathing, and may cause headaches. Chronic nasal infection can also serve as a nidus for pulmonary infection.[3]

CF has such a close association with the development of polyps and persistent sinus opacification in children that the presence of either in a child should suggest a search for CF.[4,5] The reported incidence of nasal polyposis in patients with CF varies from 6%[6–9] to 26%[10,11] in comparison with 0.5% in non-CF patients with atopy.[12] The onset of polyps in patients with CF before age 5 years is uncommon, although polyps are seen in patients as young as age 2 years.[11] The average age at which first-time polyp disease manifests is 8.5 to 10 years[4,13] (Table 72–1).

Table 72–1. AGE AT ONSET OF NASAL POLYPS IN CYSTIC FIBROSIS

Age (Years)	Total No. of Patients	Nasal Polyps No.	%
0–4	605	16	2.6
5–9	555	61	11.0
10–14	475	51	10.7
15–19	348	25	7.2
20–24	196	4	2.0
>25	87	0	0

Adapted from Stern RC, Boat TF, Wood RE, et al: Treatment and prognosis of nasal polyps in cystic fibrosis. Am J Dis Child 136:1067–1070, 1982. Copyright 1982, American Medical Association, used with permission of the publisher.

Ear diseases to which pediatric patients with CF are susceptible include acute otitis media, chronic otitis media, mastoiditis, cholesteatoma, and chronic eustachian tube dysfunction. The normal pediatric population has a 5% to 7% rate of conductive hearing loss and otitis media, usually resulting from eustachian tube dysfunction from involvement of the upper respiratory tract.[14] The reported incidence of serous otitis media in patients with CF ranges from 3%[6] to 13%;[15, 16] one patient in Cepero and colleagues' study[6] required tympanostomy tubes. Bak-Petersen and Larsen examined 111 patients; 35% had one or more episodes of acute otitis media, and none had chronic otitis media.[17] There was no correlation between the incidence of nasal polyps and otitis media.[17] Ralli and Gagliardi found that although 92% of patients with CF had significant nasal obstruction, only 18% had ear involvement.[16]

Although many patients with CF receive ototoxic drugs such as aminoglycosides (gentamicin or tobramycin) during hospitalization for treatment of acute exacerbations of chronic pulmonary disease, only 1 patient of 80 in one study had a sensorineural loss,[15] and 1 patient of 41 had a sensorineural loss in another study.[14] The mean hearing thresholds were better than 10 decibels in 80 randomly selected patients with CF.[15]

Several authors examined the association between allergy and polyps in CF patients. Caplin and co-workers[12] examined 3000 atopic patients with skin or respiratory allergy and found that only 0.5% had nasal polyps; however, among patients with aspirin allergy, there was a 95% incidence of nasal polyposis. In one study of patients with CF, the incidence of allergy was reported to be the same as in the general population without CF.[18] Neely and associates found no correlation between the presence of allergies and the presence of polyps in 93 patients with CF.[10]

Stern and colleagues[11] demonstrated a higher incidence of allergy in a group with CF and nasal polyps than in a group without polyps; however, allergy treatment with nasal steroids or hyposensitization did not seem to prevent recurrence.[11]

PATHOPHYSIOLOGY

The pathophysiology of nasal polyps is not well understood in patients with or without CF. Factors that are commonly considered as possible contributing causes of polyps include infection, allergy, immunologic factors, altered secretions, and abnormal cilia.[9, 19] Polyps do seem to regrow more quickly in the presence of poor nasal hygiene or infection (L. Gage-White, personal experience). A study of cilia in patients with CF showed normal beating action.[1] Abnormal mucus has also been reported[4] as well as abnormal properties of some glycoproteins in mucus from CF patients.[20] Sweat from CF patients has increased levels of sodium and chloride, in comparison with that from patients without CF.[21, 22] Altered ion transport in exocrine epithelial tissues has been demonstrated in CF with impairment of conductance of chloride ions.[23-25] Within the respiratory mucosa, the permeability of the apical epithelia to chloride is reduced.[26] The ion defect in CF is associated with alteration in the hydration of the periciliary fluid of respiratory mucus. Dehydration of respiratory mucus contributes to mucus stasis and obstruction of the sinus ostia in patients with CF, leading to the diminished clearance of secretions, inflammatory changes, and bacterial colonization and infection.

There is disagreement about whether the polyps removed from patients with CF are histologically unique. Tos and colleagues compared the histologic features of polyps from patients with CF with those of polyps from non-CF patients.[27] In blinded studies, it was impossible to distinguish the two groups. In 90% of CF polyps and 84% of others, there were fewer than 0.5 gland/sq mm. The glands were identical in shape, size, number, and architecture.[27]

However, Oppenheimer and Rosenstein, using special stains, concluded that polyps from allergic patients and patients with CF differ histologically. Although both had sparse hyperplastic glands and focal squamous metaplasia, the polyps from atopic patients had neutral-staining mucin and a thick basement membrane, whereas those from patients with CF had acidic mucins, a delicate basement membrane, and few eosinophils.[28] Magid and associates noted markedly increased amounts of granular substances and a decreased vascularity in CF polyps in comparison with normal nasal mucosa.[1] Singh and Hampaiah also noted eosinophilic staining material in the glandular ducts of polyps from patients with CF.[29] The glands in sinus mucosa from CF patients contain an excessive amount of eosinophilic substances.[30] Rulon and colleagues' work supported Heerup and Kettel's theory that inflammatory processes in the mucous membrane compress the vessels, leading to edema and stasis.[30]

Tos and Bak-Petersen,[31] using special stains, studied 54 temporal bones from a non-CF population for goblet cells. They noted in all age groups that there were more goblet cells at the pharyngeal end of the eustachian tube than at the tympanic end. Also there were fewer goblet cells in the middle ear in all age groups. This may explain why there is less ear disease than sinus disease in patients with CF, inasmuch as the middle ear and eustachian tube have less mucus to clear out than do the sinuses.

CLINICAL MANIFESTATIONS

Chronic rhinitis may develop in patients with CF, especially when anatomic abnormalities or polyps occlude the nasal passages. The most common organisms cultured from the noses and sinuses of pediatric patients without CF are *Haemophilus influenzae, Streptococcus pneumoniae,* and *Branhamella catarrhalis.*[11] In contrast, *Pseudomonas aeruginosa* and methicillin-resistant *Staphylococcus aureus* are the most common offenders in patients with CF.[11] Chronic rhinitis/sinusitis may be controlled through the use of nasal rinses and systemic antibiotics; sometimes surgery is needed for restoring normal airflow in patients with CF and nasal polyposis.

Symptoms of sinusitis and polyposis include nasal obstruction, persistent rhinorrhea, headache, and chronic pulmonary exacerbation. In the past, there was some reluctance to surgically treat chronic sinusitis or nasal polyps in patients with CF. Patients who are symptomatic should receive aggressive medical treatment and be evaluated for surgery if medical management fails. Improved diagnostic capabilities with computed tomographic (CT) scans and endoscopic rhinoscopy in addition to improved surgical techniques such as functional endoscopic sinus surgery have enabled surgeons to better manage the nasal and sinus diseases of patients with CF.

Radiography is rarely useful in diagnosing nasal or sinus disease in CF children because the maxillary, ethmoid, and sphenoid sinuses are well developed, but opaque, in 92%[7, 32] to 100%[10] of children over 8 months of age with CF. Adams and colleagues reported that in 99% of patients with CF, opacification of sinuses was visible on radiographs, but only 1% had clinical symptoms.[5] Cuyler and Monaghan reported opacity of one or more sinuses on CT examination in 100% of 10 children with CF, even when the nasal examination was negative.[33] In another study of 187 patients with CF, the sphenoid sinus was opaque in 86%, not pneumatized in 13%, and clear in only 1%.[8] One third of patients had opaque frontal sinuses, one third were too young to be expected to have normal pneumatization, and the remaining one third showed delayed pneumatization.[8] Initially, opacity of maxillary and ethmoid sinuses in patients with CF is secondary to retained, thickened secretions. Later, it may be secondary to polyps.[4] The secretions in both nose and sinuses tend to be thick and do not wash out easily.

TREATMENT

Indications for nasal or sinus surgery in patients with CF generally include nasal obstruction from polyps, bony anatomic abnormalities from expanding polyps, persistent rhinorrhea, and suspected compromise of pulmonary status from recurrent sinus infection.[11, 30] The decision to treat surgically must be based on symptoms because sinus radiographs are abnormal in more than 90% of patients with CF.[8]

Possible complications of sinus surgery in any patient include excessive bleeding, blindness, cerebrospinal fluid leakages, and central nervous system infections as well as pulmonary complications related to general anesthesia.

Additional operative complications such as postoperative pneumonia or atelectasis may be secondary to inspissated mucus plugs or chronic suppurative bronchitis. Some authors have recommended 2 to 5 days' preoperative admission for intravenous antibiotics directed toward endobronchial bacterial infection and chest physical therapy and bronchial drainage.[7] Others believe that an inpatient preoperative regimen is not necessary if the patient is stabilized and endobronchial infection is under control. One study, in which all patients were admitted 1 day before surgery, showed that only 2% of anticipated surgical procedures were delayed because of pulmonary complications.[13] In general, if the patient's pulmonary status is already optimal on an outpatient basis, same-day sur-

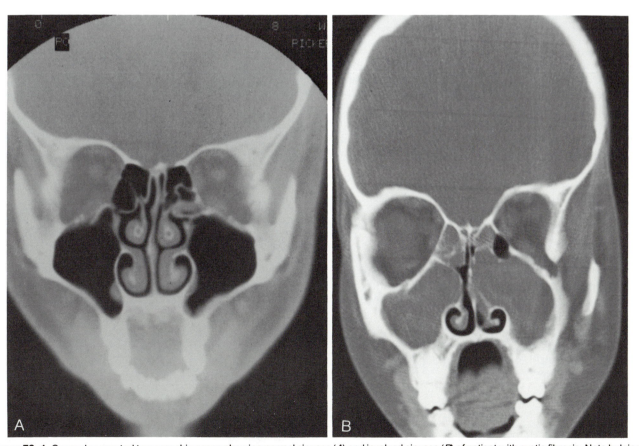

Figure 72–1. Coronal computed tomographic scans showing normal sinuses (A) and involved sinuses (B) of patient with cystic fibrosis. Note bulging of maxillary wall on left, touching septum.

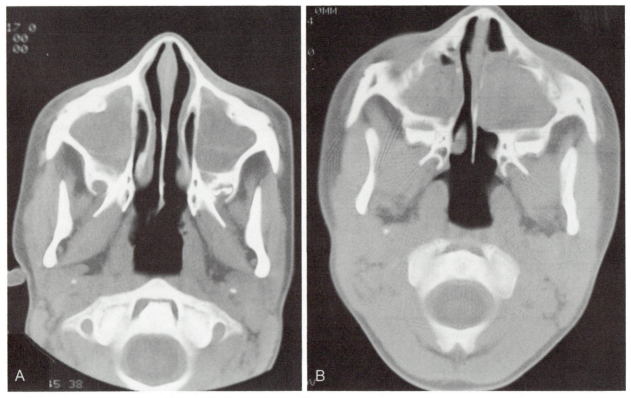

Figure 72–2. Axial computed tomographic scan showing involved maxillary sinuses without expansion (*A*) and complete filling of the maxillary sinus with bulging toward septum (*B*).

gery is possible. If the pulmonary status is not optimal, it must be improved a few days before surgery.

Many authors have agreed that the recurrence rate of nasal polyps is lower in patients with CF if more extensive surgery is performed concurrently with polypectomy, rather than only "plucking" operations, and have recommended a combined nasal-sinus procedure as the initial procedure of choice. Endoscopically controlled surgery permits safer and more thorough opening of the sinuses in patients with CF, with no additional bleeding or risk.[34] Recurrence rates vary from 87%[7] to 58%[13] for polypectomy alone and from 45%[7] to 16%[6] for polypectomy combined with an ethmoidectomy. Recurrence may be noted as early as 6 weeks postoperatively. Many patients require more than three procedures, and some require as many as ten.[11]

One of the most striking features observed at surgery on patients with CF is the large number of polyps pushing the middle turbinate against the septum and the thickened, mustard-like secretions that usually fill the maxillary sinuses (Figs. 72–1, 72–2). Culture of this material typically reveals *Pseudomonas aeruginosa*.

Postoperatively, 95% of patients with CF require nasal packing for control of hemorrhage. Patients are discharged on the day of pack removal.[13] The management team for the perioperative period should consist of a pulmonologist, a surgeon, and an anesthesiologist.[13]

The treatment of ear disease in patients with CF is the same as in non-CF patients. The criteria for insertion of ventilating tubes (i.e., persistent or recurrent middle ear infection) and for mastoidectomy (i.e., cholesteatoma or chronic drainage) are the same in all patients. The main difference in the management of ear disease in patients with CF is the need for scrupulous attendance to bronchopulmonary hygiene and control of endobronchial infection preoperatively and postoperatively.

Understanding the special problems and the physiologic characteristics of these patients increases the likelihood of a favorable outcome for CF patients with upper airway problems.

REFERENCES

1. Magid SL, Smith CC, Dolowitz DA: Nasal mucosa in pancreatic cystic fibrosis. Arch Otolaryngol 86:212–216, 1967.
2. Sade J: Pathology and pathogenesis of serous otitis media. Arch Otolaryngol 84:297–305, 1966.
3. Umetsu DT, Moss RB, King VV, et al: Sinus disease in patients with severe cystic fibrosis: Relation to pulmonary exacerbation. Lancet 335:1077–1078, 1990.
4. Berman JM, Colman BH: Nasal aspects of cystic fibrosis in children. J Laryngol Otol 91:133–139, 1977.
5. Adams GL, Hilger P, Warwick WJ: Cystic fibrosis. Arch Otolaryngol 106:127–132, 1980.
6. Cepero R, Smith RJ, Catlin FI, et al: Cystic fibrosis—An otolaryngologic perspective. Otolaryngol Head Neck Surg 97:356–360, 1987.
7. Jaffe BF, Strome M, Khaw KT, et al: Nasal polypectomy and sinus surgery for cystic fibrosis—A 10 year review. Otolaryngol Clin North Am 10:81–90, 1977.
8. Ledesma-Medina J, Osman MZ, Girdany BR: Abnormal paranasal sinuses in patients with cystic fibrosis of the pancreas—Radiological findings. Pediatr Radiol 9:61–64, 1980.
9. Shwachman H, Kulczycki LL, Mueller HL: Nasal polyps in patients with cystic fibrosis. Am J Dis Child 102:768–769, 1961.

10. Neely JG, Harrison GM, Jerger JF, et al: The otolaryngologic aspects of cystic fibrosis. Trans Am Acad Ophthalmol Otolaryngol 76:313–324, 1972.
11. Stern RC, Boat TF, Wood RE, et al: Treatment and prognosis of nasal polyps in cystic fibrosis. Am J Dis Child 136:1067–1070, 1982.
12. Caplin I, Haynes JT, Spahn J: Are nasal polyps an allergic phenomenon? Ann Allergy 29:631–634, 1971.
13. Reilly JS, Kenna MA, Stool SE, et al: Nasal surgery in children with cystic fibrosis: Complications and risk management. Laryngoscope 95:1491–1493, 1985.
14. Kulczycki LL, Butler JS, McCord-Dickman D, et al: The hearing of patients with cystic fibrosis. Arch Otolaryngol 92:54–59, 1970.
15. Forman-Franco B, Abramson AL, Gorvoy JD, et al: Cystic fibrosis and hearing loss. Arch Otolaryngol 105:338–342, 1979.
16. Ralli G, Gagliardi M: Functional rhinopharyngotubal study on patients affected with cystic fibrosis. Acta Otorhinolaryngol Belg 37:95–103, 1983.
17. Bak-Pedersen K, Larsen PK: Inflammatory middle ear diseases in patients with cystic fibrosis. Acta Otolaryngol 360(Suppl.):138–140, 1979.
18. Rachelefsky GS, Osher A, Dooley RE, et al: Coexistent respiratory allergy and cystic fibrosis. Am J Dis Child 128:355–359, 1974.
19. Samter M: Formation of nasal polyps. Arch Otolaryngol 73:334–341, 1961.
20. Lethem MI, James SL, Marriott C: The role of mucous glycoproteins in the rheologic properties of cystic fibrosis sputum. Am Rev Respir Dis 142:1053–1058, 1990.
21. Yankaskas JR, Stutts MJ, Cotton CU, et al: Cystic fibrosis airway epithelial cells in primary culture: Disease-specific ion transport abnormalities. Prog Clin Biol Res 254:139–149, 1987.
22. Darling RC, diSant'Agnese PA, Perera GA, et al: Electrolyte abnormalities of the sweat in fibrocystic disease of the pancreas. Am J Med Sci 225:67–70, 1953.
23. Quinton PM: Chloride impermeability in cystic fibrosis. Nature 301:421–422, 1983.
24. Boucher RC, Cotton CU, Gatzy JT, et al: Evidence for reduced Cl^- and increased Na^+ permeability in cystic fibrosis human primary cell cultures. J Physiol 405:77–103, 1988.
25. Quinton PM, Bijman J: Higher bioelectric potentials due to decreased chloride absorption in the sweat glands of patients with cystic fibrosis. N Engl J Med 308:1185–1189, 1983.
26. Knowles M, Gatzy J, Boucher R: Relative ion permeability of normal and cystic fibrosis nasal epithelium. J Clin Invest 71:1410–1417, 1983.
27. Tos M, Mogensen C, Thomsen J: Nasal polyps in cystic fibrosis. J Laryngol Otol 91:827–835, 1977.
28. Oppenheimer EH, Rosenstein BJ: Differential pathology of nasal polyps in cystic fibrosis and atopy. Lab Invest 40:445–449, 1979.
29. Singh K, Hampaiah M: Nasal polypi and fibro-cystic disease. J Laryngol Otol 85:185–188, 1971.
30. Rulon JT, Brown HA, Logan GB: Nasal polyps and cystic fibrosis of the pancreas. Arch Otolaryngol 78:192–199, 1963.
31. Tos M, Bak-Pedersen K: Goblet cell population and the normal middle ear and eustachian tube of children and adults. Ann Otol Rhinol Laryngol 85(Suppl 25):44–50, 1976.
32. Gharib R, Allen RP, Joos HA, et al: Paranasal sinuses in cystic fibrosis—incidence of roentgen abnormalities. Am J Dis Child 108:499–502, 1964.
33. Cuyler JP, Monaghan AJ: Cystic fibrosis and sinusitis. J Otolaryngol 18:173–75, 1989.
34. Duplechain JK, White JA, Miller RH: Pediatric sinusitis. Arch Otolaryngol 117:422–426, 1991.

VII Immunologic Disorders

73 ALLERGIC BRONCHOPULMONARY ASPERGILLOSIS

ROBERT W. WILMOTT, M.D. / RICHARD M. KRAVITZ, M.D.

Allergic bronchopulmonary aspergillosis (ABPA) is a relatively uncommon pulmonary disease in childhood, although it has been reported in children with cystic fibrosis (CF) from England[1] and several CF centers in the United States.[2, 3] Very few cases of ABPA have been reported in children with asthma, in contrast to adults, in whom it is a common complication.[4]

The mold *Aspergillus* is a ubiquitous saprophytic fungus, with a worldwide distribution that is commonly encountered in farmhouses, stables, barns, grain dusts, and decaying vegetable matter. Infection in humans has been reported from most countries, and disease is most commonly associated with infection with *Aspergillus fumigatus*.

A. fumigatus causes five types of disease in humans, according to the type of immune response associated with the infection. *A. fumigatus* may act as an allergen in children with allergic asthma or hay fever by invoking a type I immunoglobulin E– (IgE-) mediated response. It may produce invasive aspergillosis in immunodeficient children, such as those with chronic granulomatous disease, and cause disseminated infection. Children and, more commonly, adults with pulmonary cavities such as those caused by tuberculosis or a congenital pulmonary cyst may acquire a mycetoma if the cavity becomes colonized by *Aspergillus*. Such patients exhibit very high titers or precipitating antibodies (Table 73–1). Normal persons exposed to very high levels of *Aspergillus* spores in the air may acquire an allergic lung disease: extrinsic allergic alveolitis. This disease has been described for *A. fumigatus* and *A. clavatus* (maltworker's disease).

Patients with diseased airways may acquire colonization of the airway and then a hypersensitivity reaction to the mold with immunologic damage that results from a combination of type I and type III immune reactions.[5] This is the proposed mechanism for allergic bronchopulmonary aspergillosis.

INCIDENCE

ABPA occurs in both rural and urban environments. There appears to be a seasonal incidence that has been correlated with spore counts,[6] and it was suggested that an increase in spore counts may be conducive to the development of the disease. However, other studies of patients

Table 73–1. THE IMMUNOLOGIC FEATURES OF THE LUNG DISEASES ASSOCIATED WITH *ASPERGILLUS FUMIGATUS*

| Diseases | Skin Tests | | Bronchial Challenge | | Precipitins |
	Immediate (Prick)	Late (Intradermal)	Immediate	Late	
Commensal	−	−	−	−	−
Asthma	+	−	+	−	−
ABPA	+	+	+	+	+ (1–3 lines)
Mycetoma	±	±	−	−	+ + (3–8 lines)
Mycetoma and ABPA	+	+	+	+	+ + (3–8 lines)

Modified from Turner-Warwick M: Immunology of the lower respiratory tract. *In* Brostoff J (ed): Clinical Immunology—Allergy in Paediatric Medicine, pp. 163–176. Oxford, England: Blackwell, 1974.
ABPA, allergic bronchopulmonary aspergillosis. −, absent; ±, weak; +, present; + +, strong.

known to have ABPA have shown no significant differ-ence in the degree of spore exposure,[7] and studies of sugar cane workers have shown that only a small proportion of persons exposed to very high levels of *A. fumigatus* spores acquire the disease.[8] Thus it is difficult to conclude that the exposure to heavy concentrations of the spores has a strong relationship to the incidence of ABPA. Alterna-tively, there have been cases in which smoking marijuana contaminated with *A. fumigatus* appeared to be directly related to the development of ABPA, and in CF, it is the authors' impression that children in whom ABPA devel-ops tend to come from a rural setting with exposure to farm buildings or moldy vegetation. When ABPA was ini-tially recognized, the damp British climate was thought to explain an apparent discrepancy between the incidences in the United Kingdom and the United States.[9] This does not appear to be a valid assumption because many cases of ABPA have been diagnosed in the United States since 1970. A study of skin prick tests and precipitating anti-bodies showed no difference in results between a large asthma clinic in England and one in the United States.[10] Another study addressing the question of a difference in exposure between the United Kingdom and the United States showed that the mold counts in Cardiff, Wales, and in St. Louis, Missouri, were essentially the same.[11]

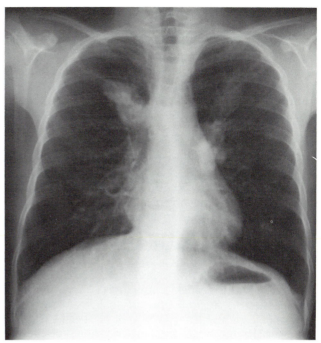

Figure 73–1. Chest radiograph from a 9-year-old girl with cystic fibrosis and allergic bronchopulmonary aspergillosis shows the typical changes of proximal bronchiectasis with mucoid impaction. (Courtesy of Donald R. Kirks, M.D.)

PATHOPHYSIOLOGY

Gross pathologic examination of ABPA reveals bron-chiectasis of the central airways with a typical cylindric configuration. These airways may become occluded by "mucoid impaction" or plugged by impacted mucus and hyphae (Fig. 73–1). Airway occlusion may lead to obstructive atelectasis of a segment or lobe and saccular bronchiectasis may develop in such lesions if atelectasis persists. The characteristic pattern of distribution in ABPA is that the disease is more severe in the upper lobes than in the lower lobes.

On microscopic examination, the airway walls show a heavy infiltration with plasma cells, lymphocytes, and eosinophils. The airway may also be occluded by mucus containing hyphal elements and inflammatory cells, par-ticularly eosinophils. The bronchial mucosa commonly undergoes squamous metaplasia, and sometimes a gran-ulomatous bronchitis is seen. Bronchiolitis obliterans and bronchocentric granulomatosis have been demonstrated in some patients.[12]

PATHOGENESIS

There is no clear consensus concerning the mecha-nisms of the lung disease in ABPA. However, it is appar-ent that both reaginic antibody (IgE) and precipitating antibodies (IgG) are involved. An important component of the disease is persistent colonization of the airway with *A. fumigatus* and failure to clear the organism. It is likely that a pre-existing airway abnormality predisposes the patient to ABPA, and this would explain the predilection of the disease for patients with asthma and CF. In ABPA, the disease process may begin with the inhalation and

trapping of the short chain spores of *A. fumigatus* in viscid secretions retained in the constricted airways, according to Slavin.[13] Slavin indicated that the size of the spores and the broad range of temperatures at which they grow make them well suited for colonization of the human bronchial tree. Once *A. fumigatus* has developed a foothold on the airway, it appears to persist and grow with constant shed-ding of antigens that stimulate the host's immune system. The antigens are of two main types: those that produce a strong precipitin reaction with a weak IgE response and those that produce a strong IgE reaction with a weak pre-cipitin response.[14]

The initial immune mechanism of ABPA is thought to be an IgE response to the mold that has colonized the air-way with the production of an allergic inflammatory response. This appears to lead to further sensitization of the patient with the production of increased titers of IgG.[13] These antibodies may form antigen-antibody com-plexes, resulting in stimulation of phagocytic cells and release of inflammatory mediators such as prostaglan-dins, leukotrienes, and lymphokines. These mediators, in turn, cause further accumulation of inflammatory cells that release lysosomal enzymes such as elastase with resul-tant damage to the airway.

It is likely that there is also a cellular contribution to the immunopathologic processes of ABPA. This is suggested by the presence of granulomas in pathologic specimens and the fact that patients have a positive lymphocyte pro-liferation response to the organism.[15] However, it is pos-sible to demonstrate this response only with whole blood; the same findings cannot be demonstrated with purified cells. To investigate whether there is a genetic contribu-tion to ABPA, human lymphocyte antigen (HLA) typing has been performed, and the results show no significant HLA linkage.[16]

The detailed pathogenesis of ABPA is only partially understood. Many immunologic mechanisms appear to be involved, and the primary abnormality is the failure to clear the mold from the airways that leads to a chain of immunologic reactions that result in permanent airway damage.

CLINICAL MANIFESTATIONS

The clinical criteria for the diagnosis of ABPA include (1) intermittent airflow obstruction, (2) transient pulmonary infiltrates, (3) sputum eosinophilia, (4) peripheral blood eosinophilia, (5) a positive immediate response to the skin prick test, (6) a positive delayed reaction to intradermal testing, (7) the presence of precipitating antibodies to *A. fumigatus,* (8) an increased serum IgE value, (9) proximal cylindric bronchiectasis, and (10) a positive specific reaction to *A. fumigatus* on an IgE antibody test (radioallergosorbent test [RAST]). It has been suggested that a certain number of these criteria should be present in order to establish the diagnosis of ABPA, but this approach is probably not valid for pediatric cases. In childhood, ABPA usually occurs in children with CF, in whom many of the criteria could be caused by CF itself.[3] In addition, it appears that children with CF may have ABPA and respond clinically to corticosteroids without having all the typical criteria. It is difficult to establish firm criteria for the diagnosis of ABPA in CF. The presence of a positive immediate wheal-and-flare reaction is not very specific, although it is a prerequisite for the diagnosis of ABPA. However, 25% of asthmatic patients and 35% of CF patients have positive immediate skin test reactions to *A. fumigatus.*[17] A survey of 75 CF patients showed that it was possible to recognize four groups. The first group (11%) fulfilled typical clinical and laboratory criteria for ABPA. The second group (13%) had typical criteria, except that the total IgE was in the normal range. It was suggested that this group might represent a clinical variant of ABPA. In the third group of patients (53%), there were no clinical criteria for ABPA, although there was evidence of immunologic sensitization such as positive skin tests or increased specific antibody levels. Seventeen patients (23%) had no evidence of an immunologic response of any type.[18]

In adults, ABPA is characterized by a history of asthma associated with fever, fatigue, increased expectoration of sputum that contains brown "plugs," increased wheezing, and new infiltrates on the chest radiograph. The disease usually affects young asthmatic adults; most cases occur before the age of 40 years. In pediatrics, the picture is complicated by the fact that ABPA rarely affects children with asthma and is most commonly seen in children with CF who may appear to have merely a worsening of their pulmonary status or a pulmonary exacerbation. However, there is a report of three children with asthma in whom ABPA developed before 2 years of age.[19] Physical examination reveals signs of chronic lung disease from CF or asthma, such as hyperaeration of the lungs, expiratory wheezing, a chronic productive cough, and rales. Chron-

ically ill patients may exhibit many coarse crackles, digital clubbing, and weight loss.

DIFFERENTIAL DIAGNOSIS

Several diseases can cause pulmonary infiltrates in children with asthma or CF. The most important considerations are consolidation caused by a pneumonic process, CF, asthma, and tuberculosis.

The differential diagnosis of ABPA should include the following:

- Bacterial pneumonia.
- Inhaled foreign body.
- CF (with or without ABPA).
- Immotile cilia syndrome.
- Tuberculosis.
- Severe asthma with mucoid impaction of the airways.
- Sarcoidosis.
- Pulmonary infiltrates with eosinophilia syndrome.
- Carcinoma (in adults).

CLINICAL STAGING

Five clinical stages have been described in patients with ABPA: acute stage, remission, recurrent exacerbation, corticosteroid-dependent asthma, and fibrosis (honeycomb lung).[20] Patients usually present with the acute stage and have many of the typical features of the disease. If they go into remission, the infiltrates clear, symptoms are reduced, and the IgE levels decline by up to 35% within 6 weeks. Exacerbations are associated with a recurrence of the initial symptoms and a twofold increase in serum IgE levels.

The next stage of ABPA is reached when patients need continuous corticosteroids to either control their asthma or prevent a recurrence of ABPA. In the fibrotic state, severe upper lobe fibrosis is visible on the chest radiograph, which may be associated with honeycombing. The lesions may not respond to corticosteroids, although patients may require steroids in order to maintain a bronchodilator response, and severe wheezing may develop if they are discontinued. Pulmonary fibrosis is a severe complication of ABPA and may result in pulmonary hypertension and cor pulmonale.

RADIOGRAPHIC FEATURES

Many characteristic radiographic changes are associated with CF and have been extensively reviewed by McCarthy and colleagues[21] (Table 73–2). The most common lesion is a large, homogeneous shadow in one of the upper lobes with no change in the positions of the fissures. The shadow may be triangular, lobar, or patchy and in many patients shifts to another site. Tram-line shadows are pairs of fine parallel lines radiating from the hila; they are thought to represent thickened airway walls from inflammatory edema. Another characteristic finding in

Table 73–2. THE RADIOGRAPHIC FEATURES OF ALLERGIC BRONCHOPULMONARY ASPERGILLOSIS

Homogeneous consolidation
  (patchy, segmental, triangular, or oblong)
Air-fluid levels in proximal bronchi
Tram-line shadows
  (two parallel hairline shadows radiating from a hilum)
"Toothpaste" shadows
  (secretions in ectatic bronchi)
Gloved-finger shadows
  (secretions in a dilated bronchus with an occluded blunt end)
Ring shadows
  (small, circular lesions representing bronchiectasis)
Atelectasis (segment, lobe, whole lung)
Contracted upper lobes with honeycomb lung
  (an advanced, irreversible lung disease)

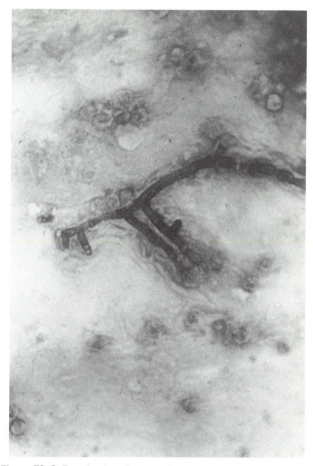

Figure 73–2. Examination of sputum from a child with unexplained infiltrates demonstrated the presence of fungal hyphae. The patient was subsequently found to have cystic fibrosis.

advanced cases is mucoid impaction, which is caused by impacted secretions in dilated bronchi (see Fig. 73–1). Other characteristic lesions include massive atelectasis and proximal bronchiectasis. However, several adult patients have been reported with normal chest radiographs,[22] and so radiographic abnormalities are not invariably present.

LABORATORY INVESTIGATION

Laboratory tests that support the diagnosis of ABPA are those that demonstrate a hypersensitivity reaction to the mold, such as a positive RAST test and the presence of *Aspergillus* precipitins. Precipitins are usually only weakly positive in comparison with the strong reactions seen in patients with a mycetoma. The culture of *A. fumigatus* from the sputum provides circumstantial evidence that a patient may have ABPA and may be one of the first clues to the diagnosis (Fig. 73–2). However, this is not a specific finding because some normal persons and many persons with other diseases have a small number of spores in the sputum, probably as a result of passive inhalation. The presence of hyphae in the sputum is much more suggestive of ABPA. In these cases, fungal elements are usually seen in association with large numbers of eosinophils.

The presence of sputum or peripheral blood eosinophilia is also suggestive of ABPA. The peripheral blood eosinophil count is usually higher than 1000/cu mm, and values higher than 3000/cu mm are common.

A very characteristic laboratory finding in ABPA is the increased serum IgE level. Very high values have been observed, sometimes reaching as high as 30,000 IU/ml. In children with ABPA as a complication of CF, the serum IgE value characteristically exceeds 800 IU/ml. Much of this IgE is not specific to *Aspergillus* but is instead the result of polyclonal B cell activation.[13] It has been proposed that the increase in IgE synthesis is caused by stimulation of helper T cells by factors elaborated by the organism or, alternatively, by specific inhibition of suppressor T cells.[23] Whatever the mechanism of the increased serum values, the IgE level is a very helpful marker of disease activity that can be used to observe outpatients for "flare-ups."[13]

Serum precipitins to *A. fumigatus* are often weakly pos-

itive in patients with ABPA. The usual pattern is that the immunoelectrophoresis shows one to three precipitin lines, sometimes to only one extract, whereas patients with an aspergilloma show high-titer, multiple-precipitin reactions to all antigen extracts. Standardization of the antigenic extracts has been difficult, but there has been some success with purification of the major antigenic components, which should lead to improved diagnosis.[24]

TREATMENT

Most cases of ABPA require treatment with systemic corticosteroids. The treatment of choice is oral prednisone,[25] although its mechanism of action is unclear. The simple explanation for its action is that the anti-inflammatory action of corticosteroids reduces the damaging host response. It is interesting, however, that steroids also seem to have a fungicidal effect with clearance of the mold from the sputum. The usual starting dose is 0.5 mg/kg/day, taken each morning, and this dose is maintained for 2 to 4 weeks while the chest radiographs are checked for resolution of the pulmonary infiltrates (Fig. 73–3). After this induction period, the dose should be reduced to 0.5 mg/kg given on alternate days for 3 months. The dose of prednisone should then be slowly tapered over a further 3

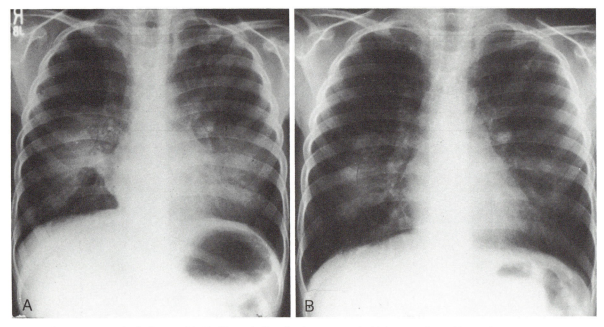

Figure 73–3. *A,* Chest radiograph of a 5-year-old girl with cystic fibrosis who presented with increased coughing and wheezing as a result of allergic bronchopulmonary aspergillosis. The radiograph showed new infiltrates in the right middle lobe and the lingula. *B,* Follow-up radiograph shows a significant reduction in the size of the infiltrates after 4 weeks of therapy with oral prednisone.

months while the chest radiographs and the serum IgE level are checked for evidence of a recurrence. The serum IgE level should be checked every 2 months initially, and if the level increases abruptly, daily steroids should be prescribed again. The patient should be observed over a long term for any recurrence with serial IgE levels and chest radiographs every 6 months. After 2 years, it should be possible to reduce the frequency of these investigations if the patient remains in remission. The efficacy of inhaled corticosteroids has been evaluated because the theoretical advantage of these drugs is reduced systemic absorption. Unfortunately, a trial of topical beclomethasone showed that it was not effective in preventing recurrences of ABPA in patients with asthma.[26]

Immunotherapy is not used in the treatment of ABPA because it has been associated with severe systemic reactions.[12] It has also been shown that cromoglycate and antifungal agents are ineffective therapies. Although the role of inhaled spores in the genesis of ABPA is unclear, it is reasonable to advise patients with ABPA to avoid exposure to barns, moldy basements, compost heaps, and stored grain.

PROGNOSIS

The prognosis for children with ABPA is good if the disease is detected early and treatment is started. It is important that a diagnosis is made before permanent changes in airway function and bronchiectasis have developed. According to results of studies on pulmonary function testing,[27] there should be no progression of the disease in such patients. However, relapses can occur many years later, and long-term follow-up is important. Symptoms

are not a reliable guide to therapy, and it is important to reevaluate the special studies at regular intervals until a long-term remission is firmly established.

REFERENCES

1. Mearns M, Longbottom J, Batten J: Precipitating antibodies to *Aspergillus fumigatus* in cystic fibrosis. Lancet 1:538–539, 1967.
2. Nelson L, Callerame ML, Schwartz R: Aspergillosis and atopy in cystic fibrosis. Am Rev Respir Dis 120:863–873, 1979.
3. Laufer P, Fink JN, Bruns T, et al: Allergic bronchopulmonary aspergillosis in cystic fibrosis. J Allergy Clin Immunol 73:44–48, 1984.
4. Henderson AH: Allergic aspergillosis: Review of 32 cases. Thorax 23:501–512, 1968.
5. McCarthy DS, Pepys J: Allergic broncho-pulmonary aspergillosis. Clin Allergy 1:415–432, 1971.
6. Radin RC, Greenberger PA, Patterson R, Ghory A: Mould counts and exacerbations of allergic bronchopulmonary aspergillosis. Clin Allergy 13:271–275, 1983.
7. Vernon DR, Allan DF: Environmental factors in allergic bronchopulmonary aspergillosis. Clin Allergy 10:217–227, 1980.
8. Mehta SK, Sandhu RS: Immunological significance of *Aspergillus fumigatus* in cane-sugar mills. Arch Environ Health 38:41–46, 1983.
9. Hinson KFW, Moon AJ, Plummar NS: Bronchopulmonary aspergillosis: A review and a report of eight new cases. Thorax 7:317–333, 1952.
10. Schwartz HJ, Citron KM, Chester EH, et al: A comparison of the prevalence of sensitization of aspergillus antigens among asthmatics in Cleveland and London. J Allergy Clin Immunol 62:9–14, 1978.
11. Mullins J, Hutcheson PS, Slavin RG: *Aspergillus fumigatus* spore concentrations in the United Kingdom and U.S.A. compared. Clin Allergy 14:351–354, 1984.
12. Ricketti AJ, Greenberger PA, Mintzer RA, Patterson R: Allergic bronchopulmonary aspergillosis. Arch Intern Med 143:1553–1557, 1983.
13. Slavin RG: Allergic bronchopulmonary aspergillosis. Clin Rev Allergy 3:167–182, 1985.

14. Longbottom JL: Allergic bronchopulmonary aspergillosis: Reactivity of IgE and IgG antibodies with antigenic components of *Aspergillus fumigatus* (IgE/IgG antigen complexes). J Allergy Clin Immunol 72:668–675, 1983.
15. Rosenberg M, Patterson R, Mintzer R, et al: Clinical and immunologic criteria for the diagnosis of allergic bronchopulmonary aspergillosis. Ann Intern Med 86:405–414, 1977.
16. Morris MJ, Faux JA, Ting A, et al: HLA-A, B and C and HLA-DR antigens in intrinsic and allergic asthma. Clin Allergy 10:173–179, 1980.
17. Pitcher-Wimott RW, Levinsky RJ, Gordon I, et al: Pseudomonas infection, allergy and cystic fibrosis. Arch Dis Child 57:582–586, 1982.
18. Zeaske R, Bruns WT, Fink JN, et al: Immune responses to Aspergillus in cystic fibrosis. J Allergy Clin Immunol 82:73–77, 1988.
19. Imbeau SA, Cohen M, Reed CE: Allergic bronchopulmonary aspergillosis in infants. Am J Dis Child 131:1127–1130, 1977.
20. Patterson R, Greenberger PA, Radin RC, Roberts M: Allergic bronchopulmonary aspergillosis: Staging as an aid to management. Ann Intern Med 96:286–291, 1982.
21. McCarthy DS, Simon G, Hargreave FE: The radiological appearances in allergic bronchopulmonary aspergillosis. Clin Radiol 21:366–375, 1970.
22. Rosenberg M, Mintzer R, Aaronson D, et al: Allergic bronchopulmonary aspergillosis in three patients with normal chest X-ray films. Chest 72:597–600, 1977.
23. Wang JL, Patterson R, Rosenberg M, et al: Serum IgE and IgG antibody activity against *Aspergillus fumigatus* as a diagnostic aid in allergic bronchopulmonary aspergillosis. Am Rev Respir Dis 117:917–927, 1978.
24. Pulmonary aspergillosis [Editorial]. Lancet 1:864–865, 1988.
25. Safirstein BH, D'Souza MF, Simon G, et al: Five-year follow-up of allergic bronchopulmonary aspergillosis. Am Rev Respir Dis 108:450–459, 1973.
26. Wang JL, Patterson R, Roberts M, Ghory AC: The management of allergic bronchopulmonary aspergillosis. Am Rev Respir Dis 120:87–92, 1979.
27. Nichols D, Dopico GA, Braun S, et al: Acute and chronic pulmonary functional changes in allergic bronchopulmonary aspergillosis. Am J Med 67:631–637, 1979.

74 CHRONIC GRANULOMATOUS DISEASE

DANIEL R. AMBRUSO, M.D. / RICHARD B. JOHNSTON, JR., M.D.

Chronic granulomatous disease (CGD) is a syndrome composed of a heterogeneous group of inherited disorders of phagocytic cells manifested by recurrent bacterial and fungal infections. Monocytes and neutrophils from patients with CGD ingest organisms normally but have defective oxidative metabolism that causes impaired intracellular microbicidal activity. This inability to kill phagocytosed microorganisms permits their sequestration and protection from extracellular killing mechanisms and antibiotics. Phagocytic cells die and release the organisms, causing further microbial proliferation and accumulation of phagocytes, leading to the abscesses and granulomas that characterize the disorder. Any organ can be infected, but significant morbidity and mortality follow pulmonary involvement. This chapter reviews the pathophysiologic processes, the clinical manifestations, and some aspects of the management of CGD, with emphasis on pulmonary complications.

PATHOPHYSIOLOGY

Phagocytosis by neutrophils, eosinophils, monocytes, and macrophages is accompanied by an extraordinary series of oxygen-related biochemical processes. Oxygen is pulled from the surrounding medium into the cell by the action of an enzyme and enzyme system termed nicotinamide adenine dinucleotide phosphate (NADPH) oxidase.[1] This oxygen is used, not in oxidative phosphorylation, but rather in formation of superoxide anion by the transfer of an electron from NADPH. Superoxide anion interacts in a rapid, spontaneous dismutation reaction to produce hydrogen peroxide (H_2O_2). These two oxygen products interact with other cell constituents, including iron and myeloperoxidase, to produce the highly reactive compounds such as hydroxyl radical hypochlorous acid and chloramines.[2-5] Phagocytosis is also associated with stimulation of glucose oxidation through the hexose monophosphate shunt, which results from accumulation of $NADP^+$ from activation of the glutathione peroxidase cycle by H_2O_2 and, probably, from the oxidation of NADPH by the initiating oxidase. Together, these events constitute the "respiratory burst." Accumulating evidence has shown that the initiating sequence of the respiratory burst is directed by an oxidase enzyme system consisting of more than one component. Constituents include cytochrome b_{558}, a flavoprotein, a quinone located in specific granules in resting cells[6-10] and cytosolic proteins, the NADPH binding protein, the p47-phox, the p67-phox, and guanine nucleotide-binding regulatory proteins.[11-14] Although it has not been completely defined, data from several studies suggest that this complex of enzymes or "respiratory chain" must be assembled by moving components from specific granules and cytosol to the plasma membrane.[8, 15]

A direct relationship between the bactericidal activity of phagocytic cells and this respiratory burst has been shown. This finding was also substantiated by the work of Klebanoff and Waltersdorph,[3] who showed that H_2O_2, myeloperoxidase, and halide ion constitute a potent microbicidal system (reviewed by Johnston[16]). Other killing systems have been described. Superoxide (O_2^-) and H_2O_2 are, by themselves, weakly bactericidal, but they can interact to form hydroxyl radical, a highly active oxidant, which may be required for efficient bactericidal activity.[2, 3] Other reactive chemical species produced in association with the respiratory burst have also been implicated in bactericidal activity, including hypochlorous acid and chloramines.[4, 5]

The importance of the respiratory burst in the physiologic processes of phagocytes has been proved by studies of neutrophils and monocytes from patients with CGD. Cells from these patients do not undergo the normal phagocytosis-associated oxygen consumption, stimulation of the hexose monophosphate shunt, nitroblue tetrazolium (NBT) dye reduction, chemiluminescence, or production of O_2^-. However, other aspects of phagocyte function are generally normal, including motility, binding of the particle to be phagocytosed, ingestion, and degranulation.[17]

It is clear that CGD represents a heterogeneous group of biochemical defects in function of the respiratory burst, and the multicomponent model for the oxidase apparatus allows a tentative classification with patients grouped according to various processes or components. The majority of patients have abnormalities in oxidase components. Patients in whom cytochrome b_{558} is missing or nonfunctional or who have decreased flavoprotein and cytochrome b_{558} have been described.[6, 7, 18–21] Because the cytochrome b_{558} is a heterodimer with subunits of 91 kD and 22 kD (gp91-phox and p22-phox), deficiency of this protein can be subclassified: the more common X-linked variant (gp91-phox deficient, Xb^0 variant) and the rare autosomal variant (p22-phox deficient, Ab^0 variant). Studies suggested the presence of both subunits, which is necessary for a stable protein; the absence of one subunit results in undetectable levels of the other.[22] Rare variants have been reported in which a defect in the 91-kD subunit results in a complete cytochrome b molecule which is detectable by spectroscopy but functions abnormally.[23] Other variants of cytochrome b_{558} may also exist.

Segal and colleagues first demonstrated that a group of patients with cytochrome b_{558}–positive CGD lacked phosphorylation of a 47-kD cytosolic protein.[24] Advances in development of assay systems that use subcellular fractions and that can evaluate the contributions of membrane-associated and cytosolic components have enabled investigators to further characterize these patients as having cytosolic cofactor deficiency but normal membrane contribution to the oxidase activity.[13] Subsequent studies defined the existence of two cytosolic proteins of 47 (p47-phox) and 67-kD (p67-phox) molecular weight, which are oxidase components. Although most autosomal, cytochrome b_{558}–positive (Ab^+) patients are missing p47-phox, a small number are deficient in p67-phox.[13]

Additional patients have an oxidase system that requires a remarkably high concentration of NADPH to function normally.[25–27] The relationship between cytochrome b_{558} flavoprotein and abnormal Km for the oxidase has not been completely defined, although there has been at least one case report of absent cytochrome b function and elevated levels of Km.

Deficiency of glucose-6-phosphate dehydrogenase (G6PD) in leukocytes, which occurs in some patients with erythrocyte deficiency, has been considered a variant of CGD. Patients with granulocyte G6PD levels of less than 1% suffer a slightly milder form of disease than most patients with CGD, but similar infections occur because of an inability to generate oxygen by-products. The defect is thought to result from deficiency of NADPH, which is needed as substrate for the initiating oxidase.[28] These patients also have hemolytic anemia.

Attention has been focused on the deficiency of Kx antigen in CGD.[29, 30] This antigen appears on both erythrocytes and leukocytes; on erythrocytes it is the precursor for the Kell blood group antigen. Synthesis of Kx on both cell lines is ordered by an X-linked gene. Some patients affected with the X-linked form of CGD do not have Kx antigen on their leukocytes, whereas Kx may or may not appear on their erythrocytes. Boys with CGD who lack Kx on their erythrocytes also have a hemolytic anemia. This could explain, at least in part, the anemia sometimes associated with CGD. Although this association of CGD and Kx antigen deficiency raised the possibility that absence of a membrane structure on neutrophils in CGD could be involved in their abnormal function, studies have suggested that expression of CGD and Kx antigen are controlled by two closely linked but distinct genes of the X chromosome.

Several aspects of metabolism of phagocytic cells have been found to be normal in patients with CGD and include changes in cyclic adenosine monophosphate (cAMP) after stimulation, activity of natural killer cells, arachidonic acid metabolism and production of leukotriene B_4, and changes in free cytosolic calcium after stimulation.[31–36] Alternatively, change in polarization across the plasma membrane after stimulation is abnormal in neutrophils from patients with CGD.[37, 38]

CLINICAL MANIFESTATIONS

Table 74–1 shows the relative frequencies of the most common signs and symptoms of CGD. Two patterns emerge from these findings. Involvement of the reticuloendothelial system is evident by the presence of purulent lymphadenitis, hepatomegaly, splenomegaly, and hepatic or perihepatic abscesses. The inability of neutrophils and monocytes to kill invading microorganisms leads to pneumonitis, infectious dermatitis, and perianal abscesses. Septicemia and meningitis may occur as a result of inability of both the reticuloendothelial system and circulating phagocytes to localize microbial invasion. The eczematoid or seborrheic dermatitis, diarrhea, rhi-

Table 74-1. MAJOR SIGNS AND SYMPTOMS IN 189 PATIENTS WITH CHRONIC GRANULOMATOUS DISEASE

Finding	Number of Patients Involved
Marked lymphadenopathy	156
Pneumonitis	151
Dermatitis	140
Onset by 1 year	127
Hepatomegaly	126
Suppuration of nodes	119
Splenomegaly	105
Hepatic-perihepatic abscess	80
Osteomyelitis	59
Onset with dermatitis	45
Onset with lymphadenitis	41
Facial dermatitis	39
Persistent diarrhea	38
Perianal abscess	35
Persistent rhinitis	33
Septicemia or meningitis	32
Ulcerative stomatitis	30
Conjunctivitis	29
Death from pneumonitis	27

From Johnston RB Jr: Biochemical defects of polymorphonuclear and mononuclear phagocytes associated with disease. *In* Sbarra AJ, Strauss RR (eds): The Reticuloendothelial System, vol. 2. New York: Plenum Press, 1980.

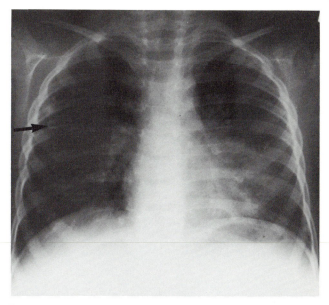

Figure 74-1. Consolidation of the left lingula. Note the calcifications *(arrow)* throughout the lung, presumably at sites of old, resolved granuloma.

nitis, and polyarthritis may represent a response to low-grade infection or microbial products. Esophagitis, narrowing of the gastric antrum, and cystitis are usually related to submucosal granulomas. Inflammatory renal complications are rare but have been reported.[39, 40] CGD has been seen in association with immunoglobulin A deficiency[41] and syndromes resembling lupus erythematosis.[42]

The onset of symptoms and signs usually occurs in infancy. Of the 160 patients whose ages at onset have been reported, 127 exhibited the first symptoms by 1 year of age and 145 by 2 years of age. Fifteen had evidence of disease within the first week of life. Of 60 deaths reported, 45 occurred before 7 years of age and 51 before 12 years. In rare instances, the initial diagnosis has been made in adulthood, and survival into the sixth decade has been noted. These cases may represent milder variants of the disease.[43] Although female carriers of X-linked CGD are usually asymptomatic, a number of reports have indicated that some carriers may exhibit a more severe defect in bactericidal activity and can have recurrent infections.[44–47]

PULMONARY COMPLICATIONS

Acute or chronic pulmonary infection is a prominent feature of chronic granulomatous disease. Not only is pneumonitis frequent and radiographic changes common, but also pulmonary disease is associated with significant mortality rates. Pulmonary disease was the primary cause of death in 31 of 53 deaths.[48] The onset of pulmonary infection may be heralded by the usual signs and symptoms: fever, cough, tachypnea, pleuritic pain, and abnormal auscultatory findings. However, in a sig-

nificant proportion of patients, few, if any, symptoms are reported in spite of extensive radiographic pulmonary infiltrates.[49]

Both pulmonary and other lesions of CGD are caused by intracellular survival and continued proliferation of phagocytosed bacteria with formation of abscesses and granulomas. Infections are prolonged in spite of prompt treatment with appropriate antibiotics, and they require prolonged antimicrobial therapy. Residual granulomas or calcifications may remain after resolution of the acute process.

Several patterns of pulmonary disease can be found in CGD.[49–53] Radiographic pulmonary findings include peribronchial, segmental, or lobar pneumonias (Fig. 74–1). These are usually associated with enlarged hilar nodes and sometimes with pleural thickening or empyema. The pneumonia can develop into an abscess that encapsulates and then undergoes necrosis and cavitation. These encapsulating pneumonias may assume a spherical form (Fig. 74–2). Hilar adenopathy tends to persist in spite of resolution of the original pneumonic processes. Infection may be diffuse as well as local, and multiple microabscesses can have a miliary appearance (Fig. 74–3). Diffuse interstitial fibrosis with honeycombing of the lung has been described.[54]

The microbial agents associated with pulmonary infections are the same as those that cause infections in other parts of the body. Of note is the increase in reported cases of pneumonitis resulting from *Aspergillus* species, *Nocardia* species, and *Pneumocystis carinii*.[55–63] Pulmonary aspergillosis may spread to involve pleura and adjacent soft tissues and bone; in one case it was associated with bronchial artery malformation. In a review of infections in 245 patients with CGD, 50 (20%) acquired fungal infection, of which 39 (78%) had documented *Aspergillus*

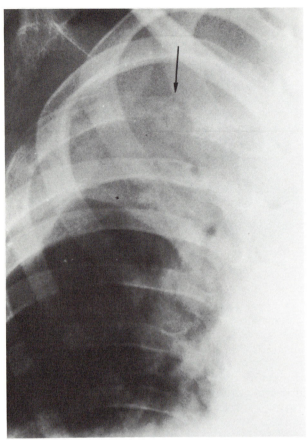

Figure 74–2. Several lung abscesses have undergone necrosis and cavitation and have given the appearance of encapsulating pneumonias in the left lung *(arrows)*. There is also a diffuse reticulonodular pattern throughout the lungs. (From Johnston RB Jr, McMurry JS: Chronic familial granulomatosis: Report of five cases and review of the literature. Am J Dis Child 114:370–378, 1967. Copyright 1967, American Medical Association, used with permission of the publisher.)

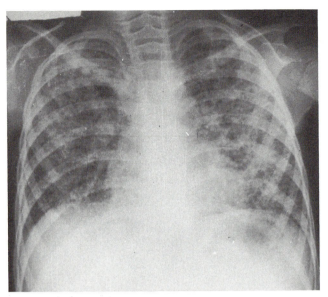

Figure 74–3. Diffuse reticulonodular infiltrates giving a miliary appearance. (Courtesy of Dr. Paul Quie, University of Minnesota.)

as the causative agent. Of patients with *Aspergillus,* 80% had pneumonia; 33% of those with pneumonia exhibited spread of infection to the chest wall.[58] Other agents reported in association with pneumonitis include *Acremonium strictum,*[64] *Candida albicans,*[58] and atypical and bacille Calmette-Guérin strains of mycobacteria.[65, 66]

LABORATORY FINDINGS AND PATHOLOGY

Except for the abnormal function of phagocytes and increased levels of immunoglobulins, all other studies of the immune system are generally normal. Other laboratory tests also reflect acute or chronic infection, including leukocytosis, an elevated erythrocyte sedimentation rate, and anemia. Although the anemia is that of chronic infection or inflammation, evidence of hemolytic anemia with acanthocytosis suggests absence of the Kx antigen as described previously. Radiologic manifestations of disease in organs other than the lung have been reviewed elsewhere.[51–53]

Information about infecting organisms has been reviewed in detail.[48] *Staphylococcus aureus* has been the

most frequently involved organism, followed by *Klebsiella-Aerobacter, Escherichia coli,* and other gram-negative enteric organisms.

Tissue specimens from infected sites show granulomas that are typical of those seen in infections resulting from intracellular parasites, such as mycobacteria or *Brucella* species. However, these granulomas often contain histiocytes that have a yellow or tan pigmented lipid material in their cytoplasm.[17]

A simple test for screening for CGD is the histochemical NBT test (reviewed by Johnston and co-authors[47]). Normal neutrophils that are stimulated reduce NBT, a yellow water-soluble dye in formazan, a purple insoluble substance. This reaction depends on the interaction between superoxide produced by the cell and the dye. More than 95% of neutrophils from normal adults and older children reduce the dye after appropriate stimulus (endotoxin or particulate stimulus). Stimulated neutrophils from patients with CGD do not reduce NBT, whereas carriers for this disease may show intermediate levels of reduction. Assessment by this test enables quantification of percentages of abnormal cells, which is important in screening affected patients as well as carriers.

Variations of this basic assay have been described.[47, 67] In addition, microassays for hexose monophosphate shunt activity and luminal amplified chemiluminescence have been described as screening assay for CGD.[68] Evaluation of erythrocyte G6PD would be helpful in ruling out the possibility of this enzyme deficiency as a cause of the disease. Bactericidal assays with staphylococci or *E. coli* are necessary for proving the diagnosis. Quantitative assays for the phagocytosis-associated respiratory burst such as measurement of hexose monophosphate shunt activity, superoxide anion, or H_2O_2 production are other tests that may be used to further evaluate a patient with suspected CGD.

Classification into one of the molecular variants can be accomplished with quantification of cytochrome b_{558} by spectroscopic technique. If adequate numbers of cells can be collected from a patient, preparation of subcellular fractions can be harvested, and determination of the plasma membrane and cytosolic contributions to oxidase activity may be completed. Further definition of cytosolic cofactors requires phosphorylation techniques on immunoblotting with specific antibodies (reviewed by Clark and colleagues[13]).

Prenatal diagnosis of CGD is possible by performing NBT slide test or chemiluminescence on fetal blood obtained by fetoscopy.[69, 70] Although a less invasive technique of measuring NBT dye reduction by fetal amniocytes was described,[71] it was not confirmed by a subsequent study.[70]

MANAGEMENT

In spite of increased understanding of the molecular defect in CGD, specific therapy to reverse the abnormality is still not available, and vigorous, supportive therapy is the basis for management of patients with the disease.[72] This approach begins with aggressive attempts at obtaining material for culture from localized areas of infection. Removal of an infected node or even lung biopsy may be warranted. Prolonged treatment with antibiotics specific for the infecting organisms is important, and treatment may be necessary for months in order to eliminate sequestered microorganisms. Aggressive surgical intervention of localized infected areas can be therapeutic as well as diagnostic. At surgery, the infected site should be aggressively debrided with prolonged drainage to prevent loculation and sequestration of infected areas. In patients with fever but no definite focus for infection, an empiric trial of antibiotics for several days may be necessary, during which time aggressive attempts to identify an infected site (including chest radiographs, ultrasonography of the liver, liver and bone scans, and other radionucleotide scans) should be performed. Gallium scans were helpful in localizing infection in three patients with CGD in whom other techniques failed to localize the infection.[73] Postural drainage may be helpful in patients with persistent lung disease. Careful blood typing at the time of diagnosis should identify those patients with McCloud's phenotype and the absence of Kx antigen on white cells and helps in avoiding alloimmunization.

Several approaches to the long-term therapy of CGD have been tried with variable success (reviewed by Johnston[72]). Prolonged administration of antistaphylococcal drugs or sulfonamides has decreased the frequency of infections.[74-77] Several in vitro studies have documented an increase in intracellular levels of antibiotics in neutrophils beyond plasma levels achieved by these drugs in association with enhanced killing of S. aureus. The drugs that show this effect include trimethoprim-sulfamethoxazole, rifampin, clindamycin, methicillin, and gentamicin.[78-83] The exact mechanism of action for enhanced killing by these antibiotics is not known, but in one study with trimethoprim-sulfamethoxazole, changes in bacterial killing were not associated with inhibition of bacterial catalase, enhanced oxidative metabolism, or synergism with nonoxidative mechanisms of bactericidal activity.[79]

Bone marrow transplantation with human lymphocyte antigen–identical siblings has been described as a hopeful solution for CGD. However, in early summaries of five patients who underwent transplantation, two had partial to complete correction of neutrophil abnormalities, and one of the five has survived without significant, durable neutrophil engraftment.[84, 85] Although several uncontrolled studies of granulocyte transfusions in severe infections have not demonstrated clear-cut efficacy over aggressive conventional therapy as noted previously, individual patients may benefit from granulocyte transfusions. It appears that such therapy should be reserved for specific clinical settings, including failure of aggressive, conventional medical and surgical therapy and rapidly progressing, life-threatening generalized infections. Granulocytes collected by standard techniques[86] should be given at a dose of 1×10^9 granulocytes per kilogram of body weight. It may be necessary to repeat the transfusions over a period of days to weeks in order to support resolution of the infection. Results of in vitro trials in selected patients suggested that human recombinant interferon (INF-γ) could reverse the defect in CGD.[87] In a large double-blind, placebo-controlled trial of INF-γ, no significant changes in functional or biochemical characteristics of neutrophils were noted, but the treatment group experienced a 70% decrease in serious infections in comparison with the patients given placebo.[88] INF-γ thus represents another management strategy for patients with CGD.

REFERENCES

1. Babior MB: Oxidants from phagocytes: Agents of defense and destruction. Blood 64:959–966, 1984.
2. Ambruso DR, Johnston RB Jr: Lactoferrin enhances hydroxyl production by human neutrophils, neutrophil particulate fractions, and an enzymatic generating system. J Clin Invest 67:352–360, 1981.
3. Klebanoff SJ, Waltersdorph AM: Pro oxidant activity of transferrin and lactoferrin. J Exp Med 172:1293–1303, 1990.
4. Weiss SJ, Klein R, Slivka A, Wei M: Chlorination of taurine by human neutrophils: Evidence of hypochlorous acid generation. J Clin Invest 70:598–607, 1982.
5. Weiss SJ, Lampert MB, Test ST: Long-lived oxidants generated by human neutrophils: Characterization and bioactivity. Science 222:625–628, 1983.
6. Gabig TG, Lefker BA: Deficient flavoprotein component of the NADPH-dependent O_2 generating oxidase in the neutrophils from three male patients with chronic granulomatous disease. J Clin Invest 73:701–705, 1984.
7. Borregaard N, Cross AR, Herlin T, et al: A variant of X-linked chronic granulomatous disease in normal nitroblue tetrazolium slide test and cytochrome b. Eur J Clin Invest 13:243–247, 1983.
8. Tauber AI, Borregaard N, Simons E, Wright J: Chronic granulomatous disease: A syndrome of phagocyte oxidase deficiencies. Medicine 62:286–309, 1983.
9. Cross AR, Jones OT, Garcia R, Segal AW: The association of FAD with cytochrome b-245 of human neutrophils. Biochem J 208:759–763, 1982.
10. Cross AR, Jones OT, Harper AM, Segal AW: Oxidation-reduction properties of the cytochrome b found in plasma membrane fraction of human neutrophils: A possible oxidase in the respiratory burst. Biochem J 194:599–606, 1981.
11. Bellavite P: The superoxide-forming enzymatic system of phagocytes. Free Radic Biol Med 4(4):225–261, 1988.
12. Babior BM: The respiratory burst oxidase. Hematol Oncol Clin North Am 2(2):201–212, 1988.
13. Clark RA, Malech HL, Gallin JI, et al: Genetic variants of CGD:

Prevalence of deficiencies of two cytosolic components of the NADPH oxidase system. N Engl J Med 321:647–652, 1989.

14. Smith RM, Curnutte JT: Molecular basis of chronic granulomatous disease. Blood 77:673–686, 1991.

15. Ambruso DR, Bolscher BG, Stokman PM, et al: Assembly and activation of the NADPH: O_2 oxidoreductase in human neutrophils after stimulation with phorbol myristate acetate. J Biol Chem 265:924–930, 1990.

16. Johnston RB Jr: Oxygen metabolism and the microbicidal activity of macrophages. Fed Proc 37:2759–2764, 1978.

17. Johnston RB Jr, Newman SL: Chronic granulomatous disease. Pediatr Clin North Am 24:365–376, 1977.

18. Segal AW, Jones OT, Webster D, Allison AC: Absence of newly described cytochrome b from neutrophils of patients with chronic granulomatous disease. Lancet 2:446–449, 1978.

19. Borregaard N, Johansen KS, Taudorff E, Wandall JH: Cytochrome b is present in neutrophils from patients with chronic granulomatous disease. Lancet 1:949–951, 1979.

20. Gabig TG: The NADPH-dependent O_2^- generating oxidase from human neutrophils. J Biol Chem 258:6352–6356, 1983.

21. Segal AW, Cross AR, Garcia RC, et al: Absence of cytochrome b-245 in chronic granulomatous disease. N Engl J Med 308:245–251, 1983.

22. Parkos CA, Dinauer MC, Walker LE, et al: Primary structure and unique expression of the 22-kilodalton light chain of human neutrophil cytochrome b. Proc Natl Acad Sci USA 85:3319–3323, 1988.

23. Dinauer MC, Curnutte JT, Rosen H, Orkin SH: A missense mutation in the neutrophil cytochrome b heavy chain in cytochrome positive x-linked chronic granulomatous disease. J Clin Invest 84(6):2012–2016, 1989.

24. Segal AW, Heyworth PG, Cockcroft S, Barrowman MM: Stimulated neutrophils from patients with autosomal recessive chronic granulomatous disease fail to phosphorylate an M_r-44,000 protein. Nature 316(6048):547–549, 1985.

25. Lew PD, Southwick FS, Stossel TP, et al: A variant of chronic granulomatous disease: Deficient oxidative metabolism due to a low affinity NADPH oxidase. N Engl J Med 305:1329–1333, 1981.

26. Shurin SB, Cohen HJ, Whitin JC, Newburger PE: Impaired granulocyte superoxide production and prolongation of the respiratory burst due to a low affinity NADPH-dependent oxidase. Blood 62:564–571, 1983.

27. Seger RA, Tiefenauer L, Matsunaga T, et al: Chronic granulomatous disease due to granulocytes with abnormal NADPH oxidase activity and deficient cytochrome b. Blood 61:423–428, 1983.

28. Baehner RL, Johnston RB Jr, Nathan DG: Comparative study of the metabolic and bactericidal characteristics of severely glucose-G-phosphate dehydrogenase deficient polymorphonuclear leukocytes and leukocytes from children with chronic granulomatous disease. J Reticuloendothel Soc 12:150–162, 1974.

29. Marsh WL: The Kell blood group, Kx antigen, and chronic granulomatous disease. Mayo Clin Proc 52:150–152, 1977.

30. Densen P, Wilkinson-Kroovand S, Mandell GL, et al: Kx: Its relationship to chronic granulomatous disease and genetic linkage with Xg. Blood 58:34–37, 1981.

31. Feinmark SJ, Uden A, Palmblad J, Malmsten C: Leukotriene biosynthesis by polymorphonuclear leukocytes from two patients with chronic granulomatous disease. J Clin Invest 72:1839–1843, 1983.

32. Henderson WR, Klebanoff SJ: Leukotriene production and inactivation by normal, chronic granulomatous disease and myeloperoxidase deficient neutrophils. J Biol Chem 258:13522–13527, 1983.

33. Herlin T, Borregaard N: Early changes in cyclic AMP and calcium efflux during phagocytosis by neutrophils from normals and patients with chronic granulomatous disease. Immunology 48:17–26, 1983.

34. Kay HD, Smith DL, Sullivan G, et al: Evidence for non-oxidative mechanism of human natural killer cell cytotoxicity by using mononuclear effector cells from healthy donors and from patients with chronic granulomatous disease. J Immunol 131:1784–1788, 1983.

35. Lew PD, Wollheim C, Seger RA, Pozzan T: Cytosolic free calcium changes induced by chemotactic peptide in neutrophils from patients with chronic granulomatous disease. Blood 63:231–233, 1984.

36. Smith DM, Walsh CE, DeChatelet LR, Waite M: Arachidonic acid metabolism in polymorphonuclear leukocytes from patients with chronic granulomatous disease. Infect Immun 40:1230–1233, 1983.

37. Whitin JC, Chapman CE, Simons ER, et al: Correlation between membrane potential changes and superoxide production in human granulocytes stimulated with phorbol myristate acetate. Evidence for defective activation in chronic granulomatous disease. J Biol Chem 255:1874–1878, 1980.

38. Seligmann BE, Gallin JI: Use of lipophilic probes of membrane potential to assess human neutrophil activation. Abnormality in chronic granulomatous disease. J Clin Invest 66:493–503, 1980.

39. van Rhenen DJ, Koolen MI, Feltkamp-Vroom TM, Weening RS: Immune complex glomerulonephritis in chronic granulomatous disease. Acta Med Scand 206:233–237, 1979.

40. Johansen KS, Borregaard N, Koch C, et al: Chronic granulomatous disease presenting as xantho granulomatous pyelonephritis. J Pediatr 100:98–100, 1982.

41. Gerba WM, Miller DR, Pahwa S, et al: Chronic granulomatous disease and selective IgA deficiency. Am J Pediatr Hematol Oncol 4:155–160, 1982.

42. Schmidt WF III, Poncz M, Russell MO, Schwartz E: Unusual manifestations of chronic granulomatous disease. Am J Dis Child 135:376–377, 1981.

43. Dilworth JA, Mandell GL: Adults with chronic granulomatous disease of "childhood." Am J Med 63:233–243, 1977.

44. Moellering RC Jr, Weinberg AN: Persistent salmonella infection in a female carrier for chronic granulomatous disease. Ann Intern Med 73:595–601, 1970.

45. Miyasaki S, Shin N, Goya N, Nakagawara A: Identification of a carrier mother of a female patient with chronic granulomatous disease. J Pediatr 89:784–786, 1976.

46. Mills EL, Rholl KS, Quie PG: X-linked inheritance in females with chronic granulomatous disease. J Clin Invest 66:332–340, 1980.

47. Johnston RB III, Harbeck RJ, Johnston RB Jr: Recurrent severe infections in a girl with apparently variable expression of mosaicism for chronic granulomatous disease. J Pediatr 106:50–55, 1985.

48. Johnston RB Jr: Biochemical defects of polymorphonuclear and mononuclear phagocytes associated with disease. In Sbarra AJ, Strauss RR (eds): The Reticuloendothelial System, vol. 2. New York: Plenum Press, 1980.

49. Johnston RB Jr, McMurry JS: Chronic familial granulomatosis: Report of five cases and review of the literature. Am J Dis Child 114:370–378, 1967.

50. Caldicott WJ, Baehner RL: Chronic granulomatous disease of childhood. AJR 103:133–139, 1968.

51. Wolfson JJ, Quie PG, Laxdal SD, Good RA: Roentgenologic manifestations in children with a genetic defect in polymorphonuclear leukocyte function. Radiology 91:37–48, 1968.

52. Gold RH, Douglas SD, Preger L, et al: Roentgenographic features of neutrophil dysfunction syndromes. Radiology 92:1045–1054, 1969.

53. Sutcliffe J, Chrispin AR: Chronic granulomatous disease. Br J Radiol 43:110–118, 1970.

54. Fleming GM, Kleinerman J, Doershuk CF, Perrin EV: Chronic granulomatous disease of childhood: An unusual case of honeycomb lung. Chest 68:834–837, 1975.

55. Raubitschek AA, Levin AS, Stites DP, et al: Normal granulocyte infusion therapy for aspergillosis in chronic granulomatous disease. Pediatrics 51:230–233, 1973.

56. Idriss ZH, Cunningham RJ, Wilfert CM: Nocardiosis in children: Report of three cases and review of the literature. Pediatrics 55:479–484, 1975.

57. Bujak JS, Kwon-Chung KJ, Chusid MJ: Osteomyelitis and pneumonia in a boy with chronic granulomatous disease of childhood caused by a mutant strain of Aspergillus nidulans. Am J Clin Pathol 61:361–367, 1974.

58. Cohen MS, Isturiz RE, Malech HL, et al: Fungal infection in chronic granulomatous disease. The importance of the phagocyte in defense against fungi. Am J Med 71:59–66, 1981.

59. Wiseman NE, Reed MH: Bronchopulmonary arterial malformation occurring in aspergillus lung infection complicating chronic granulomatous disease. J Pediatr Surg 16:457–460, 1981.

60. Gaisie G, Bowen A, Quattromani FL, Oh FS: Chest wall invasion by Aspergillus in chronic granulomatous disease of childhood. Pediatr Radiol 11:203–206, 1981.

61. Adinoff A, Johnston RB Jr, Dolen J, South MA: Chronic granulo-

matous disease and *Pneumocystis carinii* pneumonia. Pediatrics 69:133–134, 1982.

62. Chudwin DS, Wara DW, Cowan MJ, Ammann AJ: Aspergillus pneumonia in chronic granulomatous disease: Recurrence and long-term outcome. Acta Paediatr Scand 71:915–917, 1982.

63. Casale TB, Macher AM, Fauci AS: Concomitant pulmonary aspergillosis and nocardiosis in a patient with chronic granulomatous disease of childhood. South Med J 77:274–275, 1984.

64. Boltansky H, Kwon-Chung KJ, Macher AM, Gallin JI: *Acremonium strictum*-related pulmonary infection in a patient with chronic granulomatous disease. J Infect Dis 149:653, 1984.

65. Esterly JR, Sturner WG, Esterly NB, Windhorst DB: Disseminated BCG in twin boys with presumed chronic granulomatous disease of childhood. Pediatrics 48:141–144, 1971.

66. Chusid MJ, Parrillo JE, Fauci AS: Chronic granulomatous disease: Diagnosis in a 27 year-old man with *Mycobacterium fortuitum.* JAMA 233:1295–1296, 1975.

67. Johansen KS: Nitroblue tetrazolium slide test. Acta Pathol Microbiol Immunol Scand [C] 91:349–354, 1983.

68. Chusid MJ, Shea ML, Sarff LD: Determination of post-transfusion granulocyte kinetics by chemiluminescence in chronic granulomatous disease. J Lab Clin Med 95:168–174, 1980.

69. Newburger PE, Cohen NJ, Rothchild SB, et al: Prenatal diagnosis of chronic granulomatous disease. N Engl J Med 300:178–181, 1979.

70. Matthay KK, Golbus MS, Wara DW, Mentzer WC: Prenatal diagnosis of chronic granulomatous disease. Am J Med Genet 17:731–739, 1984.

71. Fikrig SM, Smithwick EM, Suntharalingam K, Good RA: Fibroblast nitroblue tetrazolium test and in-utero diagnosis of chronic granulomatous disease. Lancet 1:18–19, 1980.

72. Johnston RB Jr: Management of patients with chronic granulomatous disease. *In* Gallin JI, Fauci AS (eds): Advances in Host Defense Mechanisms, vol. 3. New York: Raven Press, 1983.

73. Papanicolaou N, Curnutti JT, Nathan DG, Treves S: Gallium-67 scintigraphy in children with chronic granulomatous disease. Pediatr Radiol 13:137–140, 1983.

74. Philippart AI, Colodny AH, Baehner RL: Continuous antibiotic therapy in chronic granulomatous disease: Preliminary communication. Pediatrics 50:923–925, 1972.

75. Johnston RB Jr, Wilfert CM, Buckley RH, et al: Enhanced bactericidal activity of phagocytes from patients with chronic granulomatous disease in the presence of sulfisoxazole. Lancet 1:824–827, 1975.

76. Kobayashi Y, Amano D, Ueda K, et al: Treatment of seven cases of chronic granulomatous disease with sulfamethoxazole-trimethoprim. Eur J Pediatr 127:247–254, 1978.

77. Weening RS, Kabel P, Pijman P, Roos D: Continuing therapy with sulfamethoxazole-trimethoprim in patients with chronic granulomatous disease. J Pediatr 103:127–130, 1983.

78. Seger RA, Baumgartner S, Tiefenauer LX, Gmunder FK: Chronic granulomatous disease: Effect of sulfamethoxazole-trimethoprim on neutrophil microbicidal function. Helv Paediatr Acta 36:579–588, 1981.

79. Gmunder FK, Seger RA: Chronic granulomatous disease: Mode of action of sulfamethoxazole-trimethoprim. Pediatr Res 15:1533–1537, 1981.

80. Jacobs RF, Wilson CB: Activity of antibiotics in chronic granulomatous disease leukocytes. Pediatr Res 17:916–919, 1983.

81. Zimmerli W, Lew PD, Suter S, et al: *In vitro* efficacy of several antibiotics against intracellular *S. aureus* in chronic granulomatous disease. Helv Paediatr Acta 38:51–61, 1983.

82. Silva J Jr, Dembinski S, Schaberg D: Effects of subinhibitory antibiotics on bactericidal activity of chronic granulomatous disease granulocytes in vitro. J Antimicrob Chemother 12(Suppl. C):21–27, 1983.

83. Hoger PH, Seger RA, Schaad UB, Hitzig WH: Chronic granulomatous disease: Uptake and intracellular activity of phosphomycin in granulocytes. Pediatr Res 19:38–44, 1985.

84. O'Reilly RJ, Brochstein J, Dinsmore R, Kirkpatrick D: Marrow transplantation for congenital disorders. Semin Hematol 21:188–221, 1984.

85. Kamani N, August CS, Douglas SD, et al: Bone marrow transplantation in chronic granulomatous disease. J Pediatr 105:42–46, 1984.

86. Gallin JI, Buescher ES, Seligmann BE, et al: NIH conference. Recent advances in chronic granulomatous disease. Ann Intern Med 99:657–674, 1983.

87. Ezekowitz RAB, Denauer MD, Jaffe HS, et al: Partial correction of the phagocyte defect in patients with X-linked chronic granulomatous disease by subcutaneous interferon gamma. N Engl J Med 319:146–151, 1988.

88. Gallin JI, Malech HL, Weening RS, et al: A controlled trial of interferon gamma to prevent infection in chronic granulomatous disease. N Engl J Med 324:509–516, 1991.

75 IMMUNODEFICIENCY AND LUNG DISEASE

DALE T. UMETSU, M.D., Ph.D.

The mechanisms by which the respiratory tract defends itself against infection involve several integrated systems. These systems include anatomic barriers as well as a variety of cells and serum proteins collectively known as the immune system. To simplify the understanding of these mechanisms, the host defense can be divided into five compartments: (1) the anatomic/mucociliary system, (2) the B cell compartment (humoral/antibody–mediated immunity), (3) the T cell compartment (cellular-mediated immunity), (4) the complement system, and (5) the phagocytic compartment. Defects may occur in one or more of these integrated compartments, leading to recurrent infection.

ANATOMIC/MUCOCILIARY COMPARTMENT

Anatomic integrity is essential in the protection against infection in the respiratory tract. Defects in the anatomic/mucociliary compartment that result in recurrent infection are listed in Table 75–1. These causes of recurrent

Table 75–1. ANATOMIC/MUCOCILIARY CAUSES OF RECURRENT INFECTION

Anatomic Defects in the Upper Airways
Aspiration syndromes
  Gastroesophageal reflux, poor gag reflex, ineffective cough
Cleft palate, eustachian tube dysfunction
Adenoidal hypertrophy
Nasal polyps
Anatomic Defects in the Tracheobronchial Bronchial Tree
Tracheal esophageal fistula
Pulmonary sequestration, bronchogenic cysts, vascular ring
Tumor, foreign body, or enlarged nodes
Physiologic Defects in the Upper and Lower Airways
Primary ciliary dyskinesia syndromes, Young's syndrome
Cystic fibrosis
Allergic disease (allergic rhinitis, asthma)
Chronic smoke exposure

infection must not be overlooked in the evaluation of children with recurrent infection.

B CELL COMPARTMENT

B cells are a class of lymphocytes that differentiate into plasma cells and secrete immunoglobulin. They are also characterized by the presence of cell-surface immunoglobulins, cell-surface receptors for the Fc region of immunoglobulin G (IgG) molecules, receptors (CR1 and CR2) for activated complement components (C3b and C3d, respectively), by the expression of the CD19 antigen, and by the expression of major histocompatibility (MHC) class I and class II antigens. Activation, proliferation, and differentiation of B cells are promoted by the interaction of B cells with antigen, T lymphocytes, and their lymphokines. Antibody secreted by B cells can bind specifically to the stimulating antigen (e.g., glycoproteins, carbohydrates, or toxins from microbes or parasites), resulting in inactivation or agglutination of the antigen, in opsonization of the antigen for phagocytosis, or in activation of complement, causing cytolysis of the pathogen.

IMMUNOGLOBULIN

Immunoglobulin molecules (antibodies) are proteins composed of two identical heavy chains and two identical light chains. Each polypeptide chain is composed of a variable region and a constant region. The constant regions of heavy chains (Fc region of the antibody) have several biologic functions, including the binding of C1q components of complement and binding to receptors for Fc on macrophages, B cells, neutrophils, and eosinophils. Functional and antigenic differences present on the constant region of the heavy chain allow immunoglobulins to be divided into five major isotypes: IgG, IgM, IgA, IgD, and IgE (Table 75–2). Antigenic differences on the constant regions of light chains allow division of antibody light chains into two types: κ and λ. Either type can combine with any type of heavy chain to form a functional immunoglobulin molecule.

Immunoglobulin G. IgG is the major immunoglobulin in blood and is the major immunoglobulin produced in secondary responses. IgG diffuses well into tissues and crosses the placenta.

Minor functional and antigenic differences on the heavy-chain polypeptide of IgG allow further subdivision of IgG into four subclasses (see Table 75–2). In general, the antibody responses to polysaccharide antigens reside in the IgG_2 subclass (with some IgG_1 produced), whereas responses to protein antigens reside in the IgG_1 and IgG_3 subclasses.[1, 2] IgG_1 and IgG_3, after binding to the target, activate complement well and opsonize foreign antigens for phagocytosis. All subclasses can agglutinate bacteria, viruses, and particulate antigens.

Immunoglobulin M. IgM circulates in the blood as a pentamer composed of five immunoglobulin units arranged in a circle joined by a molecule called the J chain. Monomeric IgM, with a distinct transmembrane Fc region, is expressed on the surface of B cells. Primary responses are initiated with production of IgM, which fixes complement very efficiently.

Immunoglobulin A. IgA is present in secretions in relatively high amounts, which suggests that it is important in mucosal immunity. IgA is also present in blood as a dimer composed of two immunoglobulin units joined by a small peptide called the J chain. When secreted, IgA is actively transported through the epithelium of serous glands, acquiring another 60-kD peptide called the secretory piece, which may confer resistance to proteolysis. The IgA_1 subclass is found primarily in serum, whereas the IgA_2 subclass is found primarily in secretions. Secretory IgA can neutralize viruses and agglutinate microbial organisms, but IgA can activate complement only via the alternate pathway. IgA is, therefore, poor at opsonizing organisms for phagocytosis.

Immunoglobulin E. IgE is responsible for type 1 immediate hypersensitivity (allergic) responses. IgE is present in minute amounts in blood but has the capacity to bind to Fc receptors on mast cells and basophils. Cross-linking of two or more IgE molecules on the surface of these cells by allergen results in degranulation with the release of preformed mediators such as histamine, eosinophil chemotactic factor, neutrophil chemotactic factor, and platelet activating factor.[3] These events also trigger the synthesis and release of other mediators such as leukotrienes. These mediators together cause allergic reactions by increasing vascular permeability and causing smooth muscle contraction and by producing an allergic inflammatory response through the recruitment of eosinophils, neutrophils, and mononuclear cells.

Immunoglobulin D. IgD is present in very small amounts in blood as well as on the surface of B cells. Its role is not well understood.

DEVELOPMENT OF ANTIBODY RESPONSES

Normal full-term infants acquire virtually all of their IgG from transplacental transfer of maternal antibody during the third trimester. Neonates are capable of syn-

Table 75–2. PROPERTIES OF IMMUNOGLOBULINS

| Ig | Serum Con (mg/dl)* | Molecular Weight | Crosses Placenta | Fixes C' | Binds to | | Serum Half-Life† |
					Mast Cells	Macrophages	
G1	900	146,000	+	+ +	−	+ +	23.0
G2	300	146,000	±	±	−	+	23.0
G3	100	170,000	+	+ +	−	+ +	9.0
G4	50	146,000	+	−	+	±	23.0
M	150	970,000	−	+ + +	−	−	5.0
A	300	160,000	−	−	−	−	7.0
D	3	180,000	−	−	−	−	2.8
E	0.05	188,000	−	−	+ + +	−	2.3

The degree of each function is denoted by + or −, whereby − indicates no function and + + + indicates a high degree of function.
*Approximate adult serum concentrations.
†Serum half-life in days.

thesizing IgM and some IgA but do not begin to synthesize IgG until about 3 to 6 months of age. As the maternal antibody is slowly catabolized, a normal physiologic nadir in serum IgG levels occurs at 4 to 7 months of age (Fig. 75–1). Because premature infants may not have received the normal amount of maternal IgG in utero, they may suffer from a more prolonged hypogammaglobulinemia at 2 to 9 months of age.

Even after infants begin to produce IgG at 6 months of age, the immune system continues to mature over a period of several years. The ability to respond to bacterial antigens is not consistently acquired until after approximately 2 years of age. Adult levels of IgG are not present until about 5 to 7 years of age, whereas adult levels of IgA are not acquired until 10 to 14 years of age.

At the molecular level, synthesis of the heavy chain of IgM begins after a series of gene rearrangements of chromosome 14.[4] First, in precursor B cells in the bone mar-

row, one of several dozen "diversity-region" (D) genes is selected and is joined to one of six "joining-region" (J_H) genes, deleting the intervening DNA and forming a DJ_H segment (Fig. 75–2). Next, one of several hundred "variable-region" (V_H) genes is selected and brought in apposition by recombination with the DJ_H segment, forming a $V_H DJ_H$ rearranged segment. Transcription of the $V_H DJ_H$ segment can then occur and includes the nearest constant-region gene (in immature B cells, this is C_μ, the constant region for IgM). The messenger RNA (mRNA) is modified and then translated into the heavy-chain protein. After light-chain gene rearrangement, transcription, and translation, which occur in a manner similar to that with heavy-chain genes, a functional IgM antibody can be expressed on the surface of the B cell. The B cell then leaves the bone marrow and can interact with specific antigen and helper T cells.

A particular antibody response is initiated by the introduction of foreign antigen, which is captured by antibody on the surface of antigen-specific B cells. The binding of antigen to immunoglobulin on the surface of B cells results in aggregation of the immunoglobulin receptors and causes partial activation of the B cell. The captured antigen is phagocytized by the B cell, is processed in lysosomes, and is then re-expressed on the surface of the B cell in association with MHC class II (HLA-D) antigens. Antigen-specific helper T cells can recognize the processed antigen on the surface of the B cell and are activated to produce a variety of lymphokines (interleukin [IL]-2, IL-3, IL-4, IL-5, IL-6, and interferon γ) (Table 75–3).[5] These lymphokines act on the partially activated B cell to effect B cell proliferation and differentiation into an antibody-secreting cell.

The maturation of antibody responses during the course of a particular immune response results in the expansion in the number of antigen-specific B cells, a switch in the heavy-chain constant region from IgM to IgG (or to IgA or IgE), an increase of the affinity of the antibody for antigen, and immunologic memory. Regulation of antibody maturation and isotype switch is not fully understood but involves gene rearrangements and somatic mutation and is thought to be controlled by helper/inducer T cells and their products. For example, production of IgE antibody by B cells is thought to be spe-

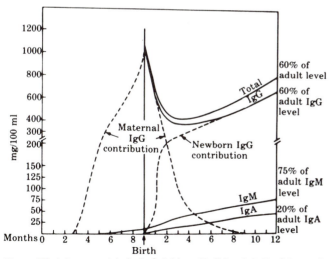

Figure 75–1. Immunoglobulin (IgG, IgM, and IgA) levels in the fetus and infant in the first year of life. The IgG of the fetus and the newborn is solely of maternal origin. The maternal IgG disappears by the age of 9 months, by which time the endogenous synthesis of IgG by the infant is well established. The IgM and IgA of the neonate are entirely endogenously synthesized because maternal IgM and IgA do not cross the placenta. (From Stiehm ER: Immunologic Disorders in Infants and Children. Philadelphia: WB Saunders, 1989.)

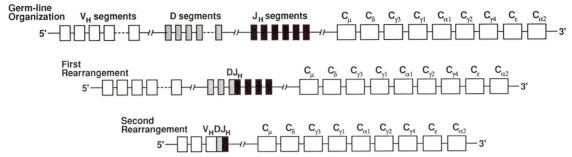

Figure 75-2. Organization and rearrangement of immunoglobulin H-chain genes. In the germ-line configuration, the immunoglobulin H-chain genes are organized with a large library of V_H regions, followed by a library of D regions, a library of J_H regions, and a cluster of constant-region genes. In the first rearrangement, a D segment joins to a J_H segment, with the deletion of the intervening DNA. In the second rearrangement, a V_H segment joins the DJ_H segment, again with deletion of intervening DNA, forming a V_HDJ_H segment. Because any V_H gene can combine with any D or J_H gene, these gene rearrangements greatly increase the possible diversity of the variable region of immunoglobulin. In addition, between the V_H-D and D-J_H joints, a few random nucleotides may be inserted, forming N regions, which further increases the possible diversity of the variable-region segment.

cifically enhanced by the presence of IL-4, whereas production of IgA responses is thought to be specifically enhanced by the presence of IL-5 and transforming growth factor β in mice.[6] At the molecular level, isotype switch occurs with deletional recombination, which places the V_HDJ_H segment adjacent to a heavy-chain constant region gene that lies downstream (in the 3′ direction on chromosome 14), such as $C_{\gamma3}$ or C_ϵ (constant-region genes for IgG_3 or IgE, respectively) (see Fig. 75–2).

SECRETORY IMMUNOGLOBULIN AND MUCOSAL IMMUNITY

Although all immunoglobulin isotypes are found in bronchial secretions, IgA is found in higher concentrations in respiratory secretions than in serum, especially in secretions from upper airways. There IgA may account for about 10% of the total protein. Secretions from lower airways contain higher amounts of IgG than do secretions from upper airways.[7]

IgA and IgE antibodies are synthesized locally in the lung by plasma cells in the mucosa of the respiratory tract. IgA is produced in plasma cells adjacent to secretory cells in the mucosa and is actively transported through the epithelium of the serous glands (see previous discussion of IgA). IgA in secretions is increased by the presence of parasympathomimetic agents, which increase glandular secretion. In contrast, IgG and IgM diffuse into tissue from blood, and IgG in secretions is enhanced by vasodilatation resulting from vasoactive mediators such as histamine or anaphylatoxins released during allergic or infectious inflammatory reactions.

After local viral infection (e.g., with rhinovirus or myxovirus), secretory IgA with viral neutralizing activity is seen in bronchial secretions, usually before it is seen in serum. Some viruses may stimulate local IgE synthesis (respiratory syncytial virus, parainfluenza), which may then lead to bronchospasm via mast-cell degranulation. Other viruses (adenovirus, poliomyelitis, measles) that often produce more systemic infection result in both systemic and local synthesis of IgA.

Table 75-3. INTERLEUKINS AND THEIR FUNCTION

Interleukin	Source	Function
IL-1	Macrophages	Costimulatory effect on T cells; enhances antigen presentation to T cells; induces fever
IL-2 (TCGF)	T cells	T cell growth factor; B cell growth and differentiation factor
IL-3	T cells	Growth factor of mast cells, eosinophils, multipotential stem cells, erythroid and myeloid progenitors
IL-4 (BSF-1, BCGF-I)	T cells	Growth factor for B cells and some T cells; increases MHC class II expression on B cells; enhances IgE synthesis and mast cell growth
IL-5 (BCGF-II)	T cells	Enhances Ig secretion, B cell proliferation, eosinophil differentiation; enhances IgA synthesis
IL-6 (BSF-2)	T cells Macrophages Fibroblasts	Enhances immunoglobulin synthesis and antiviral activity; enhances synthesis of acute-phase reactants
IL-7	Stromal cells	Enhances differentiation of pre-B cells
IL-8	T cells	Neutrophil-activating protein; T lymphocyte and neutrophil chemotactic factor
IL-10	T cells	Inhibits the synthesis of IFN γ, and IL-2 in T cells
IFN γ	T cells	Antiviral activity; activates macrophages; increases MHC class II expression on macrophages, fibroblasts, and endothelial cells; inhibits IgE synthesis; enhances murine IgG2a synthesis
TNF α (cachectin)	Macrophages	Causes necrosis of tumors; causes wasting of chronic disease, endotoxic shock, and bone resorption
TNF β (lymphotoxin)	T cells	Mediates cytotoxic T cell killing of target cells; activates macrophages; B cell growth factor?

TCGF, T cell growth factor; BSF, B cell–stimulating factor; BCGF, B cell growth factor; IFN, interferon; TNF, tumor necrosis factor; MHC, major histocompatibility; Ig, immunoglobulin.

IgA is thought to be involved in inhibiting systemic absorption of microbial organisms, allergens, or other antigens from mucosal surfaces. Absence of IgA (IgA deficiency) is thus associated with food allergy, possibly because of increased absorption of large-molecular-weight food antigens.

T CELL COMPARTMENT

T cells are another class of lymphocytes characterized by the expression of the CD3 (OKT3 or Leu-4) cell-surface antigen that associates with antigen-specific T cell receptors. T cells are involved in many immune mechanisms either directly (e.g., causing cytolysis of virus-infected cells or effecting B cell activation and differentiation) or by recruiting, by means of their soluble products (lymphokines), macrophages, neutrophils, eosinophils, basophils, and mast cells. T cells are the major cell type responsible for immunity to intracellular organisms (viruses, tuberculosis, *Brucella*) and to fungal organisms, and for causing graft-versus-host disease.

SUBSETS OF T CELLS

T cells can be divided into two major subsets. One T cell subset, called helper/inducer T cells, is characterized by the presence of the cell-surface antigen CD4 (OKT4, or Leu-3). CD4+ T cells secrete lymphokines such as IL-2, IL-3, IL-4, IL-5, and interferon γ (see Table 75–3)[5] and play a central role in regulating immune response. Further subdivision of CD4+ T cells appears to occur; each CD4+ subclass secretes a somewhat restricted profile of lymphokines.[6, 8] Some subsets of CD4+ T cells are involved in inducing B cells to synthesize immunoglobulin, and these CD4+ T cells secrete IL-4, IL-5, and IL-6. Other subsets of CD4+ T cells may be involved in producing delayed-type hypersensitivity responses (e.g., tuberculin test reactivity) and contact sensitivity responses (e.g., poison ivy dermatitis), and these CD4+ T cells secrete IL-2 and interferon γ but not IL-4, IL-5, or IL-6.

CD4+ T cells also help in the development and maturation of the other major T cell subset, the cytotoxic/suppressor T cell subset, which is characterized by the presence of the cell-surface antigen CD8 (OKT8, Leu-2). CD8+ T cells are effector cells that bind and destroy target cells, such as virus-infected cells or tumor cells. Some CD8+ T cells secrete lymphokines such as IL-2 and interferon γ but in quantities below those of CD4+ T cells. CD8+ cells may also play a role in suppressing or limiting immune responses by inhibiting B cell and CD4+ T cell function.

Large granular lymphocytes (LGL) or null cells (non-T, non-B) are a heterogeneous group of mononuclear cells that lack specific markers for B cells or for T cells. LGL include cells with natural killer activity that have cytolytic activity against a number of virally infected and transformed target cells to which they have not been previously sensitized. Also included in this group are (1) mononuclear cells, which have receptors for the Fc portion of IgG

and are cytolytic for target cells only in the presence of IgG specific for antigens expressed on the target cells (antibody-dependent cell cytotoxicity), and (2) lymphokine-activated killer cells, which are LGL capable of proliferating to IL-2 and of recognizing a wide variety of tumor cells but not normal cells.

Tumor-infiltrating lymphocytes (TIL) are CD3+ T cells that can be removed from solid tumors and expanded *in vitro* in the presence of IL-2.[9] When transferred back into the initial donor with IL-2, TIL home in on and cause regression of the target tumor. TIL may express CD4 or CD8 antigens.

DEVELOPMENT OF T CELLS

The T cell receptor for antigen is similar to immunoglobulin on B cells in that the T cell receptor confers antigen specificity to the T cell. The T cell receptor is composed of two polypeptide chains, α and β, that contain both constant and variable regions and arise after deletional recombination events of T cell receptor V, D, J, and C region genes. These events are similar to those seen with immunoglobulin genes, and in fact the primary sequences of T cell receptor genes show remarkable similarity to the sequences of immunoglobulin genes. A second type of T cell receptor, found on a minor subset of T cells, expresses γδ polypeptide chains. The immunologic function of this receptor is not known, but it is thought to be involved in immunity to certain types of bacteria. Rearrangement of T cell receptor genes and the maturation of T cells occur in the thymus, where the T cell receptor repertoire is determined. There, approximately 90% of the developing T cells are eliminated in processes known as negative selection (elimination of [autoreactive] T cells with receptors that react too strongly with self-antigens) and positive selection (elimination of T cells with receptors that do not recognize self-MHC antigens at all). The T cells that leave the thymus are thus those that can later recognize foreign but not self-peptides in association with self-MHC antigens (see later discussion).

ACTIVATION OF T CELLS

A major difference between B cells and T cells is that the T cell receptor cannot be secreted and must recognize antigen as part of a complex with MHC antigens. T cells therefore recognize peptide fragments of the antigen, which are bound to MHC antigens on the cell surface of antigen-presenting cells (Fig. 75–3). CD4+ T cells recognize peptides derived from extracellular foreign antigens complexed with MHC class II antigens (HLA-DR, HLA-DP, or HLA-DQ), which are expressed on the surface of cells specializing in antigen presentation (monocytes, macrophages, B cells, dendritic cells, or Langerhans cells of the skin). The CD4+ antigen itself is thought to be involved with this recognition step by binding to nonpolymorphic determinants on class II MHC antigens on the antigen-presenting cell, thus stabilizing the T cell receptor-peptide–MHC interaction (see Fig. 75–3). In contrast, CD8+ T cells recognize peptides derived from

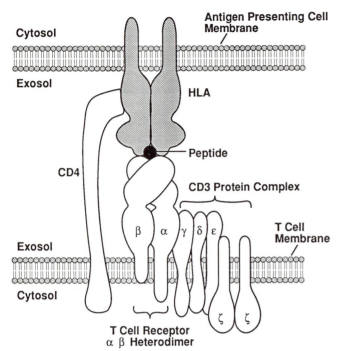

Figure 75–3. The interaction of the T cell receptor with antigen. The alpha and beta chains of the T cell receptor are anchored in the T cell membrane and are associated with the CD3 protein complex ($\gamma\delta\epsilon\zeta$ polypeptide chains). The T cell receptor recognizes antigen peptides complexed to major histocompatibility (MHC) molecules (class II, human lymphocyte antigen [HLA]-D, on antigen-presenting cells; or class I, HLA-A, HLA-B, or HLA-C, on any tissue [target] cell). CD4 molecules on CD4+ T cells bind to nonpolymorphic regions of MHC class II molecules, whereas CD8 molecules on CD8 T cells bind to nonpolymorphic regions of MHC class I molecules. The signal generated in the T cell is transduced by the CD3 protein complex. (After Krensky AM, Weiss A, Crabtree G, et al: T-lymphocyte antigen in transplant rejection. N Engl J Med, 322:510, 1990. Reprinted with permission from the *New England Journal of Medicine*, vol. 322, pp. 510–517, 1990.)

endogenously synthesized (e.g., viral) proteins complexed with MHC class I antigens (HLA-A, HLA-B, HLA-C), which are expressed on all somatic cells except erythrocytes. The CD8 antigen on the T cell binds to nonpolymorphic determinants of class I MHC antigens on target cells, stabilizing the T cell–target cell interaction. Further stabilization of the T cell–target cell interaction is mediated by leukocyte functional antigen (LFA-1) (on both CD4+ and CD8+ T cells) binding to its ligands, intercellular adhesion molecules (ICAM) 1 and 2, on the target cells, and by CD2 (sheep erythrocyte receptor) on T cells binding to its ligand, LFA-3, on target cells. Recognition by the T cell receptor of the peptide/MHC complex on the antigen-presenting or target cell results in aggregation of the T cell receptor. In the presence of additional stimuli provided by the antigen-presenting cell, aggregation of the T cell receptor leads to phosphorylation of multiple membrane and cytoplasmic proteins, hydrolyzation of membrane phosphatidylinositides into inositol phosphates and diacylglycerol, an increase in intracellular free calcium, and T cell activation (reviewed by Krensky and colleagues[10]). The T cell then goes on to proliferate and produce lymphokines, especially IL-2. Although poorly understood, stimulation with antigen also leads to the development of immunologic memory by the expansion of antigen-specific T cells, which have the potential to respond more quickly on restimulation with the production of a wider array of lymphokines, including IL-2, IL-4, IL-5, and interferon gamma.

COMPLEMENT COMPARTMENT

The complement system is a series of about 25 plasma proteins that, when triggered, act in a sequential cascade to amplify the initial stimulus dramatically. The products of complement activation have potent chemotactic, vasoactive, opsonizing, and lytic activity. These activities are antigen-nonspecific; however, complement usually functions in an antigen-specific manner when activated by antigen-specific antibody.

The most abundant and critical complement component is C3, which is present in plasma at levels of about 1 mg/ml. C3 is activated by the classical pathway (via antigen-antibody coated target, C1, C4, and C2) or via the alternate pathway (C3, factor B, factor D, and properdin). From the activation of C3, the complement cascade proceeds with the activation of C5, C6, C7, C8, and C9. The biologic functions of complement are then mediated through these activation products. These functions include the following processes:

1. *Opsonization*: C3b, iC3b (the serum-inactivated C3 fragment), and a more extensively degraded C3 fragment all opsonize antigens or microbes and facilitate phagocytosis by binding to receptors (CR1, CR2, and CR3, respectively) on phagocytic cells (neutrophils, monocytes, macrophages, and B cells).

2. *Chemotaxis*: C5a is a potent neutrophil and eosinophil chemotactic agent. It also causes vasodilatation and increased vascular permeability.

3. *Activation of neutrophils*: C3a and C5a stimulate the neutrophil respiratory burst associated with the production of oxygen metabolites.

4. *Anaphylatoxins*: C3a and C5a are anaphylatoxins that trigger mast-cell and basophil degranulation, resulting in further amplification of the response.

5. *Membrane attack complex*: The assembly of C5b through C9 forms a membrane attack complex that produces large transmembrane channels in bacteria or cells leading to cell lysis.

THE PHAGOCYTIC COMPARTMENT

Phagocytic cells engulf and digest microorganisms. Polymorphonuclear neutrophils (PMNs) are nondividing, antigen-nonspecific, short-lived phagocytic cells and are the predominant white cell in the blood. Tissue macrophages are long-lived phagocytic cells that develop from monocytes in the blood and are present throughout connective tissue, particularly in the lung (alveolar macrophages), liver (Kupffer's cells), spleen, and lymph nodes and in the skin (Langerhans cells). Macrophages are essential for host defense against many microorganisms that are capable of proliferating within cells of the host (mycobacteria and protozoa).

CHEMOTAXIS, PHAGOCYTOSIS, KILLING

Although PMNs are present in large numbers in the blood vessels and capillaries, there are few PMNs in the normal lung itself. In response to chemotactic factors such as C5a, however, neutrophils and eosinophils accumulate in the lung. Chemotaxis is aided by vasodilatation caused by C3a and C5a (anaphylatoxins), and in allergic-type reactions by mast cell mediators such as histamine, neutrophil chemotactic factor, and eosinophil chemotactic factor. The presence of large numbers of neutrophils and eosinophils in the lung is associated with late-phase reactions and increased bronchial hyperreactivity.

Phagocytosis is initiated by the recognition of foreign antigen by the phagocyte. Because phagocytic cells have receptors for complement (CR1, CR2, and CR3) and for the Fc portion of immunoglobulin, phagocytosis is greatly enhanced by opsonization of the microorganism with immunoglobulin and complement. Phagocytosis also initiates mechanisms that generate superoxide and hydrogen peroxide, which aid in the killing of ingested organisms. Hydrolytic enzymes in lysosomal granules, which combine with the phagosome, help digest the microorganism.

ANTIGEN PRESENTATION BY MACROPHAGES

Macrophages are important in presenting antigen and activitating T cells and are also most effectively activated by factors secreted by T cells. Thus macrophages conceptually belong in the T cell compartment. When confronted with foreign antigen, macrophages phagocytize and process the antigen, present it in association with MHC antigens to T cells, and secrete IL-1 and IL-6 (see Table 75–3). The macrophage–T cell interaction results in the secretion of interferon γ and other lymphokines by the T cell and in the activation of the macrophage. This allows the macrophage to effectively kill intracellular organisms such as mycobacteria, *Listeria, Leishmania, Toxoplasma*, and other intracellular parasites.

Although these antigen-presenting functions are similar in all tissue macrophages, alveolar macrophages, which are the only resident phagocyte normally present in the alveoli, may not present antigen as effectively as other tissue macrophages because they do not effectively produce IL-1. The long-lived alveolar macrophages, however, can migrate through the pores of Kohn, enter the lung lymphatic channels, travel to regional lymph nodes, or be transported to the upper airways by the mucociliary escalator and deliver antigen to lymphoid organs elsewhere.

IMMUNODEFICIENCY STATES

Clinical problems that require evaluation of the immune system include chronic or recurrent infection or infection with unusual pathogens. However, because infection is a common occurrence in children, initiation of evaluation should take into consideration the accrual of morbidity (e.g., presence of failure to thrive, bronchi-

Table 75–4. INITIAL SCREENING TESTS FOR IMMUNODEFICIENCY

Chest radiograph
Complete blood count with differential and erythrocyte sedimentation rate
Serum IgG, IgM, IgA, IgE
Serum titers to diphtheria, tetanus, or common viruses (influenza, rubella, rubeola) and isohemagglutinins in patients who are not blood group AB+
Delayed hypersensitivity skin tests (diphtheria, tetanus toxoid, *Candida*)
Total hemolytic complement (CH_{50}) or C3, C4

Ig, immunoglobulin.

ectasis, pulmonary scarring and restrictive lung disease, chronic ear drainage). Other signs and symptoms suggestive of immunodeficiency in the face of recurrent infection include persistent atypical rashes, chronic diarrhea, paucity of lymph nodes and tonsils, lymphadenopathy, chronic conjunctivitis, unusual reactions to live vaccines, and delay in umbilical cord detachment.

The evaluation of recurrent infection should be systematic with analysis of all compartments of host defense: the anatomic/mucociliary, B cell, T cell, phagocytic, and complement compartments. Initiation of immune evaluation can begin with screening tests (Table 75–4), and more sophisticated tests should be reserved for more precise immunologic evaluation. Secondary causes of immunodeficiency (e.g., acquired immunodeficiency syndrome [AIDS]; malnutrition; toxins; immunosuppressive drugs; uremia; diabetes mellitus) should not be overlooked. Specific primary immunodeficiencies are discussed next.

DISORDERS IN ANTIBODY PRODUCTION

Antibody deficiency states are the most common of the primary immunodeficiency diseases. Patients with antibody deficiency states generally have recurrent sinopulmonary infections—otitis media, sinusitis, pneumonia, and bacteremia caused by encapsulated bacteria such as *Streptococcus pneumoniae, Haemophilus influenzae* (both type B and nontypable strains), and staphylococci—and have fewer problems with fungal or viral (except enteroviral) infections. However, patients with X-linked agammaglobulinemia may acquire chronic echovirus encephalitis, have multiple bouts of chickenpox, or develop poliomyelitis with vaccination. Antibody deficiency states classically do not become manifest until after 6 months of age after the decay of transplacentally acquired maternal antibody (in full-term infants).

Immunologic Findings

Patients with these disorders have decreased serum antibody levels. Because normal levels vary with age, with a physiologic nadir occurring at 4 to 7 months of age, the serum immunoglobulin levels must be interpreted in the context of age (see Fig. 75–1). Total protein levels are useful in interpreting low immunoglobulin levels. Low albumin levels suggest low synthetic rates for all proteins or increased loss of proteins (e.g., protein-losing enteropathy or loss through skin disease). High levels of immunoglobulin suggest intact immunity (as in chronic granulomatous disease, immotile cilia syndrome, or cystic fibrosis). Very high levels suggest AIDS. When levels of immunoglobulin are normal, borderline low, or elevated, their function can be assessed by measurement of specific antibody titers to antigens to which the patient has been exposed, such as tetanus and diphtheria toxoids; polio, influenza, and rubella or rubeola viruses; and *S. pneumoniae* or *H. influenzae* bacteria.

X-Linked Agammaglobulinemia

This disorder is characterized by the absence or severe reduction of serum immunoglobulin, absence of circulating B cells, and absence of plasma cells in all lymphoid tissue. After maternal antibody is consumed (after the first few months of life), affected patients acquire sinopulmonary infections, bacteremia, and meningitis with encapsulated and gram-negative bacteria. Fungal infections are rare because T cell function is thought to be intact. Although viral infections are not generally problematic, enterovirus (poliovirus and echovirus) and hepatitis viruses may cause fatal disease. *Pneumocystis carinii* occasionally produces disease in these patients, whereas *Giardia lamblia* is a frequent cause of diarrhea.[11]

IgG levels are generally less than 100 mg/dl, and levels of IgA and IgM are undetectable. B cells cannot be detected in peripheral blood, although the number of pre–B cells (containing intracytoplasmic IgM heavy chains) is increased in the bone marrow, which suggests a maturation block in B cell development (e.g., block in V_HDJ_H recombination).

Treatment consists of replacement gamma globulin, which significantly reduces the frequency of sinopulmonary infections. The dose of intravenous gamma globulin is 400 mg/kg every 3 to 4 weeks.[12] Side effects of intravenous gamma globulin include fever, chills, and, in rare instances, anaphylaxis and are less frequently seen at slower infusion rates. Prophylactic courses of antibiotics with low threshold for use are also helpful in the therapy of these patients.

Common Variable Agammaglobulinemia or Acquired Agammaglobulinemia

This heterogeneous and not uncommon disorder is characterized by initially normal immune function with the subsequent development of recurrent sinopulmonary and skin infections or chronic bronchiectasis, usually after age 6 years and in the second or third decade of life.[13] The disorder often is familial, but apparently it is not X-linked or autosomally inherited. Lymphoid hyperplasia is often seen as is a spruelike malabsorption syndrome, sometimes caused by *G. lamblia*. Common variable agammaglobulinemia is also associated with pernicious anemia in 30% of patients, polyarthritis, systemic lupus erythematosus (SLE), idiopathic thrombocytopenic purpura, leukemia, lymphoma, and gastrointestinal tumors.

Common variable agammaglobulinemia is diagnosed when serum IgG levels are below age-related normal lev-

els in the presence of recurrent infections or chronic bronchitis. Titers to common antigens are low as are isohemagglutinins. However, autoantibodies, such as rheumatoid factor, are frequently present. Coombs positive hemolytic anemia, pernicious anemia, leukopenia, and thrombocytopenia are not uncommon. B cells are present in low or high numbers,[14] and T cell function, although initially normal, tends to deteriorate with time.

The treatment for this disorder is the same as for X-linked agammaglobulinemia, with replacement gamma globulin and prophylactic courses of antibiotics.

Transient Hypogammaglobulinemia of Infancy

This disorder, which affects children under 3 years of age, is characterized by a prolongation and accentuation of the physiologic nadir of serum levels of IgG that normally occurs at 4 to 7 months of age.[15] The exact level of serum gammaglobulin (IgG) that distinguishes normal children from patients with transient hypogammaglobulinemia may be difficult to define, resulting in differences in reported frequency and treatment of this disorder. In some cases, familial incidence is observed. Although these patients appear to have high frequency of sinopulmonary infections secondary to viral and bacterial agents, severe infections are rare, and these children have normal growth and development. Food allergy has been associated with this disorder.

In general, only serum IgG is affected; IgM and IgA levels are normal. Antibody responses to antigens such as diphtheria and tetanus toxoid are normal, and circulating B cells are normal in number. The B cells themselves in these patients are normal, but helper T cell function is thought to be delayed in maturation.[16]

Although the prognosis is generally excellent and all patients appear to recover spontaneously, in severe cases replacement therapy with gamma globulin is sometimes helpful in reducing the frequency of infections. This disorder, however, must be distinguished from other antibody deficiency states that present in infancy and require distinct types of therapy.

Selective IgG Subclass Deficiency

Patients with selective IgG subclass deficiency have recurrent sinopulmonary infection associated with normal total levels of serum IgG but with selective deficiencies of IgG_2, IgG_3, or IgG_4.[17] Patients with IgG_2 subclass deficiency can make antibody, but the spectrum of the response is decreased.[18] Titers to bacterial polysaccharide antigens (*H. influenzae*, pneumococcal antigens, meningococcal antigens) are low even after immunization, and this is thought to be because antibody responses to polysaccharides reside predominantly in the IgG_2 subclass (with some in IgG_1).[1,2] Although titers to protein antigens such as tetanus or diphtheria toxoids are normal, the absence of protective titers to polysaccharide antigens is thought to result in recurrent infection. IgG_2 subclass deficiency is associated with IgG_4 subclass deficiency, IgA deficiency, Wiskott-Aldrich syndrome, and ataxia telangiectasia.

Selective IgG₃ deficiency is also associated with recurrent sinopulmonary infection, but the mechanism for recurrent infection is not clear. Affected patients have normal responses to common protein and polysaccharide antigens.

Treatment for this syndrome includes prophylactic antibiotics, immunization with pneumococcal vaccine polyvalent (Pneumovax) for diagnostic and possible therapeutic purposes, and, in severe cases, replacement gamma globulin.

Antibody Deficiency With Normal Immunoglobulins (Poor Responsiveness to Polysaccharide Antigens)

Another group of patients with recurrent infection has been identified by the presence of a selective inability to produce antibody to polysaccharide antigens, such as that from *S. pneumoniae* or *H. influenzae* type B.[19–21] Total serum levels of IgG and IgG subclasses in these patients are normal. In addition, patients who have this heterogeneous syndrome usually have normal titers against protein antigens such as tetanus or diphtheria toxoids but are unable to produce sufficient antibody to polysaccharide antigens unless these antigens are covalently coupled to protein carrier antigens, such as diphtheria toxoid. Because the presence of antibody to the capsular polysaccharides of bacteria confers protection against infection by the particular bacteria, the inability to respond to polysaccharide antigens results in the susceptibility to bacterial infection. In severe cases, replacement gamma globulin therapy appears to reduce the frequency of infection.

Selective IgA Deficiency

Selective deficiency of IgA (serum levels <10 mg/dl) with normal total levels of IgG and IgM is seen in the general population with a frequency of about 1 in 700. Although IgA is important in mucosal immunity, the precise role of IgA is unclear because a large proportion of persons with IgA deficiency are asymptomatic. However, approximately half of persons with IgA deficiency have recurrent sinopulmonary infections, usually in association with IgG₂ subclass deficiency,[22] and IgA deficiency occurs in families with other hypogammaglobulinemia syndromes. In addition, IgA deficiency is associated with low levels of serum IgE, with food allergies, with ataxia-telangiectasia, and with collagen-vascular diseases such as rheumatoid arthritis, SLE, dermatomyositis, pernicious anemia, Sjögren's syndrome, pulmonary hemosiderosis, and hemolytic anemia. IgA deficiency may also occur secondary to defects involving the secretory component or as a reaction to drugs such as phenytoin.[23]

Because of the considerable heterogeneity in this syndrome, the diagnosis of IgA deficiency in a particular patient depends not only on the serum level of IgA but also on the history (e.g., for recurrent infection or collagen-vascular disease) and on the results of related diagnostic studies, such as IgG subclass levels, complete blood count (CBC), and erythrocyte sedimentation rate. In cases of IgA deficiency with recurrent infection and IgG subclass deficiency, treatment with aggressive antimicrobial therapy or with replacement gamma globulin is indicated. Patients with undetectable levels of IgA can acquire IgE antibodies directed against IgA and may therefore be at risk for anaphylaxis with the administration of blood products or gamma globulin that contain IgA.[24] In such patients, highly purified IgG (Gammagard, Hyland) may be administered safely.

Immunodeficiency With Increased IgM (Dysgammaglobulinemia)

This usually X-linked antibody deficiency state is characterized by elevated levels of IgM (and sometimes of IgD) but decreased levels of serum IgG and IgA in association with recurrent sinopulmonary and skin infections.[25] T cell function may be somewhat abnormal, with an inability of T cells to effect isotype switch. Patients also acquire autoimmune and lymphoproliferative diseases. Treatment for hyper-IgM syndrome includes antimicrobial therapy and replacement gamma globulin.

DISORDERS OF T CELL IMMUNITY (CELL-MEDIATED IMMUNODEFICIENCY)

Patients with defects in T cell immunity generally have infections with fungi and with microorganisms that proliferate intracellularly in somatic cells and in macrophages (e.g., viruses or mycobacteria). Effector (e.g., cytolytic and helper) T cells do not develop in these patients, and macrophages cannot be activated to kill intracellular microorganisms. The pathogens seen in these patients include viruses (especially herpes), protozoa (*P. carinii* and *Toxoplasma*), fungi *(Candida)*, mycobacteria or *M. tuberculosis,* and *Listeria.* In severe T cell deficiency, B cell function (e.g., antibody production), which requires T cell help, is also impaired.

Immunologic findings include lymphopenia, absence of thymic shadow on chest radiographs, and absence of delayed hypersensitivity reactions. T cell numbers may be decreased, and the helper/suppressor ratio (CD4 to CD8 T cell ratio) may be reversed. Functional T cell studies—proliferation to mitogens (phytohemagglutinin, pokeweed mitogen, or concanavalin A) or antigens (tetanus toxoid or diphtheria toxoid)—are also abnormal.

DiGeorge's Syndrome (Thymic Hypoplasia)

DiGeorge's syndrome is the result of dysmorphogenesis of the third and fourth nasopharyngeal pouches. Patients with DiGeorge's syndrome have hypoplasia or aplasia of the thymus and the parathyroid glands, complex cardiac malformations (truncus arteriosus and interrupted aortic arch type B, transposition, atrial and ventricular septal defects), esophageal atresia, bifid uvula, short philtrum, mandibular hypoplasia, hypertelorism, and low-set notched ears. Many patients present for cardiac evaluation and develop hypocalcemia perioperatively.[26]

The severity of the clinical and pathologic manifestations varies considerably, from severe forms with complete thymic aplasia with an immunodeficiency resembling that of severe combined immunodeficiency to only latent hypoparathyroidism, which may also be seen in relatives of patients with DiGeorge's syndrome. Most patients have partial T cell function, which improves as they mature.[27] Mature T cells are decreased in peripheral blood, whereas immature T cells are found in increased numbers. Levels of serum immunoglobulins are often normal for age, although IgA levels may be diminished and IgE levels may be elevated.

Treatment for these patients depends on the severity of the immunodeficiency. Aggressive antibiotic therapy for infections is useful. Administration of thymopoietin or recombinant IL-2 may be beneficial, and in complete aplasia, bone marrow transplantation may be indicated.

Severe Combined Immunodeficiency

Severe combined immunodeficiency (SCID) is a disorder characterized by deficiency of both the B and T cell arms of the immune system, resulting in profound hypogammaglobulinemia and absence of T cell function. The syndrome occurs in autosomal recessive or X-linked recessive forms, and affected infants have chronic infections and pneumonia (often resulting from *P. carinii*), with failure to thrive beginning in the first few months of life. A nondescript morbilliform rash secondary to chronic graft-versus-host disease from maternal lymphocytes, with oral thrush and with diarrhea, is also common.

Laboratory evaluation usually reveals lymphopenia and severely reduced IgG levels. B cells and T cells are usually absent.

Defects at several levels in the immune system can result in SCID. In some patients, SCID is caused by abnormal lymphocyte development from stem cells. In others (30% to 50%) with the autosomal recessive form, SCID may be caused by deficiency of the enzyme adenosine deaminase.[28] Diagnosis of this variant form is made by examination of red blood cells for the enzyme. Point mutations or deletions of segments of the adenosine deaminase gene on chromosome 20 result in an enzyme defect that causes the accumulation of the substrate deoxyadenosine. This substrate is perferentially toxic to T lymphoblasts. Most patients with adenosine deaminase deficiency present with severe infections within the first 6 months of life. However, those with some residual enzyme activity present later, after 1 year of age.

Purine-nucleoside phosphorylase deficiency, caused by a genetic defect on chromosome 14, is a second known cause of SCID and is characterized by a progressive impairment of T cell immunity, lymphopenia, and normal levels of immunoglobulins.[29] Patients initially may have residual enzyme activity and thus have relatively normal immunity, but accumulation of toxic deoxyribonucleotides in lymphoid tissues results in decreasing T cell function.

A third form of SCID is the bare lymphocyte syndrome. Patients with this syndrome lack MHC class I or class II antigens. Because MHC antigens play a crucial role in antigen presentation to both T and B cells, lack of these cell-surface markers results in severe recurrent infection. In the more common form, class I antigens are not detectable on somatic cells, although class II antigens are expressed normally on antigen-presenting cells. In some other cases, class II antigens are absent; in still other cases, both class I and class II antigens are absent. T cell–proliferative responses to mitogens, which do not require MHC antigens for presentation to T cells, are normal in these patients, but proliferative responses to classical antigens such as tetanus toxoid are severely impaired.

Other causes of SCID have been described and include defects in the expression of T cell receptor–associated proteins (CD3), defects in T cell receptor signal transduction, defects in the synthesis of IL-2 and other lymphokines, and defects in the expression of receptors of IL-2 or IL-1.

The treatment for SCID is bone marrow transplantation, preferably with marrow from histocompatible siblings. Graft rejection usually does not occur, because of the absence of a host immune system; however, patients are very susceptible to graft-versus-host disease. In the case of adenosine deaminase deficiency, weekly intramuscular injections of bovine adenosine deaminase conjugated to polyethylene glycol has been successfully used in more than 20 patients to reconstitute immune function.[30] Gene transfer of the normal gene for ADA with the use of retrovirus vectors is currently being studied as a definitive therapy for patients with ADA deficiency.

Wiskott-Aldrich Syndrome

This syndrome is a triad of recurrent infections, thrombocytopenia, and a skin disease indistinguishable from atopic dermatitis caused by mutations of a gene in band p11.2 on the X chromosome. Elevated IgE and IgA levels are often noted, but IgM levels are decreased, and IgG levels are normal. Responses to polysaccharide antigens are poor, and isohemagglutinins are usually absent. T cells progressively decline in number and function. Platelets are small in size and few in number, which results in severe bleeding. A 115-kD glycoprotein is absent from cell surface of lymphocytes and platelets.[31] Two thirds of patients die from infection and one third die of hemorrhage, with a mean survival of about 6 years.

In severe cases, the treatment includes bone marrow transplantation. In less severe cases, splenectomy may improve thrombocytopenia.

Ataxia-Telangiectasia

Ataxia-telangiectasia is an autosomal recessive disorder characterized by progressive cerebellar ataxia with degeneration of Purkinje cells, thymic hypoplasia associated with IgA deficiency, and IgG$_2$ subclass deficiency of variable severity along with low IgE levels.[32] T cell function is variably depressed with frequent absence of delayed-type hypersensitivity skin reactions, and patients acquire, to some degree, recurrent and chronic sinopulmonary infections. Telangiectasias occur initially in the bulbar conjunctivae and later spread to the skin. Ataxia-telangiectasia is associated with insulin-resistant diabetes mellitus, gonadal agenesis, premature aging, malignant tumors, elevated levels of serum alpha$_1$-fetoprotein and carcinoembryonic antigen, and hypersensitivity of fibroblasts and lymphocytes to ionizing radiation as a result of defects in DNA repair mechanisms.[33] The gene for ataxia-telangiectasia has been localized to chromosome 11q22-23, with an estimated carrier frequency of 0.5% to 5%. The incidence of neoplasms is thought to be increased fivefold among heterozygotes.

There is no uniformly helpful therapy for this disease, but antimicrobial therapy and gamma globulin replacement therapy (with IgA-deficient preparations) should be pursued.

Hyper-IgE Syndrome

Hyper-IgE syndrome is a triad of recurrent infections with extremely elevated serum IgE levels and skin lesions almost resembling atopic dermatitis.[34] Patients with hyper-IgE syndrome acquire deep-seated skin infections that usually heal with scar formation. Bronchiectasis with fungal infection, meningitis with opportunistic infectious agents, and coarse facies are associated with this syndrome. The exact immunologic defect is not clear, but patients exhibit a variety of immunologic problems of varying severity. These include problems with neutrophil chemotaxis, decreased delayed-type hypersensitivity, and decreased antibody production to specific antigens. A dysregulation of subsets of CD4+ T cells has been proposed to exist in these patients, with the presence of elevated numbers of T cells that produce IL-4. The diagnosis is suggested by the clinical presentation with deep-seated infections and confirmed by the presence of elevated IgE and by the presence of IgE binding to *S. aureus*.

AIDS

AIDS is caused by infection with the human immunodeficiency virus and is discussed in Chapter 21.

DISORDERS OF PHAGOCYTIC CELLS

Phagocytic cell disorders can be grouped into disorders of cell numbers and disorders of cell function.

Disorders of Numbers. These include cyclic neutropenia, Kostmann's syndrome, Shwachman-Diamond syndrome, and autoimmune neutropenia. Neutropenia usually results in furunculosis, subcutaneous abscesses, sinopulmonary infection, and bacteremia.[35] Staphylococci and enteric bacteria are the most common pathogens. Treatment for neutropenia syndromes was traditionally limited to frequent courses of antibiotics or, in severe cases, to bone marrow transplantation. The emergence of recombinant DNA technology and treatment programs with the use of recombinant granulocyte-colony stimulating factor may be a major therapeutic advance for some of these syndromes.

Loss of the splenic phagocytic function, either by surgical removal of the spleen or as a result of infarction (as in sickle-cell disease), especially in young children, results in susceptibility to septicemia and meningitis with pyogenic bacteria such as the pneumococcus.

Disorders of Function. Defects in chemotaxis or bactericidal activity generally result in subcutaneous abscesses, furunculosis, pneumonia, sinusitis, and otitis media. *S. aureus* is the most common pathogen.

Immunologic Findings

The CBC may show neutropenia. Tests for neutrophil function include the nitroblue-tetrazolium (NBT) test for chronic granulomatous disease; the Rebuck skin window, which is used for examining neutrophil chemotaxis; and zymosan uptake, which is used for examining phagocytic function. Bone marrow is useful for evaulating neutropenia, and examination of neutrophils and monocytes for expression of leukocyte adhesion molecules is necessary for ruling out leukocyte adhesion defects.

Chronic Granulomatous Disease

Chronic granulomatous disease (CGD) is usually inherited in an X-linked manner, although 20% to 30% of cases are inherited as autosomal recessive.[36] CGD is caused by a defect in a membrane-associated nicotinamide adenine dinucleotide phosphate (NADPH) oxidase in phagocytic cells, resulting in the failure of phagocytic cells to produce superoxide and kill ingested bacteria. The larger subunit of a phagocyte-specific cytochrome, which is part of the oxidase complex heterodimer, is abnormal in these patients. In the X-linked form, the gene for the cytochrome b subunit, which is located in band p21 of the X chromosome, is absent, truncated, or mutated. In the autosomal recessive form of CGD, other components of the NADPH oxidase system are affected. Phagocytes from patients with CGD fail to generate activated oxygen derivatives after phagocytosis that are required for efficient microbial killing and acquire severe, recurrent infections with catalase-positive bacteria and fungi (*Staphylococcus, Klebsiella, Serratia, Salmonella, Aspergillus, Candida*) as well as granulomas at sites of chronic inflammation. Invasive *Aspergillus* lung infections are a particular problem in these patients. Infections often start around the ears and nose. Hepatosplenomegaly is common, as are pulmonary lymphadenopathy, bronchopneumonia, empyema, and lung abscess. Gastrointestinal obstruction secondary to granulomas is also common as well as perianal fistulas, vitamin B_{12} malabsorption, steatorrhea, and osteomyelitis. Because of chronic stimulation of the immune system, hypergammaglobulinemia is often noted.

Diagnosis is made by the presence of an inability of neutrophils to reduce NBT from colorless to blue and by the inability of neutrophils to kill staphylococci.

Treatment with chronic antibiotic prophylaxis (especially trimethoprim/sulfamethoxazole) and aggressive intravenous antibiotic therapy with surgical drainage of abscesses has led to a marked improvement in survival with decreased morbidity. Treatment with subcutaneous recombinant interferon γ, which enhances gene expression of the cytochrome b mRNA and of superoxide production and may activate monocytes and macrophages, has been shown to result in decreased frequency of infections.[37] Bone marrow transplantation has also been curative in a few patients.

Leukocyte Adhesion Defects

Patients with the autosomal recessive leukocyte adhesion deficiency disease have leukocytes that lack a cell-surface glycoprotein required for cell adhesion, phagocytosis, and leukocytosis.[38] Three heterodimer cell membrane markers, LFA-1 (or CD11a, on all leukocytes), Mac-1 (CR3 or CD11b on phagocytic cells and granular lymphocytes), and p150/95 (CD11c on some activated lymphocytes including cytolytic T cells) share a common beta-chain subunit, which is absent or markedly reduced in these patients. The syndrome has been variously known as LFA-1, Mac-1, or p150/95 glycoprotein deficiency, leukocyte-cell adhesion molecule (leu-CAM) deficiency, Mo-1 deficiency, or leukocyte adhesion deficiency. Lack of expression of these glycoproteins results in decreased chemotaxis and in bacterial infections of the skin, oral and urogenital orifices, and intestinal and respiratory tracts. Infections progressively enlarge, and ulcerative and necrotic skin lesions heal very slowly, leaving dysplastic scars.

Infections may start at birth, classically with delay in umbilical cord loss and omphalitis. *S. aureus* and gram-negative enteric bacteria are the frequent causative organisms, but fungi (*Candida* and *Aspergillus*) are also seen, whereas viral infections are much less frequent. Purulent discharge is absent at the site of infections because of abnormal chemotaxis. In severe disease without expression of these proteins, patients die within the first few years of life. With reduced but measurable expression of these proteins, patients may live longer.

Diagnosis of this rare disease is made by the demonstration of the absence of leu-CAM. Treatment for this disease includes frequent antibiotics, transfusion of granulocytes, and bone marrow transplantation.

Chédiak-Higashi Disease

Chédiak-Higashi disease is an autosomal recessive disease associated with partial albinism, hypopigmentation, and recurrent infection with abnormal-appearing granules in neutrophils. Anemia, hypersplenism, and platelet function abnormality also occur in these patients. Death may occur as a result of infection, bleeding, or respiratory failure from lymphohistiocytic and reticular cell infiltrates. Other similar neutrophil disorders in which there exists deficiency of specific granules, of myeloperoxidase, or of alkaline phosphates have been described.

DISORDERS OF COMPLEMENT IMMUNITY

Disorders of complement are generally rare diseases resulting from the deficiency (absence or limited function) of any one of the complement components (Table 75–5). Such deficiencies can result in recurrent pyogenic infection (recurrent sinopulmonary infections), recurrent neisserial infection, or collagen-vascular disease.[39] Inappropriate activation of complement also results in diseases such as SLE or hemolytic anemia in which cell damage is caused by complement components activated by immune complexes deposited on cell surfaces.

Immunologic Findings

Complement function can be assessed by determining the total hemolytic activity in serum (CH_{50}, which measures the ability of serum to lyse antibody-coated sheep cells). A low CH_{50} suggests a deficiency in a complement component. Serum levels and function of specific complement components can also be determined.

C3 Deficiency

The major complement deficiency that gives rise to recurrent infections are those that severely affect C3 levels. C3 plays a pivotal role in the complement cascade and in opsonization; therefore, C3 deficiency results in severe recurrent sinopulmonary infections.

C2 Deficiency

C2 deficiency is the most common of the complement-component deficiencies, with an estimated prevalence of 1 per 10,000. Some patients with this deficiency have collagen-vascular diseases, a few have recurrent bacteremic disease, and many are asymptomatic.

C5, C6, C7, and C8 Deficiencies

Patients with deficiency of these components of complement are rare and have increased susceptibility to neisserial infection, including recurrent meningococcal meningitis.

CR1 Deficiency

The major site of CR1 (C3b receptor) is on erythrocytes. Because a reduction in the number of CR1 receptors is associated with circulating immune complexes or with complement-mediated hemolytic anemias, it is thought that CR1 receptors function to remove circulating immune complexes.

CR3 Deficiency

CR3 is a two-chain membrane protein on neutrophils and monocytes that recognizes iC3b, the serum-inactivated C3 fragment. Loss of CR3 results in abnormal phagocytosis. CR3 deficiency also is associated with loss of other leukocyte adhesion molecules that share a common beta-chain subunit (see Leukocyte Adhesion Defects).

C1 Esterase Inhibitor

Absence of C1 esterase inhibitor results in persistent consumption of C2 and C4 by C1 esterase. Release of vasoactive complement fragments occurs, resulting in vasodilatation and nonpruritic angioedema. Episodes occur typically after trauma, stress, or anxiety and last 24

Table 75–5. INHERITED DEFICIENCIES IN COMPLEMENT AND COMPLEMENT-RELATED PROTEIN

Deficient Protein	Observed Pattern of Inheritance at Clinical Level	Reported Major Clinical Correlates*
C1q	Autosomal recessive	Glomerulonephritis, SLE
C1r	Probably autosomal recessive	Syndrome resembling SLE
C1s	Found in combination with C1r deficiency	SLE
C4	Probably autosomal recessive (two separate loci: C4A and C4B)†	Syndromes resembling SLE
C2	Autosomal recessive, HLA-linked	SLE, discoid lupus erythematosus, juvenile rheumatoid arthritis, glomerulonephritis
C3	Autosomal recessive	Recurrent pyogenic infections, glomerulonephritis
C5	Autosomal recessive	Recurrent disseminated neisserial infections, SLE
C6	Autosomal recessive	Recurrent disseminated neisserial infections
C7	Autosomal recessive	Recurrent disseminated neisserial infections, Raynaud's phenomenon
C8 β chain or C8 α-γ chains	Autosomal recessive	Recurrent disseminated neisserial infections
C9	Autosomal recessive	None identified
Properdin	X-linked recessive	Recurrent pyogenic infections, fulminant meningococcemia
Factor $\overline{D}$ C1 inhibitor	Autosomal dominant	Hereditary angioedema, increased incidence of several autoimmune diseases‡
Factor H	Autosomal recessive	Glomerulonephritis
Factor I	Autosomal recessive	Recurrent pyogenic infections
CR1	Autosomal recessive§	Association between low numbers of erythrocyte CR1 and SLE
CR3	Autosomal recessive‖	Leukocytosis, recurrent pyogenic infections, delayed umbilical cord separation

From Frank MM: Complement in the pathophysiology of human disease. N Engl J Med 316:1528, 1987. Reprinted with permission from *The New England Journal of Medicine*, vol. 316, p. 1528, 1987.

SLE, systemic lupus erythematosus; HLA, human lymphocyte antigen.

*Many people with complement deficiencies, especially of C2 and the terminal components, are clinically well. A substantial number of patients with defects in C5 and C9 have had autoimmune disease.

†The deficiency in persons lacking C4a or C5b is referred to as "q0" (quantity zero). Thus such a deficiency can be designated C4aq0 or C4bq0. Persons with such deficiencies are reported to have a higher than normal incidence of autoimmune diseases. Similarly, heterozygous C2-deficient persons are reported to have an increased incidence of autoimmune disease.

‡Approximately 85% of cases involve silent alleles, and 15% involve alleles encoding for dysfunctional variant C1-inhibitor protein.

§Homozygosity for a low (not absent) numerical expression of CR1 on erythrocytes is detectable *in vitro* and appears to be associated with SLE. An acquired defect in the number of CR1 receptors may also be operative.

‖Low but not absent levels of leukocyte CR3 are detectable in both parents of most CR3-deficient children.

to 72 h. Angioedema can occur in any tissue and may not pose serious problems. However, edema of the upper airway can be life-threatening, requiring emergency tracheostomy. Edema in the bowel can cause acute abdominal pain, sometimes confused with appendicitis. An acquired form of the disease also occurs in association with lymphoproliferative disease.

Diagnosis is suggested by family history (autosomal dominant state), by the presence of angioedema without pruritus (lack of urticaria), and by the presence of chronically decreased C4 levels and decreased C2 levels during acute attacks. C1 inhibitor protein is markedly reduced or, if present, is nonfunctioning. In the acquired form, C1q levels are also reduced. Treatment consists of avoiding precipitating factors or pretreatment (e.g., before surgery) with danazol, a semisynthetic androgen that increases serum levels of C1 inhibitor. Purified C1 inhibitor is also effective for treatment of acute attacks.

REFERENCES

1. Makela O, Mattila P, Rautonen N, et al: Isotype concentrations of human antibodies to *Haemophilus influenzae* type b polysaccharide in young adults immunized with the polysaccharide as such or conjugated to a protein (diphtheria toxoid). J Immunol 139:1999–2004, 1987.
2. Siber GR, Schur PH, Aisenberg AC, et al: Correlation between serum IgG2 concentrations and the antibody response to bacterial polysaccharide antigens. N Engl J Med 303:178–182, 1980.
3. Serafin WE, Austen KF: Mediators of immediate hypersensitivity reactions. N Engl J Med 317:30–34, 1987.
4. Tonegawa S: Somatic generation of antibody diversity. Nature 302:575–581, 1983.
5. Strober W, James SP: The interleukins. Pediatr Res 24:549–557, 1988.
6. Coffman RL, Seymour BW, Lebman DA, et al: The role of helper T cell products in mouse B cell differentiation and isotype regulation. Immunol Rev 102:5–28, 1988.
7. Underdown BJ, Schiff JM: Immunoglobulin A: Strategic defense initiative at the mucosal surface. Ann Rev Immunol 4:389–417, 1986.
8. Janeway CA Jr, Carding S, Jones B, et al: CD4+ T cells: Specificity and function. Immunol Rev 101:39–80, 1988.
9. Rosenberg SA, Packard BS, Aebersold PM, et al: Use of tumor-infiltrating lymphocytes and interleukin-2 in the immunotherapy of patients with metastatic melanoma. N Engl J Med 319:1676–1680, 1988.
10. Krensky AM, Weiss A, Crabtree G, et al: T-lymphocyte-antigen interactions in transplant rejection. N Engl J Med 322:510–517, 1990.
11. Rosen FS, Cooper MD, Wedgwood RJ: The primary immunodeficiencies. N Engl J Med 311:235, 300–310, 1984.
12. Cunningham-Rundles C, Siegal FP, Smithwick EM, et al: Efficacy of intravenous immunoglobulin in primary humoral immunodeficiency disease. Ann Intern Med 101:435–439, 1984.
13. Hermans PE, Diaz-Buxo JA, Stobo JD: Idiopathic late-onset immunoglobulin deficiency. Am J Med 61:221–237, 1976.
14. Geha RS, Schneeberger E, Merler E, et al: Heterogeneity of

"acquired" or common variable agammaglobulinemia. N Engl J Med 291:1–6, 1974.

15. Rieger CH, Nelson LA, Peri BA, Lustig JV: Transient hypogammaglobulinemia of infancy. J Pediatr 91:601–603, 1977.

16. Siegel RL, Issekutz T, Schwaber J, et al: Deficiency of T helper cells in transient hypogammaglobulinemia of infancy. N Engl J Med 305:1307–1313, 1981.

17. Schur PH, Borel H, Gelfand EW, et al: Selective gamma-G globulin deficiencies in patients with recurrent pyogenic infections. N Engl J Med 283:631–634, 1970.

18. Umetsu DT, Ambrosino DM, Quinti I, et al: Recurrent sinopulmonary infection and impaired antibody response to bacterial capsular polysaccharide antigen in children with selective IgG-subclass deficiency. N Engl J Med 313:1247–1251, 1985.

19. Rothbach C, Nagel J, Rabin B, Fireman P: Antibody deficiency with normal immunoglobulins. J Pediatr 94:250–253, 1979.

20. Ambrosino DM, Siber GR, Chilmonczyk BA, et al: An immunodeficiency characterized by impaired antibody responses to polysaccharides. N Engl J Med 316:790–793, 1987.

21. Ambrosino DM, Umetsu DT, Siber GT, et al: Selective defect in the antibody response to Haemophilus influenzae type B in children with recurrent infections and normal serum IgG subclass levels. J Allergy Clin Immunol 81:1175–1179, 1988.

22. Oxelius VA, Laurell AB, Lindquist B, et al: IgG subclasses in selective IgA deficiency: Importance of IgG2-IgA deficiency. N Engl J Med 304:1476–1477, 1981.

23. Seager J, Jamison DL, Wilson J, et al: IgA deficiency, epilepsy, and phenytoin treatment. Lancet 2:632–635, 1975.

24. Burks AW, Sampson HA, Buckley RH: Anaphylactic reactions after gamma globulin administration in patients with hypogammaglobulinemia. N Engl J Med 314:560–564, 1986.

25. Goldman AS, Ritzmann SE, Houston EW, et al: Dysgammaglobulinemic antibody deficiency syndrome: Increased γM-globulins and decreased γG- and γA-globulins. J Pediatr 70:16–27, 1967.

26. Freedom RM, Rosen FS, Nadas AS: Congenital cardiovascular disease and anomalies of the third and fourth pharyngeal pouch. Circulation 46:165–172, 1972.

27. Pabst HF, Wright WC, LeRiche J, Stiehm ER: Partial DiGeorge syndrome with substantial cell-mediated immunity. Am J Dis Child 130:316–319, 1976.

28. Giblett ER, Anderson JE, Cohen F, et al: Adenosine-deaminase deficiency in two patients with severely impaired cellular immunity. Lancet 2:1067–1069, 1972.

29. Giblett ER, Ammann AJ, Wara DW, et al: Nucleoside-phosphorylase deficiency in a child with severely defective T-cell immunity and normal B-cell immunity. 1:1010–1013, 1975.

30. Hershfield MS, Buckley RH, Greenberg ML, et al: Treatment of adenosine deaminase deficiency with polyethylene glycol-modified adenosine deaminase. N Engl J Med 316:589–596, 1987.

31. Parkman R, Remold-O'Donnell E, Kenney DM, et al: Surface protein abnormalities in lymphocytes and platelets from patients with Wiskott-Aldrich syndrome. Lancet 2:1387–1389, 1981.

32. Oxelius VA, Berkel AI, Hanson LA: IgG2 deficiency in ataxia-telangiectasia. N Engl J Med 306:515–517, 1982.

33. Waldmann TA, Misiti J, Nelson DL, Kraemer KH: Ataxia-telangiectasia: A multisystem hereditary disease with immunodeficiency, impaired organ maturation, X-ray hypersensitivity, and a high incidence of neoplasia. Ann Intern Med 99:367–379, 1983.

34. Buckley RH, Wray BB, Belmaker EZ: Extreme hyperimmunoglobulinemia E and undue susceptibility to infection. Pediatrics 49:59–70, 1972.

35. Johnston RB Jr: Recurrent bacterial infections in children. N Engl J Med 310:1237–1243, 1984.

36. Curnutte JT, Babior BM: Chronic granulomatous disease. Adv Human Genet 16:229–297, 1987.

37. Ezekowitz RA, Dinauer MC, Jaffe HS, et al: Partial correction of the phagocyte defect in patients with X-linked chronic granulomatous disease by subcutaneous interferon gamma. N Engl J Med 319:146–151, 1988.

38. Fischer A, Lisowska-Grospierre B, Anderson DC, Springer TA: Leukocyte adhesion deficiency: Molecular basis and functional consequences. Immunodeficiency Rev 1:39–54, 1988.

39. Frank MM: Complement in the pathophysiology of human disease. N Engl J Med 316:1525–1530, 1987.

VIII Management

76 ANTIHISTAMINES
DIANE E. SCHULLER, M.D.

An understanding of the appropriate use of antihistamines, with emphasis on possible benefits and side effects, is important for the management of children with lung disease. As many as 65% of children with bronchial asthma have allergic components serving as "trigger factors."[1] Furthermore, such children may also experience other disorders requiring antihistamine use, such as allergic rhinitis, conjunctivitis, urticaria, and atopic dermatitis. Children with other pulmonary diseases such as cystic fibrosis also appear to have an increased incidence of concomitant allergies (ranging from 24% to 59%).[2, 3]

PATHOPHYSIOLOGY

To appreciate the therapeutic action of antihistamines, it is essential to review the current knowledge of histamine, the compound to which antihistamine therapy is directed. The role of histamine in anaphylaxis was first observed by Dale and Laidlaw.[4] Histamine, a beta-imidazolylethylamine, is stored preformed in the cytoplasmic granules of mast cells and basophils. The mast cells are located around blood vessels, nerves, and lymphatic channels in the connective tissue of all organs, especially the upper and lower respiratory tracts.[5] They constitute as much as 2% of alveolar tissue and are located in the connective tissue beneath the airway basement membrane, near the submucosal blood vessels and glands, and throughout the muscle bundles as well.[6]

Inhalation of an allergen by an atopic patient results in the bridging of membrane-bound immunoglobulin E (IgE) antibodies to the antigen located on mast cells. This triggers the degranulation of the human lung and nasal mucosal mast cells with intracellular solubilization of granule contents. Granular and cell membranes fuse to form channels to the outside, through which solubilized granule contents (i.e., histamine) are extruded.[7, 8] Histamine then appears in the blood; levels peak within 5 min and return to base line in 15 to 30 min.[9] Elevations in plama or tissue histamine levels have been demonstrated in bronchial asthma[10, 11] as well as antigen- and exercise-induced asthma.[12] Once released, histamine acts on specific receptors to induce the physiologic consequences observed. Ash and Schild noted that at least two different types of histamine receptors existed.[13] Conventional antihistamines failed to antagonize all of the observed effects of histamine (e.g., gastric acid secretion) and failed to inhibit totally the vascular response (vasodilation and increased capillary permeability). Black and colleagues[14] established the existence of H_1 and H_2 receptors. With a ratio of H_1 to H_2 receptors in the vascular response of 10:1, a combination of both receptor antagonists would be indicated for complete antagonism of histamine release in the role of anaphylaxis.

Stimulation of the H_1 receptor by histamine has major physiologic consequences on hyperreactive airways, causing bronchospasm through smooth muscle contraction in asthmatic patients.[15] Casale and co-workers demonstrated three classes of H_1 receptors in human peripheral lung tissue that may vary in histamine-binding capacities.[16] Stimulation of the H_1 receptor also increases vascular permeability and airway obstruction.[17] Even minor mucosal swelling can lead to a dramatic decrease in airway caliber (i.e., a decrease in airway diameter of only 5% during turbulent airflow can result in a 29% increase in airway resistance).[18] Neural reflexes are secondarily influenced by histamine exposure with indirect stimulation of irritant receptors and the cholinergic nervous system.[19] After upper airway infections, increased histamine responsiveness is believed to be secondary to further stimulation of irritant receptors exposed by denuding airway epithelium[20] (Table 76–1).

Histamine also appears to increase alpha$_2$-adrenergic responses, augmenting contractile responses to norepinephrine.[21] The importance of this role in asthma is evidenced by the ability of phentolamine and phenoxybenzamine to inhibit histamine-induced bronchoconstriction in asthmatic subjects.[22]

Another effect of histamine relevant to bronchial asthma is the release of neuropeptides (e.g., vasoactive intestinal peptide [VIP] through cholinergic stimulation), which has been found by several investigators to cause bronchodilation in some asthmatic subjects.[23] Thus there may exist a negative feedback loop in which histamine causes release of VIP, which could reduce further release of histamine and induce bronchial relaxation. Finally, stimulation of the H_1 receptor has been demonstrated to increase cyclic guanosine monophosphate production

Table 76–1. PHYSIOLOGIC CONSEQUENCES OF HISTAMINE RELEASE ON THE LUNG

H₁ Receptor Stimulation
Bronchospasm in hyperreactive airways
Increased vascular permeability and airway obstruction
Indirect stimulation of irritant receptors and cholinergic nervous system
Increased alpha₂-adrenergic responses
Release of neuropeptides
Increased cyclic guanosine monophosphate production and prostaglandin F₂ₐ

H₂ Receptor Stimulation
Role is controversial: relaxation at high concentrations and bronchoconstriction at lower concentrations
Increased cyclic adenosine monophosphate levels inhibiting neutrophil lysosomal enzyme release and eosinophilic migration
Inhibition of histamine release from basophils
Inhibition of delayed hypersensitivity reactions and cytotoxic T lymphocytes

H₃ Receptor Stimulation
Interacts with histamine at perivascular nerve terminals
May produce vasodilation by inhibition of sympathetic tone

and prostaglandin (PGF_2) generation, both of which may markedly exacerbate bronchial asthma.[24, 25]

As an aside, stimulation of the H_1 receptor by histamine causes a tachycardia resulting from decreased atrioventricular (AV) node connection time and secondary influences of vasodilation plus adrenal catecholamine secretion.[26] The vasodilation-associated symptoms of flushing, headache, and hypotension, as well as some component of tachycardia, have been shown to be secondary to combined H_1 and H_2 stimulation. Therefore, the treatment of the hypotension of anaphylaxis should include both H_1 and H_2 antagonists.[27]

H_2 receptors also play a role in modulating pulmonary disease. Stimulation of the H_2 receptor directly increases airway mucus secretion in humans through direct stimulation of mucous glands; reflex vagal stimulation and possibly augmentation of alpha-adrenergic responsiveness may also play a role.[28] However, the viscosity of the secretions appears to be a reflection of H_1 receptor stimulation, which increases water secretion into the lumen, modulating the viscosity of the released mucus.

The role of H_2 receptors in the bronchial airways is controversial; both bronchodilating[29] and bronchoconstrictive effects have been reported.[30, 31] Histamine stimulates gastric acid secretion through H_2 receptors linked to cyclic adenosine monophosphate (cAMP) in oxyntic cells.[32] Stimulation of H_2 receptors on neutrophils and eosinophils by histamine results in a rise in cAMP levels, with subsequent inhibition of neutrophil lysosomal enzyme release and eosinophilic migration.[33] H_2 receptors also function to inhibit histamine release from human basophils (*in vitro*),[34] delayed hypersensitivity skin test reaction,[35] and *in vivo* generated cytotoxic T lymphocytes.[36] In addition, lymphocytes with histamine-bearing H_2 receptors have been shown to interfere with the maturation of antigen-stimulated B lymphocytes (i.e., antibody secretion from more mature plasma cells and immunoglobulin production by human blood mononuclear cells)[37–39] (see Table 76–1).

An additional receptor, H_3, that serves to inhibit histamine release in the cerebral cortex has been demonstrated.[40] Further studies demonstrated the presence of this receptor at the presynaptic site of the autonomic nervous system,[41] thus involving peripheral areas, interacting with histamine at perivascular nerve terminals. The presence of H_3 receptors in the lung and skin is important. The H_3 receptors appear to be more sensitive to histamine than the H_2 receptors, and so they may have an important function in the physiologic control of circulation. They may produce vasodilation by inhibition of sympathetic tone (see Table 76–1).

The mechanism of action of antihistamines, the competitive inhibition and binding of the antihistamine to the histamine molecule, is readily reversible.[42] They do not repair tissue damage and thus do not reduce the edema and inflammation already produced by histamine exposure, but they block further untoward effects. Most of the antihistamines (the exception being topical azatadine[43]) have been thought not to impair the release of histamine and other mediators, but two studies[44, 45] showed that low concentrations of H_1 receptor antagonists have mast cell–stabilizing characteristics and result in dose-related inhibition of mediator release. However, high concentrations of antihistamines may actually cause release of histamine, even in the absence of antigen.[44]

The biochemical and pharmacologic effects of these "classical" antihistamines include direct receptor blockade of histamine, with inhibition of vasodilation and decrease in the capillary permeability. Effects on the heart include inhibition of both the negative inotropic effect (i.e., decreased contractility) and negative chronotropic effect (decrease in AV conduction), which would otherwise lower the ventricular fibrillation threshold and alter the AV conduction block and contraction failure induced by histamine.[46, 47] Blockade of H_1 receptors in the central nervous system (CNS) is responsible for the sedative effects of antihistamines.[48] The effects of inhibition of nonvascular smooth muscle contraction in the respiratory tract vary with the species studied.[43] An indirect effect of antihistamine use is the inhibition of tachycardia, which may develop from activation of the baroreceptor reflex and catecholamine release in response to histamine (Table 76–2).

In addition to the H_1 receptor blockade, antihistamines cause blockade of cholinergic, muscarinic receptors in a dose-dependent manner (especially diphenhydramine and promethazine).[43] These agents also possess local anesthetic activity.[49] Indirect cardiovascular effects include stabilization of heart tissue (prolongation of the refractory period).[50] An alpha-adrenergic blockade is produced by promethazine, as exemplified by a sudden drop in blood pressure when the drug is given by rapid intravenous injection.[51]

All antihistamines have similar structures, which include an ethylamine chain or ring. Many classical H_1 antagonists are categorized according to the group that connects to the ethylamine radical. The majority contain one or more heterocyclic or aromatic rings connected by a nitrogen, carbon, or oxygen linkage to the tertiary nitrogen of the ethylamine group. These multiple aromatic or

Table 76-2. BIOCHEMICAL AND PHARMACOLOGIC EFFECTS OF CLASSIC H₁ ANTIHISTAMINES

Direct (Receptor Blockade)
Inhibition of vasodilation
Decrease in capillary permeability
Heart effects
    Inhibition of negative inotropic effect
    Inhibition of negative chronotropic effect
Inhibition of nonvascular smooth muscle contraction
Central nervous system blockade (may cause side effects)
Respiratory tract effects (vary with species)
Histamine release possible with high concentrations

Indirect
Tachycardia
    Baroreceptor reflex
    Catecholamine release

Unrelated to Receptor Blockade
Blockade of cholinergic muscarinic receptors (dose dependent)
Local anesthesia
Heart effects (membrane stabilization)
Alpha-adrenergic receptor blockade (promethazine [Phenergan])

heterocyclic rings and alkyl substitutes make the agent lipophilic, free to cross the blood-brain barrier. The classical antihistamines have been classified in six categories on the basis of structure and linkage atom. The type and prevalence of side effects and application in therapy also vary according to class structure. The degree of bioavailability, rate and degree of absorption, degree and rapidity of metabolism, activity of metabolites, dose-dependent side effects, and process of elimination are very important factors in selectivity and effectiveness of the drug (Table 76-3).

ADVERSE REACTIONS

Adverse reactions can be classified according to the body system affected (Table 76-4). The effects on the CNS can be divided into stimulation, depression, neuropsychiatric, and peripheral reactions. Stimulation phenomena include a sudden onset of chills and both early- and delayed-onset dyskinesia. Favis reported the development of intermittent jaw spasm and inability to open the mouth after ingestion of doxylamine (Nyquil).[52] Late-onset dyskinesia has also been reported.[53, 54] Tardive dyskinesia has been observed with the use of phenothiazines[42]; these reactions appeared to be idiosyncratic and may have been secondary to chronic ingestion of large doses.[55] Acute dystonia has been reported in children after administration of diphenhydramine (Benadryl) and was considered an idiosyncratic reaction.[56]

Table 76-3. CLASSIFICATION OF ANTIHISTAMINIC DRUGS AND LISTING OF THEIR SIDE EFFECTS

Class	Examples	Side Effects
Ethylenediamines	Antazoline (Antistine) Methapyrilene Pyrilamine* Tripelennamine (PBZ)	Incidence 20%–35%; GI reactions common (give with meals); moderate CNS effect (physiologic depression > stimulation); epileptogenic; strong smooth muscle stimulant (GI and GU effects); potent sensitizer in topical form; cross sensitivity to aminophylline
Ethanolamines	Bromdiphenhydramine Carbinoxamine (Rondec) Clemastine (Tavist) Dimenhydrinate (Dramamine) Diphenhydramine (Benadryl) Doxylamine (Nyquil) Phenyltoloxamine*	Incidence 50%; marked CNS effect (depression > stimulation); significant anticholinergic and antimuscarinic properties; few GI reactions; epileptogenic; masking of antibiotic ototoxicity possible
Alkylamines	Brompheniramine (Dimetane) Chlorpheniramine (Chlor-Trimeton) Dexbrompheniramine Dexchlorpheniramine (Polaramine) Dimethindene (Foristral, Triten) Pheniramine* Pyrrobutamine (Pyronil) Triprolidine (Actidil)	Low incidence; mild CNS effects (less depression, occasional stimulation)
Phenothiazines	Methdilazine (Tacaryl) Promethazine (Phenergan) Trimeprazine (Temaril)	Marked CNS effects (especially depression); pronounced antimuscarinic activity; photosensitivity; possibility of hyperpigmentation, lenticular and corneal opacities, and chronic jaundice from long-term use of methdilazine and trimeprazine
Piperazines	Buclizine (Bucladin-S Softab) Cyclizine (Marezine) Hydroxyzine* Meclizine (Antivert)	Low incidence; less CNS effect than phenothiazines; least muscarinic effect (cholestatic jaundice reported with cyclizine)
Piperidines	Azatadine (Optimine) Cyproheptadine (Periactin)	Moderate CNS effect (depression); moderate anticholinergic effect; weight gain and increased appetite and linear growth with cyproheptadine; antiserotonin effects reported

GI, gastrointestinal; CNS, central nervous system; GU, genitourinary.
*Various trade name preparations are commercially available.

Table 76–4. SIDE EFFECTS OF ANTIHISTAMINES BY BODY SYSTEM AFFECTED

Neurologic
Stimulatory
Chills
Dyskinesia
Dystonia
Epileptogenic symptoms
Euphoria
Hyperreflexia
Hypertension
Insomnia
Irritability
Headaches
Muscle twitching
Nervousness
Tachycardia
Tremor
Vagal stimulation

Depressive
Ataxia
Coma
Delirium
Dizziness
Drowsiness
Fatigue
Lassitude
Narcolepsy
Somnolence
Weakness

Neuropsychiatric
Confusion
Delusions
Decrease in mental efficiency
Impaired judgment
Hallucinations
"High," "kicks"
Hysteria
Mental depression
Nightmares

Peripheral
Areflexia
Paralysis
Paresthesias
Toxic neuritis

Special-Sense Organs
Ears
Labyrinthitis
Tinnitus
Vertigo

Eyes
Blurred vision
Dilated pupils
Diplopia
Hypermetropia

Gastrointestinal
Anorexia
Cardiospasm
Constipation

Diarrhea
Heartburn
Nausea
Vomiting

Cardiovascular
Cerebral edema
Electrocardiographic changes
Hypertension
Hypotension
Palpitations
Shocklike state
Syncope
Tachycardia
Vasovagal phenomena

Respiratory
Bronchospasm
Dryness of respiratory passages
Nasal stuffiness

Genitourinary
Dysuria
Frequency
Irritative symptoms
Spasmodic retention
Upper nephron nephrosis

Skin and Mucous Membranes
Dermatitis
Dry mouth
Increase in perspiration
Photoallergic reaction
Urticaria

Hematologic
Agranulocytosis
Bone marrow depression
Hemolytic anemia
Neutropenia
Platelet dysfunction
Thrombocytopenia

Endocrine
Increase in appetite
Abnormal B_{12} assay
Early menses
Gynecomastia
Increase in libido
Hypoglycemia
Glycosuria
Decrease in lactation
Abnormal glucose tolerance curve
Interaction with oral contraceptives
Pheochromocytoma stimulation
Secretion in breast milk

Teratogenicity
Cleft palate
Chromatid breakage

The use of antihistamines in epileptic patients has been of concern. Diphenhydramine and tripelennamine (PBZ) may increase electroencephalographic (EEG) abnormalities and may even induce seizures.[57, 58] With antihistamine overdose, tonic-clonic convulsions may occur. Other CNS adverse effects include insomnia, irritability, nervousness, tachycardia, and tremor, which are believed to result from cholinergic blockade.[59] Peripheral neurologic adverse reactions include areflexia, paralysis, paresthesias, and toxic neuritis.[59]

Sedation and drowsiness are well-known adverse effects of antihistamines. Ethanolamines and phenothiazines have the most marked sedative effects, whereas ethylenediamines have moderate effects and alkylamines have mild effects.[60] Even with therapeutic doses, coma has been reported.[61] Delirium and psychosis have been reported with antihistamines.[62–67]

Antihistamines have multiple potential side effects on special-sense organs.[7] For instance, they may mask ototoxicity when used with ototoxic antibiotics.[51] They may also cause blurred vision and hyperopia.[51, 68] Gastrointestinal side effects are most common with ethylenediamines.[60]

Potentially serious side effects are possible in the cardiovascular system.[60] These may include electrocardiographic changes, hypertension, palpitations, and tachycardia. Also possible are vasovagal phenomena, such as ventricular depression, bradycardia, and transient vasodepression.

Antihistaminic side effects on the respiratory system include dryness of the respiratory passages and nasal stuffiness.[60] A more serious side effect, bronchospasm, was initially reported in patients already diagnosed as asthmatic. As a result, for many years, avoidance of antihistamines in asthmatic patients was recommended. However, in the early 1970s, the American College of Allergists reported that chlorpheniramine was safe for use in patients with asthma.[69] Subsequent research confirmed the safety of antihistamine use in patients with known bronchospasm.[70] However, several studies showed that a subset of asthmatic children may have decreased pulmonary function if they receive antihistamines without concurrent bronchodilator therapy.[71, 72]

Other adverse reactions to antihistamines may involve the hematologic, endocrine, and genitourinary systems and the skin and mucous membranes (see Table 76–4).

NEW H$_1$ RECEPTOR ANTAGONISTS

A new generation of H$_1$ receptor antagonists lack any direct chemical relationship to histamine but have as a common structure an aromatic nitrogen in the form of a piperidine, piperazine, or pyridine structure. Their structures are more polar; this limits passage through the blood-brain barrier and reduces or eliminates CNS-related side effects.

TERFENADINE

Terfenadine was the first of this new generation of H$_1$ antihistamines to be released for clinical use in the United States. Terfenadine is highly specific for H$_1$ receptors, has no alpha- or beta-adrenergic receptor activity, and is free of serotonin or acetylcholine antagonism.[73] It does not readily cross the blood-brain barrier, in clinical dosage, but it binds to both peripheral and central H$_1$ receptors with equal affinity. The incidence of sedation, headache, dizziness, nervousness, and dry mouth appears similar to that seen with placebo and significantly less than that seen with the classic H_1 antagonists in controlled studies.[73-76] Terfenadine does not significantly impair psychomotor function or driving performance and does not appear to potentiate the CNS effects of alcohol or tranquilizers such as diazepam.[77]

Terfenadine is rapidly metabolized (99%) on first pass through the liver by the cytochrome P450 oxidative enzymes, leaving minimal unchanged terfenadine (<10 ng/ml) levels. One of the two major metabolites (carboxylic acid derivative) is pharmacologically active, providing 30% of the antihistaminic activity. The use of terfenadine is contraindicated in patients with significant hepatic dysfunction. QT prolongation and rare serious cardiac events (including death, cardiac arrest, torsades de pointes, and other ventricular arrythmias) have been reported.[78] Metabolite peak concentrations lower than normal and a serum half-life longer than normal have been observed.[79]

Drug interactions have been observed between terfenadine and ketaconazole and related products (fluconazole, itraconazole, metronidazole, and miconazole). In one case report,[80] syncope, a prolonged QT_c interval (655 msec), torsades de pointes, and marked elevation of plasma terfenadine concentration[81] after use of ketaconazole with terfenadine were noted. A study of ketaconazole given to 12 healthy subjects taking terfenadine confirmed reduced clearance (30%), prolonged plasma half-life, and QT_c prolongation.[82] Similar observations have been made with the combination of terfenadine and macrolide antibiotics such as erythromycin (troleandomycin, azithromycin, and clarithromycin).[81] Honig[83] studied nine subjects receiving terfenadine and erythromycin together for 7 days. Unchanged terfenadine became detectable in three subjects, and the mean concentration and time to peak concentration of the metabolite were increased.

Adverse cardiac effects, including prolongation of the QT_c interval, arrhythmias, and torsades de pointes have been reported in overdose states.[84-87] ECG studies in patients with allergic rhinitis who were given single doses of terfenadine (60, 180, and 300 mg), acrivastine (8, 25, and 50 mg) diphenhydramine (50 mg), or placebo showed a significant QT interval prolongation for 180 mg and 300 mg of terfenadine as well as for diphenhydramine.[88]

Because studies suggest that terfenadine may have a place in the management of patients with bronchial asthma, especially if allergies are also present, it is important to determine whether interaction occurs between terfenadine and other asthmatic medications. In a pharmacokinetic evaluation of terfenadine in conjunction with theophylline, no significant difference in serial theophylline levels was found when the terfenadine-theophylline therapy was compared with theophylline therapy alone.[89]

ASTEMIZOLE

Another new-generation H_1 antihistamine developed and studied since 1979 is astemizole, an amino piperidinyl-benzimidazole derivative possessing potent H_1 blocking activity. Studies indicate no significant *in vivo* effect related to cholinergic, serotonergic, noradrenergic, and dopaminergic systems either centrally or peripherally.[90-91] It also crosses the blood-brain barrier poorly and appears to have a more selective affinity for peripheral H_1 receptors at the usual dosage.[91] Studies demonstrated no significant CNS depression with doses ranging between 10 and 60 mg, whereas triprolidine (10 mg)[92] and chlorpheniramine[83] produced significant changes. No potentiation of the CNS effects of either alcohol or diazepam has been observed with astemizole use.[91]

With multiple-dose administration of astemizole (10 mg/day), steady-state concentrations of unchanged astemizole were attained in 1 to 2 weeks, whereas steady-state concentrations of astemizole and its metabolites were not reached until 4 to 8 weeks after administration. The recommended dose of astemizole is 10 mg/day (5 mg or 0.2 mg/kg in children); giving a loading dose of 20 to 30 mg/day for 7 days or initially 30 mg tapered to 20 mg and then to 10 mg over several days permits a steady-state concentration to develop more rapidly.[94] However, the astemizole dose of 10 mg/day should not be exceeded because of potential serious adverse effects. After long-term administration (2 weeks to 5 months), the apparent elimination half-life of astemizole and its metabolites ranges from 18 to 20 days. Although the long duration of action would be of value in providing protection should a dose of medication be missed, it could have negative implications if skin testing is required or if side effects develop.

Side effects recorded in multiple astemizole-placebo controlled studies indicate no difference from placebo with regard to sedation, headache, dry mouth, or gastrointestinal complaints; however, increased appetite and weight gain are noted side effects.[94] Astemizole has demonstrated no toxic effects as measured by electrolyte imbalance and kidney function or on the hematologic system.[94] No mutagenic effects or carcinogenic potential has been observed in any of the standard tests to which it has been subjected.[91]

Astemizole is metabolized primarily in the liver, and its use is contraindicated in patients with significant liver disease. Cardiotoxicity from overdose (ingestion of a few tablets) has been reported with prolongation of the QT_c interval and the presence of U waves. Larger doses can lead to severe ventricular arrhythmias, commonly of the torsades de pointes variety.[95-98] Unfortunately, the worst cardiac effects appear late and last long because of the slow elimination. There appear to be no interactions between astemizole and other drugs.[99]

A survey of 50 double-blind trials provided a clinical profile as to the efficacy of astemizole.[100] In 30 studies of patients with seasonal allergic rhinitis, favorable results were observed in 66% of astemizole-treated patients, in comparison with 49% for clemastine, 56% for ketotifen, and 30% for placebo.

Holgate and associates investigated the effect of astemizole in a dose of 10 mg/day for 2 weeks on the immediate airway response to inhaled antigen in a group of nine patients with allergic asthma.[101] In comparison with a controlled airway response to antigen challenge, pretreatment with astemizole attenuated the early component of bronchoconstriction 1 to 15 min after challenge by 40% to 80% but had little effect after this time. This suggested that the release of mast cell–derived histamine in the airways makes a major contribution to the initial phase of immediate bronchoconstriction but that the release of other mediators is more important in producing the later component of this reaction. In another study, pretreatment with astemizole for 2 weeks was also shown to have a protective effect on exercise-induced bronchospasm, but this, paradoxically, was more prominent 1 week after the drug was stopped rather than during the active treatment period.[102] Holgate and colleagues[101] compared the effects of long-term astemizole and placebo on the seasonal symptoms of hay fever and asthma. Although astemizole was highly effective with hay fever symptoms, it also afforded some protection from the seasonal symptoms of asthma.

LORATADINE

Loratadine is another newly developed H_1 antagonist that is a piperidine compound related to azatadine. The conversion of the basic tertiary amino structure of azatadine to a neutral carbonate structure results in a compound that retains significant antihistamine activity but renders it lipid-insoluble, thereby limiting potential CNS and autonomic nervous system effects such as sedation and anticholinergic side effects.[103] It has been shown to preferentially block peripheral rather than central H_1 receptors in vivo[104] and to have a very low potency for binding to alpha-adrenergic receptors. At doses 300 times in excess of its usual antihistaminic dose, loratadine exhibits no depressant activity on CNS function.[106] In addition, it does not appear to interact pharmacologically with centrally depressant drugs such as ethanol, barbiturates, or benzodiazepines. Assessment of objective performance has demonstrated no declines in psychomotor function or the appearance of sedation while patients were receiving loratadine.

An extensive review of the use of loratadine in 2000 patients indicates that it is safe, nonsedating, and well tolerated.[92] Complaints of sedation, headache, fatigue, and dry mouth were similar to those accompanying the use of placebo and terfenadine. Loratadine in a dose of 10 mg once a day is comparable in efficacy with terfenadine in 60 mg twice a day for control of allergic rhinitis.[107] In a different study in which clemastine was compared with loratadine and placebo, clemastine showed significantly greater sedation effects.[108] The incidence and profile of adverse experiences did not change as the studies were extended from 2 weeks to 6 months.

CETIRIZINE

In further development of new nonsedating antihistamines, a principal metabolite of hydroxyzine, cetirizine, was discovered (produced by the carboxylation of a side-chain alcohol). It passes the blood-brain barrier with difficulty and binds to CNS H_1 receptors very poorly.[109] It also fails to bind to serotonin, dopamine, or alpha-adren-

ergic receptors and exhibits no significant anticholinergic activity. At a dose of 10 mg/day, it appears to be effective in relieving allergic symptoms and is well tolerated.[110]

ACRIVASTINE

Acrivastine is a nonsedating H_1 antagonist that is an analog of triprolidine formed by the attachment of an acrylic acid ortho to the pyridine ring nitrogen, thus reducing CNS activity while retaining H_1 receptor antagonist potency. In vivo and in vitro studies demonstrated greater potency than the parent compound triprolidine in blocking histamine-induced wheal-and-flare responses (data on file at Burroughs-Wellcome Co.). It appears to have minimal CNS effects in doses below 25 mg/kg in animals (8 to 16 mg is the usual dose in humans). Although studies of CNS effects show no significant impairment of adaptive tracking, auditory vigilance, or reaction times with clinical dosing of acrivastine,[111] EEG recordings showed that 8-mg and 16-mg doses were mildly sedating, whereas diphenhydramine at 50 mg was severely sedating. Combination of 4 mg, 8 mg, and 16 mg of acrivastine with 60 mg of pseudoephedrine did not differ from placebo with regard to sedation.[112] It appears to be effective in the treatment of allergic rhinitis.[113]

MEQUITAZINE

Mequitazine is an H_1 antagonist used in Europe. It does not readily cross the blood-brain barrier and does not cause sedation at the usual recommended dosage of 5 mg twice daily.[114] Plasma concentrations peak approximately 6 h after ingestion, and the drug is eliminated from the body 38 h after oral intake. At the 5-mg twice-daily dosage, sedation is not reported, presumably as a result of a greater affinity for peripheral H_1 receptors than for central H_1 receptors. However, some anticholinergic activity is noted, and a dose of 10 mg is associated with some central effects. This results in a narrow therapeutic range beyond which side effects may occur.[115]

AZELASTINE

Azelastine is a synthesized phthalazinone derivative that has exhibited a broad spectrum of antiallergic and antiasthmatic activities after oral or aerosol administration.[116, 117] Azelastine appears to be a unique type of drug with effectiveness in allergic rhinitis as well as bronchial asthma. The mechanisms of action appear to be the inhibition of synthesis and antagonism of the chemical mediators of airway hyperreactivity,[118] perhaps through antagonism of calcium-dependent steps necessary in the process of mediator release.

KETOTIFEN

Ketotifen is a unique oral therapeutic agent with antihistaminic properties. It possesses the ability to stabilize mast cells and to inhibit the release of histamine and other mediators. It is a benzocycloheptathiophene derivative that structurally resembles cyproheptadine and azadatine[119] except that the typical benzene ring has been replaced by a five-member sulfur-containing thiophene ring. In addition to the properties mentioned, it also possesses the ability to enhance beta-receptor mediator responses[120] and to prevent anaphylaxis.[121] Ketotifen has been in worldwide use; results indicate that its addition to the therapeutic regimen of asthma therapy allowed gradual reduction in the use of concomitant bronchodilator or steroid therapy while improving lung function. Principal side effects reported included transient drowsiness (19%). It appears to be a prophylactic asthma agent with no immediate effect appreciated by patients. The effects of ketotifen on beta-adrenoceptor action deserve special recognition. Both ketotifen and corticosteroids have been shown to restore or prevent beta-adrenergic tachyphylaxis. Ketotifen prevented the induction of more beta-adrenergic tachyphylaxis, whereas at the end of 2 weeks of therapy, baseline specific airway conductance significantly increased; these findings imply restoration of beta-adrenergic sensitivity.

In summary, ketotifen (like azelastine) will probably be most useful in the treatment of patients with chronic, mild asthma who may also have other allergic disorders such as urticaria, food allergy, or allergic rhinoconjunctivitis.

OXATOMIDE

Oxatomide is a new diphenylmethyl piperazine derivative that has also been shown to inhibit mast-cell histamine release[122] and antagonize the mediators of allergic reactions (histamine, leukotrienes, and so on).[123]

Unusual adverse neurologic reactions to oxatomide use in children commencing 30 to 60 h after initiation of therapy in five children and 8 days later in one patient have been reported.[124] All six children experienced acute dystonic reactions and altered consciousness (lasting up to 3 days). In three patients for whom plasma levels were obtained, the levels greatly exceeded the normal range (40 to 100 ng/ml) despite their use of recommended dosing of 1 mg twice daily. All children recovered after discontinuation of the drug. The authors concluded that it is important to be aware of potential neurologic reactions from oxatomide.

ROLE OF COMBINED H₁ AND H₂ ANTAGONISTS

An important concept that has emerged is the necessity for simultaneous blockade of both H_1 and H_2 vascular receptors in order to inhibit fully the actions of histamine. The histamine-induced wheal response on skin testing involves both H_1 and H_2 receptors, and responses are more effectively reduced by simultaneous use of both types of antagonist than by either alone.[125] The role of the H_1 receptor appears most important in the immediate vascular response to histamine (within 1 min of the start of an intravenous infusion); the H_2 receptors have a more prominent role in the sustained response (when infusions exceed 2 to 3 min).[126] Treatment with an H_1 receptor antagonist delays the vasodilator response to histamine, although a response develops with time during continuous exposure. Although an H_2 receptor antagonist has little effect on the immediate vasodilator response to histamine, it becomes important as the response fades substantially with continuous histamine exposure. It therefore seems logical therapeutically to block simultaneously both H_1 and H_2 histamine-mediated effects (i.e., conditions involving acute inflammation, urticaria, and vascular shock).

Tricyclic antidepressants are potent blockers of both H_1 and H_2 receptors. The tricyclic antidepressant with the greatest antihistaminic activity is doxepin HC1 (approximately 775 times more potent than diphenhydramine as an H_1 blocker and 56 times more potent than cimetidine as an H_2 receptor antagonist[127, 128]). Unfortunately, it also exhibits antimuscarinic, antiserotonergic, and antiadrenergic properties.[129]

Extensive modification of the cimetidine molecule has resulted in the development of a potent H_1 and H_2 antagonist, icotidine, which lacks sedative effects and, like other H_2 antagonists, has difficulty penetrating the blood-brain barrier.[130] This was further proved through the use of icotidine labeled with radioactive carbon, which demonstrated negligible penetration into the brain. Therefore, icotidine is likely to have significant usefulness in the future in conditions requiring complete histamine antagonism, especially anaphylactoid reactions and skin conditions such as chronic urticaria and mastocytosis.[131]

REFERENCES

1. Pearlman D, Bierman CW: Allergic Diseases of Infancy, Childhood and Adolescence. Philadelphia: WB Saunders, 1980.
2. Warner JO, Taylor BW, Norman AP, et al: Association of cystic fibrosis with allergy. Arch Dis Child 51:507–511, 1976.
3. Rachelefsky GS, Osher A, Dooley RE, et al: Coexistent respiratory allergy and cystic fibrosis. Am J Dis Child 128:355–359, 1974.
4. Dale HH, Laidlaw PP: Histamine shock. J Physiol 52:355, 1919.
5. Metcalfe DD, Kaliner MA, Donlon MA: The mast cell. Crit Rev Immunol 3:23–74, 1981.
6. Fox B, Bull TB, Guz A: Mast cells in the human alveolar wall: An electron microscopic study. J Clin Pathol 34:1333–1342, 1981.
7. Friedman MM, Kaliner MA: In situ degranulation of human nasal mucosal mast cells, ultrastructural features and cell-cell associations. J Allergy Clin Immunol 76:70–82, 1985.
8. Caulfield JP, Lewis RA, Hein A, Austen KF: Secretion in dissociated human pulmonary mast cells. J Cell Biol 85:299–312, 1980.
9. Kaplan AP, Beaven MA: In vivo studies of the pathogenesis of cold urticaria, cholinergic urticaria and vibration-induced swelling. J Invest Dermatol 67:327–332, 1976.
10. Lee TH, Nagakura T, Pappeorgiou N, et al: Exercise-induced late asthmatic reactions with neutrophil chemotactic activity. N Engl J Med 308:1502, 1982.
11. Durham SR, Lee TH, Cromwell O, et al: Immunologic studies in allergen-induced late phase asthmatic reactions. J Allergy Clin Immunol 74:49, 1984.
12. Wasserman SI: Mediators of immediate hypersensitivity. J Allergy Clin Immunol 72:101–119, 1983.
13. Ash AS, Schild HO: Receptors mediating some actions of histamine. Br J Pharmacol 27:427–439, 1966.
14. Black JW, Duncan WA, Durant CJ, et al: Definition and antagonism of histamine H₂ receptors. Nature 236:385–390, 1972.

15. Eiser NM, Mills J, Snashall PD, Guz A: The role of histamine receptors in asthma. Clin Sci 60:363–370, 1981.

16. Casale TB, Rodbard D, Kaliner MA: Characterization of histamine H_1 receptors on human peripheral lung. Biochem Pharmacol 34:3285–3292, 1985.

17. Wasserman SI: The lung mast cell: Its physiology and potential relevance to defense of the lung. Environ Health Perspect 35:153–164, 1980.

18. Dubois AB: Resistance to breathing. *In* Fenn WO, Rahn H (eds): Handbook of Physiology, Section 3, Respiration, Vol. 1, pp. 451–462. Washington, DC: American Physiological Society, 1964.

19. Yu DY, Galant SP, Gold W: Inhibition of antigen induced bronchoconstriction by atropine in asthmatic patients. J Appl Physiol 32:823–828, 1972.

20. Empey DW, Laitinen LA, Jacobs L, et al: Mechanisms of bronchial hyperreactivity in normal subjects after upper respiratory tract infection. Am Rev Respir Dis 113:131–139, 1976.

21. Barnes PJ, Skoogh BE, Brown JK, et al: Activation of alpha-adrenergic response in tracheal smooth muscle: A postreceptor mechanism. J Appl Physiol 54:1469–1476, 1983.

22. Kerr JW, Govindaraj M, Patel KR: Effect of alpha-receptor blocking drugs and disodium cromoglycate on histamine hypersensitivity in bronchial asthma. Br Med J 2:139–141, 1970.

23. Mojarad TL, Grode C, Cox C, et al: Differential responses of human asthmatics to inhaled vasoactive intestinal peptide. Am Rev Respir Dis 131:A281, 1985.

24. Platshon LF, Kaliner MA: The effects of the immunologic release of histamine upon human lung cyclic nucleotide levels and prostaglandin generation. J Clin Invest 62:1113–1121, 1978.

25. Sertl K, Casale T, Wescott S, et al: Delineation of lung cells bearing histamine H_1 receptors by immunohistologic analysis employing monoclonal anti-cGMP anti-serum. Am Rev Respir Dis 131:A7, 1985.

26. Levi R, Owen DDA, Trzeciakowski J: Actions of histamine on the heart and vasculature. *In* Ganellin CR, Parsons ME (eds): Pharmacology of Histamine Receptors, pp. 236–297. Boston: Wright PSG, 1982.

27. Kaliner M, Shelhamer JH, Ottesen EA: Effects of infused histamine: Correlation of plasma histamine levels and symptoms. J Allergy Clin Immunol 69:283–289, 1982.

28. Shelhamer JH, Marom Z, Kaliner M: Immunologic and neuropharmacologic stimulation of mucous glycoprotein release from human airways *in vitro*. J Clin Invest 66:1400–1408, 1980.

29. Nathan RA, Segall N, Glover GC, Schocket AL: The effects of H_1 and H_2 antistamines on histamine inhalation challenges in asthmatic patients. Am Rev Respir Dis 120:1251–1258, 1979.

30. Schachter EN, Brown S, Lach E, et al: Histamine blocking agents in healthy and asthmatic subjects. Chest 82:143–147, 1982.

31. Koga Y, Iwatsuki N, Hashimoto Y: Direct effects of H_2 receptor antagonists on airway smooth muscle and on responses mediated by H_1 and H_2 receptors. Anesthesiology 66:181–185, 1987.

32. McNeil JH, Verma SC: Stimulation of rat gastric adenylate cyclase by histamine and histamine analogues and blockade by burinamide. Br J Pharmacol 52:104–106, 1974.

33. Beaven MA: Histamine: Its role in physiological and pathological processes. Monogr Allergy 13:1–113, 1978.

34. Tung R, Kagey-Sobotka L, Plaut M, Lichtenstein LM: H_2 antistamines augment antigen-induced histamine release from human basophils *in vitro*. J Immunol 129:2113–2115, 1982.

35. Rocklin RE: Modulation of cellular immune responses *in vivo* and *in vitro* by histamine receptor-bearing lymphocytes. J Clin Invest 57:1051–1058, 1976.

36. Schwartz A, Askenase PW, Gershon RK: Histamine inhibition of the *in vitro* induction of cytotoxic T cell responses. Immunopharmacology 2:179–190, 1980.

37. Fallah HA, Maillard JL, Voisin GA: Regulatory mast cells 1: Suppressive action of their products on an *in vitro* primary immune reaction. Ann Immunol 126:669–682, 1975.

38. Melmon KL, Bourne HR, Weinstein Y, et al: Hemolytic plaque formation by leukocytes *in vitro*. J Clin Invest 53:13–21, 1974.

39. Lima M, Rocklin RE: Histamine modulates *in vitro* IgG production by pokeweed mitogen-stimulated human mononuclear cells. Cell Immunol 64:324–336, 1981.

40. Arrang JM, Garbarg M, Schwartz JC: Auto-inhibition of brain histamine release mediated by a novel class (H_3) of histamine receptor. Nature 302:832–837, 1983.

41. Ishikawa S, Sperelakis N: A novel class (H_3) of histamine receptors on perivascular nerve terminals. Nature 327:158–160, 1987.

42. Douglas WW: Histamine and 5 hydroxytryptamine (serotonin) and their antagonists. *In* Gilman AG, Goodman LS, Rall TW, Murad F (eds): The Pharmacologic Basis of Therapeutics, 7th ed, pp. 605–638. New York: Macmillan, 1985.

43. Naclerio RM, Meier HL, Adkinson NF Jr, et al: *In vivo* demonstration of inflammatory mediator release following nasal challenge with antigen. Eur J Respir Dis Suppl 128:26–32, 1983.

44. Church MK, Gradidge CF: Inhibition of histamine release from human lung *in vitro* by antihistamines and related drugs. Br J Pharmacol 69:663–667, 1980.

45. Lichtenstein LM, Gillespie E: The effects of the H_1 and H_2 antihistamines on "allergic" histamine release and its inhibition by histamine. J Pharmacol Exp Ther 192:441–450, 1975.

46. Levi R, Guo ZG: Roles of histamine in cardiac dysfunction. *In* Uvnas B, Tasaka K (eds): Advances in Histamine Research: Advances in the Biosciences, vol. 33, pp. 213–222. New York: Pergamon Press, 1982.

47. Levi R, Owen DAA, Trzeiciakowski J: Actions of histamine on heart and vasculature. *In* Ganellin CR, Parsons ME (eds): Pharmacology of Histamine Receptors, pp. 236–297. Boston: John Wright PSG, 1982.

48. Garbarg M, Schwartz JC: Histamine receptors in the brain. New Engl Reg Allergy Proc 6:195–200, 1985.

49. Landau SW, Nelson WA, Gay LN: Antihistaminic properties of local anesthetics and anesthetic properties of antihistaminic compounds. J Allergy 22:19–30, 1951.

50. Dutta NK: Some pharmacologic properties common to antihistaminic compounds. Br J Pharmacol 4:281, 1949.

51. American Medical Association Department of Drugs: AMA Drug Evaluation, 5th ed. Chicago: American Medical Association, 1983.

52. Favis GR: Facial dyskinesia related to antihistamine. N Engl J Med 294:730, 1976.

53. Thach BT, Chase TN, Bosma JF: Oral facial dyskinesia associated with prolonged use of antihistaminic decongestants. N Engl J Med 293:486–487, 1975.

54. Davis WA: Dyskinesia associated with chronic antihistamine use. N Engl J Med 294:113, 1976.

55. Farnebo LO, Fuxe K, Hamberger B, et al: Effect of some antiparkinsonian drugs on catecholamine neurons. J Pharm Pharmacol 22:773–777, 1970.

56. Lavenstein BL, Cantor FK: Acute dystonia: An unusual reaction to diphenhydramine. JAMA 236:291, 1976.

57. Churchill JA, Gammon GD: The effect of antihistaminic drugs on convulsive seizures. JAMA 236:291, 1976.

58. King G, Weeks SD: Pyribenzamine activation of the electroencephalogram. Electroencephalogr Clin Neurophysiol 18:503–507, 1965.

59. Wyngaarden JB, Seevers MH: The toxic effect of antihistaminic drugs. JAMA 145:277, 1951.

60. Simons FE, Simons KJ: H_1 receptor antagonists: Clinical pharmacology and use in allergic disease. Pediatr Clin North Am 30:899–914, 1983.

61. Lee JH, Turndorf H, Poppers PJ: Physostigmine reversal of antihistamine-induced excitement and depression. Anesthesiology 43:683–684, 1975.

62. Borman MC: Danger with Benadryl of self medication and large dosage. JAMA 133:394, 1947.

63. Nigro SA: Toxic psychosis due to diphenhydramine hydrochloride. JAMA 203:301–302, 1968.

64. Gott PH: Cyclizine toxicity: Intentional drug abuse of a proprietary antihistamine. N Engl J Med 279:596, 1968.

65. Sachs BA: The toxicity of Benadryl: A report of a case and review of the literature. Ann Intern Med 29:135–144, 1948.

66. Leighton KM: Paranoid psychosis after abuse of Actifed. Br Med J 284:789–790, 1982.

67. Roman D: Schizophrenia-like psychosis following "Mandrax" overdose. Br J Psychiat 121:619–620, 1972.

68. Crews SJ: Toxic effects on the eye and visual apparatus resulting from the systemic absorption of recently introduced chemical agents. Trans Ophthalmol Soc UK 82:387, 1962.

69. Drug Committee of the American College of Allergists: An investigation of the possible disadvantages of antihistamines in allergic asthma. Ann Allergy 30:95–97, 1972.
70. Karlin JM: The use of antihistamines in asthma. Ann Allergy 30:342–347, 1972.
71. Schuller DE: Adverse effects of brompheniramine on pulmonary function in a subset of asthmatic children. J Allergy Clin Immunol 72:175–179, 1983.
72. Schuller DE: The spectrum of antihistamines adversely affecting pulmonary function in asthmatic children. J Allergy Clin Immunol 71(Suppl. 1, Pt. II):47, 1983.
73. Sorkin EM, Heel RC: Terfenadine: A review of its pharmacodynamic properties and therapeutic efficacy. Drugs 29:34–56, 1985.
74. Buckley CE, Klemawesch SJ, Lucas SK: Treatment of allergic rhinitis with a new selective H_1 antihistamine—terfenadine. New Engl Reg Allergy Proc 6:63–70, 1985.
75. Buckley CE, Buchman E, Falliers CJ, et al: Terfenadine treatment of fall hay fever. Ann Allergy 60:123–128, 1988.
76. Pastorello EA, Ortolani C, Gerosa S, et al: Antihistaminic treatment of allergic rhinitis: A double-blind study with terfenadine versus dexchlorpheniramine. Pharmacotherapeutica 5:69–75, 1987.
77. Moser L, Huther KJ, Koch-Weser J, et al: Effects of terfenadine and diphenhydramine alone or in combination with diazepam or alcohol on psychomotor performance and subjective feelings. Eur J Clin Pharmacol 14:417–423, 1978.
78. Venturini E, Borghi E, Maurini V, et al: Prolongation of the QT interval and hyperkinetic ventricular arrhythmia probably induced by the use of terfenadine in a patient with hepatic cirrhosis. Recenti Prog Med 83:21–22, 1992.
79. Data on file at Marion Merrell Dow.
80. Monahan BP, Ferguson CL, Killeavy S, et al: Torsades de pointes occurring in association with terfenadine use. JAMA 264:2788–2790, 1990.
81. Mathews DR, McNutt B, Okerholm R, et al: Torsades de pointes occurring in association with terfenadine use. JAMA 266:2375–2376, 1991.
82. Eller MG, Okerholm RA: Pharmacokinetic interaction between terfenadine and ketoconazole [Abstract PI-29]. Clin Pharmacol Ther 49(2):130, 1991.
83. Honig PK, Zamani K, Woosley RL, et al: Erythromycin changes terfenadine pharmacokinetics and electrocardiographic pharmacodynamics [Abstract PII-41]. Clin Pharmacol Ther 51:156, 1992.
84. Davies AJ, Harindra V, McEwan A, Ghose RR: Cardiotoxic effect with convulsions in terfenadine overdose. Br Med J 298:325, 1989.
85. Bastecky J, Kvasnicka J, Vortel J, et al: Severe intoxication with antihistamines complicated by ventricular tachycardia. Vnitr Lek 36:266–269, 1990.
86. Guilbaud JC, Moin M, Sader R: A case of rhythm disorder during terfenadine poisoning. Reanim Soins Intensifs Med Urgence 7:233–234, 1991.
87. MacConnell TJ, Stanners AJ: Torsades de pointes complicating treatment with terfenadine. Br Med J 302:1469, 1991.
88. Sanders RI, Dockhorn RJ, Alderman JL, et al: Cardiac effects of acrivastine compared to terfenadine. J Allergy Clin Immunol 89:183, 1992.
89. Luskin A, Luskin SS, Fitzsimmons WE, MacLeod CM: Pharmacokinetic evaluation of the terfenadine-theophylline interaction. J Allergy Clin Immunol 81:320, 1988.
90. Niemegeers CJE, Awouters F: Antihistamines and astemizole: In vivo pharmacological analysis. In Astemizole, A New, Non-Sedative Long Acting H_1 Antagonist. Medicine Publishing Foundation Symposium Series 11, pp. 1–8. Oxford, England: Medical Education Services, 1984.
91. Laduron PM, Janssen PF, Gommeren W, et al: In vitro and in vivo binding characteristics of a new long-acting histamine H_1 antagonist, astemizole. Mol Pharmacol 21:294–300, 1982.
92. Richards DM, Brogden RN, Heel RC, et al: Astemizole, a review of its pharmacodynamic properties and therapeutic efficacy. Drugs 28:38–61, 1984.
93. Nicholson AN, Stone BM: Performance studies with the H_1 histamine receptor antagonists, astemizole and terfenadine. Br J Clin Pharmacol 13:199–202, 1982.
94. Bateman DM, Rawlins RD: Clinical pharmacology of astemizole. In Astemizole, A New, Non-Sedative Long Acting H_1 Antagonist. Medicine Publishing Foundation Symposium Series 11, pp. 43–53. Oxford, England: Medical Education Services, 1984.
95. Craft TM: Torsades de pointes after astemizole overdose. Br Med J 292:660, 1986.
96. Snook J, Boothman BD, Watkins J, Colin JD: Torsades de pointes ventricular tachycardia associated with astemizole overdose. Br J Clin Pract 42:257–259, 1988.
97. Simons FE, Kesselman MS, Giddins NG, et al: Astemizole-induced torsades de pointes. Lancet 2:624, 1988.
98. Stratmann HG, Kennedy HL: Torsades-de-pointes associated with drugs and toxins. Recognition and management. Am Heart J 113:1470–1482, 1987.
99. Rombaut N, Heykants J, Bussche GV: Potential interaction between the H_1 antagonist astemizole and other drugs. Ann Allergy 57:321–324, 1986.
100. Vanden Bussche G, Emanuel MB, Rombaut N: Clinical profile of astemizole: A survey of 50 double-blind trials. Ann Allergy 58:184–188, 1987.
101. Holgate ST, Emanuel MB, Howarth PH: Astemizole and other H_1 antihistaminic drug treatment of asthma. J Allergy Clin Immunol 76:375–380, 1985.
102. Clee MD, Ingram CG, Reid PC, Robertson AS: The effect of astemizole on exercise-induced asthma. Br J Dis Chest 78:180–183, 1984.
103. Hilbert J, Radwanski E, Weglein R, et al: Pharmacokinetics and proportionality of loratadine. J Clin Pharmacol 27:694–698, 1987.
104. Ahn HS, Barnett A: Selective displacement of ^3H mepyramine from peripheral versus central nervous system receptors by loratadine, a nonsedating antihistamine. Eur J Pharmacol 127:153–155, 1986.
105. Kreutner W: Non-sedating antihistamines: Basic and clinical pharmacology. Syllabus of 44th Annual Congress of American College of Allergists, 1987.
106. Friedman HM: Loratadine: A potent non-sedating and long acting H_1 antagonist. Am J Rhinology 1:95, 1987.
107. DelCarpio J, Kabbash L, Turenne Y, et al: Efficacy and safety of loratadine, terfenadine and placebo in the treatment of seasonal allergic rhinitis. J Allergy Clin Immunol 84:741–746, 1989.
108. Dockhorn R, Bergner A, Connell JT, et al: Safety and efficacy of loratadine: A new non-sedating antihistamine in seasonal allergic rhinitis. Ann Allergy 58:407–411, 1987.
109. Snyder SH, Snowman AM: Receptor effects of cetirizine. Ann Allergy 59(6, Pt. II):4–8, 1987.
110. Mansmann HC Jr, Altman RA, Berman BA, et al: Efficacy and safety of cetirizine therapy in perennial allergic rhinitis. Ann Allergy 68:348–353, 1991.
111. Coleman RM, Seidel W, Bliwise N, et al: Direct measurement of antihistamine sedation in man. J Allergy Clin Immunol 75(Pt. I, Suppl.):167, 1985.
112. Coleman RM, Dement W, Poe SH, et al: Effect of acrivastine and pseudoephedrine on daytime sleepiness. Ann Allergy 55(2, Pt. II):232, 1985.
113. Bojkowski CJ, Gibbs TG, Hellstern KH, et al: Acrivastine in allergic rhinitis: A review of clinical experience. J Int Med Res 17(Suppl 2):54B–68B, 1989.
114. Uzan A, LeFur G, Malgouris C: Are antihistamines sedative via a blockade of brain H_1 receptors? J Pharm Pharmacol 31:701–702, 1979.
115. Uzan A, LeFur G: Mequitazine et vigilance. Allergol Immunopathol (Paris) 11:27, 1979.
116. Diamantis W, Harrison JE, Melton J: In vivo and in vitro H_1 antagonist properties of azelastine. Pharmacologist 23:149, 1981.
117. Chand N, Nolan K, Diamantis W, Sofia RD: Inhibition of acute bronchial anaphylaxis by azelastine in aerosol-sensitized guinea pig asthma model. Ann Allergy 55:393, 1985.
118. Chand N, Pillar J, Diamantis W, Sofia RD: Inhibition of allergic and nonallergic histamine release by azelastine and lipoxygenase inhibitors. J Allergy Clin Immunol 75:194, 1985.
119. Craps LP: Immunologic and therapeutic aspects of ketotifen. J Allergy Clin Immunol 76:389–393, 1985.
120. Pauwels R, Van Der Straeten M: Ketotifen prevents bronchial beta-adrenergic tachyphylaxis in normal humans. J Allergy Clin Immunol 79:185, 1987.

121. Martin U, Baggiolini M: Dissociation between the antianaphylactic and the antihistaminic actions of ketotifen. Arch Pharmacol 316:186–189, 1981.
122. Borgers M, DeBrabaner M, Van Reempts J, et al: Morphological evaluation of oxatomide—A new antiallergy drug in guinea pig anaphylaxis. Int Arch Allergy Appl Immunol 56:507, 1978.
123. Awouters F, Niemegeers CJE, Van den Berk J, et al: Oxatomide, a new orally active drug which inhibits both the release and the effects of allergic mediators. Experimentia 33:1657–1659, 1977.
124. Casteels-Van Daele M, Eggermont E, Casaer P, et al: Acute dystonia reactions and long lasting impaired consciousness associated with oxatomide in children. Lancet 1:1204, 1986.
125. Marks R, Greaves MW: Vascular reactions to histamine and compound 48/80 in human skin: suppression by a histamine H_2 receptor blocking agent. Br J Clin Pharmacol 4:367–369, 1977.
126. Chipman P, Glover WE: Histamine H_2 receptors in the human peripheral circulation. Br J Pharmacol 56:494–496, 1976.
127. Richelson E: Tricyclic antidepressants and histamine H_1 receptors. Mayo Clin Proc 54:669–674, 1979.
128. Green JP, Maayani S: Tricyclic antidepressant drugs block histamine H_2 receptors in the brain. Nature 269:163–165, 1977.
129. Richelson E: Antimuscarinic and other receptor-blocking properties of antidepressants. Mayo Clin Proc 58:40–46, 1983.
130. Howey CA, Owen DAA: Inhibition of vascular responses to histamine by SKF 93319—a new antagonist at H_1 and H_2 receptors. Br J Pharmacol 80:438, 1983.
131. Ganellin CR, Blakemore RC, Brown TH, et al: Icotidine, an antagonist of histamine at both H_1 and H_2 receptors. NER Allergy Proc 7:126, 1986.

77 ANTIBIOTICS IN PEDIATRIC PULMONARY INFECTIONS

HILLEL JANAI, M.D. / HARRIS R. STUTMAN, M.D.

The most common dilemma confronting the physician who has a patient with a presumed bacterial infection of the respiratory tract is the selection of an antimicrobial agent. The causative organism is often unknown initially, and an accurate diagnostic approach is vital. The clinical syndrome should be considered carefully; the most likely pathogens should be identified; and, after appropriate microbiologic specimens are obtained, antibiotic therapy should be considered. Empiric therapy should be aimed against pathogens that are the likeliest cause of infection or cause the most significant morbidity and mortality. Risk versus benefit should be considered. Once the pathogenic organism is identified, the initial antimicrobial regimen often can be changed to more specific, less toxic, and less costly therapy.

In most cases, antibacterial administration is not an emergency procedure; therefore, every effort should be made to complete all microbiologic diagnostic procedures (Gram's stains, cultures) before therapy is begun. Ill-considered empiric therapy may mask clinical syndromes, leading to delayed diagnosis and interfering with accurate microbiologic identification. The problems of antimicrobial chemotherapy do not end with the definitive microbiologic diagnosis. Specific factors such as pathophysiologic processes and topographic anatomy of the infectious process, host factors, specific antibiotic properties (pharmacokinetics), and epidemiologic characteristics should be considered when medication is selected. The antibiotic chosen for empyema might differ from that chosen for pneumonia even though the causative organisms are identical. When the host is immunodeficient or when other factors such as hepatic or renal disease exist, the choices of both the antibiotic and the dosage may need adjustment.

The pharmacokinetics of an antibiotic include the rate of absorption, body distribution, metabolism, and excretion. The goal is to maximize antimicrobial activity at the site of infection. Antibiotics differ in tissue penetration and pH stability, properties relevant in the treatment of loculated infections. Drug concentration at the site of infection should optimally be higher than the minimal bactericidal concentration of the offending pathogens for the entire dosing interval. (Table 77–1 describes sputum and pleural fluid concentrations of antibiotics used commonly in respiratory tract infections.)

The route of administration is affected by several considerations. The intravenous route is the most rapid way to achieve high levels in blood and other compartments, but intramuscular administration of certain drugs (ceftriaxone) can achieve the same goals.[1] Furthermore, chloramphenicol, trimethoprim, and isoxazolyl penicillins are bioavailable via oral administration. Other factors that influence concentration levels in infected tissue are serum levels, degree of protein binding, and the molecular weight and electric charge of the antimicrobial agent. The more protein bound the molecule is, the less antibacterial activity will be obtained at local sites. Local environmental conditions (low pH, anaerobic conditions) in an abscess, for example, may adversely affect the bioactivity of some antimicrobial agents, especially aminoglycosides, despite adequate tissue concentrations.

Epidemiologic data on resistance patterns of common bacterial pathogens are often helpful. The increased usage of broad-spectrum antibiotics has led to selective patterns

Table 77-1. ANTIMICROBIALS AND THEIR CONCENTRATION IN SPUTUM AND PLEURAL FLUID

Antibiotic	Route	Sputum: Serum Ratio (%)	Pleural Fluid: Serum Ratio (%)
Aminoglycosides			
Amikacin	IV	16	8–42
Gentamicin	IV		0–59
Tobramycin	IV/IM	3–66	
Cephalosporins			
Cefotaxime	IV	2–10	26
Cefuroxime	IV		30
Cephalothin	IV		116
Cefazolin	IV	2	11–30
Ceftazidime	IV		22
Penicillins			
Amoxicillin	PO	5–16	36
Ampicillin	PO	3–7	49
Penicillin V	PO		67–86
Carbenicillin	IV	1	
Cloxacillin	PO	11	
Ticarcillin	IV	1	14
Tetracyclines			
Doxycycline	PO	17	36
Tetracycline	PO	20–30	
Others			
Clindamycin	PO	60	92
Erythromycin	PO	33–90	
	IV	51–89	
Vancomycin	IV		41

Adapted from Lorian V (ed): Extravascular antimicrobial distribution in man. *In* Antibiotics in Laboratory Medicine, 3rd ed, pp. 880–960. Baltimore: Williams & Wilkins, 1991.

IV, intravenous; IM, intramuscular; PO, per os. The variability of concentrations may be a result of the presence of inflammation, different protein binding, and other localized factors.

of resistance that may vary among geographic locales. For example, in Spain, resistance of *Haemophilus influenzae* to ampicillin is approximately 70% of isolates, and resistance to chloramphenicol is increasing. This is not yet the case in the United States, where *H. influenzae* resistance to ampicillin is present in 20% to 30% of isolates.

Prescribing the adequate antimicrobial agent is only the first step in therapeutics. Monitoring clinical and laboratory efficacy of treatment as well as side effects is also an important consideration. Repeated cultures should be obtained, whenever feasible, to document improvement and sterilization. Serum drug concentrations are often helpful for proving that levels are within the therapeutic range and that toxic concentrations are being avoided. Certain questions should routinely be addressed before antimicrobial therapy is started (Table 77–2).

SPECIFIC ISSUES CONCERNING ANTIMICROBIAL THERAPY

DURATION OF THERAPY

Duration of therapy is an important and frequently overlooked issue. A short course of therapy may be inadequate and lead to relapse. Conversely, an overly prolonged course may expose the patient to more side effects

Table 77-2. QUESTIONS TO ASK BEFORE PRESCRIBING AN ANTIBIOTIC

1. What is the clinical and microbiologic syndrome (e.g., pneumonia, empyema, lung abscess)?
2. Were all appropriate microbiologic studies obtained (cultures, Gram's stains, specific antigen determinations)?
3. What is the anatomic site of the infection?
4. What are the most likely pathogens?
5. What is the spectrum of activity of the antimicrobial agent to be used?
6. What concentrations of the antimicrobial agent must be achieved in order to kill or inhibit the presumptive pathogen?
7. What are the relevant pharmacokinetic properties of the antimicrobial agent (half-life, metabolism, rate of excretion)?
8. What is the best route of administration for this clinical syndrome?
9. What are the potential side effects?
10. Is this choice cost effective?

and promote the emergence of resistant pathogens. Therefore, strict clinical guidelines and carefully documented follow-up are helpful. In general, three factors are important: (1) host, (2) causative pathogen, and (3) clinical syndrome. The more immunocompromised the host is, the longer that therapy is required. For more invasive organisms *(Staphylococcus aureus, Streptococcus pneumoniae)* and patients with a greater tendency to suffer relapse (those with group B *Streptococcus, Salmonella,* and *Brucella* infections), a longer course of therapy is preferred. For pneumonias resulting from aspiration, which are often caused by multiple organisms, and those associated with empyema, surgical drainage and prolonged therapy may be required in order to prevent relapse.

MECHANISMS OF ACTION/DRUG COMBINATIONS

Antibiotics kill or inhibit bacterial growth by different mechanisms, and the understanding of these mechanisms of action (Table 77–3) is crucial in both tailoring therapy

Table 77-3. MECHANISMS OF ACTION OF ANTIMICROBIAL AGENTS

Cell Wall Synthesis Inhibitors
Beta-lactams*
Vancomycin
Teicoplanin
Protein Synthesis Inhibitors
Aminoglycosides†
Macrolides‡
Tetracyclines
Chloramphenicol
Folate Metabolism Inhibitors
Sulfonamides
Trimethoprim
DNA Gyrase Inhibitors
Quinolones
Impairment in DNA Structure and Function
Metronidazole

*Include penicillins, cephalosporins, monobactams, and carbapenems.
†Include gentamicin, tobramycin, and amikacin.
‡Include erythromycin and clindamycin.

and predicting side effects. For example, treatment of *Mycoplasma* or *Chlamydia* pneumonia should not be attempted with antibiotics that affect cell wall synthesis (penicillins and cephalosporins) because these organisms lack cell wall components. Similarly, antimetabolite antibiotics, such as trimethoprim and sulfonamides, that inhibit two steps in folate synthesis should not be prescribed for children with existing folate deficiency.

Mechanisms of action should also be considered in combination therapy. In certain mixed infections and in immunocompromised hosts, a combination of antibiotics may be prescribed. Some combinations may be synergistic, and the drugs may augment each other's antibacterial activity. For example, the combination of ceftazidime (a cephalosporin) and tobramycin (an aminoglycoside) has synergistic activity against *Pseudomonas,* which causes infection in patients with cystic fibrosis and in neutropenic hosts. Some antibiotics produce antagonistic effects. The combination of tetracycline or chloramphenicol (which inhibits protein synthesis) with a β-lactam (which interferes with cell wall synthesis) can be antagonistic and related to therapeutic failure. Therefore, when a decision for a combination therapy is made, knowledge of the mechanisms of action and of *in vitro* and *in vivo* activity are essential. Risks associated with combination therapy may include increased toxicity, *in vivo* antagonism, and selection of resistant organisms.

PROPHYLAXIS

Prophylactic antibiotic treatment in pulmonary infections is limited. The major risks of such treatment are microbial resistance and drug toxicity. The most common uses for prophylactic therapy are for prevention of (1) *Pneumocystis carinii* pneumonia in immunocompromised patients with trimethoprim-sulfamethoxazole (TMP-SMZ), (2) tuberculosis with isoniazid (discussed separately), and (3) pertussis (if the patient is not fully immunized) with erythromycin. In cases of recurrent lung infection such as cystic fibrosis, immotile cilia syndrome, and bronchiectasis, careful consideration of prophylaxis should be based on clinical and laboratory data with thorough evaluation of the risks involved and the potential benefits to be gained.

ORAL ANTIBIOTIC THERAPY FOR SEVERE BACTERIAL INFECTIONS

Promotion of antibacterial activity at the site of infection and achieving levels above the minimal bactericidal concentration of the pathogen are the goals of treatment. The pharmacokinetics of most drugs are well known, and predictable levels can be estimated in the absence of metabolic derangement or organ failure. If adequate antibiotic concentrations can be achieved orally, this route is preferred. Antibiotics that are often effective when given orally include chloramphenicol, cloxacillin, and TMP-SMZ; cephalosporins also are occasionally effective. Reduced hospitalization time, lower cost, and fewer complications (phlebitis, catheter-related infection, and so

Table 77–4. RELEVANT VARIABLES IN OBSERVING RESPONSES TO ANTIMICROBIAL THERAPY

Clinical
Reduction of fever
General well-being (reduction in symptoms: shortness of breath; pain; sputum production)
Stabilization of other vital signs (respiratory rate and blood pressure)
Laboratory
Eradication of bacteria or reduction of bacterial count in infected site
Improvement of radiologic signs (radiograph, CT scan, MRI scan)
Reduction in non-specific inflammatory markers (sedimentation rate, C-reactive protein, and peripheral white blood cell counts)
Improvement in lung functions

CT, computed tomographic; MRI, magnetic resonance imaging.

forth) are major advantages. In serious infections treated orally on an ambulatory basis, monitoring of serum killing power and urine drug bioactivity are warranted. Compliance and other factors (mainly gastrointestinal absorption) may affect this route of treatment.

Pneumonias, lung abscesses, bronchiectasis, and sinusitis can all be adequately treated orally if the causative organism has been presumptively identified, susceptibility patterns have been determined, and an orally bioavailable drug is available. In children with more severe infection, an initial course of intravenous or intramuscular antibiotics can often be followed by completion of therapy with other antibiotics.

ANTIBIOTIC THERAPY FAILURE

Monitoring of clinical symptoms and of laboratory findings is essential for ensuring response (Table 77–4). Therapy failure is defined as persistence of clinical symptoms and of laboratory findings of infection despite appropriate antibiotic therapy. If previous considerations are made (see Table 77–2), the risks for failure are minimized (Table 77–5). The reasons for therapy failure are assessed by careful analysis of other factors that may mimic inadequate therapy. Changing antibiotic regimens without these considerations is apt to increase the risks of drug toxicity and resistance without appreciable benefit. Drug fever and a prolonged natural course of the disease

Table 77–5. GUIDELINES FOR INTERPRETING A LACK OF RESPONSE TO ANTIBIOTIC THERAPY

Factors That May Cause Antibiotic Failure
Incorrect diagnosis
Inappropriate antimicrobial dosage or dosing interval
Decreased absorption or increased metabolism of medication
Undrained abscess or aspiration of a foreign body
Inadequate antibiotic activity at the site of infection
Antagonistic antibiotic combinations
Development of resistance to or tolerance of medication
Secondary infection with a different (resistant) pathogen
Factors That May Mimic Antibiotic Failure
Natural (prolonged) course of disease
Drug fever
Poor compliance with treatment regimen
Immunodeficiency

Table 77–6. RESPIRATORY CLINICAL SYNDROMES AND INITIAL ANTIBIOTIC THERAPY

Syndrome	Causative Organisms	First Choice	Second Choice
Sinusitis	Streptococcus pneumoniae, Haemophilus influenzae, Staphylococcus aureus, Branhamella catarrhalis	Cefuroxime or amoxicillin/ clavulanic acid, cefprozil	Cefaclor or erythromycin/ sulfisoxazole; in children over 8 years, doxycycline
Acute epiglottitis	H. influenzae	IV chloramphenicol (ampicillin if organism is sensitive)	Cefuroxime, cefotaxime, or ceftriaxone
Bacterial tracheitis	S. aureus, H. influenzae, Streptococcus species	IV nafcillin and chloramphenicol	Cefuroxime for penicillin- and cephalosporin-allergic patients; vancomycin and chloramphenicol
Pertussis	Bordetella pertussis	Erythromycin	Chloramphenicol or tetracycline
Diphtheria	Corynebacterium diphtheriae	Erythromycin and antitoxin	Penicillin G
Pneumonia			
Neonatal	Group B Streptococcus, gram-negative bacilli	Ampicillin and aminoglycoside	Ampicillin and cefotaxime or ceftriaxone
Ages >1 month to <3 months	Gram-negative bacilli, H. influenzae, Streptococci	Cefotaxime or ceftriaxone	
	Chlamydia trachomatis	Erythromycin	Ampicillin or amoxicillin
Ages >3 months to <5 years	S. pneumoniae, H. influenzae	Cefuroxime or amoxicillin/ clavulanic acid	Ampicillin and chloramphenicol or cefaclor; cefaclor, erythromycin, and sulfisoxazole (Pediazole)
Age >5 years	Mycoplasma pneumoniae, S. pneumoniae	Erythromycin	Chloramphenicol
Aspiration pneumonia	Oral anaerobes, gram-negative bacilli, gram-positive cocci	Clindamycin and aminoglycoside	Penicillin G and cefotaxime or ceftriaxone
Lung abscess	S. aureus, Klebsiella pneumoniae, oral anaerobes, Streptococcus species	Cefotaxime (or ceftriaxone) and clindamycin (or penicillin G)	Ticarcillin/clavulanate, ampicillin/ sulbactam

IV, intravenous. When causative pathogen is identified, therapy should be modified according to site of infection, susceptibility pattern, and drug toxicity profiles.

may mimic therapeutic failure, and poor compliance with the treatment regimen may cause other mimicking effects; these possibilities should be ruled out before a decision to change antibiotics is made.

SPECIFIC ANTIMICROBIAL AGENTS

The primary properties of antibiotics used in pulmonary infections include an *in vitro* spectrum of activity, *in vivo* applications, routes of administration, absorption and excretion rates, and common side effects. Guidelines for treatment of pulmonary infections are summarized in

Table 77–7. MONITORING FOR ANTIMICROBIAL TOXICITY (OTHER THAN DRUG CONCENTRATION)

Drug	Suggested Monitoring	Frequency
Aminoglycosides	Urinalysis	Twice weekly
	BUN, creatinine	Twice weekly
	Audiometry	If therapy is prolonged
Vancomycin	BUN, creatinine	Twice weekly
Chloramphenicol	CBC, reticulocytes	Twice weekly
Trimethoprim-sulfamethoxazole	CBC, differential	Weekly
	Urinalysis	Weekly
Sulfa drugs	Urinalysis	Weekly
Antistaphylococcal penicillins	Urinalysis, liver enzymes	Weekly
Acylpenicillins and ureidopenicillins	Electrolytes	Twice weekly
All antibiotics	*Clostridium difficile* toxin (stool)	Onset of diarrhea

Modified from Stutman HR, Marks MI: Antimicrobial therapy. Semin Pediatr Infect Dis 2:3–17, 1991.
BUN, blood urea nitrogen; CBC, complete blood count.

Table 77–6, and guidelines for monitoring therapeutic drug levels and toxicity are summarized in Table 77–7.

PENICILLINS

The penicillins remain the drugs of choice for many pediatric respiratory infections because of their high bactericidal activity, low toxicity, and low cost.

Penicillin G is the drug of choice in respiratory infections caused by groups A and B beta-hemolytic streptococci, anaerobic streptococci, oral anaerobic flora, and *Actinomyces israelii.* S. pneumoniae has traditionally been susceptible to penicillin G. Relative resistance to penicillin G (minimal inhibitory concentration, 0.1 to 1 mg/l) has been documented, especially in the pediatric population (10% to 20%).[2] Totally resistant strains have been reported most frequently from countries other than the United States. Every isolate should therefore be tested for relative resistance and, if resistance is present, the penicillin dose should be adjusted or an alternative effective drug chosen. Although high-dose penicillin therapy may suffice, alternative agents are usually available and should be considered for most serious infections. Penicillin G has retained its activity against certain strains of S. aureus that do not produce β-lactamase (5% to 10% of isolates) and is occasionally useful against this organism.

Penicillin is commonly administered (1) orally (penicillin G and penicillin V [phenoxymethyl]), (2) intravenously (aqueous penicillin G), and (3) intramuscularly (procaine penicillin G, benzathine penicillin).

The oral forms of penicillin, especially penicillin V, are well absorbed from the gastrointestinal tract, although serum levels of penicillin V reach only 40% of those of intramuscular aqueous penicillin G. The oral prepara-

Table 77–8. PENICILLINS FOR RESPIRATORY INFECTIONS

Drug	Dose	Frequency (Hours)	Indications
Oral: Phenoxymethyl	50–250 mg/kg/day	4–6	Mild to moderate infections of the upper respiratory tract by susceptible organisms (*Streptococcus pneumoniae*, group A *Streptococcus*)
Intravenous: Aqueous penicillin G Newborns	50,000–250,000 µg/kg/day 50,000–250,000 µg/kg/day	4–6 8–12	Neonatal pneumonia caused by group B *Streptococcus;* severe pneumonias caused by sensitive *S. pneumoniae*, oral anaerobes, and *Actinomyces israelii*
Intramuscular: Procaine	100,000–600,000 µg/kg/day	12–24	Infections with penicillin-susceptible organisms when intravenous access is limited

tions have a role in treating minor to moderate infections and in the completion of therapy for severe infections. In community-acquired pneumonias in which the child appears to be nontoxic and the microbiologic agent is likely to be susceptible to penicillin, treatment goals may be achieved by the oral preparation. Parenteral aqueous penicillin G is used for moderate to severe pneumonia and empyema caused by susceptible pathogens. Administration is preferred by the intravenous route, and frequent administration is usually necessary.

The uses for intramuscular procaine penicillin are limited. Peak serum levels are lower than those achieved with the oral preparation, and its use should be limited to patients who cannot tolerate oral drugs (because of vomiting and diarrhea) and without venous access. Benzathine penicillin has no role in the treatment of acute pulmonary infections.

Penicillin toxicity is rare. Hypersensitivity to penicillin, however, is not rare and may be a life-threatening process. A thorough history for allergy to penicillin should be obtained before the drug is prescribed. However, a positive family history of penicillin allergy should not be considered a contraindication. Careful monitoring of vital signs should be performed when penicillin preparations are administered to patients with such family histories. Skin tests for penicillin allergies are rarely used because of the variety of alternatives to penicillin for hypersensitive patients.[3] Penicillins are also occasionally associated with hemolytic anemia, interstitial nephritis, and neurologic syndromes, especially when large parenteral doses are used. Guidelines for usage in treating respiratory tract infections are summarized in Table 77–8.

AMINOPENICILLINS

Ampicillin and amoxicillin are the two principal representatives of extended-spectrum aminopenicillins. Bacampicillin and cyclacillin have similar spectra of activity. These drugs maintain the *in vitro* spectrum of penicillin G and, in addition, cover some enteric bacilli, non–β-lactamase–producing strains of *H. influenzae* and *Listeria monocytogenes*. Strains of *S. pneumoniae* that are relatively resistant to penicillin G (by a change in penicillin-binding proteins) often remain susceptible to ampicillin. Ampicillin is the only drug in this group that is available in the United States in parenteral prepara-

tions. Amoxicillin (which has relatively good gastrointestinal absorption) has been widely used for the treatment of community-acquired pneumonia, sinusitis, and otitis media caused by susceptible organisms. Side effects are minimal and include diarrhea (5% to 15% of patients) and diaper rash (often related to *Candida* overgrowth) and a variety of hypersensitivity reactions, principally dermatologic. Guidelines for usage in treating respiratory tract infections are summarized in Table 77–9.

BROAD-SPECTRUM PENICILLINS

Broad-spectrum penicillins retain traditional gram-positive activity and have variable effectiveness against gram-negative enteric bacilli (including *Pseudomonas*), enterococcus, and *Bacteroides fragilis.* Their role in the treatment of pediatric pulmonary infections is usually limited to use in patients with cystic fibrosis who are undergoing pulmonary exacerbation (a broad-spectrum penicillin with aminoglycoside is often used) and in immunosuppressed, neonatal, and hospitalized patients with suspected gram-negative pneumonia. Certain patients with aspiration pneumonia caused by multiple organisms may benefit from use of a broad-spectrum penicillin effective against gram-negative bacilli, enterococcus, and oral anaerobic flora. Side effects are uncommon and may include diarrhea, allergic phenomena, phlebitis, coagulopathies (vitamin K–related), neutropenia, and hypokalemia. Because all those compounds contain high sodium concentrations (2 to 6 mEq/l), careful electrolyte monitoring is required. Guidelines for usage in respiratory tract infections are summarized in Table 77–9.

BETA-LACTAMASE RESISTANT PENICILLINS (ANTISTAPHYLOCOCCAL)

After the introduction of penicillin G, resistance related to the bacterial production of β-lactamase developed rapidly among *S. aureus* strains. Methicillin was the first β-lactamase–resistant penicillin compound, but staphylococci-associated toxicity and inadequate coverage of *Streptococcus* species led to later development of oxacillin and nafcillin (parenterally administered) and cloxacillin and dicloxacillin (orally administered). These agents have fairly limited spectra, being primarily active only against

Table 77-9. AMINOPENICILLINS AND BROAD-SPECTRUM PENICILLINS FOR RESPIRATORY INFECTIONS

Drug	Route of Administration	Dose (mg/kg/day)	Frequency (Hours)	Indications
Ampicillin	PO	40–160	6	Mild to moderate respiratory tract infections caused by susceptible organisms: (1) otitis media, (2) sinusitis, (3) pneumonia, (4) epiglottitis
	IV	100–200	4–6	
Amoxicillin	PO	25–100	8	Same as for ampicillin
Ticarcillin	IV, IM	300–600	4–6	1. Moderate to severe lung infections caused by susceptible gram-positive, gram-negative, and anaerobic bacteria 2. Pulmonary exacerbations of cystic fibrosis (usually in combination with an aminoglycoside) 3. Chronic otitis media (*Pseudomonas aeruginosa*)
Azlocillin	IV	300–600	4	Same as for ticarcillin
Newborn aged <7 days		50–150	12	
Newborn aged >7 days		200	4–8	
Mezlocillin	IV	300	4	Same as for ticarcillin
Birth weight >2000 g		75	6–12	
Birth weight <2000 g		75	8–12	
Piperacillin	IV	300	4	Same as for ticarcillin

PO, per os; IV, intravenous; IM, intramuscular.

S. aureus and *Staphylococcus pyogenes.* Usage in pulmonary infections is therefore limited to definite *S. aureus* pneumonias and pulmonary exacerbations of cystic fibrosis that are caused by the same pathogen. Soon after the introduction of these antibiotics, resistance among certain staphylococci, mediated by a change in the bacterial penicillin-binding proteins, was described. The incidence of methicillin-resistant *S. aureus* in the United States remains low, although outbreaks have been reported from surgical intensive care units and neonatal nurseries. Drug toxicity is uncommon, although eosinophilia, interstitial nephritis, neutropenia, abnormal liver function tests, and rashes resulting from each of these

agents have been reported. The oral preparations have an unpleasant taste and may pose problems in administration to younger children. Guidelines for usage in treating respiratory tract infections are summarized in Table 77-10.

BETA-LACTAMASE INHIBITORS (COMBINATIONS)

Clavulanic acid and sulbactam are β-lactamase inhibitors with poor antibacterial activity.[4] Combinations of a β-lactam and a β-lactamase inhibitor extend the spectrum

Table 77-10. ANTISTAPHYLOCOCCAL PENICILLINS AND BETA-LACTAMASE INHIBITOR-CONTAINING COMBINATIONS FOR RESPIRATORY INFECTIONS

Drug	Dose (mg/kg/day)	Frequency (Hours)	Indications
Nafcillin	150	4–6	1. Respiratory infections caused by *Staphylococcus aureus* (pneumonia, lung abscess, tracheitis) 2. Cystic fibrosis, pulmonary exacerbations caused by *S. aureus*
Birth weight <2500 g	75	8	
Birth weight >2500 g	100	8	
Oxacillin	150	4–6	Same as for nafcillin
Cloxacillin	50–100	4–6	Same as for nafcillin
Dicloxacillin	25–80	4–6	Same as for nafcillin
Amoxicillin/clavulanate	25–50	8	Mild to moderate respiratory infections caused by susceptible organisms: (1) otitis media, (2) sinusitis, (3) bronchitis, (4) pneumonia

Ticarcillin with clavulanate (Timentin) and ampicillin with sulbactam (Unasyn) have not been approved by the United States Food and Drug Administration for patients under 12 years of age.

of activity of the principal β-lactam to include activity against β-lactamase–producing organisms. A number of combination compounds are currently marketed. Augmentin (amoxicillin and potassium clavulanate) extends the effectiveness of amoxicillin to include β-lactamase–producing *H. influenzae*, *Branhamella catarrhalis*, and *S. aureus*. Clinical trials have shown it to be effective in mild to moderate infections of the respiratory tract. Unasyn, a parenterally administered combination of ampicillin and sulbactam, extends the spectrum of ampicillin to include *S. aureus* and *H. influenzae* (β-lactamase producers), and it may therefore be used in more severe infections of the respiratory tract.[5] Timentin (ticarcillin and clavulanic acid) extends the spectrum of ticarcillin to include *Klebsiella* and *Staphylococcus* organisms.[6] This compound can often be used as a single drug in aspiration and hospital-acquired pneumonias that are caused by susceptible organisms. Side effects of these three agents are comparable with those of other β-lactams. Diarrhea, skin rashes, and eosinophilia are the most common. Oral formulations have been associated with a significant degree (15% to 25% of patients) of gastrointestinal upset, nausea, and vomiting. Guidelines for usage in treating respiratory tract infections are summarized in Table 77–10.

CEPHALOSPORINS

The cephalosporins also inhibit bacterial cell wall synthesis. Cephalosporins were initially developed as alternatives to penicillin for penicillin-allergic patients. However, later development enhanced antibacterial activity, spectrum of activity, and tissue penetration. Today cephalosporins are considered empiric drugs of first choice in certain clinical syndromes when antimicrobial identification is not established and susceptibility is still unknown. Most of the cephalosporins are excreted in unchanged form by the kidney; the exceptions are ceftriaxone and cefoperazone, which undergo significant biliary clearance. Toxic side effects are uncommon and mild. There is 5% to 15% allergic cross-reactivity between penicillins and cephalosporins, although this appears to be less common in the pediatric age group.[7]

First-generation cephalosporins have anti–gram-positive activity similar to that of penicillin G with the addition of β-lactamase–producing *S. aureus*. Their spectrum also includes activity against many (70%) strains of *Escherichia coli* and *Proteus mirabilis*. They have little activity against *H. influenzae*, which limits their use in pediatric pulmonary infections in children under 4 years of age. The second-generation cephalosporins have gram-positive antimicrobial activity similar to that of the first-generation drugs but with enhanced anti–*H. influenzae* activity (cefaclor, cefuroxime). Cefaclor has been used widely in pediatric respiratory infections such as otitis media, sinusitis, and pneumonia with relative success and minor toxic side effects. Its high cost makes it less attractive than other compounds. Cefuroxime, available in oral and intravenous preparations, has a major role in respiratory infections caused by common pediatric pathogens.[8,9] It is active against *S. pneumoniae*, *H. influenzae*, and *S. aureus*. It has a wide margin of safety and it is often used in initial treatment of moderate to severe pneumonia and epiglottitis.

Extended-spectrum cephalosporins are of limited usefulness in pediatric pulmonary infections. Cefotaxime, a representative of this group, has excellent gram-negative activity and somewhat reduced gram-positive potency.[10-12] Therefore, unless a patient is suspected of having a severe gram-negative infection of the respiratory tract (such as immunocompromised patients), its use is not recommended. Other extended-spectrum cephalosporins have interesting features; for example, ceftazidime[13] has enhanced activity against *Pseudomonas aeruginosa*, and ceftriaxone has a prolonged half-life and is effective when given once daily.[14] Most of the cephalosporins exhibit excellent distribution into body fluids. Levels of these drugs in the middle ear, the sinuses, and sputum are in most cases much higher than the inhibitory concentrations of causative pathogens for prolonged periods. Wide use of these antibiotics has, however, led to the development of resistant organisms. Outbreaks of infections caused by resistant organisms have occurred in intensive care units when extended-spectrum cephalosporins were used routinely. Therefore, evaluation of risks versus benefits should always be made before broad-spectrum antibiotic treatment is started.

There is an approximately 5% to 15% risk of allergic reactions in patients allergic to penicillin. Other toxic side effects are skin rashes and eosinophilia. Serum sickness (associated with cefaclor), neutropenia (cefotaxime), gallbladder deposits (ceftriaxone), and thrombophlebitis (cefuroxime) have been reported. Guidelines for usage of cephalosporins in treating respiratory tract infections are summarized in Table 77–11.

AMINOGLYCOSIDES

Aminoglycosides have been used extensively, and both efficacy and toxicity have been well established. This class of antibiotics includes streptomycin, kanamycin, gentamicin, tobramycin, amikacin, and netilmicin. Their spectrum includes activity against most gram-negative enteric aerobic bacilli, and many of these drugs have excellent activity against *P. aeruginosa*.[15] The three aminoglycosides most commonly used in pediatrics are gentamicin, tobramycin, and amikacin. Their antimicrobial spectra are similar, although activity against *P. aeruginosa* may differ slightly. Aminoglycosides have *in vitro* activity against *S. aureus*, but their *in vivo* efficacy is doubtful, and they should not be used to treat gram-positive infections. Interestingly, aminoglycosides have been shown to induce a synergistic effect in combination with penicillin against enterococcus, even though enterococcus is usually resistant to aminoglycosides alone. Guidelines for usage and in treating respiratory tract infections for desired serum levels are summarized in Table 77–12.

Use of aminoglycosides in treating pediatric pulmonary infections is limited to immunocompromised patients, patients with cystic fibrosis, neonates with pneumonias caused by gram-negative bacilli, and aspiration

Table 77–11. CEPHALOSPORINS FOR RESPIRATORY INFECTIONS

Drug	Route of Administration	Dose (mg/kg/day)	Frequency (Hours)	Indications
First Generation				
Cephalothin	IV	75–150	6	Respiratory infections caused by susceptible organisms (*Staphylococcus aureus* pneumonia in patients with penicillin allergy)
Cefazolin	PO	50–100	8	Same as for cephalothin
Cephalexin	PO	50–100	6	Same as for cephalothin
Second Generation				
Cefuroxime	IV	100–150	6–8	1. Epiglottitis (caused by *Haemophilus influenzae*); 2. Bacterial tracheitis (caused by *H. influenzae* or *S. aureus*); 3. Sinusitis;
Cefprozil	PO	15–30	12	4. Pneumonia (*Streptococcus pneumoniae, H. influenzae,* and *S. aureus*)
Cefuroxime axetil	PO	10–25	12	Mild to moderate respiratory infections; otitis media, sinusitis, community-acquired pneumonia
Cefaclor	PO	40–60	8	Same as for cefuroxime axetil
Cefadroxil	PO	40	12	Same as for cefuroxime axetil
Third Generation				
Cefotaxime	IV	50–200	6	Initial therapy for severe respiratory infections with suspected gram-negative pathogens *(Klebsiella pneumoniae, Escherichia coli)*
Newborn		100	12	
>7 days of age		150	8	
Ceftriaxone	IV, IM	50–100	12–24	Initial therapy for severe respiratory infections caused by susceptible organisms, especially if IV access is limited
Ceftazidime	IV	100–150	8	If *Pseudomonas aeruginosa* is suspected as causative pathogen
Newborn		50	12	

IV, intravenous; PO, per os; IM, intramuscular.

Table 77–12. ANTIMICROBIALS OTHER THAN BETA-LACTAMS FOR RESPIRATORY INFECTIONS THAT REQUIRE SERUM CONCENTRATION MONITORING

Drug	Dose (mg/kg/day)	Frequency (Hours)	Suggested Target (Peak) Serum Levels (mg/l)	Indications
Gentamicin (IV, IM)	5	8	6–10	1. Initial therapy for gram-negative pneumonia and lung abscesses 2. Combined with ampicillin for initial therapy of neonatal pneumonia
Newborn aged ≤7 days	5	12		
Tobramycin (IV, IM)	8–10	8	6–10	Same as for gentamicin
Newborn aged ≤7 days				
Loading dose	5			
Maintenance	5–7.5	12–24		
Newborn aged >7–<30 days	5–7.5	8–12		
Amikacin (IV, IM)	15–20	6–8	15–25	Gram-negative respiratory infections with organisms resistant to gentamicin and tobramycin
Newborn aged ≤7 days				
Loading dose	10			
Maintenance	15	12		
Chloramphenicol				
IV	75–100	6	12–20	Respiratory infections caused by susceptible organisms: (1) epiglottitis *(Haemophilus influenzae)*, (2) lung abscesses, (3) rickettsial lung infections
PO	50–75	6		
Newborn aged ≤14 days	25	24		
Newborn aged >14 days	50	12		
Vancomycin	30–50	12	25–40	1. Staphylococcal respiratory infections in patients allergic to penicillins and cephalosporins 2. Methicillin-resistant *Staphylococcus pneumoniae* infections 3. Highly resistant *S. pneumoniae* infections
Newborn (IV over 30–60 min)				
Weight ≤800 g	18	36		
Weight >800–1200 g	24	24		
Weight >1200–2000 g	36	12–18		
Weight >2000 g	45	12		

IV, intravenous; IM, intramuscular; PO, per os.

pneumonia caused by gram-negative bacilli.[16] Bacterial resistance rarely occurs during therapy. When a choice of an aminoglycoside is to be made, specific hospital susceptibility patterns may be helpful. At the authors' hospital, gentamicin remains a drug of choice for suspected gram-negative pneumonia. Some disadvantages include poor diffusion through biologic membranes and diminished antibacterial activity in anaerobic, acidic conditions, as in lung abscesses or purulent secretions. Common side effects include nephrotoxicity and ototoxicity, although toxicity has not been a common problem in the pediatric age group, especially when monitoring is thorough. Nephrotoxicity of the aminoglycosides is related to high peak levels (for gentamicin, >10 μg/ml), high trough levels (>2 μg/ml), and prolonged administration. Nephrotoxicity is usually reversible, but ototoxicity is often irreversible and related to direct vestibular damage. In adults, tobramycin and amikacin appear to be less nephrotoxic than gentamicin. Guidelines for therapy monitoring are summarized in Table 77–7.

CHLORAMPHENICOL

Chloramphenicol has been used widely for many years, and although aplastic anemia occurs in rare instances (1 in 40,000 patients), it is still a useful drug in treating pediatric patients. Chloramphenicol has a broad spectrum of activity and has bactericidal activity against most gram-positive bacteria and *H. influenzae*. It is bacteriostatic against most gram-negative bacilli and is also active against *Chlamydia* and *Rickettsia*. Among the pediatric pathogens, its important activity is against β-lactamase–producing *H. influenzae* and anaerobic bacteria. Chloramphenicol is available in intravenous, intramuscular, and oral solutions. Oral bioavailability is superior to the parenteral route and is therefore preferred.[17] Chloramphenicol is metabolized by the liver and may interfere with the metabolism of other drugs (mainly antiepileptic agents) by altering their regular expected levels. Therefore, careful drug monitoring is mandatory. Although dose-related anemia occurs, it is reversible. The newer cephalosporins have replaced chloramphenicol for many indications, although its oral bioavailability continues to make it attractive in selected cases. Guidelines for usage in treating respiratory tract infections and for desired serum levels are summarized in Table 77–12.

VANCOMYCIN

Vancomycin is a parenterally administered glycopeptide antibiotic with excellent activity against gram-positive bacteria. Its usefulness in treating pulmonary infections is limited to hospitalized patients with penicillin allergy or with resistant organisms. Methicillin-resistant *S. aureus* pneumonia is an emerging problem in some pediatric intensive care units, and vancomycin is one of the few drugs that are effective against these pathogens. Resistant or moderately resistant strains of *S. pneumoniae* are also becoming widespread, and vancomycin exhibits good activity against these organisms.

Penetration of vancomycin into most body fluids is acceptable; the exception is the central nervous system. Vancomycin can cause nephrotoxicity[18] and ototoxicity and, when administered rapidly, the "red man syndrome" with skin flushing and hypotension.[19] As with other antibiotics, side effects are seen less commonly in children than in adults. Vancomycin may potentiate nephrotoxicity of aminoglycosides, and serum levels should be monitored and adjusted (see Table 77–8) to avoid toxicity.[20] Teicoplanin, a drug with similar structure and antibacterial properties but with potentially less toxic side effects, has been introduced; data concerning its effectiveness in children are as yet limited. Guidelines for usage of vancomycin in treating respiratory tract infections and for desired serum levels are summarized in Table 77–12.

ERYTHROMYCIN

Erythromycin belongs to the macrolide antibiotic group. It is effective against many important respiratory pathogens, including gram-positive cocci such as *S. pneumoniae*, beta-hemolytic streptococci, and *S. aureus*. Furthermore, erythromycin is effective against *Mycoplasma pneumoniae*, *Corynebacterium diphtheriae*, *Bordetella pertussis*, and *Legionella pneumophila*. *Chlamydia trachomatis* is usually sensitive, and treatment of *Chlamydia* pneumonia with erythromycin is common.[21] Erythromycin is the drug of choice for prophylaxis in exposure to pertussis and may be useful in the treatment of pertussis infections.[22] *H. influenzae* is variably sensitive. Several oral preparations are available: erythromycins base, stearate, ethylsuccinate, and estolate salts. Most of them are well tolerated (if taken after meals) and although the estolate preparation has been associated with cholestatic jaundice, this phenomenon is uncommon in children. Intravenous preparations are also available for situations in which oral therapy is not feasible (e.g., vomiting, short bowel), but the intravenous procedure is very irritating to veins, and the drugs must be administered cautiously.

Erythromycin is metabolized primarily in the liver and may increase serum concentrations of theophylline preparations and anticoagulants. The primary side effects are gastrointestinal (abdominal pain, nausea, and vomiting). Guidelines for usage in treating respiratory tract infections are summarized in Table 77–13.

CLINDAMYCIN

Clindamycin is effective against streptococci, staphylococci, and many anaerobic bacteria, including *B. fragilis*. Although it is a bacteriostatic drug, clindamycin is effective in severe infections caused by susceptible organisms. The major side effect (rare in children) is pseudomembranous enterocolitis related to overgrowth and toxin production by *Clostridium difficile*.[23] It is metabolized by the liver and may interfere with metabolism of other drugs (theophylline and phenytoin). In pulmonary infections, its major role is as an alternative to penicillin in hypersensitive patients. In lung infections with anaer-

Table 77-13. ANTIMICROBIALS FOR RESPIRATORY INFECTIONS

Drug	Dose (mg/kg/day)	Frequency (Hours)	Indications
Erythromycin			1. Respiratory infections caused by *Mycoplasma pneumoniae*, *Bordetella pertussis*, *Corynebacterium diphtheriae*, *Chlamydia trachomatis*, *Legionella pneumophila*
PO	30–50	6	
IV (slow infusion)	40–70	6	2. Mild to moderate respiratory tract infections from gram-positive organisms *Staphylococcus pneumoniae*, group A *Streptococcus*
Clindamycin			1. *Staphylococcus aureus* infection in patients allergic to penicillins and cephalosporins
IV	15–40	6	
PO	10–30	6	2. Aspiration pneumonia and lung abscesses (caused by anaerobic organisms)
Infants	15–20	6	
Trimethoprim (TMP) and sulfamethoxazole (SMZ)			*Pneumocystis carinii* pneumonia: (1) IV, 20 TMP/100 SMZ mg/kg/day every 8 h; (2) for prophylaxis; 4 TMP/10 SMZ mg/kg/day every 12 h
PO	5–10 TMP,	12	Erythromycin and sulfisoxazole (Pediazole) for mild to moderate respiratory infections caused by common pediatric pathogens
IV	25–50 SMZ		(group A *Streptococcus*, *S. aureus*, *S. pneumoniae*, *Haemophilus influenzae*)
Loading dose	2 TMP, 5 SMZ	12	
Maintenance	1 TMP, 5 SMZ		
Tetracycline (PO)	20–40	6	1. First choice in rickettsial respiratory tract infections
			2. Mild to moderate sinus infections
			3. Second choice for *Mycoplasma* infection
Chlortetracycline (IV)	12	12	Same as for tetracycline
Doxycycline (PO)	5	12–24	Same as for tetracycline

PO, per os; IV, intravenous.

obic organisms, clindamycin is commonly used, although penicillin G has a nearly comparable spectrum of activity against anaerobic organisms in the respiratory tract. Guidelines for usage in treating respiratory tract infections are summarized in Table 77–13.

SULFONAMIDES/TRIMETHOPRIM

The sulfonamides have a limited role as single agents in pulmonary infections, with the exception of TMP-SMZ, the drug of choice for *P. carinii* pneumonia in immunocompromised patients.[24] This combination has good activity against most gram-negative bacteria other than *Pseudomonas* species and good bactericidal activity against gram-positive cocci, including *S. aureus*. The combination has no activity against group A streptococci. TMP-SMZ is well absorbed orally and has a prolonged half-life, allowing twice-a-day dosing for mild to moderate infections. The most common side effects are dermatologic (skin rashes) and hematologic (neutropenia, anemia, and thrombocytopenia). Reactions with severe Stevens-Johnson syndrome have been described. Another combination containing sulfisoxazole and erythromycin (Pediazole) is often used in mild to moderate respiratory infections due to streptococci, penicillin-resistant *H. influenzae*, and *B. catarrhalis*. Guidelines for usage in treating respiratory tract infections are summarized in Table 77–13.

TETRACYCLINES

Tetracyclines are effective against a broad spectrum of microorganisms. They have bacteriostatic activity against many gram-positive and gram-negative bacteria, *Rickettsia*, *Chlamydia*, and *Mycoplasma*. They are well absorbed from the gastrointestinal tract, and some tetra-

cyclines (doxycycline) are reabsorbed through the enterohepatic circulation, which prolongs their activity. Because tetracyclines are complexed to calcium, they may be deposited in growing teeth and cause staining. Therefore, their usage is very limited in children under 9 years of age.[25] Their main indication, in children over 8 years of age, is for pneumonias caused by *Rickettsia* (Rocky Mountain spotted fever, Q fever) or *Chlamydia* (psittacosis). Guidelines for usage in treating respiratory tract infections are summarized in Table 77–13.

NEWER ANTIBIOTICS

MONOBACTAMS

Aztreonam is the only monobactam currently available for clinical use. It is effective against most gram-negative aerobic bacteria (including *P. aeruginosa*).[26] It has no activity against gram-positive or anaerobic bacteria and is not yet approved by the United States Food and Drug Administration for use in pediatric patients.[27] Aztreonam is less toxic than aminoglycosides and may therefore replace aminoglycosides in the treatment of serious respiratory infections caused by susceptible gram-negative organisms. It can be given safely to penicillin-allergic patients because of the lack of cross-sensitivity. It is given in doses of 120 to 160 mg/kg/day in divided doses every 6 to 8 h for gram-negative pneumonias and lung abscesses.

CARBAPENEMS

Imipenem is the first representative of this group of antibiotics.[28] It is still investigational in the pediatric age group. Imipenem has a very wide spectrum of activity. Its only obvious role is in pulmonary mixed aerobic/anaerobic infections.[29] Imipenem is combined with cilastatin, a renal dipeptidase inhibitor (Primaxin) to prolong its half-life and minimize nephrotoxicity. The dose is 90 mg/kg/day, and it is used only for severe infections of the respiratory tract that are highly resistant organisms susceptible to imipenem

QUINOLONES

Quinolones (ciprofloxacin and norfloxacin) are carboxylic acid derivatives and are not yet approved for use in pediatric patients. They have a wide spectrum of activity, including activity against gram-positive and gram-negative bacteria. They are active against *P. aeruginosa,* methicillin-resistant *S. aureus,* and some mycobacteria. They are well absorbed by the oral route, but because arthropathic side effects have been reported in the young of some animal species, experience in children is very limited.[30] These antibiotics and newer congeners may be used in the future for the oral treatment of pediatric pulmonary infections caused by susceptible organisms. A logical use would be for patients with cystic fibrosis who are undergoing exacerbation of bronchopulmonary infections.[31] Until further toxicity data are available, however, their use in pediatric patients is not recommended.

REFERENCES

1. Ceftriaxone sodium (Rocephin). Med Lett 27:37, 1985.
2. Jackson MA, Shelton S, Nelson JD, McCracken GH: Relatively penicillin-resistant pneumococcal infections in pediatric patients. Pediatr Infect Dis 3:129–132, 1984.
3. Mendelson LM, Ressler C, Rosen JP, et al: Routine elective penicillin allergy skin testing in children and adolescents: Study of sensitization. J Allergy Clin Immunol 73:76–81, 1984.
4. Neu HC, Fu KP: Clavulanic acid, a novel inhibitor of β-lactamases. Antimicrob Agents Chemother 14:650, 1978.
5. Ampicillin/sulbactam (Unasyn). Med Lett 29:79–81, 1987.
6. Gooch WM III, Swenson E, Higbee MD: Use of ticarcillin disodium plus clavulanate potassium in the management of acute bacterial infections in children. Am J Med 79:184–187, 1985.
7. Anderson JA: Cross-sensitivity to cephalosporins in patients allergic to penicillin. Pediatr Infect Dis 5:557–561, 1986.
8. Jones RN, Thornsberry C: *In vitro* antimicrobial activity, physical characteristics and other microbiological features of cefuroxime: A new study and review. Therapy Today 3:1–8, 1983.
9. Cefuroxim axetil. Med Lett 30:57–59, 1988.
10. Jones R, Barry AL, Thornsberry C: Antimicrobial activity of desacetylcefotaxime alone and in combination with cefotaxime: Evidence of synergy. Rev Infect Dis (Suppl) 4:366–373, 1982.
11. Jones FN, Thornsberry C: Cefotaxime: A review of *in vitro* antimicrobial properties and spectrum of activity. Rev Infect Dis (Suppl) 4:300–315, 1982.
12. Meyers BR: Clinical experience with cefotaxime in the treatment of patients with bacteremia. Rev Infect Dis (Suppl) 4:411–415, 1982.
13. Gentry LO: Antimicrobial activity, pharmacokinetics, therapeutic indications and adverse reactions of ceftazidime. Pharmacotherapy 5:254–267, 1985.
14. Yogev R, Shulman ST, Chadwick EG, et al: Once daily ceftriaxone for central nervous system infections and other serious pediatric infections. Pediatr Infect Dis 5:298–303, 1986.
15. Levy J, Smith AL, Kenny MA, et al: Bioactivity of gentamicin in purulent sputum from patients with cystic fibrosis or bronchiectasis: Comparison with activity in serum. J Infect Dis 148:1069–1076, 1983.
16. Davey PG, Barza M: The inoculum effect with gram-negative bacteria *in vitro* and *in vivo.* J Antimicrob Chemother 20:639–644, 1987.
17. Kauffman RE, Thirumoorthi MC, Buckley JA, et al: Relative bioavailability of intravenous chloramphenicol succinate and oral chloramphenicol palmitate in infants and children. J Pediatr 99:963–967, 1981.
18. Odio C, McCracken GH Jr, Nelson JD: Nephrotoxicity associated with vancomycin-aminoglycoside therapy in four children. J Pediatr 105:491–493, 1984.
19. Garrelts JC, Peterie JD: Vancomycin and the "red man's syndrome" [Letter]. N Engl J Med 312:245, 1985.
20. Meyer RD: Risk factors and comparisons of clinical nephrotoxicity of aminoglycosides. Am J Med (Suppl 6B) 80:119–125, 1986.
21. Hammerschlag MR, Cummings C, Roblin PM, et al: Efficacy of neonatal ocular prophylaxis for the prevention of chlamydial and gonococcal conjunctivitis. N Engl J Med 320:769–772, 1989.
22. Hoppe JE, Haug A: Treatment and prevention of pertussis by antimicrobial agents (Part II). Infection 16:148–152, 1988.
23. McFarland LV, Stamm WE: Review of *Clostridium difficile*-associated diseases. Am J Infect Control 14:99–109, 1986.
24. Pachl MS: Treatment of prophylaxis of *Pneumocystis carinii* pneumonia. AIDS (Suppl) 2:143–250, 1988.
25. Committee on Infectious Diseases, American Academy of Pediatrics: Report of the Committee on Infectious Diseases, 22nd ed, pp. 167, 407. Elk Grove Village, IL: American Academy of Pediatrics, 1991.
26. Meyer RD: Risk factors and comparisons of clinical nephrotoxicity of aminoglycosides. Am J Med (Suppl 6B) 80:119–125, 1986.
27. Brogden RN, Heel RC: Aztreonam: A review of its antibacterial activity, pharmacokinetic properties and therapeutic use. Drugs 31:96–130, 1986.
28. Jacobs RF: Imipenem-cilastatin: The first thienamycin antibiotic. Pediatr Infect Dis 5:444–448, 1986.
29. Neu HC: Clinical perspectives on imipenem. J Antimicrob Chemother 12(Suppl D):149–153, 1983.
30. Douidar SM, Snodgrass WR: Potential role of fluoroquinolones in pediatric infections. Rev Infect Dis 2:878–889, 1989.
31. Stutman HR: Summary of a workshop on ciprofloxacin use in patients with cystic fibrosis. Pediatr Infect Dis 6:982–995, 1987.

78 HOME INTRAVENOUS ANTIBIOTIC USE

SCOTT DAVIS, M.D.

Since 1980, physicians and other health care providers have had to examine the social, psychological, economic, and personal costs to individuals and to a society faced with the medical needs of a growing number of people with chronic diseases. The result of this examination has been a gradual return to home-based care for some patients previously bound to the hospital by their treatment needs. The availability of home care has increased dramatically as new treatment regimens have developed, technologic advances have simplified medical equipment, and knowledge acquired over time has demonstrated what is necessary in order to safely administer sophisticated treatment regimens in a nonhospital setting.

Hemodialysis was one of the earliest forms of parenteral therapy to be used when home-based hemodialysis became an alternative to hospital-based care.[1] Since then, home intravenous therapy programs have expanded to include treatment for a variety of patients (e.g., those with debilitating gastrointestinal diseases requiring parenteral hyperalimentation,[2, 3] cancer patients receiving chemotherapy,[4] patients with hemophilia who require coagulation factor replacement,[5] and patients needing long-term antibiotic therapy). These programs have enabled patients to avoid prolonged or repeated hospitalizations.

HIVAT PROGRAMS

An estimated 30% to 50% of all hospitalized patients in the United States receive antibiotic therapy,[6] and a growing number of these patients require prolonged intravenous therapy. Because of the high cost of inpatient antibiotic treatment, physicians have begun to consider home intravenous antibiotic therapy (HIVAT) for some patients. The reasons for this consideration include an expected lower cost of treatment, improved efficiency in use of acute-care hospital beds, early return of patients to work and school, and intangible psychological and sociological advantages.[7]

A relatively small and mostly anecdotal body of literature details the current knowledge of the benefits and risks of HIVAT. In available studies, investigators have described HIVAT programs as safe, acceptable to patients, and both medically sound and cost effective.[8–19] Most HIVAT programs are characterized by careful selection of patients, in-hospital instruction, close monitoring of HIVAT patients after discharge, and an organized interdisciplinary team to direct individualized care. The association between an interdisciplinary approach to care and successful home therapy has been a consistent finding in both HIVAT[10, 11, 13, 14] and other types of home parenteral therapy.[20–22] Together, the members of an interdisciplinary team are responsible for providing the services that contribute to the safety and efficacy of HIVAT: (1) availability of 24-h on-call service, (2) management of intravenous access, (3) monitoring of clinical progress and complications, (4) therapeutic drug monitoring, and (5) delivery, storage, and documentation of antibiotics.

The rapid growth of home infusion companies that provide nursing support and the services of a pharmacist to physicians requesting HIVAT for their patients will undoubtedly change the character of the "team" concept. Interaction of physicians with members of the company team may be excellent if the physician prescribes such therapy frequently. However, the potential for poor communication with a breakdown in selection, in education, or in follow-up of patients may be greater when individual physicians prescribe HIVAT infrequently or a non–hospital-based program is used.

In addition to modifying the role of an interdisciplinary team in HIVAT programs, commercial companies may impose their interests on the selection process. In hospital-based HIVAT programs, the initial referral for home parenteral therapy commonly originates with the individual patient's physician. On receiving the referral, the HIVAT team initiates an assessment of the eligibility and suitability of the patient for home therapy. The rise of commercial home care companies, pressures from a variety of third-party payers, and utilization review companies may alter the traditional process of referral by the physician. Nearly all the referrals to one major home health care company came from hospitals or physicians in 1985, but that company estimated that by 1990, 40% of referrals would come from insurance companies and corporations.[23] Cost-containment pressures may have a negative impact on the selection process by removing the final decision for selection of patients for HIVAT from physicians or HIVAT teams.

SELECTION OF PATIENTS

There appear to be only two essential criteria for establishing eligibility for HIVAT: patients must require pa-

Table 78–1. SELECTION OF PATIENTS FOR HOME
INTRAVENOUS ANTIBIOTIC THERAPY

Eligibility Criteria
Patient must require parenteral antibiotic therapy
Patient must be medically stable
Patient must desire or be willing to accept home therapy

Suitability Criteria
Availability of responsible caretaker
Training program successfully completed by caretaker
Good home/family support for patient
Appropriate duration of therapy
Antibiotics appropriate for home use
Proper home environment and equipment
Availability of local medical care
Adequate intravenous access
Appropriate reimbursement coverage
Compliance of patient

renteral antibiotic therapy and should be medically stable. From a practical standpoint, the latter means that the patient's illness does not require frequent daily monitoring by health care personnel or other medical treatment that can be administered only in the hospital. Many HIVAT programs would add patient's motivation and desire for home therapy as a third eligibility criterion.[9, 11, 14, 18, 24] Even normally compliant patients may not administer parenteral antibiotics in a safe and timely manner if they are not highly motivated. However, as HIVAT gradually becomes accepted as a standard of care, some third-party payers may disregard patient's motivation as a necessary component of home therapy. These funding agencies may choose to pay a nurse to administer the antibiotics in the patient's home because of cost containment pressures.

Once the physician or the HIVAT team determines that a patient is eligible for home therapy, the suitability for HIVAT should be assessed (Table 78–1). The rejection rate of eligible patients may be as high as 50% in some institutions and populations of patients.[13] The criteria used to screen eligible patients for their suitability for HIVAT vary, depending on the availability of responsible caretakers to administer the intravenous antibiotics. To function as a responsible caretaker, a person must have the background and ability necessary to successfully complete a training program. The home care setting should be scrutinized carefully in order to determine whether the proposed caretaker will be able to administer parenteral therapy for the desired length of time. Some persons may have the ability and desire to assist with HIVAT but may be unable to do so because of other commitments at home or at work.

Some suitability factors should be examined, regardless of who will administer the antibiotics. The expected duration of treatment should be long enough to warrant the time and expense of training and the seemingly small additional risk inherent in HIVAT. Some programs restrict HIVAT to patients who require at least 2 weeks of additional therapy.[25] Shorter periods of HIVAT may be considered when nurses are available to administer the antibiotic or the prospective caretaker is familiar with intravenous antibiotic administration (e.g., a parent of a patient with cystic fibrosis). In both cases, the shorter training period necessary to provide for safe home therapy may justify a shorter duration of home therapy. Patients who need short, repeated courses of intravenous antibiotics should be considered HIVAT candidates because subsequent episodes do not require the caretaker to undergo a complete period of instruction. A suitable home environment for HIVAT requires little in the way of specific equipment.[24] Clean areas should be available for storage of drug administration and intravenous care supplies. Most antibiotics require refrigeration in order to maintain potency for more than a few hours. Data on the stability of various antibiotics at room temperature, in a refrigerator, and in a freezer are available in the medical or pharmaceutical literature.[26] There should be a telephone at the location where antibiotics are to be administered, in case problems develop. All patients receiving HIVAT should have ready access to local medical care. A local physician or medical institution from which the patient and family can seek medical attention should be identified, and communication with this local medical source should be established before the HIVAT is initiated.

Certain types of parenteral antibiotics and antibiotic dosing regimens lend themselves to administration in the home setting. Patients who are being treated with a single antibiotic that is administered infrequently are more likely to be suitable candidates for and complete a HIVAT program than are patients being treated with two or more antibiotics with frequent dosing intervals. Reports in the literature suggest that patients have successfully completed courses of parenteral antibiotics administered as often as every 4 h,[10] although in most studies, antibiotics were administered every 6 to 8 h[8, 17] or the dosing interval was not specified.[11-16]

The availability of venous access is an essential part of a successful HIVAT course.[27] Poor venous access can result in increased complications, rehospitalization, or inadequate treatment because of premature termination of therapy. Many patients, once they have returned home, are reluctant to return to the hospital to finish therapy. The choice of access mode is dependent on how irritating the antibiotic is to veins, the quantity and condition of the patient's peripheral veins, and the expected duration of therapy.[28]

The advent of indwelling central catheters that can be maintained for extended periods of time has helped ensure long-term venous access for patients who require repeated or prolonged parenteral therapy.[29, 30] Such catheters allow patients with poor venous access to participate successfully in HIVAT programs.[31, 32] The newest type of central catheter, totally implantable vascular access device (IVAD), has been found to provide a safe means of vascular access in a variety of clinical situations.[33-35] Most patients prefer these catheters to the older Broviac and Hickman catheters because IVADs require no daily care when not in use and are cosmetically more acceptable. When shorter durations of treatment are planned or frequent, repeated courses of therapy are unlikely, peripherally placed central venous catheters have been reported to be a safe and effective alternative means of vascular access.[36, 37] If peripheral venous access is used in the home setting, an appropriate and timely mechanism for restarting intravenous lines should be established before initiation of HIVAT (e.g., a local physician's office, an emergency room, or a home care nursing service).

It is necessary for patients to have adequate reimbursement coverage so they are not financially penalized for receiving treatment at home. The proportion of plans offering home health benefits rose from 46% in 1974 to 90% in 1983.[38] However, Medicare and Medicaid have been slow to reimburse health care providers for HIVAT services. The Medicare Catastrophic Coverage Act of 1988 mandated coverage for home intravenous drugs and their associated services, but it was subsequently repealed. This act listed several indications for antibiotic drugs that were specifically excluded from Medicare coverage; among these indications were respiratory tract infections.[39] Whether certain respiratory infections such as acute pulmonary exacerbations in patients with cystic fibrosis will ultimately be included under Medicare coverage remains to be determined.

ANTIBIOTIC ADMINISTRATION

The initial methods of home intravenous antibiotic administration were somewhat more complicated than those used currently. Patients were often expected to learn how to mix individual doses of an antibiotic agent from vials of powder.[13] The reconstituted antibiotics were then administered manually through a syringe or injected into a "minibag" for infusion by gravity. Most home care programs have now changed to premixed antibiotic solutions that are delivered every few days to the patient. Besides the obvious reduction in safety concerns occasioned by the use of pharmacy-prepared antibiotic doses, training requirements for patients are simplified.

Several types of drug delivery systems used in the hospital have been adapted for home use, and new ones have been developed specifically for home use. Gravity infusion delivery systems are used in the home setting primarily because of their simplicity and low cost. However, many of the drawbacks of this type of delivery system seen in the hospital are amplified in the home setting. Patients using gravity infusion cannot ambulate easily, and this may interfere with one of the main advantages of home therapy: a patient's ability to return to work or school. Gravity infusions also require careful monitoring because the equipment has no safety features for monitoring flow.

Some of the problems with gravity infusion have been solved through the use of infusion pumps similar or identical to the kind used in hospitals. Advantages of this type of delivery system include precise control of flow and alarms that signal an occlusion in the catheter or the completion of an antibiotic dose. Unfortunately, several drawbacks make the operation of these machines more difficult for caretakers with no medical experience. Significant training time is necessary because patients or caretakers must learn to change tubing, program the machines, and identify possible problems. The machines are capable of mechanical failures, and this can be a problem particularly if a home care agency has to travel long distances to a patient's home with a replacement pump. The daily cost

of pump rental and ancillary supplies can be extremely high, particularly if a backup unit is kept at the patient's home. Antibiotic administration with infusion pumps, as with gravity infusion, restricts the patient's ability to ambulate, to attend school, or to work.

The problems encountered with traditional hospital intravenous antibiotic delivery systems in the home setting have led to the development of new systems that are classified as ambulatory infusion devices. Two of the earliest such devices were peristaltic and syringe pumps. The main advantage of these pumps is that a patient's movement is unrestricted during antibiotic administration. Other advantages include the ability to deliver antibiotic at a set rate, the presence of some alarms for signaling catheter occlusion or infusion completion, and the need for a relatively limited amount of training for the patient. The major disadvantage of the syringe pump systems is that infusion volume is limited. Doses of the newer cephalosporin and penicillin derivatives usually must be diluted in a large volume of fluid if administered through peripheral veins, in order to avoid chemical phlebitis. Syringe pumps are an impractical delivery system for such antibiotics if peripheral access is used. Peristaltic pumps can accommodate larger fluid volumes, but many are not recommended for use with peripheral venous access because of the pressure developed by the pump.[26] These pumps, although generally more reliable than the larger and more complex hospital infusion pumps, still can malfunction and leave patients without any means of administering the antibiotics.

The most recent generation of new infusion pumps eliminates many of the disadvantages of previous pumps by using stored mechanical energy as the driving force for antibiotic infusion. Examples of such devices are seen in Figure 78–1*A* and 78–1*B*. In these devices, the antibiotic is instilled into a distensible bladder under pressure. The rate of antibiotic delivery is determined by the characteristics of special intravenous tubing attached to the device. Because these pumps have fewer parts, they should be more reliable than other ambulatory pumps. They do not depend on batteries or electricity and therefore can be used almost anywhere. Their small size and light weight allow them to be used easily in most school or work settings. To begin an antibiotic infusion, a patient needs only to attach a needle to the pump's tubing, insert the needle into the intravenous catheter, and release a clamp. The ease with which antibiotic administration can be accomplished reduces the training time significantly. Computerized pumps of several types are also available for HIVAT.

EFFICACY

The growing acceptance of HIVAT is based on very few well-controlled scientific studies. Most of the papers published during the 1970s and 1980s on the clinical efficacy of HIVAT have been anecdotal reports (see Table 78–1). Only one prospective clinical trial has been performed, and this involved the use of a case control rather than a randomized design. The available information suggests that HIVAT is as effective as intravenous antibiotic ther-

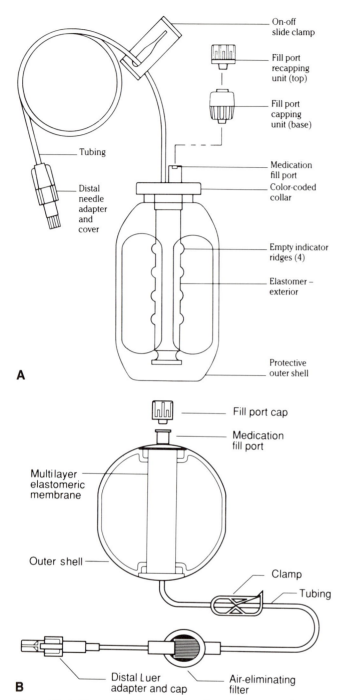

On-off
slide clamp

Fill port
recapping
unit (top)

Fill port
capping
unit (base)

Tubing

Distal
needle
adapter
and
cover

Medication
fill port
Color-coded
collar

Empty indicator
ridges (4)

Elastomer –
exterior

Protective
outer shell

A

Fill port cap

Medication
fill port

Multilayer
elastomeric
membrane

Outer shell

Clamp

Tubing

Distal Luer
adapter and cap

Air-eliminating
filter

B

Figure 78–1. Disposable infusion devices for administration of intravenous antibiotics in the home. *A,* Intermate; *B,* Homepump.

apy administered in the hospital. Early case reports[8-14] suggested a success rate ranging from 68% to 96%. The majority of patients described in these reports had bone and joint infections. Most of the treatment failures involved complicated osteomyelitis that required additional surgical intervention.

One of the earliest studies on the use of HIVAT included 127 HIVAT courses for pulmonary exacerbations in 62 patients with cystic fibrosis.[8] In 68% of these exacerbations, patients were able to avoid hospitalization.

Over the next decade, several anecdotal reports describing the use of HIVAT in smaller groups of patients with cystic fibrosis appeared in the literature.[15, 31, 32, 40, 41] Donati and colleagues reported data from the first prospective controlled trial of HIVAT in patients with cystic fibrosis.[17] They analyzed 41 home and 41 hospital treatments for patients with exacerbations of pulmonary disease caused by cystic fibrosis. The patients in each group were matched according to sex, age, pulmonary function tests, and arterial blood gas values. Both groups had a significant increase in pulmonary function tests, and there was no difference in these values between groups either at the beginning or at the end of treatment. The needs for retreatment during the study period were similar in both groups. Donati and colleagues concluded that home parenteral antibiotic therapy for patients with cystic fibrosis is as effective as similar therapy in the hospital.

The study by Donati and colleagues had some flaws. The reporting of dosing frequency of antibiotics was ambiguous as to how many home patients received antibiotics every 6 or every 8 h and which specific antibiotics were administered. The home patients in this study received daily nursing visits, and Donati and colleagues acknowledged that this high level of support may have played an important role in the success of patients treated at home. Therefore, it may not be possible to extend these results to HIVAT programs in which follow-up is not as intensive. Of more importance, these investigators did not indicate the statistical power (beta error) of their observations, in view of the relatively small size of their study sample.

SAFETY

When considering the treatment of a patient at home with a regimen once performed only in the hospital, a physician must remember Hippocrates' admonition, "Primum non nocere" ("first, do no harm"). Unfortunately, the lack of data from controlled clinical trials hampers investigators' ability to judge the safety of HIVAT. In only two studies in which a case control design was used have investigators reported on the incidence of complications related to HIVAT.[9, 17]

No deaths or major complications directly related to HIVAT have been reported to date.[8-19] The reported complications of HIVAT generally can be divided into four groups: (1) infiltrated or nonfunctioning intravenous catheter access lines or catheters, (2) adverse drug experience, (3) laboratory abnormalities, and (4) premature discontinuation of therapy. The most common type of complication reported was drug reaction, such as rashes, fevers, arthralgias, and gastrointestional symptoms. The incidence of these complications ranged from 5% to 17%.[9-11, 13, 14, 16, 18] Clinically significant phlebitis was uncommon; reported incidences ranged from 1% to 6% in the larger studies.[11, 13, 14] These complicatons were generally believed to be secondary to irritation from the antibiotics and not results of catheter infection. None of the affected patients required discontinuation of therapy or readmission to the hospital. In two studies, investigators

Table 78–2. COMPARISONS OF COST FACTORS FOR HOME INTRAVENOUS ANTIBIOTIC THERAPY

Study	Design*	No. Subjects	Age Range (Years)	Principal Diseases†	Dosing Interval	Days of Outpatient Therapy		Success Rate		Cost Saving per Day of Outpatient Treatment
						Range	Mean	No.	%	
Rucker and Harrison (1974)[8]	CS	62	7–27	CF	Every 8 h	?	—	87/127	69	?
Stiver et al. (1978)[9]	HCC	23	12–78	OS, SA	Every 3–5 h while awake or every 8 h	8–40	23	18/23	78	$97
Kind et al. (1979)[10]	CS	15	3–61	OS, EN, SA	Every 4–8 h	7–24	17	12/14	86	$95
Poretz et al. (1982)[11]	CS	150	3–86	OS, SA, PY	?	4–49	20	137/150	91	$142
Stiver et al. (1982)[12]	CS	95	4–81	OS, SA, EN, CF	?	8–46	22.9	85/95	89	$135
Rehm and Weinstein (1983)[13]	CS	48	10–77‡	OS, AB, EN, SA	?	2–42	18.8	42/48	87	$305
Goldenberg et al. (1984)[14]	CS	89	1.5–18	OS, SA, AB, SI	?	4–59	18	85/89	96	$200
Winter et al. (1984)[15]	CS	10	17.1–40.5§	CF	?	5–10	6.6	10/10	100	?
Manzella et al. (1985)[16]	CS	45	3.5–78‖	OS, EN	?	3–99	20.5	?	—	$162
Donati et al. (1987)[17]	PCC	26	13–39	CF	Every 6–8 h	?	—	26/26	100	$471
Graves et al. (1987)[18]	CS	37	3–77	OS, EN, SA	?	?	23	?	—	$121
Strandvik et al. (1988)[19]	CS	31	4–67	CF	?	?	—	31/31	100	?

*CS, case series; HCC, historical case control; PCC, prospective case control. †CF, cystic fibrosis; OS, osteomyelitis; SA, septic arthritis; EN, endocarditis; PY, pyelonephritis; AB, abscess; SI, sinusitis. ‡Mean, 41 years. §Mean, 23.1 years. ‖Mean, 45 years.

reported the occurrence of laboratory abnormalities such as eosinophilia, leukopenia, neutropenia, and elevated creatinine levels.[9, 14]

In the studies dealing with HIVAT only for patients with cystic fibrosis,[8, 15, 17, 19] very few complications were noted. Rucker and Harrison mentioned that some patients experienced mild thrombophlebitis after 7 to 8 days and required changing the intravenous catheter site.[8] Donati and colleagues described premature termination of therapy in three patients; this was the only complication among their 26 patients treated with HIVAT.[17]

The true incidence of complications from HIVAT remains unknown because of the retrospective nature of most reports on HIVAT, the dependency on patients and their families to report complications, and the lack of routine laboratory screening for complications. However, the lack of any reports of deaths or major complications arising directly from HIVAT despite its increasingly widespread use suggests that the incidence of major complications is probably very low. The appearance of previously unknown drug interactions should prompt caution when new parenteral antibiotics are used in the home setting.

COST

The cost-benefit advantages of home therapy in comparison with hospital therapy have been and will continue to be one of the principal driving forces behind the growth of HIVAT and home health care programs. In detailed analyses of health care, three categories of costs and benefits are usually considered: direct, indirect, and intangi-

ble. Because of the difficulty in determining indirect costs such as loss of income from work and intangible costs such as pain and inconvenience, studies of HIVAT costs have dealt almost exclusively with the direct costs.

In all studies on HIVAT, investigators have reported a significant reduction in daily costs with the use of home therapy (Table 78–2). The magnitude of the potential savings is illustrated best in the prospective study by Donati and colleagues,[17] in which 41 home treatments in 26 patients were compared with 41 hospital admissions in 38 patients. The cost saving per day of outpatient over inpatient therapy was $471. Over the 18-month study period, the cost of home care was $370,000 less than similar care in the hospital. Donati and colleagues estimated that home intravenous therapy could save $960,000 if half of their patients with cystic fibrosis over the age of 12 received therapy for pulmonary exacerbations at home.

Although all the studies listed in Table 78–2 seem to support Donati and colleagues' estimate of significant annual savings in care cost to patients when HIVAT is used,[17] some caution must be exercised in extrapolating these savings to larger populations. Acceptance of home parenteral therapy by patients and physicians is growing, and as a result, the market for such therapy was estimated to triple from $869 million in 1986 to nearly $2.8 billion in 1990.[23] New and established health care companies aggressively market home parenteral therapy programs. These programs undoubtedly appeal to hospitals and physicians who do not have the desire or resources to establish their own hospital program. The HIVAT companies rely on charges for preparation and delivery of antibiotics as their primary source of income. Costs for the delivery of the same HIVAT regimen differ tremendously among home care vendors.[42] Because some companies have been noted to approach or exceed the daily charges for continued hospitalization, it is important to obtain an estimate of daily cost for HIVAT when choosing among home care vendors.[28]

The duration and frequency of intravenous antibiotic treatments administered to patients with cystic fibrosis could rise as HIVAT becomes more prevalent, and they could substantially reduce the expected overall savings from administering parenteral antibiotics to these patients at home rather than in the hospital. Cost is not the only motivation for using HIVAT. The increased use of parenteral antibiotics has been reported to improve patients' health and survival.[43] Thus even if the net savings from using HIVAT instead of parenteral antibiotic therapy in the hospital were reduced to zero, other patient-derived benefits would support the use of HIVAT.

PROFESSIONAL LIABILITY ISSUES

Although the use of HIVAT is increasing rapidly in many parts of the United States, it is still unclear whether this method of delivery represents the "standard of care" in any region of the nation. As more patients are treated in the home with parenteral antibiotics, some will undoubtedly suffer adverse outcomes or complications that will lead to litigation. Few legal precedents are available in this area of medical jurisprudence, and some attorneys and physicians see HIVAT as a major source of medical litigation in the future.[28]

Most published reports on HIVAT generally acknowledge the importance of several general principles of therapy such as careful selection and thorough education of patients. However, there are no uniform guidelines or a published consensus on the specific practical aspects of HIVAT care. Although it seems that initiation of HIVAT in the hospital is the safest and most prudent course to follow, some patients receive their first dose of antibiotics in the home setting without medical supervision. No investigators have critically examined the risks of administering the first dose of parenteral antibiotics in the home with or without medical supervision. Likewise, there is no clear definition of what constitutes appropriate follow-up care while patients receive parenteral antibiotics at home. In published reports, some authors have described daily visits by team members,[17] whereas others have mentioned visits to or by medical personnel every few days[12] or as seldom as once a week.[13]

Patients treated with HIVAT are at risk for the same complications as patients receiving parenteral antibiotics in the hospital. These problems range from severe, life-threatening adverse drug reactions to premature hospital discharge or inadequate follow-up by the physician. For these reasons, some clinicians have suggested that "informed consent" be obtained from a patient before the initiation of home therapy.[28] Irrespective of whether formal informed consent is obtained, physicians must outline the possible complications and their outcomes in the home environment. Patients and their families must understand that their agreement to participate in HIVAT reflects their agreement to share the risks associated with HIVAT therapy.

REFERENCES

1. Merril JP, Schupak E, Cameron E, Hampers CL: Hemodialysis in the home. JAMA 190:468–70, 1964.
2. Jeejeebhoy KN, Langer B, Tsallas G, et al: Total parenteral nutrition at home: Studies in patients surviving four months to five years. Gastroenterology 71:943–53, 1976.
3. Byrne WJ, Ament ME, Burke M, Fonkalsrud E: Home parenteral nutrition. Surg Gynecol Obstet 149:593–599, 1979.
4. Plasse T, Ohnuma T, Bruckner H, et al: Portable infusions pumps in ambulatory cancer chemotherapy. Cancer 50:27–31, 1982.
5. Rabiner SF, Telfer MC: Home transfusion for patients with hemophilia A. N Engl J Med 283:1011–1015, 1970.
6. Kasmer RJ, Hoisington LM, Yukniewicz S: Home parenteral antibiotic therapy, part I: An overview of program design. Home Healthcare Nurse 5(1):12–18, 1987.
7. Smego RA: Home intravenous antibiotic therapy. Arch Intern Med 145:1001–1002, 1985.
8. Rucker RW, Harrison GM: Outpatient intravenous medications in the management of cystic fibrosis. Pediatrics 54:358–360, 1974.
9. Stiver HG, Telford GO, Mossey JM, et al: Intravenous antibiotic therapy at home. Ann Intern Med 89:690–693, 1978.
10. Kind AC, Williams DN, Persons G, Gibson JA: Intravenous antibiotic therapy at home. Arch Intern Med 139:413–415, 1979.
11. Poretz DM, Eron LJ, Goldenberg RI, et al: Intravenous antibiotic therapy in an outpatient setting. JAMA 248:336–339, 1982.
12. Stiver HG, Trosky SK, Cote DD, Oruck JL: Self-administration of intravenous antibiotics: An efficient cost-effective home care program. Can Med Assoc J 127:207–211, 1982.
13. Rehm SJ, Weinstein AJ: Home intravenous antibiotic therapy: A team approach. Ann Intern Med 99:388–392, 1983.
14. Goldenberg RI, Poretz DM, Eron LJ, et al: Intravenous antibiotic therapy in ambulatory pediatric patients. Pediatr Infect Dis 3:514–517, 1984.
15. Winter RJ, George RJ, Deacock SJ, et al: Self-administered home intravenous antibiotic therapy in bronchiectasis and adult cystic fibrosis. Lancet 1:1338–1339, 1984.
16. Manzella JP, Klaus B, McConville JH, Brenner T: Home intravenous antibiotic therapy. Pa Med 88:52–54, 1985.
17. Donati MA, Guenette G, Auerbach H: Prospective controlled study of home and hospital therapy of cystic fibrosis pulmonary disease. J Pediatr 111:28–33, 1987.
18. Graves G, Jackson JP, Maxwell A, Woods T: Home intravenous antibiotic therapy in Arkansas. J Arkansas Med Soc 84:55–57, 1987.
19. Strandvik B, Hjelte L, Widen B: Home intravenous antibiotic treatment in cystic fibrosis. Scand J Gastroenterol (Suppl 143):119–120, 1988.
20. Blagg CR, Daly SM, Rosenquist BJ, et al: The importance of patient training in home hemodialysis. Ann Intern Med 73:841–847, 1970.
21. Schreiber MJ, Vidt DG: Organizational aspects of continuous ambulatory peritoneal dialysis (CAPD). Cleve Clin Q 48:237–243, 1981.
22. Srp F, Steigler E, Montague N, et al: Patient preparation for cyclic home parenteral nutrition: A team approach. Nutr Support Service 1:30–34, 1981.
23. Lutz S: Home I.V. therapy companies target insurers, HMOs for future growth. Mod Healthcare 17(6):96, 99, 1987.
24. Harris WL: Home parenteral antibiotic therapy. Topic Hosp Pharm Management 4:43–55, 1984.
25. Manzella JP, McConville JH: Home intravenous antibiotic therapy. Pa Med 88:52–54, 1985.
26. Kasmer RJ, Hoisington LM, Yukniewicz S: Home parenteral antibiotic therapy, part II: Drug prescription and administration considerations. Home Healthcare Nurse 5(1):19–29, 1987.
27. Goldenberg RI: Pitfalls in the delivery of outpatient intravenous therapy. Drug Intell Clin Pharm 19:293–296, 1985.
28. McCue JD: Outpatient i.v. antibiotic therapy: Practical and ethical considerations. Hosp Pract 23:208–211, 1988.

29. Broviac JW, Cole JJ, Scribner SH: A silicone rubber atrial catheter for prolonged parenteral alimentation. Surg Gynecol Obstet 136:602–606, 1973.
30. Hickman RO, Buckner CD, Clift RA, et al: A modified right atrial catheter for access to the venous system in marrow transplant recipients. Surg Gynecol Obstet 148:871–875, 1979.
31. Splaingard ML, Pokorny WJ, Harrison GM: Experience with Broviac catheters for home hyperalimentation and antibiotic administration in patients with cystic fibrosis. Cystic Fibrosis Club Abstracts 1982:140, 1982.
32. Davis SH, Waring WW: Antibiotics administered at home through a central venous catheter in patients with cystic fibrosis. Clin Res 32:908A, 1984.
33. Bothe A, Piccione W, Ambrosino JJ, et al: Implantable central venous access system. Am J Surg 147:565–569, 1984.
34. Wallace J, Zeltzer PM: Benefits, complications, and care of implantable infusion devices in 31 children with cancer. J Pediatr Surg 22:833–838, 1987.
35. Schultz WH, Ware R, Filston HC, Kinney TR: Prolonged use of an implantable central venous access system in a child with severe hemophilia. J Pediatr 114:100–101, 1989.
36. Zanni RL, Shutack JG, Schuler PM, et al: Peripherally inserted central venous catheters for treatment of cystic fibrosis. Pediatr Pulmonol 1:328–332, 1985.
37. Dietrich KA, Lobas JG: Use of single Silastic catheter for cystic fibrosis pulmonary exacerbations. Pediatr Pulmonol 4:181–184, 1988.
38. Weinstein SM: Regulatory concerns: Home care. NITA 10:175–184, 1987.
39. Grimaldi PL: Medicare covers home IV drug therapy. Nurs Manage 20:14, 17, 1989.
40. Camerini-Otero CS, Fink RJ: Home antibiotic therapy in cystic fibrosis via a central venous catheter. Cystic Fibrosis Club Abstracts 1980:57, 1980.
41. Isenberg JN, Osher AB: Potential value of antibiotics and parenteral nutrition through a central venous catheter in cystic fibrosis. Cystic Fibrosis Club Abstracts 1978:55, 1978.
42. Kane RE, Jennison K, Wood C, et al: Cost savings and economic considerations using home intravenous antibiotic therapy for cystic fibrosis patients. Pediatr Pulmonol 4:84–89, 1988.
43. Szaff M, Hoiby N, Flensborg EW: Frequent antibiotic therapy improves survival of cystic fibrosis patients with chronic *Pseudomonas aeruginosa* infections. Acta Paediatr Scand 72:651–657, 1983.

79 BETA-ADRENERGIC AGONISTS IN THE TREATMENT OF ASTHMA

R. MICHAEL SLY, M.D.

Asthma is a chronic pulmonary disease characterized by increased irritability (hyperreactivity) of the lower airways and manifested by recurrent episodes of generalized airway obstruction that is usually reversible either spontaneously or after appropriate treatment. Accordingly, appropriate use of pharmacologic agents, including beta-adrenergic agonists, is essential for optimal management of asthma.

MECHANISMS OF ACTION

A beta-adrenergic agonist such as isoproterenol can interact with beta-adrenergic receptors on smooth muscle cells and mast cells. The beta-adrenergic receptors are coupled to adenylate cyclase by a guanine nucleotide-binding complex. Stimulation causes formation of cyclic adenosine monophosphate (cAMP) from adenosine triphosphate. Activation of cAMP-dependent protein kinase in smooth muscle regulates activity of phosphoprotein substrates that change the distribution of intracellular and extracellular calcium ions. Phosphorylation of myosin light chain kinase by cAMP-dependent protein kinase changes the myosin light-chain-kinase to a form that cannot bind calmodulin at the concentration of calcium ions present in the resting cell. This change causes dephosphorylation of myosin light-chain kinase by intrinsic phosphatase activity, resulting in smooth muscle relaxation.[1]

In the mast cells, increases in concentration of cAMP inhibit release of mediators induced by subsequent interaction of antigen with immunoglobulin (IgE) antibody. The clinical relevance of this action is uncertain, but albuterol inhibits anaphylaxis in human lungs at concentrations similar to those necessary for relaxation of human bronchial smooth muscle.[2]

Other mechanisms of possible clinical relevance include increased mucociliary clearance and reversal of mediator-induced increased microvascular permeability.[3–5]

BETA-ADRENERGIC AGONISTS

The Chinese used ma huang, derived from the plant *Ephedra equisetina*, for more than 5000 years before Chen and Schmidt identified the active constituent, ephedrine.[6] In 1900, Solis-Cohen described the use of tab-

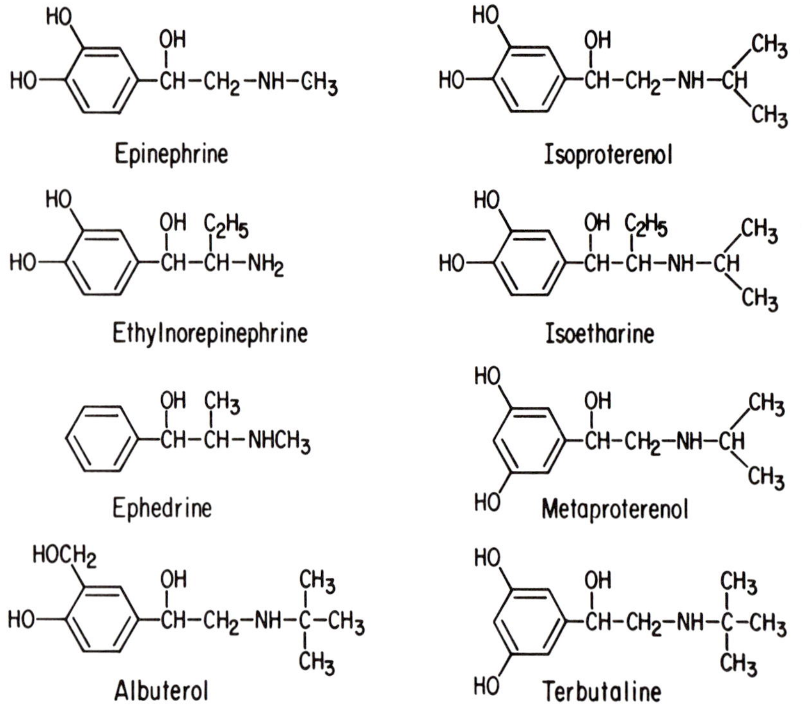

Figure 79–1. Chemical structures of some beta-adrenergic agonists.

lets prepared from desiccated adrenal glands for the treatment of asthma.[7] Later, Takamine isolated the active compound, epinephrine (adrenaline).[8] In 1940, Konzett described isoproterenol, which he found to be more effective than epinephrine in the treatment of asthma.[9]

Isoproterenol has several limitations, including substantial cardiac stimulation. Inactivation by intestinal and hepatic sulfatases follows oral administration, so inhalation is the usual route of administration; this drug can also be given by intravenous infusion. Duration of bronchodilation is relatively short after inhalation of isoproterenol, and catechol-O-methyltransferase metabolizes it rapidly to 3-methoxyisoproterenol, a weak beta-adrenergic blocking agent.[10]

Inhalation of isoproterenol has elicited increased airway obstruction within 15 to 60 min in a few asthmatic patients, sometimes after brief improvement.[11, 12] The same phenomenon can follow intravenous administration.[13] The mechanism is unknown. Tolerance is one possible explanation, but lack of bronchodilation or bronchoconstriction after inhalation of isoproterenol has been reported in some asthmatic patients who had not received this drug during the previous year.[14]

Inhalation of isoproterenol can cause decreases in arterial oxygen tension (Pa_{O_2}) in approximately half of asthmatic patients evaluated. Decreases are usually no more than 5 to 10 mm Hg but in rare instances have been as much as 15 mm Hg and very rarely have been as much as 25 mm Hg.[15] The decrease is maximal in 5 min and resolves over the next 15 min.[16, 17] The greatest decreases have generally occurred in patients with the highest initial Pa_{O_2} values, who could best tolerate some decrease, but during severe airway obstruction with hypoxemia any further decrease in Pa_{O_2} would be undesirable.

This effect is probably caused by aggravation of the ventilation/perfusion imbalance characteristic of acute asthma. Alveolar hyperinflation and increased perfusion of poorly ventilated areas of lung in which vessels are constricted by hypoxemia may be caused by preferential distribution of increased cardiac output as isoproterenol causes relaxation of vascular smooth muscle.[17] The decrease in arterial Pa_{O_2} in response to treatment can be minimized or prevented by supplemental oxygen.

Because of these shortcomings of isoproterenol, pharmacologists and biochemists sought safer, more effective beta-adrenergic agonists. Removal of two methyl groups from the N-alkyl substituent of isoproterenol leaves epinephrine, a compound characterized by increased alpha-adrenergic activity but some decrease in beta-adrenergic activity (Fig. 79–1). Elimination of the remaining terminal methyl group leaves norepinephrine, which has very little activity on beta-adrenergic receptors. However, addition of another methyl group to the N-alkyl substituent of isoproterenol, as in terbutaline, confers increased activity on the beta2-adrenergic receptors that predominate in respiratory smooth muscle.

Isoetharine was the first clinically important beta-adrenergic agonist with some selectivity for beta2-adrenergic receptors. In this agonist, the alpha-alkyl substitution resulted in increased selectivity (see Fig. 79–1). As a bronchodilator, isoetharine is more potent than epinephrine but less potent than isoproterenol.[18] Its selectivity, however, allows use of doses that more than compensate for its lesser potency.[19] The usefulness of isoetharine, like that of isoproterenol, is limited by a relatively short duration of action.

The changes in the positions of the phenolic hydroxyl groups of metaproterenol and terbutaline and the substi-

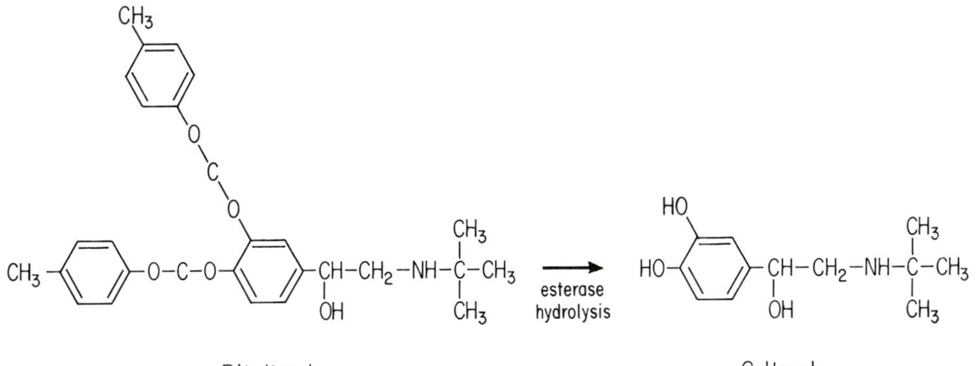

Figure 79-2. Chemical structures of bitolterol and the active catecholamine colterol.

Bitolterol

esterase hydrolysis

Colterol

tution of CH_2OH for one of those groups in albuterol prevents inactivation by catechol-O-methyltransferase, producing a duration of action that is much longer than that of isoproterenol (see Fig. 79-1). The longer duration of action for terbutaline than for metaproterenol is a result of decreased susceptibility to the action of monoamine oxidase because of the larger N-alkyl substituent.[20] Activity after oral administration is a further advantage of metaproterenol, terbutaline, and albuterol over isoproterenol.

Bitolterol is a pro-drug that requires hydrolysis by an esterase that is more abundant in the lungs than in the heart in order to form the active catecholamine colterol (Fig. 79-2).[21]

EPHEDRINE

Ephedrine is an orally effective drug with predominantly indirect action on alpha- and beta-adrenergic receptors and little direct effect on these receptors. Its effect is caused primarily by release of norepinephrine from sympathetic nerve endings. The major route of metabolism of ephedrine is by demethylation to norephedrine (phenylpropanolamine), which has pharmacologic activity similar to that of ephedrine.[22] Because of its indirect action, there can be dangerous interactions with monoamine oxidase inhibitors, which increase the amount of norepinephrine at sympathetic nerve endings.

Administration of ephedrine to normal subjects can suppress metabolic and cardiovascular responses to intravenous epinephrine,[23] and continual treatment of patients with asthma who require doses higher than 60 mg for bronchodilation can induce tolerance to its therapeutic action.[24] Continual treatment of asthmatic children with smaller doses for as long as 8 weeks, however, does not cause tolerance.[25]

As a bronchodilator, ephedrine is much less potent than several other beta-adrenergic agonists, although it offers the advantage of activity as a nasal decongestant for patients who may have concurrent allergic rhinitis.[26,27] Its usefulness is also limited by side effects common to other beta-adrenergic agonists, including insomnia, nervousness, irritability, tachycardia, palpitations, tremor, anorexia, nausea, vomiting, epigastric pain, headache, and vertigo, as well as drowsiness on occasion.

EPINEPHRINE

Epinephrine is also active on both alpha- and beta-adrenergic receptors. Actions of epinephrine and norepinephrine are terminated by uptake into nerve terminals, uptake at extraneuronal sites, and metabolic transformation, but most administered epinephrine is first methylated by catechol-O-methyltransferase to metanephrine and then acted upon by monoamine oxidase.[28] Because of gastrointestinal and hepatic inactivation, epinephrine must be administered by inhalation or subcutaneous injection.

Its alpha-adrenergic activity suggests the possibility of an advantage over other beta-adrenergic agonists in the treatment of acute asthma: reversal of a mediator-induced increase in microvascular permeability by bronchial arteriolar vasoconstriction and possible inhibition of neurotransmission in cholinergic ganglia or cholinergic nerves in the airways. Inhalation of 1 mg of nebulized epinephrine and 2.5 mg of nebulized albuterol, however, elicits similar improvement in peak expiratory flow rate in patients with acute asthma.[29] The possibilities of effects that would have been detectable only through more sensitive measurements of airway obstruction or through effects that might have been evident more than 25 min after treatment remain. Arterial Pa_{O_2} increases after inhalation of epinephrine but decreases slightly after inhalation of albuterol, which is consistent with prevention of increased ventilation/perfusion mismatching by pulmonary vasoconstriction after inhalation of epinephrine.

The chief limitation of epinephrine is its relatively short duration of action of approximately 30 min after inhalation or subcutaneous injection.[29] Apparently longer duration of bronchodilation after inhalation may be a result of failure of bronchoconstriction to recur after it is alleviated.[30] Subcutaneous injection of 1:200 aqueous epinephrine suspension (Sus-Phrine) may improve pulmonary function for 4 to 6 h because of reduced solubility of 80% of the drug found in suspension.

Anxiety, hypertension, precordial discomfort, cardiac arrhythmias, pallor, and side effects that may follow treatment with ephedrine may also follow treatment with epinephrine, more commonly after subcutaneous injection than after inhalation. Subarachnoid hemorrhage and hemiplegia have followed subcutaneous injection of 0.5 ml of 1:1000 aqueous epinephrine.[31]

ETHYLNOREPINEPHRINE

Ethylnorepinephrine hydrochloride (Bronkephrine) is an effective bronchodilator with less alpha-adrenergic activity than epinephrine. As a consequence, somewhat fewer side effects may follow its use than the use of epinephrine, and it may be safer to use in patients with hypertension and in infants, in whom accuracy of dosage may be more critical than in older children. It must be administered by subcutaneous injection. Bronchodilation occurs within 5 to 10 min after injection and persists for 1 to 2 h.[31]

ISOPROTERENOL

Isoproterenol is inactivated by catechol-O-methyltransferase. Bronchodilation peaks 5 to 15 min after inhalation and may continue for 60 to 90 min, which is somewhat longer than after epinephrine because isoproterenol is not taken up by sympathetic neurons to the same extent as epinephrine.[31] Inactivation by intestinal and hepatic sulfatases necessitates administration by inhalation or, occasionally, by intravenous infusion.

Administration by intravenous infusion causes comparable, dose-related increases in forced expiratory flow in 1 sec (FEV_1) and in heart rate, in terms of percentage change from baseline values.[13] Despite associated cardiac effects, intravenous infusions of isoproterenol have been used successfully in the treatment of children with respiratory failure resulting from status asthmaticus.[32, 33] Sudden death has occurred in asthmatic patients receiving intravenous isoproterenol.[34] Myocardial ischemia occurred in a 14-year-old boy who received as little as 0.11 μg/kg/min.[35] Myocardial ischemia, chest pain, hypotension, and congestive heart failure occurred in a 17-year-old girl who received 2.5 μg/kg/min.[36] Fatal asthma has been reported in a 14-year-old patient treated with intravenous isoproterenol with associated myocardial contraction band necrosis, a lesion associated with intracranial catastrophes and severe emotional stress as well as with administration of large doses of adrenergic agents.[37] These observations indicate that it is more prudent to deliver beta-adrenergic agonists by inhalation than by intravenous infusion.

Inhaled isoproterenol can also cause tachycardia, palpitations, headache, tremor, and insomnia, but side effects are less common and less extreme than those of epinephrine, especially if epinephrine has been administered by subcutaneous injection.

ISOETHARINE

Inhalation of nebulized isoetharine elicits peak bronchodilation within 15 to 30 min and significant bronchodilation for 1.5 to 2 h (3 h in one study) in asthmatic patients.[38, 39] Tachycardia can follow inhalation of isoetharine, but it is much less common than after inhalation of isoproterenol.

METAPROTERENOL

Metaproterenol is an effective bronchodilator after inhalation or oral administration. Peak bronchodilation occurs 60 to 120 min after inhalation, but significant bronchodilation occurs within 1 min.[40–42] Significant bronchodilation continues for at least 4 to 5 h. Peak bronchodilation occurs 1.5 to 2 h after oral administration, and bronchodilation may continue for at least 3 to 4 h, but at usual doses, improvement may not exceed the improvement that follows usual inhalation doses during the first 3 h.[42, 43]

Adverse effects, including nervousness, tremor, palpitations, nausea, and vomiting, are more common after oral administration than after inhalation.[44] Tachycardia occurs in approximately 7% of patients after oral administration and in 3.7% after inhalation. Tachycardia is the most common side effect, and it is considerably less common after oral administration than after inhalation of isoproterenol.

Metaproterenol inhibits exercise-induced asthma for 30 min after inhalation in most patients and for 1 h in many but usually affords no protection longer than that despite continued bronchodilation.[45, 46] Oral metaproterenol is protective for 1 h but not for 2 h (see Chapter 68).[45, 47]

ALBUTEROL (SALBUTAMOL)

Albuterol causes significant bronchodilation within 1 min after inhalation that peaks after 0.5 to 2 h and continues for up to 6 h after treatment.[40, 48–50] Improvement may occur by 15 min after oral administration but peaks after 1 to 3 h, which is when plasma albuterol concentration peaks.[51, 52] Bronchodilation may continue as long as 6 to 8 h after oral administration (12 h after Repetab).

Inhalation of albuterol rarely causes side effects, but tremor may occur in 3% of patients, headache in 1%, and dizziness in 1%.[44] Slight increases in heart rate may occur within 5 min after inhalation, but even at doses as high as 680 μg delivered by metered-dose inhaler, brief increases in heart rate do not usually exceed 10% of baseline values.[53] Oral albuterol also has little effect on pulse rate,[54] but tremor may occur in 25% to 35% of patients.[44] Intravenous administration of albuterol causes increases in pulse rate of more than 20 beats per minute.[55–57] Bronchodilation after intravenous administration is no better than that after inhalation in patients with severe acute asthma; accordingly, inhalation therapy, which has much less cardiac effect, is a more prudent choice of treatment.

Administration of albuterol by intravenous injection (250 μg) or by subcutaneous or intramuscular injection (500 μg) can cause decreases in serum potassium concentration of 0.6 mEq/l or more.[58] A constant intravenous infusion of albuterol may decrease serum potassium concentrations even more than intravenous injection.[59] Usual doses by inhalation may not affect serum potassium levels, although very large doses of 1200 to 2400 μg cause dose-dependent decreases in serum potassium levels in healthy men.[60] The hypokalemia is a result of cellular uptake. The clinical significance is uncertain, but such changes may increase the risk of cardiac arrhythmias. A reduced likelihood of inducing significant hypokalemia may be another advantage of inhaled albuterol over intravenous or subcutaneous albuterol. Epinephrine, terbutaline, and fenoterol can also cause hypokalemia.

Although numerous studies have confirmed that albuterol has a much larger duration of action than isoproterenol, few investigators have compared inhaled albuterol directly with metaproterenol. Findings from the few comparisons have suggested a longer duration of action for albuterol on the basis of doses that have not elicited comparable peak bronchodilation.[40, 48] It is not known whether longer lasting bronchodilation would follow inhalation of albuterol than metaproterenol at doses that cause equivalent peak bronchodilation. The chief established advantage of inhaled albuterol over metaproterenol is the much longer inhibition of exercise-induced asthma after inhaled albuterol (4 h in most patients and 6 h in many) than after metaproterenol (only 0.5 h for most patients).[45, 46, 61, 62]

Inhalation and intravenous administration of albuterol have caused fewer and less extreme decreases in arterial Pa_{O_2} than has isoproterenol, but noninvasive oximetry has revealed decreases of 5% to 13% in arterial oxygen saturation in half of 18 asthmatic children treated with nebulized albuterol in addition to intravenous aminophylline.[50, 55, 63–65]

Benzalkonium chloride, a preservative in solutions of albuterol and metaproterenol for nebulization (but not in metered-dose inhalers), can cause bronchoconstriction in some asthmatic patients.[66] Although this bronchoconstrictive effect usually is overcome by the bronchodilating effect of the beta-agonist, nebulization of terbutaline, which contains no preservatives, merits consideration whenever bronchodilating responses to nebulized albuterol or metaproterenol are insufficient.

Inhalation of either hypertonic or hypotonic aerosols can also cause bronchoconstriction in asthmatic patients.[67] Inhalation of nebulized albuterol diluted with cromolyn nebulizer solution, which is hypotonic, may afford less protection against exercise-induced airway obstruction in occasional asthmatic patients than does isotonic albuterol.[68] Accordingly, dilution of albuterol with preservative-free saline before nebulization is preferable.

TERBUTALINE

Inhalation of terbutaline causes significant bronchodilation within 1.5 min that approaches peak levels within 15 min, peaks within 2 h, and is sustained at this level for 5 to 6 hours.[69–74] In most studies of inhaled terbutaline, investigators have obtained responses similar to those to albuterol, but some authors have indicated somewhat better responses to albuterol during the first hour and longer duration of effect after terbutaline.[70] At doses that elicit comparable peak levels of bronchodilation, terbutaline causes longer lasting bronchodilation than does inhaled metaproterenol.[71] Terbutaline may be somewhat less likely than albuterol to cause temporary hypoxemia

resulting from aggravation of ventilation/perfusion imbalance.[72]

Oral terbutaline causes significant improvement in pulmonary function within 30 min and peak bronchodilation after 1.5 to 4 h, which is when serum concentrations also peak.[75–81] Bronchodilation may continue for as long as 7 h.[76] Improvement in pulmonary function is dose dependent. Some authors have recommended an initial dose of 50 μg/kg for children, increased if necessary to 100 μg/kg;[79] other authors have found doses as high as 250 μg/kg (maximum, 5 mg) safe and more effective than the usually recommended dose of 75 μg/kg.[82]

Administration of terbutaline by subcutaneous injection causes significant bronchodilation within 5 min that is maintained for as long as 4 h.[81, 83–86] Serum concentrations peak after 30 min and then decrease, with a biologic half-life of 3.6 h.[81] Durations of response to equivalent doses of epinephrine and terbutaline have been the same in some studies,[85, 86] whereas bronchodilation has continued 1 h longer after terbutaline than after epinephrine in others.[83, 84] Apparent continuation of bronchodilation may be partly a result of failure of bronchoconstriction to recur after it has been alleviated.

Intravenous administration of terbutaline causes dose-dependent improvement in pulmonary function that is comparable with the improvement that follows inhalation of nebulized terbutaline.[87] Increases in pulse rate follow intravenous administration but not inhalation of doses that cause comparable bronchodilation. Accordingly, as in the case of albuterol, inhalation is the preferable method of administration.

Intravenous or subcutaneous administration of terbutaline to asthmatic patients or healthy men can cause decreases in serum potassium levels and increases in plasma insulin and blood glucose concentrations, as can albuterol.[87, 88] Similar responses follow oral administration, but after continual treatment with oral terbutaline for 12 days, little or no change in potassium levels and only minimal changes in insulin and glucose levels follow oral doses of terbutaline.[88]

The occurrence and degree of tremor, the most common side effect of terbutaline, depend on the serum terbutaline concentration; tremor is much more common after intravenous, subcutaneous, and oral administration than after inhalation.[81] Tremor lessens progressively with continual treatment and may virtually resolve within 2 weeks.[88] Toleration of tremor varies widely among patients.[89]

Tachycardia and palpitations are also more common after systemic administration than after inhalation.

BITOLTEROL

Inhalation of bitolterol causes significant bronchodilation within 5 min that peaks after 30 to 90 min and may be maintained for at least 8 h.[90–92] An apparently longer duration of action after bitolterol inhalation than after albuterol delivered by metered-dose inhaler may be caused by somewhat greater peak bronchodilation after bitolterol at the doses studied.[90] Side effects after delivery by metered-dose inhaler include tachycardia, tremor, and headache, but these are rare and similar in frequency to those observed after albuterol.[90] Tremor occurs in 22% to 30% of patients treated with the nebulizer solution at a dose of 1 mg, however.[91, 92] With continual treatment, the proportion of patients reporting tremor decreases after 60 days and is negligible by 90 days.[91]

USE WITH THEOPHYLLINE

Concurrent administration of oral theophylline and inhaled or intravenously injected terbutaline has an additive effect on pulmonary function when both drugs are administered at modest dosages.[93, 94] This approach can avoid or minimize side effects that might follow administration of either drug at full dosage in some patients. When isoproterenol is administered by inhalation at doses large enough to cause maximal bronchodilation, however, addition of theophylline orally or by intravenous infusion does not further enhance bronchodilation in patients with acute asthma.[95] Response to treatment with a combination of albuterol and intravenous aminophylline is better than that to either drug alone in children with status asthmaticus when albuterol dosage is less than maximal.[96]

Combination treatment with 200 μg of inhaled albuterol and with slow-release theophylline enhances suppression of histamine-induced bronchospasm in asthmatic patients, in comparison with either drug alone.[97] Slow-release theophylline doubled the provocation dose, causing a 20% drop in FEV_1 (PD_{20}) 2 to 6 h after treatment. Inhaled albuterol caused a sevenfold increase in PD_{20} after 30 min, which diminished to a threefold increase after 2 h, but its suppressive effect was gone within 4 h. The combination caused a twentyfold increase in PD_{20} after 30 min and more than a sixfold increase after 2 h with an effect similar to that of slow-release theophylline alone after 4 and 6 h.[97]

Combination of a beta-agonist with theophylline is also more effective in inhibiting exercise-induced asthma than either alone, at least at modest doses.[98]

TOLERANCE

Incubation in isoproterenol of bronchial strips from 7 of 12 subjects who did not have asthma induced tachyphylaxis in response to the relaxant effect of isoproterenol after histamine had caused contraction.[99] Furthermore, treatment with oral terbutaline for as few as 6 days can reduce by 85% the number of beta-adrenergic receptors on polymorphonuclear leukocytes of asthmatic and normal persons.[100] Restoration of the usual number of receptors occurred within 7 days after discontinuation of terbutaline, but during that week, symptoms of asthma worsened, and additional treatment with other drugs was required.

Possible tolerance to the bronchodilating effects of beta-agonists is more relevant to management of asthma. Several investigators have found that modest decreases in peak bronchodilation and in duration of bronchodilation follow administration of a beta-agonist after continual treatment for a few weeks.[101-105] Maximal tolerance or subsensitivity may occur within 2 weeks without further progression as treatment continues.[101] Treatment with beta-agonists induces less tolerance in patients receiving concurrent treatment with oral or inhaled corticosteroids.[104] Intravenous corticosteroids can restore beta-adrenergic responsiveness within 1 h.[106]

Some investigators have found no evidence of tolerance to bronchodilation in asthmatic subjects treated with oral or inhaled beta-agonists for 1 to 12 months.[91, 107-109] In different studies of inhaled bitolterol, investigators have found both tolerance and lack of tolerance.[91, 92] Because of conflicting reports, the clinical importance and frequency of tolerance are uncertain.

Tolerance of tremor and of cardiac and metabolic effects of beta-agonists is common even without tolerance of bronchodilating effects.[88, 107]

BRONCHIAL HYPERRESPONSIVENESS

Beta-agonists can ameliorate bronchial hyperresponsiveness for as long as they elicit bronchodilation.[97] Although a larger dose of nebulized histamine or methacholine is necessary to cause a 20% decrease in FEV_1, measurement of responses to further increases in dosage of histamine or methacholine has disclosed increases in the slope of the dose-response curve.[110] This suggests that treatment with a beta-agonist may predispose a patient to increasing bronchoconstriction after an especially potent bronchoconstrictive stimulus. Pretreatment with an inhaled corticosteroid, however, limits the extent of bronchoconstriction induced by histamine or methacholine as well as increasing the threshold.[111]

Salmeterol, which can elicit bronchodilation for as long as 12 h after inhalation and inhibits both early- and late-phase asthmatic responses to allergenic challenge, may prevent the increased airway responsiveness associated with allergenic challenge for as long as 34 h after inhalation of the drug.[112] Such prevention suggests the possibility that this beta-agonist has an anti-inflammatory effect.

DELIVERY BY INHALATION

Inhalation is the route of choice for delivery of beta-adrenergic agonists because of rapid onset of bronchodilation and minimal side effects. Optimal use of a metered-dose inhaler requires a slow inhalation from functional residual capacity to total lung capacity, followed by breath holding for 10 sec. Rapid inhalation favors impaction of the drug particles in the oropharynx.[113] Slow inhalation (0.5 l/sec) can increase pulmonary deposition of the delivered dose twenty-fivefold in comparison with rapid inhalation (2 l/sec). Breath holding for 10 sec can increase pulmonary deposition to 14% of the delivered dose, in comparison with 7% with breath holding for only 4 sec.

The bronchodilator particles delivered by metered-dose inhalers have a mass median diameter of only 3 μm, but each is surrounded by a propellant particle that increases the mass median diameter to 36 μm, a size that renders delivery to the lower airways impossible. Furthermore, the particles leave the inhaler at a speed of 30 m/sec. By the time they have traveled 10 cm, however, their speed is much slower, and the mass median diameter is only 12 μm because of evaporation of propellant. Accordingly, some authors have recommended holding the inhaler a few centimeters from the open mouth when it is used. This technique requires a steady hand and accurate aim. Use of a spacer tube or chamber is more practical.[114] Use of a chamber such as Aerochamber, Inhal-Aid, or InspirEase also obviates the need for synchronization of inhalation with actuation of the canister, permitting effective delivery to children as young as 3 years of age as well as the 50% of adults who do not use metered-dose inhalers properly.[115–117] For children who can use metered-dose inhalers properly, however, addition of an Aerochamber does not usually enhance bronchodilation significantly after delivery of a bronchodilator.[118] Use of a larger, pear-shaped extension cone with a volume of 750 ml can significantly improve responses even in children trained in proper use of the metered-dose inhaler.[119] This device is not available commercially in the United States. Children who use metered-dose inhalers incorrectly achieve better responses to bronchodilator delivery by using InspirEase than by using Aerochamber.[120] Inhalation from a plastic storage bag fitted with a mouthpiece after actuation of the bronchodilator inhaler inside the bag can be as effective as use of InspirEase.[120] Among unselected asthmatic adults, InspirEase is also somewhat more effective than Aerochamber, but the clinical importance of the small differences is uncertain.[121]

Treatment of acute asthma in children with terbutaline delivered from a metered-dose inhaler with a cone-shaped spacer (Nebuhaler) can be as effective as delivery from an electric compressor nebulizer when equivalent doses are used (0.1 mg/kg).[122] Significantly greater improvement in FEV$_1$ ($>$75%) followed use of the spacer than of the nebulizer (55% to 60%). Delivery of terbutaline from a metered-dose inhaler with the cone-shaped spacer has also been found to be as effective as nebulization of equivalent doses in adults with chronic stable asthma.[123] Other authors have found that adults with stable asthma require four times as large a dose of terbutaline by nebulization as by metered-dose inhaler with the cone-shaped spacer for comparable bronchodilation.[124] Six to eight times as much terbutaline by compressor nebulization as by metered-dose inhaler without any spacer is required for equivalent degrees of bronchodilation.[125] These differences in required doses are consistent with observations that nebulizers deliver only 1% to 2% of the nebulized solution to the lower airways, whereas metered-dose inhalers can deliver 8% to 13% of the dose to the lungs.[114, 126]

Response to a bronchodilator delivered by metered-dose inhaler may be poorer than to one delivered by nebulization when airway obstruction is extreme.[127] In adults with acute asthma, delivery of 200 μg of albuterol by metered-dose inhaler every 15 min until there is no further significant improvement in FEV$_1$ causes sufficient bronchodilation that subsequent administration of 5 mg by compressor nebulization elicits no further improvement.[128]

Inhalation of albuterol delivered by metered-dose inhaler with an Aerochamber during four tidal breaths after each of two 100-μg doses elicits improvement in FEV$_1$ similar to that after continuous nebulization of 2.5 mg in adults with stable asthma.[129] Such observations have suggested the possibility of administration by metered-dose inhaler as a cost-saving measure even for hospitalized patients. Delivery of bronchodilator aerosols with intermittent positive pressure has no advantage over simple nebulization alone.[125]

Treatment of acute asthma in children with nebulized bronchodilators is as effective as treatment with epinephrine by subcutaneous injection.[130, 131] A parallel study in which the effects of inhaled fenoterol were compared with those of subcutaneous injection of epinephrine—0.01 mg/kg (maximum, 0.3 mg of 1:1000 aqueous epinephrine) followed 25 min later by 0.025 mg/kg of aqueous epinephrine suspension (Sus-Phrine) (maximum, 0.75 mg)—in children and adolescents with acute asthma disclosed significantly more improvement in pulmonary function and clinical scores after inhalation therapy.[130] Even the patients with the most severe airway obstruction initially, as indicated by FEV$_1$ of less than 30% of predicted normal levels, responded better to inhaled fenoterol than to injected epinephrine. In the treatment of acute asthma, clinicians often administer more than one injection of 1:1000 aqueous epinephrine before administering Sus-Phrine, but the single injection followed by Sus-Phrine in this study caused adverse effects twice as often as the inhaled fenoterol.[130]

Adverse effects of treatment were also far more common after subcutaneous injection of epinephrine than after inhalation of nebulized albuterol in another study of acute asthma in children and adolescents.[131] Side effects, which included nausea, vomiting, tremor, headache, palpitations, pallor, and excitation, occurred in 10 of 20 children who received epinephrine but in none of 20 treated with albuterol. The dose of epinephrine was 0.01 mg/kg, but the maximal dose was 0.4 mg, somewhat higher than usual. The 0.5% albuterol solution was nebulized at doses of 0.02 ml/kg (maximum, 1 ml). Treatment with either epinephrine or albuterol was repeated once after 30 min if necessary. Both drugs caused significant improvement, and there was no significant difference in clinical or spirometric responses between the two drugs.

In only a single study have researchers compared responses to treatment of acute asthma with the same drug administered by subcutaneous injection and inhalation.[132] Adults with acute asthma received epinephrine either by subcutaneous injection (1:1000 aqueous solution, 0.3 mg at 20-min intervals for three times; total dose, 0.9 mg) or by inhalation from a metered-dose inhaler (0.16 mg at 10-min intervals six times; total dose, 0.96 mg). Epinephrine by each route elicited significant improvement in peak expiratory flow rate 1 h after initiation of therapy, and there was no significant difference between the two groups. Significant improvement also followed administration by either route among the patients with the most extreme airway obstruction, as indicated by initial peak expiratory flow rates no higher than 120 l/min. Among these patients, significantly more improvement followed treatment by injection than by inhalation. The investigators concluded that parenteral administration may be more effective than inhalation when extreme airway obstruction limits delivery of drug by inhalation. Administration of larger doses by inhalation might have been more effective, however, and only a small fraction of the doses delivered from the metered-dose inhalers reached the lungs. Side effects were much more common after subcutaneous injection than after inhalation. Palpitations or tremors occurred after injections in 77% of the patients but occurred after inhalation in only 17%.

Because of rapid onset of action, effectiveness, convenience, and relative freedom from side effects, the inhalational route is the route of choice for delivery of beta-adrenergic agonists.

MORTALITY

An association between increased mortality from asthma and introduction of metered-dose inhalers that delivered epinephrine or isoproterenol in England and Wales in 1961 suggested the possibility of an adverse effect of the inhaled beta-agonists.[133] Rates of death from asthma increased from 2.60 per 100,000 of the general population in 1960 to 4.35 by 1965 and then fell to 4.24 in 1966.[134] Rates of mortality from asthma rose in all age groups but were highest among children 10 to 14 years old, among whom the rate increased from 0.33 in 1959 to 2.46 in 1966. Deaths from asthma fell in all age groups after March 1967, and the total number of annual deaths from asthma decreased after the peak in 1965. Total sales of metered-dose inhalers, however, did not decrease until 1967, 2 years after the peak mortality rate. Analysis of 174 deaths in one 6-month period suggested that 84% of the asthmatic patients who died at 5 to 34 years of age had used pressurized bronchodilator aerosols, and excessive use was inferred in at least 17%.[134] Isoprenaline Forte, marketed as an inhaler that delivered 400 μg of isoproterenol with each actuation instead of the usual 80 μg, accounted for approximately 30% of the nebulizer sales in England and Wales during the epidemic of deaths from asthma.

In Australia mortality from asthma increased in 1964, decreased after 1966, and had returned to the 1963 base line by 1968.[135] Sales of bronchodilator inhalers, including sales of Isoprenaline Forte, increased progressively from 1961 to 1970, however. Accordingly, these data did not implicate use or misuse of aerosolized bronchodilators as a cause of increased mortality from asthma.

There was also an increase in mortality from asthma in New Zealand that began in 1965 and peaked in 1966, but mortality rates there have never returned to the 1960–1964 base line.[136] A second increase in mortality there began in 1975–1976 and continued to a peak in 1980, after which mortality decreased somewhat.[137] That decrease began the year after sales of antiasthmatic drugs and beta-agonist inhalers nearly doubled in New Zealand.[138] This suggests that previous increases in mortality there were more likely attributable to undertreatment than to overtreatment.

Rates of death from asthma in the United States did not increase until 1979. The recording of an increase from 0.8 per 100,000 of the general population in 1977 and 1978 to 1.2 per 100,000 in 1979 may have been attributable entirely to implementation of the Ninth Revision of the International Classification of Diseases, which accounted for an increase in the number of deaths attributed to asthma by an estimated 35%.[139] This revision cannot account for subsequent increases to 1.6 per 100,000 by 1985 and for increases from 0.1 in 1979 to 0.3 in 1980–1984 among children aged 10 to 14 years.[140, 141] The increase in mortality has been associated with an increasing rate of beta-agonist inhaler sales, which nearly doubled between 1976 and 1983.[137] Studies of deaths from asthma in children in the United States and New Zealand have implicated inadequacies, delays in treatment, and psychosocial dysfunction rather than overtreatment.[142, 143]

It is possible that overreliance on beta-agonist metered-dose inhalers that had previously afforded rapid relief of symptoms fostered delays in seeking additional therapy until it was too late. Despite numerous possible adverse effects of treatment with beta-adrenergic agonists, however, they probably have contributed to fatalities only rarely.[144, 145] Uncertainty about the causes of the increases in rates of mortality from asthma thus indicates a need for close supervision of patients with severe asthma.

CLINICAL USE

ACUTE ASTHMA

Inhalation of adequate doses of a selective, long-acting beta-adrenergic agonist is the treatment of choice for acute asthma in most circumstances. Nebulized albuterol at 20- to 30-min intervals is of established benefit (Table 79–1).[146, 147] Even larger doses of 0.3 mg/kg (maximum, 10 mg) repeated at hourly intervals for a total of three doses may be safe in most children with acute asthma.[148] It is prudent to measure serum potassium concentrations when large doses are administered frequently and to supply supplemental potassium when indicated. When response is inadequate, addition of an antimuscarinic agent such as ipratropium bromide may produce further bronchodilation.[149] When side effects limit the beta-agonist to less than maximal dosage, addition of intravenous aminophylline or theophylline can enhance bronchodilation.[96]

The inhaled beta-agonist should be nebulized with oxygen to prevent aggravation of hypoxemia and to reverse hypoxemia.[50, 63–65] Intermittent positive pressure is neither necessary nor advisable because of potential aggravation of bronchoconstriction and increased risk of pneumothorax.[125]

Epinephrine or terbutaline administered by subcutaneous injection is an acceptable alternative to albuterol by inhalation, but treatment by injection is less desirable because of the increased frequency of side effects (see Table 79–1 for dosages).[130–132] Treatment by subcutaneous injection is indicated for patients who are apneic and when severe airway obstruction mandates immediate therapy and an injudicious delay may be required in initiation of inhalation therapy. It is wise for patients who

Table 79–1. BETA-ADRENERGIC AGONISTS

Drug	Route	Dose
Albuterol	Inhalation	0.15 mg/kg every 4 h (or immediately and 0.05–0.15 mg/kg every 20–30 min as necessary for acute asthma) (0.5% solution, 5 mg/ml; for dilution to 3 ml with normal saline before nebulization; 0.083% solution, 2.5-mg unit dose, requires no dilution) (maximum, 5 mg)
		180 μg every 4–6 h (metered-dose inhaler)
	Oral	0.1 mg/kg three to four times per day (maximum, 16 mg every 12 h as Repetab)
Bitolterol mesylate	Inhalation	740–1110 μg every 8 h (metered-dose inhaler)
Ephedrine	Oral	0.5–1.0 mg/kg every 4–6 h (maximum, 50 mg every 4 h)
Epinephrine, 1:1000, aqueous	Subcutaneous injection	0.01 ml/kg (maximum, 0.3 ml) every 20 min, three times if necessary; may repeat in 4 h
Epinephrine, 1:200, aqueous suspension (Sus-Phrine)	Subcutaneous injection	0.005 ml/kg (maximum, 0.3 ml); may repeat in 8 h
Ethylnorepinephrine (Bronkephrine)	Subcutaneous injection	0.01–0.02 ml/kg (maximum, 0.5 ml); may repeat in 20 min
Isoetharine, 1% solution	Inhalation	0.01 ml/kg (maximum, 0.5 ml), diluted in saline and nebulized, every 4–8 h
Isoproterenol, 1:200	Inhalation	0.005–0.01 ml/kg (maximum, 0.5 ml), diluted in saline and nebulized, every 4–8 h
Metaproterenol	Inhalation	0.1–0.3 ml (5% solution), diluted in saline and nebulized, every 4–6 h
		1.0–2.5 ml (0.4% solution and 0.6% solution, unit dose, equivalent to 0.2 or 0.3 ml of 5% solution) every 4–6 h
		1.3–1.95 mg every 4–6 h (metered-dose inhaler)
	Oral	0.5 mg/kg every 6–8 h (maximum, 20 mg four times per day)
Terbutaline	Inhalation	0.1 mg/kg every 4–6 h (maximum, 6 mg)
		400 μg every 4–6 h (metered-dose inhaler)
	Subcutaneous injection	0.01 mg/kg (maximum, 0.25 mg); may repeat in 20 min (maximum, 0.5 mg in 4 h)
	Oral	0.075 mg/kg or 2.5 mg every 6 h three times per day (maximum, 5 mg every 6 h three times per day)

have severe asthma to keep injectable epinephrine (EpiPen Auto-Injector) at home and in their automobiles for such emergencies in order to provide temporary relief until they reach the physician's office or the emergency room.[150]

INTERMITTENT ASTHMA

Most asthmatic children have only intermittent airway obstruction (fewer than six times per year) and require only intermittent treatment, at least if pulmonary function returns to normal between episodes of symptoms.[151, 152] Such patients need a convenient, safe, rapidly effective bronchodilator with relatively long duration of action for immediate relief and a bronchodilator with long duration of action for continued use during the several days during which obstruction may persist and symptoms may recur. An inhaled, selective beta-adrenergic agonist is indicated for immediate relief. Albuterol is the best choice because of its long-lasting inhibition of exercise-induced asthma (up to 6 h).[61, 62] Use of a chamber facilitates delivery of drug from the metered-dose inhaler for children, most of whom use metered-dose inhalers improperly.[115, 116, 120] For patients unable to inhale a beta-agonist from a chamber, nebulization of albuterol, metaproterenol, or terbutaline by an electric-powered air compressor such as the DeVilbiss #561 is effective (see Table 79–1 for dosages).

A long-acting oral beta-agonist such as the 4-mg albuterol (Repetab) or a slow-release theophylline preparation is most appropriate for continued bronchodilation for the 3 to 5 days after symptoms resolve, during which continued obstruction is likely. Significant tolerance of the beta-agonist is not likely to develop during these few days. Side effects may be less likely to occur from oral long-acting beta-agonists than with large doses of theophylline. Young children unable to swallow tablets or capsules are usually able to swallow the beads from a slow-release theophylline capsule such as Slo-bid Gyrocaps.

FREQUENT OR CONTINUAL ASTHMA

Asthmatic children who have had frequent symptoms or frequent significant airway obstruction require continual treatment. Inhaled cromolyn, an oral beta-agonist, or slow-release theophylline may be appropriate. Cromolyn most rarely causes side effects, but it is not a bronchodilator. Albuterol (Repetab) is the most convenient of the available oral beta-agonists because of the 12-h duration of action. The disadvantage of continual treatment with a beta-agonist is the potential for tolerance, but this may not occur in every patient, can sometimes be managed by modest increases in dosage, and may be minimized by concurrent treatment with an inhaled corticosteroid.[104] The disadvantage of theophylline is the occurrence of side effects at doses only slightly in excess of those that may be needed for optimal response.

Treatment of asthmatic adults with inhaled 400 μg of fenoterol powder four times each day for 24 weeks has provided poorer control of symptoms of asthma in 70% of patients than has intermittent treatment as required for relieving symptoms.[153] The relevance of these observations to treatment with other beta-agonists remains to be determined. Inhaled fenoterol causes more tachycardia and more extreme hypokalemia than either albuterol or terbutaline at doses that elicit comparable bronchodilation.[154] Results of three case-control studies have implicated prescription of fenoterol as a risk factor for death from asthma in New Zealand while also indicating a significantly reduced risk of death in patients for whom albuterol had been prescribed.[155]

Regular treatment with inhaled albuterol at the somewhat larger than usual dose of 400 μg four times a day for 12 months and 40 μg of ipratropium bromide four times a day for another 12 months has been associated with an increased rate of decline in FEV_1 in asthmatic patients, but there was no associated increase in symptoms of asthma and no increase in bronchial hyperresponsiveness.[156] Furthermore, other investigators have observed improvement in pulmonary function after prolonged treatment with albuterol.[157]

Patients with the most severe asthma and the greatest likelihood of fatal asthma are those for whom the largest amounts of bronchodilators, including beta-agonists for inhalation, have been prescribed.[158] Excessive use of beta-agonist inhalers necessitates evaluation of other approaches to management.

Inhalation of a short-acting beta-agonist can enable asthmatic patients to tolerate larger doses of inhaled allergen without immediate asthmatic responses.[159] Increased exposure to allergen can elicit late-phase asthmatic responses in patients in whom less exposure causes no late-phase reactions. Long-acting beta-agonists, however, can prevent both immediate and late-phase responses.[112]

Adrenal corticosteroids have usually been used only after failure of adequate response to other drugs, but inhaled corticosteroids such as beclomethasone are effective in reversing bronchial hyperresponsiveness, unlike beta-agonists and theophylline.[160, 161]

Continual treatment to lessen the frequency of symptoms and to improve pulmonary function can reverse bronchial hyperresponsiveness, at least when treatment includes inhaled corticosteroids or cromolyn.[162]

Patients also require an inhaled beta-agonist for relief of acute symptoms, regardless of which drug or drugs are prescribed for continual treatment.

EXERCISE-INDUCED ASTHMA

Inhaled albuterol is the treatment of choice for prevention of exercise-induced asthma.[61, 62] It is unknown whether bitolterol or terbutaline inhibits exercise-induced asthma as long as 4 to 6 hours after treatment as albuterol does.

CONCLUSION

Appropriate use of beta-adrenergic agonists is essential for optimal management of asthma. Administration by inhalation minimizes the numerous possible adverse effects. Some beta-agonists introduced more recently than isoproterenol have longer durations of action, fewer side effects, and ample activity after oral administration. Increases in mortality from asthma emphasize the importance of early treatment of airway obstruction with adequate doses of beta-agonists and prompt recognition of

the need for additional treatment when that becomes necessary.

REFERENCES

1. Krall JF: Receptor-mediated regulation of tension in smooth muscle cells. *In* Jenne JJ, Murphy S (eds): Drug Therapy for Asthma: Research and Clinical Practice, pp. 97–128. New York: Marcel Dekker, 1987.
2. Butchers PR, Fullarton JR, Skidmore IF, et al: A comparison of the anti-anaphylactic activities of salbutamol and disodium cromoglycate in the rat, the rat mast cell and in human lung tissue. Br J Pharmacol 67:23–32, 1979.
3. Wanner A: Clinical aspects of mucociliary transport. Am Rev Respir Dis 116:73–125, 1977.
4. Persson CG, Erjefalt I, Grega GJ, et al: The role of beta-receptor agonists in the inhibition of pulmonary edema. Ann N Y Acad Sci 384:544–557, 1982.
5. Persson CG: Role of plasma exudation in asthmatic airways. Lancet 2:1126–1129, 1986.
6. Chen KK, Schmidt CF: The action and clinical use of ephedrine. JAMA 87:836–842, 1926.
7. Solis-Cohen S: The use of adrenal substance in the treatment of asthma. JAMA 34:1164–1166, 1900.
8. Takamine J: Adrenaline: The active principle of the suprarenal gland. Scot Med Surg J 10:131–138, 1902.
9. Konzett H: Neues zur Asthmatherapie. Klin Wochenschr 19:1303–1306, 1940.
10. Conolly ME, Davies DS, Dollery CT, et al: Metabolism of isoprenaline in dog and man. Br J Pharmacol 46:458–472, 1972.
11. Keighley JF: Iatrogenic asthma associated with adrenergic aerosols. Ann Intern Med 65:985–995, 1966.
12. Reisman RE: Asthma induced by adrenergic aerosols. J Allergy 46:162–177, 1970.
13. Paterson JW, Evans RJ, Prime FJ: Selectivity of bronchodilator action of salbutamol in asthmatic patients. Br J Dis Chest 65:21–38, 1971.
14. Trautlein J, Allegra J, Field J, Gillin M: Paradoxic bronchospasm after inhalation of isoproterenol. Chest 70:711–714, 1976.
15. Gazioglu K, Condemi JJ, Hyde RW, et al: Effect of isoproterenol on gas exchange during air and oxygen breathing in patients with asthma. Am J Med 50:185–190, 1971.
16. Ingram RH Jr, Krumpe PE, Duffell GM, et al: Ventilation perfusion changes after aerosolized isoproterenol in asthma. Am Rev Respir Dis 101:364–370, 1970.
17. Wagner PD, Dantzker DR, Iacovoni VE, et al: Ventilation perfusion inequality in asymptomatic asthma. Am Rev Respir Dis 118:511–524, 1978.
18. Lands AM, Luduena FP, Grant JI, et al: The pharmacologic action of some analogs of 1-(3,4-dihydroxyphenyl)-2-amino-1-butanol (ethylnorepinephrine). J Pharmacol Exper Ther 99:45–56, 1950.
19. Herschfus JA, Bresnick E, Levinson L, et al: A new sympathomimetic amine ("Neosuprel") in the treatment of bronchial asthma. Ann Allergy 9:769–773, 1951.
20. Persson H, Olsson T: Some pharmacological properties of terbutaline, 1-(3,5-dihydroxyphenyl)-2-(T-butylamino)-ethanol: A new sympathomimetic beta-receptor-stimulating agent. Acta Med Scand 512(Suppl):11–19, 1970.
21. Shargel L, Dorrbecker SA, Levit M: Physiological disposition and metabolism of n-t-butylarterenol and its di-p-toluate ester (bitolterol) in the rat. Drug Metab Dispos 4:65–71, 1976.
22. Paterson JW, Woolcock AJ, Shenfield GM: Bronchodilator drugs. Am Rev Respir Dis 120:1149–1188, 1979.
23. Nelson HS: The effect of ephedrine on the response to epinephrine in normal men. J Allergy Clin Immunol 51:191–198, 1973.
24. Herxheimer H: Dosage of ephedrine in bronchial asthma and emphysema. Brit Med J 1:350–352, 1946.
25. Tinkelman DG, Avner SE: Ephedrine therapy in asthmatic children. JAMA 237:553–557, 1977.
26. Kennedy MCS, Jackson SLO: Oral sympathomimetic amines in treatment of asthma. Br Med J 2:1506–1509, 1963.

27. Lal S, Bhalla KK, Davey AJ: Slow release salbutamol and Tedral in the treatment of reversible airways obstruction. Postgrad Med J 47(Suppl):89–92, 1971.

28. Weiner N, Taylor P: Neurohumoral transmission: The autonomic and somatic motor nervous systems. *In* Gilman AG, Goodman LS, Rall TW, Murad F (eds): The Pharmacological Basis of Therapeutics, 7th ed, pp. 66–99. New York: Macmillan, 1985.

29. Coupe MO, Guly U, Brown E, Barnes PJ: Nebulised adrenaline in acute severe asthma: Comparison with salbutamol. Eur J Respir Dis 71:227–232, 1987.

30. Sly RM, Badiei B, Faciane J: Comparison of subcutaneous terbutaline with epinephrine in the treatment of asthma in children. J Allergy Clin Immunol 59:128–135, 1977.

31. Weiner N: Norepinephrine, epinephrine, and the sympathomimetic amines. *In* Gilman AG, Goodman LS, Rall TW, Murad F (eds): The Pharmacological Basis of Therapeutics, 7th ed, pp. 145–180. New York: Macmillan, 1985.

32. Wood DW, Downes JJ, Scheinkopf H, et al: Intravenous isoproterenol in the management of respiratory failure in childhood status asthmaticus. J Allergy Clin Immunol 50:75–81, 1972.

33. Cotton EK, Parry W: Treatment of status asthmaticus and respiratory failure. Pediatr Clin North Am 22:163–171, 1975.

34. Kurland G, Williams J, Lewiston NJ: Fatal myocardial toxicity during continuous infusion intravenous isoproterenol therapy of asthma. J Allergy Clin Immunol 63:407–411, 1979.

35. Matson JR, Loughlin GM, Strunk RC: Myocardial ischemia complicating the use of isoproterenol in asthmatic children. J Pediatr 92:776–778, 1978.

36. Page R, Gay W, Friday G, Fireman P: Isoproterenol-associated myocardial dysfunction during status asthmaticus. Ann Allergy 57:402–404, 429–430, 1986.

37. Drislane FW, Samuels MA, Kozakewich HN, et al: Myocardial contraction band lesions in patients with fatal asthma: Possible neurocardiologic mechanisms. Am Rev Respir Dis 135:498–501, 1987.

38. El-Shaboury AH: Controlled study of a new inhalant in asthma and bronchitis. Br Med J 2:1037–1040, 1964.

39. Spector SL, Hudson L, Petty TL: Effect of Bronkosol and its components on cardiopulmonary parameters in asthmatic patients. J Allergy Clin Immunol 59:371–376, 1977.

40. Choo-Kang YF, Simpson WT, Grant IW: Controlled comparison of the bronchodilator effects of three beta-adrenergic stimulant drugs administered by inhalation to patients with asthma. Br Med J 2:287–289, 1969.

41. Beardshaw J, MacLean L, Chan-Yeung M: Comparison of the bronchodilator and cardiac effects of hydroxyphenylorciprenaline and orciprenaline. Chest 65:507–511, 1974.

42. Lee HS: Comparison of oral and aerosol adrenergic bronchodilators in asthma. J Pediatr 99:805–807, 1981.

43. Geumei AM, Miller WF, Miller J, et al: Bronchodilator effect of a new oral beta adrenoceptor stimulant, Th 1165a: A comparison with metaproterenol sulfate. Chest 70:460–465, 1976.

44. Leifer KN, Wittig HJ: The beta-2 sympathomimetic aerosols in the treatment of asthma. Ann Allergy 35:69–80, 1975.

45. Konig P, Eggleston PA, Serby CW: Comparison of oral and inhaled metaproterenol for prevention of exercise-induced asthma. Clin Allergy 11:597–604, 1981.

46. Sly RM, Heimlich EM, Ginsburg J, et al: Exercise-induced bronchospasm: Evaluation of metaproterenol. Ann Allergy 26:253–258, 1968.

47. Sly RM, Mayer J: Exercise-induced bronchospasm: Evaluation of metaproterenol syrup. Ann Allergy 27:158–163, 1969.

48. Riding WD, Dinda P, Chatterjee SS: The bronchodilator and cardiac effects of five pressure-packed aerosols in asthma. Br J Dis Chest 64:37–45, 1970.

49. Jenkinson SG, Light RW, George RB: Comparison of albuterol and isoproterenol aerosols in bronchial asthma. Ann Allergy 39:423–425, 1977.

50. Littner MR, Tashkin DP, Siegel SC, Katz R: Double-blind comparison of acute effects of inhaled albuterol, isoproterenol and placebo on cardiopulmonary function and gas exchange in asthmatic children. Ann Allergy 50:309–316, 1983.

51. Walker SR, Evans ME, Richards AJ, et al: The clinical pharmacology of oral and inhaled salbutamol. Clin Pharmacol Ther 13:861–867, 1972.

52. Grimwood K, Johnson-Barrett JJ, Taylor B: Salbutamol: tablets, inhalational powder, or nebuliser? Br Med J 282:105–106, 1981.

53. Spector SL, Garza Gomez M: Dose-response effects of albuterol aerosol compared with isoproterenol and placebo aerosols. J Allergy Clin Immunol 59:280–286, 1977.

54. Connolly NM: Dosage of oral salbutamol in asthmatic children. Arch Dis Child 46:869–871, 1971.

55. Fitchett DH, McNicol MW, Riordan JF: Intravenous salbutamol in management of status asthmaticus. Br Med J 1:53–55, 1975.

56. Lawford P, Jones BJM, Milledge JS: Comparison of intravenous and nebulised salbutamol in initial treatment of severe asthma. Br Med J 1:84–86, 1978.

57. Bloomfield P, Carmichael J, Petrie GR, et al: Comparison of salbutamol given intravenously and by intermittent positive-pressure breathing in life-threatening asthma. Br Med J 1:848–850, 1979.

58. Rohr AS, Spector SL, Rachelefsky GS, et al: Efficacy of parenteral albuterol in the treatment of asthma: Comparison of its metabolic side effects with subcutaneous epinephrine. Chest 89:348–351, 1986.

59. Elegbeleye OO, Williams KO, Femi-Pearse D: Comparison of the metabolic effects of salbutamol administered in a one minute bolus and a continuous infusion in patients with bronchial asthma. Isr J Med Sci 14:455–458, 1978.

60. Scheinin M, Koulu M, Laurikainen E, et al: Hypokalaemia and other non-bronchial effects of inhaled fenoterol and salbutamol: A placebo-controlled dose-response study in healthy volunteers. Br J Clin Pharmacol 24:645–653, 1987.

61. Higgs CM, Laszlo G: The duration of protection from exercise-induced asthma by inhaled salbutamol and a comparison with inhaled reproterol. Br J Dis Chest 77:262–269, 1983.

62. Berkowitz R, Schwartz E, Bukstein D, et al: Albuterol protects against exercise-induced asthma longer than metaproterenol sulfate. Pediatrics 77:173–178, 1986.

63. Palmer KN, Legge JS, Hamilton WF, et al: Comparison of effect of salbutamol and isoprenaline on spirometry and blood gas tensions in bronchial asthma. Br Med J 2:23–24, 1970.

64. Warrell DA, Robertson DG, Howes JN, et al: Comparison of cardiorespiratory effects of isoprenaline and salbutamol in patients with bronchial asthma. Br Med J 1:65–70, 1970.

65. Tal A, Pasterkamp H, Leahy F: Arterial oxygen desaturation following salbutamol inhalation in acute asthma. Chest 86:868–869, 1984.

66. Zhang YG, Wright WJ, Tam WK, et al: Effect of inhaled preservatives on asthmatic subjects: II. Benzalkonium chloride. Am Rev Respir Dis 141:1405–1408, 1990.

67. Eschenbacher WL, Boushey HA, Sheppard D: Alteration in osmolarity of inhaled aerosols causes bronchoconstriction and cough, but absence of a permeant anion causes cough alone. Am Rev Respir Dis 129:211–215, 1984.

68. Soferman R, Kivity S, Topilsky M: The effect of osmolarity of respiratory salbutamol solutions on exercise-induced asthma in children. Pediatr Asthma Allergy Immunol 4:193–198, 1990.

69. Glass P, Dulfano MJ: Evaluation of a new beta$_2$ adrenergic receptor stimulant, terbutaline, in bronchospasm: III. Aerosol administration. Curr Ther Res 18:425–432, 1975.

70. Hartnett BJ, Marlin GE: Comparison of terbutaline and salbutamol aerosols. Aust N Z J Med 7:13–15, 1977.

71. Chester EH, Doggett WE, Montenegro HD, et al: Bronchodilating effect of terbutaline aerosol. Clin Pharmacol Ther 23:630–634, 1978.

72. Capecchi V, Cavalli F, Falcoone F, Fasano E: Comparison of terbutaline and salbutamol aerosols in patients with bronchial asthma. Int J Clin Pharmacol Biopharm 16:310–312, 1978.

73. Eriksson NE, Lindgren SB: The rapidity of bronchodilation. A comparison of isoprenaline, terbutaline and rimiterol. Scand J Respir Dis 59:30–36, 1978.

74. Ritchie D, Erban A, McLennan L, et al: Dose of terbutaline respirator solution in children with asthma. N Z Med J 90:332–334, 1979.

75. Geumei A, Miller WF, Paez PN, Gast LR: Evaluation of a new oral β_2-adrenoceptor stimulant bronchodilator, terbutaline. Pharmacology 13:201–211, 1975.

76. Tashkin DP, Meth R, Simmons DH, Lee YE: Double-blind comparison of acute bronchial and cardiovascular effects of oral terbutaline and ephedrine. Chest 68:155–161, 1975.

77. Fuhrmann CF: Terbutaline in bronchospastic disease: A comparison study. Curr Ther Res 22:659–665, 1977.
78. Blumberg MZ, Tinkelman DG, Ginchansky EJ, et al: Terbutaline and ephedrine in asthmatic children. Pediatrics 60:14–19, 1977.
79. Ardal B, Beaudry P, Eisen AH: Terbutaline in asthmatic children: a dose-response study. J Pediatr 93:305–307, 1978.
80. Ripe E, Hornblad Y, Tegner K: Oral administration of terbutaline in asthmatic patients. Eur J Resp Dis Suppl 134:171–179, 1984.
81. Van den Berg W, Leferink JG, Maes RA, et al: The effects of oral and subcutaneous administration of terbutaline in asthmatic patients. Eur J Respir Dis Suppl 134:181–193, 1984.
82. Dinwiddie R, Gewitz M, van der Laag H, Frame MH: Plasma terbutaline levels in asthma. Arch Dis Child 58:223–224, 1983.
83. Da Costa JL, Goh BK: A comparative trial of subcutaneous terbutaline, Th1165a and adrenaline in bronchial asthma. Med J Aust 2:588–591, 1973.
84. Schwartz HJ, Trautlein JJ, Goldstein AR: Acute effects of terbutaline and epinephrine on asthma. J Allergy Clin Immunol 58:516–522, 1976.
85. Sly RM, Badiei B, Faciane J: Comparison of subcutaneous terbutaline with epinephrine in the treatment of asthma in children. J Allergy Clin Immunol 59:128–135, 1977.
86. Spiteri MA, Millar AB, Pavia D, Clarke SW: Subcutaneous adrenaline versus terbutaline in the treatment of acute severe asthma. Thorax 43:19–23, 1988.
87. Kung M, White JR, Burki NK: The effect of subcutaneously administered terbutaline on serum potassium in asymptomatic adult asthmatics. Am Rev Respir Dis 129:329–332, 1984.
88. Bengtsson B: Plasma concentration and side-effects of terbutaline. Eur J Respir Dis Suppl 134:231–235, 1984.
89. Jenne JW, Ridley DJ, Marcucci RA, et al: Objective and subjective tremor responses to oral beta$_2$ agents on first exposure. Am Rev Respir Dis 126:607–610, 1982.
90. Orgel HA, Kemp JP, Tinkelman DG, Webb DR Jr: Bitolterol and albuterol metered-dose aerosols: Comparison of two long-acting beta$_2$-adrenergic bronchodilators for treatment of asthma. J Allergy Clin Immunol 75:55–62, 1985.
91. Pinnas JL, Bernstein IL, Bronsky EE, et al: Multicenter study of bitolterol and isoproterenol nebulizer solutions in nonsteroid-using patients. J Allergy Clin Immunol 79:768–775, 1987.
92. Nathan RA, Bernstein IL, Bronsky EA, et al: Comparison of the bronchodilator effects of nebulized bitolterol mesylate and isoproterenol hydrochloride in steroid-dependent asthma. J Allergy Clin Immunol 79:822–829, 1987.
93. Svedmyr K: Effects of oral theophylline combined with oral and inhaled β$_2$-adrenostimulants in asthmatics. Allergy 37:119–127, 1982.
94. Billing B, Dahlqvist R, Garle M, et al: Separate and combined use of terbutaline and theophylline in asthmatics. Eur J Respir Dis 63:399–409, 1982.
95. Fanta CH, Rossing TH, McFadden ER Jr: Treatment of acute asthma. Is combination therapy with sympathomimetics and methylxanthines indicated? Am J Med 80:5–10, 1986.
96. Edmunds AT, Godfrey S: Cardiovascular response during severe acute asthma and its treatment in children. Thorax 36:534–540, 1981.
97. Joad JP, Ahrens RC, Lindgren SD, Weinberger MM: Relative efficacy of maintenance therapy with theophylline, inhaled albuterol, and the combination for chronic asthma. J Allergy Clin Immunol 79:78–85, 1987.
98. Shapiro GG, McPhillips JJ, Smith K, et al: Effectiveness of terbutaline and theophylline alone and in combination in exercise-induced bronchospasm. Pediatrics 67:508–513, 1981.
99. Davis C, Connolly ME: Beta agonist resistance in human bronchial muscle. Clin Sci Mol Med 52:28p, 1977.
100. Galant SP, Duriseti L, Underwood S, Insel PA: Decreased beta-adrenergic receptors on polymorphonuclear leukocytes after adrenergic therapy. New Engl J Med 299:933–936, 1978.
101. Nelson HS, Raine D Jr, Doner HC, et al: Subsensitivity to the bronchodilator action of albuterol produced by chronic administration. Am Rev Respir Dis 116:871–878, 1977.
102. Jenne JW, Chick TW, Strickland RD, Wall FJ: Subsensitivity of beta responses during therapy with a long-acting beta-2 preparation. J Allergy Clin Immunol 59:383–390, 1977.
103. Nelson HS: Beta-adrenergic agonists. Chest 82:33S–38S, 1982.
104. Weber RW, Smith JA, Nelson HS: Aerosolized terbutaline in asthmatics: Development of subsensitivity with long-term administration. J Allergy Clin Immunol 70:417–422, 1982.
105. Repsher LH, Anderson JA, Bush RK, et al: Assessment of tachyphylaxis following prolonged therapy of asthma with inhaled albuterol aerosol. Chest 85:34–38, 1984.
106. Ellul-Micallef R, Fenech FF: Intravenous prednisolone in chronic bronchial asthma. Thorax 30:312–315, 1975.
107. Larsson S, Svedmyr N, Thiringer G: Lack of bronchial beta adrenoreceptor resistance in asthmatics during long-term treatment with terbutaline. J Allergy Clin Immunol 59:93–100, 1977.
108. Tashkin DP, Conolly ME, Deutsch RI, et al: Subsensitization of beta-adrenoceptors in airways and lymphocytes of healthy and asthmatic subjects. Am Rev Respir Dis 125:185–193, 1982.
109. Tattersfield AE: Bronchodilator drugs. Pharmacol Ther 17:299–313, 1982.
110. Bel EH, Zwinderman AH, Timmers MC, et al: The protective effect of a beta$_2$ agonist against excessive airway narrowing in response to bronchoconstrictor stimuli in asthma and chronic obstructive lung disease. Thorax 46:9–14, 1991.
111. Bel EH, Timmers MC, Zwinderman AH, et al: The effect of inhaled corticosteroids on the maximal degree of airway narrowing to methacholine in asthmatic subjects. Am Rev Respir Dis 143:109–113, 1991.
112. Twentyman OP, Finnerty JP, Harris A, et al: Protection against allergen-induced asthma by salmeterol. Lancet 336:1338–1342, 1990.
113. Newhouse MT, Ruffin RE: Deposition and fate of aerosolized drugs. Chest 73(Suppl):936–943, 1978.
114. Newman SP, Moren F, Pavia D, et al: Deposition of pressurized suspension aerosols inhaled through extension devices. Am Rev Respir Dis 124:317–320, 1981.
115. Hodges IG, Milner AD, Stokes GM: Assessment of a new device for delivering aerosol drugs to asthmatic children. Arch Dis Child 56:787–789, 1981.
116. Chang B, Sly RM, Eby D, Middleton HB: Response to delivery of albuterol aerosol by Inhal-Aid to young children. Pediatr Asthma Allergy Immunol 1:159–164, 1987.
117. Shim C, Williams MH Jr: The adequacy of inhalation of aerosol from canister nebulizers. Am J Med 69:891–894, 1980.
118. Rachelefsky GS, Rohr AS, Wo J, et al: Use of a tube spacer to improve the efficacy of a metered-dose inhaler in asthmatic children. Am J Dis Child 140:1191–1193, 1986.
119. Rivlin J, Mindorff C, Reilly P, Levison H: Pulmonary response to a bronchodilator delivered from three inhalation devices. J Pediatr 104:470–473, 1984.
120. Lee H, Evans HE: Evaluation of inhalation aids of metered dose inhalers in asthmatic children. Chest 91:366–369, 1987.
121. Crimi N, Palermo F, Cacopardo B, et al: Bronchodilator effect of Aerochamber and InspirEase in comparison with metered dose inhaler. Eur J Respir Dis 71:153–157, 1987.
122. Fuglsang G, Pedersen S: Comparison of Nebuhaler and nebulizer treatment of acute severe asthma in children. Eur J Respir Dis 69:109–113, 1986.
123. Cushley MJ, Lewis RA, Tattersfield AE: Comparison of three techniques of inhalation on the airway response to terbutaline. Thorax 38:908–913, 1983.
124. Stauder J, Hidinger KG: Terbutaline aerosol from a metered dose inhaler with a 750-ml spacer or as a nebulized solution. Respiration 44:237–240, 1983.
125. Weber RW, Petty WE, Nelson HS: Aerosolized terbutaline in asthmatics: Comparison of dosage strength, schedule, and method of administration. J Allergy Clin Immunol 63:116–121, 1979.
126. Asmundsson T, Johnson RF, Kilburn KH, et al: Efficiency of nebulizers for depositing saline in human lung. Am Rev Respir Dis 108:506–512, 1973.
127. Choo-Kang YF, Grant IW: Comparison of two methods of administering bronchodilator aerosol to asthmatic patients. Br Med J 2:119–120, 1975.
128. Tarala RA, Madsen BW, Paterson JW: Comparative efficacy of salbutamol by pressurized aerosol and wet nebulizer in acute asthma. Br J Clin Pharmacol 10:393–397, 1980.
129. Gervais A, Begin P: Bronchodilatation with a metered-dose inhaler plus an extension, using tidal breathing vs jet nebulization. Chest 92:822–824, 1987.

130. Ben-Zvi Z, Lam C, Hoffman J, et al: An evaluation of the initial treatment of acute asthma. Pediatrics 70:348–353, 1982.
131. Becker AB, Nelson NA, Simons FE: Inhaled salbutamol (albuterol) vs. injected epinephrine in the treatment of acute asthma in children. J Pediatr 102:465–469, 1983.
132. Pliss LB, Gallagher EJ: Aerosol vs. injected epinephrine in acute asthma. Ann Emerg Med 10:353–355, 1981.
133. Inman WHW, Adelstein AM: Rise and fall of asthma mortality in England and Wales in relation to use of pressurized aerosols. Lancet 2:279–285, 1969.
134. Speizer FE, Doll R, Heaf P: Observations on recent increase in mortality from asthma. Br Med J 1:335–339, 1968.
135. Gandevia B: Pressurized sympathomimetic aerosols and their lack of relationship to asthma mortality in Australia. Med J Aust 1:273–277, 1973.
136. Jackson RT, Beaglehole R, Rea HH, Sutherland DC: Mortality from asthma: A new epidemic in New Zealand. Br Med J 285:771–774, 1982.
137. Sly RM: Effects of treatment on mortality from asthma. Ann Allergy 56:207–212, 1986.
138. Keating G, Mitchell EA, Jackson R, et al: Trends in sales of drugs for asthma in New Zealand, Australia, and the United Kingdom, 1975–81. Br Med J 289:348–351, 1984.
139. Sly RM: Increases in deaths from asthma. Ann Allergy 53:20–25, 1984.
140. Sly RM: Mortality from asthma in children 1979–1984. Ann Allergy 60:433–443, 1988.
141. Sly RM: Mortality from asthma, 1979–1984. J Allergy Clin Immunol 82(5 Pt 1):705–717, 1988.
142. Sears MR, Rea HH, Fenwick J, et al: Deaths from asthma in New Zealand. Arch Dis Child 61:6–10, 1986.
143. Strunk RC, Mrazek DA, Fuhrmann GS, et al: Physiologic and psychological characteristics associated with deaths due to asthma in children. JAMA 254:1193–1198, 1985.
144. Sly RM, Anderson JA, Bierman CW, et al: Adverse effects and complications of treatment with beta-adrenergic agonist drugs. J Allergy Clin Immunol 75:443–449, 1985.
145. Sly RM, Cohn J, Jenne JW: Toxicity of beta-adrenergic drugs. In Jenne JW, Murphy S: Drug Therapy for Asthma: Research and Clinical Practice, pp. 953–996. New York: Marcel Dekker, 1987.
146. Robertson CF, Smith F, Beck R, Levison H: Response to frequent low doses of nebulized salbutamol in acute asthma. J Pediatr 106:672–674, 1985.
147. Schuh S, Parkin P, Rajan A, et al: High- versus low-dose, frequently administered, nebulized albuterol in children with severe, acute asthma. Pediatrics 83:513–518, 1989.
148. Schuh S, Reider MJ, Canny G, et al: Nebulized albuterol in acute childhood asthma: Comparison of two doses. Pediatrics 86:509–513, 1990.
149. Beck R, Robertson C, Galdes-Sebaldt M, Levison H: Combined salbutamol and ipratropium bromide by inhalation in the treatment of severe acute asthma. J Pediatrics 107:605–608, 1985.
150. Bateman JR, Clarke SW: Sudden death in asthma. Thorax 34:40–44, 1979.
151. Williams HE, McNicol KN: The spectrum of asthma in children. Pediatr Clin North Am 22:43–52, 1975.
152. Mansmann HC Jr: The evaluation, control, and modification of continuing asthma. Clin Chest Med 1:339–360, 1980.
153. Sears MR, Taylor DR, Print CG, et al: Regular inhaled beta-agonist treatment in bronchial asthma. Lancet 336:1391–1396, 1990.
154. Wong CS, Pavord ID, Williams J, et al: Bronchodilator, cardiovascular, and hypokalaemic effects of fenoterol, salbutamol, and terbutaline in asthma. Lancet 336:1396–1399, 1990.
155. Grainger J, Woodman K, Pearce N, et al: Prescribed fenoterol and death from asthma in New Zealand, 1981–7: A further case-control study, Thorax 46:105–111, 1991.
156. van Schayck CP, Dompeling E, van Herwaarden CLA, et al: Bronchodilator treatment in moderate asthma or chronic bronchitis: Continuous or on demand? A randomised controlled study. Br Med J 303:1426–1431, 1991.
157. Hilton CJ, Fuller RW: Bronchodilator treatment in asthma: Continuous or on demand? [Letter]. Br Med J 304:121, 1992.
158. Spitzer WO, Suissa S, Ernst P, et al: The use of β-agonists and the risk of death and near death from asthma. N Engl J Med 326:501–506, 1992.
159. Lai CKW, Twentyman OP, Holgate ST: The effect of an increase in inhaled allergen dose after rimiterol hydrobromide on the occurrence and magnitude of the late asthmatic response and the associated change in nonspecific bronchial responsiveness. Am Rev Respir Dis 140:917–923, 1989.
160. Kerrebijn KF, van Essen-Zandvliet EE, Neijens HJ: Effect of long-term treatment with inhaled corticosteroids and beta-agonists on the bronchial responsiveness in children with asthma. J Allergy Clin Immunol 79:653–659, 1987.
161. Dutoit JI, Salome CM, Woolcock AJ: Inhaled corticosteroids reduce the severity of bronchial hyperresponsiveness in asthma but oral theophylline does not. Am Rev Respir Dis 136:1174–1178, 1987.
162. Woolcock AJ, Yan K, Salome CM: Effect of therapy on bronchial hyperresponsiveness in the long-term management of asthma. Clin Allergy 18:165–176, 1988.

80 CROMOLYN SODIUM: BASIC MECHANISMS AND CLINICAL USAGE

SHIRLEY MURPHY, M.D.

Cromolyn sodium is unique in its mechanism of action and wide range of clinical applications. Although cromolyn sodium has been approved since 1973 for use in the United States for the treatment of asthma, its wide clinical applications and diverse mechanisms of action are just starting to be appreciated. This review focuses on both the basic scientific and clinical aspects of cromolyn sodium.

Cromolyn sodium was discovered as a result of pharmaceutic research carried out in the United Kingdom in the mid-1950s with the naturally occurring antispasmodic agent khellin. In 1956, Roger Altounyan, a physician, a clinical pharmacologist, and an asthmatic patient, joined the research team and evaluated the newly synthesized compounds. Using inhalation challenges on himself, he observed that khellin derivatives in which the 2-methyl group had been replaced by a carboxylic acid moiety had no bronchodilator properties, but when taken prophylactically, they inhibited the bronchoconstriction induced by antigen inhalation.[1] On January 19, 1965, FPL 670 was synthesized. This chrome-2-carboxylate, known as sodium cromoglycate or cromolyn sodium, offered the best protection for Altounyan's antigen-induced bronchospasm and became available for use in the treatment of asthma in the United Kingdom in 1968 and in the United States in 1973.

CHEMISTRY

Cromolyn sodium is synthesized by linking two monochromone nuclei with a shared alkyl residue. It is a white, hydrated powder that is a lipophobic, highly polar, acidic molecule with a molecular weight of 500 D and is a highly ionized acid salt with a pKa of 2. Cromolyn sodium exists almost exclusively in the ionized form at physiologic pH. Because of this, cromolyn sodium is not absorbed from the gastrointestinal tract. However, the local administration of polar drugs, such as cromolyn sodium, directly to the lung surface may be an advantage inasmuch as the absorption from the lung surface is delayed and the action prolonged. Another advantage of the ionized state is that cromolyn sodium cannot partition into cells to interfere with intracellular function. Because cromolyn sodium exists in an ionized form, it is not metabolized and is excreted unchanged in the urine and bile. Thus the existence of cromolyn sodium in the ionized form at physiologic pH explains the almost complete absence of unwanted side effects.[2]

PHARMACOKINETICS

Detailed studies in both animals and human volunteers have shown that after intravenous administration, cromolyn sodium is cleared rapidly from plasma and excreted unchanged; about 50% of the total dose is excreted in the urine and the rest in the biliary tract. Oral absorption of cromolyn sodium is less than 1%. Regardless of the route of administration, metabolism of the drug has not been detected. When 1 mg of cromolyn sodium solution is injected, via a bronchoscope, into a second-order bronchus, the pharmacokinetic properties are as follows:[3] initial half-life (in minutes) is 1.9 ± 0.4; terminal half-life (in minutes) is 64 ± 10; time of maximal concentration (in minutes) is 15 ± 4; maximal concentration (in ng/ml^{-1}) is 9.0 ± 0.7; area under the curve (AUC_{0-240}) (ng/ml^{-1}/min) is 804 ± 112.

Studies with the Spinhaler turboinhaler delivery system have shown that approximately 10% of the dose of a 20-mg capsule reaches the airways. From this delivery device, the amount reaching the airways is related directly to the inspiratory flow rates, and the drug shows absorption rate–limited disposition kinetics after inhalation.[3] Instil-

lation of 1 mg of cromolyn sodium directly into a second-order bronchus in asthmatic patients yields plasma concentration time curves similar to those seen in normal volunteers at high inspiratory flow rates.

MECHANISM OF ACTION

Despite intensive research in many laboratories since the early 1970s, a precise mechanism that explains the clinical activity of cromolyn sodium has not been completely delineated (Table 80-1). The primary mode of action of cromolyn sodium was thought for many years to be stabilization of mast cells and thus prevention of subsequent release of mediators after appropriate challenge. Early laboratory studies with antigen challenge of tissues presensitized with reaginic (immunoglobulin E [IgE]) antibodies demonstrated that cromolyn sodium inhibited the release of biologically active chemical mediators.[4] In rats sensitized with sera containing antibodies with reaginic properties, cromolyn sodium inhibited passive cutaneous anaphylactic reactions induced by antigen challenge. In human dispersed lung mast cells, cromolyn sodium showed a concentration-related inhibition of up to 30% histamine release at 1:1000 μmol and inhibited the release of prostaglandin D_2 by 85%.[5] Cromolyn sodium appears to be more effective in inhibiting IgE-dependent histamine release from mast cells recovered from the lung by bronchoalveolar lavage than from mast cells dispersed from human lung tissue by enzymatic digestion.[6] This suggests that the mast cells of the bronchial lumen, sometimes referred to as mucosal mast cells, represent a separate subpopulation of lung mast cells that are more sensitive to the inhibitory effects of cromolyn sodium.

Antigen challenge studies in humans have further emphasized the role of cromolyn sodium in stabilizing mast cells. Inhalation of ragweed in ragweed-sensitive asthmatic patients results in bronchospasm and the simultaneous release of quantifiable amounts of neutrophil chemotactic factor into the sera of patients. Previously administered cromolyn sodium blocks both the antigen-induced bronchospasm and the serum rise of chemotactic activity.[7] Neutrophil chemotactic activity has a molecular weight of 500,000 D and is considered to be of mast cell origin.

In a clinical study, cromolyn sodium therapy for 4 weeks (20 mg four times a day) in asthmatic patients

Table 80-1. PROPOSED MECHANISMS OF ACTION OF CROMOLYN SODIUM

Stabilizes mast cells[4-6]
Blocks NCF-A release[7]
Decreases number of lung inflammatory cells[8]
Inhibits protein kinase C[11]
Inhibits activation of inflammatory cells[12]
Decreases bronchial hyperreactivity[22, 37]
Blocks early and late asthmatic reactions[22]
Decreases airway permeability[13]
Inhibits neuronal reflexes within the lung[14, 17]
Prevents down-regulation of beta$_2$-receptors[15]
Inhibits bronchoconstrictor effects of tachykinins[16]

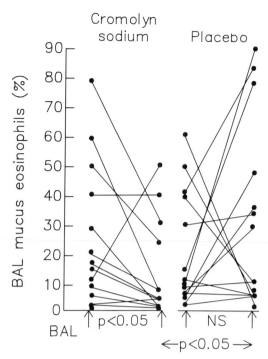

Figure 80–1. Cromolyn sodium (40 mg four times per day for 4 weeks) not only significantly improved asthma symptoms, but also reduced lung inflammation, as measured by a significant reduction in eosinophils recovered by bronchoalveolar lavage (BAL). (Adapted from Diaz P, Galleguillos FR, Gonzalez MC, et al: Bronchoalveolar lavage in asthma: The effect of disodium cromoglycate (cromolyn) on leukocyte counts, immunoglobulins, and complement. J Allergy Clin Immunol 74:41–48, 1984.)

resulted in a significant decrease in the number of eosinophils recovered in bronchoalveolar lavage fluid[8] (Fig. 80–1). Thus cromolyn sodium may block the release of other mast cell mediators such as eosinophil chemotactic factor and leukotriene B_4 that recruit eosinophils into tissue sites.

Several theories of the exact cellular site of biochemical action of cromolyn sodium have been proposed and investigated, but none has been definitely established. Because cromolyn sodium is highly ionized at physiologic pH values, it remains in the extracellular fluid. Therefore, it is most likely that its effects are mediated by interaction with a cell surface receptor. Cromolyn sodium that has been covalently conjugated to fluorescent polyacrylamide beads has been shown to bind to mast cell membranes, and Mazurek and co-workers[9] showed that cromolyn sodium, when coupled to an insoluble resin, inhibited mast cell mediator release. A specific binding site for cromolyn on the membrane of rat basophil leukemia cells has been reported.[9] Although these findings are evidence of the existence of a membrane receptor for the action of cromolyn sodium, isolation and reconstitution of this receptor have not been accomplished.

Anti-IgE and compound 48/80–stimulated histamine secretion from rat peritoneal mast cells is accompanied by the phosphorylation of four intracellular membrane proteins of approximate molecular weights of 78, 68, 59, and 42 kD. Cromolyn sodium induces the phosphorylation of a protein with a molecular weight of 78 kD.[10] Phosphorylation of this specific protein occurs 30 to 60 sec after stimulation of rat peritoneal mast cells and coincides with the termination of the entire secretory process. Thus cromolyn sodium may activate a naturally occurring cell mechanism that is thought to inhibit mast cell mediator release.

A further postulate is that cromolyn sodium inhibits cell activation by inhibiting the action of protein kinase C, an enzyme that requires calcium and phosphatidylserine for full expression of its activity. Protein kinase C has a molecular weight of 78 kD, similar to that of the protein inhibited by cromolyn sodium. Investigators using the control of melanosome movement in the *Anolis carolinesis* lizard showed that cromolyn inhibited protein kinase C activity in this model.[11]

Although cromolyn is classically known for its mast cell stabilization properties, new information suggests it has an effect on other inflammatory cells. Cromolyn sodium at low concentrations (10.8 mol/l) and in a time-dependent manner directly inhibits the *in vitro* activation of human neutrophils, eosinophils, and monocytes.[12] This effect on mast cells and other inflammatory cells may be the mechanisms by which cromolyn sodium has been shown to decrease airway permeability in experimental animal models of asthma[13] and also may explain its effect on blocking the late asthmatic response and decreasing airway hyperreactivity.

A further proposed mechanism of action is that cromolyn may inhibit neuronal reflexes within the lung. This theory had its origins in experiments in dogs in which reflex-induced bronchoconstriction that followed stimulation of C fiber sensory nerve endings with capsaicin (extract of red pepper) was blocked by prophylactic treatment with cromolyn.[14] Also, the ability of cromolyn sodium to block sulfur dioxide challenge, a nonimmunologically driven system, has added to the attractiveness of this mode of action.

Cromolyn sodium has also been shown to prevent the down-regulation of beta$_2$-receptors on lymphocytes, which occurs with chronic usage of beta$_2$-agonists[15] and also to inhibit the bronchoconstrictor effect of tachykinins.[16]

CLINICAL PHARMACOLOGY

Early bronchial challenge studies demonstrated the protective effect of cromolyn sodium in inhibiting bronchoconstriction induced by a variety of allergens. Inhalation of 20 to 40 mg of cromolyn sodium before challenge provides protection 30 min and 5 h later but not 24 h later. The effect of antigen challenge on decreasing mucociliary clearance is also blocked by pretreatment with cromolyn sodium. Cromolyn sodium has been shown to inhibit sulfur dioxide–induced bronchoconstriction in a dose-dependent manner.[17] In addition, cromolyn sodium is protective against exposure to toluene diisocyanate, western red cedar, laboratory animals, and metabisulfite; pretreatment with cromolyn sodium partially or completely blocks aspirin (acetylsalicylic acid) challenge.[18]

The effectiveness of cromolyn sodium in blocking exercise-induced asthma was first shown in 1968.[18] Total inhibition has been demonstrated in 66% of patients, and significant protection in 87%.[19] In addition, 40 mg of cromolyn sodium has been shown to prevent bronchoconstriction induced by hyperventilation of cold air.[20]

The effective dose of cromolyn sodium needed for blocking challenges appears to vary with the challenge, and the duration of effective blockage may also be dependent on dosage. In challenge with sulfur dioxide, it has been shown that 40 mg is more protective than 20 mg and 200 mg is more protective than 40 mg.[17] During exercise challenge, 150 min after the drug has been administered, 20 mg is as effective as 40 mg. However, 270 min after drug administration, 40 mg and 20 mg provide partial protection, but 2 mg is no longer protective.[21]

LATE ASTHMATIC RESPONSE

One of the important mechanisms of cromolyn sodium is its ability to block the early and late responses. This was first demonstrated by J. Pepys and has been confirmed in rabbit and sheep models of asthma.[18] A study by Cockcroft and Murdock[22] further extended this finding. Single-dose albuterol (200 μg), beclomethasone dipropionate (200 μg), and cromolyn sodium (10 mg) were inhaled 10 min before allergen challenge in a blinded crossover trial and were examined with regard to inhibition of the allergen-induced early and late asthmatic responses. The allergen-induced increase in bronchial responsiveness to inhaled histamine was also measured. Albuterol effectively blocked the early asthmatic response but did not affect the late asthmatic response. Beclomethasone did not have an effect on the early asthmatic response but did block the late asthmatic response; only cromolyn sodium blocked both the early and late responses[22] (Fig. 80–2).

Only the drugs that blocked the late asthmatic response—cromolyn sodium and beclomethasone—prevented the increase in nonspecific bronchial hyperreactivity, which occurred 7 h after the challenges[22] (Fig. 80–3). Cromolyn sodium was the more potent drug in this test, significantly protecting 100% of patients, in comparison with 60% protected by beclomethasone.

Many investigators have studied the long-term effects of cromolyn sodium on reducing nonspecific bronchial reactivity. Cromolyn sodium has been shown to prevent the seasonal rise in airway reactivity that occurs in asthmatic patients during the pollen season and also to decrease nonspecific reactivity in long-term clinical trials.[18] By decreasing nonspecific reactivity, cromolyn sodium actually modulates the basic disease process in asthma, and by decreasing the inflammatory response in the airways, it makes the airways more stable over time.

CLINICAL TRIALS

More than 5700 scientific articles on cromolyn sodium have been published in the scientific literature. This review focuses on several aspects of the clinical uses of cromolyn sodium in asthma, including (1) forms of cromolyn available for use in pediatrics, (2) comparison of

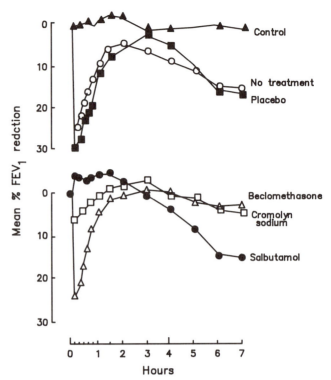

Figure 80–2. Effect of various pharmacologic agents on blocking the early and late asthmatic responses after antigen inhalation. Albuterol (salbutamol) blocked only the early asthmatic response, and beclomethasone blocked only the late asthmatic response. Cromolyn sodium blocked both the early and late responses. FEV$_1$, forced expiratory volume in 1 sec. (Adapted from Cockcroft DW, Murdock KY: Comparative effects of inhaled salbutamol, sodium cromoglycate, and beclomethasone dipropionate on allergen-induced early asthmatic responses, late asthmatic responses, and increased bronchial responsiveness to histamine. J Allergy Clin Immunol 79:734–740, 1987.)

cromolyn with other pharmacologic agents used to treat pediatric asthma, (3) safety of cromolyn sodium, and (4) guidelines for optimal use of cromolyn sodium in pediatric patients.

DELIVERY FORMS OF CROMOLYN SODIUM

Three forms of delivery of cromolyn sodium are available for use in the United States: a capsule containing 20 mg of the drug in powdered form delivered by turboinhaler (the Spinhaler); 1% solution containing 20 mg of cromolyn sodium in 2 ml of distilled water, administered by compressor-driven nebulizer; and a pressurized metered-dose inhaler that delivers 1 mg per actuation, of which approximately 800 μg reaches the airways.

SPINCAPS

The Spinhaler was developed in order to overcome coordination problems in aerosol therapy. Its effectiveness is confirmed by the number of asthma medications that are available worldwide in which the turboinhaler

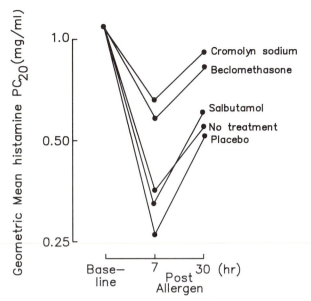

Figure 80–3. Effect of pharmacologic agents on decreasing bronchial hyperreactivity that occurs after the late asthmatic response. Only cromolyn sodium and beclomethasone decreased the allergen-induced increase in bronchial hyperreactivity. PC_{20}, provocation dose causing a 20% drop in FEV_1. (Adapted from Cockcroft DW, Murdock KY: Comparative effects of inhaled salbutamol, sodium cromoglycate, and beclomethasone dipropionate on allergen-induced early asthmatic responses, late asthmatic responses, and increased bronchial responsiveness to histamine. J Allergy Clin Immunol 79:734–740, 1987.)

method of delivery is used. The Spinhaler is a small, open plastic tube containing a plastic propellerlike part that rotates at high speed when air is inhaled through the device. Twenty milligrams of powdered cromolyn sodium mixed with 20 mg of lactose contained in a standard gelatin capsule is inserted into a cup in the propeller. Two perforations are made in the capsule by means of a simple piercing mechanism: vertically sliding a plastic sleeve down once. When air is inhaled through the mouthpiece, the turbovibratory action of the propeller causes the powdered drug to be dispersed into the inspired air through perforations in the capsule wall. The air stream inside the Spinhaler and the action of the propeller cause the active drug and lactose to break up, and the resultant fine particles of cromolyn sodium pass with the inspired air into the respiratory tract. The remaining larger lactose particles are retained in the mouth and upper airways.

Release of the drug occurs early in inhalation and continues while adequate airflow is maintained, providing distribution of cromolyn sodium over the surface of the airways. The extent to which the powder is deposited into the airways is determined both by the flow rate of air drawn through the device and by the length of breath holding. The Spinhaler can be used successfully by almost any patient over the age of 4 years. Being a breath-activated system, it requires little coordination, and no spacer devices are necessary. Moreover, the system contains no fluorocarbons, which could induce coughing.

The powdered form of cromolyn delivered by Spinhaler is the oldest form of cromolyn sodium and thus has been used in thousands of clinical trials. The first large trial in the United States was conducted in 1969 by the American Academy of Allergy and Immunology. This placebo-controlled crossover study demonstrated the short-term (4-week) therapeutic effectiveness and safety of 20 mg cromolyn sodium four times per day via Spinhaler.[23]

Among the early placebo-controlled double blind trials in childhood asthma was a 4-week crossover trial in 54 children with severe chronic asthma.[24] Symptoms of wheezing, breathlessness, feelings of tightness in the chest, and coughing were significantly diminished in the patients during the period of active drug therapy, in comparison with the period of placebo treatment. Twenty percent of the subjects became essentially asymptomatic while receiving cromolyn sodium, and an additional 65% experienced improvement in symptoms.

In another study, 38 children with chronic asthma were given cromolyn sodium or placebo in a double-blind crossover trial of 8 weeks' duration. A statistically significant difference ($p < .005$) in physicians' ratings in favor of cromolyn sodium therapy was found for both sequences.[25] Subsequently, 33 of these children received cromolyn sodium prophylactically for at least 12 months. During that year, in comparison with the previous year, they experienced improved performance in physical exercise, less school absenteeism, reduced hospitalizations, and improvement in sleep patterns. Also, 26 patients experienced a decrease in frequency of asthma attacks, 25 experienced a reduced need for bronchodilators, and improvement was observed in peak expiratory flow rates measured during seasons of airborne pollen and mold.

Twenty-four investigators from nine countries participated in one of the largest worldwide clinical trials for asthma. In this double-blind comparative study, a baseline period of 8 weeks was followed by a treatment period of 52 weeks in which either cromolyn sodium or placebo was added to existing bronchodilator therapy.[26] Treatment was by inhalation either through a metered-dose inhaler (2 mg four times per day) or by Spinhaler (20 mg powder four times per day) with appropriately matched placebo treatments. Of the 397 patients (aged 5 to 63 years and most of whom were adults) who entered the double-blind phase, 283 completed the study. The most common reason for attrition was noncooperation (50 patients); six cromolyn sodium–treated patients were excluded because of uncontrolled asthma. There were no statistically significant differences between the cromolyn sodium–treated patients who used the metered-dose inhaler and those who used the Spinhaler. There was a statistically significant decrease in chronic symptoms of asthma in the cromolyn sodium–treated patients, in comparison with the placebo-treated patients, by weeks 8, 16, and 32 and at the end of the study year. Significant differences in favor of cromolyn sodium were particularly evident in the subset of patients with moderate and severe asthma. There was also a significant increase in evening peak flow rates in patients who received cromolyn sodium. The results of this large international study confirmed those of earlier clinical trials of cromolyn sodium, reaffirming the benefit of adding cromolyn sodium to existing bronchodilator therapy in order to provide significant further improvement in asthma symptoms and pulmonary function.[26]

NEBULIZER SOLUTION

Cromolyn sodium has been available in the United States as a 1% nebulizer solution since 1982. This formulation contains 20 mg of cromolyn sodium in 2 ml of purified water with no preservatives and is packaged in unit-dose 2-ml ampules. Cromolyn sodium nebulizer solution must be delivered with a power-operated nebulizer or may be nebulized with oxygen at a high flow rate. It may be inhaled through either a mouthpiece or a face mask. The face mask has the potential of delivering cromolyn sodium to the entire upper airway, which may be an advantage in patients with concurrent allergic rhinitis, sinusitis, and recurrent otitis media.

Cromolyn sodium nebulizer solution has been demonstrated to be physically and chemically compatible with metaproterenol sulfate solution, isoproterenol hydrochloride solution, isoetharine hydrochloride (0.25% inhalation solution), epinephrine hydrochloride solution, terbutaline sulfate (sterile aqueous solution), albuterol solution, and 20% acetylcysteine solution for up to 60 min.[27] Similarly, cromolyn sodium does not adversely affect the stability of the individual bronchodilator/mucolytic drugs in the admixtures. Thus it is possible to mix cromolyn sodium nebulizer solution with a number of medications simultaneously to simplify delivery.

Inhalation of isotonic and hypotonic cromolyn sodium nebulizer solution was studied in 21 asthmatic subjects with methacholine and exercise challenges.[28] Prechallenge treatment with isotonic cromolyn sodium resulted in significantly more reduction in exercise-induced bronchospasm than did pretreatment with hypotonic cromolyn sodium. In addition, the dose of methacholine required for inducing a decrease of more than 20% in forced expiratory volume in 1 sec (FEV_1) was significantly higher after pretreatment with isotonic cromolyn sodium nebulizer solution than after placebo or hypotonic solution of cromolyn sodium. The investigators concluded that nebulized isotonic cromolyn sodium provides better protection against exercise- and methacholine-induced bronchoconstriction than does the standard solution. The standard solution is made isotonic by adding 0.2 ml of 10% saline to the commercial cromolyn sodium nebulizer solution.

Cromolyn sodium nebulizer solution is especially useful for children under 4 years of age, for patients who are unable to tolerate the powder formulation because of extremely hyperreactive airways, for patients with more severe asthma who benefit from bronchodilator/cromolyn sodium mixtures, for patients with virus-induced wheezing, and for asthmatic patients during acute exacerbations of asthma when a bronchodilator may be added directly to the solution.

In a number of studies, investigators have compared cromolyn sodium nebulizer solution with cromolyn sodium in a capsule delivered by Spinhaler. The two forms have equal clinical efficacy.[29, 30]

Cromolyn sodium as a 1% solution (20 mg) has been studied in several clinical trials in very young asthmatic patients. Hiller and co-workers[31] studied 17 asthmatic children under 5 years of age in a double-blind, placebo-controlled, randomized 2-month crossover trial. Daily symptom scores kept by the parents showed improvement in 11 children during active treatment.

Mellon and colleagues[32] studied 1% cromolyn sodium nebulizer solution in 19 young asthmatic children who required daily oral bronchodilators. During the 8-week active treatment phase, significant reductions in asthmatic symptoms, asthma severity (as assessed by physicians), and concomitant bronchodilator usage were observed in 16 of 19 children. These 16 patients continued to receive cromolyn sodium nebulizer solution for at least 1 year after completion of the study. During the interval of cromolyn maintenance, there was a marked reduction in the number of emergency room visits ($p < .01$), corticosteroid courses, and hospitalizations.

In an open study, 50 children under 4 years of age with severe chronic asthma were treated with nebulized cromolyn sodium (20 mg inhaled for 10 min four times per day) for 6 months.[33] Thirty-three of these children showed marked improvement with no attacks occurring during the treatment period, and 13 showed partial improvement. There was also a marked decrease in the use of other medications and in the number of hospital admissions.

PRESSURIZED METERED-DOSE INHALER

Cromolyn sodium became available in the United States as a pressurized metered-dose aerosol unit in 1986. Each canister contains micronized cromolyn sodium and sorbitan trioleate, with dichlorotetrafluoroethane and dichlorodifluoromethane as propellants. Each metered spray of 1 mg delivers approximately 800 μg of cromolyn sodium to the patient; most of the individual particles of cromolyn sodium have a diameter no more than 5 μm. The recommended dosage is two inhalations four times per day at regular intervals. For the prevention of acute bronchospasm that follows exercise, exposure to cold dry air, or environmental agents, the usual dose is two metered-dose sprays 10 to 15 min before exposure to the precipitating factor (Fig. 80–4).

The pressurized aerosol (two inhalations four times per day) has been shown to be equivalent to 20 mg cromolyn sodium delivered by Spinhaler four times per day.[26] The pressurized aerosol is also as effective as the powder formulation in attenuating exercise-induced asthma despite the tenfold dosage differential.

Several well-controlled short-term evaluations of cromolyn sodium delivered by pressurized metered-dose inhaler (2 mg four times per day) have been conducted. Rubin and colleagues[34] compared cromolyn sodium with matching placebo in a 12-week, double-blind crossover trial in 31 asthmatic adults in Israel. Patients who received cromolyn sodium showed significant decreases in breathlessness at rest ($p < .001$), in breathlessness on exertion ($p < .05$), and in morning peak expiratory flow rates ($p < .05$). Use of bronchodilators significantly decreased ($p < .001$) during cromolyn sodium therapy.

Forty-six children (aged 4 to 13 years) with moderately severe asthma received either cromolyn sodium delivered by pressurized aerosol (2 mg four times per day) or pla-

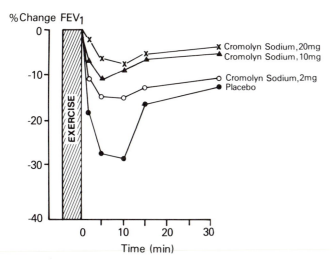

Figure 80–4. Effect of different dosages of cromolyn sodium on blocking exercise-induced asthma. At 30 min, there is no significant difference between dosages. Mean percentage change in FEV_1 (from base line after administration of the drug) was over 30 min after exercise, with different doses of cromolyn sodium aerosol.

cebo in a 12-week, double-blind crossover trial.[35] Asthma severity and pulmonary function tests after 3 and 6 weeks of treatment showed significant improvement in the cromolyn sodium–treated group. Objective assessment of peak expiratory flow rates twice a day also showed clear superiority of cromolyn sodium over placebo.

The efficacy and safety of cromolyn sodium by metered-dose inhaler was evaluated in a multicenter, double-blind, placebo-controlled, parallel group study.[36] One hundred fifty-five patients aged 8 to 58 years whose asthma was well controlled by cromolyn sodium capsules taken by Spinhaler in addition to beta$_2$-agonists were studied. The investigation began with a 2-week control interval with cromolyn sodium capsules, followed by a 4-week single-blind period with placebo capsules. Subjects in whom the asthma significantly worsened while they were receiving placebo therapy then entered a 10-week double-blind phase in which they were randomly assigned to receive either active cromolyn sodium or placebo by metered-dose inhaler. Significant differences ($p < .05$) in favor of cromolyn sodium treatment were noted at all time points for daily asthma symptoms, physicians' assessments at each clinic visit, and FEV_1 at each clinic visit. Concomitant bronchodilators were used less often by the cromolyn sodium–treated patients. The investigators concluded that cromolyn sodium by metered-dose inhaler is highly effective for controlling asthmatic symptoms, improving lung function, and decreasing the need for concomitant bronchodilators.[36]

COMPARISON WITH OTHER PHARMACOLOGIC AGENTS

THEOPHYLLINE

The primary indication for both cromolyn sodium and theophylline is mild to moderate chronic asthma. In addition, both drugs are indicated as adjunctive therapy for

chronic, severe, steroid-dependent asthma. However, in the treatment of non–steroid-dependent patients with chronic asthma, clinical trials have shown that 60% to 70% of patients can be adequately controlled with the use of either agent as first-line therapy. As a result, six double-blind comparisons of cromolyn sodium and theophylline have been performed.[37–42]

In the study of longest duration (3 months), Furukawa and associates[37] compared cromolyn sodium with sustained-release theophylline in 46 asthmatic children in a double-blind parallel design. There was no placebo group, and so each treatment was compared against a prestudy baseline value. The two agents were not significantly different from each other in that both improved symptom scores, improved pulmonary functions, and decreased the need for supplemental medications. However, the patients treated with theophylline experienced more side effects and required more office visits. Of importance was that only the patients treated with cromolyn sodium had a significant decrease in bronchial hyperreactivity, as assessed through methacholine challenge.

The most recent study was a double-blind, two-way crossover trial with 4-week treatment periods of cromolyn sodium and sustained-release theophylline.[38] No significant differences between treatments were found in symptom scores, pulmonary functions, exercise and histamine bronchial provocation tests, and additional drug consumption. In addition, the patients were administered a series of psychological tests during the third week of each study period. The four children with IQ scores of <105 performed significantly worse on the tests of visual-spatial planning while taking theophylline than while taking cromolyn sodium.

In summary, in the short-term management of chronic asthma, cromolyn sodium and theophylline are equally effective. However, theophylline therapy is associated with a higher frequency of gastrointestinal and central nervous system side effects.[39–42] Cromolyn sodium has an advantage over theophylline in its ability to decrease the bronchial hyperreactivity and thus possibly alter the course of the disease.

BETA$_2$-AGONISTS

Although usually prescribed for the relief of acute bronchospasm, beta$_2$-agonists are sometimes used as continuous maintenance medications for chronic asthma. The wisdom of this use has been questioned.

To evaluate whether the potency of a selective inhaled beta$_2$-agonist negates the need for cromolyn sodium, 27 patients aged 6 to 12 years with mild to moderate asthma who required long-term medication were assessed for the therapeutic effects of inhaled cromolyn sodium or terbutaline or both by nebulizer.[43] Patients received cromolyn sodium (20 mg) or terbutaline (0.1 mg/kg up to 4 mg) or the combination three times per day. Each patient underwent the three treatment regimens each in randomized order and for periods of 8 weeks in a double-blind crossover manner. Daily diary-recorded mean scores demonstrated better symptom control with cromolyn sodium than with terbutaline ($p < .05$). Evening peak flow measurements were higher with the combination and with cromolyn sodium alone than with terbutaline alone ($p <$ .01). With methacholine challenge, less bronchial hyperreactivity occurred with the combination and cromolyn sodium alone than with terbutaline alone ($p < .02$). The investigators concluded that the effectiveness of the nebulizer regimen for children with chronic asthma was better when cromolyn was used alone or in combination with terbutaline than when the beta$_2$-agonist was used alone.[43]

CORTICOSTEROIDS

Cromolyn sodium was initially approved by the Food and Drug Administration for use in steroid-dependent asthmatic patients as a corticosteroid-sparing drug. This resulted from the observation in several early clinical studies that corticosteroid dosage could be reduced in some patients.[44, 45] In fact, the first clinical trial of cromolyn sodium was perfomed with 12 patients with allergic, severe asthma who had not been able to control their asthma with high doses of oral steroids.

In a double-blind crossover trial, Friday and coworkers[46] gave 20 mg of inhaled cromolyn sodium or a placebo four times per day for two 4-week periods to 36 children with chronic intractable asthma, 23 of whom were corticosteroid dependent. In the very short treatment period, cromolyn sodium was not statistically superior to the placebo in the patients with severe asthma; however, 36 patients noted subjective improvement from the cromolyn sodium and entered a 12-month open-ended clinical trial. Of the 18 steroid-dependent patients who completed 12 months of cromolyn sodium therapy, 7 discontinued use of corticosteroids, 10 decreased the dosage, and 1 patient required increased amounts of corticosteroids.

It has been suggested that the combination of inhaled cromolyn sodium and inhaled corticosteroid may be more effective than either drug alone. Toogood and associates[47] assessed the usefulness of adding cromolyn sodium to patients dependent on beclomethasone therapy. Thirty patients whose asthma was well controlled on high-dose beclomethasone (mean 1040 μg per day) but whose morning cortisol levels averaged 10 μg/dl were randomly assigned to receive placebo or cromolyn sodium (20 mg four times per day) in addition to beclomethasone and other regular asthma medications. After 4 weeks, the beclomethasone dosage was halved, and both groups were monitored subjectively and objectively for more than 6 months. The distributions of good, fair, and poor risk-benefit responses were the same in both groups ($p = .20$). There was no discernible beclomethasone-sparing effect or other clinical advantage of adding cromolyn sodium to the established beclomethasone requirement. However, Toogood and associates noted that a high percentage of these patients with severe asthma had previously failed to respond to an adequate trial of cromolyn sodium therapy.

In an 8-week double-blind study of bronchial hyperreactivity in non-atopic asthmatics, Lowhagen and Rak[48] treated 40 adults with intrinsic asthma with cromolyn sodium, budesonide, cromolyn sodium plus budesonide, or placebo. A mean decrease in sensitivity to histamine provocation was seen after both cromolyn sodium and

budesonide but not after placebo. The combination of cromolyn sodium and budesonide produced no additional effect.

Svendsen and colleagues,[49] in a crossover study, administered beclomethasone or cromolyn sodium to 38 atopic asthmatic patients for 8 weeks. The study was performed out of season, and only the patients receiving beclomethasone were shown to have a decrease in bronchial reactivity. In acute single-dose studies, however, both drugs appear to protect equally well against antigen-induced increases in bronchial hyperresponsiveness to histamine.[22] Cromolyn sodium has an advantage over corticosteroids inasmuch as it inhibits both the early and late asthmatic responses, whereas beclomethasone blocks only the late obstructive response.[22] Thus a single dose of cromolyn sodium, but not a topical steroid, provides marked protection against isolated exposure to pollens, animal dander, industrial pollutants, exercise, and cold air.

Two additional controlled trials failed to show added benefit from combined cromolyn sodium and corticosteroid therapy.[50, 51] Bias in selection of patients could have resulted in a cromolyn sodium–unresponsive subset of asthmatic patients. Also, airway deposition of the drug in the formulation of cromolyn sodium used (capsule given by Spinhaler) and the dosage (20 mg four times per day) could have influenced these results because of poor compliance by patients. Despite these potential problems, it appears that the steroid-sparing effect of cromolyn sodium is not as marked as originally thought.[45]

SAFETY

Parenteral administration of cromolyn sodium in mice, rats, guinea pigs, hamsters, and rabbits has shown that the median lethal dose is approximately 4000 mg/kg. By inhalation, even in long-term studies, it has been impossible to achieve toxic levels of cromolyn sodium in a range of mammalian species.[52] In a prospective study of 375 patients, investigators reported side effects in only 2%.[53] All such effects were mild and were readily reversible.

Cromolyn sodium has a pregnancy category B rating. There have been no reports of drug-related fetal malformations. Cromolyn sodium was used as therapy for 296 asthmatic women throughout their pregnancies in France. Malformations were reported in 4 newborns (1.35%), which represents a frequency of less than that reported for the population as a whole (2% to 4%).[54]

In thirteen articles published from 1975 to 1987, researchers described type 1–like adverse reactions to cromolyn sodium. Together, these reactions compromised 19 cases. The presence of IgE antibodies to cromolyn sodium was demonstrated in one case by passive transfer of the patient's serum to a recipient and in two cases by a positive skin test, and in one case, serum contained cromolyn sodium–specific IgE antibodies.[55]

REFERENCES

1. Altounyan REC: Inhibition of experimental asthma by a new compound—disodium cromoglycate (Intal). Acta Allergol 22:487, 1967.

2. Cox JSG: Review of chemistry, pharmacology, toxicity, metabolism, specific side-effects, antiallergic properties *in vitro* and *in vivo* of disodium cromoglycate. *In* Pepys J, Franland AW (eds): Disodium Cromoglycate in Allergic Airway Disease, p. 13. London: Butterworth's, 1970.

3. Richards R, Dickson CR, Renwick AG, et al: Absorption and disposition kinetics of cromolyn sodium and the influence of inhalation technique. J Pharmacol Exper Ther 241:1028–1032, 1987.

4. Cox JS: Disodium cromoglycate (FPL670) (Intal): A specific inhibitor of reaginic antibody/antigen mechanisms. Nature 216:1328–1329, 1967.

5. Church MK, Hiroi J: Inhibition of IgE-dependent histamine release from human dispersed lung mast cells by anti-allergic drugs and salbutamol. Br J Pharmacol 90:421–429, 1987.

6. Flint KC, Leung KB, Pearce FL, et al: Human mast cells recovered by bronchoalveolar lavage: Their morphology, histamine release and the effects of sodium cromoglycate. Clin Sci 68:427–432, 1985.

7. Atkins PC, Norman ME, Zweiman B: Antigen-induced neutrophil chemotactic activity in man: Correlation with bronchospasm and inhibition by disodium cromoglycate. J Allergy Clin Immunol 62:149–155, 1978.

8. Diaz P, Galleguillos FR, Gonzalez MC, et al: Bronchoalveolar lavage in asthma: The effect of disodium cromoglycate (cromolyn) on leukocyte counts, immunoglobulins, and complement. J Allergy Clin Immunol 74:41–48, 1984.

9. Mazurek N, Berger G, Pecht I: A binding site on mast cells and basophils for the antiallergic drug cromolyn. Nature 286:722–723, 1980.

10. Theoharides TC, Sieghart W, Greengard P, Douglas WW: Anti-allergic drug cromolyn may inhibit histamine secretion by regulating phosphorylation of a mast cell protein. Science 207:80–82, 1980.

11. Lucas AM, Shuster S: Cromolyn inhibiton of protein kinase C activity. Biochem Pharmacol 36:562–565, 1987.

12. Kay AB, Walsh GM, Moqbel R, et al: Disodium cromoglycate inhibits activation of human inflammatory cells *in vitro*. J. Allergy Clin Immunol 80:1–8, 1987.

13. Erjefalt I, Persson CG: Anti-asthma attenuates inflammatory leakage of plasma into airway lumen. Acta Physiol Scand 128:653–654, 1986.

14. Harries MG: Bronchial irritant receptors and a possible new action for cromolyn sodium. Ann Allergy 46:156–158, 1981.

15. Kusenbach G, Reinhardt D: Effect of sodium cromoglycate on alpha and beta$_2$ receptors of platelets and lymphocytes. Atem Lungenkrkh 12:86–88, 1986.

16. Joos G, Pauwels R, Van Der Straeten M: The effect of sodium cromoglycate and nedocromil sodium on neuropeptide-induced bronchoconstriction in the rat. Presented at the annual meeting of the European Academy of Allergology, April 22–26, 1987.

17. Myers DJ, Bigby BG, Boushey HA: The inhibition of sulfur dioxide-induced bronchoconstriction in asthmatic subjects by cromolyn is dose dependent. Am Rev Respir Dis 133:1150–1153, 1986.

18. Murphy S: Cromolyn sodium. *In* Jenne J, Murphy S (eds): Drug Therapy for Asthma: Research and Clinical Practice, pp. 669–717, New York: Marcel Dekker, 1987.

19. Schoeffel RE, Anderson SD, Lindsay DA: Sodium cromoglycate as a pressurized aerosol (Vicrom) in exercise-induced asthma. Aust N Z J Med 13:157–161, 1983.

20. Breslin FJ, McFadden ER, Ingram RH: The effects of cromolyn sodium on the airway response to hyperpnea and cold air in asthma. Am Rev Respir Dis 122:11–16, 1980.

21. Patel KR, Kerr JW: The dose-duration effect of sodium cromoglycate in exercise-induced asthma. Clin Allergy 14:87–91, 1984.

22. Cockcroft DW, Murdock KY: Comparative effects of inhaled salbutamol, sodium cromoglycate, and beclomethasone dipropionate on allergen-induced early asthmatic responses, late asthmatic responses, and increased bronchial responsiveness to histamine. J Allergy Clin Immunol 79:734–740, 1987.

23. Bernstein IL, Siegel SC, Brandon ML, et al: A controlled study of cromolyn sodium sponsored by the Drug Committee of the American Academy of Allergy. J Allergy Clin Immunol 50:235–245, 1972.

24. McLean WL, Lozano J, Hannaway P, et al: Cromolyn treatment of asthmatic children. Am J Dis Child 125:332–337, 1973.

25. Hyde JS, Isenberg PD, Floro LD: Short- and long-term prophylaxis with cromolyn sodium in chronic asthma. Chest 63:875–880, 1973.

26. Eigen H, Reid JJ, Dahl R, et al: Evaluation of the addition of cromolyn sodium to bronchodilator maintenance therapy in the long-term management of asthma. J Allergy Clin Immunol 80:612–621, 1987.

27. Lesko LJ, Miller AK: Physical-chemical compatibility of cromolyn sodium nebulizer solution—Bronchodilator inhalant solution admixtures. Ann Allergy 53:236–238, 1984.

28. Weiner P, Saaid M, Reshef A: Isotonic nebulized disodium cromoglycate provides better protection against methacholine- and exercise-induced bronchoconstriction. Am Rev Respir Dis 137:1309–1311, 1988.

29. Bundgaard A, Pedersen JZ, Schmidt A, Bach-Mortensen N: Should stable asthma be treated with nebulizer or pressurized metered-dose spray? Ugeskr Laeger 143:2878–2880, 1981.

30. Corkey C, Mindorff C, Levison H, Newth C: Comparison of three different preparations of disodium cromoglycate in the prevention of exercise-induced bronchospasm. Am Rev Respir Dis 125:623–626, 1982.

31. Hiller EJ, Milner AD, Lenney W: Nebulized sodium cromoglycate in young asthmatic children. Arch Dis Child 52:875–876, 1977.

32. Mellon MH, Harden K, Zeiger RS: The effectiveness and safety of nebulizer cromolyn solution in the young childhood asthmatic. Immunol Allergy Pract 4:168–172, 1982.

33. Zareceansky S, Nadel G, Yahav J, Katznelson D: Treatment of asthmatic patients under four years of age with sodium cromoglycate. Harefuah 105:257–258, 1983.

34. Rubin AE, Alroy G, Spitzer S: The treatment of asthma in adults using sodium cromoglycate pressurized aerosol: A double-blind controlled trial. Curr Med Res Opin 8:553–558, 1983.

35. Geller-Bernstein C, Levin S: Sodium cromoglycate pressurized aerosol in childhood asthma. Curr Ther Res 34:345–349, 1983.

36. Blumenthal MN, Selcow J, Spector S, et al: A multicenter evaluation of the clinical benefits of cromolyn sodium aerosol by metered-dose inhaler in treatment of asthma. J Allergy Clin Immunol 81:681–687, 1988.

37. Furukawa CT, Shapiro GC, Bierman CW, et al: A double-blind study comparing the effectiveness of cromolyn sodium and sustained-release theophylline in childhood asthma. Pediatrics 74:453–459, 1984.

38. Springer C, Goldenberg B, Ben-Dov I, Godfrey S: Clinical, physiologic, and psychologic comparison of treatment by cromolyn or theophylline in childhood asthma. J Allergy Clin Immunol 76:64–69, 1985.

39. Hambleton G, Weinberger M, Taylor J, et al: Comparison of cromoglycate (cromolyn) and theophylline in controlling symptoms of chronic asthma: A collaborative study. Lancet 1:381–385, 1977.

40. Edmunds AT, Carswell F, Robinson P, Hughes AO: Controlled trial of cromoglycate and slow-release aminophylline in perennial childhood asthma. Br Med J 281:842, 1980.

41. Glass J, Archer LN, Adams W, Simpson H: Nebulized cromoglycate, theophylline, and placebo in preschool asthmatic children. Arch Dis Child 56:648–651, 1981.

42. Newth CJ, Newth CV, Turner JA: Comparison of nebulized sodium cromoglycate and oral theophylline in controlling symptoms of chronic asthma in pre-school children: A double-blind study. Aust N Z J Med 12:232–238, 1982.

43. Shapiro GG, Furukawa CT, Pierson WE, et al: Double-blind evaluation of nebulized cromolyn, terbutaline and the combination for childhood asthma. J Allergy Clin Immunol 81:449–454, 1988.

44. Smith JM, Devey GF: Clinical trial of disodium cromoglycate in the treatment of asthma in children. Br Med J 2:340–344, 1968.

45. Chai H, Molk L, Falliers CJ, Miklich D: Steroid-sparing effects of disodium cromoglycate (DSC) in children with severe clinical asthma. *In* Serafini U (ed): New Concepts in Allergy and Clinical Immunology, pp. 385–391. Amsterdam: Excerpta Medica, 1971.

46. Friday GA, Facktor MA, Bernstein RA, Fireman P: Cromolyn therapy for severe asthma in children. J Pediatr 83:299–304, 1973.

47. Toogood JH, Jennings B, Lefcoe NM: A clinical trial of combined cromolyn/beclomethasone treatment for chronic asthma. J Allergy Clin Immunol 67:317–324, 1981.

48. Lowhagen O, Rak I: Effect of sodium cromoglycate and budesonide on bronchial hyperreactivity in non-atopic asthmatics. Respiration 46(Suppl 1):105, 1984.

49. Svendsen UG, Frolund L, Madsen F, et al: A comparison of the effects of sodium cromoglycate and beclomethasone dipropionate on pulmonary function and bronchial hyperreactivity in subjects with asthma. J Allergy Clin Immunol 80:68–74, 1987.

50. Dawood AG, Hendry AT, Walker SR: The combined use of beta-methasone valerate and sodium cromoglycate in the treatment of asthma. Clin Allergy 7:161–165, 1977.
51. Hiller EJ, Milner AD: Betamethasone 17 valerate aerosol and disodium cromoglycate in severe childhood asthma. Br J Dis Chest 69:103–106, 1975.
52. Cox JS, Beach JE, Blair AM: Disodium cromoglycate (Intal). Adv Drug Res 5:115–196, 1970.
53. Settipane GA, Klein DE, Boyd GK et al: Adverse reactions to cromolyn. JAMA 241:811–813, 1979.
54. Wilson J: Use of sodium cromoglycate during pregnancy. J Pharm Med 8(2, Suppl):45–51, 1982.
55. Wass U, Plaschke P, Bjorkander J, Belin L: Assay of specific IgE antibodies to disodium cromoglycate in serum from a patient with an immediate hypersensitivity reaction. J Allergy Clin Immunol 81:750–757, 1988.

81 GLUCOCORTICOIDS

H. WILLIAM KELLY, PHARM.D. / SUSANNAH B. WALKER, M.D. / GAIL G. SHAPIRO, M.D.

MECHANISM OF ACTION OF STEROIDS

It has long been recognized that the anti-inflammatory action of glucocorticoids is of prime therapeutic importance in certain pulmonary diseases. Since the early 1970s, their biochemical and anti-inflammatory mechanisms of action have become better known. The actions of steroids on modulating the immune system interactions are still being elucidated.

This chapter is an overview of how steroids may influence such disease processes as asthma, hypersensitivity pneumonitis, and allergic bronchopulmonary aspergillosis.

BIOCHEMICAL MECHANISMS

The biologic activity of glucocorticoids appears to be caused by changes in DNA expression and subsequent protein synthesis. Glucocorticoids passively diffuse into cells, interacting with intracellular receptors to form hormone-receptor complexes. They then undergo conformational changes so that binding sites with a high affinity for nuclei and DNA are exposed. There is some debate over whether the activation process involves dissociation of the nonactivated complexes into subunits[1] or whether activation is associated with a change in charge of the steroid-receptor complex, perhaps with a dephosphorylation reaction.[2]

Activated hormone receptor complexes are translocated to the cell nucleus and interact rapidly with chromatin within seconds to minutes. It is not known how steroid hormones induce the modification of chromatin structure to allow RNA polymerase to transcribe sequences over a large segment of DNA.

Many of the peripheral tissue effects of steroids depend on RNA and protein synthesis. Qualitative differences in steroid-receptor complexes and genes affected by them in differentiated cells may determine the cellular responses of different tissues to steroids.[3] Although initiation of messenger RNA synthesis is rapid, there may be a time lag of 1 to 4 h or more before the steroid-induced protein effects become detectable in human cells[3] (Table 81–1).

The more potent steroids such as triamcinolone acetonide and dexamethasone seem to induce higher steady-state concentrations of hormone-receptor–activated, nucleus-bound complexes.[1] In addition, the affinity of binding to intracellular receptors is positively correlated with the potency of the steroid.[4]

Not all steroid-induced effects are explained by the time frame required for the hormone-receptor interaction and subsequent protein synthesis. For example, elevation of cyclic adenosine monophosphate (cAMP) occurs within minutes of the exposure of human lymphocytes to pharmacologic concentrations of corticosteroids in vitro.[5] This action may be related to the important effects of steroids on beta-adrenergic receptors. They facilitate the formulation of a high-affinity receptor, leading to increased coupling with and activation of adenylate cyclase.[6] They stimulate the synthesis of new receptors to restore lymphocyte receptor density[7] and potentiate the action of

Table 81–1. BIOCHEMICAL MECHANISMS OF ACTION OF STEROIDS

Nuclear
Passive diffusion of steroids into cells
Formation of activated hormone receptor complexes
Translocation of complex to nucleus
Modification of conformation of chromatin by complex
RNA polymerase transcription
Messenger RNA and protein synthesis

Nonnuclear
Possible effect on cAMP-dependent protein kinases
Inhibition of Ca^{++} influx

cAMP, cyclic adenosine monophosphate.

endogenous catecholamines by interfering with the extra-neuronal uptake and inactivation of catecholamines.[8,9] In addition, glucocorticoids may enhance the effectiveness of cAMP by affecting cAMP protein kinase.[3]

Another important nonnuclear mechanism of action is through alterations in calcium flux. Corticosteroids appear to produce major changes in cellular metabolism by regulating calcium influx into cells. For example, rapid inhibition of secretion of adrenocorticotropic hormone (ACTH) from pituitary cells results from steroid-induced inhibition of calcium entry.[10]

Both nuclear and nonnuclear sites of control may be involved in the steroid inhibition of prostaglandin production because the influx of extracellular Ca^{++} is a rate-limiting step in arachidonate production, as is the steroid influence on nuclear phosphorylation reactions.

ANTI-INFLAMMATORY MECHANISMS OF GLUCOCORTICOSTEROIDS

Corticosteroids cause a redistribution of leukocytes so that they are less available at inflammatory sites. Also, steroids inhibit leukotriene synthesis and prostaglandin synthesis by preventing arachidonic acid release from phospholipids. By altering soluble mediator release and thus the cellular environment, steroids influence interactions between different cell types.

EFFECT ON LEUKOCYTE DISTRIBUTION AND FUNCTION

In vivo administration of glucocorticoids in humans causes a redistribution of cells in the circulation. The effect of corticosteroids on leukocyte distribution and function has been well summarized by other authors.[11-14] The relative proportion and the absolute number of neutrophils in the circulation increase to a maximum between 4 and 6 h after steroid administration and return to normal by 24 h. The corticosteroid-induced neutrophilia involves not only sequestration within the intravascular space but also an increased bone marrow release of cells into the peripheral stream. Other cell types, including eosinophils, basophils, monocytes, B lymphocytes, and the various subclasses of T lymphocytes, show some degree of sensitivity to this effect, which results in a decrease in number and proportion of these circulating cells.

Although some of the effect may merely be a dilutional one secondary to the increased concentration of neutrophils, other mechanisms may be involved. Many authors have suggested that some alteration of the cellular surface of all these cells, possibly by new protein synthesis, may modify their selective binding to the endothelial cell walls[11-13] with subsequent changes, as mentioned, in traffic patterns. Glucocorticoids have direct effects on the endothelial cells themselves, which include decreasing capillary permeability by constricting the microvasculature.[15] The bone marrow may be the modulating pool that plays the largest role in regulating the cellular composition of the intravascular compartment.[11]

The peak steroid effect on eosinophils and basophils seems to be later (after approximately 8 h) than that on neutrophils, and the return to normal numbers of these cells is delayed (72 h, as opposed to 24 h for neutrophils). Non-recirculating lymphocytes, predominantly B cells, which live out their life span in the vascular compartment, seem relatively unaffected by glucocorticoids.[11] Monocytes seem to be the cell type most quantitatively affected by the redistribution effect, falling in number from 300 to 400 to less than 50 per cubic millimeter.[13] Because macrophages are critical both for antigen presentation to lymphocytes for subsequent stimulation of lymphokine production and for their phagocytic capacity, this depletion has an important dampening effect on the inflammatory response.

Not only are leukocyte traffic patterns altered so that cells fail to accumulate at the site of inflammation, but glucocorticoids alter the function of these cells as well. Glucocorticoids diminish granulocyte, eosinophil, and monocyte responses to chemotactic stimuli and alter eosinophil and granulocyte adherence.

Secretion of soluble mediators, such as interleukin-1 and plasminogen activator, by monocytes is suppressed.[11-13] Phagocytosis and bactericidal action are subsequently inhibited. Tissue destruction, which occurs after the secretion of proteolytic enzymes such as collagenase and elastase, is thereby prevented. The ability of macrophages to respond to lymphokines such as migration inhibition factor and macrophage activation factor may be blocked, which may lead to a dampening of the delayed hypersensitivity response.

Steroids appear to inhibit T lymphocyte responsiveness to a variety of stimuli. Steroids inhibit T cell response *in vivo* to concanavalin A, phytohemagglutinin, pokeweed mitogen, and specific antigens such as streptokinase-streptodornase and tetanus toxoid. Autologous and allogeneic mixed leukocyte reactions are inhibited by glucocorticoids.[11] In mixed leukocyte reactions, glucocorticoids inhibit interleukin-1–stimulated production of interleukin-2 by T cells.[16]

Data suggest that high-dose steroid therapy depresses B cell function and that immunoglobulin synthesis declines slightly with high-dose therapy. Serum levels of immunoglobulins G and A decrease to a greater extent than that of immunoglobulin M. The mechanism may involve both a decreased rate of catabolism and a decreased rate of production. Immunoglobulin E (IgE) levels may increase transiently, possibly because of a decrease in T suppressor cells.[11]

STEROID EFFECTS OF ARACHIDONIC ACID METABOLISM

Many of the anti-inflammatory actions of glucocorticoids are caused by their inhibitory influences on the formation of arachidonic acid metabolites. Investigators have demonstrated an inhibition of the production of leukotriene B_4, thromboxane B_2, and prostaglandins F_2 and E_2 by corticosteroids (prednisone), but synthesis of thromboxane A_2 and of leukotriene E_4 was not suppressed in macrophages.[17] Oxygenated derivatives of arachidonic acid include the leukotrienes, which are mediators in immediate hypersensitivity reactions and inflammatory reactions. Several reviews have summarized the biosynthesis, metabolism, and function of the biologically active leukotrienes.[17, 18]

In modulating a hypersensitivity reaction, steroids first actually cause a release of stored inhibitors. They then induce the formation of peptides that inhibit the action of several phospholipases (including A_2, C, and D) on the release of fatty acids from esterified phospholipid stores.[19] This serves to inhibit production of arachidonic acid metabolites, thus quelling further activity. The extent of this suppressive action depends on receptor occupation by steroids and on RNA and protein synthesis. The phospholipase inhibitor induced by steroids has been termed macrocortin[19] or lipomodulin.[20] Whether the two are identical or whether macrocortin is a phosphorylated fragment of lipomodulin is not clear.[20] There seem to be two sets of one or more inhibitory proteins that lead to distinct inhibition of membrane-bound and lysosomal phospholipase A_2.[21]

Blackwell and co-workers, in the experimental model of carrageenan-induced pleurisy in rats, showed conclusively that monoclonal antibody to macrocortin abrogated the acute local anti-inflammatory effect of dexamethasone, whereas a control immunoglobulin with no antimacrocortin activity had no effect.[19] Evidence that similar actions occur in humans is accumulating; for example, an autoantibody to lipomodulin has been found in serum from patients with lupus erythematosus.[22]

The phospholipase inhibitor effect may vary with cell type. Dexamethasone inhibits some phospholipases in human lung fragments but seems to have no effect on human lung parenchymal mast cell phospholipase.[23]

MODULATION OF SOLUBLE MEDIATOR RELEASE

Corticosteroids modulate the release of soluble mediators that play an important role in immunoregulation. Glucocorticoids may directly interfere with interleukin-1 stimulation of interleukin-2 production by T cells[11] or may block the transcription of the interleukin-2 message.[24] Corticosteroids inhibit the production of plasminogen activator, collagenase, and elastase.[13] They can augment the Sendai virus–induced production of interferon in tumor cell lines in humans.[11]

Dexamethasone has been shown to inhibit the IgE-dependent release of histamine by human basophils. The inhibition was thought to occur after the binding of anti-IgE antibody to cell surface IgE but before the opening of calcium channels, because calcium ionophore A23187–induced release of histamine was not inhibited by the 24-h incubation with steroid.[25] In this study, cell surface IgE Fc receptor numbers did not show any drug-induced change. Because 5-lipoxygenase products 5-hydroperoxyeicosatetraenoic acid and 5-hydroxyeicosatetraenoic acid enhance antigen-induced histamine release from basophils,[26] steroids might modulate the actions of these compounds through their effects on arachidonic acid metabolism.

Glucocorticoid modulation of IgE-mediated histamine release has been studied in mast cells from both mouse and human lungs. Contrasting results have been obtained, possibly because of a species difference or because of a heterogeneity in the type of mast cell studied. Dexamethasone pretreatment of mouse mast cells results in inhibition of antigen-induced histamine release and degranulation, apparently by inhibiting biochemical processes that lead to Ca^{++} channel opening.[27] The steroid did not inhibit the release of histamine, prostaglandin D_2, or thromboxane B_2 in response to anti-IgE stimulation of human lung parenchymal mast cells, but it did significantly inhibit the release of prostaglandin E_2, prostaglandin $F_{2\alpha}$, and 6-keto–prostaglandin $F_{1\alpha}$.[23]

GLUCOCORTICOID THERAPY IN ASTHMA

EFFECT ON AIRWAYS HYPERREACTIVITY

Patients with asthma manifest paroxysmal or continuous airway obstruction. The types of stimuli, sites of airway obstruction, factors that induce airway hyperreactivity, and the response to treatment vary among individuals. Two types of responses may occur in asthmatic patients after experimental challenges to inhaled antigens or after environmental exposures to antigens or chemicals. Early asthmatic responses develop in an allergic patient within minutes of exposure to a stimulus such as inhaled pollen or inhaled methacholine or histamine. Early responses are of short duration and are not followed by an increase in nonspecific airway hyperreactivity; the pre-existing level of nonspecific bronchial hyperreactivity determines the magnitude of the early response.[28] Late asthmatic reactions may follow an early response, beginning some 4 to 6 h later, or may occur alone. These reactions may occur after allergen inhalation,[29] after occupational exposures to chemicals such as toluene diisocyanate, after viral infection, or after exposure to inhaled pollutants such as ozone.[28] A significant increase in bronchial responsiveness, which may last several weeks and may be of variable magnitude, occurs in susceptible persons after a late response.

The late reaction appears to involve inflammation secondary to invasion of inflammatory cells, whereas the early reaction may be a function predominantly of reversible smooth muscle contraction produced by the release of preformed mediators such as histamine. Bronchoalveolar lavage fluid from subjects who showed late reactions after inhalation of house dust mite allergen contained significant numbers of eosinophils as well as an elevated eosinophil cationic protein/albumin ratio during the early part of the late reaction.[30] The eosinophilia was not present in patients with only early asthmatic reactions.[30] How steroids might influence eosinophil migration and activation in this situation is not known. However, it has long been known that corticosteroid prechallenge treatment effectively decreases the late reaction[31-34] and that steroids inhibit eosinophil ingress in late-phase skin reactions.[35] As a result, corticosteroid therapy significantly reduces nonspecific bronchial hyperre-activity when administered chronically to asthmatic patients.[36-39]

The data concerning whether corticosteroids are effective in immediate asthmatic responses have been in apparent conflict.[32] Corticosteroids neither inhibit the release of histamine from human lung parenchymal mast cells[23] nor relax bronchial smooth muscle[3] and therefore have no acute inhibitor effect on the early asthmatic response.[33] However, because of their ability to decrease bronchial hyperreactivity, chronic administration of corticosteroids produces a significant attenuation of the early asthmatic response to allergen[32] or mediators[34] in a dosage- and time-dependent manner. Results of one study indicated that topical corticosteroid therapy may produce greater inhibition of bronchial responsiveness than do oral corticosteroids in dosages that produced equivalent effects on baseline pulmonary function tests.[40] This finding may have important implications for the treatment of chronic asthma and warrants further study.

EFFECT ON PULMONARY GAS EXCHANGE AND AIRWAY OBSTRUCTION

To document the efficacy of any drug in acute asthma, responsiveness of patients to therapy, severity of asthma, dosages and types of medications used for care both before randomization and during the study all have to be standardized in carefully randomized, double-blind manner. Although there is general agreement that glucocorticoids are of value in the treatment of acute asthma that is refractory to bronchodilator therapy, there has been some controversy regarding this point.

In a double-blind, randomized trial of 45 children hospitalized for status asthmaticus, corticosteroid therapy produced greater and more rapid improvement in hypoxemia than did placebo.[41] A significant amount of the improvement occurred within the first 3 h of treatment. In contrast to the beta-adrenergic bronchodilators, corticosteroids seem to improve the ventilation/perfusion imbalance, possibly as a result of bronchodilation of the small airways, leading to a more uniform ventilation distribution in relation to perfusion. Steroids improve arterial oxygen tension and lead to a decrease in alveolar-arterial oxygen tension difference and in the venous admixture effect.[42] An increase in effective pulmonary blood flow accompanies alteration of the ventilation/perfusion ratio.[43]

Fanta and associates[44] evaluated 20 adult asthmatic patients who had severe obstruction at admission to the hospital. By the end of 24 h, all those who received corticosteroids had significantly greater resolution of airway obstruction, whereas in 56% of the patients treated with placebo, pulmonary mechanics had deteriorated or were unchanged after 24 h. In a double-blind, placebo-controlled study of children hospitalized for status asthmaticus, Younger and colleagues[45] reported a higher magnitude and a higher rate of improvement in forced expiratory flow between 25% and 75% of vital capacity (FEF_{25-75}) with intravenous methylprednisolone. In another double-blind trial of children with acute exacer-

bations of asthma who did not require hospitalization, significantly more children who received placebo showed persistently abnormal forced expiratory volume in 1 sec and FEF_{25-75} values and wheezing on auscultation at the time of reevaluation on day 7.[46]

Corticosteroids did not have a direct relaxing effect on bronchial smooth muscle.[47] Their influence on airway obstruction is thought to reside in their anti-inflammatory effect and their ability to improve the smooth muscle responsiveness to beta$_2$-adrenergic agonists. It has long been recognized that asthmatic patients may have desensitization or down-regulation (decreased number) or both of adrenergic receptors with decreased cAMP response to beta$_2$-agonist stimulation and that steroids can prevent and reverse this phenomenon.[47, 48]

The time course of the maximal corticosteroid effect on airway obstruction may depend on the population studied: for example, patients with chronic, stable asthma as opposed to patients experiencing status asthmaticus. In patients with chronic, stable asthma, a single intravenous dose of corticosteroid improves the responsiveness to aerosolized isoproterenol within 1 h.[3] Pulmonary function tests in patients with stable asthma begin to show improvement in 1 to 3 h after administration of single doses of intravenous, oral, or inhaled corticosteroids, with a maximal effect after 6 to 9 h.[47] In acute asthma, there is a lag time of at least 6 h before any measurable effects on airway obstruction are seen, and it may take 24 to 48 h to produce maximal benefit.[44-47]

STRUCTURE AND EFFECT OF GLUCOCORTICOIDS

The endogenous adrenocorticosteroids, principally cortisol (hydrocortisone), have both glucocorticoid (anti-inflammatory) and mineralocorticoid (salt retention) effects. The antiasthmatic effects of corticosteroids reside in the glucocorticoid activity. Figure 81-1 illustrates the basic four-ring hydrocortisone molecule and the locations of chemical modifications that have led to synthetic ana-

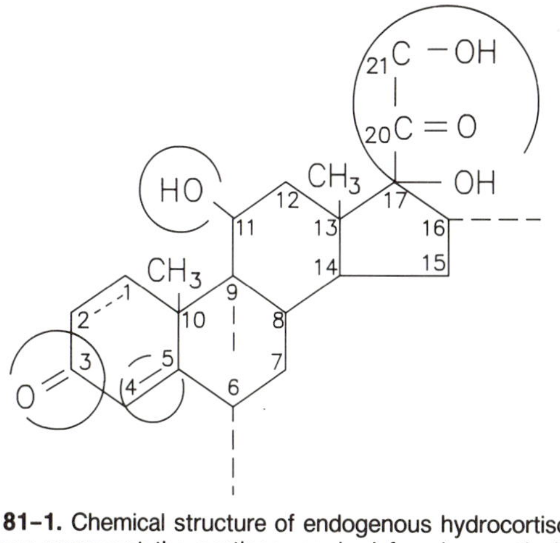

Figure 81-1. Chemical structure of endogenous hydrocortisone. Circled areas represent the portions required for glucocorticoid effect. Dashed lines indicate where chemical modifications that enhance glucocorticoid activity are made. Addition of various esters to 16, 17, or 21 carbon can enhance topical activity.

Table 81–2. GLUCOCORTICOID COMPARISON CHART

Drug	Relative Potency*	Relative Sodium-Retaining Potency	Systemic Bioavailability (%)	Duration of Biologic Activity (Hours)	Dosage per Inhalation (μg)	Plasma Elimination Half-Life (Hours)	Equivalent Dose (mg)
Systemic							
Hydrocortisone	1	1		8–12		1.5–2.0	20
Prednisone	4	0.8		12–36		2.5–3.5	5
Prednisolone	4	0.8		12–36		2.5–3.6	5
Methylprednisolone	5	0.5		12–36		3.3	4
Triamcinolone	5	0		12–36		2.5–3.3	4
Betamethasone	25	0		36–54		5–7	0.75
Dexamethasone	25	0		36–54		3.4–4.0	0.75
Aerosol							
Beclomethasone-17,21-dipropionate (Forte)	0.3–0.5		5		42 / 250†	15	
Budesonide	1.0		10		50	2.0–2.8	
Flunisolide	0.05		20		250	1.6	
Triamcinolone-16,17-acetonide	0.2		Unknown		100	0.5–1.0	

*Anti-inflammatory for systemic drugs, topical for aerosols.   †Forte formulation not available in the United States.

logs with greater and more selective glucocorticoid activity. The various chemical alterations also affect the pharmacokinetics of the compounds. Table 81–2 is a comparison of the pharmacokinetics and pharmacodynamics of the glucocorticoids frequently used in asthma therapy.

The addition of a 1,2 double bond to hydrocortisone produces prednisolone, which has a fourfold greater glucocorticoid activity.[49] All of the synthetic glucocorticoids have this addition. The addition of halogen substituents (chlorine or fluorine) on the 6α, the 9α, or both positions further enhances systemic glucocorticoid activity and prolongs the biologic activity (e.g., dexamethasone).[49] Alteration of the $16\alpha,17\alpha$–acetyl positions by acetonide (flunisolide or triamcinolone acetonide) or esterification (beclomethasone-17,21-dipropionate) is required for specifically enhancing topical activity.[47] Local activity is enhanced by increased penetration of the ester into cells and rapid conversion to relatively inactive compounds by lung esterases or liver metabolism. For example, beclomethasone dipropionate is rapidly converted to beclomethasone upon absorption from the lung; this conversion decreases the potency of the compound by five hundredfold.

Glucocorticoids may be administered parenterally, orally, or topically by inhalation. The most appropriate route depends on the clinical status of the patient. Systemic glucocorticoid administration is most appropriate for the treatment of acute asthmatic symptoms; aerosol administration, for chronic prophylaxis. Agents with selective glucocorticoid activity and a short to intermediate duration of action, such as methylprednisolone or prednisone, are preferred for systemic administration.[50] Agents with increased topical activity (i.e., beclomethasone dipropionate, triamcinolone acetonide, flunisolide, and budesonide) should be the only agents administered by aerosolization.[50] The potent systemic agents, such as methylprednisolone and dexamethasone, produce an antiasthmatic effect when administered by aerosolization, but because of their excellent absorption, they are no more bronchoselective than when they are administered systemically.[47]

GLUCOCORTICOIDS FOR ACUTE ASTHMA

The use of glucocorticoids for the therapy of acute exacerbations of asthma has been controversial. Studies have yielded conflicting results and have been critically reviewed.[51, 52] Kattan and co-workers[53] found no benefit to intravenous hydrocortisone in 10 children hospitalized for acute asthma in comparison with 9 controls in a nonblinded study. However, two double-blind, placebo-controlled trials demonstrated an increased rate and an increased extent of recovery of pulmonary functions and decrease in relapse rates for methylprednisolone therapy of acute, severe asthma in children.[45, 46] It is difficult to compare studies because of differences in study design and baseline drug therapies for the population of patients.[45, 46, 53] In addition, a number of patients with status asthmaticus who do not receive corticosteroids respond as well to other therapies (e.g., aminophylline and beta₂-agonists) as do patients who receive corticosteroids.[44] The difference is a more uniform response rate in the patients receiving corticosteroids. Therefore, it is not surprising that in studies of a small number of patients an effect of corticosteroids in acute asthma may not be detected.

Storr and collaborators[54] evaluated the effect of a single oral dose of prednisolone in 140 children admitted to the hospital for acute asthma in a double-blind, placebo-controlled study. One third of the patients receiving prednisolone were discharged within 5 h, in comparison with only two of the patients receiving placebo. In the remaining patients, those who received prednisolone experienced more rapid resolution of symptoms and shorter durations of hospitalization than did those receiving placebo. In a study in adult asthmatic patients, investigators reported a significantly lower hospitalization rate among patients receiving a single intravenous dose of methyl-prednisolone in the emergency room than among those receiving placebo.[55]

Harris and associates[56] provided a further evaluation of the ability of a short course of oral prednisone to prevent the progression of asthma requiring emergency care in young asthmatic patients. They found that patients who started a week-long course of oral prednisone at the beginning of an asthma attack that was not fully responsive to a nebulized beta-agonist required significantly less emergency intervention over a two-week period. As in the study by Fanta and associates,[44] a number of placebo-treated patients recovered at the same rate and extent as those who received glucocorticoids. There were no clinically distinguishing features in either study that could be used to predict which subjects in the placebo groups would respond or not respond. Brunette and colleagues[57] extended these findings by administering a short course of oral prednisone (1 mg/kg/day) to asthmatic children at the first sign of an infection of the upper respiratory tract. During the first year of the study, these children and a group of controls experienced acute asthma exacerbations in association with viral respiratory infections. During the second year, the patients who received treatment had significantly fewer episodes of wheezing, acute exacerbations, emergency room visits, and hospitalizations.

The precise dosage of glucocorticoids for acute exacerbations of asthma has not been established. Studies have generally failed to show an added benefit to administering very high doses of corticosteroids in status asthmaticus.[51, 58-60] There is no evidence for clinical superiority of one glucocorticoid over any other.[41, 50] The moderately potent, intermediate-duration agents such as prednisolone and methylprednisolone may be preferable because they produce less sodium retention than does hydrocortisone and less adrenal suppression than does dexamethasone at the same degree of glucocorticoid activity.[49] Parenteral administration is unnecessary but may be required in children who vomit in association with the asthma attack.[60, 61]

Airway obstruction may reverse within a few days;[58] however, full restoration of normal pulmonary functions generally takes several days to 2 weeks. Patients may exhibit an increased bronchial hyperreactivity for 2 to 4 weeks after an episode of status asthmaticus. It is usually recommended that patients be given prednisone (1 to 2 mg/kg/day) for 7 to 10 days after resolution of an episode of status asthmaticus. Tapering the dosage over a longer schedule of 7 weeks does not significantly decrease the rate of re-exacerbation or readmission in comparison with tapering over 1 week, but it has produced an increased number of adverse effects.[62] The relapse rate can be as high as 50% in the 12 weeks after a severe episode; therefore, these patients require close follow-up after discharge from the hospital.

GLUCOCORTICOIDS FOR CHRONIC ASTHMA

Patients who require frequent bursts of steroids for control of asthma symptoms or who are not able to discon-

tinue corticosteroids without inciting an acute exacerbation should receive chronic corticosteroids, if other asthma medications are optimal. Inhaled topical glucocorticoids are the preferred agents for prophylaxis of chronic asthma. The inhaled glucocorticoids can produce the same improvement in most patients with asthma with significantly fewer long-term side effects than can systemic corticosteroids and may produce greater reduction in bronchial hyperreactivity.[40, 50] The exceptions are patients unable to take aerosol corticosteroids with the aid of a spacer device (e.g., infants and young children), patients with allergic bronchopulmonary aspergillosis, and children who are noncompliant with a regimen involving the use of inhalers. If alternate-day steroids are used, agents with a short duration of activity, such as prednisone or prednisolone, are preferred.

Although there are some differences between the preparations of inhaled steroids, there is no convincing evidence that the properties of any agent, including duration of action (i.e., dosing interval), are clinically superior to those of any other. Most authors recommend that patients receive a short burst (5 to 7 days) of systemic steroids at the beginning of treatment with inhaled steroids.[3, 50]

In patients attempting to withdraw from systemic corticosteroid therapy and replace it with inhaled steroids, severe asthma relapse and sudden death are significant risks.[63, 64] Frequent follow-up, preferably in association with home peak flow monitoring, for a prolonged time (up to 1 year) is required after discontinuation of systemic glucocorticoids.[50] Severe asthma relapse has been reported to occur as late as 4 to 8 months after withdrawal of systemic glucocorticoids.[63, 64] Unfortunately, tests of the hypothalamus-pituitary-adrenal (HPA) axis function are not predictive of sudden death or asthma relapse in these patients.[50] There is some controversy concerning the optimal dosing schedule for inhaled steroids.[65-68] Many studies have demonstrated an equivalent antiasthmatic effect with twice-a-day and four-times-a-day dosing when the drugs are administered in the same daily dose in patients with stable asthma.[65-67] However, Toogood and co-authors[68] reported an improved antiasthmatic effect and decreased systemic effects by increasing the frequency and not increasing the daily dosage. It currently seems reasonable to attempt to control the patients on twice-a-day or three-times-a-day administration in order to improve convenience and compliance. If, however, a patient becomes unstable on this regimen, it may be more prudent to increase the frequency of administration, as opposed to the daily dosage.

The use of a spacer device improves the clinical efficacy and decreases local side effects of inhaled corticosteroids, presumably by improving the amount of drug deposition to the lungs.[69, 70] The use of an inhaled beta$_2$-agonist before the inhaled steroid may produce an improved response.[71]

CLINICAL PROBLEMS WITH GLUCOCORTICOIDS

The adverse effects from chronic glucocorticoid use include HPA axis suppression, growth retardation in children, Cushing's syndrome (buffalo hump, moon facies, striae atrophicae, acne, hirsutism, peripheral muscle wasting, and central obesity), fluid retention, hypertension, hypokalemia, osteoporosis, avascular necrosis of bone, hyperglycemia, myopathy, behavioral disturbances, increased risk of infections, and posterior subcapsular cataracts.[3, 49, 72] The development of these problems is both dose and duration dependent. Every effort should be made to maintain patients on the lowest systemic dose possible. Inhaled steroids, alternate-day prednisone, daily single-morning-dose prednisone, and daily multiple-dose prednisone produce respectively increasing risks of toxicity. However, regardless of the route or method of administration, increasing dosages increase the risk of significant side effects.

It is generally assumed that short bursts of high-dose corticosteroids are not harmful.[3, 50, 51] Results of dose comparison studies seem to confirm this opinion.[51, 58, 59] Although they generally do not produce acute adverse effects, high doses of hydrocortisone may aggravate preexisting heart failure or hypertension. Short bursts of prednisone have been associated with facial flushing. Excessive doses (1 to 2 g of methylprednisolone) may produce cardiac arrhythmias and sudden death through electrolyte shifts.[50] Very high doses of methylprednisolone (4 mg/kg every 6 h) resulted in tetraplegia in a 10-year-old girl being treated for acute asthma.[73] Generalized myopathy has been associated with hydrocortisone doses exceeding 1.0 g/day.[50] Effects on the central nervous system are more common with doses of prednisone higher than 2 mg/kg/day.[50]

In general, therapy for more than 5 days at doses that exceed usual physiologic cortisone production causes some aberration in endogenous cortisol production. A study in asthmatic children showed a blunted responsiveness of the HPA axis 3 days, but not 10 days, after completion of a 5-day course of 2 mg/kg/day of prednisone.[74] In another study of children receiving prednisone at doses of 40 mg/sq m to 100 mg/sq m daily for 5 to 30 days, it took 1 to 7 days or more to completely recover from HPA axis suppression;[75] there was no correlation between dose or duration of therapy and the time required for recovery. Shapiro and colleagues[46] found no difference in the cosyntropin responsiveness between placebo and 32 mg of methylprednisolone tapered down over 8 days in asthmatic outpatients treated for an acute exacerbation of asthma.

The number of short bursts of systemic steroids that constitutes chronic steroid use is not precisely known. At least eight short courses (10 days or less) of steroids per year produced decreases in trabecular bone density and increases in the risk of fracture that were similar to those increases and decreases produced by chronic daily or alternate-day steroid therapy over 1 year.[76] However, Dolan and co-workers[77] investigated the effect of multiple bursts (less than 7 days) of high-dose prednisone (1 to 2 mg/kg/day) for acute exacerbations on the HPA axis in 23 children with chronic asthma. Each child was studied at least 16 days after the last burst. Only patients who had received four or more bursts in the previous year demonstrated a subnormal response of the HPA axis to hypoglycemic stress or ACTH.

In patients requiring chronic systemic steroids, converting the regimen to a single morning dose every other day that is equivalent to the total dose for both days of a relatively short-acting glucocorticoid (such as prednisone) reverses the HPA axis suppression and produces less risk of infection and fewer Cushingoid changes.[3, 50] Long-acting glucocorticoids, such as dexamethasone, are not appropriate for alternate-day therapy. Even with alternate-day steroid therapy, the adverse effects are dose related, and some effects such as osteopenia and posterior-subcapsular cataracts may not be preventable.[50] In addition, patients with a high daily dose requirement may not achieve adequate control on alternate-day therapy. Wyatt and collaborators[78] found no greater HPA axis suppression with 20 to 40 mg of prednisone administered every other day than with 400 to 800 μg/day of inhaled beclomethasone in asthmatic children. However, the patients receiving alternate-day steroids exhibited more weight gain and facial edema.

The toxicities of inhaled steroids have been reviewed.[79] If given in sufficient quantity, inhaled steroids provide enough systemic activity to produce most of the systemic toxicities previously discussed. In children, the equivalent of 400 μg/day of beclomethasone dipropionate produces some suppression of the HPA axis.[78, 79] However, results of a study on the use of the newer high-dose inhalers (250 μg/inhalation for beclomethasone dipropionate and 200 μg/inhalation for budesonide) suggested that children could receive doses up to 2000 μg/1.73 sq m/day without risk of adrenocortical suppression.[80] Inhaled steroids produce additive suppression with alternate-day steroids. Osteoporosis, growth suppression, cataracts, and psychological problems have all been associated with inhaled steroid use; however, weight gain, hypertension, and hyperglycemia have not.[79]

In addition to the usual toxicities, inhaled steroids present problems specific to the aerosol route of administration. These include irritation, cough, fungal infection (such as oral thrush), and dysphonia (hoarseness). Initial concerns about possible atrophy of bronchial mucosa similar to the skin atrophy seen with dermal application have been largely dispelled by results of long-term follow-up studies in asthmatic patients. Epithelial damage has not been noted in bronchoscopic biopsy specimens of the bronchial mucosa after 10 years of beclomethasone dipropionate therapy.[81, 82]

Throat cultures positive for *Candida* species are much more common than for clinical thrush, which is reported to occur in 4.5 to 13% of cases.[79] Esophagitis secondary to *Candida* infection has been reported more rarely.[50] The incidence of clinical thrush is directly related to the dose and dosing frequency.[50] Switching to a twice-a-day dose can decrease the incidence of thrush.[83] Routine mouth washing after inhalation can remove as much as 98% of the steroid deposited in the mouth and may be useful in decreasing the incidence of oral thrush but appears to have no effect on HPA axis suppression.[79, 84] The use of a spacer device also significantly decreases the incidence of fungal infection.[69] If necessary, it can be controlled by oral nystatin and rarely necessitates withdrawal of the steroid. Coughing and wheezing are usually caused by irritation in patients with unstable asthma and can be largely avoided by administration of an inhaled bronchodilator before administration of the steroid. Dysphonia occurs in 5% to 50% of patients and is unrelated to the often coexisting candidiasis.[79] Dysphonia is associated with deformity of the bilateral adductor vocal cord and probably represents a localized myopathy.[85] Voice rest and a temporary decrease in drug dosage alleviate the dysphonia.

If a clinician is concerned with HPA axis suppression in a child who has received frequent bursts, high alternate-day doses, or inhaled steroid doses, the corticotropin stimulation tests probably provide the safest and most accurate assessment.

The corticotropin test is performed in the following manner. Cosyntropin (Cortrosyn) is dissolved in sterile saline and injected intramuscularly after a baseline, early morning fasting cortisol level is obtained. Patients must not take any steroid before this baseline level is established on the day of the test; 0.25 mg is the dose for children over the age of 2 years, and 0.125 mg is the dose for children under 2 years of age. A postinjection cortisol level is assessed after 30 min. The basal plasma cortisol value should exceed 5 μg/100 ml, and the 30 min level should be increased at least 7 μg/100 ml over the basal level. Alternatively, a level may be drawn 45 to 60 min after injection, in which case the plasma cortisol should be approximately double the baseline value.

Some asthmatic patients appear to be resistant to the effects of corticosteroids.[86] The resistance is not a result of altered pharmacokinetics of the corticosteroids in these patients.[50, 87] Steroid resistance in asthma is as yet unexplained and appears to fluctuate in degree over time. It may reflect differing pathogenesis of asthma or a change in the number of glucocorticoid receptors or in their drug-binding affinity.[50] More investigations are needed in order to explain steroid-resistant asthma.

The administration of a number of drugs may interfere with or enhance the effects of glucocorticoids in asthma. Rifampin, phenobarbital, phenytoin, primidone, and ephedrine increase glucocorticoid metabolism.[47] Therefore, patients taking these enzyme inducers may require an increased dosage of glucocorticoid. The macrolide antibiotics erythromycin[88] and troleandomycin[89] inhibit methylprednisolone metabolism by cytochrome P-450 metabolic enzymes. Troleandomycin has been used in conjunction with methylprednisolone as a steroid-sparing agent, but there is little evidence that it does anything other than decrease methylprednisolone clearance.[50] In addition, it has potential for liver toxicity. Thus there seems to be little reason to use troleandomycin to enhance methylprednisolone.

REFERENCES

1. Munck A, Holbrook N: Glucocorticoid-receptor complexes in rat thymus cells. J Biol Chem 259:820–831, 1984.
2. Lan N, Karin M, Nguyen T, et al: Mechanisms of glucocorticoid hormone action. J Steroid Biochem 20:77–88, 1984.
3. Morris HG: Mechanisms of action and therapeutic role of corticosteroids in asthma. J Allergy Clin Immunol 75:1–13, 1985.
4. Ballard PL: Delivery and transport of glucocorticoids to target cells. Monogr Endocrinol 12:25–48, 1979.
5. Parker CW, Huber MG, Baumann ML: Alterations in cyclic AMP metabolism in human bronchial asthma: III. Leukocyte and lymphocyte responses to steroids. J Clin Invest 52:1342–1348, 1973.
6. Davies AO, Lefkowitz RJ: Agonist-promoted high affinity state of the beta-adrenergic receptor in human neutrophils: Modulation by corticosteroids. J Clin Endocrinol Metab 53:703–708, 1981.
7. Davies AO, Lefkowitz RJ: Corticosteroid-induced differential regulation of beta-adrenergic receptors in circulating human polymorphonuclear leukocytes and mononuclear leukocytes. J Clin Endocrinol Metab 51:599–605, 1980.
8. Shenfield GM, Hodson ME, Clarke SW, Paterson JW: Interaction of corticosteroids and catecholamines in the treatment of asthma. Thorax 30:430–435, 1975.
9. Ellul-Micallef R, Fenech FF: Effect of intravenous prednisolone in asthmatics with diminished adrenergic responsiveness. Lancet 2:1269–1271, 1975.
10. Johnson LK, Longenecker JP, Baxter JD, et al: Glucocorticoid action: A mechanism involving nuclear and nonnuclear pathways. Br J Dermatol 107(Suppl 23):6–23, 1982.
11. Cupps TR, Fauci AS: Corticosteroid-mediated immunoregulation in man. Immunol Rev 65:133–155, 1982.
12. Claman HN: Corticosteroids and lymphoid cells. N Engl J Med 287:388–397, 1972.
13. Claman HN: Glucocorticosteroids I: Anti-inflammatory mechanisms. Hosp Pract 18:123–134, 1983.
14. Boggs DR, Athens JW, Cartwright GE, Wintrobe MM: The effect of adrenal glucocorticosteroids upon the cellular composition of inflammatory exudates. Am J Pathol 44:763–773, 1964.
15. Axelrod L: Inhibition of prostacyclin production mediates permissive effect of glucocorticoids on vascular tone. Lancet 1:904–906, 1983.
16. Gillis S, Crabtree GR, Smith KA: Glucocorticoid-induced inhibition of T cell growth factor production: II. The effect on the in vitro generation of cytolytic T cells. J Immunol 123:1632–1638, 1979.
17. Lewis RA, Austen KF: The biologically active leukotrienes. J Clin Invest 73:889–897, 1984.
18. Samuelsson B: Leukotrienes: Mediators of immediate hypersensitivity reactions and inflammation. Science 220:568–575, 1983.
19. Blackwell GJ, Carnuccio R, DiRosa M, et al: Suppression of arachidonate oxidation by glucocorticoid-induced antiphospholipase peptides. Adv Prostaglandin Thromboxane Leukotriene Res 11:65–71, 1983.
20. Hirata F: Lipomodulin: A possible mediator of the action of glucocorticoids. Adv Prostaglandin Thromboxane Leukotriene Res 11:73–78, 1983.
21. Ghiara P, Meli R, Parente L, et al: Distinct inhibition of membrane-bound and lysosomal phospholipase A_2 by glucocorticoid-induced proteins. Biochem Pharmacol 33:1445–1450, 1984.
22. Hirata F, del Carmine R, Nelson CA, et al: Presence of auto-antibody for phospholipase inhibitory protein, lipomodulin in patients with rheumatic diseases. Proc Natl Acad Sci USA 78:3190–3194, 1981.
23. Schleimer RP, Schulman ES, MacGlashan DW, et al: Effects of dexamethasone on mediator release from human lung fragments and purified human lung mast cells. J Clin Invest 71:1830–1835, 1983.
24. Munck A, Mendel DB, Smith LI, Orti E: Glucocorticoid receptors and actions. Am Rev Respir Dis 141 (Suppl): S2–S10, 1990.
25. Schleimer RP, MacGlashan DW, Gillespie E, Lichtenstein L: Inhibition of basophil histamine release by anti-inflammatory steroids. J Immunol 129:1632–1636, 1982.
26. Peters SP, Kagey-Sobotka A, MacGlashan DW, et al: The modulation of human basophil histamine release by products of the 5-lipoxygenase pathway. J Immunol 129:797–803, 1982.
27. Daeron M, Sterk AR, Hirata F, Ishizaka T: Biochemical analysis of glucocorticoid induced inhibition of IgE-mediated histamine release from mouse mast cells. J Immunol 129:1212–1218, 1982.
28. Dolovich J, Hargreave F: The asthma syndrome: Inciters, inducers, and host characteristics. Thorax 36:641–644, 1981.
29. Cockcroft DW, Ruffin RE, Dolovich J, Hargreave FE: Allergen-induced increase in non-allergic bronchial reactivity. Clin Allergy 7:503–513, 1977.
30. de Monchy JG, Kauffman HF, Venge P, et al: Bronchoalveolar eosinophilia during allergen-induced late asthmatic reactions. Am Rev Respir Dis 131:373–376, 1985.
31. Booij-Noord H, de Vries K, Sluiter HJ, et al: Late bronchial obstruc-

tive reaction to experimental inhalation of house dust extract. Clin Allergy 2:43–61, 1972.

32. Burge PS: The effects of corticosteroids on the immediate asthmatic reaction. Eur J Respir Dis (Suppl) 122:163–166, 1982.

33. Cockcroft DW, Murdock KY: Comparative effects of inhaled salbutamol, sodium cromoglycate, and beclomethasone dipropionate on allergen-induced early asthmatic responses, late asthmatic responses, and increased bronchial responsiveness to histamine. J Allergy Clin Immunol 79:734–740, 1987.

34. Kraan J, Kroeter GH, van der Mark TW, et al: Dosage and time effects of inhaled budesonide on bronchial hyperreactivity. Am Rev Respir Dis 137:44–48, 1988.

35. Askenase PW: Role of basophils, mast cells, and vasoamines in hypersensitivity reactions with a delayed time course. Prog Allergy 23:199–320, 1977.

36. Kerrebijn KF, van Essen-Zandvliet EEM, Neijens HJ: Effect of long-term treatment with inhaled corticosteroids and beta-agonists on the bronchial responsiveness in children with asthma. J Allergy Clin Immunol 79:653–659, 1987.

37. Dutoit JI, Salome CM, Woolcock AJ: Inhaled corticosteroids reduce the severity of bronchial hyperresponsiveness in asthma but oral theophylline does not. Am Rev Respir Dis 136:1174–1178, 1987.

38. Juniper EF, Frith PA, Hargreave FE: Long-term stability of bronchial responsiveness to histamine. Thorax 37:288–291, 1982.

39. Sotomayor H, Badier M, Vervloet D, Orehek J: Seasonal increase of carbachol airway responsiveness in patients allergic to grass pollen: Reversal by corticosteroids. Am Rev Respir Dis 130:56–58, 1984.

40. Jenkins CR, Woolcock AJ: Effect of prednisone and beclomethasone dipropionate on airway responsiveness in asthma: A comparative study. Thorax 43:378–384, 1988.

41. Pierson WE, Bierman CW, Kelley VC: A double-blind trial of corticosteroid therapy in status asthmaticus. Pediatrics 54:282–288, 1974.

42. Ellul-Micallef R, Borthwick RC, McHardy GJ: The effect of oral prednisolone on gas exchange in chronic bronchial asthma. Br J Clin Pharmacol 9:479–482, 1980.

43. Winfield CR, McAllister WAC, Collins JV: Changes in effective pulmonary blood flow with prednisolone. Thorax 35:238, 1980.

44. Fanta CH, Rossing TH, McFadden ER: Glucocorticoids in acute asthma: A critical controlled trial. Am J Med 74:845–851, 1983.

45. Younger RE, Gerber PS, Herrod HG, et al: Intravenous methylprednisolone efficacy in status asthmaticus of childhood. Pediatrics 80:225–230, 1987.

46. Shapiro GG, Furukawa CT, Pierson WE, et al: Double-blind evaluation of methylprednisolone versus placebo for acute asthma episodes. Pediatrics 71:510–514, 1983.

47. Ellul-Micallef R: Pharmacokinetics and pharmacodynamics of glucocorticosteroids. In Jenne JW, Murphy S (eds): Drug Therapy for Asthma: Research and Clinical Practice, pp. 463–516. New York: Marcel Dekker, 1987.

48. Hui KKP, Conolly ME, Tashkin DP: Reversal of human lymphocyte beta adrenoceptor desensitization by glucocorticoids. Clin Pharmacol Ther 32:566–571, 1982.

49. Haynes RC, Murad F: Adrenocorticotropic hormone: Adrenocortical steroids and their synthetic analogs; inhibitors of adrenocortical steroid biosynthesis. In Gilman AG, Goodman LS, Rall TW, Murad F (eds): The Pharmacological Basis of Therapeutics, 7th ed, pp. 1459–1489, New York: Macmillan, 1985.

50. Toogood JH: Corticosteroids. In Jenne JW, Murphy S (eds): Drug Therapy for Asthma: Research and Clinical Practice, pp. 719–759. New York: Marcel Dekker, 1987.

51. Fiel SB: Should corticosteroids be used in the treatment of acute, severe asthma? I. A case for the use of corticosteroids in acute, severe asthma. Pharmacotherapy 5:327–331, 1985.

52. Mok J, Kattan M, Levison H: Should corticosteroids be used in the treatment of acute severe asthma? II. A case against the use of corticosteroids in acute, severe asthma. Pharmacotherapy 5:331–335, 1985.

53. Kattan M, Gurwitz D, Levison H: Corticosteroids in status asthmaticus. J Pediatr 96:596–599, 1980.

54. Storr J, Barry W, Barrell E, et al: Effect of a single oral dose of prednisolone in acute childhood asthma. Lancet 1:879–882, 1987.

55. Littenberg B, Gluck EH: A controlled trial of methylprednisolone in the emergency treatment of acute asthma. N Engl J Med 314:150–152, 1986.

56. Harris JB, Weinberger MM, Nassif E, et al: Early intervention with short courses of prednisone to prevent progression of asthma in ambulatory patients incompletely responsive to bronchodilators. J Pediatr 110:627–633, 1987.

57. Brunette MG, Lands L, Thibodeau LP: Childhood asthma: Prevention of attacks with short-term corticosteroid treatment of upper respiratory tract infection. Pediatrics 81:624–629, 1988.

58. Haskell RJ, Wong BM, Hansen JE: A double-blind, randomized clinical trial of methylprednisolone in status asthmaticus. Arch Intern Med 143:1324–1327, 1983.

59. Raimondi AC, Figueroa-Casas JC, Roncoroni AJ: Comparison between high and moderate doses of hydrocortisone in the treatment of status asthmaticus. Chest 89:832–835, 1986.

60. Ratto D, Alfaro C, Sipsey J, et al: Are intravenous corticosteroids required in status asthmaticus? JAMA 260:527–529, 1988.

61. Harrison BD, Stokes TC, Hart GJ, et al: Need for intravenous hydrocortisone in addition to oral prednisolone in patients admitted to hospital with severe asthma without ventilatory failure. Lancet 1:181–184, 1986.

62. Lederle FA, Pluhar RE, Joseph AM, Niewoehner DG: Tapering of corticosteroid therapy following exacerbation of asthma: A randomized, double-blind, placebo-controlled trial. Arch Intern Med 147:2201–2203, 1987.

63. Maunsell K, Pearson RSB, Livingstone JL: Long-term corticosteroid treatment of asthma. Br Med J 1:661–665, 1968.

64. Mellis CM, Phelan PD: Asthma deaths in children—A continuing problem. Thorax 32:29–34, 1977.

65. Nyholm E, Frame MH, Cayton RM: Therapeutic advantages of twice-daily over four times daily inhalation budesonide in the treatment of chronic asthma. Eur J Respir Dis 65:339–345, 1984.

66. Berglund E, Lofdahl CG, Svedmyr N: Dosing of inhaled corticosteroids and therapeutic goals in asthmatic patients. Eur J Respir Dis 65:319–320, 1984.

67. Meltzer EO, Kemp JP, Welch MJ, Orgel HA: Effect of dosing schedule on efficacy of beclomethasone dipropionate aerosol in chronic asthma. Am Rev Respir Dis 131:732–736, 1985.

68. Toogood JH, Baskerville JC, Jennings B, et al: Influence of dosing frequency and schedule on the response of chronic asthmatics to the aerosol steroid, budesonide. J Allergy Clin Immunol 70:288–298, 1982.

69. Toogood JH, Baskerville J, Jennings B, et al: Use of spacers to facilitate inhaled corticosteroid treatment of asthma. Am Rev Respir Dis 129:723–729, 1984.

70. Greenough A, Pool J, Gleeson JGA, Price JE: Effect of budesonide on pulmonary hyperinflation in young asthmatic children. Thorax 43:937–938, 1988.

71. Clark RA, Anderson PB: Combined therapy with salbutamol and beclomethasone inhalers in chronic asthma. Lancet 2:70–72, 1978.

72. Shapiro GG: Corticosteroids in the treatment of allergic disease: Principles and practice. Pediatr Clin North Am 30:955–971, 1983.

73. Kaplan PW, Rocha W, Sanders DB, et al: Acute steroid-induced tetraplegia following status asthmaticus. Pediatrics 78:121–123, 1986.

74. Zora JA, Zimmerman D, Carey TL, et al: Hypothalamic-pituitary-adrenal axis suppression after short-term, high-dose glucocorticoid therapy in children with asthma. J Allergy Clin Immunol 77:9–13, 1986.

75. Spiegel RJ, Oliff AI, Bruton J, et al: Adrenal suppression after short-term corticosteroid therapy. Lancet 1:630–633, 1979.

76. Adinoff AD, Hollister JR: Steroid-induced fractures and bone loss in patients with asthma. N Engl J Med 309:265–268, 1983.

77. Dolan LM, Kesarwala HH, Holroyde JC, Fischer TJ: Short-term, high-dose, systemic steroids in children with asthma: The effect on the hypothalamic-pituitary-adrenal axis. J Allergy Clin Immunol 80:81–87, 1987.

78. Wyatt R, Waschek J, Weinberger N, Sherman B: Effects of inhaled beclomethasone dipropionate and alternate-day prednisone on pituitary-adrenal function in children with chronic asthma. N Engl J Med 299:1387–1392, 1978.

79. König P: Inhaled corticosteroids—Their present and future role in the management of asthma. J Allergy Clin Immunol 82:297–306, 1988.

80. Prahl P, Jensen T, Bjerregaard-Andersen H: Adrenocortical func-

tion in children on high-dose steroid aerosol therapy. Allergy 42:541–544, 1987.

81. Thiringer G, Eriksson N, Malmberg R, et al: Bronchoscopic biopsies of bronchial mucosa before and after beclomethasone dipropionate therapy. Scand J Respir Dis (Suppl) 101:173–177, 1977.

82. Lundgren R, Söderberg M, Hörstedt P, Stenling R: Morphological studies of bronchial mucosal biopsies from asthmatics before and after ten years of treatment with inhaled steroids. Eur Respir J 1:883–889, 1988.

83. Toogood JH, Jennings B, Baskerville J, et al: Dosing regimen of budesonide and occurrence of oropharyngeal complications. Eur J Respir Dis 65:35–44, 1984.

84. Toogood JH, Jennings B, Greenway RW, Chuang L: Candidiasis and dysphonia complicating beclomethasone treatment of asthma. J Allergy Clin Immunol 65:145–153, 1980.

85. Williams AJ, Baghat MS, Stableforth DE, et al: Dysphonia caused by inhaled steroids: Recognition of a characteristic laryngeal abnormality. Thorax 38:813–821, 1983.

86. Carmichael J, Paterson IC, Diaz P, et al: Corticosteroid resistance in chronic asthma. Br Med J 282:1419–1422, 1981.

87. Mortimer O, Grettve L, Lindstrom B, et al: Bioavailability of prednisolone in asthmatic patients with a poor response to steroid treatment. Eur J Respir Dis 71:372–379, 1987.

88. LaForce CF, Szefler SJ, Miller MF, et al: Inhibition of methylprednisolone elimination in the presence of erythromycin therapy. J Allergy Clin Immunol 72:34–39, 1983.

89. Szefler SJ, Brenner M, Jusko WJ, et al: Dose- and time-related effect of troleandomycin on methylprednisolone elimination. Clin Pharmacol Ther 32:166–177, 1982.

82 THEOPHYLLINE USE IN PEDIATRIC PULMONARY DISEASE

ELLIOT F. ELLIS, M.D.

Theophylline was introduced in clinical medicine for the treatment of asthma in 1937.[1] The drug was widely used for 20 years after its introduction; however, with reports of adverse reactions, including death, there was a pronounced decline of theophylline prescribing, particularly for children. In the mid-1960s and the early 1970s, when the pharmacokinetics of the drug began to be elucidated, an increase in the use of theophylline occurred, and it became the most commonly prescribed drug for the treatment of asthma. This trend is now being reversed; doubts are being raised, even about its bronchodilator activity in certain clinical settings.

Theophylline is a methylated xanthine, closely related to naturally occurring caffeine and theobromine. Two theophylline derivatives, dihydroxypropyl theophylline (dyphylline) and enprophylline, merit some comment. Dyphylline has been promoted as being safer than theophylline because it is eliminated principally through the kidneys, and its disposition is unaffected by the multiple factors that influence the biotransformation of theophylline in the liver.[2] Unfortunately, dyphylline has substantially less bronchodilator activity than theophylline. Because of its water solubility, dyphylline is rapidly excreted from the body; it has an elimination half-life of approximately 2 h. Enprophylline (3-propylxanthine), in contrast, has excellent bronchodilator activity, surpassing that of theophylline, and is free of theophylline's potential to cause seizures.[3] Unfortunately, in clinical trials in Europe and the United States, enprophylline caused headaches in an unacceptably high percentage of subjects and is currently not marketed in the United States.

MECHANISM OF ACTION

Xanthines are known to relax airway and other smooth muscles; however, the degree of relaxation of airway smooth muscle is less than that achieved with inhaled adrenergic agents in acute bronchoconstriction. Studies suggest that the bronchodilator, antiallergic, and anti-inflammatory effects of xanthines occur through multiple molecular mechanisms of action.[4] Theophylline has a variety of effects, including antagonism of prostaglandins, effects on intracellular calcium flux, and the property of causing increased binding of 3',5'–cyclic adenosine monophosphate (cAMP) to 3',5'-cAMP–binding protein.[5] Antagonism of adenosine receptors explains theophylline's potential to cause seizures but not its bronchodilator activity because enprophylline, which does not bind to adenosine receptors, is a good bronchodilator.

Evidence both from animal studies and in humans has suggested that in addition to its bronchodilator properties, theophylline also possesses some anti-inflammatory activity.[6–8] In studies that provide evidence for anti-inflammatory action of theophylline, investigators have reported attenuation of response to nonspecific agents used in airway challenge studies in asthma such as methacholine, carbachol, histamine, and hypotonic saline. Theophylline also causes a serum concentration–dependent protection against exercise challenge in asthmatic patients. Response to exercise and airway reactivity are closely linked. Alternatively, other authors have, in similar studies, not found any evidence of an anti-inflammatory effect of theophylline as reflected in decreased bronchial responses to the same agents and in prevention of an allergen-induced increase in airway reactivity.[9, 10]

PHARMACOKINETICS

ABSORPTION

Rapid-Release Formulations. Theophylline is rapidly absorbed from orally and rectally administered formulations and from orally administered uncoated tablets or liquid preparations.[11] The speed of absorption, but not the extent of absorption, is affected to a clinically insignificant degree by concurrent ingestion of food or antacid. For intravenous use, aminophylline continues to be the preferred product. The dose administered needs to be corrected for the fact that aminophylline is 80% to 85% theophylline. A marketed intravenous preparation of theophylline adds nothing but cost when used as an alternative to aminophylline.

Slow-Release Formulations. Slow-release theophylline formulations are indicated for patients in whom elimination half-lives are less than 6 h and for enhancing compliance because less frequent dosing is required. Various products differ in terms of bioavailability.[12] The ideal product releases the drug at a constant rate over the dosing interval. Slow-release formulations vary in the rate of the drug released (from slow to slower to ultraslow). With the ultraslow products, the rate of drug release is typically so slow that the drug may be out of the gut before it is completely absorbed; the studies with these drugs generally have shown relatively incomplete bioavailability. There is a diurnal variation in theophylline absorption, which results in higher morning trough concentrations. It has been surmised that host factors, in addition to the drug itself, are responsible for some of the erratic absorption patterns. To minimize fluctuation in serum concentration over a dosing interval, the patient's theophylline elimination characteristics (slow or fast) should ideally be matched to the product's release characteristics (slow, slower, or ultraslow). Most children over the age of 6 to 8 years can be successfully treated with 12-h dosing intervals with some slow-release preparations (e.g., Slo-bid Gyrocaps or Theo-Dur Tablets). Patients with exceptionally rapid theophylline clearance require 8-h dosing intervals to prevent serum concentration fluctuation greater than 100%.

Food taken concurrently with theophylline has an important effect on the rate of drug release with some products and minimal or no effect with others. Once-a-day products are more vulnerable to variations in intestinal pH and mobility. The best example of the food effect on slow-release theophylline absorption has been reported with Theo-24; when given with a high-fat-content meal (50% carbohydrate, 20% protein, and 30% fat), about half of the dose of Theo-24 is absorbed in a 4-h period (usually beginning 6 to 8 h after ingestion), and peak concentrations average two to three times higher than those observed when this drug was given during fasting.[13] This phenomenon of "dose dumping" (defined as more than 50% of the total dose being absorbed in less than 2 h) is a particular hazard with once-a-day products, in which the total dose is given at one time. Antacids may affect the rate of drug absorption from products with pH-dependent dissolution in contrast to absorption of formulations whose dissolution is not pH-dependent (e.g., Slo-bid Gyrocaps, Theo-Dur Tablets).

DISTRIBUTION

The pharmocokinetics of theophylline can be characterized by the use of a linear, two-compartment open model, because the multicompartment characteristics of theophylline are not very pronounced. After intravenous administration, theophylline distributes rapidly from the plasma to its site of action in the tissues; this distributive phase is virtually complete within 30 min. The volume of distribution averages about 0.45 l/kg in children and adults (within reasonable parameters of ideal body weight). Theophylline also passes through the placenta and into breast milk. Theophylline crosses the blood-brain barrier, and concentrations in the central nervous system in children are about 50% of the serum concentration (90% in premature infants). Salivary concentrations are approximately 60% of serum levels.

METABOLISM

Theophylline is eliminated from the body principally by biotransformation in the liver to inactive (with the exception of 3-methylxanthine) metabolites. The enzymes responsible for the metabolism of theophylline (and many other drugs) belong to the cytochrome P-450 family of oxidases located in the smooth endoplastic reticulum of the liver. Theophylline metabolism is age-dependent. In infants, drug biotransformation is slow as a result of immaturity of hepatic microsomal enzymes[14] and slowly increases during the first year of life. By 8 to 12 months of age, clearance rates approach those seen in early childhood. From 1 to 9 years of age, the rate of theophylline metabolism accelerates.[15] There is a gradual decline in the rate of theophylline biotransformation during the adolescent and early adult years. At about 16 years of age, the metabolic rate approximates that seen in young adults. After 1 year of age, approximately 10% of the drug is excreted unchanged in the urine. In premature infants and normal newborns during the first month of life, 45% to 50% of an administered dose of theophylline is cleared by the kidney unaltered. At all ages, a small amount (approximately 6%) of theophylline is N-methylated to caffeine. This minor conversion becomes clinically relevant only in premature infants, in whom caffeine has an extremely long half-life (mean, 96 h), which results in its accumulation and pharmacologic effect.[16]

Because liver microsomal enzyme activity is not only dependent on age but also subject to the inducing and inhibiting action of a large variety of unrelated environmental conditions and disease factors, it is not surprising that there is an individual variation over time in the rate of metabolism of theophylline and resultant serum concentration. Individual variations in theophylline metabolism, however, are small unless there are changes in disease factors (e.g., fluctuating cardiac function) or changes in concurrent drug therapy.[17] Other factors affecting theophylline clearance include cigarette smoking, marijuana smoking, and diet.[18] There is a dose-related increase in theophylline clearance; heavy smokers metabolize theophylline twice as fast as nonsmokers. Smokers of marijuana also have accelerated theophylline metabolism. Ingestion of a high-protein, low-carbohydrate diet accelerates theophylline metabolism, presumably by increasing liver enzyme activity. Dietary intake of methylxanthines, caffeine in particular, affects theophylline metabolism by acting as a competitive substrate for theophylline-metabolizing enzymes. The ingestion of charcoal-broiled meat, presumably because of a stimulating effect on liver enzyme function of polycyclic hydrocarbons produced during the charcoaling process, has been reported to increase metabolism of theophylline. This is seldom a clinically significant problem.

Although the data are conflicting, the effect of obesity on theophylline clearance appears to be negligible. Because theophylline distributes poorly into fat, dosage should be based on ideal body weight.

Theophylline metabolism is affected by various disease states including hepatic disease, cardiac disease, and viral illnesses.[19] Hepatic dysfunction is a major cause of altered theophylline biotransformation. Patients with decompensated cirrhosis, acute hepatitis, and possibly cholestasis have reduced theophylline clearance. A correlation between slow hepatic metabolism and serum albumin and bilirubin concentration has been made in patients with cirrhosis. Cardiac disease, presumably causing decreased liver microsomal enzyme function by passive congestion of the liver secondary to congestive heart failure, may have a profound effect on theophylline metabolism. When heart failure is treated, theophylline clearance increases. Acute viral illnesses associated with fever have been reported to prolong theophylline half-life.[20] Symptoms of nausea, vomiting, and headache are commonly observed in children during many viral infections; however, when these symptoms develop in a child receiving theophylline, the physician must consider the possibility of theophylline intoxication. If fever is high and sustained (e.g., higher than 102°F for more than 24 h), the dosage should be reduced in a patient whose theophylline serum concentration was previously maintained within the therapeutic range.

Drug interactions are another factor in altering theophylline elimination.[19] The most important drug interaction is the effect of cimetidine in decreasing theophylline clearance. The macrolide group of antibiotics may also have a similar effect on theophylline biotransformation. The degree of effect differs among agents in this class of drugs. Troleandomycin has the most profound effect, followed by erythromycin estolate. Phenytoin and rifampin, drugs known for their P-450 enzyme-inducing properties, appear to acclerate theophylline metabolism. The effect of phenobarbital is variable; some studies have shown no effect, and others have revealed a stimulatory effect on theophylline metabolism, especially when phenobarbital,

Table 82-1. THEOPHYLLINE CLEARANCE

Factors	Decreased	Increased
Age	Premature infants; neonates and up to 6 months	Ages 1–16 years
Diet	Dietary methylxanthines High carbohydrate	Low carbohydrate High protein Charcoal-broiled meats
Habits		Cigarette smoking (tobacco or marijuana)
Drugs	Troleandomycin Erythromycin salts Quinolone antibiotics Oral contraceptives	Phenytoin Phenobarbital Carbamazepine Isoproterenol (intravenous) Rifampin
Disease	Liver disease, congestive heart failure, acute pulmonary edema, chronic obstructive pulmonary disease, sustained fever with viral illness	

in doses producing therapeutic serum concentrations, is given for 4 weeks or longer (Table 82-1).

THERAPEUTIC DRUG MONITORING

The rationale for therapeutic monitoring of theophylline serum concentration is that it is a major determinant of both efficacy and toxicity.[21] Theophylline has a narrow therapeutic index. Serum concentration may be affected by many factors that affect liver microsomal enzyme function and alter elimination kinetics.

During the treatment of an acute exacerbation of asthma, a serum theophylline level should be drawn before administration of an intravenous loading dose of aminophylline if the patient has been receiving theophylline. In this circumstance, the initial bolus may need to be reduced by 25% to 50%, depending on the result. For a patient who is admitted to the hospital and receives a constant infusion of theophylline after the bolus, it is important to obtain a 1-h level and adjust the serum concentration to the therapeutic range. Thereafter, serum theophylline levels should be monitored every 12 to 24 h.

The indications for monitoring theophylline serum concentrations and management of chronic asthma are subject to some controversy. Some authors believe that all patients with chronic asthma should be monitored at regular intervals during the initial phase of theophylline adjustment. These intervals vary, and it is assumed that theophylline clearance is stable. Other clinicians reserve monitoring for patients who do not obtain optimal symptom control after an appropriate dose is given and for patients in whom adverse effects develop. In the event of symptoms associated with theophylline toxicity, immediate determination of serum theophylline concentration is mandatory.

To properly interpret serum theophylline concentration in clinical situations, a significant amount of information must be provided with a sample, such as characteristics of the patient (age, weight), formulation of the drug (rapid release or slow release), dosage, duration of therapy (to ensure steady state for maintenance-dose adjustment), dosing interval, exact timing of previous dose, exact timing of blood collection, concurrent drug therapy, and presence of fever or other disease states such as congestive heart failure or liver dysfunction. With a rapid-release theophylline product (liquid or tablet), a sample obtained 2 h after the dose approximates the peak concentration. The determination of the trough concentration (the sample obtained immediately before the next dose) does not provide much additional information except to show the magnitude of the peak-trough difference. Because of a circadian effect on theophylline absorption, specimens should be drawn during the same dosing interval when more than one measurement is being compared. Various slow-release products differ in their release characteristics (e.g., Theo-Dur Tablets or Slo-bid Gyrocaps reach peak serum concentration approximately 3 to 7 h after the morning dose). Slow-release products that have pH-dependent dissolution characteristics (e.g., Theolair and Theo-24) release drugs at variable rates, depending on whether they are given during fasting or with a meal. Intersubject and intrasubject variability in absorption of slow-release products may be the reason for a theophylline serum level to be inconsistent or lower than the expected level for a particular dose. Another reason for inconsistent levels of theophylline is poor compliance by patients.

PHARMOCODYNAMICS

It is now recognized that there is a linear relationship between the logarithm of serum theophylline concentration and improvement in forced expiratory volume in 1 sec (FEV_1). This relationship was first shown in children by Maselli and colleagues,[22] who showed a strong correlation between the intensity of bronchodilator effect (improvement in FEV_1) and the logarithm of the amount of drug in the tissue compartment. It was evident from this study that the effect on pulmonary function was not seen until 30 min after the bolus injection of intravenous aminophylline; this lag represented the time for the drug to be distributed from the plasma to the site of action in the tissues. Because the bronchodilator effect increases and then falls rapidly after a bolus, it is logical to give intravenous aminophylline by constant infusion rather than by repeated-bolus injection after the initial bolus dose. Mitenko and Ogilvie also studied the log serum concentration–bronchodilator relationship in a group of adult asthmatic patients and showed a proportionality between the log of the serum concentration and the bronchodilator effect over the 5- to 20-μg/ml range.[23] Subjects with severe asthma (status asthmaticus) have a rather flat serum concentration–bronchodilator effect curve over the range of 5 to 20 μg/ml. Patients with mild asthma who may have a nearly normal FEV_1 may also have a flat dose-response curve because their airways are capable of little additional improvement. In patients with moderate asthma, with an FEV_1 of 50% to 60% of the predicted level, the serum concentration–response curve is steep.

THEOPHYLLINE TOXICITY

Like its bronchodilator activity, adverse effects are related to the logarithm of the serum concentration.[24] Hendeles and associates[25] demonstrated a relationship between serum concentration and symptoms of theophylline toxicity. Few toxic symptoms were noted when the steady-state serum concentration was less than 14.6 μg/ml. Adverse effects appeared as the serum concentration rose beyond 20 μg/ml. These included gastrointestinal, central nervous system, and cardiovascular effects (Fig. 82–1). Of all adverse effects, those involving the gastrointestinal tract are most common. Vomiting, particularly if persistent, is very suggestive of theophylline toxicity. Hematemesis has been reported primarily in children, although its exact pathogenesis is not clear. Gastrointestinal symptoms occur most often as a result of a central effect of an excessive serum theophylline concentration on the medulla rather than because of a local irritative effect on the stomach. Relaxation of cardioesophageal smooth muscle may lead to gastroesophageal reflux; theophylline-induced gastroesophageal reflux may cause worsening of asthma by reflex stimulation of neural receptors in the distal esophagus or by aspiration of stomach contents into the upper airway and lung.

Theophylline stimulates the nervous system at various levels: the medulla (increased respiratory rate and sensitivity to carbon dioxide [CO_2], nausea and vomiting, vagal effect causing bradycardia), the cerebral cortex (restlessness, agitation, tremor, irritability, headache, seizures, difficulty in concentration, behavioral disturbances), the hypothalamus (hyperthermia), and even the spinal cord (hyperreflexia). The mechanism of theophylline's effect on the nervous system is not known. Although seizures are a prominent manifestation of theophylline toxicity and are often difficult to control, they themselves do not necessarily lead to death or to irreversible brain damage. Serum concentration associated with seizure activity varies substantially. The combination of seizures and cardiorespiratory arrest leads to the most disastrous conse-

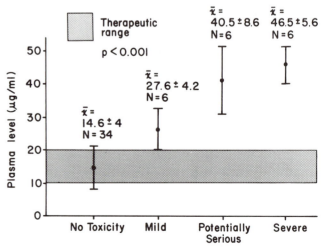

Figure 82–1. Relationship between serum concentration and theophylline toxicity in hospitalized adults. (Modified from Hendeles L, Bighley L, Richardson RH, et al: Frequent toxicity from IV aminophylline infusions in critically ill patients. Drug Intell Clin Pharm 11:12–18, 1977.)

quences of theophylline intoxication. Such children who are resuscitated and survive show signs of severe anoxic brain injury, much like those who have been resuscitated after drowning or strangulation.

Theophylline may cause behavioral disturbances in some children treated with the drug. In some instances, these effects appear to be related to dose and serum concentration, and in others, no such relationship exists. Concern about the effects of theophylline on behavior, particularly learning, was raised by Rachelefsky and co-workers;[26] however, there were many commentaries and critiques of this study. Furukawa and associates,[27] in two studies of theophylline in asthmatic children, also interpreted their results to suggest that theophylline may impair learning and behavior. It is of interest that one important abnormal finding in their initial report was not substantiated in their second study.[27] Creer and McLoughlin,[28] after a critical review of the subject, commented that there is no definitive evidence that theophylline produces any type of learning disability. A similar conclusion was reached by the U.S. Food and Drug Administration Pulmonary/Allergy Drug Advisory Committee in 1987 after a review of studies published until that time.

Theophylline has both inotropic and chronotropic effects on the heart. Although a number of opposing factors (direct effect on pacemaker tissue, effect on catecholamine release, peripheral vagolytic action, stimulation of the medullary center) confound the effects of theophylline on heart rate, the net result is usually tachycardia. Tachycardia is an almost constant finding in cases of significant theophylline intoxication. In the therapeutic range, the effect of theophylline on the heart rate is modest, in the rate of 3 to 16 beats per minute. The arrhythmogenic potential of theophylline has been shown in experimental animals, but data in humans are less clear. Metabolic effects, principally hypokalemia and hyperglycemia, are observed in cases of severe theophylline toxicity.

CLINICAL USE OF THEOPHYLLINE

Apnea of Prematurity. Theophylline stimulates the medullary respiratory center by increasing sensitivity to CO_2. This effect is used to advantage in the treatment of apnea of prematurity. The dose of theophylline may be calculated as follows: mg/kg/24 h = (0.2) age in weeks + 5. Because of the long theophylline half-life in premature and young infants (up to 24 h), theophylline dosing twice or even once a day suffices. Theophylline may be given on a trial basis for 2 weeks and may be continued or stopped, depending on the clinical circumstances.

Asthma. Although intravenous aminophylline has been standard treatment for status asthmaticus since the early 1940s, the value of aminophylline in the emergency room setting for acute asthma has been questioned.[29] Various authors suggested that theophylline adds little in terms of bronchodilator activity while increasing adverse effects when optimal therapy with aerosolized beta$_2$-agonists is used to treat status asthmaticus. In the initial study of the use of intravenous theophylline in the treatment of acute asthma, theophylline was compared with subcuta-

neous epinephrine administration in an emergency department. The bronchodilator effect of theophylline was inferior to that achieved by the sympathomimetic drugs. Subsequent studies generally confirmed the observation that in acute asthma in an emergency room setting, the bronchodilator effect of aminophylline is inferior to that of optimal administration of aerosolized beta-agonists.

At present, the published data support the addition of intravenous aminophylline in the treatment of patients who fail optimal aerosolized beta-agonist therapy and who require hospital admission. For example, Pierson and associates showed clinical benefit and pulmonary function improvement in status asthmaticus in a double-blind study of intravenous aminophylline in children with status asthmaticus.[30] An emergency department study of adults with acute airway obstructive disease showed a threefold decrease in hospital admission rates for subjects treated with aminophylline in comparison with placebo recipients.[31] Sakamoto and colleagues reported on results of a study of intravenous aminophylline administration in 12 asthmatic patients with acute episodes varying from mild or moderate to severe. They found progressive improvement in FEV_1 over the range of 5 to 15 μg/ml; the greatest bronchodilator effect was observed in patients whose initial airway obstruction was of a milder degree.[32] Extrapulmonary effects of theophylline in both improving diaphragmatic function and delaying the onset of muscle fatigue may also be useful in some patients with acute asthma who do not respond properly to optimal aerolized bronchodilator therapy.

For intravenous therapy with aminophylline, some simple calculations can be used to determine the correct loading and maintenance therapy doses. With drugs like theophylline that are distributed rapidly from the plasma to the tissues, there is a relationship among plasma concentration (C_p), dose (D), and volume of distribution (V_d) so that

$$C_p = \frac{D}{V_d}.$$

If an average V_d of 0.5 l/kg is assumed, it is easy to determine that for each milligram per kilogram (ideal body weight) infused, there will be an increase of approximately 2 mg/l (2 μg/ml) in peak plasma concentration. The loading dose (aminophylline) needed to achieve a given theophylline plasma concentration is determined as follows:

$$\text{Loading dose (D)} = \frac{(V_d)(C_p)}{0.8}.$$

In this equation, it is assumed that the patient has not previously been receiving theophylline. If the child has been taking theophylline as an outpatient, the loading dose should be reduced, unless an immediate serum theophylline determination is available. Once the observed level of theophylline is known, it can be subtracted from the desired level and multiplied by the volume of distribution:

$$D = \frac{V_d(C_p \text{ desired} - C_p \text{ initial})}{0.8}. \tag{1}$$

The dose of aminophylline required in order to maintain a desired steady state of serum theophylline concentration (C_{pss}) may be calculated as follows:

$$\text{Constant infusion rate} = \frac{(Cl)(C_{pss})(\tau)}{0.8}$$

where Cl is the clearance l/h/kg, C_{pss} is the average plasma concentration at steady state, and τ is the dosing interval. A theophylline level determined from a serum sample obtained 1 h after the loading dose is useful in determining the need for an additional minibolus loading dose. Equation 1 can be used to calculate the subsequent loading dose if needed. In children, a subsequent determination 4 h after the initiation of constant infusion shows the trend of the serum concentration; the rate can either be increased or be decreased as needed. Additional samples after 12 and 24 h guide further intravenous dosing.

To convert the intravenous dose to an equivalent oral dose, the hourly dose is multiplied by the dosing interval to be used for oral therapy. It is important to correct the aminophylline dose for the theophylline equivalent by multiplying the aminophylline dose by 0.8 to obtain a theophylline equivalent dose. In this calculation it is assumed that the oral product is completely absorbed.

When theophylline is used for the management of chronic asthma, it is most effectively administered as one of the sustained-release formulations. Use of sustained-release products minimizes the peak-and-trough fluctuation of serum concentration. Depending on an individual child's serum theophylline clearance, an 8- or 12-h dosing interval is appropriate. In general, the younger the child (under 9 years of age), the more likely it is that an 8-h dosing interval will be required to minimize peak-and-trough fluctuations in theophylline concentration. Determination of theophylline serum concentration during the initial weeks of treatment is useful in adjusting the dose and dosing interval. Sustained-release theophylline products that are completely absorbed and whose bioavailability is insignificantly affected by concomitant food administration are preferred.[12] Once-a-day dosing is inappropriate in most children, who, because of their relatively rapid theophylline clearance, show unacceptable peak-and-trough differences in theophylline concentration and may become symptomatic toward the end of the 24-h dosing interval. With pellet formulations, the beads should be added to moist food (e.g., applesauce) to ensure their dissolution. Sustained-release tablets should not be crushed because this destroys their slow-release properties. An algorithm for initial dosing and final dosage adjustment based on serum concentration measurement was given in a review of safety and efficacy of theophylline in children with asthma.[33] Because adverse affects of theophylline become manifest as the serum concentration of 20 μg/ml is approached, it is best to aim for 8 to 15 μg/ml range in the majority of patients. It is important to treat the patient and not the theophylline level.

REFERENCES

1. May CD: History of the introduction of theophylline into the treatment of asthma. Clin Allergy 4:211–217, 1974.
2. Simons FER, Simons KJ, Bierman CW: The pharmacokinetics of dihydroxypropytheophylline: A basis for rational therapy. J Allergy Clin Immunol 56:347–355, 1975.
3. Lunell E, Svedmyr N, Andersson KE, Persson CG: Effects of enprofylline, a xanthine lacking adenosine receptor antagonism, in patients with chronic obstructive lung disease. Eur J Clin Pharmacol 22:395–402, 1982.
4. Howell RE: Multiple mechanisms of xanthine action on airway reactivity. J Pharmacol Exper Ther 225:1008–1013, 1990.
5. Krzanowski JJ, Polson JB: Mechanism of action of methylxanthines in asthma. J Allergy Clin Immunol 82:143–145, 1988.
6. Pauwels R, VanRenterghem D, Van der Straeten M, et al: The effect of theophylline and enprofylline on allergen-induced bronchoconstriction. J Allergy Clin Immunol 76:583–590, 1985.
7. Magnussen H, Reuss G, Jorres R: Theophylline has a dose-related effect on the airway response to inhaled histamine and methacholine in asthmatics. Am Rev Respir Dis 136:1163–1167, 1987.
8. McWilliams BC, Menendez R, Kelly HW, et al: Effects of theophylline on inhaled methacholine and histamine in asthmatic children. Am Rev Respir Dis 130:193–197, 1984.
9. Cockcroft DW, Murdock KY, Gore BP, et al: Theophylline does not inhibit allergen-induced increase in airway responsiveness to methacholine. J Allergy Clin Immunol 83:913–920, 1989.
10. Dutoit JI, Salome CM, Woolcock AJ: Inhaled corticosteroids reduce the severity of bronchial hyper-responsiveness in asthma but oral theophylline does not. Am Rev Respir Dis 136:1174–1178, 1987.
11. Hendeles L, Weinberger M, Bighley L: Absolute bioavailability of oral theophylline. Am J Hosp Pharm 34:525–527, 1977.
12. Hendeles L, Iafrate RP, Weinberger M: A clinical and pharmacokinetic basis for the selection and use of slow-release theophylline products. Clin Pharmacokinet 9:95–135, 1984.
13. Hendeles L, Weinberger M, Milavetz G, et al: Food-induced "dose-dumping" from a once-a-day theophylline product as a cause of theophylline toxicity. Chest 87:758–765, 1985.
14. Tserng KY, King KC, Takieddine FN: Theophylline metabolism in premature infants. Clin Pharmacol Ther 29:594–600, 1981.
15. Ellis EF, Koysooko R, Levy G: Pharmacokinetics of theophylline in children with asthma. Pediatrics 58:542–547, 1976.
16. Bory C, Baltassat P, Porthault M, et al: Metabolism of theophylline to caffeine in premature newborn infants. J Pediatr 94:988–993, 1979.
17. Ginchansky E, Weinberger M: Relationship of theophylline clearance to oral dosage in children with chronic asthma. J Pediatr 91:655–660, 1977.
18. Jusko WJ, Gardner MJ, Mangione A, et al: Factors affecting theophylline clearances: Age, tobacco, marijuana, cirrhosis, congestive heart failure, obesity, oral contraceptives, benzodiazepines, barbiturates, and ethanol. J Pharm Sci 68:1358–1366, 1979.
19. Hendeles L, Weinberger M: Theophylline: A "state of the art" review. Pharmacotherapy 3:2–44, 1983.
20. Kraemer MJ, Furukawa CT, Koup JR, et al: Altered theophylline clearance during an influenza B outbreak. Pediatrics 69:476–480, 1982.
21. Ellis EF, Hendeles L: In Taylor WJ, Deirs Caviness MH (eds): A Textbook for the Clinical Application of Therapeutic Drug Monitoring, pp. 185–201. Irving, TX: Abbott Laboratories, 1986.
22. Maselli R, Casal GL, Ellis EF: Pharmacologic effects of intravenously administered aminophylline in asthmatic children. J Pediatr 76:777–782, 1970.
23. Mitenko PA, Ogilvie RI: Rational intravenous doses of theophylline. N Engl J Med 289:600–603, 1973.
24. Ellis EF: Theophylline toxicity. J Allergy Clin Immunol 76:297–301, 1985.
25. Hendeles L, Bighley L, Richardson RH, et al: Frequent toxicity from IV aminophylline infusions in critically ill patients. Drug Intell Clin Pharm 11:12, 1977.
26. Rachelefsky GS, Wo J, Adelson J, et al: Behavioral abnormalities and poor school performance due to oral theophylline usage. Pediatrics 78:1133–1138, 1986.
27. Furukawa CT, DuHamel TR, Weimer L, et al: Cognitive and behavioral findings in children taking theophylline. J Allergy Clin Immunol 81:83–88, 1988.
28. Creer TL, McLoughlin JA: Editorial: The effects of theophylline on cognitive and behavioral performance. J Allergy Clin Immunol 83:1027–1029, 1989.

29. Littenberg B: Aminophylline treatment in severe, acute asthma. JAMA 259:1678–1684, 1988.
30. Pierson WE, Bierman CW, Stamm SJ, et al: Double-blind trial of aminophylline in status asthmaticus. Pediatrics 48:642–646, 1971.
31. Wrenn K, Slovis CM, Murphy F, et al: Aminophylline therapy for acute bronchospastic disease in the emergency room. Ann Intern Med 115:241–247, 1991.
32. Sakamoto Y, Kage J, Horai Y: Effect of theophylline on improvement of the pulmonary function in the treatment of acute episodes of asthma: The influence of the severity of acute asthma. Ann Allergy 63:21–27, 1979.
33. Hendeles L, Weinberger M, Szefler S, et al: Safety and efficacy of theophylline in children with asthma. J Pediatr 120:177–183, 1992.

83 ANTIVIRAL THERAPY FOR PULMONARY INFECTIONS

RUSSELL B. VAN DYKE, M.D.

The 1970s and 1980s were periods of remarkable advances in the field of antiviral chemotherapy. Therapy for viral infections, once considered in the realm of fantasy, has now become a part of routine medical care. With these advances in therapy has come a need for rapid viral diagnosis because antiviral agents must be administered as early in the course of an infection as possible to produce maximal benefit. Therefore, all clinicians should have access to a clinical laboratory that performs rapid viral diagnosis.

Because viruses are intracellular pathogens that use the metabolic machinery of the cell for their own replication, it is difficult to find agents that inhibit growth of the virus without inhibiting cell growth as well. Thus many agents that are effective inhibitors of viral replication prove too toxic to be used in humans. Many antiviral agents were first developed in the search for inhibitors of cellular replication to be used in the treatment of malignancies. Successful antiviral therapy has resulted from the identification of agents that selectively target a step in the replication of the virus, thus limiting toxicity to uninfected cells. As exemplified by the development of agents against herpes simplex virus, carefully designed and conducted placebo-controlled clinical trials can rapidly establish the clinical usefulness of candidate antiviral agents.

TREATMENT OF INFLUENZA VIRUSES

AMANTADINE AND RIMANTADINE

The caged carbocyclics, a class of antiviral drugs with activity against influenza A virus, were developed in the 1960s. Amantadine, a member of this group, has been available since the late 1960s. However, this drug continues to be underused because most clinicians do not appreciate its value in the prevention and treatment of influenza A infections. It remains the only proven treatment for influenza A; at present, there is no approved therapy for influenza B.

Amantadine was first licensed in the United States in 1966 (as Symmetrel) for the prevention of the Asian influenza. At that time, it was the first antiviral drug approved for systemic use. In 1976, it was approved for both prophylaxis and therapy for all strains of influenza A. With activity against only influenza A virus, amantadine has the narrowest spectrum of any antiviral agent currently available. Rimantadine is a structural analog of amantadine that is not currently available in the United States but is widely used in the Soviet Union. Its activity is similar to that of amantadine with less frequent side effects.

Chemistry and Mechanism of Action

Amantadine (alpha$_1$-adamantanamine hydrochloride) and rimantadine (alpha-methyl-1-adamantanamine hydrochloride) are synthetic caged amines with similar structures. Their mechanism of action is believed to involve interference with uncoating of the viral genome after entry of the virus into the cell and perhaps, in addition, inhibition of transcription of viral RNA.[1]

Pharmacology and Toxicity

Amantadine is well absorbed orally; 90% of the dose is excreted unchanged in the urine.[2] It is available only in oral preparations, as a capsule or as syrup. It has a long serum half-life, ranging from 12 to 18 h in adults; the half-life is increased in the elderly and in the presence of renal insufficiency. Consequently, the dose must be modified in patients with impaired renal function. Rimantadine has a longer serum half-life than amantadine (24 to 36 h in adults) and is largely metabolized; less than 15% is excreted unchanged in the urine. As a consequence, renal impairment has less of an effect on the pharmacokinetics of rimantadine than on those of amantadine. The pharmacokinetics of rimantadine are similar in children and adults.

Side effects are seen in 2% to 10% of patients receiving oral amantadine. Most common are mild central nervous system symptoms such as insomnia, difficulty concentrating, drowsiness, dizziness, and nervousness. Amantadine has been reported to induce seizures in children with underlying neurologic deficits who received large doses (6.6 mg/kg/day).[3] It should be used with caution in these children and at a reduced dosage. Gastrointestinal side effects such as anorexia and nausea are seen in approximately 2% of children. These side effects abate with discontinuation of the drug.

Central nervous system complaints are less common with rimantadine,[4] although gastrointestinal toxicity may be more common.[5]

Efficacy Studies

The major use of amantadine is in the prevention of disease caused by influenza A. Most studies demonstrate that amantadine is more effective in preventing clinical disease than in preventing infection. During outbreaks of influenza A, the incidence of infection and disease in unimmunized adults is reduced by 70% to 90% among those given amantadine prophylaxis.[6, 7] Similar results have been found in teenagers.[8] Rimantadine has been shown to have efficacy similar to that of amantadine but with fewer side effects.[6, 9] In children, rimantadine prophylaxis resulted in an 87% reduction in the infection rate and an 85% reduction in the rate of disease caused by influenza A, with minimal adverse effects.[10, 11] Results of studies in adults suggest that a reduced dose of amantadine (100 mg/day) may be as effective as the usual dose (200 mg/day) for prophylaxis with fewer side effects.[12]

The role of amantadine and rimantadine in the therapy for influenza A infection is less firmly established than its prophylactic use. Studies in young adults in which either amantadine or rimantadine was compared with placebo demonstrated that when given within 24 to 48 h of onset of symptoms, both drugs result in a reduction in the duration of fever and respiratory symptoms by 24 to 48 h and a more rapid return to school.[13, 14] One comparative trial of acetaminophen and rimantadine in children demonstrated a significantly more rapid reduction in fever and improvement in symptom score among children receiving rimantadine, with a shortening of the illness by approximately 1 day.[15] However, a similar study demonstrated no benefit from rimantadine therapy.[16] It remains to be shown whether the early administration of amantadine prevents complications in children at risk, such as those with underlying cardiac disease, pulmonary disease, or immunodeficiency.

The emergence of amantadine- and rimantadine-resistant influenza virus has been reported among patients receiving these drugs.[17, 18] In a study of rimantadine in children, resistance emerged rapidly during a 5-day course of therapy. After the completion of therapy, virus shedding was, in fact, greater among those receiving rimantadine than among those receiving acetaminophen.[15] Transmission of rimantadine-resistant influenza A virus from patients receiving rimantadine therapy to family members receiving rimantadine prophylaxis has been reported.[19] Viral resistance may represent an increasing problem with greater use of these drugs, particularly in closed environments such as nursing homes and residential homes for children.

The administration of amantadine by the aerosol route has been studied as a means of delivering the drug directly to the site of infection in the respiratory tract. Preliminary results have not been encouraging.[20]

Use of Amantadine

Immunization remains the mainstay in the effort to prevent influenza in children at increased risk of complications.[21] Immunization has the advantage of preventing infection with both influenza A and influenza B. Because of annual variation in the antigenic makeup of the circulation strains of virus (antigenic drift), immunization must be repeated each year. Annual immunization is recommended for children with chronic pulmonary disease (such as cystic fibrosis, bronchopulmonary dysplasia, bronchiectasis, and moderate to severe asthma), hemodynamically significant cardiac disease, and sickle cell disease and other hemoglobinopathies and for children receiving immunosuppressive therapy.[22] Other children to be considered for immunization include those with other chronic illness such as renal or metabolic diseases, malignancies, and diabetes and those requiring long-term aspirin therapy, in whom there is an increased risk of the development of Reye's syndrome. The vaccine should not routinely be given to infants under 6 months of age. Recommendations for influenza immunization are published annually in the *Morbidity and Mortality Weekly Report* from the Centers for Disease Control, which should be consulted for complete recommendations.[23]

There are several situations in which prophylaxis with amantadine should be considered. All require the knowledge that influenza A is circulating in the community. First, children who qualify for the influenza vaccine but who fail to be vaccinated or cannot be vaccinated may be given prophylaxis with amantadine. Likewise, immunosuppressed persons, who may have an inadequate response to the vaccine, may benefit from prophylaxis. In addition, if the vaccine is not fully effective against the circulating strain of influenza A, amantadine can be given to immunized persons to provide additional protection. This can occur because the specific antigenic strains to be included in the vaccine must be chosen early each year to allow for production of vaccine by fall. On occasion, this guess is wrong and the vaccine produced is not fully effective, as occurred in 1986. The efficacy of immunization and amantadine prophylaxis is additive, and particularly high-risk children may benefit from both modalities. An alternative strategy for prophylaxis in the child who has not been immunized is to administer the vaccine and at the same time begin a 14-day course of amantadine. This will protect the child until he or she makes an antibody response to the vaccine. Amantadine does not interfere with the antibody response to the influenza vaccine.

Amantadine should be considered for the treatment of children with severe influenza A infections, particularly if they are at an increased risk for complications, whether they have received the influenza vaccine or not. Early initiation of therapy requires the ability to make a rapid and specific diagnosis of influenza A because amantadine is of no value in treating influenza B or other respiratory virus infections. If it is known that influenza A is circulating in the community, it is reasonable to initiate empirical treatment in a child with symptoms consistent with influenza while awaiting confirmation of the diagnosis by laboratory means. Obviously, it is necessary for the physician to maintain close contact with both the viral diagnostic laboratory and public health officials in the community.

The dosage of amantadine for prophylaxis and therapy is the same: 4.4 to 8.8 mg/kg/day orally in two divided doses. The lower dosage, 4.4 mg/kg/day with a maximal daily dose of 150 mg, is recommended for children under 9 years of age to minimize toxicity. For older children and adults, the maximal daily dose is 200 mg. For prophylaxis, the drug should be administered during the 4- to 6-week period that influenza A is circulating in the community. For therapy, it should be started as soon as possible after the onset of symptoms and continued for 2 to 5 days or until symptoms have resolved. The dose must be reduced in children with renal impairment or a seizure disorder. Dosage modifications for patients with reduced renal function have been published.[24] Little information is available on the use of amantadine in children under 1 year of age.

It is anticipated that rimantadine is likely to become licensed in the United States in the near future. Because of fewer side effects than amantadine, it will be the preferred drug. Dosage recommendations will be made at that time.

RIBAVIRIN AEROSOL THERAPY FOR INFLUENZA

Ribavirin has activity against both influenza A and B; small-particle aerosol therapy with ribavirin has been evaluated in the treatment of influenza A and B infections in otherwise healthy young adults.[25-27] Treated subjects demonstrated a reduction in fever, symptom score, and titer of virus in nasal wash samples in comparison with control subjects. A multicenter trial of ribavirin aerosol therapy in children with influenza is currently underway. The use of ribavirin in children and adults with influenza is investigational at this time. Because the aerosol is delivered for 12 to 18 h per day, hospitalization is required, making this form of therapy impractical in most instances.

TREATMENT OF RESPIRATORY SYNCYTIAL VIRUS

Respiratory syncytial virus (RSV) is the major cause of lower respiratory tract infection, including bronchiolitis and pneumonia, in infancy and childhood. In high-risk children, such as those with congenital heart disease or bronchopulmonary dysplasia, the rates of morbidity and mortality from RSV infections are substantial. Because no vaccine is available, it is not possible to prevent RSV infections. The availability of ribavirin aerosol therapy now makes possible the treatment of this difficult and common pediatric infection. Controversy about the use of ribavirin results in part from the fact that there exists a new delivery system—continuous small-particle aerosol therapy for treatment of pulmonary infections—in addition to a new antiviral agent.

Table 83–1. *IN VITRO* ANTIVIRAL ACTIVITY OF RIBAVIRIN

Virus	Inhibitory Concentration (TCID$_{50}$) (μg/ml)
Influenza A and B	0.1–25
Respiratory syncytial virus	3–10
Parainfluenza 1 and 3	3–32
Measles	0.003–10
Mumps	10
Lassa fever	1–10
Herpes simplex 1 and 2	0.3–>100
Adenovirus	10–>250
Human immunodeficiency virus-1	50

TCID$_{50}$, median tissue culture-inhibitory doses.

RIBAVIRIN

Ribavirin is a broad-spectrum antiviral agent with activity against a variety of DNA and RNA viruses (Table 83–1) It is currently licensed in the United States only for the treatment of RSV by aerosol delivery. However, it has been shown to be life-saving in the treatment of Lassa fever.[28] In addition, it has been or is currently being evaluated in the treatment of a variety of other viral infections, including influenza virus, parainfluenza virus, herpes simplex virus, human immunodeficiency virus (HIV), measles, and rabies.[29]

Chemistry and Mechanism of Action

Ribavirin, a synthetic analog of the naturally occurring nucleosides guanosine and adenosine, consists of a ribose sugar attached to triazole carboxamide. Any change in the structure of the molecule results in loss of antiviral activity. The mechanisms of action of ribavirin[29] have been studied most carefully for influenza viruses, and three mechanisms have been proposed, all of which may contribute to the activity of the drug. The possibility that the drug may act at several sites in the replication of the virus may account for the fact that resistant virus has not been identified *in vivo* and is difficult to develop *in vitro*.

Ribavirin triphosphate blocks influenza virus replication by inhibiting viral RNA-dependent RNA polymerase. In addition, ribavirin triphosphate inhibits formation of the 5'-terminal methylated cap structure of cellular messenger RNA (mRNA) and may be incorporated into this cap structure in place of guanosine. This 5' cap structure is required for efficient binding of mRNA to polysomes, and its absence results in impaired translation of mRNA. Influenza virus uses a short segment of cellular mRNA, containing the 5' cap, as primer for synthesis of viral mRNA. Viruses lacking a cap structure on their mRNA are not inhibited by ribavirin. Finally, ribavirin monophosphate inhibits the enzyme inosine monophosphate dehydrogenase, leading to a depletion of the intracellular guanosine triphosphate pool.

Pharmacology and Toxicity

The objective of small-particle aerosol therapy is to deliver a high concentration of ribavirin directly to the site of virus replication in the respiratory epithelium while limiting toxicity resulting from systemic absorption of the drug. The aerosol is produced by a Collison generator, provided by the manufacturer of the ribavirin, which produces particles with a mean diameter of 1.3 μm. Particles of this size maximize delivery of medication to the lower respiratory tract. With aerosol therapy, extremely high ribavirin concentrations are achieved in lower respiratory tract secretions obtained from intubated patients (300 to 27,000 μg/ml), whereas plasma concentrations are very low (0.2 to 2 μg/ml).[30] The plasma half-life ranges from 5 to 13 h with aerosol therapy, and plasma levels increase with increasing duration of therapy. With prolonged therapy, plasma levels as high as 15 μg/ml have been achieved. The half-life of ribavirin in respiratory secretions is approximately 2 h after discontinuation of aerosol therapy.

With parenteral administration of ribavirin, the major toxicity is anemia. Ribavirin accumulates in peripheral red blood cells, resulting in their shortened half-life.[31] In rare instances, indirect hyperbilirubinemia is seen. With aerosol therapy, hematologic toxicity has not been observed, but ribavirin does accumulate in red blood cells. Rash and conjunctivitis are occasionally seen with aerosol therapy, presumably resulting from a direct effect of the medication. Some patients have been noted to have a deterioration in their pulmonary status with the initiation of ribavirin aerosol therapy, which resolves with discontinuation of treatment. This may be more common when the drug is delivered directly to the lower respiratory tract through an endotracheal tube or a tracheostomy and may be caused by irritation of the airway by the aerosol vehicle (water) or by the drug itself. Ribavirin aerosol therapy has been shown to produce dyspnea in animals and in human adults with chronic obstructive lung disease and asthma.[32]

Ribavirin is teratogenic in rodents and causes fetal death in rabbits but is not teratogenic in humans.[33] It does not appear to be incorporated into cellular DNA. Concern has been raised about environmental exposure to ribavirin among personnel caring for children who receive aerosol therapy in the hospital. Ribavirin was detected in red blood cells from a single exposed hospital employee in one study,[34] whereas none was found in a second study.[35] Environmental air sampling reveals that concentrations of ribavirin in the air surrounding patients being treated are sufficient to be of concern. Techniques must be employed to limit environmental exposure. In addition, employees should be made aware of the potential risk of exposure during the care of patients, and employees who are pregnant or who plan on conceiving a child in the immediate future should avoid exposure to the drug.

Efficacy Studies

A number of studies have demonstrated clinical efficacy of ribavirin aerosol therapy in the treatment of RSV bronchiolitis or pneumonia, including five placebo-controlled, randomized clinical trials[36–40] and an additional study with historical controls[41] (Table 83–2). Each demonstrated a modest improvement in clinical symptoms in the ribavirin-treated patients, with a greater improvement in symptoms of the lower rather than the upper respiratory tract. A significant improvement in blood oxygenation was demonstrated in the three studies in which blood gases were evaluated. However, a significant reduction in virus titer and a shorter duration of virus shedding from the respiratory tract was noted in only two of the five reports in which virologic studies were performed. Children with underlying risk factors for severe RSV infections, such as congenital heart disease or bronchopulmonary dysplasia, have been shown to have a clinical response to ribavirin similar to that of otherwise healthy children.[38] However, it has not been demonstrated that early initiation of ribavirin therapy in these high-risk children decreases morbidity or mortality rates, prevents respiratory failure, or reduces the duration of mechanical ventilation. Likewise, it is not known whether treatment of the otherwise healthy infant reduces the duration of hospitalization or prevents the long-term pulmonary complications associated with RSV infections. The clinical value of ribavirin aerosol therapy in the treatment of RSV infections has been questioned.[42, 43]

A single study suggests that RSV-infected children who require mechanical ventilation benefit from administration of ribavirin aerosol therapy through the endotracheal tube.[44] This mode of administration is potentially hazardous because the medication can clog tubing, valves, and filters and result in malfunction of the ventilator. Techniques for the safe administration of ribavirin to children receiving mechanical ventilation have been developed and published.[45, 46] However, this method of administration remains experimental and should be undertaken only by clinicians with experience in it.

USE OF RIBAVIRIN SMALL-PARTICLE AEROSOL THERAPY

Candidates for ribavirin aerosol therapy include children hospitalized with a documented or suspected lower respiratory tract infection caused by RSV who are moderately or severely ill or who are at risk for a complicated course. As with any antiviral agent, it is desirable to initiate therapy as early in the course of infection as possible to obtain maximal benefit. Therefore, therapy can be started before laboratory confirmation of the presence of RSV. Children at increased risk for complications of RSV, including those with congenital heart disease (particularly with pulmonary hypertension), bronchopulmonary dysplasia, immunodeficiency, and immunosuppres-

Table 83–2. CLINICAL TRIALS OF RIBAVIRIN FOR RESPIRATORY SYNCYTIAL VIRUS INFECTIONS

Reference	Improved Symptoms	Improved Oxygenation	Antiviral Effect
Hall et al.[36]	+	+	+
Taber et al.[37]	+	NT	None
Hall et al.[38]	+	+	+
Barry et al.[39]	+	NT	None
Rodriguez et al.[40]	+	+	None
Conrad et al.[41]	+	NT	NT

NT, not tested.

sion, and premature infants, should be treated. In addition, children in whom severity of illness may require hospitalization for more than 4 days may be considered for treatment because therapy might be expected to shorten their hospital stay. Suggested criteria for treatment include rising arterial carbon dioxide concentration and hypoxemia of less than 65 mm Hg on room air.[47]

For aerosol administration, one vial (6 g) of ribavirin is dissolved in 300 ml of water (20 mg/ml) and delivered as a small-particle aerosol by mask or hood by the Collison aerosol generator. The usual course of therapy is 12 to 18 h/day for 3 to 7 days, depending on the child's clinical response. Care should be taken to minimize exposure of hospital personnel to the aerosol, as mentioned previously.

TREATMENT OF RHINOVIRUSES

Rhinoviruses are the major cause of the common cold; however, they rarely cause lower respiratory tract disease. Despite continuing efforts to develop scientific therapy, effective treatment of rhinovirus infections is not available. The topical application of interferon alpha$_2$ to the nose has been shown to be effective in preventing rhinovirus infection.[48] This modality remains experimental, and local toxicity, such as nasal irritation and stuffiness, will probably limit its acceptance. Interferon is not effective for treatment of established rhinovirus infections.

TREATMENT OF HERPESVIRUS INFECTIONS

Herpesviruses are extremely common human pathogens but symptomatic infection of the lower respiratory tract with these agents is uncommon. When it does occur, it is usually in an immunosuppressed patient. Effective antiviral therapy for herpes simplex virus and varicella-zoster virus has been available since vidarabine was licensed in 1975. More recently, acyclovir has become the drug of choice for most types of infection with these two viruses. Effective therapy for cytomegalovirus has been much more difficult to develop, although the licensure of ganciclovir for cytomegalovirus retinitis in immunosuppressed patients represents a first step. No effective therapy is available for Epstein-Barr virus infections.

VIDARABINE (ADENINE ARABINOSIDE)

Vidarabine is a synthetic purine analog that inhibits viral replication by interfering with viral DNA synthesis. After being phosphorylated to the triphosphate form by cellular kinases, it inhibits viral DNA polymerase to a greater extent than cellular DNA polymerase. It is also incorporated into the newly synthesized DNA, resulting in termination of the growing DNA chain. Finally, it also inhibits viral RNA synthesis. It has been shown to be teratogenic and mutagenic in animals. Vidarabine has activity against both herpes simplex virus and varicella-zoster virus.

Vidarabine is not absorbed orally. Because it is relatively insoluble, it must be infused in a large volume of fluid over 12 h at a concentration of no higher than 0.5 mg/ml. It is rapidly deaminated to arabinosyl hypoxanthine, which is largely excreted in the urine. Renal dysfunction results in a prolongation of the half-life and accumulation of the drug. Administration of allopurinol, which interferes with the metabolism of arabinosyl hypoxanthine, can cause arabinosyl hypoxanthine to accumulate to toxic levels. The most common side effects of vidarabine are nausea, vomiting, and diarrhea, seen in approximately 20% of adults. Central nervous system abnormalities, including tremors, paresthesias, ataxia, seizures, confusion, weakness, dysarthria, and even coma may be seen in 2% to 10%. Suppression of the bone marrow is uncommon.

ACYCLOVIR

Acyclovir is an acyclic analog of guanosine. Like vidarabine, it inhibits viral DNA synthesis when in the triphosphate form. Unlike vidarabine, however, it is not phosphorylated by cellular enzymes. Rather, it requires a viral enzyme (viral thymidine kinase) to be phosphorylated to the monophosphate form; cellular enzymes then convert it to the active triphosphate form. Acyclovir-triphosphate inhibits viral DNA polymerase and also is incorporated into the growing DNA chain, resulting in chain termination. Therefore, only virus-infected cells can convert acyclovir to its active form. Acyclovir is active against herpes simplex virus types 1 and 2 and varicella-zoster virus because they code for a viral thymidine kinase. In contrast, neither cytomegalovirus nor Epstein-Barr virus codes for thymidine kinase, and acyclovir has little activity against these viruses. Unfortunately, strains of herpes simplex virus and varicella-zoster virus that have lost thymidine kinase activity and are therefore resistant to acyclovir can develop during treatment. This has been an increasing problem in immunosuppressed patients, such as those with acquired immunodeficiency syndrome (AIDS) who are receiving chronic oral acyclovir therapy.[49] Alternative drugs for the treatment of acyclovir-resistant virus include vidarabine and foscarnet.[50, 51]

Acyclovir is absorbed orally and is largely excreted in the urine. With impaired renal function, serum levels increase. Toxicity is uncommon; rapid infusion in patients who are poorly hydrated can cause a transient decrease in renal function. Nausea and vomiting are rarely seen.

GANCICLOVIR

Ganciclovir (dihydroxy-propoxymethyl-guanine) is an acyclovir derivative with increased activity against cytomegalovirus. It is phosphorylated to the triphosphate form preferentially in cytomegalovirus-infected cells, where it inhibits viral DNA synthesis in a manner similar to that of acyclovir. It is not absorbed well orally and must be given parenterally. Unfortunately, it is much more toxic than acyclovir. The most common adverse effect is bone marrow suppression, which is often dose-limiting. Neutropenia is seen in as many as 25% to 50% of treated patients and thrombocytopenia in 10% to 20%. Bone marrow suppression is dose related and reversible on discontinuation of the drug. Hepatic, renal, and central nervous system toxicity is occasionally seen. In animals, toxic effects include bone marrow suppression, atrophy of intestinal mucosa, inhibition of spermatogenesis, and testicular atrophy. Ganciclovir is incorporated into both viral and cellular DNA; it has both carcinogenic and teratogenic potential.[52]

Because of toxicity, the use of ganciclovir has been limited to life-threatening or sight-threatening cytomegalovirus infections. Unfortunately, the disease frequently recurs once the drug is discontinued, and prolonged maintenance therapy is necessary for controlling the disease. Ganciclovir has been approved in the United States for the treatment of sight-threatening cytomegalovirus retinitis in immunocompromised patients. All other uses of ganciclovir remain investigational. Experience with the use of ganciclovir in children is limited.[53]

TREATMENT OF HERPES SIMPLEX VIRUS INFECTIONS

Herpes simplex virus is a rare cause of disease of the lower respiratory tract. Tracheobronchitis and pneumonia are occasionally seen in immunocompromised patients such as transplant recipients and AIDS patients.[54] Pneumonia is more often seen in neonates as a feature of disseminated herpes simplex virus infection. Acyclovir is the drug of choice for treating most infections resulting from herpes simplex virus, including infection of immunocompromised hosts, and has been shown to be superior to vidarabine in the treatment of herpes encephalitis.[55] Pneumonia resulting from herpes simplex virus should be treated with intravenous acyclovir in a dose of 30 mg/kg/day in three divided doses. Oral acyclovir is not appropriate for the treatment of a life-threatening infection such as herpes pneumonia. Parenteral acyclovir in a dose of 15 mg/kg/day can be used for the treatment of mucocutaneous herpes in immunocompromised children. Oral therapy (200 mg five times per day), although not yet approved for use in children, can be considered for mild mucocutaneous disease in immunocompromised children.

Vidarabine is effective in the treatment of disseminated neonatal herpes simplex virus infection in neonates.[56] Surprisingly, acyclovir has not been shown to be superior to vidarabine in this disease;[57] therefore, either can be used. Vidarabine is administered as a single 12-h infusion per day in a dose of 30 mg/kg/day for 10 to 21 days. Acyclovir is administered three times per day at 30 mg/kg/day for 10 to 21 days.

TREATMENT OF VARICELLA-ZOSTER VIRUS INFECTIONS

Varicella pneumonia is most often seen in immunosuppressed patients with primary varicella-zoster virus infection, although it does occur in normal hosts as well. In immunosuppressed hosts with primary varicella, vidarabine decreases the incidence of visceral dissemination from 55% to 5%, with a reduction in mortality rates from 15% to 0%.[58] Acyclovir has been shown to have a similar efficacy.[59] In immunosuppressed patients, the risk of dissemination is lower with recurrent disease (herpes zoster) than with primary infection (varicella). Both vidarabine and acyclovir have been shown to halt progression of herpes zoster in immunosuppressed patients.[60, 61] When compared directly in severely immunosuppressed patients with varicella-zoster infections, acyclovir was superior to vidarabine in preventing cutaneous dissemination and speeding of healing.[62] Immunosuppressed patients with varicella-zoster virus infections should be treated with acyclovir in a dose of 1500 mg/sq m/day in three divided doses. There is generally no reason to treat varicella in normal children. In children with symptomatic pneumonia, parenteral acyclovir should be considered; oral acyclovir has not been shown to be effective in treating pneumonia and should not be used.

TREATMENT OF CYTOMEGALOVIRUS PNEUMONIA

Cytomegalovirus pneumonia has a high mortality in immunosuppressed patients, such as transplant recipients and patients with AIDS. Treatment with a variety of antiviral agents, including vidarabine, acyclovir, interferons, and foscarnet, has been unsuccessful. Preliminary uncontrolled studies with ganciclovir suggest that it may have a role in the treatment of life-threatening cytomegalovirus pneumonia in immunosuppressed patients, including recipients of kidney, heart, and liver transplants.[63-67] The results of treating cytomegalovirus pneumonia with ganciclovir in bone marrow transplant patients remain extremely poor.[68] However, the use of hyperimmune anticytomegalovirus immunoglobulin in combination with ganciclovir in bone marrow transplant patients appears to offer some promise.[69] Controlled trials of ganciclovir and immunoglobulin for the treatment of cytomegalovirus pneumonia are needed.

The early initiation of ganciclovir therapy in high-risk patients with subclavial cytomegalovirus disease may offer the best promise for the treatment of this highly lethal disease.[70, 71]

Antiviral therapy has not been shown to benefit infants with a congenital cytomegalovirus infection. Clinical trials of ganciclovir for the treatment of congenital cytomegalovirus are currently under way.

The ability to prevent cytomegalovirus infection in transplant recipients would result in a major reduction in morbidity and mortality rates. Two approaches have been used: immunoprophylaxis and chemoprophylaxis. Cytomegalovirus immunoglobulin has been shown to prevent cytomegalovirus disease in seronegative recipients of seropositive kidneys.[72] Unfortunately, in bone marrow transplant patients, the efficacy of passive immunoprophylaxis has not been clearly demonstrated.[73] Although not effective in treating cytomegalovirus, acyclovir appears to be effective in preventing infection. In bone marrow allograft recipients seropositive for cytomegalovirus, intravenous acyclovir prevents both infection and disease caused by reactivation of latent virus.[74] Acyclovir was administered from 5 days before transplantation until 31 days after transplantation in this study. Children who are seronegative for cytomegalovirus and who receive a transplant from a seropositive donor should receive acyclovir prophylaxis.

TREATMENT OF HUMAN IMMUNODEFICIENCY VIRUS INFECTIONS

Pulmonary disease in children with HIV infection may manifest as an opportunistic infection or lymphoid interstitial pneumonitis (LIP), a lymphocytic infiltration of the lung.[75] It is unclear whether LIP results from infection of the lung with HIV, Epstein-Barr virus, or a combination of the two. The genome of both of these viruses has been found in the lungs of children with LIP.[76, 77]

Zidovudine (formally known as azidodeoxythymidine [AZT]) is the drug of choice for the treatment of HIV infections.[78] Limited data with the use of zidovudine in children suggest that treatment may result in weight gain, resolution of organomegaly and lymphadenopathy, and an increase in the well-being of the child. Improvement of neurologic abnormalities has been seen with the administration of zidovudine by continuous infusion.[79] It is suggested that LIP may respond to zidovudine therapy.[80] However, steroids are currently the treatment of choice for children with symptomatic LIP.[81] Clinical trials of zidovudine in children with symptomatic HIV infections are currently under way. Toxicity of zidovudine consists mainly of anemia, neutropenia, and thrombocytopenia.

PROSPECTS FOR THE FUTURE

The age of effective antiviral therapy is still in its infancy, and major advances can be expected in the next several years. The number of new antiviral drugs being developed and tested will continue to increase, and agents for treating infections such as cytomegalovirus pneumonia, for which there is no satisfactory therapy at present will become available. The problem of the emergence of viruses resistant to agents currently in use will be solved with the development of new agents with different mechanisms of action. Combination antiviral therapy, an approach well established in antibacterial therapy, will become increasingly common in order to improve efficacy and to prevent the development of resistant virus. At present, clinical trials of combinations of agents for the treatment of HIV infection are under way. Antiviral agents will also be combined with biologic response modifiers, such as interferons, in order to boost the immune response of the hosts.

REFERENCES

1. Davies WL, Grunert RR, Hall RF, et al: Antiviral activity of 1-adamantanamine (amantadine). Science 144:862–863, 1964.
2. Oxford JS, Galbraith A: Antiviral activity of amantadine: A review of laboratory and clinical data. Pharmacol Ther 11:181–262, 1980.
3. Aoki FY, Sitar DS: Clinical pharmacokinetics of amantadine hydrochloride. Clin Pharmacokinet 14:35–51, 1988.
4. Hayden FG, Gwaltney JM, Van de Castle RL, et al: Comparative toxicity of amantadine hydrochloride and rimantadine hydrochloride in healthy adults. Antimicrob Agents Chemother 19:226–233, 1981.
5. Bektimirov TA, Douglas RG, Dolin R, et al: Current status of amantadine and rimantadine as anti-influenza-A agents. Bull WHO 63:51–54, 1985.
6. Dolin R, Reichman RC, Madore HP, et al: A controlled trial of amantadine and rimantadine in the prophylaxis of influenza A infection. N Engl J Med 307:580–584, 1982.
7. Smorodintsev AA, Karpuhin GI, Zlydnikov DM, et al: The prospect of amantadine for prevention of influenza A2 in humans: Effectiveness of amantadine during influenza A2/Hong Kong epidemic of January-February, 1969 in Leningrad. Ann NY Acad Sci 173:44–61, 1970.
8. Payler DK, Purdham PA: Influenza A prophylaxis with amantadine in a boarding school. Lancet 1:502–504, 1984.
9. La Montagne JR, Galasso GJ: Report of a workshop on clinical studies of the efficacy of amantadine and rimantadine against influenza virus. J Infect Dis 138:928–931, 1978.
10. Clover RD, Crawford SA, Abell TD, et al: Effectiveness of rimantadine prophylaxis of children within families. Am J Dis Child 140:706–709, 1986.
11. Crawford SA, Clover RD, Abell TD, et al: Rimantadine prophylaxis in children: A follow-up study. Pediatr Infect Dis J 7:379–383, 1988.
12. Sears SD, Clements ML: Protective efficacy of low-dose amantadine in adults challenged with wild-type influenza A virus. Antimicrob Agents Chemother 31:1470–1473, 1987.
13. Van Voris LP, Betts RF, Hayden FG, et al: Successful treatment of naturally occurring influenza A/USSR/77 H1N1. JAMA 245:1128–1131, 1981.
14. Younkin SW, Betts RF, Roth FK, et al: Reduction in fever and symptoms in young adults with influenza A/Brazil/78 H1N1 infection after treatment with aspirin or amantadine. Antimicrob Agents Chemother 23:577–582, 1983.
15. Hall CG, Dolin R, Gala CL, et al: Children with influenza A infection: Treatment with rimantadine. Pediatrics 80:275–282, 1987.
16. Thompson J, Fleet W, Lawrence E, et al: A comparison of acetaminophen and rimantadine in the treatment of influenza A infection in children. J Med Virol 21:249–255, 1987.
17. Mast EE, Davis JP, Harmon MW, et al: Emergence and possible transmission of amantadine-resistant viruses during nursing home outbreaks of influenza A (H3N2). [abstract no. 65]. In Program and Abstracts of the 29th Interscience Conference on Antimicrobial Agents and Chemotherapy, Sept. 18, 1989, Houston, p. 111. Washington, DC: American Society for Microbiology, 1989.
18. Belshe RB, Smith MH, Hall CB, et al: Genetic basis of resistance to rimantadine emerging during treatment of influenza virus infection. J Virol 62:1508–1512, 1988.
19. Hayden FG, Belshe RB, Clover RD, et al: Emergence and apparent transmission of rimantadine-resistant influenza A virus in families. N Engl J Med 321:1696–1702, 1989.
20. Hayden FG, Hall WJ, Douglas RG: Therapeutic effects of aerosolized amantadine in naturally acquired infection due to influenza A virus. J Infect Dis 141:535–542, 1980.
21. Immunization Practices Advisory Committee: Prevention and control of influenza: Part 1. Vaccines. MMWR 38:297–311, 1989.
22. Committee on Infectious Diseases, American Academy of Pediatrics: Report of the Committee on Infectious Diseases. Elk Grove Village, IL: American Academy of Pediatrics, 1988.
23. Centers for Disease Control: Prevention and control of influenza: Recommendations of the Immunization Practices Advisory Committee. MMWR 41(No. RR-9):1–17, 1992.
24. Advisory Committee on Immunization Practices: Prevention and control of influenza. MMWR 37:361–373, 1988.
25. Knight V, McClung HW, Wilson SZ, et al: Ribavirin small-particle aerosol treatment of influenza. Lancet 2:945–949, 1981.
26. McClung HW, Knight V, Gilbert BE, et al: Ribavirin aerosol treatment of influenza B viral infection. JAMA 249:2671–2674, 1983.
27. Wilson SZ, Gilbert BE, Quarles JM, et al: Treatment of Influenza A (H1N1) virus infection with ribavirin aerosol. Antimicrob Agents Chemother 26:200–203, 1984.

28. McCormick JB, King IJ, Webb PA, et al: Lassa fever: Effective therapy with ribavirin. N Engl J Med 314:20–26, 1986.
29. Gilbert BE, Knight V: Biochemistry and clinical applications of ribavirin. Antimicrob Agents Chemother 30:201–205, 1986.
30. Connor JD, Hintz M, Van Dyke R, et al: Ribavirin pharmacokinetics in children and adults during therapeutic trials. In Smith RA, Knight V, Smith JAD (eds): Clinical Applications of Ribavirin, pp. 107–123. New York: Academic Press, 1984.
31. Catlin DH, Smith RA, Samuels AI: 14C-ribavirin: Distribution and pharmacokinetic studies in rats, baboons, and man. In Smith RA, Kirkpatrick W (eds): Ribavirin: A Broad Spectrum Antiviral Agent, pp. 83–98. New York: Academic Press, 1980.
32. Light B, Aoki FY, Serrette C: Tolerance of ribavirin aerosol inhaled by normal volunteers and patients with chronic obstructive airways disease. In Smith RA, Knight V, Smith JAD (eds): The Clinical Applications of Ribavirin, pp. 97–105. New York: Academic Press, 1984.
33. Hillyard IW: The pre-clinical toxicology and safety of ribavirin. In Smith RA, Kirkpatrick W (eds): Ribavirin: A Broad Spectrum Antiviral Agent, pp. 59–71. New York: Academic Press, 1980.
34. Centers for Disease Control: Assessing exposures of health-care personnel to aerosols of ribavirin—California. MMWR 37:560–563, 1988.
35. Rodriguez WJ, Bui RH, Connor JD, et al: Environmental exposure of primary care personnel to ribavirin aerosol when supervising treatment of infants with respiratory syncytial virus infections. Antimicrob Agents Chemother 31:1143–1146, 1987.
36. Hall CB, McBride JT, Walsh EE, et al: Aerosolized ribavirin treatment of infants with respiratory syncytial viral infection: A randomized double-blind study. N Engl J Med 308:1443–1447, 1983.
37. Taber LH, Knight V, Gilbert BE, et al: Ribavirin aerosol treatment of bronchiolitis associated with respiratory syncytial virus infection in infants. Pediatrics 72:613–618, 1983.
38. Hall CB, McBride JT, Gala CL, et al: Ribavirin treatment of respiratory syncytial viral infection in infants with underlying cardiopulmonary disease. JAMA 254:3047–3051, 1985.
39. Barry W, Cockburn F, Cornall R, et al: Ribavirin aerosol for acute bronchiolitis. Arch Dis Child 61:593–597, 1986.
40. Rodriguez WJ, Kim HW, Brandt CD, et al: Aerosolized ribavirin in the treatment of patients with respiratory syncytial virus disease. Pediatr Infect Dis J 6:159–163, 1987.
41. Conrad DA, Christenson JC, Waner JL, Marks MI: Aerosolized ribavirin treatment of respiratory syncytial virus infection in infants hospitalized during an epidemic. Pediatr Infect Dis J 6:152–158, 1987.
42. Wald ER, Dashefsky B, Green M: In re ribavirin: A case of premature adjudication? J Pediatr 112:154–158, 1988.
43. Ray CG: Ribavirin: Ambivalence about an antiviral agent. Am J Dis Child 142:488–489, 1988.
44. Smith DW, Frankel LR, Mathers LH, et al: A controlled trial of aerosolized ribavirin in infants receiving mechanical ventilation for severe respiratory syncytial virus infection. N Engl J Med 325:24–29, 1991.
45. Frankel LR, Wilson CW, Demers RR, et al: A technique for the administration of ribavirin to mechanically ventilated infants with severe respiratory syncytial virus infection. Crit Care Med 15:1051–1054, 1987.
46. Outwater KM, Meissner HC, Peterson MB: Ribavirin administration to infants receiving mechanical ventilation. Am J Dis Child 142:512–515, 1988.
47. American Academy of Pediatrics Committee on Infectious Diseases: Ribavirin therapy of respiratory syncytial virus. Pediatrics 79:475–478, 1987.
48. Hayden FG, Albrecht JK, Kaiser DL, et al: Prevention of natural colds with contact prophylaxis with intranasal alpha-2-interferon. N Engl J Med 314:71–75, 1986.
49. Erlich KS, Mills J, Chatis P, et al: Acyclovir-resistant herpes simplex virus infections in patients with the acquired immunodeficiency syndrome. N Engl J Med 320:293–296, 1989.
50. Chatis PA, Miller CH, Schrager LE, Crumpacker CS: Successful treatment with foscarnet of an acyclovir-resistant mucocutaneous infection with herpes simplex virus in a patient with acquired immunodeficiency syndrome. N Engl J Med 320:297–300, 1989.
51. Safrin S, Crumpacker C, Chatis P, et al: A controlled trial comparing foscarnet with vidarabine for acyclovir-resistant mucocutaneous herpes simplex in the acquired immunodeficiency syndrome. N Engl J Med 325:551–555, 1991.
52. Fletcher CV, Balfour HH: Evaluation of ganciclovir for cytomegalovirus disease. DICP 23:5–12, 1989.
53. Gudnason T, Belani KK, Balfour HH Jr: Ganciclovir treatment of cytomegalovirus disease in immunocompromised children. Pediatr Infect Dis J 8:436–440, 1989.
54. Ramsey PG, Fife KH, Hackman RC, et al: Herpes simplex virus pneumonia: Clinical, virologic, and pathologic features in 20 patients. Ann Intern Med 97:813–820, 1982.
55. Whitley RJ, Alford CA, Hirsch MS, et al: Vidarabine versus acyclovir therapy in herpes simplex encephalitis. N Engl J Med 314:144–149, 1986.
56. Whitley RJ, Nahmias AJ, Soong SJ, et al: Vidarabine therapy of neonatal herpes simplex virus infection. Pediatrics 66:495–501, 1980.
57. Whitley R, Arvin A, Prober C, et al: A controlled trial comparing vidarabine with acyclovir in neonatal herpes simplex virus infection. N Engl J Med 324:444–449, 1991.
58. Whitley R, Hilty M, Haynes R, et al: Vidarabine therapy of varicella in immunosuppressed patients. J Pediatr 101:125–131, 1982.
59. Prober CG, Kirk LE, Keeney RE: Acyclovir therapy of chickenpox in immunosuppressed children. A collaborative study. J Pediatr 101:622–625, 1982.
60. Whitley RJ, Ch'ien LT, Dolin R, et al: Adenine arabinoside therapy of herpes zoster in the immunosuppressed. N Engl J Med 294:1193–1199, 1976.
61. Balfour HH Jr, Bean B, Laskin O, et al: Acyclovir halts progression of herpes zoster in immunocompromised patients. N Engl J Med 308:1448–1453, 1983.
62. Shepp DH, Dandliker PS, Meyer JD: Treatment of varicella-zoster virus infection in severely immunocompromised patients: A randomized comparison of acyclovir and vidarabine. N Engl J Med 314:208–212, 1986.
63. Collaborative DHPG Treatment Study Group: Treatment of serious cytomegalovirus infections with 9-(1,3-dihydroxy-2-propoxymethyl)guanine in patients with AIDS and other immunodeficiencies. N Engl J Med 314:801–805, 1986.
64. Laskin OL, Cederberg DM, Mills J, et al: Ganciclovir for the treatment and suppression of serious infections caused by cytomegalovirus. Am J Med 83:201–207, 1987.
65. Hecht DW, Snydman DR, Crumpacker CS, et al: Ganciclovir for treatment of renal transplant-associated primary cytomegalovirus pneumonia. J Infect Dis 157:187–190, 1988.
66. Keay S, Bissett J, Merigan TC: Ganciclovir treatment of cytomegalovirus infections in iatrogenically immunocompromised patients. J Infect Dis 156:1016–1021, 1987.
67. Maj M, Jery J, Sutker W, et al: DHPG (ganciclovir) improves survival in CMV pneumonia. Transplant Proc 21:2263–2265, 1989.
68. Shepp DH, Dandliker PS, de Miranda P, et al: Activity of 9-[2-hydroxy-1-(hydroxymethyl) ethoxymethyl] guanine in the treatment of cytomegalovirus pneumonia. Ann Intern Med 103:368–373, 1985.
69. Reed EC, Bowden RA, Dandliker PS, et al: Treatment of cytomegalovirus pneumonia with ganciclovir and intravenous cytomegalovirus immunoglobulin in patients with bone marrow transplants. Ann Intern Med 109:783–788, 1988.
70. Goodrich JM, Mori M, Gleaves CA, et al: Early treatment with ganciclovir to prevent cytomegalovirus disease after allogeneic bone marrow transplantation. N Engl J Med 325:1601–1607, 1991.
71. Schmidt GM, Horak DA, Niland JC, et al: A randomized, controlled trial of prophylactic ganciclovir for cytomegalovirus pulmonary infection in recipients of allogeneic bone marrow transplants. N Engl J Med 324:1005–1011, 1991.
72. Snydman DR, Werner BG, Heinze-Lacy B, et al: Use of cytomegalovirus immune globulin to prevent cytomegalovirus disease in renal-transplant recipients. N Engl J Med 317:1049–1054, 1987.
73. Meyers JD: Prevention of cytomegalovirus infection after marrow transplantation. Rev Infect Dis 11(Suppl. 7):S1691–S1705, 1989.
74. Meyers JD, Reed EC, Shepp DH, et al: Acyclovir for prevention of cytomegalovirus infection and disease after allogeneic marrow transplantation. N Engl J Med 318:70–75, 1988.

75. Rubinstein A, Morecki R, Silverman B, et al: Pulmonary disease in children with acquired immune deficiency syndrome and AIDS-related complex. J Pediatr 108:498–503, 1986.

76. Andiman WA, Eastman R, Martin K, et al: Opportunistic lymphoproliferations associated with Epstein-Barr viral DNA in infants and children with AIDS. Lancet 2:1390–1393, 1985.

77. Chayt KJ, Harper ME, Marselle LM, et al: Detection of HTLV-III RNA in lungs of patients with AIDS and pulmonary involvement. JAMA 256:2356–2359, 1986.

78. Fischl MA, Richman DD, Greico MH, et al: The efficacy of azidothymidine [AZT] in the treatment of patients with AIDS and AIDS-related complex. N Engl J Med 317:185–191, 1987.

79. Pizzo PA, Eddy J, Falloon J, et al: Effect of continuous intravenous infusion of zidovudine (AZT) in children with symptomatic HIV infection. N Engl J Med 319:889–896, 1988.

80. Epps SC, Wilfert CM, Weinhold KJ, et al: Improvement of lymphoid interstitial pneumonitis in a child treated with azidothymidine [Abstract no. THP 234]. Presented at the 3rd International conference on AIDS, Washington, DC, June 1987.

81. Rubinstein A: Pediatric AIDS. Curr Probl Pediatr 16:361–409, 1986.

84 ENVIRONMENTAL CONTROL AS A MODALITY OF MANAGEMENT FOR THE PULMONARY PATIENT

HERBERT C. MANSMANN, JR., M.D.

The need to modify the environment is based on the long-recognized fact that the environment often affects the health of humans. Physicians concerned with children and their environment have the unique opportunity to influence the future of the human race by studying air pollutants and communicating these concerns to the patients and their parents. Although a comprehensive review of the nature of indoor allergens and air pollutants is beyond the scope of this chapter, it is necessary for clinicians to appreciate the magnitude of the problem and to know how to remove allergens and pollutants from a patient's environment. There are many satisfactory reviews of the characteristics of indoor allergens,[1–3] including house dust mite (HDM)[4] and domestic cat allergens.[5] These reviews help to provide an appreciation of the immunochemical and technologic advances to aid in the diagnosis and evaluation of the various avoidance treatment modalities. There are also several reviews on indoor and outdoor air pollution.[6–11]

Unfortunately, convincing data on the use of immunochemical techniques are not available for measuring specific pollutants or induced antibodies to them. Since 1980, there have been dramatic advances in the management of the environment of allergic asthmatic patients. These methods, in addition to an increased understanding of nonspecific bronchial hyperreactivity, make environmental control a necessary modality of care that should be appreciated by all physicians who manage pediatric pulmonary patients.

INDOOR INHALANT ALLERGENS

Although many substances are known to induce allergic symptoms in susceptible atopic patients, only a few of these are discussed in this chapter.

HOUSE DUST MITE

The common HDM, *Dermatophagoides* species, is a common environmental allergen; the HDM causes considerable distress to patients who have developed a hypersensitivity to mite allergens. It has been proposed that a concentration of 2 μg of group I mite allergens (*D. pteronyssimus* and *D. farinae*) per gram of dust (equivalent to 100 mites per gram of dust) should be considered a risk factor for sensitization and the development of allergic asthma.[12] A concentration of 10 μg of mite allergen (equivalent to 500 mites) per gram of dust is considered a risk factor for the precipitation of acute allergic asthma in mite-allergic patients.[4, 13] In a study of allergic asthma in mite-sensitive patients, the mean level of mite allergen in the patients' homes was 13.6 μg/g of dust, whereas the concentration in hospital rooms (where the patients were improving) was only 0.2 μg/g of dust.[4] The prevalence of asthma at high altitude is only half that at sea level. Interestingly, the proportion of patients with a positive skin test for HDM allergen and who live at high altitude is only 10.2%, in comparison with 27.5% for those at sea level ($p < .001$).

Children with HDM-sensitive asthma enrolled in a crossover randomized trial in which the mattresses on their beds were covered with impervious plastic bags and new pillows and blankets were provided; these environmental modifications resulted in only modest clinical improvement but statistically significant improvement in peak expiratory flow rate after 1 month.[14] It must be remembered that although living rooms contain fewer mites than bedroom dust, small children often sleep and play in family rooms or living rooms with rugs, a common source of HDMs.[15]

CAT

Approximately 25% of American homes have at least one cat. It has been estimated that approximately 6 million Americans have positive skin tests for cat allergen (Fel d I).[16] The presence of serum immunoglobulin E (IgE) antibodies to cat allergen has been demonstrated to be a significant risk factor for acute attacks of asthma that result in visits to an emergency room.[12] Ten to sixty percent of airborne cat allergen in houses is in the form of particles 2.5 μm or less in diameter, which thus remain airborne for many hours after disturbance.[5] Although cat allergen has long been recognized in cat saliva, it has been demonstrated that the skin of cats is also an important source of cat allergen.[17]

VEGETABLE GUM

Vegetable gums have been known for years as important occupational allergens. Gums are used as a sizing material for paper products and textiles. Acacia gum is used in the printing industry. Karaya and tragacanth gums are used by hairdressers. Gums are present in many foods such as salad dressings, soups, ice cream, preserved foods, cheese products, and baby food. They are used in the pharmaceutical industry in emulsions, lotions, and creams. Guar gum is used in carpet manufacturing to bind colors to rug fibers[18] and must be considered a potential allergen for children who play on living room rugs. Symptomatic patients often improve after new rugs have been cleaned with carpet-cleaning machines with liquids; this cleaning procedure apparently removes the unbound guar gum from the carpet.

AIR POLLUTANTS

Although it is almost impossible to avoid most irritants all of the time, the exposure can be significantly reduced by awareness of some of the common triggers of asthma (Table 84–1). It is also likely that these nonspecific factors may be important for many patients with bronchial hyperreactivity, regardless of the cause. Typical sources of air-pollution exposure for children are shown in Table 84–2. Three of the air pollutants are discussed in more detail. Occupational exposure can be a potential cause of exacerbation of asthma. Assessment of occupational exposure as a potential cause or exacerbation of respiratory symptoms should be considered for all adolescents who work.[19–22]

NITROGEN DIOXIDE

Nitrogen oxides come from so-called clean-burning appliances such as gas ranges. About 60% of American homes use gas, for example, for cooking and heating, and vent flues from gas furnaces, clothes dryers, and space heaters should be checked frequently to ensure adequate ventilation. Unvented kerosene space heaters should be used only in emergencies. Cigarette smoke contributes to the levels of nitrogen oxides;[23] 4.0 parts per million (ppm) of nitrogen dioxide produces bronchoalveolar evidence of inflammation.[24] Because inhalation of 0.30 ppm of nitrogen dioxide can potentiate exercise-induced asthma, it is likely that this level could induce bronchial hyperreactivity.[25] It has been shown that short-term, low-level nitrogen dioxide inhalation by asthmatic patients caused a significant increase ($p < .001$) in specific airway resistance.[26]

SULFUR DIOXIDE

Asthmatic patients have marked symptomatic bronchoconstriction if the atmospheric concentration of sulfur dioxide approaches 1 ppm, even though this concentration does not appear to affect normal airways.[27] Results of one study have suggested that prolonged exposure to low levels of atmospheric sulfur dioxide is associated with childhood asthma and bronchial hyperreactivity.[28] These effects are greatly potentiated by exercise at concentrations higher than 0.4 ppm, whereby asthma occurs after as brief an exposure as 2 min.[29, 30] This concentration can be achieved in homes heated with kerosene space heaters. Current Occupational Safety and Health Administration regulations permit exposure of up to 5 ppm in the workplace as a time-weighted average during an 8-h work shift.

OZONE

Ozone is produced by the incomplete combustion of hydrocarbons. Although a layer of ozone high in the earth's atmosphere is important as a filter for intense ultraviolet rays from the sun, the product itself is considered an atmospheric pollutant at lower altitudes. Normal subjects have significant decreases in forced vital capacity and forced expiratory volume in 1 sec (FEV_1) with continuous heavy exercise[31] after 1 h of exposure to ozone (0.21 ppm). All subjects reported symptoms of pharyngeal and tracheal irritation, cough, throat soreness, and wheezing on deep inspiration. Acute low-dose exposure to ozone has been shown to induce bronchial hyperreactivity in both normal and asthmatic subjects, equal to that seen with methacholine and histamine.[32] Ozone concentrations from 0.03 to 0.3 ppm have been correlated with the inability of some runners to improve their running times.[33]

Table 84-1. SOME COMMON CAUSES OR TRIGGERS (PRECIPITATORS) OF
RESPIRATORY SYMPTOMS

Fumes

Traffic odors	Garage	Motorboat	Gasoline stations
Fuel oil	Oil furnace	Lighter fluid	Bus stations
Refineries	Machinery	Kerosene	Dry-cleaners

Smokes

Charcoal	Tobacco	Trash fire	Fireplace
Incense	Leaf fire	Wood fire	Coal smoke
Cigarette	Cigar	Pipe	

Wood Products

Lumber	Sawdust	Sanding dust	Christmas tree
Evergreen			

Paint Odors

Lacquer	Shellac	Enamel	Varnish
Paint remover	Stains	Color set	Spray paint
Oil paint	Latex paint	Thinner	

Household Products

Bleaches	Starch	Toilet soap	Shoe polish
Detergents	Bubble bath	Soap powder	Furniture polish
Dyes	Ammonia	Floor wax	Lysol
Chalk	Cedar bags	Cedar closet	Room deodorants
Coarse paper	Magazines	Paper tissue	Newspaper
Perfumes	Glue	Insect sprays	Mops and solutions
Fabrics (wash and wear)	Silk	Moth-balls (crystals)	Fabric softener (Bounce)
Cleaners (especially those containing carbon tetrachloride)			

Cosmetics

Face powder	Face creams	Shampoos	Nail polish
Deodorants	Hair sprays	Rouge	Hair-waving materials
Sachets	Antiseptics	Shaving cream	Rubbing alcohol
Bath powder	Astringents	Mouthwashes	Nail polish remover
Perfume	Cologne	After-shave lotion	

Office and Industry

Ink	Stencils	Paper	Various chemicals
Asphalt	Metal shops	Tar	Carbon paper
Smoke	Paints	Mill dust	Typewriter ribbon
Duplicators	Formaldehyde	Perfumes	Photographic materials
Rubber goods (tires, sheeting, hose, etc.)			Warehouse dusts
Fumes from galvanizing plant			
Sulfuric acid and hydrochloric acid fumes			

Food Smells

Coffee	Onion	Beans	Frying odors
Beer	Flour	Starch	Vinegar
Spices	Egg	Fish	

BENEFITS OF ENVIRONMENTAL CONTROL

The primary aim of environmental control in respiratory disease is to break the vicious cycle of the induction, enhancement, and incitement of bronchial hyperresponsiveness. The prevention of the induction of specific IgE-mediated sensitization would be an ideal prophylactic measure. Most induction occurs before the manifestation of symptoms. The enhancement and incitement of bronchial hyperreactivity are the consequences of recurrent or continuous exposure to allergen, air pollutants, and some infections.

A large number of asthmatic children have immediate hypersensitivity to common allergens. This has been demonstrated by the presence of significantly higher allergen-specific IgE titers than in nonasthmatic subjects and by an increase in allergen-specific and nonspecific bronchial hyperreactivity. Marked improvement in symptoms and a reduction in bronchial hyperreactivity have been demonstrated by prolonged periods of avoidance of specific allergen (Table 84-3). Increased hyperreactivity is seen after 2 weeks of intense pollen exposure.[34]

Two months or more of hospitalization of HDM-sensitive asthmatic adults resulted in clinical improvement in eight of nine subjects.[35] At the end of the study, two of

Table 84-2. TYPICAL SOURCES OF AIR-POLLUTION EXPOSURE OF CHILDREN

Source	Home	School	Transportation (School Bus/ Automobile)
Tobacco Smoke			
CO	+	+	+
VOC	+	+	+
Building Materials			
Formaldehyde	+	+	±
Radon	+	+	o
Furnishings			
VOC	+	+	+
Formaldehyde	+	+	±
Insulations			
Asbestos	+	+	o
Air Conditioning			
Biologic agents	+	+	+
Heating Systems			
Gas stoves			
CO	+	+	o
NO₂	+	+	o
Kerosene stoves			
CO	+	±	o
NO₂	+	±	o
SO₂	+	±	o
Wood-burning stoves/ fireplace			
CO	+	±	o
PAH	+	±	o
Copying Machines			
VOC	+	+	o
Automobile			
CO	±	±	+
NO₂	±	±	+
VOC	±	±	+
Ozone	+	+	+

Modified from Samet JM, Marbury MC, Spengler JD: Health effects and sources of indoor air pollution. Part 1. Am Rev Respir Dis 136:1486–1508, 1987.

+, present; ±, equivocal; o, none. CO, carbon monoxide; VOC, volatile organic compounds; NO₂, nitrous dioxide; SO₂, sulfur dioxide; PAH, polycyclic aromatic hydrocarbons.

the eight were off all medication, five were receiving low-dose albuterol (salbutamol), and only two required inhaled corticosteroids. Five patients had progressive improvement over 6 to 16 weeks, and their bronchial provocation with histamine showed an eightfold or greater increase in the provocation dose, causing a 30% drop in FEV₁. In a 6-week study of HDM-sensitive asthmatic children in British Columbia, 10 controls were compared with 10 subjects who used zippered vinyl cov-

ers on pillows, mattresses, and box springs and received instructions on cleaning the bedroom. There were marked differences between the groups in subjective as well as objective asthma. The experimental subjects experienced statistical improvement in the number of days of wheezing, the use of medications, and peak expiratory flow rates.[36]

METHODS OF ENVIRONMENTAL CONTROL

Indoor air in the home can be modified in a number of ways to reduce the concentration of allergens or pollutants. Some of these ways are listed in Table 84-4. Control of outdoor air pollution or pollutants in the work environment is a far more complex problem. At present, the only way of dealing with a smog alert is to stay inside, and the only way of avoiding occupational pollutants is to change the working area. Some specific means of cleaning indoor air in the home are discussed next.

HOUSE DUST MITE MEASURES

All methods of reducing the number of mites in the bedroom include sealing the pillows, mattresses, and box springs in an impervious material such as a plastic or rubberized fabric. It has been shown that increasing the temperature of the bedding by keeping an electric blanket on at all times significantly reduces HDM concentrations.[37] Acrosan is a powder applied to upholstered furniture and carpets that has been demonstrated to remove a large percentage of HDM and their larvae. Other acaricidal chemicals have been used in Europe, but little information is available about the safety and efficacy of these products. All chemicals used in the home must be free of side effects such as primary toxicity, skin and eye irritation, and delayed-contact hypersensitivity. They also must be shown to be free of the potential to induce asthma, malignancies, or genetic defects.[38]

Once killed, the HDM products must be removed from the house. In one review of residential air-cleaning devices the investigators were unable to recommend any indications for their effective use.[39] Other reports have been more optimistic.[5] In any event, there are no substitutes for good hygiene and other measures such as HDM precautions (Table 84-5).

Table 84-3. AVOIDANCE RESULTS IN DECREASED BRONCHIAL HYPERREACTIVITY

Study	Year	Allergen	Avoidance	Provocator
Altounyan[50]	1970	Grass*	Postseason	Histamine
Kerrebijn[51]	1970	HDM†	High-altitude sanatorium	Histamine
Chan-Yeung[52]	1977	WRC‡	Change occupation	Methacholine
Cartier et al.[53]	1980	Ragweed*	Postseason	Methacholine
Platts-Mills[35]	1982	HDM	Hospitalization 6–16 weeks	Histamine
Murray and Furguson[36]	1983	HDM	Pillow, mattress, and box spring covers for 1 month	Histamine
Dorwood et al.[54]	1988	HDM	Liquid nitrogen	Histamine

*Pollen. †HDM, house dust mite. ‡WRC, western red cedar sawdust.

Table 84–4. MODALITIES FOR MODIFYING THE INDOOR ENVIRONMENT

Air Cleaners

Electrostatic: Small particles pass between charged plates and are removed with an electric spark. The grids can be washed repeatedly, and the devices are very efficient. Sometimes arcing can be associated with the distinct smell of ozone.

High-efficiency particulate air-filter systems (HEPA): Particles pass through a space-age filter. The filter becomes more efficient as particles build up but eventually has to be replaced. Efficiency of up to 99% of particles has been claimed.

Water impingement: These devices, usually less expensive than the two just mentioned, pass the air stream through water. Although the water becomes very dirty, this is not as efficient as the electrostatic or HEPA method.

Containment Methods

Mattresses and pillows can be enclosed in zippered bags made of plastic with the zipper sealed with duct tape. A more expensive but more comfortable product is made of rubberized fabric.

Miticides and Fungicides

There are a number of sprays marketed to reduce dust, mold, and mites. More information can be obtained about these from the sources listed below.

Avoidance

No smoking should be permitted in the house or automobile at any time.

Resources

More information about these methods can be obtained from the following sources:

American Academy of Allergy
611 E. Wells St.
Milwaukee, WI 53202
(414) 272-6071
Information hotline: 1-800-822-ASMA

Allergy and Asthma Foundation of America
1717 Massachusetts Ave., Suite 305
Washington, DC 20036
(202) 265-0265
Information hotline: 1-800-7-ASTHMA

Mothers of Asthmatics, Inc.
19875 Main St., Suite 210
Fairfax, VA 22030
(703) 385-4403

Table 84–5. BEDROOM HOUSE DUST MITE ELIMINATION

1. Encase mattress and box spring in plastic or with a more comfortable fabric from a special company; the zipper should be sealed with adhesive tape
2. Pillows must be made of synthetic fiber and encased or washed monthly in very hot water; replace yearly
3. All bedding must be washed in very hot water ($>54°C$) every 7–10 days (caution: water at this temperature can scald children)
4. Feather-, kapok-, and silk-filled pillows, sleeping bags, and quilts must be avoided
5. Replace carpets with polished flooring

PHILOSOPHY OF ENVIRONMENTAL CONTROL MEASURES

PATIENT COMPLIANCE, EDUCATION, AND MOTIVATION

Physicians cannot successfully influence their patients to be compliant for a specific task unless they themselves become adequately informed, have a positive attitude, and are able to communicate this information and attitude to their patients. Compliance requires education about removing the common allergens and irritants from the environment. The less common causes often require that patients also become their own detectives. An index of suspicion can be converted into a documented confirmation with proper guidance. Most patients at first resent the additional restrictions imposed on them by avoidance measures; however, once they have experienced symptomless periods, they become more compliant in preventing additional symptoms. The consequences of omissions and commissions, in regard to a specific trial of avoidance, must often be learned firsthand. Avoidance has always been the major technique in environmental control programs. Motivation is necessary for implementing and sustaining preventive measures.

In most situations, patients become motivated if results are seen. For example, after a period of avoidance is accomplished by the substitution of a polyester pillow for a feather pillow, reexposure to a feather pillow results in recurrence of allergic symptoms.

Patients should be made aware that the most common causes of therapeutic failure in the management of respiratory allergy are pets in the home and continued exposure to nonspecific triggers such as tobacco smoke. Although medications play an important role in the management of patients, they are often insufficient, and compliance in environmental control is necessary for controlling symptoms.

IMMEDIATE GOALS

Fortunately, most patients soon learn to appreciate whether an immediate change in environment proves helpful. The symptoms associated with short exposure are often self-limiting, but each episode contributes to late-phase reactions and bronchial hyperreactivity. By trial and error, patients know that a moldy, musty-smelling

CAT ALLERGEN REMOVAL

It has long been known that patients with cat allergy develop sensitivity rapidly on entering a house with a cat. This is because the allergen is a glycoprotein that fixes to particles, mostly in the range of less than 2.5 μm. These can remain airborne for many hours once the environment is disturbed. In nine houses with one to six cats, the amount of airborne cat allergen without disturbance was 2.9 to 19.7 ng/cu m. There was no correlation between the allergen level and the number of cats.[5] Two types of vacuum cleaners were evaluated: a water-impingement type (in which the air stream is washed in water) and a vacuum cleaner with a high-efficiency particulate air (HEPA) filter. The HEPA filter performed far better than the water-impingement machine in cleaning the air, although with both devices, the concentration of cat allergen increased after the rugs had been vacuumed.

basement or summer home usually causes symptoms to develop. Thus avoidance has become a well-recognized, logical, and necessary form of therapy, often instituted by atopic patients before they see a physician. The physician's role is to adequately evaluate the evidence that environmental changes are associated with clinical improvement. If the history appears sufficient for drawing such a conclusion, continued avoidance should be recommended.

When symptoms have an insidious onset, the problem is more difficult. The history often takes longer to evolve into a recognizable pattern. Patients should be instructed on how to evaluate a cause-and-effect situation by keeping a diary. This record should include time of day, place, exposure to suspected substances, duration of exposure, organ systems involved, specific symptoms, medications taken, and their effect on the symptoms. In the interim, patients should be evaluated to determine their atopic status. If immediate hypersensitivity is a possibility, environmental control should be phased in, starting with the bedroom.

LONG-TERM GOALS

The prevention of recurrent symptoms and future sensitization are equally important long-term goals in atopic children (e.g., the avoidance of exposure of an atopic child to common household environmental allergens). Feathered particles, because of their small size, produce the sunbeams that are seen whenever a feather pillow is fluffed in direct sunlight. These particles can also act as nonspecific irritants. Although the goals of preventing symptoms in all such situations are identical, it seems prudent either to implement adequate environmental control measures or to develop a protocol to prove that such measures do or do not reduce symptoms. There is a pressing need for scientific clinical assessments of the effects of environmental control measures on the frequency and severity of respiratory symptoms regardless of the cause. Limited data concerning the benefits of avoidance on bronchial hyperreactivity clearly show reversibility after avoidance.

PROPHYLAXIS OF RESPIRATORY ALLERGIES

Although prophylaxis is also a long-term goal, it is discussed separately so that special attention can be devoted to it. The usefulness of environmental controls for HDM and cat allergens have been published with aeroallergen quantification.[5, 40]

The predisposition for acquiring allergic disease is genetic, whereas the expression of the atopy and allergic disease is dependent on exposure. In a 10-year study involving 93 children evaluated between the ages of 1 and 11 years,[41] house dust samples were collected in 1978 and again in 1989. These samples were analyzed for HDM allergen (Dep p I). Of 17 subjects with active asthma, 16 were atopic, as determined by positive skin tests and specific serum IgE antibodies ($p < .005$), and all were sensitive to HDM ($p < .001$). There was a trend ($p = .062$) for children exposed to higher levels of HDM at the age of 1 year to exhibit more sensitization at age 11 years. All but one of the children had been exposed to 10 μg of Dep p I per gram of dust at 1 year of age ($p = .05$). In addition, the age of the first episode of wheezing was inversely related to the level of exposure to HDM at the age of 1 year for all children ($p = .015$) but especially for the atopic children ($p = .001$).[42]

The prevention of sensitization to pets requires special consideration. Emotional deprivation and trauma are often cited as reasons for noncompliance with a recommendation to remove pets from the home. If the household has never had a pet, intermittent exposure to the neighbors' or grandparents' pets can be a joyful experience and is probably insufficient for inducing sensitization in most children. This solution is better than the psychological trauma of having to remove a new pet from the patient's home once symptoms occur. If the animal has already been in the home, physicians should make every effort to persuade the family of an atopic child to remove the animal from the living quarters but keep the pet on the outside property, such as a garage, provided that exposure of the patient is minimized. Once continuous exposure no longer exists, patients frequently acquire acute symptoms on exposure. If symptoms develop, it is much easier to document the cause, and avoidance is less of a problem.

An interesting question arises with regard to whether physicians would be legally liable if they failed to warn the parents of an atopic child of possible future sensitization in the light of current belief or knowledge. Data from the Children's Asthma Research Institute and Hospital show that nearly 50% of patients who lost all symptoms of asthma on admission and remained asthma free without medication (rapid remitters) had dogs or cats at home.[43] It has been suggested by some authors that in cases of severe asthma resulting from household pets, failure to eliminate exposure to household pets could be considered a form of child abuse or neglect.[44]

If prophylaxis is to work, compliance is essential. If the risk exists, clinical experience suggests that education of the parents about the cost and benefit of environmental control is a part of completing the medical examination.

ABUSE OF ENVIRONMENTAL CONTROL

Environmental illness is an intellectual challenge, a medical enigma, and both an ethical and a legal dilemma for physicians, patients, and the patients' families. Some patients have true chemical sensitivities, whereas others, often called "universal reactors," do not. Patients in this latter group exhibit no objective evidence, signs, or symptoms of disease related to the specific chemical.[45] Results of all standardized laboratory tests are normal, and yet the patients are frequently skin tested and treated by unapproved and unproven techniques at great expense in terms of money and emotional dependency.[46] These patients have been forsaken by the medical establishment, inasmuch as insufficient attention has been paid to their needs.[47] They are permitted, and in many cases encouraged, to continually search for a cure when supportive therapy and often psychiatric intervention are indicated.[48, 49]

A practical approach to the evaluation of suspected environmental chemical exposure has been described.[45] Most such chemicals should be considered nonallergic triggers, but evaluations such as challenges should be reserved for medical centers fully knowledgeable and equipped to handle toxic as well as immunologic reactions.

REFERENCES

1. Reed CE, Swanson MC: Indoor allergens: Identification and quantification. Environ Int 12:115–120, 1986.
2. Yuninger JW: Allergens: Recent advances. Pediatr Clin North Am 35:981–993, 1988.
3. Lehrer SB, Salvaggio JF: Allergens: Standardizations and impact of biotechnology—A review. Allergy Proc 11:197–208, 1990.
4. Platts-Mills TAE, Chapman MD: Dust mites: Immunology, allergic disease, and environmental control. J Allergy Clin Immunol 80:755–775, 1987.
5. Luczynska CM, Li Y, Chapman MD, et al: Airborne concentrations and particle size distribution of allergen derived from domestic cats (Felis domesticus). Am Rev Respir Dis 141:361–367, 1990.
6. Samet JM, Marbury MC, Spengler JD: Health effects and sources of indoor air pollution. Part 1. Am Rev Respir Dis 136:1486–1508, 1987.
7. Koenig JQ: Pulmonary reaction to environmental pollutants. J Allergy Clin Immunol 79:833–843, 1987.
8. Samet JM, Marbury MC, Spengler JD: Respiratory effects of indoor air pollution. J Allergy Clin Immunol 79:685–700, 1987.
9. Samet JM, Marbury MC, Spengler JD: Health effects and sources of indoor air pollution. Part II. Am Rev Respir Dis 137:221–242, 1988.
10. Bardana EJ Jr, Montanaro A, O'Hollaren MT: Building-related illness. A review of available scientific data. Clin Rev Allergy 6:61–89, 1988.
11. Nero AV Jr: Controlling indoor air pollution. Sci Am 258(5):42–48, 1988.
12. Pollart SM, Platts-Mills TA: Mites and mite allergy as risk factors for asthma. Ann Allergy 63:364–365, 1989.
13. Chapman MD, Pollart SM, Luczynska CM, et al: Hidden allergic factors in the etiology of asthma. Chest 94:185–190, 1988.
14. Burr ML, Neale E, Dean BV, et al: Effect of a change to mite-free bedding on children with mite-sensitive asthma: A controlled trial. Thorax 35:513–514, 1980.
15. Maunsell K, Wraith DG, Cunnington AM: Mites and house dust allergy in bronchial asthma. Lancet 1:267–270, 1968.
16. Gergen PJ, Turkeltaub PC, Kovar MG: The prevalence of allergic skin test reactivity to eight common aeroallergens in the U.S. population: Results from the second National Health and Nutrition Examination Survey. J Allergy Clin Immunol 80:669–679, 1987.
17. Dabrowski AJ, Van Der Brempt X, Soler M, et al: Cat skin as an important source of Fel d I allergen. J Allergy Clin Immunol 86:462–465, 1990.
18. Malo JL, Cartier A, L'Archeveque J, et al: Prevalence of occupational asthma and immunological sensitization to guar gum among employees at a carpet-manufacturing plant. J Allergy Clin Immunol 86:562–569, 1990.
19. Newman Taylor AJ: Occupational asthma. Thorax 35:241–245, 1980.
20. Bates DV: Occupational lung disease. In Bates DV (ed): Respiratory Function in Disease, 3rd ed, pp. 291–336. Philadelphia: WB Saunders, 1989.
21. Piyamahunt A, Bernstein DI, Bernstein IL: Wheezing at work does not always establish the diagnosis: Is your patient's asthma caused by occupational exposure? J Respir Dis 11(8):672–688, 1990.
22. Selner JC: Helping asthmatic patients control their environment. J Respir Dis 7(1):83–104, 1986.
23. Anonymous: Wellness Letter, University of California, Berkeley 4(5):6–7, 1988.
24. Sandström T, Andersson MC, Kolmodin-Hedman B, et al: Bronchoalveolar mastocytosis and lymphocytosis after nitrogen dioxide exposure in man: A time-kinetic study. Eur Respir J 3:138–143, 1990.
25. Bauer MA, Utell MJ, Morrow PE, et al: Inhalation of 0.30 ppm nitrogen dioxide potentiates exercise-induced bronchospasm in asthmatics. Am Rev Respir Dis 134:1203–1208, 1986.
26. Orehek J, Massari JP, Gayrard P, et al: Effect of short-term, low-level nitrogen dioxide exposure on bronchial sensitivity of asthmatic patients. J Clin Invest 57:301–307, 1976.
27. Sheppard D: Sulfur dioxide and asthma. A double-edged sword? J Allergy Clin Immunol 82:961–964, 1988.
28. Tseng RY, Li CK: Low level atmospheric sulfur dioxide pollution and childhood asthma. Ann Allergy 65:379–383, 1990.
29. Sheppard D, Saisho A, Nadel JA, et al: Exercise increases sulfur dioxide–induced bronchoconstriction in asthmatic subjects. Am Rev Respir Dis 123:486–491, 1981.
30. Balmes JR, Fine JM, Sheppard D: Symptomatic bronchoconstriction after short-term inhalation of sulfur dioxide. Am Rev Respir Dis 136:1117–1121, 1987.
31. Folinsbee LJ, Bedi JF, Horvath SM: Pulmonary function changes after 1 hr continuous heavy exercise in 0.21 ppm ozone. J Appl Physiol 57:984–988, 1984.
32. Holtzman MJ, Cunningham JH, Sheller JK, et al: Effects of ozone on bronchial reactivity in atopic and non-atopic subjects. Am Rev Respir Dis 120:1059–1067, 1979.
33. Adams WC, Schelegle ES: Ozone and high ventilation effects on pulmonary functions and endurance performance. J Appl Physiol 55:805–812, 1983.
34. Lowhagen O, Rak S: Modification of bronchial hyperreactivity after treatment with sodium cromoglycate during pollen season. J Allergy Clin Immunol 75:460–467, 1985.
35. Platts-Mills TA, Mitchell EB, Nock P, et al: Reduction of bronchial hyperreactivity during prolonged allergen avoidance. Lancet 2:675–678, 1982.
36. Murray AB, Furguson AC: Dust-free bedrooms in the treatment of asthmatic children with house dust or house dust mite allergy: A controlled trial. Pediatrics 71:418–422, 1983.
37. Mosbech H, Korsgaard J, Lind P: Control of house dust mites by electrical heating blankets. J Allergy Clin Immunol 81:706–710, 1988.
38. Thompson PJ, Stewart GA: House-dust mite reduction strategies in the treatment of asthma. Med J Aust 151:408, 411, 1989.
39. Nelson HS, Hirsch SR, Ohman JL Jr, et al: Recommendations for the use of residential air cleaning devices in the treatment of allergic respiratory diseases. J Allergy Clin Immunol 82:661–669, 1988.
40. Tovey ER, Chapman MD, Wells CW, et al: The distribution of dust mite allergen in the houses of patients with asthma. Am Rev Respir Dis 124:630–635, 1981.
41. Murray AB, Morrison BJ: The effects of cigarette smoke from the mother of bronchial responsiveness and severity of symptoms in children with asthma. J Allergy Clin Immunol 77:575–581, 1986.
42. Sporik R, Holgate ST, Platts-Mills TA, et al: Exposure to house-dust mite allergen (Der p I) and the development of asthma in childhood. A prospective study. N Engl J Med 323:502–507, 1990.
43. Falliers CJ: Treatment of asthma in a residential center: A fifteen-year study. Ann Allergy 28:513–521, 1970.
44. Franklin W, Kahn RE: Severe asthma due to household pets: A form of child abuse or neglect. New Engl Reg Allergy Proc 8:259–261, 1987.
45. Selner JC, Staudenmayer H: The practical approach to the evaluation of suspected environmental exposures: Chemical intolerance. Ann Allergy 55:665–673, 1985.
46. Selner JC, Condemi J: Unproven diagnostic and therapeutic techniques for allergy. In Middleton E, Reed CE, Ellis EF (eds): Allergy Principles and Practice, 3rd ed, pp. 1571–1597. Philadelphia: CV Mosby, 1988.
47. Quill TE: Somatization disorder: One of medicine's blind spots. JAMA 254:3075–3079, 1985.
48. Brodsky CM: Multiple chemical sensitivities and other "environmental illness": A psychiatrist's view. Occup Med 2:695–704, 1987.
49. Brodsky CM: The psychiatric epidemic in the American workplace. Occup Med 3:653–662, 1988.
50. Altounyan REC: Change in histamine and atropine responsiveness as a guide to diagnosis and evaluation of therapy in obstructive airways disease. In Pepys J, Frankland AW (eds): Disodium Cromoglycate in Allergic Airways Disease, pp. 47–53. London: Butterworths, 1970.
51. Kerrebijn KF: Endogenous factors in childhood CNSLD: Methodological aspects in population studies. In Orie NGM, van der Lende

R (eds): Bronchitis III, pp. 38–48. The Netherlands: Royal Vangor-
cum Assen, 1970.
52. Chan-Yeung M: Fate of occupational asthma. A follow up study of
patients with occupational asthma due to Western Red Cedar
(Thuja plicata). Am Rev Respir Dis 116:1023–1029, 1977.
53. Cartier A, Bandouvakis J, Ryan G, et al: Asthma and increased non-

allergic bronchial responsiveness to methacholine during natural
exposure to ragweed pollen. Am Rev Respir Dis 121(Suppl.):61,
1980.
54. Dorward AJ, Colloff MJ, MacKay NS, et al: Effect of house dust
mite avoidance measures on adult atopic asthma. Thorax 43:98–
102, 1988.

85 PASSIVE SMOKING

JOHN E. VAN WYE, M.D.

Passive smoking is defined as the exposure of non-smokers to the products of tobacco combustion in the environment. The 1980s was a period of increasing public sentiment as well as legislation regarding the rights of nonsmokers to live and work in a smoke-free environment. In addition, a burgeoning scientific literature on the health effects of passive smoking has developed; more than 500 articles have been published in medical journals since 1970; the majority have appeared since 1985. The *Oxford English Dictionary* added the phrase *passive smoking* to its newly revised addition,[1] and landmark reports by both the U.S. Surgeon General[2] and the National Academy of Sciences[3] reached similar conclusions about the health hazards of environmental tobacco smoke, helping to solidify both scientific and public opinion that this is an important area for continued research as well as public health intervention.

This review summarizes the available evidence regarding the health effects of passive smoking, particularly with regard to the pediatric population. Such effects include a number of extrapulmonary as well as pulmonary manifestations, which may be further subdivided into effects on acute respiratory illnesses, chronic respiratory symptoms, and changes in lung function.

PREVALENCE

No definitive data regarding the number of children involuntarily exposed to tobacco smoke are available. Approximately 30% of adult Americans are active smokers,[4] and surveys have found that 53% to 76% of homes in the United States contain at least one smoker.[5] Thus 30 million American children under 15 years of age may be chronically exposed to cigarette smoke. Within this population, however, the degree of exposure varies widely, depending primarily on the number of cigarettes smoked indoors, the proximity of exposure, the type of ventilation in the home, and the amount of time that a child spends indoors. Such variability has made the performance and interpretation of long-term epidemiologic studies particularly difficult and in some cases has even led to conflict-

ing results. In future studies, researchers need to measure and document more reliably the degree of exposure to tobacco smoke in order to reach the most meaningful conclusions.

COMPOSITION OF ENVIRONMENTAL TOBACCO SMOKE

Environmental tobacco smoke consists of two major components: mainstream smoke and sidestream smoke. Mainstream smoke is the smoke drawn through the tobacco product, filtered by the smoker's lungs, and then exhaled into the environment. Sidestream smoke, which comprises an estimated 85% of the smoke in an average room during cigarette smoking, is emitted from the burning end of the cigarette between puffs and enters directly into the environment.[6] According to the National Academy of Sciences report, more than 3800 compounds have been identified in tobacco smoke; both mainstream smoke and sidestream smoke contain measurable quantities of gaseous and particulate matter, many of which are known toxins or carcinogens.[3] As shown in Table 85–1,[2, 7] the concentrations of these compounds are appreciably higher in sidestream than in mainstream smoke because sidestream smoke is not filtered by either the cigarette or the smoker's respiratory tract.

Air-sampling surveys documented significant increases in these products of tobacco consumption under normal indoor conditions in the presence of smokers. Smoking in enclosed rooms can produce carbon monoxide levels higher than the national air-quality standard of 9 parts per million, and even one smoker in an average home can significantly elevate indoor levels of suspended particulate matter.[2] Repace and Lowrey, for instance, found that nonsmokers' homes contain approximately 40 μg/cu m of suspended particulates and that this level can rise to as high as 700 μg/cu m in the presence of smokers.[8] These particles are extremely small, ranging between 0.1 and 1.0 μm in diameter, in comparison with other common inhalants (Table 85–2[7, 9]). Because of their small size, these

Table 85–1. SELECTED CONSTITUENTS OF ENVIRONMENTAL TOBACCO SMOKE (PER CIGARETTE) WITH RATIO OF SS TO MS COMPONENTS

Constituents	MS	SS/MS Ratio
Gases		
Carbon monoxide	10–23 mg	2.5–4.7
Carbon dioxide	20–40 mg	8–11
Hydrogen cyanide	400–500 μg	0.1–0.25
Ammonia	50–130 μg	40–170
Acetic acid	330–810 μg	1.9–3.6
Formic acid	210–490 μg	1.4–1.6
Benzene*	12–48 μg	20–100
Dimethylnitrosamine†	10–40 ng	20–100
Nitrosopyrrolidine†	6–30 ng	6–30
Particulates		
Total particulate matter*	15–40 mg	1.3–1.9
Tar*	5–40 mg	2.1–3.4
Nicotine	1–2.5 mg	2.6–3.3
Phenol	60–140 μg	1.6–3.0
Aniline	360 ng	30
Benzo(a)pyrene‡	20–40 ng	2.5–3.5
Benz(a)anthracene†	20–70 ng	2–4
2-Naphthylamine*	1.7 ng	30
4-Aminobiphenyl*	4.6 ng	31

Data from U.S. Department of Health and Human Services: The Health Consequences of Involuntary Smoking: A Report of the Surgeon General, DHEW publication no. DHHS-CDC-87-8398. Washington, DC: U.S. Government Printing Office, 1986; Corn M: Characteristics of tobacco sidestream smoke and factors influencing its concentration and distribution in occupied spaces. Scand J Respir Dis 91:21–36, 1974.
MS, mainstream; SS, sidestream.
*Human carcinogen.
†Animal carcinogen.
‡Suspected human carcinogen.

particles are not appreciably filtered by the nose, and up to 40% of those inhaled are deposited in the lungs.[10]

MEASURING SMOKE EXPOSURE

To best evaluate any relationship between passive smoking and disease, it is necessary to objectively determine the degree to which a population has been exposed to environmental tobacco smoke. Many investigators have estimated exposure to smoke simply on the basis of questionnaires, which are limited by reporting bias and other inaccuracies. In addition, variables such as type of ventilation, proximity of exposure, and time spent indoors may affect the true level of exposure. Thus considerable effort has been focused on identifying sensitive and specific markers in order to measure long-term exposure to environmental tobacco smoke.

Previously used markers, such as carboxyhemoglobin and thiocyanate, are very sensitive in identifying exposure to smoke, but they lack specificity; in addition, the short half-life (4 h) of carboxyhemoglobin limits its usefulness in assessing chronic smoke exposure.[11] Nicotine is an extremely sensitive and specific marker but has wide fluctuations of blood and urine levels in those exposed because of rapid and extensive tissue uptake as well as a short (1- to 2-h) elimination half-life.[2] Cotinine, the major metabolite of nicotine, is specific for tobacco, has a long half-life (15 to 40 h in adults, 37 to 160 h in infants), and

can be quantified at low levels in blood, urine, or saliva.[12] Therefore, it has emerged as the most widely accepted marker for both active and passive smoking. Numerous studies have shown a strong correlation, including a dose-response relationship, between urinary cotinine levels and level of exposure to environmental tobacco smoke in all age groups.[13-17] Future epidemiologic studies must incorporate such an objective measurement of exposure to establish more precisely the relationship between passive smoking and disease.

EXTRAPULMONARY MANIFESTATIONS OF PASSIVE SMOKING

This review focuses primarily on the pulmonary consequences of passive smoking; however, a number of extrapulmonary manifestations have been described and deserve comment.

INCREASED PREVALENCE OF SMOKING IN CHILDREN OF SMOKERS

Parental smoking is a significant predictor of smoking by children themselves. Children of smoking parents are approximately twice as likely to become smokers themselves and are therefore at risk for the known hazards of active smoking.[11, 18, 19]

EFFECTS ON GROWTH

The deleterious effects of passive exposure to tobacco begin in utero. Carbon monoxide preferentially moves to the fetus because fetal hemoglobin has 1.8 times more affinity for it than does adult hemoglobin.[19] Fetal oxygen-carrying capacity may thus be reduced by up to 40% by maternal smoking.[20] In addition, nicotine itself may contribute to fetal hypoxia by vasoconstriction of maternal blood supply to the placenta.[21] Perhaps as a result, infants born to smoking mothers are shorter and weigh an average of 200 g less than infants of nonsmoking mothers; the birth weight decreases proportionally with the number of cigarettes that the mother smokes.[22-25] This effect has been shown to be independent of gestational age and other potentially confounding factors. A similar but lesser effect on birth weight (24- to 100-g reduction) has been dem-

Table 85–2. DIAMETER OF COMMON INHALANTS

Inhalant	Diameter (μ)
Cigarette smoke	0.1–1.0
Coal mine dust	5
Fungal spore	10
Grass pollen	30

Data from Corn M: Characteristics of tobacco sidestream smoke and factors influencing its concentration and distribution in occupied spaces. Scand J Respir Dis 91:21–36, 1974; Hirsch SR: Airway mucus and the mucociliary system. In Middleton E, Reed CE, Ellis EF (eds): Allergy Principles and Practice, 2nd ed, p. 395. St. Louis: CV Mosby, 1983.

onstrated with passive exposure of nonsmoking mothers to environmental tobacco smoke.[22, 24–26] In addition, the subsequent physical growth of children may be affected by parental smoking. Both in utero exposure and childhood exposure to tobacco smoke have been related to lower attained heights (0.5- to 1.5-cm deficit, with a dose-response effect noted), even after birth weight, gestational age, social class, and parental height are controlled.[27–30] It is unclear which of the two exposures—prenatal or postnatal—contributes more to this effect.

SUDDEN INFANT DEATH SYNDROME

Several studies suggested a relationship between parental smoking and sudden infant death syndrome (SIDS).[31–34] Mothers of SIDS victims are 1.5 to 2.0 times more likely to have smoked during and after pregnancy than are mothers of control infants matched for gestational age and socioeconomic status.[31–33] In addition, paternal smoking in the absence of maternal smoking appears to be a risk factor for SIDS in infants over 8 weeks of age.[34] This relationship appears to be dose responsive; the incidence of SIDS increases with the number of cigarettes smoked daily by the father. The relative contribution of prenatal versus postnatal exposure is not known, and any proposed mechanisms for the apparent association between passive smoking and SIDS remain speculative.

CANCER

Active smoking has been unequivocally linked to a variety of human cancers, particularly carcinoma of the lung. Both mainstream smoke and sidestream smoke contain a wide variety of carcinogens, most of which are more highly concentrated in sidestream smoke.[2] Passive smokers, like active smokers, have increased activity of enzymes that metabolize certain carcinogens[35] and increased levels of urinary mutagens.[36, 37] It is not surprising, then, that environmental tobacco smoke has been linked to human cancer. Both the U.S. Surgeon General and the National Academy of Sciences, after reviewing the data from approximately 15 studies worldwide (primarily assessing the nonsmoking spouses of smokers), concluded that the relative risk for lung carcinoma is significantly elevated, probably on the order of 1.3 to 2.0 times, in passive smokers compared with 10.9 times for active smokers.[2, 3, 6, 38]

Children may be particularly sensitive to the carcinogenic potential of environmental tobacco smoke. In one population-based, case-control study, investigators found that household exposure to 25 or more smoker years during the first two decades of life more than doubled the risk of lung cancer in nonsmoking adults.[39]

The carcinogenic potential of in utero exposure to tobacco smoke and the association between passive smoking and other cancers have been analyzed in few studies; data are insufficient for making definitive conclusions. However, results of studies have suggested an increased risk for cancers of the paranasal sinuses,[40]

brain,[40–42] breast,[43, 44] cervix,[43, 45] and hematopoietic tissue.[41, 43, 46, 47] Biologic plausibility is called into question with some of these sites because they are not associated with active smoking, and active smokers generally receive more exposure to environmental tobacco smoke than do passive smokers. Results of three studies suggested a dose-response relationship between in utero, as well as childhood, exposure to tobacco smoke and the subsequent development of cancer, particularly leukemia.[41, 46, 47] In these cases, however, the effect of passive smoking after birth cannot readily be distinguished from any potential genetic or transplacentally mediated effects.

CARDIAC FUNCTION

A causal association between active cigarette smoking and cardiovascular disease is well established.[48] In six studies, investigators evaluated the relationship between passive smoking and heart disease (primarily in the nonsmoking spouses of smokers),[49–54] and all but one group[52] found an association. Three studies showed statistical significance,[49, 51, 54] including a dose-response relationship, with relative risks reported in the 1.2 to 1.5 range. Although it is difficult to completely factor out the many other risk factors for arteriosclerotic heart disease, these results do suggest a small but measurable risk for such disease among nonsmokers who live with smokers. No data are yet available regarding the potential relationship between passive smoking in childhood and subsequent development of coronary artery disease.

Other investigators suggested that passive smoking impairs exercise performance[55] and aggravates angina pectoris,[56] presumably by reducing oxygen-carrying capacity secondary to increased carboxyhemoglobin and, in the case of angina, by increasing myocardial oxygen demand secondary to nicotine-induced tachycardia.

IMMUNOLOGIC EFFECTS

Active cigarette smoking is associated with increased levels of total immunoglobulin E (IgE).[57–59] Serum IgE levels in smokers are approximately 10 to 30 IU higher than in nonsmokers, although the levels in both groups are within the normal range. Whether this difference represents increased sensitization to specific antigens that have more easily penetrated the damaged respiratory mucosa of smokers, or, rather, some nonspecific activation of IgE production by tobacco by-products is unknown. Attempts to correlate the increased total IgE production in smokers with sensitivity to specific aeroallergens or increased atopy in general have been mostly unsuccessful.[60] Tobacco smoke itself functions as an irritant rather than an allergen;[61, 62] the only true allergic reactions to tobacco have occurred with occupational exposure to unburned tobacco leaves.[63]

A few investigators suggested that passive smoking may also influence the IgE immune system. A Swedish study reported that maternal, but not paternal, smoking caused a significant increase in cord blood IgE,[64] although this association was not found in a subsequent group of infants in Michigan.[65] Analysis of the effect of paternal smoking on total IgE levels later in childhood has also yielded mixed results; one group reported a strong association[66] but two groups found no effect.[67,68] When the prevalence of atopy in children, as defined by positive skin tests or enzyme-linked immunosorbent assay for aeroallergen-specific IgE, was analyzed in relation to parental smoking, two groups found a strong association (particularly with maternal smoking),[69,70] but two others found none.[68,71] A limitation of many of these studies is failure to consider the effect of a family history of atopy, because hereditary factors may mask the presumably weaker effect of tobacco smoke. At this time, no definitive conclusions regarding the influence of passive smoking on the subsequent development of atopy may be drawn.

Exposure to cigarette smoke clearly affects other arms of the immune system, as demonstrated in active smokers and animal models of passive smoking. Nonspecific host defenses are depressed in the respiratory tract because of increased epithelial permeability[72] and impaired mucociliary transport.[73,74] An inflammatory cell infiltrate develops in the pulmonary interstitium and peribronchial areas.[75,76] In addition, cellular immunity appears to be adversely affected because of decreased natural killer cell number and activity, possibly contributing to the elevated risk of malignancy in this population.[2,77,78] However, the extent to which these changes occur in humans chronically exposed to environmental tobacco smoke is not yet known.

EYES, EARS, NOSE, AND THROAT

Most of the public consciousness regarding passive smoking, as well as the increasing tendency to separate smokers from nonsmokers in public areas and transport systems, is related to the acute irritant effects of environmental tobacco smoke on the eyes and upper respiratory tract. Although it is not yet known which of the many gaseous and particulate components of smoke are primarily responsible for these effects, numerous investigators documented consistent symptoms and signs in a dose-response manner both in population surveys and experimental exposure chambers. Passive smokers most frequently report eye irritation (69%), followed by headache (32%), nasal irritation or congestion (29%), and cough (25%).[79] Such symptoms are generally reported even more frequently by atopic patients.[79,80] More recent studies, through the use of exposure chambers as well as measurements of various gaseous and particulate constituents of smoke in natural environments, documented a clear-cut dose-response relationship between smoke concentration and subjective eye, nose, and throat irritation as well as eye-blink rate.[81,82] Another investigator found a significant association between maternal smoking and sore throats in children even after controlling for parental respiratory infections.[83]

Perhaps more serious than these various irritant phenomena is the now well-documented association between parental smoking and middle ear effusions in children. Numerous investigators documented that chronic exposure to indoor environmental tobacco smoke is associated with increased frequency of acute otitis media, chronic ear effusions, tympanostomy tube insertion, and tonsillectomy and adenoidectomy.[84-90] Passive smoking appears to have at least an additive, if not synergistic, effect on atopy in this regard and seems to be a significant risk factor for such disease even after exposure to infectious diseases at home is controlled for. The potential mechanisms by which parental smoking leads to an increased frequency of middle ear disease in children include a direct irritant effect of tobacco smoke on the eustachian tube and an increased frequency of respiratory infections resulting from either a direct effect of tobacco or increased respiratory infections in adult smokers in the home.

Although not yet studied formally, it is reasonable to suspect that the incidence of sinusitis may also be higher in children exposed to environmental tobacco smoke, because the anatomy and pathophysiologic features of the middle ear and paranasal sinuses are very similar with regard to infection. If true, such an association would imply the existence of a mechanism by which passive smoking may impair lower airway function, in view of the well-known relationship between sinusitis and reactive airway disease.[91]

PULMONARY MANIFESTATIONS OF PASSIVE SMOKING

ACUTE RESPIRATORY ILLNESSES

Since 1974, investigators in numerous prospective,[92-105] cross-sectional,[106-109] and case-control[110-112] studies have evaluated the effect of parental smoking on the frequency and severity of acute respiratory illness in childhood. Despite varying methodologies and geographic locales, investigators have consistently demonstrated a higher incidence of lower respiratory tract infections, as well as acute exacerbations of asthma, among the children of smokers than among those of nonsmokers. In general, the association is dose related, more related to maternal than to paternal smoking, and stronger in infants and younger children than in older children. Significant confounding variables, including birth weight, the incidence of parental respiratory infections, family size, and crowding, were controlled for in some but not all of these studies; the effect persisted even after these variables were taken into account. As before, the relative contributions of prenatal and postnatal exposure to environmental tobacco smoke in this regard are not known. The strongest findings to date of studies on the relationship between passive smoking and acute respiratory illness are summarized as follows. With the exception of otitis media and sore throat, as previously presented, data on the relationship between passive smoking and upper respiratory tract infections are inadequate; in addition, no data have yet been published on the relationship between passive smoking and acute respiratory infections in adults.

The Jerusalem Perinatal Study[92] observed more than 10,000 infants in Israel during the first 12 months of life and found a 38% higher ($p < .001$) hospital admission rate for pneumonia and bronchitis among infants whose mothers reported smoking at a prenatal visit than among infants of nonsmoking mothers. A significant dose-response effect was noted; the admission rate increased by 70% among infants born to mothers smoking 11 to 20 cigarettes per day and by 234% among infants of mothers who smoked more than 20 cigarettes per day ($p < .001$ for trend). This effect persisted even after corrections for birth weight and socioeconomic class. The effect of paternal smoking was not assessed, nor was the effect of parental respiratory symptoms, and the infants were observed only for the first year of life.

British investigators[93, 94] observed a cohort of 2205 infants over the first 5 years of life and found the incidence of pneumonia and bronchitis in the first year of life to be increased by 46% if one parent smoked and by 125% if both parents smoked ($p < .0005$). This effect persisted after control for parental respiratory symptoms, infants' birth weight, social class, and family size; however, no such relationship was demonstrated after the first year of life.

A similar longitudinal study of 1265 infants in New Zealand[96–98] demonstrated a significant effect of maternal smoking on the incidence of pneumonia and bronchitis in the first 2 years of life; no effect was seen from ages 2 to 6, and at no age did paternal smoking affect the incidence of infection of the lower respiratory tract. After controls for birth weight, socioeconomic class, and family size, the incidence of such infection was increased by 27% among children of mothers smoking 1 to 10 cigarettes per day and by 60% among children of mothers who smoked more than 10 cigarettes per day ($p < .01$).

In the United States, Ware and colleagues[99] prospectively observed more than 10,000 first- and second-graders for 2 years in six cities, assessing the effect of parental smoking on the incidence of illness of the lower respiratory tract during the first 2 years of life as well as acute respiratory illness during the study period. After adjusting for parental illness and socioeconomic status, they found a 20% to 35% increase in these illnesses in association with maternal smoking during both time periods; there was a significant dose-response effect noted, and paternal smoking was associated with smaller but still significant increases.

Two cross-sectional studies from the United States[107, 108] also confirmed the increased incidence of chest illness before the age of 2 years in children passively exposed to smoke, and in a well-controlled study from Michigan[109] of more than 3000 children between 0 and 19 years of age, investigators found an increased incidence of bronchitis at all ages among the offspring of smokers (relative risk is approximately 1.4, $p < .05$), with a significant dose-response effect noted.

Two well-controlled, prospective studies from the People's Republic of China[101, 102] involving more than 3000 infants from birth to 18 months of age revealed an 80% to 100% increase in hospital admissions for pneumonia and bronchitis among infants from families with at least one smoker in the home. A significant dose-response effect was noted, and the association was even stronger in the first 6 months of life. These studies were unique in that they were performed in a population in which extremely few women smoke. In fact, none of the mothers studied were smokers, which thereby rules out any antenatal exposure to tobacco (other than "third-hand" smoke resulting from mothers' passive smoking) as a significant cause of subsequent respiratory illness.

Investigators have linked passive smoking to an increased incidence of respiratory syncytial virus (RSV) infection. Pullan and Hey[110] retrospectively studied a group of children hospitalized with RSV in infancy and found significant differences between the smoking habits of their mothers and the smoking habits of mothers of infants admitted for other illnesses. McConnochie and Roghmann[111] found the incidence of bronchiolitis in infants under the age of 2 years to be more than twice as high ($p = .004$) among those exposed to cigarette smoke at home; maternal smoking was a stronger risk factor than paternal smoking. Hayes and colleagues[112] found that 90% of infants hospitalized for RSV on American Samoa lived with a cigarette smoker, in comparison with 53% of controls ($p = .02$); this association remained strong even after adjustments for family size. Groothuis and associates[104] prospectively evaluated 30 children under the age of 2 years with bronchopulmonary dysplasia, 16 of whom became infected with RSV during the 4-month study period. Of those 16, 15 were exposed to environmental tobacco smoke at home, in comparison with only 7 of the 14 noninfected infants ($p < .01$). However, the authors did not control for number of family members in the home; therefore, the significance of the results is somewhat uncertain.

An association has also been demonstrated between passive smoking and exacerbations of asthma, as reflected by acute care visits. Evans and associates[106] demonstrated a significant ($p < .01$) increase of 63% in asthma-related visits to the emergency room by children of smokers; Wissow and Warshaw[105] found that childhood asthmatic patients passively exposed to tobacco smoke at home have greater seasonal exacerbations of wheezing that mandate acute care than do unexposed children ($p < .05$). It is unclear whether this relationship between acute-care asthma visits and parental smoking is the result of a direct irritant effect of sidestream smoke on the lungs, an increased susceptibility to infection, or socioeconomic factors such as an increased prevalence of poverty (and diminished access to preventive medical services) among smokers.

In summary, numerous studies of varying methodology from different locales have demonstrated a consistent and significant association between parental smoking and increased rates of acute illness of the lower respiratory tract. In general, the effect is dose related and most significant in the first 1 to 2 years of life; maternal smoking makes a greater contribution than paternal smoking. The mechanisms for this association are not known, and in general the researchers in the studies cited have controlled for any potentially confounding variables. Younger infants and children appear to be more susceptible to these effects than do older children, perhaps because of intrinsic immaturity of their pulmonary defense systems, more time spent in proximity to their parents (particularly mothers), or some transient effect of prenatal exposure to tobacco smoke.

The long-term consequences of this increased incidence of lower respiratory tract illness in early childhood remain unknown. Many investigators demonstrated a striking relationship between bronchiolitis in infancy and recurrent wheezing in later childhood;[113] therefore, passive smoking may indirectly predispose infants to longer term pulmonary problems. However, a relationship between early childhood respiratory infections and obstructive lung disease in adulthood is not currently well established, and further investigation is required.[114]

CHRONIC RESPIRATORY SYMPTOMS

Investigators in a number of cross-sectional studies have examined the relationship between parental smoking and children's respiratory symptoms, particularly cough and wheeze. Although not all investigators have found a significant association, the bulk of the available evidence does suggest a causal and dose-related effect of parental (particularly maternal) smoking and chronic respiratory symptoms in children, especially in those who are younger or who have a personal or family history of atopy or asthma.

Charlton,[115] in an analysis of 7000 nonsmoking children aged 8 to 19 years, found the prevalence of frequent cough to increase directly with the number of smokers at home. This correlation was strongest in the younger children; 33%, 41%, and 50%, respectively, of children aged 8 to 11 years in households with no, one, and two smoking parents ($p < .0001$) reported frequent cough. No attempt was made, however, to control for parental respiratory illnesses or symptoms.

Ware and colleagues,[99] in a prospective study of 10,000 American children aged 6 to 9 years, also found a dose-response relationship between parental smoking and frequent cough; the relative risk of cough increased by 30%, 46%, and 112%, respectively, as mothers smoked 6 to 15, 26 to 35, and 36 to 45 cigarettes per day ($p = .0001$). This relationship remained significant even after control for parental respiratory illnesses; paternal smoking had a similar but lesser effect. Similar studies from England[103] and Sweden[116] also confirmed the relationship between passive smoking and frequent cough, especially in younger children.

Interestingly, the investigators in two studies who did not find such an association[117, 118] examined an older group of children, which suggests that children under 10 to 12 years of age are most vulnerable to such effects. Despite this, however, teenage passive smokers have not consistently been found to be symptom-free, as shown by Tsimoyianis and colleagues,[119] who demonstrated a fourfold higher incidence of cough among a group of 12- to 17-year-old high school athletes exposed to household smoking. Unfortunately, no researchers to date have attempted to determine the cause of the cough in these young passive smokers. Theoretical possibilities include a direct irritant effect of tobacco smoke, an increased incidence of respiratory tract infection, exacerbation of asthma, and sinusitis.

A number of investigators have also examined the relationship between passive smoking and persistent wheezing in childhood. Again, this relationship appears to be stronger in younger children; in addition, those with a personal or family history of atopy or asthma appear to be more vulnerable.

Geller-Bernstein and colleagues[120] prospectively evaluated 80 atopic infants from Israel from 6 months to 5 years of age and found that the incidence of recurrent wheezing persisting to age 5 years was significantly ($p < .01$) related to parental smoking. In a similar prospective study in England, Cogswell and others[121] observed 73 infants born to atopic parents and found that by age 5 years, the children with recurrent wheezing were twice as likely to come from smoking families ($p < .05$). This differential increased to threefold when a subgroup of atopic children was analyzed separately. Murray and Morrison[122] found the prevalence of asthma (defined by recurrent wheezing) in a group of Canadian children aged 1 to 17 years with atopic dermatitis to be 79% among those exposed to maternal smoking, in comparison with 52% among those not so exposed ($p = .001$). Paternal smoking played a significant but lesser role. Confirming that passive smoking is particularly asthmagenic for children already at risk for such disease, McConnochie and Roghmann[123] found that maternal, but not paternal, smoking was predictive of wheezing (31.8% versus 14.7%; $p = .03$) among a group of American children aged 6 to 10 years with a family history of atopy; no such relationship was found among the children from nonatopic families.

Although it thus seems clear that passive smoking predisposes children already at risk for atopic disease toward recurrent wheezing, less settled is the relationship between asthma and passive smoking in a general population of children. Nevertheless, several large studies have begun to shed light on this question.

Neuspiel and colleagues,[124] in a prospective analysis of almost 10,000 British children from birth to age 10 years, found the prevalence of asthma to be increased by 11% among the children of smoking mothers and by 49% when the mothers smoked more than 14 cigarettes daily ($p < .05$), even after adjusting for a number of confounding variables. No effect was observed for paternal smoking. In their cross-sectional analysis of 650 children aged 5 to 9 years in East Boston, Weiss and co-workers[125] found a dose-response relationship between the number of household smokers and persistent wheeze; wheezing was found among 1.9%, 6.9%, and 11.8% of children, respectively, in households with no, one, and two smoking parents ($p < .05$). This effect persisted after control for parental respiratory illness. Ware and colleagues,[99] in their similarly well-controlled, prospective study of 10,000 children aged 6 to 9 years from six American cities, found the relative risk of wheezing to increase by 11%, 39%, and 131%, respectively, as mothers smoked 6 to 15, 26 to 35, and 36 to 45 cigarettes per day ($p < .0001$). Several other excellent, well-controlled, cross-sectional studies from both the United States[107, 109, 126, 127] and abroad[103, 116] demonstrated similar findings in groups of children with a mean age of approximately 8 years; many have shown a dose-response effect, and most have shown maternal smoking to be a more significant predictor than paternal smoking of recurrent wheezing.

To date, four cross-sectional studies, all from the

United States,[108, 117, 118, 128] failed to find a relationship between parental smoking and wheezing in unselected children. Because the mean age of the population in these studies was somewhat higher (approximately 12 years), this may reflect an increased vulnerability of the younger child to the adverse effects of environmental tobacco smoke.

In summary, numerous studies of differing methodologies and locales have consistently documented an increased incidence of both cough and persistent wheeze among young children chronically exposed to environmental tobacco smoke. Children with a personal or family history of atopy seem particularly prone to such adverse effects. The mechanism by which passive smoking is associated with these symptoms remains unknown. One possible explanation is that bronchiolitis in infancy (shown earlier in this review to be increased by passive smoking) predisposes children to recurrent postinfancy wheezing.[113] Other possibilities include a direct irritant effect of tobacco smoke, alterations in the IgE immune system, or (although not currently documented) an increased incidence of infections of the upper respiratory tract, such as sinusitis.

ALTERATIONS OF PULMONARY FUNCTION

Perhaps of more significance to the overall respiratory health of children than the findings just described regarding acute infections or chronic symptoms is the possible relationship between passive smoking and pulmonary function. Because active smoking has been clearly associated with both acute and chronic airflow obstruction, as well as with bronchial hyperreactivity,[129-132] it is reasonable to hypothesize similar but lesser effects on patients passively exposed to cigarette smoke. A number of studies have addressed this question, both cross-sectionally and prospectively. Although not all have shown consistent effects, the bulk of the evidence suggests that passive smoking in childhood may be associated with slightly decreased lung function, increased bronchial hyperreactivity, and decreased long-term growth of lung function.

The acute effects of passive smoking on pulmonary function and bronchial hyperreactivity, assessed through the use of experimental exposure chambers, have been studied only in adults. To date, seven such investigations have been performed on small numbers of volunteers and generally reveal a measurable decrease in airflow and increase in nonspecific bronchial hyperreactivity associated with passive smoking over a 1- to 2-h period; these effects seem more pronounced in asthmatic subjects.

Pimm and associates[133] placed 20 nonsmoking, healthy adults in an exposure chamber with environmental tobacco smoke for 2 h. Flow at 25% of the vital capacity decreased significantly ($p < .05$) with smoke exposure (by 5% in men and 7% in women). No other consistent changes in pulmonary function were seen. Dahms and colleagues[134] studied 10 adults with asthma and 10 normal controls passively exposed to smoke in a chamber for 1 h. The asthmatic subjects experienced a mean decline from their baseline forced vital capacity (FVC), forced expira-

tory volume in 1 sec (FEV_1), and forced expiratory flow between 25% and 75% of vital capacity (FEF_{25-75}) of approximately 20% ($p < .01$ for each parameter), but the controls exhibited no change in pulmonary function with this exposure. In three other studies of only asthmatic subjects, small but statistically significant declines in FVC[135] and FEV_1[136, 137] were seen with acute exposure to tobacco smoke. Only one group of investigators[138] found no significant acute effect on the pulmonary function of asthmatic subjects passively exposed to smoke.

In addition to its deleterious effect on flow rates, acute exposure to cigarette smoke appears to increase nonspecific bronchial hyperreactivity. Knight and Breslin[136] exposed six adults with asthma to environmental smoke for 1 h. Bronchial reactivity, as assessed by histamine-inhalation testing, increased significantly 4 h after smoke exposure. In a similar trial, Menon and colleagues[139] found that 5 of 10 asthmatic subjects and 1 of 5 controls experienced at least a twofold increase in airway reactivity to methacholine 6 h after smoke exposure. Only one group[135] did not find an increase in nonspecific bronchial responsiveness in asthmatic subjects acutely exposed to smoke; however, in this study, methacholine-challenge testing was performed immediately after smoke exposure rather than several hours later as in the previously mentioned studies. Together, these findings suggest that acute exposure to tobacco smoke, particularly in asthmatic patients, may lead to a state of increased nonspecific bronchial reactivity; such hyperreactivity likely develops over a period of several hours, perhaps because of smoke-induced airway inflammation.

With regard to the pulmonary function and airway reactivity of children passively inhaling cigarette smoke, no such studies of acute exposure have been performed. However, a large amount of cross-sectional data on these parameters in children with regard to parental smoking has been published, and the vast majority of investigators have documented a small but statistically significant decline in flow rates associated with chronic smoke exposure. Most have also demonstrated a crude dose-response effect and have found maternal smoking more contributory than paternal smoking to this decline.

Tager and co-authors,[140] in their analysis of 456 randomly selected children aged 5 to 9 years in East Boston, found an inverse dose-response relationship ($p < .05$) between the FEF_{25-75} and the number of smoking parents in the household after controlling for height, weight, and respiratory infections. In comparison with values for children with two nonsmoking parents, the FEF_{25-75} values were 0.156 and 0.355 standard deviation units lower for children with one and two smoking parents, respectively. A less consistent relationship was found between parental smoking and function of the large airways. Tashkin and colleagues,[118] studying a group of 971 nonsmoking, nonasthmatic children aged 7 to 17 years in Los Angeles, found that maternal but not paternal smoking was associated with decreased peak flow and decreased FEF_{25} in younger boys ($p < .05$) and with decreased FEF_{25-75} in older girls ($p < .05$), but they noted that the apparent effect on older girls may have been confounded by underreporting of active smoking. Nonetheless, two other groups of investigators[117, 119] analyzing populations of unselected children aged 7 to 17 also found statistically significant reductions in the function of small but not of large airways in association with passive smoking.

Other studies, some longitudinal and involving larger numbers of children, documented that passive smoking is associated with dysfunction of both large and small airways. Burchfiel and colleagues,[109] in their analysis of more than 1300 nonsmoking children aged 10 to 19 years in Michigan, found approximately 5% reductions in the FEV_1 and FVC of boys ($p < .01$) and the FEF_{50} of girls ($p < .05$) in households in which both parents smoked in comparison with nonsmokers' households; smaller and less significant reductions were seen in households in which only one parent smoked. These associations were independent of family size, parental respiratory symptoms, and socioeconomic status. In a similarly well-controlled study of 571 children aged 8 to 16 from China, Chen and Li[141] also found reductions of approximately 5% in the FEV_1 and FEF_{25-75} of children from smokers' households and noted a consistent dose-response. O'Connor and colleagues[142] performed spirometry on 265 nonasthmatic children aged 6 to 21 years and found reductions of 7% and 15%, respectively, of the FEV_1 and FEF_{25-75} in association with maternal smoking ($p < .001$). Paternal smoking was associated with smaller and less significant reductions of these parameters. Three other groups of investigators[143-145] also confirmed this general finding of a small but statistically significant reduction in the pulmonary function of children passively exposed to parental, especially maternal, smoking.

In addition to decreased flow rates and volumes, increased nonspecific airway hyperreactivity has been associated with passive smoke exposure in childhood. Young and colleagues found significantly more sensitivity to inhaled histamine in 4-week-old infants of smoking parents than in those of nonsmoking parents.[146]

Perhaps more significant than these extensive cross-sectional data demonstrating slight airway obstruction and hyperreactivity in children with smoking parents are the findings of two large longitudinal studies assessing the impact of passive smoking on the long-term growth of children's lung function. Tager and colleagues[147] observed a cohort of 1156 children aged 5 to 9 years for 7 years to determine the impact of parental smoking on the growth of pulmonary function in children. They found, after controlling for the previous level of FEV_1 and change in height, that the expected increase in FEV_1 over 1-, 2-, and 5-year periods was reduced by 10.7%, 9.5%, and 7.0%, respectively, in children whose mothers smoked (p = .015). A similar negative effect was also observed in the analysis of FEF_{25-75} (p = .058). No effect was seen for paternal smoking, and the results were independent of socioeconomic status and type of cooking fuel used in the home.

Another prospective study by Berkey and co-workers[148] found similar results in 7834 children seen annually from the ages of 6 to 10 years. After adjustments for socioeconomic status, maternal smoking was associated with a significant (p = .05) reduction in the FEV_1 growth rate, leading to a projected cumulative deficit of approximately 3% by young adulthood. A similar but lesser trend was seen for paternal smoking.

Interestingly, the two groups of investigators who found no effect of parental smoking on the pulmonary function of children[126, 149] studied children from Arizona, a state remarkable for its temperate climate. Extensive analysis of the data from this population, as well as from the population exhibiting negative effects of passive smoking on lung function, revealed no differences in methodology to account for the conflicting results.[150, 151] It is likely that differences in degree of exposure to environmental tobacco smoke are responsible for the disparity between the two populations in this regard, thus underscoring the importance of more accurate measurement of exposure in future studies.

Although passive smoking, as noted previously, seems to be associated with small reductions in the pulmonary function of nonasthmatic children, it appears to have more pronounced effects on children with asthma. Murray and Morrison,[152, 153] in their evaluation of more than 200 asthmatic children between the ages of 7 and 17 years, found a 13% reduction in the FEV_1 and a 23% reduction in the FEF_{25-75} associated with maternal, but not paternal, smoking ($p < .005$); a consistent dose-response effect was demonstrated as well. In bronchial challenge testing, these investigators also found a fourfold greater responsiveness to aerosolized histamine associated with maternal smoking ($p = .002$). Interestingly, these negative effects of passive smoking were stronger during the cold season, when the children spent more time indoors and therefore likely had more exposure to cigarette smoke. O'Connor and colleagues,[142] using cold-air inhalation challenge, also demonstrated increased nonspecific bronchial responsiveness associated with maternal smoking in asthmatic children, although no such effects were found in nonasthmatics. Other investigators, however,[70, 107] found small but statistically significant increases in bronchial reactivity to nonspecific stimuli even in nonasthmatic children chronically exposed to parental cigarette smoke.

In summary, many well-controlled cross-sectional and prospective studies have found small reductions in pulmonary function, decreased rates of lung function growth, and increased nonspecific bronchial reactivity in children chronically exposed to parental smoking. These effects seem more pronounced in children with underlying reactive airway disease. The pathophysiologic basis for such effects remains unclear, although possibilities include a direct, toxic effect—prenatal or postnatal or both—on developing lung tissue with subsequent decreased growth and function; an increased incidence of respiratory infection in early life that causes either direct damage to the lungs or a tendency toward future reactivity of the airways; and a smoke-induced chronic inflammatory state that leads to alterations in pulmonary functions and bronchial responsiveness.

The long-term significance of such relatively small changes in lung function, particularly in children without underlying asthma, remains unclear. However, in contrast to the situation with infections of the lower respiratory tract, in which passive smoking appears to play a significant role only in the first 1 or 2 years of life, pulmonary mechanics seem to be affected by smoke exposure also at older ages, as documented in the acute-exposure studies described earlier. In addition, ongoing exposure to environmental tobacco smoke, either at home or work, has been well documented to be associated with small but statistically significant reductions in the pulmonary function of adults, particularly in the small airway function of persons who have been exposed for a period of at least 10 to 15 years.[53, 154–158] Thus it is conceivable that chronic exposure to environmental tobacco smoke beginning in infancy and continuing through adulthood could have a cumulative and quite significant impact on respiratory function. Unfortunately, no investigators to date have performed such an analysis of the potential additive relationship between passive smoking in childhood and either passive or active smoking in adulthood; in addition, more accurate and quantitative assessment of the amount of environmental smoke that a given study population has chronically inhaled is needed in order to make more meaningful conclusions.

OPPORTUNITIES FOR INTERVENTION

Although many issues remain unresolved, one clear implication of these findings is that smoking presents a public health threat broader than generally appreciated. It endangers not only the health of those who choose to actively smoke but also the health of those who passively smoke. Unfortunately, those most susceptible to the adverse effects of passive smoking—young children—have the least control over their environment. Therefore, health care professionals must serve as their advocates by promoting both personal behavior and legislation aimed at reducing the prevalence of tobacco smoking. Intermediate measures, such as segregation of smokers and nonsmokers in public places, or special air ventilation and filtration systems, are less effective interventions for reasons now discussed.

PUBLIC ATTITUDES AND LEGISLATION

Fortunately, public opinion regarding environmental tobacco smoke has changed dramatically since the late 1960s. The nonsmokers' rights movement has presented increasing challenges to the previously strong social support system for smoking, and public opinion surveys have demonstrated overwhelming antismoking sentiment. A 1986 study by the Centers for Disease Control,[159] for instance, revealed that 88% of respondents (93% of people who never smoked, 89% of former smokers, and 79% of current smokers) believed that environmental tobacco smoke was harmful to health, in comparison with 58% (69% of nonsmokers and 40% of smokers) in 1978. In addition, a majority of nonsmokers and even some smokers are annoyed by environmental smoke, and public opinion polls document strong and growing support for restricting or banning smoking in a wide range of public places.

Fueled by this sentiment, such restrictions have been enacted through private initiative and governmental action at all levels; local and state governments, in particular, have been enacting smoking ordinances at an increasing rate since 1980. However, nine states, mostly in the tobacco-growing southeastern section of the United States, still have no antismoking legislation, and a strong protobacco lobby stands behind such inaction.[38] In addition, such legislation, even if enacted, does little to help the young children and nonsmoking spouses who receive the bulk of their exposure at home.

For these reasons, the American Academy of Pediatrics, in a position statement by the Committee on Environmental Hazards,[5] advocated "vigorous and immediate action" to reduce the involuntary exposure of children to tobacco smoke, emphasizing that physicians should (1) seek a history of passive smoking in children with respiratory infections, symptoms, or alterations in pulmonary function; (2) increase their efforts to inform patients and parents about the hazards of both active and passive smoking; (3) take the lead in urging state and local governments to pass more clean-air legislation; (4) encourage the Congress and the Federal Trade Commission to ban all advertising for tobacco products, sponsor advertisements regarding the dangers of tobacco, strengthen the warnings on cigarette packages to include the hazards of passive smoking, and increase the federal excise tax on tobacco products; and (5) urge Congress to dismantle the tobacco price support program.

SMOKING CESSATION AND PREVENTION

Obviously, the most successful method of reducing environmental tobacco smoke would be further reduction of active smoking in the population through both smoking cessation and smoking prevention. Although most smokers have tried to quit and nearly 90% would like to quit, smoking cessation is extremely difficult; the rate of spontaneous quitting is currently less than 1% per year.[160, 161] If physicians simply tell smoking patients and smoking parents on routine visits that both active smoking and passive smoking cause disease and urge them to quit, the success rate increases to about 5%. Formal and comprehensive smoking-cessation programs, involving behavioral therapy, counseling by physicians, and sometimes pharmacologic intervention, can achieve a 1-year success rate of about 20% to 30%.[161, 162] To aid the health care provider in counseling patients and parents about these issues, the National Institutes of Health, in cooperation with the American Lung Association and the American Thoracic Society, published a primer on smoking cessation that is readily available.[163]

For the many parents who are unable to stop smoking, there arises the question regarding methods of minimizing exposure of their children to environmental tobacco smoke. Unfortunately, because the particulate matter in smoke is so small, it remains airborne for long periods and is rapidly and easily distributed throughout an entire home. Thus as Greenberg and co-authors[17] demonstrated, simply smoking in another room does not significantly reduce the amount of exposure that a child ultimately receives. Similarly, separation of smokers from nonsmokers in settings such as commercial airliners has been shown to have little effect on the exposure of nonsmokers to tobacco smoke.[164]

Air-cleaning devices, including both electrostatic devices and high-efficiency particulate air (HEPA) filter systems, may be effective in removing some of the particulate, but little of the gaseous, components of smoke. However, even the high-volume devices are quickly outpaced by continued smoking, and the filters must be cleaned or changed frequently. In addition, many of these devices produce ozone, a respiratory irritant that may intensify asthma in some patients.[165–167] HEPA filters may remove particles larger than 0.5 μm in diameter, but cigarette smoke contains many particles smaller than this.[167] There are no data showing that any of these devices improve the health or symptoms of children chronically exposed to cigarette smoke. Thus neither smoking in a different room nor using any number of air-cleaning devices is an adequate substitute for not smoking at all or only smoking outdoors. Parents, particularly those with young infants or children of any age with respiratory complaints, should be strongly advised in this regard.

In view of the relatively poor success rate of smoking-cessation efforts, as well as frequent lack of compliance with the recommendations just listed, smoking prevention remains the single most important area for intervention. Recognizing this fact, three major agencies—the American Cancer Society, the American Lung Association, and the American Heart Association—have joined to sponsor the Tobacco-Free Young America Project, aimed at achieving a tobacco-free generation of children by the year 2000.[160] Methods used include school curricula emphasizing the negative effects of cigarette smoking, the creation of tobacco-free schools, mass media promotions, and efforts toward more restrictive legislation regarding the advertising and purchasing of tobacco products.

Because most smokers acquired the habit in their teens, physicians caring for children have a special opportunity to contribute to the solution of the passive smoking problem. A well-thought-out approach for physicians, emphasizing age-appropriate interventions, has been proposed.[19] For infants, intervention should be directed toward the parents, inquiring about their smoking habits during well-baby visits and educating them about the adverse health effects of passive smoking. This information should be reinforced at times of acute respiratory illness or symptoms in the infant. For older children, beginning at school age, the physician should teach children that smoking is a harmful and addictive behavior. For adolescents, the physician may provide continued education as well as encouragement of patients to remain nonsmokers in an environment that often includes social pressure to smoke.

REFERENCES

1. The Oxford English Dictionary, 2nd ed. Oxford, England: Oxford University Press, 1989.
2. U.S. Department of Health and Human Services: The Health Consequences of Involuntary Smoking: A Report of the Surgeon General, DHEW publication no. DHHS-CDC-87-8398. Washington, DC: U.S. Government Printing Office, 1986.
3. National Research Council, Committee on Passive Smoking: Environmental Tobacco Smoke: Measuring Exposures and Assessing Health Effects. Washington, DC: National Academy Press, 1986.
4. Weiss ST: Passive smoking and lung cancer: What is the risk? Am Rev Respir Dis 133:1–3, 1986.
5. American Academy of Pediatrics, Committee on Environmental Hazards: Involuntary smoking: A hazard to children. Pediatrics 77:755–757, 1986.
6. Fielding JE, Phenow KJ: Health effects of involuntary smoking. N Engl J Med 319:1452–1460, 1988.
7. Corn M: Characteristics of tobacco sidestream smoke and factors influencing its concentration and distribution in occupied spaces. Scand J Respir Dis [Suppl] 91:21–36, 1974.
8. Repace JL, Lowrey AH: Indoor air pollution, tobacco smoke, and public health. Science 208:464–472, 1980.
9. Hirsch SR: Airway mucus and the mucociliary system. In Middleton E, Reed CE, Ellis EF (eds): Allergy Principles and Practice, 2nd ed, p. 395. St. Louis: CV Mosby, 1983.
10. Stober W: Lung dynamics and uptake of smoke constituents by nonsmokers: A survey. Prev Med 13:589–601, 1984.
11. Weiss ST, Tager IB, Schenker M, Speizer FE: The health effects of involuntary smoking. Am Rev Respir Dis 128:933–942, 1983.
12. Pattishall EN, Strope GL, Etzel RA, et al: Serum cotinine as a measure of tobacco smoke exposure in children. Am J Dis Child 139:1101–1104, 1985.
13. Wald NJ, Boreham J, Bailey A, et al: Urinary cotinine as marker of breathing other people's tobacco smoke. Lancet 1:230–231, 1984.
14. Matsukura S, Taminato T, Kitano N, et al: Effects of environmental tobacco smoke on urinary cotinine excretion in nonsmokers: Evidence for passive smoking. N Engl J Med 311:828–832, 1984.
15. Greenberg RA, Haley NJ, Etzel RA, Loda FA: Measuring the exposure of infants to tobacco smoke: Nicotine and cotinine in urine and saliva. N Engl J Med 310:1075–1078, 1984.
16. Labrecque M, Marcoux S, Weber JP, et al: Feeding and urine cotinine values in babies whose mothers smoke. Pediatrics 83:93–97, 1989.
17. Greenberg RA, Bauman KE, Glover LH, et al: Ecology of passive smoking by young infants. J Pediatr 114:774–780, 1989.
18. Borland BL, Rudolph JP: Relative effects of low socio-economic status, parental smoking and poor scholastic performance on smoking among high school students. Soc Sci Med 9:27–30, 1975.
19. Perry CL, Silvis GL: Smoking prevention: Behavioral prescriptions for the pediatrician. Pediatrics 79:790–799, 1987.
20. Longo L: The biological effects of carbon monoxide on the pregnant woman, fetus and newborn infant. Am J Obstet Gynecol 129:69–103, 1977.
21. International Agency for Research on Cancer: Environmental Carcinogens: Methods of Analysis and Exposure Measurement: Vol. 9. Passive Smoking. Oxford, England: Oxford University Press, 1987.
22. Martin TR, Bracken MB: Association of low birth weight with passive smoke exposure in pregnancy. Am J Epidemiol 124:633–642, 1986.
23. Brooke OG, Anderson HR, Bland JM, et al: Effects on birth weight of smoking, alcohol, caffeine, socioeconomic factors, and psychosocial stress. Br Med J 298:795–801, 1989.
24. Rubin DH, Krasilnikoff PA, Leventhal JM, et al: Effect of passive smoking on birth-weight. Lancet 2:415–417, 1986.
25. Schwartz-Bickenbach D, Schulte-Hobein B, Abt S, et al: Smoking and passive smoking during pregnancy and early infancy: Effects on birth weight, lactation period, and cotinine concentrations in mother's milk and infant's urine. Toxicol Lett 35:73–81, 1987.
26. Haddow JE, Knight GJ, Palomaki GE, McCarthy JE: Second-trimester serum cotinine levels in nonsmokers in relation to birth weight. Am J Obstet Gynecol 159:481–484, 1988.
27. Butler NR, Goldstein H: Smoking in pregnancy and subsequent child development. Br Med J 4:573–575, 1973.
28. Berkey CS, Ware JH, Speizer FE, Ferris BG: Passive smoking and height growth of preadolescent children. Int J Epidemiol 13:454–458, 1984.
29. Rona RJ, Chinn S, Du Ve Florey C: Exposure to cigarette smoking and children's growth. Int J Epidemiol 14:402–409, 1985.
30. Fogelman KR, Manor O: Smoking in pregnancy and development into early adulthood. Br Med J 297:1233–1236, 1988.
31. Steele R, Kraus AS, Langworth JT: Sudden, unexpected death in infancy in Ontario. Can J Public Health 58:359–364, 1967.
32. Naeye RL, Ladis B, Drage JS: Sudden infant death syndrome. Am J Dis Child 130:1207–1210, 1976.

33. Bergman AB, Wiesner LA: Relationship of passive cigarette-smoking to sudden infant death syndrome. Pediatrics 58:665–668, 1976.

34. Nicholl JP, O'Cathain A: Cigarette smoking and early neonatal death. Br Med J 297:487–488, 1988.

35. Manchester DK, Jacoby EH: Sensitivity of human placental monooxygenase activity to maternal smoking. Clin Pharmacol Ther 30:687–692, 1981.

36. Bos RP, Theuws JL, Henderson PT: Excretion of mutagens in human urine after passive smoking. Cancer Lett 19:85–90, 1983.

37. Sandler DP, Comstock GW, Helsing KJ, Shore DL: Deaths from all causes in non-smokers who lived with smokers. Am J Public Health 79:163–167, 1989.

38. Byrd JC, Shapiro RS, Schiedermayer DL: Passive smoking: A review of medical and legal issues. Am J Public Health 79:209–215, 1989.

39. Janerich DT, Thompson WD, Varela LR, et al: Lung cancer and exposure to tobacco smoke in the household. N Engl J Med 323:632–636, 1990.

40. Hirayama T: Cancer mortality in nonsmoking women with smoking husbands based on a large-scale cohort study in Japan. Prev Med 13:680–690, 1984.

41. Sandler DP, Everson RB, Wilcox AJ, Browder JP: Cancer risk in adulthood from early life exposure to parents' smoking. Am J Public Health 74:487–492, 1985.

42. Preston-Martin S, Yu MC, Benton B, Henderson BE: N-nitroso compounds and childhood brain tumors: A case-control study. Cancer Res 42:5240–5245, 1982.

43. Sandler DP, Wilcox AJ, Everson RB: Cumulative effects of lifetime passive smoking on cancer risk. Lancet 1:312–315, 1985.

44. Horton AW: Indoor tobacco smoke pollution: A major risk factor for both breast and lung cancer? Cancer 62:6–14, 1988.

45. Slattery ML, Robison LM, Schuman KL, et al: Cigarette smoking and exposure to passive smoke are risk factors for cervical cancer. JAMA 261:1593–1598, 1989.

46. Neutel CI, Buck C: Effect of smoking during pregnancy on the risk of cancer in children. J Natl Cancer Inst 47:59–63, 1971.

47. Stjernfeldt M, Lindsten J, Berglund K, Ludvigsson J: Maternal smoking during pregnancy and risk of childhood cancer. Lancet 1:1350–1352, 1986.

48. U.S. Department of Health and Human Services: The Health Consequences of Smoking: Cardiovascular Disease: A Report of the Surgeon General, DHHS publication no. 84-50204. Washington, DC: U.S. Government Printing Office, 1983.

49. Garland C, Barrett-Connor E, Suarez L, et al: Effects of passive smoking on ischemic heart disease mortality of nonsmokers: A prospective study. Am J Epidemiol 121:645–650, 1985.

50. Gillis CR, Hole DJ, Hawthorne VM, Boyle P: The effect of environmental tobacco smoke in two urban communities in the west of Scotland. Eur J Respir Dis 65(Suppl. 133):121–126, 1984.

51. Hirayama T: Passive smoking—A new target of epidemiology. Tokai J Exp Clin Med 10:287–293, 1985.

52. Lee PN, Chamberlain J, Alderson MR: Relationship of passive smoking to risk of lung cancer and other smoking-associated diseases. Br J Cancer 54:97–105, 1986.

53. Svendsen KH, Kuller LH, Martin MJ, Ockene JK: Effects of passive smoking in the multiple risk factor intervention trial. Am J Epidemiol 126:783–795, 1987.

54. Helsing KJ, Sandler DP, Comstock GW, Chee E: Heart disease mortality in nonsmokers living with smokers. Am J Epidemiol 127:915–922, 1988.

55. McMurray RG, Hicks LL, Thompson DL: The effects of passive inhalation of cigarette smoke on exercise performance. Eur J Appl Physiol 54:196–200, 1985.

56. Aronow WS: Effect of passive smoking on angina pectoris. N Engl J Med 299:21–24, 1978.

57. Gerrard JW, Heiner DC, Ko CG, et al: Immunoglobulin levels in smokers and non-smokers. Ann Allergy 44:261–262, 1980.

58. Burrows B, Halonen M, Barbee RA, Lebowitz MD: The relationship of serum immunoglobulin E to cigarette smoking. Am Rev Respir Dis 124:523–525, 1981.

59. Warren CP, Holford-Strevens V, Wong C, Manfreda J: The relationship between smoking and total immunoglobulin E levels. J Allergy Clin Immunol 69:370–375, 1982.

60. Burrows B, Halonen M, Lebowitz MD, et al: The relationship of serum immunoglobulin E, allergy skin tests, and smoking to respiratory disorders. J Allergy Clin Immunol 70:199–204, 1982.

61. Taylor G: Tobacco smoke allergy: Does it exist? Scand J Respir Dis [Suppl] 91:50–55, 1974.

62. Lehrer SB, Barbandi F, Taylor JP, Salvaggio JE: Tobacco smoke "sensitivity"—Is there an immunologic basis? J Allergy Clin Immunol 73:240–245, 1984.

63. Gleich GJ, Welsh PW, Yunginger JW, et al: Allergy to tobacco: An occupational hazard. N Engl J Med 302:617–619, 1980.

64. Magnusson CG: Maternal smoking influences cord serum IgE and IgD levels and increases the risk for subsequent infant allergy. J Allergy Clin Immunol 78:898–904, 1986.

65. Johnson C, McCullough J, Blocki S, et al: An epidemiologic study of parental smoking and cord blood IgE and IgD. J Allergy Clin Immunol 83:266, 1989.

66. Kjellman NI: Effect of parental smoking on IgE levels in children. Lancet 1:993–994, 1981.

67. Cogswell JJ, Mitchell EB, Alexander J: Parental smoking, breast feeding, and respiratory infection in development of allergic diseases. Arch Dis Child 62:338–344, 1987.

68. Ownby DR, McCullough J: Passive exposure to cigarette smoke does not increase allergic sensitization in children. J Allergy Clin Immunol 82:634–638, 1988.

69. Weiss ST, Tager IB, Munoz A, Speizer FE: The relationship of respiratory infections in early childhood to the occurrence of increased levels of bronchial responsiveness and atopy. Am Rev Respir Dis 131:573–578, 1985.

70. Martinez FD, Antognoni G, Macri F, et al: Parental smoking enhances bronchial responsiveness in nine-year-old children. Am Rev Respir Dis 138:518–523, 1988.

71. Suoniemi I, Bjorksten F, Haahtela T: Dependence of immediate hypersensitivity in the adolescent period on factors encountered in infancy. Allergy 36:263–268, 1981.

72. Hulbert WC, Walker DC, Jackson A, Hogg JC: Airway permeability to horseradish peroxidase in guinea pigs: The repair phase after injury by cigarette smoke. Am Rev Respir Dis 123:320–326, 1981.

73. Wanner A: Clinical aspects of mucociliary transport. Am Rev Respir Dis 116:73–125, 1977.

74. Park SS, Kikkawa Y, Goldring IP, et al: An animal model of cigarette smoking in beagle dogs: Correlative evaluation of effects on pulmonary function, defense, and morphology. Am Rev Respir Dis 115:971–979, 1977.

75. Ludwig PW, Schwartz BA, Hoidal JR, Niewoehner DE: Cigarette smoking causes accumulation of polymorphonuclear leukocytes in alveolar septum. Am Rev Respir Dis 131:828–830, 1985.

76. Stecenko A, McNicol K, Sauder R: Effect of passive smoking on the lung of young lambs. Pediatr Res 20:853–858, 1986.

77. Sopori ML, Gairola CC, DeLucia AJ, et al: Immune responsiveness of monkeys exposed chronically to cigarette smoke. Clin Immunol Immunopathol 36:338–344, 1985.

78. Tollerud DJ, Clark JW, Brown LM, et al: Association of cigarette smoking with decreased numbers of circulating natural killer cells. Am Rev Respir Dis 139:194–198, 1989.

79. Speer F: Tobacco and the nonsmoker: A study of subjective symptoms. Arch Environ Health 16:443–446, 1968.

80. Weber A, Fischer T: Passive smoking at work. Int Arch Occup Environ Health 47:209–221, 1980.

81. Muramatsu T, Weber A, Muramatsu S, Akermann F: An experimental study on irritation and annoyance due to passive smoking. Int Arch Occup Environ Health 51:305–317, 1983.

82. Weber A: Annoyance and irritation by passive smoking. Prev Med 13:618–625, 1984.

83. Willatt DJ: Children's sore throats related to parental smoking. Clin Otolaryngol 11:317–321, 1986.

84. Kraemer MJ, Richardson MA, Weiss NS, et al: Risk factors for persistent middle-ear effusions. JAMA 249:1022–1025, 1983.

85. Said G, Zalokar J, Lellouch J, Patois E: Parental smoking related to adenoidectomy and tonsillectomy in children. J Epidemiol Community Health 32:97–101, 1978.

86. Iversen M, Birch L, Lundqvist GR, Elbrond O: Middle ear effusion in children and the indoor environment: An epidemiological study. Arch Environ Health 40:74–79, 1985.

87. Black N: The aetiology of glue ear: A case control study. Int J Pediatr Otorhinolaryngol 9:121–133, 1985.

88. Pukander J, Luotonen J, Timonen M, Karma P: Risk factors affecting the occurrence of acute otitis media among 2-3-year-old urban children. Acta Otolaryngol 100:260–265, 1985.

89. Hinton AE, Buckley G: Parental smoking and middle ear effusions in children. J Laryngol Otol 102:992–996, 1988.

90. Richardson MA: Upper airway complications of cigarette smoking. J Allergy Clin Immunol 81:1032–1035, 1988.

91. Rachelefsky GS, Katz RM, Siegel SC: Chronic sinus disease with associated reactive airway disease in children. Pediatrics 73:526–529, 1984.

92. Harlap S, Davies AM: Infant admissions to hospital and maternal smoking. Lancet 1:529–532, 1974.

93. Colley JR, Holland WW, Corkhill RT: Influence of passive smoking and parental phlegm on pneumonia and bronchitis in early childhood. Lancet 2:1031–1034, 1974.

94. Leeder SR, Corkhill RT, Irwig LM, et al: Influence of family factors on the incidence of lower respiratory illness during the first year of life. Br J Prev Soc Med 30:203–212, 1976.

95. Rantakallio P: Relationship of maternal smoking to morbidity and mortality of the child up to the age of five. Acta Paediatr Scand 67:621–631, 1978.

96. Fergusson DM, Horwood LJ, Shannon FT: Parental smoking and respiratory illness in infancy. Arch Dis Child 55:358–361, 1980.

97. Fergusson DM, Horwood LJ, Shannon FT, Taylor B: Parental smoking and lower respiratory illness in the first three years of life. J Epidemiol Community Health 35:180–184, 1981.

98. Fergusson DM, Horwood LJ: Parental smoking and respiratory illness during early childhood: A six-year longitudinal study. Pediatr Pulmonol 1:99–106, 1985.

99. Ware JH, Dockery DW, Spiro A, et al: Passive smoking, gas cooking, and respiratory health of children living in six cities. Am Rev Respir Dis 129:366–374, 1984.

100. Pedreira FA, Guandolo VL, Feroli EJ, et al: Involuntary smoking and incidence of respiratory illness during the first year of life. Pediatrics 75:594–597, 1985.

101. Chen Y, Li W, Yu S: Influence of passive smoking on admissions for respiratory illness in early childhood. Br Med J 293:303–306, 1986.

102. Chen Y, Li W, Yu S, Qian W: Chang-Ning epidemiological study of children's health: Passive smoking and children's respiratory diseases. Int J Epidemiol 17:348–355, 1988.

103. Somerville SM, Rona RJ, Chinn S: Passive smoking and respiratory conditions in primary school children. J Epidemiol Community Health 42:105–110, 1988.

104. Groothuis JR, Gutierrez KM, Lauer BA: Respiratory syncytial virus infection in children with bronchopulmonary dysplasia. Pediatrics 82:199–203, 1988.

105. Wissow LS, Warshow M: Passive smoking exacerbates seasonal variation in acute visits for asthma. Am J Dis Child 142:401, 1988.

106. Evans D, Levison MJ, Feldman CH, et al: The impact of passive smoking on emergency room visits of urban children with asthma. Am Rev Respir Dis 135:567–572, 1987.

107. Ekwo EE, Weinberger MM, Lachenbruch PA, Huntley WH: Relationship of parental smoking and gas cooking to respiratory disease in children. Chest 84:662–668, 1983.

108. Schenker MB, Samet JM, Speizer FE: Risk factors for childhood respiratory disease: The effect of host factors and home environmental exposures. Am Rev Respir Dis 128:1038–1043, 1983.

109. Burchfiel CM, Higgins MW, Keller JB, et al: Passive smoking in childhood: Respiratory conditions and pulmonary function in Tecumseh, Michigan. Am Rev Respir Dis 133:966–973, 1986.

110. Pullan CR, Hey EN: Wheezing, asthma, and pulmonary dysfunction 10 years after infection with respiratory syncytial virus in infancy. Br Med J 284:1665–1669, 1982.

111. McConnochie KM, Roghmann KJ: Parental smoking, presence of older siblings, and family history of asthma increase risk of bronchiolitis. Am J Dis Child 140:806–812, 1986.

112. Hayes EB, Hurwitz ES, Schonberger LB, Anderson LJ: Respiratory syncytial virus outbreak on American Samoa. Am J Dis Child 143:316–321, 1989.

113. McConnochie KM, Roghmann KJ: Bronchiolitis as a possible cause of wheezing in childhood: New evidence. Pediatrics 74:1–10, 1984.

114. Samet JM, Tager IB, Speizer FE: The relationship between respiratory illness in childhood and chronic air-flow obstruction in adulthood. Am Rev Respir Dis 127:508–523, 1983.

115. Charlton A: Children's coughs related to parental smoking. Br Med J 288:1647–1649, 1984.

116. Andrae S, Axelson O, Bjorksten B, et al: Symptoms of bronchial hyperreactivity and asthma in relation to environmental factors. Arch Dis Child 63:473–478, 1988.

117. Schilling RSF, Letai AD, Hui SL, et al: Lung function, respiratory disease, and smoking in families. Am J Epidemiol 106:274–283, 1977.

118. Tashkin DP, Clark VA, Simmons M, et al: The UCLA population studies of chronic obstructive respiratory disease: Relationship between parental smoking and children's lung function. Am Rev Respir Dis 129:891–897, 1984.

119. Tsimoyianis GV, Jacobson MS, Feldman JG, et al: Reduction in pulmonary function and increased frequency of cough associated with passive smoking in teenage athletes. Pediatrics 80:32–36, 1987.

120. Geller-Bernstein G, Kenett R, Weisglass L, et al: Atopic babies with wheezy bronchitis. Allergy 42:85–91, 1987,

121. Cogswell JJ, Mitchell EB, Alexander J: Parental smoking, breast feeding, and respiratory infection in development of allergic diseases. Arch Dis Child 62:338–344, 1987.

122. Murray AB, Morrison BJ: Passive smoking increases the frequency of asthma in children who have had atopic dermatitis. J Allergy Clin Immunol 83:195, 1989.

123. McConnochie KM, Roghmann KJ: Breast feeding and maternal smoking as predictors of wheezing in children ages 6 to 10 years. Pediatr Pulmonol 2:260–268, 1986.

124. Neuspiel DR, Rush D, Butler NR, et al: Parental smoking and post-infancy wheezing in children: A prospective cohort study. Am J Public Health 79:168–171, 1989.

125. Weiss ST, Tager IB, Speizer FE, Rosner B: Persistent wheeze: Its relation to respiratory illness, cigarette smoking, and level of pulmonary function in a population sample of children. Am Rev Respir Dis 122:697–707, 1980.

126. Dodge R: The effects of indoor pollution on Arizona children. Arch Environ Health 37:151–155, 1982.

127. Gortmaker SL, Walker DK, Jacobs FH, Ruch-Ross H: Parental smoking and the risk of childhood asthma. Am J Public Health 72:574–579, 1982.

128. Lebowitz MD, Burrows B: Respiratory symptoms related to smoking habits of family adults. Chest 69:48–50, 1976.

129. Chiang ST, Wang BC: Acute effects of cigarette smoking on pulmonary function. Am Rev Respir Dis 101:860–868, 1970.

130. Gerrard JW, Cockcroft DW, Mink JT, et al: Increased nonspecific bronchial reactivity in cigarette smokers with normal lung function. Am Rev Respir Dis 122:577–581, 1980.

131. Tager IB, Munoz A, Rosner B, et al: Effect of cigarette smoking on the pulmonary function of children and adolescents. Am Rev Respir Dis 131:752–759, 1985.

132. Tager IB, Segal MR, Speizer FE, Weiss ST: The natural history of forced expiratory volumes: Effect of cigarette smoking and respiratory symptoms. Am Rev Respir Dis 138:837–849, 1988.

133. Pimm PE, Silverman F, Shephard RJ: Physiological effects of acute passive exposure to cigarette smoke. Arch Environ Health 33:201–213, 1978.

134. Dahms TE, Bolin JF, Slavin RG: Passive smoking: Effects on bronchial asthma. Chest 80:530–534, 1981.

135. Wiedemann HP, Mahler DA, Loke J, et al: Acute effects of passive smoking on lung function and airway reactivity in asthmatic subjects. Chest 89:180–185, 1986.

136. Knight A, Breslin AB: Passive cigarette smoking and patients with asthma. Med J Aust 142:194–195, 1985.

137. Stankus RP, Menon PK, Rando RJ, et al: Cigarette smoke-sensitive asthma: Challenge studies. J Allergy Clin Immunol 82:331–338, 1988.

138. Shephard RJ, Collins R, Silverman F: Passive exposure of asthmatic subjects to cigarette smoke. Environ Res 20:392–402, 1979.

139. Menon P, Stankus R, Rando R, et al: Increased methacholine sensitivity after exposure to environmental tobacco smoke. J Allergy Clin Immunol 83:245, 1989.

140. Tager IB, Weiss ST, Rosner B, Speizer FE: Effect of parental cigarette smoking on the pulmonary function of children. Am J Epidemiol 110:15–26, 1979.

141. Chen Y, Li W: The effect of passive smoking on children's pulmonary function in Shanghai. Am J Public Health 76:515–518, 1986.
142. O'Connor GT, Weiss ST, Tager IB, Speizer FE: The effect of passive smoking on pulmonary function and nonspecific bronchial responsiveness in a population-based sample of children and young adults. Am Rev Respir Dis 135:800–804, 1987.
143. Hasselblad V, Humble CG, Graham MG, Anderson HS: Indoor environmental determinants of lung function in children. Am Rev Respir Dis 123:479–485, 1981.
144. Vedal S, Schenker MB, Samet JM, Speizer FE: Risk factors for childhood respiratory disease: Analysis of pulmonary function. Am Rev Respir Dis 130:187–192, 1984.
145. Spinaci S, Arossa W, Bugiani M, et al: The effects of air pollution on the respiratory health of children: A cross-sectional study. Pediatr Pulmonol 1:262–266, 1985.
146. Young S, Le Souef PN, Geelhoed GC, et al: The influence of a family history of asthma and parental smoking on airway responsiveness in early infancy. N Engl J Med 324:1168–1173, 1991.
147. Tager IB, Weiss ST, Munoz A, et al: Longitudinal study of the effects of maternal smoking on pulmonary function in children. N Engl J Med 309:699–703, 1983.
148. Berkey CS, Ware JH, Dockery DW, et al: Indoor air pollution and pulmonary function growth in preadolescent children. Am J Epidemiol 123:250–260, 1986.
149. Lebowitz MD, Armet DB, Knudson R: The effect of passive smoking on pulmonary function in children. Environ Int 8:371–373, 1982.
150. Tager IB, Segal MR, Munoz A, et al: The effect of maternal cigarette smoking on the pulmonary function of children and adolescents: Analyses of data from two populations. Am Rev Respir Dis 136:1366–1370, 1987.
151. Lebowitz MD, Holberg CJ: Effects of parental smoking and other risk factors on the development of pulmonary function in children and adolescents: Analysis of two longitudinal population studies. Am J Epidemiol 128:589–597, 1988.
152. Murray AB, Morrison BJ: The effect of cigarette smoke from the mother on bronchial responsiveness and severity of symptoms in children with asthma. J Allergy Clin Immunol 77:575–581, 1986.
153. Murray AB, Morrison BJ: Passive smoking and the seasonal difference of severity of asthma in children. Chest 94:701–708, 1988.
154. White JR, Froeb HF: Small-airways dysfunction in nonsmokers chronically exposed to tobacco smoke. N Engl J Med 302:720–723, 1980.
155. Kauffmann F, Tessier JF, Oriol P: Adult passive smoking in the home environment: A risk factor for chronic airflow limitation. Am J Epidemiol 117:269–280, 1983.
156. Kentner M, Triebig G, Weltle D: The influence of passive smoking on pulmonary function—A study of 1,351 office workers. Prev Med 13:656–669, 1984.
157. Brunekreef B, Fischer P, Remijn B, et al: Indoor air pollution and its effect on pulmonary function of adult nonsmoking women: Passive smoking and pulmonary function. Int J Epidemiol 14:227–230, 1985.
158. Masi MA, Hanley JA, Ernst P, Becklake MR: Environmental exposure to tobacco smoke and lung function in young adults. Am Rev Respir Dis 138:296–299, 1988.
159. Passive smoking: Beliefs, attitudes and exposures—United States, 1986. MMWR 37:239–241, 1988.
160. Eriksen MP, LeMaistre CA, Newell GR: Health hazards of passive smoking. Annu Rev Public Health 9:47–70, 1988.
161. Benowitz NL: Pharmacologic aspects of cigarette smoking and nicotine addiction. N Engl J Med 319:1318–1330, 1988.
162. Mason RJ: Should chest physicians be passive on smoking? Am Rev Respir Dis 133:4, 1986.
163. U.S. Department of Health and Human Services: Clinical Opportunities for Smoking Intervention: A Guide for the Busy Physician, NIH publication no. 86-2178. Washington, DC: U.S. Government Printing Office, 1986.
164. Mattson ME, Boyd G, Byar D, et al: Passive smoking on commercial airline flights. JAMA 261:867–872, 1989.
165. Lefcoe NM, Ashley MJ, Pederson LL, Keays JJ: The health risks of passive smoking: The growing case for control measures in enclosed environments. Chest 84:90–95, 1983.
166. Olander L, Johansson J, Johansson R: Tobacco smoke removal with room air cleaners. Scand J Work Environ Health 14:390–397, 1988.
167. Kemp JP, Meltzer EO: Gaining control of the allergic child's environment. Am J Asthma Allergy Pediatr 1:22–31, 1987.

86 PERIOPERATIVE MANAGEMENT OF PEDIATRIC PATIENTS: PHYSIOLOGIC CONSIDERATIONS

GLENNA B. WINNIE, M.D.

EFFECTS OF GENERAL ANESTHESIA ON PULMONARY FUNCTION

In early studies, researchers examining changes in pulmonary physiology in patients under general anesthesia found that compliance of the lung and of the total respiratory system diminished markedly during anesthesia and muscle paralysis.[1,2] At that time, it was hypothesized that a change in distribution of inspired gas caused the observed decrease in pulmonary compliance. It has since been shown that shape and motion of the chest wall are altered during general anesthesia; these changes occur during spontaneous breathing and with muscle paralysis and mechanical ventilation.[3, 4] Anesthesia is associated with alteration in the distribution of the inspired gases,[5, 6] a decrease in functional residual capacity (FRC), and development of airway closure in dependent lung units. The reduction in FRC is associated with a shift of the pressure-volume curve of the lung to the right at low lung volumes. Other changes observed include increased lung recoil pressure, decreased closing capacity, altered gas exchange, and ventilation/perfusion ($\dot{V}/\dot{Q}$) mismatching.[7, 8] Inhalational agents can also impair regulation of pulmonary blood flow, causing $\dot{V}/\dot{Q}$ mismatch and impairment in gas exchange.[9]

The normal physiology of the chest wall must be described in order to compare the alterations induced by general anesthesia. The chest wall can be defined as the rib cage and the diaphragm and its actions are intimately coupled with those of the abdominal contents. The chest wall participates in ventilation and acts to stabilize the thoracic contents. The efficiency of diaphragmatic function depends on the action of the muscles that stabilize the rib cage against the changes in its shape induced by diaphragmatic contraction. In the erect position, contraction of the diaphragm everts the ribs; the interaction between rib cage and diaphragm may be less efficient in the supine position. During quiet breathing, the phasic activity of the diaphragm provides ventilation. Although phasic activity of respiratory muscles determines ventilatory function, the tonic activity of these muscles changes their baseline length between phasic contractions. There is evidence that the reduction in FRC observed during general anesthesia is a result of suppression of the tonic activity of the diaphragm;[10] this evidence is further supported by findings that muscle paralysis does not induce further change in FRC after general anesthesia.[11]

The chest wall and lungs function as a unit, and changes in the shape or motion of the chest wall affect the configuration of the lungs and vice versa. Alterations in pulmonary function induced by changes in the chest wall have been well described. Chest wall and abdominal restriction in spontaneously breathing, conscious, seated adults causes a reduction in lung compliance, a decrease in lung volumes, an increase in elastic recoil pressure of the lung, a change in distribution of inspired gases, a decrease in arterial oxygen tension, and an increase in intrapulmonary shunting.[12] Schmid and Rehder[13] also noted that the distribution of inspired gas may be changed by an altered pattern of expansion of the chest in awake persons. Halothane anesthesia suppresses intercostal muscle function more than diaphragmatic function, causing a decrease in rib cage expansion and subsequent paradoxical ventilation with alteration in distribution of inhaled gas.[6, 14]

Nonproportional changes in chest wall shape alter the distribution of inspired gas, regional lung volumes, and pleural pressure, whereas proportional changes in chest wall configuration do not change these parameters. Therefore, some of the observed effects of general anesthesia are caused by its influence on the shape and motion of the chest wall, with secondary changes in the shape of the lung. Compensatory mechanisms, including collat-

eral ventilation and mechanical interdependence of the lung parenchyma, may reduce the changes in gas distribution that result from nonproportional changes in chest wall shape.

General anesthesia and paralysis affect the distribution of inspired gases by causing alterations in diaphragmatic mechanics.[3] During normal spontaneous ventilation in the awake state, inspired gas volume is preferentially distributed to the dependent lung areas because regional ventilation parallels lung compliance. Compliance varies with differing alveolar volumes as determined by the pleural pressure gradient, which is affected both by gravity and by the abdominal contents and diaphragm. During spontaneous ventilation in the awake state and supine position, most diaphragmatic movement occurs at the dependent level of the diaphragm. With induction of anesthesia, there is loss of tonic activity of the diaphragm, causing a cephalad shift in its end-expiratory position. This cephalad shift of the diaphragm is greater in dependent areas, and diaphragmatic movement remains greater in the dependent areas. With paralysis, a cephalad shift in diaphragmatic position similar to the shift seen with anesthesia is observed. However, there is a reversal of the pattern of diaphragmatic movement, in which most of diaphragmatic movement occurs in the nondependent areas where abdominal pressure is least. Positive end-expiratory pressure (PEEP) administered during either anesthesia or paralysis does not return the diaphragm to its awake FRC position, and large mechanical breaths do not duplicate the pattern of displacement seen with spontaneous ventilation. However, stimulation of the phrenic nerve during anesthesia produces diaphragmatic movement similar to that seen in spontaneous ventilation, with greater movement in the dependent part of the diaphragm. Phrenic nerve stimulation also produces a significantly greater improvement in gas exchange than does the application of PEEP to the same increase in lung volume.[15]

VENTILATION/PERFUSION MISMATCH INDUCED BY ANESTHESIA

The changes in regional distribution of inspired gases caused by the changes in chest wall mechanics after induction of general anesthesia are not accompanied by appropriate changes in perfusion. Therefore, anesthesia is associated with $\dot{V}/\dot{Q}$ mismatching. This causes impairment of oxygenation because of the development of low $\dot{V}/\dot{Q}$ ratios in certain areas and retention of carbon dioxide as a result of the presence of high $\dot{V}/\dot{Q}$ ratios in other regions. Hypoxic pulmonary vasoconstriction is also impaired during anesthesia with certain agents, including nitrous oxide and isoflurane; this effect is weaker with halothane and enflurane.[16, 17] Other mechanisms contribute to increased $\dot{V}/\dot{Q}$ mismatch during anesthesia, because similar changes in $\dot{V}/\dot{Q}$ can occur in awake persons when the diaphragm is voluntarily relaxed during passive inflation of the lungs.[18] Atelectasis, described in the following section, may also contribute to ventilation/perfusion abnormalities.

ATELECTASIS

Atelectasis, or closure of lung units, is a common intraoperative and postoperative event. Microatelectasis may occur at the subsegmental level or more distally and may not be apparent on chest radiographs. Macroatelectasis, the localized collapse of a segment, a lobe, or an entire lung, can be observed radiographically. Studies with computed tomography have shown that areas of atelectasis develop in dependent lung regions promptly after induction of anesthesia. The atelectatic areas are perfused, and the amount of right-to-left shunting is correlated with the size of the areas of atelectasis.[19] Both atelectasis and shunting increase when muscle paralysis is added to anesthesia with spontaneous breathing. Addition of PEEP decreases the size of the areas of atelectasis but does not affect the degree of shunting.[20] Extensive atelectasis tends to develop more commonly during surgery in patients who are obese or who have a low and wide thorax. The atelectasis may persist longer than 24 h after the termination of anesthesia.

In his review of pulmonary complications associated with surgery, Tisi[21] noted that atelectasis is the result of failure of normal mechanisms to maintain the stability of lung units in the perioperative period. In addition to the changes in chest wall mechanics discussed earlier, the other factors that may contribute to the development of atelectasis include retained secretions, lack of or a decrease in sighing, and a decrease in expiratory reserve volume (ERV).

Mucociliary clearance is adversely affected by general anesthesia (to be described), and even patients with normal production of secretions are at risk for secretion retention and atelectasis. If a bronchus becomes occluded, perfusion continues in the pulmonary segment. Rate of absorption of the gas distal to the site of occlusion is a function of the nature of the gas, and nitrogen is absorbed more slowly than oxygen. Air, which consists of approximately 78.6% nitrogen, 0.04% carbon dioxide, and 20.8% oxygen, requires more time for resorption than do gas mixtures that contain higher concentrations of oxygen.[22] Therefore, the patient receiving supplemental oxygen is at increased risk for development of atelectasis. Even in normal volunteers, there is a marked increase in the alveolar-to-arterial oxygen tension gradient while breathing 100% oxygen in the supine position. This finding is consistent with intrapulmonary shunting caused by diffuse atelectasis in terminal lung units, although there is no radiographic evidence of macroatelectasis.[23]

Changes that occur in the ventilatory pattern after surgery may promote the development of atelectasis. After laparotomy, there is an approximately 20% decrease in tidal volume by the first postoperative day. This decrease is accompanied by a compensatory increase in respiratory rate with no change in minute ventilation. The ventilatory pattern returns to normal in the second postoperative week. Sighing, defined as a breath of more than three times the average tidal volume, occurs approximately 10 times per hour in normal women and 9 times per hour in normal men. However, chest wall splinting as a result of pain, residual anesthetic agents, and narcotic analgesics given for postoperative pain may decrease or ablate sighing.

In anesthetized dogs breathing spontaneously or ventilated with a pump, pulmonary compliance decreased by approximately one third within 1 to 2 h after periodic hyperinflations were stopped, and postmortem examination of the lungs suggested that the decreased compliance was caused by atelectasis. In these animals, FRC decreased approximately 10% when hyperinflations were stopped and decreased an average of 13% after forced deflation.[24] Similar changes in compliance have been measured in humans; after a series of deep breaths, breathing at close to tidal volume for 30 min leads to a decrease in compliance of 26% to 40%. Two or more deep breaths to maximal inspiration can increase compliance, but a forced expiration can eliminate the previous increase.[25]

Changes in static lung volumes after surgery are well described and may be caused by the changes in ventilatory pattern described earlier. In 1933, Beecher demonstrated the following spirometric changes after laparotomy: (1) vital capacity decreases by approximately 45% by 1 to 2 days after surgery and returns to preoperative levels within 1 to 2 weeks after surgery; (2) upper abdominal procedures are accompanied by a greater decrease in vital capacity than are lower abdominal procedures; and (3) residual volume and FRC decrease postoperatively and are at their lowest levels on the fourth postoperative day.[26] Total lung capacity and its subdivisions are decreased after abdominal surgery, and changes occurring after upper abdominal surgery are greater than those after lower abdominal surgery, although operations on an extremity do not affect lung volumes.[27] Expiratory reserve volume decreases by approximately 60% after upper abdominal surgery and by 25% after lower abdominal surgery. Such a decrease in ERV may bring the end-tidal point lower than the closing volume and promote atelectasis.

Anesthesia may change closing volume, the lung volume at which airways in the dependent portions of the lung become compressed and close because the pressure surrounding the airways is higher than the pressure within them. In normal adults, closing volume is higher than the residual volume and lower than the end-tidal point. It is not changed by the supine position in persons aged 7 to 40 years. Any situation in which closing volume is higher than the end-tidal point places the patient at risk of atelectasis caused by closure of airways during a portion of tidal breathing. The decreases in FRC and ERV that are induced by anesthesia and occur in the postoperative period may lead to atelectasis by this mechanism. Obese patients, elderly patients, smokers, and patients with chronic obstructive lung disease have increased closing volume and are therefore at increased risk of postoperative atelectasis. In comparison with adults, normal infants have an increased closing volume that is higher than the end-tidal point (Fig. 86–1). Chest wall changes induced by anesthesia can increase the closing volume to above the tidal end-inspiratory level and cause subsequent closure of dependent airways throughout tidal breathing.

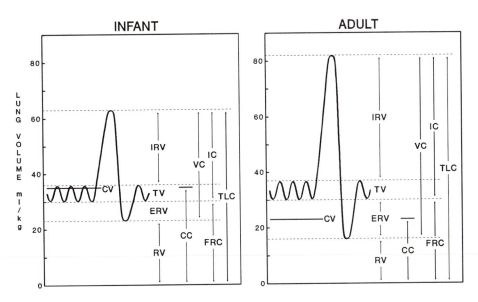

Figure 86–1. Lung volumes in infants in comparison with adults. Note location of closing volume. IRV, inspiratory reserve volume; TV, tidal volume; ERV, expiratory reserve volume; RV, residual volume; CV, closing volume; CC, closing capacity; VC, vital capacity; IC, inspiratory capacity; FRC, functional residual capacity; TLC, total lung capacity. (Data from Nelson NM: The onset of respiration. *In* Avery GB (ed): Neonatology: Pathophysiology and Management of the Newborn, 3rd ed, p. 188. Philadelphia: JB Lippincott, 1987.)

EFFECTS OF ANESTHESIA ON PULMONARY DEFENSE MECHANISMS

Several nonspecific defense mechanisms protect the respiratory tract from the effects of exposure to particulate matter and infectious agents. The most important of these mechanisms are mucociliary clearance, phagocytosis by alveolar macrophages, mechanical barriers, and cough. The first two defense mechanisms can be profoundly altered by anesthesia, and the normal upper airway barriers are completely bypassed in intubated patients. Therefore, it is not surprising that the two most common postoperative complications are atelectasis and pneumonia. The following sections concern the effects of anesthesia on mucociliary clearance and alveolar macrophage function.

MUCOCILIARY CLEARANCE

Mucociliary clearance is decreased in humans undergoing surgery under general anesthesia and remains depressed in the postoperative period. This is especially true in patients undergoing abdominal operations or who remain under prolonged anesthesia.[28] The depression in mucociliary clearance associated with surgery has several components. Factors that can affect clearance include mechanical disruption of the epithelium and mucus blanket by endotracheal tube or suction catheter, drying and cooling of the airway, hyperoxia, and anesthetic and anticholinergic agents. Pre-existing conditions may alter the character of the mucociliary transport system, for example, cystic fibrosis, bronchopulmonary dysplasia, asthma, bronchitis secondary to smoking, and other pulmonary diseases increase the risk of pulmonary complications after surgery.

Mechanical Disruption. Airway manipulations that occur during the course of surgery include intubation and suctioning. Suction catheters can cause denudation of the respiratory epithelium, edema, and formation of inflammatory exudates. Similarly, the endotracheal tube can damage the epithelium of the larynx and trachea.[29] Endotracheal tubes with low-pressure, high-compliance cuffs cause less epithelial damage than those with high-pressure, low-compliance cuffs. However, inflation of either type of endotracheal tube cuff in the subglottic area leads to a decrease in tracheal mucus velocity in the distal trachea within 1 h.[30] Rigid bronchoscopy and touching the respiratory tract epithelium with objects such as cotton swabs can cause desquamation of the mucosa and subsequent impairment of mucociliary clearance.

Temperature and Humidity. The movement of the mucociliary blanket is little affected by changes in atmospheric humidity or temperature, inasmuch as the upper airway structures normally warm and humidify the inspired air so that it reaches body temperature and is completely saturated by the time it reaches the carina. The optimal temperature range for ciliary activity appears to be body temperature, with a drop in ciliary beat frequency as temperature falls from 40°C to 20°C.[31]

Exposure of tracheal epithelium to dry air causes submucosal inflammation, sloughing of ciliated epithelial cells, and ultrastructural changes in these cells.[32] Breathing dry air at room temperature through an endotracheal tube leads to marked decrease in tracheal mucus transport in dogs, and in most dogs breathing air at 50% relative humidity, mucociliary clearance slows down.[33] Rabbits ventilated with dry gas for 6 h exhibit a precipitous fall in body temperature, desquamation of the respiratory epithelium with damage to the basement membrane, and bronchial plugging. Rabbits ventilated with humidified gas at the same temperature exhibit only a slight fall in body temperature and no histologic changes in the airways.[34] Humans who breathe dry gas for 3 h exhibit significant damage to ciliated respiratory epithelial cells. In contrast, inspiration of warm, humidified gas can prevent hypothermia and postoperative complications in infants and children.[35]

Hyperoxia. The effects of oxygen on respiratory tract epithelium are dependent on the species studied, the length of exposure, and the concentration of oxygen used. However, it is clear that oxygen has deleterious effects on mucociliary transport (clearance). In anesthetized dogs, both increased length of exposure and a higher concentration of inspired oxygen are associated with a proportional decrease in tracheal mucus velocity.[36] Although the time frame varies among animal species, the earliest changes are observed in mitochondria and in the ciliated epithelial cells, with development of acute tracheobronchitis. A decrease in mucociliary clearance may be one of the earliest changes induced by oxygen in humans, inasmuch as normal subjects breathing 90% to 95% oxygen for 6 h exhibit a decrease in tracheal mucus velocity to 50% of baseline levels.[37] Thus an increased concentration of inspired oxygen during and after surgery may contribute to stasis of pulmonary secretions and consequently increase the risk of atelectasis and infection.

Anesthetic Agents. General anesthesia decreases mucociliary clearance in animals and in humans, but it is difficult to separate the effects of airway manipulation, hyperoxia, and changes induced by other medications from the effects of specific anesthetic agents. For example, in women undergoing a 90-min gynecologic operation with halothane and nitrous oxide anesthesia, there is a progressive decrease in tracheal mucus velocity.[38] In dogs already anesthetized with thiopental, halothane slows tracheal mucus clearance; this effect is concentration dependent and reversible when administration of halothane is discontinued.[39] Tracheal explant cultures from ferrets show a reversible inhibition of ciliary activity when exposed to halothane. There is no change in ciliary activity with exposure to 2% halothane, but ciliostasis develops with 3% halothane, and ciliary activity ceases almost completely with exposure to 4% and 5% halothane.[40] Intravenous administration of pentobarbital or thioamylal decreases tracheal mucus clearance in sheep.[41]

Other agents used in the perioperative period can affect mucociliary clearance. Topical application of 2% tetracaine effectively stops mucociliary function in humans, although 4% lidocaine does not have this effect.[41] Because atropine inhibits production of tracheobronchial secretions, it is not surprising that it decreases mucus transport. When atropine or hyoscine is administered orally to normal persons, mucociliary clearance is impaired. This effect is not observed with inhaled ipratropium in therapeutic doses. Opiates that have been shown to impair mucociliary clearance include codeine, normethadone, and morphine. Codeine causes a dose-dependent depression of ciliary beat frequency.[42]

ALVEOLAR MACROPHAGE FUNCTION

Alveolar macrophages reside in the alveoli and terminal bronchioles and constitute one of the major nonspecific host defenses against inhalation of both particulate matter and infectious agents. Their functions are to ingest inhaled particles by phagocytosis, transport the particle through the lung, and detoxify or neutralize the inhaled and ingested material. Halothane, methoxyflurane, and cyclopropane depress the bactericidal activity of pulmonary alveolar macrophages,[40] placing postoperative patients at increased risk of pulmonary infection.

PREVENTION AND TREATMENT OF PERIOPERATIVE COMPLICATIONS

Understanding the physiologic changes that occur in the intraoperative and postoperative periods enables physicians to anticipate the potential pulmonary complications. Meticulous medical management of fluids and the airway and judicious administration of oxygen can help prevent complications. Initiation of appropriate therapy in the pre- and postoperative periods can lower the incidence of complications, even among patients who are at high risk.

CHEST PHYSIOTHERAPY

Different methods of chest physiotherapy have been used since the 1940s to lower the incidence of the common postoperative complications of atelectasis and pneumonia. In 1954, Thoren reported that postural drainage accompanied by breathing and coughing exercises decreased the incidence of atelectasis after cholecystectomy: atelectasis developed in 12% of patients given preoperative instruction and treatment, in comparison with 27% of patients instructed postoperatively and 42% of the control group, who were given no instructions.[41] The literature has subsequently contained numerous studies on the efficacy of diverse forms of chest physiotherapy, including chest percussion and postural drainage, various coughing exercises, incentive spirometry, intermittent positive-pressure breathing (IPPB), and continuous positive airway pressure (CPAP). These studies have yielded conflicting results; however, the patients studied and the methods used have varied widely. Some studies do not contain appropriate control groups, and few studies contain untreated controls.

The bulk of the evidence supports the use of some form of respiratory therapy to prevent postoperative complications. In a study of three groups of patients randomly assigned to IPPB to 15 cm H_2O, resistance breathing, or incentive spirometry four times a day after an upper abdominal operation, there were no differences in incidence of postoperative fever, atelectasis, or pneumonia.[42] Celli and associates,[43] in a carefully designed study, compared the following conditions among patients who underwent abdominal surgery (1) no postoperative treatment; (2) IPPB to 15 cm H_2O for 15 min, four times per day; (3) incentive spirometry with a minimum of 10 breaths, each held for 3 sec and until at least 70% of preoperative vital capacity was achieved, four times per day; and (4) deep-breathing exercises, with increasingly deep inhalations until total lung capacity was reached, followed by breath holding and then a forced triple cough, repeated at least 10 times over 15 min, four times per day. For patients who had undergone upper abdominal surgery, all three treatment groups had shorter hospital stays. There were no differences in incidence of radiographic abnormalities between groups. Significant pulmonary complications were defined as three or more of the following: cough, sputum production, dyspnea, chest pain, fever, and tachycardia. These occurred among fewer patients in the three treatment groups (21% to 22%) than in the control group (48%). Respiratory failure developed in 9% of control patients, in comparison with 7% of IPPB patients, 0% of incentive spirometry patients, and 5% of the deep-breathing exercise patients. The side effects of bloating and abdominal distension developed in 18% of patients receiving IPPB, whereas patients in the other groups experienced no such complications.[43] Resolution of pneumonia in nonsurgical adult patients has not been hastened by chest physiotherapy and IPPB.[44]

CPAP and positive expiratory pressure (PEP) by face mask also successfully decrease postoperative pulmonary complications. In a study of patients who underwent upper abdominal surgery, Ricksten and colleagues[45] compared three patient groups: (1) control patients who took 30 maximal inhalations with the aid of a Triflo deep-breathing exerciser (a type of incentive spirometer) every waking hour; (2) patients who received CPAP by face mask for 30 breaths to 10 to 15 cm H_2O every waking hour, and (3) patients who received PEP by face mask for 30 breaths with expiratory resistance to create a peak PEP of 10 to 15 cm H_2O every waking hour. All patients performed deep-breathing exercises and forced expiratory maneuvers for 30 to 40 min twice per day. The alveolar-to-arterial oxygen (A-a) difference was increased in all groups after surgery and was highest on the first postoperative day. On the second postoperative day, this difference was less in the PEP group than in the incentive spirometry group, and on the third postoperative day both the CPAP and the PEP groups had lower alveolar-to-arterial oxygen differences than did the incentive spirometry group. On the third postoperative day, forced vital capacity was higher and the incidence of radiographic evidence of atelectasis was lower in the PEP and CPAP groups than in the incentive spirometry group.

Ricksten and colleagues concluded that deep-breathing exercises with the use of an incentive spirometer are not as efficacious as periodic face mask administration of CPAP or PEP with regard to gas exchange, maintenance of lung volumes, and prevention and treatment of atelectasis after upper abdominal surgery.[43] Nasal CPAP has also been reported as an effective modality for treatment of atelectasis when chest physiotherapy and IPPB have failed.

Several other modalities have been compared with standard chest physiotherapy for prevention or treatment of postoperative atelectasis. In a prospective randomized trial, Jaworski and co-workers examined the role of routine postlobectomy fiberoptic bronchoscopy in prevention of atelectasis and found no advantage of bronchoscopy over conventional bronchodilator aerosols combined with postural drainage and chest percussion.[46] Fiberoptic bronchoscopy does not hasten the resolution of acute atelectasis in comparison with a regimen of incentive spirometry, chest percussion, postural drainage, and bronchodilator aerosols in a randomized study.[47] A minitracheostomy has been advocated for treatment of postoperative atelectasis and retention of secretions in

patients in whom atelectasis is unresponsive to nasal CPAP and chest physiotherapy.[48]

Although various forms of chest physiotherapy are important treatment modalities for postoperative patients, physicians must be aware of potential complications of physiotherapy. Pain exacerbated by chest percussion may contribute to cardiovascular instability in certain patients. Bronchospasm may develop in asthmatic patients if they are placed in a head-down position. Adult postoperative patients with cardiovascular complications may have a drop in arterial oxygen tension (Pa_{O_2}) during chest physiotherapy given with IPPB.[40] Adult patients hospitalized with acute nonsurgical pulmonary disease have been reported to sometimes exhibit a decrease in Pa_{O_2} during postural drainage and chest percussion, which is thought to be secondary to increased $\dot{V}/\dot{Q}$ mismatch. Patients most likely to experience this decrease are those with few or thick secretions. Although in an early study a drop in Pa_{O_2} occurred in intubated neonates after chest physiotherapy, Pa_{O_2} significantly increased after postural drainage and chest percussion in a controlled study of neonates with respiratory distress.[49] Drops in Pa_{O_2} can be prevented by administration of 100% oxygen during chest percussion. Thus increased supplemental oxygen may be necessary for patients who require chest physiotherapy but in whom arterial oxygen saturation decreases in association with the therapy.

OXYGEN

Postoperative hypoxia may occur secondary to $\dot{V}/\dot{Q}$ mismatch, atelectasis, fluid overload, or respiratory depression secondary to analgesia. Although high concentrations of inspired oxygen can cause tracheobronchitis, a decrease in mucociliary transport, and an increase in atelectasis, supplemental oxygen is usually indicated in the immediate postoperative period. Jones and collaborators, comparing the effects of breathing either room air or 28% oxygen after anesthesia and surgery, found that oxygen did not change the number of episodes of central apnea, obstructive apnea, or upper airway obstruction, but it did eliminate episodes of arterial desaturation to less than 80% oxygen saturation.[50] Adequate oxygenation is particularly important in children in order to help prevent muscle fatigue and episodes of respiratory instability. Increased levels of supplemental oxygen may be necessary in certain patients during chest physiotherapy (see the earlier Chest Physiotherapy section).

PAIN MANAGEMENT

Physicians are responsible for controlling postoperative pain as well as possible without significantly depressing ventilation. Unrelieved pain can compromise pulmonary function through chest wall splinting, decrease in coughing, and exacerbation of bronchospasm. It can also contribute to cardiovascular instability in postoperative patients (for a discussion of postoperative pain control, see Chapter 87).

MANAGEMENT OF CHILDREN AT HIGH RISK FOR PERIOPERATIVE COMPLICATIONS

Because of the physiologic changes associated with anesthesia, infants and children are at high risk for complications after surgery. The factors that place children at higher risk than adults include small airway size, increased peripheral airway resistance, immaturity of the ventilatory center, relative muscle weakness with inability to recruit intercostal muscles, and earlier diaphragmatic fatigue. Other considerations include high chest wall compliance and high closing volume, which place children and even healthy adolescents at higher risk for atelectasis than adults. Pre-existing disease of the respiratory tract further increases the risk of postoperative pulmonary complications. In the remainder of this chapter, the assessment and treatment of children with specific pulmonary diseases are described.

CHILDREN WITH INFECTIONS OF THE UPPER RESPIRATORY TRACT

Elective surgery should not be performed in children with acute infections of the upper or lower respiratory tract. Mucosal damage associated with infections of the respiratory tract can impair mucociliary clearance, placing the child at increased risk for atelectasis, $\dot{V}/\dot{Q}$ mismatch, and hypoxia. Secondary bacterial infection may occur. Increased reactivity of the airways is well documented in patients with infections of the upper respiratory tract, including rhinovirus infection and influenza type A infection.[51] The increased airway reactivity persists for at least 3 weeks but resolves by 5 to 6 weeks in most patients. It is thought that the epithelial damage induced by the infection exposes airway receptors to inhaled irritants and causes increased bronchoconstriction through a vagal reflex.

The history of an infection of the upper respiratory tract during the month before anesthesia, without overt abnormalities on physical examination immediately before surgery, has been associated with atelectasis and hypoxia during anesthesia in children.[52] Therefore, it is recommended that elective surgery not be performed during an infection of the upper respiratory tract and that it be deferred for at least 2 weeks thereafter. However, if patients have a history of a recently resolved infection of the upper respiratory tract, a chest radiograph should be obtained and surgery deferred if the radiograph is abnormal. Further studies are required before definite recommendations can be made with regard to children who present for elective surgery with a history of a recent infection of the respiratory tract, a normal examination, and a normal radiograph. Current practice is to proceed with anesthesia.

PREMATURE INFANTS

Premature infants and infants with bronchopulmonary dysplasia are at higher risk of postoperative pulmonary complications than are term infants. Steward reported that 33% of preterm infants undergoing herniorrhaphy experienced perioperative pulmonary complications, in comparison with 2.6% of full-term infants undergoing herniorrhaphy.[53] The most frequent complication was apnea, which was demonstrated by 18% of the infants and occurred as late as 12 h postoperatively. Atelectasis, aspiration pneumonia, stridor, excessive secretions, coughing, and cyanosis were also observed. The patients who had apnea were under 10 weeks of age and had body weights of less than 3000 g at the time of operation. History of apnea or history of respiratory distress syndrome was not predictive of which infants would experience this complication.

In a prospective study of infants receiving general anesthesia, Liu and associates found that premature infants with a history of apnea required postoperative ventilatory support for apnea more frequently than all other infants, even in comparison with other premature infants.[54] The infants requiring respiratory support were under 41 weeks of conceptual age and under 4 months of postnatal age, whereas those who did not require support were over 46 weeks of conceptual age and over 4 months of postnatal age. Mayhew and colleagues reported that 17% of infants with a history of prematurity experienced postoperative pulmonary complications after herniorrhaphy.[55] Four of the 35 patients developed postoperative apnea and required ventilatory support; three of these four children had bronchopulmonary dysplasia, and all of them had a history of apnea. Three of these children were under 44 weeks of conceptual age; however, the fourth child, who had bronchopulmonary dysplasia, was 72 weeks of conceptual age and 44 weeks of postnatal age.

In view of these considerations, it is recommended that nonessential surgery be delayed for preterm infants until they are over 44 weeks of conceptual age. Also, if such surgery cannot be delayed, even asymptomatic preterm infants should be admitted to the hospital and receive monitoring for apnea and bradycardia for at least 18 h postoperatively. The hospital should be equipped to mechanically ventilate infants postoperatively.

ASTHMA

Asthma, or reactive airways disease, is characterized by episodes of airway obstruction associated with bronchospasm, airway inflammation, and increased mucus secretion. Children with asthma are at increased risk for perioperative complications, including laryngospasm, bronchospasm, excessive secretions, $\dot{V}/\dot{Q}$ mismatch, hypoxia, atelectasis, and intraoperative arrhythmias.

Preoperative Assessment. Preoperative assessment of asthmatic patients is important for determining the severity of hyperreactivity of the airways and the adequacy of control of the airway obstruction. Pattern of symptoms, history of hospitalization for treatment of pulmonary disease and allergies, and medication history are determined. History of steroid use is of particular importance for evaluating both disease severity and appropriate use of steroids in the perioperative period. Previous experience with anesthetics should be reviewed and complications discussed. Elements of the physical examination that are to be emphasized include assessments for chest hyperinflation, chest retractions, prolonged expiratory time, adventitious sounds such as wheezes or rales (crackles), adequacy and symmetry of aeration, and digital clubbing. Pulmonary function tests are useful for determining the degree of airway obstruction, if a child is able to perform them; however, normal preoperative spirometry does not ensure an uncomplicated perioperative course. Pulse oximetry, a noninvasive method for determining adequacy of oxygenation, can be performed on patients of any age. A preoperative chest radiograph is obtained if there are abnormalities of physical examination, pulmonary function tests, or oximetry or if the previous radiograph obtained for the patient was abnormal. The value of a chest radiograph for a child who is currently asymptomatic is controversial. The planned operation and postoperative management should be explained to patients during the preoperative period because emotional stress can precipitate bronchospasm.

Premedication. Because bronchospasm may develop with induction of anesthesia or intubation in asthmatic patients, optimal control of bronchospasm before surgery is desirable. Patients with poorly controlled reactive airways disease may require hospitalization before elective operation in order to optimize treatment and pulmonary status. Aerosolized beta$_2$-agonists, theophylline, corticosteroids, and, in patients with retained secretions, chest physiotherapy are effective therapeutic modalities. However, the most appropriate ways to use theophylline or steroids in the perioperative period have not been established.

Ventricular arrythmias and cardiac arrest have been associated with halothane anesthesia in patients receiving theophylline. However, in the only case in a child in which theophylline level was documented, the level was 21.6 μg/ml 1 h after the arrest.[56] Cardiac arrhythmias on induction are nevertheless rare in children, and asthma can be associated with bronchospasm, increased secretions, cough, hypoxemia, and atelectasis during anesthesia. Therefore, a therapeutic theophylline level should be achieved preoperatively in patients who require theophylline. The anesthesiologist should be prepared to administer aminophylline intraoperatively, if bronchospasm develops.

Indications for steroids are also not clear. Patients who are currently receiving either oral or inhaled steroids should receive intravenous steroids, beginning either before surgery or close to the time of induction of anesthesia. Five milligrams of hydrocortisone hemisuccinate per kilogram or an equivalent drug may be given every 6 to 8 h for at least 24 h to prevent perioperative adrenal insufficiency and for prophylaxis against bronchospasm.

There is no consensus on whether children who have received a course of steroids in the year before surgery should also receive such a course of medication. Support for administration of steroids in this situation includes evidence that high-dose steroids given for 5 days can cause transient adrenal suppression in adults and that such suppression may persist for up to 1 year.[57] Whether asthmatic patients who have not received steroids in the year before surgery should receive perioperative steroids for prophy-

laxis against bronchospasm has not been examined, and clinical judgment must be used at present. Narcotic premedication should be avoided in asthmatic patients because it can be associated with histamine release.

Intraoperative Management. Anesthesia in asthmatic patients can precipitate bronchospasm by several mechanisms, including airway irritation and histamine release caused by agents such as thiopental, methohexital, atropine, and neuromuscular blocking agents. Patients with severe asthma should have an intravenous catheter in place at the time of induction, and it should be possible to establish access quickly in all patients.

Halothane is the most widely used inhalational agent because it causes bronchodilation and is less irritating than enflurane or isoflurane. However, because cardiac arrhythmias may occur with halothane and theophylline, isoflurane may be preferable for patients receiving that drug; adequate preoxygenation may decrease the risk of arrhythmia. Intravenous induction with thiopental or diazepam may be used and is indicated when severe bronchospasm may delay induction of anesthesia by an inhalational agent. Ketamine may be used, but it may cause seizures in patients receiving theophylline and can cause bronchorrhea and release of endogenous catecholamines. Both the establishment of deep anesthesia before intubation and the use of intravenous atropine or lidocaine to block reflex bronchoconstriction can help prevent bronchospasm at the time of intubation.

During anesthesia, the patient must be closely monitored. Cardiac monitoring should be initiated before induction and continued into the postoperative period for patients with severe asthma.[58] Warmed, humidified gases should be used throughout the procedure. Ventilation must be controlled. Manual ventilation offers the advantage of easy detection of changes in pulmonary compliance and allows for appropriate compensation for those changes. During mechanical ventilation, a volume-limited ventilator should be used, and peak airway pressure must be monitored. Adequacy of gas exchange can be assessed by oximetry, end-tidal carbon dioxide monitoring, and measurement of arterial or venous blood gases; breath sounds should also be continuously monitored.

Increased pulmonary resistance during anesthesia is most commonly caused by bronchospasm, but mucus plugging and pneumothorax must be considered as possible etiologic factors. If bronchospasm occurs, the anesthesiologist can deepen anesthesia and increase the inspired oxygen concentration, because airway stimulation under light anesthesia may be precipitating the bronchospasm. Further treatment includes intravenous aminophylline, inhalation of a beta$_2$-agonist, and intravenous hydrocortisone or equivalent intravenous corticosteroid. Intravenous isoproterenol and subcutaneous terbutaline may be used but may precipitate arrhythmias; lidocaine and ketamine have also been used with success.

Postoperative Management. The pathophysiologic features of asthma predispose patients to atelectasis, as a result of retained secretions, and to secondary pneumonia. Bronchospasm may contribute to the $\dot{V}/\dot{Q}$ mismatch and hypoxemia originally induced by anesthesia. Inadequate control of pain may lead to emotional stress and subsequent bronchospasm. Therefore, goals of postoperative management include control of bronchospasm, clearance of secretions, maintenance of adequate oxygenation and ventilation, and control of pain. Humidified oxygen should be administered in the postoperative period. Inhalation of bronchodilator aerosols every 4 h for the first postoperative day and four times per day for the next 2 days is usually adequate for preventing or treating bronchospasm in many patients with mild asthma. Aerosols should be followed by chest physiotherapy in young children; incentive spirometry may be adequate in children who can perform the maneuver. Patients with more severe asthma may require treatment with theophylline and steroids, as discussed earlier. For further information on pain control, see Chapter 87.

NEUROMUSCULAR DISEASE

The perioperative care of patients with neuromuscular disease can be extremely challenging, inasmuch as these patients are at high risk for postoperative pulmonary complications, including atelectasis, pneumonia, respiratory failure, need for prolonged ventilation, tracheostomy, and death. Patients may have dyscoordinated swallowing, aspiration, weak cough, and difficulty clearing secretions, and there is an increased frequency of infections of the lower respiratory tract among these patients. They may have respiratory muscle weakness that is not apparent on general examination and may develop respiratory failure when work of breathing is increased. Chronic respiratory muscle weakness can lead to secondary abnormalities in pulmonary mechanics, which include reduced lung volumes, microatelectasis, $\dot{V}/\dot{Q}$ mismatch, scoliosis, decreased compliance of the chest wall even in the absence of scoliosis, and decreased pulmonary compliance.[59] Patients may be hypoxemic or may develop hypoxemia only during sleep; hypoventilation may be a result of muscle weakness or may be caused by central hypoventilation. Therefore, such patients should undergo careful evaluation in preparation for surgery.

Preoperative assessment of patients with any form of neuromuscular disease includes a thorough history, a physical examination, and laboratory studies. The history should include frequency and severity of respiratory tract infections and pulmonary complications, if any, of previous surgery. A history consistent with reactive airways disease should be carefully sought because even mildly increased airway obstruction in the postoperative period may lead to respiratory failure in a patient with severe respiratory muscle weakness. The physical examination should include assessment of the gag reflex, cough, adequacy of aeration, and the presence of adventitial lung sounds. General muscle strength should be assessed, as should the patient's physical and intellectual capability for cooperating with postoperative pulmonary therapy. Laboratory investigations include a chest radiograph, measurements of arterial blood gases or mixed venous gas measurements and oximetry, and a complete blood count.

Pulmonary function tests, including those for lung volumes, should be taken in all children who are able to per-

form them, and pre- and postbronchodilator tests should be performed in patients with adequate strength who have a history or examination suggestive of reactive airways disease. Maximal inspiratory and expiratory mouth pressures should be determined because they are frequently decreased more than the lung volumes and flows, and they do not correlate with general muscle strength.[60] The patient's pulmonary status should be at its best before elective surgery, and the patient should be educated in the techniques of respiratory care that will be used postoperatively.

Patients with neuromuscular disease are at risk for several anesthetic complications unrelated to their pulmonary status, which include malignant hyperthermia and cardiac arrhythmias. Excessive potassium release and myoglobinuria may also occur. Skeletal muscle contraction may be sustained in patients with myotonic muscular dystrophy, in response to administration of succinylcholine.[60]

With vigilant care, it is possible to minimize the frequency of postoperative pulmonary complications even in patients with severe neuromuscular disease. Many patients with severe muscle weakness require ventilatory support for 24 to 48 h after major surgical procedures. However, more prolonged mechanical ventilation may be associated with disuse atrophy and further respiratory muscle weakness, thereby increasing the risk of ventilator dependency. Patients with significant neuromuscular weakness may not be able to perform incentive spirometry effectively. Therefore, chest physiotherapy and suctioning are important for clearance of secretions and prevention of atelectasis and should be done every 2 to 4 h during the first 24 h after surgery, depending on the type of surgery and the severity of lung disease; the frequency may be reduced if a patient tolerates extubation for 24 h without complications.

Patients with severe neuromuscular disease represent the major group in which IPPB may be helpful if a patient is unable to perform a deep inspiratory maneuver. To minimize work of breathing in weak patients with neuromuscular disease, oxygen saturation should be maintained above 95% with humidified oxygen. Although it has not been rigorously studied, the author's very weak patients have less postoperative atelectasis and respiratory failure if the hematocrit is maintained above 35%; the increased oxygen-carrying capacity associated with the higher hematocrit subjectively improves muscle strength during the immediate postoperative period (personal observations). Because hypoxemia and decreased pulmonary compliance can develop in the presence of increased lung water, careful attention should be paid to fluid balance, particularly after major operations such as scoliosis repair. Even minimal airway obstruction caused by bronchospasm should be treated with bronchodilator aerosols and systemic therapy if necessary. Atelectasis should be managed aggressively; therapy may include bronchodilator aerosols, mucolytic aerosols, vigorous chest physiotherapy and suctioning, and IPPB. Bronchoscopy may be necessary for removing secretions and for obtaining bronchial washings for culture. Antibiotic therapy for secondary pneumonia can then be directed against the specific pathogens, although normal mouth flora and anaerobes may be the etiologic agents in these weak patients, many of whom frequently aspirate saliva in the perioperative period.

CYSTIC FIBROSIS

The genetic defect in cystic fibrosis causes increased viscosity of an increase in secretions of the respiratory tract with secondary chronic infection of the respiratory tract infection. Patients with advanced pulmonary disease have bronchiectasis and bronchiolectasis, and many patients also have bronchial hyperreactivity. Patients with severe disease develop hypoxemia and cor pulmonale, and hypercapnia may be present in the terminal stages. Because of the pathophysiologic processes of cystic fibrosis, these patients are at increased risk for pulmonary complications in the perioperative period. Careful management can lead to a successful outcome even in patients with severe lung disease; in one study, seven of eight patients with a forced expiratory volume in 1 sec of less than 25% of the level predicted before development of a pneumothorax survived thoracotomy with pleurodesis.[61]

REFERENCES

1. Butler J, Smith BH: Pressure-volume relationships of the chest in the completely relaxed anaesthetised patient. Clin Sci 16:125–146, 1957.
2. Howell JBL, Peckett BW: Studies of the elastic properties of the thorax of supine anaesthetized paralysed human subjects. J Physiol (London) 136:1–19, 1957.
3. Froese AB, Bryan AC: Effects of anesthesia and paralysis on diaphragmatic mechanics in man. Anesthesiology 41:242–255, 1974.
4. Grimby G, Hedenstierna G, Lofstrom B: Chest wall mechanics during artificial ventilation. J Appl Physiol 38:576–580, 1975.
5. Rehder K, Knopp TJ, Sessler AD: Regional intrapulmonary gas distribution in awake and anesthetized-paralyzed prone man. J Appl Physiol 45:528–535, 1978.
6. Rehder K, Sessler AD, Rodarte JR: Regional intrapulmonary gas distribution in awake and anesthetized-paralyzed man. J Appl Physiol 42:391–402, 1977.
7. Juno P, Marsh HM, Knopp TJ, Rehder K: Closing capacity in awake and anesthetized-paralyzed man. J Appl Physiol 44:238–244, 1978.
8. Rehder K, Knopp TJ, Sessler AD, et al: Ventilation-perfusion relationship in young healthy awake and anesthetized-paralyzed man. J Appl Physiol 47:745–753, 1979.
9. Rehder K: Anaesthesia and the respiratory system. Can Anaesth Soc J 26:451–462, 1979.
10. Muller N, Volgyesi G, Becker L, et al: Diaphragmatic muscle tone. J Appl Physiol 47:279–284, 1979.
11. Westbrook PR, Stubbs SE, Sessler AD, et al: Effects of anesthesia and muscle paralysis on respiratory mechanics in normal man. J Appl Physiol 34:81–86, 1973.
12. Caro CG, Butler J, DuBois AB: Some effects of restriction of chest cage expansion on pulmonary function in man: An experimental study. J Clin Invest 39:573–583, 1960.
13. Schmid ER, Rehder K: General anesthesia and the chest wall. Anesthesiology 55:668–675, 1981.
14. Jones JG, Faithfull D, Jordan C, et al: Rib cage movement during halothane anaesthesia in man. Br J Anaesth 51:399–407, 1979.
15. Heneghan CP, Jones JG: Pulmonary gas exchange and diaphragmatic position: Effect of tonic phrenic stimulation compared with that of increased airway pressure. Br J Anaesth 57:1161–1166, 1985.
16. Mathers J, Benumof JL, Wahrenbrock EA: General anesthetics and regional hypoxic pulmonary vasoconstriction. Anesthesiology 46:111–114, 1977.
17. Sykes MK, Davies DM, Chakrabarti MK, et al: The effects of halothane, trichloroethylene and ether on the hypoxic pressure response and pulmonary vascular resistance in the isolated, perfused cat lung. Br J Anaesth 45:655–663, 1973.
18. Chevrolet JC, Martin JG, Flood R, et al: Topographical ventilation and perfusion distribution during IPPB in the lateral posture. Am Rev Respir Dis 118:847–854, 1978.
19. Brismar B, Hedenstierna G, Lundquist H, et al: Pulmonary densities during anesthesia with muscular relaxation: A proposal of atelectasis. Anesthesiology 62:422–428, 1985.
20. Tokics L, Hedenstierna G, Strandberg A, et al: Lung collapse and gas exchange during general anesthesia: Effects of spontaneous breathing, muscle paralysis, and positive end-expiratory pressure. Anesthesiology 66:157–167, 1987.
21. Tisi G: Preoperative evaluation of pulmonary function: Validity, indications and benefits. Am Rev Respir Dis 119:293–310, 1979.
22. Dale WA, Rahn H: Rate of gas absorption during atelectasis. Am J Physiol 170:606–615, 1952.
23. Prys-Roberts C, Nunn JF, Dobson RH, et al: Radiographically undetectable pulmonary collapse in the supine position. Lancet 2:399–401, 1967.
24. Mead J, Collier C: Relation of volume history of lungs to respiratory mechanics in dogs. J Appl Physiol 14:669–678, 1959.
25. Dripps RD, Deming MVN: Postoperative atelectasis and pneumonia: Diagnosis, etiology and management based upon 1,240 cases of upper abdominal surgery. Ann Surg 124:94–110, 1946.
26. Beecher HK: Effect of laparotomy on lung volume: Demonstration of a new type of pulmonary collapse. J Clin Invest 12:651–658, 1933.
27. Anscombe AR, Buxton R: Effect of abdominal operations on total lung capacity and its subdivisions. Br Med J 2:84–87, 1958.
28. Gamsu G, Singer MM, Vincent HH, et al: Postoperative impairment of mucous transport in the lung. Am Rev Respir Dis 114:673–679, 1976.
29. Hilding AC: Laryngotracheal damage during intratracheal anesthesia. Ann Otol Rhinol Laryngol 80:565–581, 1971.
30. Sackner MA, Hirsch J, Epstein S: Effect of cuffed endotracheal tubes on tracheal mucous velocity. Chest 68:774–777, 1975.
31. Mercke U, Hakansson CH, Toremalm NG: The influence of temperature on mucociliary activity: Temperature range 20 degrees C to 40 degrees C. Acta Otolaryngol (Stockh) 78:444–450, 1974.
32. Burton JDK: Effect of dry anesthetic gases on the respiratory mucous membrane. Lancet 1:235–238, 1962.
33. Forbes AR: Humidification and mucus flow in the intubated trachea. Br J Anaesth 45:874–878, 1973.
34. Marfatia S, Donahoe PK, Hendren WH: Effect of dry and humidified gases on the respiratory epithelium in rabbits. J Pediatr Surg 10:583–592, 1975.
35. Rashad KF, Benson DW: Role of humidity in prevention of hypothermia in infants and children. Anesth Analg 46:712–718, 1967.
36. Sackner MA, Hirsch JA, Epstein S, Rywlin AM: Effect of oxygen in graded concentrations upon tracheal mucous velocity: A study in anesthetized dogs. Chest 69:164–167, 1976.
37. Sackner MA, Landa J, Hirsch J, Zapata A: Pulmonary effects of oxygen breathing: A 6-hour study in normal men. Ann Intern Med 82:40–43, 1975.
38. Lichtiger M, Landa JF, Hirsch JA: Velocity of tracheal mucus in anesthetized women undergoing gynecologic surgery. Anesthesiology 42:753–756, 1975.
39. Forbes AR: Halothane depresses mucociliary flow in the trachea. Anesthesiology 45:59–63, 1976.
40. Manawadu BR, LaForce FM: Impairment of pulmonary antibacterial defense mechanisms by halothane anesthesia. Chest 75:242–243, 1979.
41. Thoren L: Post-operative pulmonary complications: Observations on their prevention by means of physiotherapy. Acta Chir Scand 107:193–205, 1954.
42. Jung R, Wight J, Nusser R, Rosoff L: Comparison of three methods of respiratory care following upper abdominal surgery. Chest 78:31–35, 1980.
43. Celli BR, Rodriguez KS, Snider GL: A controlled trial of intermittent positive pressure breathing, incentive spirometry, and deep breathing exercises in preventing pulmonary complications after abdominal surgery. Am Rev Respir Dis 130:12–15, 1984.

44. Graham WG, Bradley DA: Efficacy of chest physiotherapy and intermittent positive-pressure breathing in the resolution of pneumonia. N Engl J Med 299:624–627, 1978.
45. Ricksten SE, Bengtsson A, Soderberg C, et al: Effects of periodic positive airway pressure by mask on postoperative pulmonary function. Chest 89:774–781, 1986.
46. Jaworski A, Goldberg SK, Walkenstein MD, et al: Utility of immediate postlobectomy fiberoptic bronchoscopy in preventing atelectasis. Chest 94:38–43, 1988.
47. Marini JJ, Pierson DJ, Hudson LD: Acute lobar atelectasis: A prospective comparison of fiberoptic bronchoscopy and respiratory therapy. Am Rev Respir Dis 119:971–978, 1979.
48. Pedersen J, Schurizek BA, Melsen NC, Juhl B: Minitracheotomy in the treatment of postoperative sputum retention and atelectasis. Acta Anaesthesiol Scand 32:426–428, 1988.
49. Finer NN, Boyd J: Chest physiotherapy in the neonate: A controlled study. Pediatrics 61:282–285, 1978.
50. Jones JG, Jordan C, Scudder C, et al: Episodic postoperative oxygen desaturation: The value of added oxygen. J R Soc Med 78:1019–1022, 1985.
51. Aquilina AT, Hall WJ, Douglas RG, Utell M: Airway reactivity in subjects with viral upper respiratory tract infections: The effects of exercise and cold air. Am Rev Respir Dis 122:3–10, 1980.
52. McGill WA, Coveler LA, Epstein BS: Subacute upper respiratory infection in small children. Anesth Analg 58:331–333, 1979.
53. Steward DJ: Preterm infants are more prone to complications following minor surgery than are term infants. Anesthesiology 56:304–306, 1982.
54. Liu LM, Cote CJ, Goudsouzian NG, et al: Life-threatening apnea in infants recovering from anesthesia. Anesthesiology 59:506–510, 1983.
55. Mayhew JF, Bourke DL, Guinee WS: Evaluation of the premature infant at risk for postoperative complications. Can J Anaesth 34:627–631, 1987.
56. Richards W, Thompson J, Lewis G, et al: Cardiac arrest associated with halothane anesthesia in a patient receiving theophylline. Ann Allergy 61:83–84, 1988.
57. Fung DL, Schatz M: Surgery in allergic patients. In Bierman CW, Pearlman DS (eds): Allergic Diseases From Infancy to Adulthood, 2nd ed, pp. 748–759. Philadelphia: WB Saunders, 1988.
58. Hilman BC: Surgery in allergic patients. In Bierman CW, Pearlman DS (eds): Allergic Diseases of Infancy, Childhood and Adolescence, pp. 755–760. Philadelphia: WB Saunders, 1980.
59. Smith PE, Calverley PM, Edwards RH, et al: Practical problems in the respiratory care of patients with muscular dystrophy. N Engl J Med 316:1197–1205, 1987.
60. Kafer ER: Respiratory and cardiovascular functions in scoliosis and the principles of anesthetic management. Anesthesiology 52:339–351, 1980.
61. Penketh A, Knight RK, Hodson ME, Batten JC: Management of pneumothorax in adults with cystic fibrosis. Thorax 37:850–853, 1982.

87 SURGICAL ASPECTS OF PULMONARY DISEASES

PATRICIA C. MOYNIHAN, M.D. / MARK SMITH, M.D.

Pediatric thoracic surgeons are involved with the diagnosis and treatment of congenital and acquired pulmonary disease in various pediatric age groups. To understand pulmonary and bronchial malformations, a thorough knowledge of the embryogenesis of the respiratory system is mandatory. The acquired lesions requiring surgical procedures have decreased in incidence because of the development of effective antibiotics and immunizations. Whether the disease process is congenital or acquired, surgeons must have a complete understanding of the pathophysiologic changes affecting patients.

It is essential for surgeons performing thoracic surgery on pediatric patients to have a thorough knowledge of bronchopulmonary anatomy. Anatomic variations, particularly those of the pulmonary vessels, are not infrequent. Knowledgeable and experienced surgeons can conserve healthy lung tissue and operate safely.

It is not within the scope of this chapter to discuss the embryogenesis of all pulmonary and bronchial malformations or the cause of acquired pulmonary lesions, because they are discussed in other chapters of this book. Instead, the authors provide a brief review of the surgical anatomy and the indications for surgery, including techniques of various methods of pulmonary resections.

SURGICAL ANATOMY OF THE LUNGS

HILAR STRUCTURES

The primary structures of the hilum exiting from the mediastinum and passing to the lungs are the right and left divisions of the main bronchi, the pulmonary arteries, and the superior and inferior pulmonary veins. (The divisions of the right and left main stem bronchi and divisions of the vessels are described later.) If the various bronchi are used as a fixed reference point, the complex relationship of the pulmonary vessels and their courses can be understood.

The right and left pulmonary ligaments lie below the hilum. As a reflection of the pleura, they leave the mediastinum and extend to the lowermost medial tip of each lung. The hilum on the right is just anterior to the superior vena cava, a portion of the right atrium, the pericardiophrenic vessels, and the phrenic nerve. The azygos vein is just posterior to the right hilum and curves up and around the right main stem bronchus.

On the left, the pericardial sac lies anteriorly over the hilum and is traversed by the phrenic nerve. Superiorly, the aortic arch curves around the hilum and descends posteriorly as the thoracic aorta. Posteriorly, in both hila, are the vagus nerves and bronchial arteries.

LUNG SEGMENTS

The right and left lungs are similar despite the fact that there are three lobes on the right and two on the left. Bronchopulmonary segments function as individual units, which are subdivisions of the lungs. Each segment has a bronchus, a pulmonary artery, and a pulmonary vein.

Terminology for the segments and their bronchi proposed by Jackson Huber has been used internationally. In general, 10 segments are recognized on the right side and 8 on the left. This discrepancy is attributable to the common stem bronchus origins of the apical and posterior segmental bronchi of the left upper lobe and the anterior and medial segmental bronchi of the left lower lobe. It is important for surgeons to retain the concept that there are 10 segments on each side because segmentectomies are often performed. The left apical and posterior segments can easily be resected separately; however, there is no practical value in separating the left anterior and medial basal segments (Fig. 87–1).

BRONCHIAL TREE

If the bronchi are regarded as fixed reference points, the complex relationships of pulmonary vessels are easy to understand and remember. Complete knowledge of bronchial anatomy is required in order to interpret bronchograms, nuclear scans, and other contrast studies of the lungs.

The trachea divides at the carina into the right and left main stem bronchi (Fig. 87–2). The left main stem bronchus is longer and has a more acute angle than the right. It branches into an upper-lobe bronchus, which provides a bronchus and segmental bronchi to the upper lobe and a bronchus with bronchi to the lingula. The left lower-lobe bronchus is very short and branches into the various segmental bronchi.

The right main stem bronchus is relatively short; the upper-lobe bronchus branches a short distance from the trachea. It has a posterosuperior origin and divides into three segmental bronchi. Continuation of the right main stem is called the intermediate bronchus. It, in turn, is the origin for the segmental bronchi to the middle and lower lobes.

PULMONARY VESSELS

The pulmonary artery gives off segmental branches, which lie close to the segmental bronchi on either the superior or the lateral surfaces and have the same names as the bronchi. They continue into the lung segments with the bronchi and branch with the subsegmental bronchi. They terminate along the borders of the intersegmental planes and rarely cross these planes.

The courses of the pulmonary veins differ in that they occupy an intersegmental position. Therefore, they can drain the segments in which they lie. In general, the veins lie on the medial or inferior sides of the bronchi and have the same names.

The right pulmonary artery leaves the pericardial sac and is anterior and inferior to the right main stem bronchus. After entering the fissure, it continues inferolaterally and provides branches to the middle and lower lobes. Proximal to the fissure, a large superolateral artery branches off the right pulmonary artery to supply the upper lobe.

The right superior pulmonary vein has a position anterior and slightly inferior to the pulmonary artery. All the tributaries of the right upper and middle lobes flow into the superior pulmonary vein. The right inferior pulmonary vein is posterior and inferior to the superior pulmonary vein. All of the tributaries flow from the right lower lobe.

A three-dimensional concept of the right lung requires visualization of all the structural components and their relationships to one another. With the patient in the lateral position, three views can be obtained: the anterior view (Fig. 87–3), the fissure view (Fig. 87–4), and the posterior view (Fig. 87–5).

As the left pulmonary artery leaves the pericardial sac, it is superior and somewhat anterior to the left main bronchus. Then it curves posteriorly around the upper-lobe bronchus and continues inferolaterally into the interlobar fissure. The apical posterior trunk arises just as the main artery begins its posteroinferior curve. The anterior segmental artery arises, most commonly from the anteromedial side of the main artery, within the fissure. As the main artery continues its inferior course, it gives off branches to the lingula and superior segments of the left lower lobe. The main artery then branches into the basal segmental arteries, which parallel their segmental bronchi.

The most anterior principal structure of the left pulmonary hilum is the left superior pulmonary vein. All of its tributaries come from the left upper lobe and the lingula. The left inferior pulmonary vein is inferior and posterior to the superior pulmonary vein. It lies between the layers of the reflected pleura at the top of the pulmonary ligament. It drains the principal tributaries of the entire left lower lobe.

A three-dimensional concept of the left lung with its structures and relationships to one another can be visualized with the patient in a lateral position. The anterior (Fig. 87–6), fissure (Fig. 87–7), and posterior (Fig. 87–8) views can be seen.

SURGICAL RESECTIONS

WEDGE RESECTION OR OPEN-LUNG BIOPSY

Wedge resection in children is usually performed to remove pulmonary metastases (Fig. 87–9). Osteosarcoma, Wilms' tumor, and Ewing's sarcoma all spread preferentially to the lungs, and resection of these lesions combined with radiation or chemotherapy may prolong survival. Reviewing survival after resection of pulmonary

ANTERIOR VIEW

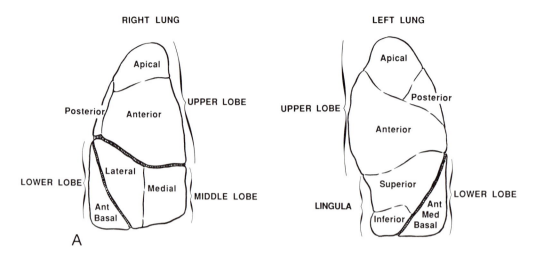

MEDIAL VIEW

LATERAL VIEW

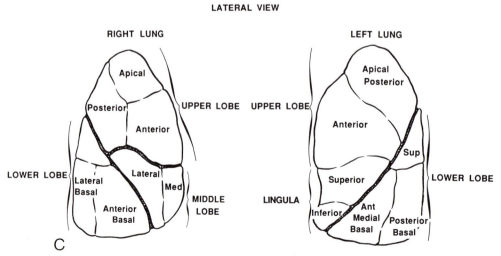

Figure 87–1. Lung segments. *A*, Anterior view. Ant, anterior; Med, medial. *B*, Medial view. Ant, anterior; Lat, lateral; Post, posterior; Sup, superior; Inf, inferior. *C*, Lateral view. Med, medial; Sup, superior; Ant, anterior.

LEFT LUNG (Fissure View)

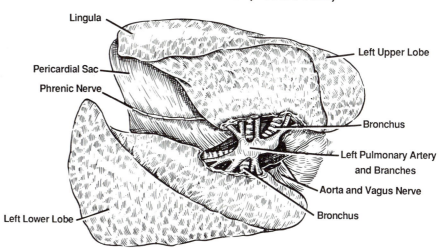

Figure 87–7. Fissure view of left lung. The fissure is open to expose the interlobar position of the left pulmonary artery. All the upper lobes and lingular branches and most of the lower lobe branches are seen. The bronchus and its divisions lie posteriorly.

as opposed to less than 30% yield with aspiration needle biopsy.[3] Wedge biopsy is often required to diagnose opportunistic infections resulting from fungi, *Pneumocystis carinii,* or cytomegalovirus in immunocompromised patients. Open-lung biopsy changed the presumptive diagnosis in 36% of patients operated on at the Mayo Clinic in one series and dictated subsequent treatment in 91% of patients.[4].

In addition, pediatric or thoracic surgeons often see children with retained foreign bodies (e.g., needles, straight pins, and spring coils from ballpoint pens). On rare occasions, these objects can migrate into a tertiary bronchus and require a wedge resection (Fig. 87–10). When indicated, this procedure may be performed rapidly with minimal morbidity and mortality.

Technique

Wedge resection is performed for peripheral lesions with no regard to intersegmental planes. Large lesions or lesions buried deeply in the lung parenchyma, whose excision would compromise the ventilation of the remaining lobar tissue, are best removed by lobectomy or segmentectomy. Wedge resection is easily performed with the use of either a mechanical stapling device or a clamp-and-suture technique.

The clamp-and-suture technique is accomplished by placing Kelly clamps around the lesions, leaving a margin of normal tissue in the specimen to be resected. The lesion is then excised with a knife, and a cuff of tissue is left in order to prevent the clamps from slipping. The lung parenchyma is closed with a 3-0 chromic suture with a running interlocking stitch (Fig. 87–11).

The authors prefer to use GIA staplers because of the ease and rapidity with which these procedures may be performed as well as the decreased incidence of parenchymal air leakage postoperatively (Fig. 87–12). These staple lines are not oversewn. The chest cavity is then filled with saline, covering the suture line, and the lung is reinflated with 20 to 30 cm of water to check for air leakages. A chest

LEFT LUNG (POSTERIOR VIEW)

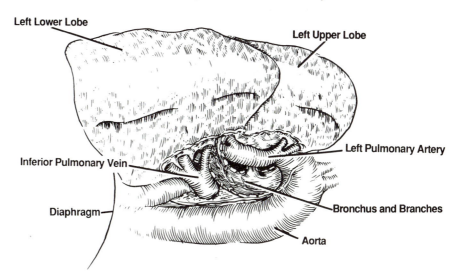

Figure 87–8. Posterior view of left lung. The lung is retracted anteriorly. The relationship of the left pulmonary artery to the left upper lobe bronchus is clearly seen in this view. The left inferior pulmonary vein lies posterior and inferior to the left lower lobe bronchus.

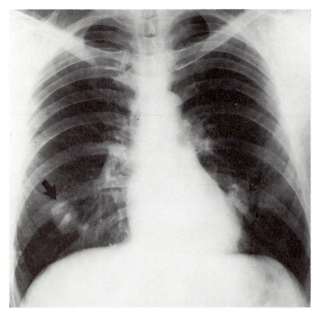

Figure 87–9. Preoperative chest radiograph of 10-year-old girl with metastatic osteogenic sarcoma *(arrow)* from the right femur. A median sternotomy was performed with a wedge resection of the right lower lobe lesion and a left lower lobe lobectomy.

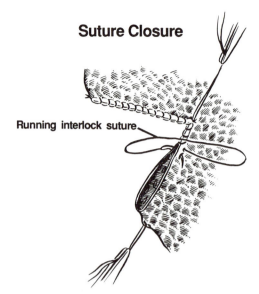

Figure 87–11. Illustration of wedge (open biopsy) resection. The Kelly clamps have been removed. Lung parenchyma is being closed with a running interlocking 3-0 chromic suture.

tube is placed through a separate stab incision and held in place with a pursestring suture. The ribs are reapproximated with polyglactin 910 (2-0 Vicryl), and the muscle layers are closed with 2-0 or 3-0 Vicryl. The skin incision is closed with a running subcuticular suture. Once the chest cavity is closed, positive airway pressure is reapplied to reinflate the lung. The chest tube is removed, and the pursestring suture is tied. Wedge resections are performed through lateral incisions with the patient in the oblique position.

Open-lung biopsy is performed with the same technique except that the chest is opened with a limited anterolateral incision with the patient in an oblique position. The side to be operated on is elevated by means of a rolled sheet.

SEGMENTAL RESECTION

Segmentectomy is the procedure of choice for removing a benign, localized lesion. This concept has evolved from the demonstration that bronchopulmonary seg-

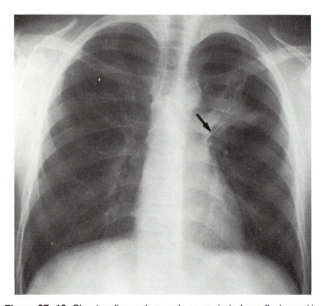

Figure 87–10. Chest radiograph reveals an aspirated needle *(arrow)* in left upper lobe of 10-year-old girl with fever and productive cough. An attempt at removal through rigid bronchoscopy was unsuccessful. A left thoracotomy and wedge resection were required.

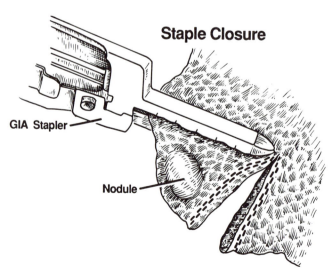

Figure 87–12. Wedge (open biopsy) resection. A nodule near the edge of the lung can be excised by two applications of the GIA stapler. The overlapping staple line ensures hemostasis and no bronchial leakages. No sutures are required.

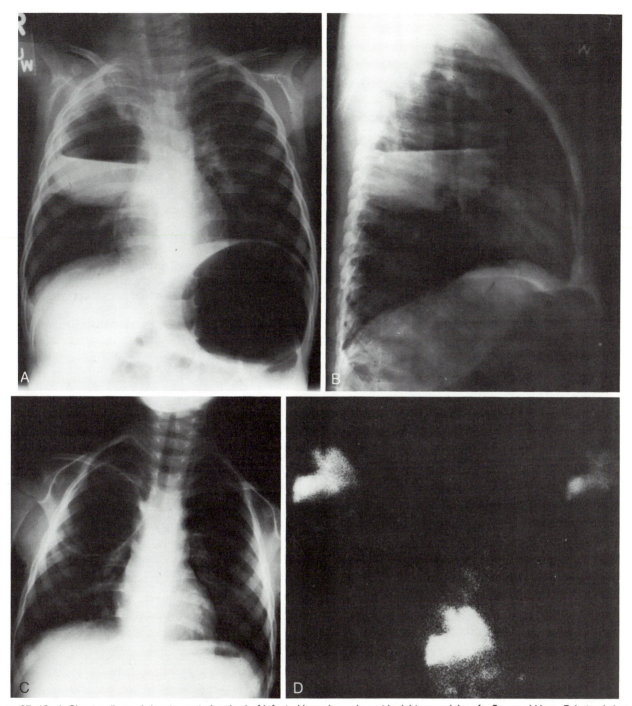

Figure 87–13. *A*, Chest radiograph (posteroanterior view) of infected bronchogenic cyst in right upper lobe of a 5-year-old boy. *B*, Lateral view of chest radiograph, demonstrating posterior location of cyst. *C*, Note discrete thin wall of cyst after antibiotic therapy on chest radiograph (postero-anterior view). *D*, Preoperative xenon 133 scan confirms location of cyst in posterior segment of right upper lobe. A segmentectomy was performed.

ments are distinctive anatomic units of each lung. The advantage of this technique is that only the segment or segments that contain diseased tissue need to be removed. Thus healthy functioning pulmonary tissue is preserved.

The surgeon must have a thorough knowledge of the anatomic relations of the tertiary hilar structures and the possibility of anomalous origins. Segmentectomy is indicated for any benign lesion that has a segmental distribution. Indications for segmental resection include simple

lung cysts, hamartomas, occasional lung abscesses and intralobar bronchogenic cysts (Fig. 87–13).

Technique

Segmental resection with the classical anatomic approach has become antiquated since the development of stapling devices.[5] Use of the stapling technique now allows the surgeon to perform a segmentectomy or resec-

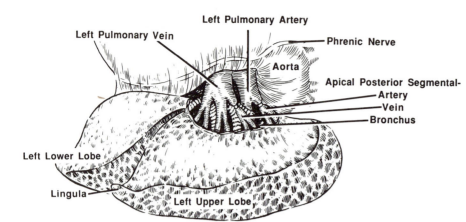

Figure 87–14. Segmental resection (left apical posterior segment). The lung is retracted posteriorly. The mediastinal pleura is opened. The apical-posterior artery and vein are divided between ligatures. The TA-30 stapler is applied across the base, and the pulmonary tissue and bronchus are divided. On occasion, additional sutures are required in order to close bronchial leakages.

tion of less than a segment unit safely. Often it is necessary to excise certain segments together because they are frequently involved in the disease process as groups. These segments include the superior and inferior lingular segments, the lateral and medial segments of the middle lobe, and all of the basal segments of the lower lobes.

Initially the hilar pleura is incised. After the arteries and veins have been carefully identified, they are ligated and divided (Fig. 87–14). Then the appropriate-sized TA stapler is applied, and the bronchi and pulmonary tissue are divided and excised. Warm saline solution is placed in the chest cavity, and the lung is expanded with positive pressure to check for possible bronchial air leakage. On occasion, additional sutures may be required to close air leakages. A chest tube is placed in an interspace below the incision in the midaxillary line. The chest is then closed in layers with polyglactin 910 (2-0 or 3-0 Vicryl). The skin is closed with a continuous subcuticular suture.

LOBECTOMY

Lung bud anomalies such as lobar emphysema, intralobar bronchogenic cysts, cystic adenomatoid malformation, lobar sequestration, bronchial atresia, and tracheal bronchus are probably the most common indications for lobar resection in children. Many of these patients have respiratory insufficiency or recurrent localized infections and require removal of the affected area.[6] On occasion, these lesions[7,8] manifest as asymptomatic lesions that may be excised electively.

Lobar emphysema or lobar overinflation is caused by persistent air trapping and should not be resected unless it causes respiratory compromise or becomes infected. Many affected infants show no progression of the disease and require only observation.[9] The left upper lobe and right middle lobe are most often affected. Some infants have progressive air trapping and increasing respiratory distress and require a lobectomy (Fig. 87–15).

Bronchogenic cysts are usually solitary lesions more often on the right side than the left. Intrapulmonary lesions that communicate with the bronchial tree are always symptomatic.[10] The presence of multiple cysts suggests a cystic adenomatoid malformation.[11] Large lesions without bronchial communication may be symptomatic

as a result of bronchial compression. These cysts should be excised whether they are symptomatic or not because of the possibility of bronchial communication and subsequent infection.[12]

Congenital cystic adenomatoid malformation is characterized by marked overgrowth of the terminal bronchioles with an adenomatoid appearance, an increased amount of elastic tissue, and the presence of a cuboid or cylindric epithelium.[13] These lesions manifest with respiratory distress in infancy or subsequently with infection and should be resected (Fig. 87–16).

In pulmonary sequestration, an area of lung tissue is supplied by an anomalous systemic artery. Such areas are usually intralobar and in the left lower chest. Up to 20% of the intralobar variety have bronchial connections.[7] Patients with pulmonary sequestration of the extralobar variety may have respiratory distress as a result of Bochdalek's hernia or congestive heart failure from shunting of blood through a large aberrant vessel. These lesions often remain asymptomatic and are diagnosed at a later date. Intralobar sequestration usually manifests as a result of recurrent infections and may be difficult to differentiate from cystic adenomatoid malformation or bronchiectasis.[14] Diagnosis is usually made on the basis of clinical findings combined with chest radiographs. The authors rarely perform arteriography for definitive diagnosis because of its invasive nature and the additional risk to patients. A large aberrant arterial supply arising from the descending aorta is demonstrated by a aortogram in Figure 87–17 in a child with left extralobar sequestration.

Tracheal bronchus is an aberrant bronchus to the right upper lobe that arises from the trachea.[15] Almost 30% of affected patients acquire recurrent pneumonias and require resection of the right upper lobe.

Bronchiectasis has decreased in incidence as an indication for pulmonary resection. In a Mayo Clinic study during the 1960s and 1970s in 170 children who required lobectomies for bronchiectasis, the predisposing cause was viral or bacterial infection in 65% of cases (Fig. 87–18). Five percent of children with cystic fibrosis have recurrent localized bronchopneumonia that usually affects the right upper lobe, and they may benefit from resection of the affected lobe. Infrequently, bronchopneumonia develops as a result of a bronchial adenoma or a primary parenchymal tumor.

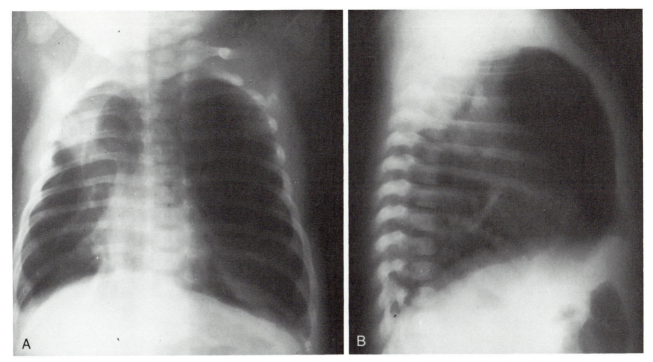

Figure 87–15. Congenital lobar emphysema as seen in the anterior (*A*) and lateral (*B*) radiographic views of the chest. Hyperinflation of left upper lobe with compressive atelectasis of contralateral upper lobe and ipsilateral lower lobe. There is anterior mediastinal herniation of left upper lobe.

Retained foreign bodies are also a cause of bronchiectasis in lower lobes (Fig. 87–19). Enlarged lymph nodes can produce bronchiectasis because of their extrinsic blockage of a bronchus. A classic example is the right middle-lobe syndrome (Fig. 87–20).[16]

Technique

Right Upper Lobe. The operative exposure for a right upper lobectomy is through a posterolateral incision with the patient in the lateral position. The fifth or sixth inter-

space is usually entered for exposure of the hilum. The right lung is then retracted posteriorly, and the mediastinal pleura overlying the pulmonary artery and the right superior pulmonary vein is incised posterior to the phrenic nerve and pericardium. The right pulmonary artery lies posterior to the right superior pulmonary vein

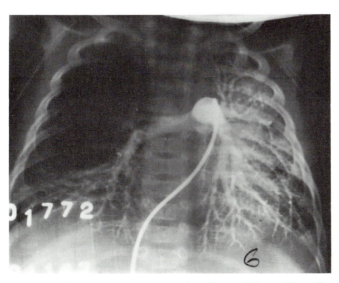

Figure 87–16. Pulmonary arteriogram in a 7-year-old boy with cystic adenomatoid malformation of right upper lobe. Note compressive displacement of pulmonary vessels.

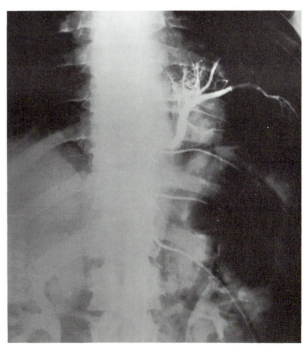

Figure 87–17. Aortogram in a 6-year-old girl with an extralobar sequestration on the left side. The large aberrant arterial supply arises from the descending aorta just above the diaphragm.

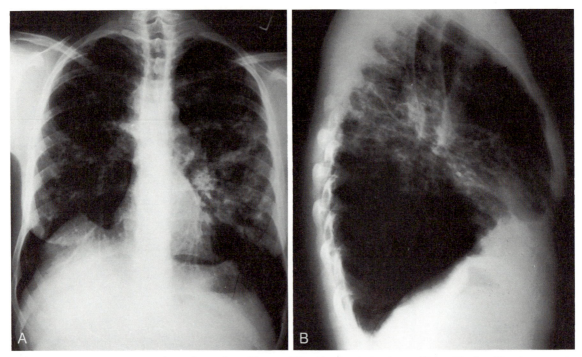

Figure 87–18. Chronic *Pseudomonas aeruginosa* disease in an 18-year-old female. *A*, anterior chest radiographic view. Note honeycomb pattern of densities in both upper-lobe fields and tenting deformities of the diaphragm on both sides. *B*, Lateral view confirms the disease distribution and is consistent with saccular bronchiectasis more advanced in the left upper lobe and lingula, which required resection.

and is partially obscured. The anterior and apical segmental arteries are identified and ligated with 2-0 or 3-0 silk ties. Suture ligatures are also placed before division of the vessels. The right upper lobe is then retracted anteriorly,

and the interlobar fissure is incised and separated by means of a combination of sharp and blunt technique to identify the posterior segmental artery. The posterior segmental artery may not be present, or it may arise from a middle lobar artery. Therefore, before ligation, it must be differentiated from a middle lobar artery. The upper lobe

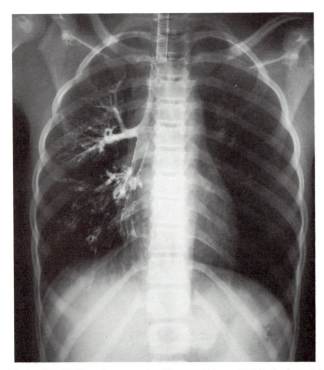

Figure 87–19. Bronchogram of a 12-year-old boy with tubular bronchiectasis of right middle and lower lobe secondary to a retained foreign body. A glass bead was previously removed through rigid bronchoscopy. The boy later required resection of both lobes.

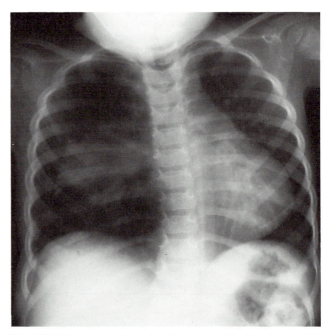

Figure 87–20. Chest radiograph of 6-year-old girl with severe pectus excavatum and right middle-lobe syndrome. She had frequent pulmonary infections and required in-hospital therapy. After simultaneous repair of the pectus and a right middle-lobe resection, she has remained asymptomatic.

is then retracted posteriorly, and the branches of the right superior pulmonary vein are identified and ligated with 3-0 silk ties. Care is taken to identify the inferior vein supplying the anterior segment of the upper lobe as well as the posterior segmental vein, which may be missed if they lie deep in the interlobar fissure.

The upper lobe bronchus is then exposed and divided with a manual suture technique or a TA-30 bronchial stapling device, depending on the age and the size of the child.

The authors perform pulmonary resection in infants and young children by using sutures. Stay sutures are placed in the bronchus just proximal to the level to be incised after the bronchus is grasped distally. As the bronchus is excised, it is closed with a running permanent suture. Care is taken not to damage the blood supply to the bronchial stump, which might result in subsequent necrosis. The authors use the TA-30 staples whenever possible in older children because of the ease and rapidity with which lobectomy may be performed, although either technique is acceptable.

After bronchial closure, the bronchial stump is covered with saline, and positive pressure is applied in order to check for air leakage. When all air leakages are eliminated, the anterior and posterior pleura are sutured over the hilar structures or a pleural flap is rotated over the divided bronchus.

A chest tube is then placed into the chest 2 to 3 interspaces below the wound and directed into the posterior chest. The wound is then closed in the manner described previously in the section on wedge resection or open-lung biopsy. The chest tube is left in place for at least 1 day postoperatively until the lung is reinflated and less than 20 to 25 ml of drainage is noted from the chest tube.

Right Middle and Right Lower Lobes. Right middle and lower lobectomies are performed through the same incision and position as right upper lobectomies. Right middle lobectomy is performed by reflecting the lobe anteriorly and dissecting out the interlobar fissure to identify the interlobar artery. The right middle lobar arteries

are ligated after it is determined that a branch of a middle lobar artery does not supply the right upper lobe. The lung is retracted posteriorly, the mediastinal pleura overlying the right pulmonary artery and the superior pulmonary vein is incised, and the right middle lobar vein is identified and ligated. The middle-lobe bronchus is divided in one of the two techniques mentioned previously.

In resection of the right lower lobe, the inferior pulmonary ligament is ligated and divided and the posterior hilar pleura opened to mobilize the right lower lobe for removal. The inferior pulmonary vein is isolated, and superior segmental and basal branches are exposed before ligature and division. Dissection is then performed in the oblique fissure, as in right middle lobectomy, until the middle lobe and posterior segmental arteries are identified. Then the basal and superior segmental arteries to the right lower lobe are ligated and divided just distal to the distal middle lobar artery. The lower lobe bronchus is divided after the middle-lobe bronchus, which arises anteriorly, is identified, and care is taken not to endanger its lumen.

Left Upper Lobe. Left upper and lower lobectomies are performed with patients in a right lateral position. The chest is entered in the fifth interspace through a routine posterolateral incision. To perform a left upper lobectomy, the lung is retracted posteriorly and inferiorly, and the pleura overlying the left pulmonary artery and superior pulmonary vein is incised. The artery and vein are then identified, and the apical and posterior segmental arteries are dissected free, ligated, and divided (Fig. 87–21). The lobe is retracted anteriorly, and an opening is made in the interlobar fissure, exposing the pulmonary artery. Once the lingular artery and the anterior segmental artery are identified, they are ligated and divided. (The lingular artery is not divided if the lingula is not to be excised.) The lobe is again retracted posteriorly and the lingular, anterior segmental, apical segmental, and posterior segmental veins are ligated and divided. The bronchus may then be divided and the lobe removed. If the lingula is to remain, care must be taken not to occlude the

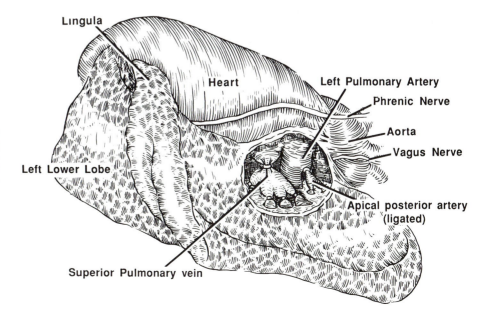

Figure 87–21. Lobectomy. The hilar pleura is open. The bronchus of the left pulmonary artery and the superior pulmonary vein to the left upper lobe are ligated and divided. The bronchus is just posterior to the vessels.

Lingula

Heart

Left Pulmonary Artery

Phrenic Nerve

Aorta

Vagus Nerve

Left Lower Lobe

Apical posterior artery (ligated)

Superior Pulmonary vein

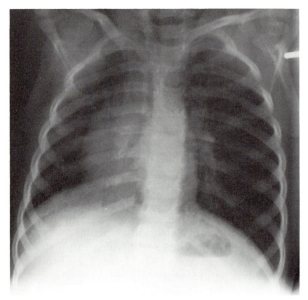

Figure 87-22. Chest radiograph of hypoplastic right lung. The heart is displaced into the right hemithorax and the left lung is hyperinflated. Because of continued shift of mediastinal contents and abnormal right pulmonary vasculature, a pneumonectomy was required.

lingular bronchus when the upper lobe bronchial stump is closed.

Left Lower Lobe. The pulmonary ligament is divided first to facilitate left lower lobectomy after the lobe is retracted anteriorly. The inferior pulmonary vein is identified, ligated, and divided. The bronchus of the right lower lobe is dissected, and the superior segmental bronchi are identified. The left lower lobe is retracted posteriorly to enable dissection in the interlobar fissure. The superior segmental, basal, and lingular arteries are identified. The superior segmental artery usually branches from the pulmonary artery proximal to the level of the lingular artery. The vessels going to the lower lobe are tied and transected. The lobes are then separated, and the relationship between the origin of the lingular bronchus and the superior segmental bronchus of the lower lobe is determined. If the left lower-lobe bronchus cannot be divided proximal to the origin of the superior segmental bronchus without danger of encroachment on the lingular bron-

chus, the superior segmental bronchus and main basal bronchus should be divided separately.

PNEUMONECTOMY

Complete lung resection may be safely performed in children. By the 16th week of intrauterine life, the bronchial tree is fully developed, but alveolar development continues as late as 8 years of age.[16] After pneumonectomy in children, the ipsilateral lung continues to increase in volume and actual mass.[17]

The indication for pneumonectomy in children is essentially the same as that for lobectomy. The extent of disease dictates the type of resection to be performed in those children with acquired lung disease. Pneumonectomies performed in children do not appear to restrict normal growth or development.[18]

On occasion, pneumonectomy is indicated in young children with an atretic lung or a hypoplastic lung (Fig. 87-22).

Right Pneumonectomy

After the chest is opened, the inferior pulmonary ligament is ligated and transected, and the lower lobe is mobilized to expose the inferior pulmonary vein, which may be divided. The lung is then retracted posteriorly, and the pleura overlying the hilum is opened, exposing the superior pulmonary vein and the pulmonary artery. The artery is dissected free and is ligated at or just distal to the level of the bifurcation; an adequate cuff is left to prevent slippage of the ligatures. The right superior pulmonary vein is dissected free, ligated, and divided (Fig. 87-23). The only remaining attachment of the right lung at this point is the right main stem bronchus, which may be divided in one of the two techniques described in the section on lobectomy, depending on the age and the size of the child. The bronchus is also similarly closed and covered with a pleural flap. For older children, the authors prefer using the TA-30 stapler to divide and ligate the bronchus (Fig. 87-24). Then additional interrupted nonabsorbable sutures may be used to ensure hemostasis and eliminate air leakages from the bronchial stump (Fig. 87-25).

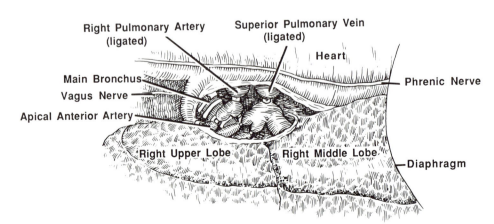

Figure 87-23. Right pneumonectomy. The right inferior pulmonary ligament and inferior pulmonary vein have been ligated and divided. The lung is now retracted posteriorly; the pleura is open, exposing the right pulmonary artery and superior pulmonary vein. The main bronchus will then be divided and oversewn.

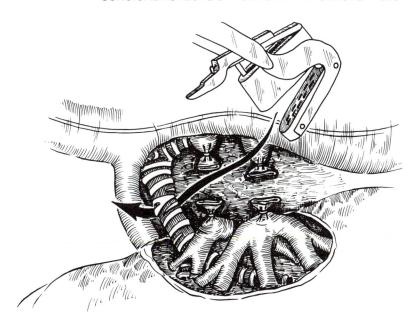

Figure 87–24. In older children, the TA-30 stapler is used in dividing and ligating the main bronchus. The bronchial stump should be at least 0.5 cm in length.

Left Pneumonectomy

Left lobectomy is performed in the same manner as a right pneumonectomy. The inferior pulmonary ligament and the inferior pulmonary vein are divided. After the lung is retracted posteriorly and the pleura overlying the hilum is incised, the pulmonary artery is ligated and divided before division of the superior pulmonary vein. The left main stem bronchus may then be easily divided.

COMPLICATIONS

Minor air leakages are common in the postoperative period, especially after segmental resections. These air leakages usually seal within a few days. Persistence of a leakage or a large increase in the amount of air leakage

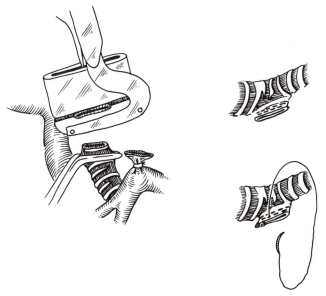

Figure 87–25. Securement of bronchial stump by interrupted, nonabsorbable sutures before the stump is covered with pleura.

suggests the development of a bronchopleural fistula. After the removal of a lobe, early postoperative bronchopleural fistulas are generally a result of technical error and can easily be prevented by adequate initial closure. The late development of a bronchopleural fistula is either bronchial stump infection or inadequate blood supply to the bronchial stump. On rare occasions, bronchopleural fistula develops because of a malignancy in the stump. Early in the postoperative period, a patient may exhibit respiratory insufficiency and collapse of the remaining lung fields with a sudden increase in the air leakage in the chest tube. Days to weeks after surgery, a new air pocket may be noted on chest radiograph, which is suggestive of a bronchopleural fistula. Bronchoscopy should be performed to visualize the stump. Definitive diagnosis may be obtained by either administering a small amount of contrast at the level of the amputated bronchus or by performing a nuclear ventilation scan. Multiple treatment modalities may be used to seal the fistula, depending on the cause and severity of the leakage.

Some leakages close after being placed on suction, but many require operative intervention. A second thoracotomy may be performed and is the treatment of choice. To identify the leakage, the surgeon covers the bronchial stump with saline, and the anesthesiologist applies positive pressure to the lungs. The leakage may then be sutured closed and covered with a pleural, pericardial, or muscle flap. On occasion, the authors have been able to avoid a second thoracotomy by visualizing the bronchial stump by means of rigid bronchoscopy and patching the leak with fibrin glue. This glue is made by combining thrombin with a mixture of cryoprecipitate and Ca^{++}. If infection and breakdown of the bronchial stump occurs because of excessive length, thoracotomy should be performed with reamputation of the stump.

One easily preventable complication is torsion of one of the remaining lobes or segments. Failure to recognize this can result in necrosis of additional pulmonary parenchyma, necessitating immediate thoracotomy, usually with resection of the involved segment. This can be prevented by placing one or two stay sutures between remaining adjacent lobes before closing the chest.

Vigorous postoperative pulmonary therapy should prevent the development of mechanical airway obstruction resulting from the accumulation of secretions or blood clots. When the remaining lobes fail to re-expand properly, bronchoscopy should be performed to rule out torsion, to mobilize secretions, and to reinflate the collapsed pulmonary parenchyma.

The phrenic nerve should be visualized before lobectomy is performed to prevent accidental injury to the nerve, resulting in diaphragmatic paralysis. Meticulous dissection, with ligation of all pulmonary vessels being transected, should prevent major blood loss. Before the chest is closed, the patient should be inspected for bleeding from the intercostal vessels, which can result in significant postoperative hemorrhage.

REFERENCES

1. Lembke J, Havers W, Doetsch N, et al: Long-term results following surgical removal of pulmonary metastasis in children with malignomas. Thorac Cardiovasc Surg 34:137–139, 1986.
2. Putnam JB, Roth JA, Wesley MN, et al: Survival following aggressive resection of pulmonary metastases from osteogenic sarcoma: Analysis of prognostic factors. Ann Thorac Surg 36:516–523, 1983.
3. Burt ME, Flye MW, Webber BL, et al: Prospective evaluation of aspiration needle, cutting needle, transbronchial, and open lung biopsy in patients with pulmonary infiltrates. Ann Thorac Surg 32:146–153, 1981.
4. Stillwell PC, Cooney DR, Telander RL, et al: Limited thoracotomy in the pediatric patient. Mayo Clin Proc 56:673–677, 1981.
5. Steichen FM, Ravitch MM: Stapling in Surgery. Chicago: Year Book Medical Publishers, 1984.
6. Sieber WK: Lung cysts, sequestration, and bronchopulmonary dysplasia. In Welch KJ, Randolph JG, Ravitch MM, O'Neill JA, Rowe MI (eds): Pediatric Surgery, 4th ed, pp. 645–654. Chicago: Year Book Medical Publishers, 1986.
7. Gdanietz K, Vorpahl K, Piehl G, Hock A: Clinical symptoms and therapy of lung separation. Prog Pediatr Surg 21:86–97, 1987.
8. DeLorimier AA: Congenital malformations and neonatal problems of the respiratory tract. In Welch KJ, Randolph JG, Ravitch MM, O'Neill JA, Rowe MI (eds): Pediatric Surgery, 4th ed, pp. 631–642. Chicago: Year Book Medical Publishers, 1986.
9. Eigen H, Lemen RJ, Waring WW: Congenital lobe emphysema: Long-term evaluation of surgically and conservatively treated children. Am Rev Respir Dis 113:823–831, 1976.
10. Ramenofsky ML, Leape LL, McCauley RG: Bronchiogenic cyst. J Pediatr Surg 14:219–224, 1979.
11. Sieber WK: Lung cysts, sequestration, and bronchopulmonary dysplasia. In Welch KJ, Randolph JG, Ravitch MM, O'Neill JA, Rowe MI (eds): Pediatric Surgery, 4th ed, pp. 645–654. Chicago: Year Book Medical Publishers, 1986.
12. Jones JC, Almond CH, Snyder HM, et al: Congenital pulmonary cysts in infants and children. Ann Thorac Surg 3:297–306, 1967.
13. Stocker JT, Drake RM, Madewell JE: Cystic and congenital lung disease in the newborn. Perspect Pediatr Pathol 4:93–154, 1978.
14. Landing BH: Congenital malformations and genetic disorders of the respiratory tract. Am Rev Respir Dis 120:151–185, 1979.
15. McLaughlin FJ, Strieder DJ, Harris GB, et al: Tracheal bronchus: Association with respiratory morbidity in childhood. J Pediatr Surg 106:751–755, 1985.
16. Bradham RR, Sealy WC, Young WG Jr: Chronic middle lobe infection: Factors responsible for its development. Ann Thorac Surg 2:612–616, 1966.
17. Davies G, Reid L: Growth of the alveoli and pulmonary arteries in childhood. Thorax 25:669–681, 1970.
18. Buhain WJ, Brody JS: Compensatory growth of the lung following pneumonectomy. J Appl Physiol 35:898–902, 1973.

88 HEART-LUNG AND LUNG TRANSPLANTATION

JAMES THEODORE, M.D. / DAVID ROSS, M.D. / VAUGHN STARNES, M.D. / NORMAN LEWISTON, M.D.

Heart-lung transplantations (HLT) and lung transplantations appear to be quite promising as effective therapeutic modalities for the treatment of selected patients with terminal cardiopulmonary or pulmonary disease. Survival and rehabilitation rates now achieved in a number of centers strongly support the claim for clinical efficacy of such surgery in patients with primary pulmonary hypertension, pulmonary hypertension associated with congenital heart disease, cystic fibrosis (CF), and bronchiectasis.[1] Among the Stanford University recipients are two patients who, when this chapter was written, had survived for more than 8 years and were living essentially normal lives. The enhancement of results through proper selection of patients, refinements of operative technique, improved preservation of donor organs, and advances in surveillance technique for the early detection of rejection and infection holds even more promise for these procedures.

B. A. Reitz, N. E. Shumway, and associates performed the first successful HLT in humans in March 1981 after success of this procedure in primates. This began a successful clinical series of such surgery for patients with end-stage pulmonary hypertension of the primary type or the type associated with congenital heart disease. In November 1983, Cooper and colleagues began the first series of successful single-lung transplantations, establishing the clinical usefulness of this procedure in patients with end-stage pulmonary fibrosis.[2, 3] Before the first successful

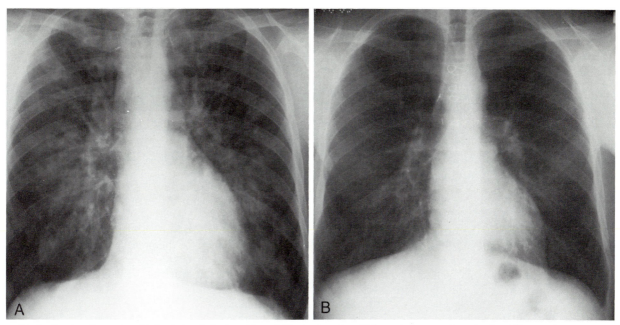

Figure 88–1. Chest radiographs obtained shortly before (*A*) and 10 months after (*B*) heart-lung transplantation in a 29-year-old man with cystic fibrosis.

HLT, lung transplantation had been a clinical failure. Of the first 39 patients on whom this procedure was tried, only two survived: one for 6 months and one for 10 months. Most of the recipients died of respiratory failure, pulmonary sepsis, pulmonary rejection, or complications of the bronchial anastomosis within days or weeks.[2, 4]

In retrospect, a number of factors may have contributed to the early failures. Some of these include difficulty in obtaining suitable donor lungs, inadequate lung-preservation techniques, a high percentage of poor-risk candidates operated on while they were in extremis, operative techniques in use at that time, and difficulties in the early diagnosis and treatment of lung rejection. The nature of the immunosuppression during the early clinical trials undoubtedly also contributed to the complications. The toxic effects of this therapy (with the use of only azathioprine and corticosteroids pushed to tolerable dosage) probably played significant roles in the impairment in healing of the bronchial anastomosis and without question contributed to the increased susceptibility of the transplanted lung to infection. Although new operative designs were of importance, the development of better immunosuppressive regimens, especially the availability of cyclosporin A, was the critical factor that ultimately led to clinical success.

Since the first successful surgery in 1981, nearly 1000 patients have undergone heart-lung, single-lung, or double-lung transplantations. Analysis of 32 patients who had undergone HLT over a 3-year period at Stanford (1986 to 1989) shows survival rates of 73%, 73%, and 65% at 1, 2, and 3 years, respectively.[5] It is anticipated that survival and rehabilitative success of HLT and lung transplantation will continue to improve with time.

The ability of the transplanted lung to maintain function during rest and exercise has a direct bearing on the clinical usefulness of this procedure. The transplanted heart and lungs function surprisingly well despite denervation, disruption of the pulmonary lymphatic and bronchial arterial systems, and ischemia of the allografts at the time of surgery (Fig. 88–1; Table 88–1). Standard measurements of pulmonary function indicate that the long-term functions of the transplanted lung are well maintained, as is the integrated dynamic function of the heart and lungs during exercise. Gas exchange at rest and exercise remains essentially normal despite the persistence of a mild restrictive abnormality, thought to be caused by chest wall factors as the result of surgery. The dramatic clinical improvement seen in patients after HLT is further substantiated by measured increases in posttransplantation exercise capacity. Although circulatory limitations of maximal exercise may persist, the transplanted heart and lungs perform sufficiently well to support normal life.[6]

The denervated transplanted lung shows bronchial hyperresponsiveness to cholinergic stimulation (methacholine inhalation) and the loss of an "airway reflex" (i.e., the absence of bronchodilatation normally associated

Table 88–1. PULMONARY FUNCTION BEFORE AND 10 MONTHS AFTER HEART-LUNG TRANSPLANTATION IN A 29-YEAR-OLD MAN WITH CYSTIC FIBROSIS

Pulmonary Function	Before Transplant (% Predicted)	After Transplant (% Predicted)
FVC	1.27 l (25%)	4.62 l (94%)
FEV_1	0.55 (14%)	4.01 (101%)
FEF_{25-75}	0.17 l/sec (4%)	5.84 l/sec (134%)
Pa_{O_2}	36 mm Hg	95 mm Hg
Pa_{CO_2}	66 mm Hg	34 mm Hg

FVC, forced vital capacity; FEV_1, forced expiratory volume in 1 sec; FEF_{25-75}, forced expiratory flow between 25% and 75% of vital capacity; Pa_{O_2}, arterial oxygen tension; Pa_{CO_2}, arterial carbon dioxide tension.

with deep inspiration after bronchoconstriction).[7, 8] Both of these changes may provide indexes for lung denervation. The bronchial hyperresponsiveness may be related to muscarinic denervation hypersensitivity. Despite this, the transplanted lungs do not manifest clinical asthma. In general, however, lung denervation does not appear to affect adversely gross ventilatory control and the overall function of the respiratory system.[9, 10]

Unilaterally transplanted lungs also function sufficiently well to support the activities of daily life. Pulmonary function and exercise are sufficiently improved after unilateral lung transplantation in patients with pulmonary fibrosis.[11] Overall pulmonary function (the combined functioning of the diseased fibrosed lung and the unilateral transplanted lung) shows significant improvement in total lung capacity, the timed forced expiratory volumes, lung diffusing capacity for carbon monoxide, and levels of arterial blood gases. The blood gases are maintained at essentially normal values. Oxygen saturations and work performance during exercise also are improved.[2, 11]

For patients without pulmonary hypertension or cardiac disease but requiring the removal of both lungs, the choice between HLT or double-lung transplantation becomes an issue of preference of the surgical team. There have been enough airway complications after the transplantation of both lungs as a block that most surgeons now perform the Noirclerc procedure, which is in essence a bilateral single-lung transplantation. One lung is transplanted with a bronchial anastomosis, and then the other lung is inserted on the other side with a bronchial anastomosis. Proper healing requires wrapping of the anastomosis with a pedicle of omentum, a procedure not required for HLT. A double-lung transplantation, however, permits the use of a donor heart for another recipient. This is a matter of extreme importance in an era when only a few centers performing lung transplantation are competing for donor organs with more than 150 centers able to transplant hearts. One solution to this is the so-called domino operation in which the native heart of the recipient of the HLT is transplanted into another patient. The success rate of this procedure compares favorably with those of other transplantations.

Single-lung transplantation is useful in patients with pulmonary hypertension, patients with Eisenmenger's complex who can undergo successful repair of the cardiac septal defect, and patients with "dry" lung disease who have essentially normal cardiac function. It is contraindicated in CF, bronchiectasis, and other conditions with chronic infection because the remaining lung will spill infection into the recipient lung.

INDICATIONS AND CONTRAINDICATIONS FOR TRANSPLANTATION

Criteria for the selection of patients are under constant review and are evolving with the acquisition of clinical information. Although complete sets of objective criteria covering all situations are ideal, such "lists" still remain incomplete, permitting the entry of subjective elements into the selection process. This may account for some of the differences in selection criteria that are found between programs and undoubtedly represent variations that are influenced by local attitudes and experience. Nonetheless, even with the differences, the overall guidelines for patient selection tend to be generally uniform in principle if not in specifics.[12] Several criteria should serve as general guidelines in considering patients for HLT or lung transplantation.

AGE OF PATIENT

The upper age limit may vary with the nature of the disease and the operation being considered. As a rule, younger patients have increased likelihood of survival and of rehabilitation after transplantation because there is a lesser tendency for the presence of multiple-organ failure, degenerative vascular disease, and other complicating factors. Muscle wasting, loss of stamina, and overall reserve are usually less of a problem in younger candidates.

At Stanford University, the upper age limit for lung transplantation is 50 years, with two exceptions. Patients with emphysema are considered eligible for HLT up to age 55 years, and the upper age limit for patients undergoing single-lung transplantation for pulmonary fibrosis is 60 years. In the latter case, the surgery does not require cardiopulmonary bypass and entails less risk. There are no lower age limits for either procedure.

CLINICAL STATUS

General Considerations

The patient should have end-stage cardiopulmonary or pulmonary disease with a poor prognosis for long-term survival and have a functional classification of no less than New York Heart Association class III or its equivalent. Except for the presence of severe cardiac and pulmonary disease, the candidate should be a healthy and relatively vigorous person who would benefit from the transplantation procedure. In keeping with this general rule, the patient should be free of significant systemic disease, have well-preserved renal and hepatic function, be properly nourished, be free of psychiatric illness and be emotionally stable with a strong family support system, should have no history of alcohol or substance abuse, be a nonsmoker (for at least 1 to 2 years, depending on the cause of the primary disorder), and be firmly committed to the idea of undergoing transplantation.

Specific Considerations

End-Stage Disease
End-stage disease does not imply terminal disease in this particular setting. Patients in the terminal phases of their disease associated with tissue wasting, inadequate nutrition, and multiple organ failure rarely, if ever, have the reserve capacity to benefit from transplantation. Many of these patients do not survive the currently long waiting period (approximately 12 months), nor do they

survive the rigorous demands of the postoperative period associated with these procedures.

Prognosis

Although imprecise, the criteria for a life expectancy of 2 years are intended to take into account the period of time that patients must wait for transplantation. It is impossible to predict when surgery will take place because this is primarily dependent on the availability of suitable donor organs. The aim is to provide a margin of safety to ensure that the patients are still in good condition for transplantation whenever the allografts become available. In essence, a "transplant window" needs to be defined for each prospective candidate (i.e., a period of time in which the patient is capable of withstanding surgery that is not premature or too late to be of real benefit).

General Physical Condition

Despite the presence of severe underlying cardiopulmonary or pulmonary disease, the overall physical condition of prospective transplantation candidates should otherwise be relatively good with the preservation of muscle mass, good muscle tone, and sound nutrition. The candidates should be as physically active as their underlying disease permits. In fact, physical activity should be encouraged to levels that are reasonably tolerable in order to maintain muscle mass and overall strength in anticipation of transplantation. Patients showing signs of cachexia are poor candidates for transplantation. Conversely, marked obesity also is a relative contraindication for transplantation. In general, vascular diseases, operative risk, and postoperative complication rates are much higher in obese patients than in their leaner counterparts. Furthermore, and aside from the effects of their underlying heart and lung disease, most obese patients are in poor physical condition as a result of a sedentary lifestyle. This condition impairs early mobilization and rehabilitation after surgery.

Although cachexia and obesity are considered to be relative contraindications, underweight and moderate overweight states do not necessarily preclude transplantation if the patient is willing to rectify the condition. It is important that these steps be made before the acceptance of the patient for surgery. Failure to achieve acceptable weight renders candidates less suitable for transplantation. In those who are moderately overweight, the ability to lose weight can also be used as a test for determining the patient's degree of motivation and commitment to the procedure.

Contraindications

The ultimate objective of transplantation is to return the patient to as normal a life as possible. In keeping with this principle, any set of conditions that preclude long-term survival, recovery, or rehabilitation should be considered contraindications for this procedure. Although these criteria may appear to be excessively stringent at times, the shortage of donor organs warrants a prudent approach in limiting transplantation to the most suitable candidates.

The conditions addressed next serve as a general guide for defining the types of clinical disorders that preclude transplantation in a given patient (Table 88–2).

Systemic Disease. Patients selected to undergo transplantation should be free of significant systemic or mul-

Table 88–2. DISEASES FOR WHICH HEART-LUNG OR LUNG TRANSPLANTATION HAS BEEN PERFORMED

Pulmonary Vascular Disease
Primary pulmonary hypertension
Eisenmenger's syndrome (atrial and ventricular septal defects, patent ductus arteriosus, truncus, other complex anomalies)
Pulmonary hypertension secondary to thromboembolic disease
Cardiomyopathy with pulmonary hypertension
Obstructive Lung Disease
Emphysema (idiopathic)
Emphysema (alpha$_1$-antitrypsin deficiency)
Cystic fibrosis
Bronchiectasis
Bronchopulmonary dysplasia
Posttransplantation obliterative bronchiolitis
Bronchiolitis obliterans organizing pneumonia
Restrictive Lung Disease
Idiopathic pulmonary fibrosis
Sarcoidosis
Asbestosis
Eosinophilic granulomatosis
Desquamative interstitial pneumonitis
Lymphangioleiomyomatosis

tisystem disease. All abnormalities present in prospective candidates should be evaluated with regard to cause, nature and extent of involvement, degree of reversibility, and possible impact on the posttransplantation state.

Active Infection. The presence of any type of active infection is a contraindication to transplantation. Risks of massive infection of the transplanted lung and the development of widely spread sepsis are considerable, particularly during the early stages of induction of immunosuppression. This is so important that children who have coryza at the time of donor availability must have negative fluorescent antibody viral studies of the upper airway before the procedure can be considered.

Notable exceptions to this guideline are the patients with CF whose airways are chronically colonized with pathogens, most typically *Pseudomonas aeruginosa* and *Staphylococcus* species. Successful HLT in such patients can be performed if the infected areas are confined within the respiratory axis and there is no evidence of active clinical infection. Patients with chronic infection outside the respiratory axis are at considerably greater risk for the development of sepsis, and transplantation should not be performed. Patients who have latent infectious disease with the potential for reactivation and dissemination are more difficult to assess, and their suitability for transplantation must be determined on a case-by-case basis.

Severe Impairment of Renal or Hepatic Function. A sufficient renal reserve must be present at the time of surgery to avoid possible renal failure or shutdown as a consequence of cyclosporin A nephrotoxicity. Acceptable function requires a creatinine clearance of 50 ml/min/1.73 sq m, with no hematuria or proteinuria in the urine sediment. In addition, there should be no significant systemic hypertension.

The demands placed on the liver by transplantation also are great, and the functional reserve must be sufficient to meet the critical need of the early posttransplantation period. Hepatic impairment can lead to excessive bleeding, hepatic failure, and renal failure. Cyclosporin A is metabolized primarily by the liver; impairment of hepatic clearance can lead to plasma levels of this drug that can cause renal toxicity. The constant exposure of the liver to a wide variety of drugs, biologic products, and infectious agents with hepatotoxic effects places it at increased risk during the entire posttransplantation period.

Mild abnormalities of hepatic function resulting from cor pulmonale and right ventricular failure are acceptable for transplantation if the total bilirubin level is less than 2.5 mg/dl. As a rule, total bilirubin appears to be the most reliable index of liver damage from passive congestion with heart failure. Marked abnormalities of hepatocellular function such as elevated levels of liver enzymes, prolonged prothrombin times, or signs of portal hypertension preclude transplantation, even though the bilirubin might be in an acceptable range.[13]

Social and Psychiatric Function. Patients with a history of alcoholism, drug abuse, or significant mental illness are considered unsuitable for transplantation. Aside from any associated medical complications, it is quite doubtful that such patients have the commitment, motivation, self-discipline, sense of responsibility, and emotional stability to cope with the demands of the posttransplantation medical regimen.

Depending on the circumstances, a history of smoking may or may not exclude a candidate for transplantation. As a general principle, active smoking is a contraindication. All candidates with a history of smoking must have stopped for at least 1 year before consideration for transplantation. In addition, patients with smoking-related disease should receive extensive evaluation to rule out significant vascular disease, particularly of the carotid arteries, and any possible malignancy of the upper and lower respiratory tracts.

Previous Therapies. Although oral corticosteroid usage no longer is an absolute contraindication to transplantation, there is clear evidence that tracheal or bronchial anastomotic healing can be affected. Every effort should be made to discontinue this drug or to reduce the dosage to as low a level as possible. If a patient is taking corticosteroids at the time of surgery, a generous omental wrap of the anastomosis should be considered.

Previous thoracic surgery also is no longer a contraindication to transplantation. Although there are some reports of successful lung transplantation after surgical and chemical pleurodesis, the pleural scarring still is a possible source of postoperative complications. If a patient who may ultimately become a transplant candidate requires an open-lung biopsy or acquires a pneumothorax, consultation with a transplantation center may avoid later difficulties.

HEART-LUNG TRANSPLANTATION PROCEDURE

The recipient operation is performed through a median sternotomy unless there is a high probability of pleural adhesions. In this instance, a "clam shell" incision may be used, which is in effect a bilateral lateral incision with a trans-sternal cross incision. Before heparinization, any pleural or pericardial adhesions are lysed with electrocautery. The patient is then heparinized; the ascending aorta, superior vena cava, and inferior vena cava are cannulated, and cardiopulmonary bypass and cooling are begun. The heart is excised at the midatrial level and at the immediate aortic supravalvar level in exactly the same manner as for cardiac transplantation. The pulmonary artery is divided near its bifurcation.

A left phrenic nerve pedicle is constructed from pericardium. The left atrium is then divided vertically, and the left-sided pulmonary veins are reflected toward the left pleural space with care to avoid the esophagus and the vagus nerve. The left inferior pulmonary ligament is divided, and the hilar structures are dissected. The pulmonary artery is divided proximally and the left main stem bronchus is stapled. The lung is then removed, with division distal to the staple line except in cases of CF, in which two staple lines are placed to avoid contamination.

A right-sided phrenic nerve pericardial pedicle is then fashioned from the level of the diaphragm to the level of the pulmonary artery. The right-sided pulmonary veins are reflected toward the right hemithorax. The right inferior pulmonary ligament is divided and the right lung removed as described previously. The pulmonary artery remnant is excised with care to avoid injury to the recurrent laryngeal nerve. Large bronchial vessels are secured with metallic clips. The bronchial stumps are dissected up to the level of the carina, where the trachea is divided.

After ascertainment of adequate hemostasis, the graft is brought into the field. The trachea is divided two rings above the carina, and then the graft is implanted. The lungs are introduced into the thorax below the phrenic nerve pedicles. The tracheal anastomosis is then performed. Ventilation is begun with room air and half-normal tidal volumes. Catheters are placed in the left atrial appendage and both pleural spaces, and cooling is begun. The donor right atrium is excised from the inferior vena cava toward the base of the right atrial appendage; care should be taken to avoid injury to the sinoatrial node. The right atrial anastomosis is then performed, and systemic warming is begun.

Finally, the aortic anastomosis is constructed. Air is evacuated from the graft and the aortic cross-clamp is removed. After gradual resuscitation of the heart, the patient is weaned from cardiopulmonary bypass. Pacing wires and drainage tubes are placed. Postoperative catecholamine support is ordinarily instituted with isoproterenol.

LUNG TRANSPLANTATION

The left lung is transplanted whenever possible because of the relatively favorable length of pulmonary artery on that side and better accessibility of the left atrium. The presence of previous left thoracotomy or pleural adhesions may make right-lung transplantation a better choice.

The patient is positioned in the right lateral decubitus position. The operation is commenced with a 4-cm vertical midline abdominal incision. If an omental wrap is deemed necessary, an omental pedicle is developed and placed in the upper abdomen near the diaphragm. A left posterolateral thoracotomy is performed. Through the use of blunt dissection posterior to the xyphoid process, a tunnel is created just anterior to the diaphragm, and the omental pedicle is brought through this tunnel.

The pericardium is entered, and a pericardial phrenic nerve pedicle is constructed from the level of the diaphragm to the level of the pulmonary artery. The ductus ligamentum is divided. The pulmonary artery is then clamped, and contralateral pulmonary arterial and right ventricular hemodynamics are observed during a 5-min period of unilateral pulmonary artery clamping. If right ventricular performance is well preserved, the transplantation is continued without cardiopulmonary bypass; if it is not, bypass procedures are instituted.

The pulmonary artery is then clamped, and both pulmonary veins are ligated and divided. The left main bronchus is clamped and divided. An atrial cuff is prepared by incising between the two pulmonary veins. The donor lung is then placed in the field. The atrial, pulmonary arterial, and bronchial anastomoses are performed, in that order. The lung is then inflated gently. The omental pedicle is brought posteriorly and tacked around the bronchial anastomosis. After careful inspection for hemostasis, the chest is closed.

MANAGEMENT OF THE HEART-LUNG TRANSPLANT RECIPIENT

After discharge from the hospital, the patient must be observed closely as an outpatient. Immunosuppression is almost always produced with an oral combination of cyclosporine, prednisone, and azathioprine. The differentiation of opportunistic infection and allograft rejection is often difficult. No signs or symptoms are deemed pathognomonic for rejection. The chest radiograph is also neither sensitive nor specific in separating opportunistic infection, pulmonary rejection, and interstitial edema. The probability of a normal radiograph in the presence of rejection at Papworth Hospital, in Cambridge, England, was reported as 0.67, and thus radiographs are "unacceptably insensitive."[14]

Infection is a persistent threat to the HLT recipients and is a more common occurrence than among recipients of the isolated heart transplant.[15, 16] Pulmonary allograft infection, which is most frequently caused by bacteria (72%), occurred in 79% of HLT recipients in a series at Stanford University, in comparison with a 22% incidence of bacterial pneumonia in similarly immunosuppressed cardiac transplant patients.[15] The reason for this increased susceptibility is not clear; however, it is most likely to be multifactorial. In addition to the effects of thoracotomy and cardiopulmonary bypass on respiratory mechanics, the pulmonary allograft may be adversely affected by lung denervation, bronchial arterial and lymphatic interruption, abnormalities in mucociliary clearance, and alterations in local immunologic defense.

Bacterial pneumonia occurs most commonly in the early postoperative period; however, it can occur at any time. In the experience at Stanford University with an immunosuppressive regimen that included OKT3-cyclosporin A–azathioprine-prednisone, the average linearized bacterial infection rate during the first 3 months was 0.93 infections per 100 patient days. This rate markedly diminished in the subsequent months after transplantation. Gram-negative rods of the *Enterobacteriaceae* family and *Staphylococcus aureus* were the most common bacterial pathogens. *Legionella pneumophila* has also afflicted transplant patients during hospital outbreaks.[15] In addition, *P. aeruginosa* has been recovered frequently from patients in whom obliterative bronchiolitis (OB) developed. Recurrent infection in this group of patients is often reminiscent of diseases such as chronic bronchiectasis or cystic fibrosis and is treated in a similar manner.

Pneumonia resulting from cytomegalovirus (CMV) does not generally occur before 2 months after transplantation. This infection is associated with high morbidity and mortality rates and may predispose the pulmonary allograft to chronic rejection and obliterative bronchiolitis. Disagreement exists among transplant centers regarding the actual incidence of CMV infection in HLT patients. At the University of Pittsburgh, the incidence has been reported as 85% to 90%, whereas at Stanford University, seroconversion was noted in only 13% of patients with negative pretransplantation serologic tests.[16–18] The lower rate of primary CMV infection in the latter series has been attributed to the avoidance of CMV-positive allografts and blood products in seronegative recipients. The HLT patient may be particularly susceptible to CMV pneumonitis, inasmuch as the University of Pittsburgh noted that pulmonary involvement developed during a CMV infection in 80% of this group, in comparison with 9% of cardiac transplant patients.[17] A primary infection with this herpesvirus is associated with a significantly higher risk for pneumonia than is latent reactivation.

The incidence of *Pneumocystis carinii* pneumonia in HLT recipients varies among centers and may be attributed to environmental differences. The Pittsburgh group noted a 90% probability of contracting this protozoan infection without chemoprophylaxis (trimethoprim-sulfamethoxazole), usually within 2 to 6 months after transplantation.[19] Many but not all patients have fever, nonproductive cough, an increased difference in alveolar-arterial oxygen pressure, and interstitial radiographic infiltrates. The diagnosis is confirmed by Gomori's methenamine silver staining of bronchoalveolar lavage (BAL) fluid and transbronchoscopic biopsy specimens. Treatment with either trimethoprim-sulfamethoxazole or pentamidine isethionate is usually effective.

Nocardia species were previously responsible for infection in 13% of heart-transplant patients at Stanford University who received immunosuppression with azathioprine; however, this rate has decreased to 3% with the introduction of cyclosporin A.[18] A solitary pulmonary nodule/abscess associated with possible central nervous system or skin involvement should suggest this diagnosis. The treatment is high doses of sulfasoxazole with possible addition of minocycline.

Fungal opportunistic infections resulting from *Aspergillus fumigatus, Candida albicans,* and *Cryptococcus neoformans* pose a considerable risk and high associated mortality rates. Surveillance cultures are routinely performed for these pathogens, and low threshold is maintained for aggressive therapy with amphotericin B. Similarly, preoperative serologic tests for *Histoplasma capsulatum, Coccidioides immitis,* and *Toxoplasma gondii* are performed and may identify patients at risk for reactivation when immunocompromised. Patients with positive tuberculin skin tests also should be treated with isoniazid prophylaxis when the status of infection is not known.

Approximately one half of all transplant patients shed herpes simplex virus in the postoperative period, whereas the remaining half manifest symptoms of stomatitis or esophagitis or genital lesions. Topical or oral acyclovir is prescribed for mild herpes labialis or genital herpes lesions. More severe cases or herpes esophagitis generally require parenteral acyclovir. Herpes zoster may similarly occur after transplantation and should certainly be treated if there exists evidence of cutaneous dissemination or visceral involvement. Herpes pneumonia is uncommon in HLT recipients; however, a high index of suspicion and prompt treatment may be life-saving.

De novo systemic hypertension is a frequent concomitant of cyclosporin A immunosuppression in transplant recipients.[20, 21] Cyclosporin A is similarly responsible for significant nephrotoxicity, which is characterized by decreased glomerular filtration rate, tubular dysfunction, and diminished renal perfusion in transplant patients.[22, 23] Systemic hypertension is usually treated with a combination of a diuretic and either a calcium-channel blocker or an angiotensin-converting enzyme inhibitor in order to maximize renal perfusion. Prevention of nephrotoxicity is attempted with strict attention to blood pressure control and to achieving cyclosporin A levels in the lower therapeutic range.[24-26] Previous attempts to completely substitute azathioprine for cyclosporin A in cardiac transplant patients with progressive nephrotoxicity led to high rates of allograft rejection; therefore, this is not generally recommended in HLT patients at Stanford University.[26]

Hypercholesterolemia is also a frequent occurrence in transplant recipients. Pharmacologic intervention is unfortunately limited because bile acid–binding resins frequently interfere with cyclosporin A absorption, and lovastatin (Mevacor) may produce myositis, rhabdomyolysis, and acute renal failure in patients taking cyclosporin A.[27]

Transplant recipients have an increased predisposition to B cell lymphomas and lymphoproliferative lesions.[28] Many of these neoplasms possess the genomes of Epstein-Barr virus (EBV), and their occurrence is frequently associated with serologic evidence of EBV infection.[29, 30] The appropriate management is controversial; however, a reduction in immunosuppression and acyclovir therapy have produced tumor regression in certain patients.

Pulmonary deterioration associated with pathologic evidence of OB has proved to be the most serious long-term complication in HLT recipients.[31] This unfortunate sequela previously occurred in approximately 50% of the patients at Stanford University with a mean onset of 13 months (range, 3 to 47 months) after transplantation. The remnants of obliterated small bronchioles may be histologically identifiable only by elastin staining in either surgical or transbronchoscopic biopsy specimens. Pulmonary function testing demonstrates a progressive obstructive ventilatory defect that is usually heralded by a disproportionate decrease in forced expiratory flow between 25% and 75% of vital capacity (FEF_{25-75}). OB is considered a manifestation of chronic pulmonary allograft rejection, which in some cases may be provoked by an opportunistic pneumonia with *P. carinii* or CMV.

Allograft rejection is stimulated by the expression of major histocompatibility complex class II (MHC II) antigens and affected by activated T lymphocytes.[32] Therefore, these pathogens may induce MHC II antigen expression and enhance alloreactivity.[33] Treatment of OB is attempted with augmented immunosuppression, which may decrease the rate of decline in pulmonary function.[34]

Transbronchoscopic biopsy specimens obtained through a fiberoptic bronchoscope may be invaluable for discerning pulmonary allograft rejection.[14, 35] The transplant group at Papworth Hospital, in Cambridge, England, reported a sensitivity of 84% and a specificity of 100% with this modality.[14] The enhanced sensitivity in this study was attributed to the much larger biopsy specimens obtainable with an alligator forceps and to the presence of small vessels, which could be assessed in the specimens.

The characteristic histologic abnormality in pulmonary allograft rejection is described as a perivascular lymphocytic infiltration combined with an "acute-on-chronic" bronchiolar mucosal inflammation. At Stanford University, routine endomyocardial and transbronchoscopic biopsies are performed approximately every 1 to 2 weeks in the early postoperative period and when allograft rejection is clinically suspected. Cardiac allograft rejection, however, is extremely rare in HLT recipients more than 6 months after surgery.[36] The frequency of biopsies decreases thereafter, but a constant vigil is maintained for evidence of allograft rejection or opportunistic infection. Interestingly, substantial myocyte necrosis on endomyocardial biopsy specimens, which establishes the diagnosis of "moderate" cardiac rejection of the cardiopulmonary allograft, has been noted to occur asynchronously in association with a normal lung biopsy specimen and vice versa.[37]

Surveillance of pulmonary function is deemed requisite for all pulmonary transplant recipients and is achieved by the performance of spirometry and maximum expiratory flow-volume loops. In the experience at Stanford University, alteration in flow parameters, specifically FEF_{25-75}, may be a sensitive marker in detecting pulmonary allograft rejection.[31] When a significant reduction occurs in these expiratory-flow parameters, transbronchoscopic biopsies are immediately performed to confirm allograft rejection and rule out possible concomitant infection.

BAL is an extremely safe and useful technique in the diagnosis of opportunistic infection, especially with *P. carinii* and CMV.[38] BAL can also be used to monitor HLT recipients for evidence of allograft rejection as well as infection. The number of BAL-derived cells from HLT recipients is much higher than normal.[18] Furthermore, during acute pulmonary allograft rejection, the cellular recovery has been noted to increase approximately two- to threefold from baseline levels, thereby reflecting an active alveolitis.

In summary, the diagnosis of pulmonary rejection, in

contrast to cardiac rejection, is imprecise and requires further investigation. Transbronchoscopic biopsy with BAL is the current procedure of choice for diagnosing possible pulmonary allograft rejection and ruling out opportunistic infection.

PROBLEMS SPECIFIC FOR CHILDREN AND ADOLESCENTS

As with cardiac transplantation, most of the early experience with HLT and lung transplantation has been in adults. The group at Papworth Hospital, in Cambridge, England, reported their experience on HLT in five children under the age of 15 years and believed that the experience in children was similar to that seen with adults.[39] The Stanford University group performed HLT or lung transplantation on 12 children. The techniques were similar to those for adults, but a higher incidence of OB was noted (72% versus 22%). As younger patients are considered for transplantation, the long-term effects of corticosteroid and other immunosuppressive therapy on growth must be considered. Experience with children who have undergone heart transplantation shows that growth velocity resumes if prednisone therapy can be terminated or at least tapered to an alternate-day regimen. There is not enough experience with HLT to determine whether this option is a realistic expectation. The use of total lymphocytic irradiation as an adjuvant to immunosuppression may be of value in this regard.

In addition to the problems associated with HLT and lung transplantation that were discussed previously, experience with these procedures in children and adolescents has uncovered some additional problems with this age group.

CYSTIC FIBROSIS

Current evidence suggests that patients with CF do as well after HLT as do other patients.[40] There have been as yet no reports of recurrence of the genetic disease in the transplanted lungs. There are, however, a number of problems that are unique to this disease process.

Need for Increased Dosage of Cyclosporin A

This important immunosuppressive drug is extremely lipophilic. It is, in fact, delivered in liquid form in olive oil. The pancreatic insufficiency of CF patients requires a dosage of this drug approximately four to five times higher than for other patients in spite of replacement therapy with pancrelipase. The extremely high cost of this drug (up to $100 per day for some CF patients) may in time affect the acceptability of these patients as transplantation candidates.

Residual Organisms in the Sinuses

In spite of eradication of the residual bronchial flora with the transplantation, the sinuses still contain CF and as such usually are packed with a thick gel of CF mucus and *P. aeruginosa.* The maxillary and ethmoid sinuses

seem to be the major offenders. The mucous drainage from these sinuses tends to drip down the posterior pharynx and causes recurrent bronchitic symptoms, especially with viral infections of the respiratory tract. There is some experience with the use of nasal antral windows and repeated flushing of the maxillary sinuses with a solution of tobramycin.[41] The authors' experience is that this seems to be necessary in the CF patients after transplantation and has shown utility in the treatment of recurrent bronchitis.

Diabetes Mellitus After Pulse Corticosteroid Therapy for Rejection

One of the important modalities in the treatment of pulmonary rejection is pulse therapy with large doses of methylprednisolone. Because the pancreatic status of many CF patients is precarious preoperatively, the large dosages of corticosteroid frequently render patients insulin-dependent. There has been some benefit in the use of oral hypoglycemic agents for maintenance regulation of blood sugar, with occasional need for insulin during periods of increased prednisone doses.

Underlying Liver and Kidney Disease Because of CF

The presence of cholestatic disease in most patients with CF and the need for repeated courses of aminoglycoside antimicrobials before transplantation render the CF patient at increased risk for drug toxicity. Extreme care should be exercised in the selection of CF patients, especially those with any elevation of total bilirubin levels or with borderline low creatinine clearances.

Need for Change in Attitude About Health Care

Among the important mechanisms by which older CF patients cope with the specter of chronic illness is the denial of symptoms and demands for control in areas of their health care. Such attitudes actually are fostered by persons who care for large CF populations. Unfortunately, these lifelong habits may be hard to change after transplantation when strict adherence to a complicated medical regimen is vital. Selection teams are urged to stress this about-face, which is required in the posttransplantation period, and to reinforce it throughout the waiting period.

DETECTION OF REJECTION

As mentioned, considerable weight is placed on monitoring pulmonary function values, especially FEF_{25-75} and arterial oxygen pressure, for early signs of pulmonary rejection. Standard methods of pulmonary function testing are appropriate for patients 6 years of age or older, but younger patients just are not sufficiently coordinated to execute a forced vital capacity maneuver. This will become an important factor as younger patients are selected for transplantation. Computerized analysis of the partial forced expiratory volume curve or of the tidal volume curve may be of benefit, although there is virtually no experience with this technique in the posttransplant patients.[42] In addition, the passage of an alligator forceps for bronchial biopsy and passage of a biotome for myocardial biopsy are higher risk procedures for small children, although experience has shown these procedures to be possible for younger children.[43] Physicians managing pediatric patients who have undergone transplantation frequently must make decisions on the basis of clinical judgment and intuition alone, whereas for an adult transplant recipient, biopsy material might have been available to aid in decision making.

DONOR ORGAN AVAILABILITY

A fairly stringent size requirement for transplanted lungs means that the pool of available donor organs for children may be quite limited. The mean waiting period for a donor organ for a child at the Stanford University center was about twice that for adults. One expediency has been the use of a living-donor lobe transplantation from parent to child. Although the ethics surrounding this are somewhat complex, it has been successful.[44] The advantages cited are a closer immunologic match (four of six loci in the Stanford patients) and a more rapid availability of an organ for a desperately ill child. Although this may become an option for selected patients in the future, it is unlikely that it will replace cadaver donor organs in general acceptability.

REFERENCES

1. Theodore J, Lewiston N: Lung transplantation comes of age. N Engl J Med 322:772–774, 1990.
2. Cooper J, Pearson F, Patterson GA, et al: Technique of successful lung transplantation in humans. J Thorac Cardiovasc Surg 93:173–181, 1987.
3. Toronto Lung Transplant Group: Unilateral lung transplantation for pulmonary fibrosis. N Engl J Med 314:1140–1145, 1986.
4. Veith F, Kamholz S, Mollenkopf F, et al: Lung transplantation 1983. Transplantation 35:271–278, 1983.
5. McCarthy P, Starnes V, Theodore J, et al: Improved survival after heart-lung transplant. J Thorac Cardiovasc Surg 99:54–60, 1990.
6. Theodore J, Jamieson S, Burke C, et al: Pulmonary function status of the post-transplanted lung. Chest 86:349–357, 1984.
7. Glanville A, Burke C, Theodore J, et al: Bronchial hyper-responsiveness after human cardio-pulmonary transplantation. Clin Sci 73:299–303, 1987.
8. Glanville A, Yeend RA, Theodore J, et al: Effect of single respiratory manoeuvres on specific airway conductance in heart-lung transplant recipients. Clin Sci 74:311–317, 1988.
9. Theodore J, Robin E, Morris A, et al: Augmented ventilatory response to exercise in pulmonary hypertension. Chest 89:39–44, 1986.
10. Theodore J, Morris A, Burke C, et al: Cardiopulmonary function at maximum tolerable constant work rate exercise following human heart-lung transplantation. Chest 92:433–439, 1987.
11. Toronto Lung Transplant Group: Experience with single lung transplantation for pulmonary fibrosis. JAMA 269:2258–2262, 1988.
12. Marshall S, Kramer M, Lewiston N, et al: Selection and evaluation of recipients for heart-lung and lung transplantation. Chest 98:1488–1494, 1990.
13. Kramer M, Marshall S, Tiroke A, et al: Clinical significance of hyperbilirubinemia in patients with pulmonary hypertension undergoing heart-lung transplantation. J Heart Lung Transplant 10:317–321, 1991.
14. Higenbottam T, Stewart S, Penketh A, et al: Transbronchial lung biopsy for the diagnosis of rejection in heart-lung transplant patients. Transplantation 46(4):532–539, 1988.
15. Brooks RG, Hofflin JM, Jamieson SW, et al: Infectious complications in heart-lung recipients. Am J Med 79:412–422, 1985.
16. Dummer JS, Montero CG, Griffith BP, et al: Infections in heart-lung transplant recipients. Transplantation 41:725–729, 1986.
17. Gryzan S, Paradis IL, Hardesty RL, et al: Bronchoalveolar lavage in heart-lung transplantation. Heart Transplant 4(4):414–416, 1988.
18. Hofflin JM, Potasman I, Baldwin JC, et al: Infectious complications in heart transplant recipients receiving cyclosporine and corticosteroids. Ann Intern Med 106:209–216, 1987.
19. Dummer JS, Hardy A, Poorstattar A, et al: Early infections in kidney, heart, and liver transplant recipients on cyclosporine. Transplantation 36:259–267, 1983.
20. Thompson ME, Shapiro AP, Johnson AM, et al: The contrasting effects of cyclosporin-A and azathioprine on arterial blood pressure and renal function following cardiac transplantation. Int J Cardiol 11:219–229, 1986.
21. Rottembourg J, Mattei MF, Cabrol A, et al: Renal function and blood pressure in heart transplant recipients treated with cyclosporine. J Heart Transplant 4(4):404–408, 1985.
22. Calne RY, White DJ, Thiru S, et al: Cyclosporin A in patients receiving renal allografts from cadaver donors. Lancet 2:1323–1327, 1978.
23. Myers BD, Ross J, Newton L, et al: Cyclosporine associated chronic nephropathy. N Engl J Med 311:699–705, 1984.
24. Imoto EM, Glanville AR, Baldwin JC, et al: Kidney function in heart-lung transplant recipients: The effect of low-dosage cyclosporine therapy. J Heart Transplant 6(4):204–213, 1987.
25. Moyer TP, Post GR, Sterioff S, et al: Cyclosporine nephrotoxicity is minimized by adjusting dosage on the basis of drug concentration in blood. Mayo Clin Proc 63:241–247, 1988.
26. Hunt SA, Stinson EB, Oyer PE, et al: Results of "immunoconversion" from cyclosporine to azathioprine in heart transplant recipients with progressive nephrotoxicity. Transplant Proc 19(1):2522–2524, 1987.
27. Corpier C, Jaros P, Suki W, et al: Rhabdomyolysis and renal injury with lovastatin use. Report of two cases in cardiac transplant recipients. JAMA 260:239–241, 1988.
28. Penn I: Tumor incidence in human allograft recipients. Transplant Proc 11:1047–1051, 1979.
29. Hanto D, Gajl-Peczalska KJ, Frizzera G, et al: EBV induced polyclonal and monoclonal B-cell lymphoproliferative diseases occurring after renal transplantation: Clinical, pathologic, and virologic findings and implications for therapy. Ann Surg 198:356–369, 1983.
30. Ho M, Miller G, Atchison RW, et al: Epstein-Barr virus infections and DNA hybridization studies in post-transplantation lymphoma and lymphoproliferative lesions. J Infect Dis 152:876–886, 1985.
31. Theodore J, Starnes V, Lewiston N: Obliterative bronchiolitis. Clin Chest Med 11:309–321, 1990.
32. Pober JS, Collins T, Gimbrone MA, et al: Inducible expression of class II major histocompatibility complex antigens and the immunogenicity of vascular endothelium. Transplantation 41:141–146, 1986.
33. Burke CM, Glanville AR, Theodore J, et al: Lung immunogenicity, rejection, and obliterative bronchiolitis. Chest 92:547–549, 1987.
34. Glanville AR, Baldwin JC, Burke CM, et al: Obliterative bronchiolitis after heart-lung transplantation: Apparent arrest by augmented immunosuppression. Ann Intern Med 107:300–304, 1987.
35. Starnes V, Oyer P, Theodore J, et al: Evaluation of heart-lung transplant recipients with prospective, serial transbronchial biopsies and pulmonary function studies. J Thorac Cardiovasc Surg 98:683–690, 1989.
36. Glanville AR, Imoto E, Baldwin JC, et al: The role of right ventricular endomyocardial biopsy in the long-term management of heart-lung transplant recipients. J Heart Transplant 6(6):357–361, 1987.
37. Griffith BP, Hardesty RL, Trento A, et al: Asynchronous rejection of heart and lungs following cardiopulmonary transplantation. Ann Thorac Surg 40:488–493, 1985.
38. Griffith BP, Hardesty RL, Trento A, et al: Heart-lung transplantation: Lessons learned and future hopes. Ann Thorac Surg 43:6–16, 1987.
39. Whitehead B, Helms P, Elliott M, de Leval M: Pulmonary function following heart-lung transplantation in children. Am Rev Respir Dis 143:A456, 1991.

40. de Leval MR, Smyth R, Whitehead B, et al: Heart and lung transplantation for terminal cystic fibrosis. J Thorac Cardiovasc Surg 101:633–642, 1991.
41. Lewiston N, King V, Umetsu D, et al: Cystic fibrosis patients who have undergone heart-lung transplantation benefit from maxillary sinus antrostomy and repeated sinus lavage. Transplant Proc 23:1207–1208, 1991.
42. Morgan W, Geller D, Tepper R, et al: Partial expiratory flow-volume curves in infants and young children. Pediatr Pulmonol 5:232–243, 1988.
43. Palazzo R, Hertz M, Maynard R, et al: Transbronchial biopsy in young children after lung transplantation: Technique and diagnostic yield. Am Rev Respir Dis 143:A459, 1991.
44. Starnes V, Stoehr C, Theodore J, Lewiston N: Deciding to perform a living-donor lung transplantation: The paradigm. Am Rev Respir Dis 143:A463, 1991.

89 THORACENTESIS AND TUBE THORACOSTOMY

WILLIAM Y. TUCKER, M.D.

Thoracentesis and tube thoracostomy are two procedures commonly used to remove fluid and air from the pleural space. Both techniques can be used for diagnostic and therapeutic benefit. Because both are invasive procedures, serious complications can result from their use. Careful planning and awareness of pertinent anatomy are necessary to avoid problems with either procedure and to ensure that definite diagnostic and therapeutic value is obtained.

Certain aspects of chest wall anatomy are pertinent to either performing a thoracentesis or placing a chest tube in the pleural space (Fig. 89–1). The neurovascular bundle in each anatomic segment courses just beneath the rib in the interspace. Avoidance of the neurovascular bundle is important in both procedures and can be accomplished by directing the needle or tube along the superior rim of the rib bordering the inferior aspect of the interspace to be used. When choosing a site for a thoracentesis or for the placement of a chest tube, the physician also needs to keep in mind the internal structures that may be damaged if the needle or tube is advanced too far into the pleural space. Avoidance of the heart and great vessels is critical. Care must be taken in choosing a site for entering the pleural space in which the diaphragm will not be punctured and no injury will be caused to intra-abdominal structures.

Both thoracentesis and tube thoracostomy are painful invasive procedures that provoke considerable anxiety in children. Careful explanation to small children, with a showing of care and concern, is important in preparing them for these procedures. Adequate sedation is necessary in infants and children to allow the procedure to be performed as comfortably as possible for them. Under certain circumstances, general anesthesia may be needed in order to accomplish either thoracentesis or the insertion of a chest tube successfully. Adequate local anesthesia, obtained by the infiltration of lidocaine, is extremely important for making the procedure as painless as possible.

THORACENTESIS

Thoracentesis is used primarily to remove fluid from the pleural space. It can be used for either diagnostic or therapeutic purposes. As a basic rule, when thoracentesis is performed for therapeutic reasons, as much fluid as possible should be removed in order to provide a therapeutic benefit to the patient from the procedure.

As with any procedure, the proper equipment must be collected and arranged before the procedure (Fig. 89–2).

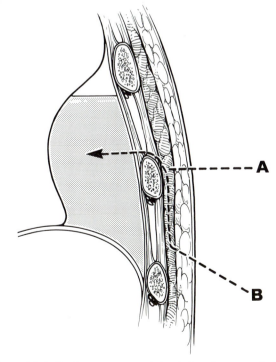

Figure 89–1. Pertinent anatomy relating to inserting a needle (proper path A) or tube (proper path B) into the pleural space.

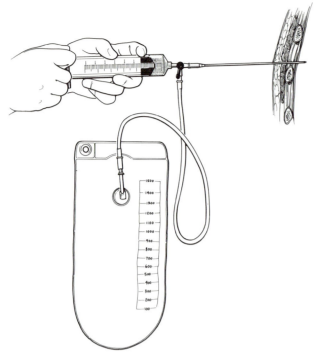

Figure 89–2. Thoracentesis needle and equipment in place.

Many companies offer prepackaged thoracentesis equipment that includes all the equipment necessary for performing the procedure. The site for the thoracentesis must be chosen carefully. In general, the proper place to insert the needle is into the center of the pleural fluid collection to be sampled. Pleural fluid, in the pediatric population, is rarely loculated and fixed in one position in the pleural space; rather, it is free in the pleural cavity and gravitates to the most dependent area of the pleural cavity. Thus the fluid changes location in the pleural space in accordance with the patient's position.

Thoracentesis is best performed in most infants and small children in the supine position. For a large pleural fluid collection to be sampled in this position, the thoracentesis should be performed laterally, in the midaxillary line, at the fifth, sixth, or seventh intercostal space. In older children and adolescents who are cooperative, a sitting position is a good choice for performing thoracentesis. The patient sits on a straight-back chair, leaning over and bracing against the back of the chair. The thoracentesis can then be performed in the posterior axillary line, usually in the sixth, seventh, or eighth intercostal space. The midaxillary and posterior axillary lines are two preferred sites for thoracentesis, and their use provides the least likelihood of damaging internal structures.

Thoracentesis should be accomplished with meticulous sterile technique. The skin is prepared with an iodine-containing solution, and the site is surrounded with sterile towels to avoid any contamination of the instruments advanced into the pleural space.

Local anesthesia is obtained by infiltrating lidocaine in the skin and raising a wheal at the site where the needle will be advanced through the skin. The needle is then progressively advanced through the subcutaneous tissue and chest wall tissue at the center of the rib beneath the inter-

space to be penetrated (see Fig. 89–1). Lidocaine is infiltrated along the path of the advancing needle. The needle is advanced until the resistance of the rib is met. The needle is then "walked" superiorly against the rib edge to the superior border. At that time, it can be advanced inward while lidocaine is injected. A large wheal of lidocaine should be placed just outside the parietal pleura to anesthetize this area. Puncture of the pleura is extremely painful, and adequate anesthesia must be obtained at this point. The needle is advanced through the pleura while aspirating with the syringe. The appearance of the suspected fluid in the syringe indicates that the pleura has been entered in the proper place. If the thoracentesis is performed purely for diagnostic purposes, the syringe may be changed and fluid withdrawn with the same needle to obtain a sample for analysis.

If fluid is to be withdrawn for both diagnostic and therapeutic benefit to the patient, the anesthetizing needle is withdrawn. The thoracentesis catheter is then inserted into the pleural space, following the same pathway as used with the anesthetizing needle. For complete drainage of the pleural space, it is best to insert a plastic catheter in the pleural space along the tract of the anesthesia. Once the catheter is in place and fluid can be freely aspirated, the tube is maintained in position with a small clamp at the skin. This provides stability in maintaining the tube in the pleural space in the right position. The catheter is connected to an aspirating syringe via a stopcock, which is also connected to the collection container (see Fig. 89–2). Fluid is then aspirated into the syringe. The stopcock is turned, and the syringe is emptied into the collection system. The stopcock can then be turned back to aspirate additional amounts of fluid from the pleural space. Commercially available thoracentesis sets contain a valve that fits between the catheter, the syringe, and the collection system to provide the proper direction of flow while the fluid is aspirated and the syringe is subsequently emptied. Fluid is evacuated until none can be obtained on aspiration. Many patients cough and sense pleuritic chest pain as the lung expands against the parietal pleura and chest wall. This is an indication that nearly all the fluid has been removed.

Each patient should have a chest radiograph immediately after thoracentesis is completed. The most common complications of thoracentesis are pneumothorax and hemothorax. If care has been taken to insert the needle in the proper position in the interspace, it is unlikely that hemothorax will result. If it does, however, urgent treatment is needed because it is a serious complication. A pneumothorax may occur with chest tube placement. A small pneumothorax that is stable and asymptomatic can be watched without the need for chest tube insertion.

TUBE THORACOSTOMY

Chest tubes are inserted to remove fluid and air from the pleural space and re-expand the lung. Pneumothoraces of various causes are the common reasons for removal of air from the pleural space. Hydrothorax and hemothorax are reasons for the use of a chest tube to remove fluid. The hydrothorax may be chyle, a large exudate, or transudate. Nearly all cases of pediatric empyema can successfully be treated with chest tube drainage of the exudate and appropriate antibiotics. Rarely is a thoracotomy necessary to treat childhood empyema.

As with thoracentesis, tube thoracostomy requires complete preparation before the procedure. The patient needs to be prepared psychologically and sedated appropriately. Appropriate equipment needs to be selected and on hand for the procedure.

Chest tubes come in a variety of sizes. In general, small tubes are much more comfortable for patients and much easier to insert than are large tubes. The small French chest tube sizes, ranging from 10 to 20, are adequate for removing air from the pleural space in cases of pneumothoraces. Many of the small tube sizes in this range also adequately drain fluid from the chest. Only in cases in which blood or thick purulent materials need to be drained do larger sizes of chest tubes become necessary. The chest tube size used is also determined by the size of the patient. In very tiny infants, a 10 or 12 French chest tube is almost always required, regardless of the fluid type that is to be drained. Older children can obviously accommodate larger chest tube sizes if they are necessary for thick fluid or blood.

Several sites for insertion of a chest tube are safe and appropriate, depending on the nature of the fluid or air to be drained. If air is to be removed from the pleural space, the chest tube should be placed anteriorly and superiorly, where the air tends to collect. Tubes placed posteriorly and inferiorly in the pleural space, in a rather dependent position, do not successfully remove air. The classic position for insertion of a chest tube for a spontaneous pneumothorax is in the second intercostal space in the midclavicular line (Fig. 89–3A). This site is ideal in male patients for placing the tube in the proper superior location to remove air. It is not an appropriate insertion site in female patients because the tube may traverse breast tissue and would leave an unsightly scar on the superior portion of the breast and anterior chest wall. The author prefers to use the third or fourth intercostal space in girls, the approach being posterior to the pectoralis major muscle in the anterior axillary line (see Fig. 89–3B). This allows positioning of the tip of the tube in the apex of the pleural space and affords adequate removal of air. In very small infants, the second intercostal space and the third or fourth intercostal space in the locations described earlier allow little room to insert a tube without danger to mediastinal and axillary structures. In these small infants, it is probably more appropriate to place the tube in the midaxillary line in the fifth or sixth intercostal space, while directing the tube superiorly after it is inserted (see Fig. 89–3C).

For the removal of fluid from the pleural space, insertion in the fifth or sixth intercostal space in the midaxillary line in the lateral position is best (see Fig. 89–3C). The tube should be directed posteriorly and dependently in order to have the best access to the fluid. For the drainage of fluid, the tube should be placed through the intercostal space that is at the level of the bottom of the fluid collection. In general, the lower and more posterior placement of the chest tube is recommended. In no instance should a tube be placed more posterior than the posterior axillary line. It is extremely uncomfortable for recumbent patients to lie on a tube that exits the chest between the

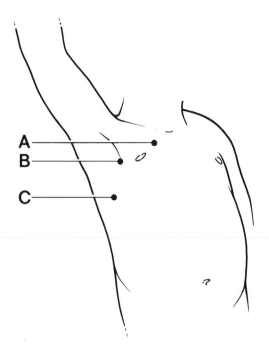

Figure 89–3. Preferred sites for chest tube insertion: the second intercostal space anteriorly (A), the third or fourth intercostal space beneath the pectoralis major muscle in the anterior axillary line (B), and the fifth or sixth intercostal space laterally (C).

posterior axillary line and the spine. If fluid and air coexist in the pleural space, an anteriorly and superiorly placed tube cannot be expected to drain the fluid, although it drains the air quite adequately.

For tube insertion, patients are generally positioned in the supine position. If the second intercostal space anteriorly or the third or fourth intercostal space behind the pectoralis muscle is chosen, elevation of the patient's head makes the insertion much more convenient for the patient and the physician inserting the chest tube. The path of the chest tube from the skin into the pleural space should be oblique, creating a small, subcutaneous tunnel (see Fig. 89–1). This is important at the time of tube removal, particularly in very small children and infants. It provides for a subcutaneous tract that is easily closed and sealed so that air is not sucked into the chest as the tube is removed. If the tube is inserted through the skin directly over the opening in the intercostal space, it is likely in a small, thin infant that the hole left by the tube will not seal and that air will be sucked into the chest and result in a pneumothorax. Thus when the interspace is located for tube insertion, penetration of the skin should be 2.5 to 3.75 cm away from the site of penetration of the intercostal space.

Meticulous sterile technique must be used to avoid introducing infection into the pleural space. The area is prepared, as in thoracentesis, with an iodine-containing solution and surrounded with drapes of sterile towels. The skin at the site of tube insertion is infiltrated with a wheal of lidocaine. The anesthetic needle is then advanced along the proposed tract, up and over the rib, and into the appropriate interspace. Along the way, lidocaine is infiltrated in advance of the path of the needle to ensure adequate local anesthesia. As the needle is passed over the superior edge of the rib, a large wheal of anesthesia should be infiltrated in the intercostal muscle and adjacent to the pleura. The author does not insert a chest tube without confirmation that the tube will go directly into the pleural space that contains the fluid or air that must be evacuated. As the anesthetic infiltration is completed, the needle should be advanced into the pleural space and negative pressure applied to the syringe plunger. Aspiration of the suspected fluid or air confirms entrance into the pleural space in the proper location to drain the fluid or air. If pleural fluid is not obtained on aspiration, the chest tube should not be inserted at this site; another site should be chosen.

The skin is incised transversely at the proposed site. The incision in the skin should be long enough only to allow insertion of the tube without binding against the skin edges. There are basically two techniques for inserting chest tubes into the pleural space. Each has advantages and disadvantages.

One technique is to use a chest tube sheathed over a sharp, pointed trocar that is used to puncture the intercostal space and pleura (Fig. 89–4). After the skin incision is made, fine scissors or a hemostat is used to bluntly dis-

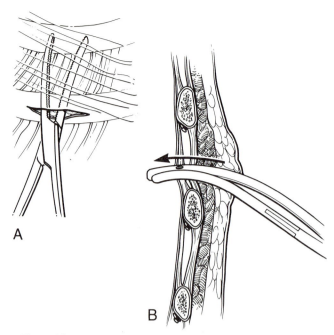

Figure 89–5. Method of inserting chest tube using blunt dissection.

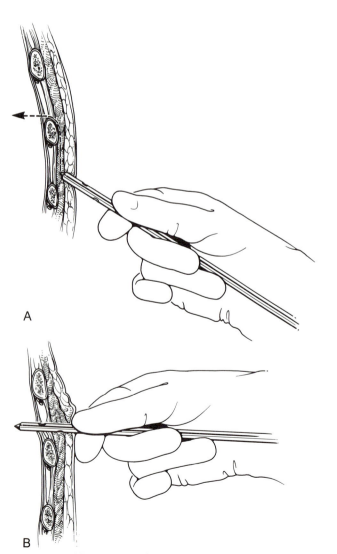

Figure 89–4. Method of inserting chest tube with trocar.

sect a tract in the subcutaneous tissue from the skin incision to the superior surface of the rib and interspace. The trocar, sheathed in the chest tube, is then inserted in the tract and carefully directed just over the superior rim of the rib. The trocar, with the chest tube, is used to puncture the pleura and is advanced a short distance into the collection of fluid or air. It is important that the chest tube and trocar be grasped firmly several centimeters back from the tip, as illustrated in Figure 89–4. This prevents dangerous advancement of the trocar into internal structures once the "give" of the parietal pleura is felt. With the trocar and chest tube minimally into the collection, the trocar is held in place and the chest tube advanced off the trocar so that all holes are within the pleural cavity. The trocar is removed from the chest tube. The chest tube is anchored to the skin with sutures and tape and connected to an appropriate drainage system. Although the trocar method of introducing a chest tube is quicker and simpler than other techniques, it can be extremely dangerous. If the sharp tip of the trocar is allowed to advance too far into the thoracic cavity, it can severely damage vital structures and cause serious complications.

The second method of insertion is somewhat safer but slightly more difficult. Anesthesia is obtained, and the finder needle is used to locate the fluid collection in the pleural space, as with the use of the trocar method. A skin incision is made in a similar manner and the subcutaneous tunnel bluntly dissected with a hemostat or a Kelly clamp (Fig. 89–5). The clamp itself is advanced over the superior rim of the rib and used to puncture the pleural surface. The clamp is spread to create an opening large enough to accommodate the tube. The tube is grasped with the clamp, directed through the tunnel into the pleural space, and advanced into the cavity. The clamp is withdrawn, leaving the tube, which is then advanced into the pleural space until all the side holes are within the cav-

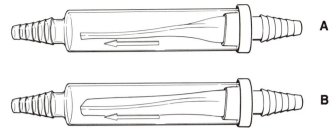

Figure 89-6. Heimlich valve: closed (*A*) and open (*B*).

ity. Again, the tube is secured in place with sutures and tape and connected to the proper drainage system. In this method, fluid invariably escapes onto the drapes when the pleural space is entered with the blunt clamp, and air is sucked into the chest; this causes a minor pneumothorax. There is little need to be concerned about this because the tube is soon connected to a drainage system that evacuates the fluid and air. After the tube is secured and connected to closed drainage, a chest radiograph should be obtained to confirm the proper position of the tube.

It is important to understand the closed thoracic drainage systems that are available for pleural evacuation. The purpose of a closed drainage system is to promote fluid evacuation and lung expansion. Each allows egress of fluid and air and prevents air from passing through the tube into the pleural space during phases of respiration with negative pleural pressure.

The simplest method of closed drainage is the Heimlich valve (Fig. 89-6), a simple, enclosed, one-way flutter valve. During the positive-pressure phase of respiration, air and fluid are allowed to escape through the Heimlich valve into a collection bag. During the negative-pressure phase of respiration, the valve closes, preventing air from reentering the pleural space. The Heimlich valve is a reliable and simple technique for closed pleural drainage. It works especially well for treatment of a pneumothorax. However, it does not allow monitoring of the amount of air escaping from the chest.

The classic closed thoracic suction drainage system has three basic components (Fig. 89-7). The first bottle in the system is simply a trap for collection of fluid, allowing monitoring and quantification of the drainage. The second bottle is the water seal. It provides a one-way valve that permits air to escape from the pleural space and prevents air from returning. As air is evacuated, it bubbles freely from the open end of the long tube beneath the surface of the water. The third bottle in the system is the suction regulator. Standard wall suction generates far too much pressure to be safe for the intrathoracic space and is also difficult to regulate. The third bottle provides a precise and constant negative pressure to the pleural space. Regardless of the wall suction level, the negative pressure applied to the pleural space is equal to the depth of the long tube beneath the water surface in the third bottle (see Fig. 89-7, length B). When wall suction is applied to the system, air bubbles freely from the tip of the long tube, which is open to the air beneath the surface. However, because it takes some negative pressure to pull air through the tube under the fluid in the second bottle, the effective negative pressure applied to the pleural space is equal to the depth of the tube at B minus the depth of the tube at A (see Fig. 89-7). Bubbling from the tube in the water seal bottle indicates a continued air leakage into the pleural space. If the chest tube is known to be in the proper place and is unobstructed, cessation of bubbling in the water seal bottle is a reliable indication that the pulmonary air leakage has sealed.

A complete understanding of a closed thoracic drainage system and attention to detail when using it is necessary for successful application in clinical practice. There must be no leakages in the system; otherwise, the one-way valve effect of the water seal bottle and the effect of the negative vacuum in the system are destroyed and lost. All connections must be sealed airtight, and the chest tube exit site from the chest must also be sealed to prevent air from leaking into the system or pleural space. Any dependent fluid-filled loops of tubing in the system, including the tube coming from the patient's chest to the trap bottle,

Figure 89-7. Classical setup for three-bottle, closed-tube suction drainage.

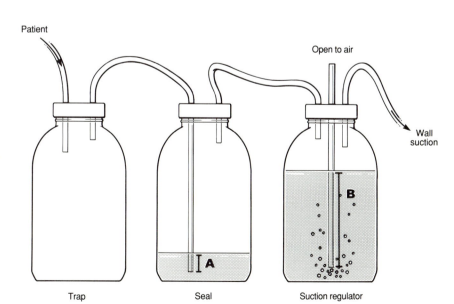

will oppose the suction created by the regulator. The tubing should not hang in a dependent loop at the bedside or between bottles. Several prepackaged commercially manufactured systems are available. Although altered in form and arrangement, they work on the same principles as the three-bottle system. Choosing a system is a matter of personal preference.

An important consideration in the management of a patient with a chest tube is the decision as to when to remove the tube. The basic principle about timing of tube removal is that when the tube stops draining either air or fluid, it is time to consider removal. Even if the chest radiograph reveals a continued collection of pleural fluid but the tube is not draining, it should be removed and possibly replaced with a second tube. If a tube is placed for management of pneumothorax alone, when no air leakage can be detected from the chest in the water seal bottle, it is time to plan removal of the chest tube. When bubbling stops in the water seal bottle, the wall suction should be discontinued. The tube is then left connected to the system on water seal drainage for 24 h. A chest radiograph after that time that shows no pneumothorax, combined with the absence of air bubbles in the water seal bottle, constitutes a significant indication that the tube may be removed safely.

Some physicians prefer to clamp chest tubes for a period of time and then obtain a chest radiograph to rule out the development of pleural fluid accumulation or pneumothorax before chest tube removal. There is some danger of tension pneumothorax developing after clamping. The author does not use chest tube clamping and believes that chest tubes should not be clamped even during transportation of patients because it is much safer for gas or fluid to be expelled freely from the chest through the water seal bottle than to be trapped within the chest by a clamped chest tube.

The chest tube should be removed during forced expiration if possible. Frequently, with children and infants, it is impossible for them to cooperate with or understand the procedure to the degree necessary for them to force

expiration at the time of tube removal. The sutures and tape are freed. The physician places a finger over the tube in the subcutaneous tunnel, and during forced expiration, the tube is quickly withdrawn. The finger over the subcutaneous tunnel is depressed to occlude the tunnel so that air cannot be sucked into the pleural space after the tube is removed. The skin incision is closed with a simple suture, and a large coating of povidone-iodine ointment is applied to the incision along with an occlusive dressing to further protect it from leaking air into the pleural space. Within several days, the skin is sealed and the dressing can be removed without any danger of a recurrent pneumothorax. As soon as the tube has been removed, a chest radiograph should be obtained to ensure that the lung is fully expanded. Appropriate observation and therapeutic intervention are undertaken if a pneumothorax is present.

The most serious complication of chest tube insertion is hemothorax with active bleeding into the pleural space. This most commonly results from injury to the intercostal artery and vein during insertion of the tube. It can also result from injury to other intrathoracic structures such as the lung, the heart, or the great vessels. When the chest tube is inserted and connected to the closed drainage system and if a large amount of blood is drained, the possibility of these injuries should be suspected. If the tube continues to drain blood from the pleural space, appropriate surgical intervention and transfusion therapy may be necessary.

REFERENCES

1. Julian JS, Pennell TC: A review of the basics of closed thoracic drainage. NC Med J 48(3):127–131, 1987.
2. Ravitch MM, Steichen FM: Atlas of General Thoracic Surgery. Philadelphia: WB Saunders, 1988.
3. Sabiston DC, Spencer FC: Gibbon's Surgery of the Chest, 5th ed. Philadelphia: WB Saunders, 1990.
4. Shields TW: General Thoracic Surgery, 3rd ed. Philadelphia: Lea & Febiger, 1989.

90 AIRWAY MANAGEMENT

KEITH CLARK, M.D. / JOHN S. DONOVAN, M.D.

Airway distress in children may be caused by many conditions that can involve various sites in the airway from the nose to the lung. Sometimes the specific cause is clear after a history and physical examination, but invasive procedures such as endoscopic examination are often required for confirming the diagnosis. To diagnose and treat airway problems, the physician should understand the anatomy and physiology of the pediatric airway and

the pathophysiology of conditions that may cause airway obstruction. Knowledge of respiratory dynamics, airflow, and abnormal respiratory sounds is essential for this understanding.

Several factors contribute to the rapid deterioration seen in children with acute upper airway obstruction. First, a significant decrease in the cross-sectional area of the pediatric glottic passage occurs with minimal swelling

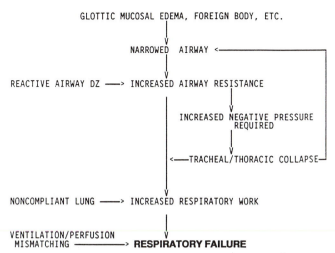

Figure 90–1. Factors in the progression from airway obstruction to respiratory failure.

of the laryngeal mucosa. This narrowing results in a dramatic increase in airway resistance. Second, the highly compliant pediatric trachea and rib cage are prone to collapse when exposed to high negative inspiratory pressures. A narrowed airway creates increased airway resistance, which leads to progressively greater negative inspiratory pressures. Unfortunately, the more negative pressures also result in tracheal and thoracic collapse that narrows the airway further. The cycle continues until the patient's respiratory workload is too high to maintain adequate ventilation and respiratory failure occurs (Fig. 90–1). In reactive airway disease, bronchiolitis, and noncompliant lung parenchyma (e.g., lobar pneumonia), the workload for respiratory muscles can increase. Finally, ventilation/perfusion mismatching in the alveoli can contribute to poor oxygenation in a child laboring to breathe with partial airway obstruction. Consequently, there is a vicious cycle leading to increased airway resistance, collapse of the compliant pediatric airway, increased respiratory workload, and finally respiratory collapse.

PATHOPHYSIOLOGY

AIRWAY FLUID DYNAMICS

The laryngeal airway may be modeled as a sharp constriction in a straight tube. The pressure in the laryngeal airway can be related to the density and mean velocity of the flowing air with the Bernoulli equation (Fig. 90–2):

$$P_1 + (p_1 \times v_1^2) = (p_2 \times v_2^2)$$

where P_1 is pressure at position 1, p_1 is density at position 1, and v_1 is mean velocity at position 1.

As the velocity through the glottis increases, the pressure at the glottis is decreased. Thus the compliant soft tissues of the larynx may prolapse and cause further narrowing of the airway. As the cross-sectional airway is narrowed further, there must be a corresponding increase in velocity and an additional decrease in pressure to maintain the same airflow. The sudden narrowing of the airway

at the glottis causes eddy currents downstream in the subglottis region, which add turbulence that disrupts the airflow, reduces efficiency of breathing, and places additional respiratory work demands on the child. The combination of increased airway resistance, collapse of the compliant pediatric airway, and increased respiratory work can lead to respiratory collapse.

LARYNGEAL ANATOMY

The larynx is the narrowest portion of the entire airway and as a result is particularly vulnerable to obstruction (Figs. 90–3, 90–4).[1] In the neonate, the addition of only 1 mm of mucosal edema/mass encroaches on the glottis and results in a dramatic decrease in the airway cross-sectional area.

The average newborn subglottic diameter measures 4.5 to 5.0 mm; a diameter of less than 3.5 to 4.0 mm is suggestive of subglottic stenosis.[2] A 1-mm circumferential narrowing in a 4.5-mm diameter subglottis would reduce the airway's cross-sectional area by 69% and would result in immense increases in airway resistance and respiratory work.

The mucosa of the epiglottis is rigidly adherent to the posterior (laryngeal) surface and loosely attached anteriorly. Edema occurring in the aryepiglottic fold or the epiglottis can extend laterally into the soft pharyngeal tissues. Consequently, supraglottic edema may become much more extensive than subglottic edema before it produces actual respiratory obstruction. Supraglottic edema causes laryngeal obstruction by extravasation of fluid anteriorly and laterally to the epiglottic cartilage, with a resultant curl inward and backward to occlude the larynx in a trapdoor manner.[3] This process does not typically extend down to the vocal cords or the subglottic tissues. However, many children with supraglottitis may have localized subglottic edema that is radiographically indistinguishable from croup.[4] Because the subglottic space is

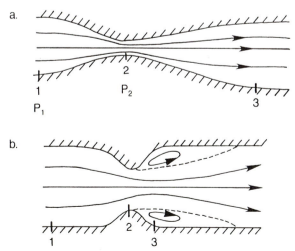

Figure 90–2. A gradually narrowing airway still allows laminar flow (more efficient) (a). A more abrupt narrowing of a glottis causing eddy currents and turbulence (less efficient) (b). (From Pedley TJ: Gas flow and mixing in the airway. In West JB (ed): Bioengineering Aspects of the Lung, pp. 163–193. New York: Marcel Dekker, 1977.)

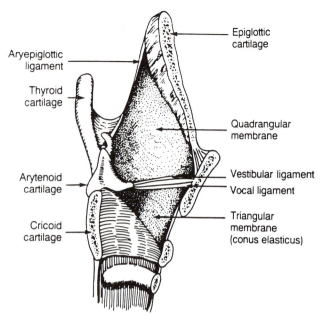

Figure 90–3. Schematic drawing of sagittal section of larynx. (From Graney D: Anatomy. *In* Cummings CW, Fredrickson JM, Harker LA, et al (eds): Otolaryngology—Head and Neck Surgery, p. 1731. St. Louis: CV Mosby, 1986.)

surrounded by the rigid cricoid cartilage, subglottic edema occurs at the expense of the airway and leads to stridor and chest retractions.

LARYNGEAL REFLEXES

A complex mechanism keeps the airway and the digestive passages separated. Feeding difficulties that cause aspiration, cyanosis, or regurgitation suggest that the sphincteric mechanism of the larynx either is malfunctioning or is being flooded. To initiate a swallow, the pharynx must be able to sense any food or liquid bolus; therefore, a superior laryngeal nerve injury compromising this sensation would promote aspiration. The glottis must be able to close completely (true vocal cord [TVC] adduction) when stimulated. Hence a paralyzed TVC does not adequately protect the lower airway. A well-coordinated pattern of proximal contraction and distal relaxation of pharyngeal musculature is needed to propel the bolus into the esophagus and to prevent pooling in the hypopharynx. Insufficient or uncoordinated relaxation of the cricopharyngeal muscles can result in pooling and aspiration. The structures that separate the digestive system from the respiratory system must remain intact. For example, a posterior laryngotracheal cleft may allow ingested material to enter the trachea (Fig. 90–5).

An active cough reflex is the most reliable defense mechanism against noxious agents. The cough reflex is triggered predominantly by sensitive receptors in the larynx and subglottic space and secondarily by additional cough receptors in the small airways, the large airways, and the nasopharynx. Closure of the larynx during coughing or during a Valsalva maneuver may help improve airway dynamics or gas exchange.

Reflex closure of the airway to prevent aspiration of food and liquids is an important function of the larynx. This reflex is clinically observed as a strong, prolonged closure of the larynx, elicited by the sensory nerve endings in the pharyngeal and laryngeal mucosa. However, the

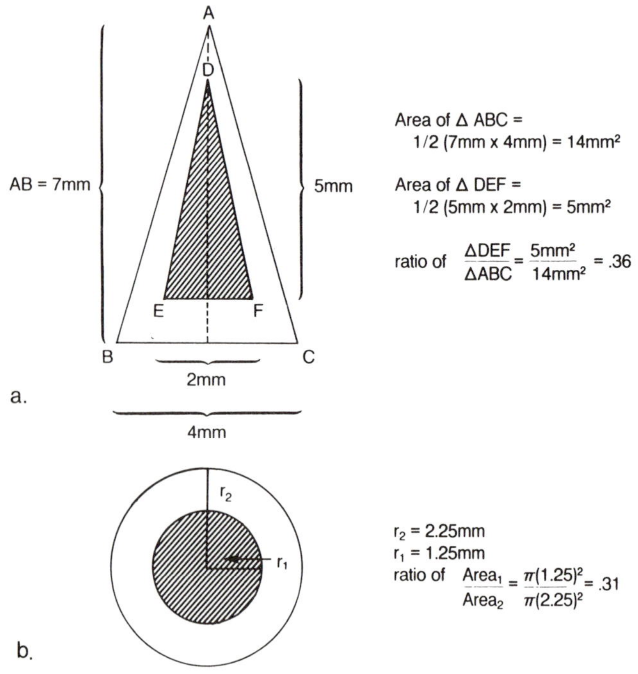

Area of △ ABC = 1/2 (7mm x 4mm) = 14mm²

Area of △ DEF = 1/2 (5mm x 2mm) = 5mm²

ratio of $\dfrac{\triangle DEF}{\triangle ABC} = \dfrac{5mm^2}{14mm^2} = .36$

r_2 = 2.25mm
r_1 = 1.25mm
ratio of $\dfrac{Area_1}{Area_2} = \dfrac{\pi(1.25)^2}{\pi(2.25)^2} = .31$

Figure 90–4. Coronal section of larynx. Note the sudden narrowing of the airway at both the false and true vocal folds. (From Pedley TJ: Gas flow and mixing in the airway. *In* West JB (ed): Bioengineering Aspects of the Lung, pp. 163–193. New York: Marcel Dekker, 1977.)

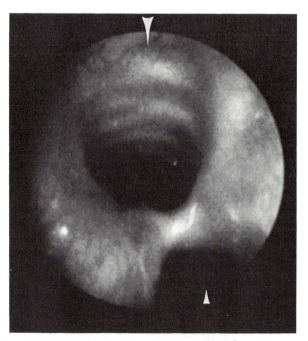

Figure 90–5. Endoscopic view of a tracheoesophageal cleft (*large arrowhead* points to trachea; *small arrowhead,* to esophagus). A 2-year-old boy presented with a chronic cough and recurrent aspiration pneumonia. A barium swallow demonstrated aspiration of barium into the larynx and trachea.

immaturity of a newborn's sensory nerve endings contributes to the weakness of the neonatal laryngeal reflex. The weakness of the laryngeal reflex at birth explains not only the ease with which intubation or bronchoscopy can be performed in an awake neonate but also the frequency of aspiration.

In the canine model, sections of the peripheral recurrent laryngeal nerve fibers studied between birth and 2 months of age showed (1) an increase in myelination and conduction velocity, (2) a shorter latency period between superior laryngeal nerve stimulation and TVC adduction, and (3) a decreased threshold for superior laryngeal nerve stimulation to elicit ipsilateral TVC adduction.[5] These findings are consistent with the temporal sequence of the laryngeal reflex's functional development. The threshold of the laryngeal reflex may be decreased by either hyperventilation or hyperoxia. Conversely, hypoventilation and hypercapnia raise the threshold of the reflex.[6] Whereas general anesthesia raises the threshold but never abolishes it, local anesthesia acts on the afferent nerve to temporarily eliminate the laryngeal reflex. Finally, the presence of a tracheostomy tube may suppress the glottic closure reflex and allow aspiration.[7]

Stimulation of the larynx may also result in changes in other organs, particularly those of the cardiovascular system. Arrhythmia, bradycardia, cardiac arrest, hypotension, and respiratory depression can result from vagal stimulation. These responses to laryngeal stimulation may be increased by light general anesthesia, hypoxia, or hypercapnia.[5]

STRIDOR

Stridor is the harsh, high-pitched, loud sound produced when air flows rapidly through a narrowed passage. Acute-onset stridor with airway obstruction requires immediate investigation because there is a potential for rapidly progressive airway obstruction. In the absence of airway obstruction, a prompt but less urgent investigation of stridor can be made. The intensity of stridor is not necessarily correlated with the seriousness of the child's condition. For example, a child with croup may have an alarming degree of stridor and retractions but may have better respiratory function than a child with life-threatening acute supraglottitis who has mild chest retractions and minimal stridor.

The earliest blood gas abnormality found in a child with acute airway obstruction is hypoxemia. Often this is not related to alveolar hypoventilation but is more likely caused by ventilation/perfusion mismatching in the lung. This mismatch is thought to occur as a result of several factors. Peripheral airway resistance is higher in children than in adults; thus edema or secretions in these small airways result in a greater increase in airway resistance and a more profound disturbance in gas exchange.[8] Irritation of the larynx and trachea is thought to cause reflex bronchoconstriction of distal airways.[9] Furthermore, impairment in the ability to cough causes retention of secretions in both large and small bronchi[10] and plugging of bronchioles.

ABNORMAL CRY/VOICE

Important diagnostic information can sometimes be obtained by listening carefully to the child's voice, cry, or cough. The voice can be characterized as normal, rough or hoarse, muffled, breathy, or high pitched. A rough voice suggests the presence of any mass that interferes with the normal vibratory pattern of the vocal cords. Mass effect can be produced by such lesions as a cyst, hemangioma, neoplasm, or laryngitis. Furthermore, the severity of the voice change does not always correspond to the seriousness of the underlying disease. Disorders of the supraglottic structures such as acute supraglottitis, supraglottic cyst, or retropharyngeal abscess usually produce a muffled voice. Breathy vocal quality results from lesions that interfere with normal vocal cord approximation, such as vocal cord paralysis, recurrent respiratory papillomatosis, vocal process granulomas, vocal nodules, or a foreign body. Aphonia (the inability to vocalize) is unusual and suggests severe laryngitis, the presence of a foreign body lodged within the larynx, or a psychogenic disorder. Unilateral and bilateral vocal cord paralysis in children can cause hoarseness and airway distress. The left recurrent laryngeal nerve is at extreme risk for injury during cardiac surgery in the area where it loops around the arch of the aorta. Thus hoarseness after repair of a patent ductus arteriosus, double aortic arch, or pulmonary artery anomalies should suggest a possible vocal cord paralysis. Foreign bodies in the larynx or esophagus may provoke hoarseness and airway blockage because of swelling.

A complete history and a thorough physical examination of a child with an abnormal voice are required in addition to a proper inspection of the larynx. Fortunately, an etiologic diagnosis can be made in most cases after the vocal cords have been adequately examined. Through the use of topical nasal anesthesia and a flexible fiberoptic nasopharyngoscope, the larynx can be easily examined in children of all ages. Recall the old adage that 'any patient with hoarseness of 2 weeks' or longer duration should undergo a visualization of the vocal cords.

PROGRESSIVE AIRWAY OBSTRUCTION

It is important to identify lesions that cause progressive airway obstruction, such as congenital cysts, laryngeal stenosis, laryngeal hemangiomas, and recurrent respiratory papillomatosis (RRP) (Fig. 90-6). Laryngeal hemangiomas and lymphangiomas are usually not symptomatic at birth, but during the first months of life, they enlarge dramatically. Progressive hoarseness suggests neoplasia, which usually compromises the airway gradually over weeks or months. RRP is the most common neoplasm of the larynx in children and is caused by human papillomavirus types 6 and 11 infection of the upper respiratory tract mucosa.[11, 12] RRP causes wartlike growths anywhere in the upper respiratory tract, but these growths are most common on and around the larynx. The papillomas can enlarge over weeks and months to fill the larynx until potentially fatal airway obstruction occurs (Fig. 90-7). Papillomas may also cause wheezing and should be considered in the differential diagnosis of asthma that is unre-

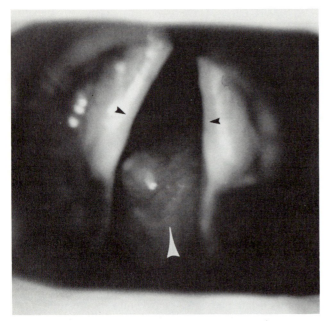

Figure 90–6. A view through the laryngoscope of a subglottic laryngeal cyst (*white arrow* points to the cyst; *black arrows,* to the vocal cords). The patient was misdiagnosed for 3 years as suffering from asthma before endoscopy was performed.

sponsive to therapy or associated with progressive airway obstruction. Treatment requires laser excision of the papillomas, but there is a very high recurrence rate; consequently, monthly removal is commonly necessary.

CLINICAL MANIFESTATIONS

A number of congenital and hereditary syndromes involve tracheal, esophageal, or oropharyngeal structures and may produce difficult problems in airway management.[14] Clinical signs associated with congenital anomalies of the larynx include respiratory obstruction, stridor, retractions, abnormal cry, dyspnea, tachypnea, aspiration, and sudden death. Extrathoracic causes of airway distress include intracranial hemorrhage, a large abdominal mass, and neuromuscular disease. Intrathoracic causes include diaphragmatic hernia, pulmonary cysts, pneumomediastinum and pneumothorax, respiratory distress syndrome, meconium aspiration, and cardiac abnormalities. Esophageal atresia, constriction, and fistula must also be considered. Hereditary or congenital anomalies, expressed by external deformities such as craniofacial anomalies, may be associated with internal anomalies such as webs, cysts, fistulas, atresias, or duplications.

VOCAL CORD PARALYSIS

Congenital vocal cord paralysis is the second most common congenital laryngeal anomaly.[13] Flexible fiberoptic laryngoscopy is an excellent way of documenting abnormalities of vocal cords. Vocal cord paralysis, when unilateral, may result in a hoarse cry with minimal respiratory distress. The abduction of the unaffected TVC is usually sufficient to provide an adequate airway because

gravity allows the paralyzed cord to drop away from the midline of the larynx. Infants with unilateral vocal cord paralysis tend to sleep peacefully when lying on the side of the paralyzed cord. Infants with laryngeal cysts or masses may behave in a similar manner.

Patients with bilateral vocal cord paralysis, alternatively, have a clear but weak cry in addition to dyspnea, stridor, and occasionally evidence of extensive central neuropathy. Bilateral congenital paralysis is seen more often than unilateral TVC paralysis in infants with respiratory distress or dysphonia.[13] About half of bilateral TVC paralysis cases are associated with other anomalies of the larynx or associated neurologic or cardiac systems.[13] Associated cardiac anomalies include septal defect of either atrium or ventricle, coarctation of the aorta, and transposition of the great vessels. Neurologic anomalies found in association with bilateral TVC paralysis include cerebral agenesis, cranial nerve palsies, and benign congenital hypoplasia.[13]

Laryngeal anomalies occurring with bilateral TVC paralysis include congenital subglottic stenosis and laryngomalacia.[13] Some patients with Arnold-Chiari malformation can have bilateral vocal cord paralysis; the TVC paralysis does not develop until the first month or two of life because the mechanism of TVC paralysis in this entity requires increasing intracranial pressure, which results in the extrusion of the brainstem through the foramen magnum and ultimately stretches the vagus nerves over the jugular foramen. Airway management in cases of bilateral vocal cord paralysis often requires tracheotomy initially and later vocal cord lateralization if no recovery of function occurs (Fig. 90–8).

LARYNGOMALACIA

Congenital flaccid larynx (laryngomalacia) is the most common congenital laryngeal anomaly and accounts for

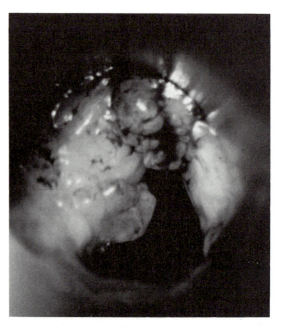

Figure 90–7. A view through the laryngoscope of papillomas growing on the left true vocal cord and the anterior commissure, causing hoarseness.

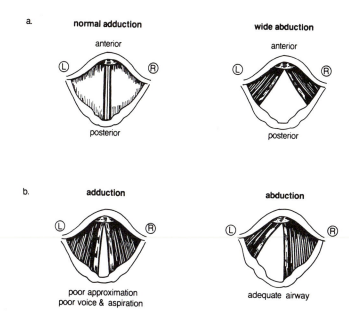

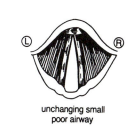

Figure 90-8. Schematics contrasting active vocal cord range of motion when vocal cord movement is normal and with unilateral and bilateral vocal cord paralysis. A normally functioning glottis (*a*) has excellent approximation of the true vocal cords (TVCs) with adduction and a wide airway with abduction. A paralyzed right TVC (*b*) results in a poor approximation during adduction but an adequate airway. Bilateral TVC paralysis (*c*) exhibits a small airway that does not change appreciably during respiration.

two thirds of laryngeal problems in newborns.[13] The diagnosis can be made by direct observation of the larynx during respiration. Holinger and Konior[15] clearly illustrated the anatomic abnormalities that, by themselves or in

combination, may obstruct the airway (Fig. 90-9). First, the aryepiglottic folds, cuneiform cartilages, and epiglottis may be drawn into the larynx during inspiration. Second, the epiglottis may be curled or folded onto itself in an omega shape. In addition, the arytenoid cartilages may collapse anteriorly into the airway during inspiration. Finally, the epiglottis may be drawn posteriorly toward the posterior pharyngeal wall and thus obstruct the airway. Severe respiratory distress is unusual; however, retractions and labored respiration with loud inspiratory stridor are common. The stridor is worse when a patient is in the supine position with the neck flexed and during episodes of crying and infections of the upper respiration tract. Cyanosis is usually not present. Therapy consists of reassurance and close follow-up to be sure the child thrives. This clinical problem usually improves as the supporting cartilage matures. Surgical intervention with excision of excessive supraglottic tissue may be successful in carefully selected patients.[16] Tracheotomy is sometimes needed when feeding and respiratory difficulties are severe.

NASAL ABNORMALITIES

The neonate is an obligate nasal breather. Therefore, any condition that causes nasal obstruction results in respiratory distress: nasal valve stenosis, choanal atresia, nasal septal fracture, nasopharyngeal masses, and nasal encephaloceles or gliomas.

CHOANAL ATRESIA

Choanal atresia or stenosis is caused by the persistence of soft tissue or bone in the posterior nasal airway.[17] The persistence of the body or membranous plate results in a lack of adequate communication between the nose and the pharynx, leaving the neonate unable to breathe through the nose except when crying. Unilateral involvement may cause few symptoms and go unrecognized until nasal secretions are increased. Bilateral choanal atresia and stenosis must be recognized and treated early for the newborn to survive. Associated anomalies include esoph-

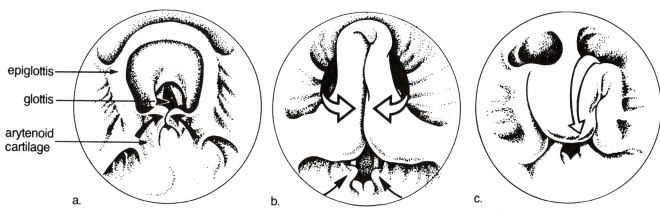

Figure 90-9. Mechanisms of airway obstruction in congenital floppy supraglottis (laryngomalacia): anterior arytenoid cartilage collapse (*a*), aryepiglottic fold medial collapse (*b*), and inferior "curling" of the epiglottis (*c*). (From Holinger L, Konior RJ: Surgical management of severe laryngomalacia. Laryngoscope 99:136–142, 1989.)

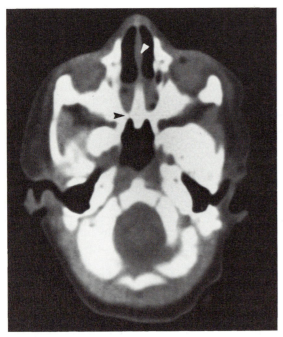

Figure 90-10. An axial computed tomogram of a bilateral choanal atresia. *White arrow*, nasal septum; *black arrow*, bony atretic plate.

ageal atresia, congenital heart disease, and colobomas. These children cannot suck or swallow normally without a patent nasal airway. During feeding, the infant becomes cyanotic, and apneic episodes can occur. The diagnosis can be made by finding obstruction to the passage of a catheter through the nose to the nasopharynx or by transnasal fiberoptic examination and can be confirmed by computed tomography (Fig. 90–10). The passage of a catheter alone through the nose to the nasopharynx can be misleading because of curling of the tube in the nose or the presence of choanal stenosis (i.e., the nasal airway is large enough to pass the catheter but too small for an adequate airway). The best method for depicting the abnormality is computed tomography. Approximately 90% of all infants with choanal atresias have a bony atretic plate.

Airway management can be accomplished with an oral airway or a McGovern nipple, a nipple with a breathing hole cut in the top. Sometimes intubation is necessary until surgery. There is no place for tracheotomy in the treatment of children with isolated choanal atresia.

ABNORMALITIES OF OROPHARYNX AND ORAL CAVITY

TONGUE

A relatively large or posteriorly displaced tongue can lead to airway obstruction. Congenital macroglossia may be either idiopathic or associated with syndromes such as trisomy 21. Glossoptosis, or posterior displacement of the tongue, occurs with any form of micrognathia: examples include Pierre Robin syndrome, Turner's syndrome, and

mandibulofacial dysostosis (Treacher Collins syndrome). Tonsillar and adenoidal hypertrophy are common and lead to partial upper airway obstruction and may cause obstructive sleep apnea. Finally, if there is an emergency airway problem in children with macroglossia or micrognathia, intubation may be difficult because of the posterior position of the tongue in the oropharynx. Fiberoptic transnasal intubation might be helpful in these cases.

PIERRE ROBIN SYNDROME

The Pierre Robin syndrome includes high arched or cleft palate, micrognathia, mandibular hypoplasia, and glossoptosis. Infants with severe forms of the Pierre Robin syndrome encounter airway difficulty because the small mandible displaces the tongue into an abnormally posterior position. The diagnosis is easily made on physical examination with findings of micrognathia and oropharyngeal stridor, especially by prone positioning or tongue retraction. In mild cases, placing the child in the prone position allows the tongue to fall forward out of the airway. Often airway control is needed only during the first year of life because the airway obstruction in the Pierre Robin syndrome usually improves by 4 to 6 months of age. When severe respiratory distress persists, tracheotomy should be performed. Alternative measures, such as glossopexy (lip-tongue adhesion), are often unsuccessful in severe cases. It has been argued that the reported success of these alternative measures was achieved because the children had a mild form of the disease and probably would have done well with no treatment at all. Chronic severe airway obstruction can cause pulmonary edema and cor pulmonale.

TONSILLAR AND ADENOIDAL HYPERTROPHY

Severe airway obstruction can develop in children with adenotonsillar hypertrophy during acute tonsillitis.[18] Severe tonsil- and adenoid-related obstruction caused by bacterial infection (retropharyngeal abscess) can be successfully managed by a nasopharyngeal airway because there is less danger of precipitous occlusion of the larynx without warning.[19] Tonsillectomy or adenoidectomy is not ordinarily performed during acute infection because of increased operative blood loss unless urgent obstructive symptoms are present.

Operation is clearly indicated in circumstances in which massive hypertrophy of the tonsils or adenoids results in unquestionable dysphagia, extreme discomfort in breathing, or, even more extreme, alveolar hypoventilation or cor pulmonale.[20] Oropharyngeal stridor while the patient is awake and frequent episodes of obstructive apnea during sleep indicate the presence of alveolar hypoventilation. The syndrome of obstructive sleep apnea is now recognized to be very common. Surgical intervention can be helpful in milder cases of tonsil and adenoid hypertrophy, even when sleep apnea is not a primary feature.[21]

PERITONSILLAR AND RETROPHARYNGEAL ABSCESS

Abscess in the peritonsillar space causes medial displacement of the soft palate, uvula, and tonsil. Patients usually have severe throat pain and a muffled "hot-potato" voice. Patients with a peritonsillar abscess require surgical drainage in addition to antimicrobial therapy. Studies have shown equivalence of the efficacy of needle aspiration in comparison with stab incision and drainage.[22] Infections of the peritonsillar space occur more commonly in older than in younger children. Children usually require general anesthesia for adequate drainage of the abscess while the airway is being protected from aspiration of purulent material.

Cellulitis and abscess in the retropharyngeal space share many features with peritonsillar infections; in contrast, infections of the retropharyngeal space are more common than peritonsillar infections in younger children. Most affected children are under the age of 5 years and exhibit a sudden onset of fever, dysphagia, neck rigidity, and noisy breathing. Many are unable to swallow, and they drool continually. Direct and mirror examination of the pharynx may reveal localized bulging of the posterior wall of the pharynx. The presenting signs, together with examination of the pharynx, usually allow the diagnosis to be made easily. On radiographs, the retropharyngeal abscess may appear as an abnormal widening of the posterior pharyngeal soft tissue.[23] Some researchers have stated that an anteroposterior thickness of prevertebral soft tissue should not be greater than the anteroposterior diameter of the adjacent cervical vertebral body.[24] Care should be taken during examination of the retropharynx to have suction available and to position the patient so as to prevent aspiration of pus if an abscess ruptures.

LUDWIG'S ANGINA

Ludwig's angina is an uncommon infection in children, but it has occurred in infants as young as 12 days old.[25] Ludwig's angina is a gangrenous cellulitis of the sublingual and submandibular spaces. Most of these infections appear to begin from a focus within the mouth, either traumatic or infectious. The patient initially has a tender swelling of the floor of the mouth. If untreated, the cellulitis spreads rapidly, pushing the tongue superiorly and anteriorly. Extensive swelling can obstruct the airway and spread into the deep spaces of the neck. Incision and drainage are not feasible because this process is not an abscess; rather, therapy should include maintenance of the airway and antimicrobial therapy directed against bacteria suspected on Gram's stain or on the basis of results of microbiologic cultures. Intubation or tracheotomy may become necessary as a result of airway compromise.

TUMORS

Obstructing congenital tumors may develop in the pharynx. Examples are Tornwaldt's cyst, bronchial cleft

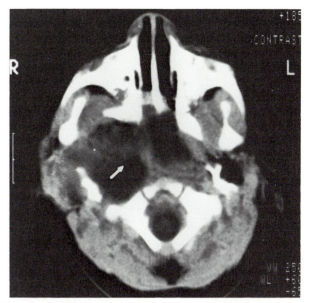

Figure 90–11. Axial computed tomogram of a nasopharyngeal teratoma obstructing the nasopharynx. The necrotic center *(arrow)* appears as a central radiolucency.

cyst, teratomas, chordomas, craniopharyngiomas, cystic hygromas, and hemangiomas (Fig. 90–11). Intubation may be possible for acute management, but tracheotomy is often required for long-term management.

FOREIGN BODY ASPIRATION

Hypopharyngeal foreign bodies should be removed as soon as possible because they may become displaced into the larynx or trachea and cause obstruction or laryngeal spasm. Placement of an oral airway during induction of general anesthesia can cause accidental dislodgment with subsequent complete airway obstruction. If vomiting occurs, proper suctioning around the foreign body may not be possible, and aspiration may occur. Because of these potential problems, hypopharyngeal foreign bodies should be removed in the operating room while the patient is awake, if possible.

Extrinsic pressure on the trachea from a foreign body in the cervical segment of the esophagus can definitely result in respiratory distress. A coin in the esophagus usually becomes oriented in the coronal plane, whereas a coin in the trachea commonly orients sagittally (Figs. 90–12A, 90–12B). However, when an esophageal coin becomes oriented sagittally, it is more likely to narrow the tracheal lumen by anteriorly displacing the posterior membranous wall of the trachea. An acute onset of stridor and hoarseness may result from the presence of a foreign body lodged at or near the glottis and causing vocal cord edema or dysfunction (Figs. 90–13A, 90–13B). Similarly, the sudden onset of wheezing in a healthy child without any other symptoms of pulmonary disease should suggest the presence of a bronchial foreign body. Direct laryngoscopy and bronchoscopy must be seriously considered in both of these cases; there is no place for conservative medical management. The rigid bronchoscope offers distinct

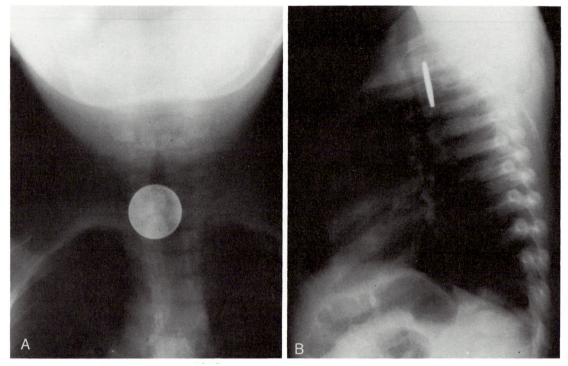

Figure 90–12. Anteroposterior (*A*) and lateral (*B*) radiographs of a coin in the upper esophagus oriented in the coronal plane.

advantages over flexible bronchoscopes for the removal of foreign bodies from the tracheobronchial tree. (For discussion of respiratory foreign bodies, rigid bronchoscopy, and flexible fiberoptic bronchoscopy, see Chapters 56, 11, and 12, respectively).

TRACHEOMALACIA

Tracheomalacia can be a difficult diagnostic and management problem. The tracheal collapse during inspira-

tion can be seen during fluoroscopy but may be missed during rigid bronchoscopic examination. This commonly occurs when a child's deep inspiratory efforts are not observed because the procedure is performed while the patient is under general anesthesia and no spontaneous inspirations are viewed. Severe tracheomalacia may require stenting of the trachea with a tracheostomy tube or tracheal reconstructive procedures. Some surgeons have had success with aortopexy, which entails suspension of the anterior trachea from the fascia of the aorta.[26, 27]

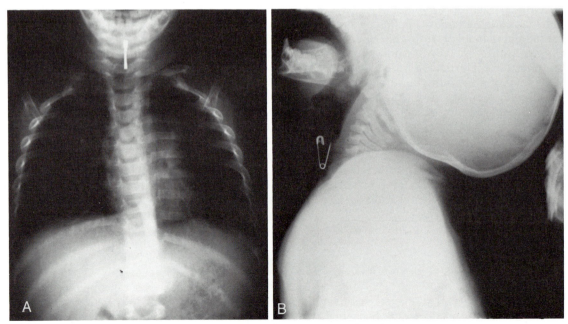

Figure 90–13. Anteroposterior (*A*) and lateral (*B*) radiographs of a safety pin lodged in the larynx.

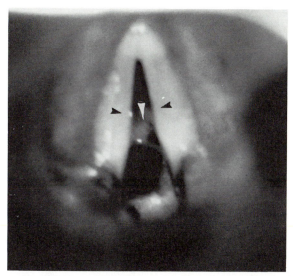

Figure 90–14. A 7-year-old patient who had been intubated for repair of a patent ductus arteriosus at 3 years of age presented with a diagnosis of asthma. Endoscopy revealed a tracheal web *(white arrow)* between the vocal cords *(black arrows)*. Note the small cross-sectional area of the airway at the web.

Primary tracheomalacia with functional or structural abnormalities of the tracheal cartilages should be distinguished from secondary tracheomalacia produced by extrinsic compression from a vascular ring. Cartilaginous rings may be congenitally absent, small and malformed, or functionally inadequate, causing obstruction of the tracheal airway. Clinical symptoms of tracheomalacia include wheezing, cough, stridor, dyspnea, tachypnea, and cyanosis. This functional stridor is worse in the supine position with the neck flexed, during crying, and with infections of the upper or lower respiratory tract. Improvement is usually noted after 6 to 12 months with maturity of the supporting cartilages.

LARYNGEAL STENOSIS FROM ENDOTRACHEAL TUBES

Laryngeal and tracheal injuries from prolonged intubation are being seen more frequently because more patients are recovering from illnesses that require mechanical ventilation. Unfortunately, injury to the larynx and trachea caused by prolonged intubation is unrecognized until extubation, after irreversible damage may have occurred (Fig. 90–14).

Factors responsible for airway obstruction from endotracheal tubes include trauma during tube insertion, long-term intubation, intubation with a tube that is large in relation to larynx size, tube composition and shape, chemical irritants on the tube, infection, excess movement of the tube within the larynx, and cuff characteristics of the tube.[28] Polyvinyl chloride (PVC) is the most suitable plastic material for endotracheal tubes because it is soft and molds to the contour of the airway at body temperature.[27] Cuffed tubes are usually not used in children unless they are necessary for maintaining positive end-expiratory pressure. If a cuffed tube is not positioned properly in the trachea, the cuff may lie within the larynx itself, where it can cause recurrent laryngeal nerve paralysis or subglottic stenosis.

Immediate postextubation hoarseness and croupy cough are common. However, if the voice does not return to normal in several days, the larynx should be visualized. The child who becomes dysphonic or aphonic after intubation may have suffered an arytenoid dislocation, especially if the intubation was difficult. Prolonged intubation or the use of an overly large tube may cause laryngeal stenosis. This scarring begins with mucosal ulcerations at the cricoid ring. When the cricoid cartilage becomes exposed, perichondritis results and granulation tissue forms. This granulation tissue matures into fibrous scar tissue, which narrows the lumen.

Glottic stenosis from endotracheal tubes usually results from scarring in the interarytenoid area, the area on which the tube exerts maximal pressure.[29] (The stenosis may be in the form of a fibrous band between the arytenoids and cause more extensive posterior commissure scarring.) This can limit the mobility of the vocal cords and produce vocal cord pseudoparalysis.

The duration of intubation of the infected or previously scarred larynx should be minimized because these children seem to be at greatest risk for the development of laryngeal trauma and subsequent stenosis. Tracheotomy should be considered when extended intubation is necessary, depending on the age of the child. The normal neonatal larynx can tolerate intubation for 1 or 2 months, whereas children under the age of 1 year can probably tolerate it for several weeks. Children up to 5 years of age can be intubated only for approximately 14 days before laryngeal stenosis becomes more likely. In children over 5 years of age, intubation should be limited to 5 to 7 days to avoid risks of laryngeal stenosis.

Although neonates tolerate extended periods of intubation with PVC tubes, these tubes can also injure the neonatal larynx.[30] Autopsy examinations have revealed a high incidence of laryngeal cricoid ulceration in neonates who died after prolonged intubation.[31] The ability of neonates to tolerate long periods of intubation may be attributable to resiliency of the cricoid cartilage. As the cricoid cartilage grows, its matrix increases in amount, becoming less hydrated, more fibrous, and more rigid.[30]

Subglottic stenosis after prolonged intubation of a premature infant may not become apparent for many months after successful extubation. This is because of a combination of the failure of the damaged subglottic area to grow in pace with the child's respiratory needs and a worsening of the cicatricial process as granulation tissue matures into scar tissue. Minor degrees of obstruction may be asymptomatic for years and be evident only when the child experiences a respiratory tract infection.

Mild cases of stenosis can be treated by serial dilatation supplemented by laser excision, but external laryngeal surgery is often required.[32] The best form of treatment, however, is prevention.[33]

DIAGNOSTIC APPROACHES

HISTORY

Many diseases causing respiratory distress manifest with a specific group of symptoms, and a careful history can narrow the differential diagnosis. The presence of congenital anomalies, time of onset and progression of the problem, character of the cry, problems with feeding, history of upper respiratory tract infection, and history of intubation are some essential items to include in the history.

If stridor has been present from birth, the most likely causes are congenital floppy larynx (laryngomalacia), subglottic stenosis, vocal cord paralysis, tracheomalacia, and a vascular ring.[2, 34] Bilateral vocal cord paralysis is most often seen in children with neurologic abnormalities, especially Arnold-Chiari malformation and hydrocephalus. Trauma caused by forceps delivery has been known to cause vocal cord paralysis or nasal fracture, either of which may alter respiration.

Respiratory obstruction manifesting several weeks after birth is suggestive of a laryngeal web or congenital subglottic stenosis. After several months, a subglottic hemangioma or laryngeal cyst should be suspected. A history of respiratory distress with feeding during the neonatal period suggests the possibility of aspiration from a tracheoesophageal fistula, a posterior laryngotracheal cleft, or gastroesophageal reflux. A history of maternal venereal condylomas in a child with gradually developing voice change and airway obstruction is suggestive of recurrent respiratory papillomatosis.

Any history of intubation raises the possibility of subglottic or tracheal stenosis. The onset of respiratory distress immediately after extubation is suggestive of atelectasis or mucus plugging in the lower respiratory tract. If several hours have passed since extubation, the obstruction is more likely related to traumatic edema of the glottis or subglottis. The child who becomes dysphonic or totally aphonic after extubation may have suffered an arytenoid dislocation. If recognized, the dislocated arytenoid can be reduced by direct manipulation in the operating room. Manipulation must be performed early; otherwise, the dislocation will be permanent. Distress several weeks after intubation may indicate early subglottic stenosis. If distress begins several months later, a large vocal process granuloma is a possibility. The physician must always consider a foreign body aspiration into either the esophagus or respiratory tract as a cause of respiratory distress.

PHYSICAL EXAMINATION

Evaluation of a child with respiratory distress should include assessment of heart rate, respiratory pattern and rate, movement of air, skin color, quality of the voice (including cough and cry), level of child's activity, swallowing ability (presence of aspiration or drooling), and relative ease of breathing. The normal child has an effortless, barely perceptible breathing pattern. Obvious physical findings of respiratory distress are flaring of the nasal alae during inspiration, circumoral pallor, stridor, and suprasternal or intercostal retractions.

The anterior nasal passage, oral cavity, and oropharynx can be easily examined by direct visualization. In older, cooperative children, the nasopharnyx and hypopharynx can be visualized indirectly with the use of a headlight and laryngeal mirror. The entire nasal passage, nasopharynx, hypopharynx, and larynx of any child can be examined with the fiberoptic nasopharyngoscope. Nasopharyngoscopy, laryngoscopy, bronchoscopy, and esophagoscopy can be performed with the patient under general anesthesia when necessary. In children with a severely compromised airway, such as with foreign body aspiration, general anesthesia can be associated with increased risks.

TRANSNASAL FIBEROPTIC LARYNGOSCOPY

The flexible fiberoptic laryngoscope has allowed examination of children with airway problems without resorting to general anesthesia. Transnasal fiberoptic examination is very well tolerated by older children. The nose is topically anesthetized and decongested, and the laryngoscope (outer diameter of 3 mm) is passed through the nose to directly view the nasal passage, nasopharynx, oropharynx, hypopharynx, and larynx. The lesion can be observed or photographed while the patient is speaking, coughing, or breathing. Because the patient is fully awake, active airway physiology, both voluntary and reflex, may be observed. For instance, TVC adduction/abduction can be evaluated during both a high-pitched "eee" and a deep breath, respectively.

DIRECT LARYNGOSCOPY, BRONCHOSCOPY, ESOPHAGOSCOPY

The indications for endoscopy are both diagnostic and therapeutic. The endoscopist and the anesthesiologist must work together efficiently. A gentle instrumentation technique minimizes postoperative edema. Cool mist, corticosteroids, and racemic epinephrine aerosol can be used for the occasional case of postendoscopy edema. The child should be observed in the hospital after the procedure until the airway is stable.

Direct laryngoscopy in the operating room is the primary technique for definitive diagnosis and management of laryngeal disease. This may be performed in infants without general anesthesia; however, modern anesthetic techniques make general anesthesia in infants quite safe. When the child is anesthetized, the endoscopist may proceed more slowly, and the procedures may be performed more precisely.

Rigid bronchoscopy provides excellent lighting and magnification of the trachea and bronchi when combined with the Hopkins optical system. The rigid system allows concurrent ventilation of the child through a side-arm attachment, which is an advantage over flexible bronchoscopes. In addition, the rigid bronchoscope allows passage of instruments for biopsy, excision, dilatation, and removal of foreign bodies (see Chapter 11).

Rigid esophagoscopy allows not only for foreign body removal but also for a more complete evaluation of the anterior esophagus and posterior larynx. For example, a rigid esophagoscope withdrawn slowly and properly (retrograde esophagoscopy) spreads the esophageal mucosa to reveal a tracheoesophageal fistula or posterior laryngeal cleft not seen on barium swallow or even with laryngoscopy, bronchoscopy, or flexible esophagoscopy.

RADIOLOGY

Many techniques are available for imaging the airway, from plain films to computed tomography and magnetic resonance imaging. On a lateral view of plain radiographs, shadows cast by the soft tissue parts contrast clearly with the air in the lumen of the larynx, especially on the lateral neck views. Superimposition of the cervical vertebrae is present in the posteroanterior view, making interpretation more difficult. Lateral neck films should be taken with the head extended to avoid widening of the normal retropharyngeal soft tissue shadow.

MONITORING OF AIRWAY PROBLEMS

No single parameter will determine whether a child requires airway intervention unless the child is in severe distress. Physical findings that should be considered include heart and respiratory rate, color, and the presence of sweating, stridor, or retractions. Oxygen saturation can be noninvasively monitored by an oximeter, which provides a good way of monitoring oxygenation. Arterial blood gas measurements are also helpful but require arterial puncture. Some authors recommend using a "croup score" to evaluate respiratory distress resulting from upper airway obstruction.[35]

MANAGEMENT

Both racemic epinephrine aerosol and cool mist are helpful when airway obstruction is caused by inflammation or edema, as seen in postintubation or inflammatory croup. Any child who receives racemic epinephrine should be closely observed because the effects of this drug last for only approximately 1 to 2 h. Racemic epinephrine can be administered every half hour, if necessary. The benefits of corticosteroids are controversial.[34] Helium and oxygen mixture (Heliox) may also be useful as a temporizing measure. The physical properties of helium increase the rate of airflow through large airways with turbulent airflow. Breathing a less dense gas such as helium can substantially decrease the airway resistance in large airways and reduce the work of breathing when there is obstruction in large airways and severe compromise of respiration.[36]

MASK VENTILATION

The majority of cases of acute airway obstruction can be successfully managed by mouth-to-mouth or bag-mask ventilation. It is important to have an appropriate-sized mask that can fit over the nose and mouth with a good seal to provide positive pressure without significant air leakages. It is also important to avoid excessive pressure on the floor of the mouth. The importance of thrust-

ing the mandible anteriorly (chin lift) cannot be overemphasized, especially if any cervical spine damage is possible. Suctioning of the oral cavity and oropharynx plus the use of a nasal trumpet or oral airway is often necessary. Only when these noninvasive measures fail should surgical approaches, such as cricothyroidotomy, be used.

CRICOTHYROIDOTOMY

The cricoid cartilage is usually palpable through the skin, even in small infants in whom the cricothyroid membrane may not be evident. A cut is made vertically through the skin over the cricoid cartilage, and the airway is opened horizontally through the cricothyroid membrane just superior to the cricoid cartilage. It is helpful for the surgeon to immobilize the larynx and trachea between two fingers while performing this technique. Early formal conversion to a tracheotomy is recommended.

PERCUTANEOUS CATHETER VENTILATION

The use of a large-bore needle or plastic catheter (intravenous type) for transtracheal ventilation is possible but difficult. This technique may improve the airway enough to allow a more orderly management of a child with severe obstruction. However, this technique is advocated only for resuscitation and is not considered the technique of choice. In children, the softness of the cartilage and the mobility of the trachea make placement of a needle quite difficult. The large-bore needle is placed through the cricothyroid membrane, and its position is confirmed by aspiration of air. Positive-pressure oxygen is then connected to the needle or catheter. Although the risk of local damage from this technique may be small, adjacent structures are vulnerable; even the spinal cord has been reported to be injured. Furthermore, this technique can cause pneumothorax if excessive air pressures are delivered.

INTUBATION

Endotracheal Tube Size

Most important, tubes should not fit too tightly; in fact, a slight leakage around the larynx is optimal. It is imperative that an oversized tube never be used to create a seal for assisted ventilation.

Nasotracheal Versus Orotracheal Intubation

The oral route is generally recommended for assisted ventilation in newborns. Nasotracheal intubation offers several advantages in older children: (1) The tube is easier to secure, (2) there is less chance of posterior glottic pressure necrosis because the tube enters the larynx with less curvature, (3) oral hygiene is easier, and (4) it is more comfortable. The disadvantages are (1) the difficulty in placing the tube through the nose, (2) possible pressure necrosis of the septum or nasal alae, and (3) the potential to cause sinusitis or otitis media. Nasotracheal intubation should not be performed when there is nasal or maxillofacial trauma because of the possibility of displacing any mobile bony fragments intracranially or causing tears in the dura mater with resultant cerebrospinal fluid leakages.

The following equipment is needed to nasotracheally intubate a child: a laryngoscope, endotracheal tubes in appropriate sizes, waterproof tape, tincture of benzoin, suction catheters for the endotracheal tubes, a larger bore catheter to suction the nose and mouth, lubricant, topical anesthetic, topical decongestant, and a Magill forceps or small-diameter fiberoptic scope. The nose must be decongested and topically anesthetized with phenylephrine hydrochloride (Neo-Synephrine) and tetracaine hydrochloride (Pontocaine) or lidocaine (Xylocaine). With the use of gentle, constant pressure, the lubricated endotracheal tube is passed along the floor of the nose parallel to the palate (not the nasal dorsum) until it bends into the pharynx. The larynx is then viewed through the laryngoscope with the child in the "sniffing position" (neck flexed and head extended). As the assistant advances the nasal tube, it is guided into the larynx with the Magill forceps. Alternatively, the flexible fiberoptic scope can be passed through the nasoendotracheal tube and advanced into the trachea. The assistant then slides the tube over the scope into the trachea while the endoscopist constantly confirms that the fiberoptic scope is not inadvertently withdrawn from the trachea. Before the scope is withdrawn, it is easy to check the position of the tube in the trachea. After coating the skin with tincture of benzoin, the tube should be secured with waterproof tape at the nose. Necrosis of the septum or skin of the nose can be avoided if the tube is taped into place so that it exits straight out of the nose.

For orotracheal intubation, similar equipment and drugs are required with endotracheal tubes of appropriate size and length (see Tables 92–2 and 92–3 in Chapter 92, on tracheostomy). The child who requires assisted ventilation without positive end-expiratory pressure can be maintained with a properly sized noncuffed tracheostomy tube with some adjustment of tidal volume settings to compensate for loss of air past the tracheostomy tube. However, when positive end-expiratory pressure is necessary, the tracheostomy tube must provide an airtight seal in the trachea. In older children, a cuffed tube can be used. Smaller children can be safely managed over the short term with a noncuffed tube that is carefully fitted to the size of the tracheal lumen. A cuffed infant-sized tracheostomy tube has become available. Oversized tubes are, of course, contraindicated.

TRACHEOTOMY

Tracheotomy is not an emergency procedure; the procedure is performed in the operating room after the airway has been secured. Indications, technique, and complications of tracheotomy are discussed in Chapter 92.

CRICOID SPLIT

Before the advent of the anterior cricoid-split procedure, many neonates receiving prolonged mechanical ventilation underwent tracheotomy when they failed extubation. With the advent of the cricoid-split procedure, a number of neonatal tracheotomy procedures can now be avoided. After an anterior cricoid-split procedure, 60% to 80% of these children can be successfully extubated. The cricoid split not only avoids the tracheotomy but also increases the diameter of the subglottic airway and hence treats the stenosis.

A vertical incision is made in the midline through the cartilage and mucosa of the first tracheal ring, cricoid cartilage, and lower portion of the thyroid ala. The child is then intubated with an endotracheal tube that is just smaller than the child's trachea. With the endotracheal tube in place, a significant gap can be visualized between the cut edges of the cricoid cartilage, which indicates the amount of enlargement of the cricoid ring. The incision is allowed to heal secondarily. A suture closure is not necessary. The endotracheal tube is removed 2 weeks later in the operating room. If the child inadvertently becomes extubated between 7 and 14 days after the procedure, an endotracheal tube a size smaller is placed. If the child fails the first extubation, another attempt is made after 2 weeks with placement of a smaller endotracheal tube; extubation is then attempted again several days later.

REFERENCES

1. Graney D: Anatomy. *In* Cummings CW, Fredrickson JM, Harker LA, et al (eds): Otolaryngology—Head and Neck Surgery, pp. 1729–1740. St Louis: CV Mosby, 1986.
2. Fearon B, Cotton RB: Subglottic stenosis in infants and children. The clinical problem and experimental surgical correction. Can J Otol 1:281–289, 1972.
3. Holinger PH, Johnston KC: Factors responsible for laryngeal obstruction in infants. JAMA 143:1229–1231, 1950.
4. Shackelford, GD, Siegel MJ, McAlister WH: Subglottic edema in acute epiglottitis in children. AJR 131:603–605, 1978.
5. Sasaki CT, Suzuki M, Horiuchi M: Postnatal development of laryngeal reflexes in the dog. Arch Otolaryngol 103:138–143, 1977.
6. Suzuki M: Laryngeal reflexes. *In* Hirano M, Kirchner JA, Bless DM (eds): Neurolaryngology, Recent Advances, pp. 142–155. Boston: College-Hill, 1987.
7. Sasaki CT, Suzuki M, Horiuchi M, Kirchner JA: The effect of tracheostomy on the laryngeal closure reflex. Laryngoscope 87:1428–1433, 1977.
8. Hogg JC, Williams J, Richardson JB, et al: Age as a factor in the distribution of lower-airway conductance and in the pathologic anatomy of obstructive lung disease. N Engl J Med 282:1283–1287, 1970.
9. Widdicombe JG, Sterling GM: The autonomic nervous system and breathing. Arch Intern Med 126:311–329, 1970.
10. Levison H, Tabachnik E, Newth CJ: Wheezing in infancy, croup, and epiglottitis. Curr Probl Pediatr 12:1–65, 1982.
11. Irwin BC, Hendrickse WA, Pincott JR, et al: Juvenile laryngeal papillomatosis. J Laryngol Otol 100:435–445, 1986.
12. Steinberg BM, Gallagher T, Stoler M, Abramson AL: Persistence and expression of human papillomavirus during interferon therapy. Arch Otolaryngol Head Neck Surg 114:27–32, 1988.
13. Faw KD, Spector GJ: Congenital malformations of the larynx. *In* Ballenger JJ (ed): Diseases of the Nose, Throat, Ear, Head, and Neck, 13th ed, pp. 412–431. Philadelphia: Lea & Febiger, 1985.
14. Cotton RT, Reilly JS: Stridor and airway obstruction. *In* Bluestone CD, Stool SE, Scheetz MD (eds): Pediatric Otolaryngology, 2nd ed, pp. 1098–1111. Philadelphia: WB Saunders, 1990.

15. Holinger L, Konior RJ: Surgical management of severe laryngomalacia. Laryngoscope 99:136–142, 1989.
16. Zalzal GH, Anon JB, Cotton RT: Epiglottoplasty for the treatment of laryngomalacia. Ann Otol Rhinol Laryngol 96:72–76, 1987.
17. Hengerer AS, Strome M: Choanal atresia: A new embryologic theory and its influence on surgical management. Laryngoscope 92:913–921, 1982.
18. Grundfast KM, Wittich DJ: Adenotonsillar hypertrophy and upper airway obstruction in evolutionary perspective. Laryngoscope 92:650–658, 1982.
19. Snyderman NL, Stool SE: Management of airway obstruction in children with infectious mononucleosis. Otolaryngol Head Neck Surg 90:168–170, 1982.
20. Brown OE, Manning SC, Ridenour B: Cor pulmonale secondary to tonsillar and adenoidal hypertrophy: Management considerations. Int J Pediatr Otorhinolaryngol 16:131–139, 1988.
21. Potsic WP, Pasquariello PS, Baranak CC, et al: Relief of upper airway obstruction by adenotonsillectomy. Otolaryngol Head Neck Surg 94:476–480, 1986.
22. Spires JR, Owens JJ, Woodson GE, Miller RH: Treatment of peritonsillar abscess. Arch Otolaryngol Head Neck Surg 113:984–986, 1987.
23. Barratt GE, Koopmann CF, Coulthard SW: Retropharyngeal abscess—a ten year experience. Laryngoscope 94:455–463, 1984.
24. Seid AB, Dunbar JS, Cotton RT: Retropharyngeal abscesses in children revisited. Laryngoscope 89:1717–1724, 1979.
25. Barkin RM, Bonis SL, Eighammer RM, et al: Ludwig angina in children. J Pediatr 87:563–565, 1975.
26. Blair GK, Cohen R, Filler RM: Treatment of tracheomalacia: Eight years' experience. J Pediatr Surg 21:781–785, 1986.
27. Greenholz SK, Karrer FM, Lilly JR: Contemporary surgery for tracheomalacia. J Pediatr Surg 21:511–514, 1986.
28. Hawkins DB: Noninfectious disorders of the lower respiratory tract. In Bluestone CD, Stool SE (eds): Pediatric Otolaryngology, pp. 1161–1171. Philadelphia: WB Saunders, 1990.
29. Hengerer AS, Strome M, Jaffe BF: Injuries to the neonatal larynx from long-term endotracheal tube intubation and suggested tube modification for prevention. Ann Otol Rhinol Laryngol 84:764–770, 1975.
30. Conner GH, Maisels MJ: Orotracheal intubation in the newborn. Laryngoscope 87:87–91, 1977.
31. Hawkins DB: Hyaline membrane disease of the neonate—prolonged intubation in management—effects on the larynx. Laryngoscope 88:201–224, 1978.
32. Cotton RT, Myer CM: Contemporary surgical management of laryngeal stenosis in children. Am J Otolaryngol 5:360–368, 1984.
33. Strome M: Subglottic stenosis: Therapeutic considerations. Otolaryngol Clin North Am 17:63–68, 1984.
34. Holinger PH, Brown WT: Congenital webs, cysts, laryngoceles, and other anomalies of the larnyx. Ann Otol Rhinol Laryngol 76:744–752, 1967.
35. Super DM, Cartelli NA, Brooks LJ, et al: A prospective randomized double-blind study to evaluate the effect of dexamethasone in acute laryngotracheitis. J Pediatr 115:323–329, 1989.
36. Orr JB: Helium-oxygen gas mixtures in the management of patients with airway obstruction. Ear Nose Throat J 67:866–869, 1988.

91 CARDIOPULMONARY RESUSCITATION IN THE PEDIATRIC PATIENT

ROBERT KATZ, M.D. / LORRY ROBERT FRANKEL, M.D.

EPIDEMIOLOGY

The epidemiologic features of cardiac arrests in children are different from those of adults. The most common cause of cardiac arrest in adults is a primary cardiac event, whereas in children it is usually the result of a progressive deterioration in respiratory and circulatory function.[1] Although the causes of arrest in children may be diverse, the final sequence of events is usually profound hypoxemia and acidosis followed by circulatory collapse. For this reason, successful resuscitation in this setting is unusual; thus health care professionals must be able to recognize and treat children who are critically ill before actual cardiac arrest occurs.

According to most studies of cardiopulmonary arrest in infants and children, one half to two thirds of the episodes occur in patients under 1 year of age, and most of these children are no more than 6 months of age.[2] Unlike adults, the causes of arrest in children are diverse and include overwhelming infections, trauma, sudden infant death syndrome, airway obstruction, and other miscellaneous problems.[3]

The outcome of cardiopulmonary arrest in children depends in part on the cause of the arrest and the location (i.e., in hospital versus out of hospital). In general, outcomes in studies involving respiratory arrest alone are better than those of cardiac or cardiopulmonary arrest. Even in-hospital nonrespiratory arrests have a very poor outcome. Out-of-hospital cardiac arrest is associated with a very high mortality rate; 90% or more of the victims die. Of the few out-of-hospital cardiac arrest survivors, almost all have extremely poor neurologic outcomes.[4]

BASIC CARDIOPULMONARY RESUSCITATION (AIRWAY, BREATHING, CIRCULATION)

Basic life support requires skills but no specific equipment and can be performed in most locations and under most circumstances. If the victim is found to be unresponsive and has no respiratory effort and no palpable pulse, he or she should be quickly assessed in a systematic manner. This should include assessment of (1) the airway, (2) breathing and ventilation, and (3) circulation.

AIRWAY

The airway should be opened by head-tilt/chin-lift maneuver or, when neck injury is suspected, by the jaw-thrust maneuver. After the airway is opened, the rescuer should look, listen, and feel for breathing activity. If the child is breathing, the patency of the airway must be maintained. If the victim is not breathing, the rescuer must breathe for the victim.

BREATHING

In the case of the nonbreathing victim, the rescuer should deliver two slow breaths with a pause between them. The appropriate amount of air is one that causes the chest to rise; because of wide variations in sizes of victims, it is impossible to make precise recommendations in regards to the volume of each breath. If the chest does not rise with ventilation, airway obstruction must be suspected. At this point, the head-tilt/chin-lift maneuver should be repeated because improper positioning is the most likely cause of obstruction. If ventilation is still not successful, obstruction by a foreign body must be suspected.

The management of the infant with an obstructed airway is an area of considerable controversy.[5] Recent guidelines suggested that during basic life support, attempts at clearing the airway should be considered for (1) children in whom the aspiration of a foreign body is witnessed or strongly suspected and (2) unconscious nonbreathing children in whom the airway remains obstructed despite the usual maneuvers to open it. The recommended procedure for clearing the airway is different in infants and older children (over 1 year of age). In infants, four back blows followed by four chest compressions is still the method of choice. The infants should be in the head-down position during these maneuvers. In older children, the application of 6 to 10 abdominal thrusts (Heimlich's maneuver) with the child held upright by the rescuer is the currently recommended procedure.[6]

CIRCULATION

After it is established that ventilation is present or after the two breaths are given by the rescuer, the circulatory system should be assessed. The pulse should be checked by palpation of the carotid artery in older children and the brachial artery in infants. If a pulse is present but spontaneous breathing is absent, ventilations are continued at a rate of 20 breaths/min for an infant and 15 breaths/min for a child. If a pulse is not present, chest compressions should be started.

Studies of Finholdt and associates documented that the heart in an infant is lower in relation to external chest landmarks than previously thought.[7] Thus as in adults, compression of the lower half of the sternum is now the recommended technique for performing cardiopulmonary resuscitation (CPR) in infants.[6, 7] Chest compressions in infants should be one finger's breadth below the intermammary line. Beyond 1 year of age, the compression location should be one finger's breadth above the xiphosternal junction.

Compressions should be given at a rate of 80 to 100 per minute; they should always be accompanied by ventilations. At the end of every fifth compression, one slow breath of 1- to 1.5-sec duration should be administered. The victim should be reassessed at the end of 1 min of CPR and every few minutes thereafter.

ADVANCED PEDIATRIC LIFE SUPPORT

After basic CPR, advanced life support provides the compromised patient with further sophisticated techniques and specialized equipment that improve on ventilation and circulation and it is hoped, outcome. Studies have identified areas that allow the persons who care for a child in the near-arrest or arrested state faster routes of vascular access and methods to improve oxygen delivery. These techniques require special instruction and are designed to be safely administered by all potential first-line responders (e.g., physicians, nurses, and paramedics in the field).

RESPIRATORY SUPPORT

Advanced methods of respiratory support can improve the patient's ability to oxygenate and ventilate and include oxygen delivery devices for the spontaneously breathing patient, bag-valve-mask ventilation, and intubation needed for nonbreathing patients.

The Spontaneously Breathing Patient

Oxygen delivery may be achieved with the use of nasal cannulas, masks, hoods, or tent devices. Humidification of the oxygen delivery is important; however, care must be taken when child is placed in a mist tent not to lose the ability to carefully observe and monitor the child in this potential "sea of fog" (Table 91–1).

Although the nasal cannula may be the easiest method of oxygen delivery to use in an infant or small child who is in only moderate distress, a variety of problems may arise with its use. First, the amount of oxygen actually being delivered to the patient may not be clear. This is dependent on oxygen flow rate, nasal resistance, oropharyngeal resistance, inspiratory flow rate, and patient's tidal volume. Second, high flow rates (>5 to 6 l/min) may be irritating to the nares. Thus the use of nasal cannulas has limitations for children who are in severe respiratory distress and need oxygen concentrations higher than 30%.

In children who require higher oxygen concentrations, the use of an oxygen hood allows for fraction of inspired oxygen (FI_{O_2}) concentrations higher than that achieved

Table 91–1. SUMMARY OF EQUIPMENT NEEDED FOR RESPIRATORY SUPPORT IN THE SPONTANEOUSLY BREATHING PATIENT

Devices	Achievable $F_{I_{O_2}}$	Comments
Nasal cannula	.21–.30	Flow dependent
Oxygen hood	Up to .5	Problems with hypothermia, difficulty maintaining $F_{I_{O_2}}$
Oxygen tent	Up to .5	Mist ("sea of fog")
Mask		Difficult to titrate $F_{I_{O_2}}$
Simple	.6	
Partial rebreathing	.6	
Non-rebreathing	.9–1.0	
Venturi mask	.25–.6	Can titrate $F_{I_{O_2}}$ more exactly
Face tent	<.4	Allows access to face and oral cavity

$F_{I_{O_2}}$, fraction of inspired oxygen.

with the nasal cannula. Usually, children under 6 months of age benefit from oxygen hoods. Oxygen concentrations of less than 50% can be achieved with high gas-flow rates. Also the oxygen hood makes it possible for the bedside personnel to have access to a patient's chest, abdomen, and extremities for examination and procedures. However, a few problems may arise with the oxygen hood:[8]

1. Thermoregulation may be problematic if the temperature of the gases is not regulated and thus cold oxygen is delivered.

2. Oxygen may escape from the hood if a good seal is not present.

3. The oxygen concentration within the hood may vary as much as 20% from the top to bottom.

The oxygen tent is usually used for children who are over the age of 1 year and who require an $F_{I_{O_2}}$ approximating 50% to 60%. However, it may be difficult to maintain the desired oxygen concentration in the tent because of room air entry, which occurs any time the tent is opened for care of the patient. Thus patients who require this level of oxygen may require more aggressive therapy such as intubation and positive-pressure ventilation. Also, with humidification, it may become difficult for the patient to be visualized through the heavy mist.

Although oxygen masks allow for the delivery of oxygen to hypoxic children, they are not well tolerated by infants and small children. They are, however, extremely useful in older children who are cooperative. A number of oxygen masks are currently used in pediatrics: the simple oxygen mask, the partial rebreathing mask, the non-rebreathing mask, the Venturi mask, and the face tent.

The simple mask can deliver oxygen concentrations from 25% to 60% but require a flow rate of 6 l/min to maintain the higher oxygen concentration and to prevent rebreathing of exhaled carbon dioxide. The partial rebreathing mask contains an added reservoir, which maintains a somewhat higher concentration of oxygen because it allows for mixing of both the inspired and expired oxygen, the first third of which is rich in oxygen. Delivered oxygen concentration may reach 60%. The non-rebreathing masks allow for the inspiration of gas with an $F_{I_{O_2}}$ approximating 1.0. This is due to the incorporation of valves that prevent entrainment of room air

during inspiration. The Venturi mask allows for more control of the $F_{I_{O_2}}$ so that it can be titrated from 25% to 60%.[9] Finally, the face tent is well tolerated in older children and allows for the delivery of an $F_{I_{O_2}}$ less than .4. An advantage of this device is that it permits access to the oral cavity for the patient and thus allows suctioning and other respiratory treatments and oral hygiene.[10]

The Obtunded But Spontaneously Breathing Patient

For such patients, the concern is about the inability to clear the airway of secretions. Two commonly used tools that help clear the upper airway of secretions are oropharyngeal and nasopharyngeal airway devices. These are soft plastic or rubber instruments that are placed in either the oral cavity or the nasal passage. They enable clearing of the airway of secretions or prevent the tongue from flopping into the airway and causing obstruction. Sizes vary depending on the age and size of the child. Special technique is required for their insertion in order to avoid pushing the tongue into the airway and hence causing further airway obstruction. Care should also be taken to avoid laceration of the tongue, nasopharynx, or oropharynx. The oropharyngeal and nasopharyngeal devices are placed in unconscious or obtunded patients who are having trouble maintaining patency of the airway. These airways may be helpful in patients with drug overdoses, in postoperative patients, in patients who are still under the effects of anesthesia, and in patients who are heavily sedated for a procedure. The nasopharyngeal tube is better tolerated and allows for better access to the airway for suctioning.[11]

Management of Respiratory Failure or Arrest

Apnea and respiratory failure must be promptly recognized in order to avoid an unnecessary life-threatening complication. Careful inspection, auscultation, and assessment may require blood gas determination for correct diagnosis and prompt therapeutic intervention (i.e., bag-valve-mask ventilation or intubation for mechanical ventilation). Again, the basic approach is not dissimilar from that used in basic life support.

First, the airway must be assessed to determine whether it is patent. If it is, the patient may need assistance with bag-valve-mask technique before intubation. It is important that the appropriate-sized mask be used for effective bag-valve-mask ventilation. The mask should fit snugly over the nose and lips to form a tight seal and thus prevent the leak of gas and pressure. It is preferable to use a mask that is clear so that it is possible to assess whether the patient vomits or whether the airway is occluded during the resuscitative efforts and thus requires suctioning. Finally, the mask must be connected to a fresh gas source that provides high concentrations of oxygen and gas-flow rates.

During bag-valve-mask ventilation, the child's head must be positioned by means of the head-tilt/chin-lift maneuver. Compression or hyperextension of the neck occludes the airway and thus must be avoided. The neutral sniffing position without hyperextension of the head seems best for infants and toddlers. On occasion, cricoid pressure (Sellick's maneuver) is required for occluding the esophagus to prevent the regurgitation of gastric contents during resuscitative events. Also, this may aid in the direct visualization of the glottic opening required for intubation. Care must be taken to avoid unnecessary tracheal compression as well. Effective bag-valve-mask ventilation enables the resuscitators to restore adequate oxygenation and ventilation for the patient before intubation.

Endotracheal intubation provides an artificial airway that enables delivery of high concentrations of oxygen and positive-pressure ventilation and cycling of the respirations so that gas exchange can occur in the most effective method possible. Appropriate endotracheal intubation requires an understanding of the skills needed, knowledge of the physiologic effects of positive-pressure ventilation, the equipment required for safe intubation, and preparedness in case of adverse reactions caused by instrumentation of the airway.

Only clinicians skilled in the technique of endotracheal intubation should perform the procedure. Because the pediatric airway may be compromised by swelling secondary to infection or trauma, clinicians must be adept at manipulating a smaller than expected airway when intubating pediatric patients.

It is critically important that the correct equipment be available for this life-saving procedure. Appropriate-sized endotracheal tubes (2.5 to 7.0-mm internal diameter) are required, as are a functioning laryngoscope with different size blades (00 to 4) and light bulbs firmly attached to the laryngoscope. The child should be in a physiologic state in which the child will not fight the procedure and thus hinder intubation and acquire airway injury. Pharmacologic agents (sedatives and muscle relaxants) may facilitate the procedure and are ideal methods for clinicians skilled in intubation (see Table 91–2.). Selection of the appropriate-sized tube can be aided by a simple formula that requires knowledge of the child's age:

$$\text{Tube size (mm of internal diameter)} = \frac{\text{age in years} + 16}{4}$$

Table 91–2. PHARMACOLOGIC AGENTS USED TO FACILITATE INTUBATION

Agents	Dose (mg/kg intravenous)
Neuromuscular Blocking Agents	
Depolarizing agent: succinylcholine	1–2
Nondepolarizing agent	
Pancuronium	0.1–0.2
Vecuronium	0.05–0.1
Metocurine	0.2–0.4
Sedatives	
Narcotics	
Morphine	0.05–0.1
Fentanyl	.001–.01
Benzodiazepines	
Diazepam	0.1–0.2
Midazolam	0.05–0.1
Ketamine	0.5–2.0
Thiopental	2–4

Alternatively, the appropriate-sized tube is approximately the size of the child's nares or the fifth finger.

In most of the acute situations, the oral route is preferred over the nasal route for the insertion of the endotracheal tube. The nasal route requires special technique and skill with the use of the Magill forceps. When attempting to secure the airway with an endotracheal tube, the clinician should preoxygenate the patient with bag-valve-mask ventilation. The airway should be secured within 30 sec because the patient may be predisposed to hypoxemia and bradycardias with prolonged attempts at intubation. On occasion, it may be necessary to use a stylet to make the flexible endotracheal tube more rigid, which may help with oral intubation. During the procedure, the patient's heart rate should be monitored and, if possible, oxygen saturation via pulse oximetry should be performed.

After intubation, the clinician must first assess for appropriate tube placement and then secure the endotracheal tube. Auscultation in the patient's axilla is used to ascertain whether the tube is in good position. If breath sounds are equal bilaterally and the patient's vital signs remain unchanged or improved, the tube is most likely in good position. However, in infants and newborns, esophageal intubations may result in transmission of breath sounds throughout the chest wall. Other indicators of poor endotracheal tube placement include unequal breath sounds, oxygen desaturation, and abdominal distension, which may indicate an esophageal intubation. The tube should be secured with waterproof tape, which adheres better to the tube and skin.

Once the patient's airway has been secured, a chest radiograph should be performed to confirm endotracheal tube placement. Also, the chest radiograph shows the extent of lung disease, if present. The patient is then initially hand ventilated at a pressure that ensures adequate minute ventilation. The chest wall should move with adequate distending pressure and at a rate that allows for adequate lung filling and alveolar emptying. In addition, all patients should receive 100% FI_{O_2} until oxygen saturations or arterial blood gas levels allow for a decrease in inspired oxygen concentration. Arterial blood gas levels also enable clinicians to determine ventilator settings appropriate for the clinical situation. Finally, the patient needs to be appropriately monitored for heart rate, oxygen saturations, and, if possible, carbon dioxide (CO_2) tension (transcutaneously or via an end-tidal CO_2 apparatus).

CARDIOVASCULAR SUPPORT

Newer methods have been developed to allow for rapid access to the vascular compartment for infusion of life-saving fluids and medication. Also, a variety of pediatric centers have developed protocols that aid in the timing of vascular access.

Vascular Access

Establishing vascular access quickly for the administration of medications and fluids is a crucial step during the

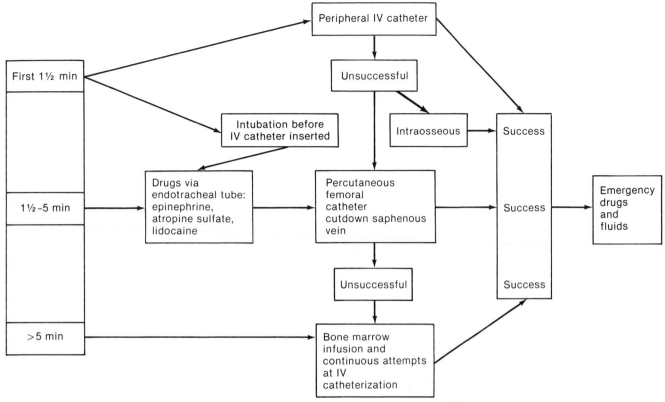

Figure 91–1. Protocol for emergency intravascular access during pediatric resuscitations. Current recommendations from the American Heart Association: If resuscitation is unsuccessful after 90 sec, an intraosseous catheter should be inserted for fluids and medications. IV, intravenous.

management of children who have suffered cardiac arrest. However, because of technical factors (chiefly the small size of a child), obtaining successful vascular access is often very difficult. Several studies have documented the difficulty in rapidly obtaining vascular access in children in the emergency situation.[12] Because of these difficulties, an organized approach with definite priorities may result in more rapid establishment of vascular access. Kanter and colleagues evaluated one such protocol and found that vascular access was obtained sooner when the vascular access protocol was followed than when it was not (Fig. 91–1).[13]

While vascular access is being established, atropine, lidocaine, and epinephrine may be administered via the endotracheal tube. Although some studies suggested that larger doses should be given if the endotracheal route is used, the current guidelines recommend that the same doses be used that are administered intravenously.[6, 14] A useful approach is to dilute the drug with 1 to 2 ml of saline and inject the resuscitation drugs through a small feeding tube placed distally in the endotracheal tube, thereby permitting more of the drug to reach the alveolar spaces rather than being suspended in the endotracheal tube.

Attempts at obtaining vascular access should begin with a brief attempt at cannulating a peripheral vein. If this is not successful within 90 sec, one of two options may be used: central venous access via percutaneous cannulation of the femoral vein (if the physician is familiar with the technique) or the now preferred intraosseous route.

The femoral route may be the preferred method of obtaining access to the central circulation because attempts to use the subclavian or internal jugular veins require interruption of chest compressions. These latter routes are technically more difficult and are associated with more potential complications.

For less experienced physicians, intraosseous cannulation is an easy and rapid method of obtaining access to the circulation. The technique consists of placing a needle into the tibial bone marrow space. It has been used effectively for blood, fluids, and medications, including vasoactive drug infusions.[15–17] A standard 16- or 18-gauge hypodermic needle, a spinal needle with a stylet, or a bone marrow needle is inserted into the proximal medial tibial surface 1 to 3 cm below the tibial tuberosity. The needle should be directed perpendicular or slightly inferior to avoid the epiphyseal plate (Fig. 91–2). Either the distal femur or proximal tibia are the preferred sites. Complications include infection, extravasation, and bleeding. The sternum should not be used because it is easily completely traversed, and this may lead to injury to the heart and lungs.[14]

Table 91–3 lists the equipment required for obtaining vascular access in children of different ages and weights.[13]

Medications

Drugs used with CPR are listed in Table 91–4. The use of medications during a cardiac arrest in children is complicated by the need to adjust drug dose to body weight.

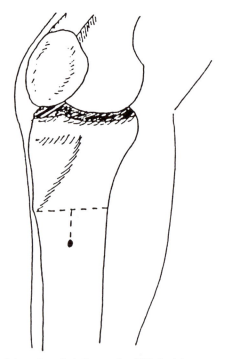

Figure 91–2. Insertion site in the proximal tibia for intraosseous infusion.

This can be simplified by the availability of drug tables that are precalculated for a range of weights.[13]

Oxygen. During a resuscitation, a number of factors contribute to severe progressive hypoxemia and tissue hypoxia. Because even optimal performance of CPR provides only a fraction of the cardiac output, tissue oxygen delivery is markedly compromised. CPR is additionally complicated by right-to-left intrapulmonary shunting. Oxygen in the highest concentration available is indicated in all cardiac arrest situations. In addition, it should be given in any condition in which hypoxemia is suspected and in any condition of respiratory difficulty that may lead to a cardiac arrest.

Epinephrine. This is an endogenous catecholamine with both alpha- and beta-adrenergic receptor–stimulating actions.[18] It appears that the most important action of epinephrine when used in the arrest setting is to increase diastolic blood pressure through alpha-adrenergic–mediated vasoconstriction. This improves coronary perfusion with increased oxygen delivery to the heart. Additional effects of epinephrine include improvement of myocardial contractility with the stimulation of spontaneous contraction and enhancement of the susceptibility of the heart to electrical defibrillation.

Epinephrine is indicated in all forms of cardiac arrest. The recommended dose is 0.01 mg/kg of the 1:10,000 solution (0.1 ml/kg), which may be given by the intravenous, intraosseous, or endotracheal route. This dose may be repeated at 5-min intervals because the duration of action is short. In the absence of clinical data to dictate the optimal endotracheal dose, it is recommended to give at least the same dose as that used intravenously with a minimal dose of 0.5 ml of the 1:10,000 solution.

Epinephrine should not be added to bicarbonate infusions because catecholamines are inactivated by an alkaline solution. Careful monitoring of patients receiving epinephrine is necessary because side effects may include postresuscitation hypertension and tachyarrhythmias.

Sodium Bicarbonate. During cardiac arrest, hypoxia-induced anaerobic metabolism results in the generation of lactic acid. This is compounded by ventilatory failure, which causes hypercapnia and respiratory acidosis. Thus during a cardiac arrest, the acidotic state is usually of mixed respiratory and metabolic origins. The contribution of these factors is best assessed by analysis of arterial blood gases.

Because the major causes of cardiac arrest in children are respiratory in nature, the achievement of adequate ventilation is essential for managing both the acidemia and hypoxemia of the arrested state. Sodium bicarbonate (HCO_3) buffers hydrogen (H^+) by a simple acid-base reaction:

$$HCO_3 + H^+ \rightarrow H_2CO_3 \rightarrow H_2O + CO_2$$

In the presence of a fixed or inadequate minute ventilation, blood pH does not improve significantly after sodium bicarbonate administration unless the increased CO_2 that is produced can be eliminated.[19] In fact, the rapid infusion of bicarbonate in cardiac arrest–like setting has been shown to transiently increase arterial CO_2 pressure, which decreases intracellular pH and worsens cell function.[20]

Because of these concerns, the use of sodium bicarbonate has been de-emphasized in the most recent recommendations.[6] The first steps in caring for a patient after cardiac arrest should always be securing the airway,

Table 91–3. EQUIPMENT FOR VENOUS ACCESS IN INFANTS AND CHILDREN*

| Age (Years) | Weight (kg) | Butterfly Needles (Gauge) | Over-the-Needle Catheters (Gauge) | Intracatheters | | Central Venous Catheters† | | |
				Catheter (Gauge)	Needle (Gauge)	French Size	Length (cm)	Diameter (mm)
<1	<10	21, 23, 25	20, 22, 24	22	19	3.0	8–12	0.46 (.018)
1–12	10–40	16, 18, 20	16, 18, 20	18	16	4.0	8–12	0.53 (.021)
>12	>40	16, 18, 20	14, 16, 18	16	14	5.0	8–20	0.89 (.035)

*For intraosseous route, a 16- or 18-gauge bone marrow needle is needed.

†Newer central venous catheters in 4 French and 5 French have multiple lumens so that one catheter may provide two venous access ports; one for volume therapy and the other for inotropic therapy.

Table 91-4. DRUGS USED IN CARDIOPULMONARY RESUSCITATION*

Drug	Dose	Supplied	Remark
Epinephrine hydrochloride	0.01 mg/kg (0.1 ml/kg)	1:10,000 (0.1 mg/ml)	Most useful drug in cardiac arrest, IV or ET
Sodium bicarbonate	1 mEq/kg (1 ml/kg)	1 mEq/l (8.4% sol)	Infuse slowly and only when ventilation is adequate
Atropine sulfate	0.02 mg/kg (0.2 ml/kg)	0.1 mg/ml	Minimum dose of (0.1 mg/or 1 ml); use for bradycardia after assessing ventilation, IV or ET
Calcium chloride	20 mg/kg	100 mg/ml	Use only for hypocalcemia, calcium blocker: overdose, hyperkalemia, hypermagnesemia; give slowly
Lidocaine hydrochloride	1 mg/kg	10 mg/ml (1%) 20 mg/ml (2%)	IV or ET for ventricular tachycardia or fibrillation
Bretylium tosylate	5 mg/kg (0.1 ml/kg)	50 mg/ml	Use if lidocaine not effective
Epinephrine infusion	0.1–1.0 µg/kg/min	1:1000	Titrate infusion to desired hemodynamic effect
Dopamine hydrochloride infusion	2–20 µg/kg/min	250 mg/vial, lyophilized	Titrate to desired hemodynamic response: little vasoconstriction, even at high unknown rates
Dobutamine infusion	5–20 µg/kg/min	1 µg/5 ml	Titrate to desired hemodynamic effect; vasodilator
Lidocaine infusion	20–50 µg/kg/min	40 µg/ml (4%)	Use lower infusion dose with shock, liver disease
Amrinone	Load 1 mg/kg 5–10 µg/kg/min	5 mg/ml	Watch for hypotension and thrombocytopenia

IV, intravenous; ET, endotracheal; sol, solution.
*For IV push medications listed, preparation is available in prefilled syringes.

hyperventilation, and ensuring that adequate chest compressions are delivered. Sodium bicarbonate may be administered if a child remains acidemic after all these maneuvers are performed and has a persistent metabolic acidosis. The dose is 1 mEq/kg of the 8.4% solution. This may be given intravenously or via the intraosseous route (not through the endotracheal tube). Subsequent doses of sodium bicarbonate should be guided by the results of serial arterial blood gas measurements. If these are not readily available, 0.5 mEq/kg may be given every 10 min while the victim remains in a state of cardiac arrest.

The use of sodium bicarbonate may lead to many potential complications, including metabolic alkalosis, which shifts the oxyhemoglobin dissociation curve to the left, thus impairing oxygen delivery to the tissue. Potassium shifts intracellularly, and decreased plasma ionized calcium levels can be observed. Hypernatremia and water overload are also potential problems because 1 mEq/kg of sodium is delivered with 1 mEq/kg of bicarbonate. The standard 8.4% solution of sodium bicarbonate is extremely hyperosmolar (2000 osm/l) in comparison with plasma (280 osm/l). Repeated doses can, therefore, result in symptomatic hypernatremia and hyperosmolality.[21] Catecholamines may become inactivated, and calcium salts may precipitate in bicarbonate solutions; therefore, the intravenous catheter should be flushed with saline before and after the administration of bicarbonate.

Atropine. Atropine sulfate is a parasympatholytic drug that accelerates sinus or atrial pacemakers and increases atrioventricular conduction. Because of these actions, atropine is useful in the treatment of bradycardia accompanied by poor perfusion or hypotension. In small infants (<6 months of age), cardiac output is rate dependent; heart rates below 80 beats/min in a distressed infant need to be treated, even if blood pressure is normal. It is important to remember that in an emergency, bradycardia usually results from hypoxemia; therefore, treatment should initially be directed at oxygenation and ventilation rather than the administration of atropine.

If, in spite of adequate ventilation, bradycardia persists, atropine should be administered by the intravenous, intraosseous, or endotracheal route. The dose of atropine is 0.02 mg/kg; the minimal dose is 0.1 mg. A minimal dose is important because paradoxical bradycardia may result from the lower dose. This may be repeated at 5-min intervals to a maximum of 1.0 mg in a child and 2.0 mg in an adolescent. With these dosages, tachycardia is not uncommon after the administration of atropine. However, this is usually well tolerated by the pediatric patient.

Glucose. Glucose is a key and often forgotten agent in the resuscitation of infants and children. It is a major substrate for the neonatal myocardium, and optimal cardiac work may not be possible in the presence of hypoglycemia. Small infants and chronically ill children have limited glycogen stores that are rapidly depleted with stress, and the resultant hypoglycemia may clinically mimic hypoxia, poor perfusion, diaphoresis, tachycardia, and hypotension.

A rapid bedside glucose test should be obtained during resuscitation and glucose should be administered intravenously or intraosseously in a dose of 0.5 to 1.0 g/kg if hypoglycemia (serum glucose less than 60 mg/dl) is present. This should be delivered in a solution of 25% dextrose in water ($D_{25}W$) or less. Because glucose is supplied as $D_{50}W$, it must be diluted 1/1 with sterile water. The administered dose of $D_{25}W$ is 2 to 4 ml/kg.

Calcium. Calcium is essential to the process of excitation-contraction coupling and produces an inotropic action on the heart, particularly when the patient is hypocalcemic. Its use in the cardiac arrest setting was based on anecdotal reports of a beneficial effect in electromechanical dissociation (EMD) and after cardiopulmonary bypass.

However, several studies cast doubt on its efficacy in either EMD or asystole.[10, 22] This lack of efficacy, combined with the fact that results of other studies suggested that calcium entry into the cell may be involved in cell death, led to a revision of the guidelines regarding the use of calcium in the cardiac arrest setting. It is no longer recommended as a routine drug for EMD or asystole.[6, 23]

Calcium is indicated when hypocalcemia has been documented or is suspected and should be considered for the treatment of hyperkalemia or hypermagnesemia. Calcium is also indicated for the treatment of hypotension from calcium-channel blocker overdoses.

Calcium is available in three different salts. Calcium chloride is the only form that should be considered in resuscitation because it directly delivers ionized calcium. The gluconate and gluceptate salts must be metabolized in the liver to release ionized calcium. The dose of calcium chloride is 20 mg/kg (0.2 ml/kg) in the 10% solution. It is recommended that this initial dose be repeated only once in 10 min and that further doses be based on measured calcium deficiency.

Rapid calcium administration may produce significant bradycardia. Patients receiving digoxin are predisposed to severe arrhythmias, including sinus arrest, after calcium administration. Calcium solution is sclerosing to veins and may produce a severe local chemical burn if it infiltrates. Therefore, calcium chloride should be administered in a central vein to avoid this problem.

Lidocaine. This is used in the unusual circumstance of ventricular tachycardia or ventricular fibrillation in pediatric patients. Ventricular fibrillation is seen in fewer than 10% of pediatric cardiac arrests, the most frequent rhythms being asystole or bradyarrhythmias.[22] When fibrillation is present in a child, the clinician should look for a metabolic cause such as abnormalities in calcium, potassium, or blood glucose as well as hypothermia, infection such as myocarditis, and drug-related causes (i.e., tricyclic antidepressant overdose).

Lidocaine should be administered to pediatric patients with ventricular tachycardia or ventricular fibrillation and also to hemodynamically unstable patients who have ventricular couplets of frequent premature beats.

The recommended dose is 1 mg/kg (by intravenous, intraosseous, or endotracheal route). If required for suppressing the abnormal rhythm, a second dose may be repeated in 10 to 15 min. Under these circumstances, a lidocaine infusion should be started. This is prepared by adding 120 mg of lidocaine to 100 ml of D_5W and delivered at a rate of 1 to 2.5 ml/kg/h (20 to 50 μg/kg/min). In the presence of shock or known liver disease, the infusion should be run at 20 μg/kg/min to minimize possible toxicity from impaired lidocaine clearance.

Toxic reactions to lidocaine include myocardial depression and central nervous system symptoms such as drowsiness, disorientation, or frank seizures. Treatment consists of terminating the lidocaine infusion and appropriate use of anticonvulsants, if seizures are present.

Bretylium Tosylate. This is an antiarrhythmic agent with complex pharmacologic action.[24, 25] After administration, there is an initial brief increase in blood pressure and heart rate, followed later by a fall in both, probably because of sympathetic nervous system inhibition. From experience with adults, it is recommended as a second-line drug after lidocaine for treatment of ventricular fibrillation. The dose is 5 mg/kg intravenously and is followed by another attempt at defibrillation. If necessary, the dose

may be increased to 10 mg/kg and the countershock repeated.

Bretylium may also be helpful in ventricular tachycardia that has not been successfully treated with lidocaine. In this setting, the drug should be administered in a dose of 5 mg/kg over 8 to 10 min because rapid administration may cause nausea and vomiting in conscious patients. Besides these side effects, the most common toxic reaction is hypotension, which generally responds to head-down positioning and fluid administration.

MEDICATIONS FOR POSTRESUSCITATION STABILIZATION

This section is a brief review of the indications and doses of the more commonly used vasoactive drugs that may be necessary when hemodynamic instability persists after CPR. Table 91-5 lists a method of preparing infusions of the vasoactive drugs discussed next.

DOPAMINE

Dopamine is an endogenous catecholamine with multiple actions.[26] When infused at 2 to 5 μg/kg/min, dopamine usually increases cardiac contractility and cardiac output with few changes in heart rate, blood pressure, or systemic vascular resistance. In addition, at this low dose, dopamine selectively increases renal and mesenteric blood flow by stimulation of dopaminergic receptors. As the infusion rate is increased above 10 to 15 μg/kg/min, the selective blood flow effects are lost, and peripheral vasoconstriction may occur because of stimulation of alpha-adrenergic receptors.

Dopamine is indicated in the treatment of hypotension or poor peripheral perfusion in pediatric patients in whom a stable rhythm is present or has been restored. This usually requires doses of 5 to 15 μg/kg/min. Because an attenuated response to dopamine has been documented in young pediatric patients, higher doses may be required. However, if it is ineffective at doses higher than 20 μg/kg/min, another agent such as epinephrine should be substituted.

Dopamine may produce tachycardia, hypertension, and arrhythmias. It should be given through a central vein

Table 91-5. METHOD TO PREPARE VASOACTIVE DRUG INFUSION*

Drug	Concentration	Infusion Rate
Epinephrine Norepinephrine Isoproterenol	0.6 × weight (kg)	1 ml/h delivers 0.1 μg/kg/min
Dopamine Dobutamine Amrinone	6 × weight (kg)	1 ml/h delivers 1 μg/kg/min
Lidocaine	60 × weight (kg)	1 ml/h delivers 10 μg/kg/min

*Dose in milligrams to add to diluent to make final volume of 100 ml. Diluent may be 5% dextrose in water, 5% dextrose in .2 water normal saline, 5% dextrose in normal saline, or 5% dextrose in lactated Ringer's solution.

if possible. A secure large-bore peripheral intravenous cannula may be a suitable alternative. Extravasation of dopamine can cause severe local tissue effects.

DOBUTAMINE

Dobutamine was synthesized by sequential systematic alterations of the chemical structure of isoproterenol.[27] It has a selective effect on beta$_1$-adrenergic receptors, which during infusion results in an increase in myocardial contractility with little change in mean arterial pressure or systemic vascular resistance. Unlike dopamine, its inotropic action does not depend on releasable stores of catecholamines, and it has no selective effect on renal blood flow or urine output. There is a paucity of published experiences with dobutamine in children, although in one study it appeared to be less effective in infants under 12 months of age.[28] Because of its lack of vasoconstrictive effect, it may not increase blood pressure as effectively as dopamine.

EPINEPHRINE

Epinephrine interacts directly with both alpha- and beta-adrenergic receptors. Lower infusion rates (0.3 μg/kg/min) are primarily associated with beta-adrenergic effects, whereas at higher doses, alpha-adrenergic effects predominate.[18, 26] At low doses, epinephrine causes an increase in myocardial contractility, an elevation of systolic blood pressure, but a fall in diastolic pressure. As the infusion is increased beyond 0.3 μg/kg/min, increased alpha-adrenergic effects are noted, primarily vasoconstriction and elevation of diastolic pressure.

Epinephrine is indicated for the treatment of hypotension or poor perfusion after restoration of spontaneous circulation. It may be effective in restoring adequate circulation in situations in which dopamine and dobutamine have failed. In addition, it is useful for the treatment of bradycardia accompanied by hemodynamic compromise and, according to some authors, is preferred over isoproterenol. The major limitation to the use of epinephrine is that, at higher doses, it is a potent vasoconstrictor, and blood flow to vital organs may be compromised when these higher doses are used.

Initial infusion rates of 0.1 to 0.3 μg/kg/min are used, and when possible, doses above 0.5 μg/kg/min are avoided. Epinephrine can cause significant tachycardia, tachyarrhythmias, and hypertension. As with dopamine, administration through a central catheter is preferred because extravasation may cause severe local ischemia.

ISOPROTERENOL

Isoproterenol is a pure beta-adrenergic agonist and therefore produces an increase in heart rate, conduction velocity, and cardiac contractility. Peripheral vasodilation occurs because of its action on beta$_2$-adrenergic receptors. If the effective circulating fluid volume is adequate, cardiac output should increase during an infusion of isoproterenol.

Isoproterenol may be used for the treatment of hemodynamically significant bradycardia that results from heart block and that is resistant to atropine or recurs shortly after atropine has been given. However, isoproterenol may cause a drop in diastolic blood pressure, which may compromise coronary perfusion and thus decrease myocardial oxygen delivery. In addition, isoproterenol increases myocardial oxygen demand by increasing myocardial contractility and heart rate. The net result of these two effects may be myocardial ischemia in the postarrest setting. As a result, epinephrine infusion (see later discussion) may be preferable to achieve an increase in heart rate.[6]

Isoproterenol has a very short half-life after intravenous infusion and must be administered as a constant infusion. Initial infusion rates are 0.05 to 0.1 μg/kg/min. The infusion rate should be increased every 5 min up to 1.0 μg/kg/min as needed. Tachycardia is the toxic effect that limits the dose; heart rates over 180 in children and over 200 in infants mandate a decrease in the infusion rate.

AMRINONE

Amrinone increases myocardial contractility and decreases systemic and pulmonary vascular resistances. It is a phosphodiesterase inhibitor that produces an increase in intracellular cyclic adenosine monophosphate in the myocyte and in vascular smooth muscle. Its experience in pediatrics is limited: it has been shown to be of value in treating states of low cardiac output commonly found with congestive heart failure or cardiomyopathy. Initial loading dose is 1 mg/kg and is followed by a continuous infusion of 5 to 10 μg/kg/min. Adverse side effects include hypotension and thrombocytopenia.[29]

DEFIBRILLATION AND CARDIOVERSION

Defibrillation is the untimed (asynchronous) depolarization of the myocardium used in the treatment of ventricular fibrillation. Because ventricular fibrillation is uncommon in pediatric patients, electrical defibrillation should not be used without documentation that the dysrhythmia is, in fact, present. As always, attention must first be directed toward the principles of basic life support: securing the airway and providing adequate ventilation and chest compressions.

The largest electrode size that allows good chest wall contact over its entire area while avoiding accidental contact with other electrodes is preferred. The infant paddle measures 4.5 cm in diameter. There are 8.0-cm and 13.0-cm paddles for older children. Electrode gel or cream should be placed between the skin and the electrode to ensure optimal delivery of the charge to the heart. The paddles must be placed so that the heart is situated between them. The standard placement is one paddle on the upper right chest below the clavicle and the other to the left of the left nipple in the anterior axillary line.[6]

The correct energy dose of the defibrillation is not definitely established. Guidelines recommend a dose of 2 J/kg. If unsuccessful, the energy dose should be doubled and repeated twice as necessary. Ongoing attention to the adequacy of basic CPR is essential during this process, and correctable metabolic causes should be sought before defibrillation is attempted again. Lidocaine or bretylium may be used in resistant cases of ventricular defibrillation again.

Cardioversion is the timed (synchronous) depolarization of the myocardium used in the treatment of rapid arrhythmias when they cause hemodynamic compromise (poor perfusion or hypotension). The required energy dose is less than that for defibrillation: Initial doses of 0.1 to 0.2 J/kg are recommended.[6] The dose may be increased in a stepwise manner until the rhythm has been converted.

REFERENCES

1. Eisenberg M, Bergner L, Hallstrom A: Epidemiology of cardiac arrest and resuscitation in children. Ann Emerg Med 12:672–678, 1983.
2. Torphy DE, Minter MG, Thompson BM: Cardiorespiratory arrest and resuscitation of children. Am J Dis Child 138:1099–1107, 1984.
3. Gillis J, Dickson D, Rieder M, et al: Results of inpatient pediatric resuscitation. Crit Care Med 14:469–474, 1986.
4. O'Rourke PP: Outcome of children who are apneic and pulseless in the emergency room. Crit Care Med 14:466–471, 1986.
5. Day RL: Differing opinions on the emergency treatment of choking. Pediatrics 71:976–978, 1983.
6. Standards and Guidelines for Cardiopulmonary Resuscitation (CPR) and Emergency Cardiac Care (ECC). JAMA 255:2954–2972, 1986.
7. Finholdt DA, Kettrick RG, Wagner HR, et al: The heart is under the lower third of the sternum. Implications for external cardiac massage. Am J Dis Child 140:646–649, 1986.
8. McPherson SP, Spearman CB: Gas regulation, administration and controlling devices. In Respiratory Therapy Equipment, 3rd ed, p. 74. St. Louis: CV Mosby, 1985.
9. Caset J, Sanchis J: Diluting effects of the breathing pattern. Eur J Respir Dis 65:58–62, 1984.
10. Textbook of Pediatric Advanced Life Support. Dallas: American Heart Association, 1988.
11. McPhersen SP, Spearman CB: Artificial airway. In Respiratory Therapy Equipment, 3rd ed, pp. 164–165. St. Louis: CV Mosby, 1985.
12. Rosetti V, Thompson BM, Aprohamian C, et al: Difficulty and delay in intravascular access in pediatric arrest. Ann Emerg Med 13:406–411, 1984.
13. Kanter RK, Zimmerman JJ, Strauss RH, et al: Pediatric emergency intravenous access. Am J Dis Child 140:132–136, 1986.
14. Chernow B, Holbrook P, D'Angona S, et al: Rapid epinephrine absorption after intratracheal administration. Anesth Analg 63:829–832, 1984.
15. Rosetti VA, Thompson BM, Miller J, et al: Intraosseous infusions: An alternative route of pediatric intravascular access. Ann Emerg Med 14:885–890, 1985.
16. Berg RA: Emergency infusion of catecholamines into bone marrow. Am J Dis Child 138:810–812, 1984.
17. Fiser PH: Intraosseous infusion. N Engl J Med 322:1579–1581, 1990.
18. Otto CW, Yakaitis RW, Blitt CD: Mechanism of action of epinephrine in resuscitation from asphyxial arrest. Crit Care Med 9:321–326, 1981.
19. Ostrea EM Jr, Odel GB: The influence of bicarbonate administration on blood pH in a "closed system": Clinical implications. J Pediatr 80:671–675, 1977.
20. Graf H, Leach W, Arieff AL: Metabolic effects of sodium bicarbonate in hypoxic lactic acidosis in dogs. Am J Physiol 249:F630–F635, 1985.
21. Mattar JA, Weil MH, Shubin H, Stein L: Cardiac arrest in the critically ill. II. Hyperosmolar states following cardiac arrest. Am J Med 56:162–168, 1974.
22. Zaritsky A: Cardiopulmonary resuscitation in children. Clin Chest Med 8:4:561–569, 1987.
23. Steuven HA, Thompson B, Aprahamian C, et al: Lack of effectiveness of calcium chloride in refractory electromechanical dissociation. Ann Emerg Med 14:626–630, 1985.
24. Kock-Weser J: Drug therapy: Bretylium. N Engl J Med 300:173–179, 1979.
25. Dronen SC: Antifibrillatory drugs: The case for bretylium tosylate. Ann Emerg Med 13(Pt 2):805, 1984.
26. Zaritsky A, Chernow B: Use of catecholamines in pediatrics. J Pediatr 105:341–351, 1985.
27. Leier CV, Unverferth DR: Drugs five years later: Dobutamine. Ann Intern Med 99:490–495, 1983.
28. Perkin RM, Levin DL, Webb R, et al: Dobutamine: A hemodynamic evaluation in children with shock. J Pediatr 100:977–981, 1982.
29. Mayer JE, Walsh E, Castenanda AR: Intensive care management of pediatric cardiac surgical patient. In Fuhrman BP, Shoemacher WC (eds): Critical Care: State of the Art, p. 345. Fullerton, CA: Society of Critical Care Medicine, 1989.

92 TRACHEOTOMY

KEITH CLARK, M.D. / JOHN S. DONOVAN, M.D.

Tracheotomy may be necessary in the management of upper airway obstruction, for prolonged mechanical ventilation, or to facilitate suctioning in children unable to clear their secretions. Although tracheotomy should be considered a safe procedure in children, the decision to perform this procedure is a difficult one. Many medical, emotional, and social factors must be weighed when considering a tracheotomy in an infant or a child. Some of these factors include the severity and speed of progression of the disease, age of the child, and availability of post-tracheotomy care. In addition to the complications, which occur most frequently in children under 1 year of age, safe postoperative management is time consuming and requires the attention of appropriately trained care-

Table 92-1. INDICATIONS FOR TRACHEOTOMY

Upper Airway Obstruction
Foreign body
Laryngeal or pharyngeal cysts/neoplasms
Macroglossia/micrognathia
Epiglottitis
Retropharyngeal abscess
Severe laryngotracheomalacia
Bilateral true vocal cord paralysis
Subglottic stenosis
Facial or laryngeal trauma
Laryngeal edema after burns

Prolonged Intubation
Bronchopulmonary dysplasia
Guillain-Barré syndrome
Coma with respiratory dysfunction
Respiratory distress syndrome

Pulmonary Toilet
Chronic aspiration
Neuromuscular diseases (e.g., poliomyelitis)
Tracheoesophageal fistula
Chronic bronchorrhea (e.g., cystic fibrosis)

From Stool SE, Eavey R: Tracheotomy. *In* Bluestone CD, Stool SE (eds): Pediatric Otolaryngology, p. 1322. Philadelphia: WB Saunders, 1990.

takers. All the patients' caretakers must be well trained in the proper care of the tracheostomy, including methods of airway humidification, endotracheal suctioning, and tracheostomy tube changing. They must be comfortable with suctioning and changing the tube. Portable suctioning equipment, an Ambu bag, and extra tracheostomy tubes should be carried with the child at all times. The parents or other caretakers should keep an adequate supply of suction catheters, saline, and other necessary supplies at home and have a written list of the proper supplies. It is also advisable to instruct the parents in cardiopulmonary resuscitation.

The general indications for tracheotomy are included in Table 92-1 and include (1) obstruction of the upper airway, (2) prolonged mechanical ventilation, and (3)

facilitation of suctioning in patients unable to clear their airway secretions (such as patients with chronic aspiration or poor cough mechanism).

TECHNIQUE

Tracheotomy is the creation of a temporary opening in the trachea with maintenance of the normal continuity between the hypopharynx and glottis (Fig. 92-1). In contrast, tracheostomy is the surgical creation of a permanent opening by fashioning skin flaps to connect the neck skin to the tracheal mucosa.

If tracheotomy is the preferred method for securing the airway, first the child should be intubated with either an endotracheal tube or a rigid bronchoscope, and then the tracheotomy should be performed over the indwelling tube. The most important consideration is repetitive identification of the trachea by palpation as the procedure progresses.

The incision in the tracheal wall should be made vertically (in children) with a knife at a level that places the tube well below the subglottic area and allows the tracheostomy tube to rest on the neck without undue tilting or twisting. In small infants or neonates, the incision may extend as low as the sixth tracheal ring, whereas in larger children the incision is properly placed through tracheal ring three or four. The vertical incision through the trachea needs to be just long enough to admit the tube, and no cartilage is excised. Cautery of the tracheal cartilages must be used judiciously when the tracheal incision is made, in order to avoid cartilage necrosis.

It is helpful to place stay sutures in the tracheal wall at the edges of the incision to retract the cartilage rings when the tube is passed into the trachea. These sutures are then brought out laterally through the incision. They can be left in place during the early postoperative period to help replace the tube, if it is accidentally removed. The tube must be fixed in place with tracheostomy ties around the neck. This may be accomplished by simply tying the tracheostomy tube around the neck with one adult finger

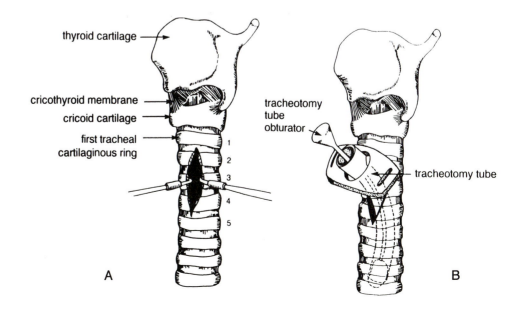

Figure 92-1. Tracheotomy technique. Schematic of the proper midline incision through the tracheal rings (*A*) shows that no cartilage has been removed. Position of the tracheotomy tube during cannulation is shown in *B*. The stylet is removed immediately after placement.

thyroid cartilage

cricothyroid membrane
cricoid cartilage
first tracheal cartilaginous ring

tracheotomy tube obturator

tracheotomy tube

A

B

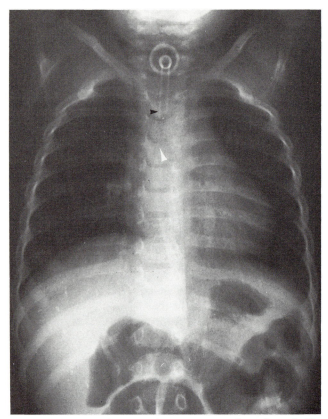

Figure 92–2. Posttracheotomy chest anteroposterior radiograph. The tracheostomy tube should be visible inside the trachea. Also, the clinician must check for any pneumothorax, pneumomediastinum, or significant subcutaneous emphysema (*white arrow,* carina; *black arrow,* distal tip of tracheostomy tube).

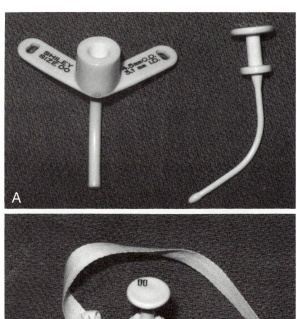

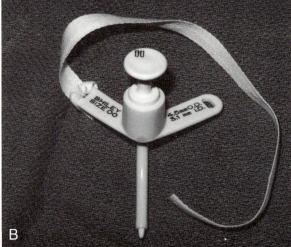

Figure 92–3. One example of a noncuffed 00 tracheostomy tube and stylet (*A*) shows that the stylet's distal end is rounded for atraumatic placement. The proper position of the stylet when the tracheotomy tube is inserted is shown in part *B*. Both tracheostomy ties may be easily secured to the tube before insertion to decrease the manipulation of the tube in the tracheal lumen.

under the tie. Thus when the finger is removed, the ties are snug but do not occlude any major vessel. A postoperative chest radiograph confirms proper positioning of the tip of the tracheostomy tube above the carina and serves to identify a pneumothorax resulting from the procedure (Fig. 92–2).

TRACHEOSTOMY TUBES

The ideal tracheostomy tube is pliable, nonreactive, easy to clean and change, and available in a variety of sizes (Fig. 92–3). The tube size should be smaller than the tracheal lumen, even when assisted ventilation is required. Oversized tubes may traumatize the trachea and lead to stenosis. A properly sized tube can be easily selected by comparing the tracheal lumen to the tracheostomy tube at the time of the procedure (Tables 92–2, 92–3). As a rule, the tracheostomy tube should be large enough to allow the child adequate air movement without traumatizing the tracheal walls. The belief that the largest possible tracheostomy tube is helping the child is unfounded; in reality, the trauma from an oversized tube will lead to tracheal stenosis.

HUMIDIFICATION AND SUCTIONING

Humidification of inspired air is required because the child with a tracheotomy no longer breathes through the nose. Nebulized air should be delivered to the tracheostomy tube via a tracheotomy collar. Secretions must be suctioned from the tube as necessary, which may be as frequently as once an hour at first. Temporarily removing the inner cannula during suctioning allows for a larger-diameter endotracheal catheter to be used. Several milliliters of saline may be instilled into the tracheostomy tube to thin the secretions before suctioning. The catheter should then be gently but quickly threaded through the tracheotomy into the trachea until resistance is met. Next, the thumb occludes the catheter's side port, and the catheter is slowly rotated and pulled out of the trachea and tube (this should require just a few seconds). The patient will cough and experience tachypnea; consequently, short rest periods should interrupt the suctioning. The episodic suctioning should be continued until the secretions are removed.

CLEANING AND CHANGING THE TUBE

The tube should not be changed for the first time until at least the third postoperative day. This is done in the hospital by the surgeon who performed the tracheotomy.

Table 92–2. APPROXIMATE SIZE OF ENDOTRACHEAL AND TRACHEOTOMY TUBES FOR INFANTS AND CHILDREN (BASED ON OUTER DIAMETER OR CIRCUMFERENCE [FRENCH NO.])

	Endotracheal*	Shiley	Aberdeen	Holinger
Premature	11–13	00		00
Newborn	14	0	3.5	0
Newborn–3 mos.	15–16	0	3.5	1
3–10 mos.	17	1	4.0	2
10–12 mos.	18	2	4.5	3
13–24 mos.	20	3	5.0	3
2–3 yrs.	22	4	5.0	4
4–5 yrs.	24	4	5.0	4
6–7 yrs.	26	4	5.0	4
8–9 yrs.	28	4	6.0	5
10–11 yrs.	30	6	6.0	6
12 and over	32	6	7.0	6

From Stool SE, Eavey R: Tracheotomy. In Bluestone CD, Stool SE (eds): Pediatric Otolaryngology, p. 1325. Philadelphia: WB Saunders, 1990.

*Usually a larger-size tracheotomy than an endotracheal tube may be used because the trachea is larger than the subglottic region. The outer diameter or circumference will determine the size tube that may be used.

A tube that is removed before that time can be very difficult to replace. The tube may be changed from daily to every 3 days.

Changing a tracheostomy tube is an easy procedure that must be learned by everyone caring for the child, including the family. The parents should exhibit an obvious competence and understanding of tracheostomy care before the child is discharged from the hospital. The tracheostomy site should be cleaned at least twice a day to minimize any chronic granulation tissue formation; the site may be cleaned with half-strength hydrogen peroxide on cotton applicators and gauze. Scissors and a clean tracheostomy tube should be kept by the patient at all times for emergency changing. The spare tracheostomy tubes are easily cleaned with pipe cleaners and gauze for the lumen and soap and water for the outside surfaces. The tubes may also be sterilized in boiling water as needed.

Ruben and colleagues[1] showed that a coordinated effort among otolaryngologists, pediatricians, nurses, and social workers drastically decreases postdischarge complications in patients with tracheotomies. First, the fatality rate of pediatric tracheotomy patients was significantly reduced to 0.13 deaths per 100 months of tracheotomy home care. Second, the time from tracheotomy to actual hospital discharge, if no other medical or social problems intervened, was reduced to as little as 2 weeks. Follow-up of a child with a tracheotomy should include examination with a fiberoptic bronchoscope to determine the health of the trachea and to rule out the presence of an impending tracheoinnominate artery fistula.

DECANNULATION

Decannulation is usually easy if the child has a normal airway. First, laryngoscopy and bronchoscopy are performed to evaluate the condition of the airway and feasibility of decannulation. Often the granulation tissue that forms at the superior aspect of the tracheotomy site makes decannulation difficult; this granulomatous tissue should be removed endoscopically. The weaning process begins at home with occlusion of the tube for successively longer periods of time. Smaller sized tracheostomy tubes should be used during the weaning period because they increase the cross-sectional area available for airflow to the nose and mouth. It must be remembered that occluding the tracheotomy adds the larynx, pharynx, and oral-nasal cavity to the airway, and so respiratory dead space and airway resistance increase accordingly. Every patient must

Table 92–3. APPROXIMATE GAUGE EQUIVALENTS FREQUENTLY USED IN ENDOTRACHEAL AND TRACHEOTOMY TUBES (BASED ON NEAREST INNER DIAMETER MEASUREMENT)

Endotracheal*			Shiley†				Aberdeen‡			Holinger§			
ID	OD	FR	ID	OD	FR	Size	ID	OD	FR	ID	OD	FR	Size
2.0	2.9	8											
2.5	3.5	10								2.5	4.0	13	00
3.0	4.2	12	3.1	4.5	14	00				3.5	5.0	15	0
3.5	4.9	15	3.4	5.0	15	0	3.5	5.0	15	3.5	5.5	17	1
4.0	5.5	16	3.7	5.5	17	1	4.0	6.7	20	4.0	6.0	18	2
4.5	6.1	18	4.1	6.0	18	2	4.5	6.7	20	4.5	7.0	21	3
5.0	6.8	20	4.8	7.0	21	3	5.0	7.3	22	5.0	8.0	25	4
5.5	7.4	22	5.0	8.5	26	4				5.5	9.0	27	5
6.0	8.0	24					6.0	8.7	26	6.0	10.0	30	6
6.5	8.7	26											
7.0	9.5	29	7.0	10.0	30	6	7.0	10.7	32				
7.5	10.0	30											
8.0	10.7	32											

From Stool SE, Eavey R: Tracheotomy. In Bluestone CD, Stool SE (eds): Pediatric Otolaryngology, p. 1325. Philadelphia: WB Saunders, 1990.

*The endotracheal tubes are marked with the internal diameter, usually with the outer diameter, and with the length.

†The Shiley tube is manufactured by Shiley Laboratories, Irvine, CA. The tube is stamped with the size and inner and outer diameters. The larger sizes are supplied with a low-pressure cuff.

‡This tube is the Aberdeen design, known also as the Great Ormond Street Tube. It is manufactured by J.G. Franklin & Sons, Ltd., High Wycombe, England. The tube is stamped with the inner diameter.

§The Holinger design is manufactured by several companies; therefore, the sizes may vary, and the internal diameter may show considerable variation. These measurements were made on tubes produced by the Pilling Company, Fort Washington, PA.

∥The French number is obtained by multiplying the outside diameter in millimeters by 3.

Table 92-4. COMPLICATIONS OF TRACHEOTOMY

Early
Hemorrhage
Accidental decannulation
Pneumomediastinum, pneumothorax, subcutaneous emphysema
Mucus plugging
Tracheitis
Chondritis of tracheal cartilage ring
Mediastinitis
Dysphagia, aspiration
Pulmonary edema

Delayed
Granulation tissue in lumen or at stoma
Stoma stenosis
Tracheoinnominate artery fistula
Mucus plugging
Tracheitis
Tracheal stenosis
Tracheoesophageal fistula
Scar after decannulation
Dysphagia, aspiration

tolerate total occlusion of the tracheostomy tube for 24 h to be considered for decannulation. It has been suggested that a child may become psychologically dependent on the tracheotomy and will avoid any cannula pluggings.[3] In the authors' experience, the majority of decannulation failures are caused by persistent airway obstruction and not psychologic dependence.

COMPLICATIONS OF TRACHEOTOMY

Mucus plugging, inadvertent decannulation, hemorrhage, pneumothorax, wound infection, tracheitis or bronchitis, and pneumonia can complicate the early post-operative period (Table 92–4).[2] Mortality is uncommon but is seen more often in patients under 1 year of age. The most common problem is mucus plugging, which can be greatly decreased by providing humidified air by tracheotomy collar, frequent endotracheal suctioning, and cleaning of the tube. When suctioning fails to clear a tube partially obstructed by mucus, the tube should be changed immediately. The parents must be thoroughly instructed to recognize the signs of mucus plugging: retractions, agitation progressing to inactivity, cyanosis, and flaring of the alae nasi. Inadvertent decannulation should not happen if the tracheostomy tube is properly secured by ties and if no tension is placed on the tracheostomy tube. The avoidance of tension on the tracheostomy tube cannot be overemphasized.

On occasion, pulmonary edema develops in a child with prolonged severe upper airway obstruction soon after either a tracheotomy or intubation.[4] This is thought to be caused by abrupt changes in the distribution of pulmonary blood flow.

Tracheal stenosis can occur either at the tracheotomy site or near the tip of the tracheostomy tube. This begins with trauma to the mucosa with exposure of cartilage and progresses to chondritis with ultimate loss of cartilage and cicatricial narrowing of the trachea. Tracheal stenosis can be difficult to treat. Proper tracheotomy technique, tracheostomy tube size, and care of the tracheostomy tube help avoid this complication.

TRACHEAL GRANULATION TISSUE FORMATION

The presence of a tracheostomy tube often causes granulation tissue to grow around the tube both outside on the neck and inside the tracheal lumen. External granulation

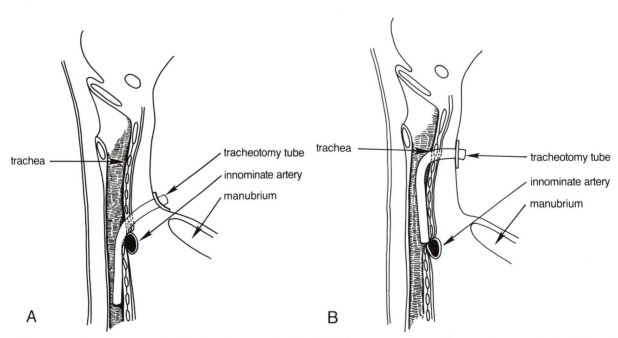

Figure 92-4. Tracheoinnominate artery fistulas. A tracheotomy placed too inferiorly may cause the tracheotomy tube to erode directly through the innominate artery (*A*). The end of the tracheotomy tube may also rub directly on the innominate artery (*B*).

tissue formation can be minimized by thorough cleaning of the neck several times a day and, when necessary, can be easily managed by cautery with silver nitrate. Large amounts of granulation tissue inside the tracheal lumen can be the cause of delayed decannulation because the mass of abnormal tissue obstructs the lumen when the tube is removed. Fenestrated tubes should be avoided because the sharp edges of the fenestration tend to traumatize the superior edge of the tracheotomy and can induce profuse amounts of granulation tissue within the trachea. It is frequently necessary to examine the trachea of children who are ready for decannulation while they are under anesthesia in order to remove granulation tissue.

TRACHEOINNOMINATE ARTERY FISTULA

After the tracheotomy tract has healed, any blood seen in or around the tracheostomy tube should prompt immediate examination. The trachea must be examined with the fiberoptic bronchoscope to rule out an impending tracheoinnominate artery fistula. Granulation tissue within the tract is usually the source of bleeding; however,

granulation tissue on the anterior wall of the trachea suggests the possibility of a tracheoinnominate fistula (Fig. 92-4). Rupture of a tracheoinnominate fistula causes profuse and often fatal bleeding into the trachea and lungs. If a tracheoinnominate fistula does occur, it is possible to control the bleeding temporarily by placing a cuffed endotracheal tube through the tracheotomy site and inflating the cuff to tamponade the artery. Thoracotomy and ligation of the innominate artery are then performed immediately in the operating room.

REFERENCES

1. Ruben RJ, Newton L, Tornsay D, et al: Home care of the pediatric patient with a tracheotomy. Ann Otol Rhinol Laryngol 91:633–640, 1982.
2. Neal GD, Gates G: Complications of tracheostomy and intubation. *In* Johns ME (ed): Complications in Otolaryngology—Head and Neck Surgery: Volume 2. Head and Neck, pp. 103–109. Toronto: BC Decker, 1986.
3. Elliot CH, Olson RA: Variations in conditioning procedures for the decannulation of tracheostomy dependent children: Clinical and theoretical implications. Health Psychol 1:389–397, 1982.
4. Galvis AG, Stool SE, Bluestone CD: Pulmonary edema following relief of acute upper airway obstruction. Ann Otol Rhinol Laryngol 89:124–128, 1980.

93 OXYGEN THERAPY
LUCILLE A. LESTER, M.D.

Oxygen therapy in children, as in adults, is indicated for the reversal of hypoxemia and the prevention of major complications associated with tissue hypoxia. The administration of oxygen to infants and children has changed from an empiric therapy of limited scope to a wide range of techniques for supporting oxygenation that have a sound clinical as well as scientific basis.[1] The efficacy and safety of short-term (acute) and long-term (chronic) oxygen therapy have been significantly improved by the realization that oxygen, like any drug, should be administered in a prescribed dose and with objective monitoring of its effects and possible toxicity. Technologic advances in the 1980s resulted in the development of simple and accurate noninvasive methods of monitoring oxygen use, particularly in infants, and should lead to decreases in complications and toxicity (an improved risk/benefit ratio).

In this overview of oxygen therapy, consideration is given first to the normal physiologic processes of gas exchange and oxygenation in children, particularly as to how they differ from those in adults, and to the pathophysiologic processes of hypoxia. Specifics of oxygen therapy in various commonly encountered respiratory disor-

ders in children are then discussed. Emphasis is placed on understanding the mechanism of hypoxia in each of the conditions as a basis for a rational approach to treatment with oxygen. Oxygen delivery systems, monitoring methods, and prevention of toxicity are also discussed, and a separate section on the topic of cor pulmonale associated with childhood respiratory problems is included.

GAS EXCHANGE PROPERTIES OF THE LUNG IN NORMAL CHILDREN

The rational use of oxygen therapy is based on a thorough understanding of the respiratory physiologic processes of gas exchange and oxygen transport.

The principal function of the lung is to perform gas exchange, to replenish the blood with oxygen, and to eliminate carbon dioxide. Pulmonary gas exchange is accomplished by a number of processes:

1. Ventilation, which includes both the volume and the distribution of air ventilating the alveoli.

2. Diffusion, by which oxygen and carbon dioxide move across alveolar-capillary membranes.

3. Pulmonary-capillary blood flow, which must be adequate in volume and distributed evenly to all ventilated alveoli.[2]

The efficacy of gas exchange that takes place in any lung unit is determined by the ratio of ventilation ($\dot{V}$) to perfusion ($\dot{Q}$), and the $\dot{V}/\dot{Q}$ "mismatch," or inequality, is the most common cause of hypoxemia and hypercapnia.[3]

The growing and developing lungs of an infant or a child have certain anatomic characteristics that render them uniquely susceptible to certain types of $\dot{V}/\dot{Q}$ inequalities and thus to hypoxemia. The pattern of conducting airway branching is complete at 16 weeks of gestation, and that of respiratory airway branching is complete at birth, but the linear dimensions of the airways grow as the lungs enlarge.[4] Before the age of 5 years, peripheral airways are smaller and account for a larger fraction of total airway resistance.[5] Infections or other processes such as asthma that result in airway obstruction are functionally more significant and reduce ventilation proportionally more in young children than in adults, in whom extensive disease of the small airways may go undetected.[6] Reduced collateral ventilation in infancy contributes to an increased tendency for atelectasis when airways become obstructed; reduced elastic recoil and a more compliant chest wall may also adversely affect the ventilatory component of the $\dot{V}/\dot{Q}$ relationship in infants. Responsiveness of the pulmonary vasculature to hypoxia undergoes a maturation process that permits better matching of perfusion to uneven ventilation in older children and adults than in infants.[6]

Lung injury affects airway growth and alveolar and vascular development; the final physiologic outcome is determined at least in part by how early in development the lung injury occurs. Normal lung growth occurs both by increase in alveolar number and by increase in alveolar volume until the ages of 8 to 12 years.[4] Compensatory lung growth proceeds in a similar manner after loss of lung tissue either from surgical resection or from extensive parenchymal lung damage caused by certain infections. The degree of compensation depends on the age at which the lung injury occurred and, in certain disease processes such as cystic fibrosis, on the efficacy of early intervention and treatment. Both injury and compensatory lung growth affect ventilation and perfusion and thus affect the development of as well as the ability to compensate for hypoxemia.

OXYGEN TRANSPORT

DISSOLVED VERSUS COMBINED OXYGEN

The essential components of the oxygen supply system *(in vivo)* are pulmonary gas exchange, blood flow, hemoglobin concentration, and hemoglobin affinity for oxygen.[7] After gas exchange takes place, oxygen diffuses from alveoli into pulmonary capillary blood, and this process proceeds as long as the partial pressure of oxygen in the

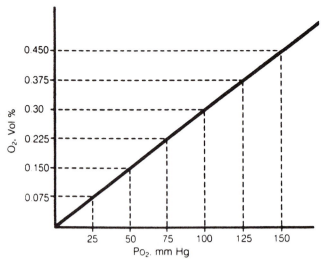

Figure 93–1. Linear relationship between the amount (vol %) of dissolved oxygen (O_2) in plasma and the corresponding partial pressure of oxygen (P_{O_2}); 0.3 vol % of oxygen dissolved in the plasma exerts a P_{O_2} of 100 mm Hg. (From Youtsey JW: Oxygen and mixed gas therapy. *In* Barnes IA, Libson A [eds]: Respiratory Care Practice, p. 132. Chicago: Year Book Medical, 1988.)

alveoli is higher than that in the blood. Oxygen molecules are then transported in the blood as dissolved oxygen and as oxygen that is physically bound to hemoglobin in red blood cells.[8] For every 760 mm Hg, 2.3 vol % of oxygen (1 ml of oxygen per 100 ml of blood) is dissolved in the plasma. There is a linear relationship between the amount of dissolved oxygen and the corresponding partial pressure of arterial oxygen (Pa_{O_2}). From a display of this relationship in Figure 93–1, it can be seen that at a Pa_{O_2} of 100 mm Hg, only 0.3 vol % of oxygen is present as dissolved oxygen. If this represented the total oxygen carrying capacity of the blood, the cardiac output would have to be inordinately large to enable normal oxygen consumption.

Because 1 g of hemoglobin is capable of combining with 1.34 ml of oxygen, 40 to 70 times more oxygen is carried by hemoglobin than by plasma, and the body can maintain normal oxygen uptake at a reasonable cardiac output (5.5 l/min in adults at rest). With a hemoglobin concentration of 15 gs, 1.34 × 15 g/dl, or 20.1 vol %, of oxygen can be bound to hemoglobin.[9]

OXYHEMOGLOBIN DISSOCIATION CURVE

Oxygen has the ability to chemically combine with hemoglobin (Hb) and form oxyhemoglobin (HbO$_2$). This reaction can be illustrated as

$$Hb + O_2 \rightleftharpoons HbO_2.$$

This reaction can move in both directions; when conditions favor the rightward movement of the reaction, hemoglobin binds with oxygen, as observed in the lung alveoli; when the reaction moves to the left, oxygen is released from the oxyhemoglobin molecule as occurs at the tissue level.

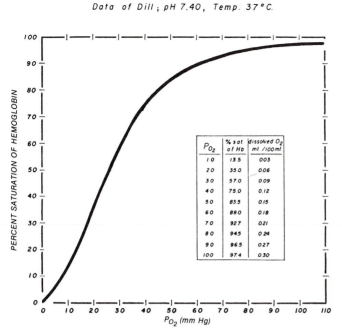

Data of Dill ; pH 7.40, Temp. 37°C.

Figure 93–2. Oxygen-hemoglobin dissociation curve. *Inset,* chart of specific O_2 saturation values with corresponding P_{O_2} and dissolved O_2. (From Comroe JH, Forster RE, Dubois AB: The Lung: Clinical Physiology and Pulmonary Function Tests, p. 142. Chicago: Year Book Medical, 1962.)

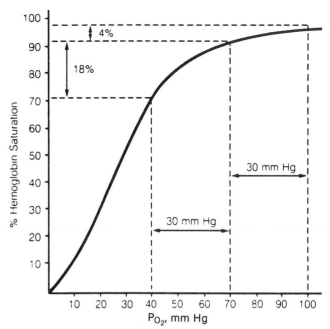

Figure 93–3. The effect of the steep portion of the oxyhemoglobin dissociation curve on equal changes in the arterial oxygen pressure (Pa_{O_2}) and resultant percentage hemoglobin saturation. Between Pa_{O_2} levels of 70 and 100 mm Hg, the change in percentage hemoglobin saturation is 4%. Between Pa_{O_2} levels of 40 and 70 mm Hg, the change in percentage hemoglobin saturation is 18%. (From Youtsey JW: Oxygen and mixed gas therapy. *In* Barnes IA, Libson A [eds]: Respiratory Care Practice, p. 132. Chicago: Year Book Medical, 1988.)

A given hemoglobin molecule can combine with more than one molecule of oxygen and can become saturated with oxygen.[8] The oxygen content or percentage saturation of hemoglobin is dependent on Pa_{O_2}; this relationship is not linear, as in the case of dissolved oxygen (see Fig. 93–1). The relationship between Pa_{O_2} and percentage of arterial oxygen saturation (Sa_{O_2}) is expressed as the oxyhemoglobin dissociation curve (Fig. 93–2). This S-shaped curve has a very steep slope between 10 and 30 mm Hg of Pa_{O_2} and is very flat between 70 and 100 mm Hg of Pa_{O_2}. A number of clinically significant facts are evident from this curve:

1. The steep slope up to 50 mm Hg of Pa_{O_2} implies that large amounts of oxygen can be released from hemoglobin with small changes in Pa_{O_2}.

2. If Pa_{O_2} decreases from 100 to 80 mm Hg as the result of cardiac or pulmonary disease, arterial blood hemoglobin continues to be saturated at 94.5%, and tissue hypoxia does not result.[10]

3. Although a 30–mm Hg decrease in Pa_{O_2} has very little effect on the curve between 70 and 100 mm Hg of Pa_{O_2} the same 30–mm Hg decrease between 70 and 40 mm Hg of Pa_{O_2} has a marked effect on the oxygen content and saturation (Fig. 93–3).

4. As Pa_{O_2} falls below 70 mm Hg, major changes in Sa_{O_2} occur with relatively little change in Pa_{O_2}, and in this lower Pa_{O_2} range, the measurement of saturation may be a more reliable measurement of oxygenation. Above 70 mm Hg of Pa_{O_2} (represented by the flat part of the curve), Sa_{O_2} changes little (83% to 98%), whereas Pa_{O_2} varies from 70 to 100 mm Hg. Pa_{O_2} may be the most accurate measure of oxygenation in this range.[11] In view of the widespread use of noninvasive oximetry to measure Sa_{O_2}, the latter

recommendation is less practical, but the clinician must be aware of this Pa_{O_2}–Sa_{O_2} relationship in order to interpret the significance of Sa_{O_2} readings.

It is important to realize that the amount of oxygen available to the tissue varies significantly with the hemoglobin level. If Pa_{O_2} is 70 and Sa_{O_2} is 93%, the oxygen content at a hemoglobin level of 10 g would be 12.5 vol %, as opposed to 18.7 vol % at a hemoglobin level of 15 g or 24.9 vol % with a hemoglobin level of 20 g.

The oxyhemoglobin dissociation curve is also dynamic in that it can shift to the left or right under certain circumstances. Acidosis (decreased pH), increase in temperature, or increase in arterial carbon dioxide tension (Bohr effect) or the increase in erythrocyte concentration of D-2,3-diphosphoglycerate (2,3-DPG) that occurs with certain anemias shifts the curve to the right.[12] This results in a *decrease* in the affinity of hemoglobin for oxygen, and therefore more oxygen is available to the tissues. The reverse process—an increase in affinity of the hemoglobin for oxygen and less oxygen available to the tissues—occurs with alkalosis, decreased arterial carbon dioxide tension, decreased temperature, and decreased level of 2,3-DPG, all of which shift the curve to the left (Fig. 93–4).

TOTAL AVAILABILITY OF OXYGEN

Oxygen carried in blood, either dissolved or bound to hemoglobin, must be delivered to the tissues for use. Factors involved in oxygen delivery include the following:

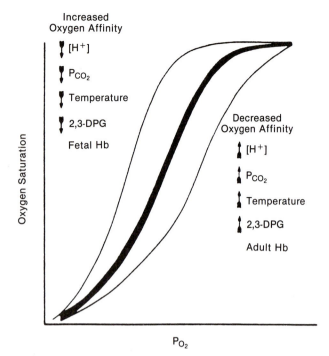

Figure 93–4. Factors affecting hemoglobin-oxygen affinity. P_{CO_2}, partial pressure of carbon dioxide; 2,3-DPG, 2,3-diphosphoglycerate. (From Hay WW: Physiology of oxygenation and its relation to pulse oximetry in neonates. J Perinatol 7:309–319, 1987.)

Table 93–1. NORMAL OXYGEN VALUES FOR ARTERIAL AND VENOUS BLOOD*

Measurement	Arterial Blood	Venous Blood	Difference
PO_2 (mm Hg)	100	40	60
O_2 saturation (%)	97	75	22
O_2 Hb (volume %)	19.5	15.1	4.4
O_2 dissolved in plasma (volume %)	0.3	0.12	0.18
O_2 content (volume %)	19.8	15.2	4.6

Modified from Burgess WR, Chernick V: Respiratory Therapy in Newborns, Infants and Children, pp. 30–58. New York: Thieme Medical Publishers, 1982.
PO_2, oxygen pressure; Hb, hemoglobin.
*Assumed Hb concentration is 15 g/dl.

1. Adequate cardiac output (dependent on cardiac function, volume status, and heart rate).
2. Adequate amount of hemoglobin.
3. Adequate saturation of hemoglobin.
4. Appropriate temperature, pH, and 2,3-DPG levels so that oxygen may be unloaded from hemoglobin.[13]

Oxygen transport can be mathematically represented as the product of cardiac output and arterial oxygen content (Ca_{O_2}). Normal tissue oxygen consumption (extraction) is about 250 ml/min, and at normal cardiac output and normal Ca_{O_2} levels, there is a significant safety margin—that is, a larger amount of oxygen delivered to tissues than is needed. If cardiac output decreases, the tissues respond by increasing oxygen extraction from the blood.

MIXED VENOUS OXYGEN CONTENT

The oxygen saturation of mixed venous blood, or the venous oxygen content ($C\overline{v}_{O_2}$), is believed by many investigators to provide the best clinical measure of delivery of oxygen to and consumption of oxygen by the tissues.[1] Ca_{O_2} determines the amount of oxygen available to be delivered to tissues, whereas $C\overline{v}_{O_2}$ indicates the amount of oxygen left in blood leaving the tissues. The difference between arterial and venous oxygen content is a measure of oxygen usage at a given time. The mean value for mixed venous oxygen tension is 39 mm Hg ± 3.4, and the value declines minimally with age.[14] A true mixed venous sample is best obtained from the pulmonary artery; this technique, however, is rarely practical except for patients in intensive care units (ICUs) who have Swan-Ganz catheters in place. A sample from the superior vena cava is an adequate representation of blood from the pulmonary artery in normal persons (children without intracardiac defects). Although regarded by many investigators as the best reflection of tissue hypoxia, the clinical usefulness of venous oxygen tension in pediatrics appears limited outside of selected ICU situations. Table 93–1 is a useful summary of normal values for all oxygen parameters of arterial and venous blood that have been discussed in this section.

PATHOPHYSIOLOGY OF HYPOXIA

HYPOXEMIA VERSUS HYPOXIA

Hypoxemia is defined as the reduction in the level of oxygen in arterial blood, whereas hypoxia is a reduction in the amount of oxygen delivered to the tissues to meet the metabolic needs of the body.[15] The terms are often used interchangeably because of the difficulty in measuring tissue oxygenation. Hypoxemia is defined as reduced values for Pa_{O_2}, Ca_{O_2}, or Sa_{O_2} and is the primary clinical indication for oxygen therapy. Hypoxia, or inadequate tissue oxygenation, is what physicians attempt to prevent by instituting oxygen therapy. Hypoxemia generally implies hypoxia at the cellular level, but in situations such as anemia or hypotension, tissue hypoxia may exist despite normal Pa_{O_2} levels.

TYPES OF HYPOXIA

It is generally useful to classify or distinguish four types of hypoxia:

1. *Hypoxic (anoxic) hypoxia* is caused by a problem of gas exchange in the lung. Such problems include ventilation/perfusion ($\dot{V}/\dot{Q}$) mismatch, decreased oxygen concentration of inspired air secondary to decreased fraction of inspired oxygen ($F_{I_{O_2}}$) or to high altitude, and alteration in diffusion at the alveolar-capillary membrane. Oxygen therapy alleviates or reverses this type of hypoxia.
2. *Anemic hypoxia* is caused by reduced oxygen-carrying capacity of the blood secondary to blood loss, decreased red blood cell production, abnormal types of hemoglobin, or carbon monoxide poisoning. In the case

Table 93–2. CLASSIFICATION OF HYPOXIA

Type	Pathology	Causes	Pa_{O_2}	Sa_{O_2}	Sv_{O_2}	Beneficial Effect of O_2
Hypoxic	↓ gas exchange in the lung	Hypoventilation V̇/Q̇ mismatch Shunt ↓ FI_{O_2} High altitude Diffusion defect	↓	↓	↓	Yes
Anemic	↓ O_2 carrying capacity	Blood loss Anemia Abnormal hemoglobin CO poisoning	Normal	Normal	↓	No (100% O_2 given in CO poisoning)
Circulatory	↓ blood flow	Congestive failure Hypotension, shock, ↓ cardiac output Cardiac arrest	↓	↓	↓	No (often used supportively)
Histotoxic	↓ O_2 use	Cyanide poisoning	Normal	Normal	↑	No

Pa_{O_2}, arterial oxygen pressure; Sa_{O_2}, arterial oxygen saturation; Sv_{O_2}, venous oxygen saturation; V̇/Q̇, ventilation/perfusion; FI_{O_2}, fraction of inspired oxygen.

of carbon monoxide poisoning, administration of 100% oxygen increases the speed at which carbon monoxide is eliminated; otherwise, oxygen therapy is not useful for this type of hypoxia because the oxygen-carrying capacity is low and additional oxygen is not supplied to the tissues.

3. *Circulatory hypoxia* is hypoxia secondary to reduced blood flow, as seen in congestive heart failure, cardiac arrest, or severe hypotension with resultant decreased cardiac output. Oxygen therapy, although given as supportive therapy, is not helpful because arterial blood is already fully saturated.

4. *Histotoxic hypoxia* is caused by inability of tissues to use oxygen that is delivered to them. Cyanide poisoning that inhibits cellular respiration is an example of this type of hypoxia, and it is not alleviated by oxygen administration because arterial blood is fully saturated.[11]

Table 93–2 summarizes the types of hypoxia, effect on oxygen values, and effect of oxygen treatment.

CAUSES OF HYPOXIA

Alveolar Hypoventilation. Hypoventilating while breathing room air always results in hypoxemia and hypercapnia; the relationship between degree of hypoventilation and level of arterial carbon dioxide tension (Pa_{CO_2}) is almost linear.[15] Hypoventilation can be the result of decreased alveolar ventilation or an increase in physiologic dead space.[8] Clinical problems in hypoventilation include depression of the respiratory center by drugs or by disease of the central nervous system, apnea in premature infants, conditions resulting in restriction of lung expansion such as musculoskeletal problems (congenital or acquired), obesity, pneumothorax, pleural effusion, and pulmonary fibrosis. Oxygen relieves hypoxia in these conditions, but normal ventilation must also be restored.

Ventilation/Perfusion Abnormalities. The 20 million alveoli in a newborn and the 300 million in an adult do not all receive the same ventilation or the same perfusion at any given time. The distribution of alveolar ventilation (V̇) and perfusion (Q̇) is uneven in the normal upright lung because of gravity and changes in hydrostatic and transmural pressures in the lung.[15] The mean value for ratio of alveolar ventilation to blood flow in adults is 0.8, and although absolute values for ventilation and perfusion are different in children, the ratio appears to hold true. Gas exchange units in the lung can be of four possible types (Fig. 93–5):

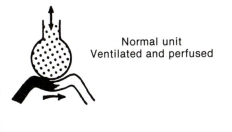
Normal unit
Ventilated and perfused

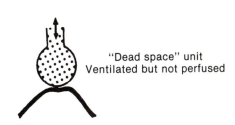
"Dead space" unit
Ventilated but not perfused

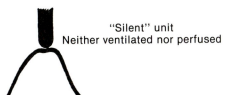
"Silent" unit
Neither ventilated nor perfused

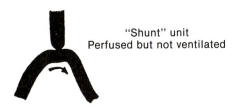
"Shunt" unit
Perfused but not ventilated

Figure 93–5. Gas exchange units of the lung (schema). (From Bendixen HH, Egbert LD, Hedley-Whyte J, et al: Respiratory Care, p. 7. St. Louis: CV Mosby, 1965.)

1. Normal units (ventilated and perfused).
2. "Silent" units (neither ventilated nor perfused).
2. "Dead space" units (ventilated but not perfused).
4. "Shunt" units (perfused but not ventilated).[16]

There is a normal distribution of all types of units in normal lungs, and pulmonary disorders that can affect ventilation, perfusion, or both result in $\dot{V}/\dot{Q}$ mismatches that fall somewhere between the extremes of dead space and shunt.

Dead space that produces disorders such as acute pulmonary emboli or pulmonary vasoconstriction results in an increased $\dot{V}/\dot{Q}$ ratio because of normal ventilation with decreased perfusion. These problems are less common in children in whom shunt-producing disorders such as asthma, atelectasis, pneumonia, cystic fibrosis (CF) or bronchopulmonary dysplasia (BPD) result in decreased ventilation with normal perfusion, or a decreased $\dot{V}/\dot{Q}$ ratio. In any type of lung disease, particularly CF or BPD, it is likely that many degrees of dead space and shunt exist simultaneously. The hypoxemia caused by $\dot{V}/\dot{Q}$ abnormalities is usually relieved by oxygen therapy; however, the hypoxemia in certain shunt-producing disorders such as atelectasis, pulmonary edema, pneumonia, and pneumothorax is not completely reversed until the efficiency of ventilation is also improved.

Arteriovenous Shunts. In the normal lung, a small amount of venous blood bypasses the ventilated lung and mixes with arterial blood, resulting in a shunt. Shunted blood in this situation comes from bronchial veins and in part from the thebesian veins from the myocardium, which drain into the left side of the heart. One to two percent of normal cardiac output constitutes the normal or physiologic shunt and results in a decrease in oxygen tension (Pa_{O_2}) of 5 mm Hg when room air is breathed.[15] If venous blood passes from the right side of the heart to the left without being exposed to ventilated alveoli, such as occurs in cyanotic congenital heart disease or in pulmonary arteriovenous malformations, the resultant shunt may be very large.[17] Although venous admixture can result from $\dot{V}/\dot{Q}$ abnormalities as well as from shunts, the hypoxemia resulting from $\dot{V}/\dot{Q}$ abnormalities disappears with oxygen administration (and ventilation improves in some cases), but hypoxemia caused by a true shunt does not. This observation forms the basis of the simple alveolar-arterial (A-a) gradient test that is recommended in the evaluation of cyanotic newborns and older patients in whom cyanosis appears to be unresponsive to oxygen administration. The procedure involves the patient's breathing 100% oxygen for 15 to 20 min and then the clinician's determining the Pa_{O_2}. With a low $\dot{V}/\dot{Q}$ ratio (indicative of a pulmonary problem), all of the nitrogen is eventually washed out of alveoli, and the arterial blood reaches full oxygenation, regardless of how poorly ventilated certain alveoli are in terms of blood flow. This should result in a Pa_{O_2} of 550 to 600 mm Hg. If venous blood is never exposed to alveolar oxygen (as in cardiac right-to-left shunts), breathing 100% oxygen does not raise the Pa_{O_2} to this level. The estimate of 550 to 600 mm Hg is calculated as follows: When $F_{I_{O_2}} = 1.0$,

$$PA_{O_2} = P_B - P_{H_2O} - PA_{CO_2}$$
$$= 760 - 47 - 40 \text{ mm Hg}$$
$$= 673 \text{ mm Hg},$$

where P_B = barometric pressure and P_{H_2O} = partial pressure of water.

Allowing for a normal physiologic shunt of 3% to 5% allows for an A-a gradient of 100 to 125 mm Hg at an $F_{I_{O_2}}$ of 1.0. Because alveolar oxygen pressure (PA_{O_2}) − A-a gradient = expected Pa_{O_2}, 673 − (100 to 125) = expected Pa_{O_2} of 548 to 573 mm Hg.[8]

If the Pa_{O_2} is less than 550 mm Hg or if the A-a gradient > 100 to 125 mm Hg at an $F_{I_{O_2}}$ of 1.0, a clinically significant shunt is present. It is possible to calculate magnitude of percentage of a shunt by determining Pa_{O_2} at a known $F_{I_{O_2}}$. Table 93–3 summarizes these shunt estimates.

Diffusion Defects. Hypoxemia may be caused by a defect in the normal rate of gas exchange across the alveolar-capillary membrane. Pulmonary edema widens the diffusion pathway, and the rate of gas transfer is reduced because of intra-alveolar and interstitial fluid. In conditions such as radiation pneumonitis or interstitial fibrosis, the alveolar wall becomes thickened and less gas permeable. Although reduced diffusion capacity can be measured by pulmonary function testing, hypoxemia in these disorders is thought to be caused primarily by an associated $\dot{V}/\dot{Q}$ mismatch.[3] Oxygen administration is beneficial in these disorders and is often required chronically.

Although the categorization of causes of hypoxia is useful for an understanding of the pathophysiologic processes and treatment of various disease states, two important facts must be recognized:

1. Disease processes that cause hypoxemia frequently occur simultaneously with other conditions that result in tissue hypoxia, particularly in critically ill children. For example, a child with pneumonia may be febrile, anemic, and hypotensive and exhibit a decrease in cardiac output secondary to sepsis. Each condition leads to more hypoxia.
2. Oxygen alone is rarely definitive treatment. It is supportive and must be used in conjunction with other definitive treatments, such as improving ventilation, treating infection, supporting blood pressure, and restoring blood volume and hemoglobin concentration as needed.

SIGNS AND SYMPTOMS OF HYPOXIA

Central and peripheral chemoreceptors are sensitive to changes in the levels of carbon dioxide and oxygen in the

Table 93–3. SHUNT ESTIMATE FROM ARTERIAL OXYGEN PRESSURE* AT VARIOUS $F_{I_{O_2}}$ LEVELS†

$F_{I_{O_2}}$	Shunt Estimate					
	5%	10%	15%	20%	30%	50%
0.21	95	80	65	60	50	42
0.35	150	110	85	65	52	45
0.40	185	180	90	70	60	47
0.60	315	235	160	105	65	52
0.80	460	475	265	180	70	55
1.00	573	475	400	290	100	60

Modified from Braun HA, Cheney FW, Loehnen CP: Introduction to Respiratory Physiology, 2nd ed. Boston: Little, Brown, 1980.
$F_{I_{O_2}}$, fraction of inspired oxygen.
*In millimeters of mercury. †Assuming that hemoglobin concentration ≥ 10 g/dl, arterial carbon dioxide pressure = 25–40 and normal = 5% shunt.

blood, and the oxygen levels (in the carotid and aortic bodies) are very sensitive to reduction in Pa_{O_2}. The onset of hypoxia may result in subtle changes in the patient's condition, and, moreover, such changes may be difficult to separate from the physiologic effects of the disease or disorder causing the hypoxia. Laboratory measurement of Pa_{O_2} quantifies the degree of hypoxemia present, but the degree of hypoxia is less easily determined and varies from organ to organ and from cell to cell. The heart and the brain are organs with high arteriovenous differences in oxygen extraction rate, and although the brain has some oxygen reserve, the heart has very little.[18] Hypoxia stimulates the rate and depth of ventilation (resulting in tachypnea) through stimulation of the aortic and carotid chemoreceptors.[19] Acute hypoxia also initially stimulates heart rate (tachycardia). Worsening or uncorrected hypoxia results in bradycardia, and cardiac arrest may occur. Pa_{O_2} of less than 30 mm Hg ($Sa_{O_2} < 50\%$) may result in hypotension, shock, and loss of consciousness,[20] and vasoconstriction and bronchoconstriction may occur in the lung as Pa_{O_2} decreases.[21] Altered cerebral function, manifested by restlessness, irritability, and headache or euphoria, occurs early in hypoxia, and these symptoms may deteriorate to the point of delirium and coma with progressive cerebral hypoxia.

Cyanosis, a condition in which the skin and mucous membranes turn bluish, is caused by an increase in the amount of reduced (unoxygenated) hemoglobin in the tissue capillaries. Peripheral cyanosis caused by vasoconstriction may be present with normal Pa_{O_2}, such as in newborns, but central cyanosis is always a clinical indication for the use of oxygen. Difficulty is encountered in attempts to correlate the degree of cyanosis with Sa_{O_2}. This difficulty is related at least in part to the fact that clinically evident cyanosis is dependent on the hemoglobin content and the rate of blood flow. Cyanosis is less evident at a hemoglobin level of 10 g than at a hemoglobin level of 15 g and may appear relatively late in patients who can increase blood flow in the presence of hypoxia.[16]

In chronic hypoxemia, numerous compensatory mechanisms may modify the signs and symptoms described earlier that occur with acute onset of hypoxia. In chronic hypoxemia, red blood cells levels of 2,3-DPG increase, shifting the oxyhemoglobin dissociation curve to the right and facilitating release of oxygen to the tissues.[22] Chronic hypoxemia may also be associated with improved tissue oxygen extraction and with increased levels of erythroprotein, which lead to increased production of red blood cells and a greater oxygen-carrying capacity.

OXYGEN THERAPY: DISEASE-SPECIFIC CONSIDERATIONS

ACUTE RESPIRATORY FAILURE

Acute respiratory failure is a term used to describe an acute abnormality of the respiratory system that results in inadequate oxygenation of arterial blood.[13] This situation may result from rapid progression or acute exacerbation of an underlying respiratory disease (asthma, BPD, CF) or it may occur de novo in an otherwise healthy child from overwhelming pulmonary infection, drowning, trauma,

drug overdose, toxic exposures, or massive aspiration. The hallmark of acute respiratory failure is the rapidity of progression, which does not permit compensatory mechanisms to maintain adequate ventilation or respiratory states.[8] The blood gas abnormalities that define acute respiratory failure are Pa_{O_2} of <50 mm Hg, Pa_{CO_2} of >50, and pH of <7.35. Because of differences in treatment and prognosis, some clinicians find it useful to distinguish between (1) type I respiratory failure, characterized by hypoxemia with normal or low arterial carbon dioxide tension (Pa_{CO_2}), and (2) type II respiratory failure, with alveolar hypoventilation ($Pa_{CO_2} > 45$ mm Hg) and pH < 7.35.

Controlled and careful administration of oxygen combined with measures to support ventilation as needed are indicated in type II respiratory failure, whereas oxygen administration may often be adequate treatment of type I respiratory failure. Type I may progress to type II respiratory failure if the cause is not treated expeditiously. Youtsey referred to this progression in terms of early and late respiratory failure, and his useful schema is presented in Figure 93–6.[8] Acute hypoxemia in acute respiratory failure is not generally well tolerated in most children because compensatory mechanisms have not had sufficient time to develop or are inadequate. The initial treatment of acute respiratory failure is supplemental inhaled oxygen. Adequate relief of hypoxemia is achieved with the attainment of Pa_{O_2} of about 60 mm Hg. The effect of a given increment of $F_{I_{O_2}}$ on Pa_{O_2} depends on the distribution of $\dot{V}/\dot{Q}$ within the lung.[3] In units with very low $\dot{V}/\dot{Q}$ ratios (0.05), small increases in $F_{I_{O_2}}$ raise the Pa_{O_2} very little, whereas in units with higher $\dot{V}/\dot{Q}$ ratios (0.10 to 0.20), slight oxygen enrichment promptly improves Pa_{O_2}. In conditions characterized by relatively few low-$\dot{V}/\dot{Q}$ units, such as airway obstructive disorders, small increases of $F_{I_{O_2}}$ rapidly improve Pa_{O_2}.[23]

In both acute and chronic respiratory failure, other measures in addition to administering oxygen must be undertaken to ensure adequate cardiac output and tissue perfusion and to provide a hemoglobin level adequate for oxygen-carrying capacity. If a patient with type II respiratory failure fails to respond to oxygen therapy, and if Pa_{CO_2} continues to rise and acidosis persists, intubation and mechanical ventilation are most often indicated.

NEONATAL RESPIRATORY DISTRESS SYNDROME

At least 60% of infants under 28 weeks of gestational age develop respiratory distress syndrome (RDS).[24] As higher percentages of premature infants cared for in neonatal ICUs weigh less than 1000 g or are born at 24 to 26 weeks of gestation, the incidence of RDS per live births can be expected only to increase. Lung immaturity, specifically the lack of adequate surfactant production, is the overriding causative factor in RDS, although additional risk factors such as maternal diabetes and caesarean birth are also recognized. The inadequate lung surfactant system results in abnormally high surface forces that lead to alveolar collapse and consolidation and, eventually, respiratory failure.[25] Other pathologic features include interstitial and intra-alveolar pulmonary edema and atelecta-

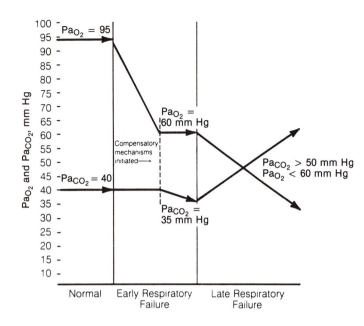

Figure 93-6. The progression of acute respiratory failure. As the Pa_{O_2} falls, compensatory mechanisms—increases in respiratory rate and volume—set in to correct and maintain the Pa_{O_2}. As these mechanisms become no longer able to maintain the blood gas levels, the patient moves into late respiratory failure, which is characterized by increasing arterial carbon dioxide pressure (Pa_{CO_2}) and decreasing Pa_{O_2}. (From Youtsey JW: Oxygen and mixed gas therapy. *In* Barnes IA, Libson A [eds]: Respiratory Care Practice, p. 132. Chicago: Year Book Medical, 1988.)

sis. Pulmonary compliance is greatly reduced, the work of breathing is increased, and hypoxemia is always present. The hypoxemia ($Pa_{O_2} < 45$ to 50 mm Hg) results in direct pulmonary vasoconstriction,[26] which may lead to pulmonary hypoperfusion as well as pulmonary hypertension. The severe hypoxemia is multifactorial. It results from $\dot{V}/\dot{Q}$ mismatch secondary to poor ventilation in many areas of the lung, from intrapulmonary shunting secondary to severe pulmonary hypertension, and at times from right-to-left shunting through a patent ductus arteriosus or a patent foramen ovale.

RDS can be a self-limited disorder if severe hypoxemia is controlled. In infants with mild RDS, administration of oxygen by hood for several days to bring the Pa_{O_2} into the range of 60 to 70 mm Hg may be all the specific therapy that is needed. These infants usually exhibit grunting, which is a form of auto–positive end-expiratory pressure (PEEP) that restricts exhalation from lungs that tend to collapse rapidly at low lung volumes. Recovery in such infants typically occurs after an abrupt and unexplained diuresis after which oxygen requirement decreases. Infants with moderate or severe RDS may need assisted ventilation in conjunction with oxygen therapy. Minimal support from continuous positive airway pressure (CPAP) by nasal prongs or face mask may be sufficient for some infants and is often begun if an $F_{I_{O_2}}$ of 60% fails to result in a Pa_{O_2} of 50 mm Hg. CPAP increases the func-

tional residual capacity, decreases the work of breathing, and improves arterial oxygenation.

There is no widespread agreement among perinatal centers on acceptable levels of Pa_{O_2} or Pa_{CO_2}, although it appears that in centers that tolerate higher Pa_{CO_2} (to 70 mm Hg) if pH is preserved at >7.2 and use CPAP in lieu of pressure ventilation, the incidence of chronic lung disease (BPD) is lower.[27] If adequate gas exchange fails to be maintained with this treatment, administration of oxygen with mechanical ventilation, usually with a continuous-flow, time-cycled, pressure-limited ventilator, is indicated. Goals of this therapy are to maintain Pa_{O_2} at 50 to 70 mm Hg in order to avoid tissue hypoxia. Care must be taken to avoid hyperoxia so that further lung injury and, in particular, retinal vascular injury may be prevented (see section on oxygen monitoring).[28, 29] Careful monitoring of blood gases is essential in these unstable infants, and weaning to the lowest level of $F_{I_{O_2}}$ required as soon as possible is desirable. Many of these infants require prolonged ventilation, and some develop chronic lung disease (see section on BPD), and so oxygen supplementation is required for many months after ventilation is no longer needed. Table 93–4 summarizes guidelines for oxygen therapy in RDS.

Numerous other disorders, some acquired and some congenital, can manifest in the neonatal period with respiratory distress that may resemble the syndrome recog-

Table 93–4. GUIDELINES FOR OXYGEN THERAPY IN RESPIRATORY DISTRESS SYNDROME

Modality	Max $F_{I_{O_2}}$	Indications			
		Pa_{O_2}	Pa_{CO_2}	pH	Mechanics
O_2 supplement	40%–60%	<50 mm Hg on room air	Normal	Stable	Adequate ventilatory efforts
O_2 + CPAP	60%–80%	<50 mm Hg on $F_{I_{O_2}}$ of 60%	≤60–65 mm Hg	≥7.2	No apnea
O_2 + mechanical ventilation	100%	<50 mm Hg on $F_{I_{O_2}}$ of 80%	≥65 mm Hg	<7.2	Apnea, severe fatigue

Max, maximum; $F_{I_{O_2}}$, fraction of inspired oxygen; Pa_{O_2}, arterial oxygen pressure; Pa_{CO_2}, arterial carbon dioxide pressure; CPAP, continuous positive airway pressure.

nized as RDS. These disorders include persistent pulmonary hypertension, persistent fetal circulation, group B streptococcal infection and sepsis, other types of neonatal pneumonitis, and meconium aspiration.[30] Oxygen is an important component of the therapy in each of these disorders; the specific needs for therapy are related to the underlying pathophysiologic processes in each of these disorders.

BRONCHOPULMONARY DYSPLASIA

BPD is a chronic lung disease that develops in 5% to 70% of premature infants treated with oxygen and mechanical pressure ventilation for severe respiratory distress syndrome.[31, 32] The incidence varies significantly with degree of prematurity and gestational age; the 70% incidence (in survivors of RDS) reported most recently has been among infants weighing less than 1000 g (very low birth weight).[33] Oxygen administered in high-flow rates is believed to play a significant role in the development of the parenchymal and airway changes that characterize this disorder, but oxygen is also a mainstay of the long-term treatment of BPD.

It has been suggested that a predisposition to develop BPD may be related to a susceptibility to oxygen injury that characterizes premature newborns. High concentrations of oxygen required in the early treatment of these infants leads to the generation of free oxygen radicals, which mediate lung damage.[34, 35] Pulmonary antioxidant systems, including superoxide dismutase, catalase, and glutathione perioxidase, are inadequately developed in premature infants,[36] and therefore pulmonary oxygen injury may aggravate the pulmonary insufficiency related to lung immaturity. Clinicians must carefully monitor oxygen use and to wean infants from oxygen to the level that permits stability in Pa_{O_2}. Even after weaning from mechanical ventilation, many of the smaller premature infants require ICU care for many months and supplemental oxygen at moderately high levels in addition to diuretics, bronchodilators, chest physiotherapy, and caloric supplementation in order to achieve up to 150% of normal recommended dietary allowance. During this time, the correct amount of oxygen is determined by the need to balance the factor of potential hypoxic lung injury against the problem of suboptimal growth and the risk of pulmonary vasoconstriction from hypoxia.

Guidelines regarding transition of care of the BPD infant to the home setting have been devised.[33, 37–40] Improvements in oxygen delivery methods (liquid oxygen systems and oxygen concentrators, described in the next section) and, in particular, the ability to monitor oxygenation noninvasively with portable pulse oximeters are partly responsible for this option. Generally accepted discharge criteria include

1. Postconceptual age of 40 to 44 weeks.
2. Appropriate growth curve with satisfactory behavior during feedings.
3. Requirement of $F_{I_{O_2}}$ of 1 l/min or less (except in unusual cases) to maintain Sa_{O_2} at 93% to 95% while the infant is awake or asleep and during feeding.

4. No changes in $F_{I_{O_2}}$ or medications required in the week before discharge from the hospital.
5. A capable and well-trained family consisting of at least two adult caregivers.[37]

After discharge, close follow-up by a team that includes physicians, nurses, and social service providers as well as respiratory therapists or technicians who maintain the oxygen equipment and supplies is necessary. Some infants cannot be discharged home and require management in a chronic disease facility until they can be weaned off oxygen. Attempts should be made to wean patients off diuretics and to achieve liberal oral intake before weaning off oxygen in either setting. Once a flow rate of 0.125 to 0.25 l/min is reached, the supplemental oxygen can be discontinued in increments; first for 1 h; next for 2, 4, and 8 h; then for all waking hours; and finally at night. At each new level, it is important to demonstrate ability to maintain an oxygen saturation range of 93% to 95% at rest and with feeding, with no increase in heart rate.[33] Attention must also be given to the presence and severity of right ventricular hypertrophy because many infants in whom this condition is severe need to be weaned more slowly. The author recommends that after an infant is weaned completely from oxygen, oxygen saturation and heart rate be recorded for 4 to 6 h with the infant asleep and off oxygen; if no significant desaturation occurs, oxygen can be discontinued. A small oxygen tank is generally held in reserve in the infant's home for 2 to 3 months because oxygen may be needed in times of respiratory viral infections.

Evidence presented by two groups strongly indicates that an oxygen saturation level of 95% is optimal for adequate growth in infants with BPD.[33, 41] This should lead to the recommendation that 95% oxygen saturation rather than the previously accepted level of 90% (Pa_{O_2} of 55)[42] be maintained to the extent possible for all infants receiving oxygen. In view of this recommendation, oxygen may have to be continued or weaning may have to be accomplished more slowly in some infants. Seventy to eighty percent of oxygen-dependent BPD infants are able to be weaned off oxygen between the ages of 1 and 2 years.

ASTHMA

Asthma is the leading cause of reversible airway obstruction in children, and during an acute attack and in periods of chronic, poorly controlled bronchospasm, significant hypoxemia is often present. McFadden and Lyons reported that 91% of 101 asthmatic patients (14 to 45 years of age) were hypoxemic with an acute attack and 70% of this group had Pa_{O_2} values of 45 to 75 mm Hg. The degree of hypoxemia was correlated with the severity of the airway obstruction but was not predictive of the rapidity of response to treatment.[43] Most children with uncomplicated asthma respond rapidly to treatment of an acute attack so that hypoxemia is not documented. Chipps and colleagues documented considerable drops in oxygen saturation during sleep in asymptomatic children at an asthma camp, which indicates that some degree of hypoxemia may not be uncommon in some children whose asthma appears to be well controlled.[44]

Hypoxemia in acute exacerbations of asthma is caused largely by $\dot{V}/\dot{Q}$ mismatch resulting from poor ventilation and relative hyperperfusion of multiple lung units.[45] Because of the nonuniformity of the airway obstruction, some alveolar units are hyperventilated in relation to their perfusion. The net result of these two processes still results in hypoxemia, inasmuch as the former situation predominates, and the desaturated blood leaving poorly ventilated areas mixes with the better oxygenated blood. In younger children or infants in whom atelectasis may result from mucus plugging of midsized and large airways, more severe hypoxemia may also be the result of shunt.

Oxygen should be promply administered to a child who is in severe respiratory distress resulting from an acute attack of asthma, and this is accomplished effectively by delivering low-flow oxygen either by a simple face mask with an $F_{I_{O_2}}$ setting starting at 40% or through a nasal cannula at 2 to 4 l/min. As soon as beta-adrenergic agents or other medications begin to relieve bronchospasm, the $F_{I_{O_2}}$ can be reduced. Hypocapnia is initially present during an acute attack because of hyperventilation, and children with asthma rarely, if ever, have chronic hypercapnia, which may be associated with other types of chronic obstructive lung diseases. They are therefore not at high risk for suppression of the hypoxic drive for respiration with the administration of oxygen. Children in extreme respiratory distress and those who do not respond promptly to treatment or whose condition worsens need arterial blood gas determinations. Pulse oximetry can be a very useful adjunct in the majority of such children and may be all that is required for monitoring oxygenation in those who respond promptly to treatment.

A significant drop in oxygen saturation has been noted in some infants immediately after administration of nebulized bronchodilators.[46] This drop has also been reported in adults[47] and can be explained by an increase in blood flow to areas with a low $\dot{V}/\dot{Q}$ ratio. The reason for this redistribution of blood flow is uncertain, but it appears that blood vessels supplying areas with a low $\dot{V}/\dot{Q}$ ratio areas preferentially dilate in response to beta-adrenergic agonists.[3] Although this factor may not be a major one in most acute asthma episodes in children, some children respond slowly to maximal treatment modalities and experience more prolonged hypoxemia. A subgroup of children with acute attacks develop hypercapnia, and some require mechanical ventilation and PEEP in order to correct hypoxemia and improve ventilation.

CYSTIC FIBROSIS

CF is a multisystem disorder characterized by progressive airway obstruction and infection (bronchiectasis) that leads to respiratory insufficiency over a variable number of years. Early in the disease course and before other pulmonary function abnormalities or significant clinical symptoms can be detected, mild hypoxemia and an increased A-a oxygen difference can be demonstrated.[48] Late or end-stage CF lung disease is characterized by severe hypoxemia, variable degrees of carbon-dioxide retention, cyanosis, and cor pulmonale. Because the airway obstruction in this disorder is focal, diffuse, and variable over time, the hypoxemia is largely caused by perfusion of units with a low $\dot{V}/\dot{Q}$ ratio. More precise physiologic studies of gas exchange have demonstrated that increased intrapulmonary shunting is a prominent cause of hypoxemia in CF patients at rest.[49] Postural hypoxemia has been documented in a group of patients with a wide range of disease severity,[50] and oxygen desaturation during sleep and during exercise has been repeatedly demonstrated.[51-56] Elevations in minute ventilation and oxygen consumption have been documented during rest and during exercise in CF patients,[57, 58] and this increased ventilation, although mechanically inefficient, appears to be an attempt to prevent oxygen desaturation.

In the clinical setting, oxygen is administered to CF patients during exacerbations of the pulmonary disease or when severe hypoxemia and cor pulmonale are present. Some very young infants with CF who acquire bronchiolitis may require oxygen supplementation or even mechanical ventilation. Outside of this group, and for many years for most patients, oxygen may be administered only during hospital treatment with parenteral antibiotics and intensive chest physiotherapy if hypoxemia is demonstrable by pulse oximetry ($Sa_{O_2} < 90\%$) or arterial blood gases. There appears to be a trend to the more liberal use of at-home nighttime oxygen in CF patients before the development of frank cor pulmonale or significant clinical symptoms related to hypoxia. This trend appears to be based in part on the awareness of the beneficial effects of nocturnal oxygen in adults with chronic obstructive pulmonary disease and is related to the availability and widespread use of pulse oximeters for detecting and monitoring treatment of hypoxemia. There is evidence that oxygen reverses pulmonary vasoconstriction and the early stages of pulmonary hypertension in CF,[59] but a 3-year study of nighttime oxygen use in patients with advanced CF lung disease showed that oxygen did not affect mortality rate, hospitalization frequency, or progression of disease.[60] Thus there are currently no uniform recommendations for the early prophylactic use of nocturnal oxygen in CF patients, and this problem must be further investigated.

INTERSTITIAL LUNG DISEASE

Interstitial lung disease (ILD) in children has numerous possible courses and in many instances is designated idiopathic. The clinical manifestations of these diseases include cough, tachypnea, dyspnea, and failure to thrive, and they result in restrictive ventilatory impairment from a decrease in effective lung volume for gas exchange. As a group, these diseases are much less common in children than the previously discussed obstructive lung diseases. Pathophysiologic processes, treatment, and prognosis are determined according to the specific cause, but the mechanisms of the production of hypoxemia have a common pathway. These diseases begin with alveolitis, and inflammatory changes in the intra-alveolar septa may progress to fibrotic changes in the collagen structure of the interstitial network, disappearance of portions of the pulmonary capillary bed, and a diminished overall alveolar-capillary surface area.[61] Small airways are involved with an inflammatory process that results in obstruction in many types of ILD, and hypoxemia results from a combination of $\dot{V}/\dot{Q}$ and diffusion-perfusion inequalities. Careful gas exchange studies have demonstrated that the $\dot{V}/\dot{Q}$ inequalities predominate at rest, and the diffusion impairment and resultant dramatic hypoxemia are more readily apparent during exercise.[3]

Supplemental oxygen is clinically indicated whenever persistent hypoxemia (Pa_{O_2} of 55 to 60 mm Hg) is exhibited. Its liberal and appropriately monitored use in infants with ILD permits better growth and development. Adequate supplementation in older children permits an increased level of activity and prevents or ameliorates cor pulmonale.

RESTRICTIVE (MECHANICAL) PROBLEMS

Any disease process that affects the muscular or skeletal structures that make up the thorax may impair chest wall mechanics and, if severe enough, result in respiratory insufficiency and hypoxemia. Congenital abnormalities of the chest wall, traumatic injury, and progressive muscular and neuromuscular diseases may at the outset or over time significantly impair gas exchange as a result of $\dot{V}/\dot{Q}$ inequalities or, in some instances, as a result of relative alveolar hypoventilation. In severe congenital deformities of the chest wall, such as asphyxiating thoracic dystrophy or severe kyphoscoliosis, pulmonary hypoplasia may coexist.[62] Oxygen and mechanical ventilation may be required for such children. Children with more slowly progressive disorders may need supplemental oxygen during intercurrent respiratory infections, which may be particularly devastating because of the children's inability to effectively cough and clear secretions. In these disorders, oxygen is rarely definitive therapy, but it is an important supportive measure.

OXYGEN THERAPY: METHODS AND MECHANICS OF ADMINISTRATION

ACUTE OXYGEN THERAPY

Oxygen therapy is always warranted in acute situations in which the Pa_{O_2} is less than 55 to 60 mm Hg or Sa_{O_2} is less than 90%. Pa_{O_2} of 60 to 70 mm Hg represents the dangerous point on the oxyhemoglobin dissociation curve at which further decreases in Pa_{O_2}, even slight ones, result in considerable decreases in the Sa_{O_2}. Further declines in Pa_{O_2} result in inability of blood to carry adequate amounts of oxygen and, consequently, in tissue hypoxia. Oxygen therapy may be indicated in unstable patients with higher Pa_{O_2} who have marked tachypnea, tachycardia, cyanosis, and dyspnea and in patients with underlying respiratory conditions who are restless, disoriented, lethargic, or comatose or are severely hypotensive from sepsis or trauma. The amount of oxygen administered and duration of use depend on measurement of Pa_{O_2} or Sa_{O_2}.

In adults it is common, for therapeutic purposes, to classify acutely hypoxemic patients on the basis of the presence or absence of hypercapnia. In patients with chronically elevated Pa_{CO_2} levels (>50 mm Hg), the administration of oxygen may eliminate the hypoxic drive for respiration and result in hypoventilation. The usual strategy in these patients is to administer oxygen at low flow rates with $F_{I_{O_2}}$ specifically controlled in order to raise Pa_{O_2} slightly (10 to 20 mm Hg). This strategy significantly increases the oxygen saturation but does not abruptly depress the hypoxic drive. This situation, although theoretically possible with chronic carbon dioxide retention (as in CF and BPD), is less commonly encountered than in adults. Nevertheless, it is generally prudent to administer the lowest possible $F_{I_{O_2}}$ that will adequately improve Pa_{O_2}.

In children, as in adults, who are acutely hypoxemic without carbon dioxide retention, oxygen can be administered more liberally with desired Pa_{O_2} levels of 70 to 90 mm Hg. If an $F_{I_{O_2}}$ of .50 to .60 fails to improve oxygenation, oxygen administered with CPAP or mechanical ventilation may be required.

CHRONIC OXYGEN THERAPY

Chronic oxygen therapy is indicated in children with known pulmonary disorders (CF, BPD, and ILD) who are stable or who have recovered from acute exacerbations but remain significantly hypoxic at rest or during minimal exercise. Central cyanosis, compensatory polycythemia, pulmonary hypertension, and demonstration of stable improvement of hypoxemia with low-flow oxygen (1 to 3 l/min) are also indications for chronic oxygen therapy.

OXYGEN DELIVERY DEVICES

A variety of delivery systems are available for administration of oxygen to children. These systems vary in efficiency, complexity, precision of oxygen delivery, expense, and tolerance by patients. Oxygen delivery devices are generally categorized as low-flow or high-flow systems. Low-flow and high-flow systems can provide either a high or a low $F_{I_{O_2}}$ to the airways (Table 93–5). A low-flow oxygen system is not intended to fulfill the total inspiratory requirements of a patient, inasmuch as each tidal volume contains a variable amount of room air. Therefore, the $F_{I_{O_2}}$ entering the airways varies in relation to the flow rate of the oxygen, the tidal volume, and the respiratory rate. A high-flow oxygen system provides flow rates that are high enough to completely satisfy the patient's inspiratory need either by high flow of gas or by controlled entrainment of ambient air.[63]

Low-Flow Oxygen Systems

Nasal Cannula. The most common oxygen delivery device for infants and children without artificial airways is the nasal cannula. It is simple, easy to use, and well tolerated by infants and young children; in particular, it provides easy access for feeding, administering medications, treatments, and chest physiotherapy. As with all low-flow systems, the $F_{I_{O_2}}$ varies greatly with the oxygen flow rate,

Table 93–5. OXYGEN DELIVERY SYSTEMS

System	O$_2$ Flow Rate (l/min)*	Approximate Inspired Oxygen Range†
Low-Flow Systems		
Nasal cannula	0.125–5.0	22%–44%
Simple mask	4–8	30%–60%
Masks with reservoirs		
Partial rebreathing	5–10	40%–100%
Non-rebreathing	5–10	60%–100%
Oxygen hoods	4–8	30%–70%
High-Flow Systems		
Venturi masks	4–6 (105)	24%*
Mechanical aerosol systems	4–6 (44)	28%
	8 (48)	35%
	8 (32)	40%
	12 (32)	50%
	12 (24)	60%

Modified in part from Block[63] and Kacmarek.[64]

F$_{IO_2}$, fraction of inspired oxygen.

*Numbers in parentheses represent total flow in liters per minute (O$_2$ flow and entrained room air).

†Actual F$_{IO_2}$ depends on ventilatory pattern; ranges apply best to adults with respiratory rate of 20/min, tidal volume of 500 ml, and inspiratory time of 1 sec. For high-flow systems, specific percentages vary slightly among manufacturers.

inspiratory flow, and minute ventilation. The smaller the tidal volume and minute ventilation, the higher the F$_{IO_2}$; conversely, the larger the tidal volume and minute ventilation, the lower the F$_{IO_2}$. Despite these well-accepted facts, 0.125-l/min flow to a small infant with a respiratory rate of 60 probably provides a substantially higher F$_{IO_2}$ than does a higher flow administered to an adult with a lower respiratory rate. This may be related in part to the size of the cannula in comparison with the diameter size of nasal passages in children and adults. There is no way of accurately measuring delivered F$_{IO_2}$ to an infant with a nasal cannula, and flow rate must be adjusted on the basis of response to therapy, preferably through the use of a noninvasive oxygen monitoring system. Flow meters deliver 0.1 l/min or less to infants, but the readily available equipment is capable of delivering 0.125 to 5 l/min of 100% oxygen, which provides F$_{IO_2}$ in the range of 22% to 44%. Even at low-flow rates, nasal patency should always be ensured. Oxygen delivered through a nasal cannula should always be humidified, especially in children with BPD or CF, in which inspissation of airway secretions causes problems. The flow rate delivered by cannula should never exceed 5 to 6 l/min because flows above this do not appreciably increase the F$_{IO_2}$ and have been associated with gastric distention and regurgitation, headache, drying and irritation of nasal mucosa, and nose bleeds.

Simple Oxygen Masks. For older children and adults, simple face masks are ideal devices for delivering F$_{IO_2}$ of 24% to 60% at flow rates of 4 to 8 l/min. Because of their construction, all masks extend anatomic dead space, and flow rates into the mask must be sufficient to eliminate accumulation of carbon dioxide in the system. Exhaled gases are expelled through exhalation ports and leakages that exist at the edge of the mask (Fig. 93–7).

Mask With Reservoir Bags. To deliver levels of inspired oxygen higher than 50% to a patient without an artificial airway, a reservoir bag can be attached to a simple face mask. The oxygen flow rate is adjusted to keep the reservoir bag continuously inflated. There are two types of reservoir mask systems: the partial rebreathing mask system and the non-rebreathing mask system. In the partial rebreathing mask system, there are no one-way valves between the mask and the reservoir bag, and open vents on the mask allow the exhaled gas to escape into the ambient air. Some of the exhaled gas in this system enters the reservoir bag and becomes part of the next inhalation (i.e., the first third of the patient's exhaled volume or anatomic dead space flows back into the reservoir); the remaining two thirds of exhaled volume is vented through exhalation ports in the mask or leakages around the mask.[64] Partial rebreathing systems can usually achieve an F$_{IO_2}$ of only .75 to .80 (see Fig. 93–7).

A non-rebreathing mask has a one-way valve between the mask and the bag, so that the patient can inhale only from the reservoir bag and can exhale through separate one-way valves on the sides of the mask. A gas inlet safety valve allows room air to enter the system if the oxygen source is accidentally disconnected. These devices are designed to deliver high F$_{IO_2}$ at low flow rates, but the flow rate must be sufficient to prevent complete collapse of the bag during inhalation. High F$_{IO_2}$ levels can be achieved with both of these masks, especially if they are tight fitting and kept in place. These devices are most suitable for short-term use (2 to 4 h) in acute situations, such as asthma without increased levels of carbon dioxide (see Fig. 93–7).

Oxygen Hoods. These hoods are clear Plexiglas domes or boxes of variable size that are placed over the head and neck of an infant to ensure an adequate and stable F$_{IO_2}$. Oxygen delivered via hood should be warmed and humidified and must be run in at flow rates to prevent accumulation of carbon dioxide (i.e., 4 to 8 l/min), which result in an F$_{IO_2}$ range of about .30 to .70.[65] Most hoods have ports that can be opened or occluded in order to vary the oxygen concentration, and F$_{IO_2}$ can be measured close to the infant's nose or mouth with an F$_{IO_2}$ analyzer. A dis-

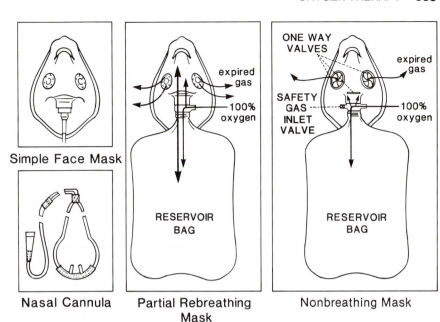

Simple Face Mask

Nasal Cannula

Partial Rebreathing Mask

ONE WAY VALVES

expired gas

SAFETY GAS INLET VALVE

100% oxygen

RESERVOIR BAG

Nonbreathing Mask

Figure 93–7. Types of oxygen administration devices used for infants and children.

advantage of the head hood is limited access to the infant, which makes nursing care procedures difficult without varying the oxygen levels. This device is most often used in infants recently weaned from mechanical ventilation with relatively high $F_{I_{O_2}}$ requirements and in infants who were previously receiving oxygen via nasal cannula but who in acute situations require a higher $F_{I_{O_2}}$.

Incubators. Supplemental oxygen can be added to an incubator to deliver an $F_{I_{O_2}}$ between .40 and .80, the higher concentration being attained by occluding air entrainment ports. Incubators are less commonly used in Level III intensive care nurseries, in which tiny, sick premature infants who require mechanical intubation and ventilation are often nursed in open radiant-heat beds. When incubators are used, $F_{I_{O_2}}$ concentration should be monitored frequently.[11]

Oxygen Tents. The oxygen tent was at one time probably the most popular method of delivering low to moderate concentrations of oxygen to young children. Well-maintained "croup tents" can provide an inspired oxygen concentration up to 50%, but manipulation in opening the tent results in an immediate drop in $F_{I_{O_2}}$. The systems described earlier are superior for more efficiently delivering a more accurate amount of oxygen, but tents are occasionally used in clinical situations such as croup, in which the major desired result is an environment of very high humidity.

High-Flow Oxygen Systems

Venturi Masks (Air Entrainment Masks). These masks are designed to deliver a specific oxygen concentration and are the optimal method for delivering controlled oxygen therapy to patients without an artificial airway who may have problems with hypercapnia. The operation of these masks is based on Bernoulli's principle, whereby oxygen flows into a jet orifice at a specific flow rate. Depending on the flow rate, the size of the jet and the size of the air entrainment ports, oxygen concentrations

between 24% and 40% can be delivered[64] (Fig. 93–8). The flow rate required for achieving a specific $F_{I_{O_2}}$ varies slightly for masks made by different manufacturers, and instructions for the specific mask being used must be followed.

Mechanical Aerosol Systems. The jet drag effect, which is the principle used in the Venturi mask system, can also be used in mechanical aerosol systems, which have the advantage of delivering particulate water to the airway. Nondisposable aerosol generators allow some variation in inspired oxygen delivered (usually 40%, 70%, or 100%), but disposable systems theoretically allow variation from 28% to 100%. These systems can be applied via aerosol mask, face hood, or tracheostomy collar and are commonly used in the author's institution to deliver carefully controlled oxygen concentrations to infants with BPD, who may have an elevation in carbon dioxide levels.

T-Tubes and Tracheostomy Collars. Subglottic stenosis resulting from prolonged or repeated intubations in premature infants with respiratory distress has unfortunately resulted in an increasing number of infants with tracheostomies. Humidified oxygen can be administered at a predictable (controlled) $F_{I_{O_2}}$ to such children through the use of a mechanical aerosol system via T-tube or tracheostomy collar. The indications for mist or humidity therapy are not the same as those for oxygen therapy, and when infants, typically those with BPD, no longer require supplemental oxygen, humidification should be supplied via a tracheostomy collar at least during sleep or with the use of a Breath-Aide device.

HOME OXYGEN USE IN CHILDREN

Feasibility and efficacy of long-term oxygen therapy were first established by Neff and Petty in 1970 in adults with chronic obstructive pulmonary disease.[66] Infants and children with a wide variety of pulmonary problems resulting in chronic hypoxemia receive supplementary

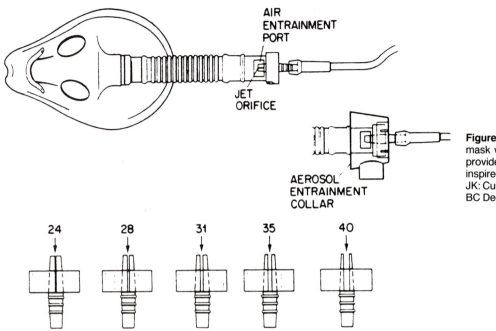

Figure 93-8. Air entrainment (Venturi) mask with various jet orifices. Each orifice provides a specific delivered fraction of inspired O_2. (From Kacmarek RM, Stoller JK: Current Respiratory Care, p. 2. Toronto: BC Decker, Inc., 1988.)

oxygen in their homes for long periods of time.[67] Children for whom oxygen therapy is prescribed are currently categorized into two groups. The first group consists of children who have serious disease but for whom there is a possibility of improvement and even recovery. In this group, which includes infants with BPD or congenital defects such as diaphragmatic hernia, the therapeutic goal is to wean patients from oxygen while enhancing nutritional status, preventing infections, and ameliorating or preventing cor pulmonale. The second group consists of patients who have chronic, progressive, and ultimately irreversible (end-stage) lung disease such as CF or ILD, for whom the goals of oxygen therapy are some improvement in quality of life, enhancement of exercise tolerance, and avoidance of discomfort.[68] In such patients, oxygen is prescribed as a late measure, and documentation of the benefits of its earlier use is needed.

Methods of oxygen delivery at home vary with age of patients, diagnosis, severity of disease, and cost and availability of equipment.[68] Nasal cannulae are most often used in infants with BPD, in whom low flow rate oxygen delivery is required. These devices are also best tolerated by older children and adults with CF or ILD. Transtracheal oxygen-using devices, such as the Scoop-2 transtracheal catheters or oxymizer reservoir cannulae, have been used for the chronic administration of oxygen in adults but have as yet been little used in children.[69] Home oxygen sources include compressed gas cylinders of various sizes and capacities, which are both stationary and portable; electrically powered oxygen concentrators, which use molecular sieve beds to purify entrained ambient air; and liquid oxygen reservoirs. Concentrators have a maximal flow of 5 l/min but are typically used for 1- to 3-l/min flows, and compressed air tanks must be available as portable units and for back-up in case of power failures. Liquid oxygen systems are most widely used in the author's center for infants and older children who require higher flow rates, for whom use is anticipated to be for

long periods, and who are on ventilators. Flow rates for these systems range between 0.5 and 5 l/min. Even at very low flow rates, humidification should be provided with all systems used in children. (Kent[69] provided detailed specifications for various commercially available systems of all three types of oxygen supply sources.)

MONITORING OXYGEN USE

OXYGEN TOXICITY

Oxygen therapy in the acute or chronic setting must be monitored with the goal of avoiding oxygen toxicity while maintaining adequate tissue oxygenation. Chronic exposure to elevated levels of inspired oxygen produced two well-characterized problems in newborns: retrolental fibroplasia and bronchopulmonary dysplasia. Acute pulmonary injury from hyperoxia more typically occurs in previously healthy patients other than newborns, and its spectrum of pathology includes atelectasis, edema, alveolar hemorrhage, inflammation, fibrin deposition, and thickening and hyalination of the alveolar membranes.[70] These changes occur either directly, through oxidation of tissue and the formation of toxic oxygen free radicals, or indirectly through regulatory effects on blood flow.[71] Three distinct clinical problems result from hyperoxia:

1. Acute tracheobronchitis, manifested by substernal chest pain, dyspnea, and cough.
2. Absorption atelectasis, which results from the elimination or washout of alveolar nitrogen and leads to a decrease in vital capacity, an increase in intrapulmonary shunting, and a decreasing Pa_{O_2}.
3. Adult respiratory distress syndrome, which is characterized by an early exudative phase (24 to 72 h) and a proliferative and potentially irreversible phase (after 72 h).[8]

Oxygen-induced lung damage demonstrates a threshold effect, and both the concentration and the duration of exposure are important variables. Specific toxic levels are difficult to define and appear to vary with the patient's age and nutritional status, the presence of underlying lung disease, and previous exposure to oxygen.[70] It appears reasonable to assume that oxygen concentrations higher than 80% produce considerable tissue damage with 36 to 48 h, concentrations of 60% to 80% also produce injury but at a slower rate, and concentrations of 50% are probably safe for prolonged periods.[72]

The clinician seeking to prevent oxygen toxicity must monitor oxygen use, and various invasive and noninvasive methods may be used.

ARTERIAL BLOOD GASES

The determination of Pa_{O_2}, Pa_{CO_2}, Sa_{O_2}, and pH from a sample of arterial blood with the use of a blood gas analyzer remains the gold standard against which all other methods of assessing blood oxygen levels must be compared, and this is the preferred method in critically ill or unstable children. Samples of blood are obtained from direct arterial puncture or from indwelling percutaneously placed catheters. Catheters containing polargraphic oxygen cathodes have been found to be accurate for direct and continuous Pa_{O_2} measurements in newborns; however, potential electrical hazards, long stabilization times, the need for frequent recalibrations, and the possible damage to arterial walls have precluded the widespread adoption of this approach.[63] Repeated arterial punctures and long-term catheter maintenance are technically difficult, and a less invasive method is far preferable in infants and young children. Measurement of capillary blood gases is feasible in infants and young children, and if samples are obtained from a warmed (arterialized) heel-stick, the correlation of capillary samples with arterial samples is good for carbon dioxide pressure and pH but unacceptably poor for oxygen pressure.

NONINVASIVE TECHNIQUES

Two systems for the noninvasive monitoring of arterial oxygenation are currently available: (1) ear or pulse oximetry and (2) transcutaneous determination of Pa_{O_2}. These measurements have been shown to be accurate and reproducible in healthy and sick newborns and in infants tested under a variety of clinical conditions.[73,74] Technical problems exist with these units with regard to electrode stability, slow response time of the oxygen sensors, the need for frequent calibration, and inconsistent results in older patients with thicker skin. The major drawback in the use of these units has been the need to frequently change the site of the electrodes because the sensors, which must be heated to 43°C to 45°C, can seriously injure the skin. Until the 1980s, this method was the noninvasive assessment most commonly used in stable newborns and in infants with BPD. More recent studies, however, have demonstrated that oxygen saturation values obtained from pulse oximetry were correlated far better with simultaneously

obtained blood gas values than were the transcutaneous Pa_{O_2} values in infants with BPD.[75,76]

Transcutaneous monitoring of oxygen saturation through ear or pulse oximetry is based on the fact that the transmission of light across a flowing hemoglobin solution is directly proportional to the oxygen saturation of the solution. In the original ear oximeter models, eight wavelengths of light in a fiberoptic bundle were passed through the warmed pinna, and the degree of transmission of the wavelengths was mathematically converted by computer into oxygen saturation values of hemoglobin in blood. Reliable values with excellent correlation with blood gas values were obtained over the range of saturations from 50% to 100%.[77] These cumbersome instruments, which were of little use in tiny infants, have essentially been replaced by the two-wavelength pulse oximeters such as the Nellcor-100 and Ohmeda Biox 3700 model oximeters, both of which provide oxygen saturation values that show excellent correlation with oxygen saturation values obtained from blood gases. Unlike the eight-wavelength ear oximeters, these units are not as reliable in the lower range of saturation,[78] and the best correlation is obtained between saturations of 70% and 95%.

Differences exist in the internal computer technology of different pulse oximeter models, and clinicians should avoid alternating or varying the oximeters for measurements in the same infants. This is particularly true at higher saturation ranges, for which the Nellcor-100 has been found to overestimate Sa_{O_2} and the Ohmeda Biox 3700 to underestimate Sa_{O_2}.[79,80] Bucher and associates recommended that type-specific alarm limits be set in order for the various models to accurately detect hypoxemia in premature newborns receiving oxygen.[80]

COR PULMONALE

The strictest definition of cor pulmonale is hypertrophy of the right ventricle that results from diseases that affect the structure or function of the lung. It occurs as a complication of any pulmonary disease in children that is associated with prolonged or chronically progressive hypoxia, notably BPD, CF, and ILD. In BPD, cor pulmonale may ameliorate and disappear with time; in CF and ILD, it is most often unremitting and may progress to right-sided heart failure. Hypoxemia, which in these disorders results primarily from $\dot{V}/\dot{Q}$ mismatch, is the single most significant cause of pulmonary vasoconstriction, although hypercapnia and acidemia may play an additive role later in the disease course. Hypoxic pulmonary vasoconstriction leads to pulmonary hypertension, which at first may be reversible or responsive to administered oxygen but, with more advanced pulmonary disease, becomes persistent and irreversible.[81] Right ventricular dilatation and right-sided heart failure occur as end-stage phenomena in children with cor pulmonale (Fig. 93–9).

Early detection of cor pulmonale in childhood pulmonary diseases is desirable because it would enable the early use of chronic oxygen therapy; however, its clinical recognition may be difficult within the symptom complex of the pulmonary pathologic processes. A right ventricular impulse at the lower left sternal border or the subxyphoid

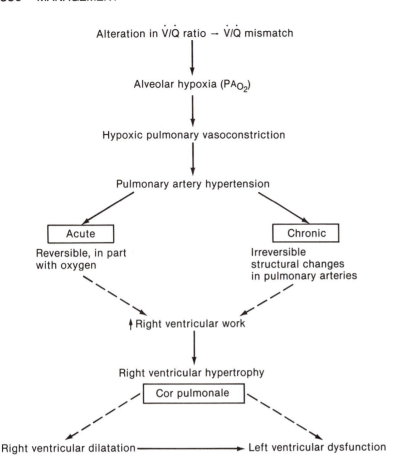

Alteration in V̇/Q̇ ratio → V̇/Q̇ mismatch

↓

Alveolar hypoxia (PA_{O_2})

↓

Hypoxic pulmonary vasoconstriction

↓

Pulmonary artery hypertension

Acute
Reversible, in part
with oxygen

Chronic
Irreversible
structural changes
in pulmonary arteries

↑ Right ventricular work

↓

Right ventricular hypertrophy

Cor pulmonale

Right ventricular dilatation ⟶ Left ventricular dysfunction

Figure 93–9. Schema: pathophysiology of cor pulmonale. V̇/Q̇, ventilation/perfusion.

area, an increased P_2 component of the second heart sound, and a tricuspid insufficiency murmur are all suggestive indications of cor pulmonale, but these signs are not consistently detectable and often are subtle. M-mode echocardiography can provide quantitative measurements of right ventricular wall thickness, right ventricular dimension, and systolic time intervals measured from the pulmonic valve tracing. Although complete imaging of these structures may be difficult if the lung is significantly

hyperexpanded, technically good images can be obtained by well-trained ultrasonographers and provide objective, reproducible evidence of cor pulmonale (Fig. 93–10). Two-dimensional echocardiography can be used for qualitative assessments of right ventricular size and function, together with Doppler estimation of pulmonary artery pressures. These methods are superior to electrocardiography for the detection of right-sided heart changes.[82, 83] In premature infants with BPD, in whom electrocardio-

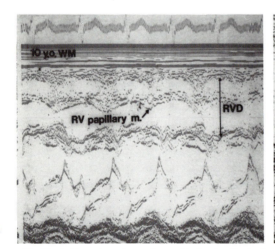

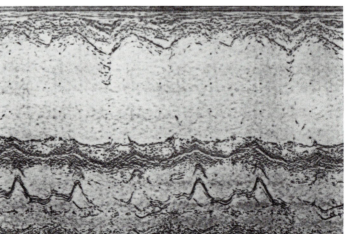

Figure 93–10. *A,* M-mode echocardiographic tracing illustrating increased right ventricular (RV) wall thickness, increased RV dimension (RVD), reversed septal motion, and prominent RV papillary muscle (m.) in a 10-year-old white male (WM) with advanced cystic fibrosis and cor pulmonale. *B,* M-mode echocardiographic tracing in an older child with severe pulmonary hypertension shows detail of the RV wall; endocardial and epicardial echoes are evident, the RV wall is thickened, and the RV is massively dilated.

graphic criteria for right ventricular hypertrophy change with age, the correlation with echocardiographic measurements of right ventricular wall thickness are not consistent. Because of the decreased expense and ready availability of electrocardiography, it is the commonly used monitor for assessing right ventricular hypertrophy and it appears to be more accurate in BPD than in diseases such as CF that are associated with severe air trapping and a vertically positioned heart (personal observation).

There is abundant clinical evidence that early discontinuation of oxygen in premature infants with BPD results in progression of cor pulmonale and, in some instances, in the development of right-to-left shunting of blood across a patent ductus arteriosus or a stretched patent foramen ovale with resultant cyanotic, or "blue," episodes. This finding supports the maintenance of adequate oxygen saturation levels (specifically, oxygen saturations of 90% to 95% in infants with BPD) and the close monitoring of these levels even after they appear to be doing well clinically without oxygen. These infants should be weaned slowly from oxygen with careful monitoring (see section on BPD), especially those with prominent right-sided heart changes. Nighttime home use of oxygen may be needed for longer periods if desaturation occurs during sleep because intermittent hypoxia appears to be a potent stimulus for the maintenance of pulmonary hypertension.

On the other end of the spectrum of disease severity and progression, it is more difficult to establish guidelines for the early use of oxygen for prevention of the progression of cor pulmonale. Nocturnal oxygen therapy trials for chronic obstructive pulmonary disease patients in the United States and the United Kingdom have demonstrated improved quality of life and prolonged survival in patients who received oxygen for some part of the day.[84,85] Results of one study of end-stage CF patients suggested that nighttime oxygen was of limited benefit,[60] although the specific cardiac effects of such treatment were not assessed.

In its early stages, hypoxic pulmonary hypertension is reversible with the administration of oxygen. Early detection of cor pulmonale may enable physicians to prevent the progression to irreversible changes of medial hypertrophy of pulmonary vessels through the educated use of oxygen. Some assessment of the presence and severity of cor pulmonale is important for the judicious use of oxygen in children.

REFERENCES

1. Mithoefer JC: Oxygen therapy. *In* Fishman AP (ed): Pulmonary Disease and Disorders, p. 1581. New York: McGraw Hill, 1980.
2. Comroe JH Jr, Forster RE, Dubois AB: The Lung: Clinical Physiology and Pulmonary Function Tests, p. 3. Chicago: Year Book Medical, 1962.
3. West JB: Ventilation-perfusion relationships. Am Rev Respir Dis 116:919–943, 1977.
4. Inselman LS, Mellins RB: Growth and development of the lung. J Pediatr 98:1–15, 1981.
5. Hogg JC, Williams J, Richardson JB, et al: Age as a factor in the distribution of lower-airway conductance and in the pathologic anatomy of obstructive lung disease. N Engl J Med 282:1283–1287, 1970.
6. Stokes DC: Effects of infection on function and development of the lung. *In* Laraya-Cuasay LR (ed): Interstitial Lung Disease in Children, p. 140. Boca Raton, FL: CRC Press, 1988.
7. Finch CA, Lenfant C: Oxygen transport in man. N Engl J Med 286:407–415, 1972.
8. Youtsey JW: Oxygen and mixed gas therapy. *In* Barnes TA, Libson A (eds): Respiratory Care Practice, pp. 131–163. Chicago: Year Book Medical, 1988.
9. O'Brodovich HM, Chernick V: The functional basis of respiratory pathology. *In* Kendig EL, Chernick V (eds): Disorders of the Respiratory Tract in Children, 4th ed, p. 30. Philadelphia: WB Saunders, 1985.
10. Comroe JH Jr, Forster RE, Dubois AB: The Lung: Clinical Physiology and Pulmonary Function Tests, p. 141. Chicago: Year Book Medical, 1962.
11. Burgess WR, Chernick V: Respiratory Therapy in Newborns, Infants and Children, pp. 30–58. New York: Thieme & Stratton, 1982.
12. Hlastala MP, Woodson RD: Saturation dependency of the Bohr effect: Interaction among H^+, CO_2 + DPG. J Appl Physiol 38:1126–1131, 1975.
13. Hudson LD: Getting oxygen to the tissues. *In* Donohue WJ (ed): Current Advances in Respiratory Care, pp. 120–127. Park Ridge, IL: American College of Chest Physicians, 1984.
14. Tisi GM: Pulmonary Physiology in Clinical Medicine, pp. 242–245. Baltimore: Williams & Wilkins, 1980.
15. Wade JF: Comprehensive Respiratory Care, pp. 150–155. St. Louis: CV Mosby, 1982.
16. Bendixen HH, Egbert LD, Hedley-Whyte J, et al: Respiratory Care, pp. 1–7. St. Louis: CV Mosby, 1965.
17. Flenley DC: Blood gas and acid base interpretation. *In* Basics of Respiratory Disease, p. 18. New York: American Thoracic Society, 1981.
18. Bendixen HH, Laver MB: Hypoxia in anesthesia, a review. Clin Pharmacol Ther 6:510–539, 1965.
19. Dempsey JA, Berssenbrugge A, Musch T, et al: The lung: Hypoxia, acid base changes and the control of breathing. Semin Respir Med 3:76–79, 1981.
20. Maker HS, Nicklas WJ: Biochemical responses of body organs to hypoxia and ischemia in extrapulmonary manifestations of respiratory disease. *In* Robin ED, Lenfant C (eds): Lung Biology in Health and Disease, pp. 107–150. New York: Marcel Dekker, 1978.
21. Fulmer JD, Snider GL: ACCP: NHLBI National Conference on Oxygen Therapy. Arch Intern Med 144:1645–1655, 1984.
22. Thomas HM 3rd, Lefrak SS, Irwin RS, et al: The oxyhemoglobin dissociation curve in health and disease. Am J Med 57:331–348, 1974.
23. Anthonisen NR: Hypoxemia and oxygen therapy. Am Rev Respir Dis 126:729–733, 1982.
24. Farzan SA: A Concise Handbook of Respiratory Diseases, 2nd ed. Reston VA: Reston Publishing, 1985.
25. Avery ME, Mead J: Surface properties in relation to atelectasis and hyaline membrane disease. Am J Dis Child 97:517–523, 1959.
26. Fishman AP: Respiratory gases in the regulation of the pulmonary circulation. Physiol Rev 41:214–280, 1961.
27. Avery ME, Tooley WH, Keller JB, et al: Is chronic lung disease in low birth weight infants preventable? A survey of eight centers. Pediatrics 79:26–30, 1987.
28. Frank L, Bucher JR, Roberts RJ: Oxygen toxicity in neonatal and adult animals of various species. J Appl Physiol 45:669–704, 1978.
29. Lucey JF, Dangman B: A reexamination of the role of oxygen in retrolental fibroplasia. Pediatrics 73:82–96, 1984.
30. Mellins RB, Jobe AH: Acute respiratory distress in the newborn infant. *In* Fishman AP (ed): Pulmonary Diseases and Disorders, 2nd ed, p. 2254. New York: McGraw-Hill, 1988.
31. Northway WH, Rosan RC, Porter DY: Pulmonary disease following respirator therapy of hyaline-membrane disease. N Engl J Med 276:357–368, 1967.
32. Northway WH Jr: Observations on bronchopulmonary dysplasia. J Pediatr 95:815–818, 1979.
33. Hudak BB, Allen MC, Hudak ML, et al: Home oxygen therapy for chronic lung disease in extremely low birth weight infants. Am J Dis Child 143:357–360, 1989.
34. Davis GM, Bureau MA: Pulmonary and chest wall mechanics in the control of respiration in the newborn. Clin Perinatol 14:551–579, 1987.

35. Freeman BA, Crapo JD: Biology of disease: Free radicals and tissue injury. Lab Invest 47:412–426, 1982.

36. Wispe JR, Roberts RJ: Development of anti-oxidant systems. *In* Merrit TA, Northway WH, Boynton BR (eds): Bronchopulmonary Dysplasia, p. 114. Boston: Blackwell Scientific, 1988.

37. Monin P, Vert P: The management of bronchopulmonary dysplasia. Clin Perinatol 14:531–549, 1987.

38. Thilo EH, Comito J, McCulliss D: Home oxygen therapy in the newborn. Costs and parental acceptance. Am J Dis Child 141:766–768, 1987.

39. Abman SH, Accurso FJ, Koops BL: Experience with home oxygen in the management of infants with bronchopulmonary dysplasia. Clin Pediatr 23:471–476, 1984.

40. Koops BL, Abman SH, Accurso FJ: Outpatient management and follow-up of bronchopulmonary dysplasia. Clin Perinatol 11:101–122, 1984.

41. Groothuis JR, Rosenberg AA: Home oxygen promotes weight gain in infants with bronchopulmonary dysplasia. Am J Dis Child 141:992–995, 1987.

42. Halliday HL, Dumpit FM, Brady JP: Effects of inspired oxygen on echocardiographic assessment of pulmonary vascular resistances and myocardial contractility in bronchopulmonary dysplasia. Pediatrics 65:536–540, 1980.

43. McFadden ER Jr, Lyons HA: Arterial-blood gas tension in asthma. N Engl J Med 278:1027–1032, 1968.

44. Chipps BE, Mak H, Schuberth KC, et al: Nocturnal oxygen saturation in normal and asthmatic children. Pediatrics 65:1157–1160, 1980.

45. Ledbetter MK, Bruck E, Farhi LE: Perfusion of underventilated compartment of the lungs in asthmatic children. J Clin Invest 43:2233–2240, 1964.

46. Prendiville A, Rose A, Maxwell DL, et al: Hypoxaemia in wheezy infants after bronchodilator treatment. Arch Dis Child 62:997–1000, 1987.

47. Knudson RJ, Constantine HP: An effect of isoproterenol on ventilation perfusion in asthmatic versus normal subjects. J Appl Physiol 22:402–406, 1967.

48. Lamarre A, Reilly BJ, Bryan AC, et al: Early detection of pulmonary function abnormalities in cystic fibrosis. Pediatrics 50:291–298, 1972.

49. Dantzker DR, Patten GA, Bower JS: Gas exchange at rest and during exercise in adults with cystic fibrosis. Am Rev Respir Dis 125:400–405, 1982.

50. Stokes DC, Wohl ME, Khaw KT, et al: Postural hypoxemia in cystic fibrosis. Chest 87:785–789, 1985.

51. Francis PWJ, Muller NL, Gurwitz D: Hemoglobin desaturation: Its occurrence during sleep in patients with cystic fibrosis. Am J Dis Child 134:734–740, 1980.

52. Tepper RS, Skatrud JB, Dempsey JA, et al: Ventilation and oxygenation changes during sleep in cystic fibrosis. Chest 84:388–392, 1983.

53. Stokes DC, McBride JT, Wall MA: Sleep hypoxemia in young adults with cystic fibrosis. Am J Dis Child 134:741–743, 1980.

54. Henke KG, Orenstein DM: Oxygen saturation during exercise in cystic fibrosis. Am Rev Respir Dis 129:708–711, 1984.

55. Versteegh FG, Neijens HJ, Bogaard JM, et al: Relationship between pulmonary function, O_2 saturation during sleep and exercise, and exercise responses in children with cystic fibrosis. Adv Cardiol 35:151–155, 1986.

56. Montgomery M, Wiebicke W, Bibi H, et al: Home measurement of oxygen saturation during sleep in patients with cystic fibrosis. Pediatr Pulmonol 7:29–34, 1989.

57. Hirsch JA, Zhang SP, Rudnick MP, et al: Resting oxygen consumption and ventilation in cystic fibrosis. Pediatr Pulmonol 6:19–26, 1989.

58. Cerny FJ, Pullano TP, Cropp GJ: Cardiorespiratory adaptations to exercise in cystic fibrosis. Am Rev Respir Dis 126:217–220, 1982.

59. Davidson A, Bossuyt A, Dab I: Acute effects of oxygen, nifedipine and diltiazem in patients with cystic fibrosis and mild pulmonary hypertension. Pediatr Pulmonol 6:53–59, 1989.

60. Zinman R, Corey M, Coates AL, et al: Nocturnal home oxygen in the treatment of hypoxemic cystic fibrosis patients. J Pediatr 114:368–377, 1989.

61. Polgar G: Pulmonary functions in children with interstitial lung disease. *In* Laraya-Cuasay LR, Hughes WT (eds): Interstitial Lung Diseases in Children, pp. 59–65. Boca Raton FL: CRC Press, 1988.

62. Wohl ME: Respiratory problems associated with chest wall abnormalities. *In* Hislop HS, Sanger JO (eds): Chest Diseases in Children, pp. 67–71. New York: American Physical Therapy Association, 1968.

63. Block ER: Oxygen therapy. *In* Fishman AP (ed): Pulmonary Diseases and Disorders, 2nd ed, pp. 2324–2328. New York: McGraw-Hill, 1988.

64. Kacmarek RM: Oxygen therapy techniques. *In* Kacmarek RM, Stoller JK (eds): Current Respiratory Care, pp. 1–8. Toronto: BC Decker, 1988.

65. Gale R, Redner-Carmi R, Gale J: Accumulation of carbon dioxide in oxygen hoods, infant cots and incubators. Pediatrics 60:453–456, 1977.

66. Neff TA, Petty TL: Long term continuous oxygen therapy in chronic airway obstruction. Ann Intern Med 72:621–626, 1970.

67. Campbell AN, Zarfin Y, Groenveld M, et al: Low flow oxygen therapy in infants. Arch Dis Child 58:795–798, 1983.

68. Sewell EM, Holsclaw D, Schidlow D, et al: The use of oxygen for children in their homes. Pediatr Pulmonol 2:72–74, 1986.

69. Kent KL: At home administration of oxygen. *In* Kacmarek RM, Stoller JK (eds): Current Respiratory Care, pp. 9–18. Toronto: BC Decker, 1988.

70. Deneke SM, Fanburg BL: Normobaric oxygen toxicity of the lung. N Engl J Med 303:76–86, 1980.

71. Phelps DL: Neonatal oxygen toxicity—Is it preventable? Pediatr Clin North Am 29:1233–1240, 1982.

72. Jenkinson SG: Oxygen toxicity. J Intensive Care Med 3:137–152, 1988.

73. Philip AG, Peabody JL, Lucey JF: Transcutaneous PO_2 monitoring in the home management of bronchopulmonary dysplasia. Pediatrics 61:655–657, 1978.

74. Huch R, Huch A, Lubbers D: Transcutaneous measurements of blood PO_2 ($TcPO_2$): Method and application in perinatal medicine. J Perinatal Med 1:183–191, 1973.

75. Solimano AJ, Smyth JA, Mann TK, et al: Pulse oximetry advantages in infants with bronchopulmonary dysplasia. Pediatrics 78:844–849, 1986.

76. Hay WW Jr, Brockway JM, Eyzaguirre M: Neonatal pulse oximetry: Accuracy and reliability. Pediatrics 83:717–722, 1989.

77. Chaudhary BA, Burki NK: Ear oximetry in clinical practice. Am Rev Respir Dis 117:173–175, 1978.

78. Fanconi S: Reliability of pulse oximetry in hypoxic infants. J Pediatr 112:424–427, 1988.

79. Praud JP, Carofilis A, Bridey F, et al: Accuracy of two wavelength pulse oximetry in neonates and infants. Pediatr Pulmonol 6:180–182, 1989.

80. Bucher HU, Fanconi S, Baeckert P, et al: Hyperoxemia in newborn infants: Detection by pulse oximetry. Pediatrics 84:226–230, 1989.

81. Lester LA: Complications of cystic fibrosis pulmonary disease. Semin Respir Med 6:285–298, 1985.

82. Riggs T, Hirschfeld S, Borkat G, et al: Assessment of the pulmonary vascular bed by echocardiographic right ventricular systolic time intervals. Circulation 57:939–947, 1978.

83. Lester LA, Egge AC, Hubbard VS, et al: Echocardiography in cystic fibrosis: A proposed scoring system. J Pediatr 97:742–748, 1980.

84. Nocturnal Oxygen Therapy Trial Group: Continuous or nocturnal oxygen therapy in hypoxemic chronic obstructive lung disease: A clinical trial. Ann Intern Med 93:391–398, 1980.

85. Medical Research Council Working Party: Long-term domiciliary oxygen therapy in chronic hypoxic cor pulmonale complicating chronic bronchitis and emphysema. Lancet 1:681–686, 1981.

94 PULMONARY OXYGEN TOXICITY

THOMAS ARTHUR HAZINSKI, M.D. / KATHLEEN A. KENNEDY, M.D.

HISTORY OF OXYGEN

Although some oxygen is produced by photolysis of water and carbon dioxide, the major source of atmospheric oxygen is from photosynthesis, which began in the seas 3.5 billion years ago. Five hundred fifty million years ago, the oxygen concentration of the earth's atmosphere rose to 10%, and sufficient ozone had been generated from oxygen to protect the land from biologically lethal solar radiation. This event enabled living organisms to leave the oceans for dry land. Today, oxygen constitutes 20.95% of the earth's atmosphere, and this concentration has not changed appreciably in the last 400 million years.[1] During evolution, hypoxic environmental niches were common, and adaptive mechanisms that could effectively regulate cellular homeostasis within the range of oxygen concentrations between 0% and 20% slowly developed. Because there has been little if any evolutionary experience with hyperoxia, it is not surprising that mammalian adaptive mechanisms are ineffective in the presence of oxygen-rich environments. It might also be expected that the first organ to manifest oxygen injury is the lung, the surface of which is in direct contact with this vital but toxic gas. Indeed, Priestly in 1775 predicted that pure oxygen "might be peculiarly salutary to the lung in certain morbid cases . . . but as a candle burns out much faster in oxygen than in common air, so we might live out too fast. A moralist may say that the air which nature has provided for us is as good as we deserve."[2]

In the century after Priestly's comment, physiologic studies demonstrated that oxygen could indeed injure the lung and eventually cause fatal pulmonary edema in virtually all mammals tested.[3] Several problems slowed progress in the understanding of the pathogenesis of pulmonary oxygen toxicity. First, the diversity of animal models has shown substantial variability in the onset and timing of biochemical and physiologic manifestation of oxygen exposure.[4] For example, hyperoxic rats acquire pulmonary vascular disease and pulmonary hypertension, whereas other species do not. At present, no single model closely resembles oxygen toxicity in humans. Indeed, humans, especially preterm infants, may be among the species most resistant to oxygen damage.[5, 6] Moreover, some of the late physiologic manifestations of oxygen toxicity observed in some species may be the result of prolonged survival; for example, rabbits succumb to fatal pulmonary edema after 60 to 70 h of oxygen exposure, whereas sheep survive 40% to 50% longer, perhaps because sheep have more efficient ways of reducing lung edema formation.

A second problem with the understanding of pulmonary oxygen toxicity is that normal lungs are rarely subjected to hyperoxia, and conclusions made on the basis of exposure of the normal lung to oxygen may be irrelevant to its clinical use in patients with pre-existing lung injury. In these instances, oxygen exposure may amplify the initial lung injury, especially when the initial injury is also mediated by free radicals.[7] Conversely, the lung's response to acute nonhyperoxic lung injury may actually protect the lung against subsequent oxygen damage. For example, tumor necrosis factor (TNF), produced by lymphoreticular cells in response to infection, can induce superoxide dismutase (SOD) activity in the lung, which in turn may reduce the oxidant stress of hyperoxia.[8]

A third problem is that methods of measuring oxidant production in vivo in specific lung cells are not yet available. Despite these limitations, research during the 1970s and 1980s clarified the physiologic, biochemical, and molecular effects of hyperoxia on lung tissue. Excellent reviews have been published,[6, 9-12] but it is sobering to note that little of clinical utility has been learned since the first comprehensive review of this subject by Clark and Lambertsen in 1971.[13] Although clinically feasible ways of reducing oxygen injury in patients are still unavailable, there is reason to hope that newer models of oxygen toxicity[14] and the powerful tools of molecular and cell biology may soon enable the development of therapeutic strategies to reduce the toxic effects of oxygen on the lung.

CLINICAL FEATURES OF PULMONARY OXYGEN TOXICITY

Although the "free radical" theory of oxygen toxicity has justifiably received the most attention as the key pathologic mechanism by which oxygen damages the lung, molecular oxygen alone can affect lung cells and their function. For example, as little as 2 h of exposure to 95% oxygen reduces ciliary beat frequency in airway epithelium, slows mucociliary clearance, and causes release of mucus from goblet cells and goblet cell destruction;[15] these changes are related to both the duration and the dose of oxygen, cannot be prevented by saturating the oxygen with water vapor, and cannot be completely mimicked by chemical oxidants.[16] Leukocytic infiltration of the submucosa eventually causes a mild tracheobronchi-

889

tis and epithelial sloughing,[17] which is expressed clinically in normal humans as substernal chest pain and cough after 2 to 4 h of oxygen breathing.[13] Oxygen breathing also causes atelectasis presumably because of the washout of nitrogen and other inert gases from lung units that lack effective collateral ventilation. Atelectasis may be focal or extensive and is expressed clinically as dyspnea after 9 to 12 h of oxygen breathing in humans. Radiographic and physiologic evidence of atelectasis can be promptly reversed by transient application of positive pressure or by breathing air, indicating that acute pulmonary edema does not account for these effects. There is some evidence that the apposition of alveolar surfaces, which occurs during atelectasis, may initiate a cascade of events leading to inflammation and fibrosis.[18] This possible aspect of pulmonary oxygen toxicity has not been examined in detail.

In laboratory animals with normal lungs, the continuous breathing of more than 95% oxygen eventually causes fatal pulmonary edema. This edema is rich in protein and forms at low vascular pressures, which indicates that it results from an increase in microvascular permeability to water and protein. The gradual development of pulmonary edema and a primary and secondary abnormality of surfactant function and production[19, 20] and control of vascular tone[21] are manifested physiologically by hypercapnia, abnormal lung mechanics, and an increase in the alveolar-arterial oxygen pressure gradient. This acute period has been termed the *exudative phase* of oxygen toxicity and is characterized histologically by endothelial and alveolar necrosis and hemorrhage, which has been termed *diffuse alveolar damage.* However, a unique feature of pulmonary oxygen toxicity *in vivo* and to some extent *in vitro* is a 24- to 48-h latency period in which there is little functional, biochemical, or histologic abnormality at the alveolar level. This is in contrast to other oxidant injuries in which the increase in microvascular permeability and inflammatory changes are immediate. This latency period has been interpreted to indicate that hyperoxic injury results from either a gradual acceleration of oxidant production or the eventual exhaustion of antioxidant defenses, or both. In either case, this latency period suggests that there is a therapeutic "window of opportunity" for preventing oxygen toxicity.

If oxygen exposure is limited or if sublethal oxygen concentrations are used, the acute exudative phase is less severe and is followed by a chronic phase characterized by alveolar type II cell hyperplasia, emphysema, inflammation, interstitial fibrosis, and, in some species, pulmonary hypertension and vascular remodeling.[22] This chronic phase is similar histologically to the pathologic lesion seen in the premature baboon model of oxygen toxicity[14] and in bronchopulmonary dysplasia (BPD) in humans.[23]

EFFECTS OF OXYGEN-DERIVED FREE RADICALS ON LUNG TISSUE

Because of its structure, molecular oxygen can accept electrons either two at a time (divalent reduction) to form water via the cytochrome *c* oxidase system or one at a time (univalent reduction) through a variety of reactions to generate a family of toxic oxidants that damage cells.

The transfer of one electron to oxygen forms superoxide ion, and the addition of a second electron generates hydrogen peroxide. Enzymatic sources of these oxidants include the xanthine oxidase reaction, aldehyde and amine oxidases, cytochrome b_5, the cytochrome P-450 monooxygenase system, and prostaglandin synthetase. Oxygen-derived oxidants are also produced within neutrophils and monocytes during the phagocytic respiratory burst and the myeloperoxidase reactions, but it is unclear whether they are released extracellularly.[24] Acute hyperoxic lung injury can occur in their absence in sheep.[25]

Nonenzymatic oxidant sources include the auto-oxidation of small molecules such as catecholamines and thiols. In the presence of iron and other metals, superoxide and hydrogen peroxide may react to form the hydroxyl radical through the Haber-Weiss and Fenton reactions. Interactions between superoxide and other radicals can result in the formation of singlet oxygen. Although hydrogen peroxide and singlet oxygen do not have unpaired electrons and therefore are technically not radicals, all of these oxygen-derived oxidants are commonly referred to as free oxygen radicals. These radicals are produced in the mitochondria, cytoplasm, endoplasmic reticulum, and cell membranes of all lung cells. They are highly reactive, usually short-lived molecules that can increase membrane permeability,[26] inhibit calcium-mediated signal transduction,[27] inactivate cytosolic and membrane-embedded enzymes,[28] cause DNA adduct formation and prevent protein-DNA interactions that regulate gene expression,[29] initiate lipid peroxidation chain reactions,[30] render harmless drugs harmful,[31] generate vasoactive metabolites of arachidonic acid,[32] and degrade carbohydrates within the extracellular matrix.[33]

These oxidants are held in check by antioxidants (small molecules and enzymes) that can react with oxidants either to eliminate them or to convert them into less potent oxidants. Substantial, albeit indirect, evidence indicates that pulmonary oxygen toxicity results primarily from the accelerated production of oxygen-derived oxidants that exceed adjacent antioxidant defenses. Oxygen-derived oxidants have been implicated in many forms of lung injury in infants and children: hyaline membrane disease, group B streptococcal sepsis/pneumonia, adult respiratory distress syndrome, neonatal asphyxia, and BPD.[34-36] Oxygen exposure may also amplify or cause secondary lung injury whenever it is used to treat other acute lung disorders such as pneumonia, bronchiolitis, and interstitial lung disease.[35] The effects of oxygen exposure on lung repair have just begun to be elucidated.[36, 37]

Oxygen exposure increases the production of oxygen-derived oxidants in the lung and eventually causes microvascular injury and fatal pulmonary edema. In this respect, oxygen-induced lung injury shares many of the features of other oxidant-mediated diseases such as radiation injury, ischemia-reperfusion, ozone injury, and chemical oxidant damage. The pathophysiologic processes of acute pulmonary oxygen toxicity have been described in developing mammals,[4, 19, 22, 28] primates,[14] and humans.[5, 13] Although oxygen breathing causes pulmonary edema in all species, the molecular mechanisms underlying the response to oxygen breathing varies widely. For example, in rats, rabbits, and mice, antioxidant enzymes are produced within 24 h of oxygen exposure, and these animals are more resistant to oxygen-induced lung injury than are guinea pigs, hamsters, and sheep.[4, 6, 37–39] In these latter species, the antioxidant defenses do not increase during oxygen exposure, and this may partially explain their increased vulnerability.

In addition, not all lung cells are equally susceptible to the oxidant stress of oxygen exposure. Alveolar type II cells appear to be resistant to oxidant injury, probably because of their abundant constitutive and rapidly inducible antioxidant enzyme pool size.[40,41] Alveolar type I cells are relatively resistant to the toxic effects of oxygen.[42] In contrast, in almost all species, the endothelial cell is particularly vulnerable to the toxic effects of oxygen. Acute pulmonary oxygen toxicity is associated with pulmonary edema and death from respiratory failure.[22, 42] The biochemical and genetic basis for endothelial cell vulnerability is unknown but may be related in part to low or poorly inducible antioxidant defenses as well as to abundant constitutive oxidant production under hyperoxic conditions.

Although the regulation of antioxidant levels has been studied extensively,[43, 44] the sites, relative importance, and regulation of specific enzymatic and nonenzymatic sources of *oxidant* production have received relatively little attention. Little is known about the biochemical and physiologic consequences of specific oxidant sources operating in the hyperoxic lung and how these sources are regulated *in vivo*.[45]

For example, in sheep, the cytochrome P-450 system may be an important source of oxidant production because inhibition of this enzyme system reduces hyperoxic lung injury.[38, 39] In baboons, apparent inhibition of the lung xanthine oxidase system with allopurinol reduces oxygen toxicity, although allopurinol also inhibits P-450.[46] Similarly, it is unknown whether the vulnerability of a cell to oxygen-induced damage is the result of unopposed oxidant production, inadequate antioxidant defenses, or both.

LUNG ENZYMATIC AND NONENZYMATIC DEFENSES AGAINST OXIDANT ATTACK

According to the free radical theory of oxygen toxicity, oxidant injury occurs when oxidants are produced at rates that exceed adjacent antioxidant defenses. Indeed, until methods are available for directly measuring free radical production in specific cells *in vivo*, the prevention or reduction of any injury by pretreatment or concurrent treatment with antioxidants is prima facie evidence that free radicals are involved. Antioxidants can be broadly categorized into enzymatic and nonenzymatic antioxidants, as shown in Table 94–1. The enzymes can be categorized into primary and secondary antioxidants.[47]

Three primary enzymatic antioxidants react directly with oxidants in cell cytoplasm: SOD, catalase, and glutathione peroxidase. To be effective, these antioxidant enzymes must be present at the site of free radical production. Two forms of SOD have been found in eukaryotic cells. The form containing copper and zinc is found in the cytoplasm and in small amounts in plasma,[48] and

Table 94–1. ENZYMATIC AND NONENZYMATIC ANTIOXIDANTS

Enzymatic Antioxidants	Nonenzymatic Antioxidants
Superoxide dismutase	Glutathione disulfide
Catalase	d-alpha-tocopherol
Glutathione peroxidase	Carotene
Glutathione reductase	Ascorbate
	Transferrin
	Ceruloplasm
Glucose-6-phosphate dehydrogenase	? Unsaturated fats

the form containing manganese is found in the mitochondria. SOD accelerates the rate of spontaneous dismutation of superoxide to hydrogen peroxide. In order for SOD to afford protection, superoxide must be removed before it reacts directly with cellular components or reacts with hydrogen peroxide to form the hydroxyl radical.

Catalase and glutathione peroxidase accelerate the reduction of hydrogen peroxide to water, thus bringing oxygen to its fully reduced state. Catalase is present primarily in the peroxisomes, whereas glutathione peroxidase is found in the cytoplasm. Like superoxide, hydrogen peroxide must be removed before it reacts with intracellular fatty acids or with superoxide to form the hydroxyl radical.

Secondary enzymatic antioxidants function by restoring peroxidized lipid membranes and oxidized protein sulfhydryl groups once the damage has already occurred. Glutathione peroxidase reduces organic hydroperoxides (as well as hydrogen peroxide) by means of glutathione as a reducing equivalent. Glutathione reductase and nicotinamide adenine dinucleotide phosphate (NADPH) are required for maintaining glutathione in its reduced state (GSH). NADPH is regenerated by the action of glucose-6-phosphate dehydrogenase (G6PD). Reduced glutathione also prevents protein sulfhydryl oxidation by competing with the proteins as a substrate for the oxidants. This concerted system of primary and secondary antioxidants is depicted in Figure 94–1. The intracellular localization of these antioxidants is depicted in Figure 94–2.

Lung antioxidant enzyme activity can be increased in rats by transient pre-exposure to either hypoxia or 85% oxygen, to bacterial endotoxin, or to TNF.[49] When lung antioxidant enzyme activity is increased by any of these methods, hyperoxic lung damage is reduced. This response may be unique to rodents, however, because similar protection by endotoxin in other species does not require comparable increases in lung antioxidant enzymes.[39] Full-term neonates of some animal species are relatively resistant to pulmonary oxygen toxicity, in comparison with adults of the same species.[50, 51] This relative protection is usually associated with an ability to increase antioxidant enzyme activity during oxygen exposure, even when the increased activity is less than the constitutive antioxidant activity in the mature animals. Premature animals of several species have been shown to be deficient in lung antioxidant enzymes in comparison with term animals.[52] However, it is equally possible that their enzymatic sources of oxidant production are also relatively underdeveloped, so that the net oxidant-antioxi-

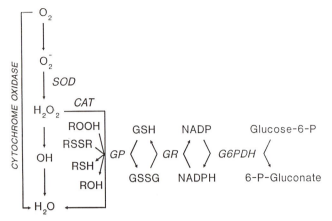

Figure 94–1. Schematic representation of oxygen (O₂) metabolites and enzymatic mechanism of inactivation. O_2^-, superoxide; SOD, superoxide dismutase; H_2O_2, hydrogen peroxide, CAT, catalase; OH, hydroxyl radical; ROOH, lipid hydroperoxide; RSSR, oxidized protein disulfide; RSH, reduced sulfhydryl protein; ROH, lipid hydroxide; GP, glutathione peroxidase; GSH, reduced glutathione; GSSG, oxidized glutathione disulfide; GR, glutathione reductase; NADP, nicotinamide adenine dinucleotide phosphate; NADPH, reduced nicotinamide adenine dinucleotide phosphate; G6PDH, glucose-6-phosphate dehydrogenase; H_2O, water.

dant balance in the premature infant is similar to that of adults.

Nonenzymatic antioxidants include a variety of intracellular substances that are susceptible to oxidation by oxygen radicals. Their role as protectors against oxidant attack depends on their ability to undergo oxidation without compromising cellular function. Vitamin E (d-alpha-tocopherol) serves this role within the lipid component of the cell membranes. The tripeptide glutathione and ascorbate (vitamin C) are soluble cytosolic antioxidants. Of these, glutathione is the most important antioxidant because of its abundance and its regulated production in all cells through a redox cycling system that requires glutathione reductase and G6PD.[53] Exposure to hyperoxia

may actually increase the requirements for glutathione synthesis because oxidized glutathione is released from the cell if produced in large amounts. Glutathione-depleted systems are markedly susceptible to oxidant stress of all varieties.

Several antioxidant enzymes depend on trace mineral cofactors for their activity, as shown in Table 94–2. The role of nutrients in free radical–mediated disease in human neonates has been reviewed.[54] The role of nutrition in ameliorating or exacerbating oxygen-induced damage in humans is still unfolding. Laboratory animals that are rendered deficient in dietary antioxidants (vitamin A, vitamin E, vitamin C, glutathione, sulfhydryl protein, selenium, or copper) are more susceptible to pulmonary oxygen toxicity than are control animals. However, attempts to enhance resistance to oxygen toxicity in normally nourished animals with pharmacologic doses of these nutrients have been largely unsuccessful.

Vitamin E, the most active form of which is alpha-tocopherol, is a fat-soluble vitamin incorporated into the lipid layer of cell membranes and functions as an intramembranous scavenger of oxygen radicals. Lipid-free radicals formed by fatty acid peroxidation are capable of initiating a chain reaction of lipid oxidation within cell membranes. Alpha-tocopherol interrupts this chain reaction by reducing the lipid radical to form a more stable alpha-tocopherol radical. In the 1960s, vitamin E received notoriety as an antioxidant when red blood cell hemolysis in premature infants was found to be caused by vitamin E deficiency.[55] Susceptibility of cell membranes to oxidation was found to depend on the amount of unsaturated fatty acids in the membrane, and the requirement for vitamin E was shown to be related to the polyunsaturated fatty acid (PUFA) and iron content of the formula.[56]

In laboratory animals, vitamin E deficiency is associated with increased susceptibility to pulmonary oxygen toxicity,[57] but attempts to enhance protection from oxygen toxicity by dietary supplementation in animals who

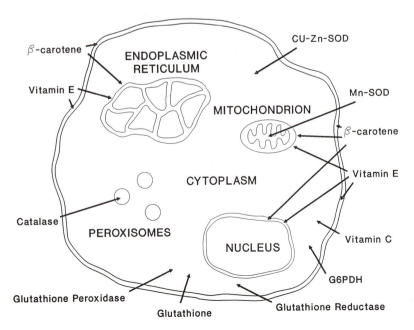

Figure 94–2. Intracellular localization of antioxidants. CU-Zn-SOD, copper-zinc superoxide dismutase; Mn-SOD, manganese superoxide dismutase; G6PD, glucose-6-phosphate dehydrogenase.

Table 94–2. NUTRIENTS AS COMPONENTS OF ENZYMATIC AND NONENZYMATIC ANTIOXIDANTS

Antioxidants	Nutrient	Function
Enzymatic		
Superoxide dismutase	Copper, zinc, manganese	Reduces superoxide to hydrogen peroxide
Catalase	Iron	Reduces hydrogen peroxide to water
Glutathione peroxidase	Selenium	Reduces lipid hydroperoxides
Glutathione reductase	Selenium	Regenerates reduced glutathione
Glucose-6-phosphate dehydrogenase	Selenium	Regenerates nicotinamide adenine dinucleotide phosphate
Nonenzymatic		
Glutathione	Sulfhydryl amino acids	Substrate for glutathione peroxidase
Tocopherol	Vitamin E	Intramembranous free radical scavenger
Carotene	Vitamin A	Intramembranous free radical scavenger
Ascorbate	Vitamin C	Regenerates reduced tocopherol

are not deficient have been unsuccessful.[58] Vitamin E is a fat-soluble vitamin with the potential for toxic effects from progressive accumulation in body tissue. Therefore, it seems prudent to exercise caution in the dietary supplementation of vitamin E to patients.

Vitamin A and its precursors may also function as antioxidants. Beta-carotene is a plant pigment precursor of vitamin A.[59] Beta-carotene can be incorporated into cell membranes and serves as an antioxidant in in vitro systems by quenching free radicals, preventing peroxidation of the membrane structural lipid.[60] In the human, vitamin A exists in several biochemical forms (retinol, retinal, retinoic acid, and retinyl esters). It is stored in the liver and circulates in plasma in the form of retinol bound to retinol-binding protein. There are also cytosolic binding proteins for intracellular vitamin A. Vitamin A is necessary for normal growth and differentiation of epithelial structures, reproductive function, and vision in the dark. The cellular mechanism of action for these physiologic functions of vitamin A has not been established, and the functional importance of the antioxidant properties of vitamin A is not known. Animals deficient in vitamin A develop necrosis and squamous metaplasia of the tracheobronchial tree, which are similar to the findings in severe BPD.

In 1985, Shenai and associates showed, in a prospective study, that premature infants in whom BPD developed had lower levels of vitamin A than did premature infants in whom chronic lung disease did not develop.[61] These studies were followed by a randomized trial of supplemental intramuscular vitamin A versus placebo in 40 infants with a birth weight of less than 1300 g who were at high risk for the development of BPD.[62]

Although there is strong evidence to support the provision of adequate vitamin A for infants of very low birth weight, the appropriate dosage and route of administration in sick, premature infants remain problematic. Because vitamin A is a fat-soluble vitamin with the potential for toxicity, further studies are needed in order to establish the optimal dosage for these infants. Although oxygen toxicity is believed to be a major factor in the early pathogenesis of BPD, the mechanism of protection by vitamin A could involve enhanced healing and differentiation of the damaged airway epithelium. The biochemical mechanism for this effect of vitamin A has not been established.

Other dietary components may function as antioxidants. For example, unsaturated fatty acids and sulfhydryl-containing amino acids are integral components of cell membranes and enzymes, respectively. Certain unsaturated fatty acids and sulfhydryl amino acids are essential nutrients for humans. Both are susceptible to oxidation by free oxygen radicals, and this damage is toxic to the cell. Moderate undernutrition[63] or selective deficiency of sulfur-containing amino acids[64] or glutathione[65] increases an animal's susceptibility to pulmonary oxygen toxicity. There has been considerable research on total protein requirements of growing infants and children, and cysteine is thought to be an essential amino acid in neonates. Much less is known about the risk of tissue glutathione depletion and cysteine requirements for optimal protection from oxidant stress in this population.

It is known that the lipid composition of the lung is affected by the lipid composition of the diet,[66] but the effect of dietary PUFA on pulmonary oxygen toxicity in humans has not been studied. This relative resistance has been associated with an ability to induce antioxidant enzyme activity, but newborn animals also have more PUFAs in their lung triglycerides than do the adult animals.[67] Increasing the PUFA content of the cell membranes in the lung might be expected to increase their susceptibility to oxygen-induced damage, but nonmembrane unsaturated fatty acids could theoretically serve as oxygen radical scavengers to protect vital constituents of the cell from oxidation. In a study by Kehrer and Autor,[66] rats who were fed a diet rich in saturated fatty acids were more susceptible to oxygen toxicity than the control animals, but rats fed a diet rich in unsaturated fats were protected. Sosenko and colleagues published a similar study in which the fatty acid composition of neonatal rat lungs was altered by maternal diet. Neonatal rats with an increased ratio of lung PUFA to saturated fatty acid were protected from the toxic effects of hyperoxia.[68]

Although it appears that pulmonary oxygen toxicity can be affected by the lipid composition of the lung and altered by diet, the mechanisms involved remain to be determined. One report suggested that intravenous lipid emulsions may aggravate lung injury in infants receiving long-term oxygen therapy.[69] The optimal fat composition of parenteral lipid solutions and infant formulas depends on considerations other than the effects on oxygen toxicity and remains to be determined in clinical trials.

Ascorbate is the only water-soluble vitamin that has antioxidant properties. Although ascorbate is known to be a powerful reducing agent, its biologic importance as an antioxidant is uncertain. Its antioxidant function may simply be to regenerate oxidized tocopherol.[70]

Transferrin and ceruloplasmin are serum proteins that have been shown to have antioxidant function *in vitro.* Their potential role as extracellular antioxidants is being explored, but some evidence suggests that these proteins (as well as glutathione) function as extracellular antioxidants in the alveolar lining fluid.[71]

Several trace minerals serve as cofactors for antioxidants. Selenium is a cofactor for glutathione peroxidase, and selenium deficiency enhances oxygen toxicity.[72] As for many of the antioxidants described previously, selenium supplementation in animals who are not deficient has not been effective in protecting them from the toxic effects of oxygen. Copper, zinc, and magnesium are cofactors for SOD. Copper deficiency has been shown to enhance oxygen toxicity in laboratory animals, but the clinical relevance of this finding in humans is unknown. Zinc and magnesium deficiency have other clinical manifestations that are more readily apparent than increased susceptibility to oxygen toxicity. Zinc deficiency can also cause retinol-binding protein deficiency, which interferes with the bioavailability of vitamin A. Although iron is a cofactor of catalase, it is also required for many oxygen radical–mediated reactions. Iron supplementation exacerbates the hemolysis seen in vitamin E deficiency; the role of iron status in pulmonary oxygen toxicity in vitamin E–replete humans is unknown.

STRATEGIES TO REDUCE PULMONARY OXYGEN TOXICITY

From this discussion, it is evident that there are at least three general strategies for reducing pulmonary oxygen toxicity *in vivo:* (1) to augment antioxidant defenses at the specific sites of increased oxidant production; (2) to render lung cells more resistant to oxidant damage; and (3) to identify and inhibit specific sources of oxidant production in cells vulnerable to oxidant attack.

AUGMENTATION OF ANTIOXIDANT DEFENSES

This first strategy has received the most attention in animal models of oxygen injury because the lung is accessible via many routes, and experimental protocols enable pretreatment with various agents hours to days before oxygen exposure. As noted, augmentation of endogenous antioxidant enzymes with endotoxin or cytokines has reduced oxygen injury in some species. Administration of antioxidants through liposomes may also reduce oxygen injury in some models. However, none of these methods enable specific adjustment of antioxidant levels at specific cellular and subcellular sites. Although these methods are useful in demonstrating that oxidants are involved in the pathogenesis of oxygen damage, clinical and laboratory

studies have already demonstrated the potential hazards of "shotgun" antioxidant therapy. For example, the administration of exogenous antioxidants may inhibit crucial oxidant pathways in granulocytes, which leads to impaired antimicrobial defenses[73] and clinical sepsis.[74] These studies strongly indicate that clinically feasible methods of reducing oxidant-induced lung injury *in vivo* must be based on site-specific regulation of the oxidant/antioxidant balance within specific cells under oxidant attack.

ENHANCED RESISTANCE TO OXIDANT ATTACK

It might be possible to adjust conditions within the hyperoxic lung that would render lung tissue at least transiently more resistant to the toxic effects of accelerated oxidant production. As noted, protein malnutrition and diets that lack unsaturated fat increase susceptibility to oxygen injury. In the first instance, protein deficiency may lead to reduced lung glutathione stores. In the second instance, diets deficient in unsaturated fat result in the synthesis of lung cell membranes, which are similarly deficient. It is thought that unsaturated fatty acids in cell membranes can function as decoys for free radical attack.[75] If this is true in humans, prompt protein supplementation and provision of unsaturated fat (e.g., with intravenous lipid emulsions) during oxygen exposure may be helpful in reducing oxygen injury. Because these interventions require cell growth, cell turnover, and long periods of supplementation to be maximally effective, it is unlikely that dietary changes could rapidly confer resistance to oxidant attack.

INHIBITION OF OXIDANT PRODUCTION

This strategy has received the least attention because it has been impossible to quantify the exact cellular and intracellular sites of oxidant production in the lungs. Results of animal studies with inhibitors of xanthine oxidase, P-450 monooxygenase, and Haber-Weiss reactions are promising, but trials in humans have not been performed. One way of limiting oxygen-derived oxidant production is to use the lowest inspired oxygen concentration that maintains normal systemic oxygen delivery within the range of normal cardiac output. Extrapolation of a few clinical reports of oxygen toxicity in humans has led to the widespread belief that there are safe and unsafe levels of oxygen, unsafe levels being defined as more than 40% to 50%. It is true that there is an approximate correlation between inspired oxygen concentration and oxygen injury, and high concentrations should obviously be avoided if possible (see Chapter 93 for a review of oxygen therapy). Some clinicians, however, resort to high inflation pressures to facilitate reduction of the inspired oxygen concentration in patients with lung disease. There is increasing evidence that excessive lung stretch and barotrauma may be just as damaging as oxidant stress.

At present, these strategies remain theoretical, and

there are currently no known safe, effective, and clinically feasible means for reducing hyperoxic lung injury.

REFERENCES

1. Levine JS: The origin and evolution of atmospheric oxygen. *In* King TE, Mason HS, Morrison M (eds): Oxidases and Related Redox Systems, pp. 111–126. New York: Alan R. Liss, 1988.
2. Priestley J: Experiments and Observations on Different Kinds of Air, vol. 2. London [publisher unknown], 1775.
3. Smith JL: The pathological effects due to increased oxygen tension in the air breathed. J Physiol 24:19–35, 1989.
4. Frank L, Bucher JR, Roberts RJ: Oxygen toxicity in neonatal and adult animals of various species. J Appl Physiol 45:699–704, 1978.
5. Hyde RW, Rawson AJ: Unintentional iatrogenic oxygen pneumonitis—response to therapy. Ann Intern Med 71:517–531, 1969.
6. Frank L: Effects of oxygen on the newborn. Fed Proc 44:2328–2334, 1985.
7. Shibamoto T, Taylor AE, Parker JC: PO_2 modulation of paraquat-induced microvascular injury in isolated dog lungs. J Appl Physiol 68:2119–2127, 1990.
8. White CW, Ghezzi P, Dinarello CA, et al: Recombinant tumor necrosis factor/cachectin and interleukin 1 pretreatment decreases lung oxidized glutathione accumulation, lung injury, and mortality in rats exposed to hyperoxia. J Clin Invest 79:1868–1873, 1987.
9. Cross CE, Halliwell B, Borish ET, et al: Oxygen radicals and human disease. Ann Intern Med 107:526–545, 1987.
10. Deneke SM, Fanburg BL: Normobaric oxygen toxicity of the lung. N Engl J Med 303:76–86, 1980.
11. Wispe J, Roberts RJ: Molecular basis of pulmonary oxygen toxicity. Clin Perinatol 14:651–666, 1987.
12. Klein J: Normobaric pulmonary oxygen toxicity. Anesth Analg 70:195–207, 1990.
13. Clark JM, Lambertsen CJ: Pulmonary oxygen toxicity: A review. Pharmacol Rev 23:37–133, 1971.
14. Delemos RA, Coalson JJ, Gerstmann DR, et al: Oxygen toxicity in the premature baboon with hyaline membrane disease. Am Rev Respir Dis 136:677–682, 1987.
15. Konradova V, Janota J, Sulova J, et al: Effects of 90% oxygen exposure on the ultrastructure of the tracheal epithelium in rabbits. Respiration 54:24–32, 1988.
16. Heino M: Morphological changes related to ciliogenesis in the bronchial epithelium in experimental conditions and clinical course of disease. Eur J Respir Dis [Suppl] 151:1–39, 1987.
17. Barnes SD, Agee CC, Peace RJ, Leffler CW: Effects of elevated PO_2 upon tracheal explants. Respir Physiol 53:285–293, 1983.
18. Burkhardt A: Alveolitis and collapse in the pathogenesis of pulmonary fibrosis. Am Rev Respir Dis 140:513–524, 1989.
19. Holm BA, Notter RH, Siegle J, Matalon S: Pulmonary physiological and surfactant changes during injury and recovery from hyperoxia. J Appl Physiol 59:1402–1409, 1985.
20. Young SL, Crapo JD, Kremers SA, Brumley GW: Pulmonary surfactant lipid production in oxygen-exposed rat lungs. Lab Invest 46:570–576, 1982.
21. Hazinski TA, Kennedy KA, France M: Effect of endotoxin pretreatment on the pulmonary vascular response to hypoxia in O_2-exposed lambs. J Appl Physiol 65:1586–1591, 1988.
22. Crapo JD, Barry BE, Foscue HA, Shelburne J: Structural and biochemical changes in rat lungs occurring during exposures to lethal and adaptive doses of oxygen. Am Rev Respir Dis 122:123–143, 1980.
23. Stocker JT: Pathology of acute bronchopulmonary dysplasia. *In* Bancalari E, Stocker JT (eds): Bronchopulmonary Dysplasia, pp. 237–278. Washington, DC: Hemisphere Publishing, 1988.
24. Henson PM, Johnston RB: Tissue injury in inflammation: Oxidants, proteinases and cationic proteins. J Clin Invest 79:669–674, 1987.
25. Raj JU, Hazinski TA, Bland RD: Oxygen-induced lung microvascular injury in neutropenic rabbits and lambs. J Appl Physiol 58(3):921–927, 1985.
26. Tate RM, Vanbenthuysen KM, Shasby DM, et al: Oxygen-radical-mediated permeability edema and vasoconstriction in isolated perfused rabbit lungs. Am Rev Respir Dis 126:802–806, 1982.
27. Elliott SJ, Schilling WP: Carmustine augments the effects of tert-butyl hydroperoxide in calcium signalling in cultured pulmonary artery endothelial cells. J Biol Chem 265:103–107, 1990.
28. Starke PE, Oliver CN, Stadtman ER: Modification of hepatic proteins in rats exposed to high oxygen concentration. FASEB J 1:36–39, 1987.
29. Deneke SM, Gershoff SN, Fanburg BL: Potentiation of oxygen toxicity in rats by dietary protein or amino acid deficiency. J Appl Physiol 54:147–151, 1983.
30. Reiter R, Burk RF: Effect of oxygen tension on the generation of alkanes and malondialdehyde by peroxidizing rat liver microsomes. Biochem Pharmacol 36:925–929, 1987.
31. Minchin RF, Boyd MR: Localization of metabolic activation and deactivation systems in the lung: Significance to the pulmonary toxicity of xenobiotics. Annu Rev Pharmacol Toxicol 23:217–238, 1983.
32. Tate RM, Morris HG, Schroeder WR, Repine JE: Oxygen metabolites stimulate thromboxane production and vasoconstriction in isolated saline-perfused rabbit lungs. J Clin Invest 74:608–613, 1984.
33. Freeman BA, Crapo JD: Biology of disease: Free radicals and tissue injury. Lab Invest 47:412–426, 1982.
34. Rojas J, Stahlman M: The effects of group B streptococcus and other organisms on the pulmonary vasculature. Clin Perinatol 11:591–599, 1984.
35. Witschi HR, Haschek WM, Klein-Szanto AJP, Hakkinen PJ: Potentiation of diffuse lung damage by oxygen: Determining variables. Am Rev Respir Dis 123:98–103, 1981.
36. Cheney FW, Huang TW, Gronka R: The effects of 50% oxygen on the resolution of pulmonary injury. Am Rev Respir Dis 122:373–379, 1980.
37. Frank L, Groseclose EE: Preparation for birth into an O_2-rich environment: The antioxidant enzymes in the developing rabbit lung. Pediatr Res 18:240–245, 1984.
38. Hazinski TA, Kennedy KA, France M, Hansen TN: Cimetidine reduces hyperoxic lung damage in lambs. J Appl Physiol 67:2586–2592, 1989.
39. Hazinski TA, Kennedy KA, France M: Effect of endotoxin pretreatment on the pulmonary vascular response to hypoxia in oxygen-exposed lambs. J Appl Physiol 65:1586–1591, 1988.
40. Forman HJ, Fisher AB: Antioxidant enzymes of rat granular pneumocytes: Constitutive levels and effect of hyperoxia. Lab Invest 45:1–6, 1981.
41. Matalon S, Holm BA, Notter RH: Mitigation of pulmonary hyperoxic injury by administration of exogenous surfactant. J Appl Physiol 62:756–761, 1987.
42. Kapanci Y, Weibel ER, Kaplan HP, Robinson FR: Pathogenesis and reversibility of the pulmonary lesions of oxygen toxicity in monkeys II. Ultrastructural and morphometric studies. Lab Invest 20:101–118, 1969.
43. Hass MA, Iqbal J, Clerch LB, et al: Rat lung Cu, Zn superoxide dismutase. J Clin Invest 83:1241–1246, 1989.
44. Visner GA, Dougall WC, Wilson JM, et al: Regulation of manganese superoxide dismutase by lipopolysaccharide, interleukin 1. FASEB J 2:2087–3091, 1988.
45. Pryor WA: Oxy-radicals and related species: Their formation, lifetimes and reactions. Ann Rev Physiol 48:657–667, 1986.
46. Jenkinson SG, Roberts RJ, Lawrence RA, et al: Induction of lung antioxidant enzymes in premature baboons treated with hyperoxia and allopurinol. Am Rev Respir Dis 139:A440, 1989.
47. Heffner JE, Repine JE: Pulmonary strategies of antioxidant defense. Am Rev Respir Dis 140:531–554, 1989.
48. Karlsson K, Marklund SL: Plasma clearance of human extracellular-superoxide dismutase C in rabbits. J Clin Invest 82:762–766, 1988.
49. Frank L, Roberts RJ: Endotoxin protection against oxygen-induced acute and chronic lung injury. J Appl Physiol 47:577–581, 1979.
50. Yam J, Frank L, Roberts RJ: Oxygen toxicity: Comparison of lung biochemical responses in neonatal and adult rats. Pediatr Res 12:115–119, 1978.
51. Frank L, Sosenko IR: Prenatal development of lung antioxidant enzymes in four species. J Pediatr 110:106–110, 1987.
52. Sosenko IR, Frank L: Guinea pig lung development: Antioxidant enzymes and premature survival in high O_2. Am J Physiol 252:R693–R698, 1987.

53. Van Asbeck BS, Hoidal J, Vercellotti GM, et al: Protection against lethal hyperoxia by tracheal insufflation of erythrocytes: Role of red cell glutathione. Science 227:756–759, 1985.
54. Kennedy KA: Dietary antioxidants in the prevention of oxygen-induced injury. Semin Perinatol 13:97–103, 1989.
55. Oski FA, Barness LA: Vitamin E deficiency: A previously unrecognized cause of hemolytic anemia in the premature infant. J Pediatr 70:211–220, 1967.
56. Williams ML, Shott RJ, O'Neal PL, et al: Role of dietary iron and fat on vitamin E deficiency anemia of infancy. N Engl J Med 292:887–890, 1975.
57. Wender DF, Thulin GE, Smith GJ, et al: Vitamin E affects lung biochemical and morphologic response to hyperoxia in the newborn rabbit. Pediatr Res 15:262–268, 1981.
58. Hansen TN, Hazinski TA, Bland RD: Vitamin E does not prevent oxygen-induced lung injury in newborn lambs. Pediatr Res 16:583–587, 1982.
59. Burton GW, Ingold KU: β-Carotene: An unusual type of lipid antioxidant. Science 224:569–573, 1984.
60. Krinsky NI, Deneke SM: Interaction of oxygen and oxy-radicals with carotenoids. J Natl Cancer Inst 69:205–210, 1982.
61. Shenai JP, Chytil F, Stahlman MT: Vitamin A status of neonates with bronchopulmonary dysplasia. Pediatr Res 19:185–188, 1985.
62. Shenai JP, Kennedy KA, Chytil F, et al: Clinical trial of vitamin A supplementation in infants susceptible to bronchopulmonary dysplasia. J Pediatr 111:269–277, 1987.
63. Frank L, Groseclose E: Oxygen toxicity in newborn rats: The adverse effects of undernutrition. J Appl Physiol 53:1248–1255, 1982.
64. Deneke SM, Gershoff SN, Fanburg BL: Potentiation of oxygen toxicity in rats by dietary protein or amino acid deficiency. J Appl Physiol 54:147–151, 1983.
65. Deneke SM, Lynch BA, Fanburg BL: Transient depletion of lung glutathione by diethylmaleate enhances oxygen toxicity. J Appl Physiol 58:571–574, 1985.
66. Kehrer JP, Autor AP: The effect of dietary fatty acids on the composition of adult rat lung lipids: Relationship to oxygen toxicity. Toxicol Appl Pharmacol 44:423–430, 1978.
67. Kehrer JP, Autor AP: Changes in the fatty acid composition of rat lung lipids during development and following age-dependent lipid peroxidation. Lipids 12:596–603, 1977.
68. Sosenko IR, Innis SM, Frank L: Polyunsaturated fatty acids and protection of newborn rats from oxygen toxicity. J Pediatr 112:630–637, 1988.
69. Hammerman C, Aramburo MJ: Decreased lipid intake reduces morbidity in sick premature neonates. J Pediatr 113:1083–1088, 1988.
70. McCay PB: Vitamin E: Interactions with free radicals and ascorbate. Annu Rev Nutr 5:323–340, 1985.
71. Pacht ER, Davis WB: Role of transferrin and ceruloplasmin in antioxidant activity of lung epithelial lining fluid. J Appl Physiol 64:2092–2099, 1988.
72. Forman HJ, Rotman EI, Fisher AB: Roles of selenium and sulfur-containing amino acids in protection against oxygen toxicity. Lab Invest 49:148–153, 1983.
73. Engle WA, Yoder MC, Baurley JL, Yu PL: Vitamin E decreases superoxide anion production by polymorphonuclear leukocytes. Pediatr Res 23:245–248, 1988.
74. Johnson L, Bowen FW, Abbasi S, et al: Relationship of prolonged pharmacologic serum levels of vitamin E to incidence of sepsis and necrotizing enterocolitis in infants with birth weight 1500 grams or less. Pediatrics 75:619–638, 1985.
75. Halliwell B, Gutteridge JM: Lipid peroxidation, oxygen radicals, cell damage, and antioxidant therapy. Lancet 1:1396–1397, 1984.
76. Bartlett D: Postnatal growth of the mammalian lung: Influence of low and high oxygen tensions. Respir Physiol 9:58–64, 1970.

95 MECHANICAL VENTILATION IN NEWBORNS

WALDEMAR A. CARLO, M.D. / RICHARD J. MARTIN, M.D.

Mechanical ventilation results in complex interactions between the ventilator and the patient. This chapter is a review of physiologic concepts that can be integrated into a rational approach to mechanical ventilation in neonates to advance the understanding of these interactions.

PULMONARY MECHANICS

Two mechanical properties of the respiratory system—compliance and resistance—largely determine the rate of gas entry and exit from the lungs.[1] Compliance is a measure of the elasticity or distensibility and can be expressed as the change in volume divided by the corresponding change in pressure. The most striking mechanical abnormality in infants with respiratory distress syndrome (RDS) is decreased compliance, which manifests as stiffness of the lungs. Resistance is a measure of the inherent capacity to resist airflow and can be expressed as the change in pressure divided by the corresponding change in flow. Pulmonary resistance is not significantly affected in infants with RDS, but it is increased in patients with bronchopulmonary dysplasia (BPD). However, endotracheal intubation with a small tube markedly increases resistance.[2]

Compliance and resistance can be evaluated together to determine their effect on airflow in and out of the lungs, inasmuch as their product (compliance × resistance) equals the time constant. The time constant is a measure of the time necessary for a lung unit (alveoli) to reach 63% of its final volume and change in pressure to equilibrate across a system. For practical purposes, pressure (and thus volume) equilibration is complete after a time longer than three to five time constants. Alveoli with short time constants fill faster than those with longer time constants. These concepts are pertinent for inspiration as well as for expiration and thus affect both tidal volume delivery and exhalation, including inadvertent end-expiratory pressure. For example, if inspiratory time is shorter than three to five time constants, tidal volume delivery is decreased.[3] Similarly, if expiratory time is shorter than three to five time constants, exhalation is incomplete, leading to an inadvertent increase in function residual capacity and in end-expiratory pressure.[4] However, it should be noted that the absolute duration of the time constant is likely to vary between inspiration and expiration largely because of differences in resistance.

One major clinical implication of the concept of time constant is that because disease states may affect compliance or resistance or both, the time constant may be altered differently by various diseases. For example, in RDS, because compliance is decreased, the time constant is short. In disease states with high resistance, such as BPD, the time constant may be prolonged. However, a very decreased compliance may counterbalance the effect of resistance because time constant is mathematically calculated as the product of compliance and resistance.

GAS EXCHANGE DURING MECHANICAL VENTILATION

Carbon dioxide (CO_2) diffuses readily from the blood into the alveoli. Thus CO_2 elimination depends largely on alveolar ventilation.[5,6] CO_2 elimination is proportional to ventilatory frequency and tidal volume (minus dead space). Increases in either frequency or tidal volume increase alveolar ventilation, increase CO_2 elimination, and thus reduce arterial CO_2 tension (Pa_{CO_2}).[4,6,7] The variables that affect minute ventilation (and thus CO_2 elimination) during pressure-limited time-cycled ventilation are illustrated in Figure 95–1.[8]

Besides fraction of inspired oxygen (FI_{O_2}), mean airway pressure is the major determinant of oxygenation in infants with RDS (Fig. 95–2).[5,7,9–14] Mean airway pressure is a measure of the average pressure to which the lungs are exposed during the respiratory cycle. Therefore, mean airway pressure is augmented by increasing peak inspiratory pressure (PIP) and positive end-expiratory pressure (PEEP). Increases in the ratio of inspiratory time to expiratory time (I:E ratio) and in inspiratory flow also increase mean airway pressure. However, increases in PIP and PEEP enhance oxygenation more than the latter changes.[13] Application of high mean airway pressures may cause lung overdistention, increase right-to-left shunting, and decrease cardiac output and thus may not be optimal for oxygen delivery. Similarly, high PEEP (more than 5 to 6 cm H_2O) may not be as effective in improving oxygenation.[15]

CONTINUOUS POSITIVE AIRWAY PRESSURE

The application of continuous positive airway pressure (CPAP) throughout the respiratory cycle constituted a

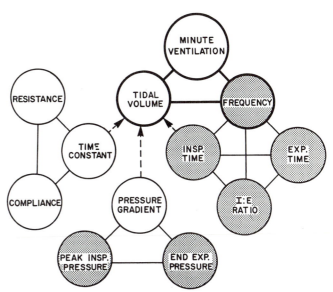

Figure 95–1. Relationship between ventilator-controlled variables (shaded circles) and pulmonary mechanics in determining minute ventilation during pressure-limited, time-cycled ventilation. The relation between the circles that are joined by solid lines is described by simple mathematic equations. Thus simple mathematic equations determine the time constant of the lungs, the pressure gradient, and inspiratory (INSP) time. These in turn determine the delivered tidal volume, and multiplication of tidal volume by the respiratory frequency yields the minute ventilation. Alveolar ventilation may be calculated from the product of tidal volume and frequency when dead space is subtracted from the former. EXP, expiratory; I:E, inspiratory:expiratory. (Adapted from Chatburn RL, Lough MD: Mechanical ventilation. *In* Lough MD, Doershuk D, Stern R [eds]: Pediatric Respiratory Therapy, 3rd ed. Chicago: Year Book Medical, 1985.)

major breakthrough in the treatment of severe RDS. Gregory and colleagues demonstrated that gas exchange in RDS can be improved significantly by applying CPAP and thereby reducing FI_{O_2}.[16] CPAP may be delivered via nasal prongs, endotracheal tube, nasopharyngeal tube, or face mask. Alternately, a continuous distending pressure

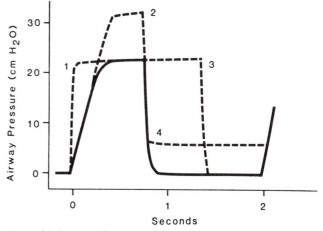

Figure 95–2. Four different ventilator-setting increases that augment mean airway pressure: 1, inspiratory flow; 2, peak inspiratory pressure; 3, inspiratory time/expiratory time (I/E) ratio; and 4, positive end-expiratory pressure. (Modified from Reynolds EOR: Pressure, waveform and ventilator settings for mechanical ventilation in severe hyaline membrane disease. Anesthesiol Clin 12:259, 1974.)

may be given by applying a negative pressure around the thorax. Access to the infant is markedly limited when a negative pressure is applied, and CPAP is generally preferred. CPAP may be used to support gas exchange in many infants with RDS. However, infants of very low birth weight often need endotracheal intubation and mechanical ventilation soon after birth.

Infants with RDS have alveolar instability secondary to surfactant deficiency, with resultant collapse of alveoli and diffuse microatelectasis, which CPAP may prevent. Furthermore, the increase in functional residual capacity that accompanies the application of CPAP is thought to decrease intrapulmonary shunting and thus improve ventilation/perfusion relationships. However, if alveolar overdistention occurs, lung compliance is decreased. Because of the Hering-Breuer reflex, the increase in functional residual capacity that accompanies the application of CPAP causes expiratory time to lengthen and respiratory rate to decrease.

The authors initiate CPAP whenever more than 70% oxygen is needed to maintain an arterial oxygen tension (Pa_{O_2}) of more than 50 to 60 mm Hg in infants with RDS, although it has been suggested that earlier use may reduce barotrauma.[17] A CPAP of 6 to 8 cm H_2O is used to initiate therapy. If this fails to improve oxygenation, a CPAP of 10 or 12 cm H_2O may be tried. These positive pressures at the airways are not transmitted completely to the pleural space because of the severely reduced lung compliance; hence venous return and cardiac output are usually not compromised. However, in infants with normal lungs, inappropriate use of CPAP is more likely to result in complications such as pulmonary air leakages, air trapping, impairment of venous return, and even decreased lung compliance. An increase in Pa_{CO_2}, as CPAP is augmented, may indicate a reduction in lung compliance. Because CPAP has a variable effect on Pa_{CO_2}, blood gases should be monitored closely. If severe respiratory acidosis ensues, assisted ventilation with endotracheal intubation is necessary. The use of CPAP during weaning from mechanical ventilation is discussed in the section on weaning from mechanical ventilation.

MECHANICAL VENTILATION

Ventilators may be classified according to how gas delivery during inspiration is limited. Thus pressure ventilators limit the PIP applied to the airways during inspiration, whereas volume ventilators limit the delivered volume. In addition to limiting pressure or volume, the inspiratory cycle may be terminated after a certain preset time or after a certain volume is reached. These ventilators are thus time or volume cycled, respectively. For safety purposes, some ventilators may also be made to cycle when a preset PIP is reached independently of their time- or volume-cycling mechanism. Because of ease of use, most neonatal ventilators are pressure-limited, time-cycle ventilators commonly called pressure ventilators.

Volume ventilators are less frequently used primarily for economic and technologic reasons. With a volume-cycled machine, delivered tidal volume is preset at 7 to 10 ml/kg. Flow rate is adjusted in order to determine the

Table 95–1. EFFECTS OF VENTILATOR-SETTING CHANGES ON BLOOD GASES

Ventilator-Setting Changes	Effects on Blood Gases	
	Pa_{CO_2}	Pa_{O_2}
↑ PIP	↓	↑
↑ PEEP	↑	↑
↑ Frequency	↓	±, ↑
↑ I/E ratio	—	↑
↑ FI_{O_2}	—	↑
↑ Flow	±, ↓	±, ↑

From Carlo WA, Chatburn R: Assisted ventilation of the newborn. *In* Carlo WA, Chatburn RL (eds): Neonatal Respiratory Care, 2nd ed, pp. 320–346. Chicago: Year Book Medical Publishers, 1988.
Pa_{CO_2}, arterial carbon dioxide pressure; Pa_{O_2}, arterial oxygen pressure; ↑, increase; ↓, decrease; ±, minimal effect; —, no consistent effect; FI_{O_2}, fraction of oxygen inspired in dry air; PIP, peak inspiratory pressure; PEEP, positive end-expiratory pressure; I/E, inspiratory time/expiratory time.

time over which the tidal volume is delivered, thus determining the I:E ratio. It must be recognized, however, that such ventilators deliver these volumes regardless of the pressure generated unless pressure limits are set. This feature assumes increasing importance in infants with severe RDS in whom compliance is so markedly diminished that delivery of a normal tidal volume requires a tremendous PIP. In this situation, a reduction in delivered tidal volume may be indicated. Another limitation of volume ventilators is that the high flow rates limit the adjustment of the I:E ratio.

The alternative is the use of a pressure ventilator, wherein flow is delivered to the patient until the predetermined PIP is reached. At this point, the pressure may be immediately allowed to return to end-expiratory levels, producing a saw-tooth pressure curve, or it may be maintained at peak levels for some time before the expiratory phase begins, producing a pressure plateau. Thus the pressure ventilator used in this way is actually time cycled and pressure limited. The ensuing discussion is specific for pressure-limited, time-cycled ventilators, but the analogies to volume ventilators are obvious.

The major effects of ventilator-setting changes on blood gases are summarized in Table 95–1. Although at times the effects of the same ventilator settings may vary and trial and error may be used, certain basic principles should serve as guidelines.[18] These principles are reviewed with a focus on the complex interrelationship between the ventilator and the mechanical characteristics of the respiratory system.

PEAK INSPIRATORY PRESSURE

The PIP in part determines the pressure gradient between onset and end of inspiration. Thus changes in PIP affect delivered tidal volume and alveolar ventilation. For a given compliance of the respiratory system, the delivered tidal volume is proportional to this pressure gradient. Therefore, an increase in PIP increases tidal volume, increases CO_2 elimination, and decreases Pa_{CO_2}.[4, 13] Furthermore, increases in PIP raise mean airway pressure and thus improve oxygenation.[7, 13] Use of an elevated PIP increases the risk of barotrauma with resultant air leakages,[19] BPD,[20] and impaired cardiac function; thus caution must be exercised when high levels of PIP are used.

POSITIVE END-EXPIRATORY PRESSURE

The use of PEEP raises mean airway pressure and thus improves oxygenation.[9, 13] PEEP may prevent alveolar collapse, increase lung volume at end expiration, and improve ventilation/perfusion relationships. However, because changes in PEEP alter the pressure gradient between inspiration and expiration, CO_2 elimination may be affected.[9] Thus elevation of PEEP may decrease tidal volume and CO_2 elimination and therefore increase Pa_{CO_2}.[4, 9, 13] Furthermore, the use of high PEEP (higher than 5 to 6 cm H_2O) may decrease lung compliance,[21, 22] which manifests as decreased tidal volume on a pressure-limited, time-cycled ventilator. Thus high PEEP (higher than 5 to 6 cm H_2O) may not be as effective in preterm infants with RDS.[15] Alveolar hypoventilation could occur with a corresponding increase in Pa_{CO_2} when high PEEP is used. In addition, use of very high PEEP may impair venous return, decrease cardiac output, and decrease oxygen transport. Although increases in both PIP and PEEP increase mean airway pressure and thus oxygenation, they usually have opposite effects on CO_2 elimination. The differential effect of PIP and PEEP on CO_2 elimination may be helpful for deciding the most appropriate ventilator-setting changes at a particular time. A minimal PEEP of 2 to 3 cm H_2O is recommended because endotracheal intubation eliminates the active maintenance of functional residual capacity that infants accomplish by vocal cord adduction.

FREQUENCY (OR RATE)

Frequency changes substantially alter alveolar ventilation and thus Pa_{CO_2}.[4, 6, 7] Use of moderately high frequencies (up to 60 breaths per minute) has enabled the use of a lower PIP and reduced the incidence of pneumothorax.[18] Nonetheless, it appears that the incidence of chronic lung disease or mortality is not altered by ventilation at these moderately high frequencies.[19] When very high frequencies are used, inspiratory time is shortened, and resultant tidal volume may decrease.[4, 21] Using a mechanical lung model simulating a neonate, investigators have demonstrated that with some pressure ventilators, minute ventilation reaches a plateau or decreases at rates higher than 75/min because of a reduction in the tidal volume.[4] In infants with RDS who are ventilated with pressure-limited, time-cycled ventilators, tidal volume delivery is maintained at a fairly constant level as long as inspiratory time is longer than approximately 0.4 sec.[21] Furthermore, if a very short expiratory time is used, expiration may be incomplete.[23] The gas trapped in the lungs would increase functional residual capacity and place the infant on the flat part of the pressure-volume curve, thus decreasing lung compliance.[23] As discussed for PEEP, the gas trapping, also known as inadvertent PEEP, that may accompany the use of a very short expiratory time would result in reduction of the effective pressure gradient and thus an elevation of Pa_{CO_2}.

Frequency changes alone (with a constant I:E ratio) usually do not alter mean airway pressure and do not substantially affect Pa_{O_2}. Nonetheless, because it takes a certain time for a pressure plateau to be reached, changes in inspiratory time that accompany frequency adjustments may affect first the airway pressure waveform and then mean airway pressure. Therefore, the decreased oxygenation observed by some investigators when high frequencies are used is likely caused by an inadvertent reduction in mean airway pressure.[5] In addition, a small increase in Pa_{O_2} may be expected as frequency is increased because of a reduction of alveolar CO_2 pressure and corresponding increase in alveolar O_2 pressure. If pulmonary artery hypertension and right-to-left shunting are prominent, the increased pH and reduced Pa_{CO_2} that accompany the use of high frequencies may reduce shunting and markedly increase Pa_{O_2} in the absence of any increase in mean airway pressure.

RATIO OF INSPIRATORY TO EXPIRATORY TIME

The major effect of changes in I:E ratio is on mean airway pressure and thus oxygenation.[7, 9, 10] Although results of a retrospective study suggested a decreased incidence of BPD with the use of reversed I:E ratios,[20] a large, well-controlled, randomized clinical trial has revealed only a reduction in the duration of high inspired oxygen concentration and PEEP exposure with reversed I:E ratios but no difference in morbidity or mortality rates.[12] Furthermore, when corrected for mean airway pressure, I:E ratio changes are not as effective in increasing oxygenation as are changes in PIP or PEEP.[13] Caution should be exercised when a very long expiratory time is used because this practice may increase the risk of air leakages[23] and impede venous return. Changes in I:E ratio do not usually alter tidal volume unless inspiratory or expiratory times become too short[5]—that is, less than three to five time constants. Thus CO_2 elimination is usually not altered by I/E ratio changes.[7, 9, 10, 12, 13]

INSPIRED OXYGEN CONCENTRATIONS

Changes in FI_{O_2} alter alveolar oxygen tension and thus oxygenation. Because both FI_{O_2} and mean airway pressure determine oxygenation, the authors attempt to balance them. During increasing support, FI_{O_2} is first increased (until approximately 60% to 70%) when additional increases in mean airway pressure may be warranted. During weaning, FI_{O_2} is first decreased (to approximately 40% to 70%) before mean airway pressure is reduced because maintenance of an appropriate pressure level may allow a substantial reduction in FI_{O_2}. Mean airway pressure should be reduced before a very low FI_{O_2} is reached. A higher incidence of air leakages has been observed when pressure is not weaned until a low FI_{O_2} is reached.[24] However, data on oxygen-related versus pressure-related lung injury are insufficient.

FLOW

Flow changes have not been well studied in infants but probably affect arterial blood gases minimally as long as a sufficient flow is used. High inspiratory flows are needed when inspiratory time is shortened, in order to maintain a square pressure waveform and deliver an adequate tidal volume.

In diseases such as meconium aspiration syndrome, asphyxia, and congenital diaphragmatic hernia, in which extrapulmonary shunting dominates the clinical picture, hyperventilation to reduce Pa_{CO_2} to 20 mm Hg (or even lower) may be necessary. The accompanying alkalosis and hypocapnia reduce pulmonary vascular resistance and right-to-left shunting. Patients with persistent fetal circulation are less likely to exhibit an increase in oxygenation in response to elevation in mean airway pressure; rather, they improve when shunting is reduced. Because lung compliance is not markedly decreased in these infants, high frequencies (up to 80 per minute) rather than high PIPs are usually safer. However, caution must be exercised when a short expiratory time is used in these infants, who usually have a normal lung compliance and a relatively long time constant. Gas trapping may occur if expiratory time is shortened too much. The use of low PEEP is also recommended in these infants. Infants who need assisted ventilation for apnea usually have normal lungs and can be ventilated with relatively low ventilator settings.

WEANING FROM MECHANICAL VENTILATION

Termination of mechanical ventilation may be attempted when the support provided by the ventilator is minimal in comparison with an infant's spontaneous breathing. Mean airway pressure and F_{IO_2} should also be relatively low. In infants with resolving RDS, weaning from assisted ventilation can usually proceed when the following settings have been achieved: PIP is less than 15 to 18 cm H_2O, frequency is less than 10 per minute, and F_{IO_2} is less than 40%. The authors administer CPAP through the endotracheal tube at the same pressure that has been used for PEEP but increase F_{IO_2} by 5% to 10%. If oxygenation and ventilation are adequate, either endotracheal CPAP may be weaned gradually to around 2 to 3 cm H_2O before extubation or nasal CPAP may be initiated. A minimal endotracheal CPAP of 2 to 3 cm H_2O should be used to maintain lung volume because tracheal intubation eliminates the laryngeal mechanism that controls expiratory airflow and lung volume.[26]

The authors prefer to restrict the use of nasal CPAP to preterm infants with resolving RDS who are at risk for atelectasis and apnea. Because very small endotracheal tubes add a high resistive load,[2] assisted ventilation may have to be continued until even lower settings are achieved in patients intubated with a 2.5-mm tube. Endotracheal CPAP should be used only for a short period before extubation because CO_2 retention may occur.[27] Infants with apnea, BPD, or extreme immaturity typically require a much slower weaning process that may last many days to weeks. In small infants, a low back-up rate of assisted ventilation elevates functional residual capacity.[28] In some infants, increasing respiratory drive with xanthines, such as theophylline, may facilitate weaning.[29]

The guidelines for ventilatory management presented in this chapter are the result of multiple individual studies, and a physiologic approach had been used to enhance understanding. Furthermore, an algorithm based on these guidelines that was tested in neonates with RDS resulted in an increased frequency of arterial blood gas correction.[30]

PATIENT-TRIGGERED VENTILATION

During neonatal mechanical ventilation, spontaneous breathing is common. Spontaneous breathing is usually beneficial because it may markedly increase minute ventilation and allow for a substantial reduction in ventilatory support. However, at times a neonate may seem to fight the ventilator, and spontaneous breathing may impair gas exchange and increase the risk of pneumothorax. In these situations, paralysis or sedation may be used to eliminate or reduce spontaneous respiratory efforts. However, this diminishes the advantages of spontaneous breathing. The technique of patient-triggered ventilation has been used to take advantage of spontaneous breathing. In this mode of ventilation, respiratory signals are used to synchronize the mechanical ventilator to the patient's breathing efforts. For example, airflow or esophageal pressure measurements are used to indicate onset of inspiration. This triggers the ventilator that has been preset to specific ventilatory settings. The availability of a back-up rate is necessary if no respiratory effort is detected for a prolonged period.

In a crossover study of infants with RDS, patient-triggered ventilation improved oxygenation.[31] However, even though both frequency and tidal volume increased, CO_2 elimination was not improved. If proved safe and efficacious by further clinical trials, this technique may reduce some of the complications resulting from mechanical ventilation.

COMPLICATIONS OF MECHANICAL VENTILATION

The introduction of mechanical ventilation into neonatal care has substantially reduced mortality rates. However, these interventions have resulted in complications previously considered rare or nonexistent.

Air leakages are among the most common complications seen during mechanical ventilation. Pneumothorax and pulmonary interstitial emphysema (PIE), which frequently occur simultaneously, are the most common types of air leakages seen in neonates.[32] As respiratory support is increased, the incidence of pneumothorax and PIE increases. Thus although the incidence of these air leakages is 8% to 10% among infants requiring hood and CPAP, respectively, 24% of infants treated with mechanical ventilation acquire a pneumothorax or PIE.[32] Pneumopericardium and pulmonary venous air embolism are

Table 95–2. TECHNIQUES FOR HIGH-FREQUENCY VENTILATION

Variable	HFPPV	Jet Ventilation	Flow Interruption	Oscillation
Frequency	60–150/min	60–600/min	300–900/min	300–3000/min
Waveform	Variable	Triangular	Triangular	Sine wave
I/E ratio	Variable	Variable	Variable	Constant (1/1)
Expiration	Passive	Passive	Passive	Active
Tidal volume	> Dead space	> or < Dead space	> or < Dead space	< Dead space
Entrainment	None	Possible	None	None

HFPPV, high-frequency positive-pressure ventilation; I/E, inspiratory time/expiratory time.

other air leakages that, although not as common, are usually life-threatening. Pneumomediastinum, on the contrary, is frequently an asymptomatic condition. Uneven alveolar ventilation and hyperinflation also occur insidiously.

A more chronic form of lung injury is BPD. Pressure and oxygen injury appear to be paramount in the pathophysiologic processes of BPD. However, the relative contributions of these factors to the development of BPD in a particular infant are unknown. Furthermore, other factors such as gestational age and weight appear to be predictive of the development of this type of lung injury. With the increased survival of smaller infants, BPD has become a common diagnosis in intensive care nurseries, occurring in about 25% of surviving infants of very low birth weight.[17]

Several complications may occur when the normal airway is bypassed. Dislodgment or occlusion of the endotracheal tube occurs commonly in neonates because of the small size of the airway and tubes. Atelectasis occurs commonly with tube malposition and in smaller infants. With prolonged endotracheal intubation, complications such as palatal groove and subglottic stenosis occur occasionally, although the latter tends to develop in infants with a relatively large tube or who have undergone frequent reintubations.[33] Necrotizing tracheobronchitis appears to occur primarily in very sick infants when humidification is less than optimal.

HIGH-FREQUENCY VENTILATION

As mentioned, mechanical ventilation frequently results in neonatal morbidity. Furthermore, RDS remains the single most common cause of neonatal mortality.[34] Interest has emerged among neonatal care providers in the use of high-frequency ventilation (HFV) because it may allow improved gas exchange while reducing barotrauma. In 1974, Heijmam and Sjöstrand first reported the application of HFV to neonates with RDS.[35] Since then, many investigators have used various devices to provide ventilation at high frequencies.

HFV encompasses new modes of ventilation that entails the use of tidal volumes that are lower and frequencies that are higher than those usual of conventional techniques. A proposed classification of the various modes of HFV is given in Table 95–2.

High-frequency positive-pressure ventilation (HFPPV) uses standard ventilators modified with low-compliance tubing and connectors so that an adequate tidal volume may be delivered despite very short inspiratory times. This technique was developed by U. Sjöstrand and co-workers in an effort to reduce cardiac side effects from mechanical ventilation.[1]

High-frequency jet ventilation (HFJV) is characterized by the delivery of gases from a high-pressure source through a small-bore injector cannula. It is possible that the fast flows out of the cannula produce areas of relative negative pressure, which entrain gases from the surroundings. This is currently the most widely used mode of HFV.

High-frequency flow interruption (HFFI) also delivers small tidal volumes by interrupting a flow (or perhaps pressure) source, but in contrast to jet ventilation, it does not involve the use of an injector.

High-frequency oscillatory ventilation (HFOV) delivers very small volumes (even less than dead space) at extremely high frequencies through the use of a piston pump or an acoustic speaker. It is unique because expiration is actively generated by the oscillator in contrast to the passive expiration that characterizes other HFVs. This characteristic may allow the use of higher frequencies without gas trapping.[36] This mode of HFV has been the mode most extensively studied.

Although gas exchange may improve during HFV, the mechanisms involved are not well understood. Gas transport by convection occurs particularly when tidal volumes are relatively large. However, adequate CO_2 elimination may occur despite tidal volumes lower than dead space,[37] and thus other mechanisms of gas transport must be involved.[38] Alveoli close to the airway obtain direct ventilation even though tidal volumes are lower than the anatomic dead space of the total respiratory system. Gas transport may occur between gas-exchanging units because some alveoli may fill or empty faster than others, a mechanism known as pendelluft.[39] Variable-velocity profiles during inspiration, turbulence, and augmented diffusion may also enhance gas exchange during HFV.[38]

CLINICAL EXPERIENCE

In a large controlled trial of neonates with RDS or pneumonia, Heicher and associates demonstrated that HFPPV markedly decreased the incidence of pneumothorax.[19] Other studies confirmed that adequate gas exchange may be achieved with HFPPV in critically ill neonates with RDS.[6, 40–41]

Jet ventilation has been used by many investigators.

Pokora and co-authors[42] first used HFJV with rates of 260 ± 50 per minute in neonates with respiratory failure; they observed reductions in the alveolar-arterial oxygen tension gradient and in Pa_{CO_2} in comparison with conventional mechanical ventilation. However, their success was adversely affected by the development of necrotizing tracheobronchitis in 44% of the infants[43,44] and fatal tracheal obstruction. The authors compared HFJV with pressure-limited, time-cycled conventional ventilation in 41 infants with RDS; these infants were randomly assigned during the first day or life either to receive HFJV at a rate of 250 per minute and I:E ratio of 1:3 to 1:4 for 48 h or to receive conventional therapy.[45] Despite comparable oxygenation in both groups, infants treated with HFJV had lower levels of Pa_{CO_2} and mean airway pressure, confirming results from smaller studies.[46-48] Furthermore, bronchoscopies did not reveal evidence of necrotizing tracheobronchitis.[49] A subsequent randomized study in which HFJV was used solely in the experimental group confirmed that HFJV resulted in improved gas exchange at lower airway pressures but did not prevent or substantially reduce rates of mortality or morbidity associated with conventional ventilation.[50]

The Bunnel Life Pulse HFJV has been evaluated in a multicenter, controlled trial in neonates with PIE.[51] Keszler and colleagues randomly assigned 144 neonates in whom interstitial emphysema developed during the first week of life to treatment either with HFJV or with "rapid rate conventional ventilation." Success criteria (resolution of PIE or improvement of emphysema with reduction in airway pressures) were met more frequently in the infants receiving HFJV (61%) than in the infants receiving conventional ventilation (38%; $p < .05$). However, mortality, air leakages, BPD, and other complications of conventional ventilation were not reduced in the neonates treated with HFJV. Spitzer and associates reported extensive experience with this jet ventilator and found evidence of the improvement in blood gases during HFJV.[52]

Gonzalez and collaborators,[53] using HFJV, demonstrated that the flow rate of the air leakage decreased markedly at the same time that HFJV allowed a reduction in the mean airway pressure. Despite improved gas exchange, survival could not be increased among infants with persistent fetal circulation and severe respiratory failure who met the criteria for high expected mortality rates.[54]

Frantz and co-workers reported the application of HFFI at frequencies of 300 to 1200 per minute in neonates with RDS with and without PIE; gas exchange was improved and resolution of RDS and PIE occurred in most infants.[55]

HFOV at rates of 480 to 1200 per minute used for 1- to 4-h periods[56] by Marchak and co-workers in neonates with RDS resulted in improvement in oxygenation. However, in the multicenter trial sponsored by the National Institutes of Health, HFOV did not result in improved gas exchange.[57] In this large, randomized study (673 preterm infants) designed to determine whether early intervention could prevent the development of chronic lung disease, HFOV did not reduce the incidence of BPD or mortality rates (Table 95-3). Furthermore, HFOV resulted in an

Table 95-3. RESULTS OF THE NATIONAL COLLABORATIVE STUDY USING HFOV

Variable	Conventional Ventilation ($n = 346$) (%)	HFOV ($n = 327$) (%)	Probability
Mortality at 28 days	17	18	.73
BPD	41	40	.79
Air leaks	38	45	.05
IVH (grade III or IV)	18	26	.02

HFOV, high-frequency oscillatory ventilation; BPD, bronchopulmonary dysplasia; IVH, intraventricular hemorrhage.

increased incidence of air leakages, intraventricular hemorrhage (grades III and IV), and periventricular leucomalacia. However, these results should be considered specific to the population studied and the type of ventilator evaluated, and they have not been reported as complications in other HFV trials. Indeed, in a preliminary report of a controlled trial, Clark and associates[58] noted that HFOV resulted in a modest reduction in the incidence of BPD ($p < .05$) and no increased complication rate. HFOV has also been used as a rescue measure in infants with persistent fetal circulation, but failure in this group of very ill infants is common.[59-61]

Several investigators successfully combined HFOV and intermittent mandatory ventilation in patients with severe respiratory failure. Boynton and colleagues[62] used an oscillator combined with intermittent mandatory ventilation as a rescue measure in neonates with respiratory failure during mechanical ventilation. They observed that oxygenation and CO_2 elimination were markedly improved during HFOV. Gaylord and associates[63] used a modification of HFFI combined with conventional ventilation in preterm infants with severe PIE and also demonstrated improved gas exchange at lower mean airway pressures and rates. Donn and collaborators[47] combined HFJV with mechanical ventilation in preterm infants, and these infants also maintained adequate blood gases at lower mean airway pressures than with mechanical ventilation. The improvement after intermittent inflations appears to be related to an increased lung volume and consequent improvement in pulmonary mechanics.[64] Intermittent inflations may prevent or resolve atelectasis, which sometimes complicates prolonged periods of HFV.

HFV may play a role in clinical conditions other than neonatal respiratory failure. In infants and children after cardiac surgery, cardiac output either improved or remained unchanged during periods of either HFJV[65] or HFFI.[66] Interestingly, cardiac output improved during HFJV in those infants who initially had poor cardiac output during conventional ventilation.[65] Regardless of the ventilatory mode, cardiac output was dependent on mean airway pressure. It is likely that the lower mean airway pressure used during HFJV may reduce the cardiovascular side effects of transpulmonary pressures.

The various HFVs are different and, accordingly, the results from clinical trials vary. However, most short-term studies revealed that improvement in gas exchange (especially a fall in Pa_{CO_2}) follows initiation of HFV. Further large trials are necessary in order to determine whether some types of HFV are able to reduce rates of morbidity associated with conventional mechanical ventilation.

REFERENCES

1. Carlo WA, Martin RJ: Principles of neonatal assisted ventilation. Pediatr Clin North Am 33:221–237, 1986.
2. LeSouef PN, England SJ, Bryan AC: Total resistance of the respiratory system in preterm infants with and without an endotracheal tube. J Pediatr 104:108–111, 1984.
3. Simbruner G, Gregory GA: Performance of neonatal ventilators: The effects of changes in resistance and compliance. Crit Care Med 9:509–514, 1981.
4. Boros SJ, Bing DR, Mammel MC, et al: Using conventional infant ventilators at unconventional rates. Pediatrics 74:487–492, 1984.
5. Boros SJ, Campbell K: A comparison of the effects of high frequency-low tidal volume and low frequency-high tidal volume mechanical ventilation. J Pediatr 97:108–112, 1980.
6. Field D, Milner AD, Hopkin IE: High and conventional rates of positive pressure ventilation. Arch Dis Child 59:1151–1154, 1984.
7. Reynolds EO: Effect of alterations in mechanical ventilator settings on pulmonary gas exchange in hyaline membrane disease. Arch Dis Child 46:152–159, 1971.
8. Chatburn RL, Lough MD: Mechanical ventilation. In Lough MD, Doershuk C, Stern R (eds): Pediatric Respiratory Therapy, 3rd ed, pp. 148–191. Chicago: Year Book Medical, 1985.
9. Herman S, Reynolds EO: Methods for improving oxygenation in infants mechanically ventilated for severe hyaline membrane disease. Arch Dis Child 48:612–617, 1973.
10. Boros SJ: Variations in inspiratory:expiratory ratio and airway pressure wave form during mechanical ventilation: The significance of mean airway pressure. J Pediatr 94:114–117, 1979.
11. Ciszek TA, Modanlou HD, Owings D, et al: Mean airway pressure—Significance during mechanical ventilation in neonates. J Pediatr 99:121–126, 1981.
12. Spahr RC, Klein AM, Brown DR, et al: Hyaline membrane disease: A controlled study of inspiratory to expiratory ratio in its management by ventilator. Am J Dis Child 134:373–376, 1980.
13. Stewart AR, Finer NN, Peters KL: Effects of alterations of inspiratory and expiratory pressures and inspiratory/expiratory ratios on mean airway pressure, blood gases, and intracranial pressure. Pediatrics 67:474–481, 1981.
14. Ratner I, Hernandez J, Accurso F: Low peak inspiratory pressures for ventilation of infants with hyaline membrane disease. J Pediatr 100:802–804, 1982.
15. Fox WW, Gewitz MH, Berman LS, et al: The Pa$_{O_2}$ response to changes in end-expiratory pressure in the newborn respiratory distress syndrome. Crit Care Med 5:226–229, 1977.
16. Gregory GA, Kitterman JA, Phibbs RH, et al: Treatment of the idiopathic respiratory distress syndrome with continuous positive airway pressure. N Engl J Med 284:1333–1340, 1971.
17. Avery ME, Tooley WH, Keller JB, et al: Is chronic lung disease in low birth weight infants preventable? A survey of eight centers. Pediatrics 79:26–30, 1987.
18. Carlo WA, Pacifico AL, Chatburn RL, et al: Efficacy of computer assisted management of respiratory failure in neonates. Pediatrics 78:139–143, 1986.
19. Heicher DA, Kasting DS, Harrod JR: Prospective clinical comparison of two methods for mechanical ventilation of neonates: Rapid rate and short inspiratory time versus slow rate and long inspiratory time. J Pediatr 98:957–961, 1981.
20. Reynolds EO, Taghizadeh A: Improved prognosis of infants mechanically ventilated for hyaline membrane disease. Arch Dis Child 49:505–515, 1974.
21. Field D, Milner AD, Hopkin IE: Inspiratory time and tidal volume during intermittent positive pressure ventilation. Arch Dis Child 60:259–261, 1985.
22. Philips JB III, Beale EF, Howard JE, et al: Effect of positive end-expiratory pressure on dynamic respiratory compliance in neonates. Biol Neonate 38:270–275, 1980.
23. Cartwright DW, Willis MM, Gregory GA: Functional residual capacity and lung mechanics at different levels of mechanical ventilation. Crit Care Med 12:422–427, 1984.
24. Primhak RA: Factors associated with pulmonary air leak in premature infants receiving mechanical ventilation. J Pediatr 102:764–768, 1983.
25. Hall RT, Rhodes PG: Pneumothorax and pneumomediastinum in infants with idiopathic respiratory distress syndrome receiving continuous positive airway pressure. Pediatrics 55:493–496, 1975.
26. Fox WW, Berman LS, Dinwiddie R, et al: Tracheal extubation of the neonate at 2–3 centimeters H$_2$O continuous positive airway pressure. Pediatrics 59:257–261, 1977.
27. Kim EH, Boutwell WC: Successful direct extubation of very low birth weight infants from low intermittent mandatory ventilation rate. Pediatrics 80:409–414, 1987.
28. Shutack JG, Fox WW, Shaffer TH, et al: Effect of low-rate intermittent mandatory ventilation on pulmonary function of low-birth-weight infants. J Pediatr 100:799–802, 1982.
29. Harris MC, Baumgart S, Rooklin AR, et al: Successful extubation of infants with respiratory distress syndrome using aminophylline. J Pediatr 103:303–305, 1983.
30. Chatburn RL, Carlo WA, Lough MD: Clinical algorithm for pressure-limited ventilation of neonates with respiratory distress syndrome. Respir Care 28:1579–1586, 1983.
31. Greenough A, Pool J: Neonatal patient triggered ventilation. Arch Dis Child 63:394–397, 1988.
32. Mandansky DL, Lawson EE, Chernick V, et al: Pneumothorax and other forms of pulmonary air leaks in newborns. Am Rev Respir Dis 120:729–737, 1979.
33. Sherman JM, Lowitt S, Stephenson C, et al: Factors influencing acquired subglottic stenosis in infants. J Pediatr 109:322–327, 1986.
34. Perelman RH, Farrell PM: Analysis of causes of neonatal death in the United States with specific emphasis on fatal hyaline membrane disease. Pediatrics 70:570–575, 1982.
35. Heijman K, Sjöstrand U: Treatment of the respiratory distress syndrome—Preliminary report. Opusc Med 19:235–244, 1974.
36. Bancalari A, Gerhardt T, Bancalari E, et al: Gas trapping with high-frequency ventilation: Jet versus oscillatory ventilation. J Pediatr 110:617–622, 1987.
37. Korvenranta H, Carlo WA, Goldthwait DA, Fanaroff AA: Carbon dioxide elimination during high-frequency jet ventilation. J Pediatr 111:107–113, 1987.
38. Chang HK: Mechanisms of gas transport during ventilation by high-frequency oscillation. J Appl Physiol 56:553–563, 1984.
39. Lehr JL, Butler JP, Westerman PA, et al: Photographic measurement of pleural surface motion during lung oscillation. J Appl Physiol 59:623–633, 1985.
40. Eyal FG, Arad ID, Godder K, et al: High-frequency positive-pressure ventilation in neonates. Crit Care Med 12:793–797, 1984.
41. Sedin G: Positive-pressure ventilation at moderately high frequency in newborn infants with respiratory distress syndrome (IRDS). Acta Anaesthesiol Scand 30:515–520, 1986.
42. Pokora T, Bing D, Mammel M, et al: Neonatal high-frequency jet ventilation. Pediatrics 72:27–32, 1983.
43. Boros SJ, Mammel MC, Coleman JM, et al: Neonatal high-frequency jet ventilation: Four years' experience. Pediatrics 75:657–663, 1985.
44. Boros SJ, Mammel MC, Lewallen PK, et al: Necrotizing tracheobronchitis: A complication of high-frequency ventilation. J Pediatr 109:95–100, 1986.
45. Carlo WA, Chatburn RL, Martin RJ: Randomized trial of high-frequency jet ventilation versus conventional ventilation in respiratory distress syndrome. J Pediatr 110:275–282, 1987.
46. Carlo WA, Chatburn RL, Martin RJ, et al: Decrease in airway pressure during high-frequency jet ventilation in infants with respiratory distress syndrome. J Pediatr 104:101–107, 1984.
47. Donn SM, Nicks JJ, Bandy KP, et al: Proximal high-frequency jet ventilation of the newborn. Pediatr Pulmonol 1:267–271, 1985.
48. Pagani G, Rezzonico R, Marini A: Trials of high frequency jet ventilation in preterm infants with severe respiratory disease. Acta Paediatr Scand 74:681–686, 1985.
49. Kercsmar CM, Martin RJ, Chatburn RL, Carlo WA: Bronchoscopic findings in infants treated with high-frequency jet ventilation versus conventional ventilation. Pediatrics 82:884–887, 1988.
50. Carlo WA, Siner B, Chatburn RL, et al: Early randomized intervention with high-frequency jet nebulization in respiratory distress syndrome. J Pediatr 117:765–770, 1990.

51. Keszler M, Donn SM, Bucciarelli RL: Controlled multicenter trial of high-frequency jet ventilation vs. conventional ventilation in newborns with interstitial emphysema. Pediatr Res 27:309A, 1990.
52. Spitzer AR, Butler S, Fox WW: Ventilatory response to combined high-frequency jet ventilation and conventional mechanical ventilation for the rescue treatment of severe neonatal lung disease. Pediatr Pulmonol 7:244–250, 1989.
53. Gonzalez F, Harris T, Black P, et al: Decreased gas flow through pneumothoraces in neonates receiving high-frequency jet versus conventional ventilation. J Pediatr 110:464–466, 1987.
54. Carlo WA, Beoglos A, Chatburn RL, et al: High-frequency jet ventilation in neonatal pulmonary hypertension. Am J Dis Child 143:233–238, 1989.
55. Frantz ID III, Werthammer J, Stark AR: High-frequency ventilation in premature infants with lung disease: Adequate gas exchange at low tracheal pressures. Pediatrics 71:483–488, 1983.
56. Marchak BE, Thompson WK, Duffy P, et al: Treatment of RDS by high-frequency oscillatory ventilation: A preliminary report. J Pediatr 99:287–292, 1981.
57. The HIFI Study Group: High-frequency oscillatory ventilation compared with conventional mechanical ventilation in the treatment of respiratory failure in preterm infants. N Engl J Med 320:88–93, 1989.
58. Clark RH, Gerstman DR, Null DM Jr, et al: High-frequency oscillatory ventilation reduces the incidence of severe chronic lung disease in respiratory distress syndrome. Am Rev Respir Dis 141:A686, 1990.
59. Cornish JD, Gerstman DR, Clark RH, et al: Extracorporeal membrane oxygenation and high-frequency oscillatory ventilation: Potential therapeutic relationships. Crit Care Med 15:831–834, 1987.
60. Kohelet D, Perlman M, Kirpalani H, et al: High-frequency oscillation in the rescue of infants with persistent pulmonary hypertension. Crit Care Med 16:510–516, 1988.
61. Bohn D, Tamura M, Perrin D, et al: Ventilatory predictors of pulmonary hypoplasia in congenital diaphragmatic hernia, confirmed by morphologic assessment. J Pediatr 111:423–431, 1987.
62. Boynton BR, Mannino FL, Davis RF, et al: Combined high-frequency oscillatory ventilation and intermittent mandatory ventilation in critically ill neonates. J Pediatr 105:297–302, 1984.
63. Gaylord MS, Quissell BJ, Lair ME: High-frequency ventilation in the treatment of infants weighing less than 1500 grams with pulmonary interstitial emphysema: A pilot study. Pediatrics 79:915–921, 1987.
64. Walsh M, Carlo WA: Sustained inflation during high-frequency oscillatory ventilation improves pulmonary mechanics and oxygenation. J Appl Physiol 65:368–372, 1988.
65. Weiner JH, Chatburn RL, Carlo WA: Ventilatory and hemodynamic effects of high-frequency jet ventilation following cardiac surgery. Respir Care 32:332–338, 1987.
66. Vincent RN, Stark AR, Lang P, et al: Hemodynamic response to high-frequency ventilation in infants following cardiac surgery. Pediatrics 73:426–430, 1984.

96 MECHANICAL VENTILATION IN PEDIATRIC PATIENTS

BENNIE McWILLIAMS, M.D.

There have been many changes in the general approach to mechanical ventilation in pediatric patients since the early 1980s for several reasons:

1. An increased understanding of pediatric pulmonary physiology and natural history of various disorders.
2. Development of ventilators into highly sophisticated systems that allow patient's interaction and control of ventilation.
3. An increased ability to assess pulmonary function in infants receiving mechanical ventilation.
4. An increasingly scientific approach to mechanical ventilation weaning and aspects of diaphragm training.
5. Improvement in the overall intensive care of pediatric patients.

This chapter is a review of the basic aspects of lung development relating to the mechanical ventilation of pediatric patients and a description of some of the newer techniques of mechanical ventilation in children.

LUNG GROWTH, DEVELOPMENT, AND FUNCTION

A basic understanding of the changes in lung structure and function from conception to maturity is important in an approach to mechanical ventilation of pediatric patients. Prenatal lung growth and development are well understood and have been reviewed elsewhere[1-5] and thus are not extensively reviewed here. Several points of normal lung development are mentioned in relation to mechanical ventilation of infants and children.

The conducting airway system is fully developed by 16 weeks of gestation and only grows in size from that time on.[4] The terminal respiratory units (respiratory bronchioles, alveolar ducts, and alveoli) grow in number until approximately 8 years of age and continue to grow in size until adulthood.[1] Because of this, the contribution of the small airways to total airway resistance is proportionally higher in infants than in older children and adults.[6] In addition, pores of Kohn,[7] which connect adjacent alveoli, do not develop until approximately 1 year of age, and canals of Lambert, which connect alveoli to larger airways, may not develop until approximately 5 years of age.[8-9] Extrapulmonary development is also significant. The chest wall of an infant is much more compliant than that of an older child or an adult.[10] In addition, the diaphragms are relatively flatter in infants than in adults, placing them at a mechanical disadvantage. These differences result in less efficient function and an increased oxygen cost of breathing in children in comparison with adults. This relative inefficiency and increased oxygen expenditure is further accentuated in pulmonary disease.

The components of respiration may be divided into ventilation and oxygenation in a model illustrated by Roussos and Macklem.[11] Ventilation deals primarily with gas movement in and out of the lungs and is considered in terms of pulmonary mechanics. Oxygenation deals primarily with gas exchange at the alveolar levels and is considered in terms of alveolar gas-exchange measurements such as arterial-alveolar gradients and shunt fractions. Although this is an oversimplification of the physiologic process, this division is useful in the approach to ventilation of children. The components of lung mechanics are basically the same for children as for adults.

Pulmonary mechanics are expressed as static and dynamic properties and are determined in the same manner in children and adults.[12] Static properties are defined by compliances of the lung, chest wall, and respiratory system. Dynamic properties are measured by resistances of the airway, chest wall, and respiratory system. In addition to the increased chest wall compliance in infants,[10] there are other differences in lung mechanics. Tepper and colleagues[5] demonstrated that infants have larger airways in proportion to their functional residual capacity, but size-corrected airflows are similar to those seen in older children and adults. To achieve gas flow into the lungs, resistive and compliant forces in the lungs must be overcome. The resistance forces that must be overcome are caused predominantly by airway resistance; compliant forces are caused predominantly by lung compliance. The product of resistance and compliance is defined as the time constant.[13] The time constant is a measure of how quickly an alveolar unit reaches equilibrium. Because there are differences in airway caliber and lung compliance with different stages of the respiratory cycle, inspiratory and expiratory time constants may be determined. In a normal lung, inspiratory and expiratory time constants are very close in value, but their difference may be accentuated in various disease states. Also, various diseases may alter the time constant, depending on the site of the pathologic process. In addition, different segments of the lung may have different time constants. In diseases causing increased airway resistance, such as asthma or bronchopulmonary dysplasia (BPD), the time constants of alveolar units increase, causing the alveolar unit to fill and empty more slowly ("slow" alveoli). In diseases resulting in decreased compliance, or "stiff" lungs, the time constant decreases, causing the alveolar unit to fill and empty quickly ("fast" alveoli). Three to five time constants are required in order to allow complete (95% to 99%) filling or emptying of an alveolar unit.[13] If three to five time constants are not allowed in expiration, air trapping occurs, resulting in intrinsic or auto–positive end-expiratory pressure (PEEP).[14, 15] Because a normal inspiratory time constant in an adult is approximately 0.5 sec, an inspiratory time of 1.5 sec is usually adequate. A normal infant may have a time constant of 0.1 sec, and an inspiratory time of 0.3 to 0.5 sec is optimal.

Factors relating to oxygenation, or gas exchange at the alveolar level, are basically the same in pediatric patients as in adults. Specific measures for improving oxygenation are discussed later.

MECHANICAL VENTILATION

TYPES OF MECHANICAL VENTILATORS

There are numerous volume ventilators on the market designed for adult patients. These usually work very well for children weighing more than 20 kg. Likewise, there are a number of ventilators available for premature and full-term infants. Table 96–1 lists some commonly used ventilators and their characteristics. For infants who weigh less than 4 to 5 kg, a time-cycled, pressure-limited ventilator, such as the Bear Cub ventilator, is typically used. In larger children, volume-limited ventilators are used. The Servo 900C is commonly used and delivers a wide range of tidal volumes (Table 96–1). In addition, it has the

Table 96–1. VENTILATORS FOR CHILDREN WEIGHING LESS THAN 20 K

Ventilator*	Inspiratory Cycling	Inspiratory Limit	Tidal Volumes (ml)	Flow Rates (Liters per Minute)	Breath Initiation	Circuitry	PEEP (cm H$_2$O)
Bear Cub BP 2001	Time	Time/pressure	0–200	3–30	IMV	Continuous flow	0–20
Baby Bird	Time	Time/pressure	0–200	0–30	IMV	Continuous flow	0–10
Servo 900C	Time/assist	Volume	0–2000	0–100	SIMV	Demand valve	0–50
Bear 5	Time/assist	Volume	50–2000	5–150	SIMV	Continuous or demand valve	0–50

PEEP, positive end-expiratory pressure; IMV, intermittent mandatory ventilation; SIMV, synchronized intermittent mandatory ventilation.
*Bear Cub and Bear 5 manufactured by Bear Medical Systems, Riverside, CA. Baby Bird manufactured by Bird Corporation/3M, St Paul, MN. Servo 900c manufactured by Siemens-Elma, Solna, Sweden.

advantage of a pressure support mode. A disadvantage is its lack of a continual flow circuit, which is needed occasionally when very small children are weaned. The Bear 5 ventilator is relatively new on the market and has the advantage of having intermittent mandatory ventilation (IMV), synchronized IMV (SIMV), pressure support, and mandatory minute ventilation. It also has both a continual mode and a demand-valve mode. It has the drawback, however, of delivering a minimal tidal volume of 50 ml, which limits its use in small children. Although there are other ventilators appropriate for use in children, these are the most commonly used in the author's institution, and they are adequate in meeting all the needs of conventional ventilation.

Mechanical ventilators have evolved from very crude instruments to highly sophisticated systems allowing advanced interaction with patients and monitoring. All ventilators in use today are either negative- or positive-pressure generated. Bulk flow of gas in and out of the lungs results from a pressure differential between mouth and alveolar pressures. Thus ventilation may be accomplished by either decreasing alveolar pressure (negative-pressure ventilation) or by increasing mouth pressure (positive-pressure ventilation).

NEGATIVE-PRESSURE VENTILATORS

Negative-pressure ventilation is the method of spontaneous breathing, and this method was used in the early ventilators.[16] Their use was expanded in the polio epidemic of the 1950s, but with the advent of positive-pressure ventilation, the use of negative-pressure ventilation decreased dramatically. Although they are not used extensively today, negative-pressure ventilators still maintain a small but important role in the management of selected diseases and conditions. This mode is discussed in more detail later.

POSITIVE-PRESSURE VENTILATORS

Although researchers studied positive-pressure ventilation in the early 1900s, its development and usage were limited until the 1950s. Since then, there have been great advances in ventilators and ventilatory techniques. Positive-pressure ventilation is currently the method used in ventilating acutely ill infants. The first step in positive-pressure ventilation is the establishment of a stable airway.

A child's airway may be stabilized by the use of a tight-fitting mask, an endotracheal tube, or a tracheostomy tube. There are, however, several points concerning artificial airways in relation to ventilated children that should be stressed. Because of the small size of a child's airway, small tubes are necessary. Also, because resistance to flow is a function of the fourth power of the radius of the tube in laminar flow and approximately the fifth power of the radius in turbulent flow,[13] the resistance to ventilation increases dramatically as tube size decreases. This increased resistance is usually overcome during positive-pressure ventilation, but it may cause difficulties in the

weaning period. When unusually small endotracheal tubes are required, as in children with subglottic stenosis, tube resistance may impair positive-pressure ventilation. To minimize laryngeal injury, uncuffed endotracheal tubes are the predominant tubes used in small children. Ideally, there should be a small air leakage during positive-pressure ventilation, which minimizes laryngeal damage.[17, 18] The presence of air leakages, however, may cause difficulties in adequately ventilating a child with a disease process causing decreased pulmonary compliance (stiff lungs). In addition, air leakages often render measurements of tidal volume or lung mechanics difficult or impossible. As the lung compliance in a mechanically ventilated child decreases, increased positive pressure is required. On occasion, this results in an increasing air leakage and inability to ventilate adequately. If this outcome is severe enough, reintubation with a larger or cuffed endotracheal tube is required. To minimize laryngeal injury, in such cases, the tube should be replaced with a smaller one or the cuff should be deflated as soon as the child's pulmonary status has improved.

In addition, small mucus plugs or debris may decrease the radius of an already small tube, thus greatly increasing tube resistance. Redding and colleagues[19] examined endotracheal tubes in intubated pediatric patients and found an overall incidence of partial endotracheal tube obstruction of 20%; 30% of the obstructed tubes had $\geq$50% obstruction of the lumen of the tubes. A 50% obstruction results in an increased resistance to airflow of four times or more. Thus adequate pulmonary toilet is essential. When a stable, ventilated child suddenly deteriorates, a plugged endotracheal tube must be suspected.

STAGES OF MECHANICAL VENTILATION

Mechanical ventilation in children may be divided into the acute, transitional or subacute, and weaning phases. The acute phase is the initial stage of stabilization in which oxygenation and ventilation are being corrected along with dysfunction of other systems. The subacute phase is the stage in which adequate oxygenation and ventilation have been achieved and the other organ systems are being corrected. The weaning phase is the transition period from mechanical ventilation to spontaneous breathing. This division, although somewhat arbitrary, is useful because each phase has different goals, objectives, and aspects unique to children.

ACUTE PHASE OF MECHANICAL VENTILATION

The goal of this phase of mechanical ventilation is the resumption of adequate oxygen delivery to the tissues. The most common approach to this phase is differentiating ventilation from oxygenation. This forms a useful framework with which to compare children and adults.

Ventilation

Ventilation involves the movement of air in and out of the lungs. In the acute phase, ventilation should be predominantly, if not completely, performed by the ventilator, and the contribution by the patient should be kept to a minimum. This allows diaphragmatic rest and return of diaphragmatic high-energy compounds to normal levels. Numerous studies demonstrated low levels of diaphragmatic high-energy compounds in respiratory failure; resting the diaphragm with mechanical ventilation enables the intracellular levels of these compounds to improve.[20, 21] In addition, many critically ill pediatric patients are uncooperative and unable to breathe synchronously with the ventilator. Thus sedation with or without muscle relaxation is often used to keep activity of patients at a minimum. This procedure improves oxygenation[22] and, in certain patients, decreases oxygen consumption.[23] Patients' contribution to ventilation is minimal or absent, and the objective is the optimal delivery of positive pressure by the ventilator.

It is helpful to consider the ventilatory cycle in terms of inspiratory and expiratory phases. The inspiratory phase of mechanical ventilation deals with aspects of the positive-pressure breath, and the expiratory phase of mechanical ventilation deals with PEEP and spontaneous ventilation.

The inspiratory phase may be divided into initiation, ending the inspiratory phase, and inspiratory pause.

Initiation. Controlled ventilation (CV), IMV, and SIMV are the most common methods of initiation of ventilation in pediatric patients. Although ventilators are usually set in the IMV or SIMV modes, they usually function as CV in the initial phases of ventilation, and it is only when the child begins spontaneous breathing that the ventilator functions as an IMV or an SIMV.

Ending the Inspiratory Phase. The inspiratory phase may be ended when a certain pressure, volume, time, or flow is achieved. Ventilators may thus be classified according to factors limiting the gas flow and ending the ventilator cycle. Most of the ventilators used in neonates and infants (time cycled, pressure limited) use IMV, whereas the ventilators used in older children and adults (time or volume cycled, volume limited) may use either IMV or SIMV.

Inspiratory Hold. The use of an inspiratory hold causes the lung to remain "held" in inspiration. Inspiratory hold is useful in diseases in which there are alveoli with increased inspiratory time constants (slow alveoli). Inspiratory holds in these circumstances allow the gas to redistribute to the slower alveoli, resulting in better gas distribution. Inspiratory holds, however, have the disadvantage of subjecting alveolar units with normal time constants to prolonged periods of positive pressure, leading to barotrauma and compromising cardiac output. The benefits gained by better gas distribution are often minimal, and because of decreased cardiac output caused by pressure support, actual oxygen delivery to the tissues may be decreased. The benefits gained by inspiratory holds are often not worth the complications; they are seldom used.

Ventilatory Parameters. The standard tidal volume used in pediatric patients is 10 to 15 ml/kg of body weight with an inspiratory time of three to five time constants, or 0.3 to 1.5 sec, depending on the child's age. Neonates are often ventilated with a somewhat smaller volume (8 to 10 ml/kg). The set tidal volume, however, may be very different from the actual volume that the child receives (corrected tidal volume). The set volume, or inspired volume, and the returned volume, or expired volume, may be measured internally (by the ventilator) or externally. In the usual situation in which the patient's respiratory quotient is slightly under 1.0, the exhaled volume is slightly less than the inspired volume. This difference in volume, however, is insignificant for clinical purposes, and in the absence of system air leakages, the inspired and expired volumes are essentially equal. In the absence of a ventilator circuit leakage, any difference in inspired and returned volumes is usually caused by endotracheal tube air leakages. Air loss may also be seen in patients with other types of air leakages such as bronchopulmonary fistulae.

The compressible volume, the volume lost to the patient in ventilatory tubing from a combination of tube expansion and gas compression, should also be taken into account. Each tubing circuit has a "compliance factor," which is used in calculating the compressible volume. In circuits for adults, the compliance factor is approximately 4 ml/cm H_2O, or for every 1 cm H_2O that the peak airway pressure rises above the PEEP value, 4 ml of gas is lost in the tubing circuit. Most pediatric ventilatory circuits have small-bore, noncompliant tubing, which minimizes compressible volume, with a compliance factor of approximately 1 ml/cm H_2O. These values, however, are estimates, and tubing compliance should be measured in each individual circuit. Compressible volumes are important in adults[24] but may be very important in the ventilation of small children with significant lung disease.[25] Because tidal volumes used in children are small and because larger children may be placed on ventilatory circuits for adults, the compressible volume may become extremely significant; it must be considered when ventilator settings are determined. Thus increases in tidal volumes and in mean airway pressure may only minimally increase the corrected tidal volume. In small children, the use of small pneumotachographic systems may be valuable in guiding ventilatory settings because all of the calculations involved in determining the corrected tidal volume may add significant error.

Ventilatory parameters may be adjusted in accordance with the pathologic process. In hyaline membrane disease (HMD), there are alveolar units with normal or decreased lung compliance, resulting in either normal or shortened time constants. Thus normal or slightly shortened inspiratory times may be used. In diseases such as meconium aspiration syndrome (MAS) or BPD, airway resistance is increased, causing increases in time constants in some areas. Thus slightly longer inspiratory times may be useful for even distribution of ventilation in these patients. The use of longer inspiratory times may, however, be limited because of the expiratory time required to prevent air trapping.

The expiratory phase of mechanical ventilation is also very important. Components that are adjusted in the expiratory phase are expiratory retard, expiratory time, and end-expiratory pressure. Expiratory retards are similar to inspiratory holds and are usually not indicated. Some ventilator circuits, especially when applied to small children with rapid ventilator rates, may have a flow resistance in exhaled valves, causing a functional expiratory retard.[26] This may result in higher expiratory pressures and impairment in ventilation as well as air trapping. Because the airways tend to collapse slightly during expiration, expiratory time constants are normally slightly longer than inspiratory time constants. In diseases involving airway obstruction, such as asthma, this difference is greatly accentuated. If the expiratory time is not at least three to five expiratory time constants in length, alveoli do not completely empty and become overdistended from residual pressure called intrinsic or auto-PEEP. This is a problem particularly in children with asthma, BPD, bronchiolitis, or other obstructive processes. Because air trapping may decrease ventilation significantly, a child with evidence of air trapping and carbon dioxide (CO_2) retention may improve with decreased ventilator rate and increased expiratory time.

The final aspect of the expiratory phase is the end-expiratory pressure. PEEP is used mainly to improve oxygenation by stabilizing alveoli. PEEP may have a variable effect on ventilation. Increasing PEEP may improve ventilation (decrease arterial CO_2 tension [Pa_{CO_2}]) by recruiting collapsed alveoli or may decrease ventilation (increase (Pa_{CO_2}) by causing overdistention of compliant alveoli. The effects of PEEP in ventilation depend on the compliance curves of individual patients.

Oxygenation

Improvement in oxygenation comes with increased fraction of inspired oxygen (FI_{O_2}) or by ventilator maneuvers. As is true in adults, ventilator manipulations are made in order to decrease FI_{O_2} to relatively nontoxic levels (0.40 to 0.60). Numerous studies have documented the relationship between oxygenation and mean airway pressure, (MAP), especially in neonates. Although this measurement is often used to monitor respiratory function in neonates and children and correlates with oxygenation, the use of MAP alone is an oversimplification. MAP is determined by a combination of positive-pressure ventilation and PEEP. These factors improve oxygenation in different ways, and each component must be considered separately. Positive-pressure breaths cause distention of alveoli, which is affected by manipulation in the inspiratory phase of mechanical ventilation.

The main components of the inspiratory phase that can be manipulated are peak inspiratory pressure (PIP), tidal volume, and inspiratory time. Usually two of these parameters are set, and the third one results from the other two and the patient's lung compliance. During volume-limited ventilation, tidal volume and inspiratory time (determined by the flow rate and tidal volume) are set, and the PIP results from the set parameters and the patient's lung mechanics. The physician may measure the PIP in volume-limited ventilators and calculate compliance, but in pressure-limited ventilation, the tidal volume is usually unknown and compliance cannot be determined.

Higher PIPs increase the distention of each alveolar unit, depending on compliance and time constant. Alveoli with low time constants ("fast" alveoli) reach equilibrium first and are more affected by barotrauma than alveoli with long time constants ("slow" alveoli). Thus when a child with airway obstruction (such as MAS, BPD, bronchiolitis, or asthma) is ventilated, high inspiratory pressures are transmitted to the normal alveoli preferentially, making them more susceptible to barotrauma. Manipulations in tidal volume have much the same effects as manipulation in PIP. Increasing the inspiratory time enables distribution of gas more evenly to the abnormal areas and improvement in oxygenation, but the normal alveoli may suffer barotrauma because of the extended exposure to high pressures. PEEP stabilizes alveoli that are already open and increases the functional residual capacity. Normally, there is a small resistance to expiration (physiologic PEEP) in spontaneously breathing children. This is important in small children because collateral ventilatory channels (pores of Kohn and channels of Lambert) are not well developed, so that alveoli in small children have a greater tendency to collapse. When a child is intubated, this physiologic PEEP is lost; consequently, every child should receive a small amount of PEEP (2 to 3 cm H_2O). Increasing PEEP improves oxygenation in children, as it does in adults. In general, PEEP levels lower than 10 cm H_2O do not cause significant impairment in cardiac output; levels higher than that may cause cardiovascular compromise. Children requiring PEEP levels higher than 10 cm H_2O should have some type of intravascular monitoring, such as a central venous or pulmonary artery catheter.

Which of the three major manipulations to improve oxygenation (tidal volume, inspiratory time, and PEEP in volume ventilation and PIP, inspiratory time, and PEEP in pressure-limited ventilation) is the best? Although no studies in pediatric patients have answered this question, there are data for neonates. Stewart and colleagues[27] found that in infants with HMD, PEEP was more efficient than PIP, tidal volume, or inspiratory time in improving arterial oxygen pressure (Pa_{O_2}) for a given increase in MAP. The complications of positive-pressure ventilation are related to MAP.[28] The components of MAP, however, seem to affect the complications differently. One of the major complications in positive-pressure ventilation is air leakage, and most evidence suggests that this complication, at least in infants with HMD, seems to result from overdistention of well-ventilated lung units.[29–31] Interstitial air from the leakage causes increased airway resistance and air trapping,[32] impairs cardiac output,[33, 34] and seems to be correlated with subsequent chronic lung disease.[35] From the interstitium, air may migrate to the subpleural space[36] to form a pneumothorax,[37, 38] pneumopericardium[39] or pneumoperitoneum;[40–42] or it may enter into the pulmonary venous system.[34, 40, 43, 44] In a study by Kolobow and associates,[45] sheep were ventilated with PIP values comparable with those used in patients with acute respiratory failure (50 cm H_2O) and exhibited severe barotrauma. Thus PIP and inspiratory time seem to result in more barotrauma than does PEEP for a given level of MAP. In addition, Heicher and associates[46] found a much higher incidence of pneumothoraces in neonates ventilated with a longer inspiratory time (1 sec) than with a short inspiratory time (0.5 sec). In a retrospective study, Primhak[47] found the inspiratory time to be the only factor related to air leakage. Thus at least in neonates and probably in older children, PEEP is the most efficient way of improving oxygenation while minimizing barotrauma.

Monitoring Pulmonary Function

Monitoring of pulmonary function during mechanical ventilation is important. Marini[48] reviewed monitoring techniques in adult patients and found that the same principles apply to infants and children. Monitoring during mechanical ventilation may be divided into assessment of gas exchange, workload, and breathing capability (Table 96-2). Gas exchange is most commonly assessed by blood gases, pulse oximetry, alveolar-arterial tension oxygen difference ($P(A-a)_{O_2}$, arterial/alveolar oxygen ratio, Pa_{O_2}/PA_{O_2}, arterial oxygen tension fraction of inspired oxygen ratio (Pa_{O_2}/Fi_{O_2}, and shunt fraction (Q_s/Q_t). With the exception of the shunt fraction, which requires a pulmonary artery catheter, these are the parameters most commonly used to assess ventilatory function in pediatric patients. Measurement of workload may be assessed by pulmonary mechanics (static and dynamic compliance and airway resistance), metabolic measurements (oxygen consumption and CO_2 production), minute ventilation, and work of breathing. Of these, static and dynamic compliances are most commonly measured and the trend, rather than the absolute values, are most important to follow. Ventilatory capability may be measured in pediatric patients by quantifying vital capacity, spontaneous tidal volume, and breathing pattern. More sophisticated tests are occasionally used in adults (inspiratory time/total time [T_i/T_{tot}], tidal volume/inspiratory time [V_T/T_i], and diaphragmatic electromyographs) but are not generally used in pediatric patients.

TRANSITIONAL PHASE OF MECHANICAL VENTILATION

Once a child is stabilized and adequate oxygenation and ventilation have been achieved, the patient moves into the subacute phase of mechanical ventilation. During this phase, the other organ systems are stabilized. Little is currently known about the effect of ventilator manipulation on subsequent weaning. Important in the transitional phase is the optimization of cardiac output and hemoglobin levels, control of any infectious process, and establishment of appropriate nutrition. Well-nourished children usually have low energy stores, and these stores are rapidly depleted in critical illness. Energy in infants who start out with subnormal energy stores[49] is more quickly depleted. Malnutrition makes critically ill infants more susceptible to infection and poor healing. In addition, malnutrition decreases the diaphragm muscle fiber cross-sectional area, resulting in decreasing diaphragm contractility and greater fatigability.[50] The effects of malnutrition on the respiratory muscle have been reviewed in detail.[51]

Table 96-2. MONITORING VENTILATED PEDIATRIC PATIENTS

Gas Exchange
Blood gases
  Arterial
  Venous
  Capillary
Pulse oximetry
$P(A-a)_{O_2}$ gradient
Pa_{O_2}/PA_{O_2} ratio
Pa_{O_2}/Fi_{O_2} ratio
Q_s/Q_t
Workload
Static compliance
Dynamic compliance
Metabolic measurements
Minute ventilation
Work of breathing
Capability
Vital capacity
Spontaneous tidal volume
Breathing pattern

$P(A-a)_{O_2}$, alveolar-arterial oxygen tension; Pa_{O_2}, arterial oxygen tension; PA_{O_2}, alveolar oxygen tension; Fi_{O_2}, fraction of inspired oxygen; Q_s/Q_t, shunt fraction.

WEANING STAGE OF MECHANICAL VENTILATION

Once the first two stages have been completed, the transition from mechanical breathing to spontaneous breathing, or the weaning phase, is begun. During the weaning phase, the emphasis shifts from dealing with lung disease and improving oxygen delivery to the tissues to enhancing the return of full diaphragmatic functioning and cessation of mechanical ventilation. It has become generally accepted that failure to wean results from diaphragmatic fatigue,[21, 52] although this concept is still questioned.[53] During the weaning phase, ways of "training" the ventilator muscles are considered.

There are numerous standard criteria for determining when and how quickly a patient can be weaned (Table 96-3). These indicators are imprecise, and in one study,[54] 63% of patients successfully extubated did not fulfill standard weaning criteria. Some authors[55] believe that these criteria prolong mechanical ventilation unnecessarily. In a study by De Troyer and associates,[56] the vital capacity seemed to be the best test for assessing neuromuscular function in acute neuromuscular disorders. Thus serial vital capacity measurements, if the patient can perform

Table 96-3. CRITERIA FOR VENTILATOR WEANING

Gas Exchange
Pa_{O_2} >60 mm Hg with Fi_{O_2} <0.35
Alveolar/arterial oxygen gradient <350 mm Hg
Pa_{O_2}/Fi_{O_2} ratio >200
Ventilation
Vital capacity >10–15 ml/kg of body weight
Negative inspiratory force <−30 mm Hg
Minute ventilation <10 l/min
Maximal voluntary ventilation more than twice/minute ventilation

Pa_{O_2}, arterial oxygen pressure/tension; Fi_{O_2}, fraction of inspired oxygen.

them, are useful for determining weanability. In infants, however, standard weaning criteria cannot be measured; the major determinants are the respiratory rate and blood gas levels.

Before specific methods of weaning are addressed, an examination of ventilator circuits is useful. Ventilator circuits may have intermittent or continual flow. In intermittent-flow circuits, there is no flow between breaths (ventilator or spontaneous breaths). When a patient attempts a spontaneous breath, he or she must decrease the pressure in the ventilator circuit and open a demand valve, which generates free gas flow. In continual-flow circuits, fresh gas is flowing all the time and the patient does not need to open any demand valves. There is less impedance to breathing in continual-flow circuits, but these circuits require high gas flows and they use a substantial amount of gas. With improvement in valve design, the differences in the work of breathing between these two systems has decreased.[57] Despite the improvements in valve design, numerous studies documented the advantage of continual-flow circuits over demand-valve circuits in decreasing both the work of breathing[58, 59] and the oxygen cost of breathing.[60] For most patients, however, intermittent-flow circuits are adequate. In patients who have difficulty weaning, changing from a demand-valve circuit to a continual-flow circuit should be considered. In infants, the work required to decrease the circuit pressure and open the demand valve to initiate a breath may be extremely demanding, and many of these patients are weaned from ventilatory support better on a continual-flow circuit. Neonates are most commonly weaned from ventilatory support with the use of continual-flow circuits.

The goal of the weaning phase is to decrease the amount of work that the ventilator performs and increase the amount of work that the patient performs. The two main methods of decreasing ventilatory support currently used are IMV (or SIMV) and T-tube or continuous positive airway pressure (CPAP) trials. When weaning with IMV, the work of breathing performed by the ventilator is gradually decreased by slowly decreasing the IMV rate while the patient spontaneously breathes more. For the majority of patients, this method is successful. In some patients, however, it has been suggested that weaning with IMV may produce a state of chronic low-grade diaphragmatic fatigue.[48] This is seen in children with BPD who tolerate weaning with IMV for several days and then deteriorate. An alternative method of weaning in these patients is use of the T-tube, or more commonly, CPAP trials. In this method, once the ventilatory rate is approximately 10 to 15 breaths per minute, the patient is placed on either a T-tube or a CPAP circuit for a specified time and then is given full ventilatory support. During CPAP trials, the patient must perform all of the work of breathing and afterwards may rest. Different schedules are used, but in general, patients begin with 5-min trials four times a day, gradually increasing until ventilatory support is discontinued. This method causes the diaphragm to have a period of work followed by complete rest. The T-tube or CPAP method of weaning has been gaining more popularity,[48] especially with knowledge of diaphragm fatigabil-

ity.[20, 52, 53] Ventilatory muscle training to offset diaphragm fatigue has successfully been used in patients with chronic lung disease.[61] The same principles have also been successfully applied to CPAP weaning in chronically ventilated adults.[48] The main disadvantage is that CPAP requires a significant amount of time from hospital staff.

Pressure support is another method of ventilator weaning that has been introduced and studied in adults.[62, 63] In this method, once the patient has triggered the demand valve to open, positive pressure is applied to the circuit. This facilitates the patient's spontaneous breath. The level of positive pressure is usually adjusted so that spontaneous breaths are full tidal volumes, known to be more physiologic and efficient.[64] This allows the patient to initiate the breath and coordinate it with the ventilator. In addition, pressure-support ventilation is more comfortable for the patients than is SIMV.[63]

Numerous studies have documented the efficacy of pressure-support ventilation in adults,[65, 66] but few investigators have examined its usefulness in children. It has, however, been used successfully in the author's institution in weaning children with severe BPD from ventilatory support. This method of weaning has several potential disadvantages in small pediatric patients. First, the work required for decreasing the pressure in the circuit and opening the demand valve is not changed when pressure support is added. As previously mentioned, this pressure is often significant in small children. Also, because infants normally have a fast respiratory rate, the response time of the system may not allow optimal coordination with pressure support. Although pressure support seems to be a good adjunct in adults and older children,[48] studies are needed in order to determine its role and usefulness in smaller children and infants. Pressure-support weaning has successfully been used with CPAP weaning.

Certain medications are often considered to facilitate ventilator weaning, such as bronchodilators and drugs to improve diaphragmatic function. Bronchodilators are helpful in controlling bronchospasm. Sympathomimetics,[67, 68] aminophylline,[69-71] caffeine,[72] digoxin,[73] and dopamine[74] have all been shown to improve diaphragmatic function. Sympathomimetics and aminophylline are occasionally used to improve diaphragmatic function in a patient who is a "difficult weaner."

Of the previously described methods of pediatric ventilatory weaning, IMV and SIMV are the most commonly used, followed by T-tube or CPAP trials. The majority of children wean successfully no matter which weaning method is used. The most important consideration in weaning a child with chronic lung disease, such as BPD, is that a consistent, slow-weaning schedule be followed. A child may require ventilatory support for over a year and still wean successfully. Patience and consistent support are indicated in these chronically ventilated patients.

HIGH-FREQUENCY VENTILATION

In the 1980s, there was increasing interest in high-frequency ventilators for neonatal and pediatric patients. High-frequency ventilators may be classified as either flow interruptors[75, 76] or high-frequency oscillators.[77] Exhalation in flow-interruptor systems occurs by means of the elastic recoil of the respiratory system, whereas it is actively facilitated in oscillators. There is a greater tendency for air trapping, development of auto-PEEP,[78] CO_2 retention, and depression in cardiac output[79] with flow-interruptor ventilators than with oscillators. Flow interruptors are usually used in the range of 1 to 5 Hz whereas oscillators are usually used in the range of 5 to 60 Hz. The mechanism of gas exchange in high-frequency ventilation has been reviewed by numerous authors[80, 81] but is still not completely understood and is probably different for high-frequency oscillation and high-frequency jet ventilation.[82]

High-frequency jet ventilation has been successfully used in neonates with HMD, pulmonary interstitial emphysema (PIE), and pulmonary air blocks.[83-85] The three main advantages of high-frequency ventilation over conventional ventilation are said to be improvement in ventilation/perfusion abnormalities, decreased depression of cardiac output, and decreased barotrauma.[86] Clinical and laboratory studies on the effects of high-frequency ventilation in gas exchange have been inconclusive.[87-91] Although high-frequency ventilation may have little advantage in preserving cardiac function in subjects with relatively normal cardiac status,[92] it may be beneficial in patients with right ventricular dysfunction.[93] Attenuation of barotrauma with high-frequency ventilation has been described in newborns,[89] but in other studies of acute respiratory failure in adults, there was no difference in the incidence of barotrauma with either modality.[94] In addition, high-frequency ventilation may cause cystic degeneration of the terminal bronchioles,[95] depression in mucociliary clearance,[96] and tracheal damage.[97] Thus severe bronchopulmonary fistulae and possibly severely compromised right ventricular functions are the main indications for using high-frequency ventilation in the pediatric intensive care unit.

EXTRACORPOREAL MEMBRANE OXYGENATION

Extracorporeal membrane oxygenation (ECMO) is a relatively new method of ventilatory support. It was introduced in 1972 in a case of acute respiratory failure in an adult,[98] but it did not gain widespread use until the early 1980s, when it was used in neonatal respiratory failure.[99-103] The concept of ECMO is relatively simple but requires a great investment in equipment, time, and expense. ECMO has been used successfully for periods ranging from several hours to weeks in neonates with HMD, MAS, diaphragmatic hernia, and persistent pulmonary hypertension.[99-103] The role of ECMO outside the neonatal period is less clear. Studies in older children and adults[104, 105] are difficult to interpret,[106] and one multiinstitutional study showed no advantage over conventional ventilation, although there are anecdotal reports of its success in children.[107] Thus although ECMO seems an attractive method of therapy that could minimize barotrauma, its role in pediatric respiratory failure is still undefined.

REFERENCES

1. Hislop A, Muir DC, Jacobsen M, et al: Postnatal growth and function of the pre-acinar airways. Thorax 27:265–274, 1972.
2. Hislop A, Reid L: Growth and development of the respiratory system. *In* Davis JA, Dopping J (eds): Scientific Foundation of Pediatrics, pp. 214–215. London: Heineman, 1974.
3. Inselman LS, Mellins RB: Growth and development of the lung. J Pediatric 98:1, 1981.
4. Reid L: The embryology of the lung. *In* DeReuck AVS, Porter R (eds): Ciba Foundation Symposium: Development of the Lung, pp. 109–124. Boston: Little, Brown, 1967.
5. Tepper RS, Morgan WJ, Cota K, et al: Physiological growth and development of the lung during the first year of life. Am Rev Respir Dis 134:513–519, 1986.
6. Hogg J, Williams J, Richardson J, et al: Age as a factor in the distribution of lower-airway conductance and in the pathological anatomy of obstructive lung disease. N Engl J Med 282:1283–1287, 1970.
7. Macklem PT: Airway obstruction and collateral ventilation. Physiol Rev 51:368–436, 1971.
8. Lambert MW: Accessory bronchiole-alveolar communications. J Pathol Bact 70:311–314, 1955.
9. Liebow AA: Recent advances in pulmonary anatomy. *In* DeReuck AVS, O'Conner M (eds): Ciba Foundation Symposium: Development of the Lung, pp. 2–28. Boston: Little, Brown, 1962.
10. Richards CC, Bachman L: Lung and chest wall compliance of apneic paralyzed infants. J Clin Invest 40:273–278, 1961.
11. Roussos C, Macklem PT: The respiratory muscles. N Engl J Med 307:786–797, 1982.
12. Murray JF: The Normal Lung. Philadelphia: WB Saunders, 1976.
13. Nunn JF (ed): Applied Respiratory Physiology, pp. 145–151. London: Butterworths, 1977.
14. Kemp J, Richardson P, Hansen T: Expiratory time constants from tidal mechanical ventilation should be used to predict inadvertent positive and expiratory pressure (IPEEP). Am Rev Respir Dis 135(Pt. 2):A240, 1987.
15. Kemp J, Richardson P, Geisler M: Expiratory time constants may be used to predict inadvertent positive and expiratory pressure (IPEEP) in normal and lavaged rabbits. Am Rev Respir Dis 135(Pt. 2):A240, 1987.
16. Woollam CH: The development of apparatus for intermittent negative pressure respiration. Anaesthesia 31:536–666, 1976.
17. Whited RE: A prospective study of laryngotracheal sequelae in long-term intubation. Laryngoscope 94:367–377, 1984.
18. Orringer MB: Endotracheal intubation and tracheostomy. Indications, techniques and complications. Surg Clin North Am 60:1447–1464, 1980.
19. Redding GJ, Fan LL, Cotton EK, et al: Partial obstruction of endotracheal tubes in children. Crit Care Med 7:227–231, 1979.
20. Rochester DF, Martin LM: Respiratory muscle rest. *In* Roussos C, Macklem PT (eds): The Thorax, vol. 29, pt. B, pp. 1303–1328. New York: Marcel Dekker, 1985.
21. Roussos C: Diaphragmatic fatigue and blood flow distribution in shock. Can Anaesth Soc J 33:S61–S64, 1986.
22. Crone RK, Favorito J: The effects of pancuronium bromide on infants with hyaline membrane disease. J Pediatr 97:991–993, 1980.
23. Palmisano BW, Fisher DM, Willis M, et al: The effect of paralysis on oxygen consumption in normoxic children after cardiac surgery. Anesthesiology 61:518–522, 1984.
24. Bartel LP, Basik JR, Powner DJ: Compression volume during mechanical ventilation: Comparison of ventilators and tubing circuits. Crit Care Med 13:851–854, 1985.
25. Mattila M: The role of the physical characteristics of the respirator in artificial ventilation of the newborn. Acta Anesthesiol Scand [Suppl.]56:1–107, 1974.
26. Marini JJ, Culver BH, Kirk W: Flow resistance of exhalation valves and positive end-expiratory pressure devices used in mechanical ventilation. Am Rev Respir Dis 131:850–854, 1985.
27. Stewart AR, Finer NN, Peters KL: Effects of alterations of inspiratory and expiratory pressures and inspiratory/expiratory ratios on mean airway pressure blood gases and intracranial pressure. Pediatrics 67:474–481, 1981.

28. Rhodes PG, Graves GR, Patel DM, et al: Minimizing pneumothorax and bronchopulmonary dysplasia in ventilated infants with hyaline membrane disease. J Pediatr 103:634–637, 1983.
29. Caldwell EJ, Powell RD, Mullooly JP: Interstitial emphysema: A study of physiologic factors involved in experimental induction of the lesion. Am Rev Respir Dis 102:516–525, 1970.
30. Macklin CC: Transport of air along sheaths of pulmonic blood vessels from alveoli to mediastinum. Arch Intern Med 64:913–926, 1939.
31. Macklin MT, Macklin CC: Malignant interstitial emphysema of the lungs and mediastinum as an important occult complication in many respiratory diseases and other conditions: An interpretation of the clinical literature in the light of laboratory experiment. Medicine 23:281–358, 1944.
32. Brooks JG, Bustamante SA, Koops BL, et al: Selective bronchial intubation for the treatment of severe localized pulmonary interstitial emphysema in newborn infants. J Pediatr 91:648–652, 1977.
33. Brazy JE, Blackmon LR: Hypotension and bradycardia associated with airblock in the neonate. J Pediatr 90:796–798, 1977.
34. Grosfeld JL, Boger D, Clatworthy HW: Hemodynamic and manometric observations in experimental air-block syndrome. J Pediatr Surg 6:339–344, 1971.
35. Watts JL, Ariagno RL, Brady JP: Chronic pulmonary disease in neonates after artificial ventilation: Distribution of ventilation and pulmonary interstitial emphysema. Pediatrics 60:273–281, 1977.
36. Plenat F, Vert P, Didier F, et al: Pulmonary interstitial emphysema. Clin Perinatol 5:351–375, 1978.
37. Hall RT, Rhodes PG: Pneumothorax and pneumomediastinum in infants with idiopathic respiratory distress syndrome receiving continuous positive airway pressure. Pediatrics 55:493–496, 1975.
38. Webb WR, Johnston JH, Geiser JW: Pneumomediastinum: Physiologic observations. J Thorac Surg 35:309–315, 1958.
39. Varano LA, Maisels MJ: Pneumopericardium in the newborn: Diagnosis and pathogenesis. Pediatrics 53:941–945, 1974.
40. Aranda JV, Stern L, Dunbar JS: Pneumothorax with pneumoperitoneum in a newborn infant. Am J Dis Child 123:163–166, 1972.
41. Donahoe PK, Stewart DR, Osmond JD, et al: Pneumoperitoneum secondary to pulmonary air leak. J Pediatr 81:797–800, 1972.
42. Leonidas JC, Hall RT, Holder TM, Amoury RA: Pneumoperitoneum associated with chronic respiratory disease in the newborn. Pediatrics 51:933–935, 1973.
43. Gregory GA, Tooley WH: Gas embolism in hyaline-membrane disease. N Engl J Med 282:1141–1142, 1970.
44. Vinstein AL, Gresham EL, Lim NO, et al: Pulmonary venous air embolism in hyaline membrane disease. Radiology 105:627–630, 1972.
45. Kolobow T, Moretti, MP, Fumagalli R, et al: Severe impairment in lung function induced by high peak airway pressure during mechanical ventilation. Am Rev Respir Dis 135:312–315, 1987.
46. Heicher DA, Kasting DS, Harrod JR: Prospective clinical comparison of two methods for mechanical ventilation of neonates: Rapid rate and short inspiratory time versus slow rate and long inspiratory time. J Pediatr 98:957–961, 1981.
47. Primhak RA: Factors associated with pulmonary air leaks in premature infants receiving mechanical ventilation. J Pediatr 102:764–768, 1983.
48. Marini JJ: The physiological determinants of ventilator dependence. Respir Care 31:271–282, 1986.
49. Pollack MM, Wiley JS, Holbrook PR: Early nutritional depletion in critically ill children. Crit Care Med 9:580–583, 1981.
50. Lewis MI, Sieck GC, Fournier M, et al: Effect of nutritional deprivation on diaphragm contractility and muscle fiber size. J Appl Physiol 60:596–603, 1986.
51. Rochester DF: Malnutrition and the respiratory muscles. Clin Chest Med 7:91–99, 1986.
52. Macklem PT: Respiratory muscles: The vital pump. Chest 78:753–758, 1980.
53. Swartz MA, Marino PL: Diaphragmatic strength during weaning from mechanical ventilation. Chest 88:736–739, 1985.
54. Tahvanainen J, Salmenpera M, Nikki P: Extubation criteria after weaning from intermittent mandatory ventilation and continuous positive airway pressure. Crit Care Med 11:702–707, 1983.
55. Millbern SM, Downs JB, Jumper LC, et al: Evaluation of criteria for discontinuing mechanical ventilatory support. Arch Surg 113:1441–1443, 1978.
56. De Troyer A, Estenne M, Heilporn A: Mechanism of active expiration in tetraplegic subjects. N Engl J Med 314:740–744, 1986.
57. Hillman K, Friedlos J, Davey A: A comparison of intermittent mandatory ventilation systems. Crit Care Med 14:499–502, 1986.
58. Gherini S, Peters RM, Virgilio RW: Mechanical work on the lungs and work of breathing with positive end-expiratory pressure and continuous positive airway pressure. Chest 76:251–256, 1979.
59. Gibney RT, Wilson R, Pontoppidan H: Comparison of work of breathing on high gas flow and demand value continuous positive airway pressure systems. Chest 82:692–695, 1982.
60. Henry WC, West GA, Wilson RS: A comparison of the oxygen cost of breathing between a continuous-flow CPAP system and a demand-flow CPAP system. Respir Care 28:1273–1281, 1983.
61. Pardy RL, Leith DE: Ventilatory muscle training. In Roussos C, Macklem PT (eds): The Thorax, vol. 29, pt. B, p. 1353. New York: Marcel Dekker, 1985.
62. MacIntyre NR: Respiratory function during pressure support ventilation. Chest 89:677–683, 1986.
63. MacIntyre N: Pressure support ventilation: Effects on ventilatory reflexes and ventilatory muscle workloads. Respir Care 32:447–453, 1987.
64. Otis AB, Fenn WO, Rahn H: Mechanics of breathing in man. J Appl Physiol 2:592–607, 1950.
65. Brochard L, Harf A, Lorino H, et al: Pressure support decreases work of breathing and oxygen consumption during weaning from mechanical ventilation. Am Rev Respir Dis 135(pt. 2):A51, 1987.
66. Brochard L, Harf A, Lorino H, et al: Optimal level of pressure support (PS) in patients with unsuccessful weaning from mechanical ventilation (MV). Am Rev Respir Dis 135(Pt. 2):A51, 1987.
67. Aubier M, Viires N, Murciano D, et al: Effects and mechanism of action of terbutaline on diaphragmatic contractility and fatigue. J Appl Physiol 56:922–929, 1984.
68. Howell S, Roussos C: Isoproterenol and aminophylline improve contractility of fatigued canine diaphragm. Am Rev Respir Dis 129:118–124, 1984.
69. Aubier M, DeTroyer A, Sampson M, et al: Aminophylline improves diaphragmatic contractility. N Engl J Med 305:249–252, 1981.
70. Dureuil B, Desmonts JM, Mankikian B, et al: Effects of aminophylline on diaphragmatic dysfunction after upper abdominal surgery. Anesthesiology 62:242–246, 1985.
71. Sigrist S, Thomas D, Howell S, et al: The effect of aminophylline on inspiratory muscle contractility. Am Rev Respir Dis 126:46–50, 1982.
72. Wittmann TA, Kelsen SG: The effect of caffeine in diaphragmatic muscle force in normal hamsters. Am Rev Respir Dis 126:499–504, 1982.
73. Aubier M, Viires N, Murciano D, et al: Effects of digoxin in diaphragmatic strength generation in patients with chronic obstructive pulmonary disease during acute respiratory failure. Am Rev Respir Dis 135:544–548, 1987.
74. Aubier M, Murciano D, Viires N, et al: Effects of digoxin on diaphragmatic strength generation in patients with chronic obstructive pulmonary disease during acute respiratory failure. Am Rev Respir Dis 135:544–548, 1987.
75. Carlon GC, Miodownik S, Ray C, Kahn RC: Technical aspects and clinical implications of high frequency jet ventilation with a solenoid valve. Crit Care Med 9:47–50, 1981.
76. Fletcher PR, Epstein MA, Epstein RA: A new ventilator for physiologic studies during high-frequency ventilation. Respir Physiol 47:21–37, 1982.
77. Bohn DJ, Miyasaka K, Marchak BE, et al: Ventilation by high-frequency oscillation. J Appl Physiol 48:710–716, 1980.
78. Beamer WC, Prough DS, Royster RL, et al: High-frequency jet ventilation produces auto-PEEP. Crit Care Med 12:734–737, 1984.
79. Chakrabarti MK, Sykes MK: Cardiorespiratory effects on high frequency intermittent positive pressure ventilation in the dog. Br J Anaesth 52:475–482, 1980.
80. Brusasco V, Knopp TJ, Rehder K: Gas transport during high-frequency ventilation. J Appl Physiol 55:472–478, 1983.
81. Chang HK: Mechanisms of gas transport during ventilation by high-frequency oscillation. J Appl Physiol 56:553–563, 1984.

82. Schuster DP, Karsch R, Cronin KP: Gas transport during different modes of high-frequency ventilation. Crit Care Med 14:5–11, 1986.

83. Carlo WA, Chatburn RL, Martin RJ, et al: Decrease in airway pressure during high-frequency jet ventilation in infants with respiratory distress syndrome. J Pediatr 104:101–107, 1984.

84. Harris TR, Christensen RD: High frequency jet ventilation treatment of pulmonary interstitial emphysema. Pediatr Res 18:326A, 1984.

85. Pokora T, Bing D, Mammel M, Boros S: Neonatal high-frequency jet ventilation. Pediatrics 72:27–32, 1983.

86. Slutsky AS, Brown R, Lehr J, et al: High frequency ventilation: A promising new approach to mechanical ventilation. Med Instrum 15:229–233, 1981.

87. Butler WJ, Bohn DJ, Bryan AC, Froese AB: Ventilation by high-frequency oscillation in humans. Anesth Analg 59:577–584, 1980.

88. Kolton M, Cattran CB, Kent G, et al: Oxygenation during high-frequency ventilation compared with conventional mechanical ventilation in two models of lung injury. Anesth Analg 61:323–332, 1982.

89. Frantz ID, Werthammer J, Stark AR: High-frequency ventilation in premature infants with lung disease: Adequate gas exchange at low tracheal pressure. Pediatrics 71:483–488, 1983.

90. Thompson WK, Marchak BE, Froese AB, Bryan AC: High frequency oscillation compared with standard ventilation in pulmonary injury model. J Appl Physiol 52:543–548, 1982.

91. Turnbull AD, Carlon G, Howland WS, Beattie EJ: High-frequency jet ventilation in major airway or pulmonary disruption. Ann Thorac Surg 32:468–474, 1981.

92. Hoff BH, Smith RB, Bunegin L, et al: High frequency ventilation in dogs with open chests. Crit Care Med 10:517–521, 1982.

93. Lucking SE, Fields AI, Mahfood S, et al: High-frequency ventilation versus conventional ventilation in dogs with right ventricular dysfunction. Crit Care Med 14:798–801, 1986.

94. Carlon GC, Howland WS, Ray C, et al: High-frequency jet ventilation: A prospective randomized evaluation. Chest 84:551–559, 1983.

95. Special conference report: High frequency ventilation for imma-

96. McEvoy RD, Davies NJHK, Hedenstierna G, et al: Lung mucociliary transport during high-frequency ventilation. Am Rev Respir Dis 126:452, 1981.

97. Carlon GC, Kahn RC, Howland WS, et al: Clinical experience with high frequency jet ventilation. Crit Care Med 9:1–6, 1981.

98. Hill JD, O'Brien TG, Murray JJ, et al: Prolonged extracorporeal oxygenation for acute post-traumatic respiratory failure (shock-lung syndrome): Use of the Bramson membrane lung. N Engl J Med 286:629–634, 1972.

99. Andrews AF, Klein MD, Toomasian JM, et al: Venovenous extracorporeal membrane oxygenation in neonates with respiratory failure. J Pediatr Surg 18:399–346, 1983.

100. Bartlett RH, Andrews AF, Toomasian JM, et al: Extracorporeal membrane oxygenation for newborn respiratory failure: 45 cases. Surgery 92:425–433, 1982.

101. Hardesty RL, Griffith BP, Debski RF, et al: Extracorporeal membrane oxygenation: Successful treatment of persistent fetal circulation following repair of congenital diaphragmatic hernia. J Thorac Cardiovasc Surg 81:556–563, 1981.

102. Kirkpatrick BV, Krummel TM, Mueller DG, et al: Use of extracorporeal membrane oxgenation for respiratory failure in term infants. Pediatrics 72:872–876, 1983.

103. Krummel TM, Greenfield LJ, Kirkpatrick BV, et al: Clinical use of an extracorporeal membrane oxygenator in neonatal pulmonary failure. J Pediatr Surg 17:525–531, 1982.

104. Lemaire F, Jardin F, Regnier B, et al: Pulmonary gas exchange during venoarterial bypass with a membrane lung for acute respiratory failure. J Thorac Cardiovasc Surg 75:839–846, 1978.

105. Zapol WM, Snider MT, Hill JD, et al: Extracorporeal membrane oxygenation in severe acute respiratory failure. JAMA 242:2193–2196, 1979.

106. Kirby RR: Membrane oxygenators: What role (if any) in acute ventilatory insufficiency. Crit Care Med 6:19–23, 1978.

107. Splaingard ML, Frazier OH, Jefferson LS, et al: Extracorporeal membrane oxygenation: Its role in the survival of a child with adrenoviral pneumonia and myocarditis. South Med J 76:1171–1173, 1983.

ture infants: Report of a conference, March 2–4. Pediatrics 71:280–281, 1983.

97 HOME VENTILATION

A. JOANNE GATES, M.D., M.B.A.

Since the 1980s, there have been increasing numbers of ventilator-dependent children and adolescents. According to a 1987 survey by the Office of Technical Assistance (OTA), there are at least 2000 ventilator-dependent children in the United States.[1] There are many reasons for the escalation in the numbers of patients who are technologically dependent for their ventilatory support. Nurseries are saving smaller infants who need ventilator support for longer periods of time, and they are surviving to go home. Patients with high spinal cord injuries are being saved at the scene by cardiopulmonary resuscitation, and they also require long-term ventilatory assistance. The care of patients with other traumatic injuries such as closed-head injuries has improved, and many of these patients are surviving with the technologic support for ventilation. Persons with other neurologic and neuromuscular disorders such as muscular dystrophy are being offered support that would not have been available in the past. Home ventilator therapy on a chronic basis is becoming more common in a variety of clinical settings; however, great differences exist in its availability and applicability and among medical practices across the country. In some states, there are many children on home ventilators, whereas in other comparably sized states there may be none.[1]

There are many benefits of home ventilation over continued ventilatory support in the hospital. Some of these include (1) reduction in the risk of nosocomial infection or the development of antibiotic resistance; (2) the opportunity to provide consistency in the caretakers, avoiding rotating teams or shifts of hospital personnel; (3) the abil-

Table 97–1. MEDICAL CONDITIONS THAT MAY CAUSE CHRONIC RESPIRATORY FAILURE OR INSUFFICIENCY IN A CHILD

Condition	Description
Cardiovascular	
Congenital	Uncorrectable or complex defects with pulmonary artery hypertension or congestive heart failure
Acquired	Myocardiopathy associated with Duchenne-type muscular dystrophy
Respiratory	
Upper	Arnold-Chiari malformation
Lower	Pulmonary hypoplasia, bronchopulmonary dysplasia
Neurologic	
Central	Congenital or acquired neurologic breathing disorder
	Congenital hypoventilation syndrome
Peripheral	Spinal cord injury
Muscular	
Congenital or acquired myopathy	
Muscular dystrophy	
Myasthenia gravis	
Skeletal	
Deformities of thoracic cage or vertebrae that restrict breathing	

ity to match the level of ventilatory support with the usual activities of daily living, and (4) the provision of a more familiar and relaxed environment with an improved quality of life.[2]

Patients who are candidates for home ventilation can be classified by diagnostic categories or by disorders of other organ systems that cause the chronic respiratory insufficiency or failure. The major pathophysiologic categories in these children include disorders of the following systems: respiratory (upper and lower respiratory tract), cardiovascular, neurologic (peripheral and central), and musculoskeletal[2] (Table 97–1). The three major diagnostic categories of patients selected for home ventilation are those with birth-related disorders, those with neurologic/neuromuscular disorders, and those with traumatic injuries. The criteria for selection are discussed in detail in the section on patient selection for home ventilation. Regardless of the cause of the chronic respiratory insufficiency or failure, medical stability is essential before the decision to consider home ventilation. The criteria for selection of an individual patient for home ventilation vary with the cause of the underlying disorder, with prognosis, and with logistic requirements for respiratory support.

SELECTION OF PATIENTS FOR HOME VENTILATION

ECONOMIC (COST AND BENEFITS) DECISIONS

The driving force for major change in health care is frequently the cost. This was certainly true in the evolution

of the care systems for ventilator-dependent children. There will be increasing demands by third-party payers to decrease costs by caring for handicapped children at home. In addition, as the home ventilator programs become more and more available and publicized, families may insist that their children with high-technologic needs receive home care. Several investigators have found per diem and total costs to be decreased.[1-10] Under pressure from parents, even Medicaid often pays, through waivers, for services that otherwise might not have been covered on the basis that home care is equal or preferable to hospital care.[11] However, home care may or may not prove to be less expensive on the basis of the number of days for which Medicaid will pay while the patient is in the hospital. In addition, 24-h private-duty nursing, if necessary, may not be a service covered by Medicaid programs. Insurance companies vary in their support of home ventilation; some encourage early discharge if less cost is involved, with 24-h nursing services. Other insurance companies prefer hospitalization because it limits their liability.

OTA reported cost data summaries demonstrating differences in costs and influences of home care nursing.[11] Many other reports support the concept that home care is less expensive than hospital care as long as some nursing care is performed by the family.[4, 5, 10, 12] Patients who are treated at home also tend to have a decreased risk of infection and decreased morbidity.[13, 14] The likelihood of being exposed to resistant organisms is reduced. Families report that there is much less family stress and turmoil when the patient is at home, despite the demands on the parents' time.[15, 16] However, when nurses and other health care providers are present in the home, there may be intrusion on family privacy and intimacy. Quality of life is defined differently among patients and families.[17, 18] However, most families express satisfaction with an improved quality of life with home ventilation.

Once the decision has been made to ventilate a child chronically, thus avoiding respiratory insufficiency failure, growth and development improve. Once the child is discharged home, in an environment in which there is more individual attention, there are often additional improvements in development and levels of functioning.

MEDICAL DECISIONS AND OBJECTIVES

The major diagnostic categories of patients selected for home ventilation are those with birth-related or congenital disorders, those with neurologic/neuromuscular disorders, and those with disorders related to traumatic injury. Patients in the first diagnostic group include those with chronic lung disease secondary to neonatal respiratory injury, known as bronchopulmonary dysplasia (BPD) (see Chapter 51). BPD is one of the most common cardiopulmonary disorders requiring long-term assisted ventilation; this need for prolonged ventilation often takes several months to define. In contrast, in children with congenital defects such as pulmonary hypoplasia or Arnold-Chiari malformation and disorders of control of breathing such as congenital hypoventilation syndrome (Ondine's curse), the need for long-term ventilation is identified earlier. Neurologic/neuromuscular disorders include static conditions (e.g., cerebral palsy or insults secondary to hypoxia) and progressive disorders (e.g., muscular dystrophy, spinal muscular atrophy, and other neuropathies or myopathies). Many affected children become candidates for home ventilation after they are placed on mechanical ventilation with an acute life-threatening event and cannot be weaned from the ventilator. Home ventilation may be an elective decision when there is deterioration as a result of increasing muscular weakness or incoordination. In the group with progressive lesions, death from respiratory failure occurs in the absence of intervention. With progressive disorders, weaning from the ventilator is unlikely, and this raises controversial issues for medical care providers and the family.

Children who sustain injury to the cervical spine at C-0 to C-3 are generally recognized from the beginning as needing chronic ventilatory support. Lower levels of injury, such as C-3 to C-7 may require varying levels, frequency, and duration of ventilatory support, depending on the exact location and the extent of the injury. For children in whom the need for long-term ventilation is almost certain at the time of injury, ventilation should be considered a modality of support and not an indication of the severity of the illness.

The first medical decision facing the physician is whether the patient will be ventilator dependent. Once the patient is designated as ventilator dependent, the objectives for optimal ventilatory support and criteria for discharge must be clearly defined. A guideline for assuming medical stability for home ventilatory support proposed by Goldberg and colleagues[2] is 1 month of clinical and physiologic stability requiring no major diagnostic interventions or changes in respiratory care that result from ventilation or oxygenation abnormalities. Specific criteria for evaluating physiologic stability may differ with the cause of the respiratory insufficiency or chronic respiratory failure. Various parameters are used in the evaluation of medical stability; these are discussed in detail in the section on evaluation. Arterial blood gases as well as noninvasive measurements of oxygen saturation (oximetry) and end-tidal carbon dioxide (CO_2) measurements are essential in the documentation of physiologic stability in children being considered for home ventilation.

The medical objectives for home ventilation in all patients are to promote age-appropriate growth, development, and cardiopulmonary function. When home ventilation is considered as an option for a ventilator-dependent child or adolescent, other essential medical decisions are included: the assessment of the family's capabilities of providing adequate (satisfactory) ventilatory support at home and the timing of when the family is ready to resume the responsibility for home ventilatory care. The family must be willing and able to learn the necessary skills for home ventilatory support.

As a part of discharge planning, it is essential to define the roles of the primary care and specialist physicians, designate a case manager, select the home health care agencies to provide nursing and respiratory therapy coverage, and establish lines of feasible communication with the hospital-based support team and community-based health care providers such as nursing agencies, durable medical equipment vendors, and visiting nurses.

MANAGEMENT

EVALUATION

Many parameters are used by physicians to determine ventilator dependence, optimal support levels, and weaning readiness. Various criteria for stability have been published in the many guidelines.[12, 13, 19] Continuing evaluation of these parameters enables the physician to monitor, reevaluate, and longitudinally manage these patients.

The first category of parameters are those for evaluating ventilation. Pulmonary function studies provide objective measurement of ventilation in patients considered for home ventilation. In general, children with a vital capacity of 30% or less need some degree of long-term ventilation (R. Spector, personal communication, 1987). Inspiratory forces and expiratory forces can be evaluated, particularly in patients whose problems include weakness. An inspiratory force less than −30 cm H_2O is preferable, although minimal, for adequate pulmonary toilet and ventilation. Sleep studies for evaluating end-tidal CO_2, pulse oximetry, and airflow help determine the need for ventilation during sleep. Disturbances during sleep are also early indicators of progressive disease requiring intervention with nighttime ventilation.[19]

Arterial blood gas levels are essential in evaluating requirements for ventilatory support. An arterial oxygen tension (Pa_{O_2}) that is acceptable in the weaning process is not acceptable under terms of optimal ventilation. Ideally, the Pa_{O_2} should be higher than 70 mm Hg, but in patients with cardiopulmonary disorders, a lower range of 60 to 65 mm Hg may be acceptable. In patients with cardiopulmonary disorders, the goal is usually to achieve an arterial CO_2 tension (Pa_{CO_2}) of 45 mm Hg or less. In those with central nervous system disorders and muscular or skeletal conditions, a Pa_{CO_2} of less than 40 mm Hg is the goal. A Pa_{CO_2} in the range of 30 to 38 mm Hg may be necessary for children with quadriplegia because they are more comfortable at those levels. (Higher levels cause them to have a continuous desire to breathe and a sensation of air hunger.) Children with chronic lung disease may tolerate a Pa_{CO_2} of up to 50 mm Hg, but it is desirable not to allow the Pa_{CO_2} to be higher than 45 mm Hg if reasonable ventilator rates can accomplish this. The patient's own respiratory rate should not exceed 30 because the child otherwise uses too much energy to maintain these higher rates. (Some patients have no ventilatory response to hypocapnia or hypoxemia, and so the respiratory rate may be unreliable.)

Growth curves should be monitored, and patients should be able to gain weight at a pace appropriate for their age. Plateaus and declines of growth usually indicate that the patient is forced to adapt to a less than ideal environment.

Electrocardiograms and echocardiograms can also be helpful in the initial evaluation and for monitoring. The electrocardiogram and echocardiogram, if abnormal initially, should improve with appropriate ventilatory support.

A complete blood count is helpful to monitor hemoglobin and hematocrit; both of these parameters must be adequate for oxygen delivery. If patients are chronically hypoxic, particularly at night, the hemoglobin should be elevated.

VENTILATION

There are several ways to provide ventilation. In some patients, particularly infants, nasal continuous positive airway pressure (CPAP) may be satisfactory, particularly if the upper airway is intact and functional. This is occasionally useful also for older patients with obstructive apnea during sleep. Negative-pressure ventilation has been recommended for patients who have muscle weakness; this requires intact airways so that the increased negative pressure does not augment upper airway collapse.[13] The effects of negative-pressure ventilation must be monitored closely. Children on negative-pressure ventilators may or may not require tracheostomies, depending on their airway control, suctioning requirements, and the need for emergency airway access. Negative-pressure ventilators include tank respirators, Port-a-Lungs, chest cuirasses, and Pulmo-Wraps. These devices are cumbersome and in many cases are considered uncomfortable.[19] There is also poor access to the patient. Emotionally, however, families seem to accept them better.

The most common mode of mechanical ventilation is positive pressure ventilation. Aversion to tracheostomies has been a great impediment to institution of positive-pressure ventilation. It does present cosmetic difficulties, but the complications are not as grave with the newer type of tracheostomy tubes. Airway safety should be an important consideration in determining whether a child needs a tracheostomy. In some children, the tracheostomy can be plugged during daytime hours and opened only at night for ventilation.

Various portable positive-pressure ventilators are available. The choice of ventilators should be based on the availability of local services for maintenance of the ventilator and response time to emergencies. The positive-pressure ventilators include the LP6; Bennett-Thompson M25A and M25B; Bear 33; Lifecare PVV, PLV-100, and PLV-102; and Puritan-Bennett Companion 2800. Other larger, less portable ventilators are also available. If larger ventilators are used and portable capabilities are lost, a major reason for considering home ventilation is lost as well.

Another modality available for children with an intact phrenic nerve and diaphragm is phrenic nerve pacing.[20] A clear airway is essential. Diaphragmatic fatigue is problematic as is infection. A tracheostomy and some ventilation are frequently required. Details of this procedure, its indications, and problems have been reviewed by Glenn and Phelps.[20]

OXYGENATION

Oxygen is frequently necessary in children with ventilatory needs; it can be introduced into the ventilatory circuit to avoid the need for pressurized gases for the ventilator. An oxygen concentrator or tanks of oxygen can be used as a source of supplemental oxygen. The oxygen flow or concentration of supplemental oxygen is determined by the Pa_{CO_2} or arterial oxygen saturation. Oxygen saturation should be higher than 90% to 92%, even at times of exertion and exercise.

TRACHEOSTOMIES

Tracheostomy care is extremely important (see Chapter 92). The more commonly used commercially available tracheostomy tubes are the Portex and Shiley. Pediatric sizes of these tubes range from 00 to 4, and these tubes do not have an inner cannula. Tracheostomy tubes larger than size 4 must have an inner cannula. Up to size 4, these tubes may or may not be fenestrated or cuffed. Once children require larger tracheostomy tubes, they may require cuffs for secretion control. Children who chronically aspirate usually require a cuffed tracheostomy tube. Cuffed tracheostomy tubes are usually avoided in order to facilitate speech development. During periods of rapid growth, the size of the tracheostomy tube may have to be increased every 6 to 12 months. The decisions about the frequency of change for tracheostomy tubes are determined by many aspects. Tracheostomy tubes may be changed every day if they are not cuffed (R. Spector, personal communication, 1987); cuffed tracheostomy tubes, for reasons of comfort, are changed less often. The presence of infection necessitates more frequent changes.

POSITIVE END-EXPIRATORY PRESSURE

The use of positive end-expiratory pressure (PEEP) makes the ventilator equipment more complex; however, most children on ventilators require it. Disposable valves with set PEEP values are available. Spring-loaded, nondisposable, variable PEEP valves are also available. Many patients with tracheomalacia or bronchomalacia benefit from higher levels of PEEP.

WEANING

The most difficult decisions for the physician to make concern weaning. The easiest arrangements to make in the home environment are pulse oximetry and checking of ventilator settings. Saturation levels higher than 90% at times of stress should be maintained, although some leeway for desaturation should be allowed. A saturation of 94% allows flexibility. End-tidal (partial) carbon dioxide tension (PET_{CO_2}) of 6.5 or a Pa_{CO_2} of 35 to 50 mm Hg may be acceptable.[12] The patient's family can monitor sleeping and awake respiratory rates, growth rates, exercise tolerance, color changes with excitation, and respiratory distress. Sputum changes can warn of impending infection.[12] Diaphoresis should be monitored and used to dictate increases or decreases in ventilatory support.[12, 13, 21] If the child does not spontaneously breathe at all during sleep and has a disease from which he or she may be recovering, further weaning can be attempted. Thorough records should be kept.[21, 22] Parents generally cannot resist the desire to decrease oxygen concentrations and increase time spent off the ventilator; this occasionally results in rapid deterioration of the patient's condition.

MEDICATIONS

Medications vary with the patient's individual disease. Those with BPD frequently require diuretics or bronchodilators. Other children may require medications for management of airway secretions. Quadriplegic patients may require medications for muscle spasm, urinary tract infection, and hypercalcemia.[23] Bronchodilators such as theophylline or aerosolized beta$_2$-agonists are commonly used, especially in patients with BPD. Chest physical therapy is usually indicated for management of airway secretions.

NUTRITION

Nutrition is a key issue in caring for children on home ventilation. Metabolic studies demonstrate the need for adequate nutrition to accomplish weaning and growth.[24, 25] These children may require caloric intake beyond their ability to consume calories and beyond predicted normal levels for their age. Caloric needs are measurable.[25] Frequently, a supplemental feeding method in addition to oral intake, such as a gastrostomy, is required; a fundoplication may be needed in order to avoid gastroesophageal reflex. Special calorie-dense formulas may be necessary, especially for children who need high-calorie intake but low fluid intake. MCT oil or Polycose may be used to increase caloric density. Tube feedings may be supplementary or may provide total nutrition. They may be given (1) as bolus feedings, (2) continuously up to 24 hours, or (3) only as supplements through the night.

MONITORING

One of the goals of home care is to avoid complexity and technology, but monitors are necessary for safety. Most of the equipment has built-in alarms that should warn of high pressures, low pressures, and loss of power. Children with tracheostomies should sleep with apnea and bradycardia monitors. Patients who are totally ventilator dependent should have constant monitoring either with personal attendants or mechanically. In patients who are totally ventilator dependent, it is essential that signal devices that they can operate in times of emergency are readily available. For quadriplegic patients with injuries of the upper spinal cord, this may mean a device triggered by an eyebrow, a puff-and-sip, or a head motion.[26]

Table 97–2. CURRICULUM FOR TRAINING

Anatomy and physiology
Tracheostomy tubes, care, and changes
Suctioning
Monitoring
Respiratory treatments
Oxygen
Go bags
Respiratory emergencies
Ventilation
Transporting
Keeping it going
Skills checklist

TRAINING

Many educational materials are required if families or other health care providers are to be adequately trained to care for complex, medically fragile children at home. The topics included in our formal training to parents are listed in Table 97–2. The training consumes time and personnel and involves several professionals; individual planning is necessary.

GAPS IN SERVICE

Despite all that is available to support children with highly technologic ventilatory needs at home, many gaps in service still exist. First, there are few alternatives to home ventilation. Home ventilation may not be possible for some families because of other obligations or because they are not capable of providing the necessary level of care. Although a medically fragile person may benefit from living at home, the author recognizes the need for caution in promotion of home ventilation and makes the following recommendations:

1. Discharge planning for a ventilator-assisted patient should be a team approach, coordinated by persons who have either been formally trained or have acquired training through extensive experience with an adequate number of ventilator patients. In discharge planning, "trial-and-error learning" is potentially dangerous to the child and family and increases the risk of liability for the professionals involved.
2. Because the population is so small, a regional approach to the care and planning appears to be more desirable than a single-case approach.
3. Local providers must be prepared to maintain the care plans developed by the regional specialists by using a case-management team approach at home.
4. Care at home must be an option and not a forced choice because of a lack of alternative placements.
5. Placement options should include long-term and out-of-home respite care settings that provide least restrictive care environments.
6. The community should support placement with maintenance of parental rights.

If the child cannot go home with the family or the family is unwilling to have the child at home, it is extremely difficult to find other facilities. Options may include foster families or institutional employees in intermediate health care facilities.

There is essentially no organized source for in-home respite care and no available facility that takes these children on an intermittent basis. Families whose children are admitted for an overnight sleep study or a weeklong rehabilitation visit are encouraged to take some days off for themselves.

It is a problem throughout the country that mental health services are not available in adequate volume or with adequate funding to provide support and counseling to families with children on home ventilation. In addition, there is a great deal of resistance by families to use these professional counseling services. It is impossible to gather the data in order to appreciate the magnitude of the problem or to allow appropriate planning for the future. Education of health care providers is also lacking so that physicians and other members of the health care team are sometimes uncomfortable and unwilling to care for children with high technologic needs.

FOLLOW-UP EVALUATIONS

Children are admitted for overnight sleep studies on a monthly to quarterly basis in order to evaluate current ventilator settings. If saturations are consistently above 90% to 92% and the P_{CO_2} is consistently in the 30s, ventilatory support is decreased.[14] If the electrocardiogram and echocardiogram are stabilized, the weaning processes are generally within the patient's tolerance. If changes in support produce signs of right-sided cardiac enlargement or other signs of deterioration, the weaning process must be slowed. It is imperative to ensure that the patient's cardiopulmonary status, growth, and development are not deteriorating secondary to attempts at weaning. Growth and development should be observed. The various parameters should be tracked, through the use of the same parameters as previously discussed, until the patient is weaned from the ventilator and the tracheostomy tube.

In addition, the child undergoes fiberoptic bronchoscopy at least once a year in order to check the airways for scarring or granulomas. Once the child has been successfully weaned from the ventilator, he or she can be weaned from the tracheostomy tube by gradually decreasing sizes as tolerated. Before final removal, fiberoptic bronchoscopy should be performed to evaluate airway dynamics and integrity. If they are clear, the tube can be removed.

PROBLEMS AND COMPLICATIONS

There are many complications for children dependent on ventilators. The first is the mortality rate. This varies between 25% and 35% among programs.[27, 28] Since the mid-1980s, 24 of 28 of the children in the author's patients on the home ventilator program have died.[28] A breakdown of the causes of death is given in Table 97–3. Children have been found asystolic with the ventilator still connected and no alarms. There is always the question, particularly because many deaths occur at night, of

Table 97–3. CAUSES OF DEATH

Cause	Number
Progression of disease	5
Unexplained arrest*	8
Disconnection	1
Hemorrhage (tracheal)	1
Inappropriate weaning	2
Unrelated illness	1
Abdominal catastrophe/sepsis	4
Sudden airway compromise†	2

*Patients, caregiver, or monitor failure. †Both patients institutionalized.

whether alarms were disarmed. Malfunctioning alarms have also been reported when equipment appears to be functional. Children also die when disease progresses to the point at which they can no longer survive even with ventilatory support.

Another major problem is professional liability. These children represent high liability risks, and there are increased risks associated with having these children at home and at school. It is the author's position that liability risks should be minimized by good initial training, good documentation of ongoing training, and repetitive written statements by the parents that they comprehend what they are being taught and understand the alternatives and liability of physicians and other health care providers who supervise home ventilation.

Families report many problems associated with ventilator-dependent children at home.[17] The obvious changes in the lifestyle leave families feeling helpless and confused. Siblings perceive varying degrees of neglect, and most families describe a sense of isolation. Financial deprivation is a common problem. Respite care is totally lacking, and funding is usually inadequate.[17]

Another problem is that care of these children is a constant emotional drain on both the family and the support system. Only patients with problems such as BPD or diaphragmatic hernias improve over time. Many, such as quadriplegic or other neurologically impaired children, never improve. They may also not die in the near future. Many families must face the fact that a child is not going to improve, and they cannot continue to support the care demands. Long-term placement may be sought at that point.[13]

Problems also exist with child abuse and neglect. This is particularly true if a family's income is supplemented or augmented by having the child at home. This keeps them from being willing to place the child outside the home, although they are unwilling or unable to provide the appropriate care.

Complications of medical requirements and primary diseases vary in accordance with the child's primary diagnosis. The most common complications are those related to the tracheostomy tube, hypoxia, and the gastrostomy tube. Children with meningomyelocele have problems associated with scoliosis, shunts, and urinary tract infections. Quadriplegic patients have many medical problems.

Another major complication results when the philosophy of optimal ventilation is not shared by all of the health care providers. Repeated attempts at weaning are counterproductive and may increase the chances of morbidity and mortality.

ETHICS

Ethical issues are implemented in managing the children who are on home ventilators. There seems to be less concern when there is a possibility of recovery, as with children with BPD or hypoplastic lungs. In children with fatal progression of disease, such as neurologic diseases, the ethical issues are more complex.[29] In children who are neurologically impaired, some professionals cannot accept long-term ventilation despite a family's wishes. Quality of life is a significant concern in patients requiring chronic ventilation. Physicians, families, and patients face choices that must be made. Options must be objectively presented to all concerned without moral judgment. Families and, if possible, the patient must be active participants in the information-gathering and decision-making processes.

REFERENCES

1. Office of Technical Assessment: Technology-Dependant Children: Hospital vs. Home Care. Technical memorandum, May 1987.
2. Goldberg AI, Faure EA, Vaughn CJ, et al: Home care for life-supported persons: An approach to program development. J Pediatr 104(5):785–795, 1984.
3. Pierce PM, Freedman SA, Frauman AC, et al: Reducing costs with a community outreach program. Pediatr Nurs 11:361–364, 1985.
4. Kahn L: Ventilator-dependent children heading home. Hospitals 58:54–55, 1984.
5. Aday LA, Wegener DH: Home care for ventilator-assisted children: Implications for the children, their families, and health policy. Children's Health Care 17(2):112–120, 1988.
6. Make BJ, Gilmartin ME: Rehabilitation and home care for ventilator-assisted individuals. Clin Chest Med 7(4):679–691, 1986.
7. Creese AL, Fielden R: Hospital or home care for the severely disabled: A cost comparison. Br J Prev Soc Med 31:116–121, 1977.
8. Burr BH, Guyer B, Todres ID, et al: Massachusetts Department of Public Health: Home care for children on respirators. N Engl J Med 309(21):1319–1323, 1983.
9. Splaingard ML, Frates RC, Harrison GM, et al: Home positive-pressure ventilation: Twenty years' experience. Chest 84(4):376–382, 1983.
10. Frates RC, Splaingard ML, Smith EO, et al: Outcome of home mechanical ventilation in children. J Pediatr 106:850–856, 1985.
11. Faure EAM, Goldberg AI (eds): Whatever Happened to Polio Patients? Proceedings of an International Symposium, Nortwestern University, Chicago, 1982. (Available from Education and Training, Rehab Institute of Chicago, 345 E. Superior St., Chicago, Il 60611).
12. Kettrick RG, Donar ME: The ventilator-dependent child: Medical and social care. Critical Care State of the Art 6:1–38, 1985.
13. O'Donohue WJ, Giovannoni RM, Goldberg AI, et al: Long-term mechanical ventilation: Guidelines for management in the home and at alternate community sites. Chest 90(Suppl.):1S–37S, 1986.
14. Gower DJ, Davis CH: Home ventilator care for high cervical cord injury. South Med J 78(8):1010–1011, 1985.
15. Kirkhart KA, Steele NF, Pomeroy M, et al: Louisiana's ventilator assisted care program: Case management services to like tertiary with community-based care. Children's Health Care 17(2):106–111, 1988.
16. Marini JJ: The physiologic determinants of ventilator dependence. Respir Care 31(4):271–282, 1986.
17. Kopacz MA, Moriarty-Wright R: Multidisciplinary approach for the patient on a home ventilator. Heart Lung 13(3):255–262, 1984.
18. Colbert AP, Schock NC: Respiratory Use in Progressive Neuromuscular Diseases [Abstract]. Unpublished survey.
19. Braun NMT: Nocturnal ventilation—A new method. Am Rev Respir Dis 135(3):523–524, 1987.
20. Glenn WW: Phelps ML: Diaphragm pacing by electrical stimulation of the phrenic nerve. Neurosurgery 17(6):974–984, 1985.
21. Fitzgerald LM, Huber GL: Weaning the patient from mechanical ventilation. Heart Lung 5(2):228–234, 1976.
22. Grossbach-Landis I: Successful weaning of ventilator-dependent patients. Top Clin Nurs 2(3):45–68, 1980.
23. Maynard FM, Imai K: Immobilization hypercalcemia in spinal cord injury. Arch Phys Med Rehabil 58:16–24, 1977.
24. Jenkinson SG: Nutritional supplementation during mechanical ventilation. Probl Pulmonary Dis 3(2):1–8, 1987.
25. Henning RJ, Shubin H, Weil MH: The measurement of the work of breathing for the clinical assessment of ventilator dependence. Crit Care Med 5(6):264–268, 1977.
26. Garrison JH: Emergency signaling for a person with quadriplegia and extraordinary regulatory risk. Arch Phys Med Rehabil 63:180–181, 1982.
27. Ventilator Program: Definitions; Guidelines; Curricula; Levels of Care and Personal Interaction. Unpublished materials, Ventilator Assisted Program, Children's Hospital, New Orleans.
28. Robert D, Gerard M, Leger P, et al: Long-term IPPV at home of patients with end stage chronic respiratory insufficiency. Chest 82(2):258–259, 1982.
29. Dunkin LJ: Home ventilatory assistance. Anaesthesia 38:644–649, 1983.

INDEX

Note: Page numbers in *italics* refer to illustrations; page numbers followed by t refer to tables.